Handbook of Mucosal Immunology

Handbook of Mucosal Immunology

Edited by

Pearay L. Ogra, M.D.
John Sealy Professor and Chairman
Department of Pediatrics
Pediatrician-in-Chief
Children's Hospital
The University of Texas Medical Branch at Galveston
Galveston, Texas

Warren Strober, M.D.
Head, Mucosal Immunology
Laboratory for Clinical Investigation
National Institute of Allergy and Infectious Diseases
National Institutes of Health
Bethesda, Maryland

Jiri Mestecky, M.D.
Professor
Departments of Microbiology and Medicine
University of Alabama-Birmingham
Birmingham, Alabama

Jerry R. McGhee, Ph.D.
Professor, Department of Microbiology
Director, Immunobiology Vaccine Center
University of Alabama-Birmingham
Birmingham, Alabama

Michael E. Lamm, M.D.
Professor and Chairman
Department of Pathology
Case Western Reserve University
University Hospitals of Cleveland
Cleveland, Ohio

John Bienenstock, FRCP, FRCPC, FRSC
Vice President and Dean
Faculty of Health Sciences
McMaster University
Hamilton, Ontario
Canada

Academic Press, Inc.
A Division of Harcourt Brace & Company
San Diego • New York • Boston • London • Sydney • Tokyo • Toronto

This book is printed on acid-free paper. ♾

Academic Press, Inc.
525 B Street, Suite 1900, San Diego, California 92101-4495

United Kingdom Edition published by
Academic Press Limited
24–28 Oval Road, London NW1 7DX

Library of Congress Cataloging-in-Publication Data

Handbook of mucosal immunology / edited by Pearay Ogra ... [et al.].
p. cm.
Includes index.
ISBN 0-12-524730-3
1. Mucous membrane. 2. Immunity. I. Ogra, Pearay L.
[DNLM: 1. Mucous Membrane--immunology. QS 532.5.M8 M94233 1994]
QR185.9.M83M84 1994
616.07'9--dc20
DNLM/DLC
for Library of Congress 93-11197
CIP

PRINTED IN THE UNITED STATES OF AMERICA
93 94 95 96 97 98 EB 9 8 7 6 5 4 3 2 1

Contents

14 Regulation of IgA B Cell Development

Warren Strober • Rolf O. Ehrhardt

15 Diversity and Function of Antigen-Presenting Cells in Mucosal Tissues

Asit Panja • Lloyd Mayer

16 Oral Tolerance and Regulation of Immunity to Dietary Antigens

Allan McI. Mowat

17 Functional Aspects of the Peptidergic Circuit in Mucosal Immunity

David W. Pascual • Andrzej M. Stanisz
Kenneth L. Bost

18 The Role of B-1 Cells in Mucosal Immune Responses

Frans G. M. Kroese • Aaron B. Kantor
Leonore A. Herzenberg

19 Lymphocyte Homing to Mucosal Effector Sites

Julia M. Phillips-Quagliata • Michael E. Lamm

Section C

Cells, Regulation, and Specificity in the Mucosal Immune System: Effector Sites

Section Editor: Jerry R. McGhee

Part a
The Normal State

20 Cytokines in the Mucosal Immune System

Deborah A. Lebman • Robert L. Coffman

PART II
Mucosal Diseases

Section E
Stomach, Intestine, and Liver
Section Editor: Pearay L. Ogra

Section F

Lungs and Airways

Section Editor: John Bienenstock

Section G

Oral Cavity, Upper Airway, and Head and Neck

Section Editor: John Bienenstock

Contributors

Numbers in parentheses indicate the pages on which the authors' contributions begin.

Rebecca Abraham (357)
Department of Pediatrics, University of Texas Medical Branch, Galveston, Texas 77555

B. Albini (457)
Departments of Microbiology and Medicine, State University of New York at Buffalo, Buffalo, New York 14214

Fernando Anaya-Velazquez (315),
IIBE, Fac. de Quim, University of Guanajuato, Guanajuato, GTO, 36000, Mexico

A. D. Befus (307)
Department of Medicine, Pulmonary and Cell Biology Research Group, University of Alberta, Edmonton, Alberta, Canada T6G 2S2

Joel M. Bernstein (625)
Departments of Otolaryngology and Pediatrics, State University of New York at Buffalo, and Division of Infectious Diseases, Children's Hospital of Buffalo, Buffalo, New York 14222

John Bienenstock (141, 529),
Departments of Medicine and Pathology, McMaster University, Hamilton, Ontario, Canada L8N 3Z5

Bengt Björkstén (561)
Department of Pediatrics, Faculty of Health Sciences, University of Linkòping, S-581 85 Linkòping, Sweden

Kenneth L. Bost (203)
Department of Microbiology and Immunology, Tulane University Medical Center, New Orleans, Louisiana 70112

C. P. Braegger (457)
Children's Hospital, H-8032 Zurich, Switzerland

Per Brandtzaeg (113, 251)
Laboratory for Immunohistochemistry and Immunopathology (LIIPAT), Institute of Pathology, University of Oslo, The National Hospital, Rikshospitalet N-0027 Oslo, Norway

R. A. Bronson (691)
Department of Obstetrics and Gynecology, Health Sciences Center, State University of New York at Stony Brook, Stony Brook, New York 11794

Jean-Claude Brouet (425)
Laboratory of Immuno-Pathology, Hôpital Saint-Louis, 75475 Paris, France

William R. Brown (513)
Gastroenterology Division, Department of Medicine, University of Colorado School of Medicine, and Department of Veterans Affairs Medical Center, Denver, Colorado 80220

B. Carlsson (653)
Department of Clinical Immunology, University of Göteborg, S-413 46 Göteborg, Sweden

John J. Cebra (151)
Department of Biology, University of Pennsylvania, Philadelphia, Pennsylvania 19104

S. J. Challacombe (607)
Department of Oral Medicine and Pathology, United Medical and Dental Schools, Guys Hospital, London SE1 9RT, England

Robert Clancy (529)
Departments of Medicine and Pathology, University of Newcastle, Newcastle, N.S.W. 2300, Australia

Robert L. Coffman (243)
DNAX Research Institute, Palo Alto, California 94304

Kenneth Croitoru (141)
Departments of Medicine, McMaster University, Hamilton, Ontario, Canada L8N 3Z5

Roy Curtiss III (373)
Department of Biology, Washington University, St. Louis, Missouri 63130

Mark T. Dertzbaugh (391)
U.S. Army Medical Research Institute of Infectious Diseases, Ft. Detrick, Frederick, Maryland 21702

Rolf O. Ehrhardt (159)
Mucosal Immunity Section, Laboratory of Clinical Investigation, National Institute of Allergy and Infectious Diseases, National Institutes of Health, Bethesda, Maryland 20892

John H. Eldridge (373)
Lederle-Praxis Biologicals, West Henrietta, New York 14586

Charles O. Elson (391)
Division of Gastroenterology, University of Alabama at Birmingham, Birmingham, Alabama 35294

Steven N. Emancipator (663)
Department of Pathology, Case Western Reserve University, University Hospitals of Cleveland, Cleveland, Ohio 44106

Peter B. Ernst (315)
Department of Pediatrics, University of Texas Medical Branch, Children's Hospital, Galveston, Texas 77555

F. M. Fusi (691)
III Department of Obstetrics and Gynecology, of the University of Milano, Istituto Scientifico Ospedale San Raffaele, Milano, Italy

Jack Gauldie (315)
Department of Pathology, McMaster University, Hamilton, Ontario, Canada L8N 3Z5

Randall M. Goldblum (643)
Departments of Pediatrics, and Human Biological Chemistry and Genetics, Children's Hospital, University of Texas Medical Branch, Galveston, Texas 77550

Armond S. Goldman (643)
Departments of Pediatrics, Microbiology, and Human Biological Chemistry and Genetics, University of Texas Medical Branch, Galveston, Texas 77550

L. Å. Hanson (653)
Department of Clinical Immunology, University of Göteborg, S-413 46 Göteborg, Sweden

Leonore A. Herzenberg (217)
The Department of Genetics, Stanford University Medical Center, Stanford, California 94305

S. T. Holgate (539)
Department of Immunopharmacology, Southampton General Hospital, Southampton S09 4XY, United Kingdom

Charles D. Howell (513)
Gastroenterology Division, Department of Medicine, University of Colorado, School of Medicine, Denver, Colorado 80220

Kimishige Ishizaka (299)
La Jolla Institute for Allergy and Immunology, La Jolla, California 92037

Graham D. F. Jackson (315)
University of New South Wales, School of Microbiology and Immunology, Kensington, NSW CP1 3NS, Australia

Stephen P. James (275)
Division of Gastroenterology, University of Maryland at Baltimore, Baltimore, Maryland 21201

D. B. Jones (539)
Departments of Immunopharmacology and Pathology, Southampton General Hospital, Southampton S09 4XY, United Kingdom

Charlotte S. Kaetzel (113)
Laboratory for Immunohistochemistry and Immunopathology (LIIPAT), Institute of Pathology, University of Oslo, The National Hospital, Rikshospitalet, N-0027 Oslo, Norway

B. Kaijser (435)
Department of Clinical Bacteriology, Institute of Medical Microbiology, Göteborg 41346, Sweden

Aaron B. Kantor (217)
Department of Genetics, Stanford University Medical Center, Stanford, California 94305

Tomohiro Kato (11)
Department of Medicine, University of California, San Francisco, and Cell Biology and Aging Section, Department of Veterans Affairs, Medical Center, San Francisco, California 94121

Mogens Kilian (127)
Institute of Medical Microbiology, University of Arhus, DK-8000, Aarhus C, Denmark

Hiroshi Kiyono (263)
Department of Oral Biology, The Immunobiology Vaccine Center, The University of Alabama at Birmingham, Birmingham, Alabama 35294

Katherine L. Knight (105)
Department of Microbiology and Immunology, Loyola University Chicago, Stritch School of Medicine, Maywood, Illinois 60153

P. Knoflach (457)
Krankenhaus Wels, Wels, A-65672 Austria

Jean-Pierre Kraehenbuhl (27, 403)
Swiss Institute for Experimental Cancer Research, and Institute of Biochemistry, University of Lausanne, CH-1066 Epalinges, Switzerland, and Children's Hospital and Harvard Medical School, Boston, Massachusetts 02115

Peter Krajči (113)
Laboratory for Immunohistochemistry and Immunopathology (LIIPAT), Institute of Pathology, University of Oslo, The National Hospital, Rikshospitalet, N-0027 Oslo, Norway

Frans G. M. Kroese (217)
Department of Histology and Cell Biology, Immunology Section, University of Groningen, 9713 EZ Groningen, The Netherlands

M. E. Lamm (113, 225, 663)
Department of Pathology, Case Western Reserve University, University Hospitals of Cleveland, Cleveland, Ohio 44106

Deborah A. Lebman (243)
Department of Microbiology and Immunology, Virginia Commonwealth University, Richmond, Virginia 23298

Leo Lefrançois (287)
Department of Medicine, Division of Rheumatic Diseases, University of Connecticut Health Center, Farmington, Connecticut 06030

Myron M. Levine (505)
Center for Vaccine Development, University of Maryland School of Medicine, Baltimore, Maryland 21201

David J. Lim (599)
Division of Intramural Research, National Institute on Deafness, and Other Communication Disorders, National Institutes of Health, Bethesda, Maryland 20892

Steven D. London (325)
Department of Microbiology and Immunology, Medical University of South Carolina, Charleston, South Carolina 29425

Britt Månsson-Rahemtulla (53)
Community and Public Health Dentistry, University of Alabama at Birmingham, Birmingham, Alabama 35294

Richard P. MacDermott[1] (439)
Gastroenterology Division, University of Pennsylvania, Philadelphia, Pennsylvania 19104

Thomas T. MacDonald (415)
Department of Pediatric Gastroenterology, The Medical College of St. Bartholomews Hospital, London EC1A 7BE, England

[1]Present address: Lahey Clinic Medical Center, Burlington, Massachusetts 01805

Lloyd Mayer (177)
Mount Sinai Medical Center, The Mount Sinai Hospital, Mount Sinai School of Medicine, New York, New York 10029

Jerry R. McGhee (263)
Department of Oral Biology, The Immunobiology Vaccine Center, The University of Alabama at Birmingham, Birmingham, Alabama 35294

Jiri Mestecky (79, 357)
Departments of Microbiology and Medicine, University of Alabama at Birmingham, Birmingham, Alabama 35294

Dean D. Metcalfe (493)
Laboratory of Clinical Investigation, National Institute of Allergy and Infectious Diseases, National Institutes of Health, Bethesda, Maryland 20892

Susanne M. Michalek (373)
University of Alabama at Birmingham, Department of Microbiology, Birmingham, Alabama 35294

Goro Mogi (599)
Department of Otolaryngology, Oita Medical University, 1-1506, Idaigaoka Oita 879-56, Japan

Allan McI. Mowat (185)
Department of Immunology, University of Glasgow, Western Infirmary, Glasgow G11 6NT, Scotland

Brian R. Murphy (333)
Respiratory Viruses Section, Laboratory of Infectious Diseases, National Institute of Allergy and Infectious Diseases, National Institutes of Health, Bethesda, Maryland 20892

D. Nadal (457, 625)
Department of Pediatrics, Division of Immunology/ Hematology, University-Children's Hospital of Zürich, H-8032 Zürich, Switzerland

James P. Nataro (505)
Center for Vaccine Development, University of Maryland School of Medicine, Baltimore, Maryland 21201

Marian R. Neutra (27, 403)
GI Cell Biology Laboratory, Children's Hospital, Boston, Massachusetts 02115

Pearay L. Ogra (357, 729)
Department of Pediatrics, The University of Texas Medical Branch at Galveston, Galveston, Texas 77550

Robert L. Owen (11)
Department of Medicine, University of California, San Francisco, and Cell Biology and Aging Section, Department of Veterans Affairs Medical Center, San Francisco, California 94121

Asit Panja (177)
Mount Sinai Medical Center, The Mount Sinai Hospital, Mount Sinai School of Medicine, New York, New York 10029

Earl L. Parr (677)
School of Medicine, Southern Illinois University, Carbondale, Illinois 62901

Margaret B. Parr (677)
School of Medicine, Southern Illinois University, Carbondale, Illinois 62901

David W. Pascual (203)
Departments of Oral Biology and Microbiology, The University of Alabama at Birmingham, University Station-BBRB-772, Birmingham, Alabama 35294

Julia M. Phillips-Quagliata (225)
Department of Pathology and Kaplan Cancer Center, New York University Medical Center, New York, New York 10016

Rao Prabhala[2] (705)
Department of Physiology, Dartmouth Medical School, Lebanon, New Hampshire 03756

Kenneth M. Pruitt (53)
Department of Biochemistry, University of Alabama at Birmingham, UAB Station, Birmingham, Alabama 35294

Firoz Rahemtulla (53)
Department of Oral Biology, University of Alabama at Birmingham, UAB Station, Birmingham, Alabama 35294

Jean-Claude Rambaud (425)
Department of Gastroenterology, Hôpital Saint-Lazare, 75010 Paris, France

A. E. Redington (539)
Department of Immunopharmacology, Southampton General Hospital, Southampton S09 4XY, United Kingdom

Hans-Christian Reinecker[3] (439)
Gastroenterology Division, University of Pennsylvania, Philadelphia, Pennsylvania 19104

Kathryn B. Renegar (347)
Department of Comparative Medicine, University of Tennessee, Memphis, Memphis 38763

Jan Richardson (705)
Department of Physiology, Dartmouth Medical School, Lebanon, New Hampshire 03756

Kenneth L. Rosenthal (373)
Molecular Virology and Immunology Program, Department of Pathology, McMaster University Health Sciences Center, Hamilton, Ontario, Canada L8N 3Z5

Michael W. Russell (127)
Department of Microbiology, University of Alabama at Birmingham, UAB Station, Birmingham, Alabama 35294

Ian R. Sanderson (41)
Harvard Medical School, Mucosal Immunology Laboratory, Combined Program in Pediatric Gastroenterology and Nutrition, Massachusetts General Hospital, Boston, Massachusetts 02115

Stefan Schreiber (439)
Department of Medicine, University of Hamburg, Z100 Hamburg, 90 Germany

Maxime Seligmann (425)
Department of Immuno-Hematology, Hôpital Saint-Louis, 75475 Paris, France

[2]Present address: Department of Microbiology, Chicago College of Osteopathic Medicine, 555 31st Street, Downers Grove, Illinois 60515

[3]Present address: Lahey Clinic Medical Center, Burlington, Massachusetts 01805

P. J. Shirlaw (607)
Department of Oral Medicine and Pathology, United Medical and Dental Schools, Guys Hospital, London SE1 9RT, England

Khushroo E. Shroff (151)
Department of Biology, University of Pennsylvania, Philadelphia, Pennsylvania 19104

Parker A. Small, Jr. (347)
Department of Immunology and Medical Microbiology, College of Medicine, University of Florida, Gainesville, Florida 32610

Phillip D. Smith (719)
Division of Gastroenterology, Department of Medicine and the Center for AIDS Research, University of Alabama, UAB Station, Birmingham, Alabama 35294

Jo Spencer (415)
Department of Histopathology, University College London, London, WC1E 6JJ, England

Andrzej M. Stanisz (203)
Intestinal Disease Research Unit, McMaster University Medical Center, Hamilton, Ontario, Canada L8N 3Z5

William F. Stenson (439)
Washington University, St. Louis, Missouri 63130

Warren Strober (159)
Mucosal Immunity Section, Laboratory of Clinical Investigation, National Institute of Allergy and Infectious Diseases, National Institutes of Health, Bethesda, Maryland 20892

David A. Sullivan (569)
Department of Ophthalmology, Harvard Medical School, and Immunology Unit, Schepens Eye Research Institute, Boston, Massachusetts 02114

C. Svanborg (71)
Department of Medial Microbiology, Clinical Immunology, Lund University, S-223 62 Lund, Sweden

Thomas B. Tomasi (3)
Roswell Park Cancer Institute, Department of Molecular Medicine, Buffalo, New York 14263

Debra A. Tristram (729)
Division of Infectious Diseases, State University of New York at Buffalo, School of Medicine and Biomedical Sciences, Children's Hospital of Buffalo, Buffalo, New York 14222

Brian J. Underdown (79, 315)
Department of Pathology, McMaster University, Hamilton, Ontario, Canada L8N 3Z5

Jean-Pierre Vaerman (99)
Catholic University of Louvain, International Institute of Cellular and Molecular Pathology, Unit of Experimental Medicine, B-1200 Brussels, Belgium

W. Allan Walker (41)
Harvard Medical School, Mucosal Immunology Laboratory, Combined Program in Pediatric Gastroenterology and Nutrition, Massachusetts General Hospital and The Children's Hospital, Boston, Massachusetts 02115

Robert C. Welliver (551)
Department of Pediatrics, State University of New York at Buffalo, Division of Infectious Diseases, Children's Hospital of Buffalo, Buffalo, New York 14222

Charles R. Wira (705)
Department of Physiology, Dartmouth Medical School, Lebanon, New Hampshire 03756

Noboru Yamanaka (625)
Wakayama Medical College, Wakayama, Sakaedani 930, Japan

Martin Zeitz (275)
Division of Gastroenterology, Medical Clinic, Klinikum Steglitz, Free University of Berlin, D-12 200 Berlin (Lichterfelde), Germany

Preface

Only 25 years ago, a multidisciplinary group of some three dozen individuals met for the first time in Vero Beach, Florida, under the auspices of the National Institute of Child Health and Human Development (NICHHD) to discuss a recently identified immunoglobulin, secretory IgA. Since that historic workshop, seven international congresses have been held to discuss secretory immunoglobulins and mucosal immunology, and there have been a number of scientific meetings on immunological mechanisms in such mucosal sites as respiratory tract, gut, genital tract, mammary glands, and periodontal tissues. The last International Congress of Mucosal Immunology, held in 1992 in Prague, Czechoslovakia, was attended by nearly 1000 participants.

The recognition that defenses are mediated via mucosal barriers dates back several thousand years. Ingestion of *Rhus* leaves to modify the severity of reactions to poison ivy is a centuries old practice among native North Americans. The modern concepts of local immunity, however, were developed by Besredka in the early 1900s, followed by the discovery of IgA in 1953 and its isolation and characterization in 1959. Studies in the early 1960s demonstrated the presence of IgA in a unique form in milk and, shortly thereafter, in other external secretions. These studies were followed by the discovery of the secretory component and the identification of the J chain. These remarkable observations were soon complemented by the characterization of the bronchus-associated lymphoid tissue (BALT) and the gut-associated lymphoid tissue (GALT), the observation of circulation of antigen-sensitized or reactive IgA B cells from BALT and GALT to other mucosal surfaces such as the genital tract and the mammary glands, and the definition of mucosal T cells. In the past decade, our concept of the mucosal immune system has been expanded to include M cells and mechanisms of mucosal antigen processing, regulatory T lymphocytes and other effector cell mechanisms, neuropeptides, and the network of interleukins and other cytokines. Finally, the biological significance of the mucosal immune system increasingly is being realized in the context of human infections acquired via mucosal portals of entry, including conventional infections as well as new syndromes such as acquired immune deficiency associated with infection by HIV.

Despite the tremendous progress made in the acquisition of new knowledge concerning the common mucosal immune system, mucosal infections, and oral immunization, no single text covering the entire spectrum of mucosal immunity was available. Therefore, this handbook was organized to develop a perspective of the basic biology of the components that constitute the framework of the common mucosal immune system, as well as of the infectious and immunologically mediated disease processes of the mucosae. Virtually all chapters have been authored by original investigators responsible for key observations on which current concepts are based.

Part I, Cellular Basis of Mucosal Immunity, provides an introductory overview and a historical perspective of the mucosal immune system (Chapter 1), followed by 10 comprehensive chapters (Section A) on development and physiology of mucosal defense (Chapters 2–11). These chapters address structure and function of mucosal epithelium, cellular basis of antigen transport, mucosal barrier, innate humoral factors, bacterial adherence, development and function of mucosal immunoglobulin, and epithelial and hepatobiliary transport. Section B (Chapters 12–19) focuses on cells, regulation, and specificity in inductive and effector sites. The inductive site chapters discuss characteristics of mucosa-associated lymphoid tissue (MALT), Peyer's patches, regulation of IgA B cell development, diversity and function of mucosal antigen-presenting cells, oral tolerance, peptidergic circuits, role of B-1 cells, and lymphocyte homing. The chapters on effector sites (Section C) present information about cytokines, mucosal Ig-producing cells, regulatory T cells, intraepithelial cells, mucosal IgE, inflammation and mast cells, cytokines in liver, cytotoxic T cells in mucosal effector sites, and immunity to viruses (Chapters 20–29). Section D addresses mucosal immunization and the concepts of mucosal vaccines. These chapters discuss passive immunization, vaccine development for mucosal surfaces, antigen delivery systems, mucosal adjuvants, and approaches for generating specific secretory IgA antibodies (Chapters 30–34).

Part II, Mucosal Diseases, addresses the secretory immune system with special reference to mucosal diseases. Section E consists of chapters on the stomach, intestine, and liver, and includes diseases of GALT and intestinal tract, α chain and related lymphoproliferative disorders, gastritis and peptic ulcer, malabsorption syndrome, food allergy, intestinal infections, and diseases of the liver and biliary tract (Chapters 35–42). Section F covers selected areas of lung and lower airway and includes chapters on BALT and pulmonary diseases, mucosal immunity in asthma, respiratory infections, and inhalant allergy (Chapters 43–46). Section G presents information on the oral cavity, upper airway, and mucosal regions in the head and neck (Chapters 47–50), as well as ocular immunity, tonsils and adenoids, and middle ear. Sections H and I are devoted to mammary glands and genitourinary tract, respectively. These sections consist of chapters on milk, immunological effects of breast feeding (Chapters 51–52), IgA nephropathy, immunology of female and male reproductive tracts, endocrine regulation of genital immunity, mucosal immunopathophysiology of HIV infection, and genital infections relative to maternal and infant disease (Chapters 53–58).

The information reviewed in the different chapters in this handbook will be of considerable interest to diverse groups of clinicians, basic and clinical immunologists, biologists, veterinarians, and public health workers interested in understanding the application of basic biology to virtually all immunological or infection-mediated disease processes of external mucosal surfaces. This handbook will be of particular importance to students of medicine and pediatrics, including individuals studying gastroenterology and pulmonology, ophthalmology, gynecology, infectious disease, otolaryngology, periodontal disease, sexually transmitted disease, and especially mucosal immunology.

Pearay L. Ogra
Jiri Mestecky
Michael E. Lamm
Warren Strober
Jerry R. McGhee
John Bienenstock

Acknowledgment

Proceeds from the sale of this book will go to the Society for Mucosal Immunology, which has sponsored this project.

PART I

Cellular Basis of Mucosal Immunity

1

Introduction: An Overview of the Mucosal System

Thomas B. Tomasi

The concept of a mucosal immune system first developed almost 30 years ago as a result of quantitative immunochemical studies of the various immunoglobulin isotypes in human mucosal fluids (Chodirker and Tomasi, 1963). The initial and most striking findings showed that external fluids that bathe mucosal surfaces contained predominantly IgA, in contrast to the low concentration of this immunoglobulin in comparison to IgG. Moreover, the IgA in saliva appeared to be different in molecular size from IgA in serum (serum IgA was primarily a 7S monomer with a smaller amount of 10S and larger polymers, whereas salivary IgA was mainly 11S). Importantly, salivary IgA was found to contain an additional component that we called the secretory piece and later termed the secretory component (SC; Tomasi *et al.*, 1965). Using antisera specific for IgA and for SC in immunofluorescent studies of the gastrointestinal tract and other tissues, large numbers of IgA cells were found in the lamina propria in close anatomical relationship with the mucosal surface, whereas SC was localized to epithelial cells. These findings suggested that the source of IgA in external secretions (secretory or SIgA) was regional and that SC was added during transport. This hypothesis was verified further by our studies showing that ^{125}I-labeled 7S IgA administered intravenously (iv) did not appear in significant amounts in saliva. However, the saliva of patients with agammaglobulinemia contained free SC, indicating that the transport of SC occurred in the absence of the specific ligand. As shown by South *et al.* (1966), the administration of large amounts of IgA to agammaglobulinemic patients resulted in the appearance of SIgA in secretions, suggesting that, if local production is diminished or absent and if enough *dimeric* IgA reaches the lamina propria from the circulation, transport will occur as in the nondeficient state. Similarly, Renegar and Small (1991) showed that polymeric IgA but not monomeric IgA or IgG1 anti-influenza antibodies promote mucosal protection in nonimmune mice. Thus, the absence of transport from serum to secretions in most tissues may be related to the saturation of local transport mechanisms by the regionally produced IgA. Later researchers demonstrated that much of the IgA in certain fluids such as the rat mammary gland (Halsey *et al.*, 1980) and especially rat bile (Fisher *et al.*, 1979) was a result of transport of polymeric 10S IgA from serum. This transport is a primary reason that 10S IgA has such a short apparent half-life in serum (Fisher *et al.*, 1979) in comparison to 7S serum IgA (Chodirker and Tomasi, 1963; Tomasi *et al.*, 1965).

There are two IgA subclasses, IgA1 and IgA2, which differ in several respects, most notably in the absence of a 13-amino-acid proline-rich region in the hinge of IgA2 that is the site of cleavage by IgA proteases. This difference confers resistance to these enzymes on the IgA2 subclass. The IgA proteases are enzymes (virulence factors) produced by a variety of bacteria that inactivate the antibody by a highly specific cleavage in the hinge region; the presence of IgA proteases in virulent strains of bacteria as shown by Plaut (1983) has great medical significance. Teleologically, therefore, having larger proportions of the IgA2 subclass in external secretions, that is, secretions that bathe the mucous surfaces these organisms colonize, would be advantageous. Moreover, after cleavage of IgA1 into Fab and Fc, the Fab portion has been suggested to coat the bacteria and protect these organisms from the destructive action of other antibodies (Kilian *et al.*, 1983).

Most of the monomeric serum IgA (90% IgA1 subclass) is produced in the bone marrow. In humans, small amounts of polymeric IgA are present in serum, probably as a result of synthesis in mucosal sites, although some polymeric IgA also is produced in the marrow. There is a catabolic site in the liver for human IgA1 which involves binding to a hepatic binding protein or the asialoglycoprotein receptor. IgA2 also is produced in bone marrow and peripheral lymphoid tissue, but the major portion appears to be synthesized in mucosal sites. SIgA is a dimer with a molecular weight of approximately 390,000 which, in addition to H and L chains, contains two additional polypeptide chains. J chain, described by Koshland (1985), is synthesized in the same cells that produce the dimeric IgA (i.e., plasma cells) and is a 15-kDa protein with one *N*-glycosylation site. This chain is not homologous to SC or Ig chains and does not appear, by sequence analysis, to be a member of the immunoglobulin superfamily. However, J chain does have a domain structure, probably a β barrel (Pumphrey, 1986), that has similarities to the classical immunoglobulin domain. J chain is involved in and probably necessary for polymer formation in B cells. J chain production occurs in pre-B cells, but its synthesis is stimulated markedly in more mature B cells by antigen contact. Complexing of J chain with the monomeric units of IgA (and IgM) to form the dimer occurs late, just prior to secretion. The complexing of J chain occurs with the penultimate cysteine in the C-terminal tail piece (an 18-amino-acid peptide characteristic of IgA and IgM). Some evidence suggests that the disulfide bridge may be formed with a sulfhydryl group in a C_H2 domain of the alpha chain. As shown by Hauptman and Tomasi (1975), J chain lends a conformation to both IgA and IgM that is required for noncovalent complexing (followed by S–S formation) to SC; SC does not interact efficiently with polymers lacking J chain, presumably because of the unique conformation of the IgA_2–J or IgM_5–J complex.

I. POLYIg RECEPTORS AND TRANSPORT

Secretory component is an 80,000 molecular weight glycoprotein that is synthesized in epithelial cells and is bonded covalently through a disulfide linkage between the fifth domain of SC and the C_H2 domain of one monomer in the human SIgA molecule. SC does not appear to cross-link the two monomeric units or bind to J chain, although the disulfide chemistry is not established completely. Bakos *et al.* (1991) showed that the binding of SC to polymeric IgA is dependent on a highly conserved N-terminal region of SC that may be the primary site of noncovalent interactions between SC and IgA. SC is a member of the immunoglobulin superfamily. This family contains over 40 different molecules present on lymphocytes and a variety of other cells. SC is a component of a larger molecule, the poly Ig receptor (poly IgR), that acts as a receptor on epithelial cells for polymeric molecules of IgA and IgM that contain J chain. The rabbit poly IgR has been cloned and sequenced by Mostov *et al.* (1984); the extracellular region is composed of five domains, four V-like domains and a C-terminal C_H-like domain close to the plasma membrane. The human poly IgR also has been cloned and shows organization similar to that of the rabbit poly IgR, with which it shares 54% homology (Krajči *et al.*, 1989). As shown in Figure 1, the poly IgR is synthesized on the rough endoplasmic reticulum (RER) as a 95-kDa protein and is then core-glycosylated to a 105-kDa molecule and transported to the Golgi complex, where the carbohydrate is trimmed and the molecule is terminally glycosylated. The 116-kDa protein then is transported in vesicles to the basal lateral surface of the mucosal cell or, in the hepatocyte, to the sinusoidal surface. The receptor has an N-terminal ectoplasmic domain on the outside acting as the receptor for ligand (IgA and IgM), a transmembrane portion, and a 103-amino-acid cytoplasmic tail. The cytoplasmic tail, as shown by Larkin *et al.* (1986), is phosphorylated on a serine residue during its intracellular journey to the membrane to give the 120-kDa mature receptor. Figure 1 illustrates how the binding of dimeric IgA (or pentameric IgM) containing J chain results in endocytosis in coated pits; the ligand–receptor complexes and unbound receptors are sorted, and the ligand–receptor complex is directed across the cells to the apical membrane by a process referred to as transcytosis. Before secretion into the lumen, the receptor is proteolyzed and SC is released from the transmembrane region and cytoplasmic tail and secreted into the lumen, either attached to its ligand or "free." The location and mechanism of proteolysis and the existence of a single specific site or multiple cleavage sites (which appears more likely from the staggered C-terminal ends) are unclear. However, in rat hepatocytes, cleavage appears to occur at the canalicular plasma membrane; the membrane-anchor domain is either internalized or secreted with SC into the bile (Solari *et al.*, 1989). The receptor is presumed to be selectively targeted to the appropriate membrane, as shown for viral and other proteins documented to undergo polarized transport. Biosynthetic studies (Schaerer *et al.*, 1990) indicate selective (rather than random) targeting of the receptor to the basolateral surface. In the Madin-Darby canine kidney (MDCK) cell line, cleavage of the receptor by an endogenous protease is delayed until after its appearance on the membrane, explaining the presence of poly IgR on the apical membrane surface. Thus, the SIgA in human external fluids consists

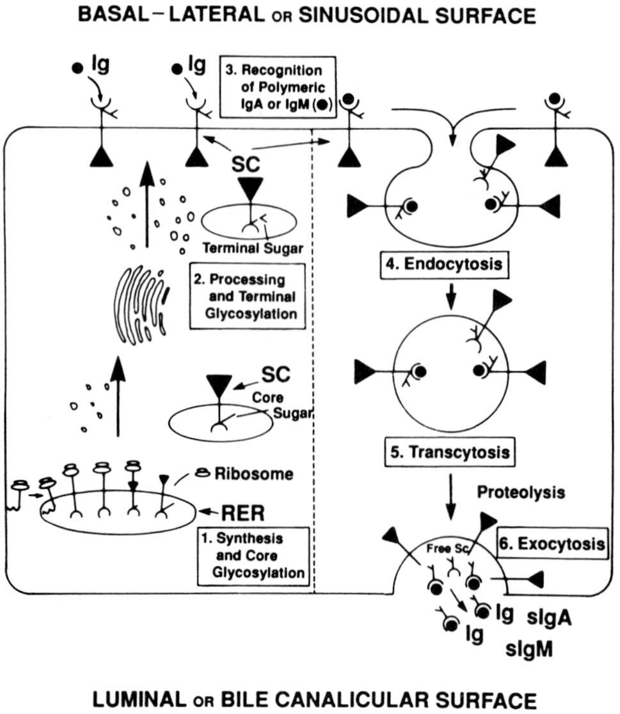

Figure 1 Model for transport of IgA and IgM across the mucosal epithelial cell or hepatocyte. The synthesis of secretory component (SC) and the steps in the transport of Ig across the cell are represented. SC is synthesized and core glycosylated on membrane-bound polysomes [rough endoplasmic reticulum (RER)] as an approximately 95,000 molecular weight transmembrane protein and is inserted cotranslationally into the RER. Further processing (including the addition of terminal sugars) may occur in the Golgi. SC then becomes integrated into the basal (and lateral) plasma membranes of the mucosal epithelial cell or the sinusoidal membrane of the hepatocyte. The transmembrane SC (Ɪ) consists of three domains: cytoplasmic (⊥), membrane-spanning (|), and ectoplasmic (Y). The ectoplasmic domain acts as the external receptor for J chain-containing polymeric Igs such as IgA and IgM (●). Endocytosis of the receptor probably occurs continuously. Transcytosis of the complexes and of SC not associated with Ig occurs in vesicles (endosomes) that probably do not fuse with lysosomes but do fuse with the plasma membrane, thus carrying the Ig–receptor complex to the luminal surface. Proteolysis occurs at an unknown stage, removing the cytoplasmic and membrane-spanning portions. The Ig is secreted covalently attached to the ectoplasmic domain (MW ~80,000).

of the J chain-containing dimer plus the covalently linked ectoplasmic domain of SC. As we first reported (Tomasi and Czerwinski, 1968), the SIgA molecule is protected from proteolysis by the secretory component, which may lend a biological advantage to SIgA functioning in a complex fluid containing many proteolytic and other degradative mechanisms.

A. Cellular Traffic

As shown by the studies of Owen and Jones (1974; Owen, 1977), antigen is taken up in significant part, although not solely, via the Peyer's patches and moves in pinocytotic vesicles across the attenuated epithelium of the patch dome (called M for microfold cells) to the lymphoid epithelium that lies immediately beneath it. Lymphoid cells in the patch consist of macrophages, dendritic cells, and T cells of several subsets [including $CD4^+$ helper (Th), $CD8^+$ suppressor (T_S), and contrasuppressor (T_{CS})], as well as B cells. The influence of T cells and various lymphokines, as described subsequently, may be involved in determining isotype specificity. In some cases, T_S cells of $CD8^+$ phenotype leave the patches to seed peripheral tissues, and are probably responsible for oral tolerance (Tomasi, 1980). After antigen presentation, by mechanisms that are not clear (but probably involve macrophages, dendritic cells, and possibly B cells), B cells become committed to antigen specificity. These cells also are predestined to a migratory journey to mucosal membranes to become IgA plasma cells. This precommitment to IgA and the migration to the lamina propria was described first by Craig and Cebra (1971). We now know that both T and B cells have homing properties and that specific receptors for homing are present at mucosal sites. From the studies of Butcher *et al.* (1980), the high endothelial venule (HEV) appears to be a site at which tissue specific receptors reside; monoclonal antibodies that block *in vitro* attachment of lymphocytes to mucosal tissues such as Peyer's patches (but not peripheral lymphoid tissues) have been described. Similarly, other monoclonal antibodies block the binding of lymphocytes to HEV in peripheral lymph nodes, but not in Peyer's patches. Interestingly, the monoclonal antibodies directed against Peyer's patch HEVs are able to inhibit homing to the lamina propria, suggesting common antigenic determinants in the Peyer's patch and lamina propria HEVs. On the lymphocyte surface, homing may involve receptors for mannose 6-phosphate and/or other sugars. In addition to the homing of Peyer's patch cells to the gut lamina propria, evidence exists for more extensive migratory patterns to and between other sites that collectively, as described by Bienenstock *et al.* (1979), are called the mucosal-associated lymphoid tissues (MALT). Central aggregates that resemble Peyer's patches have been described in the lung and elsewhere (tonsils, appendix); cells from these sites migrate to a variety of mucosal tissues and, with cells derived from Peyer's patches, give rise to the IgA in the secretions of the mammary gland, respiratory tract, gastrointestinal (GI) tract, and salivary, lacrimal, and cervical–vaginal fluids. This common mucosal system has biological and medical implications. For example, in animal models, immunization via the gut against caries-producing *Streptococcus mutans* has been shown to inhibit caries. Moreover, the important studies by Mestecky *et al.* (1978) have shown that oral immunization with killed *Streptococcus mutans* in capsules can produce significant titers of antibodies in the saliva of normal humans. This procedure could be a mechanism of vaccination in several areas, for example, generating antibodies in tears against trachoma or in vaginal secretions against organisms involved in venereal diseases, including HIV. The classical studies of Ogra and Karzon (1969) showed the importance of oral immunization in protection of mucosal surfaces of the GI tract. These studies form the basis for the concept that the content of local antibodies, particularly of the IgA class, is the first line of defense of mucosal surfaces against colonization of these surfaces by potentially pathogenic microorganisms.

II. MUCOSAL LYMPHOID CELLS

The mucosal immune system comprises three basic kinds of lymphoid tissue that are compartmentalized and, to a large degree, functionally distinct. Central or organized lymphoid tissues constitute the Peyer's patches and related aggregates in the other organs mentioned earlier. The second type of tissue is located diffusely in the various lamina propria of the mucosal system; after receiving B cells from the centralized aggregates which are already precommitted to IgA, they undergo further differentiation and give rise to IgA plasma cells. The third type of lymphoid mucosal tissue consists of cells that lie between the epithelial cells of the various membranes, the so called intraepithelial lymphocytes (IEL). This functionally heterogeneous population contains cells with antitumor activity, natural killer (NK) activity, allospecific cytotoxic T lymphocytes (CTL), precursors of CTL, and mast cells. Almost all IEL are granulated (contain sulfated proteoglycans) and about 85% are $CD8^+$. Approximately half of the $CD8^+$ cells are of thymic origin and migrate to Peyer's patches; after antigen exposure, they seed the lamina propria of the gut (Guy-Grand *et al.*, 1991). These cells also bear TCR $\alpha\beta 1$ and $CD3^+$ and their $CD8^+$ molecules have two chains: α (Lyt2) and β (Lyt3). A small percentage (~10%) of thymus-dependent $CD4^+$ cells are also present. The thymus-independent cells arise in the bone marrow and migrate directly to the gut. The high incidence of TCR γ/δ cells in IEL, their restricted specificity (selective use of $V_\gamma 7$ and a few other γ-gene segments), and their presence in athymic and germ-free mice (which lack TCR α/β) suggest that this unique T-cell subset may be directed against antigens other than conventional bacterial enteroantigens (Bandeira *et al.*, 1990). $CD8^+$, Thy 1^-, $CD5^-$ cells also have been found to be present in IEL of SCID/SCID mice (Croitoru *et al.*, 1990), which lack TCR. Therefore these T cells may arise by a different pathway or may be a unique lineage of cells. Interestingly, intestinal epithelial cells have Class I antigens encoded by TL region genes that are found uniquely in the gut (Wu *et al.*, 1991), suggesting the possibility that the TL region has evolved to generate antigen-presenting cells as a subset of

IEL TCR γ/δ cells. One hypothesis is that the γ/δ cells are directed against self-antigens (Guy-Grand *et al.*, 1991; Taguchi *et al.*, 1991), perhaps eliminating altered enterocytes, thereby maintaining the defense function of the epithelia.

A. Regulation of the Immune Mucosal Response

That T cells are required for an IgA response is well established; in fact, IgA is one of the most T-cell dependent of all the isotypes. T cells may operate in a nonspecific fashion. Immunoglobulin class is determined by the number of mitoses and the distance of the particular gene from the 3′ end of the C_H gene complex. Since the α-gene chain is located on the most 3′ end of the C_H gene complex, multiple repeated switches may occur with constant exposure to environmental antigens, as first suggested by Cebra *et al.* (1983), and could be a mechanism of the predominance of IgA in the gut. In this respect, most of the IgA antibodies in mucosal fluids are directed toward environmental substances including microbial and nonviable food antigens. The role of IgA antibodies with respect to nonviable food antigens has been shown clearly by Cunningham-Rundles *et al.* (1978) in IgA-deficient patients, who absorb large amounts of food antigens, leading to the production of immune complexes and the resulting autoimmune-like syndromes mainfested by these patients.

T cells also may operate in an isotype-specific fashion. Evidence exists for several isotype-specific T cells and T-cell factors. Some of the postulated relationships are shown in Figure 2. T cells are involved in the sequence of switching from an antigen-committed virgin IgM-bearing B cell (with or without IgD) to an IgA B cell with subsequent differentiation to an IgA-producing plasma cell. Switch T cells have been described in Peyer's patches by Kawanishi *et al.* (1983). Other cells bearing Fcα-receptors (FcαR) are capable of causing IgA-bearing cells to differentiate into plasma cells. These cells produce lymphokines as well as soluble IgA binding factors (IgA-BF) that specifically suppress or enhance the immune response of IgA. Similar factors have been identified in the IgE system by Huff and Ishizaka (1984). In the IgE system, whether the IgE-BF is suppressive or potentiating depends on the degree of glycosylation. Glycosylation in the IgE system is, in turn, dependent on factors secreted by T cells that are either glycosylation inhibiting factors (GIF) or glycosylation enhancing factors (GEF). These factors are produced by two different T-cell subsets. Thus, a complex mechanism in the IgE system determines whether the factors that bind IgE suppress or enhance. Whether such GIF and GEF molecules exist for IgA has not been determined.

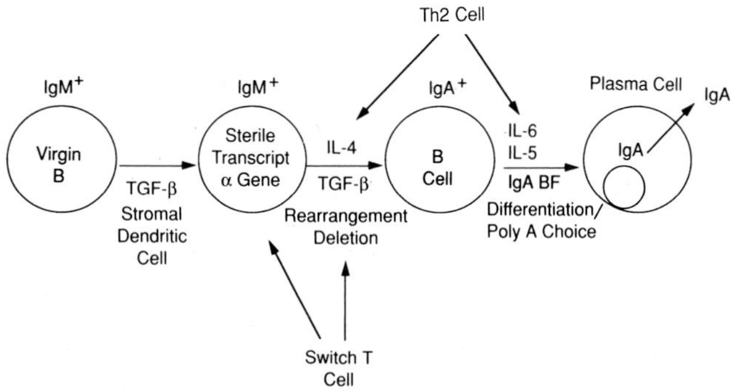

Figure 2 Production of IgA plasma cell via T cells. Postulated T switch cell may be involved in the transition of an IgM-bearing B cell to an IgA B cell. IL-4 and TGF-β may be switch factors. The differentiation from an IgA B cell to a plasma cell probably involves IL-5, IL-6, and perhaps IgA–BF.

The up-regulation of FcαR in the presence of IgA may represent a feedback mechanism, since isotype-specific suppressor cells appear in conditions such as IgA myeloma, which shows a high concentration of IgA. These cells inhibit transcription of the heavy chain mRNA of IgA as well as growth of the IgA myeloma cell. A monoclonal antibody to the FcαR that blocks binding of IgA to T cells has been described; this antibody could be helpful in eventually cloning the T-cell FcαR. Expression cloning of the Fc receptor for IgA on myeloid cells has been reported, but this receptor appears to be myeloid specific; a monoclonal antibody (My43) to it lacks reactivity with lymphocytes (Maliszewski *et al.*, 1990). In our laboratory, Crago *et al.* (1989) have shown that the FcαR on T cells may be related to secretory component. We have found that antisera to SC, but not to other cell surface antigens, inhibit IgA binding to its receptor on murine T cells and T–T hybridomas. Thus, SC and FcαR are present on different cells, but both bind the Fc region of IgA, suggesting a common evolutionary origin at least in the IgA binding site.

Evidence also suggests that interleukin 4 (IL-4; produced by Th2 cells) probably is involved at an early step and may itself be a switch factor or a factor that enhances switching by a switch T cell. This hypothesis is not unreasonable since IL-4 is known to be a switch factor for IgG1 and IgE (Snapper and Paul, 1987). The work of Berton and Vitetta (1990) has shown that IL-4 alone induces a DNase I hypersensitivity site at the 5′ end of the $\gamma 1$ switch region of resting B cells, as well as germ-line transcripts of the $\gamma 1$ gene. Thus, IL-4, probably via induction of DNA binding proteins, may enhance transcription by making the switch region more accessible to RNA polymerase and switch recombinases. The work of Strober (1990) on the CH12.LX cell line and by Shockett and Stavnezer (1991) on I.29μ suggests that the first step may involve selective isotype (or region)-specific accessibility of transcription factors to switch sites. Antigen (or mitogen) stimulation, in addition to specific factors such as transforming growth factor β (TGFβ) and IL-4, may be important in selecting the isotype switch region near which chromatin is relaxed. Other factors, perhaps derived from dendritic cells or stromal cells, also may be central to switching. Their action even may precede the lymphokine effects. Thus, the virgin IgM cell first may become unstable and show transcription of germ-line (unrearranged) C_H regions. This cell is, in a sense, poised for the isotype switch to be accomplished by recombinant enzymes that loop out the intervening sequences. Precisely how the germ-line "sterile" transcript seen in these cells and the associated deletional events occur in relation to cytokines such as TGFβ, IL-4, and "switch T cells" is unclear.

Experiments by Coffman *et al.* (1987) also have shown that IL-5, a lymphokine produced by the Th2 subset, enhances the production of IgA. IL-5 appears to act at the IgA^+ B cell and promotes both proliferation and differentiation to plasma cells. Whether IL-5 induces an IgA-BF factor and functions through this mechanism is unclear. The combination of IL-4 and IL-5 enhances the secretion of IgA from Peyer's patch B cells (Murray *et al.,* 1987).

IL-6, an autocrine growth factor for plasma cells, also is involved in IgA formation. IL-6 is produced by plasma cells, T cells, and possibly other cells. One would suspect from current data that Th2 cells (producing IL-4, 5, 6) might be more prominent in the mucosal system, which appears to be the case (Taguchi *et al.,* 1990).

Th1 cells also may play an important role in modulating the immune response at mucosal sits. The IL-2 and interferon gamma (IFN_γ) produced by Th1 may have important regulatory roles. IL-2 receptors are present on B cells and, in fact, IL-5 up-regulates these receptors and may potentiate the secretion of IgA as well as other immunoglobulins. IFN_γ has been shown to down-regulate certain immunoglobulin classes (Snapper and Paul, 1987), but whether this down-regulation occurs with IgA has not been established. IFN_γ also may affect mucosal epithelial by inducing Ia antigens. The work of Mayer and Shlien (1987) suggests that Ia^+ epithelial cells may present antigen; interestingly, the result is primarily a $CD8^+$ cell, whereas monocyte presentation produces predominantly $CD4^+$ helper cells. Thus, the predominance of interepithelial $CD8^+$ cells could be explained by this mechanism. Inflammatory cells produce large amounts of IFN_γ; increased $CD8^+$ cells frequently are seen in diseased tissues. Also interesting, as shown by Sollid *et al.* (1987), is that IFN_γ and tumor necrosis factor up-regulate the synthesis of SC by epithelial cells, which may facilitate the transport of IgA into secretions. Obviously, the interrelationship between lymphokines are very complex and represent an exciting area for future studies.

B. Molecular Mechanisms of IgA Formation

The switch and differentiation schemes outlined in preceding sections are accompanied by complex intracellular molecular events. For example, switching may involve the formation of a hypothetical intermediate B cell that contains a long primary transcript, as suggested by the work of Perlmutter *et al.* (1984) as well as by work from our laboratory (Woloschak *et al.,* 1986). Such cells would process a primary transcript of about 200 kb in length differentially into messages for IgM and IgA and produce the double-bearing IgM–IgA cells. Solid evidence suggests that the single-bearing IgA^+ B cell and IgA plasma cell have switched by a mechanism involving deletion and rearrangements. As mentioned earlier, cells and factors that induce IgA may affect chromatin structure and methylation, thereby allowing access of critical switch recombinases to the $C_H\alpha$ gene.

With respect to the differentiation of the $mIgA^+$ cell to a plasma cell, the molecular events involve the differential RNA processing of the message to that for the secreted form of the protein. This processing could be accomplished by several mechanisms: (1) termination, (2) splice site choice, and (3) choice of poly A addition sites. Some evidence exists for each of these mechanisms, although most data suggest that cleavage and polyadenylation are the most likely mechanisms, followed by appropriate splicing. Perhaps the cytokines involved in differentiation for example, IL-5 and IL-6, determine the concentration of factors (such as the endases), as suggested by Galli *et al.* (1988), that regulate the site of cleavage and poly A addition.

References

Bakos, M. A., Kurosky, A., and Goldblum, R. M. (1991). Characterization of a critical binding site for human polymeric Ig on secretory component. *J. Immunol.* **147,** 3419–3426.

Bandeira, A., Mota-Santos, T., Itohara, S., Degermann, S., Heusser, C., Tonegawa, S., and Coutinho, A. (1990). Localization of γ/δ T cells to the intestinal epithelium is independent of normal microbial colonization. *J. Exp. Med.* **172,** 239–244.

Berton, M. T., and Vitetta, E. S. (1990). Interleukin 4 induces changes in the chromatin structure of the $\gamma 1$ switch region in resting B cells before switch recombination. *J. Exp. Med.* **172,** 375–378.

Bienenstock, J., McDermott, M., and Befus, D. (1979). A common mucosal immune system. *In* "Immunology of Breast Milk" (P. L. Ogra and D. Dayton, eds.), pp. 91–104. Raven Press, New York.

Butcher, E. C., Scollay, R. G., and Weissman, I. L. (1980). Organ specificity of lymphocyte migration: Mediation by highly selective lymphocyte interaction with organ-specific determinants on high endothelial venules. *Eur. J. Immunol.* **10,** 556–561.

Cebra, J. J., Cebra, E. R., Clough, E. R., Fuhrman, J. R., Komisar, J. L., Schweitzer, P. A., and Shahin, R. D. (1983). IgA commitment: Models for B-cell differentiation and possible roles for T-cells in regulating B-cell development. *Ann. N.Y. Acad. Sci.* **409,** 25–38.

Chodirker, W. B., and Tomasi, T. B., Jr. (1963) Gamma-globulins: Quantitative relationships in human serum and nonvascular fluids. *Science* **142,** 1080–1081.

Coffman, R. L., Shrader, B., Carty, J., Mosmann, T. R., and Bond, M. W. (1987). A mouse T cell product that preferentially enhances IgA production. *J. Immunol.* **139,** 3685–3690.

Crago, S. S., Word, C. J., and Tomasi, T. B. (1989). Antisera to the secretory component recognize the murine Fc receptor for IgA. *J. Immunol.* **142,** 3909–3912.

Craig, S. W., and Cebra, J. J. (1971). Peyer's patches: An enriched source of precursors for IgA-producing immunocytes in the rabbit. *J. Exp. Med.* **134,** 188–200.

Croitoru, K., Stead, R. H., Bienenstock, J., Fulop, G., Harnish, D. G., Shultz, L. D., Jeffery, P. K., and Ernst, P. B. (1990). Presence of intestinal intraepithelial lymphocytes in mice with severe combined immunodeficiency disease. *Eur. J. Immunol.* **20,** 645–651.

Cunningham-Rundles, C., Brandeis, W. E., Good, R. A., and Day, N. K. (1978). Milk precipitins, circulating immune complexes, and IgA deficiency. *Proc. Natl. Acad. Sci. U.S.A.* **75,** 3387–3389.

Fisher, M. M., Nagy, B., Bazin, H., and Underdown, B. J. (1979). Biliary transport of IgA: Role of secretory component. *Proc. Natl. Acad. Sci. U.S.A.* **76,** 2008–2012.

Galli, G., Guise, J., Tucker, P. W., and Nevins, J. R. (1988). Poly(A) site choice rather than splice site choice governs the regulated production of IgM heavy-chain RNAs. *Proc. Natl. Acad. Sci. U.S.A.* **85,** 2439–3443.

Guy-Grand, D., Malassis-Seris, M., Briottet, C., and Vassalli, P. (1991). Cytotoxic differentiation of mouse gut thymodependent and independent intraepithelial T lymphocytes is induced locally. Correlation between functional assays, presence of perforin and granzyme transcripts, and cytoplasmic granules. *J. Exp. Med.* **173,** 1549–1552.

Halsey, J. F., Johnson, B. H., and Cebra, J. J. (1980). Transport of immunoglobulins from serum into colostrum. *J. Exp. Med.* **151,** 767–772.

Hauptman, S. P., and Tomasi, T. B., Jr. (1975). Mechanism of immunoglobulin A polymerization. *J. Biol. Chem.* **250,** 3891–3896.

Huff, T. F., and Ishizaka, K. (1984). Formation of IgE-binding factors by human T-Cell hybridomas. *Proc. Natl. Acad. Sci. U.S.A.* **81,** 1514–1518.

Kawanishi, H., Saltzman, l., and Strober, W. (1983). Mechanisms regulating IgA class-specific immunoglobulin production in murine gut-associated lymphoid tissues: I. T cells derived from Peyer's patches. *J. Exp. Med.* **157**, 433–450.

Kilian, M., Reinholdt, J., Mortensen, S. B., and Sorensen, C. H. (1983). Perturbation of mucosal immune defence mechanisms by bacterial IgA proteases. *Bull. Eur. Physiopathol. Respir.* **19,** 99–104.

Koshland, M. E. (1985). The coming of age of the immunoglobulin J chain. *Ann. Rev. Immunol.* **3,** 425–453.

Krajči, P., Solberg, R., Sandberg, M., Oyen, O., Jahnsen, T., and Brandtzaeg, P. (1989). Molecular cloning of the human transmembrane secretory component (poly-Ig receptor) and its mRNA expression in human tissues. *Biochem. Biophys. Res. Commun.* **158,** 783–789.

Larkin, J. M., Sztul, E. S., and Palade, G. E. (1986). Phosphorylation of the rat hepatic polymeric IgA receptor. *Proc. Natl. Acad. Sci. U.S.A.* **83,** 4759–4763.

Maliszewski, C. R., March, C. J., Schoenborn, M. A., Gimpel, S., and Shen, L. (1990). Expression cloning of a human Fc receptor for IgA. *J. Exp. Med.* **172,** 1665–1672.

Mayer, L., and Shlien, R. (1987). Evidence for function of Ia molecules on gut epithelial cells in man. *J. Exp. Med.* **166,** 1471–1483.

Mestecky, J., McGhee, J. R., Arnold, R. R., Michalek, S. M., and Prince, S. J. (1978). Selective induction of an immune response in human external secretions by ingestion of bacterial antigen. *J. Clin. Invest.* **61,** 731–737.

Mestecky, J., Moldoveanu, Z., Tomana, M., Epps, J. M., Thorpe, S. R., Phillips, J. O., and Kulhavy, R. R. (1989). 11th International Convocation on Immunology (B. Albini, R. J. Genco, P. L. Ogra, and M. M. Weiser, eds.). *Immunol. Invest.* **18,** 313–324.

Mostov, K. E., Friedlander, M., and Blobel, G. (1984). The receptor for transepithelial transport of IgA and IgM contains multiple immunoglobulin-like domains. *Nature* (*London*) **308,** 37–43.

Murray, P. D., McKenzie, D. T., Swain, S. L., and Kagnoff, M. F. (1987). Interleukin 5 and interleukin 4 produced by Peyer's patch T cells selectively enhance immunoglobulin A expression. *J. Immunol.* **139,** 2669–2674.

Ogra, P. L., and Karzon, D. T. (1969). Poliovirus antibody response in serum and nasal secretions following intranasal inoculation with inactivated poliovaccine. *J. Immunol.* **102,** 15–23.

Owen, R. L. (1977). Sequential uptake of horseradish peroxidase by lymphoid follicle epithelium of Peyer's patches in the normal unobstructed mouse intestine: An ultrastructural study. *Gastroenterology* **72,** 440–451.

Owen, R. L., and Jones, A. L. (1974). Epithelial cell specialization within human Peyer's patches: An ultrastructural study of intestinal lymphoid follicles. *Gastroenterology* **66,** 189–190.

Perlmutter, A. P., McDowell, J., and Gilbert, W. (1984). Antibodies of the secondary response can be expressed without switch recombination in normal mouse B cells. *Proc. Natl. Acad. Sci. U.S.A.* **81,** 7189–7193.

Plaut, A. G. (1983). The IgA1 proteases of pathogenic bacteria. *Ann. Rev. Microbiol.* **37,** 603–622.

Pumphrey, R. S. H. (1986). Computer models of the human immunoglobulins. *Immunol. Today* **7,** 206–211.

Renegar, K. B., and Small, P. A., Jr. (1991). Passive transfer of local immunity to influenza virus infection by IgA antibody. *J. Immunol.* **146,** 1972–1978.

Schaerer, E., Verrey, F., Racine, L., Tallichet, C., Reinhardt, M., and Kraehenbuhl, J.-P. (1990). Polarized transport of the polymeric immunogobulin receptor in transfected rabbit mammary epithelial cells. *J. Cell Biol.* **110,** 987–998.

Shockett, P., and Stavnezer, J. (1991). Effect of cytokines on switching to IgA and α germline transcripts in the B lymphoma 1.29μ. Transforming growth factor-β activates transcription of the unrearranged C_α gene. *J. Immunol.* **147,** 4374–4383.

Snapper, C. M., and Paul, W. E. (1987). Interferon-γ and B cell stimulatory factor-1 reciprocally regulate Ig isotype production. *Science* **236,** 944–947.

Solari, R., Schaerer, E., Tallichet, C., Braiterman, L. T., Hubbard, A. L., and Kraehenbuhl, J. P. (1989). Cellular location of the cleavage event of the polymeric immunoglobulin receptor and fate of its anchoring domain in the rat hepatocyte. *Biochem. J.,* **257,** 759–768.

Sollid, L. M., Kvale, D., Brandtzaeg, P., Markussen, G., and Thorsby, E. (1987). Interferon-γ enhances expression of secretory component, the epithelial receptor for polymeric immunoglobulins. *J. Immunol.* **138,** 4303–4306.

South, M. A., Cooper, M. D., Wollheim, F. A., Hong, R., and Good, R. A. (1966). The IgA system. I. Studies of the transport and immunochemistry of IgA in the saliva. *J. Exp. Med.* **123,** 615–627.

Strober, W. (1990). Regulation of IgA B-cell development in the mucosal immune system. *J. Clin. Immunol.* **10,** 56S–63S.

Taguchi, T., McGhee, J. R., Coffman, R. L., Beagley, K. W., Eldridge, J. H., Takatsu, K., and Kiyono, H. (1990). Analysis of T_h1 and T_h2 cells in murine gut-associated tissues. Frequencies of CD4+ and CD8+ T cells that secrete IFN-γ and IL-5. *J. Immunol.* **145,** 68–77.

Taguchi, T., Aicher, W. K., Fujihashi, K., Yamamoto, M., McGhee, J. R., Bluestone, J. A., and Kiyono, H. (1991). Novel function for intestinal intraepithelial lymphocytes. Murine CD3+, γ/δ TCR+ T cells produce IFN-γ and IL-5. *J. Immunol.* **147,** 3736–3744.

Tomasi, T. B., Jr. (1980). Oral tolerance. *Transplantation* **29,** 353–356.

Tomasi, T. B., Jr., and Czerwinski, D. S. (1968). The secretory IgA systems. *In* "Immunological Deficiency Disease in Man" (D. Bergsma, ed.), Vol. IV, pp. 270–275. The National Foundation, New York.

Tomasi, T. B., Jr., Tan, E. M., Solomon, A., and Prendergast, R. A. (1965). Characteristics of an immune system common to certain external secretions. *J. Exp. Med.* **121,** 101–124.

Woloschak, G. E., Liarakos, C. D., and Tomasi, T. B. (1986). Identification of the major immunoglobulin heavy chain poly A RNA in murine lymphoid tissues. *Mol. Immunol.* **23,** 645–653.

Wu, M., Van Kaer, L., Itohara, S., and Tonegawa S. (1991). Highly restricted expression of the thymus leukemia antigens on intestinal epithelial cells. *J. Exp. Med.* **174,** 213–218.

Section A

Development and Physiology of Mucosal Defense

Section Editor: Jiri Mestecky

(Chapters 2 through 11)

2

Structure and Function of Intestinal Mucosal Epithelium

Tomohiro Kato • Robert L. Owen

I. INTRODUCTION

The mucosal epithelial layer forms the interface between the external and the internal environments in the gastrointestinal tract. This area is the site for digestion and absorption of various essential nutrients, yet it also must function as a barrier against various harmful agents and infectious pathogens. Protecting against such agents are many nonimmunological factors including gastric acid, pancreatic juice, bile, motility, mucus, glycocalyx, and cell turnover. In addition to these physiological barriers, an immunological barrier is created and maintained by the immune defense system, which includes the gut-associated lymphoid tissue (GALT)—immunoreactive cells distributed throughout the intestinal tract—and the systemic immune system. Much has been learned about GALT, but many questions about its structure and function remain unanswered. The mucosal epithelium in GALT, which functions as the leading edge of the immunological barrier, differs in many ways from the absorptive epithelium elsewhere in the intestinal tract (Figure 1). This chapter first describes the absorptive mucosa and then the GALT mucosa.

II. INTESTINAL ABSORPTIVE EPITHELIUM

The total mucosal surface in the adult human gastrointestinal tract extends to 200–300 m^2, the largest area of the body in contact with the external environment. This mucosal surface is covered with a one-cell-thick layer, the mucosal epithelium, that is composed of columnar absorptive cells, goblet cells, undifferentiated crypt epithelial cells, Paneth cells, enteroendocrine cells, tuft cells, cup cells, and intraepithelial lymphocytes. Although not part of the epithelium, mucus on the surface of the mucosa shields the mucosal epithelial cells from direct contact with the intestinal luminal environment. Beneath the mucosal epithelium is the connective and supportive tissue called the lamina propria. In this tissue are various immunocompetent cells including dendritic cells, macrophages, and lymphocytes, which form a functional unit with the mucosal epithelial cells.

A. Structure of the Absorptive Epithelium

1. Mucosal Epithelial Cells

Absorptive epithelial cells (enterocytes)—which are about 25 μm in height, 8 μm in width, and columnar in shape—constitute the majority of the mucosal epithelium. Their surface has numerous tightly packed microvilli that are covered with glycocalyx and a thick mucus layer. The regular longitudinal cores of microvilli are interconnected by a terminal web that is composed of bundles of 20–30 interlacing actin filaments. At their apices, the enterocytes are connected with adjacent epithelial cells mainly by junctional complexes consisting of three major components: tight junctions (zonula occludens), adhesion junctions (zonula adherens), and desmosomes (macula adherens). In addition to the junctional complexes, the lateral membranes interact by means of cell adhesion molecules (CAM), gap junctions, and interdigitations (Boyer and Thiery, 1989). The tight junction, which completely encircles the apical end of absorptive cells as a belt-like band, plays a role in separating the external and internal environments, and functions as a selective barrier. The adhesion junction, located in the apical region of absorptive cells just below the tight junction, is connected to actin filaments in the cytoplasm, and is thought to anchor each cell to adjacent cells. The desmosome functions like the adhesion junction, connected to intermediate filaments in the cytoplasm. Gap junctions, which are located in the basolateral membrane in other epithelial cells and directly mediate cell-to-cell communication, also have been identified provisionally in intestinal absorptive cells (Suzuki *et al.*, 1977; Kataoka *et al.*, 1989).

The glycocalyx, which is the surface layer just above the luminal membrane of the absorptive cell, contains various enzymes and nonenzymatic proteins including disaccharidases, peptidases, receptors, and transport proteins, all of which are necessary for digestion and absorption of nutrients. The major component of the glycocalyx is carbohydrate anchored into the surface of microvilli.

The smooth endoplasmic reticulum and mitochondria are more abundant in the apical than in the basal cytoplasm. The nucleus normally is located in the basal cytoplasm below the rough endoplasmic reticulum, so enterocytes maintain a characteristic polarity. The basolateral membrane, which

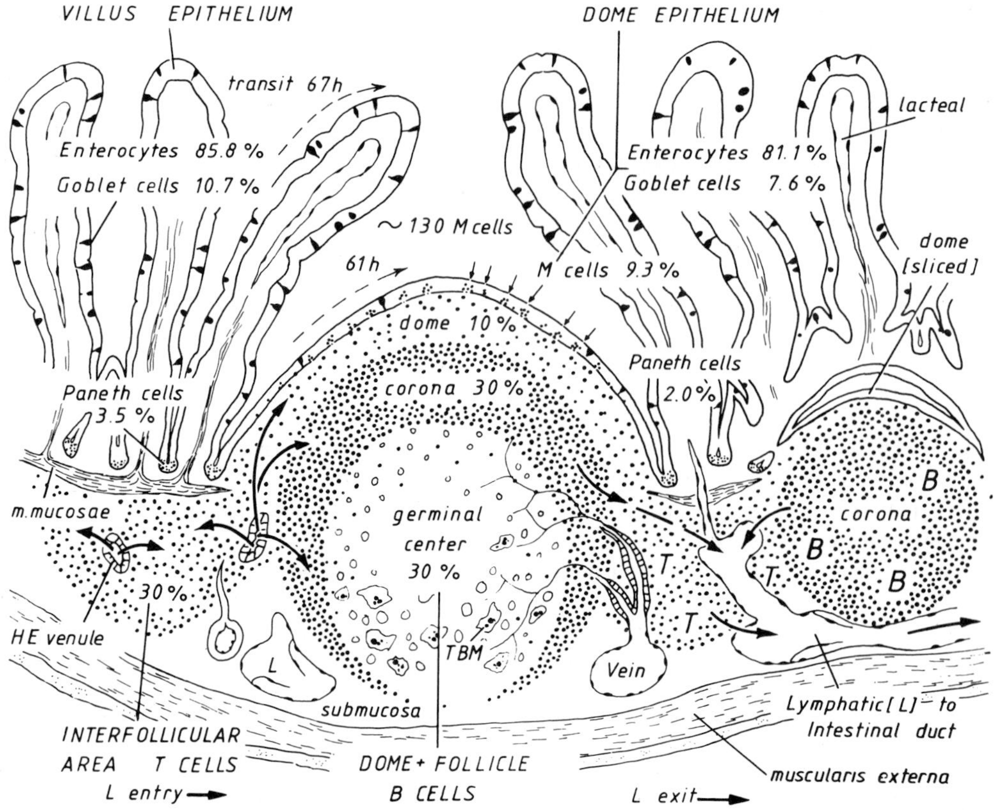

Figure 1 Diagram of an ileal Peyer's patch in the mouse. Peyer's patch lymphoid nodules are composed of three major parts: follicular area (germinal center, corona, and dome), interfollicular (parafollicular) area beneath villi, and dome epithelium. The right follicle beneath villi is sliced tangentially, through the lower slopes of the dome and the lymphocyte corona only. Curved arrows on the left show the influx of lymphocytes across postcapillary high endothelial venules (HEV), which mediate selective immigration of lymphocytes. Arrows on the right show the exit pathway of stimulated lymphocytes into submucosal lymphatics. M cells are difficult to distinguish by light microscopy, and are inferred from the location of groups of lymphoid cells (small arrows) in the follicle epithelium. Migration rates (h) and cell distribution numbers in this figure are from Smith and Peacock (1980) and Abe and Ito (1977). T, T lymphocyte; B, B lymphocyte; TBM, tingible body macrophage; m, muscularis. Diagram courtesy of E. Hamish Batten.

begins below the junctional complex, contains abundant Na^+, K^+-ATPase and adenylate cyclase and differs from the apical membrane in function. Interlocking folds are produced by adjacent cells, interdigitating their lateral membranes, which are separated by a 30-nm-wide intercellular space.

The basal membrane also is separated by a 30-nm space from the basal lamina. Junctional structures called hemidesmosomes anchor basal membrane to basal lamina. Hemidesmosomes are thought to connect with intermediate filaments of the cytoplasm, as do desmosomes. The basal lamina has numerous round or oval pores and is composed of collagen, laminin, fibronectin, and glycosaminoglycans (Hay, 1981; Ohtsuka *et al.*, 1992). Ultrastructurally, basal lamina consists of a lamina densa 20–50 nm thick that lies between two thin electron lucent layers: the lamina rata externa below and the lamina rata interna above (Dobbins, 1990). Although the function of the basal lamina is clear, researchers believe it gives polarity to the absorptive cells and guides migration of enterocytes from their crypts of origin to their eventual desquamation sites.

Goblet cells, present in both small and large intestine, increase in number from the proximal to the distal portion of the intestine and are located on villi and in crypts. The goblet cell microvilli are irregular in shape and sparse in number but contain actin filaments. The terminal web is poorly developed in goblet cells, facilitating release of mucus granules from the apical cytoplasm. Mucus granules are synthesized above the nucleus in endoplasmic reticulum and Golgi apparatus and are supported by a goblet-shaped sheath that is composed of inner and outer layers of microtubules and intermediate filaments and keeps its shape before and after release of granules (Specian and Neutra, 1984). Mucus granules are released in response to acetylcholine stimulation, but regulation of release is unclear.

Undifferentiated epithelial stem cells are located in the mid-crypts and produce daughter cells that continuously migrate upward to the crypt mouth and downward to the crypt base. These cells differentiate into absorptive cells and goblet cells above and into Paneth cells and enteroendocrine cells below. The microvilli of crypt cells are shorter and more sparse than are microvilli of mature absorptive cells. The terminal web and the junctional complex of crypt cells are undeveloped and the tight junction of these cells is structurally irregular, but its density is very high (Marcial *et al.*, 1984). In crypt cells, smooth and rough endoplasmic reticulum are sparse whereas ribosomes, mitochondria, and Golgi apparatus are relatively abundant. Small granules (0.1–1.5 μm), the functions of which are unknown, are released from crypt cells into the lumen in response to cholinergic stimuli. The undifferentiated crypt epithelial cells mature as they migrate to the summit of the villi, commonly in 3–5 days. From the crypt, cells migrate in a direct line toward the desquamation zone on the villus tip and, similarly, to the apex of the dome in GALT (Schmidt *et al.*, 1985). The migration rate is thought to depend on extraluminal and luminal factors: extraluminal factors consist of hormones, growth factors such as epidermal growth factor (EGF) and transforming growth factor (TGF), cytokines, and neural and vascular factors; luminal factors consist of nutrition, motility, and microflora (Levine, 1991). The crypt is recognized to be a major site of secretion of water and minerals into the lumen (Madara and Trier, 1987).

Paneth cells commonly are located in the crypts of the small intestine, but occasionally appear in the stomach and large intestine in some disease states. Their characteristic features are their pyramidal shape and, in the apical cytoplasm, various secretory granules that contain proteins including lysozyme, tumor necrosis factor (TNF) (Keshav *et al.*, 1990), and cryptdin (Ouellette *et al.*, 1989). These secretory granules are thought to prevent proliferation of crypt microorganisms by their strong antimicrobial action. Paneth cells also contain IgA and IgG, possibly from phagocytosis of immunoglobulin-coated microorganisms (Rodning *et al.*, 1976).

Enteroendocrine cells are distributed throughout the gastrointestinal tract. The main function of these cells is to release hormones into capillaries in the connective tissue in response to changes in the external environment. These cells contain various distinctive kinds of secretory granules and are classified structurally into closed and open types. Both commonly are located in the epithelium adjacent to the lamina propria, surrounded by other mucosal epithelial cells. Open type cells have a narrow apical surface in direct contact with the lumen, and are presumed to react to stimuli from the tissue environment and from the lumen. Closed type cells have no contact with the luminal environment (Dobbins, 1990).

Tuft cells, also called caveolated cells or fibrovesicular cells, have been discovered in the stomach, intestine, and colon of humans, dogs, mice, and rats (Nabeyama and Leblond, 1974; Owen, 1977; Blom and Helander, 1981). These cells are attached to surrounding absorptive cells by regular junctional complexes. On the surface, they have very long microvilli with filaments that are ~5 μm in length, sometimes reaching deep into the cytoplasm. Tuft cells have many caveolae or pits between the bases of microvilli that extend down to the level of the nucleus. The function of these pits is not known, but they are suspected to act as chemical sensors for the luminal milieu.

Cup cells were discovered by Madara (1982) in guinea pig, rabbit, and monkey intestine but have not yet been reported in humans. These cells stain more lightly than adjacent absorptive cells with toluidine blue stain, have abundant intermediate filaments, and have lower alkaline phosphatase activity on their surfaces than adjacent absorptive cells. Cup cells have shorter microvilli with a cuplike concavity, small mitochondria, and few vesicular bodies. The function of these cells is unknown.

Intraepithelial lymphocytes (IELs) have special characteristics that are distinct from those of other lymphocytes. The average number of IELs per 100 absorptive cells is 20 in normal adult human jejunum and decreases distally in the gut (Dobbins, 1986). These cells are located above the basal lamina in the epithelial layer and are separated from adjacent enterocytes by a 10- to 20-nm space. These lymphocyte–epithelial cell contacts have no junctional structure. Histochemically, almost all IELs are recognized to be $CD3^+$ (pan T cell). Among these cells, 5–15% express CD4 (helper/inducer phenotype) and the remaining cells express CD8 (cytotoxic/suppressor phenotype). These distributions contrast with other areas such as peripheral blood and lamina propria, where the $CD4^+$ phenotype is overwhelmingly predominant. Although the T-cell receptors that mediate antigen recognition are composed predominantly of $\alpha\beta$ chains on lymphocytes, in the intestinal epithelium the proportion of $\gamma\delta$-positive lymphocytes is much larger than in the peripheral blood and lamina propria (Jarry *et al.*, 1990). Thus, $\gamma\delta$-positive lymphocytes are thought to have a special role in the intestine. The microenvironment within the intestinal epithelium may influence the differentiation of IELs (Guy-Grand *et al.*, 1991). Although the functions of IELs are unclear, some possibilities are cytotoxicity, lymphokine secretion, regulation of renewal of mucosal epithelium, and tolerance (Cerf-Bensussan and Guy-Grand, 1991; see Chapter 24).

2. Mucus Layer and Glycocalyx

Mucus is composed of 1% mucin, 1% free protein, 1% dialyzable salts, and >95% water. Mucus contains albumin, immunoglobulin (mainly secretory IgA), α1-antitrypsin, lysozyme, lactoferrin, and EGF. In the mucus, the characteristic highly viscous and elastic substance is mucin, which is produced mainly in goblet cells as heavily glycosylated glycoprotein (Rhodes, 1990). Mucus is not digested because of its resistance to various enzymes, and is thought to protect epithelial cells from digestion by enzymes produced by intestinal flora and by pancreatic and biliary juice. The release of mucus from goblet cells is stimulated by neurogenic factors and by alterations in environmental factors, including bacterial infection, parasitic infestation, and the resident intestinal flora. Mucus secretion from goblet cells is triggered by two mechanisms: direct stimulation by immune complexes and chemical agents and indirect stimulation by mediators released by histamine and lymphokines (Snyder and Walker, 1987). Mucus can protect epithelium against the adherence of such organisms as *Entamoeba histolytica, Yersinia enterocolitica,* and enteropathogenic *Escherichia coli* by trapping microorganisms and by covering binding sites with mucin and with secretory IgA (Magnusson and Stjernström, 1982;

Chadee *et al.*, 1987; Mantle *et al.*, 1989; Sajjan and Forstner, 1990). Mucin also inhibits the epithelial attachment of such parasites as *Nippostrongylus brasiliensis* and *Trichinella spiralis* (Miller, 1987), whereas other components in mucus, including lysozyme, secretory IgA, and lactoferrin, have antibacterial activity (see Chapters 4 and 11). The glycocalyx on microvilli forms a zone for digestion and absorption. The mucus layer and rapid turnover of absorptive cells are useful for the protection and regeneration of glycocalyx, because some bacteria can digest important proteins in it by direct contact (Jonas *et al.*, 1978; see Chapter 4).

3. Resident Microflora

The resident microflora is composed of at least 400 species of bacteria of which major components are streptococci, lactobacilli, *Bacteroides*, and enterobacteria. The upper intestinal bacterial count is low in number ($<10^5$ cfu/ml) and increases distally (terminal ileum, 10^6/ml; colon, 10^{11}/ml). Intestinal bacterial numbers are regulated by the flow rate of luminal contents (intestinal motility) and by mucus and the antibacterial effects of gastric, pancreatic, and biliary juice. Some of the bacteria produce enzymes that degrade mucin, which is thought to be one of their mechanisms of survival (Rhodes, 1989). Resident microflora are known to coexist within the intestinal tract and maintain a stable environment by precluding attachment of enteropathogens (see Chapter 6). The flora can eliminate foreign pathogens by producing antimicrobial substances (colicins, short chain fatty acids; Iglewski and Gerhardt, 1978; Byrne and Dankert, 1979) and by stimulating the growth of mucosal epithelium (Thompson and Trexler, 1971). Interestingly, bacteria such as *Lactobacillus, Bacteroides,* and *Clostridium* have been reported also to exist within the intestinal mucosa. Ultrastructurally, these organisms adhere firmly to the mucus layer in crypts of the distal small intestine (Savage, 1970).

B. Absorptive Cell Function

1. Uptake and Transport of Nutrients, Minerals, Water, and Nonnutrient Materials

Digestion and absorption of nutrients is the primary function of the gastrointestinal tract. Mucosal absorptive cells have digestive and absorptive functions. The apical surface of absorptive cells consists of the glycocalyx and plasma membrane, which contains various enzymes and carriers for digestion and absorption. Sodium is important for the absorption of nutrients and other minerals because its electrical gradient regulates their movement into absorptive cells. The gradient of Na^+ is regulated mainly by secretion and absorption by Na^+,K^+-ATPase on basolateral membranes; Na^+ goes in and out with other minerals and nutrients through the brush border membrane. Water and ions are thought to pass through tight junctions (paracellular pathway) in addition to the route across epithelial cells (transcellular pathway).

Pathogens and other harmful agents including bacteria, viruses, parasites, and allergenic macromolecules are mixed with nutrient materials in the intestine. Despite protective mechanisms, these harmful agents can cross the mucosal barrier via three major routes: the transcellular route, the paracellular route across cell-to-cell junctions including tight junctions, and via M cells, which are specially differentiated epithelial cells in Peyer's patches (see subsequent discussion). Uptake mechanisms are separated into receptor-mediated and non-receptor-mediated pathways. The route of uptake of nonnutrients previously was believed to be only paracellular. However, the transcellular route through absorptive cells has been recognized to play a role in initiating mucosal and systemic infection and, possibly, in antigen presentation, since absorptive cells are the first point of contact for many luminal constituents.

For absorptive cells to function as antigen-presenting cells (APCs), uptake, endosomal degradation, processing, and presentation of antigen to immunocompetent cells (such as T cells and macrophages) restricted by major histocompatibility complex (MHC) Class II proteins would be required. This process of delivery of coherent and recognizable antigenic information also requires cytokines and, possibly, control by hormones and the nervous system. APCs must express MHC Class II proteins on their surfaces to initiate the process of presentation. Normal absorptive cells in humans and rats do, in fact, express MHC Class II proteins on their apical surfaces (Hirata *et al.*, 1986; Mayer *et al.*, 1991; see Chapter 15). $CD8^+$ IELs are reported to secrete interferon γ (IFNγ; Cerf-Bensussan *et al.*, 1984), which can stimulate absorptive cells further to express MHC Class II proteins (Hirayama *et al.*, 1987) and protect them against infection by viruses. Further, absorptive cells are reported to produce and secrete an interleukin 1 (IL-1)-like substance, which is an activator of T cells, in response to luminal antigens such as lipopolysaccharide (LPS; Santos *et al.*, 1990). These observations suggest that normal absorptive cells may function as APCs, at least under special circumstances, and that the transcellular route may play a role in immune surveillance.

2. Barrier to Entrance of Microorganisms, Particles, and Macromolecules

In the intestinal lumen, pancreatic and biliary juice, mucus, glycocalyx, intestinal motility, and resident microflora interact to limit colonization by enteropathogens. Pancreatic and biliary juices, along with secretory IgA and lysozyme, have antibacterial activities in some species (Williams *et al.*, 1975; Rubinstein *et al.*, 1985; Bassi *et al.*, 1991). Even if pathogens begin to invade the epithelium, the process may be restricted by local mechanisms and terminated as tiny lesions. Protection is provided by the epithelial cell and by the environment surrounding epithelial cells. Turnover of crypt cells increases the rate of epithelial renewal in response to the invasion of harmful pathogens that damage surface cells. Lesions will be washed by mucus and other secretions in conjunction with intestinal motility, and will be repaired by cell migration. Evidence suggests that IELs can kill virus-infected target cells and bacteria in experimental animals (London *et al.*, 1989; Tagliabue *et al.*, 1984), but no information about such a role for IELs in humans is available (see Chapter 24).

Chemical messengers including neuropeptides, gastrointestinal hormones, and lymphokines affect barrier factors. Substance P, somatostatin, and cholecystokinin (CCK) influence the production of mucin and IgA (Stanisz *et al.*, 1986; Freier *et al.*, 1987); IFNγ modulates the barrier function of absorptive cells (Madara and Stafford, 1989). Although the roles of these mediators are not elucidated completely, they are thought to contribute to the multifactorial network of nonimmunological mucosal defense mechanisms described earlier and to immunological mechanisms described in subsequent chapters (see Chapters 17, 20, 27).

III. MUCOSAL EPITHELIUM IN GUT ASSOCIATED LYMPHOID TISSUE

GALT is a general term for lymphoid tissues distributed in intestine, including aggregated lymphoid nodules in Peyer's patches, the appendix vermiformis (Uchida, 1988), colonic patches (Owen *et al.*, 1991), and solitary lymphoid nodules. In its entirety, GALT is one of the largest lymphoid organs in the body.

The typical GALT structures can be observed most easily in Peyer's patches. Peyer's patches are groups of lymphoid follicles in the small intestinal mucosa (Figures 1 and 2). Although their numbers and distribution differ among individuals and in different species, some features are characteristic: Peyer's patches are located along the antimesentric side of the small intestine and are most prominent in the terminal ileum, and the number and size of Peyer's patch follicles decrease with age.

A. Structure of the Follicle Epithelium

Morphologically, Peyer's patch nodules are separated into three major domains: the follicular area, the parafollicular area, and the follicle-associated epithelium (FAE). Histologically, intestinal lymphoid nodules differ from lymph nodes because they have no capsule, no medulla, no afferent lymphatic ducts, and no clear border. The FAE is a one-cell-thick lining layer that forms the interface between the intestinal lymphoid apparatus and the intestinal luminal environment, and is generated within the crypts that supply enterocytes to villi adjacent to lymphoid nodules. FAE is composed mainly of specially differentiated M cells, columnar epithelial cells, IELs, infrequent mucus-secreting goblet cells, and occasional tuft cells. GALT is described further in Chapter 35.

1. M Cells

By dissecting microscopy, small protruding domes can be distinguished among the villi in Peyer's patches. By scanning electron microscopy (SEM), M cells are found scattered over the dome, surrounded by absorptive cells (Figure 3).

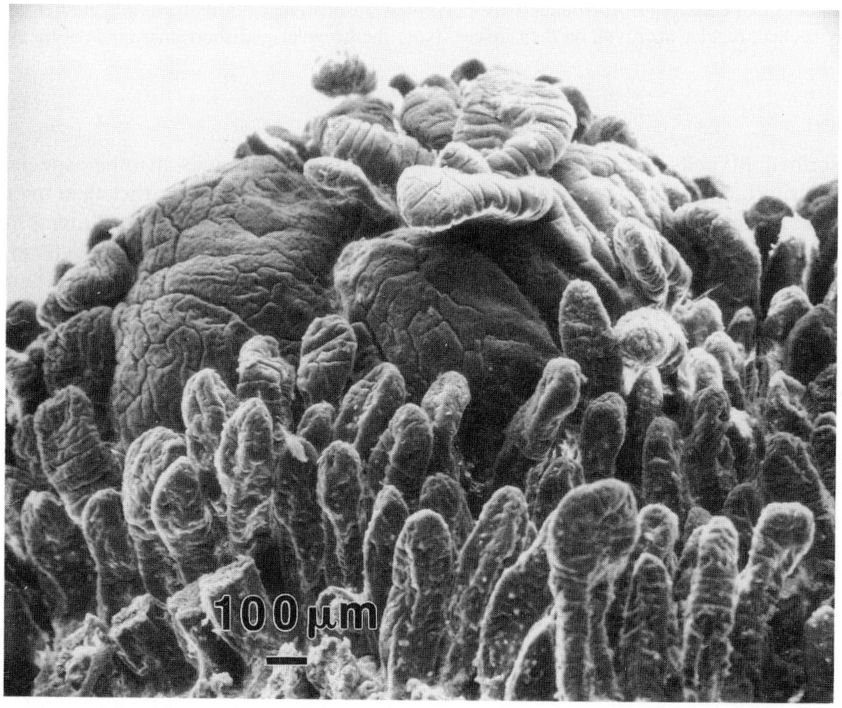

Figure 2 Scanning electron micrograph of a dome-shaped lymphoid nodule surrounded by numerous finger-shaped villi in human Peyer's patch. Note that surfaces of villi are covered with whitish-colored mucus drops that are absent over the surfaces of the lymphoid nodule. Reprinted with permission from Owen and Jones (1974). Epithelial cell specialization within human Peyer's patches: An ultrastructural study of intestinal lymphoid follicles. *Gastroenterology* **66,** 189–203. The Williams and Wilkins Company, Baltimore.

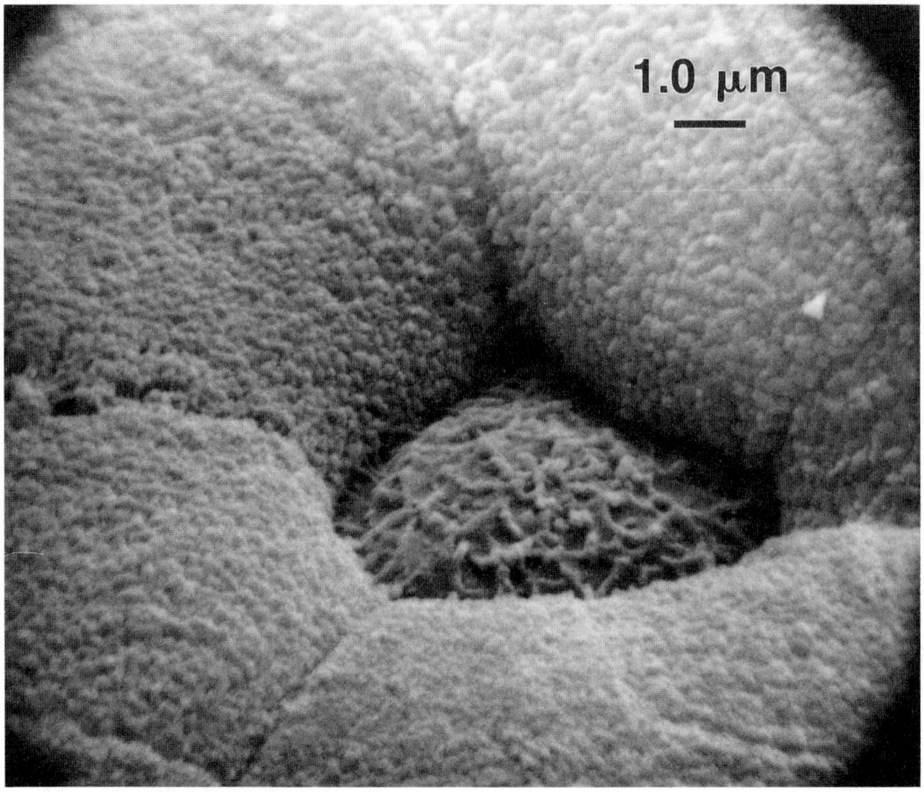

Figure 3 Scanning electron micrograph of the surface of a human Peyer's patch lymphoid nodule. The M cell in the center is surrounded by polygonal absorptive cells that possess numerous tall, closely packed, regular microvilli on their apices. Note the irregular and short microfolds of the M cell.

Since Schmedtje described M cells (which he termed lymphoepithelial cells) covering dome-shaped lymphoid follicles in the rabbit appendix (Schmedtje, 1965, 1966), similar cells have been discovered in many organs and species. Such cells were identified by Owen and Jones (1974) in human small intestine and termed M cells. M cells also have been found in nonintestinal lymphoid aggregates, including tonsil (Owen and Nemanic, 1978) and bronchi (Bienenstock and Befus, 1984; see Chapter 12; Chapters 43 and 50). M cells occupy ~50% of FAE surface area in rabbit and 10% of intestinal lymphoid follicle surface area in human and mouse.

M cells play an important role in antigen sampling, taking up particles from the intestinal lumen and transporting them to lymphocytes and macrophages enfolded in pockets in the basolateral surfaces of M cells (Trier, 1991). Figure 4 shows M cells typical of the lymphoid follicles in human ileum.

M cells have shared and unique structural features in comparison with other mucosal epithelial cells in the intestine (Figure 5). M cells have tight junctions and desmosomes in contact with adjacent columnar epithelial cells and interdigitating lateral membranes (Figure 6). The processes on their luminal surfaces are spaced more widely and often are shorter and more irregular in shape than the microvilli of absorptive cells; these processes consist of "microfolds" in humans (hence, the name "M" cell; Figure 3). Sometimes longer microfolds reach out to surround microorganisms in the intestinal lumen. M cells in other species were found to have specialized microvilli rather than microfolds. Consequently, the term M cell now denotes "membranous" or "membrane-like," reflecting the role of M cells in separating the luminal and intercellular domains yet facilitating movement from one to the other. Ultrastructurally, microfolds in human M cells and comparable M-cell microvilli in other species have fewer microfilaments such as actin and a less highly developed apical terminal web than do adjacent absorptive cells. The apical cytoplasm of M cells has closely packed mitochondria and numerous rounded, tubular, or oval microvesicles but few lysosomes (Owen *et al.*, 1988a; Figure 7).

The M cell typically has an extracellular space, called the central hollow or pocket, that invaginates its basolateral membrane and surrounds enfolded lymphoid cells (Figure 8). Within these pockets lie one or more lymphocytes, macrophages, plasma cells, or, rarely, polymorphonuclear leukocytes. Often the apical portion of the M cell is compressed into a thin membrane-like band of cytoplasm by the lymphocyte-filled pocket, which also displaces the nucleus of the M cell basally. Golgi apparatus and endoplasmic reticulum are located just above the nucleus in M cells (Figure 4). The well-developed microvesicular system, sparse lysosomes, and enfolded lymphocytes are morphological correlates of the transport function of M cells (see subsequent discussion). No connective junctions are ultrastructurally demonstrable

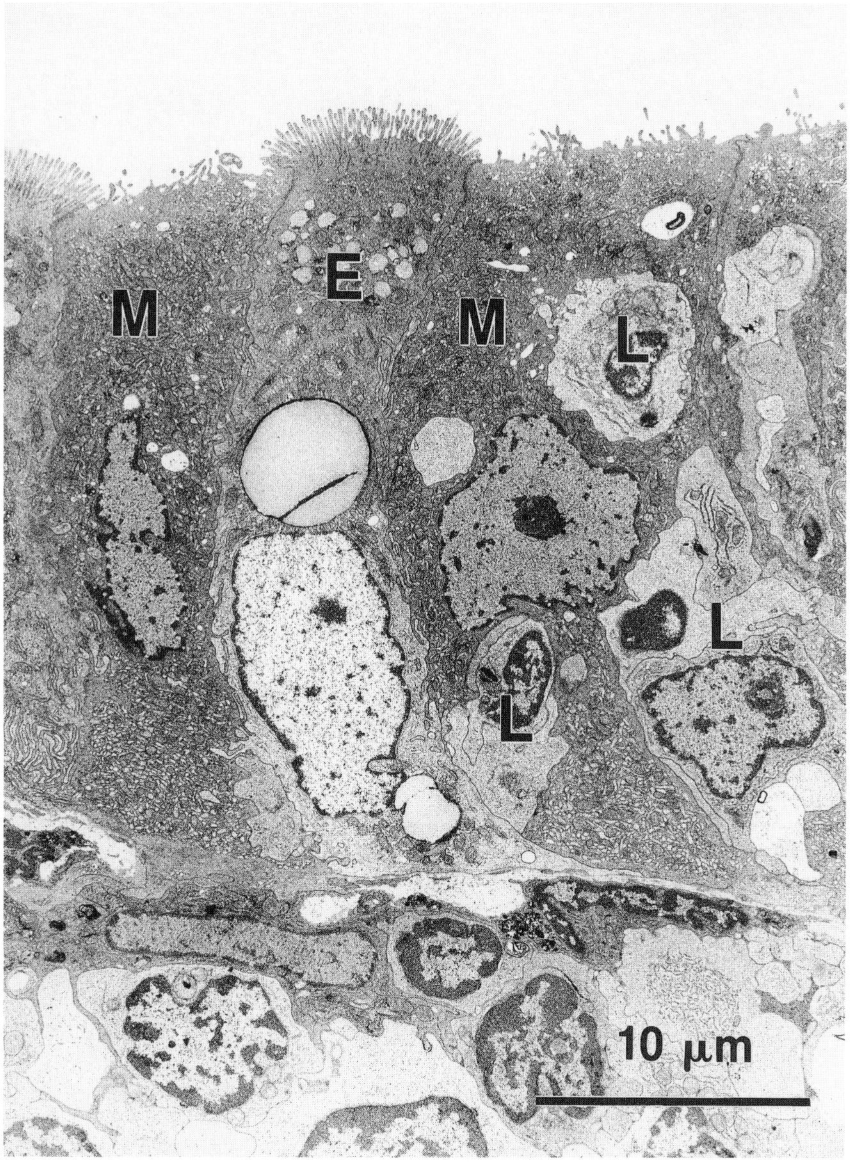

Figure 4 Transmission electron micrograph of human Peyer's patch follicle epithelium. M cells (M) are shorter than enterocytes (E), which are covered by tightly packed microvilli. The M cells on the right enfold lymphocytes (L) in their pockets, whereas the M cell on the left contains no lymphocyte.

between M cells and enfolded cells, but adhesion molecules, cytokines, and complementary cytoskeletal structures form a complex relationship. Enfolded cells intrude into the M cell from its basal or lateral surface, presumably in response to homing signals, and come in contact with surveillance information in the form of macromolecules, particles, and microorganisms transported from the intestinal lumen by M cells. This lymphoid cell traffic in and out of M cell pockets is facilitated by the numerous holes that can be observed in the basal lamina after removal of mucosal epithelium.

M cells in rabbits have been found to express an unusual pattern of intermediate filaments in their cytoplasm, that is, predominantly vimentin (Gaidar, 1989) with lesser amounts of cytokeratin (Jepson *et al.,* 1992), compared with other epithelial cells, in which vimentin is absent. This M-cell expression of intermediate filaments that is more typical of cells of mesenchymal origin than of epithelial cells may reflect the phagocytic activity, and accommodation in shape to enfolded cells, in which M cells resemble macrophages.

The layer of glycocalyx and mucus on M cells is quite sparse, compared with that on adjacent columnar cells. Consequently, the microvilli on the surface of M cells can be observed easily by SEM (Figure 3). The surface of M-cell microvilli has more esterase activity and much less alkaline phosphatase activity than the surface of microvilli of adjacent absorptive cells (Owen and Bhalla, 1983). The functional

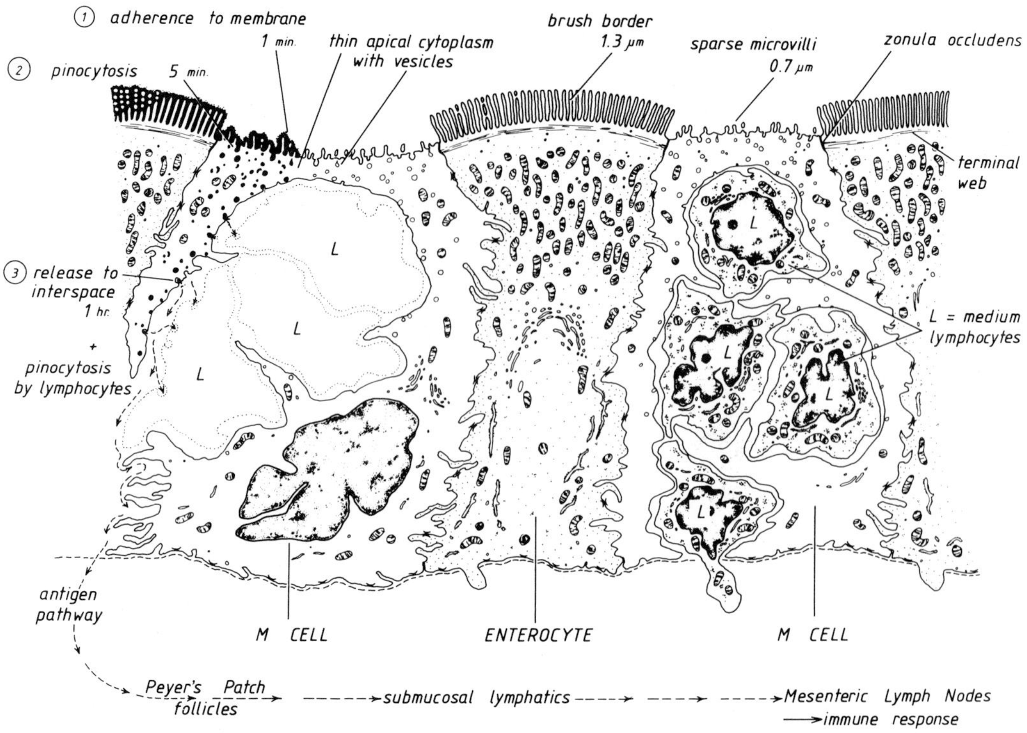

Figure 5 A diagram of the ultrastructural arrangement of enterocytes (stippled), M cells, and intraepithelial lymphocytes in follicle epithelium of Peyer's patch. On the right, four lymphocytes (L) are enfolded in the central hollow of an M cell. On the left, note the thin apical cytoplasm of the M cell, its lateral interdigitations, and three enfolded lymphocytes (L) shown only in dotted outline. Over the luminal surface, black lines show horseradish peroxidase (HRP) adhering to follicle epithelium 1 min after being injected into mouse ileum. The time sequence (1–3) shows pinocytotic transfer through the M cell into its central hollow, with some uptake by enfolded lymphoid cells (Owen, 1977). Antigens transported by M cells also pass downward through the basal lamina into the lymphoid follicles and are carried into mesenteric lymph nodes for induction of local or systemic immune responses. Diagram courtesy of E. Hamish Batten.

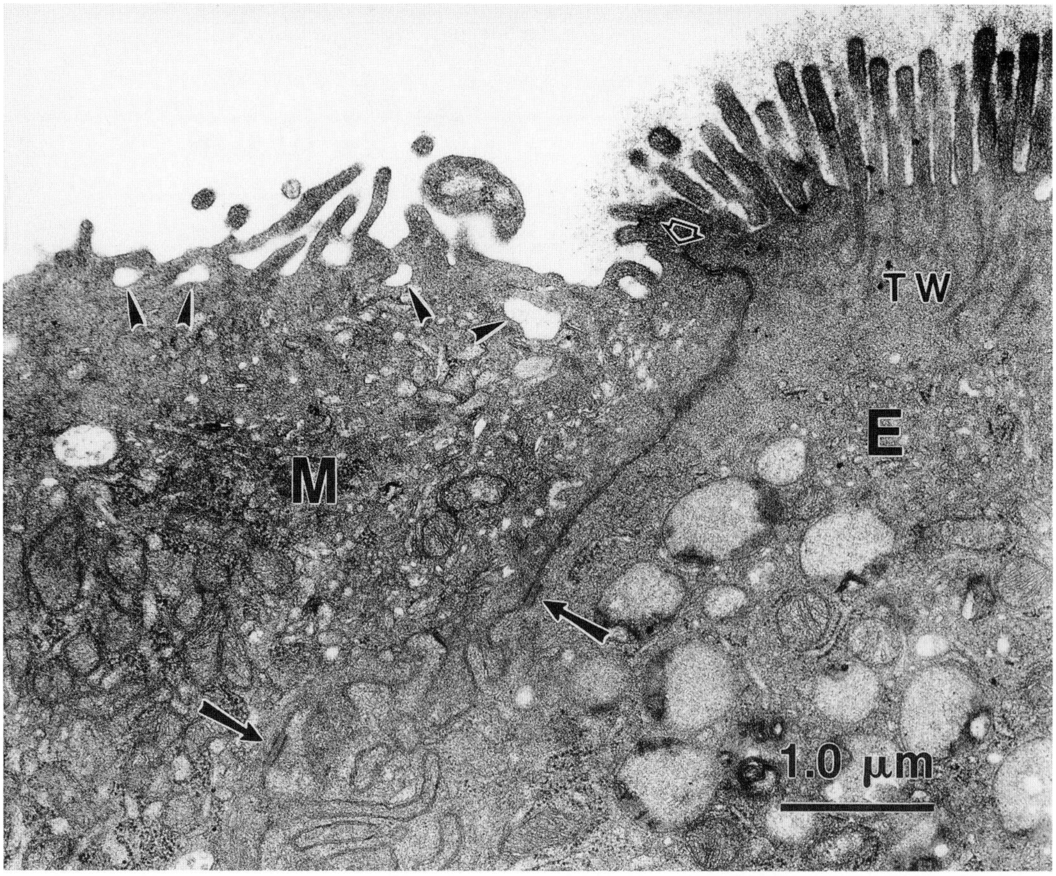

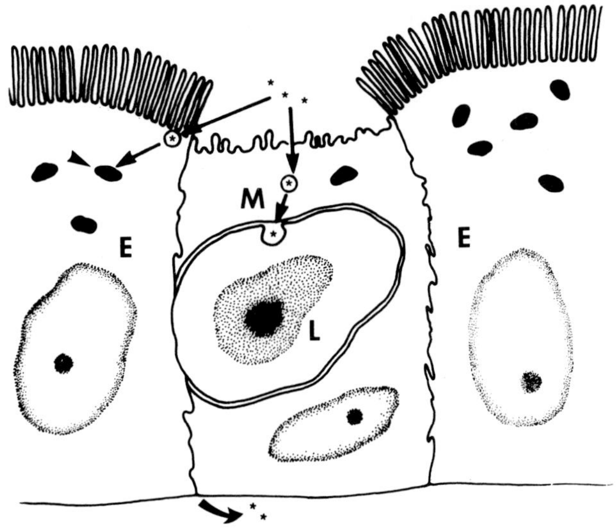

Figure 7 Diagrammatic model of uptake and transport of luminal antigens by M cells (M). The M cell has only a rare lysosome, compared with numerous lysosomes (arrowhead) in adjacent enterocytes (E). When particulate antigens (asterisks) are taken up by enterocytes, they are diverted into lysosomes and digested. In M cells, antigens escape lysosomal degradation and either are taken up by lymphoid cells (L) in the central hollow or pass into the intercellular space. Reprinted with permission from Owen *et al.*, (1986a) and Wiley-Liss.

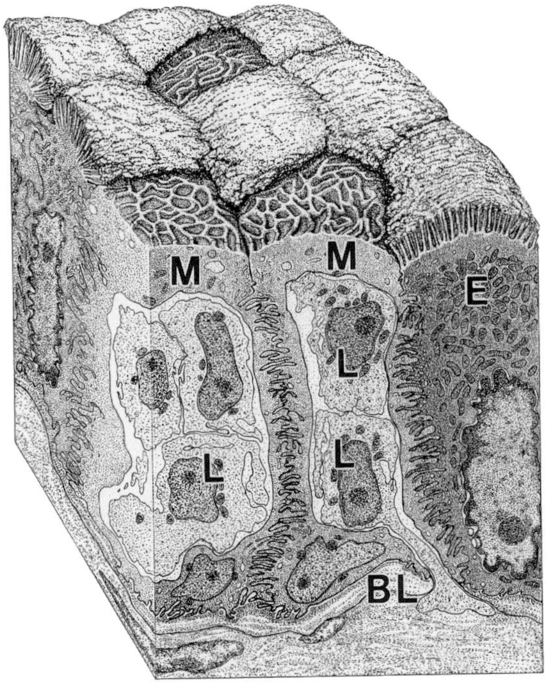

Figure 8 Three-dimensional illustration of M cells (M) interdigitating with adjacent enterocytes (E). In their central hollows, M cells enfold several lymphocytes (L), one of which is migrating through a pore in the basal lamina (BL). Reprinted with permission from Owen and Nemanic (1978).

significance of this enzymatic pattern is uncertain, but has been used to advantage by Smith and colleagues (1987) in examining patterns of M-cell distribution over follicle domes. Because of their low lysosome content, M cells can transport antigens from the intestinal lumen with little enzymatic degradation (Owen *et al.*, 1986a). The surface of M cells has been found to interact with secretory IgA in uptake of intestinal particles. The surface of the M cell has binding sites for secretory IgA (Roy and Varvayanis, 1987; Weltzin *et al.*, 1989; Kato, 1990; Figure 9), but lacks secretory component (Pappo and Owen, 1988). Immunohistochemically, the human M cell expresses MHC Class II HLA-DR antigen on its apical cytoplasm and basolateral membrane, analogous to the dendritic cell and macrophage which are known to be APCs (Nagura *et al.*, 1991). This feature of M cells, in conjunction with the fact that M cells take up complexes containing secretory IgA, suggests that these cells may function as APCs and as antigen-transporting cells. In fact, M cells from rat jejunal Peyer's patches contain acidic endosomal and prelysosomal structures but few lysosome-like structures (Figure 7) and express MHC Class II determinants, indicating that they have at least some capacity to present endocytosed antigens directly to lymphocytes (Allan *et al.*, 1992).

Putative M cells have been recognized morphologically in human fetuses by week 17 of gestation (Moxey and Trier, 1978). Although the origin of the M cell is still controversial, two theories have been proposed. One theory is that M cells develop from mature columnar epithelial cells that overlie Peyer's patches. Another theory is that M cells develop directly from undifferentiated stem cells in crypts that lie between lymphoid domes and adjacent villi (Bhalla and Owen, 1982). This theory is supported by the observations of Bye *et al.* (1984). Morphologically immature M cells, with features shared by mature M cells and crypt cells, can be identified in all regions of the follicle dome. After intraperitoneal injection of [^{3}H]thymidine into mice, only crypt cells are labeled for the first 12 hr. Radiolabeled nuclei of immature M cells are first observed near crypt mouths in mice after 24 hr and mature M cells are labeled after 48 hr. M cells are now generally accepted to derive directly from undifferentiated stem cells in the crypts surrounding the dome. Where they go is less clear, however, since more M cells are present on the edges of domes than on the apices, where desquamation and death of enterocytes generally occur.

Figure 6 Transmission electron micrograph showing the junction between a columnar enterocyte (E) and an M cell (M) in human Peyer's patch. The M cell has characteristic microfolds, absent terminal web, sparse glycocalyx, and numerous pinocytotic vesicles (arrowheads) in its apical cytoplasm compared with the adjacent enterocyte, which has thick glycocalyx, regular microvilli, and microvillus cores extending down into the termina web (TW). The interface is composed of a tight junction (open arrowhead), several desmosomes (arrows), and lateral interdigitations.

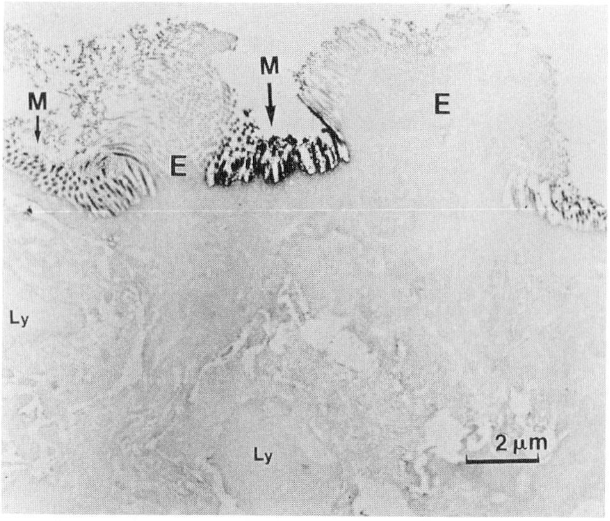

Figure 9 Immunoelectron micrograph of rabbit Peyer's patch follicle epithelium treated with anti-secretory IgA antibody and horseradish peroxidase-conjugated secondary antibody. Electron-dense areas of enzyme reaction product are prominent over the short irregular microvilli of the M cells (M) with enfolded lymphocytes (Ly), compared with the adjacent enterocytes (E). Reaction product is presumed to show binding sites of secretory IgA on M cells, which may take up IgA–antigen complexes. Reprinted with permission from Kato (1990).

The life-span of M cells is uncertain. According to the study of Bye *et al.* (1984), they migrate from the crypt to the dome base within 24 hr and to the summit of the dome within 72 hr. This life-span is essentially identical to that of the regular villus epithelium. Numbers of cells with labeled nuclei over domes gradually decrease between days 5 and 14 and no labeled cells are present by day 14 (Bye *et al.*, 1984).

GALT in specific pathogen-free (SPF) animals is poorly developed, although its basic structure is present. Exposure to the intestinal flora is essential for the complete development of GALT. M cells also need microbial exposure to proliferate. The total number of M cells is increased in mice after transfer from an SPF to a conventional environment (Smith *et al.*, 1987), whereas the ratio of M cells to FAE is reported not to be changed by such transfer (Siciński *et al.*, 1986). The invagination by lymphocytes had been considered essential to M cell development, but lymphocytes do not seem to be necessary for morphological maturation, since mature M cells can be recognized even in mice depleted of lymphocytes by total lymphoid irradiation (Ermak *et al.*, 1989).

2. Other Follicle Epithelial Cells

In addition to M cells, several other kinds of cells are present in FAE: columnar absorptive cells, IELs, and tuft cells. The structure of absorptive cells in FAE resembles that of enterocytes on villi, but these two populations of absorptive cells may differ in surface characteristics and function (Figure 5). In rabbits, secretory component is absent not only from M cells but also from absorptive cells in FAE (Pappo and Owen, 1988). The majority of IELs in FAE are $CD8^+$ T cells, as in villus epithelium (see Chapters 23, 24), but the ratio of $CD4^+$ to $CD8^+$ lymphocytes in FAE (4:10) is greater than in IELs of villi (0.6:10). Lymphocytes in FAE are often large lymphoblast forms, however, which are thought to be immature and immunologically uncommitted, compared with the mature effector IELs found among enterocytes that cover villi. FAE is involved in induction of helper T cell functions, possibly as a consequence of M-cell uptake and transport of antigens from the intestinal lumen (Bjerke *et al.*, 1988).

B. M Cell Function

Several important immunological and pathophysiological functions are recognized for M cells. M cells capture antigens from the intestinal lumen and transport them to enfolded lymphocytes and macrophages. Some of these lymphoid cells are presumed to influence IgA production directly in the germinal centers of lymphoid follicles, but this concept has been difficult to prove. Kabok *et al.* (1993) were able to induce production of antiferritin antibody by incubating isolated rabbit Peyer's patch lymphoid follicles with ferritin in organ culture for 7 days. Other stimulated lymphoid cells migrate through lymphatics to mesentric lymph nodes and via the thoracic duct to the general circulation, then ultimately return by migration and homing receptors to mucosal tissues as IgA-producing plasma cells (Figure 1).

1. Mucosal Surveillance

a. Antigen uptake. M cells take up and transport a wide variety of sizes and types of intestinal antigens and microorganisms. This unique process may depend in part on factors that include mediators released by immunocompetent cells, hormonal factors, and nervous control. To study M cell function, investigators have focused on M cells of Peyer's patches, often using ligated intestinal segments and high concentrations of organisms to facilitate detection of uptake that, under physiological conditions, would occur less frequently yet would be sufficient for induction of immunological responses. Some of the macromolecules and microorganisms for which uptake and transport by M cells has been confirmed are discussed in the following sections (see also Table I).

i. Particles and macromolecules. Native ferritin (rat; Bockman and Cooper, 1973), cationized ferritin (rabbit; Bye *et al.*, 1984), horseradish peroxidase (rabbit; Owen, 1977; von Rosen, 1981), *Ricinus communis* agglutinins I and II (rabbit; Neutra *et al.*, 1987), wheat germ agglutinin (rabbit; Neutra *et al.*, 1987), cholera toxin (guinea pig; Shakhlamov *et al.*, 1981), Picibanil (OK-432, a streptococcal biological response modifier; rabbit; Nagasaki *et al.*, 1988), and 600- to 750-nm diameter latex particles (rabbit; Pappo and Ermak, 1989) have been shown to be transported by M cells.

ii. Viruses. Reovirus type 1 and type 3 (mouse; Wolf, 1983), poliovirus type 1 (human; Siciński *et al.*, 1990), human immunodeficiency virus type 1 (HIV-1; mouse and rabbit; Amerongen *et al.*, 1991), and mouse mammary tumor virus

Table I Substances and Microorganisms Taken up by M Cells

Particles and macromolecules
Native ferritin
Cationized ferritin
Horseradish peroxidase
Ricinus communis agglutinins I and II
Wheat germ agglutinin
Cholera toxin
Picibanil (OK-432)
600- to 750-nm diameter latex particles
Viruses
Reovirus type 1 and type 3
Poliovirus type 1
Human immunodeficiency virus type 1 (HIV-1)
Mouse mammary tumor virus (MMTV)
Bacteria
Vibrio cholerae
Salmonella typhi
Bacillus Calmette–Guérin (BCG)
Mycobacterium paratuberculosis
Brucella abortus
Streptococcus pyogenes
Campylobacter jejuni
Yersinia enterocolitica
Yersinia pseudotuberculosis
Shigella flexneri
Salmonella enteritidis
Escherichia coli RDEC-1 strain
Escherichia coli 0 : 124 K : 72 strain
Parasites
Cryptosporidium

(MMTV; mouse; Neutra and Kraehenbuhl, 1992) have been shown to be transported by M cells.

iii. Bacteria. *Vibrio cholerae* (rabbit; Owen *et al.*, 1986b), *Salmonella typhi* (mouse; Kohbata *et al.*, 1986), BCG (*Bacillus* Calmette-Guérin; rabbit; Fujimura, 1986), *Mycobacterium paratuberculosis* (calf; Momotani *et al.*, 1988), *Brucella abortus* (calf; Ackermann *et al.*, 1988), *Streptococcus pyogenes* (rabbit; Nagasaki *et al.*, 1988), *Campylobacter jejuni* (rabbit; Walker *et al.*, 1988), *Yersinia enterocolitica* (mouse; Grützkau *et al.*, 1990), *Yersinia pseudotuberculosis* (rabbit; Fujimura *et al.*, 1989), *Shigella flexneri* (rabbit; Wassef *et al.*, 1989), *Salmonella enteritidis* (rabbit; Kamoi, 1991), RDEC-1 strain of *Escherichia coli* (rabbit; Inman and Cantey, 1984), and 0:124 K:72 strain of *E. coli* (rabbit; Uchida, 1987) have been shown to be transported by M cells.

iv. Parasites. *Cryptosporidium* (guinea pig; Marcial and Madara, 1986) has been shown to be taken up. Even under optimizing conditions, observation of uptake of *Giardia muris* trophozoites has not been possible, although they were found in the pocket within mouse M cells (Owen *et al.*, 1981).

M cells are also capable of reverse transport of some substances into the intestinal lumen, as demonstrated by the fact that injected horseradish peroxidase can be seen to move from the tissue into the lumen through M cells (Bockman and Stevens, 1977).

Information about M cell function in absorption of nutrients is limited; however, no absorption of lipid by M cells of mice was observed (Bye *et al.*, 1984).

Although the range of microorganisms and other particles taken up by M cells is wide, these cells also exhibit selectivity of uptake and specific characteristics impede or facilitate attachment, uptake, and transport. Viable and killed *M. paratuberculosis* are taken up by M cells. Living *V. cholerae* are taken up, transported, and presented (Figure 10), but killed *Vibrio* are scarcely taken up by M cells. When suspensions of 10^9 *Vibrio* killed by acidification, formalin treatment, ultraviolet irradiation, or heating were injected into ligated intestinal segments of rabbit intestine containing Peyer's patches, none were taken up after 180 min, although motile noninvasive but colonizing living *Vibrio* of the same strain were taken up readily by M cells when administered in the same concentration (Owen *et al.*, 1988b). Because cholera toxin stimulates a variety of cellular processes, mutant *Vibrio* that produce neither the A nor the B subunit of cholera toxin were administered and found to be taken up by M cells as efficiently as toxigenic strains. In contrast, a toxin-producing but nonmotile strain, CVD 49, was not taken up, indicating that one of the most important determinants of bacterial uptake is whether organisms can reach the M cell surface, either by motility or by lateral spread across the colonized mucosal surface (Owen *et al.*, 1988a).

Even different strains of the same microorganism have very different interactions with M cells. Among *E. coli*, the O:124 K:72 strain is taken up and presented but the O:124 RDEC-1 strain can adhere to the M cell surface without being transported. Reovirus type 1 is taken up by M cells only, but type 3 is taken up by M cells and columnar cells in FAE (Wolf *et al.*, 1983). Further, after passage through M cells, reovirus type 1 passes through the basolateral membrane of these cells to adjacent columnar epithelial cells and proliferates there, finally producing an inflammatory lesion (Weiner *et al.*, 1988).

Whether the relatively weak alkaline phosphatase activity on the apical surface of the M cell has functional significance is unclear, but the very few lysosomes and the well-developed vesicular transport system in its apical cytoplasm contribute to the function of the M cell as the gateway to the immune defense system (Figure 7). This function as a gatekeeper seems to depend on the equilibrium between the motility, colonizing potential, and invasiveness of pathogens and the defensive competence of M cells and associated macrophages. The efficiency and vigor with which M cells function as the gateway for antigen sampling contribute to a pathophysiological role of M cells as entry points for invasion by virulent pathogens. Some types of intestinal infection, particularly typhoid fever and intestinal tuberculosis, occur initially in Peyer's patches. Virulent pathogens such as *S. typhi* and *S. flexneri* invade M cells and subsequently precipitate the destruction of Peyer's patches. Thus, the M cell seems to be a target cell as well as a conduit for some virulent pathogens that cause enteritis in clinical settings.

In M cells, whether initiation of an immune response or systemic invasion occurs may depend on binding to the M-cell apical membrane and on the ability of M cells and associ-

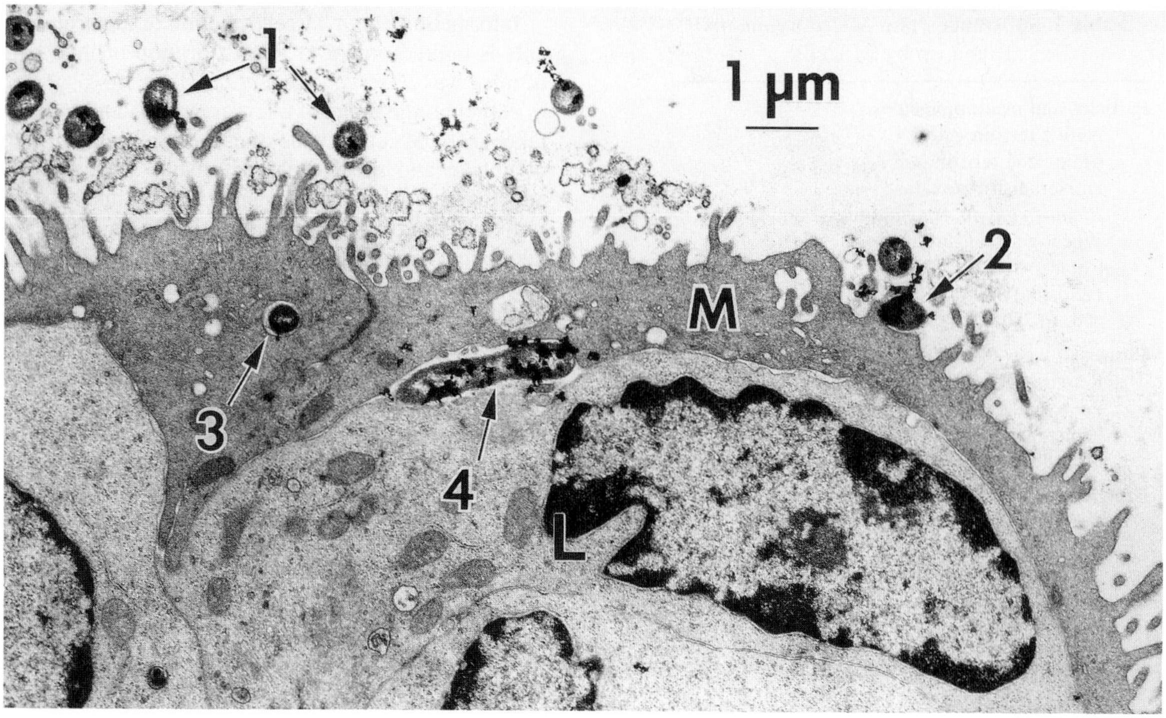

Figure 10 Transport of tritium-labeled *Vibrio cholerae* by rabbit M cells (M). Vibrios (1) lie in the mucus layer of the intestinal lumen. Vibrio 2 is adherent to M cell microvilli. After uptake, vibrio 3 is transported within a vesicle through the cytoplasm. Finally, vibrio 4 lies within the central hollow, adjacent to an enfolded lymphocyte (L). Reprinted with permission from Owen *et al.* (1988b).

ated phagocytic cells to digest and inactivate microoganisms. The apical membrane of M cells has been shown to have an enhanced capacity to bind secretory IgA, possibly because of its thin glycocalyx compared with adjacent columnar cells (Figure 9). This ability of M cells to bind secretory IgA may protect them against the luminal environment and may accelerate M-cell uptake of luminal antigens that are complexed with IgA to boost an existing immune response. The former possibility is supported by the fact that the mouse intestinal mucosa can be protected against virulent *V. cholerae* and *Salmonella typhimurium* infection by secretion of hybridoma-derived IgA specific to each bacterium (Winner *et al.*, 1991; Michetti *et al.*, 1992). The latter suggestion is supported by the fact that transport of some viruses by M cells is accelerated by monoclonal IgA antibodies directed against proteins of these viruses (Weltzin *et al.*, 1989; see Chapter 34).

The range of mechanisms for capture and uptake of various antigens from the intestinal lumen, and for antigen processing and presentation to enfolded cells, is complex and incompletely understood. Gebert and Hach (1993) have shown that M cells of the rabbit cecum selectively bind lectins specific for fucose and *N*-acetylgalactosamine. These lectins bind to the apical membrane and to the membranes of vesicles in the cytoplasm of M cells. In contrast, rabbit enterocytes selectively bind galactose-specific lectins. In rabbit jejunal Peyer's patches, M cells and enterocytes do not show differences in surface glycoconjugates. Adherence of microorganisms to glycoconjugates on M-cell surfaces may be a critical determinant of variations in microbial uptake and colonization at different levels in the gastrointestinal tract. Even binding sites that are shared by M cells and enterocytes are more accessible for microbial adherence on M cells, which lack mucus and the thick glycocalyx coat present over microvilli of enterocytes. Characterization of M-cell receptor sites that bind microorganisms and antigenic molecules may be critical for the logical development of oral immunizing agents; see Chapters 31 and 32).

b. Antigen processing. Using immunohistochemical techniques, investigators have shown that M cells express IL-1 and MHC Class II molecules (Ia antigen in mice, HLA-DR in humans; Nagura *et al.*, 1991). Previously researchers believed that no digestive mechanism was involved in transport through the M cell. However, Allan and associates (1993) showed that M cells possess acidic endosomal, prelysosomal, and lysosomal compartments and express MHC Class II determinants in their prelysosomal and lysosomal structures. These data show that M cells have some potential for processing endocytosed agents and presenting them to the enfolded immunocompetent cells. In mice, IgM plasma cells, macrophages, and T cells that express the CD8 molecule are located in close proximity to M cells and could receive such processed antigen (Jarry *et al.*, 1989). Other APCs such as dendritic cells and macrophages exist beneath the FAE.

These cells extend processes into the FAE and are thought to communicate with M cells in information processing, but their interactions and division of functions remain unclear.

Although the fact that all necessary elements for initiation of intestinal immune responses are present in Peyer's patch follicles has been clearly demonstrated, proving that M cell uptake is an essential step in this process has not been possible. Isolation and culture of M cells, which would be helpful in elucidating their various features, have not yet been accomplished.

2. Target for Migration and Homing of Lymphoblasts

Before lymphoblasts can reach FAE to be enfolded within M cells and brought in contact with various antigens in Peyer's patches, they must leave the systemic circulation via postcapillary venules (PCV) (Figure 1). This directed migration is mediated by high endothelial venules (HEV) in Peyer's patches. In homing, lymphocytes are controlled by surface markers peculiar to each mucosal site; the HEVs have receptors recognized by lymphocyte adhesion molecules such as LECAM-1 (in mouse, MEL-14 antigen) and CD 44 (Berg *et al.,* 1989; Hamann *et al.,* 1991; see Chapter 19). Factors that guide the next step of migration, that is, from HEVs in the parafollicular domain to FAE, are only now being investigated. Extracellular matrix components, arrayed along the migration pathway from HEVs to the apices of follicle domes, may provide the physical basis for this directional cell traffic (Ohtsuka *et al.,* 1992). The migratory stimulus for lymphoid cells to move from follicle domes into and out of M cell pockets is unknown.

Lymphocytes of B-cell lineage finally return to the gut mucosa as mature IgA-producing plasma cells. The migration process of these cells from GALT back to the gut is reported to require 4–6 days (Hall, 1979). B lymphocytes from GALT also can go to other mucosal sites such as mammary glands, salivary glands, bronchial tissues, and the genitourinary tract, and there become stationary plasma cells that produce IgA (Bienenstock and Befus, 1980; see Chapters 12, 13, 19, and 21).

Acknowledgments

We are grateful to Martin F. Heyworth for editorial advice and thank Anthony J. Piazza for assistance in preparing illustrations for this chapter.

References

Abe, K., and Ito, T. (1977). A qualitative and quantitative morphologic study of Peyer's patches of the mouse. *Arch. Histol. Jpn.* **40,** 407–420.

Ackermann, M. R., Cheville, N. F., and Deyoe, B. L. (1988). Bovine ileal dome lymphoepithelial cells: Endocytosis and transport of *Brucella abortus* strain 19. *Vet. Pathol.* **25,** 28–35.

Allan, C. H., Mendrick, D. L., and Trier, J. S. (1993). Rat intestinal M cells contain acidic endosomal-lysosomal compartments and express class II major histocompatibility complex determinants. *Gastroenterology* **104,** 698–708.

Amerongen, H. M., Weltzin, R., Farnet, C. M., Michetti, P., Haseltine, W. A., and Neutra, M. R. (1991). Transepithelial transport of HIV-1 by intestinal M cells: A mechanism for transmission of AIDS. *J. Acq. Immune Defic. Syndr.* **4,** 760–765.

Bassi, C., Fontana, R., Vesentini, S., Cavallini, G., Marchiori, L., Falconi, M., Corrà, S., and Pederzoli, P. (1991). Antibacterial and mezlocillin-enhancing activity of pure human pancreatic fluid. *Int. J. Pancreatol.* **10,** 293–297.

Berg, E. L., Goldstein, L. A., Jutila, M. A., Nakache, M., Picker, L. J., Streeter, P. R., Wu, N. W., Zhou, D., and Butcher, E. C. (1989). Homing receptors and vascular addressins: Cell adhesion molecules that direct lymphocyte traffic. *Immunol. Rev.* **108,** 5–18.

Bhalla, D. K., and Owen, R. L. (1982). Cell renewal and migration in lymphoid follicles of Peyer's patches and cecum—An autoradiographic study in mice. *Gastroenterology* **82,** 232–242.

Bienenstock, J., and Befus, A. D. (1980). Mucosal immunology. A review. *Immunology* **41,** 249–270.

Bienenstock, J., and Befus, D. (1984). Gut- and bronchus-associated lymphoid tissue. *Am. J. Anat.* **170,** 437–445.

Bjerke, K., Brandtzaeg, P., and Fausa, O. (1988). T cell distribution is different in follicle-associated epithelium of human Peyer's patches and villous epithelium. *Clin. Exp. Immunol.* **74,** 270–275.

Blom, H., and Helander, H. F. (1981). Quantitative ultrastructural studies on parietal cell regeneration in experimental ulcers in rat gastric mucosa. *Gastroenterology* **80,** 334–343.

Bockman, D. E., and Cooper, M. D. (1973). Pinocytosis by epithelium associated with lymphoid follicles in the bursa of Fabricius, appendix, and Peyer's patches. An electron microscopic study. *Am. J. Anat.* **136,** 455–478.

Bockman, D. E., and Stevens, W. (1977). Gut-associated lymphoepithelial tissue: Bidirectional transport of tracer by specialized epithelial cells associated with lymphoid follicles. *J. Reticuloendothel. Soc.* **21,** 245–254.

Boyer, B., and Thiery, J. P. (1989). Epithelial cell adhesion mechanisms. *J. Membrane Biol.* **112,** 97–108.

Bye, W. A., Allan, C. H., and Trier, J. S. (1984). Structure, distribution, and origin of M cells in Peyer's patches of mouse ileum. *Gastroenterology* **86,** 789–801.

Byrne, B. M., and Dankert, J. (1979). Volatile fatty acids and aerobic flora in the gastrointestinal tract of mice under various conditions. *Infect. Immun.* **23,** 559–563.

Cerf-Bensussan, N., and Guy-Grand, D. (1991). Intestinal intraepithelial lymphocytes. *Gastroenterol. Clin. North Am.* **20,** 549–576.

Cerf-Bensussan, N., Quaroni, A., Kurnick, J. T., and Bhan, A. K. (1984). Intraepithelial lymphocytes modulate Ia expression by intestinal epithelial cells. *J. Immunol.* **132,** 2244–2252.

Chadee, K., Petri, W. A., Jr., Innes, D. J., and Ravdin, J. I. (1987). Rat and human colonic mucins bind to and inhibit adherence lectin of *Entamoeba histolytica*. *J. Clin. Invest.* **80,** 1245–1254.

Dobbins, W. O., III (1986). Human intestinal intraepithelial lymphocytes. *Gut* **27,** 972–985.

Dobbins, W. O., III (1990). Biopsy interpretation—electron microscopy. *In* "Diagnostic Pathology of the Intestinal Mucosa," pp. 23–94. Springer-Verlag, New York.

Ermak, T. H., Steger, H. J., Strober, S., and Owen, R. L. (1989). M cells and granular mononuclear cells in Peyer's patch domes of mice depleted of their lymphocytes by total lymphoid irradiation. *Am. J. Pathol.* **134,** 529–537.

Freier, S., Eran, M., and Faber, J. (1987). Effect of cholecystokinin and of its antagonist, of atropine, and of food on the release of Immunoglobulin A and Immunoglobulin G specific antibodies in the rat intestine. *Gastroenterology* **93,** 1242–1246.

Fujimura, Y. (1986). Functional morphology of microfold cells (M cells) in Peyer's patches- Phagocytosis and transport of BCG by M cells into rabbit Peyer's patches. *Gastroenterol. Jpn.* **21,** 325–335.

Fujimura, Y., Ohtani, K., Kamoi, R., Kato, T., Kozuka, K., Miyashima, N., Uchida, J., Kihara, T., and Mine, H. (1989). An ultrastructural study of ileal invasion process of *Yersinia pseudotuberculosis* in rabbits. *J. Clin. Electron Microscopy* **22,** 712–713.

Gaidar, Y. A. (1989). Vimentin-positive epithelial cells in the cupolas of the aggregated lymphoid noduli (Peyer's patches) of the rabbit. *Arkh. Anat. Gistol. Embriol.* **97,** 84–88.

Gebert, A., and Hach, G. (1993). Differential binding of lectins to M-cells and enterocytes in the rabbit cecum. *Gastroenterology* **105,** in press.

Grützkau, A., Hanski, C., Hahn, H., and Riecken, E. O. (1990). Involvement of M cells in the bacterial invasion of Peyer's patches: A common mechanism shared by *Yersinia enterocolitica* and other enteroinvasive bacteria. *Gut* **31,** 1011–1015.

Guy-Grand, D., Cerf-Bensussan, N., Malissen, B., Malassis-Seris, M., Briottet, C., and Vassalli, P. (1991). Two gut intraepithelial $CD8^+$ lymphocyte populations with different T cell receptors: A role for the gut epithelium in T cell differentiation. *J. Exp. Med.* **173,** 471–481.

Hall J. (1979). Lymphocyte recirculation and the gut: The cellular basis of humoral immunity in the intestine. *Blood Cells* **5,** 479–492.

Hamann, A., Jablonski-Westrich, D., Jonas, P., and Thiele, H.-G. (1991). Homing receptors reexamined: Mouse LECAM-1 (MEL-14 antigen) is involved in lymphocyte migration into gut-associated lymphoid tissue. *Eur. J. Immunol.* **21,** 2925–2929.

Hay, E. D. (1981). Extracellular matrix. *J. Cell Biol.* **91,** 205s-223s.

Hirata, I., Austin, L. L., Blackwell, W. H., Weber, J. R., and Dobbins, W. O., III (1986). Immunoelectron microscopic localization of HLA-DR antigen in control small intestine and colon and in inflammatory bowel disease. *Dig. Dis. Sci.* **31,** 1317–1330.

Hirayama, K., Matsushita, S., Kikuchi, I., Iuchi, M., Ohta, N, and Sasazuki, T. (1987). HLA-DQ is epistatic to HLA-DR in controlling the immune response to schistosomal antigen in humans. *Nature* (*London*) **327,** 426–430.

Iglewski, W. J., and Gerhardt, N. B. (1978). Identification of an antibiotic-producing bacterium from the human intestinal tract and characterization of its antimicrobial product. *Antimicrob. Agents Chemother.* **13,** 81–89.

Inman, L. R., and Cantey, J. R. (1984). Peyer's patch lymphoid follicle epithelial adherence of a rabbit enteropathogenic *Escherichia coli* (strain RDEC-1)—Role of plasmid-mediated pili in initial adherence. *J. Clin. Invest.* **74,** 90–95.

Jarry, A., Robaszkiewicz, M., Brousse, N., and Potet, F. (1989). Immune cells associated with M cells in the follicle-associated epithelium of Peyer's patches in the rat. *Cell Tissue Res.* **255,** 293–298.

Jarry, A., Cerf-Bensussan, N., Brousse, N., Selz, F., and Guy-Grand, D. (1990). Subsets of $CD3^+$ (T cell receptor $\alpha\beta$ or $\gamma\delta$) and $CD3^-$ lymphocytes isolated from normal human gut epithelium display phenotypical features different from their counterparts in peripheral blood. *Eur. J. Immunol.* **20,** 1097–1103.

Jepson, M. A., Mason, C. M., Bennett, M. K., Simmons, N. L., and Hirst, B. H. (1992). Co-expression of vimentin and cytokeratins in M cells of rabbit intestinal lymphoid follicle-associated epithelium. *Histochem. J.* **24,** 33–39.

Jonas, A., Krishnan, C., and Forstner, G. (1978). Pathogenesis of mucosal injury in the blind loop syndrome. Release of disaccharidases from brush border membranes by extracts of bacteria obtained from intestinal blind loops in rats. *Gastroenterology* **75,** 791–795.

Kabok, Z., Ermak, T. H., and Pappo, J. (1993). Microdissected domes from gut-associated lymphoid tissues: a model for M cell transepithelial transport *in vitro*. *In* Proceedings of the 7th International Congress of Mucosal Immunology. (S. Jackson, H. Kiyono, J. R. McGhee, J. Mestecky, S. M. Michalek, M. W. Russell, J. Sterzl, and H. Tiaskalova, eds). Recent Advances in Mucosal Immunology. Plenum Press, New York.

Kamoi, R. (1991). Morphological studies of *Salmonella enteritidis* uptake by microfold cells (M cells) of the Peyer's patch. *Kawasaki Igakkaishi* **17,** 225–235. (in Japanese)

Kataoka, K., Tabata, J., Yamamoto, M., and Toyota, T. (1989). The association of gap junctions with large particles in the crypt epithelium of the rat small intestine. *Arch. Histol. Cytol.* **52,** 81–86.

Kato, T. (1990). A study of secretory immunoglobulin A on membranous epithelial cells (M cells) and adjacent absorptive cells of rabbit Peyer's patches. *Gastroenterol. Jpn.* **25,** 15–23.

Keshav, S., Lawson, L., Chung, L. P., Stein, M., Perry, V. H., and Gordon, S. (1990). Tumor necrosis factor mRNA localized to Paneth cells of normal murine intestinal epithelium by *in situ* hybridization. *J. Exp. Med.* **171,** 327–332.

Kohbata, S., Yokoyama, H., and Yabuuchi, E. (1986). Cytopathogenic effect of *Salmonella typhi* GIFU 10007 on M cells of murine ileal Peyer's patches in ligated ileal loops. An ultrastructural study. *Microbiol. Immunol.* **30,** 1225–1237.

Levine, G. M. (1991). Regulation of intestinal mucosal growth. *In* "Growth of the Gastrointestinal Tract: Gastrointestinal Hormones and Growth Factors" (J. Morisset and T. E. Solomon, eds.), pp. 175–189. CRC Press, Boca Raton, Florida.

London, S. D., Cebra, J. J., and Rubin, D. H. (1989). Intraepithelial lymphocytes contain virus-specific, MHC-restricted cytotoxic cell precursors after gut mucosal immunization with Reovirus serotype 1/Lang. *Reg. Immunol.* **2,** 98–102.

Madara, J. L. (1982). Cup cells: Structure and distribution of a unique class of epithelial cells in guinea pig, rabbit, and monkey small intestine. *Gastroenterology* **83,** 981–994.

Madara, J. L., and Stafford, J. (1989). Interferon-γ directly affects barrier function of cultured intestinal epithelial monolayers. *J. Clin. Invest.* **83,** 724–727.

Madara, J. L., and Trier, J. S. (1987). Functional morphology of the mucosa of the small intestine. *In* "Physiology of the Gastrointestinal Tract" (L. R. Johnson, ed.), pp. 1209–1249. Raven Press, New York.

Magnusson, K.-E., and Stjernström, I. (1982). Mucosal barrier mechanisms. Interplay between secretory IgA (SIgA), IgG and mucins on the surface properties and association of salmonellae with intestine and granulocytes. *Immunology* **45,** 239–248.

Mantle, M., Basaraba, L., Peacock, S. C., and Gall, D. G. (1989). Binding of *Yersinia enterocolitica* to rabbit intestinal brush border membranes, mucus, and mucin. *Infect. Immun.* **57,** 3292–3299.

Marcial, M. A., and Madara, J. L. (1986). *Cryptosporidium:* Cellular localization, structural analysis of absorptive cell–parasite membrane–membrane interactions in guinea pigs, and suggestion of protozoan transport by M cells. *Gastroenterology* **90,** 583–594.

Marcial, M. A., Carlson, S. L., and Madara, J. L. (1984). Partitioning of paracellular conductance along the ileal crypt–villus axis: A hypothesis based on structural analysis with detailed consideration of tight junction structure–function relationship. *J. Membrane Biol.* **80,** 59–70.

Mayer, L., Eisenhardt, D., Salomon, P., Bauer, W., Plous, R., and Piccinini, L. (1991). Expression of class II molecules on intestinal epithelial cells in humans: Differences between normal and inflammatory bowel disease. *Gastroenterology* **100,** 3–12.

Michetti, P., Mahan, M. J., Slauch, J. M., Mekalanos, J. J., and Neutra, M. R. (1992). Monoclonal secretory immunoglobulin A protects mice against oral challenge with the invasive pathogen *Salmonella typhimurium*. *Infect. Immun.* **60,** 1786–1792.

Miller, H. R. P. (1987). Gastrointestinal mucus, a medium for survival and for elimination of parasitic nematodes and protozoa. *Parasitology* **94,** S77–S100.

Momotani, E., Whipple, D. L., Thiermann, A. B., and Cheville, N. F. (1988). Role of M cells and macrophages in the entrance of *Mycobacterium paratuberculosis* into domes of ileal Peyer's patches in calves. *Vet. Pathol.* **25,** 131–137.

Moxey, P. C., and Trier, J. S. (1978). Specialized cell types in the human fetal small intestine. *Anat. Rec.* **191,** 269–286.

Nabeyama, A., and Leblond, C. P. (1974). "Caveolated cells" characterized by deep surface invaginations and abundant filaments in mouse gastro-intestinal epithelia. *Am. J. Anat.* **140,** 147–166.

Nagasaki, S., Kamoi, R., Kato, T., Kozuka, K., Miyashima, N., Fujimura, Y., Uchida, J., and Kihara, T. (1988). M cell transport of *Streptococcus pyogenes,* Su strain, ATCC 2106 and OK-432 from the intestinal lumen into rabbit Peyer's patches. *J. Clin. Electron Microsc.* **21,** 588–589.

Nagura, H., Ohtani, H., Masuda, T., Kimura, M., and Nakamura, S. (1991). HLA-DR expression on M cells overlying Peyer's patches is a common feature of human small intestine. *Acta Pathol. Jpn.* **41,** 818–823.

Neutra, M. R., and Kraehenbuhl, J.-P. (1992). Transepithelial transport and mucosal defence I: the role of M cells. *Trends Cell Biol.* **2,** 134–138.

Neutra, M. R., Phillips, T. L., Mayer, E. L., and Fishkind, D. J. (1987). Transport of membrane-bound macromolecules by M cells in follicle-associated epithelium of rabbit Peyer's patch. *Cell Tissue Res.* **247,** 537–546.

Ohtsuka, A., Piazza, A. J., Ermak, T. H., and Owen, R. L. (1992). Correlation of extracellular matrix components with the cytoarchitecture of mouse Peyer's patches. *Cell Tissue Res.* **269,** 403–410.

Ouellette, A. J., Greco, R. M., James, M., Frederick, D., Naftilan, J., and Fallon, J. T. (1989). Developmental regulation of cryptdin, a corticostatin/defensin precursor mRNA in mouse small intestinal crypt epithelium. *J. Cell Biol.* **108,** 1687–1695.

Owen, R. L., (1977). Sequential uptake of horseradish peroxidase by lymphoid follicle epithelium of Peyer's patches in the normal unobstructed mouse intestine: An ultrastructural study. *Gastroenterology* **72,** 440–451.

Owen, R. L., and Bhalla, D. K. (1983). Cytochemical analysis of alkaline phosphatase and esterase activities and of lectin-binding and anionic sites in rat and mouse Peyer's patch M cells. *Am. J. Anat.* **168,** 199–212.

Owen, R. L., and Jones, A. L. (1974). Epithelial cell specialization within human Peyer's patches: An ultrastructural study of intestinal lymphoid follicles. *Gastroenterology* **66,** 189–203.

Owen, R. L., and Nemanic, P. (1978). Antigen processing structures of the mammalian intestinal tract: An SEM study of lymphoepithelial organs. *Scanning Electron Microsc.* **2,** 367–378.

Owen, R. L., Allen, C. L., and Stevens, D. P. (1981). Phagocytosis of *Giardia muris* by macrophages in Peyer's patch epithelium in mice. *Infect. Immun.* **33,** 591–601.

Owen, R. L., Apple, R. T., and Bhalla, D. K. (1986a). Morphometric and cytochemical analysis of lysosomes in rat Peyer's patch follicle epithelium: Their reduction in volume fraction and acid phosphatase content in M cells compared to adjacent enterocytes. *Anat. Rec.* **216,** 521–527.

Owen, R. L., Pierce, N. F., Apple, R. T., and Cray, W. C., Jr. (1986b). M cell transport of *Vibrio cholerae* from the intestinal lumen into Peyer's patches: A mechanism for antigen sampling and for microbial transepithelial migration. *J. Infect. Dis.* **153,** 1108–1118.

Owen, R. L., Cray, W. C., Jr., Ermak, T. H., and Pierce, N. F. (1988a). Bacterial characteristics and follicle surface structure: Their roles in Peyer's patch uptake and transport of *Vibrio cholerae. Adv. Exp. Med. Biol.* **237,** 705–715.

Owen, R. L., Pierce, N. F., and Cray, W. C., Jr. (1988b). Effects of bacterial inactivation methods, toxin production, and oral immunization on uptake of *Vibrio cholerae* by Peyer's patch lymphoid follicles. *In* "Advances in Research on Cholera and Related Diarrheas" (S. Kuwahara and N. F. Pierce, eds.), pp. 189–197. KTK Scientific Publishers, Tokyo.

Owen, R. L., Piazza, A. J., and Ermak, T. H. (1991). Ultrastructural and cytoarchitectural features of lymphoreticular organs in the colon and rectum of adult BALB/c mice. *Am. J. Anat.* **190,** 10–18.

Pappo, J., and Ermak, T. H. (1989). Uptake and translocation of fluorescent latex particles by rabbit Peyer's patch follicle epithelium: A quantitative model for M cell uptake. *Clin. Exp. Immunol.* **76,** 144–148.

Pappo, J., and Owen, R. L. (1988). Absence of secretory component expression by epithelial cells overlying rabbit gut-associated lymphoid tissue. *Gastroenterology* **95,** 1173–1177.

Rhodes, J. M. (1989). Colonic mucus and mucosal glycoproteins: The key to colitis and cancer? *Gut* **30,** 1660–1666.

Rhodes, J. M. (1990). Mucus and inflammatory bowel disease. *In* "Inflammatory Bowel Diseases" (R. N. Allan, M. R. B. Keighley, J. Alexander-Williams, and C. F. Hawkins, eds.), 2d Ed., pp. 171–179. Churchill Livingstone, London.

Rodning, C. B., Wilson, I. D., and Erlandsen, S. L. (1976). Immunoglobulins within human small-intestinal Paneth cells. *Lancet* **i,** 984–987.

Roy, M. J., and Varvayanis, M. (1987). Development of dome epithelium in gut-associated lymphoid tissues: association of IgA with M cells. *Cell Tissue Res.* **248,** 645–651.

Rubinstein, E., Mark, Z., Haspel, J., Ben-Ari, G., Dreznik, Z., Mirelman, D., and Tadmor, A. (1985). Antibacterial activity of pancreatic fluid. *Gastroenterology* **88,** 927–932.

Sajjan, S. U., and Forstner, J. F. (1990). Role of the putative "link" glycopeptide of intestinal mucin in binding of piliated *Escherichia coli* serotype O157:H7 strain CL-49. *Infect. Immun.* **58,** 868–873.

Santos, L. M. B., Lider, O., Audette, J., Khoury, S. J., and Weiner, H. L. (1990). Characterization of immunomodulatory properties and accessory cell function of small intestine epithelial cells. *Cell. Immunol.* **127,** 26–34.

Savage, D. C. (1970). Association of indigenous microorganisms with gastrointestinal mucosal epithelia. *Am. J. Clin. Nutr.* **23,** 1495–1501.

Schmedtje, J. F. (1965). Some histochemical characteristics of lymphoepithelial cells of the rabbit appendix. *Anat. Rec.* **151,** 412–413. (Abstract)

Schmedtje, J. F. (1966). Fine structure of intercellular lymphocyte clusters in the rabbit appendix epithelium. *Anat. Rec.* **154,** 417. (Abstract)

Schmidt, G. H., Wilkinson, M. M., and Ponder, B. A. J. (1985). Cell migration pathway in the intestinal epithelium: An *in situ* marker system using mouse aggregation chimeras. *Cell* **40,** 425–429.

Shakhlamov, V. A., Gaidar, Y. A., and Baranov, V. N. (1981). Electron-cytochemical investigation of cholera toxin absorption by epithelium of Peyer's patches in guinea pigs. *Bull. Exp. Biol. Med.* **90,** 1159–1161.

Siciński, P., Rowiński, J., Warchoł, J. B., and Bem, W. (1986). Morphometric evidence against lymphocyte-induced differentiation of M cells from absorptive cells in mouse Peyer's patches. *Gastroenterology* **90,** 609–616.

Siciński, P., Rowiński, J., Warchoł, J. B., Jarzabek, Z., Gut, W., Szczygieł, B., Bielecki, K., and Koch, G. (1990). Poliovirus type 1 enters the human host through intestinal M cells. *Gastroenterology* **98,** 56–58.

Smith, M. W., and Peacock, M. A. (1980). "M" cell distribution in follicle-associated epithelium of mouse Peyer's patch. *Am. J. Anat.* **159,** 167–175.

Smith, M. W., James, P. S., and Tivey, D. R. (1987). M cell numbers increase after transfer of SPF mice to a normal animal house environment. *Am. J. Pathol.* **128,** 385–389.

Snyder, J. D., and Walker, W. A. (1987). Structure and function of intestinal mucin: Development aspects. *Int. Arch. Allergy Appl. Immunol.* **82,** 351–356.

Specian, R. D., and Neutra, M. R. (1984). Cytoskeleton of intestinal goblet cells in rabbit and monkey—The theca. *Gastroenterology* **87,** 1313–1325.

Stanisz, A. M., Befus, D., and Bienenstock, J. (1986). Differential effects of vasoactive intestinal peptide, substance P, and somatostatin on immunoglobulin synthesis and proliferations by lymphocytes from Peyer's patches, mesentric lymph nodes, and spleen. *J. Immunol.* **136,** 152–156.

Suzuki, H., Konno, T., Igarashi, Y., and Yamamoto, T. (1977). The occurrence of electron dense intercellular materials and gap junctions in the human intestinal epithelium. *Tohoku J. Exp. Med.* **121,** 301–313.

Tagliabue, A., Boraschi, D., Villa, L., Keren, D. F., Lowell, G. H., Rappuoli, R., and Nencioni, L. (1984). IgA-dependent cell-mediated activity against enteropathogenic bacteria: Distribution, specificity, and characterization of the effector cells. *J. Immunol.* **133,** 988–992.

Thompson, G. R., and Trexler, P. C. (1971). Gastrointestinal structure and function in germ-free gnotobiotic animals. *Gut* **12,** 230–235.

Trier, J. S. (1991). Structure and function of intestinal M cells. *Gastroenterol. Clin. North Am.* **20,** 531–547.

Uchida, J. (1987). An ultrastructural study on active uptake and transport of bacteria by microfold cells (M cells) to the lymphoid follicles in the rabbit appendix. *J. Clin. Electron Microscopy* **20,** 379–394.

Uchida, J. (1988). Electron microscopic study of microfold cells (M cells) in normal and inflamed human appendix. *Gastroenterol. Jpn.* **23,** 251–262.

von Rosen, L., Podjaski, B., Bettmann, I., and Otto, H. F. (1981). Observations on the ultrastructure and function of the so-called "Microfold" or "Membranous" cells (M cells) by means of peroxidase as a tracer. *Virchows Arch. Pathol. Anat.* **390,** 289–312.

Walker, R. I., Schmauder-Chock, E. A., Parker, J. L., and Burr, D. (1988). Selective association and transport of *Campylobacter jejuni* through M cells of rabbit Peyer's patches. *Can. J. Microbiol.* **34,** 1142–1147.

Wassef, J. S., Keren, D. F., and Mailloux, J. L. (1989). Role of M cells in initial antigen uptake and in ulcer formation in the rabbit intestinal loop model of shigellosis. *Infect. Immun.* **57,** 858–863.

Weiner, D. B., Girard, K., Williams, W. V., McPhillips, T., and Rubin, D. H. (1988). Reovirus type 1 and type 3 differ in their binding to isolated intestinal epithelial cells. *Microb. Pathogen.* **5,** 29–40.

Weltzin, R., Lucia-Jandris, P., Michetti, P., Fields, B. N., Kraehenbuhl, J. P., and Neutra, M. R. (1989). Binding and transepithelial transport of immunoglobulins by intestinal M cells: Demonstration using monoclonal IgA antibodies against enteric viral proteins. *J. Cell Biol.* **108,** 1673–1685.

Williams, R. C., Showalter, R., and Kern, F., Jr. (1975). *In vivo* effect of bile salts and cholestyramine on intestinal anaerobic bacteria. *Gastroenterology* **69,** 483–491.

Winner, L., III, Mack, J., Weltzin, R., Mekalanos, J. J., Kraehenbuhl, J.-P., and Neutra, M. R., (1991). New model for analysis of mucosal immunity: Intestinal secretion of specific monoclonal immunoglobulin A from hybridoma tumors protects against *Vibrio cholerae* infection. *Infect. Immun.* **59,** 977–982.

Wolf, J. L., Kauffman, R. S., Finberg, R., Dambrauskas, R., Fields, B. N., and Trier, J. S. (1983). Determinants of reovirus interaction with the intestinal M cells and absorptive cells of murine intestine. *Gastroenterology* **85,** 291–300.

3

Cellular and Molecular Basis for Antigen Transport in the Intestinal Epithelium

Marian R. Neutra • Jean-Pierre Kraehenbuhl

I. INTRODUCTION

The mucosal surfaces that line digestive, respiratory, and urogenital systems represent a vast surface area that is covered for the most part by a monolayer of epithelial cells. The importance of secretory antibodies in defense of these surfaces is discussed in detail elsewhere in this volume. Secretory antibodies, primarily of the polymeric IgA type, are designed to interact with their target microorganisms or antigens in external secretions, an environment that is separated by a tight epithelial barrier both from the local cellular assemblies responsible for induction of mucosal immune responses and from the widespread effector cells responsible for production of polymeric IgA antibodies. Epithelial cells thus play important roles in mucosal immune defense apart from their simple function as a barrier (for review, see Neutra and Kraehenbuhl, 1992). A minority population of epithelial cells (the M cells) is highly specialized for transport of antigens to the cells of the mucosal immune system, whereas a major population of diverse epithelial and glandular cells selectively exports polymeric immunoglobulins onto mucosal surfaces. In this chapter, we focus on the basic mechanisms of membrane traffic and the epithelial cell specializations that allow the epithelium in the intestine to function as a gatekeeper that controls access of antigens to the mucosal immune system, while still fulfilling many other complex roles such as digestion, absorption, and maintenance of an effective barrier.

A. Enterocyte Diversity and Antigen Transport

The phenotype of the intestinal absorptive cell or enterocyte changes during intestinal development of the fetus and neonate, and during differentiation of individual cells along the crypt–villus axis in adults. These changes have important effects on the capacity of the epithelium for endocytosis and transcytosis. Dramatic changes in endocytic activity occur in the entire absorptive enterocyte population during fetal and postnatal development in mammals as they pass through progressive stages of digestive function (Neutra and Louvard, 1989). The cellular heterogeneity of the epithelium that covers the normal adult intestinal mucosa and the changes in cell ultrastructure and function that occur as cells migrate along the crypt–villus axis have been reviewed in detail elsewhere (Madara and Trier, 1987, Neutra, 1988). In adults, the capacity of individual absorptive enterocytes on intestinal villi to take up intact proteins generally is very limited; endocytic activity and limited transcytosis occur, however, and may vary with the stage of cell differentiation. The functional effect of such transport may be amplified by the immense numbers of cells involved.

Transcytosis by enterocytes would deliver antigens to the basolateral surface of the epithelium that faces a diffuse lymphoid tissue called the lamina propria. This highly vascularized connective tissue contains lymphoid and phagocytic cell populations including sessile antibody-producing cells (mainly IgA-producing plasma cells) as well as various cell types capable of processing and presenting antigens, producing cytokines, and collectively initiating and modulating immune responses. The epithelium itself also harbors intraepithelial lymphocytes (IELs) that are thought to play roles in immune surveillance of foreign antigens, suppression of immune responses, or elimination of damaged or infected epithelial cells. The identity and possible functions of specific lymphoid cell populations in the mucosa and epithelium are addressed in subsequent sections of this volume (see Sections B and C).

B. M Cells and Antigen Transport

Over specific mucosal sites marked by the presence of organized lymphoid follicles, a unique epithelium occurs. The unusual phenotypes, in particular the M cells that exist only at these sites, are described in Chapter 2. Although M cells represent an exceedingly small minority in the intestinal epithelium, their functional significance is amplified greatly by their unique position over the organized lymphoid tissues that serve as inductive sites for mucosal immune responses and by their ability to transport antigens with great efficiency. Researchers generally agree that M cells play a primary role in transport of antigens to the inductive arm of the mucosal immune system. In M cells as well as in enterocytes, the immunological consequences of antigen uptake and transport are determined in part by the nature and capacity of the intracellular pathways through which antigens are directed. These pathways are driven by the basic mechanisms that govern the direction and rate of membrane traffic in all cells.

II. GENERAL MECHANISMS OF TRANSEPITHELIAL TRANSPORT

In the past several years, an explosion of new information has become available on the binding of macromolecular ligands and microorganisms to cell surfaces and on the mechanisms by which macromolecules and particles are internalized by endocytosis and phagocytosis. The nature and function of the compartments that compose endocytic pathways, directed either toward the degradative lysosomal compartment or to other destinations, have been elucidated mostly through studies on nonpolarized cells (for review, see Kornfeld and Mellman, 1989). However, attention also has been focused on the endocytic compartments involved in transport of vesicles across polarized epithelial cells (Mostov and Simister, 1985; Schaerer *et al.*, 1991; Sztul *et al.*, 1991). Most studies have exploited relatively simple model cell culture systems such as Madin–Darby canine kidney (MDCK) cells (Brandli *et al.*, 1990; Casanova *et al.*, 1990). Although the nature of specific membrane receptors and the relative importance of various intracellular vesicular pathways clearly differ among epithelial cell types, investigators generally agree that the basic mechanisms operating in one cell type, for example, MDCK, are likely to operate in other cell types such as intestinal enterocytes and M cells. Therefore, some salient findings are reviewed briefly here.

A. Maintenance of Cell Polarity

In all confluent polarized epithelial cells, the tight junctions that seal the apical poles of the cells not only provide efficient diffusion barriers for many ions, small molecules, and all macromolecules (Madara, 1988), but also prevent lateral diffusion of glycolipids and proteins between apical and basolateral domains of the plasma membrane (Dragsten *et al.*, 1981). The apical domain of epithelial cells, including intestinal cells, contains many components not present in either nonpolarized cell types or the same epithelial cells in culture prior to polarization and junction formation (Louvard *et al.*, 1985; LeBivic *et al.*, 1986; Godefroy *et al.*, 1988; Rodriguez-Boulan and Nelson, 1989; Lisanti and Rodriguez-Boulan, 1990). The basolateral cell surface is divided further into two major subdomains. The lateral subdomain is involved in cell–cell interactions via cell adhesion molecules (Nelson and Hammerton, 1989) and is enriched in Na^+,K^+-ATPase, poly Ig receptors, and other components in enterocytes (Slot and Geuze, 1984; Amerongen *et al.*, 1989). The basal subdomain is enriched in receptors that recognize extracellular matrix and basal lamina. In addition, both apical and basolateral plasma membranes can contain specialized microdomains such as microvilli, cell–cell interdigitations, and other sites stabilized by submembrane cytoskeleton and clathrin-coated pits (Mooseker, 1985; Neutra *et al.*, 1988; Nelson and Hammerton, 1989).

Maintenance of the apical and basolateral domains involves at least two types of membrane traffic. First, vesicles derived from the trans-Golgi network and containing newly synthesized, domain-specific proteins can be transported directly to either the apical or the basolateral domain (Danielson and Cowell, 1985; Caplan *et al.*, 1986; Wandinger-Ness and Simons, 1991). Second, specific components initially inserted into one domain can be re-sorted to the opposite side by "corrective" transcytosis. Studies on the biogenesis of polarized membrane proteins have shown that, in hepatocytes and intestinal enterocytes *in vivo* and in cell culture, certain proteins that are considered residents of the apical domain actually are directed initially to the basolateral domain, but are then endocytosed selectively and carried to the apical domain in transcytotic vesicles (Bartles *et al.*, 1987; Massey *et al.*, 1987; Matter *et al.*, 1990). Corrective transcytosis also may occur in the opposite direction in MDCK cells (Matlin *et al.*, 1983); if this occurs in intestinal cells *in vivo*, such traffic would be expected to provide a potential pathway for uptake of foreign proteins from the lumen.

B. Endocytosis and Sorting

The initial event in transcytosis is the endocytic uptake of either adsorbed or fluid-phase macromolecules via clathrin-coated or noncoated pits and vesicles (Anderson, 1991). Incoming vesicles fuse to form an "early endosome," a compartment of distinctive morphology consisting of clear vesicles with attached tubules (for review, see Kornfeld and Mellman, 1989). Studies using ligands tagged with pH-sensitive probes showed that this compartment acidifies to pH 6.0–6.2, a milieu in which certain ligands are released from their receptors (for review, see Maxfield and Yamashiro, 1991). In addition, various receptors may be sorted from each other in the plane of the early endosome membrane. Sorting of receptors in basolateral (sinusoidal) endosomes in hepatocytes was studied by electron microscopic (EM) immunocytochemistry. The images suggested that receptors cluster together and are removed from the endosomal tubules by selective budding of small vesicles destined for transport to three different destinations: rapid return to the same cell surface (recycling), transport along the degradative pathway (ultimately to lysosomes), or transport to the opposite membrane domain (transcytosis) (Geuze *et al.*, 1984,1987).

The basic molecular mechanisms by which sorting occurs in the endosomal membrane and the exact site at which transcytotic vesicles are formed are not known. Recycling of membrane proteins and vesicle contents can occur not only from early endosomes but also from late endosomes, a population that includes multivesicular endosomes (or transport endosomes) and pre-lysosomal compartments (Hughson and Hopkins, 1990; Rabinowitz *et al.*, 1992). This observation is consistent with the observation that vesicles all along the endosomal pathway have tubular extensions (Neutra *et al.*, 1985; Rabinowitz *et al.*, 1992). However, whether these extensions give rise to transcytotic vesicles all along the pathway, that is from early endosomes, late endosomes, and prelysosomes is not known. This idea is of interest since the origin of the vesicles would affect the degree of proteolytic processing that might occur during transcytosis.

In kidney tubular cell lines, intestinal cell lines, and enterocytes *in vivo,* distinct sets of apical and basolateral early endosomes are seen (Rodewald, 1980; Fuller and Simons, 1986; Bomsel *et al.*, 1989; Parton *et al.*, 1989; Fujita *et al.*, 1990; Hughson and Hopkins, 1990). Despite many structural and functional similarities, apical and basolateral early endosomes seem to be different functionally and compositionally because, when isolated from MDCK cells, they are unable to fuse with each other *in vitro* (Bomsel *et al.*, 1990). Both types of early endosomes can, nevertheless, fuse with common "late endosomes" isolated from the same cells (Gruenberg *et al.*, 1989; Gruenberg and Howell, 1989; Bomsel *et al.*, 1990); these fusion patterns correspond to the pathways of transfer of apical and basolateral tracer proteins observed in intact MDCK cells (Parton *et al.*, 1989) as well as in intestinal epithelial cells *in vivo* (Rodewald, 1980; Fujita *et al.*, 1990).

Although early endosomes were thought initially to lack degradative enzymes because they lack traditional lysosomal enzyme markers such as acid phosphatase, we now know that certain degradative enzymes are indeed present in very early endosome compartments (Diment and Stahl, 1985; for review; see Courtoy, 1991). In some cell types, these enzymes enter the endosome by receptor-mediated uptake from the outside, but the major source of endosomal proteases seems to be receptor-mediated delivery from the Golgi complex (Brown *et al.*, 1986; von Figura and Hasilik, 1986; Griffiths *et al.*, 1988; Kornfeld and Mellman, 1989). Whether the same enzymes are delivered to early apical and basolateral endosomes in polarized cells is not known. Uptake of extracellular enzymes may be limited to the basolateral side, since cell-surface mannose 6-phosphate receptors on MDCK cells are basolateral (Prydz *et al.*, 1990). Additional hydrolases from the Golgi continue to be delivered along the endocytic pathway; a major delivery site is the late endosome. Although lysosomes generally don't have tubular extensions and have been considered stable dead-end organelles, "resident" glycoproteins of the lysosome membrane have been shown to cycle to the plasma membrane and back via the endocytic pathway (Lippincott-Schwartz and Fambrough, 1987; Braun *et al.*, 1989). In MDCK cells, newly synthesized lysosomal membrane proteins may go to the basolateral plasma membrane on their way to the lysosome (Nabi *et al.*, 1991), implying that digested protein fragments can be re-exposed to both the external and the endosomal milieu.

C. Transcytosis

Soluble tracers and specific ligands have been used as markers of transcytosis in intact epithelial organs, but since they often enter multiple pathways, the exact transcytotic route and the identity of transcytotic vesicles is not clear. To date, a biochemical analysis of isolated transcytotic carrier vesicles from normal cells has been achieved only by immunoaffinity isolation of vesicles from hepatocytes (Sztul *et al.*, 1991). Since access to apical as well as basolateral surfaces generally is restricted in intact organs, the kinetics of internalization and the fates of endocytosed proteins have been analyzed primarily in cultured kidney or intestinal cell lines grown on permeable supports. Results derived from MDCK cells and Caco-2 or HT29 human colon carcinoma cells have revealed striking differences among these models. In MDCK cells, for example, the amount of internalization of fluid phase proteins from apical and basolateral surfaces was identical, but the subsequent fate of the proteins differed dramatically (Bomsel *et al.*, 1989). Of the horseradish peroxidase (HRP) taken up from the apical side, relatively small amounts were directed to lysosomes; most of the protein was released from the cells—half by recycling and half by transcytosis to the other side. Of the HRP taken up basolaterally, only small amounts were transcytosed to the apical side. Certain membrane proteins also were found to be transported bidirectionally across MDCK cells, indicating that single membrane vesicles may have made the entire transepithelial trip (Brandli *et al.*, 1990). The dominance of the apical-to-basolateral pathway in MDCK cells contrasts with the situation in Caco-2 cells, in which apical-to-basolateral transepithelial transport of HRP was documented by some investigators (Hidalgo *et al.*, 1989) but was found to be limited to paracellular leakage by others (Heyman *et al.*, 1990) or was not observed at all (Hughson and Hopkins, 1990). These discrepancies may have been the result of differences in the Caco-2 cell clones used. In any case, the amount, rate, and direction of transcytosis in cultured epithelial cell lines, although providing useful guidelines, may not reflect transport activity in the various enterocyte phenotypes *in vivo* accurately.

To date, only two receptor systems that mediate transcytosis have been analyzed at the molecular level. These analyses have contributed significantly to our understanding of transcytosis (Breitfeld *et al.*, 1989a; Simister and Mostov, 1989; Apodaca *et al.*, 1991; Hirt *et al.*, 1993). Both these receptor systems operate in the intestinal epithelium. The epithelial Fc receptor mediates apical-to-basolateral transcytosis of maternal immunoglobulins in small intestine of neonatal rodents, but not in neonatal humans (Rodewald, 1980; Simister and Mostov, 1989); the polymeric immunoglobulin (poly Ig) receptor mediates basolateral-to-apical delivery of IgA in a wide variety of epithelial and glandular cells (Kuhn and Kraehenbuhl, 1982; Mostov *et al.*, 1984; Kraehenbuhl and Neutra, 1992a,b). The molecular mechanisms mediating cell surface targeting and trafficking of these immunoglobulin-like receptor molecules through early endosomes and into their respective transcytotic pathways to the opposite cell surface have been studied in epithelial cell lines transfected with either wild-tye or mutated receptor cDNAs encoding them (Breitfeld *et al.*, 1989b; Hunziker and Mellman, 1989; Casanova *et al.*, 1990; Hunziker *et al.*, 1990, 1991a; Hirt *et al.*, 1993). Collectively, these studies have shown that the major portion of the targeting information required for the complex itineraries of these proteins resides in the cytoplasmic tails of the receptors, and may be contained both in specific amino acid phosphorylation sites and in motifs of secondary structure (for review, see Apodaca *et al.*, 1991; Schaerer *et. al.*, 1991).

Although scientists often assume that transcytotic vesicles directly recognize and fuse with the contralateral cell surface, studies on transfected MDCK cells expressing either the Fc receptor or the poly Ig receptor showed that transcytosed membrane proteins can recycle between early endosomes and the adjacent cell surface both at their original site of insertion and at their ultimate destination (Breitfeld *et al.*, 1989b; Hunziker *et al.*, 1990), implying that a single population of transcytotic carrier vesicles could shuttle between the apical and basolateral early endocytic compartments. If such a shuttle exists, these vesicles would be competent to fuse with early endosomes at either cell pole.

D. Epithelial Cytoskeleton and Vesicular Traffic

In epithelial cells, microtubules play an important but controversial role in cell membrane polarity and transcytosis. Researchers generally agree that microtubules serve primarily to move vesicles over "long" distances in cells, but are not required for endocytosis or exocytosis (Schroer and Kelly, 1985; Kelly, 1990). Vesicles carrying newly synthesized cell surface and secretory materials in epithelial cells move from the Golgi region toward the apical surface along microtubules that run parallel to the lateral cell membrane (Specian and Neutra, 1984; Achler *et al.*, 1989; Bacallao *et al.*, 1989). Microtubule-inhibiting drugs interfere with delivery of newly synthesized membrane components to the apical surface of enterocytes *in vivo* (Quaroni *et al.*, 1979; Pavelka *et al.*, 1983) and *in vitro* (Eilers *et al.*, 1989). The minus ends of the microtubules are oriented toward the apical cell surface of cultured epithelial cells (Bacallao *et al.*, 1989); polarized delivery of apically directed vesicles presumably involves a dynein-like motor since these vesicles move toward the minus end (Schroer and Sheetz, 1989; van der Sluijs *et al.*, 1990).

Microtubules also may play a role in transcytosis. For example, microtubules were found to be involved in transcytosis of poly Ig receptors from the basolateral to the apical membrane in transfected MDCK cells (Hunziker *et al.*, 1990). In addition, microtubule-inhibiting drugs reduced the secretion of hepatocyte proteins into bile (Goldman *et al.*, 1983). Endocytosis is not itself microtubule dependent, but movement of peripheral endosomes to more central locations and to lysosomes is mediated in polarized epithelial cells (as in nonpolarized cells) by microtubules (Gruenberg *et al.*, 1989; Bomsel *et al.*, 1990; Hughson and Hopkins, 1990). In this case, vesicles move toward the plus end of the microtubules, presumably via a kinesin-type motor (Schroer and Sheetz, 1989). In transfected MDCK cells expressing both the poly Ig receptor and the epithelial Fc receptor, microtubules were found to be required for basolateral-to-apical transcytosis, whereas apical-to-basolateral transcytosis was microtubule independent (Hunziker *et al.*, 1990). Whether some other type of molecular motor and cytoskeletal "track" facilitate apical-to-basolateral vesicular transport is unknown.

Collectively, new information on the nature of the transcytotic pathway indicates that transport of proteins from one side of an epithelium to the other is not accomplished by simple movement of a vesicle derived from one plasma membrane and subsequent fusion with the opposite side. Rather, this process probably requires a complex series of events including formation and fusion of endosomes and other membrane vesicles and participation of additional organelles and cytoskeleton. The observed alteration in basolateral endosomes that accompanies inhibition of transcytosis of the poly Ig receptor in MDCK cells by the antibiotic brefeldin A supports this general caveat (Hunziker *et al.*, 1991b). Current information about pathways of vesicular traffic must be considered in the interpretation of experiments exploring antigen transport, processing, and presentation by intestinal epithelial cells.

III. MEMBRANE TRAFFIC IN INTESTINAL ENTEROCYTES

Epithelial cells of the intestine constitutively express major histocompatibility complex (MHC) Class I determinants and also express MHC Class II determinants on their surfaces and in internal compartments. Enterocytes isolated from intestine and dispersed *in vitro* have been shown to contain MHC Class II determinants and to be capable of mediating T-cell activation when incubated with predigested antigens and sensitized T cells (Bland and Warren, 1986; Mayer and Shlien, 1987). The hypothesis has been proposed that, in the gut, antigens resulting from digestion in the lumen and transported transepithelially or degraded intracellularly in enterocyte lysosomes could associate with MHC II and be presented to lymphocytes to suppress the systemic immune response to lumenal antigens such as products of food digestion (Bland and Warren, 1986; Nedrud and Lamm, 1991; Mayer *et al.*, 1991). On the other hand, other evidence suggests that intact food antigens can be transported across the intestinal epithelium in amounts sufficient to evoke an immune response. The available evidence for these phenomena is discussed in more detail in Chapters 4, 15, and 16. In this chapter, we consider the possible functions of antigen-presenting molecular complexes in enterocytes and the significance of lymphocyte–enterocyte interactions in the light of available information on membrane traffic in enterocytes and the roles of endocytic pathways in antigen presentation.

A. Antigen Exclusion at the Apical Membrane

Intestinal absorptive cells are well equipped to face an environment rich in foreign proteins and microorganisms. The normal villus and crypt epithelium *in vivo* is sealed by continuous tight junctions that permit charge-selective passage of certain ions, water, and, under some conditions, small organic molecules such as glucose but exclude peptides or macromolecules (Madara, 1988). The apical membrane of enterocytes is a highly differentiated structure dominated by rigid, closely packed microvilli (Mooseker, 1985), each of which is coated with a thick layer of membrane-anchored and peripheral glycoproteins called the glycocalyx (Semenza, 1986). This coat impedes the passage of particles such as viruses, bacteria, and macromolecular aggregates between microvilli and can prevent their contact with the microvillus membrane (Gonnella and Neutra, 1985; Amerongen *et al.*,

1991). Lectin binding studies on tissue sections or fixed cells have shown that the glycocalyx is rich in the many saccharides that serve as receptors for lectins or microorganisms. We have shown, however, that on living enterocytes *in vivo* many lectin receptors are masked by the macromolecular assembly of the glycocalyx (Gonnella and Neutra, 1985). Although crypt cell apical membranes may be more accessible, outward fluid flow tends to inhibit passive entry at this site (Phillips *et al.*, 1987). In addition, normal enterocytes can "shed" microvillus membrane in the form of vesicles after cross-linking by lectins (Weinman *et al.*, 1989) and also can shed other adherent macromolecules (Gonnella and Neutra, 1985), perhaps by release of lipid-linked or integral membrane enzymes (Alpers, 1975). Thus, enterocyte-like cell lines and MDCK cells in culture, whose apical surfaces may be less fully differentiated, can provide misleading information concerning antigen or microbial adherence and endocytosis in the normal gut.

The structure of the brush border and glycocalyx also shields the plasma membrane microdomains at the bases of microvilli that are responsible for endocytosis (Neutra *et al.*, 1988). In adult enterocytes, the molecules that can pass between microvilli enter clathrin-coated endocytic pits at this site, which apparently is intended for uptake of physiological ligands such as intrinsic factor–cobalamin complexes (Levine *et al.*, 1984). In suckling rodents, this endocytic domain is expanded to provide access for maternal milk IgG in jejunum and other milk macromolecules in ileum (Rodewald, 1980; Gonnella and Neutra, 1984; Neutra *et al.*, 1988). Note, however, that these specialized cell types and expanded endocytic membrane domains are not present in human intestine beyond the midpoint of gestation (Moxey and Trier, 1979).

B. Membrane Traffic in Vacuolated Enterocytes

During fetal and neonatal development of the mammalian intestine, the epithelium undergoes two major bursts of cytodifferentiation (Neutra and Louvard, 1989). The first involves conversion of the undifferentiated fetal epithelium to a monolayer containing enterocytes that are specialized for active endocytosis of lumenal contents. The timing and duration of this "endocytic stage" varies widely among species (Kraehenbuhl *et al.*, 1979): in humans, for example, it begins and ends during the first half of gestation (Moxey and Trier, 1979) whereas in sheep and cattle it begins during fetal life but extends for a few days after birth (Trahair and Robinson, 1986,1989). This stage has been most studied in rats, whose endocytic enterocytes appear a few days before birth and persist through the 3-week suckling period (Kraehenbuhl *et al.*, 1979). During this stage in rats, specialized enterocytes in proximal intestine conduct receptor-mediated endocytosis and transcytosis of IgG from maternal milk (Rodewald, 1980). IgG uptake is mediated by epithelial Fc receptors that show structural similarities to MHC I, consisting of a membrane-anchored immunoglobulin-like protein associated with $\beta 2$ microglobulin (Simister and Mostov, 1989). Jejunal enterocytes contain abundant apical endosomes into which both IgG–receptor complexes and soluble proteins from the lumen are delivered after uptake from clathrin-coated pits located between microvilli (Rodewald, 1980). The apical endosomal system appears to be a sorting compartment, since proteins in the fluid content of the vesicles are directed to lysosomes whereas IgG ligand–receptor complexes enter small transport vesicles that release their content by exocytosis at the lateral cell surface (Abrahamson and Rodewald, 1981).

Enterocytes in more distal regions of suckling rat intestine, and enterocytes throughout the intestines of 10- to 20-week fetal humans and fetuses and newborns of other mammalian species, are specialized cells known as "vacuolated enterocytes" (Moxey and Trier, 1979; Trier and Moxey, 1979). These cells take up large amounts of lumenal protein into specialized apical endosomal tubules and vesicles and, hence, into large lysosomal vacuoles (Gonnella and Neutra, 1984). In humans, these cells have been suggested but not proven to conduct transfer of antibodies from amniotic fluid to the fetus (Israel *et al.*, 1989). The endocytic compartments of vacuolated enterocytes have been studied in detail in suckling rats, in which endocytosis allows for intracellular digestion of milk proteins. The apical endocytic complex of rat vacuolated enterocytes is an endosomal system in which hormone and growth factors from milk including epidermal growth factor (EGF), nerve growth factor (NGF), and prolactin are sorted into a transepithelial transport pathway (Siminoski *et al.*, 1986; Gonnella *et al.*, 1987,1989). A small change in EGF motility on gels after transport suggests that the peptide encounters an intracellular protease, either in endosomes or in transport vesicles (Gonnella *et al.*, 1987).

In both proximal and distal enterocytes of rats, an adherent protein tracer, cationized ferritin, enters transepithelial transport vesicles in small amounts (Abrahamson and Rodewald, 1981; Siminoski *et al.*, 1986), indicating that positively charged peptides or lectins could be transported across these cells in immunologically significant amounts. Soluble proteins, however, are directed efficiently to lysosomes for degradation (Abrahamson and Rodewald, 1981; Gonnella and Neutra, 1984). In other species such as humans and sheep, in which these cells are present during fetal life, transepithelial transport of proteins from amniotic fluid may be conducted by vacuolated enterocytes (Moxey and Trier, 1979; Trahair and Robinson, 1986); these cells contain a specific apical endosomal antigen called endotubin (J. F. Trahair, J. M. Wilson, and M. R. Neutra, unpublished observations). The specificity of transepithelial transport or the nature of the transport vesicles, however, is not known.

Because of their well-developed endocytic compartments, vacuolated enterocytes of suckling rats also have served as models for mapping the interaction of apical and basolateral endocytic pathways. Apical endosomal markers such as the glycoprotein "endotubin" and basolateral membrane receptors such as transferrin appear to cycle in and out of their respective plasma membrane domains and early endosome systems in intestinal cells (Wilson *et al.*, 1987; Godefroy *et al.*, 1988; Hughson and Hopkins, 1990). In vacuolated enterocytes, soluble tracers that enter apical or basolateral endosomes do not mix, but do meet in late endosomes located in the apical cytoplasm and are delivered together to the lysosomal vacuole (Fujita *et al.*, 1990). Whether the transepithelial transport vesicles that carry growth factors and possibly other proteins can transfer protein from apical to basolateral endosomes is not known, but such a pathway would provide an opportunity for interaction of endocytosed antigens with newly synthesized unoccupied MHC II (see Section B).

C. Membrane Traffic in Adult Enterocytes

In the human fetus, highly endocytic vacuolated enterocytes are replaced at about 20 weeks gestation by cells that are morphologically and functionally analogous to adult enterocytes (Moxey and Trier, 1979). This second stage of cytodifferentiation occurs much later in certain other species (at weaning in rodents and one or more days after birth in cattle, sheep, and pigs; Kraehenbuhl *et al.,* 1979). The dramatic change at this stage has been termed "closure," referring to the halt in maternal Ig transfer and disappearance of specialized endocytic epithelial cells. In humans, other more subtle maturational changes such as increased expression of brush border enzymes (and, perhaps, changes in endocytic activity) continue until after birth. Despite indirect evidence for antigen uptake in neonatal humans, the endocytic and transport activities of individual enterocytes at this age has not been documented. Confluent Caco-2 and HT29 enterocytes in culture, when fully differentiated, are analogous to enterocytes in human fetal colon during the second half of gestation (Huet *et al.,* 1987; Neutra and Louvard, 1989).

Nonspecific tracer proteins, including adherent and soluble molecules, are endocytosed in very small amounts by adult enterocytes and appear to be directed entirely to lysosomes in the apical cytoplasm. If late endosome- or lysosome-derived vesicles are shuttled back to the apical surface, no immunological consequences would ensue. If, however, they are delivered to basolateral endosomes or plasma membrane, processed antigens would be exposed to cells of the immune system, either free or associated with MHC complexes. Such vesicular shuttles operate in nonpolarized cells (Kornfeld and Mellman, 1989). Return of protein from apical endosomes to the basolateral surface was observed in Caco-2 cell monolayers (Hughson and Hopkins, 1990), but the existence of shuttles in normal enterocytes is not established. Nevertheless, transepithelial transport of intact biologically active insulin across normal adult epithelium occurs in some species, and ultrastructural evidence for a vesicular transport pathway has been obtained (Bendayan *et al.,* 1990). Although these studies suggest that transepithelial transport is highly selective, membrane-adherent proteins may be carried along.

D. Endocytosis and Transport of Cholera Toxin

Certain adherent proteins may be particularly efficient in entering apical endocytic or transcytotic pathways. Cholera toxin is of particular interest in this regard since, unlike most luminal antigens, it binds with high affinity to membrane glycolipid GM1, is endocytosed efficiently, and has profound effects on enterocyte physiology. Using confluent monolayers of polarized T84 cells in culture, Lencer *et al.* (1992) demonstrated that endocytosis and probably transport of cholera toxin beyond early apical endosomes is required for activation of basolaterally located adenylate cyclase and the resultant chloride secretory response. Others had demonstrated that cholera toxin enters a transepithelial transport pathway in enterocytes *in vivo* (Hansson *et al.,* 1984). Thus, vesicular transport in enterocytes could have important physiological consequences, and endocytic or transcytotic pathways could play a role in the unique modulatory action of cholera toxin in the mucosal immune system (Lycke and Holmgren, 1986; Czerkinsky *et al.,* 1989; Dertzbaugh and Elson, 1991). In addition, cholera toxin has been shown to enhance endocytic activity in other cell types. If this occurs in enterocytes, uptakes of bystander antigens also might be enhanced.

IV. ANTIGEN-PRESENTING COMPLEXES AND ENTEROCYTE MEMBRANE TRAFFIC

Expression of MHC Class I and II molecules by epithelial cells of the small intestine is both constitutive and cytokine regulated (Bland and Kambarage, 1991). These complexes, which act as receptors for protein antigens, are encoded by the MHC locus. As on all other cells, enterocyte MHC I consists of a highly polymorphic A chain noncovalently associated with $\beta 2$ microglobulin (for review, see Yewdell and Bennink, 1990). The MHC II complexes on enterocytes are assumed to be identical to those found on "professional" antigen-presenting cells such as B lymphocytes, macrophages, and dendritic cells, consisting of two highly polymorphic transmembrane polypeptides. The assembly of these complexes along the biosynthetic pathway and their interaction with peptides in intracellular compartments has been elucidated greatly by studies on nonpolarized cells. However, how cell polarity and the existence of two separate endocytic pathways might influence their function in intestinal epithelial cells is not yet clear. Further, the access of MHC on epithelial cells to specific T-cell populations may be restricted by the presence of a basal lamina and by the migration patterns of specific T-cell subsets.

A. MHC I

In enterocytes, MHC Class I determinants are resident noncycling molecules that are restricted to the basolateral membrane (Godefroy *et al.,* 1988), where they could interact readily with $CD8^+$ IELs. The peptides presented to IELs in the context of MHC I probably would originate in the cytosol of the epithelial cell and might represent, for example, newly synthesized viral proteins. These proteins would be degraded by cytoplasmic proteasomes and the resultant peptides transported into the lumen of the endoplasmic reticulum, probably via transporters that belong to the ABC ATPase family (Spiess *et al.,* 1990). Note that interferon γ(IFNγ), a cytokine that can induce MHC expression in many cells including enterocytes (Bland and Warren, 1986), also up-regulates proteasome production and that proteasome genes are located adjacent to the MHC region (Brown *et al.*, 1991; Glynne *et al.*, 1991). These peptides thus would associate with newly synthesized MHC Class I determinants in a compartment that also contains MHC Class II molecules, but the latter would be prevented from binding antigen at this point by the presence of the invariant chain (Roche and Cresswell, 1990). Membrane proteins destined for the basolateral cell surface of enterocytes apparently are sorted into vesicles in the trans-Golgi cisternae, and travel directly to the basolateral membrane (Hauri *et al.*, 1985; Matter *et al.*, 1990). Thus, newly synthesized MHC I determinants on infected or damaged enterocytes would induce lysis by intraepithelial $CD8^+$ T cells, which also would result in production of specific cytokines that might in turn affect epithelial cell proliferation and repair.

B. MHC II

MHC II determinants have been visualized by immunocytochemistry on basolateral surfaces as well as in intracellular vesicles and on apical membranes of intestinal cells (Mayrhofer and Spargo, 1989,1990). In nonpolarized cells (and presumably in enterocytes), Class II molecules are synthesized and assembled in the rough endoplasmic reticulum as heterotrimers that include an additional polypeptide, the invariant chain (Brodsky *et al.*, 1989). This complex travels along the secretory pathway to the Golgi, where it may be segregated spatially from MHC Class I molecules (Peters *et al.*, 1991). Whether the MHC II in enterocytes is sorted initially into the apical or basolateral secretory pathway (or both), or whether it initially enters polarized endosomes, is not known. This information will be important in determining whether MHC II picks up luminally digested antigens or peptides that have "leaked" into the interstitium.

In nonpolarized cells, MHC II enters endosomes on its way to the cell surface (Lotteau *et al.*, 1990; Peters *et al.*, 1991) where a distinct endosomal protease cleaves the invariant chain, exposing the antigen-binding cleft (Brodsky and Guagliardi, 1991). Antigens are taken up by adsorptive or fluid-phase endocytosis into common endosomes and are partially digested by endosomal proteases. The resultant peptides then are able to bind to MCH II and are transported as a complex to the cell surface, where the peptide may be presented to T helper cells that express CD4. In the intestine, how frequently enterocyte basolateral MCH II actually would interact with lamina propria $CD4^+$ lymphocytes is unclear since these cells generally are found in the lamina propria but not within the epithelium (Brandtzaeg *et al.*, 1988). Both luminal and interstitial antigens could gain access to newly synthesized MHC II if the complex is sorted in both directions, but where antigen-MHC II interaction actually occurs in enterocytes is not known. Both endocytic paths meet at the late endosome in enterocytes, but in some cells MHC II is not present in late endosomes (Peters *et al.*, 1991). The inability of isolated enterocytes *in vitro* to process proteolytically and to present intact proteins suggests that predigestion by proteases in the lumen or by other cell types in the lamina propria is required (Bland and Warren, 1986). Luminal digestion also would require movement of peptide fragments or MHC II–peptide complexes through the apical-to-basolateral transepithelial transport pathway, a phenomenon that has been suggested but not yet proven to occur. Studies on isolated cells are complicated by the fact that the membrane domains and basolateral endocytic systems of enterocytes are altered rapidly and dramatically after epithelial isolation (Amerongen *et al.*, 1989). Thus, patterns of endocytosis, transport, and proteolysis that occur *in vivo* might not be reproduced by isolated cells.

MHC receptors may mediate several distinct functions in the intestinal epithelium. As noted earlier, enterocyte MHC may restrict antigen presentation *in vitro* (Bland and Warren, 1986; Mayer and Shlien, 1987; Kaiserlain *et al.*, 1989; Pang *et al.*, 1990; Mayer *et al*, 1991), but no direct evidence is available as yet that antigens absorbed *in vivo* actually are processed and presented to intraepithelial lymphocytes. The small intestine can act as a primary lymphoid organ specifying both the immunoglobulin (Reynaud *et al.*, 1991) and the T-cell repertoire (Guy-Grand *et al.*, 1991). Thus, epithelial MHC molecules also may have an educational role, permitting positive selection of those lymphocytes that recognize "self" MHC molecules. The early development of epithelial and lamina propria cells expressing MHC II, and the early presence of thymus-independent intraepithelial T lymphocytes expressing T cell receptor complexes (TCR) ($\alpha\beta$ or $\gamma\delta$), suggests that MHC II-positive enterocytes and lamina propria cells cooperate to restrict the diversity of responses to self-antigens in the fetus and to bacterial or food antigens in the neonate. The IELs in the general intestinal epithelium are distinct from those in the follicle-associated epithelium over organized lymphoid tissue such as Peyer's patches (Brandtzaeg *et al.*, 1988; Ermak *et al.*, 1990). These lymphoid cell populations are likely to be organized to respond to transport of different types of antigens by enterocytes or M cells, or to induce very different responses (such as secretory immunity or tolerance) to the same antigen. The dramatic differences observed in epithelial membrane traffic in enterocytes and M cells presumably play a central role in these responses.

V. MEMBRANE TRAFFIC IN INTESTINAL M CELLS

A. Adherence of Macromolecules to M Cell Apical Membranes

Studies using various soluble tracers and inert particles have demonstrated rapid endocytosis and transcytosis by M cells (Bockman and Cooper, 1973; Owen, 1977; Lefevre *et al.*, 1978; Pappo and Ermak, 1989). These data suggest that uptake is nonselective, but that the hydrophobicity of particle surfaces could enhance their interaction with M-cell surfaces. Avid binding of cationized ferritin to these cells shows that simple electrostatic interactions also could play a role in binding of bacteria and inert particles (Bye *et al.*, 1984; Neutra *et al.*, 1987). Although these mechanisms clearly play roles in M-cell uptake they do not explain the M-cell selectivity of binding often observed, since both M-cell and enterocyte surfaces are rich in negatively charged carbohydrates. However, indirect evidence suggests that unique protein, glycoprotein, or glycolipid components are exposed on these cells since certain microorganisms bind selectively to M cells with high efficiency.

Adherent particles, microbes, or macromolecules are concentrated effectively by adherence and may be transcytosed by M cells up to two orders of magnitude more efficiently than nonadherent materials (Neutra *et al.*, 1987). Since adherent antigens tend to elicit strong secretory (and often systemic) immune responses (DeAizpurua and Russell-Jones, 1988) and these responses appear to be initiated in sites such as Peyer's patches, M cell adherence is thought to be a key event in induction of mucosal immunity. M cells also endocytose and transport solutes in the fluid content of endocytic vesicles (Owen, 1977); perhaps transport of very small aliquots of soluble antigens over time may play a role in immune tolerance to soluble food antigens (Mayrhofer, 1984). The exact relationship of M cell transport activity to either mucosal or systemic tolerance, however, is not clear.

B. Adherence of Microorganisms to M Cells

The pathogenic viruses that adhere selectively to M cells could provide information about the unique features of the M cell apical membrane, but the interacting viral and M cell surface molecules responsible for adherence are not yet identified. The best-known example of M cell-specific adherence is provided by the mouse pathogen reovirus (Wolf *et al.*, 1981). Processing of reovirus by proteases in the intestinal lumen is known to increase viral infectivity through cleavage of the major outer capsid protein $\sigma 3$ and through a conformational change resulting in extension of the viral hemagglutinin $\sigma 1$ (Bass *et al.*, 1988; Nibert *et al*, 1991). Our laboratory has demonstrated that proteolytic processing of the outer capsid also is required for M cell adherence: neither unprocessed virus nor capsidless cores can bind (H. Amerongen, G. Wilson, B. Fields, M. Neutra, unpublished observations). Thus, the virus uses either the protease-resistant outer capsid protein $\mu 1c$ or the extended $\sigma 1$ protein to bind to M cells, presumably at a site not involved in serotype-specific cell tropism. M cell binding might be mediated by sialic acid residues, since sialylated glycoproteins serve as viral receptors on other cell types (Paul *et al.*, 1989) and M cell surface components avidly bind wheat germ agglutinin (Neutra *et al.*, 1987). These and other viral adhesins, once identified, could serve as affinity ligands to elucidate the M cell molecules or oligosaccharides responsible for the interaction (Bass and Greenberg, 1992). Studies of other viruses that adhere to M cells, including the neurotropic poliovirus (Siciński *et al.*, 1990) and the retrovirus HIV-1 (Amerongen *et al.*, 1991), are needed to determine whether common molecular motifs are used for M cell binding.

The wide range of gram-negative bacteria that bind selectively to M cells includes *Vibrio cholerae* (Owen *et al.*, 1986b; Winner *et al.*, 1991), some strains of *Escherichia coli* (Inman and Cantey, 1983), *Salmonella* (Kohbata *et al.*, 1986), and *Shigella* (Wassef *et al.*, 1989). That each organism utilizes a unique type of binding mechanism seems unlikely, since M cells seem to be designed to capture whole classes of pathogens for immunological sampling. Lectin–carbohydrate recognition systems are widely used by bacteria to interact with eukaryotic cells, so these also may operate in M cell adherence. The participating lectin could be a bacterial adhesin such as a pilus or fimbrial protein, or an M cell membrane protein analogous to the mannose or galactose recognition proteins of hepatocytes and macrophages. These possibilities have proven difficult to test in the absence of a system for culture of polarized functional M cells.

Selective M cell adherence could be caused not by the presence of M cell-specific proteins but by the absence of "blocking" molecules. The possible blocking effect of the enterocyte glycocalyx was demonstrated in our laboratory using cholera toxin, a molecule that binds specifically to the glycolipid receptor GM1 that is present on apical membranes of M cells as well as enterocytes. When cholera toxin was applied to Peyer's patch mucosa as single toxin molecules tagged with a fluorescent probe, it bound to all cell surfaces as expected. When the toxin was applied as polyvalent complexes on 15-nm colloidal gold particles, however, the particles failed to bind to enterocytes but still bound avidly to M cells (R. Weltzin, H. Amerongen, W. Lencer, and M. Neutra, unpublished observations). These results suggest that the thick glycocalyx of enterocytes prevents movement of the colloidal gold probe to GM1 binding sites on microvillar membranes, whereas M cell GM1 is more accessible. Since viruses and bacteria also can be considered particulate polyvalent ligands, they too may find their receptors particularly accessible on M cells.

C. Binding of Immunoglobulins

M cells also have binding sites for immunoglobulins on their apical membranes. Native milk secretory IgA ingested by suckling rabbits accumulates on M cell surfaces (Roy and Varvayanis, 1987). In studies in our laboratory, monoclonal IgA or polyclonal sIgA as well as IgG antibodies were found to bind selectively to M cells and to compete with each other for binding sites (Weltzin *et al.*, 1989). Binding of immunoglobulins appears not to be mediated by known Fc receptors, since antibodies against epithelial and macrophage Fc receptors of other types failed to recognize any M cell component. This binding mechanism would allow M cells to endocytose and transport free IgA as well as IgA–antigen complexes (Weltzin *et al.*, 1989). The role of such transport is not clear; one possibility is that it promotes reuptake of small amounts of antigen into inductive sites. These antigens then might be sampled by intraepithelial or subepithelial antigen-presenting cells to boost an existing secretory immune response. Uptake of IgA also could have other modulatory effects in the mucosal immune system (Kraehenbuhl and Neutra, 1992a; also see Chapter 34).

D. Mechanisms of Antigen Uptake by M Cells

Adherent macromolecules such as cationized ferritin and lectins are taken up by M cells via clathrin-coated pits and are delivered to tubulovesicular structures in the apical cytoplasm that bear morphological resemblance to early endosomes (Neutra *et al.,* 1987). Early endosomes of other cell types contain a subset of lysosomal enzymes (Diment and Stahl, 1985; Courtoy, 1991). Endosomes of most cells generate an acidic internal milieu (Maxfield and Yamashuro, 1991), although specialized apical endosomes of some epithelial cells were found to be pH neutral (Lencer *et al.,* 1990). In M cells, acid phosphatase-containing compartments were not detected in the apical transepithelial pathway (Owen *et al.,* 1986b), but one study has shown that M-cell endosomes are acidified and that some apical vesicles bear a membrane marker typical of late endosomes and lysosomes (Allan *et al.,* 1992). Viruses appear to be unaltered during transepithelial transport (Wolf *et al.,* 1981; Amerongen *et al.,* 1991). However, whether M cell apical endosomes contain endosomal hydrolases is not known. These enzymes are potentially important because if immunogens are processed by partial proteolysis in the transepithelial pathway, such alteration could affect the specificity of the subsequent mucosal immune response. Whether M cells are able to "present" foreign antigens to cells of the immune system has been controversial, because MHC Class II molecules were detected by immunocytochemistry in rat M cells but not in other species. EM immunocytochemistry has revealed that MHC II localize in apical endosomes of rat M cells (Allan *et al.,* 1992), but the functional significance of this localization is not yet known.

Dense "mature" lysosomes are present deeper in M cells (Owen *et al.,* 1986a), but material taken up from the lumen has not been seen to enter this degradative compartment. Also striking is that transcytotic vesicle traffic in M cells is not directed toward the lateral or basal cell surfaces as it is in enterocytes. Rather, either the endosomal vesicles or the vesicles derived from them fuse directly with the modified invaginated basolateral subdomain lining the intraepithelial pocket (Owen, 1977; Neutra *et al.,* 1987). The "pocket" membrane differs from other areas of the basolateral plasma membrane because it contains very low amounts of Na^+,K^+-ATPase (Neutra *et al.,* 1986) and presumably contains adhesion molecules that serve as homing sites for a special subpopulation of lymphocytes (Ermak *et al.,* 1990). The nature of the pocket subdomain and the mechanisms by which endosomes are targeted directly to it are important areas for future study.

The exact mechanism of uptake of adherent particles, viruses, and bacteria by M cells also deserves further scrutiny. Bacteria are taken up by a process that resembles phagocytosis in macrophages. *Vibrio cholerae,* for example, forms broad areas of close interactions with M cells in which the bacterial and eukaryotic cell membranes are separated by a 10- to 20-nm gap under which cytoplasmic actin is reorganized (J. Mack, M. Mekalanos, and M. R. Neutra, unpublished observations). This result implies that specific M cell membrane components are recruited to the interaction site. Evidence from macrophages and nonpolarized cells suggests that adhesion molecules provide direct or indirect links to cytoskeletal elements and to the intracellular signaling machinery that may control local calcium flux (Odin *et al.,* 1992). For bacteria or viruses, which microbial gene products and which M cell membrane components play roles in binding and internalization are not known. The fact that adherent bacteria, viruses, and some macromolecules are released readily into the pocket at the basolateral side implies that initial binding may be accomplished through multiple low affinity interactions that can be reversed by a shift in ionic strength or pH, raising the possibility that the membranes of transport vesicles or the intraepithelial pocket may conduct active transport of protons or other ions.

VI. CONCLUSION

Design of new mucosal vaccines and rational strategies for enhancing tolerance to mucosal immunogens may be facilitated by a clearer understanding of transepithelial transport by both M cells and enterocytes. Such advances will require more information about the basic mechanisms that direct endocytosed antigens into enterocyte transepithelial pathways and about the nature of the interactions of such antigens with epithelial membrane proteins and with subepithelial and intraepithelial cells. In the case of the M cell, an important goal is elucidating the mechanisms of adherence of the pathogens that efficiently invade at this site and exploiting this information to produce "pseudopathogens" that can serve as efficient oral vaccines.

Acknowledgments

We thank the current and former members of our laboratories, especially R. Weltzin, J. Mack, L. Winner, H. Amerongen, P. Michetti, F. Apter, W. Lencer, R. Hirt, and E. Schaerer, who contributed to the published and unpublished work discussed in this chapter.

References

Abrahamson, D. R., and Rodewald, R. (1981). Evidence for the sorting of endocytic vesicle contents during receptor-mediated transport of IgG across newborn rat intestine. *J. Cell Biol.* **91,** 270–280.

Achler, C., Filmer, D., Merte, C., and Drenckhahn, D. (1989). Role of microtubules in polarized delivery of apical membrane proteins to the brush border of the intestinal epithelium. *J. Cell Biol.* **109,** 179–189.

Allan, C. H., Mendrick, D. L., and Trier, J. S. (1993). M cells contain acidic compartments and express class II MHC determinants. *Gastroenterology* **104,** 698–708.

Alpers, D. H. (1975). Protein turnover in intestinal mucosal villus and crypt brush border membranes. *Biochem. Biophys. Res. Commun.* **75,** 130–135.

Amerongen, H. M., Mack, J. A., Wilson, J. M., and Neutra, M. R. (1989). Membrane domains of intestinal epithelial cells: Distribution of Na^{+},K^{+}-ATPase and the membrane skeleton in adult rat intestine, during fetal development, and after epithelial isolation. *J. Cell Biol.* **109,** 2129–2138.

Amerongen, H. M., Weltzin, R. A., Farnet, C. M., Michetti, P., Haseltine, W. A., and Neutra, M. R. (1991). Transepithelial transport of HIV-1 by intestinal M cells: A mechanism for transmission of AIDS. *J. Acq. Immune Defic. Syndr.* **4,** 760–765.

Anderson, R. G. W. (1991). Molecular motors that shape endocytic membrane. *In* "Intracellular Trafficking of Proteins" (C. J. Steer and J. A. Hanover, eds.), pp. 13–46. Cambridge University Press, Cambridge.

Apodaca, G., Bomsel, M., Arden, J., Breitfeld, P. P., Tang, K. C., and Mostov, K. E. (1991). The polymeric immunoglobulin receptor. A model protein to study transcytosis. *J. Clin. Invest.* **87,** 1877–1882.

Bacallao, R., Antony, C., Dotti, D., Karsenti, E., Stelzer, E. H., and Simons, K. (1989). The subcellular organization of Madin–Darby canine kidney cells during formation of a polarized epithelium. *J. Cell Biol.* **109,** 2817–2832.

Bartles, J. R., Feracci, H. M., Steiger, B., and Hubbard, A. L. (1987). Biogenesis of the rat hepatocyte plasma membrane *in vivo:* Comparison of the pathways taken by apical and basolateral proteins using subcellular fractionation. *J. Cell Biol.* **105,** 1241–1251.

Bass, D. M., and Greenberg, H. B. (1992). Strategies for the identification of icosahedral virus receptors. *J. Clin. Invest.* **89,** 3–9.

Bass, D. M., Trier, J. S., Dambrauskas, R., and Wolf, J. L. (1988). Reovirus type I infection of small intestinal epithelium in suckling mice and its effect on M cells. *Lab. Invest.* **58,** 226–235.

Bendayan, M., Ziv, E., Ben-Sasson, R., Bar-On, H., and Kidron, M. (1990). Morphocytochemical and biochemical evidence for insulin absorption by the rat ileal epithelium. *Diabetologia* **33,** 197–204.

Bland, P. W., and Kambarage, D. M. (1991). Antigen handling by the epithelium and lamina propria macrophages. *Gastroenterol. Clin. North Am.* **20,** 577–596.

Bland, P. W., and Warren, L. G. (1986). Antigen presentation by epithelial cells of the rat small intestine II. Selective induction of suppressor T cells. *Immunology* **58,** 9–14.

Bockman, D. E., and Cooper, M. D. (1973). Pinocytosis by epithelium associated with lymphoid follicles in the bursa of Fabricius, appendix, and Peyer's patches. An electron microscopic study. *Am. J. Anat.* **136,** 455–478.

Bomsel, M., Prydz, K., Parton, R. G., Gruenberg, J., and Simons, K. (1989). Endocytosis in filter-grown Madin–Darby canine kidney cells. *J. Cell Biol.* **109,** 3243–3258.

Bomsel, M., Parton, R., Kuznetsov, S. A., Schroer, T. A., and Gruenberg, J. (1990). Microtubule- and motor-dependent fusion *in vitro* between apical and basolateral endocytic vesicles from MDCK cells. *Cell* **62,** 719–731.

Brandli, A. W., Parton, R. G., and Simons, K. (1990). Transcytosis in MDCK cells: Identification of glycoproteins transported bidirectionally between both plasma membrane domains. *J. Cell BIol.* **111,** 2909–2921.

Brandtzaeg, P., Sollid, L. M., Thrane, P. S., Kvale, D., Bjerke, K., Scott, H., Kett, K., and Rognum, T. O. (1988). Lymphoepithelial interactions in the mucosal immune system. *Gut* **29,** 1116–1130.

Braun, M., Waheed, A., and von Figura, K. (1989). Lysosomal acid phosphatase is transported to lysosomes via the cell surface. *EMBO J.* **8,** 3633–3640.

Breitfeld, P. P., Casanova, J. E., Simister, N. E., Ross, S. A., McKinnon, W. C., and Mostov, K. E. (1989a). Sorting signals. *Curr. Opin. Cell Biol.* **1,** 617–623.

Breitfeld, P. P., Harris, J. M., and Mostov, K. E. (1989b). Postendocytotic sorting of the ligand for the polymeric immunoglobulin receptor in Madin–Darby canine kidney cells. *J. Cell Biol.* **109,** 475–486.

Brodsky, F. M., and Guagliardi, L. E. (1991). The cell biology of antigen processing and presentation. *Annu. Rev. Immunol.* **9,** 707–744.

Brodsky, F. M., Koppelman, B., Blum, J. S., Marks, M. S., Cresswell, P., and Guagliardi, L. (1989). Intracellular colocalization of molecules involved in antigen processing and presentation by B cells. *Cold Spring Harbor Symp. Quant. Biol.* **54,** 319–331.

Brown, M. G., Driscoll, J., and Monaco, J. J. (1991). Structural and serological similarity of MHC-linked LMP and proteasome (multicatalytic proteinase) complexes. *Nature (London)* **352,** 355–357.

Brown, W. J., Goodhouse, J., and Farquhar, M. G. (1986). Mannose-6-phosphate receptors for lysosomal enzymes cycle between the Golgi complex and endosomes. *J. Cell Biol.* **103,** 1235–1247.

Bye, W. A., Allan, C. H., and Trier, J. S. (1984). Structure, distribution and origin of M cells in Peyer's patches of mouse ileum. *Gastroenterology* **86,** 789–801.

Caplan, M. J., Anderson, H. C., Palade, G. E., and Jamieson, J. E. (1986). Intracellular sorting and polarized cell surface delivery of (Na^{+},K^{+})ATPase, an endogenous component of MDCK cell basolateral plasma membranes. *Cell* **46,** 623–631.

Casanova, J. E., Breitfeld, P. P., Ross, S. A., and Mostov, K. E. (1990). Phosphorylation of the polymeric immunoglobulin receptor required for its efficient transcytosis. *Science* **248,** 742–745.

Courtoy, P. J. (1991). Dissection of endosomes. *In* "Intracellular Trafficking of Proteins" (C. J. Steer and J. A. Hanover, eds), pp. 103–156. Cambridge University Press, Cambridge.

Czerkinsky, C., Russell, M. W., Lycke, N., Lindblad, M., and Holmgren, J. (1989). Oral administration of a streptococcal antigen coupled to cholera toxin B subunit evokes strong antibody responses in salivary glands and extramucosal tissues. *Infect. Immun.* **57,** 1072–1077.

Danielson, E. M., and Cowell, G. M. (1985). Biosynthesis of intestinal microvillar proteins. Evidence for an intracellular sorting taking place in, or shortly after exit from the Golgi complex. *Eur. J. Biochem.* **152,** 493–499.

De Aizpurua, H. J., and Russell-Jones, G. J. (1988). Oral vaccination: Identification of classes of proteins that provoke an immune response upon oral feeding. *J. Exp. Med.* **167,** 440–451.

Dertzbaugh, M. T., and Elson, C. O. (1991). Cholera toxin as a mucosal adjuvant. *In* "Topics in Vaccine Adjuvant Research" (D. R. Spriggs and W. C. Koff, eds.), pp. 119–132. CRC Press, Boca Raton, Florida.

Diment, S., and Stahl, P. (1985). Macrophage endosomes contain proteases which degrade endocytosed protein ligands. *J. Biol. Chem.* **260,** 15211–15317.

Dragsten, P. R., Blumenthal, R., and Handler, J. S. (1981). Membrane asymmetry in epithelia: Is the tight junction a barrier to diffusion in the plasma membrane? *Nature (London)* **294,** 718–722.

Eilers, U., Klumperman, J., and Hauri, H. P. (1989). Nocodazole, a microtubule-active drug, interferes with apical protein delivery in cultured intestinal epithelial cells (Caco-2). *J. Cell Biol.* **108,** 13–22.

Ermak, T. H., Steger, H. J., and Pappo, J. (1990). Phenotypically distinct subpopulations of T cells in domes and M- cell pockets of rabbit gut-associated lymphoid tissues. *Immunology* **71,** 530–537.

Fujita, M., Reinhart, F., and Neutra, M. (1990). Convergence of apical and basolateral endocytic pathways at apical late endosomes in absorptive cells of suckling rat ileum. *J. Cell Sci.* **97,** 385–394.

Fuller, S. D., and Simons, K. (1986). Transferrin receptor polarity and recycling accuracy in "tight" and "leaky" strains of Madin–Darby canine kidney cells. *J. Cell Biol.* **103,** 1767–1769.

Geuze, H. J., Slot, J. W., Strous, G. J. A. M., Peppard, J., von Figura, K., Hasilik, A., and Schwartz, A. L. (1984). Intracellular receptor sorting during endocytosis: Comparative immunoelectron microscopy of multiple receptors in rat liver. *Cell* **37,** 195–204.

Geuze, H. J., Slot, J. W., and Schwartz, A. L. (1987). Membranes of sorting organelles display lateral heterogeneity in receptor distribution. *J. Cell Biol.* **104,** 1715–1723.

Glynne, R., Powis, S. H., Beck, S., Kelly, A., and Kerr, L. A. (1991). A proteasome related gene between the two ABC transporter loci in the class II region of the human MHC. *Nature (London)* **343,** 357–361.

Godefroy, O., Huet, C., Blair, L. A. C., Sahuquillo-Merino, C., and Louvard, D. (1988). Differentiation properties of a clone isolated from the HT29 cell line (a human colon carcinoma): Polarized differentiation of histocompatibility antigens (HLA) and of transferrin receptors. *Biol. Cell* **63,** 41–56.

Goldman, I. S., Jones, A. L., Hradek, G. T., and Huling, S. (1983). Hepatocyte handling of immunoglobulin A in the rat: The role of microtubules. *Gastroenterology* **85,** 130–140.

Gonnella, P. A., and Neutra, M. R. (1984). Membrane-bound and fluid-phase macromolecules enter separate prelysosomal compartments in absorptive cells of suckling rat ileum. *J. Cell Biol.* **99,** 909–917.

Gonnella, P. A., and Neutra, M. R. (1985). Glycoconjugate distribution and mobility on apical membranes of absorptive cells of suckling rat ileum *in vivo*. *Anat. Rec.* **213,** 520–528.

Gonnella, P. A., Simonski, K., Murphy, R. A., and Neutra, M. R. (1987). Transepithelial transport of epidermal growth factor by absorptive cells of suckling rat. *J. Clin. Invest.* **80,** 22–32.

Gonnella, P. O., Harmatz, P., and Walker, W. A. (1989). Prolactin is transported across the epithelium of the jejunum and ileum of the suckling rat ileum. *J. Cell Physiol.* **140,** 138–149.

Griffiths, G., Hoflack, B., Simons, K., Mellman, I., and Kornfeld, S. (1988). The mannose 6-phosphate receptor and the biogenesis of lysosomes. *Cell* **52,** 329–341.

Gruenberg, J., and Howell, K. E. (1989). Membrane traffic in endocytosis: insights from cell free assays. *Annu. Rev. Cell Biol.* **5,** 453–481.

Gruenberg, J., Griffiths, G., and Howell, K. E. (1989). Characterization of the early endosome and putative endocytic carrier vesicles *in vivo* and with an assay of vesicle fusion *in vitro*. *J. Cell Biol.* **108,** 1301–1316.

Guy-Grand, D., Malassis-Seris, M., Briottet, C., and Vassalli, P. (1991). Cytotoxic differentiation of mouse gut thymodependent and independent intraepithelial T lymphocytes is induced locally. Correlation between functional assays, presence of perforin and granzyme transcripts, and cytoplasmic granules. *J. Exp. Med.* **173,** 1549–1552.

Hansson, H. A., Lange, S., and Lonnroth, I. (1984). Internalization *in vivo* of cholera toxin in the small intestine of the rat. *Acta Pathol. Microbiol. Scand.* **92,** 15–21.

Hauri, H. P., Sterchi, E. E., Bienz, D., Fransen, J. A. M., and Marxer, A. (1985). Expression and intracellular transport of microvillus membrane hydrolases in human intestinal epithelial cells. *J. Cell Biol.* **101,** 838–851.

Heyman, M., Crain-Denoyelle, A. M., Nath, S. K., and Desjeux, J. F. (1990). Quantification of protein transcytosis in the human colon carcinoma cell line Caco-2. *J. Cell Physiol.* **143,** 391–395.

Hidalgo, I. J., Raub, T. J., and Borchardt, R. T. (1989). Characterization of the human colon carcinoma cell line (Caco-2) as a model system for intestinal epithelial permeability. *Gastroenterology* **96,** 736–749.

Hirt, R. P., Hughes, G. J., Frutiger, S., Michetti, P., Perregaux, C., Jeanguenat, N., Neutra, M. R., and Kraechenbuhl, J.-P. (1993). Transcytosis of the polymeric immunoglobulin receptor requires phosphorylation of serine 664 in the absence but not in the presence of dimeric IgA. *Cell,* in press.

Huet, C., Sahuquillo-Merino, C., Coudrier, E., and Louvard, D. (1987). Absorptive and mucus-secreting subclones isolated from multipotent intestinal cell line (HT-29) provide new models for cell polarity and terminal differentiation. *J. Cell Biol.* **105,** 345–357.

Hughson, E. J., and Hopkins, C. R. (1990). Endocytic pathways in polarized Caco-2 cells: Identification of an endosomal compartment accessible from both apical and basolateral surfaces. *J. Cell Biol.* **110,** 337–348.

Hunziker, W., and Mellman, I. (1989). Expression of macrophage-lymphocyte Fc receptors in Madin-Darby canine kidney cells: Polarity and transcytosis differ for isoforms with or without coated pit localization domains. *J. Cell Biol.* **109,** 3291–3302.

Hunziker, W., Male, P., and Mellman, I. (1990). Differential microtubule requirements for transcytosis in MDCK cells. *EMBO J.* **9,** 3515–3525.

Hunziker, W., Harter, C., Matter, K., and Mellman, I. (1991a). Basolateral sorting in MDCK cells requires a distinct cytoplasmic domain determinant. *Cell* **66,** 907–920.

Hunziker, W., Whitney, J. A., and Mellman, I. (1991b). Selective inhibition of transcytosis by Brefeldin A in MDCK cells. *Cell* **67,** 617–628.

Inman, L. R., and Cantey, J. R. (1983). Specific adherence of *Escherichia coli* (strain RDEC-1) to membranous (M) cells of the Peyer's patch in *Escherichia coli* diarrhea in the rabbit. *J. Clin. Invest.* **71,** 1–8.

Israel, E. J., Simister, N., Freiberg, E., Hendren, R., and Walker, W. A. (1989). Immunoglobulin G binding sites on the human fetal intestine. *Pediatr. Res.* **25,** 116a.

Kaiserlain, D., Vidal, K., and Revillard, J. P. (1989). Murine enterocytes can present soluble antigen to specific class II restricted CD4+ T cells. *Eur. J. Immunol.* **19,** 1513–1516.

Kelly, R. B. (1990). Microtubules, membrane traffic, and cell organization. *Cell* **61,** 5–7.

Kohbata, S., Yokobata, H., and Yabuuchi, E. (1986). Cytopathogenic effect of Salmonella typhi GIFU 10007 on M cells of murine ileal Peyer's patches in ligated ileal loops; An ultrastructural study. *Microbiol. Immunol.* **30,** 1225–1237.

Kornfeld, S., and Mellman, I. (1989). The biogenesis of lysosomes. *Annu. Rev. Cell Biol.* **5,** 483–525.

Kraehenbuhl, J. P., and Neutra, M. R. (1992a). Molecular and cellular basis of immune protection of mucosal surfaces. *Physiol. Rev.* **72,** 853–879.

Kraehenbuhl J. P., and Neutra M. R. (1992b). Transepithelial transport and mucosal defense: secretion of IgA. Trends Cell Biol. **2,** 170–174.

Kraehenbuhl, J. P., Bron, C., and Sordat, B. (1979). Transfer of humoral secretory and cellular immunity from mother to offspring. *Curr. Top. Pathol.* **66,** 105–157.

Kuhn, L. C., and Kraehenbuhl, J. P. (1982). The sacrificial receptor—Translocation of polymeric IgA across epithelia. *Trends Biochem. Sci.* **7,** 299–302.

LeBivic, A., Hirn, M., and Reggio. H. (1986). HT-29 cells are an *in vitro* model for the generation of cell polarity in epithelia during embryonic differentiation. *Proc. Natl. Acad. Sci. U.S.A.* **85,** 136–140.

LeFevre, M. E., Olivo, R., and Joel, D. D. (1978). Accumulation of latex particles in Peyer's patches and their subsequent appearance in villi and mesenteric lymph nodes. *Proc. Soc. Exp. Biol. Med.* **159,** 198.

Lencer, W. I., Verkman, A. S., Arnaout, A., Ausiello, D., and Brown, D. (1990). Endocytic vesicles which retrieve the vasopressin-sensitive water channel do not contain a functional H^+ ATPase. *J. Cell Biol.* **111,** 379–389.

Lencer, W. E., Delp, C., Neutra, M. R., and Madara J. L. (1992). Mechanism of cholera toxin action on a polarized human intestinal epithelial cell line: Role of vesicular traffic. *J. Cell Biol.* 117: 1197–1210.

Levine, J. S., Allen, R. H., Alpers, D. H., and Seetheram, B. (1984). Immunocytochemical location of intrinsic factor-cobalamin receptors in dog ileum. *J. Cell Biol.* **98,** 1110–1117.

Lippincott-Schwartz, J., and Fambrough, D. M. (1987). Cycling of the integral glycoprotein LEP 100 between plasma membrane and lysosomes: Kinetic and morphological analysis. *Cell* **49,** 669–677.

Lisanti, M. P., and Rodriguez-Boulan, E. (1990). Glycophospholipid membrane anchoring provides clues to the mechanism of protein sorting in polarized epithelial cells. *Trends Biochem. Sci.* **15,** 113–118.

Lotteau, V., Teyton, L., Peleraux, A., Nilsson, T., Karlsson, L., Schmid, S. L., Quaranta, V., and Peterson, P. A. (1990). Intracellular transport of class II MHC molecules directed by invariant chain. *Nature (London)* **348,** 600–605.

Louvard, D., Godefroy, O., Huet, C., Sahuquillo-Merino, C., Robine, S., and Coudrier, E. (1985). Basolateral membrane proteins are expressed at the surface of immature intestinal cells whereas transport of apical proteins is abortive. *In* "Current Communications in Molecular Biology. Protein Transport and Secretion" (M. J. Gething, ed.), pp. 168–173. Cold Spring Harbor Laboratory Press, Cold Spring Harbor, New York.

Lycke, N., and Holmgren, J. (1986). Strong adjuvant properties of cholera toxin on gut mucosal immune responses to orally presented antigens. *Immunology* **59,** 301–308.

Madara, J. L. (1988). Tight junction dynamics: Is paracellular transport regulated? *Cell* **53,** 497–498.

Madara, J. L., and Trier, J. S. (1987). Functional morphology of the mucosa of the small intestine. *In* "Physiology of the Gastrointestinal Tract" (L. R. Johnson, ed.), pp. 1209–1250. Raven Press, New York.

Massey, D., Feracci, H., Gorvel, J. P., Rigal, A., Soulie, J. M., and Maroux, S. (1987). Evidence for the transit of aminopeptidase N through the basolateral membrane before it reaches the brush border of enterocytes. *J. Membrane Biol.* **96,** 19–25.

Matlin, K., Bainton, D. F., Pesonen, M., Louvard, D., Genty, N., and Simons, K. (1983). Transepithelial transport of a viral membrane glycoprotein implanted into the apical plasma membrane of MDCK cells. I. Morphological evidence. *J. Cell Biol.* **97,** 627–637.

Matter, K., Brauchbar, M., Bucher, K., and Hauri, H. P. (1990). Sorting of endogenous plasma membrane proteins occurs from two sites in cultured human intestinal epithelial cells (Caco-2). *J. Cell Biol.* **60,** 429–437.

Maxfield, F. R., and Yamashiro, D. J. (1991). Acidification of organelles and the intracellular sorting of proteins during endocytosis. *In* "Intracellular Trafficking of Proteins (C. J. Steer and J. A. Hanover, eds.), pp. 157–182. Cambridge University Press, Cambridge.

Mayer, E. L., and Shlien, R. (1987). Evidence for function of IgA molecules on gut epithelial cells in man. *J. Exp. Med.* **166,** 1471–1483.

Mayer, L., Panja, A., and Li, Y. (1991). Antigen recognition in the gastrointestinal tract: death to the dogma. *Immunol. Res.* **10,** 356–359.

Mayrhofer, G. (1984). Physiology of the intestinal immune system. *In* "Local Immune Responses of the Gut" (T. J. Newby and C. R. Stokes, eds.), pp. 1–96. CRC Press, Boca Raton, Florida.

Mayrhofer, G., and Spargo, L. D. (1989). Subcellular distribution of class II major histocompatibility antigens in enterocytes of the human and rat small intestine. *Immunol. Cell Biol* **67,** 25–60.

Mayrhofer, G., and Spargo, L. D. (1990). Distribution of class II major histocompatibility antigens in enterocytes of the rat jejunum and their association with organelles of the endocytic pathway. *Immunology* **70,** 11–19.

Mooseker, M. (1985). Organization, chemistry and assembly of the cytoskeletal apparatus of the intestinal brush border. *Ann. Rev. Cell Biol.* **1,** 209–241.

Mostov, K. E., and Simister, N. E. (1985). Transcytosis. *Cell* **43,** 389–390.

Mostov, K. E., Friedlander, M., and Blobel, G. (1984). The receptor for transepithelial transport of IgA and IgM contains multiple immunoglobulin-like domains. *Nature (London)* **308,** 37–43.

Moxey, P. C., and Trier, J. S. (1979). Development of villus absorptive cells in the human fetal small intestine: A morphological and morphometric study. *Anat. Rec.* **195,** 463–482.

Nabi, I. R., LeBivic, A., Fambrough, D., and Rodriguez-Boulan, E. (1991). An endogenous MDCK lysosomal membrane glycoprotein is targeted basolaterally before delivery to lysosomes. *J. Cell Biol.* **115,** 1573–1584.

Nedrud, J. G., and Lamm, M. (1991). Adjuvants and the mucosal immune system. *In* "Tropics in Vaccine Adjuvant Research" (D. R. Spriggs and W. C. Koff, eds.), pp. 54–67. CRC Press, Boca Raton, Florida.

Nelson, W. J., and Hammerton, R. W. (1989). A membrane-cytoskeletal complex containing Na^+,K^+-ATPase, ankyrin, and fodrin in Madin–Darby canine kidney (MDCK) cells: Implications for the biogenesis of epithelial cell polarity. *J. Cell Biol.* **108,** 893–902.

Neutra, M. R. (1988). The gastrointestinal tract. *In* "Cell and Tissue Biology" (L. Weiss, ed.), pp. 641–684. Urban and Schwartzenberg, Baltimore.

Neutra, M. R., and Kraehenbuhl, J. P. (1992). Transepithelial transport and mucosal defense. *Trends Cell Biol.* 2:134–138.

Neutra, M. R., and Louvard, D. (1989). Differentiation of intestinal cells *in vitro*. *In* "Functional Epithelial Cells in Culture" (K. S. Matlin and J. D. Valentich, eds.), pp. 363–398. Liss, New York.

Neutra, M. R., Owen, L., Lodish, H., and Ciechanover, A. (1985). Intracellular transport of transferrin and asialoorosomucoid–colloidal gold conjugates to lysosomes after receptor-mediated endocytosis. *J. Histochem. Cytochem.* **33,** 1134–1145.

Neutra, M. R., Phillips, T. L., Fishkind, D. J., and Mack, J. A. (1986). Membrane domains of the intestinal M cell. *J. Cell Biol.* **103,** 466a.

Neutra, M. R., Phillips, T. L., Mayer, E. L., and Fishkind, D. J. (1987). Transport of membrane-bound macromolecules by M cells in follicle-associated epithelium of rabbit Peyer's patch. *Cell Tissue Res.* **247,** 537–546.

Neutra, M. R., Wilson, J. M., Weltzin, R. A., and Kraehenbuhl, J. P. (1988). Membrane domains and macromolecular transport in intestinal epithelial cells. *Am. Rev. Respir. Dis.* **138,** S10–S16.

Nibert, M. L., Furlong, D. B., and Fields, B. N. (1992). Mechanisms of viral pathogenesis. Distinct forms of reoviruses and their roles during replication in cells and host. *J. Clin. Invest.* **88,** 727–734.

Odin, J. A., Edberg, J. C., Painter, C. J., Kimberly, R. P., and Unkeless, J. C. (1992). Regulation of phagocytosis and (Ca^{2+}) flux by distinct regions of an Fc receptor. *Science* **254,** 1785–1788.

Owen, R. L. (1977). Sequential uptake of horseradish peroxidase by lymphoid follicle epithelium of Peyer's patch in the normal unobstructed mouse intestine: An ultrastructural study. *Gastroenterology* **72,** 440–451.

Owen, R. L., Apple, R. T., and Bhalla, D. K. (1986a). Morphometric and cytochemical analysis of lysosomes in rat Peyer's patch follicle epithelium: Their reduction in volume fraction and acid phosphatase content in M cells compared to adjacent enterocytes. *Anat. Rec.* **216,** 521–527.

Owen, R. L., Pierce, N. F., Apple, R. T., and Cray, W. C., Jr. (1986b). M cell transport of *Vibrio cholerae* from the intestinal lumen into Peyer's patches: A mechanism for antigen sampling and for microbial transepithelial migration. *J. Infect. Dis.* **153,** 1108–1118.

Pang, G., Clancy, R., and Saunders, H. (1990). Dual mechanisms of inhibition of the immune response by enterocytes isolated from the rat small intestine. *Immunol. Cell Biol* **68,** 387–396.

Pappo, J., and Ermak, T. H. (1989). Uptake and translocation of fluorescent latex particles by rabbit Peyer's patch epithelium: a quantitative model for M cell uptake. *Clin. Exp. Immunol.* **76,** 144–148.

Parton, R. G., Prydz, K., Bomsel, M., Simons, K., and Griffiths, G. (1989). Meeting of the apical and basolateral endocytic pathways of the Madin–Darby canine kidney cell in late endosomes. *J. Cell Biol.* **109,** 3259–3272.

Paul, R. W., Choi, A. H., and Lee, P. W. (1989). The alpha-anomeric form of sialic acid is the minimal receptor determinant recognized by reovirus. *Virology* **172,** 382–385.

Pavelka, M., Ellinger, A., and Gangl, A. (1983). Effect of colchicine on rat small intestinal absorptive cells. I. Formation of basolateral microvillus borders. *J. Ultrastruct. Res.* **85,** 249–259.

Peters, P. J., Neefjes, J. J., Oorschot, V., Ploegh, H. L., and Geuze, H. J. (1991). Segregation of MHC class II molecules from MHC class I molecules in the Golgi complex for transport to lysosomal compartments. *Nature (London)* **349,** 669–675.

Phillips, T. E., Phillips, T. H., and Neutra, M. R. (1987). Macromolecules can pass through occluding junctions of rat ileal epithelium during cholinergic stimulation. *Cell Tissue Res.* **247,** 547–554.

Prydz, K., Brandli, A. W., Bomsel, M., and Simons, K. (1990). Surface distribution of the mannose 6-phosphate receptors in epithelial Madin–Darby canine kidney cells. *J. Biol. Chem.* **265,** 12629–12635.

Quaroni, A., Kirsch, K., and Weiser, M. M. (1979). Synthesis of membrane glycoproteins in rat small-intestinal villus cells. Effect of colchicine on the redistrubution of L-[1,5,6-^{3}H] fucose-labelled membrane glycoproteins among Golgi, lateral, basal and microvillus membrane. *Biochem. J.* **182,** 213–221.

Rabinowitz, S., Horstmann, H., Gordon, S., and Griffiths, G. (1992). Immunocytochemical characterization of the endocytic and phagolysosomal compartments in peritoneal macrophages. *J. Cell Biol* **116,** 95–112.

Reynaud, C. A., Mackay, C. R., Miller, R. G., and Weill, J. C. (1991). Somatic generation of diversity in a mammalian primary lymphoid organ: The sheep ileal Peyer's patches. *Cell* **64,** 995–1006.

Roche, P. A., and Cresswell, P. (1990). Invariant chain association with HLA-DR moelcules inhibits immunogenic peptide binding. *Nature (London)* **345,** 615–618.

Rodewald, R. (1980). Distribution of immunoglobulin G receptors in the small intestine of the young rat. *J. Cell Biol.* **85,** 18–32.

Rodriguez-Boulan, E., and Nelson, W. J. (1989). Morphogenesis of the polarized epithelial cell phenotype. *Science* **245,** 718–725.

Roy, M. J., and Varvayanis, M. (1987). Development of dome epithelium in gut-associated lymphoid tissues: Association of IgA with M cells. *Cell Tissue Res.* **248,** 645–651.

Schaerer, E., Neutra, M. R., and Kraehenbuhl, J. P. (1991). Molecular and cellular mechanisms involved in transepithelial transport. *J. Membrane Biol.* **123,** 93–103.

Schroer, T. A., and Kelly, R. B. (1985). *In vitro* translocation of organelles along microtubules. *Cell* **40,** 729–730.

Schroer, T. A., and Sheetz, M. P. (1989). Role of kinesin and kinesin-associated proteins in organelle transport. *In* "Cell Movement" (J. R. McIntosh and F. D. Warner, eds.), pp. 295–306. Liss, New York.

Semenza, G. (1986). Anchoring and biosynthesis of stalked brush border membrane glycoproteins. *Annu. Rev. Cell Biol* **2,** 255–314.

Sicinski, P., Rowinski, J., Warchol, J. B., Jarzcabek, Z., Gut, W., Szczygiel, B., Bielecki, K., and Koch, G. (1990). Poliovirus type 1 enters the human host through intestinal M cells. *Gastroenterology* **98,** 56–58.

Siminoski, K., Gonnella, P., Bernanke, J., Owen, L., Neutra, M., and Murphy, R. A. (1986). Uptake and transepithelial transport of nerve growth factor in suckling rat ileum. *J. Cell Biol.* **103,** 1979–1990.

Simister, N. E., and Mostov K. E. (1989). An Fc receptor structurally related to MHC class I antigens. *Nature (London)* **337,** 184–187.

Slot, J. W., and Geuze, H. J. (1984). Transcytosis of IgA in duodenal epithelial cells observed by immunocytochemistry. *J. Cell Biol.* **99,** 7a.

Specian, R. D., and Neutra, M. R. (1984). The cytoskeleton of intestinal goblet cells. *Gastroenterology* **87,** 1313–1325.

Spiess, T., Bresnahan, M., Bahram, S., Arnold, D., Blanck, G., Mellins, E., Pious, D., and Demars, R. (1990). A gene in the human major histocompatibility complex class II region controlling the class I antigen presentation pathway. *Nature (London)* **348,** 744–747.

Sztul, E., Kaplin, A., Saucan, L., and Palade, G. (1991). Protein traffic between distinct plasma membrane domains: Isolation and characterization of vesicular carriers involved in transcytosis. *Cell* **64,** 81–89.

Trahair, J. F., and Robinson, P. M. (1986). The development of the ovine small intestine. *Anat. Rec.* **214,** 294–303.

Trahair, J. F., and Robinson, P. M. (1989). Enterocyte ultrastructure and uptake of immunoglobulins in the small intestine of the neonatal lamb. *J. Anat.* **166,** 103–111.

Trier, J. S., and Moxey, P. (1979). Morphogenesis of the small intestine during fetal development. *In* "Development of Mammalian Absorptive Processes" Ciba Foundation Symposium 70 (J. T. Harries, ed.), pp. 3–29. Exerpta Medica, Amsterdam.

van der Sluijs, P., Bennett, M. K., Antony, C., Simons, K., and Kreis, T. E. (1990). Binding of exocytic vesicles from MDCK cells to microtubules *in vitro*. *J. Cell Sci.* **95,** 545–553.

von Figura, K., and Hasilik, A. (1986). Lysosomal enzymes and their receptors. *Ann. Rev. Biochem.* **55,** 167–193.

Wandinger-Ness, A., and Simons, K. (1991). The polarized transport of surface proteins and lipids in epithelial cells. *In* "Intracellular Trafficking of Proteins" (C. J. Steer and J. A. Hanover, eds), pp. 575–612. Cambridge University Press, Cambridge.

Wassef, J. S., Keren, D. F., and Mailloux, J. L. (1989). Role of M cells in initial antigen uptake and in ulcer formation in the rabbit intestinal loop model of shigellosis. *Infect. Immun.* **57,** 858–863.

Weinman, M. D., Allan, C. H., Trier, J. S., and Hagen, S. J. (1989). Repair of microvilli in the rat small intestine after damage with lectins contained in the red kidney bean. *Gastroenterology* **97,** 1193–1204.

Weltzin, R. A., Lucia-Jandris, P., Michetti, P., Fields, B. N., and Kraehenbuhl, J. P. (1989). Binding and transepithelial transport of immunoglobulins by intestinal M cells: Demonstration using monoclonal IgA antibodies against enteric viral proteins. *J. Cell Biol* **108,** 1673–1685.

Wilson, J. M., Whitney, J. A., and Neutra, M. R. (1987). Identification of an endosomal antigen specific to absorptive cells of suckling rat ileum. *J. Cell Biol.* **105,** 691–703.

Winner, L. S., III, Mack, J., Weltzin R. A., Mekalanos, J. J., Kraehenbuhl, J. P., and Neutra, M. R. (1991). New model for analysis of mucosal immunity; Intestinal secretion of specific of specific monoclonal immunoglobulin A from hybridoma tumors protects against *Vibrio cholerae* infection. *Infect. Immun.* **59,** 977–982.

Wolf, J. L., Rubin, D. H., Finberg, R., Kauffman, R. S. Sharpe, A. H., Trier, J. S., and Fields, B. N. (1981). Intestinal M cells; A pathway for entry of reovirus into the host. *Science* **211,** 471–472.

Yewdell, J. W., and Bennink, J. R. (1990). The binary logic of antigen processing and presentation to T cells. *Cell* **62,** 203–206.

4

Mucosal Barrier

Ian R. Sanderson • W. Allan Walker

I. INTRODUCTION

The primary function of the small intestine is to absorb nutrients into the circulation (Field and Frizzell, 1991). During the course of this activity, the intestine is exposed to a wide variety of antigens derived from foods, resident bacteria and invading microorganisms. These antigens must be limited by a barrier that will allow absorption of nutrient molecules. In addition, the intestine transports macromolecules that are important in growth and development, for example, epidermal growth factor (EGF; Weaver and Walker, 1988; Weaver *et al.,* 1990; Carpenter and Wahl, 1991) and maternal IgG (Rodewald and Kraehenbuhl, 1984; Simister and Rees, 1985). Thus, any mechanism that acts as a barrier must also allow entry of physiologically important molecules the size of which is comparable to that of many antigens.

The lumen of the intestine is capable of harboring harmful microorganisms (Snyder, 1991); to mount an immune response against these potential pathogens, the mucosal immune system must survey antigens in the lumen. Evidence suggests that immunosurveillance by the small intestine depends on transport of antigens across the gut (Winner *et al.,* 1991). However, such transport must occur in a controlled manner to avoid harmful immune responses. Nevertheless, at times the control of antigen entry breaks down and this may lead to an excessive influx of antigens, which ultimately may cause disease (Sanderson and Walker, 1993).

1. Macromolecular Absorption

To maintain immunosurveillance, antigens are transported across the intestine in physiological amounts, but pathological transport may occur when the mucosal barrier is breached. This barrier consists of two main components (Figure 1). Extrinsic mechanisms will limit the amount of antigen reaching the surface of the intestine. The intrinsic barrier consists of the structural and functional properties of the intestine itself. Both clinical and experimental evidence suggests that antigens traverse the epithelium and enter the circulation (Warshaw and Walker, 1974; Paginelli *et al.,* 1979). For the most part, this transport is not harmful and may, at times, be beneficial.

Production of immunoglobulins directed against luminal antigens depends on immunologically intact antigen interacting with membrane-bound immunoglobulins on the surface of B cells that are located beyond the intestinal epithelium (Elson *et al.,* 1986; Kagnoff, 1989). Mechanisms that allow passage of antigen through the intestinal epithelium in controlled amounts are, therefore, an essential prelude to B-cell activation.

T-cell responses, on the other hand, are initiated by presentation of short peptides bound to major histocompatibility complexes (MHC; Unanue, 1984). Since luminal antigen can activate mucosal T cells (as occurs, for example, in celiac disease; Marsh, 1992), the intestine must process luminal antigen to peptides of the correct size to bind to MHC molecules and, in turn, interact with T-cell receptors. Antigens could be processed in two ways by the intestine: first, peptide fragments could be generated during epithelial transport; second, antigen could be processed from whole antigen that has traversed the epithelium and reached antigen-presenting cells in the mucosal immune system. In either case, uptake of antigen by the epithelium is essential. Moreover, the pathway by which the antigen or its product reaches the immune system of the gut may affect critically the type of immune reaction that ensues. Thus, an understanding of the mechanisms by which antigen is handled is central to the study of the mucosal immune response.

II. PHYSIOLOGIC TRANSPORT

Sampling of luminal antigen by the mucosa is likely to be a physiological phenomenon that will result in appropriate immune responses by the gut. These responses will include the local production of secretory IgA and mechanisms that lead to oral tolerance (Thompson and Staines, 1991). Such reactions are beneficial and are described in other chapters of this volume. At times, however, excessive antigen crosses the intestine, causing more widespread immune reactions. These reactions could result in gastrointestinal disease or even systemic illness (Sanderson and Walker, 1993).

Macromolecules cross intestinal epithelial cells in two ways of which we can be certain: they can be shuttled through absorptive cells on specific receptors, in which case only those macromolecules that bind to a receptor will pass, or they can pass through specialized epithelial cells called M cells (Chapter 2). An additional possibility is that antigenic fragments cross epithelial cells for presentation by MHC Class II molecules at the basolateral surface. Definitive evidence for this mode of uptake is still awaited, but this would constitute a third form of macromolecular transport.

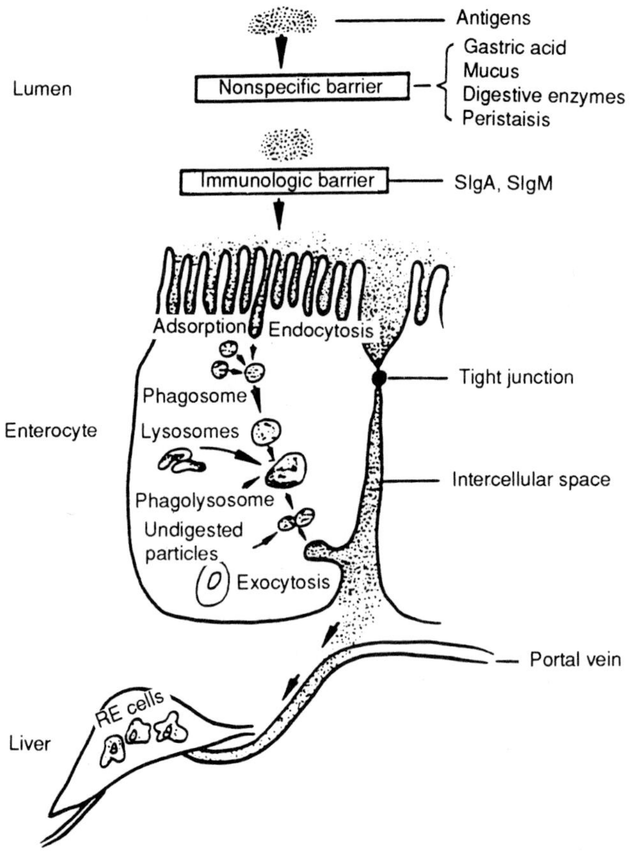

Figure 1 Barriers to macromolecular absorption. Antigen entry is prevented by nonspecific and immunologic mechanisms in the gastrointestinal tract as well as by the physical structure of the epithelium itself. [Reprinted with permission from Iyngkaran and Abidin (1981). Copyright © 1981 by Marcel Decker.]

1. Receptor Bound Transport

Most of the macromolecules that are required for transport can be made *de novo;* however, this is not always the case. For example, certain growth factors including EGF, transforming growth factor α (TGFα), and nerve growth factor (NGF) are all polypeptides that are transported across the intestine (Chu and Walker, 1991). IgG also can be transported across the intestine at times (Simister and Rees, 1985). The newborn makes very little immunoglobulin, so most circulating antibody is IgG derived passively from the mother. In humans, IgG is transferred primarily by the placenta during late gestation, whereas in many animals the transfer occurs from maternal milk through the proximal small intestine. The transfer of IgG across the gut is mediated by receptors that are similar to those present in human placenta (Sedmark *et al.,* 1991). These receptors bind the Fc portion of the immunoglobulin molecule.

Macromolecules are transferred by a mechanism that is altogether different from those that transport nutrients such as glucose and amino acids. Nutrient molecules enter the intestinal cell cytoplasm at the apical membrane and exit the basolateral membrane. Macromolecules, on the other hand, transverse the cell (Figure 2) in membrane-bound compartments that invaginate from the apical membrane. The first step in this process is attachment to receptors on the apical surface of enterocytes.

In young mice, maternal IgG absorption shows features characteristic of membrane-receptor transport: IgG is absorbed selectively (Jones and Waldmann, 1972; Guyer *et al.,* 1976) and its absorption shows saturation kinetics (Brambell, 1966). Binding is pH dependent, occurring at pH 6.5 but not at pH 7.4 (Rodewald, 1976). Since the contents of the upper jejunum are at low pH, the conditions are ideal for binding (Jones and Waldmann, 1972). Moreover, intracellular membrane and components are acidic, so binding wound be maintained after invagination of surface membrane and formation of vesicles (Abrahamson and Rodewald, 1981). The IgG receptor has been isolated, its gene has been cloned, and the nucleic acid sequence has been determined. From this sequence, the amino acid sequence has been deduced (Mostov and Simister, 1985). This receptor is a molecule homologous to MHC Class I molecules and is bound in its active form to β_2 macroglobulin. Despite the homology, the two molecules have very different functions and their assembly is different.

The machanisms involved in the transit of membrane-bound ligands to the basolateral pole of the enterocyte are still poorly understood. In electron microscopic studies, the apical membrane of absorptive cells can be seen invaginating to form endosomes (Figure 2). On the inner aspect of these developing membrane compartments appear to be regular arrays of clathrin (Shibata *et al.,* 1983; Gonnella and Neutra, 1984; Knutton *et al.,* 1974), a protein designed to form lattices around membrane vesicles. Clathrin has a central role in the

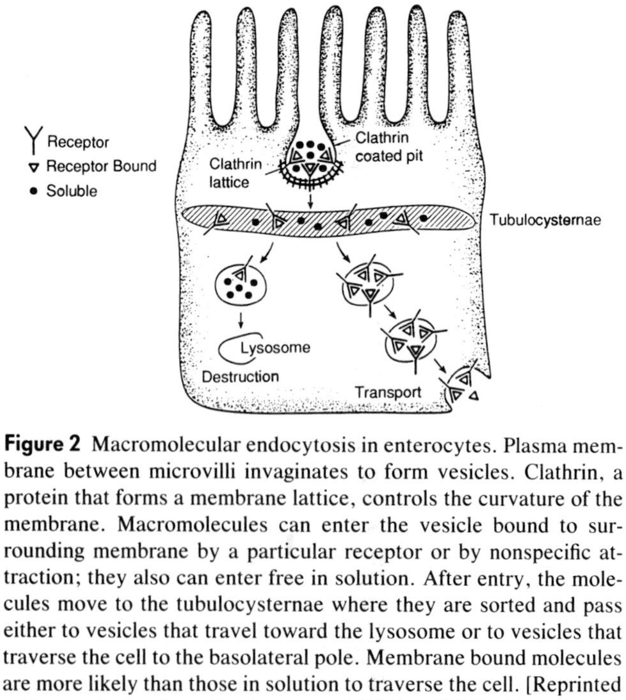

Figure 2 Macromolecular endocytosis in enterocytes. Plasma membrane between microvilli invaginates to form vesicles. Clathrin, a protein that forms a membrane lattice, controls the curvature of the membrane. Macromolecules can enter the vesicle bound to surrounding membrane by a particular receptor or by nonspecific attraction; they also can enter free in solution. After entry, the molecules move to the tubulocysternae where they are sorted and pass either to vesicles that travel toward the lysosome or to vesicles that traverse the cell to the basolateral pole. Membrane bound molecules are more likely than those in solution to traverse the cell. [Reprinted with permission from Sanderson and Walker (1993). Copyright © 1993 by American Gastroenterology Association.]

budding and fusion of membrane vesicles (Brodsky, 1984). In particular, clathrin assembly at the surface membrane of cells promotes the endocytosis of external receptors (Steinman *et al.*, 1983).

Transit further into the cell may occur by the movement of separated vesicles (Figure 2). Hopkins and colleagues (1990) have challenged this concept and favor a single transport compartment called the endosomal reticulum that extends from the cell surface. The shape and movement of these intracellular compartments will depend on the structural proteins that make up the cytoskeleton of the cell.

The Fc receptor is able to move across the epithelial cell. This transcytosis occurs in both directions. The receptor is carried with the membrane trafficking from lumen to serosa and returns by another membrane transport mechanism. Some membrane proteins contain specific amino acid sequences that direct the protein within the cell, for example, the polymeric IgA receptor (Casanova *et al.*, 1991) that transports IgA from the basolateral membrane to the apical membrane. However the amino acid sequences that determine the movement of the Fc receptor have not been elucidated.

Transfer of maternal IgG in the neonatal rodent falls markedly at weaning (after 21 days of age, a phenomenon known as closure). This event is now known to be caused by the decrease in the expression of the Fc receptor gene (Mostov and Simister, 1988). Thus, factors in breast milk may affect Fc receptor gene expression. The Fc receptor has been detected in humans in the placenta, and transfers maternal immunoglobulin *in utero* during the later stages of gestation. An observation by Israel and colleagues (1993) suggests that the Fc receptor may be present on small intestinal epithelium in the first trimester and may function early in the transfer of maternal IgG from amniotic fluid to the fetus.

2. Cells Specialized for Macromolecular Transport

Generation of secretory immune responses by the intestinal mucosa depends on transfer of antigens across the epithelium. Any loss of the molecular structure of the antibody recognition sites (the epitopes) during transport would render them unrecognizable by B cells. The passage of intact macromolecules across the gut is at variance with the role of the gut as a macromolecular barrier. For macromolecules to cross the gut in a controlled manner, specialized epithelial cells have evolved that overlie lymphoid follicles (Bockman and Cooper, 1973; Owen, 1977). These "M" cells, discussed in detail in Chapters 2 and 3, have features that facilitate controlled entry of antigens and larger particles through the intestinal epithelium.

3. Enterocytes as Antigen-Presenting Cells

Effective immune responses to antigenic proteins require the help of T lymphocytes. Stimulation of T cells, in turn, depends on exogenous antigen being presented by antigen-presenting cells (APCs; Unanue, 1984). The APC must internalize, digest, and link a small fragment of the antigen to a surface glycoprotein (the MHC Class II or HLA-D in humans) that interacts with a T-cell receptor. A number of cells of the immune system can act as APCs including B cells, macrophages, and dendritic cells. The ability of these cells to present antigen depends on the expression of MHC Class II molecules on their surface (Unanue, 1984). MHC Class II determinants are also present in epithelia of the normal small intestine, particularly on villous cells, in humans (Wiman *et al.*, 1978) and in rodents (Kirby and Parr, 1979). *In vitro* studies (Bland *et al.*, 1986; Mayer and Shlien, 1987; Kaiserlian *et al.*, 1989) have demonstrated that isolated enterocytes from rat and human small intestine can present antigens to appropriately primed T cells, raising the possibility that, in the intestine, MHC Class II molecules might present peptides from cellular membrane compartments to cells of the immune system that are localized below the epithelium. In support of this concept, MHC Class II molecules have been detected in adult rat jejunum villi in association with intracellular organelles (Mayrhofer and Spargo, 1990). Class II molecules were not detected in microvillus brush border or in vesicles at the base of microvilli. However, organelles below the terminal web and throughout the apical cytoplasm were stained specifically. Basolateral membranes clearly showed MHC Class II molecules. These molecules are, therefore, in an ideal position for binding with polypeptides that may have been taken up by and processed within the epithelial cell (Figure 3). Interestingly, the expression of MHC Class II molecules in the gastrointestinal epithelium is increased in a number of diseases. In Crohn's disease (Selby *et al.*, 1983; Mayer *et al.*, 1991), enhanced expression occurs on enterocytes from inflamed areas. Moreover, the effect of enterocytes from inflamed tissue is to stimulate helper T lymphocytes (Mayer and Eisenhardt 1990). Increased expression of MHC Class II molecules is also evident in the small intestine

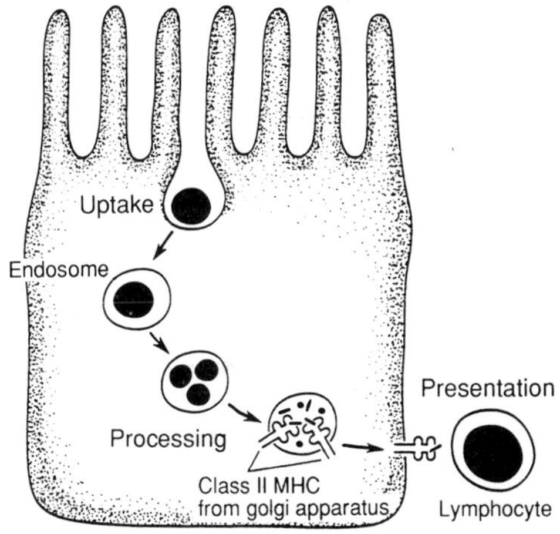

Figure 3 Model of antigen presentation by enterocyte. Macromolecules can enter membrane-bound organelle of the enterocyte. Instead of binding to the surrounding membrane or being destroyed in lysosomes, antigen is processed within the endosomal component into fragments that can bind to Class II MHC on the inner membrane of the components. Then antigens are presented on the basolateral surface of the cell. Prepared with the help of L. Mayer. [Reprinted with permission from Sanderson and Walker (1993). Copyright © 1993 by American Gastroenterology Association.]

in patients with autoimmune enteropathy (Hill *et al.*, 1991) and in graft-versus-host disease (Mason *et al.*, 1981). Certain gastrointestinal infections increase MHC Class II expression, for example, in the stomach infected with *Helicobacter pylori* (Engstrand *et al.*, 1989) and in the intestine infested with nematode parasites (Masson and Perdue, 1990). If MHC Class II molecules transport peptides derived from luminal macromolecules, these diseases will lead to an increase in the presentation of these peptides to the gastrointestinal immune systems, which may cause further inflammation and further presentation of luminal antigens, leading to a vicious cycle. Some drugs used to treat inflammatory bowel disease reduce Class II expression in epithelial cells. 5-Aminosalicylic acid (5-ASA), for example, reduces the MHC Class II expression that occurs in cultured cells that express MHC Class II in response to interferon γ (Crotty *et al.*, 1992)

III. BARRIERS PREVENTING PATHOLOGICAL TRANSPORT

Physiological passage of macromolecules is essential for the development of immune responses by the intestine, but uncontrolled penetration of antigens could initiate pathological processes that lead to gastrointestinal disease states. For antigen transport to be controlled, nonspecific entry into the circulation must be limited. This limitation is accomplished in two ways: first, by restricting the amount of antigen reaching the surface of the intestine (extrinsic barrier) and, second, by the physical characteristics of the intestine itself (intrinsic barrier) (Figure 1).

Many barrier mechanisms are not fully developed at birth. Evidence suggests that antigen transport in the neonatal period is less restricted that in adults. In animals, the changes in antigen absorption form the newborn to the adult are particularly evident, a phenomenon known as closure. Initially, the phenomenon was applied to the transport of immunoglobulins (Brambell, 1966), but significant changes in absorption have been documented for antigens that do not have specific transport receptors. Radiolabeled bovine serum albumin (BSA; Udall *et al.*, 1981a) was fed in physiological amounts to rabbits at birth and at 1 week, 2 weeks, 6 weeks, and 1 year of age and the plasma radioactivity measured. The study was designed to insure that the radioactivity measured corresponded to protein absorption. From 1 week of age, a marked fall in the transport of BSA across the intestine was detected. Moreover, in a later study (Udall *et al.*, 1981b) the development of the mucosal barrier was found to depend on the type of feeding during the neonatal period. Naturally fed (breast-fed) rabbits had lower plasma BSA levels that did formula-fed rabbits, suggesting that breast milk affects the development of the mucosal barrier. In this chapter, we review how different components of the barrier develop, particularly since a fall in antigen absorption has been demonstrated in humans also. Milk protein penetrates more readily in infants than in adults. In one study, α-lactalbumin absorption decreased with age in breast-fed babies (Axelson *et al.*, 1989). In a second study, formula-fed neonates had greater levels of β-lactoglobulin (BLG) than older infants (Roberton *et al.*, 1982).

A. Extrinsic Barrier

1. Proteolysis

Antigen access to the epithelium will be limited in many ways (Figure 1). Proteolysis will destroy the structure of antigens and thus destroy epitopes for immunological recognition. Altering the proteolytic capacity of the gastrointestinal tract affects macromolecular uptake. In everted gut sacs (Walker *et al.*, 1975) of rats who had previously undergone ligation of the pancreatic duct, transport of horse radish peroxidase (HRP) was greater that in sacs from sham-operated animals. Further, prior feeding with pancreatic extract decreased the uptake of HRP. The effects of digestion on macromolecular uptake have been confirmed elegantly by feeding rats aprotinin (a trypsin inhibitor) with lysine vasopressin (Saffron *et al.*, 1979). This peptide hormone, when fed orally, is absorbed through the intestine in sufficient quantities to have a noticeable effect on fluid retention. When given with aprotinin, however, the effects of vasopressin are more marked, implying that more has reached the surface of the intestine because of reduced proteolysis.

Experiments show that neutralizing gastric acidity (which reduces the activity of gastric enzymes) also increases antigen transport. Sodium bicarbonate given to rats orally with BSA increases BSA found in the gut (Walker *et al.*, 1975). These findings have important consequences because deficiencies of pancreatic enzymes occur in various diseases. In cystic fibrosis, in which pancreatic activity is affected severely, an increased incidence of cow milk allergy is seen, presumably because of increased antigen uptake. Also, gastric acidity (Hyman *et al.*, 1985) and pancreatic activity (Lebenthal and Lee, 1982) may be less in the newborn, which may have consequences for the development of the mucosal barrier.

2. Peristalsis

The time available for absorption will depend on the speed of luminal contents down the bowel. A common experience in clinical gastroenterology is that uptake of nutrients in patients with limited absorptive capacity (for example, in short bowel syndrome) is improved by reduced intestinal motility with agents such as loperamide (Remington *et al.*, 1983), providing good reason to believe that antigen absorption also will be limited by peristaltic action. An association between motility and antigen absorption has important implications. First, motility patterns change in development (Bisset *et al.*, 1988), which may contribute to alterations in antigen uptake with age. Second, gastrointestinal disease can affect the motility of the intestine (Mayer *et al.*, 1988) and may result in changes in antigen absorption, although such changes may be small relative to the effect that a disease has on the physical barrier created by the intestine itself. Nevertheless, antibody–antigen complex formation in the mucus coat, coupled with peristalsis, causes rapid expulsion of antigens from small intestine (Snyder and Walker, 1987).

3. Mucus Coat

a. Structure of mucus coat. The mucus coat lining the intestine is composed of a solution of glycoproteins (mucin) of molecular sizes ranging from one to several million Daltons. Intestinal mucin molecules are made up of carbohydrate side chains (70–80%) bound to a protein skeleton. This protein core has a high proportion of serine, threonine, and proline residues (Forstner, 1978; Allan, 1981); the carbohydrate moieties are attached to it by means of *N*-acetylgalactosamine. Five carbohydrates moieties (*N*-acetylgalactosamine, *N*-acetyglucosamine, fucose, galactose, and sialic acid) are arranged in side chains 2–22 sugars in length.

The exact composition of the molecules of mucin can vary greatly. Clear differences are seen among animal species. Even within localized regions of the intestinal tract, mucus molecules appear to be a heterogeneous group. At least six different mucin species have been identified after separation on DEAE–cellulose chromatography, both from rat and from human (Podolsky, 1985). Each species has distinct carbohydrate and amino acid composition. Marked changes in the composition of mucin occur with development. The mucin from the small intestine of newborn rats contains more protein than does adult rat mucin (Shub *et al.*, 1983). The carbohydrate content also changes as the animals grow. Not only does the total carbohydrate ratio increase with age, but the types of sugar moieties change also: newborn rat mucin has less fucose and *N*-acetylgalactosamine than does mucin from adult rats.

b. Function of mucus coat

i. Viscous coat. Mucus offers protection to the intestinal wall in a number of ways (Figure 4). First, it provides a mucus blanket. The physical characteristics of this blanket are determined by the chemical structure of the glycoprotein molecules themselves. The sticky quality of the mucus is an important mechanism for preventing penetration of organisms. The motility of *Entamoeba histolytica* traphozoites (Leitch *et al.*, 1985), for example, is decreased significantly by mucus. The increased viscosity that mucus provides to the luminal solution enhances the depth of the unstirred layer overlying the surface of the intestine, thus reducing the diffusion of molecules toward the intestinal surface (Strocchi and Levitt, 1991). The effect is most marked for lager molecules, and will limit absorption of antigens rather than nutrient molecules, which are smaller.

ii. Competitive binding. The carbohydrate moieties that constitute the majority of the structure of mucus are analogous to the glycoprotein and glycolipid receptors that exist on the enterocyte membrane (Gibbons, 1981). Therefore, they could act as competitors to the binding of proteins and microorganisms at the enterocyte surface. Many infectious agents adhere to epithelial cells through cell-surface appendages (fimbria, pili, and flagella; Freter, 1981) that have carbohydrate binding properties. Indeed, competition between salivary mucus glycoproteins and receptors on buccal epithelium already has been shown for binding of pathogenic streptococci (Williams and Gibbons, 1973). Further, the invasiveness of *Shigella flexneri* in primates, in part, may depend on the lack of barrier function of mucus (Denari *et al.*, 1986). Guinea pig colonic mucus inhibits invasion of HeLa cells by *Shigella,* whereas monkey colonic mucus (and, by implication, human mucus) does not.

iii. Mucin release. Release of mucus into the gastrointestinal tract will act as a barrier by generating a stream that draws luminal contents away from epithelial cells. Both nonspecific and immunological agents can initiate mucus release. The role of nonimmunological agents and their relationship to endogenous agents that alter mucus secretion are not well understood (Snyder and Walker, 1987). Cholinergic agents (Specian and Neutra, 1980) and mustard oil (Neutra *et al.*, 1982) cause goblet cell release, but a number of regulatory peptides (including histamine, serotonin, and α- and β-adrenergic agents; Neutra *et al.*, 1982) had no effect. Nevertheless, immunological phenomena cause goblet cells to release mucus (see subsequent discussion).

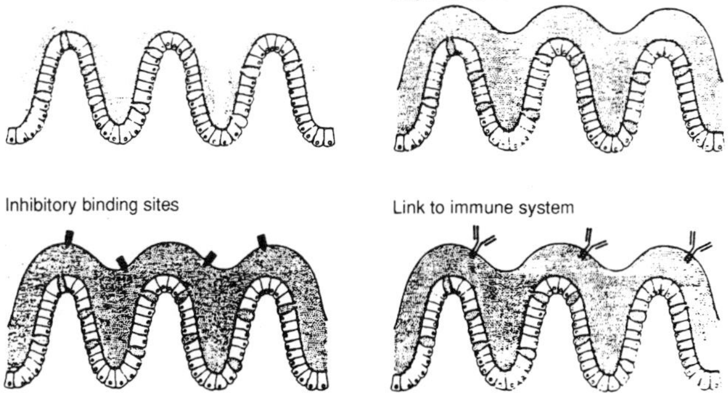

Figure 4 Four proposed mechanism for mucus protection: rate and quantity of mucus release, viscous blanket (physical barrier), competitive binding sites, and link to the intestinal immune system. [Reprinted with permission from Snyder and Walker (1981). Copyright © 1981 by Karger.]

4. Immunologic Barrier

The adequacy of immune function in the gastrointestinal tract affects the attachment and penetration of bacteria and toxins. This concept was illustrated elegantly (Winner *et al.*, 1991) by implantation of IgA-secreting hybridomas under the skin of infant mice who were then inoculated with cholera. IgA appeared in large amounts in the small intestine as secretory IgA. When hybridomas are implanted that secrete IgA that interacts with the antigen on the surface of *Vibrio cholerae,* mortality form cholera is reduced dramatically.

IgA is also likely to prevent the transfer of antigens across the gut. This hypothesis is supported by studies of patients with selective IgA deficiency. These patients have increased circulating immune complexes and precipitating antibodies to absorbed bovine milk proteins (Cunningham-Rundles *et al.*, 1978); peak concentrations occur between 1 an 2 hr after milk ingestion (Cunningham-Rundles *et al.*, 1979).

5. Combined Effects of Immunologic and Nonimmunologic Barriers

Both oral and parenteral immunization with specific antigens can reduce their uptake by the intestine (Walker *et al.*, 1972,1973). These observations may be a combined effect of immunological and nonimmunological components of the mucosal barrier. Proteolysis of intestinal antigens was considerably greater in immunized animal that in nonimmunized controls (Walker *et al.*, 1975). This enhanced proteolysis is likely to be the result of interaction of immune complexes in the mucus coat. This augmented protective process is illustrated in Figure 5.

Another example of combined protection is the increased discharge of goblet cell mucus occurring in intestinal anaphylaxis. Lake and colleagues (1980) have shown, using radiolabeled goblet cell mucus to quantitate release, that IgE-mediated mast cell discharge of histamine results in enhanced mucus release into the intestinal tract, which may explain why parasites eventually are expelled from the intestine in conjunction with mucus (Miller and Nawa, 1979). Figure 4 illustrates possible mechanisms of immune complex-mediated goblet cell mucus release on the intestinal surface.

B. Intrinsic Barrier

Once antigens have negotiated the many components of the extrinsic barrier mechanism, a considerable physical barrier to further penetration exists. This barrier is formed by the surface of the enterocytes and the tight junctions that are formed between the cells. However, this barrier is not impervious to the passage of antigens, as once was thought. The integrity of this barrier often is reduced in diseases of the gastrointestinal tract.

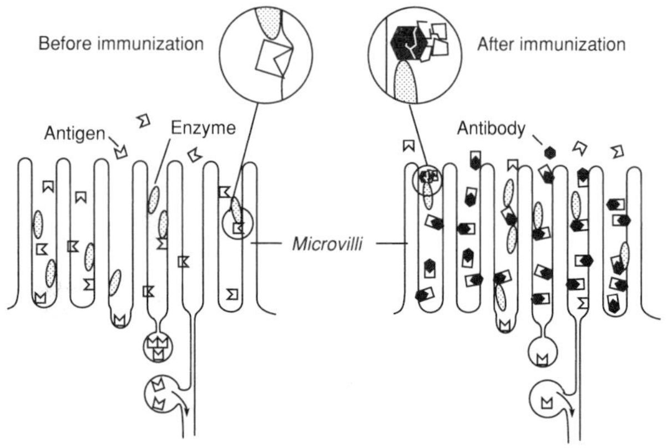

Figure 5 Schematic representation of the processing of protein antigen at the surface of the gut. Prior to immunization (*left*), a small portion of ingested protein escapes intraluminal digestion and is taken up by the enterocyte and transported to the intercellular spaces. After immunization (*right*), antibodies present on the gut surface interact with antigen to form complexes, thereby preventing or decreasing the binding of antigen to, and subsequent pinocytosis of antigen by, intestinal epithelial cells. Antigens complexed with antibodies in the mucus coat (glycocalyx) may be degraded by pancreatic enzymes absorbed to the gut surface. Consequently, less antigen is available to intestinal epithelial cells. [Reprinted with permission from Walker *et al.* (1975). Copyright © of the American Gastroenterology Association.]

1. Microvillous Structure

Microvilli could constitute a significant barrier because of their size and charge. In the intestinal epithelium of children (Phillips *et al.*, 1979) are 40 microvilli each of diameter 100 nm every 5 μm. Thus, if microvilli beat in unison, the distance between them is only 25 nm, which is the same order of magnitude as the dimensions of some macromolecules, for example, albumin at 3×13 nm. Microvilli also are negatively charged (they stain easily with ruthenium red; Jacobs, 1983); therefore a charged molecule may be inhibited significantly even if its diameter is less than 25 nm.

The site of invagination of apical plasma membrane has been demonstrated as being between microvilli (Shibata *et al.*,1983; Gonnella and Neutra, 1984; Knutton *et al.*, 1974). Thus, antigens likely must pass the microvillus "barrier" to enter the cell, a restriction that has direct relevance to disease processes, since any agent that strips off microvilli or affects their formation will alter the barrier function of the intestine. Microvillus structure is altered greatly by infections of cryptosporidia (Phillips *et al.*, 1992) or enteropathogenic *Escherichia coli* (Ulshen and Rollo, 1980).

Additional support for the concept of a microvillous barrier comes from morphological studies on M cells. The function of these cells is macromolecular transport. Unlike absorptive cells, they do not have well-developed microvilli. Since every morphological feature of these cells is in keeping with their function, microvilli are likely to constitute a significant barrier.

2. Enterocyte Surface Membrane

At the base of the microvilli, the surface of the enterocyte consists of plasma membrane. As in other cells, this membrane is composed of a lipid bilayer through which are situated membrane-bound proteins. This bilayer presents a considerable barrier to antigen transport because of its physical structure. In fact, that antigens can cross this lipid bilayer into the enterocyte cytosol is very unlikely. However, invagination of apical membranes occurs regularly, allowing macromolecules to be carried into the cell within membrane-bound compartments (Figure 2). Indeed, a large number of compartments exists beneath the apical surface of the enterocyte into which antigens can be transferred. Some of this activity is physiological and has been described in an earlier section; however, bystander molecules can be carried into the cell by this process, as was demonstrated clearly in electron micrographs that showed HRP inside membrane-bound compartments (Cornell *et al.*, 1971). Stern and Walker (1984) have shown that binding to the surface of the enterocyte is an important determinant of whether macromolecules are transported across the cell. For both BSA and BLG, absorption was nonsaturable and correlated with binding to the intestinal surface. Membrane-bound macromolecular transport can be distinguished from molecules moving freely in the lumen of compartments of the enterocyte (Gonnella and Neutra, 1984) in newborn rat ileum.

Binding to the surface of the cell depends on the structure of the antigen and the chemical composition of the microvillous membrane. Both these factors can vary. The structure of the antigen depends on the actual antigen itself. BSA binds less efficiently to the surface of the intestine than BLG and, consequently, is transported less readily (Stern and Walker, 1984). In addition, structural alterations in antigen caused by proteolysis also might affect its binding, since this activity will change the physicochemical characteristics of the molecule. For example, the gliadin fraction B3 (Stern *et al.*, 1988) binds less well to microvillous membrane protein than the pure gliadin peptide B3142.

The composition of the microvillous membrane has a marked effect on antigen binding. Plasma membrane consists of both lipids and proteins, and changes in either will affect binding to antigen. Partial digestion of microvillous membrane can alter binding to macromolecules (Stern and Gellerman, 1988). Damage to the protein in membranes is unlikely to occur in healthy individuals since the intestinal surface is protected by mucus. However, if the mucus layer is affected by, for example, resident bacteria, some digestion of the surface membrane might occur, leading to increased antigen binding and transport; such an occurrence, however, is probably rare. Changes in lipid composition, on the other hand, are encountered regularly because lipid composition changes with development. Differences in membrane composition can be detected by electron spin resonance (ESR). In this technique, the movements of the lipid-soluble probe can be followed by a spectrophotometer (Pang *et al.,* 1983). Movements of the probe in the membrane of the newborn rabbit were less confined than in membranes from adults, suggesting a more disorganized membrane structure. Indeed, chemical analysis of the membrane (Chu and Walker, 1988) demonstrated changes in the phospholipid headgroups with age, as well as alterations in protein–lipid ratios (Pang *et al.*, 1983). Changes in membrane fluidity noted by ESR were found to correlate with alterations in lectin binding (Pang *et al.*, 1985). These changes were noted to be under hormonal control, since alterations in the fluidity were affected by both cortisone and thyroxine (Israel *et al.,* 1987).

3. Intracellular Organelles and Enzymes

Antigens that enter enterocytes from the lumen are affected by a number of different factors that will influence transport to the basolateral surface. Of primary importance is the rate of vesicular passage to the basolateral membrane, which will depend on the rate of endocytosis, the proportion of vesicles being directed toward the lysosome, and the speed of travel of membrane-bound compartments. The rate of breakdown of products held in membrane compartments is determined by lysosomally derived enzymes that include proteases, such as cathepsin B and D, and enzymes that catalyze carbohydrate breakdown, such as acid phosphatase and mannosidase. The degree to which the organellar contents encounter such enzymes determines the rate of intracellular destruction of macromolecules. This encounter can be in the lysosome or in endocytic vesicles (Dinsdale and Healy, 1982). We know that such enzymes are present in intestinal epithelial cells at levels of activity that can influence macromolecular transport. In the rat (Davies and Messer, 1984), cathepsin B and D activity can be found throughout the length of intestine, particularly in the mid and distal thirds. Interestingly, this activity peaks in the second week of age and then falls progressively. The ontogeny of macromolecular transport (Udall *et al.*, 1981a) in no way reflects this pattern, emphasizing the importance of *interaction* between membrane-bound compartment flow and enzyme activity. This interaction is seen more clearly in the piglet, in which intestinal cathepsin B and D levels do not change with age (Ekstrom and Westrom, 1991) but closure can be demonstrated clearly in the second day of life.

Although cathepsins are capable of destroying macromolecular biological activity, they may not digest the protein molecule completely so the final steps in digestion of peptides may be by peptidases (Vaeth and Henning, 1982) in the cytoplasm.

4. Junctions between Cells

The physical barrier that prevents penetration of antigen across the intestinal epithelium consists of two main components: the epithelial cells (the transcellular route) and the spaces between cells (the paracellular route). The pathophysiology of this latter pathway has been reviewed (Powell, 1981; Gumbiner, 1987; Madara, 1989b,1990). The pathway consists of the tight junctions (or zonulae occludentes) and the subjunctional space.

The subjunctional space dose not act as a significant barrier since molecules as large as HRP can diffuse freely between the serosa and this space. However, the tight junctions offer a substantial barrier to diffusion of large molecules, although they are permeable to water and small ions (Frizzell and Schultz, 1972). Claude and Goodenough (1973) demonstrated a correlation between the structure of the tight junction as seen in freeze fracture preparations and passive electrical permeability in a number of epithelial preparations. The preparations, when viewed under the electron microscope, show a network resembling anastomosing strands. The composition of these strands is unknown, but they are likely to be proteins of high tensile strength. In tight epithelia (such as gall bladder), many such strands are seen, whereas in more permeable epithelia (such as mammalian proximal small intestine), few are found. The relationship between strand density and epithelial resistance has been confirmed in intestinal epithelial cells (Madara and Dharmsathaphorn, 1985), T84 cells, grow as confluent monolayers in culture. In the first 10 days after passage, the junctions become increasingly tight, as judged by transepithelial resistance. This resistance was found to correlate with the number of strands formed between cells.

The barrier formed by tight junctions is preserved even when epithelial cells themselves are extruded at the villous tip. The band from the tight junction moves away from the apex down the lateral aspect of the cell as the cell is extruded (Madara, 1990b). Eventually, younger cells beneath the extruding cell form tight junctions at the very moment that the old cell is lost. Thus, the preservation of the tight junction network is a function with importance that overrides that of epithelial cell viability.

The tight junction is a dynamic structure with resistance that varies with events taking place in the epithelium and intestinal lumen. Changes in paracellular absorption occur during active transport of nutrients by epithelial cells, particularly in relation to smaller molecules. Pappenheimer and colleagues (Madara and Pappenheimer, 1987; Pappenheimer, 1987; Pappenheimer and Reiss, 1987) have calculated that the rate of uptake of molecules smaller than 5500 Daltons from the lumen was proportional to the rate of fluid absorption—a concept known as solvent drag. The application of an alternating current across isolated intestine, with and without mucosa, gave an estimate of the impedance of the intestinal mucosa. The impedance falls with the stimulation of sodium-coupled solute transport across the enterocyte. Therefore, sodium-coupled solute transport may trigger contraction of cytoskeletal elements of the enterocyte, which in turn pulls open tight junctions. These predictions have been confirmed by electron microscopy (Madara and Pappenheimer, 1987). Sodium-dependent transport of solutes such as glucose and amino acids induces expansion of intercellular spaces associated with condensation of microfilaments of the actinomycin ring associated the tight junction. Although these observations have enormous importance for the physiology of absorption of nutrients, their impact on our understanding of macromolecular transport has yet to be fully assessed. The calculated pore radius of the open tight junction (5 nm) is similar to that of small macromolecules; sodium-assisted glucose transport will, in fact, allow the passage of polypeptides 11 amino acids long (MP-1; Atisook and Madara, 1991) but larger immunogenic proteins may not pass through this route under physiological conditions. HRP, for example, does not pass the tight junction (Atisook and Madara, 1991) even when these junctions have been rendered permeable to MP-1.

However, pathological insults to the intestine may open these pores sufficiently to allow passage of antigens. The macromolecular permeability of the gut in disease models needs to be reexamined using Pappenheimer's methodology. Macromolecular markers of different sizes, charges, and hydrophilicity all have been used independently *in vivo* in animals and humans, but the physical characteristics of these molecules have not been used to predict pore size in disease. An important model of increased permeability caused by intestinal inflammation is the effect of mast cell dependent reactions in the rat intestine following *Nippostrongylus brasiliensis* infection. Increased amounts of BSA can be detected immunologically in the circulation after infection with the organism, following mild systemic anaphylaxis (Bloch *et al.*, 1979). Similarly, transfer of ^{51}Cr-labeled EDTA and ovalbumin is enhanced (Ramage *et al.*, 1988). Estimating the physical characteristics of the paracellular pathway during inflammation should be possible.

The permeability of the tight junction can be examined *in vitro*, enabling workers to study the effects of epithelial events that are seen *in vivo*. Monolayers of epithelial cells (T84) have effective tight junctions that produce a resistance of $\sim$1500 Ω cm^2. Application of interferon γ (Madara and Stofford, 1989) reduces the resistance and allows easier permeation of large sugars. Interferon γ levels are increased in the mucosa of patients with Crohn's disease because of T-cell activation. Bowel inflammation is characterized by the transepithelial passage of polymorphonuclear neutrophils (PMNs). This phenomenon has been reproduced *in vitro* by placing chemotactic agents and PMNs on different sides of the monolayer (Nash *et al.*, 1987). The passage of neutrophils opens tight junctions, reducing the resistance of the monolayer resistance and allowing transfer of large sugars.

VI. CONCLUSIONS

The mucosal barrier, like the skin, defines the boundary between an animal and its environment. Unlike the skin, the mucosae of the gut and respiratory tract must absorb substances that are essential for life. To be selective, the intestinal mucosa has developed a complex network containing elements that are extrinsic to the intestine itself and those defined by intestinal structure. The challenges for the future lie in defining the role of these barriers in the establishment of gastrointestinal disease. Examining whether cellular elements in the mucosal immune system can recognize antigens without their needing to penetrate the intestinal epithelium will also be interesting. The observations that members of the immunoglobulin superfamily are found on the surface of the epithelium and that lymphocytes can pass into the intestinal lumen make this a tantalizing possibility.

References

Abrahamson, D. R., and Rodewald, R. (1981). Evidence for the sorting of endocytic vesicle contents during the receptor-mediated transport of IgG across the newborn rat intestine. *J. Cell Biol.* **91,** 271–280.

Allan, A. (1981). Structure and function of gastrointestinal mucus. *In* "Physiology of the Gastrointestinal Tract," Vol. 7, pp. 617–639. (L. R. Johnson, ed.) Raven Press, New York.

Atisook, K., and Madara, J. L. (1991). An oligopeptide permeates intestinal tight junctions at glucose-elicited dilatations. Implications for oligopeptide absorption. *Gastroenterology* **100,** 719–724.

Axelsson, I., Jakobsson, I., Lindberg, T., Poleberger, S., Benediktsson, B., and Raiha N. (1989). Macromolecular absorption in preterm and term infants. *Acta Paediatr. Scand.* **78,** 532–537.

Bisset W. M., Watt J. B., Rivers R. P., and Milla P. J. (1988). Ontogeny of fasting small intestinal motor activity in the human infant. *Gut* **29,** 483–488.

Bland, P. W., and Warren, L. G. (1986). Antigen presentation by epithelial cells of the rat small intestine. I. Kinetics, antigen specificity and blocking by anti-Ia antisera. *Immunology* **58,** 1–8.

Bloch, K. J., Bloch, D. B., Stern, M., and Walker, W. A. (1979). Intestinal uptake of macromolecules. VI. Uptake of protein antigen in vivo in normal rats and rats infected with *Nippostrongylus brasiliensis* or subjected to mild systemic anaphylaxis. *Gastroenterology* **77,** 1038–1044.

Bockman, D. E., and Cooper, M. D. (1973). Pinocytosis by epithelium associated with lymphoid follicles in the bursa of Fabricus, appendix, and Peyer's patches. An electron microscopic study. *Am. J. Anat.* **136,** 455–478.

Brambell, F., W. (1966). The transmission of immunity from mother to young and the catabolism of immunoglobulins. *Lancet* **2,** 1087–1093.

Brodsky, F. M. (1984). Living with clathrin: Its role in intracellular membrane traffic. *Science* **242,** 1396–1402.

Carpenter, G., and Wahl, M. I. (1991). The epidermal growth factor family. *In* "Peptide Growth Factors and Their Receptors" (M. B. Sporn and A. B. Roberts, eds.), Vol. I, pp. 69–171. Springer-Verlag, New York.

Casanova, J. E., Apodaca, G., and Mostov, K. E. (1991). An autonomous signal for basolateral sorting in the cytoplasmic domain of the polymeric immunoglobulin receptor. *Cell* **66,** 65–75.

Chu S. H., and Walker W. A. (1988). Development of the gastrointestinal mucosal barrier: Changes in phospholipid head groups and fatty acid composition of intestinal microvillus membranes form newborn and adult rats. *Pediatr. Res.* **23,** 439–442.

Chu, S. W., and Walker, W. A. (1991). Growth factor signal transduction in human intestinal cells. *Adv. Exp. Med. Biol.* **310,** 107–112.

Claude, P., and Goodenough, D. A. (1973). Fracture faces of zonulae occludentes from "tight" and "leaky" epithelia. *J. Cell Biol.* **58,** 390–440.

Cornell, R., Walker, W. A., and Isselbacher, K. J. (1971). Small intestinal absorption of horseradish peroxidase. A cytochemical study. *Lab. Invest.* **25,** 42–48.

Crotty, B., Hoang, P., Dalton, H. R., and Jewell, D. P. (1992). Salicylates used in inflammatory bowel disease and colchicine impair interferon-γ induced HLA-DR expression. *Gut* **33,** 59–64.

Cunningham-Rundles, C., Brandeis, W. E., Good, R. A., and Day, N. K. (1978). Milk precipitin circulating immune complexes and IgA deficiency. *Proc. Natl. Acad. Sci. U.S.A.* **75,** 3387–3389.

Cunningham-Rundles, C., Brandeis, W. E., Good, R. A., and Day, N. K. (1979). Bovine antigens and the formation and the circulating immune complexes in selective immunoglobulin A deficiency. *J. Clin. Invest.* **64,** 272–279.

Davies, P. H., and Messer, M. (1984). Intestinal cathepsin B and D activities of suckling rats. *Biol. Neonate* **45,** 197–202.

Denari, G., Hale, T. L., and Washington, O. (1986). Effect of guinea pig or monkey colonic mucus on *Shigella* aggregation and invasion of HeLa cells by *Shigella flexneri* 1b and 2a. *Infect. Immun.* **51,** 975–978.

Dinsdale. D., and Healy, P. J. (1982). Enzymes involved in protein transmission by the intestine of the newborn lamb. *Histochem. J.* **14,** 811–821.

Ekstrom, G. M., and Westrom, B. R. (1991). Cathespin B and D activities in intestinal mucosa during postnatal development in pigs. Relation to intestinal uptake and transmission of macromolecules. *Biol. Neonate* **59,** 314–321.

Elson, C. O., Kagnoff, M. F., Fiocchi, C., Befus, A. D., and Targan, S. (1986). Intestinal immunity and inflammation: Recent progress. *Gastroenterology* **91,** 746–768.

Engstrand, L., Scheynius, A., Pahlson, C., Grimelius, L., Schwan, A., and Gustavsson, S. (1989). Association of *Campylobacter pylori* with induced expression of class II transplantation antigen on gastric epithelial cells. *Infect. Immun.* **57,** 827–832.

Field, M., and Frizzel, R. A. (1991) Intestinal absorption and secretion. *In* "The Gastrointestinal System" (S. G. Schultz, ed.), Vol. IV. American Physiology Society, Bethesda, Maryland.

Forstner, J. (1978). Intestinal mucins in health and disease. *Digestion* **17,** 234–263.

Freter, R. (1981). Mechanisms of association of bacteria with mucosal surfaces. *Ciba. Found. Symp.* **80,** 36–55.

Frizzell, R. A., and Schultz, S. G. (1972). Ionic conductance of extracellular shunt pathway in rabbit ileum. *J. Gen. Physiol.* **59,** 318–346.

Gibbons, R. A. (1981). Mucus of the mammalian genital tract. *Br. Med. Bull.* **34,** 34–38.

Gonnella, P. A., and Neutra, M. R. (1984). Membrane-bound and fluid-phase macromolecules enter separate prelysosomal compartments in absorptive cells of suckling rat ileum. *J. Cell Biol.* **99,** 909–917.

Gumbiner, B. (1987). The structure, biochemistry, and assembly of epithelial TJs. *Am. J. Physiol.* **253,** C749–C758.

Guyer, R. L., Koshland, M. E., and Knopf, P. M. (1976). Immunoglobulin binding by mouse intestinal epithelial cell receptors. *J. Immunol.* **117,** 587–593.

Hill S. M., Milla P. J., Bottazzo G. F., and Mirakian R. (1991). Autoimmune enteropathy and colitis: Is there a generalized autoimmune gut disorder? *Gut* **32** 36–42.

Hopkins, C. R., Gibson, A., Shipman, M., and Miller, K. (1990). Movement of internalized ligand-receptor complexes along a continuous endosomal reticulum. *Nature (London)* **346,** 335–339.

Hyman, P. E., Clarke, D. D., Everett, S. L., Sonne, B., Stweard, D., Harada, T., Walsh, J. H., and Taylor, I. L. (1985). Gastric acid secretory function in preterm infants. *J. Pediatr.* **106,** 467–471.

Israel, E. J., Pang, K. Y., Harmatz, P. R., and Walker, W. A. (1987). Structural and functional maturation of rat gastrointestinal barrier with thyroxine. *Am. J. Physiol.* **252,** 762–767.

Israel, E. J., Simister N., Freiberg E., Caplan A., and Walker W. A. (1993). Immunoglobulin G binding sites on the human fetal intestine: A possible alternate for the passive transfer of immunity from mother to infant. *Immunology* **79,** 77–81.

Iyngkaran, N., and Abidin, Z. (1981). Intolerance to food proteins. In "Pediatric Nutrition" (Lifshitz, F. ed.). p. 453. Marcel Decker, New York.

Jacobs, L. R. (1983). Biochemical and ultrastructural characterization of the molecular topography of the rat intestinal microvillous membrane. Asymmetric distribution of hydrophilic groups and anionic binding sites. *Gastroenterology* **85,** 46–54.

Jones, E. A., and Waldmann, T. A. (1972). The mechanism of intestinal uptake and transcellular transport of IgG in the newborn rat. *J. Clin. Invest.* **51,** 2916–2927.

Kagnoff, M. F. (1989). General characteristics and development of the immune system. *In* "Immunology and Disease of the Gastrointestinal Tract" (M. H. Sleisenger and J. S. Fordtran, eds.), 4th Ed., pp. 114–143. Saunders, Philadelphia.

Kaiserlian, D., Vidal, K., and Revillard, J-P. (1989). Murine enterocytes can present soluble antigen to a specific class II-restricted $CD4^+$ T cells. *Eur. J. Immunol.* **19,** 1513–1516.

Kirby, W. N., and Parr, E. L. (1979). The occurrence and distribution of H-2 antigens on mouse intestinal epithelial cells. *J. Histochem. Cytochem.* **27,** 746–750.

Knutton, S., Limbrick, A. R., and Robertson, J. D. (1974). Regular structures in membranes: Membranes in the endocytic complex of ileal epithelial cells. *J. Cell Biol.* **62,** 679–694.

Lake, A. M., Bloch, K. J., Sinclair, K. J., and Walker, W. A. (1980). Anaphylactic release of intestinal goblet cell mucus. *Immunology* **39,** 173–178.

Lebenthal, E., and Lee, P. C. (1982). Alternate pathways of digestion and absorption in early infancy. *J. Pediatr. Gastroneterol. Nutr.* **3,** 1–3.

Leitch, G. J., Dickey, A. D., Udezuler, I. A., and Bailey, G. B. (1985). *Entamoeba histolytica* trophozoites in the lumen and mucus blanket of rat colons studied *in vivo*. *Infect. Immun.* **47,** 68–73.

Madara, J. L. (1990a). Maintenance of the macromolecular barrier at cell extrusion sites in intestinal epithelium: Physiological rearrangement of tight junction. *J. Membrane Biol.* **116,** 177–184.

Madara, J. L. (1990b). Pathobiology of the intestinal epithelial barrier. *Am. J. Pathol.* **137,** 1273–1281.

Madara, J. L. (1989). Loosening TJs. Lessons from the intestine. *J. Clin. Invest.* **83,** 1089–1094.

Madara, J. L., and Dharmsathaphorn, K. (1985). Occluding junction structure–function relationships in a cultured epithelial monolayer. *J. Cell Biol.* **101,** 2124–2133.

Madara, J. L., and Pappenheimer, J. R. (1987). Structural basis for physiological regulation of paracellular pathways in intestinal epithelial. *J. Membrane Biol.* **100,** 149–164.

Madara, J. L., and Stafford, J. (1989). Interferon-γ directly affects barrier function of cultured intestinal epithelial monolayers. *J. Clin. Invest.* **83,** 724–727.

Marsh, M. N. (1992). Gluten, major histocompatibility complex, and the small intestine. A molecular and immunobiologic approach to the spectrum of gluten sensitivity (celiac sprue). *Gastroenterology* **102,** 330–354.

Mason, D. W., Dallman, M., and Barclay, A. N. (1981). Graft-versus-host disease induces expression of Ia antigen in rat epidermal cells and gut epithelium. *Nature (London)* **293,** 150–151.

Masson, S. D., and Perdue, M. H. (1990). Changes in distribution of Ia antigen on epithelium of the jejunum and ileum in rats infected with *Nippostrongylus brasiliensis*. *Clin. Immunol. Immunopathol.* **57,** 83–95.

Mayer, E. A., Raybould, H., and Koelbel, C. (1988). Neuropeptides, inflammation, and motility. *Dig. Dis. Sci.* **33,** 71S–77S.

Mayer, L., and Eisenhardt, D. (1990). Lack of induction of suppressor T cells by intestinal epithelial cells from patients with inflammatory bowel disease. *J. Clin. Invest.* **86,** 1255–1260.

Mayer, L., and Shlien, R. (1987). Evidence for function of Ia molecules on gut epithelial cells in man. *J. Exp. Med.* **166,** 1471–1483.

Mayer, L., Eisenhardt, D., Salomon, P., Bauer, W., Plous, R., and Piccinini, L. (1991). Expression of class II molecules on intestinal epithelial cells in humans. Differences between normal and inflammatory bowel disease. *Gastroenterology* **100,** 3–12.

Mayrhofer, G., and Spargo, L. D. J. (1990). Distribution of class II major histocompatibility antigens in enterocytes of the rat jejunum and their association with organelles of the endocytic pathway. *Immunology* **70,** 11–19.

Miller, H. R. P., and Nawa, Y. (1979). Immune regulation of intestinal goblet cell differentiation. *Nouv. Rev. Fr. Hematol.* **21,** 31–45.

Mostov, K. E., and Simister, N. E. (1988). Transcytosis. *Cell* **42,** 389–390.

Nash, S., Stafford, J., and Madara, J. L. (1987). Effects of polymorphonuclear leukocyte transmigration of the barrier function of cultured intestinal epithelial monolayers. *J. Clin. Invest.* **80,** 1104–1113.

Neutra, M. R., O'Malley, L. J., and Specian, R. D. (1982). Regulation of intestinal goblet cell secretion. II. A survey of potential secretagogue. *Am. J. Physiol.* **242,** G380–G387.

Owen, R. L. (1977). Sequential uptake of horseradish peroxidase by lymphoid follicle epithelium of Peyer's patches in the normal unobstructed mouse intestine: An ultrastructural study. *Gastroenterology* **72,** 440–451.

Paganelli, R., Levinsky, R. J., Brostoff, J., and Wraith, D. G. (1979). Immune complexes containing food proteins in normal and atopic subjects after oral challenge and effect of sodium cromoglycate on antigen absorption. *Lancet* **1,** 1270–1272.

Pang, K. Y., Bresson, J. L., and Walker, W. A. (1983). Development of the gastrointestinal mucosal barrier: Evidence for structural differences in microvillus membranes from newborn and adult rabbits. *Biochim. Biophys. Acta* **727,** 201–208.

Pang, K. Y., Newman, A. P., Udall, J. N., and Walker, W. A. (1985). Development of the gastrointestinal mucosal barrier. VI. *In utero* maturation of the microvillus surface by cortisone. *Am. J. Physiol.* **249,** G85–G91.

Pappenheimer, J. R. (1987). Physiological regulation of transepithelial impedance in the intestinal mucosal of rat and hamster. *J. Membrane Biol.* **100,** 137–148.

Pappenheimer, J. R., and Reiss, K. Z. (1987). Contribution of solvent drag through intercellular junctions to absorption of nutrient by the small intestine of the rat. *J. Membrane Biol.* **100,** 123–136.

Phillips, A. D., France, N. E., and Walker-Smith, J. A. (1979). The structure of the enterocyte in relation to its position on the villus in childhood: An electron microscopical study. *Histopathology* **3,** 117–130.

Phillips, A. D., Thomas, A. G., and Walker-Smith, J. A. (1992). Cryptosporidium, chronic diarrhoea and the proximal small intestinal mucosa. *Gut* **33,** 1057–1061.

Podolsky, D. K. (1985). Oligosaccharide structure of isolated human colonic mucin species. *J. Biol. Chem.* **260,** 15510–15515.

Powell, D. (1981). Barrier function of epithelial cells. *Am. J. Physiol.* **231,** G272–G288.

Ramage, J. K., Stanisz, A., Scicchitano, R., Hunt, R. H., and Perdue, M. H. (1988). Effect of immunologic reactions on rat intestinal epithelium. Correlation of increased permeability to chromium 51-labeled ethylenediaminetetraacetic acid and ovalbumin during acute inflammation and anaphylaxis. *Gastroenterology* **94,** 1368–1375.

Remington, M., Malagelada, J. R., Zinsmeiste, A., and Fleming, C. R. (1983). Abnormalities in gastrointestinal motor activity in patients with short bowels: Effect of a synthetic opiate. *Gastroenterology* **85,** 629–636.

Roberton D. M., Paganelli, R., Dinwiddie, R., and Levinsky, R. J. (1982). Milk antigen absorption in the preterm and term neonate. *Arch. Dis. Child* **57,** 369–372.

Rodewald, R. (1976). pH-Independent binding of immunoglobulins to intestinal cells of the neonatal rat. *J. Cell Biol.* **71,** 666–669.

Rodewald, R., and Kraehenbuhl, J. P. (1984). Receptor-mediated transport of IgG. *J. Cell Biol.* **99,** 159s–164s.

Saffron, M., Franco-Saenz, R., Kong, A., Pepthadjopoulos, D., and Szoka, F. (1979). A model for the study of oral administration of peptide hormones. *Can. J. Biochem.* **57,** 548–553.

Sanderson, I. R., and Walker, W. A. (1993). Uptake and transport of macromolecules by the intestine: possible role in clinical disorders (an update). *Gastroenterol* **104,** 622–639.

Sedmark, D. D., Davis, D. H., Singh, U., and van de Winkel, J. G. (1991). Expression of IgG Fc receptor antigens in placenta and on endothelial cells in humans. An immunohistochemical study. *Am. J. Pathol.* **138,** 175–181.

Selby, W. S., Janossy, G., Maso, D. Y., and Jewell, D. P. (1983). Expression of HLA-DR antigens by colonic epithelium in inflammatory bowel disease. *Clin. Exp. Immunol.* **53,** 614–618.

Shibata, Y., Arima, T., and Yamamoto, T. (1983). Regular structures on the microvillar surface membrane of ileal cells in suckling at intestine. *J. Ultrastruct. Res.* **85,** 70–81.

Shub, M. D., Pang, K. Y., Swann, D. A., and Walker, W. A. (1983). Age-related changes in chemical composition and physical properties of mucus glycoproteins from rat small intestine. *Biochem. J.* **215,** 405–411.

Simister, N. E, and Rees, A. R. (1985). Isolation and characterization of an Fc receptor from neonatal rat small intestine. *Eur. J. Immunol.* **15,** 733–738.

Snyder, J. D. (1991). Bacterial infections. *In* "Pediatric Gastrointestinal Disease: Pathophysiology, Diagnosis, Management" (W. A. Walker, P. R. Durie, J. R. Hamilton, J. A. Walker-Smith, J. B. Watkins, eds.). pp. 527–537. BC Decker, Philadelphia.

Snyder, J. D., and Walker, W. A. (1987). Structure and function of intestinal mucin: Developmental aspects. *Int. Arch. Allergy Appl. Immunol.* **82,** 351–356.

Specian, R. D., and Neutra, M. R. (1980). Mechanism of rapid mucus secretin in goblet cells stimulated by acetylcholine. *J. Cell Biol.* **85,** 626–640.

Steinman, R. M., Mellman, I. S., Mueller, W. A., and Cohn, Z. A. (1983). Endocytosis and the recycling of plasma membrane. *J. Cell Biol.* **96,** 1–27.

Stern, M., and Gellermann, B., (1988). Food proteins and maturation of small intestinal microvillus membranes (MVM). I. Binding characteristics of cow's milk proteins and concanavalin A to MVM from newborn and adult rats. *J. Pediatr. Gastroenterol. Nutr.* **7,** 115–121.

Stern, M., and Walker, W. A. (1984). Food proteins and the gut mucosal barrier. I. Binding and uptake of cow's milk proteins by rat jejunum in vivo. *Am. J. Physiol.* **246,** G556–G562.

Stern, M., Gellermann, B., Belitz, H. D., and Wieser, H. (1988) Food proteins and maturation of small intestinal microvillus membranes (MVM). II. Binding of gliadin hydrolysate fractions and of the gliadin peptide B3142. *J. Pediatr. Gastroenterol. Nutr.* **7,** 122–127.

Strocchi, A., and Levitt, M. D. (1991). A reappraisal of the magnitude and implications of the intestinal unstirred layer. *Gastroenterology* **101,** 843–847.

Thompson, H. S. G., and Staines, N. A. (1991). Could specific oral tolerance by a therapy for autoimmune disease? *Immunol. Today* **11,** 396–399.

Udall, J. N., Pang, K., Fritze, L., Kleinman, R., and Walker, W. A. (1981a). Development of gastrointestinal mucosal barrier. I. The effect of age on intestinal permeability to macromolecules. *Pediatr. Res.* **15,** 241–244.

Udall, J. N., Colony, P., Fritze, L., Pang, K., Trier, J. S., and Walker, W. A. (1981b). Development of gastrointestinal mucosal barrier. II. The effect of natural versus artificial feeding on intestinal permeability to macromolecules. *Pediatr. Res.* **15,** 245–249.

Ulshen, M. H., and Rollo, J. L. (1980). Pathogenesis of escherichia coli gastroenteritis in man—another mechanism. *N. Engl. J. Med.* **302,** 99–101.

Unanue, E. R. (1984). Antigen presenting function of the macrophage. *Ann. Rev. Immunol.* **2,** 395–428.

Vaeth, G. F., and Henning, S. J. (1982). Postnatal development of peptidase enzymes in rat small intestine. *J. Pediatr. Gastroenterol. Nutr.* **1,** 111–117.

Walker, W. A., and Isselbacher, K. J. (1974). Uptake and transport of macromolecules by the intestine. *Gastroenterology* **67,** 531–550.

Walker, W. A., Isselbacher, K. J., and Bloch, K. J. (1972). Intestinal uptake of macromolecules: Effect of oral immunization. *Science* **177,** 608–610.

Walker, W. A., Isselbacher, K. J., and Bloch, K. J. (1973). Intestinal uptake of macromolecules. II. Effect of parenteral immunization. *J. Immunol.* **111,** 221–226.

Walker, W. A., Wu, M., Isselbacher, J. K., and Bloch, K. J. (1975). Intestinal uptake of macromolecules IV. The effect of duct ligation on the breakdown of antigen and antigen–antibody complexes on the intestinal surface. *Gastroenterology* **69,** 1123–1229.

Warshaw, A. L., and Walker, W. A. (1974). Intestinal absorption of intake antigenic protein. *Surgery* **76,** 495–499.

Weaver, L. T., and Walker, W. A. (1988). Epidermal growth factor and the developing human gut. *Gastroenterology* **94,** 845–847.

Weaver, L. T., Gonnella, P. A., Israel, E. J., and Walker, W. A. (1990). Uptake and transport of epidermal growth factor by the small intestinal epithelium of the fetal rat. *Gastroenterology* **98,** 828–837.

Williams, R. C., and Gibbons, R. J. (1975). Inhibition of streptococcal attachment of receptors on human buccal epithelial cells by antigenically similar salivary glycoproteins. *Infect. Immun.* **11,** 711–715.

Wiman, K., Curman, B., Forsum, U., Klareskog, L., Malmnas-Tjernlund, U., Rask, L., Tragardhl, L., and Peterson, P. A. (1978). Occurrence of Ia antigen on tissue of non-lymphoid origin. *Nature (London)* **276,** 711–713.

Winner, L. S., Mack, J., Weltzin, R. A., Mekalanos, J. J., Kraehenbuhl, J. P., and Neutra, M. R. (1991). New model for analysis of mucosal immunity: Intestinal secretion of specific monoclonal immunoglobulin A from hybridoma tumors protects agains *Vibrio cholerae* infection. *Infect. Immun.* **59,** 977–982.

5

Innate Humoral Factors

Kenneth M. Pruitt • Firoz Rahemtulla • Britta Månsson-Rahemtulla

I. INTRODUCTION

We define the innate humoral factors as those proteins that are secreted onto mucosal surfaces by exocrine glands and are able to carry out their protective functions independent of the presence of specific antibodies. The innate humoral factors are important components of mucosal defense mechanisms. Two families of proteins that function as innate humoral factors—the acidic proline-rich proteins (PRP) and the histidine-rich proteins (HRP)—have not been included in this chapter because of space limitations. The PRPs and HRPs are present in high concentrations in mucosal secretions and participate in a variety of defensive mechanisms. These proteins have been the subject of several reviews (PRP, Hay and Moreno, 1989; HRP, Oppenheim, 1989).

II. LACTOFERRIN

Lactoferrin (Lf) is found in the exocrine secretions, blood, and leukocytes of many species and has been the subject of numerous investigations. Mammalian Lfs show structural homologies and may have common antigenic determinants (Magnuson *et al.,* 1990). Lfs from different species have similar properties (Shimazaki *et al.,* 1991). A comprehensive review of the vast Lf literature is beyond the scope of this chapter. Here we focus on selected aspects of the biochemistry and biology of human Lf. Human Lf is an 80-kDa glycoprotein composed of a single polypeptide chain of 691 residues. The three-dimensional structure of this molecule has been determined from X-ray crystallographic analyses (Baker *et al.,* 1991). The complete cDNA nucleotide sequence has been reported (Powell and Ogden, 1990; Rey *et al.,* 1990) and the amino acid sequence has been determined (Metz-Boutique *et al.,* 1984; Anderson *et al.,* 1989). The amino acid sequence deduced from cDNA (Rey *et al.,* 1990) was 98% identical to the reported sequence (Anderson *et al.,* 1989). Lf binds Fe^{3+} reversibly but with great affinity ($K_B \sim 10^{20}$), but has much less affinity for Fe^{2+} ($K_B \sim 10^3$). The molecule has an absolute requirement of binding one HCO_3^- with each Fe^{3+}

Apolactoferrin (apo-Lf) and diferric Lf (both Fe^{3+} sites occupied) have different three-dimensional structures (Baker *et al.,* 1991). In the diferric form, the molecule is folded into two globular lobes, the N lobe and the C lobe, representing the N-terminal and C-terminal halves with similar three-dimensional structures. Each lobe contains one Fe^{3+} and one HCO_3^- binding site located in a deep cleft between two dissimilar domains. Thus, the molecule has a two-lobe four-domain structure. Each lobe has one site of carbohydrate attachment. Although little is known about the structure of the carbohydrate components, one report (Kawasaki *et al.,* 1992) provided evidence that the terminal sialic acid residues in these components are important structural determinants for the Lf inhibition of the binding of cholera toxin to Chinese hamster ovary cells. The two lobes are connected by a three-turn α helix. In apo-Lf, the N-lobe binding cleft is open wide whereas the C-lobe binding cleft is closed although no Fe^{3+} is bound. The molecule is quite flexible, and extensive folding is associated with the binding of Fe^{3+}. Deferric Lf has increased conformational stability and increased resistance to unfolding compared with apo-Lf (Harrington, 1992).

An isoform of Lf, hmRNase with high ribonuclease activity against retroviral-like RNAs, has been identified in human milk (Furmanski *et al.,* 1989). Lf and hmRNase comigrate on SDS–PAGE with calculated sizes of 80 kDa, stained similarly with periodic acid–Schiff reagent, had the same pI (8.7) as determined by isoelectric focusing, yielded identical peptide patterns after treatment with trypsin or papain, and had identical NH-terminal amino acid sequences (determined up to 8 residues). Monospecific rabbit antihuman Lf reacted identically with Lf and with hmRNase. In spite of these striking similarities, Lf has no RNase activity and hmRNase does not bind iron. The biological origins of these isoforms of Lf are unknown. Another example of structurally similar and functionally distinct milk proteins, found in bovine, goat, sheep, and human milk in comparable quantities, is the lactoperoxidase enzyme and a nonheme lactoperoxidase that is enzymatically inactive (Allen and Morrison, 1963; Dumontet and Rousset, 1983). These two lactoperoxidase isoforms have the same apparent molecular weight, similar amounts of carbohydrate, similar peptide maps after subtilisin or trypsin treatment, and lines of identity in immunodiffusion experiments. The origin and biological significance of these isoforms of lactoperoxidase are unknown as well.

The iron-binding properties of Lf generally have been assumed to be the basis for its biological functions. The low frequency of iron deficiency anemia in breast-fed infants has been attributed to the transport of iron to the intestinal mucosa of the infant in a readily available Lf-bound form. A human Lf receptor has been isolated from human fetal intestinal brush border membranes (Kawakami and Lönnerdal, 1991). The receptor specifically bound human Lf and showed little affinity for bovine Lf or for human transferrin. However, the data supporting the role of milk Lf in the bioavailability of iron are conflicting (Hurley and Lönnerdal, 1988). Studies of human infants (Roberts *et al.*, 1992) have failed to establish a unique role for Lf in modulating the development of infant fecal flora. Reports (reviewed by Djeha and Brock, 1992) of the effects of Lf on human T-lymphocyte proliferation are complex and conflicting. An interesting hypothesis is that the release of Lf by degranulation of neutrophils may preserve T-cell function at inflammatory sites.

In contrast to the *in vivo* studies reviewed earlier, the *in vitro* antimicrobial properties of Lf have been confirmed by numerous reports. Lf kills or inhibits the growth of many species of microorganisms. The studies summarized in Table I show that, in general, dose-dependent killing or inhibition of microorganisms is caused by apo-Lf but not by iron-saturated Lf. The specific kinetics and quantitative aspects of the dose response depend on the species of microorganism. Human and bovine Lf have similar properties. Both proteins bind to the surface of microorganisms in the apo- and iron-saturated forms. Binding may or may not be correlated with the biological effects, depending on the species of microorganism. Susceptibility of microorganisms to Lf depends on pH, growth phase, temperature, composition of the reaction medium, and methods used to determine viability. Sublethally injured cells of *Escherichia coli* apparently are able to repair damage caused by Lf when the cells are cultured on blood agar, but not when they are enumerated by the pour plate method (Rainard, 1987). Biological effects may be blocked by citrate, by iron salts, and by Ca^{2+} and Mg^{2+}. Many of the observed biological effects are consistent with the hypothesis that Lf acts by interfering with microbial iron metabolism. However, Lf binding to microbial membranes produces other effects as well, including damage to the outer membrane of gram-negative bacteria resulting in subsequent release of lipopolysaccharides (LPS), increased cell permeability (Ellison *et al.*, 1988), and increased susceptibility to hydrophobic antibiotics (Ellison *et al.*, 1990).

Many bacteria are resistant to Lf. Under conditions that inhibit the growth of *E. coli,* six isolates of *Streptococcus agalactiae* and five isolates of *Streptococcus uberis* were unaffected (Rainard, 1986). Some strains of *E. coli, Salmonella wien,* and *Staphylococcus aureus* are resistant to Lf inhibition (Dalmastri *et al.*, 1988). This resistance may be correlated with the production of enterochelins or aerobactins. Clinical isolates of *E. coli* that do not bind Lf are not inhibited by Lf (Visca *et al.*, 1990). Virulence and Lf resistance may be correlated (Arnold *et al.*, 1980).

The antibacterial properties of Lf are enhanced in the presence of other components of mucosal secretions. Suzuki *et al.* (1989) reported that the growth of *E. coli* strain 011 was inhibited moderately in the presence of egg white lysozyme alone and by bovine apo-Lf alone. No inhibition was observed in the presence of iron-saturated Lf. The combination of lysozyme with either apo-Lf or iron-saturated Lf significantly magnified the growth inhibition. However, these authors also reported that the bacteria were agglutinated by the lysozyme and iron-saturated Lf mixture. Since these authors measured growth spectrophotometrically, the observed growth "inhibition" could have been a result of a reduction in absorbance as a consequence of agglutination. Ellison and Giehl (1991) found that human lysozyme and human Lf alone were bacteriostatic for strains of *Vibrio cholerae, Salmonella typhimurium,* and *E. coli.* However, in combination, lysozyme and Lf were bactericidal for these bacteria. These authors measured the antibacterial effects by serial dilution and plating of aliquots from the reaction mixtures. Therefore, agglutination could have contributed to the observed reduction in the cfu/ml. However, transmission electron microscopic observations showed that *E. coli* cells exposed to the combination of lysozyme and Lf were enlarged and hypodense. Large amounts of cell debris were also present. The latter observations suggest that killing was a consequence of osmotically induced swelling and lysis. This possibility was confirmed by the observation that the effects of lysozyme and Lf could be partially or totally blocked by increasing the media osmolarity. The bastericidal effects were dose dependent, blocked by iron saturation of Lf, and inhibited by high concentrations of calcium. These authors also presented evidence that Lf does not chelate calcium. They concluded that Lf interacts with the outer membrane of these gram-negative bacteria, causing LPS release and increasing membrane permeability. This increase in permeability increases the access of lysozyme to the bacterial cell wall and accounts for the synergistic killing of lysozyme and Lf mixtures.

Increased killing of gram-positive microorganisms by mixtures of Lf and lysozyme also has been reported (Soukka *et al.*, 1991a). Human apo-Lf and human lysozyme alone gave a dose-dependent reduction in viable counts of a strain of *Staphylococcus mutans.* No reduction was observed with iron-saturated Lf. Mixtures of apo-Lf and lysozyme showed an additive but not synergistic reduction in viable counts. The contribution of aggregation to the reduction in viable counts was minimized by subjecting mixtures to vortexing and ultrasonic treatment before plating. The killing of *S. mutans* by Lf and lysozyme was not as dramatic as that reported for gram-negative bacteria. An additive effect of the lactoperoxidase system on apo-Lf killing of *S. mutans* has been reported (Soukka *et al.*, 1991b). These authors also reported that the lactoperoxidase system alone had a bactericidal effect on this bacterium at pH 5.5. Esaguy *et al.* (1991) reported that the 65-kDa heat-shock protein produced by *Mycobacterium leprae* and by *Mycobacterium tuberculosis* is recognized specifically by polyclonal antibodies directed against human Lf, suggesting that these Lf-mimicking bacterial proteins may be responsible for the autoimmune reactions observed in individuals suffering from leprosy and tuberculosis.

The hypothesis that Fe^{2+} and apo-Lf can generate hydroxyl radicals ($OH^{\bullet}$) via an H_2O_2 intermediate and that this reaction may contribute to the microbicidal activity of phagocytes is controversial (reviewed by Klebanoff and Waltersdorph, 1990). These authors have described a series of experiments that show that the system is more complex than generally is realized and that the results of experiments intended to generate $OH^{\bullet}$ are critically dependent on experi-

Table I Effects of Lactoferrin on Microorganisms[a]

Microorganism	Test medium	Biological effects	Comments	Reference
Actinobacillus actinomycetemcomitans	Simple broth	Bactericidal	Dose-dependent killing by Apo-HLf; Sat-HLf no effect	Kalmar and Arnold (1988)
Aeromonas hydrophila, 28 isolates from clinical specimens and foods	Phosphate-buffered saline	Not reported	Both HLf and BLf bound; specific binding proteins in a representative strain seemed to be cell porins	Kishore *et al.* (1991)
Bacillus stearothermophilus, *Bacillus subtilis*	Nutrient agar and broth	Growth inhibited	BLf inhibition reversible; suppressed by addition of Fe^{2+}	Oram and Reiter (1968)
Candida albicans	Saline	Fungicidal	Dose-dependent killing by Apo-HLf; Sat-HLf no effect	Arnold *et al.* (1980)
	0.05 m*M* KCl	Fungicidal	Dose-dependent killing by Apo-HLf; killing blocked by physiological concentrations of phosphate and bicarbonate; Sat-HLf no effect	Soukka *et al.* (1992)
Coliforms associated with mastitis (*Klebsiella pneumoniae*, *Klebsidla* spp., *Aerobacter aerogenes*, *Escherichia coli*)	Synthetic medium	Dose-dependent growth inhibition of all coliforms by apo-BLf	No growth inhibition by Sat-BLf or when Fe^{3+} or citrate was added to Apo-BLf; Apo-BLf (20 mg/ml) killed *E. coli*	Bishop *et al.* (1976)
Haemophilus influenzae	Growth medium	Bactericidal	HLf bound to cells in presence and absence of Fe	Dalmastri *et al.* (1988)
Klebsiella pneumoniae	Growth medium	Bacteriostatic	HLf bound to cells in presence and absence of Fe	Dalmastri *et al.* (1988)
Escherichia coli	Bovine milk	Bacteriostatic	BLf inhibited growth; effect blocked by citrate, enhanced by bicarboante	Reiter and Brock (1975); Reiter *et al.* (1975)
enteropathogen	Growth medium	No effect	Apo-HLf and Sat-HLf bound to cells	Arnold *et al.* (1977)
nonenteropathogen	Saline	Bactericidal	Weak dose-dependent killing by Apo-HLf; sat-HLf no effect	Arnold *et al.* (1980)
enteropathogen	Human milk	Bacteriostatic	Growth slowed for 10 hr, but resumed after 24 hr; effect abolished by addition of iron or enterobactin	Brock *et al.* (1983)
several strains differing in iron-transport systems	Growth medium	Bacteriostatic	Antimicrobial effects of Zn-Lf > Apo-Lf; strains with only enterochelin Fe transport more sensitive; strains with only aerobactin or both Fe transport sytems overcame inhibition by Zn-Lf	Valenti *et al.* (1985)

(continues)

Table I *(continued)*

Microorganism	Test medium	Biological effects	Comments	Reference
mastitic (bovine); 35 isolates	Growth medium	Bacteriostatic	All ioslates inhibited by Apo-BLf	Rainard (1986)
serum-resistant strain	Bovine milk—normal, mastitic	Basteriostatic	Apo-BLf but not Sat-BLf inhibited growth when added to ultrafiltrate from mastic milk; no inhibition when Apo-BLf added to ultrafiltrate from normal milk	Rainard (1987)
strain 803	Growth medium	Bacteriostatic	Lf bound to cells in presence and absence of Fe	Dalmastri *et al.* (1988)
UDP-galactose epimerase-deficient strain	Growth medium	Bacteriostatic	Apo-HLf but not Sat-HLf caused release of LPS from outer membrane; LPS release inhibited by Mg^{2+}, Ca^{2+}	Ellison *et al.* (1988, 1990)
K-12, four strains; clinical isolates, five strains	Minimal medium	Bacteriostatic for K-12 strains; no effect on clinical isolates	Apo-HLf and Sat-HLf bind to K-12 strains but not to clinical isolates	Visca *et al.* (1990)
Legionella pneumophila	Growth medium, human milk	Bactericidal	Dose-dependent killing by Apo-HLf in growth medium but not by Sat-HLf; human milk bactericidal, but effect blocked by addition of iron	Bortner *et al.* (1986)
	Water	Bactericidal	Susceptibility dependent on growth phase, pH; killing blocked by Ca^{2+}, Mg^{2+}; Apo-HLf, Sat-HLf both bind to cells; binding independent of killing	Bortner *et al.* (1989)
	Growth medium	Intracellular growth in monocytes inhibited	Apo-HLf completely inhibited intracellular multiplication in nonactivated monocytes; Sat-HLf had no effect	Byrd and Horwitz (1991)
Mycobacterium leprae, *Mycobacterium tuberculosis*	Western blotting (cell extracts), electron microscopy (intact cells, cell fragments)	Polyclonal antibodies against HLf, bind to cell surfaces and cytoplasmic components	Major component in both species binding HLf antibodies is 65-kDa heat-shock protein; may contribute to autoimmune disease in leprosy and tuberculosis	Esaguy *et al.* (1991)
Neisseria catharralis	Growth medium	Bacteriostatic	HLf bound to cells in presence and absence of Fe	Dalmastri *et al.* (1988)
Neisseria gonorrhoeae—40 clinical (human) isolates	Broth	Not reported	All clinical isolates expressed detectable levels of HLf receptors; no correlation between HLf receptor expression and disease state	Lee and Bryan (1989)
Neisseria gonorrhoeae FA19	Defined medium	No inhibition	Bacteria utilized iron bound to HLf; required energy and cell contact	McKenna *et al.* (1988)
Porphyromonas gingivalis, *Prevotella intermedia*,	Phosphate-buffered saline	Not reported	HLf bound to varying extents: *P. intermedia* > *P. gingivalis* > *P.*	Kalfas *et al.* (1991)

Prevotella melaninogenica: human isolates (116 strains) from diseased periodontal pockets			*melaninogenica;* specific binding to *P. intermedia*, nonspecific binding to *P. gingivalis*, *P. melaninogenica;* binding capacity affected by culture medium; binding components affected by heat, proteases	
Pseudomonas aeruginosa	Agar gel	Bacteriostatic	Apo-HLf (4%) added to agar well inhibited growth; effect abolished by addition of Fe^{2+}	Masson and Heremans (1966)
	Saline	Bactericidal	Dose-dependent killing by Apo-HLf; Sat-HLf no effect	Arnold *et al.* (1980)
clinical isolate	Growth medium	Bactericidal	HLf bound to cells in presence and absence of Fe	Dalmastri *et al.* (1988)
Salmonella wien 1 (clinical isolate)	Growth medium	Bacteriostatic	HLf bound to cells in presence and absence of Fe	Dalmastri *et al.* (1988)
Salmonella typhmurium SL696, SH4247	Growth medium	Bacteriostatic	Apo-HLf but not Sat-HLf caused release of LPS from outer membrane; LPS release blocked by Mg^{2+}, Ca^{2+}	Ellison *et al.* (1988) Ellison *et al.* (1990)
Shigella flexneri, Shigella sonnei	Growth medium	Bacteriostatic/bactericidal	HLf bound to cells in presence and absence of Fe	Dalmastri *et al.* (1988)
Staphylococcus albus	Nutrient agar gel	Bacteriostatic	HLf (0.5%) added to paper discs inhibited growth; effect abolished by addition of Fe^{2+}	Masson *et al.* (1966)
Streptococcus mitior	Saline	Bactericidal	Dose-dependent killing by Apo-HLf; Sat-HLf no effect	Arnold *et al.* (1980)
Streptococcus mutans	Growth medium	Bactericidal	Dose-dependent suppression of growth by Apo-HLf; Sat-Lf no effect; Apo-HLf binds to cells	Arnold *et al.* (1977)
five serotypes	Saline	Bactericidal	Dose-dependent killing by Apo-HLf; Sat-HLf no effect	Arnold *et al.* (1980)
	Water, glycine buffer, phosphate, HEPES buffer	Bactericidal, reversible inhibition	Growth phase-dependent sensitivity to HLf; killing in water, glycine buffer, but not phosphate or HEPES buffers;	Arnold *et al.* (1981)
	Water	Bactericidal	HLf bactericidal effects not limited to iron-deprivation	Arnold *et al.* (1982)
clinical isolate	Growth medium	Bactericidal	HLf bound to cells in presence and absence of Fe	Dalmastri *et al.* (1988)
strain 6715-13	Growth medium	Bacteriostatic	Bacteriostasis reversed by saturation of HLf with iron	Visa *et al.* (1989)
Streptococcus pneumoniae	Saline	Bactericidal	Dose-dependent killing by Apo-HLf; Sat-HLf no effect	Arnold *et al.* (1980)
Streptococcus salivarius	Saline	Bactericidal	Dose-dependent killing by Apo-HLf; Sat-HLf no effect	Arnold *et al.* (1980)

(*continues*)

Table I *(continued)*

Microorganism	Test medium	Biological effects	Comments	Reference
Staphylococcus aureus	Agar gel	Bacteriostatic	Solution of 4% Apo-HLf in agar well inhibited growth; effect abolished by addition of Fe^{2+}	Masson and Hereman (1966)
mastitic (bovine) bacteria, 10 isolates	Growth medium	Bacteriostatic	6 isolates inhibited, 4 unaffected by Apo-Lf	Rainard (1986)
mastitic (bovine) isolates: *Staphylococcus epidermidis, warneri, hominis, xylosus, hyicus,* and *chromogenes*	Phosphate-buffered saline	Not reported	Specific binding of BLf to all strains; affinity constants varied: $1–12 \times 10^6$ liter/mol; BLf binding sites 1900–4700/cell	Naidu *et al* (1990)
human clinical isolates (489 strains)	Phosphate-buffered saline	Not reported	HLF binds to 85% of isolates; binding correlated with clinical condition; binding optimal with organisms grown in agar, but abolished by strains grown on carbohydrate and salt-rich agar	Naidu *et al.* (1991)
Vibrio cholerae	Growth medium	Bactericidal	Dose-dependent suppression of growth by Apo-HLf; Sat-HLf no effect; Apo-HLf binds to cells	Arnold *et al.* (1977)
	Saline	Bactericidal	Dose-dependent killing by Apo-HLf; Sat-HLf no effect	Arnold *et al.* (1980)

[a] Abbreviations used: Apo-BLf, iron free bovine lactoferrin; Apo-HLf, iron free human lactoferrin; BLf, bovine lactoferrin; HEPES, *N*-2-hydroxyethylpiperazine-*N*′-2-ethanesulfonic acid; HLf, human lactoferrin; Sat-BLf, iron-saturated BLf; Sat-HLf, iron-saturated HLf.

mental conditions. Klebanoff and Waltersdorph reported that incubation of Fe^{2+} with apo-Lf resulted in the formation of oxidants that were toxic to *E. coli*. They obtained evidence for the formation of H_2O_2 and $OH^{\bullet}$. However, precise experimental conditions were required to obtain these results. The microorganisms must be in the early log phase of growth and the following experimental conditions must be met: pH 4.5–5.5, $[Fe^{2+}] \sim 10\ \mu M$, and $[\text{apo-Lf}] \sim 0.3\ \mu M$. These investigators explained their results in terms of the following mechanism:

$$2\,Fe^{2+} + \text{apo-Lf} + 2\,O_2 \rightarrow (Fe^{3+})_2 - \text{Lf} + 2\,O_2^{\bullet -} \quad (1)$$
$$2\,O_2^{\bullet -} + 2\,H^+ \rightarrow O_2 + H_2O_2 \quad (2)$$
$$H_2O_2 + Fe^{2+} \rightarrow Fe^{3+}OH^- + OH^{\bullet} \quad (3)$$

These authors found that the autooxidation of Fe^{2+} (reaction 1) was accelerated greatly by apo-Lf at the pH they used (5.0). Formation of $OH^{\bullet}$ was measured by electron paramagnetic resonance detection of the signal from the formation of the complex between the spin-trap DMPO (5,5-dimethyl-1-pyrrolidone-*N*-oxide) and the $OH^{\bullet}$ radical. Evidence for formation of H_2O_2 was inhibition of the generation of the DMPO–$OH^{\bullet}$ complex and of reduction of toxicity by the addition of catalase. The strict experimental conditions required for generation of $OH^{\bullet}$ and for the observation of toxicity imply that $OH^{\bullet}$ production by Lf may be restricted *in vivo*. The sensitivity of the reactions to experimental conditions may explain why some authors find that Lf enhances $OH^{\bullet}$ production (Ambruso and Johnston, 1981) whereas others report that it does not (Baldwin *et al.*, 1984). Britigan and Edeker (1991) reported that apo-Lf inhibits $OH^{\bullet}$ formation by the hypoxanthine/xanthine oxidase/$O_2^{\bullet}$/H_2O_2 system. However, diferric transferrin and, to a much lesser extent, diferric Lf, when treated by *Pseudomonas* elastase, induce $OH^{\bullet}$ radical formation by this system. Thus, at sites of *Pseudomonas aeruginosa* infection, alteration of transferrin and Lf by bacterial enzymes may contribute to tissue injury by increasing the local potential for $OH^{\bullet}$ formation. Nakamura (1990) presented evidence that the Fe^{3+} bound to diferric Lf may be reduced to Fe^{2+} by the NADPH–cytochrome P450 reductase system in the presence of superoxide dismutase, resulting in formation of $OH^{\bullet}$ through reaction of H_2O_2 with Lf Fe^{2+}. Britigan *et al.* (1991) reported that, when human monocytes were incubated with apo-Lf, cell-associated apo-Lf increased in proportion to apo-Lf concentration in the incubation medium. These investigators estimated 3.4×10^7 Lf binding sites per monocyte. Similar results were obtained with diferric Lf. These researchers stimulated $OH^{\bullet}$ formation by exposing the cells to phorbol myristic acetate (PMA) in the presence of ferric nitrilotriacetic acid. The generation of $OH^{\bullet}$ by apo-Lf-loaded monocytes was reduced by 50% compared with controls. Under these conditions, auto-oxidation of cell membranes was reduced 28% in the apo-Lf-loaded cells compared with controls. These authors suggested that Lf may protect tissue *in vivo* from phagocyte-associated $OH^{\bullet}$ generation. The various studies reviewed in this section show that apo-Lf and diferric Lf may contribute to or inhibit the formation of $OH^{\bullet}$, depending on specific reaction conditions. The chemistry of these reactions is complex and speculations relating the results of *in vitro* experiments to conditions existing *in vivo* must be considered carefully.

Several studies have been undertaken to determine directly the possible *in vivo* significance of the antimicrobial properties of Lf. Human Lf was administered to 5 human patients receiving chemotherapy for acute myelogenous leukemia (Trumpler *et al.*, 1989). The Lf did not delay the onset of enterogenic infection significantly but reduced its duration and severity. Compared with 9 matched untreated controls, Lf-treated patients had a lower incidence of bacteremia. In animal studies, calves experimentally infected with *E. coli* were treated with a preparation containing the lactoperoxidase system and Lf (Still *et al.*, 1990). Mortality and occurrence and duration of diarrhea were significantly lower in the treated animals than in infected but untreated controls. The latter study did not distinguish between the effects of the lactoperoxidase system and those of Lf. In another study (Zagulski *et al.*, 1989), the survival of mice injected with a lethal dose of *E. coli* was improved significantly when either human or bovine Lf was administered intravenously 24 hr before challenge. Different results were obtained by Czirók *et al.* (1990). These authors confirmed the *in vitro* antibacterial effects of Lf against various strains of *E. coli, S. typhimurium*, and *P. aeruginosa*. However, when mice were injected with these same organisms and injected also with Lf using different routes of injection and different time schedules, the results did not establish a consistent pattern for the ability of Lf to protect mice from the lethal effects of injected microorganisms. The latter was a complex study. Some of its conclusions did not seem to be supported clearly by the data presented.

The *in vivo* significance of the many observations of the *in vitro* antimicrobial effects of Lf has yet to be firmly established by direct observation. A comprehensive understanding of the *in vivo* significance of Lf must await the outcome of future studies. However, the evidence reviewed here suggests that the biological activity of Lf must be considered within the context of the concomitant actions of other components of mucosal secretions.

III. LYSOZYME

Human milk lysozyme appears to be identical to the forms of lysozyme found in other body fluids such as urine and pancreatic juice (Canfield *et al.*, 1971; Jollès and Jollès, 1971; Wang and Kloer, 1985). The concentration of lysozyme in human milk is higher than it is in the milk of most other species. In human milk, lysozyme concentrations are 3000 times higher than in cow milk (Parry *et al.*, 1968). Concentrations vary during lactation. The mean concentration of human lysozyme during the first few days of lactation is approximately 80 μg/ml, falls to 20–25 μg/ml at 1 month, and rises to 245 μg/ml after 6 months of lactation (Goldman *et al.*, 1982,1983).

Human lysozyme consists of a single polypeptide chain, composed of 129 amino acids, with a molecular mass of 14,600 Da and a pI of 10.5. This protein is cross-linked by four disulfide bridges that give stability to the compact, roughly ellipsoidal structure (for review, see Jolles and Jolles, 1984). Lysozyme isolated from different species and different organs of the same individual shows the same type of biological activity. However, these enzymes differ in their chemical properties (Jolles and Jolles, 1984) and specific activity (Balkejian *et al.*, 1969). Human salivary lysozyme originates from the salivary glands and oral leukocytes present in the gingival crevices (Petit and Jollès, 1963; Senn *et al.*, 1970; Raeste, 1972; Korsrud and Brandtzaeg, 1982). The salivary concentration of lysozyme ranges from 2 to 80 μg/ml. Because of its higher specific activity, human lysozyme is considered a more potent antibacterial factor for oral microorganisms than hen egg white lysozyme (Iacono *et al.*, 1980,1982). Human lysozyme exerts its antibacterial effects by hydrolyzing the peptidoglycans of the bacterial cell wall (muramidase activity) by cleaving the β(1-4) glycosidic bond between *N*-acetylmuramic acid and *N*-acetyl-D-glucosamine (Chipman and Sharon, 1969), by activating bacterial autolysins (Laible and Germaine, 1985), by aggregating bacteria (Pollock *et al.*, 1976) resulting in inhibition of bacterial adherence (Iacono *et al.*, 1980), and by inhibiting acid production by oral streptococci (Twetman *et al.*, 1986; Lumikari and Tenovuo, 1991). Originally, the antibacterial effects of lysozyme were ascribed only to the lytic activity. However, several studies (Laible and Germaine, 1985; Wang and Germaine, 1991) reported that bactericidal and autolytic activities that are independent of the enzymatic activity, as well as the cationic property (pI ~ 10.5) of the molecule, are essential for the bactericidal characteristic of the protein. Although oral streptococci are not lysed directly by lysozyme, the cell walls are damaged by exposure to lysozyme to such an extent that a subsequent addition of anions or detergents results in immediate lysis (Goodman *et al.*, 1981; Cho *et al.*, 1982; Laible and Germaine, 1985; Pollock *et al.*, 1987; Wang and Germaine, 1991). Additionally, the major monovalent anions in saliva, namely bicarbonate, fluoride, thiocyanate, and chloride, all have been demonstrated to activate bacterial lysis at neutral pH, whereas only bicarbonate triggers lysis of oral streptococci at acidic pH (Wilkens *et al.*, 1982; Pollock *et al.*, 1983). Electron microscopic studies have demonstrated that, in the absence of salt or detergent, *S. mutans* treated with high concentrations of lysozyme exhibits areas of cell wall dissolution without cell lysis (Bleiweis *et al.*, 1971; Cho *et al.*, 1982; Iacono *et al.*, 1985). Adsorption of lysozyme to oral bacteria is strongly dependent on pH and ionic strength. Bacteriolysis caused by this cationic molecule therefore may be of physiological significance in an environment such as the oral cavity in which a continuous variation in pH and in ionic strength occurs. However, note that the susceptibility of various serotypes of *S. mutans* to lysozyme varies considerably; for example, *Streptococcus rattus,* serotype b, is highly sensitive whereas *S. mutans,* serotype c, is less sensitive (Iacono *et al.*, 1980).

Several studies have demonstrated a synergistic inhibitory effect of lysozyme and other nonimmunoglobulin defense factors in saliva (Arnold *et al.*, 1984; Soukka *et al.*, 1991a,b; Lenander-Lumikari *et al.*, 1992). A combination of lysozyme and Lf had a bactericidal effect on *S. mutans* (Soukka *et al.*, 1991). Results from our laboratory (Lenander-Lumikari *et al.*, 1992) showed that lysozyme alone slightly stimulated *S. mutans* glucose uptake. Incubation with 7–15 μmol/liter HOSCN + $OSCN^-$ resulted in 20–40% inhibition of glucose uptake. However, when *S. mutans* cells were incubated with lysozyme with subsequent addition of HOSCN and $OSCN^-$, glucose incorporation was inhibited completely. The inhibition could be reversed by addition of reducing agents such as 2-mercaptoethanol and dithiothreitol, indicating dependence on the salivary peroxidase (SPO) system. The combined treatment with the peroxidase system and lysozyme did not affect the viability of the bacteria, since no differences in cfu/ml were found between treated and untreated *S. mutans*. When all the components of the SPO system were present with lysozyme in the bacterial suspension, the glucose incorporation of lysozyme-treated bacteria was inhibited totally. However, if the peroxidase enzyme was removed from the HOSCN/$OSCN^-$ preparation, the inhibition was reduced significantly and was only slightly greater than the inhibition achieved by HOSCN/$OSCN^-$ alone. A possible explanation is that, when SPO and SCN^- are present in excess in the bacterial suspension and minimal amounts of H_2O_2 are produced by *S. mutans,* the H_2O_2 produced would be sufficient for the continuous generation of HOSCN/$OSCN^-$, resulting in the observed effects on the bacteria.

The studies reviewed here show that the biological effects of lysozyme extend beyond the catalysis of the hydrolysis of cell wall components. In part because of its cationic nature, lysozyme is able to bind to bacterial cell surfaces and impair vital membrane functions. Membrane alterations may facilitate the diffusion of products of the SPO system into the cell and amplify oxidative damage to enzymes required for glucose metabolism.

IV. PEROXIDASES

Peroxidase activity has been measured in many mucosal secretions (for review, see Tenovuo, 1991): saliva, milk, tears, sweat, and mucus from cervix, intestine, and lung. The activity is derived from enzymes synthesized in exocrine glands and secreted onto mucosal surfaces by the glands. Contributions also come from polymorphonuclear leukocytes (myeloperoxidase) and eosinophils (eosinophil peroxidase). A comprehensive discussion of the numerous studies of the various members of the peroxidase family is beyond the scope of this chapter. We focus our attention on human salivary peroxidase (SPO), human lactoperoxidase (HLPO), and, for comparative purposes, bovine lactoperoxidase (LPO). The latter enzyme has been studied extensively because of its ready availability and has many properties in common with SPO and HLPO.

Peroxidases protect mucosal surfaces from microorganisms by catalyzing the peroxidation of halides (Cl^-, Br^-, I^-) and the thiocyanate ion (SCN^-) to generate reactive products that have potent antibacterial properties. Myeloperoxidase and eosinophil peroxidase will catalyze the peroxidation of Cl^-, Br^-, I^- and SCN^-. However, LPO, HLPO, and SPO will not catalyze the peroxidation of Cl^-. In the absence of halides and SCN^-, peroxidases can behave as catalases. The catalase and peroxidase activities of these enzymes also protect mucosal surfaces by preventing the accumulation of toxic products of oxygen reduction.

Preparations of LPO from bovine milk are heterogeneous (reviewed by Paul and Ohlsson, 1985). A major fraction of LPO consists of a single polypeptide chain of 78.5 kDa. Subfractions of lower molecular mass are derived by loss of carbohydrate groups and by deamidation of asparagine or glutamine residues. SPO from human saliva is also heterogeneous (reviewed by Månsson-Rahemtulla *et al.*, 1988). At least three major forms of 78, 80, and 280 kDa have been reported. Human milk contains at least two peroxidase enzymes (reviewed in Pruitt *et al.*, 1992), HLPO and myeloperoxidase (MPO). The relative amounts vary widely from sample to sample and depend on the stage of lactation. The properties of HLPO are similar to those of SPO. The MPO is derived from milk leukocytes.

The amino acid sequence of SPO has not been reported. However, Dull *et al.* (1990) used peptide sequences obtained from cyanogen bromide fragments of bovine LPO to design oligonucleotide probes for screening cDNA libraries constructed from bovine and human mammary tissue. The deduced amino acid sequence of bovine LPO was consistent with reported amino acid compositions and was homologous to those reported for myelo-, thyroid, and eosinophil peroxidases. These investigators found that HLPO was homologous to bovine LPO. The C-terminal 324 amino acids of these two peroxidases showed 84% homology. The complete amino acid sequence of bovine LPO, determined by Cals *et al.* (1991), agrees with the deduced sequence reported by Dull *et al.* (1990), except that the latter authors reported aspartate at position 9 and asparagine at position 349 whereas the former reported aspartate or asparagine and arginine, respectively, at these positions. The enzyme consists of a single polypeptide chain containing 612 amino acid residues, with 15 half-cystines and 4–5 potential *N*-glycosylation sites. The odd number of half-cystines is consistent with other evidence suggesting a disulfide bond between the heme and the peptide chain. The sequence of LPO can be aligned with human peroxidases to give the following similarities: myeloperoxidase, 55.4%; eosinophil peroxidase, 54%; and thyroid peroxidase, 44.6%. In these four enzymes, 14 of 15 of the half-cystines are located in identical positions. The sequences of SPO and HLPO are likely to show similar homologies with the other members of the peroxidase family. For comparative purposes, the amino acid compositions of LPO and SPO are listed in Table II. The compositions are generally similar, but significant differences exist. SPO apparently has fewer half-cystine, methionine, and isoleucine residues than does LPO. However, SPO has more alanine, glycine, proline, and serine residues than does LPO. These differences in amino acid composition may account for the differences in the biochemical properties of the two enzymes (Pruitt, *et al.*, 1988)

LPO and SPO also differ in carbohydrate composition (Månsson-Rahemtulla *et al.*, 1988). SPO contains 4.6% and LPO 7% total neutral sugars by weight. The weight ratio of glucosamine to galactosamine is 2 : 1 in SPO and 3 : 1 in LPO. The weight ratios of mannose : fucose : galactose in the two enzymes are 1.5 : 1.4 : 1.0 for SPO and 14.9 : 0.5 : 1.0 for LPO.

No reports have been made of higher order structural studies of SPO and HLPO. Spectroscopic circular dichroism (CD) studies of bivine LPO suggest 65% β structure, 23% α helix, and 12% unordered structure (Sievers, 1980). Bovine LPO probably has an ellipsoidal structure in solution (Paul and Ohlsson, 1985) and has properties in solution that are similar to those of other small globular proteins (Pfeil and Ohlsson, 1986). However, inferences about the higher order structure of SPO can be made based on amino acid composition (Table II) and solution properties. SPO contains 50% nonpolar side chains. These nonpolar side chains exist in part as exposed clusters on the surface of the molecule, since hydrophobic chromatography is an effective means for purification of SPO. The molecule also has exposed positive charges on its surface, as indicated by its affinity for negatively charged ion-exchange resins. The mosaic of hydrophobic and charged groups on the surface of SPO is responsible for its strong affinity for many different kinds of surfaces (Pruitt and Adamson, 1977; Pruitt *et al.*, 1979; Honka *et al.*, 1982).

Since absorbed SPO retains its enzyme activity, attachment to surfaces does not block donor access to the heme group. Thus, the surface binding sites and the heme group are not in immediate proximity on the SPO surface. This separation is consistent with the domain structure proposed for LPO by Pfeil and Ohlsson (1986). Based on their observations and on the general structural similarities between LPO and SPO and HLPO, we may suggest that SPO and HLPO have at least two structural domains that differ in stability.

The ultraviolet and visible spectra of bovine LPO and human SPO are identical (Månsson-Rahemtulla *et al.*, 1988). Therefore the two enzymes probably have the same prosthetic group located in similar environments. The prosthetic group of bovine LPO has been identified as protoheme IX (1,3,5,8-tetramethyl-2,4-divinylporphyrine-6,7-dipropionic acid; Sievers, 1979) and is covalently bound (Nichol *et al.*, 1987; Thanabal and La Mar, 1989; Modi *et al.*, 1990) to the peptide backbone via a disulfide bond at the 8-CH_2 group. The Fe^{3+} is held in the porphyrin ring by four bonds to nitrogen; the fifth and sixth axial ligands are thought to be a histidyl residue and a carboxylate ion (Sievers, 1980; Sievers *et al.*, 1983).

Peroxidase kinetics and reaction mechanisms are very complex (for review, see Pruitt and Kamau, 1991). The products of the reactions and the mechanisms depend on the particular enzyme; the particular donor; the relative concentrations of enzyme, peroxide, and donors; the pH; and the temperature. For mucosal defense mechanisms, the most significant peroxidase reactions are those related to catalase activity and to thiocyanate oxidation. The relevant enzymes are SPO (Månsson-Rahemtulla *et al.*, 1988; Pruitt *et al.*, 1988) and HLPO (Pruitt *et al.*, 1992). The actual reactions are complex and include multiple intermediates. The net reactions follow:

1. Catalase activity (occurs in the absence of sufficient donor concentrations)

$$\text{Native enzyme} + 2\ H_2O_2 \rightarrow \text{ferrous enzyme} + O_2 + H_2O_2$$

Subsequent reactions may convert the ferrous enzyme back to the native enzyme.

Table II Amino Acid Composition of Bovine Lactoperoxidase and Human Salivary Peroxidase[a]

Nonpolar side chains			Polar side chains			Basic side chains			Acidic side chains		
	LPO[b]	SPO[c]		LP	SP		LPO	SPO		LP	SP
Alanine	38	45	Serine	32	47	Arginine	39	35	Asparagine + aspartic acid	71	72
Cystine	15	10	Threonine	32	30	Lysine	33	31	Glutamine + glutamic acid	59	64
Glycine	40	47	Tyrosine	15	13	Histidine	14	11	Total	130	136
Isoleucine	27	19	Total	142	162	Total	86	77			
Leucine	69	72									
Methionine	11	3									
Phenylalanine	31	31									
Proline	42	59									
Tryptophan	14	ND[d]									
Valine	29	23									
Total	316	(309)[e]									

[a] Expressed as the nearest integer per 613 total residues.
[b] LPO, Bovine lactoperoxidase. Data from Cals *et al.* (1991).
[c] SPO, Human salivary peroxidase. Data from Månsson-Rahemtulla *et al.* (1988).
[d] ND, Not determined.
[e] Does not include tryptophan.

2. Peroxidation of SCN^- (occurs under normal *in vivo* concentrations of SCN^-)

$$\text{Native enzyme} + H_2O_2 \rightarrow \text{Compound I} + H_2O$$
$$\text{Compound I} + SCN^- \rightarrow OSCN^- + \text{native enzyme}$$

In Compound I, both oxidizing equivalents of peroxide have been transferred to the heme group. The $OSCN^-$ is in equilibrium with its conjugate acid (HOSCN, pKa = 5.3; Thomas, 1981). The net peroxidation reaction may be in an apparent state of dynamic equilibirum *in vivo* (Pruitt *et al.*, 1986) that minimizes the concentration of H_2O_2 and maximizes the concentration of HOSCN and $OSCN^-$.

Both sets of reactions consume toxic H_2O_2 and generate products that are harmless to the host. HOSCN and $OSCN^-$ inhibit the growth and metabolism of many species of bacteria (for review, see Pruitt and Reiter, 1985).

The complex dependence of rates of peroxidation on donor concentrations and on pH are consistent with the following mechanism (Pruitt *et al.*, 1988).

1. Oxidation of the native enzyme by H_2O_2 to generate Compound I. This reaction is independent of pH.
2. Oxidation of SCN by protonated Compound I to produce HOSCN and $OSCN^-$ and regenerate the native enzyme. This reaction is strongly pH dependent. Compound I must be protonated to react. A second protonation at low pH produces an inactive form.
3. Binding of SCN^- to the native enzyme to produce an inactive form. This reaction is enhanced by low pH.

The major limiting factor for SCN^- peroxidation in human saliva is the availability of H_2O_2, as has been shown by experiments in which the addition of H_2O_2 to human saliva *in vivo* (Månsson-Rahemtulla *et al.*, 1983) and *in vitro* (Tenovuo *et al.*, 1981) results in increased concentrations of HOSCN and $OSCN^-$. However, concentrations of SCN^- below 0.6 m*M* also may be limiting (Pruitt *et al.*, 1982). In human milk, the concentrations of SCN^- are usually below this level. The low peroxidase concentration in human milk also may be a limiting factor (for review, see Pruitt and Kamau 1991; Pruitt *et al.*, 1992).

The peroxidase system enhances the antibacterial effects of lysozyme and Lf (discussed previously). The reduction of bacterial acid production by the peroxidase system is enhanced in the presence of secretory IgA (Tenovuo *et al.*, 1982a), but this effect does not depend on specific antibodies.

In summary, secretory peroxidase systems in human saliva and in human milk are natural defense mechanisms that do not require specific antibodies for their effectiveness. They protect mucosal surfaces from infection by inhibiting the growth and metabolism of many species of microorganisms. They prevent damage to mucosal surfaces from toxic products of oxygen reduction by converting hydrogen peroxide into products that are nontoxic for host cells but inhibit the growth and metabolism of many species of microorganism.

A. Thiocyanate

The thiocyanate ion is a critical component of the SPO system. This anion is secreted by salivary, mammary, lacrimal, and gastric glands and can originate from several sources. The major source of SCN^- is the detoxification reaction of CN^- (Burgen and Emmelin, 1961), which occurs primarily in the liver through conversion of CN^- to SCN^- by the enzyme thiosulfate cyanide sulfur transferase. This enzyme catalyzes the transfer of a sulfur atom from thiosulfate to a cyanide ion, the result of which is the far less toxic SCN^- (for review, see Wood, 1975). Sources of cyanide are dietary, for example, from bitter almonds, cassava, or tobacco smoke. Certain vegetables of the genus *Brassica* also contain appreciable amounts of SCN^- (Weuffen *et al.*, 1984). Thiocyanate is found in parotid, submandibular, and whole saliva as well as in gingival crevicular and plaque fluids (for review, see Tenovuo, 1985) and milk (for review, see Pruitt and Kamau, 1991). Average values of SCN^- in saliva of nonsmokers has been reported to be in the range of 0.35 to 1.24 m*M*, whereas the reported range for smokers varies from 1.38 m*M* to 2.74 m*M* (Maliszewski and Bass, 1955; Courant, 1967; Tenovuo and Mäkinen, 1976; Azen, 1978; Lamberts *et al.*, 1984; Olson *et al.*, 1985). In human milk, mean values of 0.021–0.122 m*M* have been reported with large variations from sample to sample (for review, see Pruitt and Kamau, 1991).

Thiocyanate is concentrated 10 to 20-fold from plasma into the salivary glands (Edwards *et al.*, 1954; Fletcher *et al.*, 1956; Logothetopoulos and Myant, 1956; Bratt & Paul, 1983) in humans and animals. Competition experiments provide evidence that iodide, thiocyanate, perchlorate, and nitrate compete as substrates for receptors on the same protein that transports them across the salivary cells (Edwards *et al.*, 1954; Fletcher *et al.*, 1956; Stephen *et al.*, 1973). The concentrating mechanism has been shown to be energy dependent (Fletcher *et al.*, 1956). Thus, this mechanism appears to be active transport. Tenovuo *et al.* (1982b) showed that the concentration of SCN^- in whole saliva rises on initial stimulation and then gradually declines. However, in no instance does the SCN^- secretion (concentration of $SCN^- \times$ secretion rate) in whole stimulated saliva drop below that of unstimulated saliva. These observations indicate that the SCN^- transport system is able to maintain SCN^- levels despite the increased dilution resulting from stimulation. Thus, active transport of SCN^- may be increased by stimulation. Active transport of SCN^- into saliva also may provide a recycling mechanism for this important ion. Saliva is swallowed continuously so SCN^- would be brought back into the blood by the gastrointestinal transport system and concentrated again in the salivary glands. This recycling mechanism may explain the long half-life (6 days) of SCN^- in blood (Junge, 1985).

SCN^- has been demonstrated to be extremely important in protecting a variety of tissues against tissue destruction that might occur as a result of peroxidase-catalyzed oxidation of Cl^- and Br^-. For example, in a reaction that accompanies the respiratory burst of leukocytes, the oxidation of the Cl^- ion by MPO may generate toxic products. MPO, a major protein of polymorphonuclear leukocytes, will catalyze the oxidation of Cl^- by H_2O_2 to form water and a highly reactive oxidizing agent, the hypochlorite ion (OCl^-). Hypochlorite will activate latent collagenase, elastase, gelatinase, and cathepsin that are present in leukocytes, and inactivate circulating protease inhibitors, causing tissue injury (Weiss, 1989). The cytocidal hypohalous acid oxidants also can be produced by eosinophil peroxidase (EPO) through oxidation of halides (Br^-, Cl^-, and I^-) in the absence of the pseudohalide SCN^-. Although the hypohalous acid oxidants mediate the killing of bacteria and the extracellular destruction of invading helminthic parasites (Gleich and Adolphson, 1986), these oxidants are also extremely tissue destructive (Slungaard and Mahoney, 1991). However, SCN^- has been shown to be the preferred substrate for both MPO and EPO, although it is present in serum in significantly lower concentrations than the other halides (Thomas and Fishman, 1986; Slungaard and Mahoney, 1991). This preference for SCN^- results in generation of HOSCN and $OSCN^-$, which are nontoxic to human cells and tissues (Hänström *et al.*, 1983; Tenovuo and Larjava, 1984; Thomas and Fishman, 1986; Slungaard and Mahoney, 1991). Note that SCN^- is recognized as a useful therapeutic agent for the treatment of sickle-cell crises in sickle-cell anemia patients. The much greater incidence of sickle-cell anemia in African Americans than in tropical Africans has been attributed to the much greater SCN^- content of African diets compared with American diets (Agbai, 1986).

Work from our laboratory has shown that patients suffering from leukemia and undergoing chemotherapy have significantly lower SCN^- concentrations in saliva than do healthy control subjects. This reduction is correlated with a simultaneous reduction in the number of granulocytes (Månsson-Rahemtulla *et al.*, 1991). These observations have led us to hypothesize that the reduction in SCN^- concentration is related to the granulocytopenia resulting from chemotherapy and not from the disease itself. A decrease in SCN^- may cause an accumulation of H_2O_2 and subsequent damaging effects on the oral mucosa. Hydrogen peroxide has been shown to be toxic to a variety of life forms by causing lysis of normal cells, for example, red blood cells (Weiss *et al.*, 1980), endothelial cells (Sacks *et al.*, 1978), fibroblasts (Simon *et al.*, 1981), lymphoma cells (Nathan *et al.*, 1979), and gingival fibroblasts (Hänström *et al.*, 1983; Tenovuo and Larjava, 1984; Bratt *et al.*, 1991).

B. Peroxidase Antibodies

Comparative immunological studies of LPO and SPO have been published (Månsson-Rahemtulla *et al.*, 1990). In double immunodiffusion experiments, LPO and SPO showed partial identity to polyclonal antibodies raised against a highly purified preparation of LPO. However, in competitive radioimmunoassays and enzyme-linked immunosorbent assays, LPO replaced the test antigen but SPO did not. The epitopes recognized by the antibodies are present on the protein cores of LPO and SPO. *N*-Linked oligosaccharides were removed from LPO and SPO by treatment with *N*-glycanase. The deglycosylated peroxidases were subjected to SDS–PAGE and transferred to nitrocellulose on which immunodetection was performed. Deglycosylation had no effect on the binding of the antibodies to the protein cores. Structural differences in the core protein of the two enzymes were demonstrated by partial proteolytic digestion and subsequent immunodetection of the peptide fragments. The antibodies did not inhibit the catalytic activity of LPO but did cause partial inhibition of SPO enzyme activity, indicating that sites of the epitopes of the two enzyme were not identical or that they were distributed differently on the enzyme surface relative to the location of the catalytic sites (Månsson-Rahemtulla *et al.*, 1990). Ongoing studies in our laboratory using a panel of monoclonal antibodies to probe the structures of various peroxidases have indicated that substantial cross-reactivity exists. Of five monoclonal antibodies raised against SPO, four cross-react with LPO, EPO, and MPO whereas one of the three anti-LPO monoclonal antibodies cross-reacts with SPO and EPO (Månsson-Rahemtulla and Rahemtulla, 1989; Kiser *et al.*, 1991).

The studies reviewed here show that antibodies raised against a single peroxidase, for example, LPO, cannot be used for reliable quantitation of other peroxidases (SPO, MPO, EPO) in secretions (saliva and crevicular fluid) in which several peroxidases may be present. These studies also show that the secondary and tertiary structures of LPO and SPO reveal different epitopes and that, relative to the catalytic sites, these epitopes occupy different positions on the exposed surfaces of the two enzymes.

V. HIGH MOLECULAR WEIGHT GLYCOPROTEINS

Functions that have been proposed for high molecular weight glycoproteins and mucins in saliva include tissue coating and formation of intraoral pellicles, formation of a lubricating film at hard and soft tissue interfaces, selective clearance and adherence of microorganisms and viruses, heterotypic complexing with other salivary proteins, and protection of the oral mucosa against desiccation (for review, see Cohen and Levine, 1989). High molecular weight glycoproteins found in saliva are synthesized and secreted by all major and minor salivary glands. However, high molecular weight mucinous glycoproteins have been localized to cells in the labial, submandibular, and sublingual glands by specific antibodies to these glycoproteins. Further, distinct acinus populations secrete these mucinous glycoproteins (Cohen and Levine, 1989; Cohen *et al.*, 1990). All high molecular weight glycoproteins bear oligosaccharides that are O-glycosidically linked through *N*-acetylgalactosamine–serine/threonine linkages. However, mucinous glycoproteins also may contain *N*-glycosidically linked oligosaccharides (for details see Tabak, 1990,1991).

The agglutinating properties of the high molecular weight glycoproteins have been studied extensively. The first report on salivary-induced aggregation of oral bacteria was by Gibbons and Spinell (1970), who demonstrated that saliva contained a component that adhered to the tooth surface and caused agglutination of bacteria. This component later was isolated from whole saliva and partially characterized as a high molecular weight glycoprotein containing, of the dry weight of the isolated material, 33.3% protein, 19% anthrone-positive carbohydrates, and 2.9% *N*-acetylneuraminic acid. The remaining components were not chemically characterized. Glucosamine and galactosamine were detected in substantial quantities but the proportions were not reported. The amino acid composition revealed that this component was rich in threonine, serine, and proline. This glycoprotein could cause aggregation of certain oral bacteria, had a high affinity for hydroxyapatite, and had similar properties to a compound isolated from dental plaque. Based on these observations, the authors suggested that the high molecular weight salivary glycoprotein played a significant role in the initial formation of the dental plaque, as well in further development of the bacterial plaque by facilitating binding of the oral microorganisms to each other (Hay *et al.*, 1972).

Several other high molecular weight glycoproteins in saliva have the capacity to agglutinate and prevent oral bacteria from adhering to mucosal and hard tissue surfaces (Ericson *et al.*, 1976; Levine *et al*, 1978,1985; Eggert, 1980a,b,c,d; Ericson and Rundegren, 1983; Rundegren, 1986). These glycoproteins are dependent on calcium for their agglutinating activity (Gibbons and Spinell, 1970; Eggert, 1980b,c; Rundegren and Ericson, 1981). Agglutinating activity is abolished by removal of carbohydrate chains by beta elimination (Ericson *et al.*, 1976), by removal of sialic acid (Levine *et al.*, 1978), and by treatment with hydrogen peroxide (Ericson and Bratt, 1987). These high molecular weight glycoproteins may modulate the oral microbial flora by favoring attachment and subsequent proliferation of certain microorganisms or by promoting clearance of others. An important question regarding the high molecular weight glycoproteins is whether the molecules partially characterized by investigators mentioned earlier are the same or belong to a family of glycoproteins that occur in several forms originating from transcriptional, translational, and posttranslational modifications. Understanding the origin of the molecules requires a knowledge of the biochemical structure. Work by Ericson and Rundegren (1983) has demonstrated that parotid saliva contains a high molecular weight glycoprotein that can agglutinate *S. mutans* serotype c strain. The chemical characterization of this glycoprotein revealed that it was fucose rich; contained sialic acid, hexosamine, and hexose; and had a total carbohydrate content of 45%. The peptide core of this glycoprotein was rich in aspartic acid, serine, and threonine and low in proline residues. The molecular weight was estimated at 5×10^6 Da. After treatment with SDS, the molecular mass was reduced to 4.4×10^5. The purified preparation of this glycoprotein showed agglutinating activity only in the presence of calcium; 0.1 μg caused aggregation of 10^8 bacteria. Calculations based on these numbers show that only a few agglutinin molecules are required for aggregation of the bacteria. Assuming a molecular weight of 5×10^6 Da, 0.1 μg corresponds to 2×10^9 agglutinin molecules. Therefore, approximately 20 agglutinin molecules per bacterial cell can be estimated to produce aggregation of the cells. More recently, *Streptococcus sanguis* has been demonstrated to contain a receptor that binds purified salivary agglutinin. This protein is highly homologous to a surface antigen expressed by *S. mutans*. The interaction of this receptor was inhibited by neuraminidase digestion of the salivary agglutinin and also by simple sugars containing sialic acid, demonstrating that sialic acid is involved in the binding of this microorganism (Demuth *et al.*, 1988,1990).

The mucinous glycoproteins occur in at least two different forms, a high molecular weight glycoprotein designated MG1 and a low molecular weight glycoprotein MG2. Several studies have demonstrated that the two forms of mucinous glycoproteins are present in submandibular saliva obtained from a wide variety of species (reviewed in Tabak, 1990,1991). MG1 and MG2 share common properties. Both are secreted from labial, sublingual, and submandibular glands. Their amino acid compositions are similar with a preponderance of serine, threonine, and proline and a small number of aromatic amino acids. Bovine mucins (Tabak, 1990) and porcine mucins (Eckhardt *et al.*, 1987; Timpte *et al.*, 1988) contain highly repetitive sequences dominated by serine, threonine, and proline. Both MG1 and MG2 have O-glycosidically linked oligosaccharides with *N*-acetylgalactosamine, *N*-acetylglucosamine, galactose, fucose, and sialic acids. A small amount of *N*-glycosidically linked oligosaccharides has been reported to be present in submandibular mucins (Denny and Denny 1980,1982; Levine *et al.*, 1987). The oligosaccharide side chains of mucinous glycoproteins are sulfated; the sulfate groups are attached to galactose or C4 or C6 of *N*-acetylglucosamine residues (Lombardt and Winzler, 1974; Embery and Ward, 1976; Tabak and Levine, 1981; Green and Embery, 1987; Hofsoy and Jonsen, 1987). The sulfation has been confirmed by demonstration of a sulfotransferase enzyme identified in rat sublingual and submandibular glands. This enzyme catalyzes the transfer of a sulfate ester group from 3′-phosphoadenosine-5′-phosphosulfate to the oligosaccharide chains. Structural studies of the sulfated oligosaccharides have revealed the presence of a sulfate residue on the C6 of *N*-acetylglucosamine (Slomiany *et al.*, 1988,1989). Some of the oligosaccharide side chains of the mucins are related structurally to blood group antigens. The blood group reactive glycoproteins in saliva have been demonstrated to cause aggregation of several strains of oral bacteria (Williams and Gibbons, 1975; Gibbons and Qureshi, 1978; Hogg and Embery, 1979,1982; Ligtenberg *et al.*, 1990a,b).

The mucinous glycoprotein MG1 has a molecular weight in excess of 1 million Da. The molecule consists of several peptide subunits that are disulfide bridged. MG1 had 15% protein and contains only O-glycosidically linked oligosaccharides that are distributed randomly on the protein core. The nonglycosylated regions, referred to as naked regions on the molecule, are highly susceptible to proteases. Approximately 80% of the carbohydrates are located in 292 oligosaccharide side chains consisting of 4–16 monosaccharides per chain. The low molecular weight mucinous glycoprotein MG2 has a molecular weight of 200–250 kDa and an estimated protein content of 30%. The large amount of carbohydrate (approximately 69%) is present as 170 oligosaccharide chains made up of 2–7 monosaccharide residues each. The oligosaccharides are predominantly O-linked through serine/threonine–*N*-acetylgalactosamine bonds, but small amounts of asparagine-linked oligosaccharides are also present (Cohen and Levine, 1989; Tabak, 1990,1991).

The studies reviewed here show that the high molecular weight glycoproteins found in mucosal secretions are heterogeneous. The heterogeneity may arise from transcriptional variations and from translational and posttranslational modifications. These glycoproteins have high affinity for mucosal surfaces and for the surfaces of microorganisms. This affinity is based on carbohydrate components. These components are probably responsible for the calcium-dependent bacterial clearance and selection, the tissue lubricating, and the protective properties of these glycoproteins.

References

Agbai, O. (1986). Anti-sickling effect of dietary thiocyanate in prophylactic control of sickle cell anemia. *J. Nat. Med. Assoc.* **78,** 1053–1056.

Allen, P. Z., and Morrison, M. (1963). Lactoperoxidase. IV. Immunological analysis of bovine lactoperoxidase preparations obtained by a simplified fractionation procedure. *Arch. Biochem. Biophys.* **102,** 106–113.

Ambruso, E. R., and Johston, R. B., Jr. (1981). Lactoferrin enhances hydroxyl radical production by human neutrophils, neutrophil particulate fractions, and an enzymatic generating system. *J. Clin. Invest.* **67,** 352–361.

Anderson, B. F., Baker, H. M., Norris, G. E., Rice, D. W., and Baker, E. N. (1989). Structure of human lactoferrin: Crystallographic structure analysis and refinement at 2.8 Å resolution. *J. Mol. Biol.* **209,** 711–734.

Arnold, R. R., Cole, M. F., and McGhee, J. R. (1977). A bactericidal effect for human lactoferrin. *Science* **197,** 263–265.

Arnold, R. R., Brewer, M., and Gauthier, J. J. (1980). Bactericidal activity of human lactoferrin: sensitivity of a variety of microorganisms. *Infect. Immun.* **28,** 893–898.

Arnold, R. R., Russell, J. E., Champion, W. J., and Gauthier, J. J. (1981). Bactericidal activity of human lactoferrin: Influence of physical conditions and metabolic state of the target microorganism. *Infect. Immun.* **32,** 655–660.

Arnold, R. R., Russell, J. E., Champion, W. J., Brewer, M., and Gauthier, J. J. (1982). Bactericidal activity of human lactoferrin: Differentiation from the stasis of iron deprivation. *Infect. Immun.* **35,** 792–799.

Arnold, R. R., Russell, J. E., Devine, S. M., Adamson, M., and Pruitt, K. M. (1984). Antimicrobial activity of the secretory innate defense factors lactoferrin, lactoperoxidase and lysozyme. *In* "Cariology Today" (B. Guggenheim, ed.), pp. 75–88. Karger, Basel.

Azen, E. A. (1978). Salivary peroxidase activity and thiocyanate concentration in human subjects with genetic variants of salivary peroxidase. *Arch. Oral Biol.* **23,** 801–805.

Baker, E. N., Anderson, B. F., Baker, H. M., Haridas, M., Jameson, G. B., Norris, G. E., Rumball, S. V., and Smith, C. A. (1991). Structure, function and flexibility of human lactoferrin. *Int. J. Biol. Macromol.* **13.** 122–129.

Baldwin, D. A., Jenny, E. R., and Aisen, P. (1984). The efect of human serum transferrin and milk lactoferrin on hydroxyl radical formation from superoxide and hydrogen peroxide. *J. Biol. Chem.* **249,** 13391–13394.

Balkejian, A. Y., Hoerman, K. C., and Berzinskas, V. J. (1969). Lysozyme of the human parotid gland secretion: Its purification and phsiochemical properties. *Biochem. Biophys. Res. Commun.* **35,** 887–894.

Bishop, J. G., Schanbacher, F. L., Ferguson, L. C., and Smith, K. L. (1976). *In vitro* growth inhibition of mastitis-causing coliform bacteria by bovine apo-lactoferrin and reversal of inhibition by citrate and high concentrations of apo-lactoferrin. *Infect. Immun* **14,** 911–918.

Bleiweis, A. S., Craig, R. A., Coleman, S. E., and van de Rijn, I. (1971). The streptococcal cell wall: Structure, antigenic composition, and reactivity with lysozyme. *J. Dent. Res.* **50,** (*Suppl. 5*), 1118–1130.

Bortner, C. A., Miller, R. D., and Arnold, R. R. (1986). Bactericidal effect of lactoferrin on *Legionella pneumophila*. *Infect Immun.* **51,** 373–377.

Bortner, C. A., Arnold, R. R., and Miller, R. D. (1989). Bactericidal effect of lactoferrin on *Legionella pneumophila:* Effect of the physiological state of the organism. *Can J. Microbiol.* **35,** 1048–1051.

Bratt, P., and Paul, K. G. (1983). Peroxidase activity and thiocyanate accumulation in salivary glands. *Experientia* **39,** 386–387.

Bratt, P., Rahemtulla, A., Chung, T., and Rahemtulla, F. (1991). Hydrogen peroxide mediated toxicity to human gingival fibroblasts. *J. Dent. Res.* **70,** 375. (Abstract)

Britigan, B. E., and Edeker, B. L. (1991). Pseudomonas and neutrophil products modify transferrin and lactoferrin to create conditions that favor hydroxyl radical formation. *J. Clin. Invest.* **88,** 1092–1102.

Britigan, B. E., Serody, J. S., Hayek, M. B., Charniga, L. M., and Cohen, M. S. (1991). *J. Immunol.* **147,** 4271–4277.

Brock, J. H., Pickering, M. G., McDowall, M. C., and Deacon, A. G. (1983). Role of antibody and enterobactin in controlling growth of *Escherichia coli* in human milk and acquisition of lactoferrin- and transferrin-bound iron by *Escherichia coli. Infect Immun.* **40,** 453–459.

Burgen, A. S. V., and Emmelin, N. G. (1961). "Physiology of the Salivary Glands." Williams & Wilkins, Baltimore.

Byrd, T. F., and Horwitz, M. A. (1991). Lactoferrin inhibits or promotes *Legionella pneumophila* intracellular multiplication in nonactivated and interferon gamma-activated human monocytes depending upon its degree of iron saturation. *J. Clin. Invest.* **88,** 1103–1112.

Cals, M.-M., Mailliart, P., Brignon, G., Anglade, P., and Dumas, B. R. (1991). Primary structure of bovine lactoperoxidase, a fourth member of a mammalian heme peroxidase family. *Eur. J. Biochem.* **198,** 733–739.

Canfield, R. E., Kammerman, S., Sobel, J. H., and Morgan, F. J. (1971). Primary structure of lysozyme from man and goose. *Nature New Biol.* **232,** 16–17.

Chipman, D. M., and Sharon, N. (1969). Mechanism of lysozyme action. Lysozyme is the first enzyme for which the relation between structure and function has become clear. *Science* **165,** 454–465.

Cho, M.-I., Holt, S. C., Iacono, V. J., and Pollock, J. J. (1982). Effects of lysozyme and inorganic anions on the morphology of *Streptococcus mutans* BHT: Electron microscopic examination. *J. Bacteriol.* **151,** 1498–1507.

Cohen, R. E., and Levine, H. J. (1989). Salivary glycoproteins. *In* "Human Saliva: Clinical Chemistry and Microbiology" (J. O. Tenovuo, ed.), pp. 101–130. CRC Press, Boca Raton, Florida.

Cohen, R. E., Aguirre, A., Neiders, M. E., Levine, M. J., Jones, P. C., Reddy, M. S., and Haar, J. G. (1990). Immunochemistry of high molecular-weight human salivary mucin. *Arch. Oral Biol.* **35,** 127–136.

Courant, P. (1967). The effect of smoking of the antilactobacillus system in saliva. *Odontol. Rev.* **18,** 251–261.

Czirók, É., Milch, H., Németh, K., and Gadó, I. (1990). *In vitro* and *in vivo* (LD_{50}) effects of human lactoferrin on bacteria. *Acta Microbiol. Hung.* **37,** 55–71.

Dalmastri, C., Valenti, P., Visca, P., Vittorioso, P., and Orsi, N. (1988). Enhanced antimicrobial activity of lactoferrin by binding to the bacterial surface. *Microbiologica* **11,** 225–230.

Demuth, D. R., Golub, E. E., and Malamud, D. (1990). Streptococcal-host interactions: Structural and functional analysis of a *Streptococcus sanguis* receptor for a human salivary glycoprotein. *J. Biol. Chem.* **265,** 7120–7126.

Demuth, D. R., Golub, E. E., and Malamud, D. (1990). Streptococcal-host interactions: Structural and functional analysis of a *Streptococcus sanguis* receptor for a human salivary glycoprotein. *J. Biol. Chem.* **265,** 7120–7126.

Denny, P. A., and Denny, P. C. (1980). Purification and biochemical characterization of a mouse submandibular sialomucin. *Carbohydrate Res.* **87,** 265–274.

Denny, P. A., and Denny, P. C. (1982). A mouse submandibular sialomucin containing both *N*-and O-glycosidic linkages. *Carbohydrate Res.* **110,** 305–314.

Djeha, A., and Brock, J. H. (1992). Effects of transferrin, lactoferrin and chelated iron on human T-lymphocytes. *Brit. J. Haemat.* **80,** 235–241.

Dull, T. J., Uyeda, C., Strosberg, A. D., Nedwin, G., and Seilhamer, J. J. (1990). Molecular cloning of cDNAs encoding bovine and human lactoperoxidase. *DNA Cell Biol.* **9,** 499–509.

Dumontet, C., and Rousset, B. (1983). Identification, purification, and characterization of a non-heme lactoperoxidase in bovine milk. *J. Biol. Chem.* **258,** 14166–72.

Eckhardt, A. E., Timpte, C. S., Abernethy, J. L., Toumadje, A., Johnson, Jr., W. C., and Hill, R. L. (1987). Structural properties of porcine submaxillary gland apomucin. *J. Biol. Chem.* **262,** 11339–11344.

Edwards, D. A. W., Fletcher, K., and Rowlands, E. N. (1954). Antagonism between perchlorate, iodide, thiocyanate, and nitrate for secretion in human saliva. Analog with the iodide trap of the thyroid, *Lancet* **1,** 498–499.

Eggert, F. M. (1980a). The nature of secretory agglutinins and aggregating factors. I. Secretory conglutinin-like factor, secretory bacterial aggregating factors and secretory IgA antibody in human saliva and amniotic fluid. *Int. Archs. Allergy Appl. Immun.* **61,** 192–202.

Eggert, F. M. (1980b). The nature of secretory agglutinins and aggregating factors. II. Biochemical and immunochemical properties of factors in human saliva and amniotic fluid. *Int. Archs. Allergy Appl. Immun.* **61,** 203–212.

Eggert, F. M. (1980c). The nature of secretory agglutinins and aggregating factors. III Secretory conglutinin-like factor SKF detects a cross-reaction between bacteria and complement component C3. *Int. Archs. Allergy Appl. Immun.* **62,** 34–45.

Eggert, F. M. (1980d). The nature of secretory agglutinins and aggregating factors. IV. Complexing between non-mucin glycoproteins, immunoglobulins and mucins in human saliva and amniotic fluid. *Int. Archs. Allergy Appl. Immun.* **62,** 46–58.

Ellison III, R. T., and Giehl, T. J. (1991). Killing of Gram-negative bacteria by lactoferrin and lysozyme. *J. Clin. Invest.* **88,** 1081–1091.

Ellison III, R. T., Giehl, T. J., and LaForce, F. M. (1988). Damage of the outer membrane of enteric Gram-negative bacteria by lactoferrin and transferrin. *Infect. & Immun.* **56,** 2774–2781.

Ellison, R. T., III, LaForce, F. M., Giehl, T. J., Boose, D. S., and Dunn, B. E. (1990). Lactoferrin and transferrin damage of the gram-negative outer membrane is modulated by Ca^{2+} and Mg^{2+}. *J. Gen. Microbiol.* **136,** 1437–1446.

Embery, G., and Ward, C. (1976). The nature of the sulphate grouping in a rat salivary sulphated glycoprotein. *Arch. Oral Biol.* **21,** 627–629.

Ericson, T., and Bratt, P. (1987). Interactions between peroxide and salivary glycoprotein: protection by peroxidase. *J. Oral Pathol.* **16,** 421–424.

Ericson, T., and Rundegren, J. (1983). Characterization of a salivary agglutinin reacting with a serotype c strain of *Streptococcus mutans. Eur. J. Biochem.* **133,** 255–261.

Ericson, T., Carlen, A., and Dagerskog, E. (1976). Salivary aggregating factors. *In* "Microbial Aspects of Dental Caries" (H. M. Stiles, W. J. Loesche, and T. C. O'Brien, eds.), pp. 151–162. Information Retrieval, Washington, D.C.

Esaguy, N., Aguas, A. P., van Embden, J. D. A., and Silva, M. T. (1991). Mycobacteria and human autoimmune disease: Direct evidence of cross-reactivity between human lactoferrin and the 65-kilodalton protein of tubercle and leprosy bacilli. *Infect. Immun.* **59,** 1117–1125.

Fletcher, K., Honour, A. J., and Rowlands, E. N. (1956). Studies on the concentration of radioiodide and thiocyanate by slices of the salivary gland. *Biochem. J.* **63,** 194–199.

Furmanski, P., Li, Z.-P., Fortuna, M. B., Swamy, C. V. B., and Das, M. R. (1989). Multiple molecular forms of human lactoferrin. *J. Exp. Med.* **170,** 415–419.

Gibbons, R. J., and Qureshi, J. V. (1978). Selective binding of blood group-reactive salivary mucins by *Streptococcus mutans* and other oral organisms. *Infect. Immun.* **22,** 665–671.

Gibbons, R. J., and Spinell, D. M. (1970). Salivary-induced aggretation of plaque bacteria. *In* "Dental Plaque" (D. McHugh, eds.), pp. 207–216. Livingston, Edinburgh.

Gleich, G. J., and Adolphson, C. R. (1986). The eosinophilic leukocyte: Structure and function. *Adv. Immunol.* **39,** 177–253.

Goldman, A. S., Garza, C., and Nichols, B. L. (1982). Immunologic factors in human milk during the first year of lactation. *J. Pediatr.* **100,** 563–567.

Goldman, A. S., Goldblum, R. M., and Garza, C. (1983). Immunologic components in human milk during the second year of lactation. *Acta Pediatr. Scand.* **72,** 461–462.

Goodman, H., Pollock, J. J., Katona, L. I., Iacono, V. J., Cho, M.-I., and Thomas, E. (1981). Lysis of *Streptococcus mutans* by hen egg white lysozyme and inorganic sodium salts. *J. Bacteriol.* **146,** 764–774.

Green, D. R. J., and Embery, G. (1987). Isolation, chemical and biological characterization of sulphated glycoproteins synthesized by rat buccal and palatine minor salivary glands *in vivo* and *in vitro*. *Arch. Oral Biol.* **32,** 391–399.

Hänström, L., Johansson, A., and Carlsson, J. (1983). Lactoperoxidase and thiocyanate protect cultured mammalian cells against hydrogen peroxide toxicity. *Med. Biol.* **61,** 268–274.

Harrington, J. P. (1992). Spectroscopic analysis of the unfolding of transition metal ion complexes of human lactoferrin and transferrin. *Int. J. Biochem.* **24,** 275–280.

Hay, D. I., and Moreno, E. C. (1989). Statherin and the acidic proline-rich proteins. *In* "Human Saliva; Clinical Chemistry and Microbiology" (J. O. Tenovuo, ed.), Vol. I, pp. 131–150. CRC Press, Boca Raton, Florida.

Hay, D. I., Gibbons, R. J., and Spinell, D. M. (1971). Characteristics of some high molecular weight constituents with bacterial aggregating activity from whole saliva and dental plaque. *Caries Res.* **5,** 111–123.

Hofsoy, H., and Jonsen, J. (1979). *In vivo* $^{35}SO_4$-labelling of rabbit salivary components. *Arch. Oral Biol* **24,** 41–45.

Hogg, S. D., and Embery, G. (1979). The isolation and partial characterization of a sulphated glycoprotein from human whole saliva which aggregates strains of *Streptococcus sanguis* but not *Streptococcus mutans*. *Arch. Oral Biol.* **24,** 791–797.

Hogg, S. D., and Embery, G. (1982). Blood group-reactive glycoproteins from human saliva interacts with lipoteichoic acid on the oral surface of *Streptococcus sanguis* cells. *Arch. Oral Biol.* **27,** 261–268.

Honka, E., Ohlsson, P. I., and Paul, K. G. (1982). The adsorption of lactoperoxidase to glass. *Acta Chem. Scand.* **B36,** 273–274.

Hurley, L. S. and Lönnerdal, B. (1988). Trace elements in human milk. *In* "Biology of Human Milk" (L. Å. Hanson, ed.), pp. 87–88. Raven Press, New York.

Iacono, V. J., Byrnes, T. P., Crawford, I. T., Grossbard, B. L., Pollock, J. J., and MacKay, B. J. (1985). Lysozyme-mediated dechaining of *Streptococcus mutans* and its antibacterial significance in an acidic environment. *J. Dent. Res.* **64,** 48–53.

Iacono, V. J., MacKay, B. J., DiRienzo, S., and Pollock, J. J. (1980). Selective antibacterial properties of lysozyme for oral microorganisms. *Infect. & Immun.* **29,** 623–632.

Iacono, V. J., MacKay, B. J., Pollock, J. J., Boldt, P. R., Ladenheim, S., Grossbard, B. L., and Rochon, M. L. (1982). Roles of lysozyme in the host response to periodontopathic microoganisms. *In* "Host-Parasite Interactions in Periodontal Disease" (R. J. Genco and S. E. Mergenhagen, eds.), pp. 318–342. American Society for Microbiology, Washington.

Jolès, J., and Jollès, P. (1971). Human milk lysozyme: unpublished data concerning the establishment of the complete primary structure; comparisons with lysozymes of various origins. *Helv. Chim. Acta* **54,** 2668–2675.

Jolles, P., and Jolles, J. (1984). What's new in lysozyme research? Always a model sysytem, today as yesterday. *Mol. Cell. Biochem.* **63,** 165–189.

Junge, B. (1985). Changes in serum thiocyanate concentration on stopping smoking. *Brit. Med. J.* ***291,*** 22.

Kalfas, S., Andersson, M., Edwardsson, S., Forsgren, A., and Naidu, A. S. (1991). Human lactoferrin binding to *Porphyromonas gingivalis, Prevotella intermedia,* and *Prevotella melaninogenica. Oral Microbiol. Immunol.* **6,** 350–355.

Kalmar, J. R., and Arnold, R. R. (1988). Killing of *Actinobacillus actinomycetemcomitans* by human lactoferrin. *Infect. Immun.* **56,** 2552–2557.

Kawakami, H., and Lönnerdal, B. (1991). Isolation and function of a receptor for human lactoferrin in human fetal intestinal brush-border membranes. *Am. J. Physiol.* **261,** G841–846.

Kawasaki, Y., Hiroko, I., Tanimoto, M., Dosako, S., Idota, T., and Ahiko, K. (1992). Inhibition by lactoferrin and κ-casein glycomacropeptide of binding of *Cholera* toxin to its receptor. *Biosci. Biotech. Biochem.* **56,** 195–198.

Kiser, C. S., Miller, H. K., Rahemtulla, F., and Rahemtulla, B. (1991). Monoclonal antibodies specific for human salivary peroxidase. *J. Dent. Res.* **69,** 2196. (Abstract).

Kishore, A. R., Erdei, J., Naidu, S. S., Falsen, E., Forsgren, A., and Naidu, A. S. (1991). Specific binding of lactoferrin to *Aeromonas hydrophilia. FEMS Microbiol. Lett.* **83,** 115–120.

Klebanoff, S. J., and Waltersdorph, A. M. (1990). Prooxidant activity of transferrin and lactoferrin. *J. Exp. Med.* **172,** 1293–1303.

Korsrud, F. R., and Brandtzaeg, P. (1982). Characterization of epithelial elements in human major salivary glands by functional markers: Localization of amylase, lactoferrin, lysozyme, secretory component, and secretory immunoglobulins by paired immunofluorescence staining. *J. Histochem. Cytochem.* **30,** 657–666.

Laible, N. J., and Germaine, G. R. (1985). Bactericidal activity of human lysozyme, muramidase-inactive lysozyme, and cationic polypeptides against *Streptococcus sanguis* and *Streptococcus faecalis:* Inhibition by chitin oligosaccharides. *Infect. Immun.* **48,** 720–728.

Lamberts, B. L., Pruitt, K. M., Pederson, E. D., and Golding, M. P. (1984). Comparison of salivary peroxidase system components in caries-free caries-active naval recruits. *Caries Res.* **18,** 488–494.

Lee, B. C., and Bryan, L. E. (1989). Identification and comparative analysis of the lactoferrin and transferrin receptors among clinical isolates of gonococci. *J. Med. Microbiol.* **28,** 199–204.

Lenander-Lumikari, M., Månsson-Rahemtulla, B., and Rahemtulla, F. (1992). Lysozyme enhances the inhibitory effects of the peroxidase system on glucose metabolism of *Streptococcus mutans*. *J. Dent. Res.* **71,** 484–490.

Levine, M. J., Herzberg, M. C., Levine, M. S., Ellison, S. A., Stinson, M. W., Li, H. C., and van Dyke, T. (1978). Specificity of salivary-bacterial interactions: Role of terminal sialic acid residues in the interaction of salivary glycoproteins with *Streptococcus sanguis* and *Streptococcus mutans*. *Infect. Immun.* **19,** 107–115.

Levine, M. J., Tabak, L. A., Reddy, M., and Mandel, I. D. (1985). Nature of salivary pellicles in microbial adherence: Role of salivary mucins. *In* "Molecular Basis of Oral Microbial Adhesion" (S. E. Mergenhagen and B. Rosan, eds.), pp. 125–130. American Society for Microbiology, Washington, D.C.

Levine M. J., Reddy, M. S., Tabak, L. A., Loomis, R. E., Bergey, E. J., Jones, P. C., Cohen, R. E., Stinson, M. W., and Al-Hashimi, I. (1987). Structural aspects of salivary glycoproteins. *J. Dent. Res.* **66,** 436–441.

Ligtenberg, A. J. M., Veerman, E. C. I., de Graaff, J., and Nieuw Amerongen, A. V. (1990a). Influence of the blood group reactive substances in saliva on the aggregation of *Streptococcus rattus*. *Antonie van Leeuwenhoek* **57,** 97–107.

Ligtenberg, A. J. M., Veerman, E. C. I., de Graaff, J., and Nieuw Amerongen, A. V. (1990b). Saliva-induced aggregation of oral streptococci and the influence of blood reactive substances. *Arch. Oral Biol.* **35,** 141s–143s.

Logothetopoulos, J. H., and Myant, N. B. (1956). Concentration of radio-iodide and ^{35}S-thiocyanate by the salivary glands. *J. Physiol.* **134,** 189–194.

Lombardt, C. G., and Winzler, R. J. (1974). Isolation and characterization of oligosaccharides from canine submaxillary mucin. *Eur. J. Biochem.* **49,** 77–86.

Lumikari, M., and Tenovuo, J. (1991). Effects of lysozyme–thiocyanate combinations on the viability of *Streptococcus mutans* and *Streptococcus rattus* in human saliva. *Acta Odont. Scand.,* **49,** 175–181.

McKenna, W. R., Mickelsen, P. A., Sparling, P. F., and Dyer, D. W. (1988). Iron uptake from lactoferrin and transferrin by *Neisseria gonorrhoeae*. *Infect. Immun.* **56,** 785–791.

Magnuson, J. S., Henry, J. F., Yip, T-T., and Hutchens, T. W. (1990). Structural homology of human, bovine, and porcine milk lactoferrins: evidence for shared antigenic determinants. Pediatr. Res. **28,** 176–181.

Maliszewski, T. F., and Bass, D. E. (1955). "True" and "apparent" thiocyanate in body fluids of smokers and nonsmokers. *J. Appl. Physiol.* **8,** 289–291.

Månsson-Rahemtulla, B., and Rahemtulla, F. (1989). Monoclonal antibodies as probes for structural studies of peroxidases. *J. Dent. Res.* **67,** 1785. (Abstract)

Månsson-Rahemtulla, B., Pruitt, K. M., Tenovuo, J., and Le, T. M. (1983). A mouthrinse which optimizes *in vivo* generation of hypothiocyanite. *J. Dent. Res.* **62,** 1062–1066.

Månsson-Rahemtulla, B., Rahemtulla F., Baldone, D. C., Pruitt, K. M., and Hjerpe, A. (1988). Purification and characterization of human salivary peroxidase. *Biochemistry* **27,** 233–239.

Månsson-Rahemtulla, B., Rahemtulla, F., and Humphreys-Beher, M. G. (1990). Human salivary peroxidase and bovine lactoperixidase are cross-reactive. *J. Dent. Res.* **69,** 1839–1846.

Månsson-Rahemtulla, B., Techanitiswad, T., Rahemtulla, F., McMillan, T. O., Bradley, E. L., and Wahlin, Y. B. (1991). Analyses of salivary components in leukemia patients receiving chemotherapy. *Oral Surg. Oral Med. Oral Pathol.* **73,** 35–46.

Masson, P. L., and Heremans, J. F. (1966). Studies on lactoferrin, the iron-binding protein of secretions. *In* "Protides of the Biological Fluids" (H. Peeters, ed.), pp. 115–124. Elsevier, Amsterdam.

Masson, P. L., Heremans, J. F., Prignot, J. J., and Wauters, G. (1966). Immunohistochemical localization and bacteriostatic properties of an iron-binding protein from bronchial mucus. *Thorax* **21,** 538–544.

Metz-Boutique, M.-H., Jolles, J., Mazurier, J., Schoentgen, F., Legrand, D., Spik, G., Montreuil, J., and Jolles, P. (1984). Human lactotransferrin: Amino acid sequence and structural comparison with the other transferrins. *Eur. J. Biochim.* **145,** 659–676.

Modi, S., Behere, D. V., and Mitra, S. (1990). Binding of thiocyanate to lactoperoxidase: ^{1}H and ^{15}N nuclear magnetic resonance studies. *Biochemistry* **28,** 4689–4694.

Naidu, A. S., Miedzobrodzki, J., Andersson, M., Nilsson, L.-E., Forsgren, A., and Watts, J. L. (1990). Bovine lactoferrin binding to six species of coagulase-negative staphylococci isolated from bovine intramammary infections. *J. Clin. Microbiol.* **28,** 2312–2319.

Naidu, A. S., Miedzobrodzki, J., Musser, J. M., Rosdahl, V. T., Hedström, S.-Å., and Forsgren, A. (1991). Human lactoferrin binding in clinical isolates of *Staphylococcus aureus*. *J. Med. Microbiol.* **34,** 323–328.

Nakamura, M. (1990). Lactoferrin-mediated formation of oxygen radicals by NADPH cytochrome P-450 reductase system. *J. Biochem.* **107,** 395–399.

Nathan, C. F., Silverstin, S. C., Brukner, L. H., and Cohn, Z. A. (1979). Extracellular cytolysis by activated macrophages and granulocytes. II. Hydrogen peroxide as a mediator of cytotoxicity. *J. Exp. Med.* **149,** 100–113.

Nichol, A. W., Angel, L. A., Moon, T., and Clezy, P. S. (1987). Lactoperoxidase haem, an iron–porphyrin thiol. *Biochem. J.* ***247,*** 147–150.

Olson, B. L., McDonald, J. L. J., Gleason, M. J., Stookey, G. K., Schemehorn, B. R., Drook, C. A., Beiswanger, B. B., and Christen, A. G. (1985). Comparisons of various salivary parameters in smokers before and after the use of a nicotine-containing chewing gum. *J. Dent. Res.* **64,** 826–30.

Oppenheim, F. G. (1989). Salivary histidine rich proteins. *In* "Human Saliva: Clinical Chemistry and Microbiology" (J. O. Tenovuo, ed.), Vol. I, pp 151–160. CRC Press, Boca Raton, Florida.

Oram, J. D., and Reiter, B. (1968). Exhibition of bacteria by lactoferrin and other iron-chelating agents. *Biochim. Biophys. Acta* **170,** 351–365.

Paul, K-G., and Ohlsson, P-I. (1985). The chemical structure of lactoperoxidase. *In* "The Lactoperoxidase System" (K. M. Pruitt and J. O. Tenovuo, eds.), pp. 15–29. Marcel Dekker, New York.

Parry, R. M., Chandan, R. C., and Shahani, K. M. (1968). Lysozyme, lipase and ribonuclease in milk of various species. *J. Dairy Sci.* **51,** 606–607.

Petit, J. F., and Jollès, P. (1963). Purification and analysis of human saliva lysozyme. *Nature* (*London*) **200,** 168–169.

Pfeil, W., and Ohlsson, P. I. (1986). Lactoperoxidase consists of domains: A scanning calorimetric study. *Biochim. Biophys. Acta* **872,** 72–75.

Pollock, J. J., Iacono, V. J., Goodman Bicker, H., MacKay, B. J., Katona, L. I., Taichman, L. B., and Thomas, E. (1976). The binding, aggregation and lytic properties of lysozyme. *In* "Proceedings: Microbial Aspects of Dental Caries. Special Supplement to Microbiology Abstracts" (H. M. Stiles, W. J. Loesche, and T. C. O'Brien, eds.), pp. 325–352. Information Retrieval, Washington, D.C.

Pollack, J. J., Goodman, H., Elsey, P. K., and Iacono, V. J. (1983). Synergism of lysozyme, proteases, and inorganic monovalent anions in the bacteriolysis of oral *Streptococcus mutans* GS5. *Arch. Oral Biol.* **28,** 865–871.

Pollock, J. J., Lotardo, S., Gavai, R., and Grossbard, B. L. (1987). Lysozyme–protease–inorganic monovalent anion lysis of oral bacterial strains in buffers and stimulated whole saliva. *J. Dent. Res.* **66,** 467–74.

Powell, M. J., and Ogden, J. E. (1990). Nucleotide sequence of human lactoferrin cDNA. *Nucleic Acids Res.* **18,** 4013.

Pruitt, K. M., and Adamson, M. (1977). Enzyme acitivity of salivary lactoperoxidase adsorbed to human enamel. *Infect. Immun.* **17,** 112–116.

Pruitt, K. M., and Kamau, D. N. (1991). The lactoperoxidase systems of bovine and human milk. *In* "Oxidative Enzymes in Foods" (D. S. Robinson and N. A. M. Eskin, eds.), pp. 133–174. Elsevier Applied Science, London.

Pruitt, K. M., and Reiter, B. (1985). Biochemistry of the peroxidase system: Antimicrobial effects. *In* "The Lactoperoxidase System" (K. M. Pruitt and J. Tenovuo, eds.), pp. 143–178. Marcel Dekker, New York.

Pruitt, K. M., Adamson, M., and Arnold, R. (1979). Lactoperoxidase binding to streptococci. *Infect. Immun.* **25,** 304–309.

Pruitt, K. M., Tenovuo, J., Fleming, W., and Adamson, M. (1982). Limiting factors for the generation of hypothiocyanite ion, an antimicrobial agent, in human saliva. *Caries Res.* **16,** 315–323.

Pruitt, K. M., Tenovuo, J., Månsson-Rahemtulla, B., Harrington, P., and Baldone, D. C. (1986). Is thiocyanate peroxidation at equilibrium *in vivo*? *Biochim. Biophys. Acta* **870,** 285–391.

Pruitt, K. M., Månsson-Rahemtulla, B., Baldone, D. C., and Rahemtulla, F. (1988). Steady-state kinetics of thiocyanate oxidation catalyzed by human salivary peroxidase. *Biochemistry* **27,** 240–245.

Pruitt, K. M., Rahemtulla, F., Månsson-Rathemutulla, B., Baldone, D. C., and Laven, G. T. (1992). Peroxidases in human milk. *In* "Immunology of Milk and the Neonate" (J. Mestecky, C. Blair, and P. L. Ogra, eds.), pp. 137–144. Plenum Press, New York.

Raeste, A.-M. (1972). Lysozyme (muramidase) activity of leukocytes and exfoliated epithelial cells in the oral cavity. *Scand. J. Dent. Res.* **80,** 422–427.

Rainard, P. (1986). Bacteriostatic activity of bovine milk lactoferrin against mastitic bacteria. *Vet. Microbiol.* **11,** 387–392.

Rainard, P. (1987). Bacteriostatic activity of bovine lactoferrin in mastitic milk. *Vet. Microbiol.* **13,** 159–166.

Reiter, B., and Brock J. H. (1975). Inhibition of *Escherichia coli* by bovine colostrum and postcolostral milk. I. Complement-mediated bactericidal activity of antibodies to a serum susceptible strain of *E. coli* of the serotype O 111. *Immunology* **28,** 71–82.

Reiter, B., Brock, J. H., and Steel, E. D. (1975). Inhibition of *Escherichia coli* by bovine colostrum and post-colostral milk. II. The bacteriostatic effect of lactoferrin on a serum susceptible and serum resistant strain of *E. coli. Immunology* **28,** 83–95.

Rey, M. W., Woloshuk, S. L., deBoer, H. A., and Pieper, F. R. (1990). Complete nucleotide sequence of human mammary gland lactoferrin. *Nucleic Acids Res.* **18,** 5288.

Roberts, A. K., Chierici, R., Sawatzki, G., Hill, M. J., Volpato, S., and Vigi, V. (1992). Supplementation of an adapted formula with bovine lactoferrin: 1. Effect on the infant faecal flora. *Acta Pediatr.* **81,** 119–124.

Rundegren, J. (1986). Calcium-dependent salivary agglutinin with reactivity to various oral bacterial species. *Infect. Immun.* **53,** 173–178.

Rundegren, J., and Ericson, T. (1981). Effect of calcium on reaction between salivary agglutinin and serotype c strain of *Streptococcus mutans. J. Oral Pathol.* **10,** 269–275.

Sacks, T., Moldow, C. F., Craddock, P. R., Bowers, T. K., and Jacob, H. S. (1978). Endothelial damage provoked by toxic oxygen radicals released from complement-triggered granulocytes. *Prog. Clin. Biol. Res.* **21,** 719–726.

Senn, H. J., Chu, B., O'Malley, J., and Holland, J. F. (1970). Experimental and clinical studies on muramidase (lysozyme). *Acta Haemat* **44,** 65–77.

Shimazaki, K.-I., Kawano, N., and Yoo, Y. C. (1991). Comparison of bovine, sheep, and goat milk lactoferrins in their electrophoretic behavior, conformation, immunochemical properties, and lectin reactivity. *Comp. Biochem. Physiol.* **98B,** 417–422.

Sievers, G. (1979). The prosthetic group of milk lactoperoxidase is protoheme IX. *Biochem. Biophys. Acta* **579,** 181–190.

Sievers, G. (1980). Structure of milk lactoperoxidase. A study using circular dichroism and difference absorption spectroscopy. *Biochim. Biophys. Acta* **624,** 249–259.

Sievers, G., Gadsby, P. M. A., Peterson, J., and Thomson, A. J. (1983). Assignment of the axial ligands of the haem in milk lactoperoxidase using magnetic circular dichroism spectroscopy. *Biochem. Biophys. Acts* **742,** 659–668.

Simon, R. H., Scoggin, C. H., and Patterson, D. (1981). Hydrogen peroxide causes the fatal injury to human fibroblasts exposed to oxygen radicals *J. Biol. Chem.* **256,** 7181–7186.

Slomiany, A., Murty, V. L., Sarosiek, J., Carter, S. R., and Slomiany, B. L. (1988). Enzymatic sulfation of mucus glycoprotein in rat sublingual salivary gland. *Arch. Oral Biol.* **33,** 669–676.

Slomiany, B. L., Murty, V. L., Sarosiek, J., and Slomiany, A. (1989). Enzymatic sulfation of mucus glycoprotein in rat submandibular salivary glands. *Int. J. Biochem.* **21,** 165–171.

Slungaard, A., and Mahoney Jr., J. R. (1991). Thiocyanate is the major substrate for eosinophil peroxidase in physiologic fluids. Implications for cytotoxicity. *J. Biol. Chem.* **266,** 4903–4910.

Soukka, T., Lumikari, M., and Tenovuo, J. (1991a). Combined bactericidal effect of human lactoferrin and lysozyme against *Streptococcus mutans* serotype c. *Microbial Ecol. Health Dis.* **4,** 259–264.

Soukka, T., Lumikari, M., and Tenovuo, J. (1991b). Combined inhibitory effect of lactoferrin and lactoperoxidase system on the viability of *Streptococcus mutans,* serotype c. *Scand. J. Dent. Res.* **99,** 390–396.

Soukka, T., Tenovuo, J., and Lenander-Lumikari, M. (1992). Fungicidal effect of human lactoferrin against *Candida albicans. Microbiol. Let.* **90,** 223–228.

Stephen, K. W., Robertson, J. W., Harden, R. M., and Chisholm, D. M. (1973). Concentration of iodide, pertechnetate thiocyanate, and bromide in saliva from parotid, submandibular, and minor salivary glands in man. *J. Lab. Clin. Med.* **81,** 219–29.

Still, J., Delahut, P., Coppe, P., Kaeckenbeeck, A., and Perraudin, J. P. (1990). Treatment of induced enterotoxigenic colibacillosis (scours) in calves by the lactoperoxidase system and lactoferrin. *Ann. Rech. Vet.* **21,** 143–152.

Suzuki, T., Yamauchi, K., Kawase, K., Tomita, M., Kiyosawa, I., and Okonogi, S. (1989). Collaborative bacteriosatic activity of bovine lactoferrin with lysozyme against *Escherichia coli* 0111. *Agric. Biol. Chem.* **53,** 1705–1706.

Tabak, L. A. (1990). Structure and function of human salivary mucins. *Crit. Rev. Oral Biol. Med.* **1,** 229–234.

Tabak, L. A. (1991). Genetic control of salivary mucin formation. *In* "Frontiers of Oral Physiology" (D. B. Ferguson, ed.), pp. 77–94. Karger, Basel.

Tabak, L. A., and Levine, M. J. (1981). Charactrization of sulphated monosaccharides from stumptail monkey salivary mucins. *Arch. Oral Biol.* **26,** 315–317.

Tenovuo, J. O. (1985). "The Peroxidase System in Human Secretions. Marcel Dekker, New York.

Tenovuo, J. O. (1991). Salivary peroxidase. *In* "Peroxidases in Chemistry and Biology" (J. Everse, K. E. Evers, and M. B. Grisham, eds.), Vol. 1, pp. 181–197. CRC Press, Boca Raton, Florida.

Tenovuo, J., and Larjava, H. (1984). The protective effect of peroxidase and thiocyanate against hydrogen peroxide toxicity assessed by the uptake of [^{3}H]-thymidine by human gingival fibroblasts cultured *in vitro*. *Arch. Oral Biol.* **29,** 445–451.

Tenovuo, J., and Mäkinen, K. K. (1976). Concentration of thiocyanate and ionizable iodine in saliva of smokers and nonsmokers. *J. Dent. Res.* **55,** 661–663.

Tenovuo, J., Månsson-Rahemtulla, B., Pruitt, K. M., and Arnold, A. (1981). Inhibition of dental plaque acid production by the salivary lactoperoxidase antimicrobial system. *Infect. Immun* **34,** 208–214.

Tenovuo, J., Moldoveanu, Z., Mestecky, J., Pruitt, K. M., and Mänsson-Rahemtulla, B. (1982a). Interaction of specific and innate factors of immunity: IgA enhances the antimicrobial effect of the lactoperoxidase system against *Streptococcus mutans*. *J. Immunol.* **128,** 726–731.

Tenovuo, J., Pruitt, K. M., and Thomas, E. L. (1982b). Peroxidase antimicrobial system of human saliva: Hypothiocyanite levels in resting and stimulated saliva. *J. Dent. Res.* **61,** 982–985.

Thanabal, V., and La Mar, G. N. (1989). A nuclear overhauser effect investigation of the molecular and electronic structure of the heme crevice in lactoperoxidase. *Biochemistry* **28,** 7038–7044.

Thomas, E. L. (1981). Lactoperoxidase-catalyzed oxidation of thiocyanate: Equilibria between oxidized forms of thiocyanate. *Biochemistry* **20,** 3273–3280.

Thomas, E. L., and Fishman, M. (1986). Oxidation of chloride and thiocyanate by isolated leukocytes. *J. Biol. Chem.* **261,** 9694–9702.

Timpte, C. S., Eckhardt, A. E., Abernethy, J. L., and Hill, R. L. (1988). Porcine submaxillary gland apomucin contains tandemly repeated identical sequences of 81 residues. *J. Biol. Chem.* **263,** 1081–1088.

Trumpler, U., Straub, P. W., and Rosenmund, A. (1989). Antibacterial prophylaxis with lactoferrin in neutropenic patients. *Eur. J. Clin. Microbiol. Infect. Dis.* **8,** 310–313.

Twetman, S., Lindqvist, L., and Sund, M.-L. (1986). Effect of human lysozyme on 2-deoxyglucose uptake by *Streptococcus mutans* and other oral microorganisms. *Caries Res.* **20,** 223–229.

Valenti, P., Visca, P., Nicoletti, M., Antonini, G., and Orsi, N. (1985). Synthesis of siderophores by *E. coli* strains in the presence of lactoferrin–Zn. *In* "Proteins of Iron Storage and Transport" (G. Spik, J. Montreuil, R. R., Crichton, and J. Mazurier, eds.), pp. 245–249. Elsevier, Amsterdam.

Visca, P., Berlutti, F., Vittorioso, P., Dalmastri, C., Thaller, M. C., and Valenti, P. (1989). Growth and adsorption of *Streptococcus mutans* 6715–13 to hydroxyapatite in the presence of lactoferrin. *Med. Microbiol. Immunol.* **178.** 69–79.

Visca, P., Dalmastri, C., Verzili, D., Antonini, G., Chiancone, E., and Valenti, P. (1990). Interaction of lactoferrin with *Escherichia coli* cells and correlation with antibacterial activity. *Med. Microbiol. Immunol.* **179,** 323–333.

Wang, C. S., and Kloer, H. U. (1985). Purification of human lysozyme from milk and pancreatic juice. *Anal. Biochem.* **139,** 224–227.

Wang, Y.-B., and Germaine, G. R. (1991). Effect of lysozyme on glucose fermentation, cytoplasmic pH, and intracellular potassium concentrations in *Streptococcus mutans* 10449. *Infect. Immun.* **59,** 638–644.

Weiss, S. J. (1989). Tissue destruction by neutrophils. *N. Engl. J. Med.* **320,** 365–376.

Weiss, S. J., LoBuglio, A. F., and Kessler, H. B. (1980). Oxidative mechanisms of monocyte-mediated cytotoxicity. *Proc. Natl. Acad. Sci. U.S.A.* **77,** 584–587.

Weuffen, W., Franzke, C., and Thürkow, B. (1984). Zur alimentären Aufnahme, Analytik, und biologischen Bedeutun des Thiocyanats. *Nahrung* **28,** 341–355.

Wilkens, T. J., Goodman, H., MacKay, B. J., Iacono, V. J., and Pollock, J. J. (1982). Bacteriolysis of *Streptococcus mutans* GS5 by lysozyme, proteases, and sodium thiocyanate. *Infect. Immun.* **38,** 1172–1180.

Williams, R. C., and Gibbons, R. J. (1975). Inhibition of streptococcal attachment on human buccal epithelial cells by antigenically similar salivary glycoproteins. *Infect. Immun.* **11,** 711–718.

Wood, J. (1975). "Chemistry and Biochemistry of Thiocyanic Acid and its Derivatives." Academic Press, New York.

Zagulski, T., Lipinski, P., Zagulska, A., Broniek, S., and Jarzabek, Z. (1989). Lactoferrin can protect mice against a lethal dose of *Escherichia coli* in experimental infection *in vivo Br. J. Exp. Pathol.* **70,** 697–704.

6

Bacterial Adherence and Mucosal Immunity

C. Svanborg

I. INTRODUCTION

Adhesion is a key to the organized functions of multicellular organisms. Adhesion between eukaryotic cells is a prerequisite for the establishment of tissues and organs. During embryogenesis, tissues evolve from "founder" cells. The progeny remain attached to each other and show greater affinity for cells of the same origin than for other cells. Changes in adhesive properties often accompany the spread of cells to a new site and the development of new functions. Adhesion is also fundamental to the communication between cells that is required for the diversification of cellular functions. For example epithelial cells have elaborate systems for cell-to-cell adhesion. These cells are held together by tight junctions that contribute to the barrier function of the epithelium by limiting the uptake of water-soluble molecules from the lumen. These junctions also maintain the polarity of the cells by limiting the flux of membrane proteins from the apical to the basolateral part of cell.

Bacteria share with eukaryotic cells the requirement for adhesion. The tendency of bacteria to grow attached to surfaces first was observed in aquatic systems (Zobell, 1943). Bacteria that were attached to rocks in a stream multiplied faster than free-floating cells of the same species (Zobell, 1943; Gibbons, 1973). Their likelihood of trapping nutrients was calculated to be enhanced by the attached state (Zobell, 1943; Zafriri *et al.*, 1987). Subsequent studies have shown that attachment between bacteria is essential for the cooperation of cells within a colony, as well as for the exquisitely regulated interactions that make complex bacterial habitats composed of different bacterial species resemble tissues composed of several eukaryotic cell types (Savage, 1984,1988).

The attachment of bacteria to human cells and tissues lacks the seemingly altruistic quality of adhesion between eukaryotic cells on the one hand and between bacteria on the other. The pro- and eukaryotic cells are unlikely to share any expectations of the outcome of this interaction. Attachment is needed for the bacteria to remain in the human host and to enhance nutrient access. Unattached bacteria are eliminated from mucosal surfaces by the flow of secretions. Attachment also is needed to permit the establishment of the indigenous microflora for the host to benefit from its functions. For example, the microflora has been proposed as a major driving force behind the evolution of genetic polymorphisms in the human host (for review, see Svanborg-Edén and Levin, 1988).

In view of the mutual toxicity of bacteria and host cells, the consequences of attachment may be severe for both parties. Even members of the indigenous microflora contain potent toxins and activators of immunity and inflammation. Pathogens have evolved additional mechanisms to disrupt the organization and function of host tissues (Orskov and Orskov, 1983). A large group of bacteria are considered "coincidental" pathogens (Svanborg-Edén and Levin, 1988). They persist as members of the indigenous flora at one site, apparently without causing damage, but induce disease when they reach a different site within the same host.

The different mechanisms of bacterial adherence may have evolved as a way to reconcile the opposing needs of bacteria and host. The bacteria select habitats in which survival is optimal. This is achieved by the expression of surface molecules—adhesins—that selectively recognize specific habitats, permitting attaching cells to find the appropriate site in each new host and to expand their population there (Leffler *et al.*, 1983). The host directs the establishment of the indigenous flora by expressing variable receptor structures that define the different habitats. By specific attachment to these receptors, the flora is directed to these sites. The toxic effects of the flora may be reduced if the receptors are loosely associated with the cells (Svanborg-Edén *et al.*, 1988a). In contrast, pathogens express adhesins that recognize cell-bound receptors that promote the access of toxin, the invasion of bacteria, and so on. In this way, the specificity as well as the architecture of bacterial adherence will influence the outcome of host–parasite interactions.

II. MECHANISMS OF ADHERENCE

Adhesive bacterial surface proteins, adhesins, often act as lectins. They bind receptor epitopes provided by host cell glycoconjugates (for review, see Mirelman, 1986). All cells surround themselves with a shell of carbohydrates. Chemical analyses have revealed extensive differences in carbohydrate composition among species, individuals, and tissues within an individual (Berger *et al.*, 1982; Hakomori, 1983). Indeed, blood group antigens that distinguish one individual from the next are often carbohydrate in nature (Berger *et al.*, 1982; Hakomori, 1983). Bacterial cells also use carbohydrates to generate individuality. Isolates of *Escherichia coli* that share the same lipopolysaccharide and capsular polysaccharide antigens are genetically more alike than those with different carbohydrate structures (Caugant *et al.*, 1985). Polysaccharide capsules help maintain the bacterial self, both as a defense against inflammation and as a mechanism for evasion of the immune response.

The extensive variability of oligosaccharide sequences makes them suitable as receptors for diverse bacterial ligands. Early studies of toxins and viruses showed that microbial ligands can bind glycoconjugate receptors. The influenza virus hemagglutinin recognizes certain acetylneuraminic acid-containing structures (van Heyningen, 1974). Cholera toxin binds specifically to GM1 ganglioside (Paulson, 1985). The fimbriae of gram-negative *E. coli* recognize a variety of host cell glycoconjugates. Adherence consequently might be achieved by the binding of a host lectin to a bacterial glycoconjugate.

A. *Escherichia coli P Fimbriae Bind to the Globoseries of Glycolipids*

Before the identification of glycolipid receptors, the *in vitro* attachment of bacteria to a given epithelial cell type was known to predict their ability to colonize a mucosal site in the individual. This ability was demonstrated for streptococci with affinity for different mucosal compartments within the oral cavity (Gibbons and van Houte, 1971,1975) and for uropathogenic *E. coli* that attached to uroepithelial cells but not to small intestinal cells (Leffler *et al.*, 1983; Leffler and Svanborg-Edén, 1980). At the same time, biochemical analyses of intestinal epithelial glycolipids had shown that epithelial cells are highly glycosylated, and that the glycolipid composition varies extensively among species, individuals, and tissues (see Berger *et al.*, 1982; Hakomori, 1983; Leffler *et al.*, 1983; Leffler and Svanborg-Edén, 1986; and references therein). The observation of variability of bacterial attachment and epithelial glycolipid composition led us to study and identify glycolipids as receptors for P fimbriated *E. coli* (Svanborg-Edén and Leffler, 1979; Leffler and Svanborg-Edén, 1980,1986). The symbol P was chosen for two reasons: (1) P fimbriated *E. coli* are accumulated in patients with acute pyelonephritis (reviewed by Svanborg-Edén *et al.*, 1988b; Johnson, 1991). (2) The globoseries of glycolipids acts as both receptors for P fimbriae and antigens in the P blood group system (Källenius *et al.*, 1980; Bock *et al.*, 1985; Leffler and Svanborg-Edén, 1980).

The initial studies showed that the receptor activity of epithelial cells resided in the globoseries of glycolipids (Leffler and Svanborg-Edén, 1980,1986). Attachment was inhibited by pretreatment of *E. coli* with those glycolipids. The glycolipids also could induce binding to an inert surface or to a cell that lacked receptor-active glycolipids. Further, attachment was P blood group dependent. Cells from individuals of blood group p, who lack the globoseries of glycolipids, did not interact with P fimbriated *E. coli* (Källenius *et al.*, 1980; Leffler and Svanborg-Edén, 1980). Additional studies have shown variation in receptor activity among members of the globoseries of glycolipids (Leffler and Svanborg-Edén, 1981; Lund *et al.*, 1988; Lindstedt *et al.*, 1989; Strömberg *et al.*, 1990). The P fimbriae constitute a family of adhesins that recognize the globoseries of glycolipids but differ in the preferred receptor epitope.

The P fimbriae are encoded by the *pap* family of chromosomal gene clusters (Hull *et al.*, 1981). *pap* gene clusters cloned from different *E. coli* strains show extensive sequence homology except for *pap*A, which encodes the major fimbrillin subnits, and *pap*E, papF, and *pap*G sequences, which encode the adhesin (Hull *et al.*, 1981; Clegg, 1982; Väisänen-Rhen *et al.*, 1984; vanDie and Bergmans, 1984; Karr *et al.*, 1989). The adhesin complex *pap*E–*pap*G is located at the tip of the fimbriae (Lindberg *et al.*, 1987; Hanson *et al.*, 1988; Jann and Hoschützky, 1989). *pap*G is present in the periplasmic space and has been proposed to act as a chaperone stabilizing the subunits *pap*E and *pap*G during the transport from the inner membrane to the outer membrane (Huttgren *et al.*, 1989). *pap*C has been proposed to form a pore through which the pilus is assembled (Norgren *et al.*, 1987). *pap*H terminates fimbrial assembly and helps anchor the fimbriae (Tennent *et al.*, 1990). The roles of *pap*J and *pap*K are less clear. The *pap*J gene product has been suggested to facilitate the assembly of *pap*A subunits into the pilus structure (Tennent *et al.*, 1990). The *pap*K gene produce has been suggested to be a pilin-like protein located at the pilus tip (Tennent *et al.*, 1990). *pap*B and *pap*I encode regulatory proteins involved in positive transregulation of *pap*A transcription (Norgren *et al.*, 1984; Uhlen *et al.*, 1985).

The G adhesins of the $papG_{IA2}$ type dominate in the virulent *E. coli* strains that cause acute pyelonephritis (Johanson *et al.*, 1993). Their adhesins recognize most members of the globoseries of glycolipids, but appear to prefer globotetraosylceramide (Johanson *et al.*, 1992; Strömberg *et al.*, 1990). The G adhesins of the $prsG_{J96}$ type are less prevalent among clinical isolates and show no clear-cut association with disease, except possibly acute cystitis (I. M. Johanson). These adhesins prefer a receptor epitope composed of an *N*-acetylgalactosamine α-linked to a globoseries core (Karr *et al.*, 1989; Lindstedt *et al.*, 1989; Strömberg *et al.*, 1990). Although these adhesins also recognize globotetraosylceramide on thin-layer chromatogram plates, their binding to uroepithelial cells requires the Forssmann or globo-A glycolipids (Lindstedt *et al.*, 1989; Johanson *et al.*, 1992).

B. *Type 1 Fimbriae*

Type 1 or mannose-sensitive (MS) fimbrial adhesins recognize mannose-containing receptors. Their binding is blocked by solutions of D-mannose or α-methyl-D-mannoside (Duguid *et al.*, 1955,1979; Ofek *et al.*, 1985). Receptors for type 1 fimbriae are present on a variety of cells from many species (Duguid *et al.*, 1979). Type 1 fimbriae bind mannose epitopes on secreted glycoproteins such as the Tamm–Horsefall protein and secretory IgA (Orskov *et al.*, 1980; Svanborg-Edén *et al.*, 1981; Parkkinen *et al.*, 1988; Wold *et al.*, 1990). When these substances coat uroepithelial cells, they may provide receptor epitopes for bacterial surface colonization. When secreted, they may eliminate type 1 fimbriated *E. coli* strains and prevent colonization or infection. Further, type 1 fimbriae play a complex role in the interaction with human polymorphonuclear leukocytes (PMNs). The adhesion of type 1 fimbriated *E. coli* strains to PMNs may promote bacterial killing (Bar Shavit *et al.*, 1977; Öhman *et al.*, 1982; Svanborg-Edén *et al.*, 1984). The type 1 fimbriae are encoded by the *pil* or *fim* genes of four clusters (Hull *et al.*, 1981; Klemm, 1985). *fim*A encodes the fimbrial subunit protein and can be expressed independent of the *fim*H-encoded adhesin protein (Minion *et al.*, 1986). The *fim*A gene product must be present on the cells to confer the adhesive phenotype, in contrast to what has been found for the P fimbriae.

The expression of fimbriae is subject to phase variation (Brinton, 1965; Eisenstein, 1981; Rhen *et al.*, 1983; Klemm 1986). Changes in temperature, glucose concentration, and other experimental conditions may switch the fimbriae on or off (Uhlin *et al.*, 1985). Little is known about *in vivo* growth conditions that control fimbrial expression. Pere studied the expression of fimbriae in urine directly by immunofluorescence and found that the P fimbriae were expressed whereas the type 1 fimbriae occurred less frequently (Pere *et al.*, 1987).

C. Other Fimbrial–Carbohydrate Interactions

The fimbria-mediated attachment to oligosaccharide receptor epitopes is common among gram-negative bacteria (Beachey, 1981; Mirelman, 1986). *Haemophilus influenzae* attaches to the respiratory tract mucosa via fimbriae that have been suggested to recognize *N*-acetylglucosamine β(1-3)-galactose-containing glycolipids (van Alphen *et al.*, 1986; Krivans *et al.*, 1988). *Pseudomonas aeruginosa* has both fimbria-associated and independent adherence. Attachment of these cells to nasopharyngeal epithelium is fimbria-mediated and inhibited by acetylneuraminic acid. The attachment to respiratory tract cells is determined by alginate or proteins associated with the alginate that specifically recognize gangliotri- and gangliotetraosylceramide, as well as lactosylceramide (Baker and Svanborg-Edén, 1989; Baker *et al.*, 1990). The attachment of *Vibrio cholerae* to intestinal mucosa is inhibited by fucose, but the receptor epitope remains to be identified (Jones and Feter, 1976). *Neisseria gonorrhoeae* binds to a subset of lactose-containing glycolipids, as does the nonvirulent variant *Neisseria subflava* (Nyberg *et al.*, 1990). *Actinomyces naeslundii* and *Actinomyces viscosus* bind lactosyl ceramide (Strömberg and Karlsson, 1990). The adherence of *Actinomyces* to salivary pellicles was found to be sensitive to *N*-acetylgalactosamine β, but with variation in affinity for different *N*-acetylgalactosamine-containing glycoconjugates (Strömberg and Karlsson, 1990; N. Strömberg, T. Boren, A. Carlén, and J. Olsson, unpublished observations). This list might be extended considerably.

III. FUNCTIONAL CONSEQUENCES OF ADHERENCE

The simplest outcome of bacterial attachment is the mechanical association of bacteria with the receptor-bearing surface. This result may be sufficient if the attached state promotes bacterial multiplication and permits the attached cells to reach higher numbers than the unattached bacteria, which are washed away by the flow of secretions (Zobell, 1943; Gibbons, 1973; Zafriri *et al.*, 1987). Attachment is, however, also a way for pathogens to gain access to the host mucosal tissues. Further, attachment may trigger changes in the receptor-bearing target cell such as effacing lesions of microvilli, cytokine production, or invasion into or through epithelial cells (for review, see Gibbons, 1973; Beachey, 1981; Orskov and Orskov, 1983).

A. Adherence and Toxicity

The crucial role of adherence for virulence first was demonstrated in two models—diarrhea caused by K88-bearing *E. coli* in piglets (Smith and Halls, 1967; Smith and Lingood, 1972; Stirm *et al.*, 1967) and experimental cholera infection in mice (Freter, 1969). *Escherichia coli* causing diarrhea in newborn piglets carried a virulence plasmid encoding the K88 fimbrial adhesin and the exotoxin. Deletion of the plasmid abolished virulence. Mutation of genes encoding the toxin or the K88 adhesin permitted experiments to assess their relative contribution to virulence. The toxin-negative mutant colonized the intestine and caused minor discomfort, but not overt disease, in the piglets. The K88-negative mutant did not colonize or cause disease. Consequently, both adherence and toxin production are required for disease to occur.

Vaccination studies with *V. cholerae* gave similar results. Vaccinated animals were protected against cholera, but carried the same number of *V. cholerae* in their large intestine. However, the bacteria were localized in the lumen rather than adjacent to the mucosal surface (Freter, 1969). Antibodies that prevented adherence protected the animals. Similarly, piglets that received anti-K88 antibodies in milk were protected from infection (Sellwood *et al.*, 1975).

The synergy between adhesin and toxin since has been observed in a variety of models (Sansonetti, 1991; Burroughs *et al.*, 1992). Adherence is presumed to enhance toxicity by approaching the bacteria to the mucosal surface in such a manner that toxin delivery to the epithelial cells becomes more effective (Smith and Halls, 1967; Freter, 1969; Jones and Rutter, 1972; Smith and Lingood, 1972). Adherence also has been shown to enhance the effect of endotoxins. Whereas lipid A alone and P fimbriae alone can trigger a mucosal inflammatory response, the magnitude of the response is enhanced by the combination of P fimbriae and lipid A (Linder *et al.*, 1991).

B. Attaching Bacteria Elicit Mucosal Cytokine Production

Bacterial products stimulate cytokine production. Molecules such as endotoxin can activate cytokine production in a variety of cells including fibroblasts, monocytes, and lymphocytes. Indeed, many of the clinical signs of gram-negative septicemia may be prevented by compounds that inhibit tumor necrosis factor (TNF) and interleukin 1 (IL-1) (Tracey *et al.*, 1987; Michie *et al.*, 1988; Hirano *et al.*, 1990;

Starnes *et al.*, 1990). Septicemia is, however, a rare event. In most cases, the indigenous gram-negative flora and pathogens are carried at the mucosal level, where they attach and exert the majority of their effects.

The existence of a mucosal cytokine response to gram-negative bacteria first was recognized in patients and in experimental infection models. An IL-6 response occurred in mice within minutes of intravesial instillation of *E. coli* bacteria (de Man *et al.*, 1989). Even mucosal exposure to dead bacteria or isolated P fimbriae elicited an IL-6 response (Linder *et al.*, 1991). No elevation of the circulating cytokine levels was seen (de Man *et al.*, 1989; Hedges *et al.*, 1991). In humans, deliberate colonization of the urinary tract with *E. coli* bacteria caused an increase in the urinary IL-6 and IL-8 levels (Hedges *et al.*, 1991; W. Agace *et al.*, 1993). No concomitant elevation of the serum cytokines was measured, however, and no induction of symptoms was noted. Patients with natural episodes of urinary tract infection also were found to secrete IL-6 into the urine (Hedges *et al.*, 1992). Elevated urinary IL-6 levels were found in most individuals with bacteriuria, regardless of the type of bacteria that caused the infection. Children infected with P fimbriated bacteria had a higher cytokine response than other children (M. Benson, U. Jodal, Å. Karlsson, A. Andreasson, and C. Svanborg, unpublished observations), but no significant difference in mucosal cytokine production related to bacterial adherence was seen in adults. Elevated serum IL-6 levels were seen only in patients with systemic infections who had fever and acute phase reactants. These observations are consistent with the hypothesis that attaching bacteria elicit a local cytokine response and that spread of cytokines from the mucosal site of infection to systemic sites can cause some of the symptoms associated with mucosal infections.

Epithelial cells constitute one source of the mucosal cyto kines. Cytokine production was shown for epithelial cell lines in culture and for exfoliated epithelial cells. Their constitutive IL-6 secretion was up-regulated by *in vitro* stimulation with *E. coli* bacteria (Hedges *et al.*, 1990). Cytokine production by epithelial cells has since been analyzed by a variety of techniques (Kvale *et al.*, 1988; Hedges *et al.*, 1990,1992a,b; Mayer *et al.*, 1992; Moro *et al.*, 1992; W. Agace *et al.*, 1993.) Attaching bacteria elicited a higher cytokine response in epithelial cell lines than did nonattaching bacteria. The IL-6 response was stimulated even by isolated P fimbriae of the F7 type with the ability to bind the globoseries of glycolipids. These organisms triggered a significantly higher IL-6 response than the same fimbriae that had lost the receptor-binding domain (Hedges *et al.*, 1992a). Type 1 fimbriae enhanced the IL-8 response of epithelial cell lines to *E. coli* (W. Agace *et al.*, 1993). These observations suggest that the bacterial adherence properties influence the epithelial cytokine response.

Epithelial cells also respond to cytokine stimulation. Interferon γ stimulation up-regulated the expression of secretory component and HLA-II antigens in HT29 cells (Kvale *et al.*, 1988; Moro *et al.*, 1992). This secondary cytokine production may be relevant in at least two situations. First, the epithelial cell cytokines that are triggered by the bacteria and released at the local site may stimulate adjacent cells. Second, cells such as lymphocytes, granulocytes, and macrophages, which migrate to the site of infection and release their cytokines at this site, may influence the cytokine profile of the epithelial cells. Epithelial cells therefore play a more active role in the cytokine network than previously has been understood.

IV. ANTI-ADHESIVE MUCOSAL DEFENSE MECHANISMS

Early studies demonstrated that secretory IgA antibodies inhibit bacterial attachment. This property of IgA has been discussed as a major protective mechanism of mucosal antibodies (Freter, 1969; Sellwood *et al.*, 1975). Are individuals who lack mucosal antibody production or antibody responses in general overwhelmed by mucosal infections? Clinical observations in such patient groups do not support such an idea. Individuals with hypogammaglobulinemia mainly acquire recurrent upper respiratory tract infections with encapsulated bacteria. IgA-deficient individuals have an increased morbidity in mucosal infections such as traveler's diarrhea but rarely suffer from recurrent mucosal infections (World Health Organization, 1992).

This apparent contradiction probably reflects the fact that the mucosal surfaces are equipped with multiple defense systems that cooperate to control bacterial attachment. Not only sIgA antibodies but also secreted molecules of a nonimmunoglobulin nature interfere with bacterial adherence. Soluble glycoconjugates carry the same oligosaccharide epitopes as cell-bound receptors, but function as competitive inhibitors when secreted. By occupying receptor binding sites on the fimbriae, they prevent subsequent attachment to the cell-bound receptors (Holmgren *et al.*, 1981; Andersson *et al.*, 1986; Askenazi and Mirelman, 1987; Leffler and Svanborg-Edén, 1990; Schroten *et al.*, 1992).

The anti-adhesive antibodies may act in either of two ways: (1) Antibodies to the receptor binding site of the adhesin competitively inhibit receptor interactions. (2) Antibodies to bacterial surface molecules that are not directly involved in adherence may interfere with the binding. This interference is illustrated by the immune response to bacterial fimbriae. The majority of antibodies elicited by fimbriated bacteria are directed against the antigenically variable fimbrial subunit protein and interferes with attachment only at concentrations high enough to cause agglutination (Svanborg-Edén *et al.*, 1981). A minor fraction of antibodies is directed against the receptor binding lectin and, when purified, such antibodies block adherence (de Ree *et al.*, 1987; Hoschötzky *et al.*, 1989). In either case, the anti-adhesive activity of the antibody is attributed to the specificity of the antigen-combining site.

IgA also can act as a soluble receptor for bacterial adhesins (Wold *et al.*, 1990), a characteristic that is explained by mannose residues on oligosaccharide sequences on the heavy chain (Kornfeld and Kornfeld, 1976). The type 1 fimbriated *E. coli* agglutinates colostral IgA, with a higher titer for IgA2 than IgA1. Type 1 fimbriated *E. coli* also agglutinate IgA2 and IgA1 myeloma proteins, which lack specific antibody activity against *E. coli* (Wold *et al.*, 1990). The IgA2 myelomas that give the highest agglutination titer with type 1 fimbriated strains were rich in high-mannose oligosaccharides. In contrast, the concentration of such oligosaccharides was low in the less active IgA1 myeloma proteins. The agglutination was inhibited by mannose. Myeloma IgA2 as well as colostral IgA inhibits the attachment of type 1 fimbriated *E. coli* to epithelial cells, providing a mechanism for IgA to be broadly protective regardless of the antigen specificity of the antigen-combining site of the molecule.

Human milk is rich in glycoconjugates and has been used as a source for the purification of nonimmunoglobulin glycoproteins with anti-adhesive activity. Holmgren *et al.* (1981) showed that the nonimmunoglobulin fraction of human milk was able to inhibit the colonization factor antigen-mediated agglutination of human erythrocytes by *E. coli* (Andersson *et al.*, 1986). Askenazi and Mirelman (1987) found similar results for adhesion to guinea pig intestinal epithelia. Human milk was shown to inhibit the attachment of S fimbriated *E. coli* to buccal epithelial cells. The inhibition was suggested to be mediated by carbohydrate residues on secreted mucins of breast milk (Schroten *et al.*, 1992). The molecular mechanisms of these anti-adhesive interactions have, however, not been defined in detail.

Andersson *et al.* (1983) showed that human milk inhibits the adherence of the respiratory tract pathogens *Streptococcus pneumoniae* and *H. influenzae* to human respiratory tract epithelial cells. The anti-adhesive effect is retained after removal of IgA by immunoabsorption. Further, milks from IgA-deficient donors block adherence. Several anti-adhesive components have been identified, including the free oligosaccharides in the low molecular weight fraction and glycoproteins (Andersson *et al.*, 1983) that coprecipitate with casein.

V. MUCOSAL RECEPTOR REPERTOIRE

Mucosal receptor expression can influence the susceptibility of infection, as was first documented in the *E. coli* K88 piglet diarrhea model. Susceptibility to diarrhea was inherited as an autosomal recessive trait and was determined by the presence of receptors in the *E. coli*-colonized intestine of piglets that expressed the receptors. These piglets were susceptible to infection. The piglets that did not express receptors were not colonized and were resistant to infection (Sellwood *et al.*, 1975).

The double identity of the globoseries of glycolipids as blood group antigens and as receptors for P fimbriae has provided a basis to analyze the role of receptor expression in infection. Individuals of the p blood group phenotype lack a glycosyltransferase required to add the galactose α(1-4)-galactose β polysaccharide to glycoproteins and glycolipids. Cells from p individuals therefore lack functional receptors for P fimbriated *E. coli*. Unfortunately, the frequency of p individuals is too low to permit a direct evaluation of their relative morbidity and mortality in infections caused by P fimbriated *E. coli*. However, qualitative differences in receptor expression exist among P blood group positive individuals. P_1 individuals have a higher intestinal carrier rate of P fimbriated *E. coli* than P_2 individuals. Individuals of the P_1 blood group run an ~11-fold higher relative risk of attracting recurrent kidney infections than P_2 individuals (Lomberg *et al.*, 1983).

The subgroup of P fimbriated *E. coli* that carries the *prs* adhesin also shows host selectivity (Lindstedt *et al.*, 1991). One subgroup of P fimbriae requires globo-A for binding. Although all except the p individuals express the P antigen, only A_1 secretor individuals also express the globo-A glycolipid. The P fimbriae that recognize this receptor structure, attach mainly to uro-epithelial cells from A_1 secretor individuals, and mainly infect A_1 positive individuals (100% blood group A positive compared with 43% in the population at large).

References

Andersson, B., Dahmén, J., Freijd, T., Leffler, H., Magnusson, G., Noori, G., and Svanborg, C. (1983). Identification of an active disaccharide unit of a glycoconjugate receptor for pneumococci attaching to human pharyngeal epithelial cells. *J. Exp. Med.* **158,** 559–570.

Andersson, B., Porras, O., Hanson, L. Å., Lagergård, T., and Svanborg-Edén, C. (1986). Inhibition of attachment of *Streptococcus pneumoniae* and *Haemophilus influenzae* by human milk and receptor oligosaccharides. *J. Infect. Dis.* **153,** 232–237.

Askenazi, S., and Mirelman, D. (1987). Non-immunoglobulin fractoin of human milk inhibits the adherence of certain enterotoxigenic *Escherichia coli* strains to guinea pig intestinal tract. *Pediatr. Res.* **22,** 130–134.

Agace, W., Andersson, J., Andersson, U., Ceska, M., Hedges, S. and Svanborg, C. (1993). Selective cytokine production by epithelial cells following exposure to *E. coli*. *Infection Immunity,* **61,** 602–609.

Agace, W., Hedges, S., Ceska, M. and Svanborg, C. Interleukin-8 and the neutrophil response in mucosal gram-negative infections. *J. Clin. Invest.* in press.

Baker, N., and Svanborg-Edén, C. (1989). Role of alginate in the adherence of *Pseudomonas aeruginosa*. *Antibiotic Chemother.* **42,** 72–79.

Baker, N., Hansson, G. C., Leffler, H., Riise, G., and Svanborg-Edén, C. (1990). Glycosphingolipid receptors for *Pseudomonas aeruginosa*. *Infect. Immun.* **58,** 2361–2366.

Bar Shavit, Z., Ofek, I., Goldman, R., Mirelman, D., and Sharon, N. (1977). Mannose residues on phagocytes as receptors for the attachment of *Escherichia coli* and *Salmonella typhi*. *Biochem. Biophys. Res. Commun.* **78,** 455–460.

Beachey, E. H., (1981). Adhesin-receptor interactions mediating the attachment of bacteria to mucosal surfaces *J. Infect. Dis.* **143,** 325–345.

Berger, E. G., Buddecke, E., Kamerling, J. P., Kobata, A., Paulson, J. C., and Vliegenthart, J. F. G. (1982). Structure, biosynthesis and functions of glycoprotein glycans. *Experientia* **38,** 1129–1162.

Bock, K., Breimer, M. E., Brignole, A., Hansson, G. C., Karlsson, K.-A., Larson, G., Leffler, H., Samuelsson, B. E., Strömberg, N., Svanborg-Edén, C., and Thurin, J. (1985). Specificity of binding of a strain of uropathogenic *Escherichia coli* to Galα1-4Galβ-containing glycosphingolipids. *J. Biol. Chem.* **260,** 8545–8551.

Brinton, C. C. (1965). The structure function, synthesis and genetic control of bacterial pili, and a molecular model of DNA and RNA transport in gram-negative bacteria. *Trans. N.Y. Acad. Sci.* **27,** 1003–1054.

Burroughs, M., Cabellos, C., Prasad, S., and Tuomanen, E. (1992). Bacterial components and the pathophysiology of injury to the blood-brain barrier: Does cell wall add to the effects of endotoxin in Gram-negative meningitis? *J. Infect. Dis.* **165,** 82–89.

Caugant, D. W., Levin, B., Örskov, I., Örskov, F., Selander, R. K., and Svanborg-Edén, C. (1985). Genetic diversity in relation to serotype in *Escherichia coli. Infect. Immun.* **49,** 407–413.

Clegg, S. (1982). Cloning of genes determining the production of mannose-resistant fimbriae in a uropathogenic strain of *Escherichia coli* belonging to serogroup O6. *Infect. Immun.* **38,** 739–744.

de Man, P., Aarden, L., Engberg, I., Linder, H., Svanborg-Edén, C., and van Kooten, C. (1989). Interleukin-9 induced at mucosal surfaces by gram-negative bacterial infection. *Infect. Immun.* **57,** 3383–3388.

de Ree, I. M., Schwillens, P., and van den Bosch, J. F. (1987). Monoclonal antibodies raised against *pap* fimbriae recognize minor component(s) involved in receptor binding. *Microbiol. Pathogen.* **2,** 113–121.

Duguid, J. P., Dempster, G., Edmund, P. N., and Smith, I. W. (1955). Nonflagellar filamentous appendages ("fimbriae") and haemagglutinating activity in *Bacterium coli. J. Pathol. Bacteriol.* **70,** 335–348.

Duguid, J. P., Cleff, S., and Wilson, M. I. (1979). The fimbrial and nonfimbrial haemagglutinations of *Escherichia coli. J. Med. Microbiol.* **12,** 213–227.

Eisenstein, B. I. (1981). Phase variation of type 1 fimbriae in *Escherichia coli* is under transcriptional control. *Science* **214,** 337–339.

Freter, R. (1969). Studies on the mechanism of action of intestinal antibody in experimental cholera. *Texas Rep. Biol. Med.* **27,** 299–316.

Gibbons, R. J. (1973). Bacterial adherence in infection and immunity. *Rev. Microbiol.* **4,** 49–60.

Gibbons, R. J., and von Houte, J. (1971). Selective bacterial adherence to oral epithelial surfaces and its role as an ecological determinant. *Infect. Immun.* **3,** 567–573.

Gibbons, R. J., and Van Houte, J. (1975). Bacterial adherence in oral microbial ecology. *Ann. Rev. Microbiol.* **29,** 19–44.

Hakomori, S.-I. (1983). Chemistry of glycosphingolipids. *In* "Sphingolipid Biochemistry" (J. N. Kanfer and S.-I. Hakomori, eds.), vol. 3, pp. 1–165. Plenum Press, New York.

Hanson, M. S., Hempel, J., and Brinton, C. C. Jr. (1988). Purification of the *Escherichia coli* type 1 pilin and minor pilus proteins and partial characterization of the adhesin protein. *J. Bacteriol.* **170,** 3350–3358.

Hedges, S., de Man, P., Linder, H., Svanborg-Edén, C., and van Kooten, C. (1990). Interleukin-6 is secreted by epithelial cells in response to Gram-negative bacterial challenge. *In* "Advances in Mucosal Immunology" (T. MacDonald *et al.*, eds.), pp. 144–148. International Conference of Mucosal Immunity. Kluwer, London.

Hedges, S., Anderson, P., Lidin-Janson, G., de Man, P., and Svanborg, C. (1991). Interleukin-6 response to deliberate colonization of the human urinary tract with gram-negative bacteria. *Infect. Immun.* **59,** 421–427.

Hedges, S., Svanborg, C., and Svensosn, M. (1992a). Interleukin-6 response of epithelial cell lines to bacterial stimulation *in vitro. Infect. Immun.* **60,** 1295–1301.

Hedges, S., Svensson, M., Agace, W., and Svanborg, C. (1992b). Cytokines induce and epithelial cell cytokine response. 7th International Congress of Mucosal Immunology, Prague. (Abstract)

Hedges, S., Lidin-Janson, G., Martinell, J., Sandberg, T., Stenqvist, K., and Svanborg, C. (1992c). Comparison of urine and serum concentrations of interleukin-6 in women with acute pyelonephritis or asymptomatic bacteriuria. *J. Infect. Dis.* **166,** 653–656.

Hirano, T., Akira, S., Taga, T., and Kishimoto, T. (1990). Biological and clinical aspects of interleukin-6. *Immunol. Today* **11,** 443–449.

Holmgren, J., Svennerholm, A. M., and Ahren, C. (1981). Non-immunoglobulin fraction of human milk inhibits bacterial adhesion (haemagglutination) and enterotoxin binding of *Escherichia coli* and *Vibrio cholerae. Infect. Immun.* **33,** 136–141.

Hoschützky, H., Lottspeich, F., and Jann, K. (1989). Isolation and characterization of the α-Galactosyl-1,4-β-galactosyl specific adhesin (Padhesin) from fimbriated *Escherichia coli. Infect. Immun.* **57,** 76–81.

Hull, R. A., Gill, R. E., Hsu, P., Minshew, B. H., and Falkow, S. (1981). Construction and expression of recombinant plasmids encoding type 1 or D-mannose resistant pili from the urinary tract infection *Escherichia coli* isolate. *Infect. Immun.* **33,** 933–938.

Hultgren, S. J., Lindberg, F., Magnusson, G., Kihlberg, J., Tennent, J. M., and Normark, S. (1989). The *pap*G adhesin of uropathogenic *Escherichia coli* contains separate regions for receptor binding and for the incorporation into the pilus. *Proc. Nat. Acad. Sci. U.S.A.* **86.** 4357–4361.

Jann, K., and Hoschützky, H. (1989). Nature and organization of adhesins. *Curr. Top. Microbiol. Immunol.* **151,** 55–70.

Johanson, I. M., Lindstedt, R., and Svanborg, C. (1992). Roles of the *pap* and *prs* encoded adhesins in *Escherichia coli* adherence to human uroepithelial cells. *Infect. Immun.* **60,** 3416–3422.

Johanson, I. M., Plus, K., Jodal, V., Masklund, B. I., Mårild, S., Svanburg-Edén, C., and Wettergren, B. (1993). *Microbial. Pathogenesis,* in press.

Johnson, J. R. (1991). Virulence factors in *Escherichia coli* urinary tract infection. *Clin. Microb. Rev.* **4,** 80–128.

Jones, G. W., and Freter, R. (1976). Adhesive properties of *Vibrio cholerae*. Nature of the interaction with isolated rabbit brush border membranes and human erythrocytes. *Infect. Immun.* **14,** 240–245.

Jones, G. W., and Rutter, J. M. (1972). Role of the K88 antigen in the pathogenesis of neonatal diarrhoea caused by *Escherichia coli* in piglets. *Infect. Immun.* **6,** 918–927.

Källenius, G., Cedergren, B., Möllby, R., and Svensson, S. B. (1980). The pk antigen as receptors for the hemagglutination of pyelonephritis *Escherichia coli. FEMS Microbiol. Lett.* **7,** 297–302.

Karr, J. F., Nowicki, B., Truong, L. D., Hull, R. A., and Hull, S. I. (1989). Purified P fimbriae from two cloned gene clusters of a single pyelonephritogenic strain adhere to unique structures in the human kidney. *Infect. Immun.* **57,** 3594–3600.

Klemm, P. (1985). Fimbrial adhesins. *Rev. Infect. Dis.* **7,** 321–340.

Klemm, P. (1986). Two regulatory *fim* genes, *fim*B and *fim*E, control the phase variation of type 1 fimbriae in *Escherichia coli. EMBO J.* **5,** 1389–1393.

Kornfeld, R., and Kornfeld, S. (1976). Comparative aspects of glycoprotein structure. *Annu. Rev. Biochem.* **45,** 217–233.

Krivans, H. C., Roberts, D. D., and Ginsburg, V. (1988). Many pulmonary pathogenic bacteria bind specifically to the carbohydrate sequence GalNAcβ-1-4Gal found in some glycolipids. *Proc. Natl. Acad. Sci. U.S.A.* **85,** 6157–6161.

Kvale, D., Brandtzaeg, P., and Lövhaug, D. (1988). Up-regulation of the expression of secretory component and HLA molecules in a human colonic cell line by tumour necrosis factor-α and gamma-interferon. *Scand. J. Immunol.* **28,** 351–357.

Leffler, H., and Svanborg-Edén, C. (1980). Chemical identification of a glycosphingolipid receptor for *Escherichia coli* attaching to human urinary tract epithelial cells and agglutinating human erythrocytes. *FEMS Microbiol. Lett.* **8,** 127–134.

Leffler, H., and Svanborg-Edén, C. (1981). Glycolipid receptors for uropathogenic *Eschericha coli* on human erythrocytes and uroepithelial cells. *Infect. Immun.* **34,** 920–929.

Leffler, H., and Svanborg-Edén, C. (1986). Glycolipids as receptors for *Escherichia coli* lectins or adhesins. *In* "Microbial Lectins and Agglutinins" (D. Mirelman, ed.). pp. 83–111. John Wiley and Sons, New York.

Leffler, H., and Svanborg-Edén, C. (1990). Host epithelial glycoconjugates and pathogenic bacteria. *Am. J. Respir. Cell Biol.* **2,** 409–411.

Leffler, H., Svanborg-Edén, C., Schoolnik, G., and Wadström, T. (1983). Glycosphingolipids as receptors for bacterial adhesion: Host glycolipid diversity and other selected aspects. (E. C Boedekker, ed.), Vol. II, pp. 177–187. CRC Press, Boca Raton, Florida.

Lindberg, F., Lund, B., Johansson, L., and Normark, S. (1987). Localization of the receptor-binding protein adhesin at the tip of the bacterial pilus. *Nature (London)* **328,** 84–87.

Linder, H., Engberg, I., Hoschützky, H., Mattsby-Baltzer, I., and Svanborg, C. (1991). Adhesion-dependent activation of mucosal Interleukin-6 production. *Infect. Immun.* **59,** 4357–4362.

Lindstedt, R., Baker, N., Hull, R., Hull, S., Karr, J., Leffler, H., Svanborg-Edén, C., and Larson G. (1989). Binding specificities of wild-type and cloned *Escherichia coli* strains that recognize globo-A. *Infect. Immun.* **57,** 3389–3394.

Lindstedt, R., Larson, G., Falk, P., Jodal, U., Leffler, H., and Svanborg, C. (1991). The receptor repertoire defines the host range for attaching *E. coli* recognizing globo-A. *Infect. Immun.* **59.** 1086–1091.

Lomberg, H., Hanson, L. Å., Jacobsson, B., Jodal, U., Leffler, H., and Svanborg-Edén, C. (1983). Correlation of P blood group vesicoureteral reflux and bacterial attachment in patients with recurrent pyelonephritis. *N. Engl. J. Med.* **308,** 1189–1192.

Lund, B., Marklund, B.-I., Strömberg, N., Lindberg, F., Karlsson, K.-A., and Normark, S. (1988). Uropathogenic *Escherichia coli* can express serologically identical pili of different receptor binding specificities. *Mol. Microbiol.* **2,** 255–263.

Mayer, L., Kalb, T., and Panja, A. (1992). Accessory cell function by respiratory epithelium: Not the gut that breathes. 7th International Congress of Mucosal Immunology, Prague. (Abstract.)

Michie, H. R., Manogue, K. R., Spriggs, D. R., Revhaug, A., O'Dwyer, S., Dinarello, C. A., Cerami, A., Wolff, S. M., and Wilmore, D. W. (1988). Detection of circulating tumor necrosis after endotoxin administration. *N. Engl. J. Med.* **318,** 1481–1486.

Minion, F. C., Abraham, S. N., Beachey, E. H., and Gougen, J. D. (1986). The genetic determinant of adhesive function in type 1 fimbriae of *Escherichia coli* is distinct from the gene encoding the fimbrial subunit. *J. Bacteriol.* **165,** 1033–1036.

Mirelman, D. ed. (1986). "Microbial Lectins and Agglutinins." John Wiley and Sons, New York.

Moro, I., Takahashi, T., Iwase, T., Krajci, P., Brandtzaeg, P., Modoveanu, A., and Mestecky, J. (1992). Expression of SC, IL-6 and TGR-b1 in epithelial cell lines. 7th International Congress of Mucosal Immunology, Prague. (Abstract)

Norgren, M., Båga, M., Falkow, S., Lark, D., Normark, S., O'Hanley, P., Schoolnik, G., Svanborg-Edén, C., and Uhlin B.-E. (1984). Mutations in *E. coli* cistrons affecting adhesion to human cells do not abolish *pap* pili fiber formation. *EMBO J.* **3,** 1159–1165.

Norgren, M., Båga, M., Normark, S., and Tennent, J. M. (1987). Nucleotide sequence, regulation and functional analysis of the *pap* C gene required for cell surface localization of *pap* pili of uropathogenic *Escherichia coli. Mol. Microbiol.* **1,** 169–178.

Nyberg, G., Strömberg, N., Jonsson, A., Karlsson, K.-A., and Normark, S. (1990). Erythrocyte gangliosides act as receptors for *Neisseria subflava:* Identification of the Sia-1 adhesin. *Infect. Immun.* **58,** 2555–2563.

Ofek, I., Mirelman, D., and Sharon, N. (1985). Adherence of *Escherichia coli* to human mucosal cells mediated by mannose receptors. *Nature (London)* **265,** 623–625.

Öhman, L., Hed, J., and Stendahl, O. (1982). Interaction between human polymorphonuclear leukocytes and two different strains of type 1 fimbriae-bearing *Escherichia coli. J. Infect. Dis.* **146,** 751–757.

Orskov,, F., and Orskov, I. (1983). Summary of a workshop on the clone concept in the epidemiology, taxonomy, and evoluation of the Enterobacteriaceae and other bacteria. *J. Infect. Dis.* **148,** 346–357.

Orskov, F., Jann, B., Jann, K., and Orskov, I. (1980). Tamm-Horsefall protein or uromucoid is the normal urinary slime that traps type 1 fimbriated *Escherichia coli. Lancet* **1,** 8173.

Orskov, I., Orskov, F., Sojka, W. J., and Leach, J. M., (1961). Simultaneous occurrence of *E. coli* B and L antigens in strains from diseases swine. *Acta Path. Microbiol. Scand.* **53,** 404–409.

Parkkinen, J., Virkola, R., and Korhonen, T. K. (1988). Identification of factors in human urine that inhbit the binding of *Escherichia coli* adhesins. *Infect. Immun.* **56,** 2623–2630.

Paulson, J. C. (1985). Interactions of animal viruses with cell surface receptors. *In* "The Receptors" (P. M. Conn, ed.), Vol. 2, pp. 131–219. Academic Press, London.

Pere, A., Korhonen, T. K., Nowicki, B., Saxén, H., and Siitonen, A. (1987). Expression of P, type 1 and type 1 C fimbriae of *Escherichia coli* in the urine of patients with acute urinary tract infection. *J. Infect. Dis.* **156,** 567–574.

Rhen, M., Korhonen, T. K., and Mäkelä, H. (1983). P-fimbriae of *Escherichia coli* are subject to phase variation. *FEMS Microbiol. Lett.* **19,** 267–271.

Sansonetti, P. J. (1991). Genetic and molecular basis of epithelial cell invasion by shigelle species. *Rev. Infect. Dis.* **13,** 285–292.

Savage, D. C. (1984). Overview of the association of microbes with epithelial surfaces. *Microecol. Ther.* **14,** 169–182.

Savage, D. C. (1988). "The Regulatory and Protective Role of the Normal Microflora." MacMillan, London.

Schroten, H., Hanisch, F. G., Plogmann, R., Hacker, J., Uhlenbruck, G., Nobis-Bosch, R., and Wahn, V. (1992). Inhibition of adhesion of S-fimbriated *Escherichia coli* to buccal epithelial cells by human milk fat globule membrane components: A novel aspect of the protective function of mucins in the nonimmunoglobulin fraction. *Infect. Immun.* **60,** 2893–2899.

Sellwood, R., Gibbons, R. A. Jones, G. W., and Rutter, J. M. (1975). Adhesin of enteropathogenic *Escherichia coli* to pig intestinal brush borders: The existence of two pig phenotypes. *J. Med. Microbiol.* **8,** 405–411.

Smith, H. W., and Halls, S. (1967). Observations by the ligated intestinal segment and oral inoculation methods on *Escherichia coli* infections in pigs, calves, lambs and rabbits. *J. Pathol. Bacteriol.* **93,** 499–529.

Smith, H. W., and Lingood, M. A. (1972). Further observations on *Escherichia coli* enterotoxins with particular regard to those produced by atypicl piglet strains and by calf and lambs strains: The transmissible nature of these enterotoxins and of a K antigen possessed by calf and lamb strains. *J. Med. Microbiol.* **5,** 243–250.

Starnes, H. F., Pearce, M. K., Tewari, A., Yim, J. H., Zou, J.-C., and Abrams, J. C. (1990). Anti-IL-6 monoclonal antibodies protect against lethal *Escherichia coli* infection and lethal tumor necrosis factor-α challenge in mice. *J. Immunol.* **145,** 4185–4191.

Strömberg, N., and Karlsson, K.-A. (1990). Characterization of the binding of *Actinomyces naeslundii* (ATCC 12104) and *Actinomyces viscosus* (ATC 19246) to glycosphingolipids, using a solid-phase overlay approach. *J. Biol. Chem.* **265,** 11251–11258.

Strömberg, N., Marklund, B.-I., Lund, B., Ilver, D., Hamers, A., Gaastra, W., Karlsson, K.-A., and Normark, S. (1990). Host-specificity of uropathogenic *Escherichia coli* depends on differences in binding specificity to Galα1-4Galβ-containing isoreceptors. *EMBO J.* **9,** 2001–2010.

Svanborg-Edén, C., and Leffler, H. (1979). Glycosphingolipids of human urinary tract epithelial cells as possible receptors for adhering *Escherichia coli* bacteria. *Scand. J. Infect. Dis.* **24,** 144–149.

Svanborg-Edén, C., and Levin, B. (1988). Infectious disease and natural selection in human populations: A critical reexamination. *In* "Disease and Populations in Transition: Anthropological and Epidemiological Considerations" (A. Swedlund and G. Armelagosen, eds.). Bergen and Garber, South Hadley, Massachusetts.

Svanborg-Edén, C., Fasth, A., Hagberg, L., Hanson, L. Å., Korhonen, T. A., and Leffler, H. (1981). Host interaction with *Eschericha coli* in urinary tract. *In* "Bacterial Vaccines". (R. Robbins, J. Hill, and J. Sadof, eds.), pp. 113–133. Thieme-Stratton, New York.

Svanborg-Edén, C., Bjursten, L. M., and Hull, R. (1984). Influence of adhesins on the interaction of *Escherichia coli* with human phagocytes. *Infect. Immun.* **44,** 407–413.

Svanborg-Edén, C., Hull, S., Leffler, H., Norgren, S., Plos, K., and Wold, A. (1988a). Attachment of organisms to the gut mucosa. "The Regulatory and Protective Role of the Normal Microflora" (D. C. Savage, ed.), pp. 47–58. MacMillan, London.

Svanborg-Edén, C., Hansson, S., Jodal, U., Lidin-Janson, G., Lincoln, K., Linder, H., Lomberg, H., de Man P., Mårild, S., Martinell, J., Plos, K., Sandberg, T., and Stenqvist, K. (1988b). Host–parasite interaction in the urinary tract. *J. Infect. Dis.* **157,** 421–426.

Tennent, J. M., Lindberg, F., and Normark, S. (1990). Integrity of *Escherichia coli* P pili during biogenesis: Properties and role of *pap*. *J. Mol. Microbiol.* **4,** 747–758.

Tracey, K. J., Fong, Y., Hesse, D. G., Manogue, K. R., Lee, A. T., Kuo, G. C., Lowry, S. F., and Cerami, A. (1987). Anticachectin/TNF monoclonal antibodies prevent septic shock during lethal bacteremia. *Nature (London)* **330,** 662–664.

Uhlin, B.-E., Båga, M., Norgren, M., and Normark, S. (1985). Adhesion to human cells by *Escherichia coli* lacking the major subunit of a digalactoside-specific pilus-adhesin. *Proc. Natl. Acad. Sci. U.S.A.* **82,** 1800–1804.

Väisänen-Rhen, V., Elo, J., Väisänen, E., Siitonen, A., Örskov, I., Örskov, F., Svenson, S. B., Mäkelä, P. H., and Korhonen, T. K. (1984). P-fimbriated clones among uropathogenic *Escherichia coli* strains. *Infect. Immun.* **43,** 149–155.

van Alphen, L., Poole, J., and Overbeeke, M. (1986). The Anton blood group antigen is the erythrocyte receptor for *Haemophilus influenzae*. *FEMS Microbiol. Lett.* **37,** 69–71.

van Die, I., and Bergmans, H. (1984). Nucleotide sequence of the gene encoding the F72 fimbrial subunit of a uropathogenic *Escherichia coli*. *Gene* **32,** 83–90.

van Heyningen, W. R. (1974). Gangliosides as membrane receptors for tetanus toxin, cholera toxin and serotinin. *Nature (London)* **249,** 415–417.

Wold, A., Endo, T., Kobata, A., Mestecky, J., Tomana, J. M., Ohbayashi, H., and Svanborg-Edén, C. (1990). Secretory immunoglobulin A carries oligosaccharide receptors for the *E. coli* type 1 fimbrial lectin. *Infect. Immun.* **58,** 3073–3077.

World Health Organization (1992). Primary immunodeficiency diseases. Report of a WHO Scientific Group. *Immunodeficiency Rev.* **3,** 195–236.

Zafriri, D., Oron, Y., Eisenstein, B., and Ofek, I. (1987). Growth advantage and enhanced toxicity of *Escherichia coli* adherence to tissue culture cells due to restricted diffusion of products secreted by the cells. *J. Clin. Invest.* **79,** 1210–1216.

Zobell, C. E. (1943). The effect of solid surfaces on bacterial activity. *J. Bacteriol.* **46,** 39–56.

7

Mucosal Immunoglobulins

Brian J. Underdown • Jiri Mestecky

I. INTRODUCTION

Interest in mucosal immunology as a field of study accelerated in the early 1960s with the discovery of IgA and its predominance in mucosal secretions (reviewed by Heremans, 1974; Tomasi, 1968). The subject has broadened considerably since that time, but the study of the structure and function of IgA, as well as the role of other antibody types in the external secretions, are still under active investigation.

Researchers generally agree that antibodies in mucosal secretions, particularly IgA, combine with microorganisms to reduce their motility, growth, and adhesive properties within the mucosal lumen and at its surface (Williams and Gibbons, 1972; Fubara and Freter, 1973; Winner *et al.,* 1991; see Chapter 11). These functions attenuate the ability of microorganisms to attach to the epithelium and subsequently enter the internal environment of the body. More recently, evidence has been presented that indicates that, during their transport to the mucosal lumen, poly IgA (pIgA) antibodies can combine with antigens and viruses that have entered mucosal epithelial cells (Kaetzel *et al.,* 1991; Mazanec *et al.* 1992).

The function of IgA within the blood circulation and lymph is less well established. IgA antibodies are capable of neutralizing viruses and agglutinating bacteria, but the extent to which these antibodies interact with inflammatory cells and the complement system to enhance the elimination and destruction of microorganisms is still under active investigation. Evidence even suggests that in systemic *Neisseria meningitidis* infections, serum IgA1 antibodies to polysaccharide antigens actually may attenuate IgG and complement-mediated destruction of bacteria (Jarvis and Griffiss, 1991). An additional property of circulating IgA appears to be the removal of antigen via the liver (Socken *et al.,* 1981; Russell *et al.,* 1981,1983).

This chapter reviews current knowledge on the structure and function of IgA, as well as highlighting features of the other immunoglobulin isotypes as they pertain to mucosal secretions.

II. IMMUNOGLOBULINS OF THE EXTERNAL SECRETIONS

The predominance of IgA in most mucosal secretions compared with blood is now well established. Table I summarizes some of the data reported in the literature for humans. In general, IgA is present in mucosal secretions in greater concentrations than are other immunoglobulin isotypes. However, note that marked species differences exist with respect to the preponderance of IgA in certain mucosal secretions, notably bile and mammary secretions. These differences (see Section II,C) may be important in the function of the mucosal immune system in particular species and may influence approaches to the study of mucosal immunity in experimental animals.

A. Secretory IgA

The importance of immunoglobulin A in mucosal secretions was based on two important discoveries: (1) the predominance of immunoglobulin A in intestinal secretions and saliva of humans and (2) the presence of an additional antigenic structure in secretory IgA that came to be known as secretory component (SC; Brandtzaeg, 1985). Subsequently, SC was recognized to be part of the poly Ig receptor (pIgR) that transports IgA from mucosal tissue to its secretions (Mostov *et al.,* 1984). During their ground-breaking work, (Tomasi and Bienenstock, 1968) noted that the IgA in human serum was primarily monomeric whereas in mucosal secretions it was primarily polymeric. Studies of other species indicate that the proportion of serum IgA that is polymeric can vary between less than 10 and 60% (Section II,C). (A schematic representation of the various forms of human serum and secretory IgA is provided in Figures 4 and 5 and is described more fully in Sections VI and VII.)

The majority of secretory IgA in humans is derived from local synthesis and not from the circulation (Jonard *et al.,* 1984). A relatively high proportion of Ig-producing cells in the mucosal lymphoid tissue is committed to the IgA isotype (Table I). This fact, in conjunction with the presence of the specific pIgR expressed on mucosal epithelial cells (Apodaca *et al.,* 1991), accounts for the high relative concentration of IgA in mucosal secretions.

B. Other Immunoglobulins in Secretions

IgM in the external secretions also is associated with SC, which results from its transport to the secretions by the pIgR (Brandtzaeg, 1985). However, the concentration of secretory IgM is substantially lower than that of secretory IgA because

Table I Isotype Distribution of Immunoglobulin and Cells in Selected Human Fluids and Tissue[a]

Fluid	Immunoglobulin concentration (mg/ml) IgG	IgA	IgM	Tissue	Distribution of Ig+ cells[b] IgG	IgA	IgM
Serum	12.0	3.0	1.5	Bone marrow	55	30	15
Milk	0.1	1.5	0.4	Mammary gland	4	86	10
Parotid saliva	0.004	0.04	0.006	Parotid gland	5	87	6
Jejunal fluid[c]	0.005	0.05	0.002	Jejunum	3	79	18
Hepatic bile	0.09	0.07	0.02	Lacrimal gland	6	77	7
Tears	0.007	0.19	0.006				

[a] Data are from Brown *et al.*, 1975; Delacroix *et al.*, 1982,1985; Brandtzaeg, 1983a,b; Jonard *et al.*, 1984; Allansmith *et al.*, 1985; Kett *et al.*, 1986.
[b] Determined by immunofluorescence.
[c] The concentration is influenced by the amount of perfusate fluid added to the secretion. In some studies, IgG concentration ~IgA.

of the lower proportion of IgM-producing cells in mucosal tissue. IgM also may not be transported as well as pIgA because of a molecular weight restriction in SC-dependent transport (Schiff *et al.*, 1983). On the other hand, a compensatory increase of IgM is observed in mucosal tissue and secretions of IgA-deficient individuals (Plebani *et al.*, 1983). In some species such as rodents and rabbits, SC-dependent transport of IgM may not occur (Underdown *et al.*, 1992).

In most species, the concentration of IgG in mucosal secretions is approximately the same as or somewhat greater than that of IgM. IgG is thought to enter the mucosal secretions nonspecifically via paracellular transport or fluid phase endocytosis. A notable exception is found in the ungulates (i.e., sheep, goats, cows) which, in addition to pIgA, selectively transport the IgG1 isotype from serum into selected secretions such as colostrum, milk, and saliva (Cripps and Lascelles, 1976; Butler, 1983).

IgE has been detected in relatively low concentrations in the respiratory and gastrointestinal secretions and often is associated with allergic responses at the mucosae (Brown *et al.*, 1975; Mygind *et al.*, 1975; Jonard *et al.*, 1984). Little evidence suggests that IgE is transported specifically to mucosal secretions. Perhaps increases in permeability of mucosal tissue as a result of allergic reactions increase the concentration of IgE in mucosal secretions.

Several reports indicate that low concentrations of IgD are found in milk and saliva; this may reflect selective synthesis but not facilitated transport to the mucosal secretions (Leslie and Teramura, 1977).

C. Species Variability with Respect to Mucosal Immunoglobulin

The information provided in Table I reflects data for humans. Several noteworthy differences exist among species.

i. Serum. In contrast to humans and nonhuman primates, the bone marrow in other mammals synthesizes negligible amounts of IgA. Instead, gastrointestinal tissue appears to be the primary source of serum IgA as well as secretory IgA (Vaerman *et al.*, 1973). Therefore, in most mammals the level of serum IgA is approximately 10-fold less than that observed in humans and nonhuman primates. In addition, the proportion of serum IgA that is polymeric is often higher in mammals such as mice, dogs, and guinea pigs, reflecting the contribution of the gastrointestinal tissue to serum IgA as well as the degree to which the pIgR is expressed on hepatocytes (Kaartinen *et al.*, 1978; Delacroix *et al.*, 1983).

ii. Bile. As reviewed previously (Underdown and Schiff, 1986), only a few species such as rabbit, rat, chicken, and mouse express pIgR on hepatocytes and have a highly active transport system to remove pIgA from blood to bile. The bile of these species is a rich source of secretory IgA and free SC, with concentrations in the range of 0.5–1.5 mg/ml. IgA is predominantly polymeric (Lemaitre-Coelho *et al*, 1977; Rose *et al.*, 1981). In contrast, other species including humans have lower concentrations of biliary IgA; the proportion of polymer to monomer is closer to unity. The mouse appears to be intermediate with respect to the level of hepatic transport of pIgA from serum. Clearly antibody-producing cells in the liver can contribute to bile IgA (Nagura *et al.*, 1983; Manning *et al.*, 1984; Jackson *et al.*, 1984; Altorfer *et al.*, 1987).

iii. Mammary gland secretions. The ungulates such as sheep, goats, and bovines express, in addition to pIgR, a receptor for the IgG1 istoype on mammary epithelium that transports considerable amounts of IgG1 from blood to colostrum or milk (Butler, 1983). Evidence also suggests IgG1 is transported selectively into sheep saliva (Cripps and Lascelles, 1976). The secretion of large amounts of IgG1 in these species is thought to reflect the requirement of neonates to obtain serum IgG from mother's milk early in life.

D. Secretory Ig in Serum

Immunoassay of serum indicates that secretory IgA and secretory IgM can be detected at relatively low levels (~10 μg/ml) in serum (Iscaki *et al.*, 1979; Delacroix and Vaerman, 1981; Kvale and Brandtzaeg, 1986). These levels are elevated in patients with liver disease. The reasons for the elevation of secretory immunoglobulin in liver disease are not entirely known, but could be (1) release of SC from damaged biliary epithelial cells, which would complex with pIg in blood, or (2) defective clearance of secretory IgA and secretory IgM, which might enter the blood after retrograde transport from mucosal tissue.

E. Hormonal Control of Secretory Ig

Several investigators have reported hormonal control of mucosal immunoglobulin production or secretion in the reproductive tract. Estradiol in female rats regulates the mucosal immune system by controlling IgA and IgG movement from blood to tissue, as well as by influencing the number of IgA-committed cells and the expression of pIgR in the reproductive tract (McDermott *et al.*, 1980; Wira *et al.*, 1980; Sullivan and Wira, 1983; Parr and Parr, 1989). The mucosal epithelium of the male reproductive tract expresses pIgR under the influence of androgens (Parr *et al.*, 1992). Interestingly, synthesis and secretion of SC in the lacrimal gland are also under the control of androgens (Sullivan *et al.*, 1984).

III. IgA: STRUCTURE AND ARRANGEMENT OF COMPONENT CHAINS

The function of IgA in both serum and secretions depends on the primary structure of its component chains, as well as on the conformation these chains assume in monomeric and polymeric IgA.

A. α Chains

1. Domain Structure of α Chains

Mammalian α chains have three constant region domains (Cα1–Cα3) similar to the number of constant region domains in γ and δ heavy chains whereas avian α chain has four constant region domains as do μ and ε chains. Based on the similarities in structure of IgM and IgA, IgA has been proposed to have evolved after IgM but before IgG. The fact that avian μ chains have four constant region domains would be consistent with this hypothesis (Mansikka, 1992). Evolution of the mammalian α chains may have involved the loss of the avian Cα2 domain to yield a three-domain structure. The hinge region in IgA1 molecules has been suggested to consist of remnants of the avian Cα2 domain (Mansikka, 1992).

Investigators generally assume that the Cα domains are folded in a manner similar to the Cγ structure that has been determined at the atomic level by X-ray crystallographic techniques. Based on this assumption, each α chain domain is thought to be composed of seven β strands in a four–three configuration with intervening "loops" to create a β-barrel conformation typical of other members of the Ig superfamily (Williams, 1986; Hunkapiller and Hood, 1989). Unfortunately, the Fcα structure has not been determined at the atomic level by X-ray crystallography and the extent to which the arrangement of the α chain domains in Fcα mimics Fcγ is uncertain.

2. Primary Structure of α Chains

Figure 1 presents the amino acid sequences of a number of α heavy chain constant regions that have been obtained by amino acid or DNA sequence analysis. The variable region domains of the α chains are obviously important to the antigen-binding function of IgA antibodies, but will not be discussed further.

The degree of amino acid similarity among α chains of different species increases from N- to C-terminal domains; the greatest homology is observed among the Cα3 domains (Cα4 of chicken). Some of the common amino acid residues found in the Cα constant region domains are highly invariant in all immunoglobulin molecules and presumably are critical in maintaining the structural features common to all Ig isotypes. Typical examples that are cited often are the highly apolar intraheavy-chain disulfide bonds that are almost (but not uniformly) characteristic of the Ig fold and tryptophan residues, most of which also are buried strategically within each domain. Other residues are highly conserved among IgM and IgA molecules. The relatively high degree of homology between IgA and IgM presumably reflects their close evolutionary origin and the importance of certain residues in maintaining common structural and functional characteristics. One such structure is the characteristic 18-amino-acid extension or "tail" that, during synthesis of IgM and IgA, associates with J chain, a 15-kDa protein synthesized in plasma cells (Section III,B).

In humans, nonhuman primates, and rabbits, multiple α chain isotypes have been described that define IgA subclasses (for review, see Chapter 9). Two IgA subclasses have been described in humans (reviewed by Mestecky and Russell, 1986), two in hominoid primates (gorilla, and chimpanzee; Kawamura *et al.*, 1992), and 13 in lagomorphs (see Burnett *et al.*, 1989). In all other species studied, only one IgA isotype has been observed.

Within a given species, the α chains belonging to each of the subclasses are highly homologous in amino acid sequence (Figure 1). A major difference between the two human isotypes or subclasses occurs in the hinge region. IgA2 molecules lack a 13-amino-acid segment found in the hinge region of IgA1 molecules that contains five carbohydrate moieties O-linked to serine. The presence of this extended hinge region has been postulated to confer greater segmental flexibility on IgA1 molecules (Pumphrey, 1986), but renders IgA1 molecules susceptible to IgA1-specific proteases produced by bacterial pathogens at mucosal surfaces (see Chapter 12). The absence of the hinge region in IgA2 molecules makes them resistant to the IgA1-specific proteases, which presumably is advantageous to IgA2 antibody function at mucosal surfaces. Based on the criteria that IgA2 molecules do not possess the extended hinge region characteristic of IgA1 molecules and generally do not bind the lectin Jacalin (Skea *et al.*, 1988; Aucouturier *et al.*, 1989), murine IgA appears to be similar to the IgA2 isotype of humans. In addition to the differences

Cα1

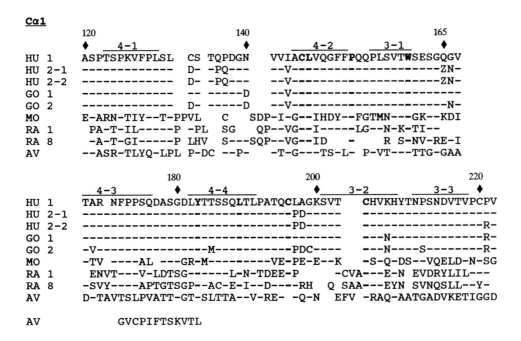

```
        120                  140                         165
        ♦    4-1               ♦        4-2        3-1     ♦
HU 1    ASPTSPKVFPLSL  CS TQPDGN   VVIACLVQGFFPQQPLSVTWSESGQGV
HU 2-1  -------------  D- -PQ---   --V---------------------ZN-
HU 2-2  -------------  D- -PQ---   --V---------------------ZN-
GO 1    -------------  -- -----D   --V------------------------
GO 2    -------------  D- -----D   --V----------------------N-
MO      E-ARN-TIY--T-PPVL   C   SDP-I-G--IHDY--FGTMN---GK--KDI
RA 1     PA-T-IL-----P -PL  SG    QP--VG--I-----LG--N-K-TI--
RA 8     -A-T-GI-----P LHV  S---SQP--VG--ID   -    R S-NV-RE-I
AV      --ASR-TLYQ-LPL P-DC --P-   -T-G---TS-L- P-VT---TTG-GAA

                    180                 200                    220
          4-3        ♦    4-4            ♦    3-2         3-3   ♦
HU 1    TAR NFPPSQDASGDLYTTSSQLTLPATQCLAGKSVT   CHVKHYTNPSNDVTVPCPV
HU 2-1  ------------------------------PD-----   -------------------
HU 2-2  ------------------------------PD-----   -----------------R-
GO 1    -------------------------------------   ---N-------------R-
GO 2    -V----------------M-----------PDC----   ---N----S--------R-
MO      -TV ----AL ---GR-M---------VE-PE-E--K   -S-Q-DS--VQELD-N-SG
RA 1     ENVT---V-LDTSG------L-N-TDEE-P     -CVA---E-N EVDRYLIL---
RA 8    -SVY----APTGTSGP--AC-E-I--D----RH  Q SAA---EYN SVNQSLL--Y-
AV      D-TAVTSLPVATT-GT-SLTTA--V-RE- -Q-N  EFV -RAQ-AATGADVKETIGGD

AV           GVCPIFTSKVTL
```

Cα HINGE

```
            223                          238
            ♦↓       ↓       ↓       ↓   ↓♦
HU 1        P S T P P T P S P S T P P T P S
HU 2-1                                P P P
HU 2-2                                P P P
CH 1        P S T P C P P T P S T P P P P P
CH 2                                  P P P
GO 1        P S T P C P P T P S T P P P P P
GO 2                                      P
OR              P R C P P T P S T P P C P P
GI 1                          T L P P C P H
GI 2                                P P S P
CR                              S E T K P C
MO                          P P T P P P I T
RA 1                        D T H S S C P P
RA 8  D C C P A N S C C T C P S S S S R N L
```

Figure 1 Amino acid sequence of α chains from various species. The isotypes shown are human IgA1 (HU 1), human IgA2 m(1) (HU 2-1), human IgA2 m(2) (HU 2-2), gorilla IgA1 (GO 1), gorilla IgA2 (GO 2), mouse IgA (MO), rabbit IgA1 (RA 1), rabbit IgA8 (RA 8), and chicken IgA (AV). The prototype sequence chosen was HU 1 and the numbering of amino acid residues was after Tsuzukida *et al.*, (1979). Sequences were aligned for maximum homology. Dashes indicate identity with the prototype sequence. In human IgA, the sites of N-glycosylation for IgA1 are residues 263 and 459. For IgA2m(1), sites of N-glycosylation are residues 166, 263, 337, and 459. For IgA2m(2), sites of N-glycosylation are residues 166, 211, 263, 337, and 459. Sites of O-glycosylation in human IgA1 are residues 224, 230, 232, 238, and 240. The bonds that are susceptible to IgA1-specific proteases are shown by arrows. Residues that are common to all IgA molecules are printed in boldface. Data are from Knight *et al.* (1984), Kratzin *et al.* (1975), Torano *et al.* (1977), Torano and Putnam (1978), Putnam *et al.* (1979), Tsuzukida *et al.* (1979), Yang *et al.* (1979), and Tucker *et al.* (1981). Where differences in the literature existed, the data base of Kabat *et al.* (1987) was used to construct the prototype sequence.

```
Cα2                                       260
                  4-1                      ♦       4-2            3-1
HU 1      PSCC  HPRLSLHRPALQDLLLGSE  ANLTCTLHGLRDASGVTFTWTPSSG  K
HU 2-1    -P--  -------------------  ------- -------A---------  -
HU 2-2    -P--  -------------------  ------- -------A---------  -
GO 1      -P--  ----------------------------------------------  -
GO 2       --   -------------------------------------A---------  -
MO        IPS-  Q-S---Q----E------D  -SI----N---NPE-AV---E--T-  -
RA 1      T--G  E-S---QP-D-R------D  -S-----R--K-PKDAV---E-TN-  N
RA 8      I-G-C E-S---Q--DIG-----RD  -S-----S--KNPEDAV---E-TN-  N
AV        -TD-DAT-Q-QVSLLPPTLEE-LVSHN-TV--VVSNAAA-D--SVS-SR---GGL

                     300                                   340
           4-4      ♦  4-3                3-3        3-3   ♦
HU 1      SAV  QGPPERDLCGCYSVSSVLPGCAEPWNHGKTFTCTAAYPESKTPLTATLSKS  G
HU 2-1    ---  ----------------------------E-------H--L------NIT--  -
HU 2-2    -    -----------------V----------E-------H--L------NIT--  -
GO 1      ---  E-------------------------------------------------  -
GO 2      --I  ------------------------KN---------H---------NIT--  -
MO        D--  -KKAVQNS--------------R--S-AS-K--VTH---G-LTGTIAKVT  V
RA 1      EP-  -QS-Q--P--------------T-TA-TE----VTH--IEGSSLTATIRKDT-
RA 8      EP-  -QRAQ---S----------SS--T-KVRTE----VTH--IEGGSLTATISKDT-
AV        D -S-TEDRQADGR -T-R-F-RV---E--G-E--G-SV R -EGVVVAEESIRK  E

Cα3                           360                             390
          4-1                  ♦          4-2         3-1      ♦
HU 1      NTFR    PEVHLLPPPSEELALNELVTLTCLARGFSPKDVLVRWLQGSQELPR
HU 2-1    ----    -Q----------------------------------------------
HU 2-2    ----    - ----------------------------------------------
GO 1      -M--    ------------------------------------------------
GO 2      -M--    ------------------------------------------------
MO        ---P    -Q----------------LS----V-A-N--E------H-NE--SP
RA 1      SLTP    -Q--------------A-------V-G--------Y-TNKGVVV-K
RA 8      VVTP    -L--------------A-------V----------S-THNGTVV-E
AV        TDTPLHA-S-YVF---A---S-Q-TA----M-SS-L-SSI-LT-T-QN-PISP

                                   420
           4-4            4-3       ♦          3-2
HU 1      EKYLTWASRQEPSQGTTTFAVTSILRVAAEDWKKGDTFSCMVGHEALPL
HU 2-1    -------------------------------------------------
HU 2-2    ------------------Y----------------E-------------
GO 1      -------------------------------------------------
GO 2      -------------------------------------------------
MO        -S--VFEPLK--GE-A--YL---V---S--T--Q--QY----------M
RA 1      DSF-V-KPLP--G-EP--Y----L-P-S----NQ--SY--V----G-AE
RA 8      DSF-V-KPLP----DP--Y----L--MS----NQ---Y-------G-AE
AV        QNF-IFGP  -KD -DFYSLY -K-K-SV---QR--V-G-V---DGI--

                 450               470
           3-3    ♦                 ♦
HU 1      AFTQKTIDRLAGKPTHVNVSVVMAEVEGTCY
HU 2-1    -------------------------------
HU 2-2    ----------------I--------A-----
GO 1      -------------------------------
GO 2      -------------------------------
MO        N---------S----N-S---I-S-GD-I--
RA 1      H------R-Q-------------V-D---V--
RA 8      H----------------------V-D---V--
AV        N-IH-S--KN---AS-------LSDADV---
```

Figure 1 (*Continued*)

noted in the hinge region, the human IgA subclasses differ at 14 amino acid positions in the α chain sequence (Figure 1).

The human IgA2 subclass exists in two allotypic forms. A major structural difference between these two allotypes concerns the arrangement of inter α-L chain disulfide bridges. In IgA2 of the A2m(1) allotype, the α and L chains are *not* covalently linked and therefore can be separated by exposure to dissociating agents without cleavage of disulfide bonds (Grey *et al.*, 1968). The absence of the L–H disulfide bond presumably relates to the exchange of cysteine at residue 133 for aspartic acid. Interestingly, this exchange does not prevent IgA2m(2) molecules from having the typical α-L disulfide-linked configuration, presumably by linking the L chain to a cysteine residue at another location in the α chain. The A2m(2) allotype differs from the A2m(1) allotype and the A1 isotype in six positions, two of which are in the Cα1 domain (residues 212 and 222) and four of which are located in the Cα3 domain (residues 411, 428, 458, and 467). Thus, the Cα3 domains of the A1 and A2m(1) chains are identical and the Cα2 domains of the A2 allotypes are identical and differ from that of A1. The A2m(1) allotype is a hybrid of A1 and A2m(2) and may have arisen by a gene conversion event (Tsuzukida *et al.*, 1979; Tucker *et al*, 1981).

The Cα1 domain is the least homologous among IgA molecules but one feature, the presence of multiple "extra" intrachain disulfide loops, is common to most IgA molecules (see Figure 4). Among the 13 rabbit α chain isotypes, the number of "extra" cysteine residues varies from 5 to 13 with 11 possible disulfide bond distribution patterns. These extra cysteines also may be present in the reduced (free SH) form (Burnett *et al.*, 1989).

The Cα2 domain of chickens is the least related domain and is thought to have been deleted in mammals (Mansikka, 1992).

The Cα2 domain of mammals (analogous to the Cα3 domain of chickens) also contains intrachain disulfide bridges not found in the other Ig isotypes (e.g., in human IgA: Cys 196–Cys 220; Cys 242–Cys 301) as well as interheavy-chain disulfide bonds that are unique to this isotype (i.e., between Cys 311 and Cys 299 on each α chain). The cysteine at residue 311 within Cα2 is involved in a disulfide bond with SC in secretory IgA (Fallgren-Gebauer *et al.*, 1992).

The Cα3 domain of mammals (Cα4 of chickens) has fewer distinguishing features, except for the extended 18-amino-acid "tail". The penultimate residue of the α chain is a cysteine that is linked covalently to J chain in IgA polymers (Garcia-Pardo *et al.*, 1981; Bastain *et al.*, 1992; Mestecky *et al.*, 1974b).

3. Carbohydrate Moiety of α Chains

Generally, carbohydrates contribute 6–7% of total molecular mass in human IgA1 and 8–10% in human IgA2 myeloma proteins (Tomana *et al.*, 1976). The higher carbohydrate content in IgA2 proteins is the result of additional *N*-linked oligosaccharide side chains [two in A2m(1) and three in A2m(2)]. However, the primary structures of carbohydrate side chains have been determined for very few myeloma proteins and the considerable variability in the content, composition, and number of oligosaccharide side chains among various myeloma proteins appears quite remarkable (Wold *et al.*, 1990). The carbohydrate side chains that have been characterized on α chains of both human subclasses demonstrate statistically significant differences in the amount fucose, mannose, and *N*-acetylglucosamine. The most striking difference is the presence of *N*-acetylgalactosamine in IgA1 proteins and its absence in IgA2. Differences in galactose and sialic acid are not significant (Baenziger and Kornfeld, 1974a,b; Tomana *et al.*, 1976; Torano *et al.*, 1977; Mestecky and Russell, 1986; Wold *et al.*, 1990).

The hinge region of IgA1 contains five short chains containing *N*-acetylgalatosamine, galactose (Baenziger and Kornfeld, 1974b), and, in some proteins, sialic acid (Field *et al.*, 1989) connected by O-glycosidic linkages to serine residues. Interestingly only a few serum proteins contain O-linked side chains, This unique property of IgA1 has been exploited in an efficient isolation of IgA1 proteins by affinity chromatography employing the lectin Jacalin (Roque-Barreira and Campos-Neto, 1985). This procedure is not absolutely specific for IgA1 proteins since a small proportion of IgA2 proteins also binds Jacalin (Aucouterier *et al.*, 1989).

The total carbohydrate content of secretory IgA is higher than that of serum IgA because of the carbohydrate-rich SC (subsequent discussion).

B. J Chain

In the early 1970s, comparative studies of the polypeptide chain composition of polymeric Ig (secretory IgA, polymeric serum IgA, and IgM) with that of IgG revealed an additional polypeptide chain in pIg with a fast electrophoretic mobility (for review, see Inman and Mestecky, 1974; Koshland, 1985). Subsequent studies revealed that this chain was glycosylated, with a molecular mass of 15–16 kDa, and was linked by disulfide bridges to the Fc fragment of polymeric IgM or IgA of secretory and serum (myeloma) origin. Based on the given criteria (molecular mass, fast electrophoretic mobility, characteristic amino acid composition, and immunochemical cross-reactivity), the presence of J chain has been established, with varying degrees of confidence, in polymeric Ig from many vertebrate species including mammals (human, monkey, rabbit, mouse, pig, dog, goat, cat, cow, horse, rat, guinea pig, and sheep), birds (chicken and pheasant), reptiles (turtle), amphibians (frog and toad), and fishes (catfish and sharks) (Kobayashi *et al.*, 1973; Inman and Mestecky, 1974; Koshland, 1985; Mikoryak *et al.*, 1988). Most recent studies using molecular biological approaches combined with immunochemical techniques revealed that J chain also is expressed in invertebrates (earthworm, slug, clam, and silkworm) and additional vertebrate species (African clawed frog, lamprey, and newt) (Takahashi *et al.*, 1993).

Sequence analyses of mouse genomic DNA reveal that J chain-encoding information is contained in four exons of a single gene located on chromosome 5; in humans, the J chain gene is on chromosome 4.

1. Domain Structure of J Chain

Despite the low degree of sequence homology with H and L chains, studies of the secondary structure of J chain have been interpreted to suggest that it folds into an eight-stranded antiparallel β barrel (with 35% β sheet and the remainder in random coil; Zikan *et al.*, 1985; Pumphrey, 1986). An alternative model suggests a two-domain model in which the first domain consists of a six-stranded antiparallel β-barrel and the second domain (folded under the first) is a two-stranded β barrel (Frutiger *et al.*, 1992).

2. Primary Structure of J Chain

The primary structure of J chain has been determined in human, mouse, and rabbit (Figure 2). J chain consists of 137 amino acid residues and displays a high degree of sequence homology (70%) among species (Koshland, 1985; Hughes *et al.*, 1990). Incomplete sequence studies of earthworm J chain reveal a high degree of homology with both human and mouse J chains (Takahashi *et al.*, 1993). These findings, in conjunction with remarkable similarity in physicochemical properties and interspecies cross-reactivities (Kobayashi *et al.*, 1973), suggest that many of the features of J chain are conserved through evolution. J chains are rich in acidic (aspartic, glutamic) amino acid residues and low in glycine, serine, and phenylalanine; tryptophan is absent (Inman and Mestecky, 1974). Six of the eight cysteine residues form three intrachain disulfide bridges; the other two residues close to the N terminus are involved in disulfide bonds that link J chain to the penultimate cysteine residues of α and μ chains (Mestecky and McGhee, 1987; Frutiger *et al.*, 1992).

3. Carbohydrate of J Chain

Approximately 8% of the molecular mass of J chain is contributed by a single carbohydrate side chain linked to asparagine residue 48 by an *N*-glycosidic bond. This chain consists of fucose, mannose, galactose, glucoamine, and sialic acid (Niedermeier *et al.*, 1972; Baenziger, 1979).

C. Secretory Component

Identification of SC as part of the transport receptor for secretory IgA began with immunohistochemical studies in which specific antisera to the (secretion-specific) "secretory piece" established its presence not only within the secretory IgA molecule but as a component of mucosal epithelial cells (South *et al.*, 1966; Brandtzaeg, 1978; Crago *et al.*, 1978; Nagura *et al.*, 1979). Subsequently, SC was isolated free in mucosal secretions as well as associated with secretory IgA. The exquisite binding specificity for polymeric but not monomeric Ig was established (Mach, 1970; Radl *et al.*, 1971; Brandtzaeg, 1974; Weiker and Underdown, 1975).

1. SC Domain Structure

In most species, SC (molecular mass, ~70 kDa) consists of five Ig-like domains with definite but relatively low homology to the λ chain variable region (Mostov *et al.*, 1984). In addition to the five-domain form, rabbits synthesize a truncated three-domain form (Frutiger *et al.*, 1987). Within the basolateral membrane of mucosal epithelial cells, SC consists of five extracellular domains, a transmembrane segment, and a cytoplasmic domain. The term poly Ig receptor was proposed to differentiate between the membrane form of the transport receptor and the cleaved soluble form known as SC (Mostov *et al.*, 1984). For a more complete discussion of the pIgR, see Chapter 10.

2. Primary Amino Acid Sequence of SC

The amino acid sequences of pIgR have been determined completely for three species and are shown in Figure 3. In addition to the intrachain disulfide bonds that are thought to be buried within each domain, several of the domains have "extra" disulfide bonds. One of these, located in the fifth domain, is susceptible to disulfide interchange. Data from Hilschmann and colleagues (Fallgren-Gebauer *et al.*, 1992) suggest that only one cysteine residue from this labile disul-

```
        1             ↑    20                   40      ■
HU      QEDERIVLVDNKCKCARITSRIIRSSEDPNEDIVERNIRIIVPLNNRENIS
MO       D--ATI-A----M-T-V-----P-T--------------V----------
RA       ---ST-------Q-V---------DPDN-S---------------T-----

                 60       ↑            80                  100
HU      DPTSPLRTRFVYHLSDLCKKCDPTEVELDNQIVTATQSNICDEDSAT ETC
MO      -------RN--------V------V----ED-V---------N--DGVP---
RA      --------E-K-N-AN---------I-----VF--S-----PD-DYS ---

                  110                130
HU      YTYDRNKCYTAVVPLVYGGETKMVETALTPDACYPD
MO      -M--------TM---R-H------QA-----S----
RA      ----------TL--ITHR-V-R--KAT----S----
```

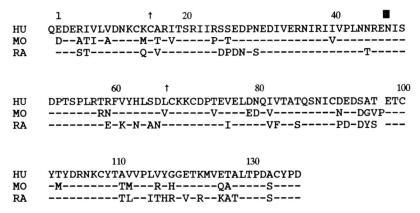

Figure 2 Amino acid sequence of J chain from human (HU), mouse (MO), and rabbit (RA). The two cysteine residues that join J chain to the penultimate amino acid cysteine residue in α chains (Cys 471) are shown by arrows. Site of N-glycosylation is shown by filled square. Data are from Max and Kornsmeyer (1985), Frutiger *et al.* (1986), Matsuuchi *et al.* (1986), and Hughes *et al.* (1990).

fide bond (see Figures 3 and 4) is linked to one Cys 311 in the Cα2 domain.

3. Carbohydrate of SC

Approximately 22% of the total molecular mass of SC is contributed by carbohydrates (Tomana *et al.*, 1978). The 5–7 oligosaccharide side chains contain *N*-acetylglucosamine, fucose, mannose, galactose, and sialic acid attached by *N*-glycosidic bonds (Mizoguchi *et al.*, 1982). Studies of rabbit SC indicate one common glycosylation site at the asparagine residue at position 400 and a second site in the N-terminal domain that varies among different allotypes (Frutiger *et al.*, 1988).

D. Structure of Monomeric and Polymeric IgA

As shown schematically in Figure 5, IgA exists in both monomeric and polymeric forms. Dimers, trimers, and tetramers are found commonly, although the dimer is the predominant form in most mucosal secretions. A distinguishing feature of pIgA, as well as of IgM (which is generally pentameric), is the presence of J chain, a polypeptide synthesized by antibody-producing cells of all isotypes, which is incorporated into pIgA and IgM just prior to their secretion from plasma cells (Parkhouse and Della Corte, 1973). Chemical analysis indicated that each polymer (IgM or IgA) contains one mole of J chain (Zikan *et al.*, 1986). In native molecules of polymeric Ig, the antigenic determinants of J chain are poorly exposed; further, J chain is highly susceptible to proteolysis. These findings may explain failure to detect J chain in some polymeric Ig. Cleavage of interchain disulfide bonds usually is sufficient to release it from Ig, suggesting that only weak noncovalent interactions exist between J chain and the Fc region of polymeric Ig.

The arrangement of disulfide bonds and the manner in which J chain is linked within the polymeric structure has been a matter of debate. Two models have been presented (Figure 5). In one model, dimeric IgA consists of two monomer subunits linked end to end with J chain attaching or bonding both monomeric subunits at one cysteine residue (471) of each monomer subunit. The two remaining Cys 471 residues link directly to each other. Direct experimental data have been presented to support this hypothesis (Bastian *et al.*, 1992). A second model (Figure 5) takes into account the fact that electron micrographs present IgA dimers that appear to be shorter than would be predicted based on the expected length of each of the monomer subunits (Svehag and Bloth, 1970), as well as data that indicate that Cys 311 could be linked to Cys 471 (Underdown and Schiff, 1986). Naturally occurring as well as genetically engineered IgM, which lacks J chain, will form polymers but these are often mixtures of various oligomeric forms including hexamers, in contrast with the majority of naturally occurring IgM polymers that are primarily pentameric, suggesting that J chain may regulate the degree of polymerization of IgM and, possibly, of IgA. In so doing, J chain may be responsible for creating a conformation within pIgA and IgM that binds pIgR (Section III,E).

E. Structure of Secretory IgA

The single most important distinguishing feature of secretory IgA with respect to serum IgA is the presence of SC. In addition to its crucial role in the transport of pIgA to mucosal secretions, SC has been shown to confer resistance to proteolysis on secretory IgA, presumably an added advantage in the gastrointestinal milieu (Brown *et al.*, 1970).

In vitro experiments convincingly demonstrated that SC binds only to polymeric IgA or IgM (Weiker and Underdown, 1975; Brandtzaeg, 1981). The discovery of J chain in these immunoglobulins led to the postulation that this small polypeptide is instrumental in SC binding. Brandtzaeg (1985) has maintained that SC binding by polymeric IgA and IgM is dependent on the presence of J chain: Pentameric IgM that lacks J chain did not bind SC efficiently and the ability of polymeric IgA to bind SC in solution or on the surface of SC-bearing epithelial cells was related to the J chain content. However, how the presence of J chain leads to such remarkable enhancement of SC binding is not clear. Previous structural studies of human SIgA cleaved by cyanogen bromide indicated that J chain and SC are bound to different fragments of the α chain and are not connected by disulfide bridges (Mestecky *et al.*, 1974a). This result does not rule out the possibility that J chain is required to create a conformation in pIg that generates the SC binding site.

Results concerning the structure of IgA, SC, and J chain indicate that both SC and J chain display immunoglobulin domain-like folding of their polypeptide chains and belong to the immunoglobulin superfamily (Mostov *et al.*, 1984; Zikan *et al.*, 1985; Pumphrey, 1986). Therefore, the mutual interactions between the Fc portion of dimeric IgA, J chain, and SC are likely to be based on the complementarities of their domain-like structures.

Binding of pIgR to pIgA begins with a high affinity noncovalent association that is followed by the formation of disulfide bonds through which SC links to only one of the IgA monomer subunits (Underdown *et al.*, 1977; Garcia-Pardo *et al.*, 1979; Figure 5). Several groups have reported association constants on the order of $10^8 M^{-1}$ for the noncovalent interaction, but these data in all likelihood underestimate the affinity of noncovalent binding (Schiff *et al.*, 1983). More important, however, is the fact that dissociation of the complex is much slower than the time required (30 min) for the pIgA–pIgR complex to cross the epithelial cell, during which time pIgA must stay bound to its receptor to insure that it reaches the apical face of the cell and is discharged into the lumen.

The heavy chains of pIgA and IgM, respectively, are likely to contribute to the binding site for pIgR (Geneste *et al.*, 1986). In some species, notably those that display pIgR on hepatic parenchymal cells, IgM binds homologous SC with little affinity (Underdown *et al.*, 1992). In these species, high affinity binding between IgM and pIgR has been argued to be detrimental to the host, since IgM would be lost via hepatic transport from the blood where it is known to function. Thus, the rat, rabbit, and chicken may have given up their ability to transport IgM in return for a highly active biliary transport system for pIgA. The exact nature of the binding site for pIgR on pIgA and IgM is still under study, but evidence

```
                  |←    pIg-binding       →|                          84
HU   KSPIFGPEEVNSVEGNSVSITCYYPPTSVNRHTRKYWCRQGARGGCITLISSEGYVSSKYAGRANL
RT      ----QD-S-I------------D-----------------N-Y-A-----N--L-KE-S---S-
RA   P-S----GE--VL--D---------T---T--S--F---EEES-R-V-- A-T--T-QE-S--QK-

                                                D1 ←|→ D2           150
HU   TNFPENGTFVVNIAQLSQDDSGRYKCGLGINSRGLSFDVSLEVSQGPGLLNDTKVYTVDLGRTVTI
RT   I-----S---I---H-T-E-T-S------TTN---F---------V-EFP---H---K-I------
RA   -D--DK-E---TVD--T-N---S----V-V-G---D-G-NVL---K-E  P-DV--KQYESY----

                                                                    214
HU   NCPFKTENAQKRKSLYKQIGLYPVLVID  SSGYVNPNYTGRIRLDIQGTGQLLFSVVINQLRLSD
RT   E-R--EG--HSK---C-KR-EACEV---  -TE--D-S-KD-AI-FMK--SRDI-Y-N-SH-IP--
RA   T---TYATR-LK--F--VEDGEL--I--SS-KEAVD-R-K---T-Q--S-TAKE-T-T-KH-Q-N-

                         D2 ←|→ D3                                  280
HU   AGQYLCQAGDDSNSNKKNADLQVLKPEPELVYEDLRGSVTFHCALGPEVANVAKFLCRQSSGENCD
RT   --L-V----EGPSAD-N-------E-----L-K---S----E-D--R----D--Y--- KNK-T--
RA   ----V--S-S-PTAEEQ-V--RL-  T-G-L-GN-G-----E---DS-D-- -VASL  RQVRGGN

                                                                    346
HU   VVVNTLGKRAPAFEGRILLNPQDKDGSFSVVITGLRKEDAGRYLCGAHSDGQLQEGSPIQAWQLFV
RT   -II------D---------T-R-DN-R---L----------H-Q-----S-LP---W-V-------
RA   --IDSQ-TID--------FT KAEN-H-----A------T-N----VQ-N--SGD- -T-LR----

      D2←|→ D4                                                      412
HU   NEESTIPRSPTVVKGVAGSSVAVLCPYNRKESKSIKYWCLWEGAQNGRCPLLVDSEGWVKAQYEGR
RT   -------N-RS-----T-G---IV----P---S-L----H--ADE-----V--GTQAL-QEG----
RA   ---IDVS---P-L--FP-G--TIR----P-R-D-HLQLY----S-TRHLLVDSG --L-QKD-T--

                                                       D4←|→D5      475
HU   LSLLEEPGNGTFTVILNQLTSRDAGFYWCLTNGDTLWRTTVEIKIIE   GEPNLKVPGNVTAVLG
RT   -A-FDQ--S-AY--------TQ-S-------D--SR----IELQVA-ATKKP-LEVT-Q-A---I-
RA   -A-F--------S-------AE-E-----VSDD-ESLT-S-KLQ-VDGEPSP    TIDKF---Q-

               ↑                                                    541
HU   ETLKVPCHFPCKFSSYEKYWCKWNNTGCQALPSQDEGPSKAFVNCDENSRLVSLTLNLVTRADEGW
RT   --FTIS--Y----Y-Q-------S-D--HI---H---ARQSS-S--QS-QI--M---P-KKE----
RA   -PVEIT------YF-S--------DH--ED--  TKLS-SGDLVKCN-NLVLT---DS-SED----

                                                                    591
HU   YWCGVKQGHFYGETAAVYVAVEE                RKAAGSRDVSLAKADAAPDEKVLDSGFR
RT   ------E-QV----T-I------  RTRGSPHINPTDANAR-KDAPEEE-          ME-SV-
RA   ----A-D--EFE-V---R-ELT-PAKVAVEPAKVPVDPA---PAPAEEK---RCPVPRRRQWYPLS

                D5←|↓                                               658
HU   EIENKAIQDPRLFAEEKAVADTRDQADGSRASVDSGSSEEQGGSSRALVSTLVPLGLVLAVGAVAV
RT   -D----NL------D-REIQNAG---QEN---GNAG-AGG-S---KV-F-----------------
RA   RKLRTSCPE---L---V--QSAE-P-S-------AS-ASG-S--AKV-I-----------A--M--

                                                                    723
HU   GVARARHRKNVDRVSIRSYRTDISMSDFENSREFGANDNMGASSITQETSLGGKEEFVATTESTTE
RT   W---V--------M--S--------G--R---DL-G------TPDT---V-E--D-IET---C---
RA   AI------R-------G----------L--------I--PS-CPDAR--A----D-LATA----V-

                                        764
HU   TKEPKKAKRSSKEEAEMAYKDFLLQSSTVAAEAQDGPQEA
RT   PE-S------------D---SA--F----I--QVH------
RA   IE-------------DL--SA-----N-I---H----K--
```

Figure 3 Amino acid sequence of poly Ig receptor from human (HU), rat (RT), and rabbit (RA). The number system is after Krajči *et al.* (1991). The location of the domains (D1–D5) are according to Eiffert *et al.* (1984,1991). The location of the proposed pIg-binding site is based on the work of Frutiger *et al.* (1986), Beale (1987), and Bakos *et al.* (1991). Up arrows represent cysteine involved in linking SC to Cα2 (Cys311) Down arrows indicate postulated site of cleavage that releases SC and secretory IgA from the apical face of the mucosal epithelial cell. Sequence data based on Eiffert *et al.* (1984), Mostov *et al.* (1984), Banting *et al.* (1989), and Krajči *et al.* (1992).

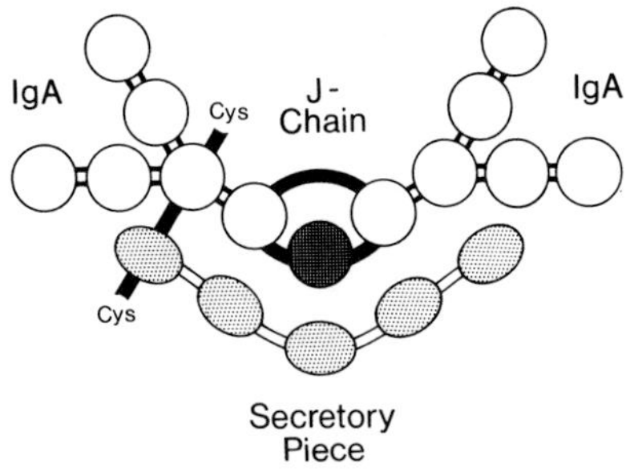

Figure 4 Model of secretory IgA according to Fallgren-Gebauer and colleagues (1992). SC is bound noncovalently to the IgA dimer (model I, Figure 5) and is linked at domain five by a disulfide-bond to Cys311 in Cα2 in only one monomer subunit. This figure was provided by N. Hilschmann and is based on the work of Fallgren-Gebauer *et al.* (1992).

suggests that both the heavy chains and the J chain are involved.

IV. BIOSYNTHESIS AND ASSEMBLY OF IgA

A. Monomeric IgA

The light and α chains that become assembled intracellularly into monomeric IgA (mIgA) molecules are synthesized on separate sets of polyribosomes and are assembled into the monomeric unit through several pathways (Heremans, 1974). Depending on the cell type studied, various types of pairings of H and L chains occur early on polyribsomes, but the final core-glycosylated molecule of mIgA is assembled in the Golgi apparatus. Additional carbohydrate residues are attached during the intracellular passage of mIgA from Golgi to the cell surface and ultimate secretion into the medium.

B. Polymeric IgA

Early investigations of the biosynthetic pathways of mouse IgA suggested that, in cells secreting polymeric IgA, a majority of intracellular IgA was present as monomers and that polymerization occurred shortly before or at the time of secretion (Parkhouse, 1971). This hypothesis is supported by subsequent comparative biochemical studies of the molecular forms of intracellular versus secreted IgA in cell lysates and tissue culture supernatants of cell derived from various human tissues, which indicated that, although small amounts of polymeric IgA were detected in some cell lysates, most intracellular IgA occurred in a monomeric form (even when the predominant form of secreted IgA was polymeric) (Buxbaum *et al.*, 1974; Moldoveanu *et al.*, 1984).

C. Distribution of Cells Synthesizing Monomeric and Polymeric IgA

Analyses of molecular forms of IgA in perfusates and supernatants of *in vitro* cultured tissue explants as well as immunohistochemical studies of mucosal tissues and glands clearly demonstrated that separate populations of pIgA- and mIgA-secreting cells exist that display a characteristic tissue distribution (for review, see Brandtzaeg, 1983a; Mestecky and McGhee, 1987; Mestecky *et al.*, 1991). Typically, the majority of IgA-producing cells in the normal human bone marrow are monomeric (they do not express J chain and do not bind SC) whereas the majority of such cells in the intestinal lamina propria produce pIgA, express J chain, and bind SC. The spleen and lymph nodes from different locations display a variable proportion of pIgA- and mIgA- secreting cells. Under pathological conditions (e.g., IgA multiple myeloma), the bone marrow may contain predominantly J chain-positive cells; concurrently, high levels of pIgA are present in blood (Mestecky *et al.*, 1980).

D. Role of J Chain in the Polymerization of Ig

The association of J chain with pIg but not mIg in serum and secretions raised the possibility that J chain either initiated or regulated the formation of polymers intracellularly. The following observations seem consistent with this hypothesis: (1) Ig-producing cells in the submucosae of the gastrointestinal and respiratory tracts, as well as in the interstitium of mammary, salivary, and lacrimal glands, prominantly display the presence of intracellular J chain and primarily secrete pIgA; (2) in contrast, IgA- or IgG-containing plasma cells from the normal bone marrow that secrete monomeric IgA are uniformly J chain negative (Brandtzaeg, 1985).

Since a small proportion of intracellular Ig is linked to J chain, this chain has been proposed to initiate polymerization by binding first to a monomeric molecule of intracellular IgA or IgM that subsequently is linked to another monomer, forming a dimeric molecule (for reviews, see Brandtzaeg, 1983a,1985; Koshland, 1985; Mestecky and McGhee, 1987).

However, Stott (1976) observed that polymeric IgM could be detected in lysates of certain mouse cell lines in a tetrameric form lacking J chain. This polypeptide, linked to monomeric IgM, was added as a last step in the process of polymerization. Site-directed mutagenesis of cysteine residues of α or μ chains involved in J chain binding, and transfection of α and L chain genes into J chain-negative cells, further disputes the necessity for J chain in polymerization (Cattaneo and Neuberger, 1987; Davis *et al.*, 1989). *In vitro* studies concerning the role of J chain in polymerization also were reported in which covalently linked IgM polymers were synthesized *in vitro* in good yield in the absence of J chain (Bouvet *et al.*, 1987).

These data suggest that J chain may not initiate polymerization but may regulate the degree and form of polymerization in pIg. In support of this hypothesis is the observation that, in the absence of J chain, polymers of Ig may form *in vitro* or *in vivo* but the preferred conformation observed under natural conditions often is not produced quantitatively. Thus, under normal conditions, J chain may act to regulate the formation of polymers which, in the case of IgA, are dimers, trimers, and tetramers and rarely become pentamers, whereas the pentamer is the preferred configuration for IgM.

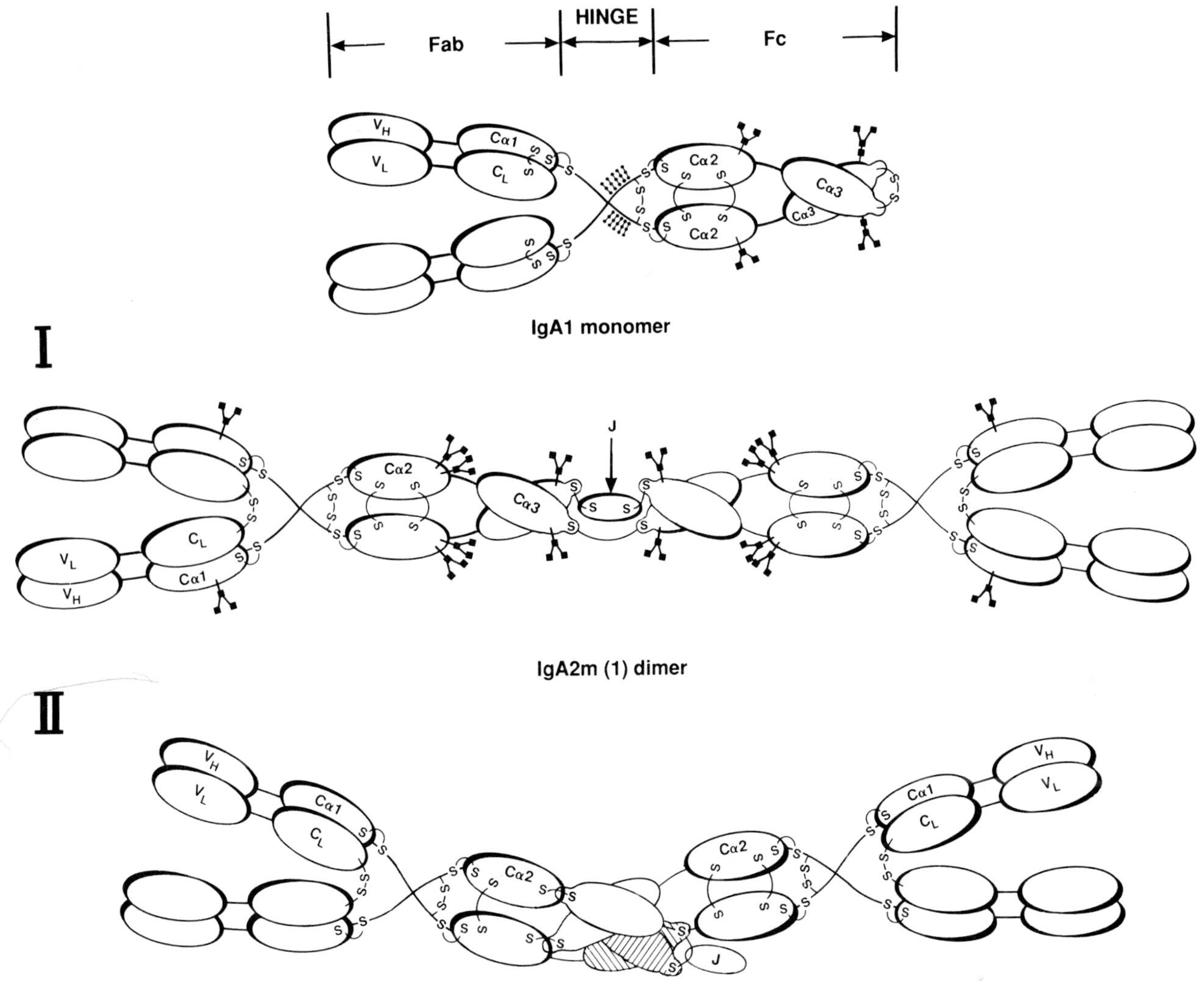

Figure 5 Schematic diagram of IgA monomer and two models of IgA dimer (I and II). The circles in the IgA1 monomer represent the O-linked carbohydrate side chains in the hinge. This region is deleted in IgA2 molecules. The squares represent N-linked carbohydrate side chains that are placed in a position consistent with their location in the Ig-domain fold. The disulfide bonds (S–S) shown in the monomer are the inter-α-L bond in IgA1 (also present in IgA2 m(2), inter-α bonds Cys241–Cys241, Cys299–Cys299, Cys311–Cys311, and Cys471–Cys471, and intraaα bonds Cys196–Cys220 and Cys242–Cys301. In models I and II of the dimer, the inter-L bond in IgA2 m(1) is shown. In model I, the monomer subunits are joined end to end with cysteine residues from J chain linking a Cys471 from each monomer; the remaining two Cys471 residues are joined directly together (Bastian *et al.* 1992). In model II, the dimer is shown forming a more compact structure based on data presented by Svehag and Bloth (1970) and Abel and Grey (1968). The monomeric subunits are joined via two Cys311 residues from the Cα2 domains of one monomer subunit to two Cys471 residues from the "extended tail" of the other monomer subunit. J chain is joined within the former monomer subunit via two Cys471 residues of the "extended tail".

E. J-Chain Expression in B Cells Not Producing Polymeric Ig

In the bone marrow of patients with multiple myeloma, J chain frequently is detected by immunofluorescent staining of plasma cells synthesizing monomeric Ig such as IgG (Mestecky *et al.*, 1980). Similarly, J chain has been detected in IgG plasma cells from inflammatory sites and in mitogen-stimulated peripheral blood lymphocytes (Mestecky *et al.*, 1980; Brandtzaeg, 1985). The expression of J chain in cells that are not engaged in the synthesis of polymers has been interpreted as a sign of clonal immaturity. Extensive studies of human cells from leukemic patients, established lymphoid cell lines, and Epstein–Barr virus (EBV)-transformed fetal bone marrow cells (depleted of surface Ig-positive cells) reveal that J chain may be expressed in the cytoplasm of lymphocytes from the earliest stages of their differentiation along the B-cell axis (McCune *et al.*, 1981; Hajdu *et al.*, 1983; Max and Korsmeyer, 1985; Kubagawa *et al.*, 1988). Thus, cells phenotypically characterized as null or pre-B cells contain J chain, frequently in the absence of μ chain. EBV-transformed fetal bone marrow cells or cells from a few patients with a clinically established diagnosis of multiple myeloma display the morphological features of plasma cells but contain no intracellular Ig; in the former, the cells exhibit a germ-line configuration or abortive VDJ rearrangement of H chain gene segments (Kubagawa *et al.*, 1988). J chain expression in B cells at early stages of differentiation is apparently different in mice in which J chain is detectable only in Ig-secreting cells but not in pre-B or B cells (Koshland, 1985).

The presence of J chain in non-pIg-producing cells is an enigma, but suggests that this protein may have an additional role in B cells that is unrelated to polymer formation. In this regard, work by Takahashi *et al.* (1993) indicates that J chain may be present in species as primitive as the earthworm.

V. IgA METABOLISM

The metabolism of IgA has not been studied extensively. In human plasma and cerebral spinal fluid, IgG is found in concentrations that are higher than those of the other isotypes. However, the levels of individual Ig isotypes in these fluids are not reflective of their biosynthetic rates. Considering the distribution in various body fluids of the major Ig isotypes and their catabolic rates, clearly IgA is synthesized in quantities (~66 mg/kg body weight/day) that exceed by far the combined daily synthesis of all other Ig isotypes (for reviews, see Mestecky *et al.*, 1986; Conley and Delacroix, 1987).

The lower concentration of IgA than IgG in human serum is the result of the more rapid catabolism of IgA (half-life of IgA is 6 days vs 20–25 days for IgG), in conjunction with the fact that cells engaged in IgA synthesis in humans are found both in mucosal (e.g., gastrointestinal tract, salivary gland) and systemic (e.g., bone marrow and, to a lesser extent, spleen and lymph nodes) tissue.

A. Liver as a Major Site of IgA Metabolism: SC-Dependent Clearance

The importance of the liver in IgA metabolism was established by a series of studies performed in animals and in humans with liver diseases. Experiments by Jackson *et al.* (1978) pointed out that the liver transported pIgA from blood to bile in rats. Vaerman and Delacroix (1984) proposed that, in rodents, the liver functions as an "IgA pump" that regulates serum levels of IgA by transporting circulating pIgA into the bile. By this mechanism, significant quantities of IgA are delivered into the intestinal tract of rodents. SC present on the surface of rat hepatocytes was identified as the receptor for pIgA, and is the most important receptor responsible for its selective and efficient transport into bile in several species in which pIgA is the primary form of circulating IgA (Underdown and Schiff, 1986).

Interactions between pIgA and hepatocytes are strongly species dependent. SC has been found on hepatocytes of many species (rat, rabbit, and mouse), but not on human hepatocytes (for reviews, see Vaerman and Delacroix, 1984; Mestecky and McGhee, 1987; Brown and Kloppel, 1989). Consequently, the extent to which SC-mediated clearance of pIgA occurs is highly species dependent.

B. Role of Other Receptors in Hepatic Clearance

IgA interactions with hepatocytes also can be mediated through hepatic receptors specific for asialoglycoproteins [asialoglycoprotein receptor (ASGP-R) or hepatic binding protein (HBP); Stockert *et al.*, 1982; Tomana *et al.*, 1988]. The presence and properties of ASGP-R have been described for hepatocytes from several species (Ashwell and Harford, 1982). ASGP-R recognizes terminal galactose residues of desialylated glycoproteins and has been proposed, in addition to SC, to play an important role in the endocytosis of IgA by hepatocytes (for reviews, see Brown and Kloppel, 1989; Mestecky *et al.*, 1991). The binding of glycoproteins, including IgA, to ASGP-R depends on Ca^{2+} and is therefore inhibitable by chelating agents. Bound IgA is internalized and the IgA-containing vesicles fuse with lysosomes, resulting in intracellular degradation.

Thus, the liver is involved in regular catabolism of immunoglobulins, including pIgA and mIgA (Moldoveanu *et al.*, 1988,1990; Tomana *et al.*, 1988). However, in humans only negligible amounts (approximatley 1 mg/kg/day) of the total IgA produced in the bone marrow, spleen, and lymph nodes (approximately 20 mg/kg/day) reach the external secretions (Conley and Delacroix, 1987).

The site of catabolism of IgA was studied in animal models (Moldoveanu *et al.*, 1988,1990). Mice and monkeys (*Macaca fuscata*) were used as representatives of species with SC-positive and SC-negative hepatocytes, respectively; however, both species display ASGP-R on hepatocytes. In both species, the liver was identified as the organ with the highest uptake of mIgA and pIgA. Although both parenchymal (hepatocytes) and nonparenchymal cells were involved in the catabolism, the hepatocytes were more active. Other tissues and organs, including muscles, kidneys, skin, and spleen, also catabolized IgA, although to a much lower degree than the liver.

VI. BIOLOGICAL SIGNIFICANCE OF THE HUMAN IgA SUBCLASSES

As described in Section III,A,2, two IgA isotypes have been described in humans (for reviews, see Mestecky and Russell, 1986; Mestecky *et al.*, 1986,1989) as well as in hominoid primates (Kawamura and Ueda, 1992; Kawamura *et al.*, 1992); 13 IgA isotypes have been reported in rabbits (Burnett *et al.*, 1989; see Chapter 9). These isotypes have been identified by sequence analysis or, in some cases, by serologic and structural studies.

Allotypic determinants specified by allelic genes have been described only in the IgA2 subclass and are now designated A2m(1) and A2m(2). The major structural difference between these two allotypes concerns the arrangement of α–L interchain disulfide bridges. In IgA2 of the A2m(1) allotype, the α and L chains are *not* covalently linked and therefore can be separated by exposure to dissociating agents without cleavage of disulfide bonds (Grey *et al.*, 1968).

Population studies of the IgA2 allotypes revealed a characteristic racial and ethnic distribution. In Caucasians, the overwhelming proportion of IgA2 is of the A2m(1) allotype, whereas in Africans and in African Americans, the A2m(2) allotype dominates (Wang and Fudenberg, 1974; van Longhem and Biewenga, 1983). Interestingly, American Indians, Australian Aborigines, and Eskimos resemble Caucasians in this respect.

A. Distribution of Human IgA Subclasses in Various Body Fluids and Tissues

Using polyclonal and monoclonal antibodies specific for human IgA1 and IgA2, several groups of investigators determined that serum IgA is represented primarily by the IgA1 subclass (~85% of total serum IgA) (for reviews see Mestecky and Russell, 1986; Conley and Delacroix, 1987). This value mirrors the proportion of IgA1- and IgA2-secreting cells in the bone marrow (Skvaril and Morell, 1974; Crago *et al.*, 1984) and, in conjunction with additional data (Alley *et al.*, 1982), indicates that almost all serum IgA originates from this source.

The proportion of IgA1 to IgA2 varies in individual secretions. Because almost all secretory IgA in humans is of local origin, this IgA1 : IgA2 ratio apparently reflects the characteristic distribution of IgA1- and IgA2-secreting cells in various tissues (Crago *et al.*, 1984; Kett *et al.*, 1986; Kutteh *et al.*, 1988). Although IgA1 cells predominate in most mucosal tissues and glands, in the large intestine and in the female genital tract the IgA2 cells equal or outnumber IgA1-positive cells. Lymph nodes contain a mixed proportion of IgA1 and IgA2 cells, depending on the source.

B. Functional Differences between IgA Subclasses

Despite the high degree of identity between the primary structures of human IgA1 and IgA2 molecules, an understanding of the functional differences among the IgA subclasses is just beginning to emerge and is related to the structural differences between the two isotypes.

The extended hinge region in IgA1 molecules renders them highly susceptible to unique IgA1-specific proteases produced by several bacterial species, including many important human pathogens (see Chapter 12). Conversely, the absence of this region in IgA2 molecules makes them resistant to the IgA1 proteases (see Chapter 12). The extended hinge theoretically confers added segmental flexibility and increased antigen-binding ability on IgA1 molecules compared with IgA2 molecules, although this hypothesis has not been demonstrated experimentally (Pumphrey, 1986).

A second and profound structural difference between the human α1 and α2 chains concerns the composition and distribution of the oligosaccharide side chains described in Section III,A,3. Human IgA1 and IgA2 myeloma proteins differ in the total amount and proportion of component carbohydrates, as well as in the number and distribution of oligosaccharide side chains (Niedermeier *et al.*, 1972; Tomana *et al.*, 1972, 1976,1978; Baenziger and Kornfeld, 1974a,b; Torano *et al.*, 1977; Baenziger, 1979; Mizoguchi *et al.*, 1982; Wold *et al.*, 1990).

Differences in the carbohydrate composition of human IgA1 and IgA2 antibodies would be expected to influence a number of important properties of these molecules, some of which have been demonstrated experimentally. For example, the removal of terminal sialic acid substantially shortens the half-life of IgA molecules in the circulation because of the exposure of galactose residues that are recognized by ASGP-R on hepatocytes (Stockert *et al.*, 1982; Tomana *et al.*, 1988). Because of the availability of terminal galactose residues, IgA1 proteins bind better than IgA2 to the asialoglycoprotein receptor expressed on hepatocytes or on the human hepatoma cell line HepG2 (Tomana *et al.*, 1988).

More recent analysis indicates that some IgA myeloma proteins, especially those belonging to the IgA2 subclass (which also is represented in the mucosal secretions), display a high degree of carbohydrate heterogeneity as well as truncated oligosaccharide side chains with terminal mannose residues (Wold *et al.*, 1990). Such proteins effectively interact with gram-negative bacteria of the family Enterobacteriaceae that express type 1 fimbrial lectin. Since IgA2-producing cells predominate in the colon and vagina (Crago *et al.*, 1984; Kett *et al.*, 1986; Kutteh *et al.*, 1988), which are colonized by gram-negative bacteria expressing mannose-specific lectins, IgA2 may function in these areas independent of specific antibody activity. This type of carbohydrate-mediated interaction could form the basis for a broad antibacterial function of secretory IgA against enterobacteria, regardless of the antigenic specificity of antibody molecules, in conjunction with other immune elements.

Mildly aggregated IgA1 proteins have been demonstrated to attach to fibronectin-coated plates in greater amounts than similarly treated IgA2 proteins (Mestecky *et al.*, 1987). Although the biological significance of these *in vitro* observations is unclear at present, one may speculate that such interactions may be important in the catabolism and distribution of IgA molecules and possibly of IgA-containing immune complexes.

IgA1 and IgA2 myeloma proteins also have been compared with respect to their ability to influence biological functions of cells, such as natural killer (NK) cells or eosinophils. Secretory IgA and IgA2, but not IgA1 myeloma proteins significantly inhibit, in a concentration-dependent fashion, the NK activity of peripheral blood HNK-1$^+$ cells against K 563 target cells (Komiyama *et al.*, 1986). In the eosinophil degranulation assay, IgA1 and IgA2 myeloma proteins and secretory IgA display a comparable activity (Abu-Ghazaleh *et al.*, 1989). Thus, IgA may be a principal immunoglobulin that mediates effector functions of eosinophils at mucosal surfaces in infections with parasites and in hypersensitivity diseases.

C. Distribution of Naturally Occurring or Vaccination-Induced IgA1 and IgA2 Antibodies Specific for Various Types of Antigens

Studies of the IgA subclass association of naturally or artificially induced serum and secretory antibodies specific for different types of antigens revealed several potentially important findings. In colostrum (Ladjeva *et al.*, 1989) or saliva (Brown and Mestecky, 1985), antibodies specific for protein antigens were found predominantly in the IgA1 subclass. In contrast, antibodies to bacterial lipopolysaccharide and lipoteichoic acid in these fluids were of the IgA2 subclass. However, in serum, such antibodies were present as IgA1 (Russell *et al.*, 1986; Moldoveanu *et al.*, 1987), suggesting that they were derived from another tissue, probably bone marrow, and were induced by a different stimulatory pathway. The differences in the IgA subclass distribution of specific antibodies were even more pronounced in response to local or systemic infection or immunization. Although low levels of IgA1 and IgA2 antibodies to influenza A virus were detected before infection, IgA1 accounted for most of the rise in antihemagglutinin levels seen after infection (Brown *et al.*, 1985). However, in serum, almost all IgA antibodies were of the IgA1 subclass before and after the infection. Systemic immunization with pneumococcal polysaccharide vaccine induced a vigorous serum response in IgG and IgA isotypes. However, when analyzed by an ELISPOT assay for specific antibody-secreting cells, IgA-producing cells predominated in the peripheral blood (Lue *et al.*, 1988). Further, examination with monoclonal anti-IgA1 and anti-IgA2 reagents revealed the predominance of IgA2 cells producing specific antipolysaccharide antibodies. Comparable results were obtained in another concurrent, although independent, study (Heilman *et al.*, 1988). Subsequent immunizations of another group of young adult volunteers with tetanus toxoid or with polysaccharides from *Haemophilus influenzae* or *N. meningitidis* led to the transient appearance of antigen-specific antibody-secreting cells in the peripheral blood (Tarkowski *et al.*, 1990). Low frequencies of IgA-secreting cells, predominantly of subclass IgA1, were detected against tetanus toxoid. In contrast, the antipolysaccharide response was dominated by IgA2-producing cells.

Collectively, these results indicate that the character of an antigen greatly influences the outcome of the immune response with respect to the IgA subclass. Similar conclusions were reached in studies of the distribution of specific IgG subclass antibodies induced by systemic immunizations with protein or polysaccharide antigens (Hammerström and Smith, 1986). The mechanisms that regulate the isotype responses to various types of antigens remain speculative. Processing of different antigens and the involvement of different types of T helper cells and lymphokines (McGhee *et al.*, 1989) represent attractive avenues for future investigations.

D. Phylogenetic Aspects of the Human IgA Subclasses

Kawamura *et al.* (1992) reported elegant work in which they obtained genomic sequences of α chain genes from a series of hominoid species (Figure 6). Their data show clearly the presence of IgA1 and IgA2 molecules in some of the hominoid species, although all features (e.g., the extended hinge in IgA1) were not always present. These authors suggest that gene conversion was a major avenue to creating the IgA subclasses in humans and their immediate predecessors.

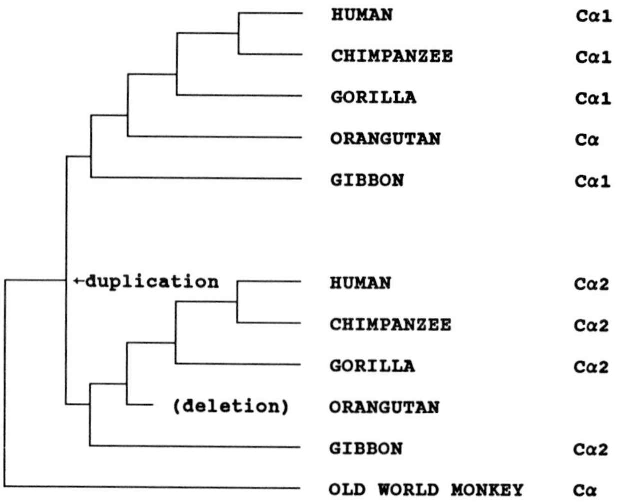

Figure 6 Primate immunoglobulins. A phylogenetic tree tracing the origins of the IgA subclasses in hominoids and humans. The model is adapted from that of Kawamura *et al.* (1992).

VII. SUMMARY

Mucosal immunoglobulins represent a family of immunoglobulin isotypes that function to protect the host from molecules and microorganisms to which the mucosal surfaces are exposed continually. Transcytosis of the major isotype, IgA, is mediated by poly Ig receptor and provides mucosal secretions with a highly avid antibody.

Functional differences among the multiple IgA isotypes are just beginning to be understood. As these unfold, vaccination strategies may have to be designed to direct immune responses toward particular IgA isotypes. Preliminary findings indicate that the IgA subclass response in humans may be antigen dependent.

Acknowledgments

Thanks to Grace Loney and Sharon Molnar for preparation of the manuscript.

References

Abel, C. A., and Grey, H. M. (1968). Studies on the structure of mouse γA myeloma proteins. *Biochemistry* **1,** 2682–2688.

Abu-Ghazaleh, R. I., Fujisawa, T., Mestecky, J., Kyle, R. A., and Gleich, G. J. (1989). IgA-induced eosinophil degranulation. *J. Immunol.* **142,** 2393–2400.

Allansmith, M. R., Radl, J., Haaijman, J. J., and Mestecky, J. (1985). Molecular forms of tear IgA and distribution of IgA subclasses in human lacrimal glands. *J. Allergy Clin. Immunol.* **76,** 569–576.

Alley, C. D., Nash, G. S., and MacDermott, R. P. (1982). Marked *in vitro* spontaneous secretion of IgA by human rib bone marrow mononuclear cells. *J. Immunol.* **128,** 2604–2608.

Altorfer, J., Hardesty, S. J., Scott, J. H., and Jones, A. L. (1987). Specific antibody synthesis and biliary secretion by the rat liver and intestinal immunization with cholera toxin. *Gastroenterology* **93,** 539–549.

Apodaca, G., Bomsel, M., Arden, J., Breitfeld, P. P., Tang, K., and Mostov, K. E. (1991). The polymeric immunoglobulin receptor. *J. Clin. Invest.* **87,** 1877–1882.

Ashwell, G., and Harford, J. (1982). Carbohydrate-specific receptor of the liver. *Annu. Rev. Bioshem.* **52,** 531–554.

Aucouturier, P., Pineau, N., Kobayashi, K., and Preud'homme, J. L. (1989). Methodological pitfalls in immunoglobulin subclass assays: An investigation of anti-Ig subclass monoclonal antibody and jacalin reactivity. *Protides Biol. Fluids* **36,** 61–69.

Baenziger, J. (1979). Structure of the oligosaccharide of human J chain. *J. Biol. Chem.* **254,** 4063–4071.

Baenziger, J., and Kornfeld, S. (1974a). Structure of the carbohydrate units of IgA1 immunoglobulin. I. Composition, glycopeptide isolation, and structure of the asparagine-linked oligosaccharide units. *J. Biol. Chem.* **249,** 7260–7269.

Baenziger, J., and Kornfeld, S. (1974b). Structure of the carbohydrate units of IgA1 immunoglobulin. II. Structure of the O-glycosidically linked oligosaccharide units. *J. Biol. Chem.* **249,** 7270–7281.

Bakos, M.-A., Kurosksy, A., and Goldblum, R. M. (1991). Characterization of a critical binding site for human polymeric Ig on secretory component. *J. Immunol.* **147,** 3419–3426.

Banting, G., Brake, B., Braghetta, P., Luzio, J. P., and Stanley, K. K. (1989). Intracellular targetting signals of polymeric immunoglobulin receptors are highly conserved between species. *Fed. Eur. Biochem. Soc.* **254,** 177–183.

Bastian, A., Kratzin, H., Eckart, K., and Hilschmann, N. (1992). Intra- and Interchain disulfide bridges of the human J chain in secretory immunoglobulin A. *Biol. Chem.* Hoppe-Seyler **373,** 1255–1263.

Beale, D. (1987). The structure of bovine secretory component. *Vet. Immunol. Immunopathol.* **17,** 37–49.

Bouvet, J.-P., Pieres, R., Iscaki, S., and Pillot, J. (1987). IgM reassociation in the absence of J chain. *Immunol. Lett.* **15,** 27–31.

Brandtzaeg, P. (1974). Characteristics of SC-Ig complexes formed *in vitro. Adv. Exp. Med. Biol.* **45,** 87–90.

Brandtzaeg, P. (1978). Polymeric IgA is complexed with secretory component (SC) on the surface of human intestinal epithelial cells. *Scand. J. Immunol.* **8,** 39–52.

Brandtzaeg, P. (1981). Transport models for secretory IgA and secretory IgM. *Clin. Exp. Immunol.* **44,** 221–232.

Brandtzaeg, P. (1983a). Immunohistochemical characterization of intracellular J-chain and binding site for secretory component (SC) in human immunoglobulin (Ig)-producing cells. *Mol. Immunol.* **20,** 941–966.

Brandtzaeg, P. (1983b). The secretory immune system of lactating human mammaray glands compared with other exocrine organs. *Ann. N.Y. Acad. Sci.* **409,** 353–382.

Brandtzaeg, P. (1985). The role of J chain and secretory component in receptor-mediated glandular and hepatic transport of immunoglobulins in man. *Scand. J. Immunol.* **22,** 111–146.

Brown, T. A., and Mestecky, J. (1985). Immunoglobulin A subclass distribution of naturally occurring salivary antibodies to microbial antigens. *Infect. Immun.* **49,** 459–462.

Brown, T. A., Murphy, B. R., Radl, J., Haajman, J. J., and Mestecky, J. (1985). Subclass distribution and molecular form of immunoglobulin A hemaglutinin antibodies in sera and nasal secretions after experimental secondary infection with influenza A virus in humans. *J. Clin. Microbiol.* **22,** 259–264.

Brown, W. R., and Kloppel, T. M. (1989). The liver and IgA: Immunological, cell biological and clinical implications. *Hepatology* **9,** 763–784.

Brown, W. R., Newcomb, R. W., and Ishizaka, K. (1970). Proteolytic degradation of exocrine and serum immunoglobulins. *J. Clin. Invest.* **49,** 1374–1380.

Brown, W. R., Borthisle, B. K., and Chen, S. T. (1975). Immunoglobulin E (IgE) and IgE-containing cells in human gastrointestinal fluids and tissues. *Clin. Exp. Immunol.* **20,** 227–237.

Burnett, R. C., Hanley, W. C., Zhai, S. K., and Knight, K. L. (1989). The IgA heavy-chain gene family in rabbit: Cloning and sequence analysis of 13 Cα genes. *EMBO J.* **8,** 4041–4047.

Butler, J. E. (1983). Bovine immunoglobulins: An augmented review. *Vet. Immunol. Immunopathol.* **4,** 43–152.

Buxbaum, J. N., Zolla, S., Scharff, M. D., and Franklin, E. C. (1974). The synthesis and assembly of immunoglobulins by malignant human plasmocytes. III. Heterogeneity of IgA polymer assembly. *Eur. J. Immunol.* **4,** 367–369.

Cattaneo, A., and Neuberger, M. S. (1987). Polymeric immunoglobulin M is secreted by transfectants of non-lymphoid cells in the absence of immunoglobulin J chain. *EMBO J.* **112,** 1401–1406.

Conley, M. E., and Delacroix, D. L. (1987). Intravascular and mucosal immunoglobulin A: Two separate but related systems of immune defense? *Ann. Int. Med.* **106,** 892–899.

Crago, S. S., Kulhavy, R., Prince, S. J. and Mestecky, J. (1978). Secretory component of epithelial cells is a surface receptor for polymeric immunoglobulins. *J. Exp. Med.* **147,** 1832–1837.

Crago, S. S., Kutteh, W. H., Moro, I., Allansmith, M. R., Radl, J., Haaijman, J. J., and Mestecky, J. (1984). Distribution of IgA1-, IgA2- and J chain-containing cells in human tissues. *J. Immunol.* **132,** 16–18.

Cripps, A. W., and Lascelles, A. K. (1976). The origin of immunoglobulins in salivary secretion of sheep. *Austr. J. Exp. Biol. Med. Sci.* **54,** 191–194.

Davies, A. C., Roux, K. H., Pursey, J., and Shulman, M. J. (1989). Intermolecular disulfide bonding in IgM: Effect of replacing cysteine residues in the μ heavy chain. *EMBO J.* **8,** 2519–2526.

Delacroix, D. L., and Vaerman, J. P. (1981). A solid phase, direct competition, radioimmunoassay for quantitation of secretory IgA in human serum. *J. Immunol. Meth.* **40,** 345–358.

Delacroix, D. L., Dive, C., Rambaud, J. C., and Vaerman, J. P. (1982). IgA subclasses in various secretions and in serum. *Immunology* **47,** 383–385.

Delacroix, D. L., Furtado-Barreira, G., de Hemptinne, B., Goudswaard, J., Dive, C., and Vaerman, J-P. (1983). The liver in the IgA secretory immune system. Dogs, but not rats and rabbits, are suitable models for human studies. *Hepatology* **3,** 980–988.

Delacroix, D. L., Marchandise, F. X., Francis, C., and Sibille, Y. (1985). α-2-Macroglobulin, monomeric and polymeric immunoglobulin A, and immunoglobulin M in bronchoalveolar lavage. *Am. Rev. Resp. Dis.* **132,** 829–835.

Eiffert, H., Quentin, E., Decker, J., Hillmeir, S., Hufschmidt, M., Klingmuller, D., Weber, M. H., and Hilschmann, N. (1984). The primary structure of the human free secretory component and the arrangement of the disulfide bonds. Hoppe–Seyler's *Z. Physiol. Chem. (Germany)* **365,** 1489–1495.

Eiffert, H., Quentin, E., Wiederhold, M., Hillemeir, S., Decker, J., Weber, M., and Hilschmann, N. (1991). Determination of the molecular structure of the human free secretory component. *Biol. Chem.* Hoppe–Seyler **372,** 119–128.

Fallgren-Gebauer, E., Gebauer, W., Bastian, A., Kratzin, H., Eiffert, H., Zimmerman, B., Karas, M., and Hilschmann, N. (1992). The covalent linkage of the secretory component to IgA. *Adv. Exp. Biol.,* in press.

Field, M. C., Dwek, R. A., Edge, C. J., and Rademacher, T. W.

(1989). O-linked oligosaccharides from human serum immunoglobulin A1. *Biochem. Soc. Trans.* **17,** 1034–1035.

Frutiger, S., Hughes, G. J., Hanly, W. C., Kingzette, M., and Jaton, J-C. (1986). The amino-terminal domain of rabbit secretory component is responsible for noncovalent binding to immunoglobulin A dimers. *J. Biol. Chem.* **261,** 16673–16681.

Frutiger, S., Hughes, G. J., Fonck, C., and Jaton, J-C. (1987). High and low molecular weight rabbit secretory components. *J. Biol. Chem.* **262,** 1712–1715.

Frutiger, S., Hughes, G. J., Hanly, W. C., and Jaton, J-C. (1988). Rabbit secretory components of different allotypes vary in their carbohydrate content and their sites of *N*-linked glycosylation. *J. Biol. Chem.* **263,** 8120–8125.

Frutiger, S., Hughes, G. J., Paquet, N., Lüthy, R., and Jaton, J.-C. (1992). Disulfide bond assignment in human J chain and its covalent pairing with immunoglobulin M. *Biochemistry* **31,** 12643–12647.

Fubara, E. S., and Freter, R. (1973). Protection against bacterial infection by secretory IgA antibodies. *J. Immunol.* **111,** 395–403.

Garcia-Pardo, A., Lamm, M. E., Plaut, A. G., and Frangione, B. (1979). Secretory component is covalently bound to a single subunit in human secretory IgA. *Mol. Immunol.* **16,** 477–482.

Garcia-Pardo, A., Lamm, M. E., Plaut, A. G., and Frangione, B. (1981). J Chain is covalently bound to both monomer subunits in human secretory IgA. *J. Biol. Chem.* **256,** 11734–11738.

Geneste, C., Iscaki, S., Mangalo, R., and Pillot, J. (1986). Both Fcα domains of human IgA are involved in *in vitro* interaction between secretory component and dimeric IgA. *Immunol. Lett.* **13,** 221–226.

Grey, H. M., Abel, C. A., Yount, W. J., and Kunkel, H. G. (1968). A subclass of human γA-globulins (γA2) which lacks the disulfide bonds linking heavy chain and light chains. *J. Exp. Med.* **128,** 1223–1236.

Hajdu, I., Moldoveanu, Z., Cooper, M. D., and Mestecky, J. (1983). Ultrastructural studies of human lymphoid cells. μ and J chain expression as a function of B cell differentiation. *J. Exp. Med.* **158,** 1993–2006.

Hammerström, L., and Smith, C. I. E. (1986). IgG subclass changes in response to vaccination. *Monogr. Allergy* **19,** 241–252.

Heilman, C., Barington, T., Sigsgaard, T. (1988). Subclass of individual IgA-secreting human lymphocytes. Investigation of *in vivo* pneumococcal polysaccharide-induced blood B cells by monolayer plaque-forming cell assay. *J. Immunol.* **140,** 1496–1499.

Heremans, J. F. (1974). Immunoglobulin A. *In* "The Antigens" (M. Sela, ed.), Vol. II, pp. 365–522. Academic Press, New York.

Hughes, G. J., Frutiger, S., Paquet, N., and Jaton, J.-C. (1990). The amino acid sequence of rabbit J chain in secretory immunoglobulin A. *Biochem. J.* **271,** 641–647.

Hunkapiller, T., and Hood, L. (1989). Diversity of the immunoglobulin gene superfamily. *Adv. Immunol.* **44,** 1–63.

Inman, F. P., and Mestecky, J. (1974). The J chain of polymeric immunoglobulins. *Contemp. Top. Mol. Immunol.* **3,** 111–141.

Iscaki, S., Genestte, C., d'Azambuja, S., and Pillot, J. (1979). Human secretory component. II. Easy detection of abnormal amounts of combined secretory component in human sera. *J. Immunol. Meth.* **28,** 331–339.

Jackson, G. D. F., Lemaitre-Coelho, I., Vaerman, J. P., Bazin, H., and Beckers, A. (1978). Rapid disappearance from serum of intravenously infected rat myeloma IgA and its secretion into bile. *Eur. J. Immunol.* **8,** 123–126.

Jackson, G. D. F., Walker, P. G., Schiff, J. M., Barrington, P. J., Fisher M. M., and Underdown, B. J. (1985). A role for the spleen in the appearance of IgM in the bile of rats injected intravenously with horse erythrocytes. *J. Immunol.* **135,** 152–157.

Jarvis, G. A., and Griffiss, J. M. (1991). Human IgA1 blockade of IgG-initiated lysis of *Neisseria meningitidis* is a function of antigen-binding fragment binding to the polysaccharide capsule. *J. Immunol.* **147,** 1962–1967.

Jonard, P. P., Rambaud, J. C., Dive, C., Vaerman, J. P., Galian, A., and Delacroix, D. L. (1984). Secretion of immunoglobulins and plasma proteins from jejunal mucosa. *J. Clin. Invest.* **74,** 525–535.

Kaartinen, M., Imir, T., Klockars, M., Sandholm, M., and Makela, O. (1978). IgA in blood and thoracic duct lymph: Concentration and degree of polymerization. *Scand. J. Immunol.* **7,** 229–232.

Kabat, E. A., Wu, T. T., Biolofsky, H., Reid-Miller, M., and Perry, H. (1987). Sequences of proteins of immunological interest. National Institutes of Health, Washington, D. C.

Kaetzel, C. S., Robinson, J. K., Chintalacharuvu, K. R., Vaerman, J. P., and Lamm, M. E. (1991). The polymeric immunoglobulin receptor (secretory component) mediates transport of immune complexes across epithelial cells: A local defense function for IgA. *Proc. Natl. Acad. Sci. U.S.A.* **88,** 8796–8800.

Kawamura, S., Saitou, N., and Ueda, S. (1992). Concerted evolution of the primate immunoglobulin α-gene through gene conversion. *J. Biol. Chem.* **267,** 7359–7367.

Kett, K., Brandtzaeg, P., Radl, J., and Haaijman, J. J. (1986). Different subclass distribution of IgA-producing cells in human lymphoid organs and various secreting tissues. *J. Immunol.* **136,** 3631–3635.

Knight, K. L., Martens, C. L., Stoklosa, C., and Schneiderman, R. D. (1984). Genes encoding α-heavy chains of rabbit IgA: characterization of cDNA encoding IgA-g subclass α-chains. *Nucleic Acids Res.* **12,** 1657–1670.

Kobayashi, K., Vaerman, J.-P., Bazin, H., Lebacq-Verheyden, A.-M., and Heremans, J. F. (1973). Identification of J-chain in polymeric immunoglobulins from a variety of species by cross-reaction with rabbit antisera to human J-chain. *J. Immunol.* **111,** 1590–1594.

Komiyama, K., Crago, S. S., Itoh, K., Moro, I., and Mestecky, J. (1986). Inhibition of natural killer cell activity by IgA. *Cell. Immunol.* **101,** 143–155.

Koshland, M. E. (1985). The coming of age of the immunoglobulin J chain. *Ann. Rev. Immunol.* **3,** 425–453.

Krajči, P., Grzeschik, K. H., Geurts van Kessell, A. H. M., Olaisen, B., and Brandtzaeg, P. (1991). The human transmembrane secretory component (poly-Ig receptor): Molecular cloning, restriction fragment length polymorphism and chromosomal sublocalization. *Human Genetics* **87,** 642–648.

Kratzin, H., Altevogt, P., Ruban, E., Kortt, A., Staroscik, K., and Hilschmann, N. (1975). The primary structure of a monoclonal IgA-immunoglobulin (IgA Tro.). II. The amino acid sequence of the H-chain, α-type, subgroup III; structure of the complete IgA-molecule. Hoppe–Seyler's *Z. Physiol. Chem.* (*Germany*) **356,** 1337–1342.

Kubagawa, H., Burrows, P. D., Grossi, C. E., Mestecky, J., and Cooper, M. D. (1988). Precursor B cells transformed by Epstein–Barr virus undergo sterile plasma-cell differentiation: J-chain expression without immunoglobulin. *Proc. Natl. Acad. Sci. U.S.A.* **85,** 875–879.

Kutteh, W. H., Hatch, K. D., Blackwell, R. E., and Mestecky, J. (1988). Secretory immune system of the female reproductive tract: I. Immunoglobulin and secretory component-containing cells. *Obstet. Gynecol.* **71,** 56–60.

Kvale, D., and Brandtzaeg, D. (1986). An enzyme-linked immunosorbent assay for differential quantitation of secretory immunoglobulins of the A and M isotypes in human serum. *J. Immunol. Meth.* **86,** 107–114.

Ladjeva, I., Peterman, J. H., and Mestecky, J. (1989). IgA subclasses of human colostral antibodies specific for microbial and food antigens *Clin. Exp. Immunol.* **78,** 85–90.

Lemaitre-Coelho, I., Jackson, G. D. F., and Vaerman, J. P. (1977). Rat bile as a convenient source of secretory IgA and free secretory component. *Eur. J. Immunol.* **8,** 588–590.

Leslie, G. A., and Teramura, G. (1977). Structure and biological functions of human IgD. XIV. The development of a solid-phase radioimmunoassay for the quantitation of IgD in human sera and secretions *Int. Arch. Allergy Appl. Immunol.* **54,** 451–456.

Lue, C., Tarkowski, A., and Mestecky, J. (1988). Systemic immunization with pneumococcal polysaccharide vaccine induces predominant IgA2 response of peripheral blood lymphocytes and increases of both serum and secretory anti-pneumococcal antibodies. *J. Immunol.* **140,** 3793–3800.

McCune, J. M., Fu, S. M., and Kunkel, H. G. (1981). J chain biosynthesis in pre-B cells and other possible precursors of B cells. *J. Exp. Med.* **154,** 138–145.

McDermott, M. R., Clark, D. A., and Bienenstock, J. (1980). Evidence for a common mucosal immunologic system. II. Influence of the estrous cycle in B immunoblast migration into genital tract and intestinal tissues. *J. Immunol.* **123,** 2536–2539.

McGhee, J. R., Mestecky, J., Elson, C. O., and Kiyono, H. (1989). Regulation of IgA synthesis and immune responses by T cells and interleukins. *J. Clin. Immunol.* **9,** 175–199.

Mach, J. P. (1970). *In vitro* combination of human and bovine secretory component with IgA of various species. *Nature (London)* **228,** 1278–1282.

Manning, R. J., Walker, P. G., Carter, L., Barrington, P. J., and Jackson, G. D. F. (1984). Studies on the origins of biliary immunoglobulins in rats. *Gastroenterology* **87,** 173–179.

Mansikka, A. (1992). Chicken IgA H Chains. *J. Immunol.* **149,** 855–861.

Matsuuchi, L., Cann, G. M., and Koshland, M. E. (1986). Immunoglobulin J chain gene from the mouse. *Proc. Natl. Acad. Sci. U.S.A.* **83,** 456–460.

Max, E. E., and Korsmeyer, J. S. (1985). Human J chain gene. Structure and expression in B lymphoid cells. *J. Exp. Med.* **161,** 832–849.

Mazanec, M. B., Kaetzel, C. S., Lamm, M. E., Fletcher, D., and Nedrud, J. G. (1992). Intracellular neutralization of virus by immunoglobulin A antibodies. *Proc. Natl. Acad. Sci. U.S.A.* **89,** 6901–6905.

Mestecky, J., and McGhee, J. R. (1987). Immunoglobulin A (IgA): Molecular and cellular interactions involved in IgA biosynthesis and immune response. *Adv. Immunol.* **40,** 153–245.

Mestecky, J., and Russell, M. W. (1986). IgA subclasses. Monogr. *Allergy* **19,** 277–301.

Mestecky, J., Kulhavy, R., Wright, G. P., and Tomana, M. (1974a). Studies on human secretory immunoglobulin A. VI. Cyanogen bromide cleavage. *J. Immunol.* **113,** 404–412.

Mestecky, J., Schrohenloher, R. E., Kulhavy, R., Wright, G. P., and Tomana, M. (1974b). Site of J chain attachment to human polymeric IgA. *Proc. Nat. Acad. Sci. USA* **71,** 544–548.

Mestecky, J., Preud'homme, J.-L., Crago, S. S., Mihaesco, E., Prchal, J. T., and Okos, A. J. (1980). Presence of J chain in human lymphoid cells. *Clin. Exp. Immunol.* **39,** 371–385.

Mestecky, J., Russell, M. W., Jackson, S., and Brown, T. A. (1986). The human IgA system: A reassessment. *Clin. Immunol. Immunopathol.* **40,** 105–114.

Mestecky, J., Tomana, M., Czerkinsky, C., Tarkowski, A., Matsuda, S., Waldo, F. B., Moldoveanu, Z., Julian, B. A., Galla, J. H., Russell, M. W., and Jackson, S. (1987). IgA-associated renal diseases: Immunochemical studies of IgA1 proteins, circulating immune complexes, and cellular interactions. *Sem. Nephrol.* **7,** 332–335.

Mestecky, J., Lue, C., Tarkowski, A., Ladjeva, I., Peterman, J. H., Moldoveanu, Z., Russell, M. W., Brown, T. A., Radl, J., Haaijman, J. J., Kiyono, H., and McGhee, J. R. (1989). Comparative studies of the biological properties of human IgA subclasses. *Protides Biol. Fluids* **36,** 173–182.

Mestecky, J., Lue, C., and Russell, M. W. (1991). Selective transport of IgA. Cellular and molecular aspects. *Gastroenterol. Clin. North Am.* **20,** 441–471.

Mikoryak, C. A., Morgolies, M. N., and Steiner, L. A. (1988). J chain in *Rana catesbeiana* high molecular weight Ig. *J. Immunol.* **140,** 4279–4285.

Mizoguchi, A., Mizuochi, T., and Kobata, A. (1982). Structures of the carbohydrate moieties of secretory component purified from human milk. *J. Biol. Chem.* **257,** 9612–9621.

Moldoveanu, Z., Egan, M. L., and Mestecky, J. (1984). Cellular origins of human polymeric and monomeric IgA: Intracellular and secreted forms of IgA. *J. Immunol.* **133,** 3156–3162.

Moldoveanu, Z., Brown, T. A., Ventura, M. T., Michalek, S. M., McGhee, J. R., and Mestecky, J. (1987). IgA subclass responses to lipopolysaccharide in humans. *Adv. Exp. Med. Biol.* **216B,** 1199–1205.

Moldoveanu, Z., Epps, J. M., Thorpe, S. R., and Mestecky, J. (1988). The sites of catabolism of murine monomeric IgA. *J. Immunol.* **141,** 208–213.

Moldoveanu, Z., Moro, I., Radl, J., Thorpe, S. R., Komiyama, K., and Mestecky, J. (1990). Catabolism of autologous and heterologous IgA in non-human primates. *Scand. J. Immunol.* **32,** 577–583.

Mostov, K. E., Friedlander, M., and Blobel, G. (1984). The receptor for transepithelial transport of IgA and IgM contains multiple immunoglobulin-like domains. *Nature (London)* **308,** 37–43.

Mygind, N., Weeke, B., and Ullman, S. (1975). Quantitative determination of immunoglobulins in nasal secretion. *Int. Arch. Allergy Appl. Immun.* **49,** 99–107.

Nagura, H., Nakane, P. K., and Brown, W. R. (1979). Translocation of dimeric IgA through neoplastic colon cells *in vitro*. *J. Immunol.* **123,** 2359–2368.

Nagura, H., Tsutsumi, Y., Hasegawa, H., Watanabe, K., Nakane, P. K., and Brown, W. R. (1983). IgA plasma cells in biliary mucosa: A likely source of locally synthesized IgA in human hepatic bile. *Clin. Exp. Immunol.* **54,** 671–680.

Niedermeier, W., Tomana, M., and Mestecky, J. (1972). The carbohydrate composition of J chain from human serum and secretory IgA. *Biochem. Biophys. Acta* **257,** 527–530.

Parkhouse, R. M. E. (1971). Immunoglobulin A biosynthesis. Intracellular accumulation of 7S subunits. *FEBS Lett.* **16,** 71–73.

Parkhouse, R. M. E., and Della Corte, E. (1973). Biosynthesis of immunoglobulin A (IgA) and immunoglobulin M (IgM). *Biochem. J.* **136,** 607–609.

Parr, M. B., and Parr, E. L. (1989). Immunohistochemical localization of secretory component and immunoglobulin A in the urogenital tract of the male rodent. *J. Reprod. Fert.* **85,** 115–124.

Parr, M. B., Ren, H. P., Russell, L. D., Prins, G. S., and Parr, E. L. (1992). Urethral glands of the male mouse contain secretory component and immunoglobulin A plasma cells and are targets of testosterone. *Biol. Reprod.* **47,** 1031–1039.

Plebani, A., Mira, E., Mevio, E., Monafo, V., Notarangelo, L. D., Avanzini, A., and Ugazio, A. G. (1983). IgM and IgD concentrations in the serum and secretions of children with selective IgA deficiency. *Clin. Exp. Immunol.* **53,** 689–696.

Pumphrey, R. S. H. (1986). Computer models of the human immunoglobulins. Binding sites and molecular interactions. *Immunol. Today* **7,** 206–211.

Putnam, F. W., Yu-Sheng, V. L., and Low, T. L. K. (1979). Primary structure of a human IgA1 immunoglobulin. *J. Biol. Chem.* **254,** 2865–2874.

Radl, J. F., Klein, M. H., van den Berg, P., de Bruyn, A. M., and Hijmans, W. (1971). Binding of secretory piece to polymeric IgA and IgA paraproteins *in vitro*. *Immunol.* **20,** 843–852.

Roque-Barreira, M. C., and Campos-Neto, A. (1985). Jacalin: An IgA-binding lectin. *J. Immunol.* **134,** 1740–1743.

Rose, M. E., Orlans, E., Payne, A. W. R., and Hesketh, P. (1981). The origin of IgA in chicken bile: Its rapid active transport from blood. *Eur. J. Immunol.* **11,** 561–564.

Russell, M. W., Brown, T. A., Claflin, J. L., Schroer, K., and Mestecky, J. (1983). Immunoglobulin A-mediated hepatobiliary transport constitutes a natural pathway for disposing of bacterial antigens. *Infect. Immun.* **42,** 1041–1048.

Russell, M. W., Brown, T. A., and Mestecky, J. (1981). Role of Serum IgA. Hepatobiliary transport of circulating antigen. *J. Exp. Med.* **153,** 968–976.

Russell, M. W., Mestecky, J., Julian, B. A., and Galla, J. H. (1986). IgA-associated renal diseases: Antibodies to environmental antigens in sera and deposition in immunoglobulins and antigens in glomeruli. *J. Clin. Immunol.* **6,** 74–86.

Schiff, J. M., Endo, Y., Kells, D. I. C., Fisher, M. M., and Underdown, B. J. (1983). Kinetic differences in hepatic transport of IgA polymers reflect molecular size. *Fed. Proc.* **42,** 1341. (Abstract)

Skea, D. L., Christopoulous, P., Plaut, A. G., and Underdown, B. J. (1988). Studies on the specificity of the IgA-binding lectin, jacalin. *Mol. Immunol.* **25,** 1–6.

Skvaril, F., and Morell, A. (1974). Distribution of IgA subclasses in sera and bone marrow plasma cells of 21 normal individuals. *Adv. Exp. Med. Biol.* **45,** 433–435.

Socken, D. J., Simms, E. S., Nagy, B., Fisher, M. M., and Underdown, B. J. (1981). Secretory component-dependent hapatic transport of IgA antibody-antigen complexes. *J. Immunol.* **127,** 316–319.

South, M. A., Cooper, M. D., Wolheim, F. A., Hong, R., and Good, R. A. (1986). The IgA system. I. Studies of the transport and immunochemistry of IgA in the saliva. *J. Exp. Med.* **123,** 615–627.

Stockert, R. J., Kressner, M. S., Collins, J. C., Sternlieb, I., and Morell, A. G. (1982). IgA interactions with the asialoglycoprotein receptor. *Proc. Natl. Acad. Sci. U.S.A.* **79,** 6229–6231.

Stott, D. I. (1976). Biosynthesis and assembly of IgM. Addition of J chain to intracellular pools of 8S and 19S IgM. *Immunochemistry* **13,** 157–163.

Sullivan, D. A., and Wira, C. R. (1983). Hormone regulation of immunoglobulins in the rat uterus: Uterine response to a single estradiol treatment. *Endocrinology* **114,** 650–658.

Sullivan, D. A., Block, K. J., and Allansmith, M. R. (1984). Hormonal influence on the secretory immune system of the eye: Androgen control of secretory component production by the rat exorbital gland. *Immunology* **52,** 239–246.

Svehag, S. E., and Bloth, B. (1970). Ultrastructure of secretory and high-polymer serum immunoglobulin A of human and rabbit origin. *Science* **168,** 847–849.

Takahashi, T., Iwase, T., Kobayashi, K., Rejnek, J., Mestecky, J., and Moro, I. (1993). Phylogeny of the immunoglobulin joining (J) chain. *Adv. Exp. Med. Biol.* in press.

Tarkowski, A., Lue, C., Moldoveanu, Z., Kiyono, H., McGhee, J. R., and Mestecky, J. (1990). Immunization of humans with polysaccharide vaccines induces systemic, predominantly polymeric IgA2-subclass antibody responses. *J. Immunol.* **144,** 3770–3778.

Tomana, M., Mestecky, J., and Niedermeier, W. (1972). Studies on human secretory immunogloulin A. IV. Carbohydrate composition. *J. Immunol.* **108,** 1631–1636.

Tomana, M., Niedermeier, W., Mestecky, J., and Skvaril, F. (1976). The differences in carbohydrate composition between the subclasses of IgA immunoglobulins. *Immunochemistry* **13,** 325–328.

Tomana, M., Niedermeier, W., and Spivey, C. (1978). Microdetermination of monosaccharides in glycoproteins by gas-liquid chromotography. *Anal. Biochem.* **89,** 110–118.

Tomana, M., Kulhavy, R., and Mestecky, J. (1988). Receptor-mediated binding and uptake of immunoblobulin A by human liver. *Gastroenterology* **94,** 762–770.

Tomasi, T. B., and Bienenstock, J. (1968). Secretory immunoglobulins *Adv. Immunol.* **9,** 1–96.

Torano, A., and Putnam, F. W. (1978). Complete amino acid sequence of the $\alpha 2$ heavy chain of a human IgA2 immunoglobulin of the A2 in (2) allotype. *Proc. Natl. Acad. Sci. U.S.A.* **75,** 966–969.

Torano, A., Tsuzukida, Y., Liu, Y.-S.V., and Putnam, F. W. (1977). Location and structural significance of the oligosaccharides in human IgA1 and IgA2 immunoglobulins. *Proc. Natl. Acad. Sci. U.S.A.* **74,** 2301–2305.

Tsuzukida, Y., Wang, C. C., and Putnam, F. W. (1979). Structure of the A2m(1) allotype of human IgA—A recombinant molecule. *Proc. Natl. Acad. Sci. U.S.A.* **76,** 1104–1108.

Tucker, P. W., Slightom, J. L., and Blattner, F. R. (1981). Mouse IgA heavy chain gene sequence: Implications for evolution of immunoglobulin hinge exons. *Proc. Natl. Acad. Sci. U.S.A.* **78,** 7684–7688.

Underdown, B. J., and Schiff, J. M. (1986). Immunoglobulin A: Strategic defense initiative at the mucosal surface. *Ann. Rev. Immunol.* **4,** 389–417.

Underdown, B. J., DeRose, J., and Plaut, A. (1977). Disulfide bonding of secretory component to a single monomer subunit in human secretory IgA. *J. Immunol.* **118,** 1816–1821.

Underdown, B. J., Switzer, I. C., and Jackson, G. D. F. (1992). Rat secretory component binds poorly to rodent IgM. *J. Immunol.* **149,** 487–491.

Vaerman, J.-P., and Delacroix, D. L. (1984). Role of the liver in the immunobiology of IgA in animals and humans. *Contr. Nephrol.* **40,** 17–31.

Vaerman, J.-P., Andre, C., Bazin, H., and Heremans, J. F. (1973). Mesenteric lymph as a major source of serum IgA in guinea pigs and rats. *Eur. J. Immunol.* **3,** 580–584.

van Longhem, E., and Biewenga, J. (1983). Allotypic and isotypic aspects of human immunoglobulin A. *Mol. Immunol.* **20,** 1001–1007.

Wang, A. C., and Fundenberg, H. H. (1974). IgA and evolution of immunoglobulins. *J. Immunogenet.* **1,** 3–31.

Weiker, J., and Underdown, B. J. (1975). Secretory component bonding to immunoglobulins A and M. *J. Immunol.* **114,** 1337–1344.

Williams, A. F. (1986). A year in the life of the immunoglobulin superfamily. *Immunol. Today* **8,** 298–303.

Williams, R. C., and Gibbons, R. J. (1972). Inhibition of bacterial adherence by secretory immunoglobulin A: A mechanism of antigen disposal. *Science* **177,** 697–699.

Winner, L., III, Mack, J., Weltzin, R., Mekalanos, J. J., Kraehenbuhl, J. P., and Neutra, M. R. (1991). New model of analysis of mucosal immunity: Intestinal secretion of specific monoclonal immunoglobulin A from hybridoma tumors protect against *Vibrio cholerae* infection. *Infect. Immun.* **59,** 977–982.

Wira, C. A., Hyde, E., Sandoe, C. P., and Spencer, S. (1980). Cellular aspects of the rat uterine IgA response to oestradiol and progesterone. *J. Steroid Biochem.* **12,** 451–459.

Wold, A. E., Mestecky, J., Tomana, M., Kobata, A., Ohbayashi, H., Endo, T., and Svanborg-Edén, C. (1990). Secretory immunoglobulin A carries oligosaccharide receptors for *Escherichia coli* type 1 fimbrial lectin. *Infect. Immun.* **58,** 3073–3077.

Yang, Ch. Y., Kratzin, H., Gotz, H., and Hilschmann, N. (1979). Die Primarstruktur eines monoklonalen IgA1 Immunoglobulins

(Myelomprotein Tro). VII. Darstellung, Reinigung und Charakterisierung der Disulfidbrücken. *Hoppe-Seyler's Z. Physiol. Chem.* **360,** 1919–1940.

Zikan, J., Novotny, J., Trapane, T. L., Koshland, M. E., Urry, D. W., Bennett, J. C., and Mestecky, J. (1985). Secondary structure of the immunoglobulin J chain. *Proc. Natl. Acad. Sci. U.S.A.* **82,** 5905–5909.

Zikan, J., Mestecky, J., Kulhavy, R., and Bennett, J. C. (1986). The stoichiometry of J chain in human secretory dimeric IgA. *Mol. Immunol.* **23,** 541–544.

8

Phylogenetic Aspects of Mucosal Immunoglobulins

Jean-Pierre Vaerman

I. INTRODUCTION

The concept of a secretory immune system is based on the well-defined secretory immune systems of human, mouse, and rabbit. Essential components of these systems are a secretory immunoglobulin isotype (IgA or IgM) and a receptor–transporter system such as the polymeric IgA (or IgM) receptor (pIgR) or secretory component (SC) and J chain. This chapter summarizes the evidence for the presence of secretory IgA and SC or pIgR in various species of mammals, birds, reptiles, amphibians, and fish but does not include data on J chain, which has been well identified in cartilaginous primitive fish (Klaus *et al.*, 1971; Hagiwara *et al.*, 1985).

Unambiguous identification of an IgA molecule requires comparison of the amino acid sequence of the constant part of the heavy chain of the putative IgA with the amino acid sequences of the prototype IgA sequences of human, mouse, and rabbit. Putative IgA molecules also can be identified clearly by cross reaction with antisera specific for the prototypic α chains. In the absence of such data, several other characteristics of the well-characterized IgA molecules have been used to identify putative IgA molecules, including (1) the predominant expression, relative to IgG, in exocrine secretions, (2) the differential expression of monomeric forms in serum, (3) the ability to associate in J chain-containing polymers with high affinity for SC and the formation of additional serological determinants by these associations, and (4) the abundant synthesis in mucosal plasmacytes.

The identification of putative SC components has been more difficult. IgA-bound SC is poorly immunogenic and few serological cross reactions have been reported. Further, free SC is sensitive to protease digestion and is about the same size as some immunoglobulin heavy chains.

II. MAMMALS

IgA has been identified in all mammals examined on the basis of immunodiffusion analysis of cross reactions using mammalian or chicken antisera specific for mammalian or chicken α chains (Vaerman *et al.*, 1969; Orlans and Feinstein, 1971; Neoh *et al.*, 1973). Researchers now accept that even primitive mammals such as insectivores (mole, Orlans and Feinstein, 1971; European hedgehog, Vaerman *et al.*, 1969), monotremes (echidna), and marsupials (opossum, quokka, Bell *et al.*, 1974) possess a typical secretory IgA immune system.

As described earlier, the identification of SC or pIgR has been more difficult. However, these components have been identified in humans, dogs (Reynolds and Johnson, 1971; Delacroix *et al.*, 1983), cows (Mach *et al.*, 1969) goats and sheep (Pahud and Mach, 1970), pigs (Bourne, 1969a,b; Baumgarth *et al.*, 1990), horses (Pahud and Mach, 1972), rabbits (Cebra and Small, 1967; O'Daly and Cebra, 1971), guinea pigs (Vaerman *et al.*, 1975a), rats (Vaerman *et al.*, 1975b; Acosta-Altamirano *et al.*, 1980), and mice (Lemaître-Coelho *et al.*, 1977a; Pierre *et al.*, 1993).

III. BIRDS

A. Galliforms

1. IgA

Lebacq-Verheyden *et al.* (1972a,b) first reported a putative analog of mammalian IgA in chicken serum and secretions. In addition to light chain-specific common determinants, this IgA expressed antigenic determinants that were distinct from IgM and IgG (or IgY). In serum, the IgA was predominantly polymeric and represented a minor component. In contrast, the IgA was abundant in intestinal fluids, especially in gall bladder bile (Lebacq-Verheyden *et al.*, 1974). The secretion : serum concentration ratio was also larger for IgA than for IgG and IgM in saliva, tears, and semen (Lebacq-Verheyden *et al.*, 1974). Finally, in contrast to fluorescent anti-μ and anti-γ antibodies, fluorescent anti-chicken α chain antibodies revealed a wealth of IgA plasmacytes in duodenal, jejunal, ileal, cecal, oviduct, and bronchial lamina propria, with fewer IgA-positive cells in the spleen (Lebacq-Verheyden *et al.*, 1974).

Bienenstock *et al.* (1972,1973a) also identified chicken IgA using antibiliary IgA antibodies that had been absorbed with IgG. These studies confirmed (Bienenstock *et al.* 1973b) the abundance of IgA in several chicken secretions and, using fluorescent-labeled antibodies, demonstrated many IgA-positive cells in the gut and other mucosae but not in the spleen. In addition, these researchers demonstrated a high level of incorporation of ^{14}C-labeled amino acids into IgA, but not IgG and IgM, molecules that were secreted during short-term cultures of intestinal and other mucosae. Independently, Orlans and Rose (1972) and Rose *et al.* (1974) described a putative chicken IgA by its antigenic differences from IgM and IgG, and by higher IgA/IgG ratios in secretions than in serum. Leslie and Martin (1973) and Katz *et al.* (1974) also identified chicken IgA using similar criteria.

IgA has been identified in galliforms other than chickens by similar immunochemical, immunohistological, and biological techniques. In addition, cross reactions with anti-chicken IgA have been shown for turkey (Goudswaard *et al.*, 1977a), pheasant, japanese quail, and guinea fowl (Parry and Aitken, 1975) but not pigeon, a member of Columbiformes in which only the former criteria were met (Goudswaard *et al.*, 1977b).

The data described were all consistent with the hypothesis of chicken IgA as a precursor of mammalian IgA. However, Hädge and Ambrosius (1983,1984,1986) used inhibition of radioimmunoassays to determine cross-reactivities and to screen for immunoglobulins resembling chicken bile IgA in concentrated serum globulins of diverse species. Since no cross-reactivities or related immunoglobulins were found, these investigators concluded that chicken bile immunoglobulin was not the precursor of mammalian IgA. These researchers termed chicken bile Ig IgB, for dominant immunoglobulin in bile of some birds, although clearly shown in chicken serum. Based on their radioimmunoassays and immunodiffusion studies, these investigators concluded that IgY is the precursor of mammalian IgA (Hädge and Ambrosius, 1987). However, these data have not been confirmed independently, weak cross reactions in sensitive radioimmunoassays must be interpreted with caution, and some of the data presented were contradictory (outlined by Ng and Higgins, 1986).

More recent data may settle this controversial point. Mansikka (1992) has obtained an amino acid sequence of the constant portion of the heavy chain that is different from IgG (or IgY) and IgM. Three nucleic acid probes including the chicken VH1 probe, a Cμ probe, and a Cγ probe were used to screen 20,000 recombinant clones from a cDNA library prepared from Harderian glands, which are rich in IgA, IgM, and IgY plasmacytes. Nine clones hybridized only with VH1. One of these clones (A1) had an insert of ~1900 base pairs. The deduced amino acid sequence showed that it encoded a leader sequence identical to the VH1 leader followed by a V region that was 92% identical to the known germ-line VH1. Most of the differences were in the three complementary determining regions. Frameworks of A1-V and germ-line VH1 differed only by three nucleotides. After a D region, A1-J was identical to the single germ-line J sequence, followed by a C region consisting of 1329 base pairs or 443 amino acids before the stop codon. A1-C fit with four immunoglobulin C domains, with correctly spaced invariant cysteine–cysteine and tryptophan residues. A1 is thus a full-length H chain cDNA that is isotypically different form μ and γ chains. The fowl Cα was 37% identical to mouse Cα; identity to mouse Cμ, Cγ1, and Cδ was much lower (29, 30, and 26%, respectively). Homology with human and rabbit α chains was high. The C terminal –Cys–Tyr sequence and the Cα2 glucosamine binding site that are typical of mammalian α chains were both present. A major difference was the presence of four C domains in chicken α chain, as in chicken γ chain, suggesting that the fowl Cα2 had been deleted from the human α chain during evolution.

These data clearly identify an IgA isotype in chickens and suggest that it is the precursor to mammalian IgA. Whether the amino acid sequence of H chains from fowl bile IgA will correspond to the nucleotide-derived sequence remains to be determined.

2. SC

Additional studies have been concerned with the association of SC with IgA and with the identification of different forms of IgA. Bienenstock *et al.* (1973b) first showed binding of radiolabeled human free SC to a chicken serum immunoglobulin that was precipitable by anti-IgA, but did not observe binding to chicken biliary IgA, suggesting the presence of SC in this chicken immunoglobulin. Rose *et al.* (1974) demonstrated that egg white contained a major 16.2S IgA that, on reduction and SDS–PAGE analysis, released a polypeptide with molecular mass of 50–70 kDa; this protein was identified tentatively as chicken SC. Antibodies that had been raised against oviduct fluid and absorbed with adult serum gave an identical reaction with egg white IgA and a soluble protein that was retained in immunoglobulin-depleted egg white and may represent SC. However, this antibody did not detect SC in chicken biliary or intestinal IgA. Leslie and Martin (1973) suggested that SC was associated with biliary IgA (~350 kDa) and not with serum IgA, but this hypothesis was not demonstrated convincingly.

Katz *et al.* (1974) found no antigenic differences between IgA in sera and secretions, and concluded that the equivalent of mammalian SC does not exist in chicken. However, other investigators continued the search. Watanabe and Kobayashi (1974) compared bile and intestinal IgA from chicken. Bile IgA resembled serum IgA from chickens, was of high molecular mass (800–900 kDa), and was without SC. In contrast, intestinal IgA resembled mammalian secretory IgA, had a molecular mass of ~400 kDa, and was associated with SC. Subsequently, Watanabe *et al.* (1975) isolated a 70-kDa glycoprotein from gut fluid that was reactive with antibodies to intestinal but not biliary IgA. Using an antibody specific for this putative free SC, prepared by immunizing with gut SIgA and absorbing with bile IgA, these researchers determined that free gut SC was deficient compared with SC in gut SIgA. However, this finding could reflect sensitivity of the antibodies to conformational changes or to proteolysis in the gut. The anti-SC reacted with IgA in intestinal but not in other secretions; labeled free SC did not combine *in vitro* with biliary IgA or IgG. In these studies, Watanabe and Kobayashi

(1974) found the molecular mass of the IgA to be 350 kDa in gut secretions but 650–710 kDa in bile, tears, saliva, oviduct fluid, and urine. In later studies, Kobayashi and Hirai (1980) stated that chicken bile and intestinal IgA had the same size (~560 kDa) and found no evidence for SC in intestinal or bile IgA by SDS–PAGE and immunodiffusion of reduced or native proteins. The interpretation of these data is complicated by the poor immunogenicity of SC in chicken IgA and the similarity in size to the reduced α chains in SDS–PAGE.

Porter and Parry (1976) isolated a putative SC with molecular mass of ~68 kDa from intestinal secretions but not from bile. Significantly, antibodies to bile IgA reacted identically with bile and intestinal IgA and partially with the 68-kDa protein. The major 15S serum IgA spurred (SC?) over the 7.5S serum IgA, as did pure bile and gut SIgA. Reduced bile IgA released a ~70-kDa protein that resembled free intestinal SC. Free SC also was identified in gut fluids from 20-day-old germ-free chicks with no IgA cells in their gut. As has been observed for mammalian SC, fluorescent labeled anti-SC antibodies stained only gut epithelium—mostly crypts in the supranuclear region, apical cytoplasm, and along basolateral membranes. However, these data seem incompatible with those of Bienenstock *et al.* (1972). Labeled human SC would not be expected to combine with polymeric chicken serum IgA bearing SC (Parry and Porter, 1978) nor with monomeric chicken serum IgA, which probably lacks J chain and thus would be unable to bind SC.

More recent experiments have concentrated on the use of functional criteria to elucidate the role of SC in galliforms. As in rats and rabbits (Lemaître-Coelho *et al.*, 1977b; Delacroix *et al.*, 1982), the levels of IgA were much higher in cannulated chicken hepatic bile than in plasma (Rose *et al.*, 1981). Again, as in rats and rabbits (Lemaître-Coelho *et al.*, 1978; Delacroix *et al.*, 1982), ligation of chicken bile ducts led to a fourfold increase in plasma IgA. Thus, the chicken liver quickly clears plasma chicken polymeric IgA by transporting it into bile. Rose *et al.* (1981) confirmed these findings by determining a high recovery in the bile of intravenously (iv) injected human labeled dimeric but not monomeric IgA, again as in rats and rabbits (Lemaître-Coelho *et al.*, 1978; Delacroix *et al.*, 1982).

Peppard *et al.* (1983) biolabeled chicken glycoproteins by iv injection of [^{14}C]fucose in bile duct cannulated chickens, followed by iv injection of human cold dimeric IgA 30 min later. The human IgA recovered in the bile was labeled, presumably by binding to chicken SC. [^{14}C]IgA collected from bile, when reinjected iv into a new recipient, did not repass into the bile. Moreover, ^{125}I-labeled human milk and chicken bile IgA injected iv were not recovered in chicken bile. Thus, as has been found in rats, IgA already combined with SC is not actively cleared by the chicken liver (Vaerman and Lemaître-Coelho, 1979; Lemaître-Coelho *et al.*, 1981).

Finally, Peppard *et al.* (1986) purified human dimeric IgA by antihuman light chain immunoadsorption chromatography after its transport into chicken bile. Approximately half this IgA had increased in size by ~80 kDa, suggesting that it had bound chicken SC. After mild reduction of this immunopurified IgA, isoelectric focusing, SDS–PAGE, transfer to nitrocellulose, and reaction with rabbit antichicken bile antibodies, these investigators identified a protein of ~80 kDa with an isoelectric point of 4.6 that is thought to be chicken SC.

The data just discussed suggest that chicken IgA and SC have been reasonably well identified, although the case for chicken SC is less clear. Unfortunately, no serological cross reactions were reported between mammalian IgA and SC and their putative chicken equivalents. SC has not been identified in galliforms other than chickens. Since nucleic acid probes are now available for human, rabbit, and rat SC/pIgR, future identification of this elusive molecule (Peppard *et al.*, 1983) will probably rely on methods involving molecular biology as well.

B. Anseriforms

Analogs to mammalian (or chicken) IgA have not been identified in anseriforms (Ng and Higgins, 1986; Higgins *et al.*, 1987). Ducks and geese also differ from chickens by the presence of a 5.7S Ig in the serum, as found in reptiles and lungfish. Hädge and Ambrosius (1988a,b) found no radioimmunoassay cross reactions between bile immunoglobulins of galliforms and anseriforms. None of the biliary anseriform immunoglobulins resemble mammalian IgA by radioimmunoassay cross reaction, but anseriform biliary immunoglobulins do resemble human and carp IgM by such criteria. Thus, the secretory immune system of anseriforms may be related more closely to that of reptiles, apparently relying on a predominance of IgM in secretions. In ducks, biliary IgM spurred (SC?) over serum IgM with anti-bile IgM antiserum but not with anti-serum IgM antiserum (Higgins *et al.*, 1987). However, gut secretions and immunohistological sections were not examined with antibodies specific for the spur, and no additional peptide was found in biliary IgM after reduction and SDS–PAGE. The ontogeny of IgM and IgY in bile and serum, and the kinetics of antiviral antibodies, additionally supports a secretory immune system in anseriforms (Ng and Higgins, 1986; Higgins *et al.*, 1987).

IV. REPTILES AND AMPHIBIANS

As in ducks, three serum immunoglobulin isotypes occur in reptiles: 19S IgM and two smaller immunoglobulins, a 7.8S IgY and a 5.7S immunoglobulin. IgM predominates in the bile and gut fluids of snakes, turtles, and bullfrogs (Portis and Coe, 1975). No evidence for SC was presented in these studies. In tortoise bile and gut secretions, IgM largely predominated over the 7.8S IgY and the 5.7S immunoglobulin; fluorescent anti-μ and anti-light chain antibodies stained similar numbers of plasmacytes in intestinal mucosae (Vaerman *et al.*, 1975c), suggesting that no other major IgA-like immunoglobulin existed in the gut.

Fellah *et al.* (1992) reported that the serum of developing axolotls lacked an IgY-like immunoglobulin (11.9S dimer, Fellah and Charlemagne, 1988). However, the gut epithelium of the immature axolotls stained both with fluorescent monoclonal anti-axolotl IgY and some anti-mammalian SC antibodies. After Western blotting with anti-mammalian SC, the axolotl stomach and intestinal extracts revealed 78-kDa and occasional 120 to 130-kDa bands that may represent axolotl SC and pIgR. These data require confirmation.

V. FISH

Oral immunization of plaice with *Vibrio anguillarum* antigens resulted in higher antibody titers in gut extracts and skin mucus than in sera, whereas the serum titers were higher than those of secretions after parenteral injections (Fletcher and White, 1973). Antibodies in mucus and serum were similar to IgM in size. In sheepshead (Lobb and Clem, 1981a,b), biliary immunoglobulin was a noncovalent dimer that was antigenically identical to serum IgM. The heavy chains were smaller (~55 kDa) than those of serum μ chains (70 kDa), but the light chains were of similar molecular mass (25 kDa). SC-like peptides were not found. Skin mucus immunoglobulins were composed of serum-like IgM and some dimers, some of which were associated covalently and, on reduction, released peptides with molecular mass of 70 kDa (H), 25 kDa (L), and 95 kDa (SC?). The only evidence for a secretory immune system in rainbow trout was the finding by St. Louis-Cormier *et al.* (1984) of serum IgM-like antibodies in mucus and immunoglobulin-containing cells in skin dermis and mucus. Local immune responses in the posterior gut of trout receiving oral human IgG were determined by immunohistology and by antibody secretion from cells of the intestine (Georgopoulou and Vernier, 1986). Oral and anal administration of *V. anguillarum* into carp (Rombout *et al.*, 1986) also suggested a local immune response, mostly in the hindgut. Oral bacteria elicited no serum antibody, whereas anal injection induced higher serum titers, with lower titers in bile and intestinal and skin mucus. Bath immunizations of catfish (Lobb, 1987) against dinitrophenyl (DNP)–albumin induced anti-DNP antibody in skin mucus of 5 of 6 fish, but induced serum antibody in only 1 of 6. The affinity-purified skin mucus antibody resembled IgM-like tetrameric serum antibody. Thus, some indication exists for a local secretory system in fish, but better characterization is required (Hart *et al.*, 1989).

VI. CONCLUSION

The emergence of a classical primary, primarily SIgA-related, secretory humoral immune system seems to have occurred first in the galliform branch of birds, but we have adopted a mammalian viewpoint for this survey. In more primitive animal species (fish, amphibians, reptiles), whether such a viewpoint is acceptable is not clear at all. A completely different set of criteria from those used for mammals and galliforms may be required to define a mucosal immune system; the cellular components could be much more important, as could nonspecific defense factors such as complement-like proteins and mucus components. Clearly, the mucosal SIgA immune system is probably efficient, with minor variations (see, for example, the huge predominance of IgG1 in ruminant milk throughout lactation), in all mammals, as well as in galliform birds. However, these are the limits of possible conclusions without too much risk of error.

References

Acosta-Altamirano, G., Barranco-Acosta, C., Van Roost, E., and Vaerman, J. P. (1980). Isolation and characterization of secretory IgA (SIgA) and free secretory component (FSC) from rat bile. *Mol. Immunol.* **17,** 1525–1537.

Baumgarth, N., Klobasa, F., and Petzoldt, K. (1990). Isolation of secretory immunoglobulin A and free secretory component from porcine whey. *In* "Advances in Mucosal Immunology" (T. T. MacDonald, S. J. Challacombe, P. W. Bland, C. R. Stokes, R. V. Heatley, and A. McI. Mowatt, eds.), pp. 545–546. Kluwer, Dordrecht, The Netherlands.

Bell, R. B., Stephens, C. J., and Turner, K. J. (1974). Marsupial immunoglobulins: An immunoglobulin molecule resembling eutherian IgA in serum and secretions. *J. Immunol.* **113,** 371–378.

Bienenstock, J., Perey, D. Y. E., Gauldie, J., and Underdown, B. J. (1972). Chicken immunoglobulin resembling γA. *J. Immunol.* **109,** 403–406.

Bienenstock, J., Perey, D. Y. E., Gauldie, J., and Underdown, B. J. (1973a). Chicken γA: Physicochemical and immunochemical characteristics. *J. Immunol.* **110,** 524–533.

Bienenstock, J., Gauldie, J., and Perey, D. Y. E. (1973b). Synthesis of IgG, IgA, IgM by chicken tissues: Immunofluorescent and ^{14}C amino acid incorporation studies. *J. Immunol.* **111,** 1112–1118.

Bourne, F. J. (1969a). IgA immunoglobulin from porcine milk. *Biochim. Biophys. Acta* **181,** 485–487.

Bourne, F. J. (1969b). IgA immunoglobulin from porcine serum. *Biochem. Biophys. Res. Commun.* **36,** 138–145.

Cebra, J. J., and Small, P. A. (1967). Polypeptide chain structure of rabbit immunoglobulins. III. Secretory γA-immunoglobulins from colostrum. *Biochemistry* **6,** 503–512.

Delacroix, D. L., Denef, A. M., Acosta, G. A., Montgomery, P. C., and Vaerman, J. P. (1982). Immunoglobulins in rabbit hepatic bile: Selective secretion of IgA and IgM, and active plasma-to-bile transfer of polymeric IgA. *Scand. J. Immunol.* **16,** 343–350.

Delacroix, D. L., Furtado-Barreira, G., de Hemptinne, B., Goudswaard, J., Rahier, J., Dive, C., and Vaerman, J. P. (1983). The liver in the IgA secretory immune system. Dogs, but not rats and rabbits, are suitable models for human studies. *Hepatology* **3,** 980–988.

Fellah, J. S., and Charlemagne, J. (1988). Characterization of an IgY-like low molecular weight immunoglobulin in the Mexican axolotl. *Mol. Immunol.* **25,** 1377–1386.

Fellah, J. S., Iscaki, S., Vaerman, J. P., and Charlemagne, J. (1992). Transient developmental expression of IgY and secretory component-like protein in the gut of the axolotl (*Ambystoma mexicanum*). *Dev. Immunol.* **2,** 181–190.

Fletcher, T. C., and White, A. (1973). Antibody production in the plaice (*Pleuronectes platessa* L.) after oral and parenteral immunization with *Vibrillo anguillarum* antigens. *Aquaculture* **1,** 417–428.

Georgopoulou, U., and Vernier, J. M. (1986). Local immunological response in the posterior intestinal segment of the rainbow trout after oral administration of macromolecules. *Dev. Comp. Immunol.* **10,** 529–537.

Goudswaard, J., Noordzij, A., Van Dam, R. H., Van der Donck, J. A., and Vaerman, J. P. (1977a). The immunoglobulins of the turkey (*Melleagris gallopavo*). Isolation and characterization of IgG, IgM and IgA in body fluids, eggs and intraocular tissues. *Poultry Sci.* **56,** 1847–1851.

Goudswaard, J., Vaerman, J. P., and Heremans, J. F. (1977b). Three immunoglobulin classes in the pigeon (*Columba livia*). *Int. Arch. Allergy* **53,** 409–419.

Hädge, D., and Ambrosius, H. (1983). Evolution of low molecular weight immunoglobulins. III. The immunoglobulin from chicken bile—not an IgA. *Mol. Immunol.* **20,** 597–606.

Hädge, D., and Ambrosius, H. (1984). Evolution of low molecular weight immunoglobulins. IV. IgY-like immunoglobulins of birds, reptiles and amphibians, precursors of mammalian IgA. *Mol. Immunol.* **21,** 699–707.

Hädge, D., and Ambrosius, H. (1986). Evolution of low molecular weight immunoglobulins. V. Degree of antigenic relationship between the 7S immunoglobulins of mammals, birds and lower vertebrates to the turkey IgY. *Dev. Comp. Immunol.* **10,** 377–385.

Hädge, D., and Ambrosius, H. (1987). Chicken immunoglobulins. *Vet. Immunol. Immunopathol.* **17,** 57–67.

Hädge, D., and Ambrosius, H. (1988a). Comparative studies on the structure of biliary immunoglobulins of some avian species. I. Physico-chemical properties of biliary immunoglobulins of chicken, turkey, duck and goose. *Dev. Comp. Immunol.* **12,** 121–129.

Hädge, D., and Ambrosius, H. (1988b). Comparative studies on the structure of biliary immunoglobulins of some avian species. II. Antigenic properties of biliary immunoglobulins of chicken, turkey, duck and goose. *Dev. Comp. Immunol.* **12,** 319–329.

Hagiwara, K., Kobayashi, K., Kajii, T., and Tomonaga, S. (1985). J chain-like component in 18S immunoglobulin of the skate *Raja kenojei,* a cartlaginous fish. *Mol. Immunol.* **22,** 775–778.

Hart, S., Wrathmell, A. B., Harris, J. E., and Grayson, T. H. (1989). Gut immunology in fish: A review. *Dev. Comp. Immunol.* **12,** 453–480.

Higgins, D. A., Shortridge, K. F., and Ng, P. L. K. (1987). Bile immunoglobulins of the duck (*Anas platyrhynchos*). II. Antibody response to influenza virus infections. *Immunology* **62,** 499–504.

Katz, D., Kohn, A., and Arnon, R. (1974). Immunoglobulins in the airway washings and bile secretions of chickens. *Eur. J. Immunol.* **4,** 494–499.

Klaus, G. G., Halpern, M. S., Koshland, M. E., and Goodman, J. W. (1971). A polypeptide chain from leopard shark 19S immunoglobulin analogous to mammalian J chain. *J. Immunol.* **107,** 1785–1787.

Kobayashi, K., and Hirai, H. (1980). Studies on subunit components of chicken polymeric immunoglobulins. *J. Immunol.* **124,** 1695–1704.

Lebacq-Verheyden, A. M., Vaerman, J. P., and Heremans, J. F. (1972a). A possible homologue of mammalian IgA in chicken serum and secretions. *Immunology* **22,** 165–175.

Lebacq-Verheyden, A. M., Vaerman, J. P., and Heremans, J. F. (1972b). Immunohistologic distribution of the chicken immunoglobulins. *J. Immunol.* **109,** 652–654.

Lebacq-Verheyden, A. M., Vaerman, J. P., and Heremans, J. F. (1974). Quantification and distribution of chicken immunoglobulins IgA, IgM and IgG in serum and secretions. *Immunology* **27,** 683–692.

Lemaître-Coelho, I., André, C., and Vaerman, J. P. (1977a). Murine secretory component. *Protides Biol. Fluids* **25,** 891–894.

Lemaître-Coelho, I., Jackson, G. D. F., and Vaerman, J. P. (1977b). Rat bile as a convenient source of secretory IgA and free secretory components. *Eur. J. Immunol.* **7,** 588–590.

Lemaître-Coelho, I., Jackson, G. D. F., and Vaerman, J. P. (1978). High levels of secretory IgA and free secretory component in the serum of rats after bile duct obstruction. *J. Exp. Med.* **147,** 934–939.

Lemaître-Coelho, I., Acosta-Altamirano, G., Barranco-Acosta, C., Meykens, R., and Vaerman, J. P. (1981). In vivo experiments involving secretory component in the rat hepatic transfer of polymeric IgA from blood into bile. *Immunology* **43,** 261–270.

Leslie, G. A., and Martin, L. N. (1973). Studies of the secretory immunologic system of fowl. III. Serum and secretory IgA of the chicken. *J. Immunol.* **110,** 1–9.

Lobb, C. J. (1987). Secretory immunity induced in catfish, *Ictalurus punctatus,* following bath immunization. *Dev. Comp. Immunol.* **11,** 727–738.

Lobb, C. J., and Clem, L. W. (1981a). Phylogeny of immunoglobulin structure and function. XI. Secretory immunoglobulins in the cutaneous mucus of the sheepshead, *Archosargus probatocephalus. Dev. Comp. Immunol.* **5,** 587–596.

Lobb, C. J., and Clem, L. W. (1981b). Phylogeny of immunoglobulin structure and function. XII. Secretory immunoglobulins in the bile of the marine teleost, *Archosargus probatocephalus. Mol. Immunol.* **18,** 615–619.

Mach, J. P., Pahud, J. J., and Isliker, H. (1969). IgA with "secretory piece" in bovine colostrum and saliva. *Nature (London)* **223,** 952–955.

Mansikka, A. (1992). Chicken IgA H chains: Implications concerning the evolution of H chain genes. *J. Immunol.* **149,** 855–861.

Neoh, S. H., Jahoda, D. M., Rowe, D. S., and Voller, A. (1973). Immunoglobulin classes in mammalian species identified by cross-reactivity with antisera to human immunoglobulins. *Immunochemistry* **10,** 805–813.

Ng, P. L. K., and Higgins, D. A. (1986). Bile immunoglobulins of the duck (*Anas platyrhynchos*). Preliminary characteristics and ontogeny. *Immunology* **58,** 323–327.

O'Daly, J. A., and Cebra, J. J. (1971). Chemical and physicochemical studies of the component polypeptide chains of rabbit secretory immunoglobulin. A. *Biochemistry* **10,** 3483–3850.

Orlans, E., and Feinstein, A. (1971). Detection of alpha, kappa and lambda chains in mammalian immunoglobulins using fowl antisera to human IgA. *Nature (London)* **233,** 45–48.

Orlans, E., and Rose, M. E. (1972). An IgA-like immunoglobulin in the fowl. *Immunochemistry* **9,** 833–838.

Pahud, J. J., and Mach J. P. (1970). Identification of secretory IgA, free secretory piece and serum IgA in the ovine and caprine species. *Immunochemistry* **7,** 679–686.

Pahud, J. J., and Mach J. P. (1972). Equine IgA and secretory component. *Int. Arch. Allergy* **42,** 175–186.

Parry, S. H., and Aitken, J. D. (1975). Immunoglobulin A in some avian species other than the fowl. *Res. Vet. Sci.* **18,** 333–334.

Parry, S. H., and Porter, P. (1978). Characterization and localization of secretory component in the chicken. *Immunology* **34,** 471–478.

Peppard, J. V., Rose, M. E., and Hesketh, P. (1983). A functional homologue of mammalian secretory component exists in chickens. *Eur. J. Immunol.* **13,** 566–570.

Peppard, J. V., Hobbs, S. M., Jackson, L. E., Rose, M. E., and Mockett, A. P. A. (1986). Biochemical characterization of chicken secretory component. *Eur. J. Immunol.* **16,** 225–229.

Pierre, P., Havaux, X. B., Langendries, A., Courtoy, P. J., Goto, K., Maldague, P., and Vaerman, J. P. (1993). Murine secretory component. *In* "Recent Advances in Mucosal Immunology" (J. McGhee, J. Mestecky, H. Tlaskalova, and J. Sterzl, eds.). Plenum Press, New York, in press.

Porter, P., and Parry, S. H. (1976). Further characterization of IgA in chicken serum and secretions with evidence of a possible homologue of mammalian secretory component. *Immunology* **31,** 407–415.

Portis, J. L., and Coe, J. E. (1975). IgM the secretory immunoglobulin of reptiles and amphibians. *Nature (London)* **258,** 547–548.

Reynolds, H. Y., and Johnson, J. S. (1971). Structural units of canine serum and secretory immunoglobulin A. *Biochemistry* **10,** 2821–2827.

Rombout, J. W., Blok, L. J., Lamers, C. H., and Egberts, E. (1986). Immunization of carp (*Cyprinus carpio*) with a *Vibrio anguillarum* bacterin: Indications for a common mucosal immune system. *Dev. Comp. Immunol.* **10,** 341–351.

Rose, M. E., Orlans, E., and Buttress, N. (1974). Immunoglobulin classes in the hen's egg: their segregation in yolk and white. *Eur. J. Immunol.* **4,** 521–523.

Rose, M. E., Orlans, E., Payne, A. W. R., and Hesketh, P. (1981). The origin of chicken IgA in chicken bile: Its active transport from blood. *Eur. J. Immunol.* **11,** 561–564.

St. Louis-Cormier, E. A., Osterland, C. K., and Anderson, P. D. (1984). Evidence for a cutaneous secretory immune system in a rainbow trout (*Salmo gairdneri*). *Dev. Comp. Immunol.* **8,** 71–80.

Vaerman, J. P., and Lemaître-Coelho, I. (1979). Transfer of circulating human IgA across the rat liver into the bile. *In* "Transmission of Proteins through Living Membranes" (W. A. Hemmings, ed.), pp. 383–398. Elsevier, Amsterdam.

Vaerman, J. P., Heremans, J. F., and Van Kerckhoven, G. (1969). Identification of IgA in several mammalian species. *J. Immunol.* **103,** 1421–1423.

Vaerman, J. P., Naccache-Corbic, M., and Heremans, J. F. (1975a). Secretory component of the guinea pig. *Immunology* **29,** 933–944.

Vaerman, J. P., Heremans, J. F., Bazin, H., and Beckers, A. (1975b). Identification and some properties of rat secretory component. *J. Immunol.* **114,** 265–269.

Vaerman, J. P., Picard, J., and Heremans, J. F. (1975c). Structural data on chicken IgA and failure to identify IgA in the tortoise. *Adv. Exp. Med. Biol.* **64,** 185–195.

Watanabe, H., and Kobayashi, K. (1974). Peculiar secretory IgA system identified in chickens. *J. Immunol.* **113,** 1405–1409.

Watanabe, H., Kobayashi, K., and Isayama, Y. (1975). Peculiar secretory IgA system identified in chickens. II. Identification and distribution of free secretory component and immunoglobulins of IgA, IgM, and IgG in chicken external secretions. *J. Immunol.* **115,** 998–1001.

9

Developmental Aspects of Mucosal Immunoglobulin Genes: Organization and Expression of IgA Heavy-Chain, Polymeric Immunoglobulin Receptor, and J-Chain Genes

Katherine L. Knight

I. INTRODUCTION

In Chapter 8, Vaerman described evidence for the presence of secretory IgA and a receptor–transporter (SC or pIgR) in various species of mammals, birds, reptiles, amphibians, and fish. Genes encoding these molecules are cloned principally from mammals. This chapter addresses the structure and expression of these genes.

II. IgA HEAVY-CHAIN GENES

Genes encoding Cα regions are cloned from the genomes of human, mouse, cow, rabbit, and several nonhuman primates including gorilla, chimpanzee, orangutan, gibbon, and Old World monkey (Tucker *et al.*, 1981; Flanagan *et al.*, 1984; Knight *et al.*, 1988; Ueda *et al.*, 1988; Burnett *et al.*, 1989; Kawamura *et al.*, 1989,1990). With the exception of rabbits, all mammals studied have one or two IgA subclasses; correspondingly, they have one or two Cα genes in their germ line. As do other C_H genes, the Cα genes of each species studied have a separate exon that encodes each domain—Cα1, Cα2, and Cα3—as diagrammed in Figure 1. The hinge region is not encoded as a separate exon, as it is in Cγ and Cδ genes, but is encoded at the 5′ end of the Cα2 exon. The hinge regions of human Cα1 and Cα2 genes contain tandem 15-bp repeat units. Kawamura *et al.* (1990) showed that the Cα1 and Cα2 genes of chimpanzee, gorilla, and gibbon have hinge structures similar to those of the human Cα1 and Cα2 genes, respectively. In contrast, the hinge region of the Cα gene of Old World monkeys does not contain the 15-bp repeat unit and, in general, its structure is markedly different from that of any hominoid Cα gene examined.

The 19-amino-acid extension found at the C-terminal end of the secreted form of α heavy chains is encoded at the 3′ end of the Cα3 exon. The transmembrane and cytoplasmic tail sequences found at the C-terminal end of the membrane form of α heavy chains are encoded by one small exon, αM, located approximately 2–4 kb downstream (3′) of the Cα3-encoding exon (Word *et al.*, 1983; S. K. Zhai, and K. L. Knight, unpublished data). Approximately 2–6 kb upstream (5′) of the Cα genes is the switch region that undergoes recombination in B lymphocytes during isotype switching.

A. Cα Genes of Mouse, Bovines, and Primates

The Cα gene of mouse is the 3′-most C_H gene of the H-chain gene cluster 5′-J_H-Cδ-Cγ3-Cγ1-Cγ2b-Cγ2a-Cε-Cα-3′ (Shimizu *et al.*, 1982). In humans, the C_H gene order differs slightly from that in mice, presumably because of the duplication of a cluster of two Cγ genes, one Cε, and one Cα gene (Figure 2). In this case, the gene order is 5′-J_H-Cμ-Cδ-Cγ3-Cγ1-pseudo Cε-Cα1-pseudo Cγ-Cγ2-Cγ4-Cε-Cα2-3′ (Flanagan and Rabbits, 1982; Hofker *et al.*, 1989). The bovine Cα gene is 3′ of Cε, but has not been linked by overlapping phage or cosmid clones to Cμ or Cγ (Knight *et al.*, 1988).

B. Cα Genes of Rabbit and Other Lagomorphs

Rabbits are highly unusual because their germ line has 13 nonallelic Cα genes (Burnett *et al.*, 1989). The 13 Cα genes span a minimum of 160 kb of DNA. Three of the Cα genes—Cα4, Cα5, and Cα6—have been linked to the Cμ, Cγ, and Cε genes by overlapping cosmid clones (Figure 3; Burnett *et al.*, 1989). The remaining 10 Cα genes are in separate or overlapping phage or cosmid clones. Isolating phage or cosmid clones that link these 10 genes to the 5′-J_H-Cμ-Cγ-Cα4-Cα5-Cα6-3′ cluster has been difficult, although multiple genomic phage and cosmid libraries were screened for clones that would link the 13 Cα genes. Clearly, some genomic DNA segments of the Cα gene cluster are difficult to clone. We suggest that, because the Cα chromosomal region seems to have a high content of repeated elements, some DNA is deleted repeatedly during construction of the genomic libraries, making cloning the entire region difficult. Another possible reason for not being able to link the 13 Cα genes together

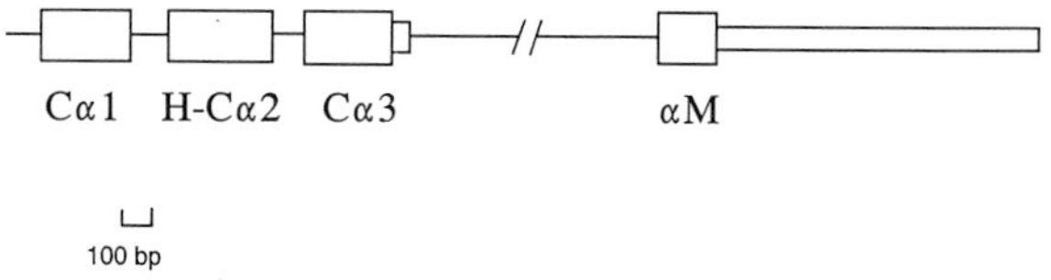

Figure 1 Intron–exon structure of Cα genes. The boxes represent the exons that encode the Cα1 domain, the hinge (H) and Cα2 domain, the Cα3 domain and secreted tail, and the membrane/cytoplasmic domain (αM). The smaller open box represents 3′-untranslated region of the RNA.

is that some of them are not within the heavy chain chromosomal region; this possibility, however, seems unlikely.

Because of the large number of Cα genes in rabbit compared with other mammals, Burnett *et al.* (1989) investigated whether multiple copies of Cα also were found in other lagomorphs. Southern blots of DNA from members of the two families of lagomorphs—Leporidae and Ochotonidae—hybridized with rabbit Cα probes revealed multiple hybridizing fragments in each sample of DNA (Figure 4). These data indicate that multiple Cα genes are found in animals throughout the order Lagomorpha and that the expansion of Cα genes occurred in a common ancestor. Similar attempts to identify multiple Cα genes in mammals that belong to an order other than Lagomorpha have been unsuccessful to date. Thus we do not yet know, in evolutionary terms, when the expansion of Cα occurred.

C. Cα Gene of Chicken

As described in Chapter 8, IgA-like molecules have been identified in chicken serum and secretions, but the evolutionary relationship between the heavy chains of these molecules and mammalian α heavy chains is not clear. Mansikka (1992) cloned a non-μ-, non-γ-encoding H chain cDNA from a library derived from mRNA of chicken Harderian gland, a tissue rich in plasma cells. On the basis of the deduced amino acid sequence, the constant region of the H chain encoded by the cDNA was 37% identical to murine Cα chains and only 29% and 30% identical to murine IgM and IgG1, respectively. The data show that chickens have a third Ig isotype that is distinct

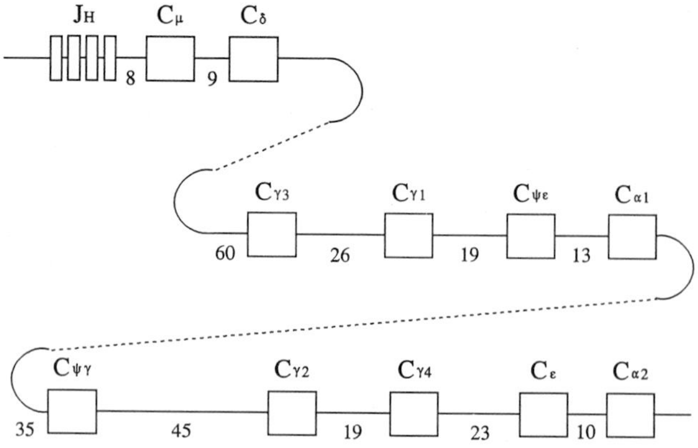

Figure 2 Organization of the human J_H and C_H Ig locus.

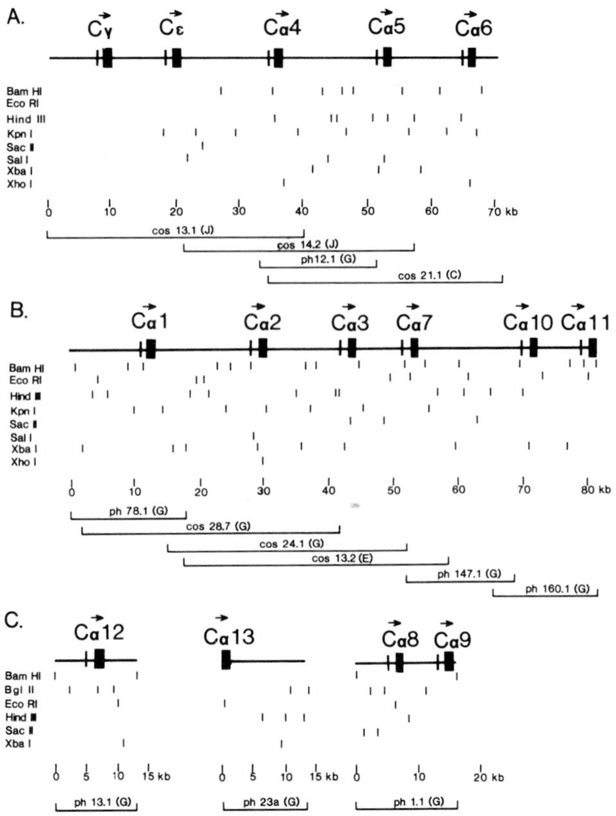

Figure 3 Organization of 13 rabbit germline Cα genes. Cα genes are indicated by solid boxes; the vertical lines to the left of each gene indicate S regions. Arrows indicate transcriptional direction. (A) Cluster 1 obtained from overlapping cosmid and phage clones (Burnett *et al.*, 1989), showing linkage of Cα4, Cα5, and Cα6 genes to the C_H genes, Cγ, and Cε. (B) Cluster 2 obtained from overlapping cosmid and phage clones. (C) Cluster of two Cα genes, Cα8 and Cα9, and two individual clones on nonoverlapping phage clones. Reprinted with permission from Burnet et. al. (1989).

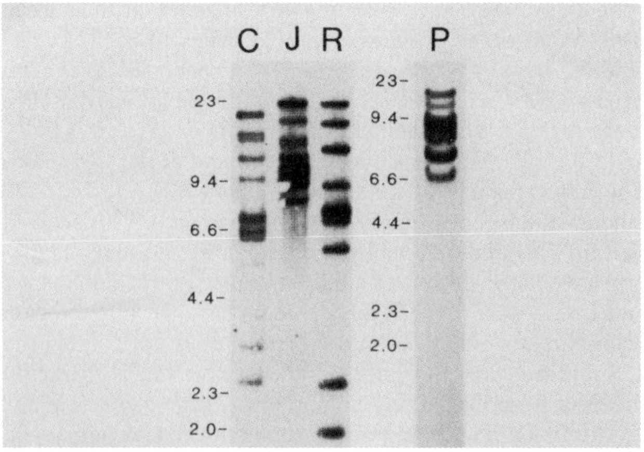

Figure 4 Southern analysis of lagomorph genomic DNA with the rabbit Cα cDNA probe. DNA samples, domestic rabbit (R), cottontail rabbit (C), jackrabbit (J), and pika (P), were restricted with *Bam* HI. Lambda *Hin* dIII size standards are indicated. Reprinted with permission from Burnett *et al.* (1989), and Oxford University Press.

from IgM and IgG, and that this isotype is most likely the homolog of mammalian IgA. Of particular interest is that these heavy chains have four C_H domains. By comparing the similarity of the sequences of each chicken $C\alpha$ domain with mammalian $C\alpha$ domains, Mansikka (1992) showed that the chicken $C\alpha 2$ domain was the least similar to mammalian α chains and concluded that the $C\alpha 2$ domain was deleted in mammals during evolution.

D. Expression of Cα Genes

In humans, IgA1 and IgA2 are expressed differentially in various tissues (Brandtzaeg *et al.*, 1986; Kett *et al.*, 1986; Mestecky and Russell, 1986). For example, IgA1 represents 80–95% of the IgA in serum whereas, in external secretions, it generally represents 30–50% of the IgA. The factors responsible for this differential expression are not known. In rabbits, the 13 germ-line $C\alpha$ genes were examined for their expressibility by nucleotide sequence analysis and by transfection studies. Burnett *et al.* (1989) analyzed the nucleotide sequences and found that each of the 13 $C\alpha$ genes was expressible. Schneiderman *et al.* (1989) ligated each of the $C\alpha$ genes to a murine VDJ gene, transfected murine L-chain-producing SP2/0 cells with each of the chimeric rabbit–mouse α heavy chain gene constructs, and showed that most, if not all, of the $C\alpha$ genes could be expressed *in vitro* in these cells. Using probes specific to each of the 13 $C\alpha$ genes, RNase protection studies of mRNA from mucosal tissues, including gut and mammary tissue, identified mRNA representing 10 of the $C\alpha$ genes (Spieker-Polet *et al.*, 1993). These data show that rabbits express 10 $C\alpha$ genes in the mucosae. Presumably, then, 10 IgA isotypes will be found in rabbit mucosal secretions. The functional significance of multiple IgA isotypes remains to be elucidated. Serologically, only two isotypes of IgA, f and g, are well defined (Knight and Hanly, 1975). The chimeric rabbit–mouse IgA molecules generated by Schneiderman *et al.* (1989), which represent each of the IgA isotypes, can be used as immunogens to develop antibodies specific to each of the 10 isotypes. Using such antibodies, or using the RNase protection assay, the relative expression of each IgA isotype in various mucosal tissues can be determined. Considering the differential expression of the two IgA isotypes IgA1 and IgA2 in various human mucosal tissues (Brandtzaeg *et al.*, 1986; Mestecky and Russell, 1986) the 10 IgA isotypes in rabbit are likely to be expressed differentially in various mucosal tissues.

III. CLASS SWITCHING

IgA expression results from class switching, by which in IgM–IgD-bearing B lymphocytes a $C\alpha$ gene is rearranged to the region downstream of the rearranged VDJ gene. During isotype switching to IgA, the $C\mu$, $C\delta$, $C\gamma$, and $C\varepsilon$ genes 5′ of the switched $C\alpha$ gene and 3′ of the VDJ gene are deleted from the germ line (Rabbits *et al.*, 1980; Yaoita and Honjo, 1980; Kataoka *et al.*, 1981; von Schwedler *et al.*, 1990). The isotype switch generally occurs by recombination between the tandem direct repeat sequences, that is, switch sequences, that are found 5′ of each C_H gene except $C\delta$ (Davis *et al.*, 1980; Obata *et al.*, 1981). Switching may be regulated by the accessibility of switch regions to a recombinase that presumably is involved in the switch recombination; such recombinases are not yet identified. The induction of IgA isotype switching has been studied extensively; of particular interest are the results of Coffman and colleagues, who showed that the addition of transforming growth factor β (TGFβ) to lipopolysaccharide (LPS)-stimulated cultures of murine splenic and Peyer's patch B cells resulted in an approximately 10-fold increase of IgA production (Coffman *et al.*, 1989; Lebman *et al.*, 1990a). In their experiments, TGFβ stimulated $SIgA^-$ cells to express IgA; the authors suggest that TGFβ acts as an isotype-specific factor for IgA. Stavnezer and her colleagues also studied isotype switching in a murine B-lymphoma cell line (I.29), which switches from IgM to IgA (Stavnezer *et al.*, 1985; Severinson *et al.*, 1990). These investigators found a germ-line $C\alpha$ transcript from unrearranged $C\alpha$ genes that spanned the $C\alpha$ gene and a region 5′ of the switch site; this sterile transcript did not have V_H or J_H gene sequences (Stavnezer *et al.*, 1988; Radcliffe *et al.*, 1990). Lebman *et al.* (1990b) cloned sterile $C\alpha$ transcripts from TGFβ-induced LPS-stimulated B cells and also found that the transcripts contain germ-line sequences 5′ to the α switch site as well as $C\alpha$ sequences. The results suggest that switching to IgA is preceded by transcription of unrearranged $C\alpha$ genes. The function of these transcripts remains unknown, but Stavnezer *et al.* (1988) suggested that transcription may promote recombination. To date, however, we do not understand how a particular C_H gene, especially $C\alpha$, would be selected for transcription nor how this transcription would promote the switch recombination process.

IV. POLYMERIC IMMUNOGLOBULIN RECEPTOR/SECRETORY COMPONENT GENES

Polymeric immunoglobulin receptor (pIgR) mediates the transport of polymeric Ig across the epithelia into secretions. Polymeric Ig binds to pIgR at the basolateral cell surface and is internalized via receptor-mediated endocytosis. The complex then is transcytosed to the apical cell surface, where the polymeric Ig is secreted with a portion of the pIgR (called SC; Brandtzaeg, 1974; Mostov and Blobel, 1982; Solari and Kraehenbuhl, 1984). Mostov *et al.* (1984) first cloned the pIgR gene from a rabbit cDNA library; subsequently, Deitcher and Mostov (1986) isolated the genomic pIgR gene from a rabbit genomic DNA library. By analyzing the deduced amino acid sequence, Deitcher and Mostov (1986) identified five extracellular domains with structural similarity to immunoglobulin domains, suggesting that pIgR is a member of the immunoglobulin superfamily (Mostov *et al.*, 1984; Hunkapiller and Hood, 1989). The sixth domain has a highly hydrophobic region and is believed to be the region that spans the cell membrane. The seventh, or cytoplasmic, domain is unusually large, having 103 amino acids. This domain does not appear to be a member of the immunoglobulin superfamily.

Two forms of SC are found in rabbit secretions, a high molecular weight form (HMW; M_r ~81,000) and a low molecular weight form (LMW; M_r ~55,000) (Mostov *et al.*, 1980; Kuhn and Kraehenbuhl, 1981; Kuhn *et al.*, 1983). Deitcher and Mostov (1986) showed that these two forms probably arise from differential RNA splicing. One unusual feature of the genomic pIgR gene is that the immunoglobulin-like domains 2 and 3 are encoded by the same exon (Deitcher and Mostov, 1986). The HMW form of SC contains all seven SC domains, whereas LMW SC contains five SC domains; domains 2 and 3 are absent because of alternative splicing of the primary RNA transcript. Hanly (1992) identified repetitive sequence elements on both the 5′ and the 3′ side of exon 2–3, and suggests that these elements may mediate the alternative splicing event resulting in LMW SC.

The human pIgR gene also has been cloned from both a cDNA library (Krajči *et al.*, 1989) and a genomic phage library (Davidson *et al.*, 1988). Analysis of human × mouse somatic cell hybrids localized the pIgR gene to the long arm of chromosome 1. The intron–exon organization of the human pIgR gene is similar to that of rabbit (Hanly *et al.*, 1989; Krajči *et al.*, 1992; W. C. Hanly, unpublished data), but no mRNA encoding LMW SC was found in human secretory tissues (Krajči *et al.*, 1989), indicating that the pIgR transcript is not alternatively spliced.

pIgR has been used as a model system to investigate intracellular protein traffic. The availability of the cloned pIgR gene allows systematic analysis of regions of the protein required for specific biological functions (for example, see Mostov *et al.*, 1986; Breitfeld *et al.*, 1989; Schaerer *et al.*, 1990; Apodaca *et al.*, 1991; Casanova *et al.*, 1991). Banting *et al.* (1989) cloned the rat pIgR gene as cDNA and showed that the cytoplasmic domain was conserved remarkably with the cytoplasmic domain of rabbit and human pIgR genes. Further comparison of the amino acid sequence similarities among species may help identify functionally important amino acid residues in the cytoplasmic domain.

V. J-CHAIN GENES

J chain, a protein of 137 amino acid residues, is associated with polymeric IgA and IgM (see review by Koshland, 1985). The J-chain gene first was cloned from a murine plasmacytoma cDNA library (Mather *et al.*, 1981; Cann *et al.*, 1982) and subsequently was cloned from murine and human genomic libraries (Max and Korsmeyer, 1985; Matsuuchi *et al.*, 1986). Analysis of human × rodent somatic cell hybrids located the human J-chain gene on the long arm of chromosome 4 (Max *et al.*, 1986); the J-chain gene in mouse is located on chromosome 5 (Yagi *et al.*, 1982). J chains are highly conserved: the sequences of these mouse and human genes are 77% identical. Analysis of the amino acid sequence and circular dichroism measurements led Zikan *et al.* (1985) to propose that the J chain may be a member of the immunoglobulin superfamily, since it has a single-domain antiparallel β pleated sheet bilayer structure. Previously, Cann *et al.* (1982) had proposed a two-domain structure for J chain, which was unlike that of an immunoglobulin-like fold. Although the data are more consistent with the single-domain structure for J chain, X-ray crystallographic analysis of J-chain-containing polymers will establish which model more accurately depicts the structure of J chain.

The J-chain gene consists of four exons distributed over 7.3 kb. Unlike immunoglobulin heavy- and light-chain genes, the J-chain gene does not undergo rearrangement during B cell differentiation (Yagi and Koshland, 1981; Matsuuchi *et al.*, 1986). A single primary transcript of the J-chain gene appears to be produced. Unlike C_H and pIgR gene transcripts, this transcript does not seem to undergo alternative splicing. However, like immunoglobulin light- and heavy-chain genes, the region 5′ of the translational start site includes a TATA sequence as well as two tissue-specific decanucleotide and pentadecanucleotide elements that are common to human and mouse Vκ genes, mouse Vλ genes, and heavy-chain enhancers (Mills *et al.*, 1983; Falkner and Zachau, 1984; Parslow *et al.*, 1984; Mage *et al.*, 1989). The presence of these elements in the J-chain gene suggests that its transcription may be controlled in a manner similar to that of light- and heavy-chain genes.

Expression of the J-chain gene during B-cell differentiation was studied in mouse and humans, but the results do not establish the stage in the differentiation pathway at which J-chain synthesis is initiated. In mouse, J chain was not found in μ heavy chain producing pre-B or B lymphoma cell lines but was highly expressed in Ig-secreting B-lineage cells (Mather *et al.*, 1981; Koshland, 1985). These data indicated that J-chain expression occurred after the synthesis of μ heavy chains. However, in human, several investigators (McCune *et al.*, 1981; Mason and Stein, 1981; Hajdu *et al.*, 1983; Max and Korsmeyer, 1985) showed that J chain was expressed in pre-B and null lymphocytic leukemias. Subsequently, Kubagawa *et al.* (1988) showed that some Epstein–Barr virus-transformed human B-cell progenitors expressed J chain in the absence of immunoglobulin gene rearrangements. These data indicate that J-chain expression precedes μ-chain expression. The discrepancy between the J-chain expression in mouse and human B-lineage cells may reflect that most data were obtained from transformed cells (Max and Korsmeyer, 1985). Additional studies using normal untransformed cells may resolve this discrepancy.

Koshland and colleagues studied the activation of the J-chain gene in mitogen-stimulated IgM-secreting murine lymphocytes (Minie and Koshland, 1986) and in a cloned murine B-cell line (BCL_1) that was stimulated by interleukin 2 (IL-2) to synthesize J-chain RNA and to secrete pentameric IgM (Blackman *et al.*, 1986). In both examples, the chromatin structure 5′ to the J-chain gene was altered. Blackman *et al.* (1986) suggest that these changes make the promoter region accessible to regulatory elements that, in turn, activate transcription of the J-chain gene. The ability to activate J-chain gene transcription by stimulating BCL_1 cells with IL-2 provides us with a model system in which to identify and characterize regulatory elements involved in signal-induced gene activation.

VI. CONCLUSIONS

A secretory immune system is present in most, if not all mammals, including primitive mammals such as insectivores, monotremes, and marsupials (see Chapter 8). Of nonmammalian species, a clear description of an IgA-like molecule has been given only for chicken. Most mammalian species seem to have one or two IgA isotypes expressed in secretions, but rabbits have at least 10 secretory IgA isotypes. The presence of 10 secretory IgA isotypes in rabbits is intriguing; evaluating their individual roles in secretory immunity will be important.

Genes encoding IgA heavy chains are cloned from several mammals, including humans, mice, rabbits, and bovines. These Cα genes are highly similar to each other and, in the future, can be used easily as probes to clone Cα genes of other mammals. In fact, the mammalian Cα probes probably can be used to identify Cα genes in nonmammalian species. For example, segments of Cα3 domains are highly conserved among mammals, and regions of the mammalian Cα3 domains are even highly similar to the chicken Cα chain. We suggest that probes derived from these conserved regions of the Cα3 domain-encoding region of mammalian Cα genes would hybridize with the Cα genes of nonmammalian species and aid in their cloning.

Genes encoding pIgR and J chain are cloned from rabbit and human and mouse and human, respectively. Experiments with the J-chain gene will help elucidate the role of J chain in polymeric immunoglobulins, including secretory IgA. Experiments with the pIgR gene will elucidate the means by which IgA is transcytosed across the epithelium.

References[1]

Apodaca, G., Bomsel, M., Arden, J., Breitfeld, P. P., Tang, K., and Mostov, K. E. (1991). The polymeric immunoglobulin receptor. A model protein to study transcytosis. *J. Clin Invest* **87,** 1877–1882.

Banting, G., Brake, B., Braghetta, P., Luzio, J. P., and Stanley, K. K. (1989). Intracellular targetting signals of polymeric immunoglobulin receptors are highly conserved between species. *Febs. Lett.* **254,** 177–183.

Blackman, M. A., Tigges, M. A., Minie, M. E., and Koshland, M. E. (1986). A model system for peptide hormone action in differentiation: Interleukin 2 induces a B lymphoma to transcribe the J chain gene. *Cell* **47,** 609–617.

Brandtzaeg, P. (1974). Mucosal and glandular distribution of immunoglobulin components: Differential localization of free and bound SC in secretory epithelial cells. *J. Immunol.* **112,** 1553–1559.

Brandtzaeg, P., Kett, K., Rognum, T. O., Soderstrom, R., Bjorkander, J., Soderstrom, T., Petrusson, B., and Hanson, L. A. (1986). Distribution of mucosal IgA and IgG subclass-producing immunocytes and alterations in various disorders. *Monogr. Allergy* **20,** 179–194.

Breitfeld, P. P., Harris, J. M., and Mostov, K. E. (1989). Postendocytotic sorting of the ligand for the polymeric immunoglobulin receptor in Madin–Darby canine kidney cells. *J. Cell Biol.* **109,** 475–486.

Burnet, R. C., Hanly, W. C., Zhai, S. K., and Knight, K. L. (1989). The IgA heavy-chain gene family in rabbit: Cloning and sequence analysis of 13 Cα genes. *EMBO J.* **8,** 4041–4047.

[1] The literature search for this chapter was completed in March, 1992.

Cann, G. M., Zaritsky, A., and Koshland, M. E. (1982). Primary structure of the immunoglobulin J chain from the mouse. *Proc. Natl. Acad. Sci. U.S.A.* **79,** 6656–6660.

Casanova, J. E., Apodaca, G., and Mostov, K. E. (1991). An autonomous signal for basolateral sorting in the cytoplasmic domain of the polymeric immunoglobulin receptor. *Cell* **66,** 65–75.

Coffman, R. L., Lebman, D. A., and Shrader, B. (1989). Transforming growth factor β specifically enhances IgA production by lipopolysaccharide-stimulated murine β lymphocytes. *J. Exp. Med.* **170,** 1039–1044.

Davidson, M. K., Le Beau, M. M., Eddy, R. L., Shows, T. B., DiPietro, L. A., Kingzette, M., and Hanly, W. C. (1988). Genetic mapping of the human polymeric immunoglobulin receptor gene to chromosome region 1q31-q41. *Cytogenet. Cell Genet.* **48,** 107–111.

Davis, M. M., Kim, S. K., and Hood, L. E. (1980). DNA sequences mediating class switching in α-immunoglobulins *Science* **209,** 1360–1365.

Deitcher, D. L., and Mostov, K. E. (1986). Alternative splicing of rabbit polymeric immunoglobulin receptor. *Mol. Cell. Biol.* **6,** 2712–2715.

Falkner, F. G., and Zachau, H. G. (1984). Correct transcription of an immunoglobulin κ gene requires an upstream fragment containing conserved sequence elements. *Nature (London)* **310,** 71–74.

Flanagan, J. G., and Rabbitts, T. H. (1982). Arrangement of human immunoglobulin heavy chain constant region genes implies evolutionary duplication of a segment containing τ, epsilon and α genes. *Nature (London)* **300,** 709–713.

Flanagan, J. G., Lefranc, M.-P., and Rabbitts, T. H. (1984). Mechanisms of divergence and convergence of the human immunoglobulin α1 and α2 constant region gene sequences. *Cell* **36,** 681–688.

Hajdu, I., Moldoveanu, Z., Cooper, M. D., Mestecky, J. (1983). Ultrastructural studies of human lymphoid cells. μ and J chain expression as a function of B cell differentiation. *J. Exp. Med.* **158,** 1993–2006.

Hanly, W. C. (1992). C-family repetitive elements within the rabbit polymeric immunoglobulin receptor (pIgR) gene may contribute to alternative splicing. *FASEB J.* **6,** p. A1227.

Hanly, W. C., Kingzette, M., and Davidson, M. K. (1989). Genomic organization of the rabbit polymeric immunoglobulin receptor gene. *FASEB J.* **3,** 5146.

Hofker, M. H., Walter, M. A., and Cox, D. W. (1989). Complete physical map of the human immunoglobulin heavy chain constant region gene complex. *Proc. Natl. Acad. Sci. U.S.A.* **86,** 5567–5571.

Hunkapiller, T., and Hood, L. (1989). Diversity of the immunoglobulin gene superfamily. *Adv. Immunol.* **44,** 1–63.

Kataoka, T., Miyata, T., and Honjo, T. (1981). Repetitive sequences in class-switch recombination regions of immunoglobulin heavy chain genes. *Cell* **23,** 357–368.

Kawamura, S., Omoto, K., and Ueda, S. (1989). Nucleotide sequence of the gorilla immunoglobulin alpha 1 gene. *Nucleic Acids Res.* **17,** 6732.

Kawamura, S., Omoto, K., and Ueda, S. (1990). Evolutionary hypervariability in the hinge region of the immunoglobulin alpha gene. *J. Mol. Biol.* **215,** 201–206.

Kett, K., Brandtzaeg, P., Radl, J., and Haaijman, J. J. (1986). Different subclass distribution of IgA-producing cells in human lymphoid organs and various secretory tissues. *J. Immunol.* **136,** 3631–3635.

Knight, K. L., and Hanly, W. C. (1975). Genetic control of α chains of rabbit IgA: Allotypic specificities on the variable and the constant regions. *Contemp. Top. Mol. Immunol.* **4,** 55–88.

Knight, K. L., Suter, M., and Becker, R. S. (1988). Genetic engineering of bovine Ig: Construction and characterization of hapten-binding bovine/murine chimeric IgE, IgA, IgG1, IgG2 and IgG3 molecules. *J. Immunol.* **140,** 3654–3659.

Koshland, M. E. (1985). The coming of age of the immunoglobulin J chain. *Ann. Rev. Immunol.* **3,** 425–453.

Krajči, P., Kvale, D., Tasken, K., and Brandtzaeg, P. (1992). Molecular cloning and exon–intron mapping of the gene encoding human transmembrane secretory component (the poly-Ig receptor). *Eur. J. Immunol.* **22,** 2309–2315.

Krajči, P., Solgerg, R., Sandberg, M., Oyen, O., Jahnsen, T., and Brandtzaeg, P. (1989). Molecular cloning of the human transmembrane secretory component (poly-Ig receptor) and its mRNA expression in human tissues. *Biochem. Biophys. Res. Commun.* **158,** 783–789.

Kubagawa, H., Burrows, P. D., Grossi, C. E., Mestecky, J., and Cooper, M. D. (1988). Precursor B cells transformed by Epstein–Barr virus undergo sterile plasma-cell differentiation: J-chain expression without immunoglobulin. *Proc. Natl. Acad. Sci. U.S.A.* **85,** 875–879.

Kuhn, L. C., and Kraehenbuhl, J.-P. (1981). The membrane receptor for polymeric immunoglobulin is structurally related to secretory component. *J. Biol. Chem.* **256,** 12490–12495.

Kuhn, L. C., Kocher, H. P., Hanly, W. C., Cook, L., Jaton, J.-C., and Kraehenbuhl, J.-P. (1983). Structural and genetic heterogeneity of the receptor mediating translocation of immunoglobulin A dimer antibodies across epithelia in the rabbit. *J. Biol. Chem.* **258,** 6653–6659.

Lebman, D. A., Lee, F. D., and Coffman, R. L. (1990a). Mechanism for transforming growth factor β and IL-2 enhancement of IgA expression in liposaccharide-stimulated B cell cultures. *J. Immunol.* **144,** 952–959.

Lebman, D. A., Nomura, D. Y., Coffman, R. L., and Lee, F. D. (1990b). Molecular characterization of germ-line immunoglobulin A transcripts produced during transforming growth factor type β-induced isotype switching. *Proc. Natl. Acad. Sci. U.S.A.* **87,** 3962–3966.

McCune, J. M., Fu, S. M., and Kunkel, H. G. (1981). J chain biosynthesis in pre-B cells and other possible precursors of B cells. *J. Exp. Med.* **154,** 138–145.

Mage, R. G., Newman, B. A., Harindranath, N., Bernstein, K. E., Becker, R. S., and Knight, K. L. (1989). Evolutionary conservation of splice sites in sterile $C\mu$ transcripts and of immunoglobulin heavy chain (IgH) enhancer region sequences. *Mol. Immunol.* **26,** 1007–1010.

Mansikka, A. (1992). The chicken IgA heavy chains: implications concerning the evolution of H chain genes. *J. Immunol.* **149,** 855–861.

Mason, D. Y., and Stein, H. (1981). Reactive and neoplastic human lymphoid cells producing J chain in the absence of immunoglobulin: evidence for the existence of "J" chain disease? *Clin Exp. Immunol.* **46,** 305–312.

Mather, E. L., Alt, F. W., Bothwell, A. L. M., Baltimore, D., and Koshland, M. E. (1981). Expression of J chain RNA in cell lines representing different stages of B lymphocyte differentiation. *Cell* **23,** 369–378.

Matsuuchi, L., Cann, G. M., and Koshland, M. E. (1986). Immunoglobulin J chain gene from the mouse. *Proc. Natl. Acad. Sci. U.S.A.* **83,** 456–460.

Max, E. E., and Korsmeyer, S. J. (1985). Human J chain gene. Structure and expression in B lymphoid cells. *J. Exp. Med.* **161,** 832–849.

Max, E. E., McBride, O. W., Morton, C. C., and Robinson, M. A. (1986). Human J chain gene: chromosomal localization and associated restriction fragment length polymorphisms. *Proc. Natl. Acad. Sci. U.S.A.* **83,** 5592–5596.

Mestecky, J., and Russell, M. W. (1986). IgA subclasses. *Monogr. Allergy* **19,** 277–301.

Mills, F. C., Fisher, L. M., Kuroda, R., Ford, A. M., and Gould, H. J. (1983). DNase I hypersensitive sites in the chromatin of human μ immunoglobulin heavy-chain genes. *Nature (London)* **306,** 809–812.

Minie, M. E., and Koshland, M. E. (1986). Accessibility of the promoter sequence in the J-chain gene is regulated by chromatin changes during B-cell differentiation. *Mol. Cell. Biol.* **6,** 4031–4038.

Mostov, K. E., and Blobel, G. (1982). A transmembrane precursor of secretory component. *J. Biol. Chem.* **257,** 11816–11821.

Mostov, K. E., Kraehenbuhl, J.-P., and Blobel, G. (1980). Receptor-mediated transcellular transport of immunoglobulin: Synthesis of secretory component as multiple and larger. *Immunochemistry* **10,** 805–813.

Mostov, K. E., Friedlander, M., and Blobel, G. (1984). The receptor for transepithelial transport of IgA and IgM contains multiple immunoglobulin-like domains. *Nature (London)* **308,** 37–43.

Mostov, K. E., de Bruyn Kops, A., and Deitcher, D. L. (1986). Deletion of the cytoplasmic domain of the polymeric immunoglobulin receptor prevents basolateral localization and endocytosis. *Cell* **47,** 359–364.

Obata, M., Kataoka, T., Nakai, S., Yamagishi, H., Takahashik N., Yamakami-Kataoka, Y., Nikaido, T., Shimizu, A., and Honjo, T. (1981). Structure of a rearranged $\gamma1$ chain gene and its implication to immunoglobulin class-switch mechanism. *Proc. Natl. Acad. Sci. U.S.A.* **78,** 2437–2441.

Parslow, T. G., Blair, D. L., Murphy, W. J., and Granner, D. K. (1984). Structure of the 5′ ends of immunoglobulin genes: A novel conserved sequence. *Proc. Natl. Acad. Sci. U.S.A.* **81,** 2650–2654.

Rabbitts, T. H., Forster, A., Dunnick, W., and Bentley, D. L. (1980). The role of gene deletion in the immunoglobulin heavy chain switch. *Nature (London)* **283,** 351–356.

Radcliffe, G., Lin, Y.-C., Julius, M., Marcu, K. B., and Stavnezer, J. (1990). Structure of germ line immunoglobulin α heavy-chain RNA and its location on polysomes. *Mol. Cell Biol.* **10,** 382–386.

Schaerer, E., Verrey, F., Racine, L., Talichet, C., Reinhardt, M., and Kraehenbuhl, J.-P. (1990). Polarized transport of the polyeric immunoglobulin receptor in transfected rabbit mammary epithelial cells. *J. Cell Biol.* **110,** 987–998.

Schneiderman, R. D., Hanly, W. C., and Knight, K. L. (1989). Expression of 12 rabbit IgA $C\alpha$ genes as chimeric rabbit-mouse IgA antibodies. *Proc. Natl. Acad. Sci. U.S.A.* **86,** 7561–7565.

Severinson, E., Fernandez, C., and Stavnezer, J., (1990). Induction of germ-line immunoglobulin heavy chain transcripts by mitogens and interleukins prior to switch recombination. *Eur. J. Immunol.* **20,** 1079–1084.

Shimizu, A., Takahashi, N., Yaoita, Y., and Honjo, T. (1982). Organization of the constant-region gene family of the mouse immunoglobulin heavy chain. *Cell* **28,** 499–506.

Solari, R., and Kraehenbuhl, J.-P. (1984). Biosynthesis of the IgA antibody receptor: A model for the transepithelial sorting of a membrane glycoprotein. *Cell* **36,** 61–71.

Spieker-Polet, H., Yam, P., and Knight, K. L. (1993). Differential expression of thirteen IgA-heavy chain genes in rabbit lymphoid tissues. *J. Immunology* **151,** in press.

Stavnezer, J., Sirlin, S., and Abbott, J. (1985). Induction of immunoglobulin isotype switching in cultured I.29 B lymphoma cells: Characterization of the accompanying rearrangements of heavy chain genes. *J. Exp. Med.* **161,** 577–601.

Stavnezer, J., Radcliffe, G., Lin, Y.-C., Nietupski, J., Berggren, L., Sitia, R., and Severinson, E. (1988). Immunoglobulin heavy-chain switching may be directed by prior induction of transcripts from constant-region genes. *Proc. Natl. Acad. Sci. U.S.A.* **85,** 7704–7708.

Tucker, P. W., Slightom, J. L., and Blattner, F. R. (1981). Mouse IgA heavy chain gene sequence: Implications for evolution of immunoglobulin hinge exons. *Proc. Natl. Acad. Sci. U.S.A.* **78,** 7684–7688.

Ueda, S., Matsuda, F., and Honjo, T. (1988). Multiple recombinational events in primate immunoglobulin epsilon and alpha genes suggest closer relationship of human to chimpanzees than to gorillas. *J. Mol. Evol.* **27,** 77–83.

von Schwedler, U., Jack, H. M., and Wabl, M. (1990). Circular DNA is a product of the immunoglobulin class switch rearrangement. *Nature (London)* **345,** 452–456.

Word, C. J., Mushinski, J. F., and Tucker, P. W. (1983). The murine immunoglobulin α gene expresses multiple transcripts from a unique membrane exon. *EMBO J.* **2,** 887–898.

Yagi, M., and Koshland, M. E. (1981). Expression of the J chain gene during B cell differentiation is inversely correlated with DNA methylation. *Proc. Natl. Acad. Sci. U.S.A.* **78,** 4907–4911.

Yagi, M., D'Eustachio, P., Ruddle, F. H., and Koshland, M. E. (1982). J-chain is encoded by a single gene unlinked to other immunoglobulin structural genes. *J. Exp. Med.* **155,** 647.

Yaoita, Y., and Honjo, T. (1980). Deletion of immunoglobulin heavy chain genes from expressed allelic chromosome. *Nature (London)* **286,** 850–853.

Zikan, J., Novotny, J., Trapane, T. L., Koshland, M. E., Urry, D. W., Bennett, J. C., and Mestecky, J. (1985). Secondary structure of the immunoglobulin J chain. *Proc. Natl. Acad. Sci. U.S.A.* **82,** 5905–5909.

10

Epithelial and Hepatobiliary Transport of Polymeric Immunoglobulins

Per Brandtzaeg · Peter Krajči · Michael E. Lamm · Charlotte S. Kaetzel

I. INTRODUCTION

Mucous membranes generally are protected by a physically vulnerable monolayer of epithelium that covers an enormous surface area, perhaps 300–400 m^2 in adult humans. Most of this area is bombarded continuously by potentially infectious agents such as bacteria, viruses, fungi, and parasites, in addition to soluble dietary and environmental substances.

The first observations suggesting that the gastrointestinal mucosa has its own humoral immune system were published at the beginning of this century (Besredka, 1919; Davies, 1922). The molecular basis for the antibody activity found in exocrine secretions was described much later when Tomasi *et al.* (1965) characterized secretory IgA (SIgA) as an IgA dimer linked to an epithelial glycoprotein of ~80 kDa. This "secretory piece" is now called the secretory component (SC) and its transmembrane counterpart (~100 kDa) often is referred to as the polymeric immunoglobulin receptor (pIgR). Both bound SC (present in SIgA) and the structurally identical free SC found in most exocrine fluids (Brandtzaeg, 1973a) are generated by cleavage from the transmembrane component (Chapter 7).

In the early 1970s, dimers and larger polymers of IgA (collectively called polymeric IgA; pIgA) first were shown to be produced mainly by plasma cells adjacent to exocrine glands, especially in the gastrointestinal mucosa (Brandtzaeg, 1973b). These cells also produce the "joining" or J chain (Brandtzaeg, 1974a,1985), a peptide of ~15 kDa that becomes incorporated into the quaternary structure of both pIgA and pentameric IgM (Mestecky and McGhee, 1987). The J chain appears to determine the pIg structure that enables SC to complex noncovalently with pIgA and pentameric IgM, thereby being crucial to their transport through SC-expressing epithelium (Brandtzaeg and Prydz, 1984).

Thus, an interesting cooperation occurs between local plasma cells and secretory epithelia in the generation of SIgA and secretory IgM (SIgM). The gut mucosa contains most Ig-producing cells and is, therefore, quantitatively the major effector organ of humoral immunity (Chapter 21). The selectivity and capacity of the SC-mediated pIg transport mechanism are remarkable (Figure 1); more SIgA (40 mg/kg body weight) than the total daily production of IgG appears in the gut lumen every day (Conley and Delacroix, 1987).

II. COMMON EPITHELIAL POLYMERIC Ig TRANSPORT MECHANISM

Various models have been proposed for the external translocation of IgA (Brandtzaeg, 1985). The common transport mechanism proposed in the early 1970s suggested that pIgA and pentameric IgM both are translocated through secretory epithelia by receptor-mediated endocytosis; this notion implied that SC performs this function as an integrated plasma membrane protein (Brandtzaeg 1973a,b,1974b,1985). The model also implied that the J chain is a key protein in this process by generating the SC binding site in the pIg structure (Brandtzaeg, 1974a,b). The obvious biological significance of the striking J-chain expression shown by immunocytes in secretory tissues (Brandtzaeg, 1985) is, therefore, that locally produced pIgA and pentameric IgM become readily available for external transport (Figure 2). This important functional goal in terms of mucosal defense is necessarily reflected by a clonal maturation stage of B cells homing to secretory sites compatible with high J-chain-expressing potency (Chapter 21).

III. EVIDENCE THAT SECRETORY COMPONENT IS A POLYMERIC Ig RECEPTOR

A. Epithelial Localization of SC, IgA, and IgM

Immunohistochemical staining of different human exocrine tissues has demonstrated firmly the widespread epithelial distribution of SC; no convincing documentation of primary SC deficiency is available (Brandtzaeg and Baklien, 1977a; Brandtzaeg, 1985). SC is expressed mainly by serous types of epithelial cells in gastrointestinal mucosa; salivary, lacrimal, and mammary glands; the exocrine pancreas; the renal tubules; and the fallopian tube and endocervix of the female reproductive tract. The most prominent expression is seen in crypt cells of the large bowel and in mammary glands during late pregnancy (Brandtzaeg, 1974b,1983). Immunoelectron-microscopic studies have substantiated that not only do serous secretory cells synthesize SC, but they also clearly express SC in the basolateral plasma membrane (Brown *et al.,* 1976).

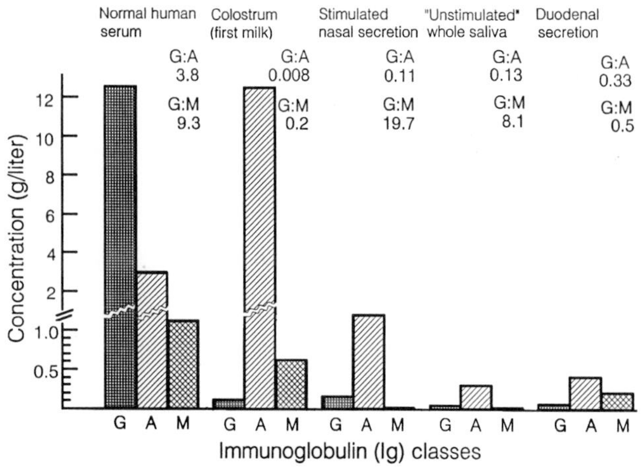

Figure 1 Average levels of IgG (G), IgA (A), and IgM (M) in various normal human body fluids. The concentration ratios (G : A and G : M) are indicated also to show the strikingly preferential appearance of IgA and, to a lesser extent, IgM in external secretions. This selectivity is particularly remarkable for colostrum, which is obtained directly from the duct opening, thus avoiding substantial contamination of IgG from interstitial fluid by leakage through surface epithelia. Modified from Brandtzaeg (1973a).

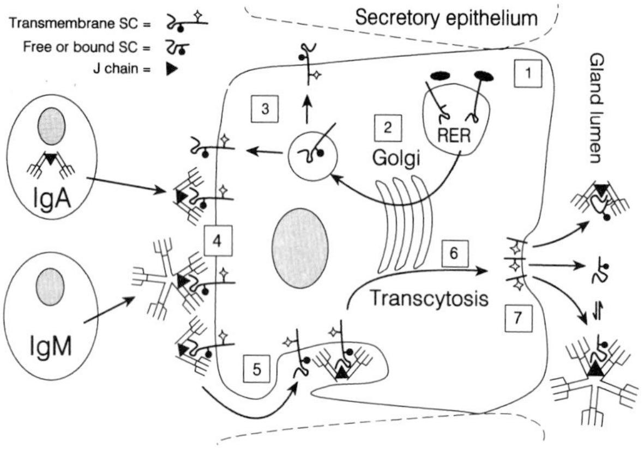

Figure 2 Model for the generation of human secretory IgA (SIgA) and secretory IgM (SIgM) via SC-mediated epithelial transport of J chain-containing pIgA and pentameric IgM produced by local plasma cells. (1) Synthesis and core glycosylation (−) of transmembrane SC in rough endoplasmic reticulum (RER) of secretory epithelial cell. (2) Terminal glycosylation (-●) in Golgi complex. (3) Phosphorylation (✧) at some later step. (4) Complexing of SC with J chain-containing pIg on basolateral cell membrane. (5) Endocytosis of complexed and unoccupied SC. (6) Transcytosis of vesicles. (7) Cleavage and release of SIgA, SIgM, and excess free SC. The cleavage mechanism and the fate of the cytoplasmic tail of transmembrane SC are mainly unknown. During the external translocation, covalent stabilization of the IgA–SC complexes regularly occurs (two disulfide bridges indicated in SIgA), whereas an excess of free SC in the secretion stabilizes the noncovalent IgM–SC complexes (dynamic equilibrium indicated for SIgM). Modified from Brandtzaeg (1985).

IgA and IgM can be traced with a distribution similar to that of SC, both in the cytoplasm and in relation to the basolateral borders of serous-type secretory epithelial cells (Brandtzaeg, 1974b,1975a; Brown *et al.*, 1976). Nevertheless, the detailed staining patterns revealed by paired immunofluorescence staining are not completely congruent; free SC is concentrated selectively in a granular pattern corresponding to the Golgi zone, whereas bound SC is seen mainly apically in the cytoplasm together with IgA and IgM (Brandtzaeg, 1974b; Poger and Lamm, 1974). Ultrastructural studies have confirmed these observations (Kraehenbuhl *et al.*, 1975; Brown *et al.*, 1976).

In the human hepatobiliary system, SC generally is found to be expressed only by the gall bladder and portal bile duct epithelia (Nagura *et al.*, 1981; Brandtzaeg, 1985; Tomana *et al.*, 1988), in contrast with the rat, rabbit, and some other species in which abundant SC expression is shown by hepatocytes (see subsequent discussion). Some reports have claimed such expression for human hepatocytes as well (Hsu and Hsu, 1980; Foss-Bowman *et al.*, 1983). Perez *et al.* (1989) reported positive staining with one of several monoclonal antibodies to SC, but in our hands this antibody reacted only with biliary duct epithelium (P. Brandtzaeg, unpublished observations).

B. Interactions between Polymeric Ig and SC

1. Binding Affinity and J-Chain Dependency

The apparent association constant (K_a) of pIg with free SC in solution is about $10^8\ M^{-1}$ (Brandtzaeg, 1985). This value is similar to that observed for a variety of antigen–antibody reactions but probably is underestimated for interactions with SC-expressing epithelial cells. In the latter case, a K_a of about $10^9\ M^{-1}$ has been suggested (Kühn and Kraehenbuhl, 1979). Both free and transmembrane SC molecules appear to depend on the presence of J chain in pIgA and pentameric IgM for the binding of these ligands (Brandtzaeg and Prydz, 1984). A crucial role of J chain in the formation of the SC binding site was, nevertheless, questioned by Schiff *et al.* (1986a), who claimed that some J chain-containing polymeric fractions of a human myeloma IgA lacked affinity for SC; however, these investigators did not formally prove the presence of J chain in the actual polymers.

Much stronger noncovalent interactions occur between pentameric IgM and SC than between pIgA (both subclasses) and SC; the K_a is several times higher for the former ligand (Brandtzaeg, 1985). Whether a "bonus effect" of a potentially higher molar J-chain content in pentameric IgM than in pIgA might explain this disparity remains to be clarified. In contrast to the notion that one J chain is found per polymer regardless of its size (Mestecky and McGhee, 1987), immunochemical quantitations have suggested the presence of two J chains in native dimeric IgA and two to four J chains in pentameric IgM (Brandtzaeg, 1985). The tendency for spontaneous dimerization shown by J chains obtained from pIgA by mild reduction could reflect that this peptide exists as a dimer in its native bound form (Brandtzaeg, 1985). Such isolated J-chain dimers show a marginal but significant affinity for free

SC. Antibody to J chain blocks the binding of SC to pIgA and pentameric IgM completely (Brandtzaeg, 1985). All these observations support the idea that the J chain contributes to the SC binding site.

2. Molecular Topography of Interactions

The reduction-sensitive "I determinant" region of SC (Brandtzaeg, 1971), apparently corresponding to its N-terminal or first Ig-like domain (Section IV,A), is likely to mediate the initial noncovalent interactions with pIg (Brandtzaeg, 1975b; Frutiger *et al.*, 1986; Geneste *et al.*, 1986a). The first binding step may depend on the highly conserved 15-37 amino-acid sequence that shows affinity not only for pIg but also for monomeric IgA and IgG (Bakos *et al.*, 1991). This step may be followed by further noncovalent interactions, apparently extending beyond the first domain at least in some species (Beale, 1989; Bakos *et al.*, 1991). Both the Cα2 and Cα3 domain of pIgA seem to take part (Geneste *et al.*, 1986b) although the exact site initially contacting the conserved SC region remains undefined. The subsequent covalent stabilization, which occurs selectively for SIgA, apparently depends on disulfide exchange reactions between one Cα2 domain and the fifth domain of SC (Figure 3). However, other possibilities have not been excluded (Mestecky and McGhee, 1987). Covalent binding between pIgA and the first domain of bovine domain of bovine SC was proposed (Beale, 1989). The disulfide appears to occur mainly in a late transcytotic compartment, at least in rat hepatocytes (Chintalacharuvu, *et al.*, 1993).

Computer-assisted analyses of human and murine J chains suggested that they may show an Ig domain-like folding despite a low degree of amino-acid sequence homology (Zikán *et al.*, 1985). Therefore, the noncovalent binding of SC to the Fc portion of pIgA and pentameric IgM may be determined by progressive complementary interdomain interactions (Figure 3), both with the J chain and with the constant region domains of α or μ chains. With regard to pIgA, such noncovalent interactions occur also secondarily to the disulfide bonding of SC and result in a remarkable "packing" of the SIgA molecule (Brandtzaeg, 1971). This topic has been further discussed by Pumphrey (1986) and by Mestecky and McGhee (1987).

3. Role of Interactions in Endocytosis of Polymeric Ig

Endocytosis of pIg by epithelial cells might start with ligand-induced active clustering of the pIg–SC complexes (Brandtzaeg, 1978; Gebhart and Robenek, 1987). However, the possibility that SC becomes clustered in coated pits even without ligand complexing was suggested by immunoelectron-microscopic studies of intestinal glands from immunodeficient patients (Nagura *et al.*, 1980). An inherent tendency

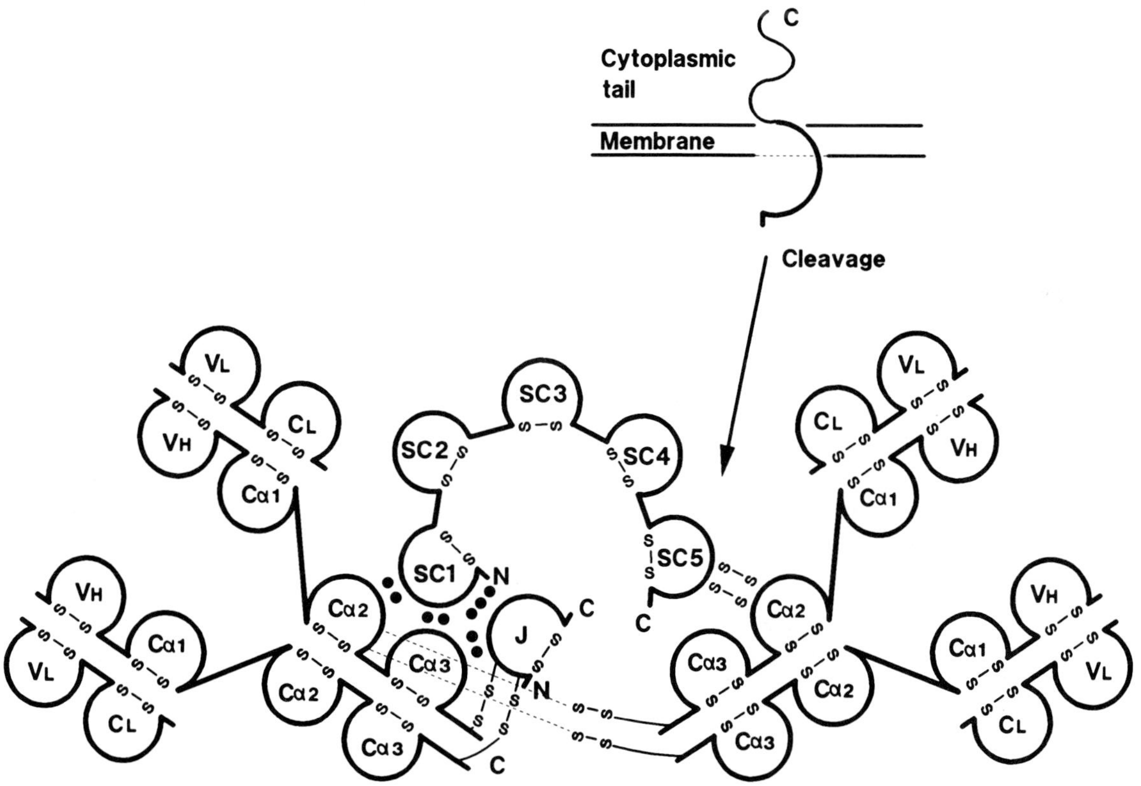

Figure 3 Putative domain interactions between J chain, Cα2, Cα3, SC1, and SC5 in the formation of human SIgA. Noncovalent interactions (⁚) are shown with only one IgA subunit. Only one J chain is depicted, although this is probably an oversimplification. Also, a recent report suggests that the J chain links the two IgA monomers (Bastian *et al.*, 1992). N, amino terminus; C, carboxyl terminus; V, variable region; CL and Cα1–3, constant regions; L, light chain; H, heavy chain; SC1–5, Ig-like domains of human SC; S–S, covalent interactions.

of SC to migrate in endocytic vesicles from the basolateral plasma membrane to the apical face of glandular cells could, in fact, explain that the concentration of free SC in secretions from subjects with hypogammaglobulinemia amounts to approximately the sum of free and bound SC secreted in normal individuals (Brandtzaeg, 1973a).

In rat hepatocytes, the pIgA–SC complexes are taken up via the same clathrin-coated pits and endosomes as other imported proteins (Geuze *et al.*, 1984). The sorting for delivery to lysosomes or transport to the bile canalicular face apparently takes place in the acidic compartment of uncoupling of receptor and ligand (CURL; Geuze *et al.*, 1984; Perez *et al.*, 1988).

IV. MOLECULAR BIOLOGY OF SECRETORY COMPONENT

A. Homology among Species and Relation to the Ig Supergene Family

Sequencing of human free SC isolated from colostrum (Eiffert *et al.*, 1984) and cloning of rabbit transmembrane SC cDNA (Mostov *et al.*, 1984) showed five extracellular homologous domains with considerable similarity to Ig domains (particularly Ig Vκ and Ig VH domains), each 100–115 residues long and stabilized by disulfide bridges between paired cysteines. Subsequent cloning of human transmembrane SC cDNA (Figure 4) made it possible to deduce the complete amino-acid sequence of this receptor (Krajči *et al.*, 1989,1991), including the peptide signal (18 residues) and 746 amino acids (the mature SC) extending 187 residues more at the C terminus than the sequence of free SC as reported by Eiffert *et al.* (1984). This extension includes the membrane-spanning segment and the cytoplasmic tail. These cloning results subsequently were confirmed by Piskurich *et al.* (1993).

The mature human SC shows an overall similarity of 56% with the 755-amino-acid-long-rabbit SC (Mostov *et al.*, 1984), 65% with the 751-amino-acid-long rat SC (Banting *et al.*, 1989), 79% with the 739-amino-acid-long bovine SC (Kulseth *et al.*, 1993), and 66% with the 753-amino-acid-long mouse SC (J. F. Piskurich, M. Hsieh, K. R. Youngman and C. S. Kaetzel, unpublished observations). As mentioned earlier (Section III,B,2), the amino-acid residues 15-37 of human SC apparently initiate its noncovalent interactions with Ig; this stretch represents a highly conserved sequence homology showing only one to five amino-acid differences among the five species; that is, the identity amounts to 78–96%, with the rat counterpart most similar to the human, followed by the mouse, bovine, and rabbit in that order. Except for this stretch, the five species show a striking increase in homology from the extracellular to the membrane-spanning and cytoplasmic parts, which is interesting in relation to the intracellular sorting of SC (Section IV,E,2).

Mostov *et al.* (1984) proposed a sixth domain in rabbit SC that includes the membrane-spanning part. However, this region shares low similarity with Ig domains and is not stabilized by a disulfide bridge. In this chapter, this region will

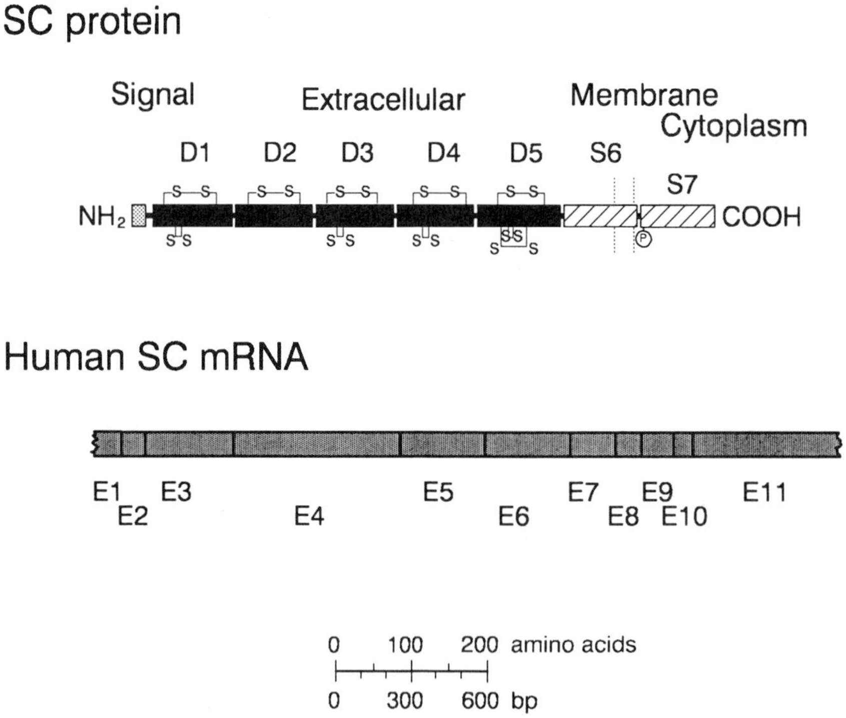

Figure 4 (*Top*) Schematic representation of extracellular homologous human SC domains (D1–D5) with their disulfide bridges (–S–S–), segment including the membrane-spanning portion (S6), and cytoplasmic segment (S7). The serine residue known to be phosphorylated in rabbit SC is indicated (Ⓟ). (*Bottom*) Schematic representation of the organization of exons (E1–E11) in human SC mRNA. Modified from Krajči *et al.* (1992a).

be referred to simply as the sixth segment, and the cytoplasmic tail will be called the seventh segment (Figure 4). Compared with the rabbit counterpart, the first part of the sixth segment in the other species lacks 12–15 amino acids, suggesting that this region has little functional importance. Conversely, the second half (positions 584–643) is well conserved, especially the postulated membrane-spanning part (rabbit positions 630–652) (Mostov *et al.*, 1984). This part constitutes a hydrophobic region that contains 23 uncharged residues (human positions 621–643), dividing transmembrane SC into an extracellular receptor portion and an intracytoplasmic tail.

Three putative cleavage sites have been proposed for rabbit SC, localized to Ala–Glu dipeptides that occur three times (positions 563–564, 597–598, and 605–606) in the sixth segment just upstream from the membrane-spanning portion (Kühn *et al.*, 1983; Mostov *et al.*, 1984). One of these is conserved in the rat and human sequences (Banting *et al.*, 1989; Krajči *et al.*, 1989), but not in those of mouse and cattle.

B. Exon–Intron Organization of the SC Gene

Cloning and characterization of the human SC gene (Figures 4 and 5) revealed its exon–intron organization in relation to the domain structure of the protein (Krajči *et al.*, 1992a). Domains 1, 4, and 5 were shown to be confined to one exon each. Domains 2 and 3, however, were found to be encoded by exon 4, corresponding to the rabbit exon that is involved in alternative splicing that results in the generation of a smaller transcript which, nevertheless, translates a functional receptor protein (Deitcher and Mostov, 1986). With this exception, the SC gene accords with the "one domain–one exon" rule characteristic of the Ig superfamily (Williams and Barclay, 1988). Also, within the cytoplasmic tail of human SC, encoded by the four distal exons (Krajči *et al.*, 1992a), a striking correspondence is seen between exon boundaries and the structural determinants proposed to be responsible for the intracellular routing of SC in the rabbit (Section IV,E,2).

C. Restriction Fragment Length Polymorphism and Chromosomal Localization of the Human SC Gene

The human SC gene exhibits a two-allelic restriction fragment length polymorphism (RFLP; Figure 6) caused by a polymorphic restriction site (for *Pvu* II) confined to its third intron (Krajči *et al.*, 1992a). This RFLP shows an autosomal codominant expression pattern and allelic frequencies of 0.63 and 0.37 among 370 unrelated Norwegians chromosomes (Krajči *et al.*, 1991,1992b).

In situ hybridization on metaphase chromosomes and discordance analysis of human–rodent somatic hybrids have assigned the human SC gene (locus *PIGR*) to region q31-q41 on chromosome 1 (Davidson *et al.*, 1988; Krajči *et al.*, 1991). Genetic linkage was demonstrated between the SC gene and the polymorphic DNA marker *pYNZ23* (locus *D1S58*), which is linked to other markers residing in 1q32 (Krajči *et al.*, 1992b). This linkage suggested a close relationship of *PIGR*

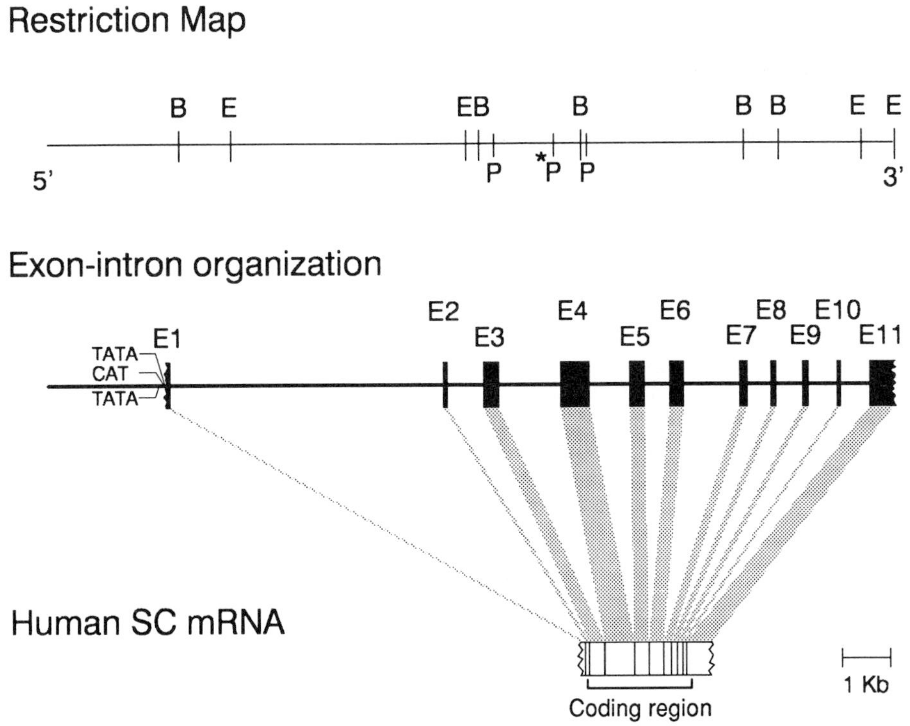

Figure 5 Schematic representation of the gene encoding human transmembrane SC. (*Top*) Partial restriction map: *Bam* HI (B), *Eco* RI (E), *Pvu* II (P) (only the three sites involved in *Pvu* II RFLP are indicated; the polymorphic site is labeled by an asterisk). (*Middle*) Exon–intron organization: E1–E11. TATA and CAT boxes are indicated. (*Bottom*) Schematic representation of SC mRNA with coding region indicated. Modified from Krajči *et al.* (1992a).

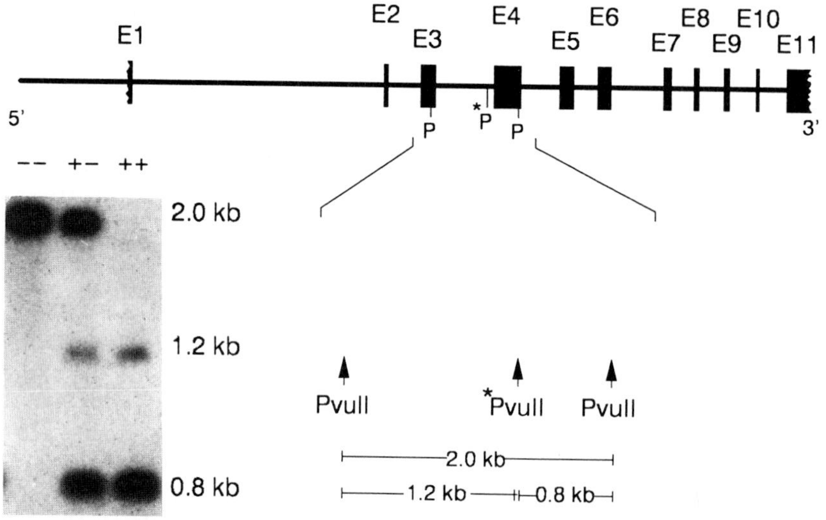

Figure 6 Schematic representation of the gene encoding human transmembrane SC. (*Top*) Exon–intron organization, with three restriction sites for *Pvu* II (P) involved in RFLP indicated. The polymorphic site is labeled by an asterisk. (*Bottom left*) Southern blot of *Pvu* II-digested genomic DNA hybridized with the 0.67-kb *Pvu* II cDNA probe, heterozygotic (+−) or homozygotic for the absence (−−) or presence (++) of the polymorphic cleavage site. (*Bottom right*) Schematic enlargement of the 2.0-kb *Pvu* II fragment of the gene showing the suggested location of the polymorphic *Pvu* II site. Modified from Krajči *et al.* (1992a).

to loci encoding the decay accelerating factor and the complement receptors CR1 and CR2, all involved in complement regulation.

D. Expression of SC mRNA

Northern blot analysis demonstrated only one human (~3.8 kb) and one rat (~3.5 kb) SC mRNA (Banting *et al.*, 1989; Krajči *et al.*, 1989,1991), whereas rabbit was shown to express two transcripts (~3.8 kb and ~3.1 kb) that are produced by alternative splicing (Mostov *et al.*, 1984; Deitcher and Mostov, 1986), as discussed earlier.

The relative distribution of SC mRNA in human exocrine tissues (Figure 7) corresponds with earlier immunohistochemical findings (Section III,A); the highest level is seen in the gut, whereas only weak expression appears in the liver, probably reflecting inclusion of biliary duct epithelium (Krajči *et al.*, 1989). Conversely, SC mRNA is expressed by hepatocytes in rabbits and rats (Mostov *et al.*, 1984; Banting *et al.*, 1989). This remarkable disparity with respect to hepatic SC correlates with the fact that about 90% of IgA in the upper duodenal fluid is derived from bile in rats but less than 15% is so derived in humans (Conley and Delacroix, 1987).

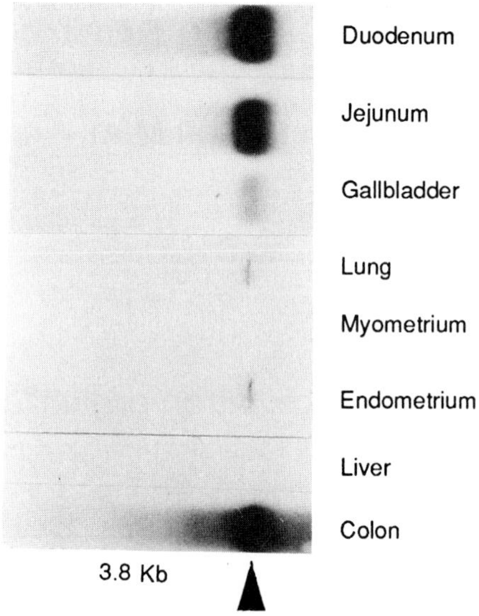

Figure 7 Northern blot analysis of SC mRNA extracted from various human tissues as indicated. Total RNA (20 μg) was separated by electrophoresis and hybridized with a nick-translated human transmembrane SC probe.

E. Intracellular Routing of SC

1. Transcytosis and Cleavage of the Polymeric Receptor

Cell biology studies first showed that rabbit SC is produced as a transmembrane protein 25–30 kDa larger than the secreted free or bound form (Mostov *et al.*, 1980). Subsequent experiments with the adenocarcinoma cell line HT-29 demonstrated that human SC also is produced as a transmembrane precursor (~95 kDa) that, following terminal glycosylation, becomes ~20 kDa larger than the ~80-kDa secreted form (Mostov and Blobel, 1982).

After synthesis and core glycosylation in the rough endoplasmic reticulum, maturation of transmembrane SC takes place in the Golgi complex (see subsequent discussion), as shown by the acquisition of *Endo* H resistance (30–60 min). This modification probably represents the rate-limiting step in its intracellular routing (Solari and Kraehenbuhl, 1984). SC becomes phosphorylated near or in the basolateral plasma membrane (Larkin *et al.*, 1986; Casanova *et al.*, 1990). Ligand-complexed or unoccupied SC then is endocytosed and transcytosed toward the luminal (or, in the liver, bile canalicular) plasma membrane (Brown *et al.*, 1976; Brandtzaeg, 1978; Crago *et al.*, 1978; Hoppe *et al.*, 1985). PIg-bound and free SC molecules finally are generated by cleavage from the membrane-spanning portion of the receptor and released into the secretions (Figure 2). The cleavage apparently takes place at the apical cell surface (Solari *et al.*, 1989; Schaerer *et al.*, 1990) and involves unknown enzymes that are sensitive to leupeptin (Musil and Baenziger, 1988). The fate of the membrane-spanning and cytoplasmic parts of SC is largely unknown, but an ~34-kDa fragment derived from them has been detected in the rat liver cytosol; smaller degradation products are released into rat bile (Solari *et al.*, 1989).

2. Signals Determining Migration and Sorting of SC

The intracellular sorting of SC is still poorly understood, but several putative determinants within its relatively long cytoplasmic tail (~15 kDa) have been identified by experiments with mutant rabbit receptor (Bomsel and Mostov, 1991). A 14-amino-acid segment (655–668) distal to the membrane-spanning segment apparently directs SC to the basolateral surface (Figure 8). Phosphorylation of serine at position 664 seems to afford the signal for sorting from basolateral early endosomes into the transcytotic pathway under the guidance of microtubules (Casanova *et al.*, 1990). Deletion of residues 670–707 causes increased degradation of receptor-bound pIg after endocytosis, whereas deletion of the C-terminal 30 amino acids (726–755) (or mutation of the tyrosine at position 668 to serine, and/or the tyrosine at position 734 to cysteine, particularly the latter) reduces the rate of internalization (Breitfeld *et al.*, 1990; Okamoto *et al.*, 1992). All these regions are highly conserved among the five species studied (Section IV, A), except that the latter tyrosine mentioned above is lacking in bovine SC. This homology suggests that the structural sorting signals possessed by the cytoplasmic tail, as well as their intracellular recognition apparatus, are quite similar. Moreover, good correspondence exists between the putative sorting determinants and the identified human exons encoding the cytoplasmic tail (Figure 8).

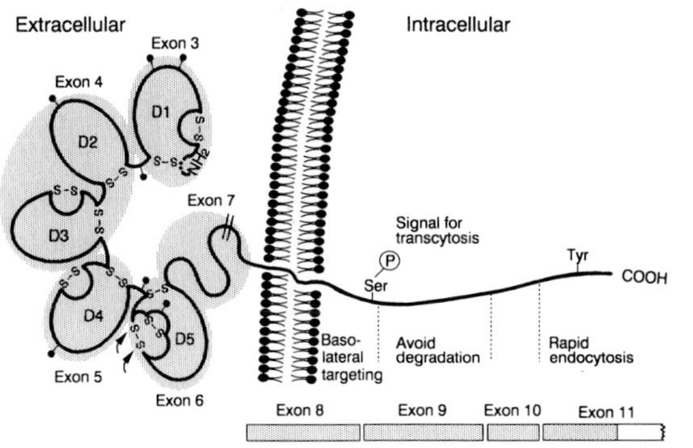

Figure 8 Schematic depiction of extracellular homologous human SC domains (D1–D5) with the membrane-spanning portion and cytoplasmic tail. The shaded areas and boxes at the bottom represent extensions of the corresponding 11 exons (Krajči *et al.*, 1992a). Exons 8–11 are lined up in relation to the different functional parts of the cytoplasmic tail recognized for rabbit SC, including the phosphorylated serine residue (Ⓟ) and the C-terminal tyrosine residue (Tyr) (Bomsel and Mostov, 1991). Carbohydrate-binding sites (–•) and disulfide bridges (–S–S–) are shown also. The amino-acid residues 15–37 of D1 (••) is likely to be involved in the initial noncovalent binding to pIg. The cysteines believed to be involved in the formation of disulfide bridges between SC and IgA are indicated by arrows (Mestecky and McGhee, 1987). A possible cleavage site for generation of free and pIg-bound SC is indicated by //.

V. MODULATION OF SECRETORY COMPONENT EXPRESSION

A. Ontogenic Aspects

Human bronchial epithelium was reported to express SC at 8 weeks gestation (Ogra *et al.*, 1972), in contrast to the somewhat later expression (18–29 weeks) observed for intestinal and salivary gland epithelium (Brandtzaeg *et al.*, 1991,1992). Occasional J-chain-positive IgA immunocytes and some epithelial IgA also can be seen in parotid glands after 30 weeks gestation, suggesting that pIg transport may take place during the fetal period (Hayashi *et al.*, 1989; Thrane *et al.*, 1991). SC shows a strikingly increased expression in salivary gland epithelium after the second postnatal week but decreases to the perinatal level in or near the 6th month (Hayashi *et al.*, 1989; Thrane *et al.*, 1991). This temporarily raised expression, which is reflected in relatively large amounts of free SC in saliva shortly after birth (Burgio *et al.*, 1980), suggests that the secretory epithelium in the immediate postnatal period is exposed to stimulatory factors that enhance constitutive SC expression (Section V,C). This result correlates with the rapid accumulation of Ig-producing cells in exocrine tissues after birth (Chapter 21). In the intestinal crypts, adult levels of SC expression and signs of external IgA and IgM transport are seen at 1–2 weeks (Brandtzaeg *et al.*, 1991,1992).

Victims of sudden infant death syndrome (SIDS) often have been claimed to have suffered from mild upper respiratory tract infection with various viruses shortly before death. In agreement with this possibility, we found a significantly elevated number of IgA, IgM, and IgG immunocytes in salivary glands of such infants (Thrane *et al.*, 1990). Intensified local immunostimulation also was supported strongly by the fact that the salivary glands from the same SIDS victims showed significantly raised numbers of interstitial leukocytes and enhanced epithelial MHC Class II and SC expression (Brandtzaeg *et al.*, 1992).

B. Aberrant Up-Regulation of SC in Vivo

Immunohistochemical observations in chronic gastritis demonstrated increased SC expression and enhanced uptake of IgA in fundic and antral glands surrounded by dense infiltrates of mononuclear cells (Valnes *et al.*, 1984). Similar epithelial features have been seen in celiac disease and sialadenitis (Brandtzaeg *et al.*, 1992), and most likely can be explained by local cytokine release (Section V,C). In keeping with this suggestion, interferon-γ (IFNγ) placed in the uterine cavity of rats induced raised levels of SC in uterine secretions (Wira *et al.*, 1991). Conversely, reduced expression of SC has been reported for regenerating and dysplastic colonic epithelium in inflammatory bowel disease (Brandtzaeg and Baklien, 1977; Rognum *et al.*, 1987).

Enhanced external pIg transport associated with mucosal immune responses probably explains why the serum levels of pIgA and IgM generally are increased only marginally despite the markedly expanded jejunal IgA- and IgM-producing cell populations in untreated celiac disease (Brandtzaeg, 1991). Nevertheless, the SC-dependent transport capacity may be insufficient in certain patients with an unusual intestinal IgA-producing cell proliferation, resulting in excessive amounts of pIgA in serum (Brandtzaeg and Baklien, 1977b; Colombel *et al.*, 1988).

C. Effect of Cytokines

Recombinant IFNγ causes a time- and concentration-dependent accumulation of SC mRNA in the human adenocarcinoma cell line HT-29, detectable 6 hr after stimulation (Krajči *et al.*, 1993; Piskurich *et al.*, 1993). A strikingly enhanced expression of SC mRNA likewise is seen by *in situ* hybridization (Krajči *et al.*, 1993). Cycloheximide abolishes this effect with a time course that suggests that regulatory proteins with a turnover shorter than 6 hr are required for accumulation of SC message (Krajči *et al.*, 1993). This retarded mRNA response is in agreement with an even longer delay (6–12 hr) observed for enhancement of the intracellular pool and membrane expression of functionally active SC (Sollid *et al.*, 1987; Kvale *et al.*, 1988a,b).

Co-incubation with 5,6-dichloro-1-β-ribofuranosyl benzimidazole (DRB), a selective inhibitor of RNA polymerase II, indicated a half-life of about 1 hr for IFNγ-induced SC mRNA (Krajči *et al.*, 1993). These findings, in conjunction with the identification of two consensus motifs for IFNγ-responsive elements upstream of the first exon of the SC gene (P. Krajči and P. Brandtzaeg, unpublished results), suggested transcriptional activation in addition to posttranscriptional stabilization of SC mRNA, as previously observed for MHC gene products (Williams, 1991).

Also, tumor necrosis factor-α (TNFα) (Kvale *et al.*, 1988a,b) and interleukin 4 (IL-4) (Phillips *et al.*, 1990) have been found to enhance SC expression in HT-29 cells; IFNγ and TNFα in combination showed an additive effect, whereas IFNγ and IL-4 acted synergistically. IL-2, IL-3, IL-5, and IL-6 have not been found to stimulate SC (Phillips *et al.*, 1990), whereas the results for IL-1 are controversial. Kvale and Brandtzaeg (1992) observed enhancing effects of IL-1 and TNFα that, in combination with IFNγ, were increased markedly in HT-29 cells differentiated by exposure to butyrate. Conversely, the effect of IL-4 alone or in combination with IFNγ was decreased in these cells, which might be more comparable to the gut epithelium *in vivo*. In addition, transforming growth factor-β (TGFβ) has been reported to enhance SC expression in the IEC-6 rat intestinal cell line (McGee *et al.*, 1991).

Although SC both in humans (Section V,A) and in rats (Buts *et al.*, 1992) clearly is expressed constitutively, the above results suggest that various cytokines may be involved in its *in vivo* modulation. IFNγ, TNFα, IL-1, IL-4, and TGFβ all are produced by activated mononuclear cells and, to some extent, by other cell types. The *in vivo* (Section V,B) and the *in vitro* results imply that macrophages and T cells, which most likely contribute to terminal differentiation of J-chain-positive B cells that appear at exocrine sites, also are involved in enhancing SC-dependent external transport of the local pIg product. Epithelial translocation of IgA and IgM can, in this way, be adapted to the degree of mucosal immunostimulation.

D. Effect of Hormones

Several *in vivo* studies have demonstrated hormonal regulation of humoral immunity in the rat uterus (Sullivan and Wira, 1983; Wira and Sullivan, 1985). Estradiol and progesterone increase IgA translocation to the uterine secretions, involving enhanced serum IgA and IgG transudation as well as SC transport (Sullivan *et al.*, 1983; Wira *et al.*, 1991). However, the IgA level is suppressed by glucocorticoids such as dexamethasone, both in cervicovaginal and in salivary secretions (Sullivan *et al.*, 1983; Wira and Rossoll, 1991), although SC production by rat hepatocytes *in vivo* is increased by this steroid hormone (Wira and Colby, 1985; Buts *et al.*, 1992). Testosterone increases the external translocation of SC and IgA by lacrimal glands in rats; both proteins are found at higher levels in tears from males than in those from females (Sullivan and Allansmith, 1987). Obviously, hormonal influence on the SIgA system is complex and may vary among different secretory sites.

VI. HEPATIC IgA TRANSPORT AND CATABOLISM

A. Role of SC in Hepatocytes and Bile Duct Epithelium

The molecular biology of SC-dependent pIgA transport has been explored in liver cells from the rat to a great extent. This model system has contributed significantly to the understanding of intracellular protein trafficking. Translocation of serum-derived pIgA into bile was described first in this species as a rapid SC-mediated process performed by the hepatocytes (Jackson *et al.*, 1978; Fisher *et al.*, 1979; Orlans *et al.*, 1979). This transport was shown to follow a vesicular pathway to the canalicular face (Mullock *et al.*, 1979; Renston *et al.*, 1980; Takahashi *et al.*, 1982; Hoppe *et al.*, 1985; Limet *et al.*, 1985), where release into bile took place by proteolytic cleavage of transmembrane SC (Mullock *et al.*, 1980; Solari *et al.*, 1986). A similar, although less efficient, SC-dependent hepatocytic pathway has been described in mice (Jackson *et al.*, 1977; Phillips *et al.*, 1984) and rabbits (Delacroix *et al.*, 1982,1984), in contrast with the situation in humans (Section III,A; Figure 7). In fact, hepatobiliary pIgA secretion appears to correlate with hepatocyte expression of SC in the species under study (Delacroix *et al.*, 1984). Transport across the biliary epithelium is likely to represent only a secondary pathway including primarily pIgA produced by plasma cells within the portal tract and gall bladder mucosa (Dooley *et al.*, 1982; Nagura *et al.*, 1983; Brandtzaeg, 1985).

Studies on hepatic transcytosis of pIgA have focused on molecular modifications of transmembrane SC during its biosynthesis and transport, as well as on the nature of the vesicular carriers. Pulse labeling of rat liver with [^{35}S]cysteine followed by immunoprecipitation with antibodies to SC revealed that newly translated and core-glycosylated SC in the endoplasmic reticulum has an M_r ~105,000 kDa (Sztul *et al.*, 1985; Buts *et al.*, 1992). After 15–30 min of chase with unlabeled cysteine, the ~105-kDa form is converted successively to two molecular species of ~115,000 and ~120,000 kDa, the former representing terminal glycosylation of SC in the Golgi complex (Sztul *et al.*, 1985; Solari *et al.*, 1986) and the latter representing phosphorylated mature SC (Larkin *et al.*, 1986). The fact that only terminally glycosylated SC is a target for phosphorylation is consistent with the demonstration that phosphorylation of a serine residue on its cytoplasmic tail is a critical signal for endocytosis and transcytosis (Section IV,E,2).

Evidence that hepatic transcytosis of SC–pIgA complexes is vesicular in the rat was obtained initially by quantitative electron-microscopic autoradiography (Renston *et al.*, 1980) and immunoelectron microscopy (Takahashi *et al.*, 1982; Courtoy *et al.*, 1983; Hoppe *et al.*, 1985). A distinct population of vesicular carriers from rat liver has been isolated using antibodies to the cytoplasmic tail of SC (Sztul *et al.*, 1991). These vesicles are enriched in the mature ~120-kDa form of SC as well as in pIgA and are depleted in elements of the secretory pathway, Golgi, sinusoidal plasma membrane, and early endosomal components. Apparently these vesicles represent a unique compartment specialized for transcytosis to the bile canaliculus. This conclusion is supported by the observation that transcytotic vesicular carriers containing mature phosphorylated SC and pIgA accumulate in the pericanalicular cytoplasm of rat hepatocytes after bile duct ligation (Larkin and Palade, 1991).

B. Role of Other IgA Binding Activities

Although hepatobiliary transport of pIgA appears to correlate best with SC expression on the hepatocytes (Delacroix *et al.*, 1984), other cell surface receptors also may participate in the uptake of IgA by the liver parenchyma. For example, purified asialoglycoprotein receptor (ASGP-R) from rat liver was shown to bind IgA from normal human serum (Stockert *et al.*, 1982). The ASGP-R recognition site on IgA appears to be the O-linked oligosaccharides in the hinge region of the IgA1 subclass. Human monomeric IgA1 as well as SIgA1 (which cannot bind SC) was as effective as pIgA from serum in binding to ASGP-R (Tomana *et al.*, 1985). Further, binding of asialoorosomucoid by rat or mouse liver *in vivo* (Schiff *et al.*, 1984), or by plasma membrane-enriched fractions from rat, monkey, and human liver (Daniels *et al.*, 1989), was inhibited by human IgA1 but not by rat IgA, which lacks O-linked oligosaccharides.

Hepatic uptake by ASGP-R generally results in delivery of the ligand to lysosomes for degradation. Nevertheless, Schiff *et al.* (1986b) demonstrated in rat liver that human IgA endocytosed via this receptor could dissociate within endosomes to become associated with transmembrane SC in this compartment, and thus be targeted to the transcytotic pathway for translocation as SIgA into bile. Because the expression of SC by human hepatocytes is extremely low or absent (Section III,A; Figure 7), endocytosis of IgA1 by ASGP-R may represent an important pathway for hepatic clearance of this major IgA subclass in human serum. Whereas the bulk of endocytosed IgA presumably would be catabolized in lysosomes, some of the pIgA could end up as biliary SIgA. However, experiments in nonhuman primates did not reveal any difference in hepatic clearance of intravenously injected human IgA1 and IgA2, although polymers were favored strikingly over monomers (Moldoveanu *et al.*, 1990). Thus an as yet undefined binding site for IgA is likely to exist on hepatocytes that is distinct from ASGP-R and has preferential affinity for pIgA, regardless of subclass. This binding site has been suggested previously on the basis of *in vitro* experiments with rat and human hepatocytes (Tolleshaug *et al.*, 1981; Brandtzaeg, 1985; Tomana *et al.*, 1988).

In addition, the carbohydrate moieties on human IgA have been shown to bind to galactosyltransferase enzymes, either in free form in colostrum and serum (McGuire *et al.*, 1989) or on the surface of hepatocytes and a variety of cultured cell lines (Tomana *et al.*, 1991). In the absence of UDP-galactose, cell-surface galactosyltransferase acts as a lectin and binds both IgG and IgM, as well as monomeric IgA, pIgA, and SIgA, with relatively high association constants. Because ligands bound to galactosyltransferase on cells are apparently not internalized (Tomana *et al.*, 1991), the possible role of this binding in the physiology of IgA remains unclear.

Kupffer cells and murine hepatocytes have been shown to express receptors for the Fc region of both monomeric IgA and pIgA (Sancho *et al.*, 1986). The contribution of these receptors to hepatic clearance of IgA is unclear, but nonparenchymal cells do contribute significantly to making the liver of nonhuman primates (and therefore probably humans) the major site of uptake and catabolism of circulating IgA (Moldoveanu *et al.*, 1990).

VII. CLEARANCE OF IgA-CONTAINING IMMUNE COMPLEXES

A. Role of the Liver

Clearance of IgA-containing immune complexes (IC) has been studied primarily with respect to systemic mechanisms relevant for circulating IC. In humans (Rifai *et al.*, 1989) and rodents (Russell *et al.*, 1981; Socken *et al.*, 1981; Harmatz *et al.*, 1982), intravenously administered IgA IC or heat-aggregated IgA are cleared primarily by the liver, presumably via the same receptors that mediate uptake of IgA (Section

VI). Thus, SC-mediated hepatobiliary transport of circulating IgA IC is probably of little or no significance in humans. Phagocytosis by Kupffer cells contributes to the clearance of IC (Rifai and Mannik, 1984); for IgA IC also containing IgG, Fcγ and complement receptors on these cells apparently are involved (Roccatello *et al.*, 1992). Because the systemic mechanisms for clearance of IgA IC are saturable (Russell *et al.*, 1981; Rifai and Mannik, 1984), high concentrations of IgA IC in the circulation may lead to their deposition in extrahepatic tissues, as has been implicated in the pathogenesis of IgA nephropathy (Emancipator and Lamm, 1989).

B. Role of Mucosal Epithelia

IgA antibodies are produced mainly by plasma cells in the lamina propria of mucous membranes (Chapter 21), where significant amounts of IgA IC most likely form when antigens penetrate the epithelial barrier. Thus, in addition to its role as SIgA performing immune exclusion, locally produced IgA antibodies within the mucosa may trap antigens derived from the environment, diet, and luminal microbiota or synthesized in the mucosal tissue during infections. Such IgA-mediated trapping would, by itself, be an antiinflammatory mechanism in competition with the formation of potentially harmful immune complexes containing IgM or IgG antibodies (Figure 9). Moreover, external transport of IgA IC by mucosal epithelia could be an efficient and potentially less harmful clearance mechanism than systemic elimination of these complexes after they reach the circulation.

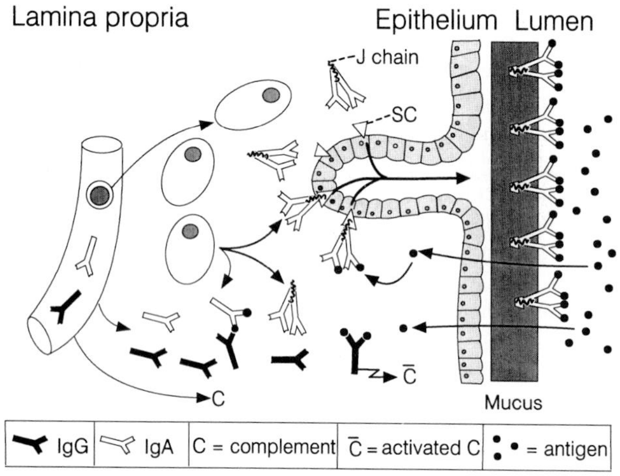

Figure 9 It is postulated that humoral immunological homeostasis is maintained in mucous membranes through a critical balance between available immunoglobulins (for simplicity, only IgG and IgA are depicted). Secretory IgA acts in a "first line" of defense by performing antigen exclusion in the mucus layer at the epithelial surface (to the right). Antigens by-passing this barrier may meet corresponding serum-derived IgG antibodies in the lamina propria. The resulting immune complexes will activate complement, and inflammatory mediators probably are formed continuously in the mucosa. An adverse inflammatory and tissue-destructive development is most likely inhibited by blocking antibody activities exerted in the lamina propria by serum-derived monomeric IgA and locally produced monomeric or dimeric IgA. Moreover, antigens may be returned efficiently in a noninflammatory way to the lumen by the SC-mediated transport mechanism after being bound to dimeric IgA antibodies.

SC-expressing epithelial cells transport vectorially *in vitro* IC with pIgA from the basolateral surface to the apical face where release occurs (Figure 9); the antigen remains undegraded and bound to the pIgA antibody throughout transcytosis (Kaetzel *et al.*, 1991). Interestingly, monomeric IgA and IgG antibodies, when cross-linked via antigen to pIgA, also can participate in SC-mediated epithelial trancystosis (Kaetzel *et al.*, submitted). Secretory epithelium might, therefore, participate *in vivo* in the clearance of IgA IC directly at sites at which they are most likely to be formed. This antiinflammatory mechanism probably is enhanced in disease states with immunological activation as a result of cytokine-induced up-regulation of SC (Section V,C). Direct clearance of locally formed IgA IC by SC-expressing epithelia could afford an important, but hitherto unappreciated, defense function mediated by pIgA.

Evidence from *in vitro* studies also suggests that IgA IC can form within secretory epithelial cells infected with virus if these cells are simultaneously transporting specific pIgA antibody (Mazanec *et al.*, 1992). In such cases, the antibody can neutralize the virus intracellularly. Although the intracellular compartment localization and efficiency of this neutralization are currently unclear, these results could reflect still another important defense function of pIgA. On the other hand, the possibility has been suggested from similar *in vitro* experiments that SC may promote viral infection of usually resistant epithelial cells by mediating uptake of virus bound to pIgA antibody (Sixbey and Yao, 1992).

VIII. CONCLUSIONS

Transmembrane SC is quantitatively the most important receptor of the immune system because it is responsible for external translocation of the major product of humoral immunity, that is, pIgA. SC also may be involved in mucosal clearance of immune complexes containing pIgA and, in rodents, in hepatic elimination of such complexes from peripheral blood. The molecular biology of SC is complicated and interesting; its function as a receptor is the best defined part of mucosal immunity and has thrown considerable light on intracellular trafficking of proteins in general. The cleavage of this receptor to release free or pIg-bound SC into the secretions is a unique process. This continuous sacrifice of large amounts of receptor protein appears biologically justified to stabilize secretory antibodies. Such stabilization is particularly successful for SIgA, in which covalent bonding takes place between SC and pIgA by disulfide exchange reaction during epithelial transcytosis; the noncovalent stabilization of SIgM apparently depends on an excess of free SC in the secretions.

Acknowledgments

Studies in the authors' laboratories have been supported by the Norwegian Cancer Society, the Norwegian Research Council, Otto

Kr. Bruun's Legacy, and USA National Institutes of Health Grants A1-26449, CA-51998, DK-43999, and HL-37117. Hege E. Svendsen is gratefully acknowledged for excellent secretarial assistance.

References

Bakos, M.-A., Kurosky, A., and Goldblum, R. M. (1991). Characterization of a critical binding site for human polymeric Ig on secretory component. *J. Immunol.* **147,** 3419–3426.

Banting, G., Brake, B., Braghetta, P., Luzio, P. J., and Stanley, K. K. (1989). Intracellular targetting signals of polymeric immunoglobulin receptors are highly conserved between species. *FEBS Lett.* **254,** 177–183.

Beale, D. (1989). Tryptic digestion of bovine secretory IgA at elevated temperature and in urea. Isolation of SC domain 1 which is covalently bound to IgA dimer and binds noncovalently to IgM. *Int. J. Biochem.* **21,** 549–554.

Bastian, A., Kratzin, H., Eckart, K., and Hilschmann, N. (1992). Intra- and interchain disulfide bridges of the human J chain in secretory immunoglobulin A. *Biol. Chem. Hoppe-Seyler* **373,** 1255–1263.

Besredka, A. (1919). De la vaccination contre les états typhoides par la voie buccale. *Ann. Inst. Pasteur* **33,** 882–903.

Bomsel, M., and Mostov, K. (1991). Sorting of plasma membrane proteins in epithelial cells. *Curr. Opin. Cell Biol.* **3,** 647–653.

Brandtzaeg, P. (1973a). Structure, synthesis and external transfer of mucosal immunoglobulins. *Ann. Inst. Pasteur Immunol.* **124C,** 417–438.

Brandtzaet, P. (1971). Human secretory immunoglobulins. III. Immunochemical and physicochemical studies of secretory IgA and free secretory piece. *Acta Path. Microbiol. Scand., Section B* **79,** 165–188.

Brandtzaeg, P. (1973b). Two types of IgA immunocytes in man. *Nature New Biol.* **243,** 142–143.

Brandtzaeg, P. (1974a). Presence of J chain in human immunocytes containing various immunoglobulin classes. *Nature (London)* **252,** 418–420.

Brandtzaeg, P. (1974b). Mucosal and glandular distribution of immunoglobulin components. Differential localization of free and bound SC in secretory epithelial cells. *J. Immunol.* **112,** 1553–1559.

Brandtzaeg, P. (1975a). Human secretory immunoglobulin M. An immunochemical and immunohistochemical study. *Immunology* **29,** 559–570.

Brandtzaeg, P. (1975b). Human secretory component. IV. Aggregation and fragmentation of free secretory component. *Immunochemistry* **12,** 877–881.

Brandtzaeg, P. (1978). Polymeric IgA is complexed with secretory component (SC) on the surface of human intestinal epithelial cells. *Scand. J. Immunol.* **8,** 39–52.

Brandtzaeg, P. (1983). The secretory immune system of lactating human mammary glands compared with other excrine organs. *Ann. N.Y. Acad. Sci.* **409,** 353–381.

Brandtzaeg, P. (1985). Role of J chain and secretory component in receptor-mediated glandular and hepatic transport of immunoglobulins in man. *Scand. J. Immunol.* **22,** 111–146.

Brandtzaeg, P. (1991). Immunologic basis for celiac disease, inflammatory bowel disease, and type B chronic gastritis. *Curr. Opin. Gastroenterol.* **7,** 450–462.

Brandtzaeg, P., and Baklien, K. (1977a). Intestinal secretion of IgA and IgM: A hypothetical model. *Ciba Found. Symp.* **46,** 77–113.

Brandtzaet, P., and Baklien, K. (1977b). Characterization of the IgA-immunocyte population and its produce in a patient with excessive intestinal formation of IgA. *Clin. Exp. Immunol.* **30,** 77–88.

Brandtzaeg, P., and Prydz, H. (1984). Direct evidence for an integrated function of J chain and secretory component in epithelial transport of immunoglobulins. *Nature (London)* **311,** 71–73.

Brandtzaeg, P., Nilssen, D. E., Rognum, T. O., and Thrane, P. S. (1991). Ontogeny of the mucosal immune system and IgA deficiency. *Gastroenterol. Clin. North Am.* **20,** 397–439.

Brandtzaeg, P., Halstensen, T. S., Huitfeldt, H. S., Krajči, P., Kvale, D., Scott, H., and Thrane, P. S. (1992). Epithelial expression of HLA, secretory component (poly-Ig receptor), and adhesion molecules in the human alimentary tract. *Ann. N.Y. Acad. Sci.* **664,** 157–179.

Breitfeld, P. P., Casanova, J. E., McKinnon, W. C., and Mostov, K. E. (1990). Deletions in the cytoplasmic domain of the polymeric immunoglobulin receptor differentially affect endocytotic rate and postendocytotic traffic. *J. Biol. Chem.* **265,** 13750–13757.

Brown, W. R., Isobe, Y., and Nakane, P. K. (1976). Studies on translocation of immunoglobulins across intestinal epithelium. II. Immunoelectron-microscopic localization of immunoglobulins and secretory component in human intestinal mucosa. *Gastroenterology* **71,** 985–995.

Burgio, G. R., Lanzavecchia, A., Plebani, A., Jayakar, S., and Ugazio, A. G. (1980). Ontogeny of secretory immunity: Levels of secretory IgA and natural antibodies in saliva. *Pediatr. Res.* **14,** 1111–1114.

Buts, J.-P., Vaerman, J.-P., and Lescoat, G. (1992). Ontogeny of the receptor for polymeric immunoglobulins in rat hepatocytes. *Gastroenterology* **102,** 949–955.

Casanova, J. E., Breitfeld, P. P., Ross, A. S., and Mostov, K. E. (1990). Phosphorylation of the polymeric immunoglobulin receptor required for its efficient transcytosis. *Science* **248,** 742–745.

Chintalacharuvu, K. R., Tavaill, A. S., Louis, L. N., Vaerman, J.-P., Lamm, M. E., and Kaetzel, C. S. (1992). Disulfide bond formation between dimeric immunoglobulin A and the polymeric immunoglobulin receptor during hepatic transcytosis. *Hepatology,* in press.

Colombel, J. F., Rambaud, J. C., Vaerman, J. P., Galian, A., Delacroix, D. L., Nemeth, J., Duprey, F., Halphen, M., Godeau, P., and Dive, C. (1988). Massive plasma cell infiltration of the digestive tract. Secretory component as the rate-limiting factor of immunoglobulin secretion in external fluids. *Gastroenterology* **95,** 1106–1113.

Conley, M. E., and Delacroix, D. L. (1987). Intravascular and mucosal immunoglobulin A: Two separate but related systems of immune defense? *Ann. Int. Med.* **106,** 892–899.

Courtoy, P. J., Limet, J. N., Quintart, J., Schneider, Y. J., Vaerman, J.-P., and Baudhuin, P. (1983). Transfer of IgA into rat bile: Ultrastructural demonstration. *Ann. N.Y. Acad. Sci.* **409,** 799–802.

Crago, S. S., Kulhavy, R., Prince, S. J., and Mestecky, J. (1978). Secretory component on epithelial cells is a surface receptor for polymeric immunoglobulins. *J. Exp. Med.* **147,** 1832–1837.

Daniels, C. K., Schmucker, D. L., and Jones, A. L. (1989). Hepatic asialoglycoprotein receptor-mediated binding of human polymeric immunoglobulin A. *Hepatology* **9,** 229–234.

Davidson, M. K., Le Beau, M. M., Eddy, R. L., Shows, T. B., DiPietro, L. A., Kingzette, M., and Hanly, W. C. (1988). Genetic mapping of the human polymeric immunoglobulin receptor gene to chromosome region 1q31 → q41. *Cytogenet. Cell Genet.* **48,** 107–111.

Davies, A. (1922). An investigation into the serological properties of dysentery stools. *Lancet* **ii,** 1009–1012.

Deitcher, D. L., and Mostov, K. E. (1986). Alternate splicing of rabbit polymeric immunoglobulin receptor. *Mol. Cell. Biol.* **6,** 2712–2715.

Delacroix, D. L., Denef, A. M., Acosta, G. A., Montgomery, P. C., and Vaerman, J.-P. (1982). Immunoglobulins in rabbit hepatic bile: Selective secretion of IgA and IgM and active plasma-to-bile transfer of polymeric IgA. *Scand. J. Immunol.* **16,** 343–350.

Delacroix, D. L., Furtado-Barreira, G., Rahier, J., Dive, C., and Vaerman, J.-P. (1984). Immunohistochemical localization of secretory component in the liver of guinea pigs and dogs versus rats, rabbits, and mice. *Scand. J. Immunol.* **19,** 425–434.

Dooley, J. S., Potter, B. J., Thomas, H. C., and Sherlock, S. (1982). A comparative study of the biliary secretion of human dimeric and monomeric IgA in the rat and in man. *Hepatology* **2,** 323–327.

Eiffert, H., Quentin, E., Decker, J., Hillemeir, S., Hufschmidt, M., Klingmüller, D., Weber, M. H., and Hilschmann, N. (1984). Die Primärstruktur der menschlichen freien Sekretkomponente und die Anordnung der Disulfidbrücken. *Hoppe-Seyler's Z. Physiol. Chem.* **365,** 1489–1495.

Emancipator, S. N., and Lamm, M. E. (1989). IgA nephropathy: Overproduction or decreased clearance of immune complexes? *Lab. Invest.* **61,** 365–367.

Fisher, M. M., Nagy, B., Bazin, H., and Underdown, B. J. (1979). Biliary transport of IgA: Role of secretory component. *Proc. Natl. Acad. Sci. U.S.A.* **76,** 2008–2012.

Foss-Bowman, C., Jones, A., Dejbakhsh, S., and Goldman, I. S. (1983). Immunofluorescent and immunocytochemical localization of secretory component and immunoglobulins in human livers. *Ann. N.Y. Acad. Sci.* **409,** 822–823.

Frutiger, S., Hughes, G. J., Hanly, W. C., Kingzette, M., and Jaton, J. C. (1986). The amino-terminal domain of rabbit secretory component is responsible for noncovalent binding to immunoglobulin A dimers. *J. Biol. Chem.* **261,** 16673–16681.

Gebhart, R., and Robenek, H. (1987). Ligand-dependent redistribution of the IgA receptor on cultured rat hepatocytes and its disturbance by cytochalasin. *Br. J. Histochem.* **35,** 301–309.

Geneste, C., Mangalo, R., Iscaki, S., and Pillot, J. (1986a). Human secretory component. IV. Antigenic regions involved in *in vitro* binding to dimeric IgA. *Immunol. Lett.* **13,** 121–126.

Geneste, C., Iscaki, S., Mangalo, R., and Pillot, J. (1986b). Both Fcα domains of human IgA are involved in *in vitro* interaction between secretory component and dimeric IgA. *Immunol. Lett.* **13,** 221–226.

Geuze, H., Slot, J. W., Strous, G. J. A. M., Peppard, J., von Figura, K., Hasilik, A., and Schwartz, A. L. (1984). Intracellular receptor sorting during endocytosis: Comparative immunoelectron microscopy of multiple receptors in rat liver. *Cell* **37,** 195–204.

Harmatz, P. R., Kleinman, R. E., Bunnell, B. W., Bloch, K. J., and Walker, W. A. (1982). Hepatobiliary clearance of IgA immune complexes formed in the circulation. *Hepatology* **2,** 328–333.

Hayashi, Y., Kurashima, C., Takemura, T., and Hirokawa, K. (1989). Ontogenic development of the secretory immune system in human fetal salivary glands. *Pathol. Immunopathol. Res.* **8,** 314–320.

Hoppe, C. A., Connolly, T. P., and Hubbard, A. L. (1985). Transcellular transport of polymeric IgA in the rat hepatocyte: Biochemical and morphological characterization of the transport pathway. *J. Cell Biol.* **101,** 2113–2123.

Hsu, S. M., and Hsu, P. L. (1980). Demonstration of IgA and secretory component in human hepatocytes. *Gut* **21,** 985–989.

Jackson, G. D. F., Lemaitre-Coelho, I., and Vaerman, J.-P. (1977). Transfer of MOPC-315 IgA to secretions in MOPC-315 tumour-bearing and normal BALB/c mice. *Protides Biol. Fluids* **25,** 919–922.

Jackson, G. D. F., Lemaitre-Coelho, I., Vaerman, J.-P., Bazin, H., and Beckers, A. (1978). Rapid disappearance from serum of intravenously injected rat myeloma IgA and its secretion into bile. *Eur. J. Immunol.* **8,** 123–126.

Kaetzel, C. S., Robinson, J. K., Chintalacharuvu, K. R., Vaerman, J.-P., and Lamm, M. E. (1991). The polymeric immunoglobulin receptor (secretory component) mediates transport of immune complexes across epithelial cells: A local defense function for IgA. *Proc. Natl. Acad. Sci. U.S.A.* **88,** 8796–8800.

Kaetzel C. S., Robinson, J. K., Lamm, M. E., The polymeric immunoglobulin receptor mediates epithelial transcytosis of monomeric IgA and IgG cross-linked through multivalent antigen to polymeric IgA: A role for monomeric antibodies in the mucosal immune system, submitted for publication.

Kraehenbuhl, J. P., Racine, L., and Galardy, R. E. (1975). Localization of secretory IgA, secretory component, and α chain in the mammary gland of lactating rabbits by immunoelectron microscopy. *Ann. N.Y. Acad. Sci.* **254,** 190–202.

Krajči, P., Solberg, R., Sandberg, M., Øyen, O., Jahnsen, T., and Brandtzaeg, P. (1989). Molecular cloning of the human transmembrane secretory component (poly-Ig receptor) and its mRNA expression in human tissues. *Biochem. Biophys. Res. Commun.* **158,** 783–789.

Krajči, P., Grzeschik, K. H., Geurts van Kessel, A. H. M., Olaisen, B., and Brandtzaeg, P. (1991). The human transmembrane secretory component (poly-Ig receptor): Molecular cloning, restriction fragment length polymorphism and chromosomal sublocalization. *Hum. Genet.* **87,** 642–648.

Krajči, P., Kvale, D., Taskén, K., and Brandtzaeg, P. (1992a). Molecular cloning and exon-intron mapping of the gene encoding human transmembrane secretory component (the poly-Ig receptor). *Eur. J. Immunol* **22,** 2309–2315.

Krajči, P., Gedde-Dahl, T., Høyheim, B., Rogde, S., Olaisen, B., and Brandtzaeg, P. (1992b). The gene encoding human transmembrane secretory component (locus PIGR) is linked to D1S58 on chromosome 1. *Hum. Genet.* **90,** 215–219.

Krajči, P., Taskén, K., Kvale, D., and Brandtzaeg, P. (1993). Interferon-γ stimulation of messenger RNA for human secretory component (poly-Ig receptor) depends on continuous intermediate protein synthesis. *Scand. J. Immunol.* **37,** 251–256.

Kühn, L. C., and Kraehenbuhl, J. P. (1979). Role of secretory component, a secreted glycoprotein, in the specific uptake of IgA dimer by epithelial cells. *J. Biol. Chem.* **254,** 11072–11081.

Kühn, L. C., Kocher, H. P., Hanly, W. C., Cook, L., Jaton, J.-C., and Kraehenbuhl, F.-P. (1983). Structural and genetic heterogenity of the receptor mediating translocation of immunoglobulin A dimer antibodies across epithelia in the rabbit. *J. Biol. Chem.* **258,** 6653–6659.

Kulseth, M.-A., Krajči, P., Myklebost, O., and Rogne, S. (1993). Cloning and characterization of two forms of bovine polymeric immunoglobulin receptor. *DNA and Cell Biol*, in Press.

Kvale, D., and Brandtzaeg, P. (1992). Butyrate enhances basal and cytokine-induced expression of HLA molecules, secretory component (SC), and ICAM-1 in intestinal epithelial cell lines. 7th International Congress of Mucosal Immunology, Prague. (Abstract)

Kvale, D., Løvhaug, D., Sollid, L. M., and Brandtzaeg, P. (1988a). Tumour necrosis factor-α upregulates expression of secretory component, the epithelial receptor for polymeric Ig. *J. Immunol.* **140,** 3086–3089.

Kvale, D., Brandtzaeg, P., and Løvhaug, D. (1988b). Up-regulation of the expression of secretory component and HLA molecules in a human colonic cell line by tumour necrosis factor-α and gamma interferon. *Scand. J. Immunol.* **28,** 351–357.

Larkin, J. M., and Palade, G. E. (1991). Transcytotic vesicular carriers for polymeric IgA receptors accumulate in rat hepatocytes after bile duct ligation. *J. Cell Sci.* **98,** 205–216.

Larkin, J. M., Sztul, E. S., and Palade, G. E. (1986). Phosphorylation of the rat hepatic polymeric IgA receptor. *Proc. Natl. Acad. Sci. U.S.A.* **83,** 4759–4763.

Limet, J., Quintart, J., Schneider, Y., and Courtoy, P. J. (1985).

Receptor-mediated endocytosis of polymeric IgA and galactosylated serum albumin in rat liver: Evidence for intracellular ligand sorting and identification of distinct endosomal compartments. *Eur. J. Biochem.* **146,** 539–548.

Mazanec, M. B., Kaetzel, C. S., Lamm, M. E., Fletcher, D., and Nedrud, J. G. (1992). Intracellular neutralization of virus by immunoglobulin A antibodies. *Proc. Natl. Acad. Sci. U.S.A.* **89,** 6901–6905.

McGee, D. W., Aicher, W. K., Eldridge, J. H., Peppard, J. V., Mestecky, J., and McGhee, J. R. (1991). Transforming growth factor-β enhances secretory component and major histocompatibility complex class I antigen expression on rat IEC-6 intestinal epithelial cells. *Cytokine* **3,** 543–550.

McGuire, E. J., Kerlin, R., Cebra, J. J., and Roth, S. (1989). A human milk galactosyl-transferase is specific for secreted, but not plasma, IgA. *J. Immunol.* **143,** 2933–2938.

Mestecky, J., and McGhee, J. R. (1987). Immunoglobulin A (IgA): Molecular and cellular interactions involved in IgA biosynthesis and immune response. *Adv. Immunol.* **40,** 153–245.

Moldoveanu, Z., Moro, I., Radl, J., Thorpe, S. R., Komiyama, K., and Mestecky, J. (1990). Site of catabolism of autologous and heterologous IgA in non-human primates. *Scand. J. Immunol.* **32,** 577–583.

Mostov, K. E., and Blobel, G. (1982). A transmembrane precursor of secretory component. The receptor for transcellular transport of polymeric immunoglobulins. *J. Biol. Chem.* **257,** 11816–11821.

Mostov, K. E., Kraehenbuhl, J. P., and Blobel, G. (1980). Receptor-mediated transcellular transport of immunoglobulin: Synthesis of secretory component as multiple and larger transmembrane forms. *Proc. Natl. Acad. Sci. U.S.A.* **77,** 7257–7261.

Mostov, K. E., Friedlander, M., and Blobel, G. (1984). The receptor for transepithelial transport of IgA and IgM contains multiple immunoglobulin-like domains. *Nature (London)* **308,** 37–43.

Mullock, B. M., Hinton, R. H., Dobrota, M., Peppard, J., and Orlans, E. (1979). Endocytic vesicles in liver carry polymeric IgA from serum to bile. *Biochim. Biophys. Acta* **587,** 381–391.

Mullock, B. M., Jones, R. S., and Hinton, R. H. (1980). Movement of endocytic shuttle vesicles from the sinusoidal to the bile canalicular face of hepatocytes does not depend on occupation of receptor sites. *FEBS Lett.* **113,** 201–205.

Musil, L. S., and Baenziger, J. U. (1988). Proteolytic processing of rat liver membrane secretory component. Cleavage activity is localized to bile canalicular membranes. *J. Biol. Chem.* **263,** 15799–15808.

Nagura, H., Nakane, P. K., and Brown, W. R. (1980). Secretory component in immunoglobulin deficiency: An immunoelectron microscopic study of intestinal epithelium. *Scand. J. Immunol.* **12,** 359–363.

Nagura, H., Smith, P. D., Nakane, P. K., and Brown, W. R. (1981). IgA in human bile and liver. *J. Immunol.* **126,** 587–595.

Nagura, H., Tsutsumi, Y., Hasegawa, H., Watanabe, K., Nakane, P. K. and Brown, W. R. (1983). IgA plasma cells in biliary mucosa: A likely source of locally synthesized IgA in human hepatic bile. *Clin. Exp. Immunol.* **54,** 671–680.

Ogra, S. S., Ogra, P. L., Lippes, J., and Tomasi, T. B. (1972). Immunohistologic localization of immunoglobulins, secretory component, and lactoferrin in the developing human fetus. *Proc. Soc. Exp. Biol. Med.* **139,** 570–572.

Okamoto, C. T., Shia S-P., Bird, C., Mostov, K. E., Roth, M. G. (1992). The cytoplasmic domain of the polymeric immunoglobulin receptor contains two internalization signals that are distinct from its basolateral sorting signal. *J. Biol. Chem.* **267,** 9925–9932.

Orlans, E., Peppard, J., Fry, J. F., Hinton, R. H., and Mullock, B. M. (1979). Secretory component as the receptor for polymeric IgA on rat hepatocytes. *J. Exp. Med.* **150,** 1577–1581.

Perez, J. H., Branch, W. J., Smith, L., Mullock, B. M., and Luzio, J. P. (1988). Investigation of endosomal compartments involved in endocytosis and transcytosis of polymeric immunoglobulin A by subcellular fractionation of perfused isolated rat liver. *Biochem. J.* **251,** 763–770.

Perez, J. H., Wight, D. G. D., Wyatt, J. I., Van Schaik, M., Mullock, B. M., and Luzio, J. P. (1989). The polymeric immunoglobulin A receptor is present on hepatocytes in human liver. *Immunology* **68,** 474–478.

Phillips, J. O., Russell, M. W., Brown, T. A., and Mestecky, J. (1984). Selective hepatobiliary transport of human polymeric IgA in mice. *Mol. Immunol.* **21,** 907–914.

Phillips, J. O., Everson, M. P., Moldoveanu, Z., Lue, C., and Mestecky, J. (1990). Synergistic effect of IL-4 and IFN-γ on the expression of polymeric Ig receptor (secretory component) and IgA binding by human epithelial cells. *J. Immunol.* **145,** 1740–1744.

Piskurich, J. F., France, J. A., Tamer, C. M., Willmer, C. A., Kaetzel, C. S., and Kaetzel, D. M. (1993). Interferon-γ induces polymeric immunoglobulin receptor mRNA in human intestinal epithelial cells by a protein synthesis dependent mechanism. *Mol. Immunol.* **30,** 413–421.

Poger, M. E., and Lamm, M. E. (1974). Localization of free and bound secretory component in human intestinal epithelial cells. A model for the assembly of secretory IgA. *J. Exp. Med.* **139,** 629–642.

Pumphrey, R. S. H. (1986). Computer models of the human immunoglobulins. Binding sites and molecular interactions. *Immunol. Today* **7,** 206–211.

Renston, R. H., Jones, A. L., Christiansen, W. D., Hradek, G. T., and Underdown, B. J. (1980). Evidence for a vesicular transport mechanism in hepatocytes for biliary secretion of immunoglobulin A. *Science* **208,** 1276–1278.

Rifai, A., and Mannik, M. (1984). Clearance of circulating IgA immune complexes is mediated by a specific receptor on Kupffer cells in mice. *J. Exp. Med.* **160,** 125–137.

Rifai, A., Schena, F. P., Montinaro, V., Mele, M., D'Addabbo, A., Nitti, L., and Pezzullo, J. C. (1989). Clearance kinetics and fate of macromolecular IgA in patients with IgA nephropathy. *Lab. Invest.* **61,** 381–388.

Roccatello, D., Picciotto, G., Ropolo, R., Coppo, R., Quattrocchio, G., Cacace, G., Molino, A., Amoroso, A., Baccega, M., Isidoro, C., Cardosi, R., Sena, L. M., and Piccoli, G. (1992). Kinetics and fate of IgA–IgG aggregates as a model of naturally occurring immune complexes in IgA nephropathy. *Lab. Invest.* **66,** 86–95.

Rognum, T. O., Brandtzaeg, P., Elgjo, K., and Fausa, O. (1987). Heterogeneous epithelial expression of class II (HLA-DR) determinants and secretory component related to dysplasia in ulcerative colitis. *Br. J. Cancer* **56,** 419–424.

Russell, M. W., Brown, T. A., and Mestecky, J. (1981). Role of serum IgA. Hepatobiliary transport of circulating antigen. *J. Exp. Med.* **153,** 968–976.

Sancho, J., Gonzalez, E., and Egido, J. (1986). The importance of the Fc receptors for IgA in the recognition of IgA by mouse liver cells: Its comparison with carbohydrate and secretory component receptors. *Immunology* **57,** 37–42.

Schaerer, E., Verrey, F., Racine, L., Tallichet, C., Reinhardt, M., and Kraehenbuhl, J.-P. (1990). Polarized transport of the polymeric immunoglobulin receptor in transfected rabbit mammary epithelial cells. *J. Cell. Biol.* **110,** 987–998.

Schiff, J. M., Fisher, M. M., and Underdown, B. J. (1984). Receptor-mediated biliary transport of immunoglobulin A and asialoglycoprotein: Sorting and missorting of ligands revealed by two radiolabeling methods. *J. Cell Biol.* **98,** 79–89.

Schiff, J. M., Fisher, M. M., and Underdown, B. J. (1986a). Secretory component as the mucosal transport receptor: Separation of physicochemically analogous human IgA fractions with different receptor-binding capacities. *Mol. Immunol.* **23,** 45–56.

Schiff, J. M., Fisher, M. M., Jones, A. L., and Underdown, B. J. (1986b). Human IgA as a heterovalent ligand: Switching from the asialoglycoprotein receptor to secretory component during transport across the rat hepatocyte. *J. Cell Biol.* **102,** 920–931.

Sixbey, J. W., and Yao, Q.-Y. (1992). Immunoglobulin A-induced shift of Epstein–Barr virus tissue tropism. *Science* **255,** 1578–1580.

Socken, D. J., Simms, E. S., Nagy, B. R., Fisher, M. M., and Underdown, B. J. (1981). Secretory component-dependent hepatic transport of IgA antibody-antigen complexes. *J. Immunol.* **127,** 316–319.

Solari, R., and Kraehenbuhl, J.-P. (1984). Biosynthesis of the IgA antibody receptor: A model for the transepithelial sorting of a membrane glycoprotein. *Cell* **36,** 61–71.

Solari, R., Racine, L., Tallichet, C., and Kraehenbuhl, J.-P. (1986). Distribution and processing of the polymeric immunoglobulin receptor in the rat hepatocyte: Morphological and biochemical characterization of subcellular fractions. *J. Histochem. Cytochem.* **34,** 17–23.

Solari, R., Schaerer, E., Tallichet, C., Braiterman, L. T., Hubbard, A. L., and Kraehenbuhl, J.-P. (1989). Cellular location of the cleavage event of the polymeric immunoglobulin receptor and fate of its anchoring domain in the rat hepatocyte. *Biochem. J.* **257,** 759–768.

Sollid, L. M., Kvale, D., Brandtzaeg, P., Markussen, G., and Thorsby, E. (1987). Interferon-gamma enhances expression of secretory component, the epithelial receptor for polymeric immunoglobulins. *J. Immunol.* **138,** 4304–4306.

Stockert, R. J., Kressner, M. S., Collins, J. C., Sternlieb, I., and Morell, A. G. (1982). IgA interaction with the asialoglycoprotein receptor. *Proc. Natl. Acad. Sci. U.S.A.* **79,** 6229–6231.

Sztul, E. S., Howell, K. E., and Palade, G. E. (1985). Biogenesis of the polymeric IgA receptor in rat hepatocytes. I. Kinetic studies of its intracellular forms. *J. Cell Biol.* **100,** 1248–1254.

Sztul, E., Kaplin, A., Saucan, L., and Palade, G. (1991). Protein traffic between distinct plasma membrane domains: Isolation and characterization of vesicular carriers involved in transcytosis. *Cell* **64,** 81–89.

Sullivan, D. A., and Allansmith, M. R. (1987). Hormonal influence on the secretory immune system of the eye: Endocrine interactions in the control of IgA and secretory component levels in tears of rats. *Immunology* **60,** 337–343.

Sullivan, D. A., and Wira, C. R. (1983). Variations of free secretory component levels in mucosal secretions of the rat. *J. Immunol.* **130,** 1330–1335.

Sullivan, D. A., Underdown, B. J., and Wira, C. R. (1983). Steroid hormone regulation of free secretory component in the rat uterus. *Immunology* **49,** 379–386.

Takahashi, I., Nakane, P. K., and Brown, W. R. (1982). Ultrastructural events in the translocation of polymeric IgA by rat hepatocytes. *J. Immunol.* **128,** 1181–1187.

Thrane, P., Rognum, T. O., and Brandtzaeg, P. (1990). Increased immune response in upper respiratory and digestive tracts in SIDS. *Lancet* **335,** 229–230.

Thrane, P. S., Rognum, T. O., and Brandtzaeg, P. (1991). Ontogenesis of the secretory immune system and innate defence factors in human parotid glands. *Clin. Exp. Immunol.* **86,** 342–348.

Tolleshaug, H., Brandtzaeg, P., and Holte, K. (1981). Quantitative study of the uptake of IgA by isolated rat hepatocytes. *Scand. J. Immunol.* **13,** 47–56.

Tomana, M., Phillips, J. O., Kulhavy, R., and Mestecky, J. (1985). Carbohydrate-mediated clearance of secretory IgA from the circulation. *Mol. Immunol.* **22,** 887–892.

Tomana, M., Kulhavy, R., and Mestecky, J. (1988). Receptor-mediated binding and uptake of immunoglobulin A by human liver. *Gastroenterology* **94,** 762–770.

Tomana, M., Zikan, J., and Mestecky, J. (1991). Galactosyltransferase as a receptor for immunoglobulins on epithelial cells and hepatocytes. *In* "Frontiers of Mucosal Immunology" (M. Tsuchiya, H. Nagura, T. Hibi, and I. Moro, eds.), Vol. 1, pp. 239–242. Elsevier Science Publishers, Amsterdam.

Tomasi, T. B., Tan, E. M., Solomon, A., and Prendergast, R. A. (1965). Characteristics of an immune system common to certain external secretions. *J. Exp. Med.* **121,** 101–124.

Valnes, K., Brandtzaeg, P., Elgjo, K., and Stave, R. (1984). Specific and nonspecific humoral defense factors in the epithelium of normal and inflamed gastric mucosa. Immunohistochemical localization of immunoglobulins, secretory component, lysozyme, and lactoferrin. *Gastroenterology* **86,** 402–412.

Williams, A. F., and Barclay, A. N. (1988). The immunoglobulin superfamily—Domains for cell surface recognition. *Ann. Rev. Immunol.* **6,** 381–405.

Williams, B. R. G. (1991). Transcriptional regulation of interferon-stimulated genes. *Eur. J. Biochem.* **200,** 1–11.

Wira, C. R., and Colby, E. (1985). Regulation of secretory component by glucocorticoids in primary cultures of rat hepatocytes. *J. Immunol.* **134,** 1744–1748.

Wira, C. R., and Rossoll, R. M. (1991). Glucocorticoid regulation of the humoral immune system. Dexamethasone stimulation of secretory component in serum, saliva, and bile. *Endocrinology* **128 (2),** 835–842.

Wira, C. R., and Sullivan, D. A. (1985). Estradiol and progesterone regulation of IgA, IgG and secretory component in cervico-vaginal secretions of rat. *Biol. Reprod.* **32,** 90–95.

Wira, C. R., Bodwell, J. E., and Prabhala, R. H. (1991). *In vivo* response of secretory component in the rat uterus to antigen, IFN-γ, and estradiol. *J. Immunol.* **146,** 1893–1899.

Zikán, J., Novotny, J., Trapane, T. L., Koshland, M. E., Urry, D. W., Bennett, J. C., and Mestecky, J. (1985). Secondary structure of the immunoglobulin J chain. *Proc. Natl. Acad. Sci. U.S.A.* **82,** 5905–5909.

11

Function of Mucosal Immunoglobulins

Mogens Kilian · Michael W. Russell

I. INTRODUCTION

A. Immunoglobulin Isotypes at Mucosal Surfaces

Although the predominant isotype of Ig-secreting cells in most human secretory tissues is IgA, significant but variable numbers of IgM, IgG, and IgD immunocytes also occur (Brandtzaeg *et al.*, 1986b; see Chapter 21). Among the immunoglobulin isotypes present on mucosal surfaces (Table I) as a result of active secretion or of transudation, secretory IgA (SIgA) is particularly stable and well suited to function in the enzymatically hostile environment that prevails at these locations. This stability is ascribed largely to the secretory component (SC) which renders the SIgA molecule less susceptible to attack by metabolic and microbial enzymes. In contrast to SIgM, the complex of polymeric IgA (pIgA) and SC is stabilized by covalent linkages (see Chapter 7), which may contribute to its resistance to proteolytic enzymes. Moreover, SIgA has been shown to bind trypsin and chymotrypsin in an antibody-independent manner that inactivates the enzymes (Shim *et al.*, 1969).

The mucosal environment in which SIgA operates is very different from the circulation and tissues in which other Igs, including plasma IgA, operate, both physicochemically and in terms of the presence or absence of ancillary factors (notably the complement system, phagocytic or other cells, and nonspecific defense factors) and of other macromolecules. The host defense problems in the two situations are completely different: mucosal surfaces are not normally sterile but are colonized by a commensal flora that must be held in check without compromising the mucosal barrier, whereas the internal presence of a microorganism indicates a potentially life-threatening invasion. SIgA and the mucosal immune system therefore can be considered as having evolved to maintain a balance with the normal microbial flora. An important aspect of this balancing act may be the role of maternal milk SIgA antibodies in promoting the establishment of an appropriate intestinal microflora in the neonate (see Chapter 52).

B. Protective Potential of SIgA Antibodies

Numerous studies in animal models and in humans have provided convincing evidence that protection against a variety of viral and bacterial mucosal pathogens can be obtained by oral or intranasal immunization (see Chapter 31). Although protection generally is correlated with levels of IgA antibodies in relevant secretions, the participation of other classes of antibody or of antiviral T cells cannot be excluded, but the protective significance and superiority of SIgA antibodies has been demonstrated in several systems. Monoclonal IgA antibodies (without SC) to Sendai virus hemagglutinin–neuraminidase passively administered to the mouse respiratory tract confer significant protection against the virus (Mazanec *et al.*, 1987). Intranasal administration of affinity-purified human SIgA antibody to M protein protects mice against nasal inoculation with group A streptococci, whereas locally applied serum opsonizing antibodies are not protective (Bessen and Fischetti, 1988). In an elegant model of mucosal immunity (Winner *et al.*, 1991), pIgA antibody to *Vibrio cholerae* lipopolysaccharide (LPS), secreted into the circulation by "backpack" tumors of mouse hybridoma cells and transported into intestinal secretions, provides serotype-specific protection against oral challenge with *V. cholerae*. In a conceptually similar model (Renegar and Small, 1991), intravenously administered monoclonal pIgA against influenza virus hemagglutinin is transported into nasal secretions of mice and protects against nasal challenge, whereas monoclonal monomeric IgA (mIgA) or IgG antibodies do not.

II. BIOLOGICAL PROPERTIES OF IgA

As for IgG and IgM antibodies, although some biological properties of IgA antibodies may be the simple consequence of antigen binding, most depend on structures within the Fc region and, in the case of SIgA, on the attached SC and on the interactions of these structures with other molecules (Kilian *et al.*, 1988). Among the unusual structural features of human IgA is the presence of O-linked oligosaccharides in the hinge region of IgA subclass 1 (see Chapter 7). Whereas the biological significance of these sugar moieties is not fully understood, they have been implicated in carbohydrate-dependent interactions of IgA with cellular receptors (Tomana *et al.*, 1988) and may impart resistance to many proteolytic enzymes. Further, such oligosaccharides, which are found more typically in mucins, probably confer a stiff and extended conformation on the peptide chain (Jentoft, 1990), limiting the segmental flexibility of IgA1 antibodies and restricting their ability to bind to adjacent epitopes. IgA2 antibody often

Table I Isotypes and Functions of Mucosal Immunoglobulins

Isotype	Occurrence	Functions
SIgA	Major form of Ig in most secretions of humans and many other mammals	Noninflammatory mucosal protection[a]
(S)IgM	Second most abundant Ig in most secretions; SIgM compensates for lack of SIgA in IgA deficiency	Probably similar to plasma IgM or SIgA; activates complement
IgG	Normally minor component, but relatively abundant in nasal and respiratory tract secretions; probably transudes from plasma; increased in pathological, especially inflammatory, conditions	Neutralization; potentially inflammatory; activates complement and phagocytes
IgA (plasma type)	Found in human bile and possibly other secretions; transudes from plasma, or transported by alternative secretion mechanisms	Possibly similar to SIgA; poor complement activation, or inhibitory[a]
IgD	Significant minor component of nasal secretions, milk	Unknown
IgE	Normally insignificant; elevated in atopic allergies and helminthic infections	Adverse hypersensitivity states (atopy); parasite expulsion

[a] See test for additional discussion.

is directed against polysaccharide antigens, which typically have repeating epitopes, but whether its hinge region (although shorter but with five consecutive proline residues) allows greater flexibility for divalent binding to adjacent epitopes is not known.

A. Molecular Mechanisms of Protection by SIgA at Mucosal Surfaces

1. Inhibition of Adherence: Agglutination

Concomitant with the recognition that adherence of a microorganism to a mucosal surface is a critical first step in colonization (see Chapter 6) has been the concept that inhibition of adherence by antibodies is a major protective function of mucosal immunity (Abraham and Beachey, 1985). Although the molecular nature of the adhesin–receptor interactions may not have been well defined, SIgA antibodies to microbial surfaces have been demonstrated to inhibit adherence to pharyngeal, intestinal, and genitourinary tract epithelia as well as to tooth surfaces (Williams and Gibbons, 1972; Tramont, 1977; Svanborg-Edén and Svennerholm, 1978; Hajishengallis *et al.*, 1992).

Whereas any antibody may be capable of inhibiting adherence, SIgA antibodies have advantageous properties that are not shared by other isotypes because of the hydrophilic and negatively charged Fc · SC part of the molecule (Kilian *et al.*, 1988; see Chapter 7). In contrast IgG, with considerably fewer carbohydrate residues, is more hydrophobic and less charged in the Fc region and may substitute the specific adhesin–receptor binding with other (less specific) hydrophobic interactions. Thus, SIgA appears to surround a microbe with a hydrophilic shell that repels attachment to a mucosal surface. Presumably SIgM, which compensates for SIgA in many IgA-deficient subjects, can exert a similar effect, but specific evidence of this ability is not available. Although pIgA and SIgA antibodies are particularly adept at agglutinating microorganisms, mIgA antibodies agglutinate and precipitate poorly (Heremans, 1974), possibly because their hydrophilic Fc (or Fc_2 · SC) regions are less able to form Fc–Fc interactions. However, information on the composition and nature of IgA antibody–antigen complexes and precipitates involving the different molecular forms of IgA has not been obtained to test this assumption.

It is speculated that SIgA may be able to form particular associations with mucins, possibly through interactions between mucin and the mucin-like hinge region of IgA1, or even by forming disulfide bonds (Clamp, 1977). Since the binding of SIgA to bacteria renders them more "mucophilic" (Magnusson and Stjernström, 1982), this mucin affinity would help entrap the microbes within the mucus layer. High molecular weight fractions of saliva contain mucins and small amounts of SIgA, suggesting an interaction between them; binding of SIgA to the salivary mucin MG2 has been reported (Biesbrock *et al.*, 1991). An interaction between the Fc_2 · SC region of SIgA and mucus also is implied by the finding that spermatozoa coated with SIgA show impaired penetration of cervical mucus, but that treatment of the coated spermatozoa with IgA protease restores this ability (Bronson *et al.*, 1987).

In addition to specific antibody-mediated inhibition of adherence, human IgA and especially IgA2, which can agglutinate *Escherichia coli* through its type 1 (mannose-dependent) pili by means of mannose-rich glycan chains, also may act in this way to inhibit type 1 pilus-dependent adherence of *E. coli* to epithelial cells (Wold *et al.*, 1990).

2. Virus Neutralization

A considerable body of evidence shows that SIgA antibodies to various viruses can neutralize them effectively and, although inhibition of viral binding to cellular receptors seems plausible, neutralization may occur by other mechanisms, depending on the epitope specificity, isotype, and concentration of antibody and the virus and cells involved (reviewed by Childers *et al.*, 1989). High concentrations of SIgA or IgM antibodies to influenza virus hemagglutinin inhibit cellular attachment, whereas IgG or lower concentrations of pIgA antibodies that permit attachment may inhibit internalization or intracellular replication (Armstrong and Dimmock, 1992). The isotype of antiviral antibody may be especially important because one mechanism of cellular uptake can be replaced by another. Human antibodies of any isotype to the surface gp340 of Epstein–Barr virus neutralize its infectivity for B cells (via complement receptor CR2), but pIgA antibodies promote infection of SC-expressing HT-29 colonic carcinoma cells, thereby changing the tissue tropism of the virus (Sixbey and Yao, 1992). The general extent of this phenomenon is unknown although potentially important, particularly in connection with HIV infection in which antibodies to gp160 may inhibit CD4-mediated uptake by T cells but promote uptake by other cells with opsonic receptors.

One publication (Mazanec *et al.*, 1992) proposes a novel mechanism of viral neutralization mediated by pIgA antibodies during SC-mediated transit through epithelial cells. This mechanism was demonstrated in an elegant *in vitro* system using Sendai virus-infected Madin–Darby canine kidney (MDCK) cells expressing the transfected SC gene. The pIgA-bearing transcytotic vesicles are suggested to interact with secretory vesicles in which the replicated virus is assembled and thereby inhibit this process. Sendai virus, like other paramyxoviruses (e.g., measles, mumps, parainfluenza, and respiratory syncytial viruses), can induce membrane fusion, which may be instrumental in the interaction of the two types of vesicle. Determining the extent to which such intracellular viral neutralization occurs *in vivo* will be important since this hypothesis implies that pIgA antibody can promote recovery from viral infections of mucosae, as well as provide initial protection against them.

3. Neutralization of Enzymes and Toxins

Antibody-mediated inhibition of enzyme or toxin activity has been demonstrated in several systems. If this effect is simply caused by steric blocking of binding to the substrate or target molecule (or cell), or by a conformational change in the antigen molecule that affects its biological function, it may be independent of the Fc region or of antibody isotype. Specific examples of SIgA antibodies that neutralize enzymes or toxins include intestinal antibodies to cholera and related heat-labile enterotoxins (Majumdar and Ghose, 1981; Lycke *et al.*, 1987); salivary antibodies to the glucosyltransferases of *Streptococcus mutans* and *Streptococcus sobrinus*, which synthesize adherent glucans from sucrose and enable these cariogenic bacteria to adhere to tooth surfaces (Smith *et al.*, 1985); and antibodies that neutralize IgA proteases (see Section III,A).

4. Immune Exclusion and Inhibition of Antigen Absorption

The intestinal uptake of antigenically intact food substances (see Chapter 4) is diminished by SIgA antibodies arising from prior enteric exposure to them (Walker *et al.*, 1972). Absorption of antigen instilled into the airway is inhibited by the simultaneous administration of IgA antibody (Stokes *et al.*, 1975). The importance of immune exclusion for the protection of the host against excessive antigenic challenge from environmental macromolecules is suggested by the findings that IgA-deficient subjects show increased absorption of food antigens and formation of circulating immune complexes (Cunningham-Rundles *et al.*, 1978), as well as statistically increased susceptibility to atopic allergies or autoimmune disease.

In contrast, enteric SIgA antibodies have been suggested to promote uptake of antigen through the M cells of Peyer's patches and, consequently, enhance the mucosal immune response to that antigen (Weltzin *et al.*, 1989). Further elaboration of the mechanism involved, especially the receptor, seems necessary to substantiate this intriguing possibility.

5. Interaction with Nonspecific Antibacterial Factors

The secretions of most mucosal surfaces contain an array of nonspecific defense systems that are highly effective in killing or inhibiting a broad range of bacteria and fungi (see Chapter 5). Because SIgA is able to interact with some of the protein components of these systems, ample opportunity exists for synergism in which SIgA antibodies might introduce an element of specificity. However, few such interactions have been described in molecular detail.

a. Lactoferrin. The bacteriostatic synergy of lactoferrin and SIgA antibodies (Stephens *et al.*, 1980) may be the result of antibody-mediated interference with alternative channels of iron uptake possessed by many mucosal organisms. Lactoferrin is a frequent contaminant of SIgA purified from secretions, but whether the implied interaction or formation of covalent complexes between lactoferrin and SIgA (Watanabe *et al.*, 1984) is important for synergy is not known.

b. Peroxidases. An enhancement of the inhibitory effect of lactoperoxidase–H_2O_2–SCN^- on *S. mutans* metabolism by myeloma IgA1 and IgA2 proteins and by SIgA but not IgG or IgM has been attributed to binding of lactoperoxidase to IgA, presumably by the Fc region, and a subsequent stabilizing effect on enzyme activity (Tenovuo *et al.*, 1982).

c. Lysozyme. Two reports of lytic activity against *E. coli* by human or porcine colostral SIgA antibody, complement, and lysozyme have not been confirmed in other studies. Although most secretions contain lysozyme, they generally lack a functional complement system, and the ability of IgA to activate complement is controversial. Thus, the significance of this lytic system remains uncertain.

B. Molecular Mechanisms of Protection by Circulatory IgA in Tissues

1. Interaction with Complement

The question of whether and how IgA activates complement is a controversial issue that has not yet been completely resolved. Early findings that IgA is incapable of binding C1q and activating the classical complement pathway (CCP) generally have been accepted; IgA molecules do not have the C1q-binding motif found in IgG. In contrast, some researchers believe that IgA activates the alternative complement pathway (ACP), but in reality the situation is more complicated. Several reports have demonstrated that artificially aggregated, chemically cross-linked, or denatured human serum polyclonal or monoclonal (myeloma) IgA or colostral SIgA can activate the ACP (Hiemstra *et al.*, 1987; for discussion, see Russell and Mansa, 1989). A chimeric human

IgA2–rat antibody produced in a mouse transfectoma cell line shows ACP activation when complexed with a haptenated protein antigen (Lucisano Valim and Lachmann, 1991). However, human monoclonal and polyclonal pIgA1 or mIgA1 antibodies, when complexed with corresponding antigen, fail to activate the ACP whereas the same antibodies, interfacially aggregated on a plastic surface or complexed with antigen after chemical cross-linking, can activate the ACP (Russell and Mansa, 1989). Naturally occurring human IgA immune complexes also fail to activate the ACP (Imai *et al.*, 1988). Note that heat-aggregated mixtures of human IgG and IgA activate the ACP in proportion to the content of IgG, and analysis of the C3b-containing complexes shows that C3b is linked to the IgG and not to the IgA component (Waldo and Cochran, 1989).

Several studies on animal (mouse, rat, rabbit) IgA antihapten antibodies have shown that, when complexed with a haptenated protein antigen, IgA antibodies activate the ACP (Pfaffenbach *et al.*, 1982; Rits *et al.*, 1988; Schneiderman *et al.*, 1990). However, certain reservations persist regarding denaturation of the IgA in purification, abnormal glycosylation of proteins produced in hybridoma or transfectoma cells, and the direct role of heavily haptenated proteins in ACP activation, all of which could materially affect the outcome. Nevertheless, human and animal IgA—which have structural differences in terms of amino acid sequence, especially in the hinge region, as well as in glycosylation (see Chapter 7) and display other important physiological differences *in vivo*—could differ also in ACP-activating properties. Additional work is necessary to clarify these issues.

In contrast, IgA antibody to the capsular polysaccharide inhibits IgG or IgM antibody-dependent complement-mediated lysis of *Neisseria meningitidis,* thereby possibly accounting for the exacerbation of meningococcal infection in certain patients (Griffiss *et al.*, 1975). Similarly, murine IgA antibodies inhibit IgG antibody-dependent complement-mediated hemolysis *in vitro* and the Arthus reaction *in vivo* (Russell-Jones *et al.*, 1980,1981). Human monoclonal and polyclonal IgA1 antibodies inhibit IgG antibody-dependent CCP activation *in vitro*. Further, Fab fragments of IgA1 antibodies possess the same inhibitory activity as intact IgA antibodies (Russell *et al.*, 1989). Fab fragments of IgA antibodies to meningococci, which produce IgA1 protease (see Section III,A), also inhibit IgG- and complement-mediated cytolysis of these bacteria (Jarvis and Griffiss, 1991).

Overall, human IgA antibodies appear to have poor to no complement-activating ability by either pathway when bound physiologically to antigen, whereas the ACP-activating properties of IgA depend on some degree of denaturation or conformational change that does not ensue directly from binding to antigen, or possibly on abnormal structure. Whether such changes can occur in physiological or pathological conditions *in vivo,* or as a result of aberrant synthesis, and thereby contribute to inflammatory conditions in which IgA is implicated (for example, IgA nephropathy; see Chapter 53) remains to be elucidated. In contrast, the anti-inflammatory property of IgA antibodies with respect to CCP may be of physiological significance in controlling inflammation at or beneath mucosal surfaces on which IgA is abundant and where maintenance of the mucosal barrier is important.

2. Interaction with Phagocytic Cells

Several studies indicate that IgA has a negative or inhibitory effect on phagocytosis, bactericidal activity, or chemotaxis by neutrophils and monocytes or macrophages (Kilian *et al.*, 1988). In some cases, results obtained with specific IgA antibody suggest that it competes with IgG antibody for binding to the target antigen, but in most experiments myeloma IgA proteins or colostral SIgA, regardless of antibody activity, were used. Other studies, particularly using neutrophils or monocytes derived from a mucosal environment (the gingival crevice) or cultured *in vitro* with purified myeloma IgA or colostral SIgA, reveal an opsonizing effect of IgA antibodies especially in synergy with IgG antibodies (Fanger *et al.*, 1983; Gorter *et al.*, 1987). Several instances of heat-stable (i.e., complement-independent) opsonization or antibody-dependent cell-mediated cytotoxicity by IgA antibodies (reviewed by Kerr, 1990), including the postphagocytotic respiratory burst and intracellular killing as well as degranulation of eosinophils (Abu-Ghazaleh *et al.*, 1989), have been reported to date. Generally, pIgA antibodies are more effective than mIgA; in some cases, the effect is demonstrably dependent on an intact Fcα region, which implies the involvement of an Fcα receptor (FcαR) on the cells (Kerr *et al.*, 1990).

An FcαR has been demonstrated on human neutrophils, monocytes/macrophages, and eosinophils (Maliszewski *et al.*, 1990; Mazengera and Kerr, 1990; Monteiro *et al.*, 1990). The M_r of the mature polypeptide chain (deduced from the cloned gene) is ~29,900, but the observed M_r of the extracted FcαR (50,000–70,000; 90,000 on eosinophils) implies extensive and possibly variable patterns of glycosylation (Monteiro *et al.*, 1992). Immunoprecipitation of the deglycosylated protein with monoclonal antibody reveals two bands of M_r 32,000 and 36,000 that could arise from differential mRNA splicing or mRNA processing, posttranslational modification, or even two separate, possibly allelic, genes. The neutrophil FcαR has an apparent affinity for mIgA ($\sim 5 \times 10^7\ M^{-1}$) that is comparable with that of FcγRII for IgG. This receptor binds both subclasses of IgA and SIgA equally. Approximately 10^4 molecules are found per cell. The FcαR is expressed constitutively on neutrophils and monocytes, but culture with IgA, phorbol esters, or calcitriol enhances expression. The report that granulocyte–monocyte and granulocyte colony-stimulating factors decrease the number and increase the affinity of FcαR on neutrophils (Weisbart *et al.*, 1988) awaits further explanation in molecular terms.

Despite some evidence to the contrary, human IgA can mediate phagocytosis and related processes by neutrophils and monocytes/macrophages and can induce postphagocytotic intracellular events, although the biological significance of this ability remains unclear. IgA-mediated killing of bacteria by intestinal T cells also has been described (Tagliabue *et al.*, 1986). The finding that activated murine $\gamma\delta$ T cells express FcαR (Sandor *et al.*, 1992) raises the possibility that

$\gamma\delta$ $CD8^+$ intraepithelial cells are involved. Since IgG antibodies strongly activate complement but IgA antibodies do not (and may inhibit IgG-mediated complement activation), the opsonizing effects of IgA and IgG antibodies *in vivo* in the presence of complement are probably different. At least with normal neutrophils, IgG antibodies effectively opsonize only at high concentration unless bound C3b enhances binding of the particle by engaging CR3 receptors, and IgM-mediated opsonization depends on complement activation. Moderate amounts of IgA antibodies that are insufficient to activate FcαR therefore may inhibit IgG (or IgM)- and C3b-mediated phagocytosis. Similar concentration-dependent properties and interactions with other agonists have been observed in the biphasic effects of IgA on chemotaxis or chemokinesis of neutrophils exposed to other chemoattractants *in vitro* (Sibille *et al.*, 1987).

At mucosal surfaces, where SIgA is the predominant Ig, however, functionally active complement and phagocytes are not normally present. Consequently, SIgA does not have the opportunity to activate either system. Where the mucosal barrier is breached or inflammation occurs, both mucosal SIgA and submucosal pIgA secreted by resident plasma cells could have an important anti-inflammatory regulatory activity in a complex interplay of immunological effectors that may provide not only immune defense but also damage-limiting capability.

3. Interaction with Epithelial Cells

IgA-mediated elimination of antigen from the circulation by hepatobiliary transport (Russell *et al.*, 1981) has been demonstrated to occur notably in certain rodents and rabbits, in which rapid active transport of pIgA from the circulation to the bile occurs by means of SC expressed on the sinusoidal surface of hepatocytes (see Chapter 9). However, despite a few reports to the contrary, it is now accepted that human hepatocytes do not express SC or transport pIgA and IgA immune complexes in this manner. Nevertheless, other receptors such as the asialoglycoprotein receptor (or possibly membrane galactosyltransferase), which normally mediates the vesicular uptake of IgA and other desialylated glycoproteins for catabolism by hepatocytes (Mestecky *et al.*, 1991), may allow a proportion of the IgA that is taken up, in conjunction with any complexed antigen, to be diverted into the biliary secretory pathway instead of the lysosomal degradative pathway. Polarized monolayer cultures of SC-expressing epithelial cells also can transport pIgA and IgA-bound antigen from the basal to the luminal surface (Kaetzel *et al.*, 1991).

III. MICROBIAL EVASION OF IgA FUNCTIONS

The importance of IgA in host–parasite relationships at mucosal membranes is revealed further by the fact that several microbial species have evolved various ways of evading its functions. The most convincing evidence in this respect involves bacterial IgA1 proteases, which have evolved independently in several mucosal pathogens and members of the normal flora of the respiratory tract, apparently with the principal function of cleaving IgA1.

A. Microbial Proteases

1. IgA1 Proteases

Since the original detection of an IgA1 protease in the oral commensal *Streptococcus sanguis* (Plaut *et al.*, 1974), comprehensive screening of numerous species of bacteria and a few fungi, parasites, and viruses has shown that IgA1 proteases are produced by limited groups of bacteria that successfully colonize or infect mucosal membranes of humans. These pathogens include the three leading causal agents of bacterial meningitis, important respiratory tract and ear pathogens, some urogenital pathogens, and anaerobic gram-negative rods implicated in the pathogenesis of periodontal diseases (Table II). In addition, three commensals of the human oral cavity and pharynx that are responsible for initiating plaque formation on teeth produce IgA1 proteases.

All known IgA1 proteases are constitutively expressed, extracellular, postproline endopeptidases (M_r ~100,000). These enzymes attack one of the Pro–Ser (type 1 proteases) or Pro–Thr (type 2 proteases) peptide bonds within the duplicated O-glycosylated octapeptide Thr–Pro–Pro–Thr–Pro–Ser–Pro–Ser present in the hinge region of the α1 chain but absent from the α2 chain (see Chapter 7). Cleavage of IgA1 thus results in monomeric Fab fragments that retain antigen-binding properties and Fc fragments or $Fc_2 \cdot SC$ when SIgA is the substrate (for reviews, see Kilian and Reinholdt, 1986; Mulks, 1985; Plaut, 1983).

Until recently, IgA1s from humans, chimpanzee, and gorilla were the only known substrates for IgA1 proteases. However, studies by Pohlner *et al.* (1987a) revealed that, during the secretion process, the 165-kDa precursor of the IgA1 protease of *Neisseria gonorrhoeae* undergoes autoproteolysis at several sites within a sequence similar but not identical to that of the hinge region of IgA1. Synthetic decapeptides based on the sequences of two of these autoproteolytic sites (B and C) are cleaved by the *N. gonorrhoeae* type 2 protease (Wood and Burton, 1991). Homology searches identified similar sequences in the CD8 molecule of cytotoxic T lymphocytes and in granulocyte–macrophage colony-stimulating factor (Pohlner *et al.*, 1987b), but cleavage of these proteins in their natural configuration has not been demonstrated. Shoberg and Mulks (1991) showed that the type 2 IgA1 protease from *N. gonorrhoeae* cleaves several proteins in preparations of cytoplasm and outer membranes of gonococci, suggesting the possibility that IgA1 proteases may play an additional role in modulating proteins of the microorganism itself.

Some of the IgA1 proteases have been cloned in *E. coli*. The genes and their products have been fully characterized (Pohlner *et al.*, 1987a; Poulsen *et al.*, 1989; Gilbert *et al.*, 1991). The IgA1 proteases from *N. gonorrhoeae, N. meningitidis*, and *Haemophilus influenzae*, which show significant sequence homology, are all serine proteinases. IgA1 prote-

Table II IgA-Cleaving Activity in Microorganisms

Disease	Species	Cleavage specificity[a]	Fragments produced
IgA1 protease			Fab and Fc (or Fc_2SC)
Meningitis and respiratory tract infections	*Haemophilus influenzae*	Pro–Ser (231–232) or Pro–Thr (235–236)	
	Neisseria meningitidis	Pro–Ser (237–238) or Pro–Thr (235–236)	
	Streptococcus pneumoniae	Pro–Thr (227–228)	
Conjunctivitis	*Haemophilus aegyptius*	Pro–Ser (231–232)	
Urethritis	*Neisseria gonorrhoeae*	Pro–Thr (237–238) or Pro–Thr (235–236)	
	Ureaplasma urealyticum	Pro–Thr (235–236)	
Periodontitis	*Prevotella* species (all)	Pro-Ser (223–224)	
	Capnocytophage species (all)	Pro-Ser (223–224)	
Initial dental plaque formation	*Streptococcus sanguis*	Pro-Thr (227–228)	
	Streptococcus oralis	Pro-Thr (227–228)	
	Streptococcus mitis	Pro-Thr (227–228)	
Miscellaneous	*Haemophilus parahaemolyticus*	Pro-Thr (235–236)	
	Gemella haemolysans	Not determined	
IgA1/A2m(1) Protease			Fab and Fc (or Fc_2SC)
Normal gut flora	*Clostridium ramosum*	Pro-Val (221–222)	
IgA-cleaving proteases with broad substrate specificity			
Urethritis	*Proteus mirabilis*	Between CH_2 and CH_3 of both IgA1 and IgA2	
	Proteus vulgaris	Not determined	
	Proteus pennei	Not determined	
	Serratia marcescens	Near hinge region of IgA1 (and IgG1 and IgG3)	
	Escherichia coli	Not determined[b]	
	Klebsiella pneumoniae	Not determined[b]	
	Acinetobacter calcoaceticus	Not determined[b]	
Periodontitis	*Porphyromonas gingivalis*		Complete degradation
	Porphyromonas asaccharolyticus		Complete degradation
Mucosal infections	*Candida albicans*	Between CH_2 and CH_3 of both IgA1 and IgA2	
	Candida tropicalis	Same	
	Torulopsis glabrata	same	

[a] Numbers refer to the residues between which the peptide bond is cleaved (see Kilian and Reinholdt, 1986).
[b] See text for additional discussion.

ases from pneumococci and the oral streptococcal species are metalloproteinases and show no homology with the serine-type IgA1 proteases. Finally, the IgA1 protease of *Prevotella* (*Bacteroides*) *melaninogenica* is a cysteine proteinase (Mortensen and Kilian, 1984). Thus, bacterial IgA1 proteases with virtually identical activity have developed convergently through at least three independent evolutionary lines, thereby attesting to their biological significance.

2. Antigenic Polymorphism of IgA1 Proteases

Among *H. influenzae, N. meningitidis,* and *N. gonorrhoeae* strains, IgA1 proteases of two distinct cleavage specificities (Pro–Ser or Pro–Thr) have been observed (Kilian and Reinholdt, 1986; Mulks, 1985). Enzyme-neutralizing antibodies reveal at least 16 antigenic variants ("inhibition types") among *H. influenzae* IgA1 proteases (Kilian *et al.*, 1983), whereas antigenic variation is less pronounced among pathogenic *Neisseria* (Lomholt *et al.*, 1992) and virtually absent among oral streptococci and *Prevotella* and *Capnocytophaga* species (Frandsen *et al.*, 1987; Reinholdt *et al.*, 1990). Sequence analyses of IgA1 protease genes (*iga*) of *H. influenzae* and *N. gonorrhoeae* have disclosed that the antigenic diversity is a result of genetic exchange and recombination between and within these species (Halter *et al.*, 1989; Poulsen *et al.*, 1992). This antigenic diversity among some of the IgA1 proteases may increase their immune escape potential.

3. Other Microbial Proteases with IgA-Cleaving Activity

Among IgA-cleaving proteases with broader substrate specificities, one is of particular interest. Fujiyama *et al.* (1985) demonstrated an EDTA-sensitive protease in *Clostridium ramosum* that cleaves a Pro–Val peptide bond present in the α chain of both IgA1 and the A2m(1) allotype of IgA2 in the transition between the C_H1 domain and the hinge region. The A2m(2) allotype of IgA2 lacks the susceptible sequence. The specificity of this *Clostridium* protease may reflect the equal proportions of the two subclasses in the lower gut, which is the natural habitat of this bacterium. Although the original IgA1/A2m(1) protease-producing strain of *C. ramosum* was isolated from a patient with ulcerative colitis, subsequent studies have not confirmed that the species plays a pathogenic role in inflammatory bowel diseases (Senda *et al.*, 1985).

Several microbial broad-spectrum proteases can degrade IgA among other proteins: strictly speaking, such enzymes should not be called IgA proteases. Their exact cleavage sites have not been determined but appear to lie outside the hinge region of IgA. Few such enzymes have been characterized; in some cases, their wide activity spectrum may be the result of several enzymes working in concert as, for example, in the case of the putative periodontal pathogen *Porphyromonas gingivalis* (*Bacteroides asaccharolyticus*), which degrades IgA1 and IgA2 as well as other immunoglobulin isotypes and many other host proteins into small fragments (Kilian, 1981). *Pseudomonas aeruginosa*, a notable opportunistic pathogen that has significant hydrolytic activity, cleaves IgA, SIgA, SC, and IgG. Among several proteases secreted by this bacterium, the elastase completely degrades the Fab fragment of IgA (Döring *et al.*, 1981; Heck *et al.*, 1990).

Of potential importance is the finding that some members of the family Enterobacteriaceae are capable of cleaving human IgA (Table II; Mehta *et al.*, 1973; Milazzo and Delisle, 1984). This activity has been detected only in fresh isolates from feces or urinary tract infections and is lost on subcultivation of the bacteria. Similar strains from culture collections have not disclosed IgA-cleaving activity, nor has restoration of lost activity been possible. Hence, nothing is known about the specificity of the enzyme(s) involved. An exception is an IgA-cleaving protease from *Proteus mirabilis*, which is stable, has a pepsin-like activity on IgA, and cleaves initially between the C_H2 and C_H3 domains, whereas it cleaves IgG initially on either side of the hinge region (Loomes *et al.*, 1990).

Protease activity that cleaves IgA of both subclasses between the C_H2 and C_H3 domains, as well as SIgA and SC, also has been demonstrated in several *Candida* species including *Candida albicans* (Table II; Reinholdt *et al.*, 1987; Rückel, 1984). Finally, trophozoites of the protozoan parasite *Entamoeba histolytica* have been noted to induce electrophoretic changes in IgA that are suggestive of proteolytic cleavage (Quezada-Cavillo and Lopez-Revillo, 1987).

4. Cleavage of IgA *in Vivo*

IgA1 proteases are not inhibited by physiological protease inhibitors. Ample evidence is available for their activity *in vivo*. Characteristic fragments of IgA (Fab, Fc, $Fc_2 \cdot SC$) have been observed in intestinal fluids, vaginal secretions of women with gonorrhoea, cerebrospinal fluid of patients with *Haemophilus* meningitis, and nasopharyngeal secretions of certain children (for review, see Kilian and Reinholdt, 1986). Further, in samples from the oral cavity including dental plaque, monomeric Fabα fragments have been demonstrated on the surface of bacteria (Ahl and Reinholdt, 1991). Frandsen *et al.* (1991) have provided evidence for cleavage of IgA1 in periodontitis patients by demonstrating serum antibodies specific for a neoepitope exposed on Fabα released from IgA1 after cleavage by *Prevotella* or *Capnocytophaga* IgA1 proteases. IgA cleavage products similar to those obtained *in vitro* and active protease have been demonstrated in the urine of patients with *P. mirabilis* urinary tract infection (Senior *et al.*, 1991).

As are other microbial enzymes, IgA1 proteases and other IgA-cleaving proteases are subject to inhibition by specific neutralizing antibodies. Antibodies capable of inhibiting the activity of IgA1 proteases can be induced in rabbits (Kilian *et al.*, 1983). Naturally occurring neutralizing antibodies to proteases from *H. influenzae*, *N. meningitidis*, *N. gonorrhoeae*, and *Streptococcus pneumoniae* have been detected in colostral SIgA and in serum IgG and IgA (Gilbert *et al.*, 1983; Kobayashi *et al.*, 1987). High titers of neutralizing antibodies to IgA1 proteases of oral streptococci also have been detected in serum from patients with subacute endocarditis caused by the respective bacteria (Reinholdt *et al.*, 1990), whereas very low inhibitory antibody activity against *S. sanguis* IgA1 protease is present in pooled colostrum (Gilbert *et al.*, 1983). Neutralizing antibodies to the IgA1/A2m(1) protease of *C. ramosum* have not been detected, even in sera of subjects whose bowels are colonized by this bacterium (Kobayashi *et al.*, 1987).

5. Biological Significance of Proteolytic IgA Degradation

Since the protective functions of IgA in its different forms depend on the integrity of the immunoglobulin molecule, any significant degradation of IgA is likely to influence its functional activity. Cleavage of IgA in the hinge region will interfere with all its Fc-dependent properties described earlier. However, the specific IgA1 and IgA1/A2m(1) proteases are uniquely adept in counteracting the effects of IgA antibodies as well as perhaps other immune effector mechanisms. Both *in vivo* and *in vitro* studies have shown that monomeric Fab fragments of antibodies, in spite of their antigen-binding activity, do not inhibit adherence and colonization of bacteria (Steele *et al.*, 1975; Reinholdt and Kilian, 1987; Ma *et al.*, 1990; Hajishengallis *et al.*, 1992). Although cross-linking and agglutination of bacteria may be a factor here, these findings indicate the importance of structures in the Fc (or $Fc_2 \cdot SC$ of SIgA) for mucosal protection. It is furthermore postulated that the binding of Fabα fragments to the surface of bacteria protects them from the host immune system by blocking access of intact antibodies of the same or other isotypes and of immunocompetent cells as, for example, in the inhibition of IgG and complement-mediated bacteriolysis described previously. These processes have been hypothesized to play a role in the pathogenesis of invasive infections caused by IgA1 protease-producing bacteria (Kilian and Reinholdt, 1987). Thus, IgA1 proteases appear to represent a subtle way of turning a specific immune response against a pathogen to its advantage, which may be effective no matter what other immune effector mechanisms remain intact.

Because cleavage of IgA by IgA1 proteases is not restricted to antibodies against the bacteria that secrete them, IgA1 proteases may affect host–parasite interactions involving other microorganisms. Further, cleavage of IgA1 may jeopardize the immune barrier of the respiratory tract to potential allergens, as suggested by the significantly increased incidence of IgA1 cleavage in nasopharyngeal secretions of children with a history of atopic diseases (Sørensen and Kilian, 1984).

The biological consequences of cleavage of IgA by proteases that remove the C_H3 domain remain unclear, partly because of our limited knowledge concerning individual Fc domains in the secondary effector functions of IgA.

B. Other Potential Evasion Strategies

1. Glycosidases

IgAs, in particular SIgA, are heavily glycosylated with both N-linked and O-linked glycan chains (see Chapter 7) that may be attacked by bacterial glycosidases. As an example, *S. pneumoniae* and certain oral streptococci are capable of stripping IgA molecules of all their carbohydrate moieties (Kilian *et al.*, 1980; Reinholdt *et al.*, 1990). Studies involving IgG have disclosed dramatic effects of carbohydrate depletion (Nose and Wigzell, 1983). However, the biological consequences of such an event for IgA remain unclear, except that the ability of IgA to agglutinate *E. coli* via lectin–carbohydrate interactions (Wold *et al.*, 1990) would be lost.

2. IgA Binding Proteins

Some strains of pathogenic streptococci of groups A (*S. pyogenes*) and B (*S. agalactiae*) are capable of interacting with IgA of both subclasses in an antibody-independent manner. The phenomenon is the result of expression of Fcα binding proteins on the streptococcal surfaces (Brady and Boyle, 1990; Lindahl *et al.*, 1990). By analogy with the IgG-binding protein A on *Staphylococcus aureus*, researchers speculate that the streptococcal IgA Fc receptors serve an immune escape function at mucosal surfaces.

IV. IgA AND HOMEOSTASIS

Despite the considerable advances that have been made in unraveling the complexities of the immune system, the biological activities and physiological functions of the major isotype of human Ig are still poorly understood. This lack of understanding is especially obvious for the circulating plasma form of IgA, which remains an enigma. The role of plasma IgA has been suggested to be that of the "discrete housekeeper," implying a background regulatory activity that is supported by a good deal of evidence. SIgA can be viewed in a similar way, except that perhaps it is the "discrete gatekeeper" whose job is to keep undesirables out. Nevertheless, clearly situations exist in which IgA function is less than discrete, since it can be involved in pathological conditions under circumstances that suggest it has a pro-inflammatory effect, for example, in IgA nephropathy and IgA immune complex-induced lung injury. Are these, however, manifestations of a derangement of normal IgA structure and function, or the exaggerated result of normal physiological IgA activity? Conversely, other mucosal diseases are associated with an apparent failure of IgA to maintain adequate anti-inflammatory control, which might be the case in inflammatory bowel disease (see Chapter 38). In this context, the balance between IgA and IgG antibodies may be the important factor (Tolo *et al.*, 1977; Lim and Rowley, 1982). An analogous situation may occur in periodontal disease, which involves chronic inflammatory destruction of the structures supporting the teeth. These situations raise the question of whether the anti-inflammatory effects of IgA can be exploited to ameliorate these conditions.

Deficiency of IgA might be expected to manifest itself in profound disturbances, but these generally do not occur. Selective IgA deficiency occurs in Western populations with a frequency as high as 1 in 400 individuals, yet the subjects usually do not suffer serious consequences, although they have statistically increased tendencies to develop upper respiratory tract and oral infections, atopy, autoimmunity, and neoplasia (Hong and Amman, 1989). However, most IgA-deficient subjects compensate by the production of secretory IgM at their mucosal surfaces, whereas noncompensators frequently suffer problems. Moreover, IgA deficiency may have much more serious consequences in populations lacking modern hygienic facilities, so the antigenic and infectious challenge to mucosal surfaces is much greater. A lower prevalence of IgA deficiency in Africa and elsewhere is consistent with this concept. Curiously, significant numbers of IgD-secreting plasma cells also occur in certain submucosae such as the nasal passages (Brandtzaeg *et al.*, 1991), but no mechanism is known for the secretion of this poorly understood isotype. Further, IgD is highly susceptible to proteolysis, thus placing it at a disadvantage in secretions in which proteases occur; apparently IgD cannot compensate for lack of IgA in IgA deficiency (Brandtzaeg *et al.*, 1986a).

IgA is a phylogenetically ancient Ig and has been found in plasma and secretions of all mammals examined. However, the concentration and relative physiological significance of this Ig vary markedly in different mammalian orders and families. Most notably in ruminants, although SIgA occurs, the dominant mucosal Ig is a subclass of IgG (IgG1) that is transported selectively into secretions by a mechanism that involves a receptor other than SC. Interestingly, ruminant IgG1 is less effective than the other IgG subclass of these animals (IgG2) in complement-mediated and opsonic effector functions, and so may share some of the noninflammatory or anti-inflammatory properties of IgA that are deemed important for mucosal protection.

References

Abraham, S. N., and Beachey, E. H. (1985). Host defenses against adhesion of bacteria to mucosal surfaces. *In* "Advances in Host Defense Mechanisms" (J. F. Gallin and A. S. Fauci, eds.), Vol. 4, pp. 63–88. Raven Press, New York.

Abu-Ghazaleh, R. I., Fujisawa, T., Mestecky, J., Kyle, R. A., and Gleich, G. J. (1989). IgA-induced eosinophil degranulation. *J. Immunol.* **142,** 2393–2400.

Ahl, T., and Reinholdt, J. (1991). Detection of immunoglobulin A1 protease-induced Fabα fragments on dental plaque bacteria. *Infect. Immun.* **59,** 563–569.

Armstrong, S. J., and Dimmock, N. J. (1992). Neutralization of influenza virus by low concentrations of hemagglutinin-specific polymeric immunoglobulin A inhibits viral fusion activity, but activation of the ribonucleoprotein is also inhibited. *J. Virol.* **66,** 3823–3832.

Bessen, D., and Fischetti, V. A. (1988). Passive acquired mucosal immunity to group A streptococci by secretory immunoglobulin A. *J. Exp. Med.* **167,** 1945–1950.

Biesbrock, A. R., Reddy, M. S., and Levine, M. J. (1991). Interaction of a salivary mucin-secretory immunoglobulin A complex with mucosal pathogens. *Infect. Immun.* **59,** 3492–3497.

Brady, L. J., and Boyle, M. D. P. (1990). Immunoglobulin A Fc-binding proteins associated with group B streptococci. *In* "Bacterial Immunoglobulin-Binding Proteins. Microbiology, Chemistry, and Biology" (M. D. P. Boyle, ed.), Vol. 1, pp. 201–224. Academic Press, San Diego.

Brandtzaeg, P., Karlsson, G., Hansson, G., Petruson, B., Björkander, J., and Hanson, L. Å. (1986a). The clinical condition of IgA-deficient patients is related to the proportion of IgD- and IgM-producing cells in their nasal mucosa. *Clin. Exp. Immunol.* **67,** 626–636.

Brandtzaeg, P., Kett, K., Rognum, T. O., Söderström, R., Björkander, J., Söderström, T., Petrusson, B., and Hanson, L. Å. (1986b). Distribution of mucosal IgA and IgG subclass-producing immunocytes and alterations in various disorders. *Monogr. Allergy* **20,** 179–194.

Brandtzaeg, P., Nilssen, D. E., Rognum, T. O., and Thrane, P. S. (1991). Ontogeny of the mucosal immune system and IgA deficiency. *Gastroenterol. Clin. North Am.* **20,** 397–439.

Bronson, R. A., Cooper, G. W., Rosenfeld, D. L., Gilbert, J. V., and Plaut, A. G. (1987). The effect of an IgA1 protease on immunoglobulins bound to the sperm surface and sperm cervical mucus penetrating ability. *Fertil. Steril.* **47,** 985–991.

Childers, N. K., Bruce, M. G., and McGhee, J. R. (1989). Molecular mechanisms of immunoglobulin A defense. *Ann. Rev. Microbiol.* **43,** 503–536.

Clamp, J. R. (1977). The relationship between secretory immunoglobulin A and mucus. *Biochem. Soc. Trans.* **5,** 1579–1581.

Cunningham-Rundles, C., Brandeis, W. E., Good, R. A., and Day, N. K. (1978). Milk precipitins, circulating immune complexes, and IgA deficiency. *Proc. Natl. Acad. Sci. U.S.A.* **75,** 3387–3389.

Döring, G., Obernesser, H. J., and Botzenhart, K. (1981). Extrazelluläre Toxine von *Pseudomonas aeruginosa* II. Einwirkung zweier gereinigter Proteasen auf die menschlichen Immunoglobuline IgG, IgA und sekretorisches IgA. *Zbl. Bakt. Hgy. 1, Abt. Orig.* **A249,** 89–98.

Fanger, M. W., Goldstine, S. N., and Shen, L. (1983). Cytofluorographic analysis of receptors for IgA on human polymorphonuclear cells and monocytes and the correlation of receptor expression with phagocytosis. *Mol. Immunol.* **20,** 1019–1027.

Frandsen, E. V. G., Reinhodt, J., and Kilian, M. (1987). Enzymatic and antigenic characterization of immunoglobulin A1 proteases from *Bacteroides* and *Capnocytophaga* spp. *Infect. Immun.* **55,** 631–638.

Frandsen, E. V. G., Reinholdt, J., and Kilian, M. (1991). Immunoglobulin A1 (IgA1) proteases from *Prevotella* (*Bacteroides*) and *Capnocytophaga* species in relation to periodontal diseases. *J. Periodont. Res.* **26,** 297–299.

Fujiyama, Y., Kobayashi, K., Senda, S., Benno, Y., Bamba, T., and Hosoda, S. (1985). A novel IgA protease from *Clostridium* sp. capable of cleaving IgA1 and IgA2 A2m(1) allotype but not IgA2 A2m(2) allotype paraproteins. *J. Immunol.* **134,** 573–576.

Gilbert, J. V., Plaut, A. G., Longmaid, B., and Lamm, M. E. (1983). Inhibition of microbial IgA proteases by human secretory IgA and serum. *Mol. Immunol.* **20,** 1039–1049.

Gilbert, J. V., Plaut, A. G., and Wright, A. (1991). Analysis of the immunoglobulin A protease gene of *Streptococcus sanguis*. *Infect. Immun.* **59,** 7–17.

Gorter, A., Hiemstra, P. S., Leijh, P. C. J., van der Sluys, M. E., van den Barselaar, M. T., van Es, L. A., and Daha, M. R. (1987). IgA- and secretory IgA-opsonized *S. aureus* induce a respiratory burst and phagocytosis by polymorphonuclear leucocytes. *Immunology* **61,** 303–309.

Griffiss, J. M., Broud, D., and Bertram, M. A. (1975). Bactericidal activity of meningococcal antisera. Blocking by IgA of lytic antibody in human convalescent sera. *J. Immunol.* **114,** 1779–1784.

Hajishengallis, G., Nikolova, E., and Russell, M. W. (1992). Inhibition of *Streptococcus mutans* adherence to saliva-coated hydroxyapatite by human secretory immunoglobulin A antibodies to the cell surface protein antigen I/II: Reversal by IgA1 protease cleavage. *Infect. Immun.* **60,** 5057–5064.

Halter, R., Pohlner, J., and Meyer, T. F. (1989). Mosaic-like organization of IgA protease genes in *Neisseria gonorrhoeae* generated by horizontal genetic exchange *in vivo*. *EMBO J.* **8,** 3737–2744.

Heck, L. W., Alarcon, P. G., Kulhavy, R. M., Morihara, K., Russell, M. W., and Mestecky, J. F. (1990). Degradation of IgA proteins by *Pseudomonas aeruginosa* elastase. *J. Immunol.* **144,** 2253–2257.

Heremans, J. F. (1974). Immunoglobulin A. *In* "The Antigens" (M. Sela, ed.), Vol. 2, pp. 365–522. Academic Press, New York.

Hiemstra, P. S., Gorter, A., Stuurman, M. E., van Es, L. A., and Daha, M. R. (1987). Activation of the alternative pathway of complement by human serum IgA. *Eur. J. Immunol.* **17,** 321–326.

Hong, R., and Amman, A. J. (1989). Disorders of the IgA system. *In* "Immunologic Disorders in Infants and Children" (E. R. Stiehm, ed.), 3d Ed., pp. 329–342. Saunders, Philadelphia.

Imai, H., Chen, A., Wyatt, R. J., and Rifai, A. (1988). Lack of complement activation by human IgA immune complexes. *Clin. Exp. Immunol.* **73,** 479–483.

Jarvis, G. A., and Griffiss, J. M. (1991). Human IgA1 blockade of IgG-initiated lysis of *Neisseria meningitidis* is a function of antigen-binding fragment binding to the polysaccharide capsule. *J. Immunol.* **147,** 1962–1967.

Jentoft, N. (1990). Why are proteins O-glycosylated? *Trends Biochem. Sci.* **15,** 291–294.

Kaetzel, C. S., Robinson, J. K., Chintalacharuvu, K. R., Vaerman, J.-P., and Lamm, M. E. (1991). The polymeric immunoglobulin receptor (secretory component) mediates transport of immune complexes across epithelial cells: A local defense function for IgA. *Proc. Natl. Acad. Sci. U.S.A.* **88,** 8796–8800.

Kerr, M. A. (1990). The structure and function of human IgA. *Biochem. J.* **271,** 285–296.

Kerr, M. A., Mazengera, R. L., and Stewart, W. W. (1990). Structure and function of immunoglobulin A receptors on phagocytic cells. *Biochem. Soc. Trans.* **18,** 215–217.

Kilian, M. (1981). Degradation of immunoglobulins A1, A2, and G by suspected principal periodontal pathogens. *Infect. Immun.* **34,** 757–765.

Kilian, M., and Reinholdt, J. (1986). Interference with IgA defence mechanisms by extracellular bacterial enzymes. *In* "Medical Microbiology" (C. S. F. Easmon and J. Jeljaszewics, ed.), Vol. 5, pp. 173–208. Academic Press, London.

Kilian, M., and Reinholdt, J. (1987). A hypothetical model for the development of invasive infection due to IgA1 protease-producing bacteria. *In* "Recent Advances in Mucosal Immunology" (J. R. McGhee, J. Mestecky, P. L. Ogra, and J. Bienenstock, ed.), Part B, pp. 1261–1269. Plenum, New York.

Kilian, M., Mestecky, J., Kulhavy, R., Tomana, M., and Butler, W. T. (1980). IgA1 proteases from *Haemophilus influenzae, Streptococcus pneumoniae, Neisseria meningitidis,* and *Streptococcus sanguis:* Comparative immunochemical studies. *J. Immunol.* **124,** 2596–2600.

Kilian, M., Thomsen, B., Petersen, T. E., and Bleeg, H. (1983). Molecular biology of *Haemophilus influenzae* IgA1 proteases. *Mol. Immunol.* **20,** 1051–1058.

Kilian, M., Mestecky, J., and Russell, M. W. (1988). Defense mechanisms involving Fc-dependent functions of immunoglobulin A and their subversion by bacterial immunoglobulin A proteases. *Microbiol. Rev.* **52,** 296–303.

Kobayashi, K., Fujiyama, Y., Hagiwara, K., and Kondoh, H. (1987). Resistance of normal serum IgA and secretory IgA to bacterial IgA proteases: Evidence for the presence of enzyme-neutralizing antibodies in both serum and secretory IgA, and also in serum IgG. *Microbiol. Immunol.* **31,** 1097–1106.

Lim, P. L., and Rowley, D. (1982). The effect of antibody on the intestinal absorption of macromolecules and on intestinal permeability in adult mice. *Int. Arch. Allergy Appl. Immunol.* **68,** 41–46.

Lindahl, G., Åkerström, B., Frithz, E., Hedén, L.-O., and Stenberg, L. (1990). Protein Arp, the immunoglobulin A receptor of group A streptococci. *In* "Bacterial Immunoglobulin-Binding Proteins. Microbiology, Chemistry, and Biology" (M. D. P. Boyle, ed.), Vol. 1, pp. 193–200. Academic Press, San Diego.

Lomholt, H., Poulsen, K., Caugant, D. A., and Kilian, M. (1992). Molecular polymorphism and epidemiology of *Neisseria meningitidis* immunoglobulin A1 proteases. *Proc. Natl. Acad. Sci. U.S.A.* **89,** 2120–2124.

Loomes, L. M., Senior, B. W., and Kerr, M. A. (1990). A proteolytic enzyme secreted by *Proteus mirabilis* degrades immunoglobulins of the immunoglobulin A1 (IgA1), IgA2, and IgG isotypes. *Infect. Immun.* **58,** 1979–1985.

Lucisano Valim, Y. M., and Lachmann, P. J. (1991). The effect of antibody isotype and antigenic epitope density on the complement-fixing activity of immune complexes: A systematic study using chimaeric anti-NIP antibodies with human Fc regions. *Clin. Exp. Immunol.* **84,** 1–8.

Lycke, N., Eriksen, L., and Holmgren, J. (1987). Protection against cholera toxin after oral immunization is thymus-dependent and associated with intestinal production of neutralizing IgA antitoxin. *Scand. J. Immunol.* **25,** 413–419.

Ma, J. K.-C., Hunjan, M., Smith, R., Kelly, C., and Lehner, T. (1990). An investigation into the mechanism of protection by local passive immunization with monoclonal antibodies against *Streptococcus mutans. Infect. Immun.* **58,** 3407–3414.

Magnusson, K.-E., and Stjernström, I. (1982). Mucosal barrier mechanisms. Interplay between secretory IgA (SIgA), IgG and mucins on the surface properties and association of salmonellae with intestine and granulocytes. *Immunology* **45,** 239–248.

Majumdar, A. S., and Ghose, A. C. (1981). Evaluation of the biological properties of different classes of human antibodies in relation to cholera. *Infect. Immun.* **32,** 9–14.

Maliszewski, C. R., March, C. J., Schoenborn, M. A., Gimpel, S., and Shen, L. (1990). Expression cloning of a human Fc receptor for IgA. *J. Exp. Med.* **172,** 1665–1672.

Mazanec, M. B., Nedrud, J. G., and Lamm, M. E. (1987). Immunoglobulin A monoclonal antibodies protect against Sendai virus. *J. Virol.* **61,** 2624–2626.

Mazanec, M. B., Kaetzel, C. S., Lamm, M. E., Fletcher, D., and Nedrud, J. G. (1992). Intracellular neutralization of virus by immunoglobulin A antibodies. *Proc. Natl. Acad. Sci. U.S.A.* **89,** 6901–6905.

Mazengera, R. L., and Kerr, M. A. (1990). The specificity of the IgA receptor purified from human neutrophils. *Biochem. J.* **272,** 159–165.

Mehta, S. K., Plaut, A. G., Calvanico, N. J., and Tomasi, T. B. (1973). Human immunoglobulin A: Production of an Fc fragment by an enteric microbial proteolytic enzyme. *J. Immunol.* **111,** 1274–1276.

Mestecky, J., Lue, C., and Russell, M. W. (1991). Selective transport of IgA: cellular and molecular aspects. *Gastroenterol. Clin. North Am.* **20,** 441–471.

Milazzo, F. H., and Delisle, G. J. (1984). Immunoglobulin A proteases in gram-negative bacteria isolated from human urinary tract infections. *Infect. Immun.* **43,** 11–13.

Monteiro, R. C., Kubagawa, H., and Cooper, M. D. (1990). Cellular distribution, regulation, and biochemical nature of an Fcα receptor in humans. *J. Exp. Med.* **171,** 597–613.

Monteiro, R. C., Cooper, M. D., and Kubagawa, H. (1992). Molecular heterogeneity of Fcα receptors detected by receptor-specific monoclonal antibodies. *J. Immunol.* **148,** 1764–1770.

Mortensen, S. B., and Kilian, M. (1984). Purification and characterization of an immunoglobulin A1 protease from *Bacteroides melaninogenicus. Infect. Immun.* **45,** 550–557.

Mulks, M. H. (1985). Microbial IgA proteases. *In* "Bacterial Enzymes and Virulence" (I. A. Holder, ed.), pp. 81–104. CRC Press, Boca Raton, Florida.

Nose, M., and Wigzell, H. (1983). Biological significance of carbohydrate chains on monoclonal antibodies. *Proc. Natl. Acad. Sci. U.S.A.* **80,** 6632–6636.

Pfaffenbach, G., Lamm, M. E., and Gigli, I. (1982). Activation of the guinea pig alternative complement pathway by mouse IgA immune complexes. *J. Exp. Med.* **155,** 231–247.

Plaut, A. G. (1983). The IgA1 proteases of pathogenic bacteria. *Ann. Rev. Microbiol.* **37,** 603–622.

Plaut, A. G., Genco, R. J., and Tomasi, T. B. (1974). Isolation of an enzyme from *Streptococcus sanguis* which specifically cleaves IgA. *J. Immunol.* **113,** 289–291.

Pohlner, J., Halter, R., Beyreuther, K., and Meyer, T. F. (1987a). Gene structure and extracellular secretion of *Neisseria gonorrhoeae* IgA protease. *Nature (London)* **325,** 458–462.

Pohlner, J., Halter, R., and Meyer, T. F. (1987b). *Neisseria gonorrhoeae* IgA protease. Secretion and implications for pathogenesis. *Antonie van Leeuwenhoek* **53,** 479–484.

Poulsen, K., Brandt, J., Hjorth, J. P., Thøgersen, H. C., and Kilian, M. (1989). Cloning and sequencing of the immunoglobulin A1 protease gene (iga) of *Haemophilus influenzae* serotype b. *Infect. Immun.* **57,** 3097–3105.

Poulsen, K., Reinholdt, J., and Kilian, M. (1992). A comparative study of serologically distinct *Haemophilus influenzae* type 1 immunoglobulin A1 proteases. *J. Bacteriol.* **174,** 2913–2921.

Quezada-Cavillo, R., and Lopez-Revillo, R. (1987). IgA protease in *Entamoeba histolytica* trophozoites. *In* "Recent Advances in Mucosal Immunology" (J. R. McGhee, J. Mestecky, P. O. Ogra, and J. Bienenstock, ed.), Part B, pp. 1283–1288. Plenum, New York.

Reinholdt, J., and Kilian, M. (1987). Interference of IgA protease with the effect of secretory IgA on adherence of oral streptococci to saliva-coated hydroxyapatite. *J. Dent. Res.* **66,** 492–497.

Reinholdt, J., Krogh, P., and Holmstrup, P. (1987). Degradation of IgA1, IgA2, and SIgA by *Candida* and *Torulopsis* species. *Acta Pathol. Microbiol. Immunol. Scand. C.* **95,** 265–274.

Reinholdt, J., Tomana, M., Mortensen, S. B., and Kilian, M. (1990). Molecular aspects of immunoglobulin A1 degradation by oral streptococci. *Infect. Immun.* **58,** 1186–1194.

Renegar, K. B., and Small, P. A. (1991). Passive transfer of local immunity to influenza virus infection by IgA antibody. *J. Immunol.* **146,** 1972–1978.

Rits, M., Hiemstra, P. S., Bazin, H., Van Es, L. A., Vaerman, J.-P., and Daha, M. R. (1988). Activation of rat complement by soluble and insoluble rat IgA immune complexes. *Eur. J. Immunol.* **18,** 1873–1880.

Rückel, R. (1984). A variety of *Candida* proteinases and their possible targets of proteolytic attack in the host. *Zbl. Bakt. Hyg. A* **257,** 266–274.

Russell, M. W., and Mansa, B. (1989). Complement-fixing properties of human IgA antibodies: Alternative pathway complement activation by plastic-bound, but not by specific antigen-bound IgA. *Scand. J. Immunol.* **30,** 175–183.

Russell, M. W., Brown, T. A., and Mestecky, J. (1981). Role of serum IgA: Hepatobiliary transport of circulating antigen. *J. Exp. Med.* **153,** 968–976.

Russell, M. W., Reinholdt, J., and Kilian, M. (1989). Anti-inflammatory activity of human IgA antibodies and their Fabα fragments: Inhibition of IgG-mediated complement activation. *Eur. J. Immunol.* **19,** 2243–2249.

Russell-Jones, G. J., Ey, P. L., and Reynolds, B. L. (1980). The ability of IgA to inhibit the complement-mediated lysis of target red blood cells sensitized with IgG antibody. *Mol. Immunol.* **17,** 1173–1180.

Russell-Jones, G. J., Ey, P. L., and Reynolds, B. L. (1981). Inhibition of cutaneous anaphylaxis and Arthus reactions in the mouse by antigen-specific IgA. *Int. Arch. Allergy Appl. Immunol.* **66,** 316–325.

Sandor, M., Houlden, B., Bluestone, J., Hedrick, S. M., Weinstock, J., and Lynch, R. G. (1992). In vitro and in vivo activation of murine γ/δ T cells induces the expression of IgA, IgM, and IgG Fc receptors. *J. Immunol.* **148,** 2363–2369.

Schneiderman, R. D., Lint, T. F., and Knight, K. L. (1990). Activation of the alternative pathway of complement by twelve different rabbit–mouse chimeric transfectoma IgA isotypes. *J. Immunol.* **145,** 233–237.

Senda, S., Fujiyama, Y., Ushijima, T., Hodohara, K., Bamba, T., Hosoda, S., and Kobayashi, K. (1985). *Clostridium ramosum,* an IgA protease-producing species and its ecology in the human intestinal tract. *Microbiol. Immunol.* **29,** 1019–1028.

Senior, B. W., Loomes, L. M., and Kerr, M. A. (1991). The production and activity *in vivo* of *Proteus mirabilis* IgA protease in infections of the urinary tract. *J. Med. Microbiol.* **35,** 203–207.

Shim, B. S., Kang, Y. S., Kim, W. J., Cho, S. H., and Lee, D. B. (1969). Self-protective activity of colostral IgA against tryptic digestion. *Nature (London)* **222,** 787–788.

Shoberg, R. J., and Mulks, M. H. (1991). Proteolysis of bacterial membrane proteins by *Neisseria gonorrhoeae* type 2 immunoglobulin A1 protease. *Infect. Immun.* **59,** 2535–2541.

Sibille, Y., Delacroix, D. L., Merill, W. W., Chatelain, B., and Vaerman, J. P. (1987). IgA-induced chemokinesis of human polymorphonuclear neutrophils: requirement of their Fc-alpha receptor. *Mol. Immunol.* **24,** 551–559.

Sixbey, J. W., and Yao, Q. (1992). Immunoglobulin A-induced shift of Epstein–Barr virus tissue tropism. *Science* **255,** 1578–1580.

Smith, D. J., Taubman, M. A., and Ebersole, J. L. (1985). Salivary IgA antibody to glucosyltransferase in man. *Clin. Exp. Immunol.* **61,** 416–424.

Sørensen, C. H., and Kilian, M. (1984). Bacterium-induced cleavage of IgA in nasopharyngeal secretions from atopic children. *Acta Path. Microbiol. Immunol. Scand. C* **92,** 85–87.

Steele, E. J., Chaicumpa, W., and Rowley, D. (1975). Further evidence for crosslinking as a protective factor in experimental cholera: properties of antibody fragments. *J. Infect. Dis.* **132,** 175–180.

Stephens, S., Dolby, J. M., Montreuil, J., and Spik, G. (1980). Differences in inhibition of the growth of commensal and enteropathogenic strains of *Escherichia coli* by lactotransferrin and secretory immunoglobulin A isolated from human milk. *Immunology* **41,** 597–603.

Stokes, C. R., Soothill, J. F., and Turner, M. W. (1975). Immune exclusion is a function of IgA. *Nature (London)* **255,** 745–746.

Svanborg-Edén, C., and Svennerholm, A.-M. (1978). Secretory immunoglobulin A and G antibodies prevent adhesion of *Escherichia coli* to human urinary tract epithelial cells. *Infect. Immun.* **22,** 790–797.

Tagliabue, A., Villa, L., De Magistris, M. T., Romano, M., Silvestri, S., Boraschi, D., and Nencioni, L. (1986). IgA-driven T cell-mediated anti-bacterial immunity in man after live oral Ty21a vaccine. *J. Immunol.* **137,** 1504–1510.

Tenovuo, J., Moldoveanu, Z., Mestecky, J., Pruitt, K. M., and Mansson-Rahemtulla, B. (1982). Interaction of specific and innate factors of immunity: IgA enhances the antimicrobial effect of the lactoperoxidase system against *Streptococcus mutans. J. Immunol.* **128,** 726–731.

Tolo, K., Brandtzaeg, P., and Jonsen, J. (1977). Mucosal penetration of antigen in the presence or absence of serum-derived antibody. An *in vitro* study of rabbit oral and intestinal mucosa. *Immunology* **33,** 733–743.

Tomana, M., Kulhavy, R., and Mestecky, J. (1988). Receptor-mediated binding and uptake of immunoglobulin A by human liver. *Gastroenterology* **94,** 762–770.

Tramont, E. C. (1977). Inhibition of adherence of *Neisseria gonorrhoeae* by human genital secretions. *J. Clin. Invest.* **59,** 117–124.

Waldo, F. B., and Cochran, A. M. (1989). Mixed IgA-IgG aggregates as a model of immune complexes in IgA nephropathy. *J. Immunol.* **142,** 3841–3846.

Walker, W. A., Isselbacher, K. J., and Bloch, K. J. (1972). Intestinal uptake of macromolecules: Effect of oral immunization. *Science* **177,** 608–610.

Watanabe, T., Nagura, H., Watanabe, K., and Brown, W. R. (1984). The binding of human milk lactoferrin to immunoglobulin A. *FEBS Lett.* **168,** 203–207.

Weisbart, R. H., Kacena, A., Schuh, A., and Golde, D. W. (1988). GM-CSF induces human neutrophil IgA-mediated phagocytosis by an IgA Fc receptor activation mechanism. *Nature (London)* **332,** 647–648.

Weltzin, R., Lecia-Jandris, P., Michetti, P., Fields, B. N., Kraehenbuhl, J. P., and Neutra, M. R. (1989). Binding and transepithelial transport of immunoglobulins by intestinal M cells: Demonstration using monoclonal IgA antibodies against enteric viral proteins. *J. Cell. Biol.* **108,** 1673–1685.

Williams, R. C., and Gibbons, R. J. (1972). Inhibition of bacterial adherence by secretory immunoglobulin A: A mechanism of antigen disposal. *Science* **177,** 697–699.

Winner, L., Mack, J., Weltzin, R., Mekalanos, J. J., Kraehenbuhl, J.-P., and Neutra, M. R. (1991). New model for analysis of mucosal immunity: intestinal secretion of specific monoclonal immunoglobulin A from hybridoma tumors protects against *Vibrio cholerae* infection. *Infect. Immun.* **59,** 977–982.

Wold, A., Mestecky, J., Tomana, M., Kobata, A., Ohbayashi, H., Endo, T., and Svanborg Edén, C. (1990). Secretory immunoglobulin A carries oligosaccharide receptors for *Escherichia coli* type 1 fimbrial lectin. *Infect. Immun.* **58,** 3073–3077.

Wood, S. G., and Burton, J. (1991). Synthetic peptide substrates for the immunoglobulin A1 protease from *Neisseria gonorrhoeae* (Type 2). *Infect. Immun.* **59,** 1818–1822.

Section B

Cells, Regulation, and Specificity in the Mucosal Immune System: Inductive Sites

Section Editor: Warren Strober

(Chapters 12 through 19)

12

Characteristics and Functions of Mucosa-Associated Lymphoid Tissue

Kenneth Croitoru · John Bienenstock

I. INTRODUCTION

Lymphoid tissue can be identified early in phylogeny in the gills and guts of species more advanced than cyclostomes (Good and Papermaster, 1964; Marchalonis, 1974). Evidence that this local immune system protects mucosal surfaces independent of circulating antibodies first was suggested by experiments in rabbits that were immunized orally with killed *Shigella* bacteria. These animals were resistant to experimentally induced bacillary dysentery (Besredka, 1927). In humans with dysentery, fecal antibodies can be detected before serum antibodies develop (Davies, 1922). Similar evidence exists for specific local immunity in other mucosal tissues such as the respiratory tract and the female reproductive tract (Amoss and Taylor, 1917; Byrne and Nelson, 1939; Tomasi and Bienenstock, 1968). We have come to appreciate that the lymphoid elements distributed in different mucosal tissues are part of a unique immune system that confers local immunity in a regulated fashion. This immunity protects a large and fragile epithelium, preventing the disruption of the normal physiological function of these mucosal tissues.

Technical advances in cellular and molecular biology over the last 10 years have changed our ability to probe and examine the nature and function of the mucosa-associated lymphoid tissue (MALT). New concepts have emerged and notions previously considered incorrect have been rekindled. In this chapter, we highlight some of these findings as a prelude to the chapters that follow in this section.

A. *Definitions*

MALT can be separated into several components (see Table I), a few of which are described here.

1. Gut-Associated Lymphoid Tissue

The gut-associated lymphoid tissue (GALT) is the most extensively studied component of MALT. This tissue consists of organized lymphoid aggregates represented by the Peyer's patches, the appendix, mesenteric lymph nodes (MLN), and solitary lymphoid nodules. In addition, the nonorganized lymphoid elements in the epithelium—the intraepithelial lymphocytes (IEL)—and in the lamina propria—the lamina propria lymphocytes (LPL)—are considered part of GALT. Collectively, this mass of lymphoid tissue easily would challenge other lymphoid organs in size (see Figure 1).

In the chicken, an additional specialized organ can be found at the end of the intestine and is referred to as the bursa of Fabricius. This organ has been shown to be the site of primary B-cell development in the chicken (Cooper *et al.*, 1966; Perey *et al.*, 1968), a function that remains difficult to localize to any one organ in mammals.

2. Bronchus-Associated Lymphoid Tissue

Burdon-Sanderson first described the lymphoid tissue in the lung in 1867 and noted that "these lymphoid follicles in the bronchial walls are therefore in every respect analogous to the lymph follicles found in other mucous membranes, e.g., tonsils, and in the intestine" (Klein, 1875). Similarities between the organized lymphoid tissue in the lung and GALT led to the term bronchus-associated lymphoid tissue (BALT; Bienenstock *et al.*, 1973a,b). As reviewed elsewhere in this book, BALT consists of lymphoid aggregates distributed in the larger passageways of the respiratory tract. As in GALT, specialized antigen sampling structures represented by lymphoid follicles with overlying follicle-associated epithelia (FAE) that contain specialized epithelial cells referred to as M cells are seen (Bienenstock and Johnson, 1976). In addition, lymphocytes are distributed in the subepithelial spaces as well as within the epithelium of the bronchi (Bienenstock, 1984). This organization suggests a functional role for BALT that is not dissimilar from that of GALT.

3. Mucosa-Associated Lymphoid Tissue

The term "mucosa-associated lymphoid tissue" (MALT) arose from the realization that not only did mucosal surfaces share organizational similarities in their lymphoid elements, but also functional ones (Bienenstock *et al.*, 1978). As discussed subsequently, MALT is characterized by the predominance of local IgA production and by the finding that activated lymphocytes derived from one mucosal surface can recirculate and localize selectively to other mucosal surfaces. This connection between different mucosal surfaces permits immunity initiated at one anatomical site to protect other mucosal sites. Therefore, the tissues that are considered part of MALT include the middle ear, parts of the urogenital tract,

Table I Components of the Mucosa-Associated Lymphoid Tissue

Intestine (GALT)
Bronchial tree (BALT)
Nasopharyngeal area (NALT)
Mammary gland
Salivary and lacrimal glands
Genitourinary organs
Inner ear

the mammary gland, the conjunctiva, the salivary glands, and the tonsils [as part of the nasopharyngeal lymphoid tissue (NALT); Kuper *et al.,* 1992], as well as BALT and GALT (see Figure 2).

II. ONTOGENY

Significant species differences exist in the ontogeny of mucosal lymphoid tissues that suggest possible differences in function. In humans, lymphoid aggregates are present at birth whereas in rodents they develop after the first few weeks of life. In humans Peyer's patches develop *in utero* and increase in size and number with the exposure to gut flora, but then decrease with age (Cornes, 1965). T and B cells are found in clusters by 14 weeks gestation and increase in number thereafter; the early B cells express IgM, IgD, and CD5 (Spencer *et al.,* 1986a). Germinal centers only develop after birth (Bridges *et al.,* 1959).

In the mouse, follicles are first identified as a cluster of reticular cells that, by day 3 after birth, become populated by lymphocytes (Joel *et al.,* 1971; Ferguson and Parrott, 1972a). Primary nodules then appear between 3 and 7 days and germinal centers between 4 and 5 weeks of age (Ferguson and Parrott, 1972a), but not in germ-free mice (Pollard and Sharon, 1970). Interestingly, no germinal centers are seen in the Peyer's patches of the nude mouse, suggesting a T-cell dependence (Parrott, 1976). Therefore, in humans a significant degree of Peyer's patch development appears to occur independent of gut flora.

In humans, lymphoid cells including $CD4^+$ T cells appear in the lamina propria by 14 weeks gestation, whereas B cells appear by 22 weeks gestation. Plasma cells, on the other hand, only develop 12 days after birth (Perkkio and Savilahti, 1980; Spencer *et al.,* 1986a), whereas plasma cells in the lamina propria appear only after day 10 in the mouse. In humans, IELs can be identified in the fetal intestine by 11 weeks gestation (Spencer *et al.,* 1986b), whereas in mice IEL are found only by the third week of life (MacDonald and Spencer, 1990). Although this event is coincident with weaning in the mouse, it is not antigen-dependent (Ferguson and Parrott, 1972b; Ferguson, 1977). On the other hand, the gut flora does influence the number and phenotype of IELs (Ferguson and Parrott, 1972a; Leigh *et al.,* 1985). Clearly, luminal antigen has a great influence on the development of several compartments of GALT in humans and in rodents.

III. FUNCTION OF MUCOSA-ASSOCIATED LYMPHOID TISSUE

The function of MALT can be divided into three main categories (Table II). The induction of the local immune response and the effector mechanisms of local immunity have been the focus of much of the experimental work on MALT. In addition, however, the role that MALT may play as a primary immune organ, as suggested long ago, has become the focus of more recent work.

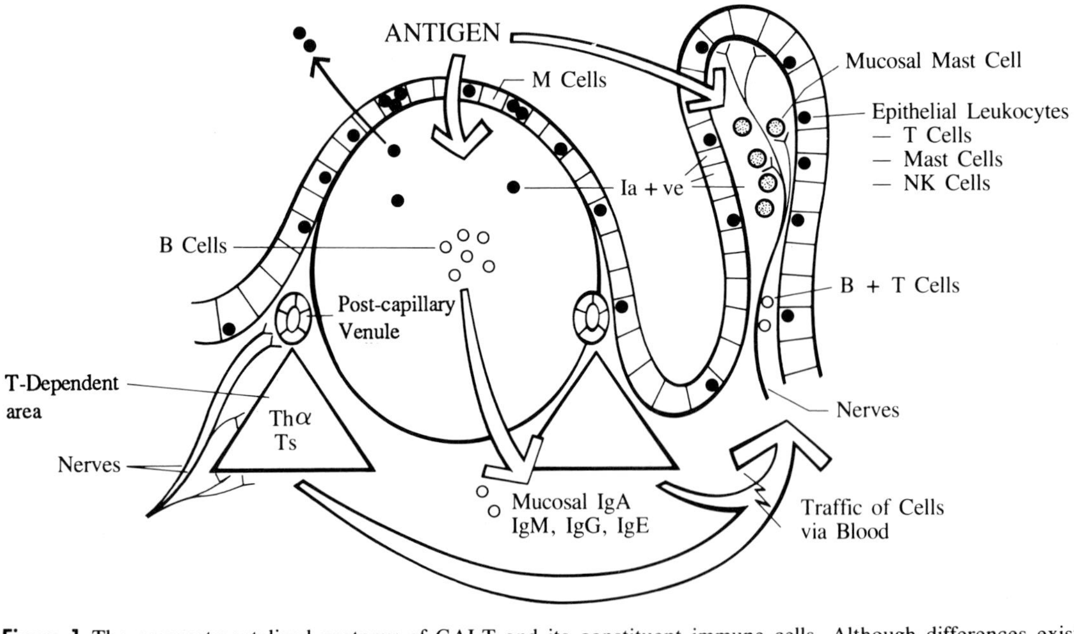

Figure 1 The compartmentalized anatomy of GALT and its constituent immune cells. Although differences exist between different tissues, the general organization of MALT is similar to that depicted for GALT.

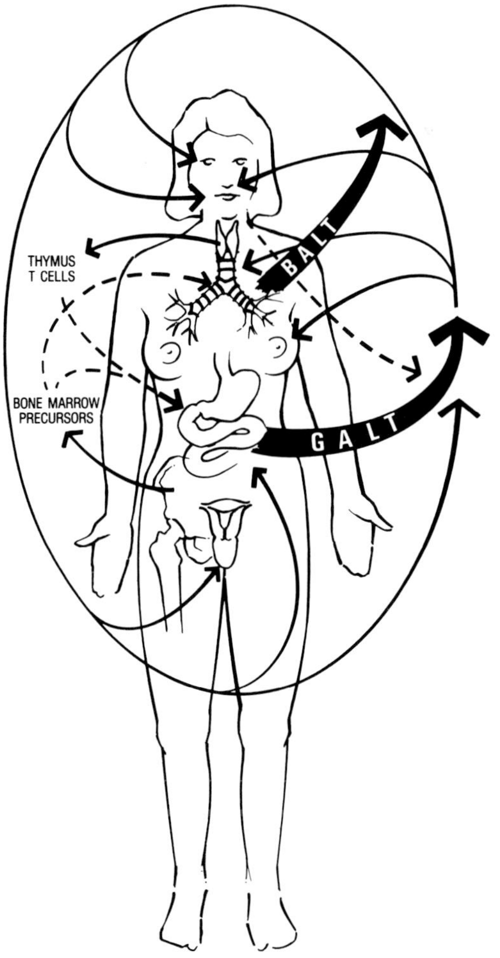

Figure 2 Lymphoid elements in GALT from the bone marrow or thymus enter the mucosa through specific high endothelial venules to occupy the different compartments. Thymic-independent mucosal T cells may arise in the fetal liver or bone marrow or develop within the intestine itself. Primary antigen exposure can occur within the Peyer's patches or possibly in the draining lymph nodes. In the Peyer's patches, B cells committed to IgA production and sensitized to foreign antigen are stimulated to proliferate. Lymphoblasts emigrate via the efferent lymphatics and mesenteric lymph nodes to the thoracic duct to recirculate via the blood stream. T lymphoblasts, detected in the thoracic duct lymph, also can recirculate. These cells can repopulate various mucosa-associated lymphoid tissues selectively undergo terminal differentiation.

A. Primary Lymphoid Development

1. Bursa of Fabricius

One of the most intriguing organs of the mucosal immune system is the bursa of Fabricius. Found in chickens, the bursa is a specialized organ that contains a major collection of lymphoid follicles in a hollow pouch-like outgrowth dorsal to the cloaca at the end of the gut. This outgrowth is attached to the cloaca by a long thin duct. The mucosal surface within this pouch is folded and contains numerous lymphoid follicles. The epithelium overlying these follicles does not lie on

Table II Functions of the Mucosa-Associated Lymphoid Tissue

Primary lymphoid development
Induction and amplification of the mucosal immune responses
Effector mechanisms of local immunity

a basement membrane and is part of a stratified network of stellate cells that forms the medulla of each follicle. This medulla is bounded by the basal lamina, and the cortex of the follicle lies outside this basal lamina. Lymphocytes infiltrate the medulla and epithelium overlying the follicle and may form clumps (Owen and Bhalla, 1983). This "lymphoepithelium" represents the site of primary B-cell development in the chicken (Owen and Bhalla, 1983). The bursa also can serve in antigen sampling.

2. Mammalian Bursa Equivalent

In mammals, the absence of a bursa or any other clearly identifiable organ of primary B-cell development has led to a search for the "mammalian bursa equivalent." The fact that the bursa of Fabricius is part of the intestine led to speculation that mammalian GALT might serve as a site of primary lymphoid development. The features of the bursa that are characteristic of a primary lymphoid organ include a follicular structure that develops independent of antigenic stimulation, the absence of fully differentiated plasma cells; the presence of rapid cellular proliferation, thymic independence, essential nature with respect to the development of follicles in other secondary lymphoid organs, and identification as the first site of immunoglobulin synthesis (Perey, 1971). Mammalian GALT does not fulfill all these characteristics.

In 1963, Archer first suggested that the rabbit appendix might represent the bursa homolog (Archer *et al.*, 1963), an idea that was supported by others (Perey *et al.*, 1970). Several groups have shown that X irradiation and removal of the appendix, Peyer's patches, and sacculus rotundus in rabbits leads to a selective defect in antibody production (Cooper *et al.*, 1966; Perey *et al.*, 1970; Heatley *et al.*, 1982). On the other hand, the lymphoid aggregates, associated with the epithelium, such as the tonsil and Peyer's patches, do not appear to have a true lymphoepithelium in which primary B-cell development occurs (Perey, 1971). Further, Peyer's patches are found in the chicken, in which the bursa is clearly the site of B-cell development (Befus *et al.*, 1980). Therefore, the existence of a mammalian bursa equivalent in the intestine remains controversial (Archer *et al.*, 1963; Fichtelius, 1966; Meuwissen *et al.*, 1969; Perey *et al.*, 1970). More recent studies now point to the fetal yolk sac, liver, spleen, and bone marrow as sites of primary B-cell development in mammals (Owen *et al.*, 1974).

However, this issue has been re-examined in the lymphoid follicles of the proximal colon in rodents and in the Peyer's patches in sheep (Perry and Sharp, 1988; Motyka and Reynolds, 1991). In sheep Peyer's patches, for example, antigen-independent B-cell proliferation and local apoptosis occur, and evidence suggests that immunoglobulin diversity is generated *in situ* (Griebel *et al.*, 1991; Motyka and Reynolds, 1991; Reynaud *et al.*, 1991). The CD5 or Ly1 B-cell lineage also has been shown to develop in lymphoid aggregates, referred to as milk spots, that are found in the omentum of human and mouse (Solvason and Kearney, 1992; Solvason *et al.*, 1992). Collectively, these data suggest that some degree of early differentiation of B-cell elements can occur in mammalian GALT. The advantage of the local development of the B-cell repertoire is not clear, although one could speculate that it might be involved in the generation of oral tolerance.

T-cell differentiation in the intestine also differs from that of peripheral thymus-derived T cell. Evidence is now emerging that suggests that intestinal T cells, particularly the IELs, can develop independent of thymic processing (Lefrancois *et al.*, 1990; Mosley *et al.*, 1990; Guy-Grand *et al.*, 1991; Barrett *et al.*, 1992; Croitoru and Ernst, 1992). Although the process of repertoire selection could occur in the intestinal mucosa (Bonneville *et al.*, 1990; Bandeira *et al.*, 1991; Rocha *et al.*, 1991), this event has not been demonstrated directly. The presence of a diffuse primary lymphoid organ in the intestinal epithelium, albeit for B cells, was suggested first by Fichtelius (1968). If the mucosal T-cell repertoire does indeed develop in the intestinal environment, the local antigenic milieu could influence the reactivity of these cells.

B. Afferent Limb of the Local Immune Response

1. Peyer's Patch

The Peyer's patches are lymphoid aggregates, first described by Johanni Conradi Peyeri in 1677 in his thesis entitled "De Glandulis Intestinorum Earumque Usu et Affectionibus Cui Fubjungitur Anatome Ventriculi Gallinacei." These clusters are found on the antemesenteric side of the distal small bowel (ileum) and colon and extend through the lamina propria and submucosa. The patches appear as mounds protruding between the intestinal villi and, on the serosal surface, as a group of small bulges. In humans, Peyer's patches increase in number and size progressively down the distal small intestine.

Peyer's patches differ from lymph nodes elsewhere in the body because they lack afferent lymphatics. This characteristic is in keeping with the notion that antigen is sampled from the lumen via the overlying epithelium. The efferent lymphatics drain to the mesenteric lymph nodes. In the normal adult, Peyer's patches contain germinal centers with B cells and internodular zones that are predominantly T cells (Faulk *et al.*, 1970; Parrott, 1976; Mayrhofer, 1984). The lymphocytes in the central areas of the follicle include IgM-, IgG-, IgA-, and IgE-producing B cells, although IgA-producing cells predominate. Interspersed are T cells, predominately CD4 helper T cells, and macrophages that function as antigen-presenting cells (APCs).

2. Antigen Uptake and Presentation

The Peyer's patches are considered a major site of initiation of the local immune response in the gut, although some researchers suggest that these clusters serve more as an amplification system in which B cells primed elsewhere are exposed to antigen (Waksman and Ozer, 1976). In this regard, investigators have suggested that the site in which priming of mucosal B-cell responses may occur is the draining lymph nodes (Craig and Cebra, 1971; Gearhart and Cebra, 1979; Cebra *et al.*, 1991). Nonetheless, in the Peyer's patches, antigen can be taken up and presented to mucosal lymphocytes. The epithelium overlying these lymphoid follicles samples and transports antigen from the lumen to the adjacent APCs and lymphoid cells (Owen and Nemanic, 1978). Referred to as the FAE, this epithelium is devoid of goblet cells and consists of specialized cuboidal cells derived from adjacent crypts (Owen and Jones, 1974; Bockman and Cooper, 1975; Bhalla and Owen, 1982). Among the FAE are further specialized cells, the M cells, that have a decreased number of small apical microvilli. The microvilli actually are replaced by microfolds, hence the name "M cell." In addition, M cells have increased numbers of cytoplasmic vesicles in which particulate antigen is transported across the cell from luminal to basement membrane surface (Owen and Jones, 1974; Owen, 1977; Smith and Peacock, 1992). Some viruses and bacteria have been shown to bind to M cells specifically (Inman and Cantey, 1971; Carter and Collins, 1974; Wolf *et al.*, 1981), making this a preferential route of entry. Given the concentration of antigen uptake at this site one should note that erosion of the FAE over the surface of Peyer's patches, (the aphthous ulcer) is the earliest lesion seen in Crohn's disease (Rickert and Carter, 1980).

The antigen transported into the Peyer's patches is then taken up by macrophages, which process and present antigen to the local T cells (MacDonald and Carter, 1982). The underlying progenitors of IgA-secreting plasma cells found in the Peyer's patches are then the first lymphocytes to be exposed to these foreign antigens (Craig and Cebra, 1975; Befus *et al.*, 1978).

3. Absorptive Epithelial Cells

The absorptive epithelial cells on the luminal two-thirds of the villi of the small bowel of rat and human express the major histocompatibility complex (MHC) Class II antigen (Scott *et al.*, 1980; Mayrhofer *et al.*, 1983). The FAE overlying the Peyer's patches, on the other hand, are devoid of MHC Class II expression (Owen, 1977), suggesting that the intestinal epithelial cells may have a role in antigen presentation distinct from that of the FAE. Interestingly, the epithelial cells have been shown to stimulate the CD8 or cytotoxic/suppressor T cell preferentially (Mayer and Schlien, 1987; Bland, 1988; Bland and Kambarage, 1991). This preference may represent a mechanism that down-regulates the local immune response, preventing unwanted inflammatory responses to food antigens and normal gut flora.

C. Effector Arm of MALT

1. Humoral Immunity—IgA

IgA, first discovered by Heremans (Heremans *et al.*, 1959), was shown to exist in the unique form of secretory IgA (SIgA) as the predominant immunoglobulin in external secretions (Chodirker and Tomasi, 1963; Tomasi *et al.*, 1965). In addition to IgA, IgG-, IgM- and IgE-secreting cells exist in the intestinal lamina propria, albeit at a much lower frequency. Phylogenetically, IgA is not found in some lower life forms such as cold-blooded animals. IgA deficiency in humans is associated variably with significant disease or morbidity, suggesting that IgA is not necessary for survival. However, IgA does represent a considerable advance in the adaptation of the local immune response to the rather hostile environment encountered in mucosal secretions. Certain functional properties of IgA make it ideal for protecting mucosal surfaces. First, IgA is more resistant to proteolytic degradation than IgG or monomeric IgA (Shuster, 1971; Underdown and Dorrington, 1974). Second, a specific mechanism exists for the transport of polymeric IgA (or IgM) from the lamina propria into the lumen via the epithelial cell receptor, secretory component (SC) (Brandtzaeg *et al.*, 1988). Finally, IgA does not activate complement via the classical pathway and, therefore, tends not to induce potentially damaging inflammatory reactions (Colten and Bienenstock, 1974), but functions to neutralize toxins and viruses (Ogra *et al.*, 1968; Holmgren *et al.*, 1975) and to prevent bacterial adherence to epithelial cells (Williams and Gibbons, 1972).

IgE-producing cells are found in the mucosal tissues, including Peyer's patches, as well. Durkin *et al.* (1981), in fact, showed that the numbers of IgE-bearing cells were increased in neonatal and germ-free mice and that, on conventionalization, this reverted to IgA synthesis.

The predominance of IgA in mucosal secretions is thought to be the result of the collection of IgA-selective regulatory T cells. For example, in the Peyer's patches, regulatory helper T cells are involved in switching IgM^+ B cells to IgA^+ B cells as well as in the terminal differentiation of IgA B cells (Kawanishi *et al.*, 1983a,b; Beagley *et al.*, 1989; McGhee *et al.*, 1989). As discussed subsequently, when these lymphocytes encounter antigen and become activated, they leave the Peyer's patches, since antigen specific Ig cannot be detected in Peyer's patches after oral immunization (Dolezel and Bienenstock, 1971). These lymphocytes recirculate back to the mucosa, occupying the lamina propria, where the B cell differentiates into IgA-secreting plasma cells (Befus *et al.*, 1978). Therefore, the presence of dimeric IgA has become synonymous with MALT.

2. Cellular Immunity

Within the epithelium, above the basement membrane, is a heterogenous population of mononuclear cells referred to as IELs. These cells include a large population of T cells expressing T-cell receptor and CD8. The nature of these cells, their function, and their lineage relationship to thymic-dependent T cells is not clear (Croitoru and Ernst, 1992). In addition, IELs contain mast cells and their precursors, as well as antitumor and antiviral natural killer (NK) cells (Arnaud-Battandier *et al.*, 1978; Tagliabue *et al.*, 1982; Schrader *et al.*, 1983; Ernst *et al.*, 1985; Carman *et al.*, 1986). This population, therefore, has both natural cytolytic activity and classical MHC-restricted cytotoxic T cells (Ernst *et al.*, 1986). The granules of IELs contain proteases that may play a role in influencing epithelial cell function (Guy-Grand *et al.*, 1991). In fact, a possible biological function of the IELs may be regulating the absorptive and secretory function of the epithelial cells in response to antigenic stimuli. This regulation could occur through the release of the contents of these granules or through the release of cytokines, and would be important to consider when examining the pathogenesis of inflammatory diseases of the bowel.

Within the lamina propria are lymphocytes with cytotoxic potential as well as T cells with the ability to produce cytokines. The cytotoxic T cells include cells that can be activated by stimulation of the T-cell receptor to produce tumor necrosis factor α (TNFα) or interferon γ (IFNγ) (Elson *et al.*, 1986; James and Strober, 1986; Deem *et al.*, 1991). These cytokines have been shown to affect epithelial cell growth and function, including the expression of MHC Class II molecules used for antigen presentation (Kvale *et al.*, 1988; Lundin *et al.*, 1990). Such interactions between elements of GALT and the structural elements of the intestine are emerging as important functions to examine in our attempt to understand the control of the physiological function of the gut.

3. Neural Control

The regulation of these effector functions is, in part, influenced by the local nervous tissue. The mucosal tissues, because they are highly innervated, have a major accumulation of neurotransmitters such as substance P, somatostatin, and vasointestinal polypeptide (VIP). These neurotransmitters have been shown to interact with and regulate the local immune response. Substance P, for example, can influence lymphocyte proliferation, antibody secretion, and even mucosal NK activity (Stanisz *et al.*, 1986; Croitoru *et al.*, 1990). Further, VIP has been shown to influence the selective trafficking of lymphocytes to mucosal tissues (Ottaway, 1984). These and other influences of neuropeptides and the local immune cells provide a mechanism for important interactions between the central nervous system and the local immune response (Stead *et al.*, 1987).

4. Lymphocyte Traffic

As discussed earlier, mucosal lymphocytes can recirculate and traffic between different mucosal tissues (see Figure 2). The MLN, for example, contains precursors for IgA plasma cells that, when adoptively transferred, will repopulate the lamina propria within 24 hr (Gowans and Knight, 1964). Thoracic duct lymphocytes also recirculate and enter the lamina propria (Gowans and Knight, 1964); this movement appears to be antigen independent (Ferguson, 1974; Halstead and Hall, 1992). Both Peyer's patch lymphocytes and BALT contain precursors for IgA-secreting plasma cells (Craig and Cebra, 1975) that could seed the intestinal lamina propria (Bienenstock *et al.*, 1978). More recent work has examined the interactions that occur between the circulating lymphocytes and the vascular endothelium in the mucosa and Peyer's patches that allow for the selective homing to mucosal tissues (Gallatin *et al.*, 1983; Navarro *et al.*, 1985; Jalkanen *et al.*, 1988).

This homing highlights the communication that exists between different mucosal sites, and allow specific antigen reactivity to extend quickly over all these tissues (Bienenstock and Dolezel, 1971). Thus, the common mucosal immune system or MALT functionally behaves as one immune organ (Bienenstock *et al.,* 1978; McDermott and Bienenstock, 1979). The value of this function is exemplified by the success of oral vaccination with poliovirus, for which immunization at one mucosal site leads to protection at a second.

One of the mysteries of mucosal immunology has been the fate of the IEL population. Considered by some as terminally differentiated cells, IELs have been speculated to cross the basement membrane in both directions (Marsh, 1975). In fact, work in *Eimeria*-infected chicken has shown that IELs containing the parasite acquired in the epithelium can return to the tissues (Lawn and Rose, 1982). On the other hand, IELs have poor migratory ability (Bacq *et al.,* 1987) and turnover at quite a different rate than the adjacent epithelium (Darlington and Rogers, 1966).

Details of the molecular interactions and adhesion molecules involved in the selective trafficking of mucosal lymphocytes are discussed in other chapters.

IV. CONCLUSION

MALT is a complex immune organ spread over a large noncontiguous tissue that is the major barrier between the external and internal environments. This organ has evolved to protect the host without inducing potentially damaging local inflammatory responses. How this tightly regulated response is altered and how the integrity of mucosal surfaces is maintained is the key to understanding these tissues, and may be the key to the treatment of disease involving these tissues.

Acknowledgments

Work described in this chapter that was done by the authors was supported by the Medical Research Council of Canada and the Canadian Foundation for Ileitis and Colitis.

References

Amoss, H. L., and Taylor, E. (1917). Neutralization of the virus of poliomyelitis by nasal washings. *J. Exp. Med.* **25,** 507–523.

Archer, O. K., Sutherland, D. E. R., and Good, R. A. (1963). Appendix of the rabbit: A homologue of the bursa in the chicken? *Nature (London)* **200,** 337–339.

Arnaud-Battandier, F., Bundy, B. M., O'Neill, M., Bienenstock, J., and Nelson, D. L. (1978). Cytotoxic activities of gut mucosal lymphoid cells in guinea pigs. *J. Immunol.* **121,** 1059–1065.

Baca, M. E., Mowat, A. M., Mackenzie, S., and Parrott, D. M. V. (1987). Functional characteristics of intraepithelial lymphocytes from mouse small intestine III. Inability of intraepithelial lymphocytes to induce a systemic graft-versus-host reaction is because of failure to migrate *in vivo*. *Gut* **28,** 1267–1274.

Bandeira, A., Itohara, S., Bonneville, M., Burlen-Defranoux, O., Mota-Santos, T., Coutinho, A., and Tonegawa, S. (1991). Extrathymic origin of intestinal intraepithelial lymphocytes bearing T-cell antigen receptor gammaδ. *Proc. Natl. Acad. Sci. U.S.A.* **88,** 43–47.

Barrett, T. A., Delvy, M. L., Kennedy, D. M., Lefrancois, L., Matis, L. A., Dent, A. L., Hedrick, S. M., and Bluestone, J. A. (1992). Mechanisms of self-tolerance of gamma/δ T cells in epithelial tissue. *J. Exp. Med.* **175,** 65–70.

Beagley, K. W., Eldridge, J. H., Lee, F., Kiyono, H., Everson, M. P., Koopman, W. J., Hirano, T., Kishimoto, T., and Mcghee, J. R. (1989). Interleukins and IgA synthesis. Human and murine interleukin 6 induce high rate IgA secretion in IgA-committed B cells. *J. Exp. Med.* **169,** 2133–2148.

Befus, A. D., O'Neill, M., and Bienenstock, J. (1978). Immediate IgA precursor cells in rabbit intestinal lamina propria. *Immunology* **35,** 901–906.

Befus, A. D., Johnston, N., Leslie, G. A., and Bienenstock, J. (1980). Gut-associated lymphoid tissue in the chicken. I. Morphology, ontogeny, and some functional characteristics of Peyer's patches. *J. Immunol.* **125,** 2626–2632.

Besredka, A. (1927). Dysentery. *In* "Local Immunization. Specific Dressings" (H. Plotz, ed.) pp. 85–107. Williams & Wilkins, Baltimore.

Bhalla, D. K., and Owen, R. L. (1982). Cell renewal and migration in lymphoid follicles of Peyer's patches and cecum—An autoradiographic study in mice. *Gastroenterology* **82,** 232.

Bienenstock, J. (1984). Bronchus-associated lymphoid tissue. *In* "Immunology of the Lung and Upper Respiratory Tract" (J. Bienenstock, ed.), pp. 96–118. McGraw-Hill, New York.

Bienenstock, J., and Dolezel, J. (1971). Peyer's patches: Lack of specific antibody-containing cells after oral and perenteral immunization. *J. Immunol.* **106,** 938–945.

Bienenstock, J., and Johnston, N. (1976). A morphologic study of rabbit bronchial lymphoid aggregates and lymphoepithelium. *Lab. Invest.* **35,** 343–348.

Bienenstock, J., Johnston, N., and Perey, D. Y. E. (1973a). Bronchial lymphoid tissue. I. Morphologic characteristics. *Lab. Invest.* **28,** 686–692.

Bienenstock, J., Johnston, N., and Perey, D. Y. E. (1973b). Bronchial lymphoid tissue. II. Functional characteristics. *Lab. Invest.* **28,** 693–698.

Bienenstock, J., McDermott, M., Befus, D., and O'Neill, M. (1978). A common mucosal immunologic system involving the bronchus, breast, and bowel. *Adv. Exp. Med. Biol.* **107,** 53–59.

Bland, P. W. (1988). MHC class II expression by the gut epithelium. *Immunol. Today* **9,** 174–178.

Bland, P. W., and Kambarage, D. M. (1991). Antigen handling by the epithelium and lamina propria macrophages. *Gastroenterol. Clin. North Am.* **20,** 577–596.

Bland, P. W., and Whiting, C. V. (1989). Antigen processing by isolated rat intestinal villus enterocytes. *Immunology* **68,** 497–502.

Bockman, D. E., and Cooper, M. D. (1975). Early lymphoepithelial relationships in human appendix. A combined light- and electron-microscopic study. *Gastroenterology* **68,** 1160.

Bonneville, M., Itohara, S., Krecko, E. G., Mombaerts, P., Ishida, I., Katsuki, M., Berns, A., Farr, A. G., Janeway, C. A., and Tonegawa, S. (1990). Transgenic mice demonstrate that epithelial homing of gamma/delta T cells is determined by cell lineages independent of T cell receptor specificity. *J. Exp. Med.* **171,** 1015–1026.

Brandtzaeg, P., Sollid, L. M., Thrane, P. S., Kvale, D., Bjerke, K., Scott, H., Kett, K., and Rognum, T. O. (1988). Lymphoepithelial interactions in the mucosal immune system. *Gut* **29,** 1116–1130.

Bridges, R. A., Condie, R. M., Zak, S. J., and Good, R. A. (1959). The morphologic basis of antibody formation development during the neonatal period. *J. Lab. Clin. Med.* **53,** 331–357.

Byrne, H. J., and Nelson, P. M. (1939). Nature of immunity to *Trichomonas foetus* infection in rabbits. *Arch. Pathol.* **28,** 761.

Carman, P. S., Ernst, P. B., Rosenthal, K. L., Clark, D. A., Befus,

A. D., and Bienenstock, J. (1986). Intraepithelial leukocytes contain a unique subpopulation of NK-like cytotoxic cells active in the defense of gut epithelium to enteric murine coronavirus. *J. Immunol.* **136,** 1548–1553.

Carter, P. B., and Collins, F. M. (1974). The route of enteric infection in normal mice. *J. Exp. Med.* **139,** 1189–1203.

Cebra, J. J., Schrader, C. E., Shroff, K. E., and Weinstein, P. D. (1991). Are Peyer's patch germinal centre reactions different from those occurring in other lymphoid tissues. *Res. Immunol.* **142,** 222–226.

Chodirker, W. B., and Tomasi, T. B. (1963). Gamma-globulin: Quantitative relationships in human serum and nonvascular fluids. *Science* **142,** 1080–1081.

Colten, H. R., and Bienenstock, J. (1974). Lack of C3 activation through classical or alternte pathways by human secretory IgA anti-blood group A antibody. *Adv. Exp. Med. Biol.* **45,** 305–308.

Cooper, M. D., Perey, D. Y., McKneally, M. S., Gabrielsen, A. E., Sutherland, D. E. R., and Good, R. A. (1966). A mammalian equivalent of the avian bursa of Fabricius. *Lancet* **i,** 1388–1391.

Cornes, J. S. (1965). Number, size, and distribution of Peyer's pathces in the human small intestine. Part I. The development of Peyer's patches. *Gut* **6,** 225–229.

Craig, S. W., and Cebra, J. J. (1971). Peyer's patches: An enriched source of precursors for IgA-producing immunocytes in the rabbit. *J. Exp. Med.* **134,** 188–200.

Craig, S. W., and Cebra, J. J. (1975). Rabbit Peyer's patches, appendix, and popliteal lymph node B lymphocytes. A comparative analysis of their membrane immunoglobulin components and plasma cell precursor potential. *J. Immunol.* **114,** 492–502.

Croitoru, K., Ernst, P. B., Bienenstock, J., Padol, I., and Stanisz, A. M. (1990). Selective modulation of the natural killer activity of murine intestinal intraepithelial leukocytes by the neuropeptide substance P. *Immunology* **71,** 196–201.

Croitoru, K., and Ernst, P. B. (1992). Leukocytes in the intestinal epithelium: An unusual immunological compartment revisited. *Reg. Immunol.* **4,** 63–69.

Darlington, D., and Rogers, A. W. (1966). Epithelial lymphocytes in the small intestine of the mouse. *J. Anat.* **100,** 813.

Davies, A. (1922). Serological properties of dysentery stools. *Lancet* **2,** 2009.

Deem, R. L., Shanahan, F., and Targan, S. R. (1991). Triggered human mucosal T cells release tumour necrosis factor-alpha and interferon-gamma which kill human colonic epithelial cells. *Clin. Exp. Immunol.* **83,** 79–84.

Dolezel, J., and Bienenstock, J. (1971). GammaA and non-gammaA responses after oral and parenteral immunization of the hamster. *Cell. Immunol.* **2,** 458–468.

Durkin, H. G., Bazin, H., and Waksman, B. H. (1981). Origin and fate of IgE bearing lymphocytes. I. Peyer's patches as a differentiation site of cells simultaneously bearing IgA and IgE. *J. Exp. Med.* **154,** 640–652.

Elson, C. O., Kagnoff, M. F., Fiocchi, C., and Befus, A. D. (1986). Intestinal immunity and inflammation: Recent progress. *Gastroenterology* **91,** 746–768.

Ernst, P. B., Befus, A. D., and Bienenstock, J. (1985). Leukocytes in the intestinal epithelium. An unusual immunological compartment. *Immunol. Today* **6,** 50–55.

Ernst, P. B., Clark, D. A., Rosenthal, K. L., Befus, A. D., and Bienenstock, J. (1986). Detection and characterization of cytotoxic T lymphocyte precurors in the murine intestinal intraepithelial leukocyte population. *J. Immunol.* **136,** 2121–2126.

Faulk, W. P., McCormick, J. N., Goodman, J. R., Yoffey, J. M., and Fudenberg, H. H. (1970). Peyer's patches: Morphologic studies. *Cell. Immunol.* **1,** 500–520.

Ferguson, A. (1974). Secretion of IgA into 'antigen-free' isografts of mouse small intestine. *Clin. Exp. Immunol.* **17,** 691–696.

Ferguson, A. (1977). Intraepithelial lymphocytes of the small intestine. *Gut* **18,** 921–937.

Ferguson, A., and Parrott, D. M. V. (1972a). The effect of antigen deprivation on thymus-dependant and thymus-independant lymphocytes in the small intestine of the mouse. *Clin. Exp. Immunol.* **12,** 477–488.

Ferguson, A., and Parrott, D. M. V. (1972b). Growth and development of "antigen-free' grafts of foetal mouse intestine. *J. Pathol.* **106,** 95–101.

Fichtelius, K. E. (1966). The mammalian equivalent to bursa fabricii of birds. *Exp. Cell Res.* **466,** 231–234.

Fichtelius, K. E. (1968). The gut epithelium-A first level lymphoid organ? *Exp. Cell Res.* **49,** 87–104.

Gallatin, W. M., Weissman, I. L., and Butcher, E. C. (1983). A cell-surface molecule involved in organ-specific homing of lymphocytes. *Nature (London)* **303,** 30.

Gearhart, P. J., and Cebra, J. J. (1979). Differentiated B lymphocytes. Potential to express particular antibodies of variable and constant regions depends on site of lymphoid tissue and antigen load. *J. Exp. Med.* **149,** 216–227.

Good, R. A., and Papermaster, B. W. (1964). Ontogeny and phylogeny of adoptive immunity. *In* "Advances in Immunology" (F. J. Dixon and J. H. Humphrey, eds.), pp. 1–115. Academic Press, New York.

Gowans, J. L., and Knight, E. J. (1964). The route of recirculation of lymphocytes in the rat. *Proc. R. Soc. London (Biol.)* **159,** 257–282.

Griebel, P. J., Davis, W. C., and Reynolds, J. D. (1991). Negative signaling by surface IgM on B cells isolated from ileal Peyer's patch follicles of sheep. *Eur. J. Immunol.* **21,** 2281–2284.

Guy-Grand, D., Cerf-Bensussan, N., Malissen, B., Malassis-Seris, M., Briottet, C., and Vassalli, P. (1991). Two gut intraepithelial $CD8^+$ lymphocyte populations with different T cell receptors: A role for the gut epithelium in T cell differentiation. *J. Exp. Med.* **173,** 471–481.

Halstead, T. G., and Hall, J. G. (1992). The homing of lymph-borne immunoblasts to the small gut of neonatal rats. *Transplantation* **14,** 339–346.

Heatley, R. V., Befus, A. D., and Bienenstock, J. (1982). *Nippostrongylus brasiliensis* infection in the rat: Effects of surgical removal of Peyer's patches, mesenteric lymph nodes and spleen. *Int. Arch. Allergry Appl. Immunol.* **68,** 397–398.

Heremans, J. F., Heremans, M.-Th., and Schultz, H. E. (1959). Isolation and description of a few properties of the β2A-globulin of human serum. *Clin. Chim. Acta* **4,** 96–102.

Holmgren, J., Svennerholm, A.-M., Ouchterlony, Ö., Andersson, Å., Wallerström, G., and Westerberg-Berndtsson, U. (1975). Antitoxic immunity in experimental cholera: Protection, and serum and local antibody responses in rabbits after enteral and parenteral immunization. *Infect. Immun.* **12,** 1331–1340.

Inman, L. R., and Cantey, J. R. (1971). Specific adherence of *Escherichia coli* (Strain RDEC-1) to membranous (M) cells of Peyer's patches in *Escherichia coli* diarrhea in the rabbit. *J. Clin. Invest.* **1,** 1983.

Jalkanen, S., Jalkanen, M., Bargatze, R., Tammi, M., and Butcher, E. C. (1988). Biochemical properties of glycoproteins involved in lymphocyte recognition of high endothelial venules in man. *J. Immunol.* **141,** 1615–1623.

James, S. P., and Strober, W. (1986). Cytotoxic lymphocytes and intestinal disease. *Gastroenterology* **90,** 235–240.

Joel, D. D., Hess, M. W., and Cottier, H. (1971). Thymic origin of lymphocytes in developing Peyer's patches of newborn mice. *Nature New Biol.* **231,** 24–25.

Kawanishi, H., Saltzman, L. E., and Strober, W. (1983a). Mechanisms regulating IgA class-specific immunoglobulin production in murine gut-associated lymphoid tissues. I. T cells derived from Peyer's patches that switch SIgM B cells to SIgA B cells *in vitro*. *J. Exp. Med.* **157,** 433–450.

Kawanishi, H., Saltzman, L., and Strober, W. (1983b). Mechanism regulating IgA class-specific immunoglobulin production in murine gut-associated lymphoid tissues. II. Terminal differentiation of postswitch SIgA-bearing Peyer's patch B cells. *J. Exp. Med.* **158,** 649–669.

Klein, E. (1875). "The Anatomy of the Lymphatic System. II. The Lung." Smith, Elder, London.

Kuper, C. F., Koornstra, P. J., Hameleers, D. M. H., Biewenga, J., Spit, B. J., Duijvestijn, A. M., van Breda Viesman, P. J. C., and Sminia, T. (1992). The role of nasopharyngeal lymphoid tissue. *Immunol. Today* **13,** 219–224.

Kvale, D., Lovhaug, D., Sollid, L. M., and Brandtzaeg, P. (1988). Tumour necrosis factor-alpha up-regulates expression of secretory component, the epithelial receptor for polymeric Ig. *J. Immunol.* **140,** 3086–3089.

Lawn, A. M., and Rose, M. E. (1982). Mucosal transport of *Eimeria tenella* in the cecum of the chicken. *J. Parasitol.* **68,** 1117–1123.

Lefrancois, L., LeCorre, R., Mayo, J., Bluestone, J. A., and Goodman, T. (1990). Extrathymic selection of TCR gamma/delta+ T cells by class II major histocompatability complex molecules. *Cell* **63,** 333–340.

Leigh, R. J., Marsh, M. N., Crowe, P., Kelly, C., Garner, V., and Gordon, D. (1985). Studies of intestinal lymphoid tissue IX. Dose dependent, gluten-induced lymphoid infiltration of coeliac jejunal epithelium. *Scand. J. Gastroenterol.* **20,** 715–719.

Lundin, K. E. A., Sollid, L. M., Bosnes, V., Gaudernack, G., and Thorsby, E. (1990). T-cell recognition of HLA class II molecules induced by gamma-interferon on a colonic adenocarcinoma cell line (HT29). *Scand. J. Immunol.* **31,** 469–475.

McDermott, M. R., and Bienenstock, J. (1979). Evidence for a common mucosal immunologic system. I. Migration of B immunoblasts into intestinal, respiratory, and genital tissues. *J. Immunol.* **122,** 1892–1898.

MacDonald, T. T., and Carter, P. B. (1982). Isolation and functional characteristics of adherent phagocytic cells from mouse Peyer's patches. *Immunology* **45,** 769.

MacDonald, T. T., and Spencer, J. (1990). Ontogeny of the mucosal immune response. *Springer Sem. Immunopathol.* **12,** 129–137.

McGhee, J. R., Mestecky, J., Elson, C. O., and Kiyono, H. (1989). Regulation of IgA synthesis and immune response by T cells and interleukins. *J. Clin. Immunol.* **9,** 175–199.

Marchalonis, J. J. (1974). Phylogenetic origins of antibodies and immune recognition. *In* "Progress in Immunology II" (L. Brent and J. Holborrow, eds.) pp. 249–259. North-Holland, Amsterdam.

Marsh, M. N. (1975). Studies of intestinal lymphoid tissue. II. Aspects of proliferation and migration of epithelial lymphocytes in the small intestine of mice. *Gut* **16,** 674–682.

Mayer, L., and Shlien, R. (1987). Evidence for function of Ia molecules on gut epithelial cells in man. *J. Exp. Med.* **166,** 1471–1483.

Mayrhofer, G. (1984). Physiology of the intestinal immune system. *In* "Local Immune Responses of the Gut" (T. J. Newby and C. R. Stokes, eds.) pp. 1–96. CRC Press, Boca Raton, Florida.

Mayrhofer, G., Pugh, C. W., and Barclay, A. N. (1983). The distribution, ontogeny and origin in the rat of Ia-positive cells with dendritic morphology of Ia antigen in epithelia, with reference to the intestine. *Eur. J. Immunol.* **13,** 112–122.

Meuwissen, H. J., Kaplan, G. T., Perey, D. Y. E., and Good, R. A. (1969). Role of rabbit gut-associated lymphoid tissue in cell replication. The follicular cortex as primary germinative site. *Proc. Soc. Exp. Biol. Med.* **130,** 300–304.

Mosley, R. L., Styre, D., and Klein, J. R. (1990). Differentiation and functional maturation of bone marrow-derived intestinal epithelial T cells expressing membrane TCR in athymic radiation chimeras. *J. Immunol.* **145,** 1369–1375.

Motyka, B., and Reynolds, J. D. (1991). Apoptosis is associated with the extensive B cell death in the sheep ileal Peyer's patch and the chicken bursa of Fabricius: A possible role in B cell selection. *Eur. J. Immunol.* **21,** 1951–1958.

Navarro, R. F., Jalkanen, S. T., Hsu, M., Sënderstrup-Hansen, G., Goronzy, J., Weyand, C., Fathman, C. G., Clayberger, C., Krensky, A. M., and Butcher, E. C. (1985). Human T cell clones express functional homing receptors required for normal lymphocyte trafficking. *J. Exp. Med.* **162,** 1075–1080.

Ogra, P. L., Karzon, D. T., Rightland, F., and McGillivary, M. (1968). Immunoglobulin response in serum and secretions after immunization with live and inactivated polio vaccine and natural infection. *N. Engl. J. Med.* **279,** 893–900.

Ottaway, C. A. (1984). *In vitro* alteration of receptors for vasoactive intestinal peptide changes the in vivo localization of mouse T cells. *J. Exp. Med.* **160,** 1054–1069.

Owen, J. J. T., Cooper, M. D., and Raff, M. C. (1974). *In vitro* generation of B lymphocytes in mouse foetal liver, a mammalian "bursa equivalent". *Nature (London)* **249,** 361–363.

Owen, R. L. (1977). Sequential uptake of horseradish peroxidase by lymphoid follicle epithelium of Peyer's patches in the normal unobstructed mouse intestine: An ultrastructural study. *Gastroenterology* **72,** 440–451.

Owen, R. L., and Bhalla, D. K. (1983). Lympho-epithelial organs and lymph nodes. *Biomed. Res. Appl. Sem.* **3,** 79–169.

Owen, R. L., and Jones, A. L. (1974). Epithelial cell specialization within human Peyer patches: An ultrastructural study of intestinal lymphoid follicles. *Gastroenterology* **66,** 189–203.

Owen, R. L., and Nemanic, P. (1978). Antigen processing structures of the mammalian intestinal tract: An SEM study of lymphoepithelial organs. *SEM Symp.* **II,** 367–378.

Parrott, D. M. V. (1976). The gut-associated lymphoid tissues and gastrointestinal immunity. *In* "Immunological Aspects of the Liver and Gastrointestinal Tract" (A. Ferguson and R. M. M. MacSween, eds.) pp. 1–32. MTP Press, Lancaster.

Perey, D. Y. E. (1971). Mammalian analogues of the bursal-thymic systems. *In* Cohen S, "Second International Convocation on Immunology, Buffalo, 1970" (S. Cohen, G. Cudhowicz, and R. T. McCluskey, eds.) pp. 13–24. Karger, Basel.

Perey, D. Y. E., Cooper, M. D., and Good, R. A. (1968). Lymphoepithelial tissues of the intestine and differentiation of antibody production. *Science* **161,** 265–266.

Perey, D. Y. E., Frommel, D., Hong, R., and Good, R. A. (1970). The mammalian homologue of the avian bursa of Fabricius. II. Extirpation, lethal X-irradiation, and reconstitution in rabbits. Effects on humoral immune responses, immunoglobulins, and lymphoid tissues. *Lab. Invest.* **22,** 212–227.

Perkkio, M., and Savilahti, E. (1980). Time of appearance of immunoglobulin-containing cells in the mucosa in neonatal intestine. *Pediatr. Res.* **14,** 953.

Perry, G. A., and Sharp, J. G. (1988). Characterization of proximal colonic lymphoid tissue in the mouse. *Anat. Rec.* **220,** 305–312.

Pollard, M., and Sharon, N. (1970). Responses of the Peyer's patches in germ-free mice to antigenic stimulation. *Infect. Immun.* **2,** 96–100.

Reynaud, C. A., Mackay, C. R., Muller, R. G., and Weill, J. C. (1991). Somatic generation of diversity in a mammalian primary lymphoid organ: The sheep ileal Peyer's patches. *Cell* **64,** 995–1005.

Rickert, R. R., and Carter, H. W. (1980). The "early" ulcerative lesion of Crohn's disease: Correlative light- and scanning electron-microscopic studies. *J. Clin. Gastroenterol.* **2,** 11–19.

Rocha, B., Vassalli, P., and Guy-Grand, D. (1991). The Vβ repertoire of mouse gut homodimeric α CD8$^+$ intraepithelial T cell receptor α/β^+ lymphocytes reveals a major extrathymic pathway of T cell differentiation. *J. Exp. Med.* **173,** 483–486.

Schrader, J. W., Scollay, R., and Battye, F. (1983). Intramucosal lymphocytes of the gut. Lyt2 and Thy1 phenotype of the granulated cells and evidence for the presence of both T cells and mast cell precursors. *J. Immunol.* **130,** 558–564.

Scott, H., Solheim, B. G., Brandtzaeg, P., and Thorsby, E. (1980). HLA-DR like antigens in the epithelium of human small intestine. *Scand. J. Immunol.* **12,** 77–82.

Shuster, J. (1971). Pepsin hydrolysis of IgA. Delineation of two populations of molecules. *Immunochem.* **8,** 405–411.

Smith, M. W., and Peacock, M. A. (1992). Microvillus growth and M-cell formation in mouse Peyer's patch follicle-associated epithelial tissue. *Exp. Physiol.* **77,** 389–392.

Solvason, N., and Kearney, J. F. (1992). The human fetal omentum: A site of B cell generation. *J. Exp. Med.* **175,** 397–404.

Solvason, N., Chen, X., Shu, F., and Kearney, J. F. (1992). The fetal omentum in mice and humans. A site enriched for precursors of CD5 B cells early in development. *Ann. N.Y. Acad. Sci.* **651,** 10–20.

Spencer, J., MacDonald, T. T., Finn, T., and Isaacson, P. G. (1986a). The development of gut associated lymphoid tissue in the terminal ileum of fetal human intestine. *Clin. Exp. Immunol.* **64,** 536–543.

Spencer, J., Dillon, S. B., Isaacson, P. G., and MacDonald, T. T. (1986b). T cell subclasses in fetal human ileum. *Clin. Exp. Immunol.* **65,** 553–558.

Stanisz, A. M., Befus, D., and Bienenstock, J. (1986). Differential effects of vasoactive intestinal peptide, substance P, and somatostatin on immunoglobulin synthesis and proliferation by lymphocytes from peyer's patch, mesenteric lymph node and spleen. *J. Immunol.* **136,** 152–156.

Stead, R. H., Bienenstock, J., and Stanisz, A. M. (1987). Neuropeptide regulation of mucosal immunity. *Immunol. Rev.* **100,** 333–359.

Tagliabue, A., Befus, A. D., Clark, D. A., and Bienenstock, J. (1982). Characteristics of natural killer cells in the murine intestinal epithelium and lamina propria. *J. Exp. Med.* **155,** 1785–1796.

Tomasi, T. B., and Bienenstock, J. (1968). Secretory immunoglobulins. *In* "Advances in Immunology" (F. J. Dixon and H. G. Kunkel, eds.), pp. 1–96. Academic Press, New York.

Tomasi, T. B., Tan, E. M., Solomon, A., and Prendergast, R. A. (1965). Characteristics of an immune system common to certain external secretions. *J. Exp. Med.* **121,** 101–124.

Underdown, B. J., and Dorrington, K. J. (1974). Studies on the structural and confromational basis for the relative resistance of serum and secretory immunoglobulin A to proteolysis. *J. Immunol.* **112,** 949–959.

Waksman, B. H., and Ozer, H. (1976). Specialized amplification elements in the immune system. The role of nodular lymphoid organs in the mucous membranes. *Prog. Allergy* **21,** 1.

Williams, R. C., and Gibbons, R. J. (1972). Inhibition of bacterial adherence by secretory immunoglobulin A: A mechanism of antigen disposal. *Science* **177,** 697–699.

Wolf, J. L., Rubin, D. J., Finberg, R., Kauffman, R. S., Sharpe, A. H., Trier, J. S., and Fields, B. N. (1981). Intestinal M cells: A pathway for entry of reovirus into the host. *Science* **212,** 471–472.

13

Peyer's Patches as Inductive Sites for IgA Commitment

John J. Cebra · Khushroo E. Shroff

I. ROLE OF GUT-ASSOCIATED LYMPHOID TISSUE IN THE INDUCTION OF A HUMORAL MUCOSAL IMMUNE RESPONSE

A. Effector Arm

For decades, researchers have appreciated that specific resistance to a variety of bacterial and viral pathogens that infect via the respiratory or gastrointestinal tract was better correlated with antibody titers in local exocrine secretions than with those in serum (Francis, 1940; Smith *et al.*, 1966; Fubara and Freter, 1973). The independent findings of Hanson (1961) and Tomasi (1965) and their co-workers that secretory IgA (sIgA) was the most prevalent Ig in the exocrine secretions of most mammalian species rapidly led to the recognition of this isotype as the principal mediator of virus neutralization and blocker of bacterial adhesion at the surfaces of the wet epithelium and, hence, as the main element of the humoral mucosal immune response. The partitioning of sIgA into exocrine secretions rather than blood could be explained in part by (1) local synthesis and secretion of IgA by plasma cells in lamina propria and the interstitia of exocrine glands at sites proximal to the appearance of sIgA in secretions and (2) the selective receptor-mediated transport of IgA dimer across epithelial cell barriers and into secretions. These mechanisms for enriching sIgA in secretions raised questions concerning (1) the origins and characteristics of the precursors for IgA plasma cells, (2) the sites of their specific antigen-dependent priming and commitment to IgA expression, and (3) the trafficking of these cells to secretory tissue and their selective lodging there, relative to plasmablasts making other isotypes of Ig.

B. Inductive Arm

Again, researchers have known for decades that a humoral mucosal immune response could be potentiated by exposure of mucosal surfaces to antigens, especially infectious replicating ones (see Smith *et al.*, 1966), although the efficacy of nonliving antigens given by this route as well as the value of parenteral priming to induce such a response have been controversial. A role for Peyer's patches, clusters of lymphoid follicles in the wall of the small intestine, in initiating this response was indicated strongly by analyses of tissues from lapine radiation chimeras (Craig and Cebra, 1971). Cells from a variety of lymphoid tissues—including spleen, peripheral blood, lymph nodes, appendix, and Peyer's patches—were adoptively transferred from donor rabbits into lethally irradiated, allogeneic recipients differing in Ig allotype (Craig and Cebra, 1971,1975). Only cells from gut-associated lymphoid tissue (GALT), appendix, or Peyer's patches gave rise to a preponderance of donor-derived IgA plasma cells in both the spleen and the gut lamina propria of the recipients. These observations, in conjunction with similar ones on comparison of lymphoid cells from different sources after *in vitro* culture with pokeweed mitogen (Jones *et al.*, 1974), suggested that Peyer's patches were enriched sources of precursors for IgA plasma cells. Subsequently, lymphoid cells containing equivalent numbers of B cells from different tissue sources were transferred into histocompatible, congeneic, sublethally irradiated murine recipients differing in Ig allotype (Cebra *et al.*, 1977; Tseng, 1981). Again, Peyer's patch cells were quantitatively most effective at transiently repopulating the intestinal lamina propria with donor-derived IgA plasma cells. However, all lymphoid cell sources tested in this histocompatible system, including peritoneal cavity cells (Kroese *et al.*, 1989), had the potential to contribute IgA plasma cells to the lamina propria of temporarily immunocompromised recipients.

The importance of Peyer's patches in the actual induction of a humoral mucosal immune response was supported by surgical construction in rabbits of pairs of externalized intestinal loops, which either had a Peyer's patch or lacked one (Robertson and Cebra, 1976). Introduction of antigens into the lumen of one loop resulted in the appearance of sIgA antibodies in both loops over a similar time course, but only if the immunized loop bore a Peyer's patch. If the immunized loop lacked a Peyer's patch, no appreciable response could be detected in the luminal secretions of either loop, irrespective of whether the nonimmunized loop contained a Peyer's patch. These observations are consistent with the importance of Peyer's patches in uptake of antigen from the gut lumen (see Chapters 2 and 3) or as a site where antigen-specific IgA-committed B cells are generated. The latter role was supported by an elegant rat model developed to analyze a humoral mucosal immune response by Pierce and Gowans (1975). Low doses (10–50 μg) of cholera toxin, one of the most efficacious nonreplicating mucosal immunogens known, was introduced intraduodenally twice with a fortnightly interval. Within 3–5 days of the challenge injection, a wave of cholera toxin-specific IgA plasmablasts was detected in thoracic duct lymph, followed by their accumulation in intestinal lamina propria. Using this model with extirpation of either Peyer's patches or mesenteric lymph nodes, researchers demonstrated that the presence of intact Peyer's patches but not mesenteric lymph nodes was required for the appearance of the IgA plasmablasts in thoracic duct lymph (Husband and Gowans, 1978).

II. PHENOTYPIC AND FUNCTIONAL STATUS OF PEYER'S PATCH B CELLS: PERTURBATIONS ASSOCIATED WITH COMMITMENT TO IgA AND INDUCTION OF A HUMORAL MUCOSAL IMMUNE RESPONSE

A. Correlation of Plasma Membrane (Surface) Phenotype of Peyer's Patch B Cells with Potential to Express Various Ig Isotypes

Adoptive transfer of subsets of Peyer's patch B cells, purified by fluorescence-activated cell sorting (FACS), to irradiated rabbit recipients indicated that the richest source of precursors for IgA plasma cells contained $sIgM^-$ sIg^+ B cells that bore allotype markers for IgA (Jones and Cebra, 1974; Craig and Cebra, 1975). Later, the potential of Peyer's patch B cells from mice not deliberately immunized was compared with that of B cells from other sources in a T-cell dependent antigen-dependent assay that scored individual B cells based on the output of antibody isotypes expressed by their clones (Gearhart and Cebra, 1979). Limited numbers of B cells from different sources were transferred into lethally irradiated mice that had been primed previously with a protein carrier to generate an excess of T_H cells in the recipients. Within 1 day, spleens were removed and cut into fragments that were cultured with various antigenic determinants conjugated to the protein carrier. The major findings were that frequencies of B cells of certain specificities were much higher than those of B cells with other specificities and that, often, B cells with specificities in the former group gave much higher proportions of clones that solely expressed IgA when taken from Peyer's patches than when taken from other lymphoid tissues (Gearhart and Cebra, 1979; Cebra *et al.*, 1980). These IgA-committed B cells from murine Peyer's patches commonly had specificities against molecules such as phosphocholine, β2-1 fructosyl-groups, and β galactosyl groups associated with bacterial antigens found on members of the intestinal flora (Cebra *et al.*, 1980). For this reason, it was not surprising to learn that Peyer's patches of gnotobiotic or neonatal mice lack IgA-committed B cells, but such cells appear after bacterial colonization of the gut (Cebra *et al.*, 1980,1986; Shahin and Cebra, 1981). Finally, separation of subsets of Peyer's patch B cells by FACS and assessment of their isotype potential by clonal analysis in splenic fragment cultures indicated that IgA-committed cells from Peyer's patches are $sIgA^+$ (Lebman *et al.*, 1987) and $sIgM^-sIgD^-$ (Gearhart and Cebra, 1981). Because such $sIgA^+$ B cells appear to arise after gut mucosal stimulation with antigen but require specific T_H cells and antigen to generate clones exclusively expressing the IgA isotype, we considered them operationally to represent IgA memory cells. Primary B cells, which can be isolated by FACS as $sIgM^+sIgD^+$ cells, yield clones in specific fragment (Gearhart and Cebra, 1981) or single B cell clonal microcultures (Schrader *et al.*, 1990) that can express any or all Ig isotypes, including IgA (see Cebra *et al.*, 1984). Such primary B cells predominate in all lymphoid tissue and probably account for the potential of all sources to contribute IgA plasmablasts to gut lamina propria via intraclonal isotype switching to IgA, emigration of IgA blasts to exocrine tissue, and selective accumulation at these sites (see Cebra *et al.*, 1977; Tseng, 1981; Kroese *et al.*, 1989).

B. Antigenic Stimulation of the Gut Mucosa Leads to Priming for a Subsequent Humoral Mucosal Immune Response

Much controversy existed for many years over whether or not a mucosal challenge with antigen (pathogen) could elicit a secondary mucosal IgA response—more sIgA sooner and of higher affinity than a primary sIgA response. Much of the confusion was likely the result of frequently ineffective priming for this humoral mucosal immune response. Study of the rat model for secondary responses to intraduodenal application of cholera toxin clearly showed that the challenge with cholera toxin resulted in a substantially increased number of specific IgA plasma cells in intestinal lamina propria over the number that appeared following initial gut exposure to cholera toxin (Pierce and Gowans, 1975). Acute intraduodenal or oral administration of cholera toxin, embryonated *Ascaris* eggs, or reovirus to mice resulted in 10- to 50-fold increases in antigen-specific B cells in Peyer's patches and a dominant contingent of specific IgA memory cells there (Fuhrman and Cebra, 1981; Clough and Cebra, 1983; London *et al.*, 1987). If the cholera toxin-primed mice were challenged intraduodenally *in vivo* with cholera toxin, a significant (2–5%) proportion of specific IgA plasma cells appeared in gut lamina propria (Fuhrman and Cebra, 1981). Although intraperitoneal priming with cholera toxin increased the frequency of cholera toxin-specific B cells in Peyer's patches as did intraduodenal priming with cholera toxin, it did not result in appreciable IgA-committed cells. A subsequent intraduodenal challenge with cholera toxin of intraperitoneally primed mice did not result in a significant appearance of specific IgA plasma cells in gut lamina propria. Thus, the appearance of IgA memory cells in Peyer's patches after intraduodenal priming correlates with an effective humoral mucosal immune response after gut mucosal challenge.

C. Generation of sIgA$^+$ Cells Within the Peyer's Patch—Is the Peyer's Patch a Source or a Sink for IgA-Committed B Cells?

In conventionally reared (non-germ-free) mice, the greatest number of sIgA$^+$ B cells is found in Peyer's patches, compared with any other organized lymphoid tissue (Butcher *et al.*, 1982; Lebman *et al.*, 1987). At least half these sIgA$^+$ B cells are dividing, compared with about 15% of all B cells (Lebman *et al.*, 1987). Thus, sIgA$^+$ B cells are being generated in Peyer's patches. Currently, researchers question whether B cells committed to switch to IgA expression elsewhere accumulate in Peyer's patches to receive proliferative and differentiative signals (Peyer's patch is a sink) or whether uncommitted primary B cells are recruited by antigen and specific T_H cells to undergo proliferation and preferential switching to IgA in the Peyer's patch microenvironment (Peyer's patch is a source)?

III. DO B CELLS PREFERENTIALLY ISOTYPE SWITCH TO THE EXPRESSION OF IgA IN PEYER'S PATCHES AND DO GERMINAL CENTERS PROVIDE THE MICROENVIRONMENT FOR THIS PROCESS, SERVING AS SITES FOR THE GENERATION OF IgA PREPLASMABLASTS AND IgA MEMORY CELLS?

A. Typical Characteristics of Germinal Centers and Their Putative Role in B Cell Differentiation

Germinal centers are histologically defined, roughly spherical regions that appear transiently at the base of B-cell follicles in lymph nodes and spleen after acute, often local, stimulation by antigens (see Kroese *et al.*, 1990). These centers consist mainly of B lymphoblasts, mostly dividing or dying by apoptosis, enmeshed in a network of follicular dendritic cells that also contain tingible-body macrophages and relatively few, mostly CD4$^+$, T cells (Rouse *et al.*, 1982; Szakal *et al.*, 1989; see Kosco, 1991). Typically, the germinal center reaction waxes and wanes over 3–4 weeks, reaching a maximum size about 10–14 days after antigenic stimulation (Coico *et al.*, 1983). However, rather large germinal centers are chronically present in all B-cell follicles of Peyer's patches in conventionally reared mammals (Butcher *et al.*, 1982; Weinstein *et al.*, 1991). The germinal center reaction appears to be dependent on CD4$^+$ T cells, does not occur in response to thymus-independent antigens in euthymic mice or to any antigen in athymic mice, and is much diminished in mice treated with anti-CD4 antibodies perinatally (Davies *et al.*, 1970; de Sousa and Pritchard, 1974; Tolaymat *et al.*, 1990). The follicular dendritic cell meshwork is particularly efficient at trapping antigen (Nossal and Ada, 1971), especially as antigen–antibody–complement complexes via FcR and complement receptors on the cell surface (Klaus and Humphrey, 1977). Follicular dendritic cells may express high levels of surface major histocompatibility complex (MHC) Class II antigens, possibly containing immunogenic peptide and passively acquired from B lymphoblasts (Humphrey *et al.*, 1984; Gray *et al.*, 1991). Follicular dendritic cells and germinal center B lymphoblasts can present antigen to T cells and stimulate them (Kosco *et al.*, 1988). A mechanism has been proposed that is analogous to positive selection in the thymus, by which dividing germinal center B lymphoblasts are rescued from apoptosis via higher affinity interactions of their sIg receptors with antigens and their CD40 molecules with ligands on the surface of follicular dendritic cells (Liu *et al.*, 1989,1991a). This hypothesis requires affinity maturation of sIg receptors on germinal center B cells and, possibly, various B-cell growth factors such as soluble CD23 provided by the follicular dendritic cells that may up-regulate expression of the *bcl*-2 gene in germinal center B cells, thus somehow forestalling apoptosis (Hockenbury *et al.*, 1990,1991; Liu *et al.*, 1991a).

Current dogma is that recirculating B cells are recruited by antigen or antigen–antibody complexes and CD4$^+$ T cells into a germinal center reaction as they pass through the corona of follicles; these B cells give rise to oligoclonal proliferation (Kroese *et al.*, 1987). Whether memory B cells rather than the more likely primary B cells can participate in germinal center reactions is still unknown (see Kroese *et al.*, 1991). Ig isotype switching appears to accompany B-cell proliferation in germinal centers; the earliest antigen-specific sIgG$^+$ cells that can be detected after antigenic stimulation bear a germinal center marker (Kraal *et al.*, 1982). The most encompassing germinal center marker for B cells of mice and several other mammalian species is the capacity to bind relatively high levels of the lectin peanut agglutinin (PNA^{high}) (Rose *et al.*, 1980). Regretably, this property is shared with other cell types such as cortical thymocytes and goblet cells, and often must be defined quantitatively rather than qualitatively by analysis using FACS.

In addition to Ig isotype switching, another molecular genetic process peculiarly associated with memory B cells has been detected among germinal center B lymphoblasts: point mutations in the productive VDJ and VJ segments encoding the variable regions of their H and L chains, respectively (Apel and Berek, 1990; Jacob *et al.*, 1991). Using either hybridomas formed by splenic PNA^{high} partners (Apel and Berek, 1990) or polymerase chain reaction products from small numbers of cells dissected from sections of splenic germinal centers (Jacob *et al.*, 1991), sequencing of gene segments for variable regions has indicated that point mutations arise with high frequency during B-cell division in germinal centers. Although hybridomas expressing variants of germ-line V-region genes that no longer bind the putative provoking antigen have been detected (Apel and Berek, 1990), variants expressing the sequences commonly associated with higher affinity antigen-specific memory cells have not yet been recovered (Jacob *et al.*, 1991).

Generally, germinal center B cells do not secrete detectable amounts of antibody, but immunohistochemical methods have revealed cytoplasmic specific antibody (Szakal and Tew, 1991; Terashima *et al.*, 1991). Nevertheless, a considerable variety of circumstantial and direct evidence indicates that preplasmablasts are generated in germinal centers and that some of these emigrate to secrete antibody elsewhere (see subsequent discussion). Certainly, adoptive transfer of germinal center B cells, enriched by binding to PNA, results in specific antibody responses in recipients (Coico *et al.*, 1983; Kraal *et al.*, 1988). However, requisite criteria for the transferred response being mediated by memory B cells—antigen and specific Th-cell dependence for restimulation—were not satisfied. Nevertheless, detection of point mutations in variable region genes from germinal center cells, especially their greater prevalence in complementarity determining regions, suggesting antigen selection (Apel and Berek, 1990), establishes the occurrence of a process in germinal centers that is required for the generation of memory B cells. Functional evidence for the development of memory B cells in germinal centers is awaited (see Cebra *et al.*, 1991).

B. Preferential Switching to IgA Expression by Peyer's Patch Germinal Center B Cells and Antigen-Specific Precursors of Antibody-Secreting Cells Is Likely the Result of the Intrinsic Influence of Their Microenvironment

Our previous working hypothesis was that the physiological status of the chronically present Peyer's patch germinal centers differed from the state of the transient centers in lymph nodes and that this disparancy could account for the apparent differences in isotype preference exhibited by B cells responding at the two sites to a new local antigenic stimulus (Cebra *et al.*, 1977). In other words, a novel antigenic stimulus of Peyer's patches would be superimposed on various prior environmental stimuli and would, perhaps, benefit from an unusual level or pattern of cytokines not ordinarily present in the lymph node germinal center microenvironment. One simple benefit might be an increased number of divisions—greater clonal burst size—without maturation to plasma cells by B cells in Peyer's patch germinal centers (Cebra *et al.*, 1977). Larger burst sizes stochastically might lead eventually, through consecutive isotype switching, to VDJ recombination to the $C\alpha$ gene, the most 3′ of the murine C_H gene cluster (Shimizu *et al.*, 1982). Alternatively, Peyer's patch germinal centers may differ intrinsically from those of lymph nodes in their content of particular kinds of antigen-presenting cells, stromal cells, or regulatory T cells and, hence, in the particular kinds of cytokines or switch factors available. To test these different hypotheses to explain IgA isotype preference in Peyer's patches, we sought to initiate acute germinal center reactions *de novo* in both Peyer's patches and lymph nodes, to analyze Ig isotype expression in germinal centers as well as the functional potential of B cells from the two types of sites to produce antibody of various isotypes within similar time intervals after local antigenic stimulation. Our approach (Weinstein and Cebra, 1991) was to initiate acute *de novo* germinal center reactions in Peyer's patches of germ-free mice by orally infecting with reovirus serotype 1 (see London *et al.*, 1987) or in lymph nodes of conventionally reared mice by footpad injection of the infectious virus. If the formerly germ-free mice infected orally with reovirus are kept in isolators under otherwise germ-free conditions, the germinal center reactions in Peyer's patches wax and wane while the intestinal virus infection is resolved completely. The germinal center reactions and antibody expression by B cells from Peyer's patches of these mice were compared with those from lymph nodes of mice injected in footpads with infectious virus. Initially, prior to, and for 3 days after oral infection, the Peyer's patch B-cell follicles of germ-free mice contain no germinal centers, unlike those of conventionally reared mice (see Figure 1). The development of germinal centers in either Peyer's patches or lymph nodes was followed after local infection using both FACS analysis for PNA^{high} B cells and immunohistochemical staining of tissue sections. Typically, germinal center B cells appeared first at day 6, reached maximum numbers by days 10–12, and declined during the period of days 14–21 after infection at both Peyer's patch and lymph node sites. The earliest and most persistent germinal center cells displayed the phenotype $PNA^{high}s\kappa^{high}$ at both sites, whereas cells with the $PNA^{high}s\kappa^{low}$ phenotype were only prevalent around the time of maximal germinal center reaction (Weinstein and Cebra, 1991). These two phenotypes of germinal center B cells have been equated with centrocytes and centroblasts, respectively (Raedler *et al.*, 1981). Whereas the time courses of the acute reactions were similar at the two sites, the two types of reactions differed conspicuously in several respects: (1) B lymphoblasts appeared with the phenotype $sIgA^+$ by day 6 and persisted through day 19 in Peyer's patches but not in lymph nodes, and most of these were $PNA^{high}sIgA^+$ and occurred in germinal centers. A very small component of $sIgG1^+$ cells was detected in lymph nodes but not in Peyer's patches. (2) On secondary local reinfection with reovirus, the germinal center reactions in Peyer's patches and lymph nodes again exhibited similar time courses, but in the lymph nodes they were exaggerated whereas in the Peyer's patches they were attenuated compared with the primary reactions. (3) More $sIgA^+$ cells that were PNA^{low} appeared in Peyer's patches and many more $sIgG1^+$ cells, both PNA^{high} and PNA^{low}, appeared in lymph nodes after reinfection, but not vice versa.

To assess the functional significance of these perturbations in subsets of Peyer's patch and lymph node B cells detected by surface phenotyping, lymphoid tissue fragment cultures (Logan *et al.*, 1991) were initiated *in vitro* using Peyer's patch or lymph node samples taken at different times during the course of the germinal center reactions after acute *in vivo* local infection with reovirus. Supernatants from the cultures were analyzed for both reovirus-specific antibody and total Ig of each isotype secreted during 7–10 days of culture. We found that acute local infection of mice with reovirus resulted in Peyer's patch fragment cultures that secreted exclusively IgA and IgM *in vitro* or in lymph node cultures that secreted IgM, IgG1, and IgG2 antibodies. Cultures initiated 3 days after infection from either source of tissue secreted only IgM, but by day 6 cultures could be initiated that progressed to the expression of non-IgM isotypes of antibody (Weinstein

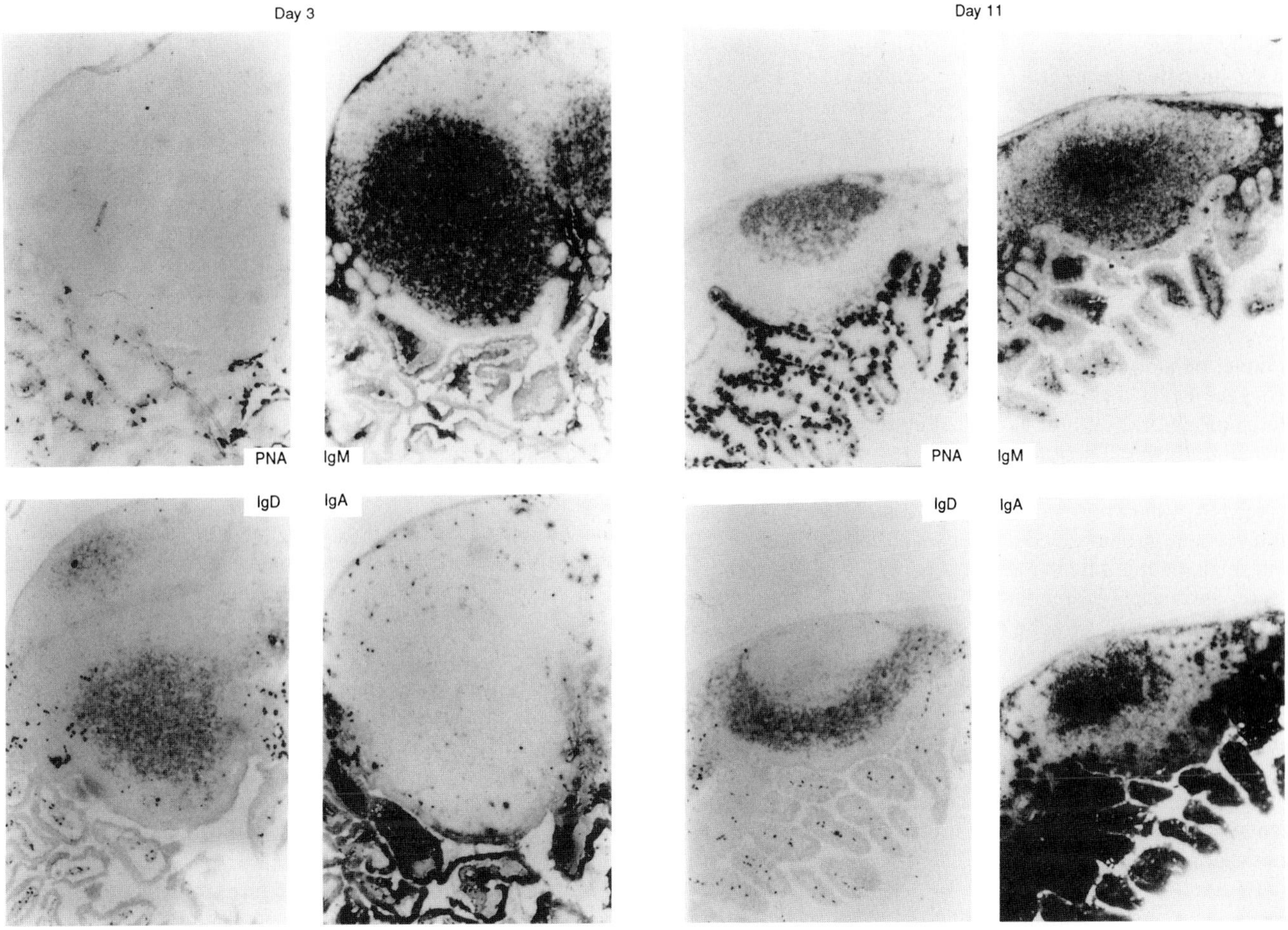

Figure 1 Consecutive sections of B-lymphocyte follicles in Peyer's patches from formerly germ-free mice after oral infection with type 1 reovirus 3 or 11 days previously. The sections were analyzed immunohistochemically using biotinylated peanut agglutinin (PNA) or biotinylated anti-IgM, -IgD, or -IgA, followed by avidin/peroxidase and its substrate (see Weinstein and Cebra, 1991, for experimental details). The sections taken at day 3 after infection are similar to those from noninfected germ-free mice.

and Cebra, 1991). In general, fragment cultures initiated after secondary local reinfections quantitatively and qualitatively reflected the secondary germinal center reactions: Peyer's patch fragment cultures produced less antibody but mostly IgA, whereas lymph node fragment cultures produced more antibody and mostly IgG1, compared with cultures initiated after primary *in vivo* local infection. The prompt switching to the expression of different non-IgM/IgD isotypes in Peyer's patches rather than lymph nodes during acute *de novo* germinal center reactions at the two types of sites suggests differences in their microenvironments as the basis for isotype preference rather than differences in the physiological states that commonly prevail in conventionally reared animals. A possible molecular basis for the observed preference for IgA expression by B cells stimulated in Peyer's patches may be the prevalence of direct IgM-to-IgA isotype switching there, compared with a perhaps more typical consecutive or sequential isotype switching in lymph nodes, eventually leading to some IgA-committed cells. Such a distinction remains to be supported, perhaps by seeking evidence for switch-γ (Sγ) footprints within the recombined S regions of IgA-expressing cells developed from or at different lymphoid sites (see Yoshida *et al.,* 1990).

C. Molecular Genetic Features and Functional Potential of Germinal Center B Cells from Peyer's Patches Also Reflect the Preference for Ig Isotype Switching to IgA in GALT

Evaluating the functional potential of germinal center B cells, including those from Peyer's patches, by *in vivo* or *in vitro* methods has proven difficult. Essential frequency analyses for specificity and isotype potential of germinal center B cells *in vitro* have been unsuccessful to date—germinal center cells usually die rapidly in culture—and assessment of their functional potential by adoptive transfer has been confounded both by the lack of homing receptors on most germinal center B cells and by the difficulty of establishing a germinal center precursor-Ig-secreting progeny relationship in the host (Reichert *et al.*, 1983; Lebman *et al.*, 1987). For instance, adoptive transfer of PNA^{high} B cells from Peyer's patches yields no clonal precursors in the splenic fragment assay, whereas all IgA memory cells that give IgA-only secreting clones are found in the PNA^{low} fraction of Peyer's patch cells (IgA memory cells) (Lebman *et al.*, 1987). Thus, we sought to assess the possible functional potential of germinal center B cells from Peyer's patches by *in situ* hybridization for mRNA encoding the various isotypes of Ig heavy chains using riboprobes (Weinstein *et al.*, 1991). We have identified a novel phenotype characteristic of germinal center B cells from the Peyer's patches of conventionally reared mice undergoing natural chronic intestinal stimulation by environmental antigens. The major subset of germinal center cells that is $PNA^{high}s\kappa^{low}$ contains levels of cytoplasmic mRNAα or mRNAμ that are easily detectable by *in situ* hybridization at levels that are intermediate between those of plasma cells and small resting B lymphocytes. About 40% of this germinal center subset has easily detectable mRNAα and about 50% contains mRNAμ. Enrichment of $sIgA^+$ and $sIgA^-$ cells by FACS led to the recovery of essentially all the cells with moderate levels of mRNAα in the $sIgA^+$ fraction of cells (48% positive). The sizes of the cytoplasmic mRNAs, determinable by Northern analysis, were similar to those encoding the membrane and secretory forms of the μ and α chains. Thus, much of the mRNA for Ig heavy chains in germinal center cells is likely to be mature, potentially productive message.

To determine whether most Peyer's patch germinal center B cells that were $sIgA^+$ and expressed mRNAα had undergone switch recombination of the VDJ gene segment to Cα gene, we determined their relative content of Cμ, Cγ1, and Cα genes. Restriction enzyme digestion and Southern analysis of genomic DNA from the $PNA^{high}s\kappa^{low}$ and the $sIgA^+$ cells prepared by FACS indicated that these subsets had lost about 25% and 80% of their Cμ and Cγ1 genes relative to Cα genes, respectively (Weinstein *et al.*, 1991). Thus, irreversible isotype switching, with deletion of intervening C_H genes, occurs in germinal centers. Most Peyer's patch germinal center cells are not expressing sIgA or mRNAα via processing of polycistronic mRNA or transplicing of mRNAs while in some intermediate, possibly reversible, stage of the switching process.

We have developed a single B cell clonal microculturing technique, using alloreactive cloned Th cells and dendritic cells, that is supportive of IgA expression (Schrader *et al.*, 1990). These cultures permit IgA expression by clones from IgA memory cells and from $sIgM^+sIgD^+$ primary B cells after intraclonal isotype switching (Schrader *et al.*, 1990; George and Cebra, 1991). However, although effective T, B, and dendritic cell interactions presumably do not require B cells to have competent homing receptors, germinal center B cells did not develop into secretory plasma cells in microculture, despite their extensive proliferation. Because proliferation and differentiation often have been observed to be seemingly antagonistic processes (see Bishop and Haughton, 1987), we assessed the effect of blocking division on Ig secretion by germinal center B cells from Peyer's patches (George and Cebra, 1991). If division of germinal center B cells is blocked by either X irradiation (1600 rad) or aphidicolin, a specific inhibitor of DNA polymerases, a high proportion of the Ig-positive microcultures (60–70%) exclusively would express IgA. About 30–40% of the division-blocked germinal center B cells responded with Ig secretion; both dendritic cells and Th cells were required for such expression. We propose that our microculture assay of germinal center B cells from Peyer's patches reveals a subset of cells, preplasmablasts, that are committed to secretion. Such cultures indicate that, although many germinal center B cells die *in situ* by apoptosis, death need not be their immediate fate if their division is blocked and they are provided with necessary supportive cells and cytokines. These cultures also emphasize the extraordinary preference for the expression of IgA by the preplasmablasts in the germinal centers of Peyer's patches.

D. Does Switch Recombination to Cα Gene Commence and Proceed in the Germinal Centers of Peyer's Patches?

The expression of transcripts initiated 5′ of Sα of the Cα gene in germ-line context has been found to precede and be predictive of subsequent recombination of an active VDJ gene segment with the Cα gene in $sIgM^+$ cell lines cultured *in vitro* to give rise to IgA-secreting progeny (Stavnezer *et al.*, 1988). Using the p5′Sα probe developed for these studies, we analyzed total cytoplasmic RNA from unfractionated, PNA^{high}, and PNA^{low} Peyer's patch cells collected at various times after acute oral infection of germ-free mice with reovirus (Weinstein and Cebra, 1991). Dot-blotting and Northern analyses showed that Cα germ-line transcripts could be detected by day 3 and persisted through at least day 12 after infection. Transcripts of 1.7 and 6.0 kb predominated that were detected readily only in the RNA from unfractionated and PNA^{high} Peyer's patch cells as early as 2–3 days before sIgA expression was observed on germinal center B cells. No germ-line Cα transcripts could be detected in cells from lymph nodes undergoing germinal center reactions. Thus, our observations on normal B cells developing *in vivo* in Peyer's patch germinal centers indicate that the switch recombination process to Cα gene proceeds at that site and likely begins there. However, we cannot formally exclude the selective accumulation of precursors already biased toward expression of Cα germ-line transcripts in the germinal centers of Peyer's patches.

E. Are Germinal Centers in Peyer's Patches a Source of IgA Memory Cells?

Analogous to the earliest appearance of $sIgG^+$ cells in the germinal centers of locally stimulated lymph nodes (Kraal *et al.*, 1982), $sIgA^+$ B cells are detected first in the developing germinal centers of Peyer's patches from orally infected germ-free mice (Weinstein and Cebra, 1991). B cells with the phenotype of IgA memory cells—$PNA^{low}sIgA^+$—appear later in the Peyer's patches of these formerly germ-free mice after acute gut mucosal infection. However, a precursor–product cell relationship still has not been established between germinal center B cells and functional memory B cells from any lymphoid source (see Cebra *et al.*, 1991), although distinct pathways leading to either preplasmablasts or memory B cells have been hypothesized for germinal center cells (Liu *et al.*, 1991a). Vλ genes from B cells isolated from perinatal ovine ileal Peyer's patches have been analyzed for variants of germ-line genes (Reynaud *et al.*, 1991). Molecular genetic analysis has indicated that variation of a sort consistent with the occurrence of point mutations begins before birth in ileal Peyer's patches but becomes extremely prevalent after birth, when clustering of changes in nucleotide sequence in the complementarity determining regions, indicating antigen selection, may be occurring. Thus, as do splenic germinal centers (Apel and Berek, 1990), ovine ileal Peyer's patch germinal centers exhibit a genetic process of change that is required for the affinity maturation of Ig receptors that characteristically has occurred in typical memory B cells.

Acknowledgments

The authors wish to thank Ethel Cebra for assistance in the production of this manuscript and Arthur Anderson for the immunohistochemical analyses shown in the figure.

References

Apel, M., and Berek, C. (1990). Somatic mutations in antibodies expressed by germinal centre B cells early after primary immunization. *Int. Immunol.* **2,** 813–819.

Bishop, G. A., and Haughton, G. (1987). Role of the interleukin 2 receptor in differentiation of a clone of LY-1$^+$ B cells. *J. Immunol.* **138,** 3308–3313.

Butcher, E. C., Rouse, R. V., Coffman, R. L., Nottenburg, C. N., Hardy, R. R., and Weissman, I. L. (1982). Surface phenotype of Peyer's patch germinal center cells: Implications for the role of germinal centers in B cell differentiation. *J. Immunol.* **129,** 2698–2707.

Cebra, J. J., Gearhart, P. J., Kamat, R., Robertson, S. M., and Tseng, J. (1977). Origin and differentiation of lymphocytes involved in the secretory IgA response. *Cold Spring Harbor Symp. Quant. Biol.* **41,** 201–215.

Cebra, J. J., Gearhart, P. J., Halsey, J. F., Hurwitz, J. L., and Shahin, R. D. (1980). Role of environmental antigens in the ontogeny of the secretory immune response. *J. Reticuloendothel. Soc.* **28s,** 61–71.

Cebra, J. J., Komisar, J. L., and Schweitzer, P. A. (1984). C_H isotype 'switching' during normal B lymphocyte development. *Ann. Rev. Immunol.* **2,** 493–548.

Cebra, J. J., Cebra, E. R., and Shahin, R. D. (1986). Perturbations in specific B cell subsets following deliberate contamination of germ-free or natural colonization of neonatal mice by intestinal bacteria. *In* "Bacteria and the Host" (M. Ryc and J. Franek, eds.), pp. 303–307. Avicenum, Prague.

Cebra, J., Schrader, C., Shroff, K., and Weinstein, P. (1991). Discussion. *Res. Immunol.* **142,** 275–276.

Clough, E. R., and Cebra, J. J. (1983). Interrelationship of primed B cells with the potential for IgE and/or IgA expression. *Mol. Immunol.* **20,** 903–915.

Coico, R. F., Bhogal, B. S., and Thorbecke, G. J. (1983). Relationship of germinal centers in lymphoid tissue to immunologic memory. VI. Transfer of B cell memory with lymph node cells fractionated according to their receptors for peanut agglutinin. *J. Immunol.* **131,** 2254–2257.

Craig, S. W., and Cebra, J. J. (1971). Peyer's patches: An enriched source of precursors for IgA-producing immunocytes in the rabbit. *J. Exp. Med.* **134,** 188–200.

Craig, S. W., and Cebra, J. J. (1975). Rabbit Peyer's patches, appendix, and popliteal lymph node B-lymphocytes: A comparative analysis of their membrane immunoglobulin components and plasma cell precursor potential. *J. Immunol.* **114,** 492–502.

Davies, A. J. S., Carter, R. L., Leuchars, E., Wallis, V., and Dietrich, F. M. (1970). The morphology of immune reactions in normal, thymectomized and reconstituted mice. III. Response to bacterial antigens: *Salmonella* flagellar antigen and pneumococcal polysaccharide. *Immunology* **19,** 945–957.

de Sousa, M., and Pritchard, H. (1974). The cellular basis of immunological recovery in nude mice after thymus grafting. *Immunology* **26,** 769–776.

Francis, T. (1940). Inactivation of epidemic influenza virus by nasal secretions of human individuals. *Science* **91,** 198–199.

Fubara, E. S., and Freter, R. (1973). Protection against enteric bacterial infection by secretory IgA antibodies. *J. Immunol.* **111,** 395–403.

Fuhrman, J. A., and Cebra, J. J. (1981). Special features of the priming process for a secretory IgA response. *J. Exp. Med.* **153,** 534–544.

Gearhart, P. J., and Cebra, J. J. (1979). Differentiated B lymphocytes: Potential to express particular antibody variable and constant regions depends on site of lymphoid tissue and antigen load. *J. Exp. Med.* **149,** 216–227.

Gearhart, P. J., and Cebra, J. J. (1981). Most B cells that have switched surface immunoglobulin isotypes generate clones of cells that do not secrete IgM. *J. Immunol.* **127,** 1030–1034.

George, A., and Cebra, J. J. (1991). Responses of single germinal-center B cells in T-cell-dependent microculture. *Proc. Natl. Acad. Sci. U.S.A.* **88,** 11–15.

Gray, D., Kosco, M., and Stockinger, B. (1991). Novel pathways of antigen presentation for the maintenance of memory. *Int. Immunol.* **3,** 141–148.

Hanson, L. Å. (1961). Comparative immunological studies of the immune globulins of human milk and of blood serum. *Int. Arch. Allergy Appl. Immunol.* **18,** 241–253.

Hockenbury, D., Nunez, G., Milliman, C., Schreiber, R. D., and Korsmeyer. (1990). Bcl-2 is an inner mitochondrial membrane protein that blocks programmed cell death. *Nature (London)* **348,** 334–336.

Hockenbury, D., Zutter, M., Hickey, W., Nahm, M., and Korsmeyer, S. J. (1991). BCL2 protein is typographically restricted in tissues characterized by apoptotic cell death. *Proc. Natl. Acad. Sci. U.S.A.* **88,** 6961–6965.

Humphrey, J. H., Grennan, D., and Sundaram, V. (1984). The origin of the follicular dendritic cell in the mouse and the mechanism of trapping of immune complexes. *Eur. J. Immunol.* **14,** 859–864.

Husband, A. J., and Gowans, J. L. (1978). The origin and antigen-dependent distribution of IgA-containing cells in the intestine. *J. Exp. Med.* **148,** 1146–1160.

Jacob, J., Kelsoe, G., Rajewsky, K., and Weiss, U. (1991). Intraclonal generation of antibody mutants in germinal centres. *Nature (London)* **354,** 389–392.

Jones, P. P., and Cebra, J. J. (1974). Restriction of gene expression in B-lymphocytes and their progeny. III. Endogenous IgA and IgM on the membranes of different plasma cell precursors. *J. Exp. Med.* **140,** 966–976.

Jones, P. P., Craig, S. W., Cebra, J. J., and Herzenberg, L. A. (1974). Restriction of gene expression in B lymphocytes and their progeny. II. Commitment to immunoglobulin heavy chain isotype. *J. Exp. Med.* **140,** 452–469.

Klaus, G. G. B., and Humphrey, J. H. (1977). The generation of memory cells. I. The role of C3 in the generation of B memory cells. *Immunology* **33,** 31–40.

Kosco, M. (1991). 37th Forum in Immunology: Germinal centres and the immune response. *Res. Immunol.* **142,** 219–282.

Kosco, M. H., Szakal, A. K., and Tew, J. G. (1988). *In vivo* obtained antigen presented by germinal center B cells to T cells *in vitro. J. Immunol.* **140,** 354–360.

Kraal, G., Weissman, I. L., and Butcher, E. C. (1982). Germinal centre B cells: Antigen specificity and changes in heavy chain class expression. *Nature (London)* **298,** 377–379.

Kraal, G., Weissman, I. L., and Butcher, E. C. (1988). Memory B cells express a phenotype consistent with migratory competence after secondary but not short-term primary immunization. *Cell. Immunol.* **115,** 78–87.

Kroese, F. G. M., Wubbena, A. S., Seijen, H. G., and Nieuwenhuis, P. (1987). Germinal centers develop oligoclonally. *Eur. J. Immunol.* **17,** 1069–1072.

Kroese, F. G. M., Butcher, E. C., Stall, A. M., Lalor, P. A., Adams, S., and Herzenberg, L. A. (1989). Many of the IgA producing plasma cells in murine gut are derived from self-replenishing precursors in the peritoneal cavity. *Int. Immunol.* **1,** 75–84.

Kroese, F. G. M., Timens, W., and Nieuwenhuis, P. (1990). Germinal center reaction and B lymphocytes: Morphology and function. *Curr. Top. Pathol.* **84,** 103–148.

Kroese, F. G. M., Seijen, H. G., and Nieuwenhuis, P. (1991). The initiation of germinal centre reactivity. *Res. Immunol.* **142,** 249–252.

Lebman, D. A., Griffin, P. M., and Cebra, J. J. (1987). Relationship between expression of IgA by Peyer's patch cells and functional IgA memory cells. *J. Exp. Med.* **166,** 1405–1418.

Liu, Y-J., Joshua, D. E., Williams, G. T., Smith, C. A., Gordon, J., and MacLennan, I. C. M. (1989). Mechanism of antigen-driven selection in germinal centres. *Nature (London)* **342,** 929–931.

Liu, Y-J., Cairns, J. A., Holder, M. J., Abbot, S. D., Jansen, K. U., Bonnefoy, J-Y., Gordon, J., and MacLennan, I. C. M. (1991a). Recombinant 25-kDa CD23 and interleukin 1alpha promote the survival of germinal center B cells: Evidence for bifurcation in the development of centrocytes rescued from apoptosis. *Eur. J. Immunol.* **21,** 1107–1114.

Liu, Y-J., Mason, D. Y., Johnson, G. D., Abbot, S., Gregory, C. D., Hardie, D. L., Gordon, J., and MacLennan, I. C. M. (1991b). Germinal center cells express bcl-2 protein after activation by signals which prevent their entry into apoptosis. *Eur. J. Immunol.* **21,** 1905–1910.

Logan, A. C., Chow, K-P. N., George, A., Weinstein, P. D., and Cebra, J. J. (1991). Use of Peyer's patch and lymph node fragment cultures to compare local immune responses to *Morganella morganii. Infect. Immun.* **59,** 1024–1031.

London, S. D., Rubin, D. H., and Cebra, J. J. (1987). Gut mucosal immunization with reovirus serotype 1/L stimulates specific cytotoxic T-cell precursors as well as IgA memory cells in Peyer's patches. *J. Exp. Med.* **165,** 830–847.

Nossal, G. J. V., and Ada, G. L. (1971). "Antigens, Lymphoid Cells, and the Immune Response." Academic Press, New York.

Pierce, N. F., and Gowans, J. L. (1975). Cellular kinetics of the intestinal immune response to cholera toxoid in rats. *J. Exp. Med.* **142,** 1550–1563.

Raedler, A., Raedler, E., Arndt, R., and Thiele, H-G. (1981). Centroblasts and centrocytes display receptors for peanut lectin. *Immunol. Lett.* **2,** 335–338.

Reichert, R. A., Gallatin, W. M., Weissman, I. L., and Butcher, E. C. (1983). Germinal center B cells lack homing receptors necessary for normal lymphocyte recirculation. *J. Exp. Med.* **157,** 813–827.

Reynaud, C-A., Mackay, C. R., Muller, R. G., and Weill, J-C. (1991). Somatic generation of diversity in a mammalian primary lymphoid organ: The sheep ileal Peyer's patches. *Cell* **64,** 995–1005.

Robertson, S. M., and Cebra, J. J. (1976). A model for local immunity. *Ricerca Clin. Lab.* **6** (Suppl. 3), 105–119.

Rose, M. L., Birbeck, M. S. C., Wallis, V. J., Forrester, J. A., and Davies, A. J. S. (1980). Peanut lectin binding properties of germinal centres of mouse lymphoid tissue. *Nature (London)* **284,** 364–366.

Rouse, R. V., Ledbetter, J. A., and Weissman, I. L. (1982). Mouse lymph node germinal centers contain a selected subset of T cells—The helper phenotype. *J. Immunol.* **128,** 2243–2246.

Schrader, C. E., George, A., Kerlin, R. L., and Cebra, J. J. (1990). Dendritic cells support production of IgA and other non-IgM isotypes in clonal microculture. *Int. Immunol.* **2,** 563–570.

Shahin, R. D., and Cebra, J. J. (1981). The rise in inulin-sensitive B cells during ontogeny can be prematurely stimulated by thymus-dependent and thymus-independent antigens. *Infect. Immun.* **32,** 211–215.

Shimizu, A., Takahashi, N., Yaoita, Y., and Honjo, T. (1982). Organization of the constant region gene family of the mouse immunoglobulin heavy chain. *Cell* **28,** 499–506.

Smith, C. B., Purcell, R. H., Bellanti, J. A., and Chanock, R. M. (1966). Protective effect of antibody to parainfluenza type 1 virus. *N. Engl. J. Med.* **275,** 1145–1152.

Stavnezer, J., Radcliffe, G., Lin, Y-C., Nietupski, J., Berggren, L., Sitia, R., and Severinson, E. (1988). Immunoglobulin heavy-chain switching may be directed by prior induction of transcripts from constant-region genes. *Proc. Natl. Acad. Sci. U.S.A.* **85,** 7704–7708.

Szakal, A. K., and Tew, J. G. (1991). Significance of iccosomes in the germinal centre reaction. *Res. Immunol.* **142,** 261–263.

Szakal, A. K., Kosco, M. H., and Tew, J. G. (1989). Microanatomy of lymphoid tissue during the induction and maintenance of humoral immune responses: Structure function relationships. *Ann. Rev. Immunol.* **7,** 91–109.

Terashima, K., Dobashi, M., Maeda, K., and Imai, Y. (1991). Cellular components involved in the germinal centre reaction. *Res. Immunol.* **142,** 263–268.

Tolaymat, N., Weber, S. P., and Cowdery, J. S. (1990). Chronic *in vivo* depletion of CD4 T cells begun *in utero* inhibits gut B cell differentiation. *Clin. Immunol. Immunopathol.* **56,** 97–107.

Tomasi, T. B., Jr., Tan, E. M., Solomon, A., and Prendergast, R. A. (1965). Characteristics of an immune system common to certain external secretions. *J. Exp. Med.* **121,** 101–142.

Tseng, J. (1981). Transfer of lymphocytes of Peyer's patches between immunoglobulin allotype congenic mice: Repopulation of the IgA plasma cells in the gut lamina propria. *J. Immunol.* **127,** 2039–2043.

Weinstein, P. D., and Cebra, J. J. (1991). The preference for switching to IgA expression by Peyer's patch germinal center B cells is likely due to the intrinsic influence of their microenvironment. *J. Immunol.* **147,** 4126–4135.

Weinstein, P. D., Schweitzer, P. A., Cebra-Thomas, J. A., and Cebra, J. J. (1991). Molecular genetic features reflecting the preference for isotype switching to IgA expression by Peyer's patch germinal center B cells. *Int. Immunol.* **3,** 1253–1263.

Yoshida, K., Matsuoka, M., Usuda, S., Mori, A., Ishizaka, K., and Sakano, H. (1990). Immunoglobulin switch circular DNA in the mouse infected with *Nippostrongylus brasiliensis:* Evidence for successive class switching from mu to epsilon via gamma1. *Proc. Natl. Acad. Sci. U.S.A.* **87,** 7829–7833.

14

Regulation of IgA B Cell Development

Warren Strober • Rolf O. Ehrhardt

I. INTRODUCTION

In this chapter, we consider the process that governs the emergence of IgA B cells in mucosal follicles and thus determines why IgA antibodies dominate the mucosal humoral immune response. This process, known as IgA switch differentiation, is the most used of the possible pathways that B cells follow as they transform into cells producing the various Ig isotypes, yet in some ways it is the most poorly understood: in contrast to the switch differentiation resulting in the various IgG isotypes and IgE, IgA switch differentiation has not been reproduced *in vitro* satisfactorily to date and the various cell–cell interactions or cytokines involved have not yet been identified clearly. IgA switch differentiation is also the most unique and seemingly the most vulnerable of the switch processes, unique because it is the only form of B-cell switching that clearly is tied to a specific site, the mucosal lymphoid environment, and vulnerable because in various congenital and acquired immunodeficiencies it is often the form that is most affected by the disease.

In summarizing the very considerable body of research that relates to IgA switch differentiation, we hope to clarify some of the advances that have informed this field and to focus on the problems that remain to be solved. Our approach is to consider first B-cell switch differentiation in general, drawing attention to the ways in which IgA switching is one example of a process that characterizes all B cells. We then turn to IgA switch differentiation in particular, dwelling on the phenomena that set this form of switching apart from other forms. In this discussion, we highlight the information that is solid and unassailable in this area, as well as the information that is uncertain and requires further support. Finally, we abstract from the studies already presented the information necessary to create as complete a picture of IgA switch differentiation as currently possible.

II. MOLECULAR FEATURES OF Ig CLASS SWITCHING

A. Switch Differentiation—S Regions

B cells undergo a complex developmental process that can be divided roughly into antigen-dependent and antigen-dependent phases (reviewed by Kishimoto and Hirano, 1989). The task of the first phase is the selection and assembly of the genes encoding the variable region of the Ig molecule, a process that allows the B cell to gain its definitive specificity. Such selection and assembly occur as a result of a random recombination process by which selected V, D, and J gene segments come together to form a single VDJ gene complex. At this point, the Ig gene has all the elements in place for VDJ–Cμ transcription: 5′ promotor, rearranged VDJ gene segment, VDJ–Cμ intron containing various enhancer sites, and, finally, the Cμ gene. A very similar series of molecular events now can take place with respect to the various segments of one of the light chain genes. The task of the second phase of B-cell development is either terminal differentiation into IgM-producing plasma cells or switch differentiation into B cells producing another Ig isotype, followed again by terminal differentiation. Switch differentiation involves a second recombination event, this time leading to replacement of the Cμ gene with a downstream (3′) C_H gene. In this way, the downstream C_H gene assumes the position formerly occupied by the Cμ gene and the new VDJ–C_H gene complex formed can be transcribed.

The process of switch differentiation, in its simplest form, involves a recombination between specialized DNA segments known as switch regions (S regions) that lie ~2 kb upstream (5′) of their respective C_H genes. These S regions are structurally similar DNA segments composed of tandem repeats of short (5-bp) units organized into 20- to 80-bp larger units, depending on the C_H gene with which they are associated. Despite this organization, rearrangement does not occur at conserved recombination splice sites (as in the case of VDJ recombination) and, thus, is not likely to involve Ig class-specific recombinases capable of recognizing particular S-region target sequences. However, the repetitive structure of the switch region implies that the recombination machinery involved in switching relies on an array of generic splice sites and end-region joining interactions.

The recombination process, involving the joining of the upstream and downstream S-region sites, would be expected to generate a loop of DNA that is excised when the S-region segments are joined. That this actually occurs was inferred initially from the molecular analysis of the S-region splice sites in clonal B cells that have undergone switching and from the fact that C_H gene order is usually, if not always, preserved, indicating that recombination is intra (not inter)-

chromosomal. However, recombination via looping-out of intervening DNA has been shown directly by the fact that switch recombination is accompanied by the elaboration of circular DNA excision products that contain the 3′ segment of the upstream S region and the 5′ segment of the downstream S region (Iwasato *et al.*, 1990; Matsuoka *et al.*, 1990; Yoshida *et al.*, 1990).

One of several insights to emerge from the study of such DNA circles is that they can contain 3′ Sγ rather than 3′ Sμ linked to a more downstream 5′ S-region segment. For example, in the case of cells undergoing IgE switch differentiation, DNA circles containing Sγ1–Sε and Sμ–Sε fragments are found, indicating that IgE switch rearrangement is accompanied by intermediate rearrangements between Sμ and Sγ_1 and Sε. Similarly, in the case of switching to IgA, circles containing Sγ–Sα as well as Sμ–Sα fragments are found, showing that switching to IgA is accompanied by intermediate rearrangement between Sμ and Sγ or Sγ and Sα (Matsuoka *et al.*, 1990; Iwasato *et al.*, 1992). Although these data indicate that the switch process may proceed by steps, they do not invalidate the concept that switch differentiation always involves the differentiation of an sIgM$^+$ B cell into a B cell expressing a single downstream isotype. Stated differently, the data do not necessarily imply that cells bearing a downstream isotype, such as one of the IgG subclasses, switch to an even more downstream isotype, such as IgE or IgA. Thus, although dual-positive B cells bearing two isotypes such as sIgM and sIgG may appear transiently during switch differentiation, no evidence exists that the dual-positive B cells actually have undergone a recombination event. As discussed subsequently, they may be producing two isotypes simultaneously as the result of a process known as transsplicing. Thus, at the moment, regarding intermediate S–S recombination as a transient intracellular phenomenon that accompanies B cell switching and acknowledging that sequential switching at the molecular level is not reflected by stepwise switching at the cellular level is best.

B. Influence of Cytokines on Switch Differentiation

A considerable body of data has now accumulated that indicates that the molecular processes just described that underlie switch differentiation are not random or "stochastic" events, but are processes that are induced by influences acting from outside the cell. This external control first became apparent when researchers discovered that, whereas lipopolysaccharide (LPS)-stimulated mouse B cells produce mainly IgG3 and IgG2b (Yuan and Vitetta, 1983; Lutzker *et al.*, 1988; Rothman *et al.*, 1990), the same cells cultured in the presence of interleukin 4 (IL-4) produced large amounts of IgG1 and decreased amounts of IgG3 and IgG2b (Isakson *et al.*, 1982). In later studies, IL-4 was shown to (1) induce purified sIgM$^+$ B cells to produce IgG1,(2) increase the precursor frequency of IgG1-secreting B cells in limiting dilution studies, and (3) induce molecular events involving the Cγ1 gene segment that precede the onset of B-cell proliferation (see below) (Vitetta *et al.*, 1985; Coffman *et al.*, 1986; Berton *et al.*, 1989; Esser and Radbruch, 1989). These studies rule out the possibility that IL-4 merely promotes the selective proliferation of B cells that already had switched to IgG1 expression, and focus attention on the ability of this lymphokine to induce IgG1 switch differentiation. Finally, note that IL-4 (at high concentrations) also induces IgE switch differentiation (Coffman and Carty, 1986; Coffman *et al.*, 1986; Lebman and Coffman, 1988). Although this effect is quantitatively small in comparison to the IgG1 effect, it is critical to IgE production since mice treated with anti-IL-4 have greatly reduced or even absent IgE responses when challenged with an IgE antibody-inducing stimulus.

In other studies, interferon γ (IFNγ) and transforming growth factor β (TGFβ) also were shown to act as switch factors. IFNγ induces mouse B cells to switch to IgG3 and IgG2a, the former when anti-IgD (coupled to dextran) is the proliferative stimulus, the latter when LPS is the proliferative stimulus (Snapper and Paul, 1987; Snapper *et al.*, 1992). Of interest is that these IFNγ effects are inhibited by IL-4 and, in turn, IL-4 effects are inhibited by IFNγ; thus, IL-4 and IFNγ appear to be two lymphokines that have opposing functions with respect to induction of switch differentiation. TGFβ, on the other hand, induces LPS-stimulated B cells to switch to IgA (Coffman *et al.*, 1989; Sonoda *et al.*, 1989). In this case, studies parallel to those conducted with IL-4 showed that TGFβ acts on purified sIgM$^+$ B cells and induces IgA-specific molecular events prior to B-cell proliferation; thus, TGFβ is promoting a true switching event rather than inducing selective IgA B-cell proliferation.

The effects of lymphokines and cytokines on switch differentiation also could be appreciated at the molecular level, since treatment of B cells with LPS plus IL-4 could be shown to enhance the occurrence of DNA circles containing Sμ–Sγ1 fragments and, correspondingly, suppress the occurrence of Sμ–Sγ3 and Sμ–Sγ2b fragments (Iwasato *et al.*, 1990,1992; Matsuoka *et al.*, 1990; Yoshida *et al.*, 1990). Similarly, treatment of cells with LPS plus TGFβ favored the occurrence of DNA circles containing Sμ–Sα (or Sγ–Sα) fragments (Matsuoka *et al.*, 1990; Iwasato *et al.*, 1992). Therefore, these data provide direct molecular evidence that cytokines induce certain types of isotype switching.

C. Role of B-Cell Activation in Switch Differentiation

The capacities of lymphokines and cytokines to act as inducers of B-cell switch differentiation, as just described, usually are demonstrated in activated B cells. Researchers generally have assumed that cell activation is a necessary (if not sufficient) condition for B-cell switch differentiation. Thus, although early molecular events of switch differentiation can be initiated by lymphokines and cytokines in resting B cells (see subsequent discussion), no evidence exists that these substances can cause resting B cells to complete the switch process, that is, undergo switch recombination in the absence of a proliferative stimulus. Also, the type of proliferative stimulus causing B-cell activation may influence certain kinds of switching, either directly or indirectly via induction of cytokine production by B cells. LPS, for instance, induces sIgM$^+$ B cells to switch to IgG3- and IgG2b-producing B cells in the absence of T cells (Yuan *et al.*, 1983; Lutzker *et al.*, 1988; Rothman *et al.*, 1990). However, whereas the switch to IgG3-producing B cells seems to be induced by the proliferative stimulus alone, the switch to IgG2b-producing cells actually is mediated via TGFβ production by the LPS-stimulated B cells (Snapper and Mond, 1993). Similarly, anti-IgD (coupled with dextran) supports IFNγ-induced switching to IgG2a and TGFβ-induced switching to IgA, but does not support IL-4-induced switching to B cells producing IgE (Snapper *et al.*, 1991). Finally, several observations show that IFNγ or TGFβ effects on B-cell differentiation vary with the type of B-cell stimulus used. For instance, IFNγ inhibits IgG3 secretion in LPS-stimulated sIgM$^+$ B-cell cultures but enhances IgG3 secretion in anti-IgD and T cell-stimulated sIgM$^+$ B-cell cultures (Snapper *et al.*, 1992); in a similar vein, TGFβ enhances IgA secretion only in LPS-stimulated sIgM$^+$ B-cell cultures, not in T cell-stimulated cultures (Ehrhardt *et al.*, 1992). Note, however, that the characteristic measured in these cases was immunoglobulin secretion rather than the number of B cells bearing the downstream isotype, so the different effects seen could relate to terminal differentiation rather than to switch differentiation. This latter point actually was proven in the TFGβ example, in which both LPS and T-cell stimulation were found to induce a similar amount of sIgA$^+$ B cells but very different amounts of IgA secretion (Ehrhardt *et al.*, 1992).

An even better case for the role of B-cell activation in switch differentiation has emerged from studies of B-cell activation via cell–cell interaction. That B cells can be activated via the latter mechanism was shown initially by the fact that activated T-cell clones or cell membranes derived from such clones induce resting B cells to proliferate and to differentiate (Kupfer *et al.*, 1986; Sanders *et al.*, 1986; Swain and Dutton, 1987; Vitetta *et al.*, 1987; Whalen *et al.*, 1988; Hodgkin *et al.*, 1990; Noelle *et al.*, 1992). Later, such proliferation and differentiation was shown to involve the binding of CD40 ligand on the T cell to the CD40 molecule on the B cell; the latter was shown to be the major signaling pathway through which T cells stimulate B cells during cognate/noncognate cell interactions (Banchereau *et al.*, 1991).

In the same studies, of more direct interest to this discussion, the activation signal delivered by the CD40 ligand was shown to be quite different from that delivered by more conventional proliferative signals. Thus, in studies of human cells, stimulation of B cells with anti-CD40 antibodies was found to lead to stimulation of B cells in such a way that they are maintained in culture for weeks rather than days. Further, it was shown whereas *Staphylococcus aureus* Cowen I (SAC) induces B cells to produce only negligible amounts of IgM, this stimulus in conjunction with anti-CD40 induces B cells to produce large amounts of IgM as well as considerable amounts of IgG and IgA; in addition, whereas SAC or anti-IgM plus TGFβ and IL-10 produces very little IgA, these stimuli given with anti-CD40 give rise to large amounts of IgA (Rousset *et al.*, 1991; Defrance *et al.*, 1992). Thus, the CD40 proliferative signal may prepare the cell for switch and/or terminal differentiation much better than anti-IgM or SAC can. This last conclusion is punctuated by the finding that patients with the hyper-IgM syndrome, whose B cells synthesize IgM but not IgG or IgA, appear to have a defective or absent CD40 ligand on their T cells, suggesting that B-cell signaling via CD40 is a necessary precondition for switch and/or terminal differentiation (Aruffo *et al.*, 1993; Cutler Allen *et al.*, 1993).

To complete the discussion of the role of proliferation signals on B-cell differentiation we mention that, in the studies with anti-CD40, mere cross-linking of CD40 was not sufficient to stimulate the B cell; the anti-CD40 had to be presented by an antigen-presenting cell (a mouse L cell transfected with a human Fc receptor gene) (Banchereau *et al.*, 1991; Rousset *et al.*, 1991), suggesting that the CD40 signal is "incomplete" without certain as yet undefined accessory signals. In this context, note that CD45 cross-linking has been shown to regulate LPS-induced IgG3 switching and that LyB-2 (CD72) cross-linking has been shown to regulate LPS plus IL-4-induced IgG1 switching (Ogimoto *et al.*, 1992). These studies provide tangible evidence that the cell–cell interactions necessary for switch differentiation involve a complex series of signals that may modify the switch and also terminal differentiation.

D. Molecular Events Accompanying Cytokine Induction of Switch Differentiation

The ability of various proliferation signals, cell–cell interations, and cytokines to influence switch differentiation raised the immediate question of how such stimuli function at the molecular level. If we assume at this point that switch differentiation is indeed a directed event, as the data on the effect of cytokines in B-cell switch differentiation strongly imply, then two broad molecular mechanisms can be suggested to explain such direction. The first is that the factors directing switch differentiation induce C_H-specific recombinases that act only on particular C_H gene segments to bring about switch rearrangement. Evidence in favor of this view derives from the analysis of DNA circles generated during switch recombination (Iwasato *et al.*, 1990; Matsuoka *et al.*, 1990; Yoshida *et al.*, 1990). Such analyses show that $S\mu$–$S\gamma 1$ breakpoints are dispersed in both the $S\mu$ and $S\gamma 1$ regions, whereas $S\mu$–$S\alpha$ breakpoints occur in the 3′ half of $S\mu$ and the 5′ half of $S\alpha$; thus, one might postulate that the recombinases mediating $C\mu \rightarrow C\gamma_1$ switches and $C\mu \rightarrow C\alpha$ switches are different because the former is promiscuous in its selection of donor and acceptor S-region splice sites whereas the latter is fastidious. However, these data also can be explained by assuming that S-region accessibility to a common recombinase is more or less complete in $C\mu \rightarrow C\gamma_1$ switching whereas it is limited in $C\mu \rightarrow C\alpha$ switching.

Evidence against the view that Ig-specific recombinases are induced by particular cytokines comes from data obtained by Marcu and his associates, showing that the presence of recombinases does not insure that recombination will occur (Ott *et al.*, 1987). In the relevant studies, these authors have demonstrated that, when Abelson virus-transformed pre-B cells are transfected with a retroviral vector containing $S\mu$ and $S\gamma 2b$ inserts separated by a selectable marker that is lost on $S\mu$–$S\gamma 2b$ recombination (thereby allowing isolation and study of cells containing recombined vector segments), authentic $S\mu$–$S\gamma 2b$ recombination occurs in cells that have not rearranged their endogenous C_H genes. Thus, the presence of a recombinase is necessary but not sufficient for recombination; further, recombinases exist in cells (pre-B cells) prior to induction by cytokines and, by implication, the latter do not act by inducing recombinase synthesis or activation.

A second possible molecular mechanism that has been proposed to explain directed switch differentiation is that directing factors acting on B cells render particular C_H gene segments accessible to recombinases (and other necessary proteins) that secondarily mediate the switch process. The earliest evidence in favor of this view was the observation that certain B-cell lines were capable of elaborating transcripts originating from a C_H gene to which the cell eventually would switch. For example, Yancopoulos *et al.* (1986) showed that, in Abelson murine leukemia virus-transformed pre-B cell lines switching to cells expressing $\gamma 2b$, the switch was preceded by transcription of an mRNA originating 2 kb upstream of the $S\gamma 2b$ region and terminating at the 3′ end of the $C\gamma 2b$ gene segment. Additional work showed that this "germ-line" or "sterile" transcript has an exon located 2 kb upstream of the $C\gamma 2b$ gene segment which, during transcription, is spliced to the C_H1 domain of the $C\gamma 2b$ gene segment. At about the same time, Stavnezer and co-workers showed that similar germ-line transcripts occur in I.29 B-cell lymphoma cells that switch under the influence of LPS to cells expressing IgA or, to a far lesser extent, IgG2a or IgE (Stavnezer *et al.,* 1985; Shockett and Stavnezer, 1991). Again, germ-line transcripts relating to each of the expressed Ig genes were found; in addition, the genes in question were shown to be hypomethylated (an indication that they were available to mRNA polymerase) and displayed DNA hypersensitivity (an indication that they were associated with exposed chromatin).

With the demonstration that transcriptional activity of downstream genes preceded class switching, a series of studies quickly followed that showed that the very factors that induce class switching at the cellular level induce germ-line transcription at the molecular level. Thus, in a series of studies involving pre-B cells (Abelson virus-transformed B-cell lines), B-cell lymphomas, and normal B cells, Lutzker *et al.* (1988) showed that various switch factors induce the production of germ-line transcripts corresponding to the Ig genes to which the cells switch. IL-4, for instance, induces IgG1 germ-line transcripts and $C\varepsilon$ germ-line transcripts in lymphoma or normal B cells; such induction is inhibited by IFNγ. Similarly, IFNγ induces $C\gamma 3$ germ-line transcripts in association with anti-IgD cell stimulation and $C\gamma 2b$ germ-line transcripts in association with LPS stimulation (Lutzker *et al.,* 1988; Gerondakis, 1990). Finally, Stavnezer and colleagues showed that TGFβ induces increased $C\alpha$ germ-line transcripts in I.29 lymphoma B cells in an amount roughly equivalent to the increase in cells induced to express IgA. Additionally, in this case, the effect of the cytokine increase was shown by nuclear run-on analysis to be the result of increased mRNA transcription rather than decreased mRNA turnover (Shockett and Stavnezer, 1991). Note that, in I.29 B cells and CH12.LX B cells, that is, cell lines that spontaneously undergo IgA switch differentiation, IL-4 also induces increased IgA switching, albeit to a lesser extent than TGFβ, and that such switching also is accompanied by increased $C\alpha$ germ-line transcription that is inhibited by IFNγ (Stavnezer *et al.,* 1985; Kunimoto *et al.,* 1988).

A common associated finding in the studies of cytokine-induced germ-line transcription just cited is that the latter temporarily precedes switch differentiation. This fact, along with the fact that germ-line transcription can be considered a marker of upstream C_H gene accessibility, strongly implies that the mechanism of cytokine-induced switch differentiation relates, at least in part, to the ability of cytokines to change the ability of recombination machinery to gain access to 5′ regulatory regions of C_H genes. Stated another way, these data strongly support the accessibility theory of directed switch differentiation.

E. Dual-Positive B Cells Occurring during Switch Differentiation

Another important advance in the understanding of Ig class switching, one that interrelates with the expanding knowledge of germ-line transcription, concerns the fact that B cells undergoing switch differentiation pass through a stage in which they can express surface IgM as well as one of the downstream Ig isotypes. This phenomenon was noted first by Perlmutter and Gilbert (1984), who reported that normal mouse spleen contains $sIgM^+$ $sIgG1^+$ dual-positive B cells that contain nuclear mRNA transcripts for both these Ig classes. Later, Snapper and Paul found that B cells stimulated by LPS and IL-4 develop (at a reasonably high frequency) into cells expressing sIgM and sIgG1 or into cells expressing surface IgM and IgE (Snapper *et al.,* 1988). Similarly, Yaoita *et al.* (1982) showed that mice stimulated with *Nippostrongylus braziliensis* (a potent inducer of T cells producing IL-4) develop cells that bear both sIgM and sIgE. These dual-positive B cells could, of course, be transient cells that are dual-isotype expressing because of the persistence of mRNA message characteristic of an earlier stage of development. This idea, however, is not supported by the finding that the downstream gene in the dual-positive cells studied by both Perlmutter and Gilbert (1984) and Yaoita *et al.* (1982) had not undergone rearrangement.

Similar and complementary results were obtained in the study of dual-positive cell lines. Chen *et al.* (1986) showed that, in a $sIgM^+sIgG1^+$ dual-positive variant of the BCL1 murine B-cell line, both the IgM and IgG1 produced by the cell had the same idiotype and utilized a single J_H gene segment; in addition, extensive analysis of the entire Ig gene in this cell showed no evidence of C_H rearrangement. Similar findings were obtained in $sIgM^+sIgG^+$ and $sIgM^+sIgE^+$ dual-positive Epstein–Barr virus (EBV)-transformed B-cell lines. Finally, Kunimoto and Strober showed that the lymphoma cell line CH12.LX, a line that spontaneously switches from sIgM cells to sIgA cells at a low frequency and increases such switching when cultured with IL-4 and/or TGFβ, gives rise to a $sIgM^+sIgA^+$ dual-positive cell during the switch process (Kunimoto *et al.*, 1988). These authors also analyzed a stable dual-positive clone of this line and showed rather unequivocally that both Cμ and Cα mRNA were utilizing the same VDJ segment, and that the Cα gene in both alleles was not juxtaposed to the rearranged VDJ segment, that is, the μ mRNA and α mRNA were arising from a single Ig gene on a single chromosome. These studies thus established that dual-positive unrearranged B cells are a regular occurrence during switch differentiation. Whether they are an obligate pathway of such differentiation remains to be seen.

The molecular mechanism explaining the occurrence of dual-positive but unrearranged B cells is not yet resolved. As mentioned earlier, Perlmutter and Gilbert (1984) showed that dual-positive cells contain nuclear mRNA for both Ig species. These authors postulated that the mRNAs may arise from alternative splicing of long mRNA transcripts that span multiple Ig genes. This view, however, seems unlikely in view of the instability of such transcripts and of the fact that certain cell lines seem precommitted to a particular isotype. Another explanation is that VDJ mRNA may be "transpliced" to C_H gene mRNA, the latter presumably arising from germ-line transcripts, as discussed previously. That transplicing does, in fact, occur is supported by several observations. First, in earlier studies rabbits were shown to be heterologous for V_H and C_H allotype Ig markers, although the V_H markers and C_H genes are encoded by different chromosomes. Second, Shimizu has shown that, in B cells of transgenic mice carrying a human Cμ transgene, a hybrid message may occur containing transgene VDJ mRNA spliced to endogenous C_H gene mRNA (Shimizu *et al.*, 1989). Since, in these studies, the transgene was *not* located in the J_H and C_H gene regions, the splice was presumed to be a transplice. One possible alternative explanation of this finding is that the trans-mRNA occurred via S–S recombination, that is, intrachromosomal splicing. Indeed, Gerstein *et al.* (1990) have presented evidence that, in hybridoma B-cell lines containing a mouse VDJ–C_H transgene on one chromosome, the transgene can give rise to mRNA that is linked to mRNA derived from endogenous Cα gene. In this case, the authors provide good evidence that this mixed product is generated by transgene isotype switching and that actual joining of VDJ of the transgene with Cα occurred at the DNA rather than at the mRNA level. Despite these findings, intrachromosomal splicing and S–S recombination do not seem to explain the trans-mRNA in the transgenic model of Shimizu *et al.*, (1989,1991), these authors have provided evidence that in, a lymphoma B cell derived from the transgenic mouse and containing the transgene, no evidence was found of S–S rearrangement.

Additional support for transplicing also comes from the studies of Nolan-Willard and colleagues (1992), who have shown, using the double-isotype expressing BCL1 lymphoma B cells mentioned previously, that the cells produce a pre-RNA in their nuclei that contains μ and γ1 linked sequences. The pre-RNA is about 15 kb long, rather than 150 kb as one might expect from a long transcript; thus, in these double-isotype producing cells, the synthesis of the linked mRNA must have occurred by a transplicing mechanism or, as the authors suggest, by "discontinuous transcription."

F. Induction and Function of Germline Transcripts

As discussed earlier, various cytokines induce germ-line transcription in the process of bringing about switch differentiation (Stavnezer-Nordgren and Sirlin, 1986; Lutzker *et al.*, 1988; Stavnezer *et al.*, 1988). The question therefore arises about the molecular mechanism involved in such induction. To begin to answer this question, Stavnezer and colleagues have analyzed the regulatory regions 5′ to the Iα gene segment in the I.29 B-cell line, that is, the start site of Cα germ-line transcript in this cell (Lin and Stavnezer, 1992). These studies have shown that, although this site contains neither a TATA box nor an Sp1 element near the possible mRNA initiation sites, it does contains DNA sequences with homology to a variety of known target sites of DNA binding proteins that are involved in regulation of transcription of mRNA, for example, AP-2, NF-III, and ATF/CRE sites. Further, in a series of studies in which the 5′ Iα sequences were fused to a reporter gene and the resulting constructs transfected into permissive B-cell lymphomas, the ATF/CRE sequence was shown to be important for constitutive expression of the germ-line transcript. On the other hand, TGFβ induction of transcription depended on the presence of sequences present at position -128 to -106 and position -41 to -30 relative to the upstream-most mRNA initiation site. This region, subsequently termed the TGF-RE, contains tandem repeats of the 5′ CACAG(G) and CCAGAC 3′ motifs. Stavnezer and colleagues suggest that up-regulation of Cα germ-line transcripts may occur as a result of TGFβ induction of a DNA binding factor that competes with suppressor factors for occupation of the TGF-RE (Lin and Stavnezer, 1992).

The ATF/CRE just mentioned binds a family of transcription factors that is involved in the induction of many different mRNAs, including the major histocompatibility complex (MHC) Class II A(α) mRNA. The TGF-RE, on the other hand, is homologous with sequences in the promotors of the mouse and human TGFβ1 genes and in the β-actin gene. Thus, the various regulatory sequences mediating TGFβ effects are not specific for Cα germ-line transcription. Indeed, these elements have been found upstream of several of the C_H genes, a fact that correlates with the discovery that TGFβ induces IgG2a switch differentiation in LPS-stimulated murine B cells (McIntyre *et al.*, 1993).

Assuming that the regulation of Cα germ-line transcripts in I.29 cells by TGFβ, as just described, can be considered a model for regulation of germ-line transcripts generally, the data just presented suggest that lymphokines and cytokines influence germ-line transcription via the induction of regulatory DNA binding factors. In this context, that different lymphokines and cytokines have different effects (induce different types of switch differentiation) seems reasonable because they induce different DNA binding factors. Indeed, even in cases in which two different cytokines induce the same germ-line transcript, for example, IL-4 and TGFβ induction of Cα germ-line transcripts, the molecular mechanism underlying induction is likely to involve a distinct array of DNA binding factors, since these cytokines have been shown to induce Cα germ-line transcripts at different rates and magnitudes.

Finally, whether induction of DNA binding factors also accounts for lymphokine and cytokine effects on the earliest steps of switch differentiation, such as accessibility itself, and whether such induction is the same as germ-line transcript induction, is still unknown.

The emerging data relative to the regulation of germ-line transcription beg the question of the function of the germ-line transcripts. One possibility is that they have no function and occur merely because of the accessibility of the region 5′ to the C_H genes to transcriptional factors and enzymes. This possibility is unlikely, however, because the germ-line transcripts have specific start sites in the I region as well as specific splice sites and, thus, seem too highly structured to be random (opportunistic) transcriptional products. Another possibility is that germ-line transcripts play a necessary role in switch recombination, either directly via the function of the germ-line transcript itself or indirectly via a translation product of the transcript. Wakatsuki and Strober addressed this possibility by transfecting plasmids producing antisense oligonucleotides specific for sequences in the Iα region into CH12.LX B cells in an attempt to down-regulate Cα germ-line transcription in such cells. These investigators found that such transfection did, in fact, down-regulate Cα germ-line transcription and, in doing so, led to a decrease in the appearance of dual-positive ($sIgM^+sIgA^+$) B cells and IgA synthesis (Wakatsuki and Strober, 1993). From this result, germ-line transcripts appear to be a necessary if not a sufficient condition for switch differentiation.

G. Molecular Mechanisms Related to Human Switch Differentiation

To this point in our discussion, we have been concerned mostly with studies relating to mouse Ig switch differentiation. We now turn our attention to what is known about switch differentiation in human cells.

The human Ig heavy-chain gene is far more complex than the murine Ig gene because it is composed of two separate units, one containing an initial group of C_H genes—Cγ3–Cγ1–ψCε–Cα1—followed by a second group of C_H genes—ψC_H–cγ2–Cγ4–Cε–Cα2—that are presumed to have arisen as a result of gene duplication events. Despite this increased complexity, the fine structure of human C_H genes is remarkably similar to that of mouse C_H genes with respect to S regions and regions upstream of the S regions extending into the I regions. This similarity includes an evolutionarily conserved region 5′ to and overlapping the human Iγ4 and Iε gene segments and the mouse Iγ2b gene segments that includes the regulatory regions of these human and mouse I region gene segments (Flanagan and Rabbitts, 1982; Hofker *et al.*, 1989).

This structural homology is reflected in important functional similarities relating to molecular events occurring during human and murine switch differentiation. In particular, human B cells that are about to undergo switch differentiation first produce germ-line transcripts initiating 5′ to the C_H gene to which the cell is switching. That these transcripts are under the transcriptional control of cytokines was shown in relation to IgE switch differentiation, for which IL-4-treated B cells, in the absence of other stimuli, were found to produce Iε germ-line transcripts, and in relation to IgA switch differentiation, for which TGFβ was shown to induce Iα germ-line transcripts (Berton *et al.*, 1989; Lebman *et al.*, 1990). The need for proliferative stimuli in such induction was studied in relation to Iε germ-line transcription. No such stimuli were found to be necessary, although T cells or other stimuli such as anti-CD40 antibody were necessary for IgE secretion (i.e., Cε switch differentiation). Whether TGFβ alone can induce Iα germ-line transcripts (in the absence of other stimuli) is less clear; however, we know that not every proliferative stimulus acts in conjunction with TGFβ to bring about IgA secretion: anti-CD40 antibody and certain antigens have this ability but anti-Ig cross-linking antibodies do not (Defrance *et al.*, 1992).

With respect to IgG subclass germ-line transcripts, studies have shown that germ-line transcripts associated with Cγ genes in the first duplication unit (Cγ3 and Cγ1) require proliferation stimuli for induction, for example, SAC or SAC plus IL-2 (alone or in combination with other cytokines), whereas the germ-line transcripts associated with the Cγ genes in the second duplication unit (Cγ2 and Cγ4) can be induced by cytokines alone (IFNγ and IL-4, respectively; Kitani and Strober, 1993, in press). Other effects of proliferation stimuli and cytokines on Iγ germ-line transcript expression were that, whereas Iγ1 germ-line transcripts were induced by SAC alone and such induction was not enhanced by cytokines, Iγ3 germ-line transcripts required both SAC and IL-4. In addition, whereas Iγ2 germ-line transcript was induced by a proliferation stimulus or by IFNγ alone, Iγ4 germ-line transcript was not induced by a proliferation stimulus and only by IL-4 alone. Thus, the germ-line transcripts associated with each of the Cγ genes are unique in their regulatory requirements. Finally, IFNγ and IL-4, as in murine systems, have opposing actions because IFNγ down-regulates both Iγ1 and Iγ4 germ-line transcripts induced by IL-4.

The new data concerning Iγ germ-line transcript regulation have certain implications regarding the two duplication units in the Ig gene region. First, the regulation of Iγ germ-line transcripts arising from the first and second duplication units appears to be governed by somewhat different mechanisms, since transcription of germ-line transcripts from C_H genes in the first unit requires a proliferation signal whereas transcription from those in the second does not (Kitani and Strober, 1993). This functional difference appears to be imbedded in a structural difference since, in human B-cell malignancies, c-*myc* translocation has been found mainly in the S regions of the first duplication unit (Hamlyn and Rabbitts, 1983; Care *et al.*, 1986).

Second, based on the capacity of Cγ genes to response to IL-4 and IFNγ induction, evolutionary relationships between human Cγ2/Cγ4 and murine Cγ3/Cγ1 can be assigned, suggesting that these gene pairs define a unit that underwent duplication or deletion during evolution. For instance, duplication of a pair of primordial Cγ genes could have led to the C_H gene format present in the mouse, whereas duplication of the entire C_H array (including the Cε and Cα genes) led to the C_H gene format in humans (Flanagan and Rabbitts, 1982; Hofker *et al.*, 1989).

Third, these studies lead to the possibility that human B cells are separable into two lineages that express either of the genes in the Cγ3/Cγ1 gene pair of the Cγ2/Cγ4 gene pair. This concept is based on the fact that human B-cell leukemia lymphoma cell lines can express simultaneously Cγ1 and Cγ3 germ-line transcripts originating from the first duplication unit exclusively (Sideras *et al.,* 1992). In addition, several groups have described switchable IgM-producing human B-cell lines that constitutively produce Cγ1 and Cγ3 germ-line transcripts and switch to IgG1 and IgG3 B cells, respectively (Sideras *et al.,* 1992; Kuze *et al.,* 1991; Mizuta *et al.,* 1991). These cells are thus similar to normal B cells that switch to IgG1 and IgG3 B cells when stimulated by SAC and IL-4 or SAC alone. The fact that these cells do not produce Cγ1 and Cγ3 germ-line transcripts when stimulated with IFNγ or IL-4 alone suggests that they represent a lineage only capable of differentiating into B cells expressing the isotypes corresponding to the C_H genes in the first duplication unit.

Fourth, and finally, the fact that lymphoma B cells can express simultaneously Cγ1 and Cγ3 germ-line transcripts from the first duplication unit leads to the further suggestion that Ig genes in a given unit are under the control of factors that affect all Ig genes in that unit. This possibility could explain the observation that human B-cell lines differ from mouse B-cell lines by the fact that the gene rearrangement of the Ig gene on the unexpressed allele frequently does not correspond to that of the Ig gene on the expressed allele. This observation now can be explained on the assumption that, in humans, the entire duplication unit rather than the specific Ig gene becomes accessible after the cell is subject to a particular induction signal. Thus, directed switch differentiation only requires that the unexpressed C_H allele be in the same duplication unit as the expressed allele.

Molecular analyses of regulatory sequences 5′ to the I gene segments in humans are only now becoming available. As in murine systems, initiation sites at I gene segments are heterogeneous and lack classic 5′ promoters. Structural studies initiated to date reveal enhancer and repressor regions in the region 5′ to the Iγ3 gene segment, as well as binding sites for known transcription factors. However, much additional work will be necessary to gain even a skeletal picture of the molecular regulation of these human I gene segments.

III. CELLULAR BASIS OF IgA B-CELL DIFFERENTIATION

A. Peyer's Patches, Loci of IgA B-Cell Development

Studies of the cellular basis of IgA B-cell differentiation can be said to begin with the landmark experiments of Craig and Cebra (1981), who showed that adoptively transferred Peyer's patch cell populations could repopulate the intestinal lamina propria and spleen of X irradiated rabbits with IgA B cells far more efficiently than could lymph node cell populations. Earlier, Rudzik and his colleagues (1975) extended these findings by showing in a very similar system that adoptively transferred bronchial lymph node cells were also very efficient in repopulating intestinal lamina propria. These findings, eventually verified in a syngeneic cell transfer system in mice, were the first to show that Peyer's patches are a major site of IgA B-cell development (Tseng, 1981). In addition, these studies presaged a great number of studies that established that IgA B cells developing in Peyer's patches and bronchial lymph nodes migrate through the draining mesenteric lymph node and also through the spleen on their way to the lamina propria of the various mucosal surfaces.

These studies establishing the origin of IgA B cells in Peyer's patches correlate with those focused on the cellular architecture of the Peyer's patches. Peyer's patches contain germinal centers characterized by a high proportion of $sIgA^+$ B cells (75–80%), whereas germinal centers in peripheral lymph nodes contain very low numbers of such cells (Butcher *et al.,* 1982). The $sIgA^+$ germinal center B cells are rapidly dividing cells that, for the most part, die by apoptosis before leaving the center. However, when their proliferation is inhibited chemically or physically or they are cultured with competent T cells, these cells develop into IgA-secreting cells (see subsequent discussion). A related finding is that Peyer's patches contain memory IgA B cells, a B-cell population specific for a particular antigen and expanding rapidly when restimulated with that antigen. The precise localization of such B cells in the patch is unknown, but suggesting that they are part of the recycling B-cell population in the germinal centers is tempting. Finally, note that memory B cells, whatever their location, should be distinguished from terminally differentiated IgA plasma cells. The latter are only rarely found in Peyer's patches and develop from the subpopulation of $sIgA^+$ B cells that escape from the Peyer's patch germinal centers and migrate to other sites such as the bone marrow or the lamina propria. The factors that allow sIgA B cells to migrate out of germinal centers, and thus to pursue a terminal differentiation pathway, are still poorly understood.

Whereas IgA B-cell development is one of the predominant features of Peyer's patches of rodents (and humans), IgM B-cell development may characterize this lymphoid site in other species. Thus, as shown by Reynolds and his colleagues, neonatal sheep contain ileal Peyer's patches that contain a rapidly proliferating $sIgM^+$ B-cell population and differ from more conventional $sIgA^+$ B cell-containing Peyer's patches in jejunal areas (Pabst and Reynolds, 1986; Reynolds, 1986; Reynolds and Kirk, 1989). These ileal patches involute as the sheep matures and contain cells that, for the most part, undergo cell death in the patch rather than migrate to other lymphoid tissues; thus, these regions may be a kind of "bursal equivalent," that is, a generation of pro-B, pre-B, and immature B cells.

Other cells found in the Peyer's patches are T cells, which are numerous in both the follicular and interfollicular areas. The follicular T cells are almost all $CD4^+$ T cells, whereas the interfollicular T cells are $CD4^+$ T cells interspersed with small numbers of $CD8^+$ T cells. A unique feature of the Peyer's patch $CD4^+$ T-cell population is that it contains a subset of $Thy1^-$ cells (about 15% of the total) located mainly, if not exclusively, in the follicles (Harriman *et al.,* 1990). The latter rarely are found in other lymphoid organs (~5%) and when they are, they are Thy^{dull} rather than Thy1$^-$. Various *in vitro* studies reveal that this population arises from Thy1$^+$ T cells as a result of cell activation; thus, their presence in Peyer's patches is an indication of a high state of T-cell activation in this lymphoid site.

Finally, Peyer's patches contain various types of dendritic cells, including interdigitating dendritic cells that are highly efficient antigen-presenting cells capable of addressing T cells, as well as follicular dendritic cells capable of addressing B cells (Spalding *et al.*, 1983; Tew *et al.*, 1990). The precise localization of these cells within the Peyer's patch is unknown although, on the basis of information from other lymphoid organs, interdigitating dendritic cells are in the interfollicular areas whereas follicular dendritic cells are in germinal centers. As we shall see, evidence is emerging that interdigitating dendritic cells may play an important role in the T-cell activation processes occurring in Peyer's patches and, secondarily, in the IgA switch differentiation process. What role, if any, follicular dendritic cells have in IgA switch differentiation is unknown.

B. B Cell- and T Cell-Centered Theories of IgA Switch Differentiation

The identification of the Peyer's patches and bronchial lymph nodes as major sites of B-cell development and IgA switch differentiation focused attention on conditions at those sites that make such development possible there but not at other lymphoid sites. Historically, two competing hypotheses describing these conditions have been proposed. In one hypothesis, IgA switch differentiation is visualized as a B cell-centered process that occurs when B cells are subjected to intense antigen-driven stimulation. In this view, although T cell interaction with B cells is assumed to occur in the usual antigen-mediated (cognate) fashion, the T cells themselves (or, indeed, other accessory cells) play no role in B-cell development other than the facilitation of B-cell activation and terminal differentiation. This theory, originally put forward by Cebra and his colleagues, took advantage of the fact that B cells entering the Peyer's patches (presumably sIgM$^+$ B cells) encounter an environment in which cells are more exposed to all sorts of antigens (and mitogens). Assuming that the latter would subject the B cells to a unique inductive influence that results in progressive switch differentiation was reasonable. In addition, the theory took advantage of the fact that, in mice, the Cα gene is the most 3′ of the C_H genes. Thus, any process that favored progressive switch differentiation would lead inevitably to the emergence of IgA B cells.

Several facts, both theoretical and experimental, now have led to the abandonment of this theory, at least in its simplest form. First, the theory does not explain the fact that direct stimulation of B cells with any of a variety of T cell-independent mitogens or antigens does not lead to significant IgA switch differentiation and IgA secretion. Second, the theory would predict that, under active stimulation leading to more 3′ switch differentiation, the Cγ2a and Cε genes, the penultimate C_H genes (and the equivalent genes in humans), also would be overexpressed in Peyer's patches; However, no evidence exists that this is true. Third, the theory presupposes intermediate switching from the various Cγ genes (or Cε gene) to the Cα gene. Although we have seen evidence that this can occur at the molecular level and, indeed, dual-positive cells appear that can switch to more downstream isotypes, no evidence exists that stable sIgG$^+$ or sIgE$^+$ B cells are switchable to more downstream isotypes such as IgA. Moreover, even progressive switching at the moelcular level occurs under the influence of cytokines, that is, not as a result of stimulation of B cells in the absence of T cells or other cells.

The latter point introduces the fourth and main problem with the B cell-centered theory of IgA switch differentiation, the fact that it is "out of synch" with the entire thrust of current concepts of isotype differentiation, which consistently relate a particular form of switch differentiation to a particular cytokine influence. In this regard, we have little reason to believe that sIgA$^+$B cells are different from B cells expressing other isotypes in being the end result of an external inductive influence. Interestingly, Cebra and his colleagues have, themselves, provided a persuasive argument against B cell-centered IgA switch differentiation. These authors have shown that *de novo* induction of a germinal center reaction in Peyer's patches by infection of germ-free mice with reovirus is sufficient to induce high numbers of Peyer's patch B cells expressing sIgA (Weinstein and Cebra, 1991). This study shows that, even in a Peyer's patch containing B cells not chronically exposed to a multitude of the antigens present in the normal gut, IgA switch differentiation in Peyer's patches is favored.

Whereas the B cell-centered theory of IgA switch differentiation clearly is untenable as originally proposed, it may contain a germ of truth. IgA switch differentiation in Peyer's patches may be B cell-centered in the sense that the B cells undergoing this process have been committed to it partially before they enter the patch and thus do not require a specific inductive influence to complete their differentiation program. One might speculate that the partially committed cells are either sIgM$^+$ B cells or dual-positive sIgM$^+$sIgA$^+$ B cells that are producing Cα germ-line transcripts and thus have an accessible region 5′ to the Cα gene segment. One might speculate further that such cells arise via random (stochastic) switch differentiation at some site of early B-cell development and then migrate to Peyer's patches via a patch-specific homing mechanism.

Several scraps of data can be marshaled to support this theory. First, the idea that some sIgM$^+$ B cells present in Peyer's patches are precommitted to IgA switch differentiation is supported by the knowledge that such B cells do, in fact, exist in the form of lymphoma B-cell lines such as CH12.LX B cells and I.29. Such cells maybe present normally in a more transient form at certain lymphoid sites and migrate from the latter to the Peyer's patches. Worth mentioning in this context is that CH12.LX B cells arose in animals subjected to systemic immunization and thus did not necessarily arise in mucosal tissues. Second, this idea is favored by the knowledge that, at least in humans, a considerable number of IgA-producing B cells develops in a lymphoid organ other than the Peyer's patch—the bone marrow. Although such bone marrow IgA B cells may have originated in Peyer's patches and are merely undergoing terminal differentiation in the bone marrow, the reverse also may be true: the bone marrow may be the site of initiation of IgA B-cell development and the Peyer's patches the site where such development is completed. Third, putative partially committed IgA$^+$ B cells, dual-positive sIgM$^+$SIgA$^+$ B cells (5–7%) are found in Peyer's patches in substantial numbers (R. Ehrhardt, Gregory R. Harriman, John K. Inman, and W. Strober, unpublished observations). Although such cells usually are thought to arise secondary to a process inductive of IgA switch differentiation, this need not be the case; these cells may be the starting point of Peyer's patch IgA B-cell development rather than the intermediate point. Finally, some data show that certain B cells bear surface receptors that allow interaction with high endothelial venules in Peyer's patches and thus would facilitate selective entry of B cells into this lymphoid site (as opposed to peripheral lymph nodes); thus, some support is available for the possibility that cells precommitted to IgA switch differentiation preferentially accumulate in Peyer's patches.

The data in favor of a resurrected B cell-centered theory of IgA B-cell differentiation cannot be considered sufficient to establish its validity. Additional evidence, such as the demonstration that at least some B cells entering Peyer's patches are, in fact, partially committed to IgA switch differentiation at the molecular level (i.e., are synthesizing Cα germ-line transcripts), will be necessary. Further, demonstrating that such partially committed B cells do not require specific inductive signals at their site of origin or in the patch will be essential; otherwise, the B-cell centeredness is more apparent than real since, in this case, only the nature or location of the external signal is changed, not its existence. Finally, why and how a cell undergoing IgA switch differentiation on a random basis also acquires a cell surface protein that enables specific homing to the Peyer's patch must be explained. These additional requirements for proof of the theory emphasize the distance that must be traveled before it is accepted; nevertheless, the theory must be kept in mind, since at least some elements untimately may prove to be true (see further discussion).

A second hypothesis concerning IgA switch differentiation and one that, as mentioned, is more consonant with processes that govern differentiation of B cells of other Ig isotypes, is that such differentiation is a directed process in which B cells in the Peyer's patch are induced to undergo IgA switch differentiation by Ig class-specific inductive cells or factors derived from such cells. Early evidence in support of an essential role of T cells in IgA B-cell differentiation was the observation that thymectomized rabbits have decreased IgA antibody responses and normal IgM and IgG responses; similarly, nude mice manifest a selective IgA deficiency (Clough *et al.*, 1971; Pritchard *et al.*, 1973). These observations in studies of whole animals eventually were related to Peyer's patch T-cell function by Elson and Strober who showed that, whereas antigen-activated T cells derived from Peyer's patches enhance LPS-driven IgA synthesis, they suppress LPS-driven IgM and IgG synthesis; on the other hand, spleen T-cell populations activated in the same way suppress LPS-driven responses of any isotype (Elson *et al.*, 1970). Since in titration studies in which increasing numbers of spleen T cells were cultured with a fixed number of Peyer's patch B cells, IgM, IgG, and IgA responses were equally susceptible to the suppressive influence of concanavalin A (Con A) activated spleen T cells, the enhancing effect of Peyer's patch T cells could not be the result of an inherent inability of Peyer's patch IgA B cells to respond to a suppressive influence. In parallel studies, Mongini *et al.* (1983) studied isotype switching of B cells using a splenic focus technique in which isotype switching in clonal B-cell populations of adoptively transferred, irradiated mice was evaluated. In this study, the addition of T cells to the inoculum of cells used to replete "indicator" mice was shown to enhance the frequency of IgA-expressing clones and such clones usually did not coexpress the various IgG subclasses. Collectively, these initial studies of IgA B-cell differentiation established the point that such differentiation is regulated by T cells in a manner that, at least in part, is distinct from that governing IgG B-cell differentiation.

From the data gathered by Elson *et al.* (1979), whether the regulatory effect of Peyer's patch T cells was operating at the level of switch differentiation or terminal differentiation could not be determined since the Peyer's patch B cells under study contained, at least in part, sIgA$^+$ B cells that already had undergone isotype switching. To address this question, Kawanishi *et al.* (1983) prepared cloned Thy1$^+$ T-cell populations from the spleen and Peyer's patches and found that LPS-stimulated sIgM$^+$ B cells cocultured with Peyer's patch T-cell clones either remained as sIgM$^+$ B cells (~36%) or differentiated into sIgA$^+$ B cells (~40–45%); very few (~3%) differentiated into sIgG$^+$ B cells. This result was in striking contrast with LPS-stimulated sIgM$^+$ B cells cultured alone or with spleen T-cell clones. In this case, the resulting cells were either sIgM$^+$ or sIgG$^+$ B cells and very few of the cells were sIgA$^+$ B cells (0.3–0.4%). Other findings emerged from these studies: (1) The Peyer's patch-derived T-cell clones did not induce LPS-stimulated sIgG$^+$ B cells to become sIgA$^+$ B cells, indicating that they were not inducing progressive and stepwise switching. (2) The Peyer's patch-derived cloned cells did not augment B-cell proliferation in general, or IgA B-cell proliferation in particular, over that induced by LPS, so their effect cannot be attributed to preferential proliferation of preformed sIgA$^+$ B cells. (3) Neither Peyer's patch-derived nor spleen-derived T-cell clones induced significant numbers of plasma cells capable of producing either IgG or IgA. In fact, both types of clones greatly decreased the occurrence of IgM or IgG plasma cells, and only the Peyer's patch-derived clone caused an increase in IgA plasma cells compared with B cells stimulated by LPS alone. This result suggested that the processes of switch differentiation and terminal differentiation are separate phenomena. Finally, sIgA$^+$ B cells (or, indeed, sIgG$^+$ B cells), once having switched, could be induced to undergo terminal differentiation into Ig-secreting plasma cells if they were cocultured with appropriate helper T cells (i.e., T cells producing cytokines that induce terminal B-cell differentiation). Collectively, the results of these studies suggested that IgA B-cell switch differentiation was indeed a Peyer's patch T cell-directed process and therefore provided an explanation why IgA switch differentiation occurs predominantly in Peyer's patches.

The general concept that switch T cells of the type described by Kawanishi and colleagues do, in fact, exist was supported by subsequent studies by Mayer and his colleagues (1985, 1986) relating to a human lymphoma T-cell line derived from a patient with the Sézary syndrome. These authors showed first that the lymphoma T cells, when cocultured with normal B cells (non-T cells) and pokeweed mitogen, induced IgG and IgA secretion but little or no IgM secretion, and induced normal $sIgM^+$ tonsillar B cells to produce IgG and IgA. They then showed that this T-cell line induced cells from patients with hyper-IgM syndrome, that is, patients with an immune defect in which only IgM is secreted (in increased amounts), to produce IgG and IgA. On the basis of these data, the investigators concluded that the lymphoma cell line was composed of "switch" T cells that induced, in this case, both IgG and IgA switching; in addition, they postulated that the patients with hyper-IgM syndrome had a defect in their switch T cells. As already mentioned, this latter hypothesis has received support from the finding that the hyper-IgM syndrome is caused by a CD40-ligand defect.

Yet other evidence for the existence of switch T cells was obtained by Benson and colleagues, who derived Con A-induced T-cell clones from gastrointestinal tissues and showed that these lines had a far greater propensity to induce IgA secretion than similar lines obtained from peripheral blood (Benson and Strober, 1988). More precisely, these researchers showed that several of these lines had a greater capacity to increase IgA production in $sIgM^+$ $sIgA^-$ B cells rather than in $sIgM^-$ $sIgA^+$B cells, suggesting that some of the lines were acting as switch T cells.

These studies in support of the concept that switch T cells present in Peyer's patches account for IgA switch differentiation (and perhaps other types of switching, as well) must be considered in light of subsequent studies that are, at best, highly equivocal in their support of this concept. Phillips-Quagliata and colleagues showed, in several studies, that T cells from various organs were equally efficient in inducing IgA responses (Al Maghazachi and Phillips-Quagliata, 1988a,b; Arny *et al.,* 1984). In one study, for example, antigen-primed peripheral lymph node T cells induced as good an IgA response as antigen-primed Peyer's patch T cells in *in vitro* cultures of hapten-primed B cells containing the T-cell priming antigen (Arny *et al.,* 1984). Similarly, in another study, this group of investigators found that (KLH)-specific T-cell clones were capable of inducing IgA responses regardless of their tissue of origin, that is, KLH-induced T cell clones derived from peripheral lymph nodes, spleen, and Peyer's patches all helped (TNP–KLH) primed B cells to produce IgA anti-TNP antibody when the latter were cultured with T-cell clones from these sources and TNP–KLH (Al Maghazachi and Phillips-Quagliata, 1988b). These data, tending to undermine the concept that IgA-specific switch T cells exist in Peyer's patches, are mitigated by the fact that the study design used makes it difficult to distinguish the effects of T cells on switch differentiation from the effects on terminal differentiation: plaque-forming cell responses were measured and the starting B-cell population contained B cells that already had expressed IgG. Further, a larger fraction of Peyer's patch T-cell clones was found to support high IgA responses than clones from other tissues, and representative Peyer's patch T-cell clones were shown to support IgA but not IgG responses when B cells were stimulated with low doses of antigen. Overall, these attempts to demonstrate IgA-specific switch T cells in Peyer's patches in an antigen-specific system were not fully convincing.

C. Role of Dendritic Cells in IgA B-Cell Differentiation

At the same time, Kawanishi and colleagues were pursuing the idea that T cells were the key cell in the Peyer's patch necessary for IgA switching, other investigators were pursuing the possibility that the Peyer's patch cell necessary for IgA-specific switching is a dendritic cell. In initial studies of the latter cell type, Spalding and co-workers (1984) showed that mixtures of periodate-activated T cells and dendritic cells (T cell–dendritic cell clusters) derived from Peyer's patches induced either whole spleen or Peyer's patch B-cell populations to produce IgA in amounts that were equal or even greater than that of IgM. In contrast, whereas T cell–dendritic cell clusters from spleen had an equal capacity to induce IgM, they induced 10 to 100-fold less IgA. These data could be explained by the ability of Peyer's patch T cell–dendritic cell clusters to induce terminal B-cell differentiation, since the B-cell population induced did not consist of purified $sIgM^+$ B cells and may have contained substantial numbers of $sIgA^+$ B cells. However, Spalding *et al.* (1986) followed these studies with ones in which the capacity of a T cell–dendritic cell clusters to induce a pre-B cell line to switch to IgA was determined. These researchers showed that T cell–dendritic cell clusters obtained from Peyer's patches induced pre-B cells to produce mainly IgA (plus small amounts of IgM and IgG), whereas clusters obtained from the spleen induced the pre-B cells to produce IgM and little or no IgG and IgA. Surprisingly, in these experiments the source of the T cells seemed less important than the source of the dendritic cells: mixtures of Peyer's patch dendritic cells with either Peyer's patch T cells or spleen cells resulted in substantial amounts of IgA secretion (and lesser amounts of IgG or IgM secretion), whereas mixtures of spleen dendritic cells and either Peyer's patch or spleen T cells, resulted in mainly IgM secretion. Thus, Spalding and co-workers suggested that either the dendritic cell rather than the T cell was the cell in Peyer's patches critical for IgA switch differentiation or the Peyer's patch dendritic cell was necessary for the activation of T cells in a manner that endows the latter with IgA switch capability.

Additional studies on the role of dendritic cells in IgA B-cell switch differentiation were performed by Cebra and colleagues. In these studies, Peyer's patch B-cell populations were primed with an antigen, enriched for cells responding to the antigen, and cultured at limiting dilution in the prescence of priming antigen, dendritic cells, and conalbumin-activated T cells of the clonal T-cell line D10, a T_H2-type T cell responsive to conalbumin (George and Cebra, 1991). These investigators found that, whereas B cells cultured with T cells alone gave rise to a small number of clones that produce only IgM antibodies, B cells cultured with T cells plus dendritic cells gave rise to clones that produced IgG and IgA antibody as well as IgM antibody (including clones producing only IgA or only IgG antibody). Moreover, additional studies showed that dendritic cell–T cell mixtures could induce purified sIgD$^+$ B cells to give rise (again under limiting dilution conditions) to clones producing mixtures of immunoglobulins, including IgA. Although these studies appear to show that dendritic cell–T cell mixtures do indeed induce isotype switching (IgA as well as IgG), the magnitude of the switch is unclear since the measurement was of the percentage of clones giving rise to IgA secretion and not the percentage of sIgA$^+$ B cells. Under these conditions, low levels of IgA switch differentiation would be considered a positive indicator for switching.

One key difference between the study by Cebra and colleagues and the earlier work by Spalding and colleagues is that, in the Cebra studies, the dendritic cell–T cell clusters inducing IgAB-cell differentiation could be derived from either the Peyer's patch or the spleen whereas, in the Spalding studies, they could be derived only from the Peyer's patch. Cebra and colleagues reasoned that this critical difference is explained by the assumption that, in the Spalding studies, the dendritic cells taken from Peyer's patches had been activated by environmental antigens (prior to isolation) and therefore were able to induce T-cell activation, whereas dendritic cells from spleen were not so activated and did not induce T-cell activation. On the other hand, in the Cebra system, antigen was added to the cultures so both spleen and Peyer's patch dendritic cells were equally stimulatory. Note, however, that this explanation of the Spalding observation fails to give an explanation for why IgA switch differentiation does not occur in the spleen during the course of an infection.

D. Role of TGFβ and Other Switch Factors in IgA B-Cell Differentiation

One question that might be raised in relation to the role of either T cells and dendritic cells in IgA B-cell differentiation is whether either of these cell types acts via a switching factor. In the earlier studies of Kawanishi *et al.* (1983), a factor inducing IgA B-cell differentiation was not found in supernatants of cloned Peyer's patch T cells, nor was IgA switch factor found in T cell–dendritic cell cluster supernatants by Spalding *et al.* or Cebra *et al.* On one hand, Spalding and colleagues emphasized that T cell–dendritic cell clusters required direct contact with B cells to achieve their effects and on the other hand, Phillips-Quagliata *et al.* did obtain evidence for the presence of an IgA switch factor (Al Maghazachi and Phillips-Quagliata, 1988a). Phillips-Quagliata and co-workers identified at least one Con A-stimulated clonal T-cell population that produced a factor that helped IgG and IgA responses but not IgM responses (Al Maghazachi and Phillips-Quagliata, 1988a). Curiously, although this clone induces B-cell differentiation, it fails to induce B cell proliferation. This observation raises an interesting question regarding the relationship of switch differentiation to B-cell proliferation.

Far more solid evidence for the presence of an IgA switch factor came with the demonstration by two groups that TGFβ could induce LPS-activated mouse splenocytes to switch from IgM to IgA production (Coffman *et al.*, 1989; Sonada *et al.*, 1989). In the relevant studies, these investigators showed that TGFβ augmented LPS-induced IgA production 10-fold or more, particularly in cultures also containing terminal differentiation factors such as IL-5 and IL-2. Thus, while IgA constitutes only 0.1% of the total Ig produced by LPS-stimulated B cells cultures in the absence of TGFβ, the percentage increases to 15–25% in LPS-stimulated cultures containing TGFβ plus IL-2. This striking finding in murine B-cell systems was confirmed by others (Kim and Kagnoff, 1990; Lebman *et al.*, 1990a,b; Ehrhardt *et al.*, 1992) and, in addition, was extended to human B-cell systems (Islam *et al.*, 1991; Nilsson *et al.*, 1991; Defrance *et al.*, 1992; van Vlasselaer *et al.*, 1992), in which B cells were stimulated with pokeweed mitogen in the presence of CD4$^+$ T cells.

From the outset, strong evidence was presented that this TGFβ effect is manifest at the level of isotype switch differentiation rather than terminal differentiation. First were the findings that TFGβ acts on sIgA$^-$ B cells rather than sIgA$^+$ B cells and that TGFβ increases the frequency of B-cell clones secreting IgA rather than the number of IgA B cells per clone. Second came evidence that TFGβ induces the production of Cα germ-line transcripts which, as noted earlier, is an early molecular step in the IgA switch process. Third, and finally, was the observation that TGFβ has no selective effect on B-cell viability and produces its maximal effect on IgA production if added early in the culture period and then removed isotype; and, in fact, TGFβ inhibits IgA production by already switched IgA$^+$ B cells (Kim and Kagnoff, 1990; Ehrhardt *et al.*, 1992). Collectively, these data establish beyond question that, under *in vitro* conditions, TGFβ does act as an IgA switch factor. The data fall short, however, of providing a clear picture of the role of this cytokine in overall IgA B-cell differentiation as it occurs *in vivo*. To approach this more fundamental question, such issues as the precise stage of B-cell differentiation at which TFGβ acts, its class and, tissue specificity, the magnitude of its effect, and, finally, its collateral properties must be explored more completely.

With respect to data on the stage of B-cell development at which TGFβ acts, the fact that this cytokine induces Cα germ-line transcripts in sIgM$^+$ B cells localizes the effect to an early stage of IgA switch differentiation. This early action does not necessarily imply, however, that TGFβ initiates IgA switch differentiation since, as discussed at some length previously, the first step of isotype differentiation involves the processes that lead to an increase in the accessibility to transcriptional enzymes of the regions 5′ to C_H genes rather than to germ-line transcription, the latter being viewed as a secondary event. Data on whether TGFβ can induce Cα accessibility (as well as Cα germ-line transcription) is equivocal at best (Lebman *et al.*, 1990a,b; Islam *et al.*, 1991; Nilsson *et al.*, 1991; Lin and Stavnezer, 1992). In murine systems, studies of TGFβ switch effects on normal B cells always have been conducted in the presence of a B-cell stimulant such as LPS, leaving open the possibility that the B-cell stimulant induces Cα accessibility (albeit at a low level) and that the action of TGFβ is limited to its effect on Cα germ-line transcription occurring after induction of Cα accessibility. In this context, the accessibility induced by the B-cell stimulant is assumed to be nonspecific with respect to Ig class and, indeed, may relate to all Ig classes; thus, the fact that TGFβ seems to have a specific effect on IgA switching could arise from the fact that it has an Ig-specific effect on Cα germ-line transcription. Also relevant to the discussion of whether TGFβ induces Cα accessibility in murine B-cell systems is the fact that TGFβ does not induce CH1 B cells, a murine lymphoma sIgM$^+$ B-cell line that is not demethylated at the Cα locus (i.e., does not have an accessible Cα locus), to produce Cα germ-line transcripts or to secrete IgA (Whitmore *et al.*, 1990). However, CH1 B cells may be inherently unswitchable, as are most immortal B-cell lines.

Data on human B cells are similar to those on murine B cells. Again, the effect of TGFβ effects on Cα germ-line transcription were evaluated on resting sIgA$^-$ B cells with a sensitive reverse transcriptase–polymerase chain reaction (RT–PCR) assay; researchers found that, whereas induction of Cα1 germ-line transcription required TGFβ plus mitogen, induction of Cα2 transcription required only TGFβ (Islam *et al.*, 1991). Thus, in this instance TGFβ may act as a factor inducing both accessibility and germ-line transcription.

A final possibility relative to TGFβ effects on early molecular events of IgA switch differentiation is that, although TGFβ induces some level of Cα accessibility, this effect is marginal and, in any case, subordinate to its effect on Cα germ-line transcription. Indirect evidence for this hypothesis comes from studies of CH12.LX B cells, a sIgM$^+$ lymphoma B-cell line mentioned earlier that is demethylated in the Cα locus (i.e., has an accessible Cα gene segment) and undergoes spontaneous switching to sIgA$^+$ B cells at low frequency (Arnold *et al.*, 1988; Kunimoto *et al.*, 1988). Presumably, such cells are "preswitched" B cells, meaning they have received an initial switch signal that set them on a pathway of IgA B-cell differentiation before they were immortalized. In studies of the effects of cytokines on these B cells, Strober and colleagues have shown that a particular subclone of these cells that switches only to IgA can be induced by LPS and IL-4, LPS and TGFβ, or LPS and IL-4/TGFβ to increase greatly Cα germ-line transcription and the frequency of switching to IgA (Kunimoto *et al.*, 1988). In this case, whereas the spontaneous switching to IgA B cells is 2%, in the presence of IL-4/TGFβ the frequency of switching is 50–70%. These data in addition to data obtained with another preswitched lymphoma B-cell line (I.29), indicate that, although TGFβ induction of IgA switch differentiation in normal B cells is modest (see subsequent discussion), this cytokine has a profound effect on already switched B cells, suggesting that the true stage at which this cytokine acts is after the initial switch event (Shockett and Stavnezer, 1991).

Additional studies relative to this point were done by Whitmore *et al.* (1990), who showed that CH12.LX B cell subclones capable of switching to a number of Ig isotypes, but mainly IgA (i.e., clones that differ to some extent from those studied by Kawanishi *et al.*, 1983, which switch only to IgA), are induced by TGFβ to switch to various Ig isotypes as well as to IgA and that, in general, TGFβ does not affect the relative frequency of IgA switching, only the absolute frequency. Thus, TGFβ appears not to have an isotype-specific effect on preswitched B cells and appears to facilitate switching to all isotypes in such cells. This result, in turn, implies that TGFβ is a general or non-isotype-specific inducer of germ-line transcription and that its IgA-specific effects on normal B cells are the result of selective antiproliferative activity on non-IgA B cells, as discussed previously. This view is supported by molecular findings that show that TGFβ-responsive elements are found in several Ig regulatory regions, not only in the IgA regulatory region, again suggesting that the primary effect of TGFβ is on regulation of germ-line transcription rather than on accessibility (Lin and Stavnezer, 1992).

A second consideration relevant to the role of TGFβ in isotype switching, one that complements the discussion on the locus of the TGFβ effect, relates to the magnitude of this effect. In the earliest studies by Lebman and colleagues relating to the ability of TGFβ to affect IgA switching, TGFβ was shown to induce only a small fraction of LPS-stimulated sIgM$^+$ B cells to switch to sIgA$^+$ B cells (3.2%). From these data one might conclude that, although TGFβ does indeed induce IgA switching, it does so only at a minor and nonphysiological rate that is in no way comparable to the rate observed at *in vivo* IgA induction sites, at which the frequency of Ig switching is at the 70–85% level (Butcher *et al.*, 1982). However, LPS is not a physiological B-cell stimulant so one can argue that, when B cells are stimulated in other ways, a more significant TGFβ-mediated IgA induction can be seen. To examine this question, Ehrhardt *et al.* (1992) stimulated highly purified sIgM$^+$sIgD$^+$ B cells (containing $<$0.2% sIgA$^+$ B cells) in a T cell-independent fashion, that is, with LPS or with anti-IgD–dextran (T cell-independent B cell mitogens), and in a T cell-dependent fashion, that is, with T cells in a cognate interaction (using a T-cell clone that recognized rabbit Ig determinants and B cells treated with IgG rabbit anti-IgM) or in a noncognate interaction (using irradiated anti-CD3-activated T-cell clones in the absence of additional mitogens or antigens), all in the presence and absence of TGFβ. These investigators found that, regardless of the method of B-cell stimulation, TGFβ induced only a small fraction of B cells (1–3%) to undergo IgA switch differentiation. Note that this low frequency of TGFβ-induced switching to IgA contrasts with the high frequency of IL-4-induced switching to IgG (Snapper and Paul, 1987) or, as mentioned, with the high frequency of switching to IgA observed in the germinal centers of Peyer's patches (Butcher *et al.*, 1982). Therefore, we must conclude that TGFβ is either a weak, that is, nonphysiological IgA switch signal or, alternatively, that TGFβ is a secondary signal that only operates effectively in the context of a more primary signal that prepares cells to respond to TGFβ with Cα germ-line transcripts and switch signals. Of these two views, the latter seems more reasonable in light of the observation already mentioned that high levels of IgA switching (20–70%) can be obtained in cultures of CH12.LX B cells, that is, B cells that are precommitted to IgA switching. However, more physiological methods of inducing high level IgA switch differentiation in normal B cells must be found before this question can be answered definitively.

Note that the magnitude of IgA switch differentiation induced by TGFβ, as assessed by the appearance of sIgA$^+$ B cells (2–3%), seems too low to account for the amount of IgA secreted after 7–10 days (20% of total Ig secreted). The reason for this paradox became apparent in studies also conducted by R. Ehrhardt, G. R. Harriman, Y. K. Inman, and W. Strober, (unpublished observations), who stimulated purified sIgA$^+$ B cells (>95% pure) in a highly efficient fashion to undergo terminal differentiation into IgA-secreting plasma cells by incubating the B cells with T cells in a cognate or noncognate fashion. In this case, an excess of 2×10^5 ng IgA were produced per 10^5 B cells, indicating that the 2000–6000 ng IgA produced in LPS-stimulated sIgM$^+$ B-cell cultures containing TGFβ really does represent the differentiation of only 2–3% of the B cells present. In view of these findings, the TGFβ-induced switching is quantitatively minor, even if the amount of IgA secreted is considered. In retrospect, this amount was only impressive when TGFβ-induced IgA secretion was compared with IgA secretion in the absence of this lymphokine.

A third consideration concerning the role of TGFβ in IgA switch differentiation concerns its overall role in physiological IgA switching as opposed to switching that occurs *in vitro*. More specifically, we must reconcile the fact that IgA B-cell development is site specific, that is, a characteristic of Peyer's patch lymphoid follicles, with the fact that TGFβ production is widespread and occurs in many, if not all, lymphoid tissues. Thus, although the data indicates that all kinds of lymphoid cells are important producers of this cytokine, no evidence suggests that such production itself creates a situation in which TGFβ plays a unique role in B-cell development in lymphoid tissues in general or in Peyer's patches in particular. Overall, the most likely conclusion to be drawn from the fact that TGFβ secretion is widespread, and probably sufficient in many tissues to support IgA switching, is that TGFβ is best viewed as a cofactor that acts on B cells that already have received signals to commit to IgA switch differentiation.

A final consideration relating to the physiological role of TGFβ in IgA switch differentiation relates to the inhibitory effect of this cytokine on lymphoid cells. Even before the effect of TGFβ on IgA switching was known, TGFβ had been shown to have a profound negative effect on both B- and T-cell proliferation, including LPS-induced B-cell proliferation (Kehrl *et al.*, 1986,1987,1991; Wahl *et al.*, 1988; Moses *et al.*, 1990). This suppressive effect was most evident for IgG and IgM secretion, but was seen also for IgA secretion. We have shown that, although TGFβ clearly enhances LPS-induced IgA synthesis, such enhancement is obtained most clearly by addition of anti-TGFβ to the culture 1–2 days after the start of the culture, suggesting that the positive effect of TGFβ on IgA B-cell switch differentiation can be mitigated subsequently by the negative effect of TGFβ on B-cell terminal differentiation (Ehrhardt *et al.*, 1992). In addition, in cells activated by other more physiological signals such as cognate or noncognate T-cell interactions, TGFβ either has no effect on overall IgA secretion or actually inhibits IgA secretion unless anti-TGFβ is added to the 48-hr cultures. Finally, B cells in cultures containing low doses of TGFβ (0.1 ng/ml) secrete more than 15 times the amount of IgA than do B cells in cultures containing high doses of TGFβ (1.0 ng/ml), despite an increase in sIgA$^+$ B cells in the high-dose TGFβ cultures. These data, plus the fact that the inhibitory effect of TGFβ is much more evident in the T-cell activation systems than in the LPS activation system, strongly suggest that IgA secretion is not a sensitive indicator of IgA switch differentiation, especially when B-cell stimulation by a factor other than LPS is used. In general, the presence of TGFβ in a lymphoid milieu is a double-edged sword. We are prompted to postulate that, if TGFβ plays a physiological role in IgA B-cell differentiation, that role requires the B cell to receive the TGFβ signal at a particular induction site (the mucosal follicle) and then to migrate rapidly to another site (the lamina propria) where TGFβ effects are, attenuated. Finally, note that the capacity of TGFβ to exert an antiproliferative effect on B cells may be one of the ways in which this cytokine influences IgA switching. The concept applicable here is that TGFβ, by preventing cells from entering the G_1 phase of the cell cycle while favoring cell–cell interaction via induction of MHC Class II determinant expression (Moses *et al.*, 1990), increases the interval of time that an isotype-nonspecific differentiation signal can be applied without leading to cell division and terminal differentiation. Thus, a greater chance exists that Cα accessibility will occur and that other, more IgA-specific differentiation effects can supervene and move the system in favor of IgA B-cell differentiation.

Evidence has appeared that another B-cell differentiation factor, IL-10, also plays a role in IgA B-cell differentiation. In the relevant studies conducted by Banchereau and colleagues, human B cells stimulated with anti-IgM plus anti-CD40 antibody in the presence of TGFβ and IL-10 were shown to produce impressive amounts of IgA (Defrance *et al.*, 1992). Since, in these studies, IgA secretion rather than the frequency of sIgA$^+$ B cells was measured, the question remains whether IL-10 is acting as a terminal differentiation factor in this case.

IV. OVERVIEW OF IgA B CELL SWITCH DIFFERENTIATION

Having discussed at some length the molecular and cellular factors involved in B-cell isotype differentiation generally, as well as the cellular and humoral factors involved in IgA B-cell switch differentiation particularly, we can draw together various pieces of evidence to create a more-or-less coherent outline of the processes that govern the emergence of IgA B cells in mucosal tissues.

IgA B-cell differentiation probably can be said to begin when inductive T cells interact with $sIgM^+$ B cells and initiate the molecular processes that lead to IgA switch differentiation. What are the characteristics of these "switch" T cells? In the first place, these cells are likely to be activated T cells that have gained the ability to bring about IgA switching after antigen-specific interaction with Peyer's patch antigen-presenting cells, (i.e., interdigitating dendritic cells). The working hypothesis here is that the dendritic cells in Peyer's patches unique in their capacity to induce IgA "switch" T cells by some as yet undefined cell–cell interaction or cytokine effect. However, we cannot rule out the possibility that the stimulatory interaction is not unique and that T cells in Peyer's patches are not intrinsically different from cells at other sites.

The bases for saying that a T cell and not a dendritic cell provides the key switch signal to B cells undergoing IgA switch differentiation are several. First, T cells alone seem able to induce isotype switch differentiation under appropriate conditions, whereas dendritic cells alone have not been shown to have this ability (Kawanishi *et al.*, 1983; Mayer *et al.*, 1986). Evidence to the contrary, such as that of Spalding *et al.*, showing that the ability of T cell–dendritic cell clusters to induce IgA switching seemed to be associated with the dendritic cell rather than the T cell, can be explained by assuming that (1) T cells from any tissue can act as IgA-specific switch cells, provided they are activated in an appropriate way, and (2) such activation is brought about by Peyer's patch dendritic cells rather than by spleen dendritic cells, because the former develop in a characteristic way in the mucosal environment. Indeed, in the studies by Cebra and colleagues, Peyer's patch *and* spleen dendritic cells were able to support IgA switch differentiation to an equal extent, presumably because external stimulation of dendritic cells was provided in this case (Schrader *et al.*, 1990; George and Cebra, 1991).

A second and perhaps more cogent reason to posit the primacy of a T-cell signal in IgA switch differentiation comes from work showing that B-cell switch differentiation, regardless of isotype specificity, occurs more readily during T cell–B cell interactions. Thus, as reviewed earlier, purified $sIgM^+sIgD^+$ B cells stimulated with conventional B-cell mitogens such as anti-IgM or SAC (in the presence of TGFβ) have been shown to produce little IgA, whereas the same cells stimulated by one of these mitogens plus anti-CD40 antibody (again in the presence of TGFβ) produce large amounts of IgA (Defrance *et al.*, 1992). These data suggest that T-cell signaling via CD40 is necessary for IgA switch differentiation and that high levels of CD40 ligand expression may, in fact, be one of the defining features of an IgA-specific switch T cell.

Although the CD40 ligand–CD40 interaction may be necessary for IgA switch differentiation, it is almost certainly not sufficient, since little evidence suggests that this interaction does anything more than prepare the cell for "generic" switch differentiation. As reviewed in the discussion on the role of cytokines in switch differentiation, a cytokine with a now well-described ability to induce IgA switch differentiation under a variety of B-cell activation conditions (Coffman *et al.*, 1989; Sonada *et al.*, 1989; Kim and Kagnoff, 1990; Lebman *et al.*, 1990a,b; Islam *et al.*, 1991; Ehrhardt *et al.*, 1992). However, in suggesting TGFβ as the directing cytokine in IgA B-cell switch differentiation, at least two caveats must be remembered. First, the magnitude of IgA switch differentiation induced by TGFβ, including that induced in B cells activated by T cells via a CD40 ligand–CD40 interaction, is quite modest ($\leq$3%). Second, TGFβ is secreted in many tissues in addition to the Peyer's patches, so this cytokine hardly can account for the unique relationship between Peyer's patches and IgA B-cell development. Based on these caveats, TGFβ is best looked on as a cofactor in IgA switch differentiation that acts opportunistically on $sIgM^+$B cells in Peyer's patches while the latter are receiving additional IgA-specific switch signals. The concept that TGFβ plays only a limited role in IgA switch differentiation leaves us with the necessity of considering other possible switch T-cell influences that account for the large-scale IgA switch differentiation actually observed in Peyer's patches. Such other influences could involve as yet undefined cell–cell interactions that are accessory to the CD40 ligand–CD40 interaction or to other cytokines.

Another point to consider in relation to other possible IgA switch differentiation signals is that these signals may consist of an inhibitory signal that negatively regulates switching to more 3′ C_H genes, rather than an enhancing signal that positively regulates Cα switching. At the moment, support for this inhibition mechanism of IgA switching is scant. One piece of evidence is that the switch T-cell clones identified by Kawanishi *et al.* (1983), despite being capable of inducing high frequency IgA switch differentiation, fail to induce IgA secretion. Similarly, although TGFβ suppresses IgA secretion (as well as IgA and IgM secretion), at the same time it induces IgM B cells to undergo switch differentiation to IgA (Ehrhardt *et al.*, 1992).

So far in this discussion, we have assumed that the B cell acted on initially by switch T cells is a completely unswitched $sIgM^+$ B cell that does not have accessible regions 5′ to the Cα gene and does not produce Cα germ-line transcripts. At this point, however, we also should consider the possibility that the B cells acted are, in reality, B cells that are partially committed to IgA switch differentiation (i.e., partially switched B cells) and, thus, are capable of responding to "switch" signals with high-frequency IgA switching. One fact in favor of this concept is that partially switched B cells already exist in the form of several B-cell lymphoma lines such as CH12.LX B cells and I.29 B cells (Arnold *et al.*, 1988; Kunimoto *et al.*, 1988; Shockett and Stavnezer, 1991). As described earlier, these B cells are largely $sIgM^+$ B cells that spontaneously switch to $sIgA^+$ B cells at a low rate. In keeping with this fact, they have accessible regulatory regions 5′ to the Cα gene segment and continually are synthesizing Cα germ-line transcripts. Other properties of these CH12.LX cells that are germane to this discussion are that (1) in undergoing isotype switch, they appear to become dual-positive $sIgM^+sIgA^+$ B cells that have not yet rearranged their productive C_H genes (and thus still retain the Cμ gene segment), and (2) CH12.LX B cells, in contrast to normal $sIgM^+$ B cells, respond to TGFβ (and, to a lesser extent, to IL-4) with high-frequency switch to $sIgA^+$ B cells. Thus, as indicated earlier, such precommitted cells are much more responsive to the switch impetus of TGFβ than are normal $sIgM^+$ B cells.

If we consider these partially switched B-cell lines models of B cells in Peyer's patches that are capable of responding to IgA-specific switch signals, we can postulate that partially switched B cells of this kind initially develop in bone marrow during the course of VDJ gene arrangement, possibly as a result of intracellular conditions occurring during this process. These cells, although still expressing surface IgM or perhaps expressing sIgM and sIgA, then migrate to Peyer's patches as a result of as yet poorly understood cell homing patterns. Alternatively, they migrate to many or most lymphoid organs, but only receive a secondary switch signal in Peyer's patches. The main evidence for this hypothesis, already alluded to previously, is that the partially switched B cells (of the CH12.LX type) respond with greater alacrity to TGFβ than do normal $sIgM^+$ B cells. Another kind of evidence relates to the fact that, to date, demonstrating high-frequency IgA switch differentiation *in vitro* has been difficult, possibly because, in the studies conducted to date, the subpopulation in Peyer's patch B cells that is susceptible to switching has not been identified. Relevant here is the fact that the switch T-cell clone studies by Kawanishi and colleagues caused 3–4 times more switching of Peyer's patch B cells than of spleen B cells, suggesting that B cells in the patches may be more "switchable" than B cells in the spleen (Kawanishi *et al.,* 1982,1983). Finally, the idea that IgA switch differentiation is initiated in the bone marrow is favored by the fact that mature IgA B cells are unusually plentiful in human and mouse bone marrow. More study of Peyer's patch B-cell populations for evidence of the presence of an "immature" partially switched B-cell population is necessary to bring this theory to more serious consideration.

In summary, this discussion has emphasized that, although we can be reasonably sure that IgA switch differentiation requires the influence of a T cell as well as the probable influence of one or more isotype-directing cytokines, much is still unknown about this differentiation process. In particular, whether the B-cell target is an uncommitted B cell or a B cell partially committed to IgA switch differentiation and whether additional as yet undefined cytokines or cell–cell interactions are necessary for either of these targets to become fully differentiated IgA B cells is still unknown. Further studies using newer *in vitro* culture techniques and cells from different lymphoid sites are necessary to decide these issues.

References

Al Maghazachi, A., and Phillips-Quagliata, J. M. (1988a). Con A-propagated, auto-reactive T cell clones that secrete factors promoting high IgA responses. *Int. Arch. Allergy Appl. Immunol.* **86(2),** 147–156.

Al Maghazachi, A., and Phillips-Quagliata, J. M. (1988b). Keyhole limpet hemocyanin-propagated Peyer's patch T cell clones that help IgA responses. *J. Immunol.* **140(10),** 3380–3388.

Arnold, L. W., Gordina, T. A., Whitemore, A. C., and Haughton, G. (1988). Ig isotype switching in B lymphocytes. Isolation and characterization of clonal variants of the murine Ly-1+ B cell lymphoma, CH12, expressing isotypes other than IgM. *Proc. Natl. Acad. Sci. U.S.A.* **85(20),** 7704–7708.

Arny, M., Kelly-Hatfield, P., Lamm, M. E., and Phillips-Quagliata, J. M. (1984). T-cell help for the IgA response: The function of T cells from different lymphoid organs in regulating the proportions of plasma cells expressing various isotypes. *Cell. Immunol.* **89,** 95–112.

Aruffo, A., Farrington, M., Hollenbaugh, D., Li, X., Milatovich, A., Nonoyama, S., Ledbbetter, J. A., Francke, U., and Ochs, H. D. (1993). The CD40 ligand, gp39, is defective in activated T cells from patients with X-linked hyper-IgM syndrome. *Cell* **72(2),** 291–300.

Banchereau, J., de Paoli, P., Valle, A., Garcia, E., and Rousett, F. (1991). Long-term human B cell lines dependent on interleukin-4 and antibody to CD40. *Science* **251,** 70–72.

Benson, E. B., and Strober W. (1988). Regulation of IgA secretion by T cell clones derived from the human gastrointestinal tract. *J. Immunol.* **140(6),** 1874–1882.

Berton, M. T., Uhr, J. W., and Vitetta, E. S. (1989). Synthesis of germline γ1 immunoglobulin heavy-chain transcripts in resting B cells: Induction by interleukin-4 and inhibition by interferon γ. *Proc. Natl. Acad. Sci. U.S.A.* **86,** 2829–2833.

Butcher, E. C., Rouse, R. V., Coffman, R. L., Nottenburg, C. N., Hardy, R. R., and Weissman I. L. (1982). Surface phenotype of Peyer's patch germinal center cells: Implications for the role of germinal centers in B cell differentiation. *J. Immunol.* **129,** 2698–2707.

Care, A., Cianetti, L., Gianpaolo, A., Sposi, N. M., Zappavigna, V., Mavilio, F., Alimera, G., Amadori, S., Mandelli, F., and Peschle C. (1986). Translocation of c-*myc* into the immunoglobulin heavy chain locus in human acute B cell leukemia: A molecular analysis. *EMBO J.* **5,** 905.

Chen, Y.-W., Word, C. J., Dev. V., Uhr, J. W., Vitetta, E. S., and Tucker, P. W. (1986). Double isotype production by a neoplastic B cell line. II. Allelically excluded production of μ and γ1 chain without C_H gene rearrangement. *J. Exp. Med.* **164,** 562.

Clough, J. D., Mims, L. H., and Strober. W. (1971). Deficient IgA antibody responses to arsonilic acid bovine serum albumin (BSA) in neonatally thymectomized rabbits. *J. Immunol.* **106,** 1624–1629.

Coffman, R. L., and Carty, J. (1986). A T cell activity that enhances polyclonal IgE production and its inhibition by interferon-gamma. *J. Immunol.* **136(3),** 949–954.

Coffman, R. L., Ohara, J., Bond, J. W., Carty, J., Zlotnick, A., and Paul, W. E. (1986). B cel stimulatory factor-1 enhances the IgE response of lipopolysaccharide-activated B cells. *J. Immunol.* **136(12),** 4538–4541.

Coffman, R. L., Lebman, D. A., and Schrader, B. (1989). Transforming growth factor β specifically enhances IgA production by lipopolysaccharide-stimulated murine B lymphocytes. *J. Exp. Med.* **170,** 1039–1044.

Craig, S. W., and Cebra, J. J. (1981). Peyer's patches: An enriched source of precursors for IgA-producing immunocytes in the rabbit. *J. Exp. Med.* **134,** 188–200.

Cutler Allen, R., Armitage, R. J., Conley, M. E., Rosenblatt, H., Jenkins, N. A., Copeland, N. G., Bedell, M. A. Edelhoff, S., Disteche, C. M., Simoneaux, D. K., Fanslow, W. C., Belmont, J., and Spriggs, M. K. (1993). CD40 ligand gene defects responsible for X-linked hyper IgM syndrome. *Science* **259,** 990–993.

Defrance, T., Vanbervliet, B., Briére, F., Durand, I., Rousett, F., and Banchereau, J. (1992). Interleukin-10 and transforming growth factor β cooperate to induce anti-CD40-activated naive human B cells to secrete immunoglobulin A. *J. Exp. Med.* **175,** 671–682.

Ehrhardt, R. O., Strober, W., and Harriman, G. R. (1992). Effect of transforming growth factor (TGF)β_1 on IgA isotype expression TGF-β_1 induces a small increase in sIgA+ B cells regardless of the method of B cell activation. *J. Immunol.* **148,** 3830–3836.

Elson, C. C., Heck, J. A., and Strober, W. (1979). T-cell regulation of murine IgA synthesis. *J. Exp. Med.* **149,** 632–643.

Esser, C., and Radbruch, A. (1989). Rapid induction of transcription of unrearranged sγ1 switch regions in activated murine B cells by interleukin 4. *EMBO J.* **8,** 4832–4888.

Flanagan, J. G., and Rabbitts, T. H. (1982). Arrangement of human immunoglobulin heavy chain constant region genes implies evolutionary duplication of a segment containing γ, ε, and α genes. *Nature (London)* **300,** 709.

George, A. and J. J. Cebra (1991). Responses of single germinal-center B cells in T-cell-dependent microculture. *Proc. Natl. Acad. Sci. U.S.A.* **88,** 11–15.

Gerondakis, S. (1990). Structure and expression of murine germline immunoglobulin heavy chian transcripts induced by interleukin 4. *Proc. Natl. Acad. Sci. U.S.A.* **87(4),** 1581.

Gerstein, R. M., W. N. Frankel, C. L. Hsieh, Durdik, J. M, Rath, S., Cottin, J. M., Nisonott, A, and Selsing, E. (1990). Isotype switching of an immunoglobulin heavy chain transgene occurs by DNA recombination between different chromosomes. *Cell* **63,** 537–548.

Hamlyn, P. H., and T. H. Rabbitts (1983). Translocation of c-myc and immunoglobulin γ 1 genes in a Burkitt lymphoma revealing a third exon in the d-myc oncogene. *Nature (London)* **304,** 190.

Harriman, G. R., N. S. Lycke, L. J. Elwood, and W. Strober (1990). T lymphocytes that express CD4 and the $\alpha\beta$-T cell receptor but lack Thy-1. *J. Immunol.* **145,** 2406–2414.

Hodgkin, P. D., L. C. Yamashita, R. L. Coffman, and M. R. Kehry (1990). Separation of events mediating B cell proliferation and Ig production by using T cell membranes and lymphokines. *J. Immunol.* **145(7),** 2025–2034.

Hofker, M. H., M. A. Walter, and D. W. Cox (1989). Complete physical map of the human immunoglobulin heavy chain constant region gene complex. *Proc. Natl. Acad. Sci. U.S.A.* **86,** 5567.

Isakson, P. C., E. Puré, E. S. Vitetta, and P. H. Krammer (1982). T cell-derived B cell differentiation factor(s). Effect on the isotype switch of murine B cells. *J. Exp. Med.* **155,** 734–748.

Islam, K. B., L. Nilsson, P. Sideras, L. Hammarström, and C. I. Edvard Smith (1991). TGF-β1 induces germ-line transcripts of both IgA subclasses in human B lymphocytes. *Int. Immunol.* **3,** 1099–1106.

Iwasato, T., A. Shimizu, T. Honjo, and H. Yamagishi (1990). Circular DNA is excised by immunoglobulin class switch recombination. *Cell* **62,** 143–149.

Iwasato, T., H. Arakawa, A. Shimizu, Honjo, T., and Yamagishi, H. (1992). Biased distribution of recombination sites within A regions upon immunoglobulin class switch recombination induced by transforming growth factor β and lipopolysaccharide. *J. Exp. Med.* **175,** 1539–1546.

Kawanishi, H., L. E. Saltzman, and W. Strober (1982). Characteristics and regularly function of murine con A-induced, cloned T cells obtained from Peyer's patches and spleen. Mechanisms regulating istoype-specific immunoglobulin production by Peyer's patch B cells. *J. Immunol.* **129,** 475–483.

Kawanishi, H., L. Saltzman, and W. Strober (1983). Mechanisms regulating IgA class-specific immunoglobulin production in murine gut-associated lymphoid tissues. I. T cells derived from Peyer's patches that switch sIgM B cells to SIgA B cells *in vitro*. *J. Exp. Med.* **157,** 437–450.

Kehrl, J. H., A. B. Roberts, L. M. Wakefield, S. Jakowlew, M. B. Sporn, and A. S. Fauci (1986).Transforming growth factor beta is an important immunomodulatory protein for human B lymphocytes. *J. Immunol.* **137,** 3855.

Kehrl, J. H., L. M. Wakefield, A. B. Roberts, S. Jakowlew, M. Alvarez-Mon, R. Derynck, M. B. Sporn, and A. S. Fauci (1987). Production of transforming growth factor beta by human T lymphocytes and its potential role in the regulation of T cell growth. *J. Exp. Med.* **163,** 1037.

Kehrl, J. H., C. Thevenin, P. Rieckmann, and A. S. Fauci (1991). Transforming growth factor-beta suppresses human B lymphocyte Ig production by inhibiting synthesis and the switch from the membrane form to the secreted form of Ig mRNA. *J. Immunol.* **146,** 4016.

Kim, P. H., and M. F. Kagnoff (1990). Transforming growth factor β1 increases IgA isotype switching at the clonal level. *J. Immunol.* **145,** 3773.

Kishimoto, T. and T. Hirano (1989). B lymphocyte activation, proliferation and immunoglobulin secretion. *In* "Fundamental Immunology" (W. E. Paul, ed.), 2d Ed. pp. 385–413. Raven Press, New York.

Kitani, A., and W. Strober (1993). Regulation of Cγ subclass germline transcripts in human peripheral blood B cells. *J. Immunol.*, in press.

Kunimoto, D. Y., G. R. Harriman, and W. Strober (1988). Regulation of IgA differentiation in CH12.LX B cells by lymphokines: IL-4 induces membrane IgM-positive CH12.LX cells to express membrane IgA and IL-5 induces membrane IgA-positive CH12.LX cells to secrete IgA. *J. Immunol.* **141,** 713–720.

Kupfer, A., S. L. Swain, C. A. Janeway, Jr., and S. J. Singer (1986). The specific direct interaction of helper T cells and antigen-presenting B cells. *Proc. Natl. Acad. Sci. U.S.A.* **83,** 6080.

Kuze, K., A. Shimizu, and T. Honjo (1991). Characterization of the enhancer region for germline transcription of the γ3 constant region gene of human immunoglobulin. *Int. Immunol.* **7,** 647.

Lebman, D. A., and R. L. Coffman (1988). Interleukin 4 causes isotype switching to IgE in T cell-stimulated clonal B cell cultures. *J. Exp. Med.* **168(3),** 853–862.

Lebman, D. A., F. D. Lee, and R. L. Coffman (1990a). Mechanism for transforming growth factor β and IL-2 enhancement of IgA expression in lipopolysaccharide-stimulated B cell cultures. *J. Immunol.* **144,** 942–959.

Lebman, D. A., D. Y. Nomura, R. L. Coffman, and F. D. Lee (1990b). Molecular characterization of germline immunoglobulin A transcripts produced during transforming growth factor type β-induced isotype switching. *Proc. Natl. Acad. Sci. U.S.A.* **87,** 3962–3966.

Lin, Y.-C. A., and J. Stavnezer (1992). Regulation of transcription of the germ-line Igα constant region gene by an ATF element and by novel transforming growth factor-β1-responsive elements. *J. Immunol.* **149,** 2914–2925.

Lutzker, S., P. Rothman, R. Pollock, R. Coffman, and F. W. Alt (1988). Mitogen- and IL-4-regulated expression of germline Ig γ2b transcripts: Evidence for directed heavy chain class switching. *Cell* **53,** 177–184.

McIntyre, T. M., Klinman, D. R., Rothman, P., Lugo, M., Dasch, J. R., Mond, J. J., and Snapper, C. M. Transforming growth factor β_1 selectivity stimulates immunoglobulin G2b secretion by lipopolysaccharide-activated murine B cells. *J. Exp. Med.* **177,** 1031–1037.

Matsuoka, M., K. Yoshida, T. Maeda, S. Usuda, and H. Sakano (1990). Switch circular DNA formed in cytokine-treated mouse splenocytes: Evidence for intramolecular DNA deletion in immunoglobulin class switching. *Cell* **62,** 135–142.

Mayer, L., D. N. Posnett, and H. G. Kunkel (1985). Human malignant T cells capable of inducing an immunoglobulin class switch. *J. Exp. Med.* **161,** 134–144.

Mayer, L., S. P. Swan, C. Thompson, H. S. Ko, Chiorazzi, N., Waldmann, T., and Roseu, F. (1986). Evidence for a defect in "switch" T cells in patients with immunodeficiency and hyperimmunoglobulinemia M. *N. Eng. J. Med.* **314,** 409–413.

Mizuta, T. R., N. Suzuki, A. Shimizu, and T. Honjo (1991). Duplicated variable region genes account for double isotype expression in a human leukemic B cell line that gives rise to single isotype-expressing cells. *J. Biol. Chem.* **266(19),** 12514–12521.

Mongini, P. K. A., W. E. Paul, and E. S. Metcalf (1983). IgG subclass IgE, and IgA anti-trinitrophenol antibody production within trinitrophenol–Ficoll-responsive B cell clones. Evidence in support of three distinct switching pathways. *J. Exp. Med.* **157,** 69–85.

Moses, H. L., E. Y. Yang, and J. A. Pietenpol (1990). TFG-β stimulation and inhibition of cell proliferation: New mechanistic insights. *Cell* **63,** 245–247.

Nilsson, L., K. B. Islam, O. Olafsson, I. Zalcberg, *et al.* (1991). Structure of TGF-β1-induced human immunoglobulin Cα1 germline transcripts. *Int. Immunol.* **3,** 1107–1115.

Noelle, R. J., D. M. Shepherd, and H. P. Fell (1992). Cognate interaction between T helper cells and B cells. VII. Role of contact and lymphokines in the expression of germ-line and mature γ_1 transcripts. *J. Immunol.* **149,** 1164–1169.

Nolan-Willard, M., M. T. Berton, and P. Tucker (1992). Coexpression of μ and γ 1 heavy chains can occur by a discontinuous transcription mechanism from the same unrearranged chromosome. *Proc. Natl. Acad. Sci. U.S.A.* **89,** 1234–1238.

Ogimoto, M., K. Mizuno, G. Tate, H. Takahashi *et al.* (1992). Regulation of lipopolysaccharide- and IL-4-induced immunoglobulin heavy chain gene activation: differential roles of CD45 and Lyb-2. *Int. Immunol.* **4,** 651–659.

Ott, D. E., F. W. Alt, and K. B. Marcu (1987). Immunoglobulin heavy chain switch region recombinant within a retroviral vector in murine pre-B cells. *EMBO J.* **6,** 577–584.

Pabst, R., and J. D. Reyonlds (1986). Evidence of extensive lymphocyte death in sheep Peyer's patches. II. The number and fate of newly-formed lymphocytes that emigrate from Peyer's patches. *J. Immunol.* **136,** 2011–2017.

Perlmutter, A., and Gilbert, W. (1984). Antibodies of secondary response can be expressed without switch recombination in normal mouse B cells. *Proc. Natl. Acad. Sci. U.S.A.* **81,** 7189.

Phillips-Quagliata, J. M., and A. Al Maghazachi (1987) T cell clones that help IgA responses. *Adv. Exp. Med. Biol.* **216A,** 101–117.

Pritchard, H., Riddaway, J., and H. S. Micklem (1973). Immune responses in congenitally thusmusless mice. II. Quantitative studies of serum immunoglobulin, the antibody responses to sheep erythrocytes, and the effect of thymus allografting. *Clin. Exp. Immunol.* **13,** 125–138.

Reynolds, J. D. (1986). Evidence of extensive lymphocyte death in sheep Peyer's patches. I. A comparison of lymphocyte production and export. *J. Immunol.* **136(6),** 2005–2010.

Reynolds, J. D., and D. Kirk (1989). Two types of sheep Peyer's patches: Location along gut does not influence involution. *Immunol.* **66(2),** 308–311.

Rothman, P., Y.-Y. Chen, S. Lutzker, S. C. Li, Stewart, V., Cottman, R., and Alt, F. W. (1990). Structure and expression of germline immunoglobulin heavy-chain ε transcripts: Interleukin-4 plus lipopolysaccharide-directed switching to Cε. *Mol. Cell. Biol.* **10,** 1672–1679.

Rousset, F., E. Gracia, and J. Banchereau (1991). Cytokine-induced proliferation and immunoglobulin production of human B lymphocytes triggered through their CD40 antigen. *J. Exp. Med.* **173,** 705–710.

Rudzik, R., R. L. Clancy, D. Y. Perey, R. P. Day, and J. Bienenstock (1975). Repopulation with IgA-containing cells of bronchial and intestinal lamina propria after transfer of homologous Peyer's patch and bronchial lymphocytes. *J. Immunol.* **114,** 1599–1604.

Sanders, V. M., J. M. Snyder, J. W. Uhr, and E. S. Vitetta (1986). Characterization of the physical interaction between antigen-specific B and T cells. *J. Immunol.* **137,** 2395.

Schrader, C. E., A. George, R. L. Kerlin, and J. J. Cebra (1990). Dendritic cells support production of IgA and other non-IgM isotypes in clonal microculture. *Int. Immunol.* **2,** 563–570.

Shimizu, A., M. C. Nussenzweig, T.-R. Mizuta, Leder, P., and Honjo, T. *et al.* (1989). Immunoglobulin double-isotype expression by trans-mRNA in a human immunoglobulin transgenic mouse. *Proc. Natl. Acad. Sci. U.S.A.* **86,** 8020–8023.

Shimizu, A., M. C. Nussenzweig, H. Han, Sanchez, M., and Honjo, T. (1991). Trans-splicing as a possible molecular mechanism for the multiple isotype expression of the immunoglobulin gene. *J. Exp. Med.* **173,** 1385–1393.

Shockett, P., and J. Stavnezer (1991). Effect of cytokines on switching to IgA and α germline transcripts in the B lymphoma I.29μ. Transforming growth factor-β activates transcription of the unrearranged C_α gene[1]. *J. Immunol.* **147,** 4374–4383.

Sideras, P., L. Nilsson, K. B. Islam, I. Z. Quintana, L. Freihff, Rosén, G. Juliusson, L. Hammarström, and C. I. Edward Smith (1992). Transcription of unrearranged Ig H chain genes in human B cell malignancies. Biased expression of genes encoded within the first duplication unit of the IgH chain locus. *J. Immunol.* **149,** 244.

Snapper, C. M., and J. J. Mond (1993). Towards a comprehensive view of immunoglobulin class switching. *Immunol. Today* **14(1),** 15–17.

Snapper, C. M., and W. E. Paul (1987). Interferon-gamma and B cell stimulatory factor-1 reciprocally regulate Ig isotype production. *Science* **236(4804),** 944–947.

Snapper, C. M., F. D. Finkelman, D. Stefany, D. H. Conrad, and W. E. Paul (1988). IL-4 induces co-expression of intrinsic membrane IgG1 and IgE by murine B cells stimulated with lipopolysaccharide. *J. Immunol.* **141,** 489–498.

Snapper, C. M., L. M. T. Peçanha, A. D. Levine, and J. J. Mond (1991). IgE class switching is critically dependent upon the nature of the B cell activator, in addition to the presence of IL-4. *J. Immunol.* **147(4),** 1163–1170.

Snapper, C. M., T. M. McIntyre, R. Mandler, *et al.* (1992). Induction of IgG3 secretion by interferon γ: A model for T cell-independent class switching in response to T cell-independent type 2 antigens. *J. Exp. Med.* **175,** 1367–1371.

Sonada, E., R. Matsumoto, Y. Hitoshi, T. Ishii, M. Sugimoto, S. Araki, A. Tominaga, N. Yamaguchi, and K. Takatsu (1989). Transforming growth factor β induces IgA production and acts additively with Interleukin 5 for IgA production. *J. Exp. Med.* **170,** 1415.

Spalding, D. M., and J. A. Griffin (1986). Different pathways of differentiation of pre-B cell lines are induced by dendritic cells and T cells from different lymphoid tissues. *Cell* **44,** 507–515.

Spalding, D. M., W. J. Koopman, J. H. Eldridge, J. R. McGhee, and R. M. Steinman (1983). Accessory cells in murine Peyer's patch. I. Identification and enrichment of a functional dendritic cell. *J. Exp. Med.* **157,** 1646–1659.

Spalding, D. M., S. I. Williamson, W. J. Koopman, and J. R. McGhee (1984). Preferential induction of polyclonal IgA secretion by murine Peyer's patch dendritic cell–T cell mixtures. *J. Exp. Med.* **160,** 941–946.

Stavnezer-Nordgren, J., and S. Sirlin (1986). Specificity of immunoglobulin heavy-chain switch correlates with activity of germline heavy chain genes prior to switching. *EMBO J* **5,** 95–102.

Stavnezer, J., S. Sirlin, and J. Abbot (1985). Induction of immunoglobulin isotype switching in cultured I.29 B lymphoma cells. Characterization of the accompanying rearrangements of heavy chain genes. *J. Exp. Med.* **161,** 577–601.

Stavnezer, J., G. Radcliffe, Y.-C. Lin, J. Nietupski, L. Berggren, R. Sitia, and E. Severinson (1988). Immunoglobulin heavy-chain switching may be directed by prior induction of transcripts from constant-region genes. *Proc. Natl. Acad. Sci. U.S.A.* **85,** 7704–7708.

Swain, S. L., and R. W. Dutton (1987). Consequences of the direct interaction of helper T cells with B cells presenting antigen. *Immunol. Rev.* **99,** 263.

Tew, J. G., M. H. Kosco, G. F. Burton, and A. K. Szakal (1990). Follicular dendritic cells as accessory cells. *Immunol. Rev.* **117,** 185–211.

Tseng, J. (1981). Transfer of lymphocytes of Peyer's patches between immunoglobulin allotype congenic mice: Repopulation of the IgA plasma cells in the gut lamina propria. *J. Immunol.* **127,** 2039–2043.

van Vlasselaer, P., J. Punnonen, and J. E. de Vries (1992). Transforming growth factor-β directs IgA switching in human B cells. *J. Immunol.* **148,** 2062–2067.

Vitetta, E. S., A. Bossie, R. Fernandez-Botran, C. D. Myers, K. G. Oliver, V. M. Sanders, and T. L. Stevens (1987). Interaction and activation of antigen-specific T and B cells. *Immunol. Rev.* **99,** 193.

Wahl, S. M., D. A. Hunt, H. L. Wong, S. Dougherty, N. McCartney-Francis, L. M. Wahl, L. Ellingsworth, J. A., Schmidt, G. Hall, A. B. Roberts (1988). Transforming growth factor-beta is a potent immunosuppressive agent that inhibits IL-1-dependent lymphocyte proliferation. *J. Immunol.* **140,** 3026.

Wakatsuki, Y., and W. Strober (1993). Effect of down-regulation of germline transcripts on IgA isotype differentiation. *J. Exp. Med.* **178,** 7.

Weinstein, P. D., and J. J. Cebra (1991). The preference of switching to IgA expression by Peyer's patch germinal center B cells is likely due to the intrinsic influence of their microenvironment. *J. Immunol.* **147,** 4126–4135.

Whalen, B. J., H.-P. Tony, and D. C. Parker (1988). Characterization of the effector mechanism of help for antigen-presenting and bystander resting B cell growth mediated by IA-restricted Th2 helper T cell lines. *J. Immunol.* **141,** 2230.

Whitmore, A. C., D. M. Prowse, G. Haughton, and L. W. Arnold (1990). Ig isotype switching in B lymphocytes. The effect of T cell-derived interleukins, cytokines, cholera toxin, and antigen on isotype switch frequency of a cloned B cell lymphoma. *Int. Immunol.* **3,** 95–103.

Yancopoulos, G. D., R. A. DePinho, K. A. Zimmerman, S. G. Lutzker, N. Rosenberg, and F. W. Alt (1986). Secondary gemonic rearrangement events in pre-B cells; V_HDJ_H replacement by a LINE-1 sequence and directed class switching. *EMBO J.* **5(12),** 3259–3266.

Yaoita, Y., Y. Kumagai, K. Okumura, and T. Honjo (1982). Expression of lymphocyte surface IgE does not require switch recombination. *Nature (London)* **297,** 697.

Yoshida, K., M. Matsuoka, S. Usuda, Mori, A., Ishizaka, K., and Sakano, H. (1990). Immunoglobulin switch circular DNA in the mouse infected with *Nippostrongylus brasiliensis:* Evidence for successive class switching from μ to ε via γ1. *Proc. Natl. Acad. Sci. U.S.A.* **87(20),** 7829–7833.

Yuan, D., and E. S. Vitetta (1983). Structural studies of cell surface and secreted IgG in LPS-stimulated murine B cells. *Mol Immunol.* **20,** 367.

15

Diversity and Function of Antigen-Presenting Cells in Mucosal Tissues

Asit Panja • Lloyd Mayer

I. OVERVIEW OF ANTIGEN PRESENTATION

The most important feature of the immune system is its ability to distinguish between self and nonself. The network of defense against nonself is maintained by an intricate communication system between specialized cells that are stationed throughout the body. These cells, T and B lymphocytes, interact to fight off foreign pathogens that gain access to the host. T cells and B cells possess specialized receptor molecules on their surfaces that are capable of recognizing and responding to foreign antigens, B cells by their surface immunoglobulin and T cells by their antigen receptor. Surface immunoglobulin (sIg) is capable of binding to antigen (Ag) in solution. However, unlike B cells, T cells can interact only with antigen that is cell bound and presented in association with products of the major histocompatibility complex (MHC) on an antigen-presenting cell (APC) (Ziegler and Unanue, 1981). One group of MHC glycoproteins, known as Class I molecules, arms the immune system to help eradicate cells that have been altered secondary to infection or malignant degeneration. These molecules are expressed on virtually all nucleated cells in the body. The other group of MHC glycoproteins, known as Class II molecules, binds processed peptides that had been taken up exogenously by APCs and presents them to helper T cells. In peripheral blood, lymph nodes, and spleen, helper T cells ($CD4^+$) recognize antigen bound to MHC Class II molecules on macrophages and B cells. Cytotoxic T cells ($CD8^+$), on the other hand, are restricted to recognizing antigen bound to MHC Class I molecules.

Given the general characteristics of this system, we must realize that regulation of immune responses depends on the nature of antigen handling by the APCs through appropriate cellular and molecular mechanisms.

A. Types of Antigen-Presenting Cells

Several distinct cell types have been documented to function as APCs for T-cell activation (Rosenthal and Shevach, 1973; Nussenzweig and Steinman, 1980; Ziegler and Unanue, 1981; Pober *et al.*, 1983; Geppert and Lipsky, 1985). Although most of our knowledge is limited to *in vitro* systems, clearly differences exist among various APCs relating to their mechanism(s) of antigen presentation as well as to other accessory functions. Monocytes and macrophages are the principal APCs located in blood, lymph nodes, spleen, and interstitium. These cells are large, with active lysosomes, endosomes, and hydrolytic enzymes. These phagocytes are not only vital for the initiation of immune responses, but also play a crucial role in T-cell activation through their ability to produce potent accessory cytokines. B cells, apart from their major function as antibody-producing cells, also possess phagocytic capacity, most effectively via interaction of specific Ag with sIg receptors. When antigen is encountered by sIg on the B cell, the antigen is internalized in an endocytic vacuole and subsequently processed and presented, complexed to MHC Class II determinants, to the helper T cell. This activated T cell in turn secretes the necessary cytokines required for B cells to become antibody-producing plasma cells. Steinman and Cohn (1973) described a novel cell isolated from the mouse spleen that appears to be one of the most potent APCs—the dendritic cell. Distinct from the macrophages and B cells, dendritic cells are irregularly shaped cells with abundant Class II antigens but no Fc receptors (Steinman and Nussenzweig, 1980). These cells are potent stimulators in a mixed lymphocyte reaction and, on a cell per cell basis, are probably the most effective APCs described to date. Dendritic cells are not phagocytic and therefore require accessory cells to process proteins into peptides that can complex with MHC molecules. These cells are ubiquitous, however, and are found within lymph nodes, spleen, thymus, and the gastrointestinal tract. Depending on location, dendritic cells are part of a family of APCs that promote local immune responses. In the skin, these are the classical Langerhans cells; in the gut, they are represented by the "veiled cells" in the Peyer's patch (see subsequent discussion).

These three cell types (B cells, monocytes, dendritic cells) constitute the group termed the "professional APCs," since they express Class II molecules, typically process and present Ag to T cells, and, as will be described, provide the conventional accessory signals required for T-cell activation. However, several investigators have described other cells capable of expressing Class II molecules (when activated) and presenting peptides to T cells. However, the results of T-cell interactions with these "nonprofessional APCs" are quite distinct from the interactions described previously. Activated human T cells are such a cell type that can express Class II molecules (Lanzarecchia *et al.*, 1988; Siliciano *et al.*, 1988). These cells are capable of taking up, processing, and presenting human immunodeficiency virus (HIV) gp120 protein to other T cells and presenting mouse monoclonal antibodies (mAbs) against the T-cell receptor (TcR), CD3, CD4, and CD8 molecules that bind to the T cell surface. However, in contrast to professional APCs, activated T cells are unable to present soluble antigen (e.g., tetanus toxoid) (Lanzavecchia *et al.*, 1988) and generally result in the induction of anergy (La Salle *et al.*, 1992). Class II Ag expression has been induced on fibroblasts, endothelial cells, and a variety of epithelial cells and, although the Class II molecules can be recognized by the T-cell receptors, these cells are either poorly stimulatory or evoke a unique type of immune response. The neoexpression of Class II molecules on epithelial cells in the thyroid or the pancreatic islets has been invoked to explain the induction of autoimmunity (Botazzo *et al.*, 1983; Piccinini *et al.*, 1987), with the presentation of self peptides to previously tolerized self-reactive T cells. Clearly this area of research is growing rapidly, and our knowledge base relating to the regulation of immune responses using such cells is expanding. One such cell, the intestinal epithelial cell, is described in greater detail in a subsequent section.

II. MECHANISMS OF ANTIGEN UPTAKE

For foreign antigen to be placed into a form that can be recognized by the T-cell Ag receptor, it must be taken up and processed within intracytoplasmic organelles. Mechanisms of antigen uptake include those that are nonspecific, random, and therefore less efficient and those mediated by receptor interactions, which have higher efficiency. First we discuss receptor-mediated uptake, which is different for various APCs.

A. sIg-Mediated Uptake of Antigen

Antigen uptake by B cells was reported first by Chesnut and Grey (1981). In this study, these investigators demonstrated the capacity of rabbit IgG-specific B cells to present processed rabbit IgG to T cells. Clearly this way of generating a specific immune response is extremely effective. If antigen-specific B cells are presenting to antigen-specific T cells, help for clonal growth or differentiation (specific or nonspecific) can be focused on these activated B cells. In such an antigen-driven system, the requirement for high concentrations of antigens needed to activate T cells would be less. Studies by Rock and colleagues (1984) have demonstrated that hapten-specific B lymphocytes are extremely efficient at presenting hapten to T cells via hapten binding to surface Ig molecules. In contrast to the nonspecific antigen uptake by B cells, maximal stimulation of responding T lymphocytes can be achieved with a minimum of antigen (Chesnut *et al.*, 1982). Thus, within a lymph node, antigen carried to the primary follicles may interact with sIg on B cells and be presented as peptides to parafollicular T cells.

B. Fc Receptor-Mediated Antigen Uptake

With the exception of dendritic cells, which are nonphagocytic, all professional APCs express Fc receptors (FcR). These receptors are specific for distinct Ig isotypes and vary in their ability to bind immune complexes. FcR appears to play a major role in the immune response by facilitating antigen uptake after binding to an immune complex. In this respect, initial evidence was provided by Cohen and coworkers (1973), who showed that cytophilic antibodies in the serum of immune animals could enhance the antigen-presenting capacity of naive macrophages. Further, a similar phenomenon was demonstrated by Celis and Chang (1984), documenting that the presence of FcR^+ APCs could reduce 10- to 100-fold the concentration requirement of hepatitis B virus surface antigen (HBsAg) to trigger an HBsAg-specific T-cell clone. This phenomenon was supported further by studies by Kehry and Yamashita (1990), in which they described that presentation of trinitrophenol (TNP) carrier conjugates by mouse B cells could be enhanced 100- to 1000-fold if TNP-specific IgE is bound to FcεRII on mouse B cells.

C. Uptake by Complement Components

Complement is the clearest example of the incorporation of the innate (nonspecific) immune system with adaptive (specific) immunity. Bacterial products can trigger the alternative pathway of complement activation, resulting in the generation of C3b fragments. C3b fragments coat bacteria, rendering them accessible to complement receptors on B cells and monocytes. Thus, in the absence of an adaptive immune response (i.e., antibody), bacteria can be opsonized by macrophages, processed, and presented to T cells, initiating a specific immune response.

Immune complexes also can bind complement (IgG and IgM), and therefore be susceptible to uptake through C3b receptors. Studies by Daha and van Es (1984) demonstrated, in a guinea pig model, that receptors for C3b are present on red blood cells, which seem to bind complement-coated immune complexes and deliver them to the Kupffer cells in the liver. Arvieux and colleagues (1988) showed that triggering of tetanus toxoid antigen-specific T cells by Epstein-Barr virus (EBV)-transformed B cells can be enhanced by binding C3b or C4b components to the antigen. Thus, through a number of interactions, complement can play an important role in Ag uptake.

D. Antigen Uptake by Phagocytosis

To this point we have discussed specific mechanisms for antigen uptake, yet a very important mechanism is the one that occurs before any immune response has been generated—nonspecific phagocytosis. As the term suggests, B cells and monocytes can sample their environment by engulfing macromolecules through pinocytosis or by uptake of molecules in clathrin-coated pits. By either mechanism, the process is relatively inefficient; only a small fraction of the antigen is taken up. However, by any of these processes, Ag is incorporated into the endosomal compartment, where processing begins in an effort to generate a specific response.

III. MECHANISMS OF ANTIGEN PROCESSING

As mentioned in the introduction, antigens must be processed before they are presented to and recognized by T cells. Conventionally, APCs (monocytes, B cells) internalize exogenous antigens through phagocytosis (a phenomenon first described by Metchnikoff in 1884) as described earlier. Within the endosome, limited proteolysis results in the generation of fragments that subsequently are expressed on the cell surface in combination with MHC Class II molecules (Germain, 1986). Endogenous Ags (viral proteins) utilize a distinct pathway described subsequently and typically associate with Class I molecules.

The numerous steps and mechanisms of these cytosolic phenomena (processing) are not completely understood. The endosomal compartment develops an acidic pH that facilitates proteolytic enzyme activity that digests pinocytosed material (Braciale *et al.*, 1987). After digestion in the endosome, the antigen fragments have one of two fates: they can bind to Class II molecules in multivesicular bodies and be recycled back to the membrane as a complex or the endosome can fuse with a lysosome, resulting in further proteolysis and loss of immunogenicity or potential recycling to the surface. The signals that direct the choice of one pathway or the other are unknown. However, Class II molecules produced in the Golgi are associated with a third chain, the invariant chain (Cresswell, 1992). This chain stabilizes the Class II molecule so it can exit the Golgi, but will dissociate in an acidic compartment allowing peptide to bind to the MHC molecule. Once dissociated, the Class II molecule is targeted to the surface. Fusion of multiple endosomes or Golgi vesicles with endosomes forms multivesicular bodies that may be important in signaling recycling.

Peptides generated by processing associate with the antigen-binding groove in the MHC. Typically, for macrophage- and B cell-derived peptides, these peptides between 8 and 14 amino acids in length (Sette and Grey, 1992). Thus, potential differences in processing machinery may alter the types of immune response generated. Association of peptides with MHC Class I molecules is different than association with Class II. Class I molecules formed in the endoplasmic reticulum (ER) associate with cytoplasmic peptides that are carried to the ER by peptide transporters (Monaco, 1992). Peptides of shorter length (compared with Class II MHC) are generally the rule (8 to 10-mers) (Braciale, 1992). Class I–peptide complexes traffic to the membrane, where they can be recognized by TcRs on $CD8^+$ T cells. One additional intracytoplasmic transporter has been identified that may be relevant in the gastrointestinal tract. The family of heat-shock proteins bind peptides and can transfer these peptides to Class I (and maybe Class II) molecules within the cell (Vanbuskirk *et al.*, 1989).

IV. ANTIGEN-PRESENTING CELLS PRESENT IN THE MUCOSAL TISSUES

Because of differences in the antigenic microenvironments of the different organs, the responsibilities of the local immune systems also must be different. To coordinate these diverse responsibilities, the mechanisms of antigen handling also must be diverse. Among the mucosal tissues, the intestinal mucosa is the largest and is exposed continuously to food antigens, viruses, bacteria, parasites, or the by-products of these organisms. For this reason, it is appropriate that antigen presentation, interactions between immunocompetent T cells and APCs, and other immunological phenomena also are very specialized.

Although other mucosal sites (lung, bladder) also are exposed chronically to Ag, the volume of antigens is much less. Therefore, let us first discuss mechanisms of antigen entry into the gastrointestinal mucosa. Early reports suggested that specialized epithelial cells, M cells, were responsible for antigen handling in the gut. M cells are believed to derive from epithelial cells and reside over Peyer's patches (Shimizu and Andrew, 1967; Wolf and Bye, 1984). Some variability has been seen in the reports that these cells express Class II molecules on their surface (Bjerke and Brandtzaeg, 1988; Bland and Kambarage, 1991). Large particulate Ags seem particularly well suited for uptake by M cells (Owen, 1977) and some viruses bind to M cells via a specific receptor (e.g., poliovirus, reovirus III) (Wolf *et al.*, 1981; Sicinski *et al.*, 1990). However, the number of M cells in the intestine is limited when compared to the vast array of immunogenic substances encountered in the lumen. M cells appear to transport antigen by transcytosis without any processing of the antigen (Owen *et al.*, 1986), so the immune response relies on macrophages lying below the M cells. Major evidence for this concept has been provided by the studies of Owen and Jones (1974) documenting that these cells lack lysosomes, an important source of proteolytic enzymes in their cytoplasm.

The transport of large macromolecules has been demonstrated clearly by many researchers. Although controversy exists over whether M cells express Class II molecules (Hirata *et al.*, 1986; Bjerke and Brandtzaeg, 1990), the general feeling is that these cells do not interact with T cells in the lamina propria. Instead, antigens pass through in pinocytotic vesicles untouched or unprocessed. One group of investigators has documented the presence of acidic vesicles (lysosomes ?) in these cells, but formal proof is still required (Allen *et al.*, 1992). M cells predominate in the small bowel, where Ag entry is greatest, but also exist in the colon and rectum. In fact, some investigators have suggested that these cells may be the site of entry for HIV (Lehner *et al.*, 1991).

The next obvious question is what happens to Ag after passage through the M cell. This question raises the issue of the role of macrophages in the gastrointestinal tract. Macrophages are quite heterogeneous, and subpopulations localize to distinct areas in the gastrointestinal tract, where they express different functional properties. Much of the information regarding intestinal macrophages comes from immunohistochemical studies, unfortunately with some degree of disparity. However, the disparate findings can be explained. Most studies come to a general consensus on location and functional properties. Researchers generally agree on the location of intestinal macrophages: the villous core of the small bowel, the subepithelial space in the crypt, under the dome (M cell) epithelium overlying Peyer's patches, and in the patch itself (Golder and Doe, 1983; Selby *et al.*, 1983; Winter *et al.*, 1983; Berken *et al.*, 1987; Harvey and Jones, 1991). Most groups report that macrophages are greater in number in the small bowel, underscoring a role in Ag sampling, detoxification via release of chemical mediators (superoxides, etc.), and scavenging of potentially harmful substances (with possible release into the lumen). This latter point has been suggested by the finding of large amounts of carbon particles in carbon-fed mice within subepithelial macrophages, and little free carbon elsewhere (including the patch) (Joel *et al.*, 1978). Several types of material have been found within macrophages, including DNA from damaged cells (Sawicki *et al.*, 1977). Colonic macrophages may be increased because of the numbers of enteric Ags that pass through or between the epithelium.

With respect to M cell transport of Ag, subepithelial macrophages take up the transported Ag and presumably "carry" it to the Peyer's patch. The actual transfer of Ag has not been elucidated, especially since the number of macrophages within the patch is limited and Ag transfer has never been visualized. Within the villous core, the observations have been more clear. Macrophages reside near plasma cells in the subepithelial layer. Non-M cell-transported Ag may be processed and presented by the macrophage, although formal proof of this behavior is required. Macrophages in the small and large bowel have been reported to be suppressive, secreting prostaglandin E_2 (PGE_2), and inhibiting immune responses (Pavli *et al.*, 1990) in a manner similar to alveolar macrophages (in a mixed lymphocyte reaction). These cells do express nonspecific esterase and acid phosphatase, consistent with conventional APCs, but the level of expression is lower than that of peripheral monocytes in some studies (Mahida *et al.*, 1989). These enzymes, however, render the cells functional as APCs.

Functionally, gut macrophages are also quite heterogeneous. Generally, they are poorly adherent to plastic although this characteristic may relate to isolation by Ficoll–hypaque (Verspaget and Beeken, 1985). These cells do adhere to fibronectin-coated plates, however, and can be enriched by this method. Gut macrophages express FcR and take up immune complexes (coated red blood cells, toxin–antitoxin complexes). Phagocytosis can stimulate the respiratory burst, which is less active than that of peripheral monocytes but present nonetheless. Finally, these cells produce complement components C3 and C4 and express complement receptors. However, as stated earlier, they may be suppressive in mixed lymphocyte reactions; macrophages within the patch are poorly stimulatory (Le Fevre *et al.*, 1979). This latter point is important because, with the potential for a large antigen load in the patch, priming but not active immune response is consistent with the histology of the patch, which differs from a reactive lymph node. Thus, in summary, much is still unknown about intestinal macrophages. Our knowledge has been limited by the lack of good reproducible methods for purification of large populations of these cells, coupled with the marked heterogeneity evident within the gut.

If the macrophages do not play a key role in immune responses in the gut, what cell fills this role? As discussed earlier, the most potent APC described to date is the dendritic cell. For these cells too, we are hampered by heterogeneity—interdigitating cells in the lymph node, Langerhans cells in the skin, and so on all fall into this category. Two populations of dendritic cells have been described in the gut. The classical dendritic cell is esterase negative, acid phosphatase negative, FcR negative, fibronectin nonadherent, and strongly DR positive with dendritic extensions that are actively involved in T-cell interactions (Sminia and Jeunssen, 1986; Nahida *et al.*, 1988; Marsetyawan *et al.*, 1990; Bland and Kambarage, 1991). This type of dendritic cell, also called the "veiled cell" in the gut, is found in the lamina propria throughout the small bowel, predominantly in subepithelial tissue. Functionally, these cells are potent stimulators of the mixed lymphocyte reaction (MLR; Mahida *et al.*, 1988). A second type of dendritic cell is the interdigitating cell found in Peyer's patches. These cells, isolated by several groups, are effective APCs but, interestingly, in one study appear to promote IgA-specific responses [possibly related to transforming growth factor β (TGFβ) production] (Spalding and Griffith, 1986; Spalding *et al.*, 1984). These cells likely prime the Ag-specific response in the patch and generate IgA-specific responses. However, these cells fail to explain the dichotomy of immune responses in the gastrointestinal tract (active immunity vs. tolerance).

We are, therefore, left with one cell (B cells have not been studied carefully for their APC function in the gut) that has been proposed as a major player in antigen presentation in the gut—the intestinal epithelial cell (IEC). Several groups studying different model systems have documented that intestinal epithelium, especially in the small bowel, constitutively expresses Class II molecules (Wiman *et al.*, 1978; Mason *et al.*, 1981; Selby *et al.*, 1981; Kaiserlian *et al.*, 1990; Mayer *et al.*, 1990). Further, subsequent studies revealed that these cells could function as APCs, processing and presenting Ag to primed T cells (Bland and Warren, 1986a,b; Mayer and Shlien, 1987; Kaiserlian *et al.*, 1989). However, the unique feature is that these cells appear to activate $CD8^+$ suppressor T cells selectively by direct activation (Bland and Warren, 1986a,b; Mayer and Shlien, 1987) or by suppression by soluble factors (PGE_2) (Santos *et al.*, 1990). Such findings concur with the phenomenon of oral tolerance, in which the mechanisms of suppressor cell activation were previously unclear. However, epithelial cells are capable of stimulating $CD4^+$ T cells as well (Kaiserlian *et al.*, 1989; Mayer and Eisenhardt, 1990) via classical Class II-mediated pathways. Under most circumstances, suppression would predominate whereas in other situations (e.g., inflammatory states), helper T cell activation could occur.

The expression of Class II molecules by IECs has been somewhat controversial. Although researchers generally agree that small bowel IECs constitutively express Class II molecules, identification of these molecules on colonocytes has been more variable. With sensitive techniques, Class II molecules can be detected with expression that may be patchy. Expression appears to relate to the presence of intraepithelial lymphocytes (IELs) (Cerf-Bensussan *et al.*, 1984) and is enhanced in states in which interferon γ is produced or passively administered (Quyang *et al.*, 1988; Steiniger *et al.*, 1989; Masson and Perdue, 1990; Zhang and Michael, 1990). The distribution of Class II molecules on the IECs is also of interest. Presumably because of the overlapping membranes on the microvillous border, Class II molecules are highly expressed on the luminal side. Intuitively, this situation makes little sense since cell interactions (i.e., T cell–IEC) do not occur in the lumen. However, Bland (1990) has suggested that the Class II molecules may serve as "peptide receptors" for predigested (or preprocessed) peptides that result from proteolysis within the stomach and upper small bowel. Peptides bound to Class II molecules then would be internalized and presented to lamina propria T cells (via fenestrations in the basement membrane) or even potentially to IELs.

Several unresolved issues remain. The first relates to the ability of IECs to take up and process large macromolecules into a form recognized by the TcR. Small di- and tripeptides (predigested) are taken up by IECs, but little evidence exists for larger macromolecular transport. However, some data suggest that at least malignant epithelial cell lines take up large proteins (tetanus toxoid, transferrin) and incorporate them into multivesicular bodies (L. P. So, K. Pelton, G. Small, and L. Mayer, unpublished observations). Bland and colleagues have shown that rat IECs take up ovalbumin, but processing is limited; fixed conventional APCs fail to present IEC-processed Ags (suggesting that distinct peptides are generated; Bland and Whiting, 1989). Further, the I–E molecules expressed on murine IECs may be altered, potentially reducing the potency of these molecules as restriction elements.

A second major issue is the fact that a Class II molecule-bearing cell stimulates $CD8^+$ T cells, especially if one assumes that IECs are stimulating IELs (typically $CD8^+$). The data on this topic are only now becoming available; some suggest a non-class II–CD8 interaction between IECs and T cells (Mayer *et al.*, 1990), and potentially a nonclassical Class I molecule such as CDld or TL, demonstrated to be present on human and murine IECs (Bleicher *et al.*, 1990; Hershberg *et al.*, 1990; Blumberg *et al.*, 1991). The interaction of a Class I-like molecule with $CD8^+$ T cells may overshadow the "typical" interaction of Class II with CD4. These speculations are just that and, although IECs are tempting cells to evoke in normal antigen presentation in the gut, no *in vivo* model has been generated and no clear evidence exists that these cells function as APCs in a physiological system.

V. SUMMARY

Given the nature of the gastrointestinal tract and its continuous Ag exposure, obviously unique systems of Ag handling must be developed. Clearly typical APCs do not function typically in the gastrointestinal tract and atypical (nonprofessional) APCs may play a more dominant role. However, a clear understanding of this entire process awaits the development of physiological model systems in which these hypotheses can be tested.

References

Allen, C. H., Mendrick, D. L., Trier, J. S. (1992). M cells contain acidic comparments and express class II MHC determinants. *Gastroenterology* **102,** A589.

Arvieux, J., Yssel, H., and Colomb, M. G. (1988). Antigen bound C3b and C4b enhance antigen-presenting cell function in activation of human T-cell clones. *Immunology* **65,** 229–235.

Beeken, W., Northwood, I., Beliveau, C., and Gump, D. (1987). Phagocytes in cell suspensions of human colon mucosa. *Gut* **28,** 976–980.

Bjerke, K., and Brandtzaeg, P. (1988). Lack of relation between HLA-DR and secretory component (SC) in follicle associated epithelium of human Peyers patches. *Clin. Exp. Immunol.* **71,** 502–507.

Bland, P. W., and Kambarage, D. M. (1991). Antigen handling by the epithelium and lamina propria macrophages. *Gastroenterol. Clin. North Am.* **20,** 577.

Bland, P. W., and Warren, L. G. (1986a). Antigen presentation by epithelial cells of the rat small intestine. I. Kinetics, antigen specificity and blocking by anti-Ia antisera. *Immunology* **58,** 1–7.

Bland, P. W., and Warren, L. G. (1986b). Antigen presentation by epithelial cells of the rat small intestine. II. Selective induction of suppressor T cells. *Immunology* **58,** 9–14.

Bland, P. W., and Whiting, C. V. (1989). Antigen processing by isolated rat intestinal villus enterocytes. *Immunology* **68(4),** 497–502.

Bleicher, P. A., Balk, S. P., Hagen, S. J., Blumberg, R. S., Flotte, T. J., and Terhorst, C. (1990). Expression of murine CD1 on gastrointestinal epithelium. *Science* **250,** 679–682.

Blumberg, R. S., Terhorst, C., Bleicher, P., McDermott, F. V., Allan, C. H., Landau, B. S., Trier, J. S., and Balk, S. P. (1991). Expression of a nonpolymorphic MHC class I-like molecule, CDld, by human intestinal epithelial cells. *J. Immunol.* **147,** 2518–2524.

Botazzo, G. F., Pujol-Burrell, R., Hanafusa, T., and Feldmann, M. (1983). Role of aberrant HLA-DR expression and antigen presentation in induction of endocrine autoimmunity. *Lancet* **2,** 1115–1118.

Braciale, T. J. (1992). Antigen processing for presentation by MHC class I molecules. *Curr. Opin. Immunol.* **4,** 59–62.

Braciale, T. J., Morrison, L. A., Sweetser, M. T., Sambrook, J., Gething, M. J., and Braciale, V. L. (1987). Antigen presentation pathways to class I and class II MHC-restricted T lymphocytes. *Immunol. Rev.* **98,** 95–114.

Brandtzaeg, P., and Bjerke, K. (1990). Immunomorphological characteristics of human Peyer's patches. *Digestion* **46,** (Suppl. 2)262–273.

Celis, E., and Chang, T. W. (1984). Antibodies to hepatitis B surface antigen potentiate the response of human T lymphocyte clones to the same antigen. *Science* **224,** 297–299.

Cerf-Bensussan, N., Quaroni, A., Kurnick, J., and Bhan, A. (1984). Intraepithelial lymphocytes modulate la expression by intestinal epithelial cells. *J. Immunol.* **132,** 2244–2251.

Chesnut, R. W., and Grey, H. M. (1981). Studies on the capacity of B cells to serve as antigen presenting cells. *J. Immunol.* **126,** 1075–1079.

Chesnut, R. W., Colon, S. M., and Grey, H. M. (1982). Antigen presentation by normal B cells, B cell tumors, and macrophages: Functional and biochemical comparison. *J. Immunol.* **128,** 1764–1768.

Cohen, B. E., Rosenthal, A. S., and Paul, W. E. (1973). Antigen-Macrophage Interaction. II. Relative roles of cytophilic antibody and other membrane sites. *J. Immunol.* **111,** 820–828.

Cresswell, P. (1992). Chemistry and functional role of the invariant chain. *Curr. Opin. Immunol.* **4,** 87–92.

Daha, M. R., and van Es, L. A. (1984). Fc- and complement receptor dependent degradation of soluble immune complexes and stable immunoglobulin aggregates by guinea pig monocytes, peritoneal macrophages, and Kupffer cells. *J. Leuk. Biol.* **36,** 569–579.

Geppert, T. D., and Lipsky, P. E. (1985). Antigen presentation by interferon γ-treated endothelial cells and fibroblasts: Differential ability to function as antigen presenting cells despite comparable Ia expression. *J. Immunol.* **135,** 3750–3762.

Germain, R. N. (1986). The ins and outs of antigen processing and presentation. *Nature (London)* **322,** 687.

Golder, J. P., and Doe, W. F. (1983). Isolation and preliminary characterization of human intestinal macrophages. *Gastroenterology* **84,** 795–802.

Harvey, J., and Jones, D. B. (1991) Human mucosal T-lymphocyte and macrophage subpopulations in normal and inflamed intestine. *Clin. Exp. Allergy* **21,** 549–560.

Hershberg, R., Eghtesady, P., Sydora, B., Brorson, K., Cheroutre, H., Madlin, R., and Kronenberg, M. (1990). Expression of the thymus leukemia antigen in mouse intestinal epithelium. *Proc. Natl. Acad. Sci. U.S.A.* **87,** 9727–9731.

Hirata, I., Austin, L. L., Blackwell, W. H., Weber, J. R., and Dobbins, W. (1986). Immunoelectron microscopic localization of HLA-DR antigen in control small intestine and colon and in inflammatory bowel disease. *Dig. Dis. Sci.* **31,** 1317.

Joel, D. D., Laissue, J. A., and LeFevre, M. E. (1978). Distribution and fate of ingested carbon particles in mice. *J. Reticuloendothel. Soc.* **24,** 477.

Kaiserlian, D., Vidal, K., and Revillard, J. P. (1989). Murine enterocytes can present soluble antigen to specific class II-restricted CD4+ T cells. *Eur. J. Immunol.* **19(8),** 1513–1516.

Kaiserlian, D., Nicolas, J. F., and Revillard, J. P. (1990). Constitutive expression of Ia molecules by murine epithelial cells: A comparison between keratinocytes and enterocytes. *J. Invest. Dermatol.* **94(3),** 385–386.

Kehry, M. R., and Yamashita, L. C. (1990). Role of the low affinity Fc epsilon receptor in B-lymphocyte antigen presentation. *Immunology* **141,** 77–81.

Lanzavecchia, A., Roosnek, E., Gregory, T., Berman, P., and Abrignani, S. (1988). T cells can present antigens such as HIV gp120 targeted to their own surface molecules. *Nature (London)* **334,** 530–532.

LaSalle, J. M., Tolentino, P. J., Freeman, G. J., Nadler, L. M., and Hafler, D. A. (1992). Early signaling defects in human T cells anergized by T cell presentation of autoantigen. *J. Exp. Med.* **176,** 177–186.

LeFevre, M. E., Hammer, R., Joel, D. D. (1979). Macrophages of the mammalian small intestine: A review. *J. Reticuloendothel. Soc.* **26,** 5.

Lehner, T., Hussain, L., Wilson, J., and Chapman, M. (1991). Mucosal transmission of HIV. *Nature (London)* **353,** 709.

Mahida, Y. R., Wu, K. C., and Jewell, D. P. (1988). Characterization of antigen-presenting activity of intestinal mononuclear cells isolated from normal and inflammatory bowel disease colon and ileum. *Immunology* **65,** 543–549.

Mahida, Y. R., Patel, S., Gionchetti, P., Vaux, D., and Jewell, D. P. (1989). Macrophage subpopulations in lamina propria of normal and inflamed colon and terminal ileum. *Gut* **30,** 826–834.

Marsetyawan, S., Biewenga, J., Kraal, G., and Sminia, T. (1990). The localization of macrophage subsets and dendritic cells in the gastrointestinal tract of the mouse and special reference to the presence of high endothelial venules. *Cell Tissue Res.* **259,** 587–593.

Mason, D. W., Dallman, M., and Barclay, A. N. (1981). Graft versus host disease induces expression of Ia antigen in rat epidermal cells and gut epithelium. *Nature (London)* **293,** 150–151.

Masson, S. D., and Perdue, M. H. (1990). Changes in distribution of la antigen on epithelium of the jejunum and ileum in rats infected with *Nippostrongylus basiliensis*. *Clin. Immunol. Immunopathol.* **57(1),** 83–95.

Mayer, L., and Eisenhardt, D. (1990). Lack of induction of suppressor T cells by intestinal epithelial cells from patients with inflammatory bowel disease. *J. Clin. Invest.* **86,** 1255–1260.

Mayer, L., and Shlien, R. (1987). Evidence for function of Ia molecules on gut epithelial cells in man. *J. Exp. Med.* **166,** 1471–1483.

Mayer, L., Eisenhardt, D., Salomon, P., Bauer, W., Plous, R., and Piccininni, L. (1990a). Expression of class II molecules on intestinal epithelial cells in man: Differences between normal and inflammatory bowel disease. *Gastroenterology* **100,** 3–12.

Mayer, L., Siden, E. Becker, S., and Eisenhardt, D. (1990b). Antigen handling in the intestine mediated by normal enterocytes. *Adv. Mucosal Immunol.* 23–28.

Monaco, J. J. (1992). Genes in the MHC that may affect antigen processing. *Curr. Opin. Immunol.* **4,** 70–73.

Nussenzweig, M. C., and Steinman, R. M. (1980). Contribution of dendritic cells to stimulation of the murine syngeneic mixed leukocyte reaction. *J. Exp. Med.* **181,** 1196.

Ouyang, Q., El-Youssef, M., Yen-Lieberman, B., Sapatnekar, W., Youngman, K., Kusagami, K., and Fiocchi, C. (1988). Expression of HLA-DR antigens in inflammatory bowel diseas mucosa: Role of intestinal lamina propria mononuclear cell derived interferon gamma. *Dig. Dis. Sci.* **33,** 1528–1536.

Owen, R. L. (1977). Sequential uptake of horseradish peroxidase by lyphoid follicle epithelium of Peyer's patches in the normal unobstructed mouse intestine: An ultrastructural study. *Gastroenterology* **72,** 440–451.

Owen, R. L., and Jones, A. L. (1974). Epithelial cell specialization within human Peyer's patches: An ultrastructural study of intestinal lymphoid follicles. *Gastroenterology* **66,** 189.

Owen, R. L., Pierce, N. F., Apple, R. T., Cray, W. C., Jr. (1986). M cell transport of *Vibrio cholerae* from the intestinal lumen into Peyer's patches: A mechanism for antigen sampling and for microbial transepithelial migration. *J. Infect. Dis.* **153,** 1108–1118.

Pavli, P., Woodhams, C. E., Doe, W. F., and Hume, D. A. (1990). Isolation and characterization of antigen-presenting dendritic cells from the mouse intestinal lamina propria. *Immunology* **70,** 40–47.

Piccinini, L. A., Goldsmith, N. K., Roman, S. H., and Davies, T. F. (1987). HLA-DP, DQ and DR gene expression in Graves disease and normal thyroid epithelium. *Tissue Antigens* **30,** 145–154.

Pober, J. S., Collins, T., Gimbrone, M. A., Jr., Cotran, R. S., Gitlin, J. J., Fiers, W., Clayberger, C., Krensky, A. M., Burakoff, S. J., and Reiss, C. S. (1983). Lymphocytes recognize human vascular endothelial and dermal fibroblast la antigens induced by recombinant immune interferon. *Nature (London)* **355,** 726–729.

Rock, K. L., Benacerraf, B., and Abbas, A. K. (1984). Antigen presentation by hapten-specific B lymphocytes. I. Role of surface immunoglobulin receptors. *J. Exp. Med.* **160,** 1102–1113. (1982).

Rosenthal, A. S., and Shevach, E. M. (1973). The function of macrophages in antigen recognition by guinea pig T lymphocytes. I. Requirement for histocompatibility macrophages and lymphocytes. *J. Exp. Med.* **138,** 1194–1212.

Santos, L. M., Lider, O., Audette, J., Khoury, S. J., and Weiner, H. L. (1990). Characterization of immunomodulatory properties and accessory cell function of small intestinal epithelial cells. *Cell. Immunol.* **127,** 26–34.

Sawicki, W., Kucharczyk, K., Szymanska, K., and Kujawa, M. (1977). Lamina propria macrophages of intestine of the guinea pig. *Gastroenterology* **73,** 1340–1344.

Selby, W. S., Poulter, L. W., Hobbs, S., and Jewell, D. P. (1981). Expression of HLA-DR antigens by colonic epithelium in inflammatory bowel disease. *Clin. Exp. Immunol.* **44,** 453–458.

Selby, W. S., Poulter, L. W., Hobbs, S., Jewell, D. P., and Janossy, G. (1983). Heterogeneity of HLA-DR-positive histiocytes in human intestinal lamina propria: A combined histochemical and immunohistological analysis. *J. Clin. Pathol.* **36,** 379–384.

Sette, A., and Grey, H. (1992). Chemistry of peptide interactions with MHC proteins. *Curr. Opin. Immunol.* **4,** 79–86.

Shimizu, Y., and Andrew, W. (1967). Studies on the rabbit appendix. 1. Lymphocyte-epithelial relations and the transport of bacteria from lumen to lymphoid nodule. *J. Morphol.* **123,** 231–250.

Sicinski, P., Rowinski, J., Warchol, J. B., Jarzabek, Z., Gut, W., Szcygiel, B., Bielecki, K., and Koch, G. (1990). Poliovirus type 1 enters the human host through intestinal M cells. *Gastroenterology* **98,** 56–58.

Siliciano, R. F., Lawton, T., Knall, C., Karr, R. W., Berman, P., Gregory, T., and Reinherz, E. L. (1988). Analysis of host-virus interactions in AIDS with anti-gp120 T cell clones: Effect of HIV sequence viration and a mechanism for CD4+ cell depletion. *Cell* **54,** 561–575.

Spalding, D. M., and Griffin, J. A. (1986). Different pathways of differentiation of pre-B cell lines are induced by dendritic cells and T cells from different lymphoid tissues. *Cell* **44,** 507.

Spalding, D. M., Williamson, S. I., Koopman, W. J., and McGhee, J. R. (1984). Preferential induction of polyclonal IgA secretion by murine Peyer's patch dendritic cell-T cell mixtures. *J Exp Med.* **160,** 941–946.

Sminia, T., and Jeurissen, S. (1986). The macrophage population of the gastro-intestinal tract of the rat. *Immunobiol.* **172,** 72–80.

Steiniger, B., Falk, P., Lohmuller, M., and van der Meide, P. H. (1989). Class II MHC antigens in the rat digestive system. Normal distribution and induced expression after interferon-gamma treatment in vivo. *Immunology* **68(4),** 507–513.

Steinman, R. M., and Cohn, Z. (1973). Identification of a novel cell type in peripheral lymphoid organs of mice. I. Morphology, quatitation, tissue distribution. *J. Exp. Med.* **137,** 1142–1162.

Steinman, R. M., and Nussenzweig, M. C. (1980). Dendritic cells: Features and functions. *Immunol. Rev.* **53,** 127–147.

Vanbuskirk, A., Crump, B. L., Margoliash, E., and Pierce, S. K. (1989). A peptide binding protein having a role in antigen presentation is a member of the HSP70 heat shock family. *J. Exp. Med.* **170,** 1799–1809.

Verspaget, H., and Beeken, W. (1985). Mononuclear phagocytes in the gastrointestinal tract. *Acta Chir. Scand. (Suppl.)* **525,** 113–136.

Wiman, K., Curman, B., Forsum, U., Klareskvg, L., Malmas-Tjernlund, U., Rask, L., Tragardh, L., and Peterson, P. A. (1978). Occurrence of Ia antigens on tissues of non-lymphoid origin. *Nature (London)* **276,** 711–713.

Winter, H. S., Cole, F. S., Huffer, L. M., Davison, C. B., Katz, A. J., and Edelson, P. J. (1983). Isolation and characterization of resident macrophages from guinea pig and human intestine. *Gastroenterology* **85,** 358–363.

Wolf, J. L., and Bye, W. A. (1984). The membranous epithelial (M) cell and the mucosal immune system. *Ann. Rev. Med.* **35,** 95–112.

Wolf, J. L., Rubin, D. H., Finberg, R., Kauffman, R. S., Sharpe, A. H., Trier, J., and Fields, B. N. (1981). Intestinal M cells: A pathway for entry of reovirus into the host. *Science* **212,** 471.

Zhang, Z. Y., and Michael, J. G. (1990). Orally inducible immune unresponsiveness is abrogated by IFN-gamma treatment *J. Immunol.* **144(11),** 4163–4165.

Ziegler, H. K., and Unanue, E. R. (1981). Identification of a macrophage antigen-processing event required for I-region-restricted antigen presentation to T lymphocytes, *J. Immunol.* **127,** 1869–1875.

16

Oral Tolerance and Regulation of Immunity to Dietary Antigens

Allan McI. Mowat

I. INTRODUCTION

The diet of all animals consists of a complex mixture of animal and vegetable products, most of which are nonself in immunological terms and, hence, are potentially antigenic. As other chapters in this volume describe, the gut-associated lymphoid tissues (GALT) are the largest in the body and contain a wide array of different effector mechanisms to counter continual bombardment by potential pathogens. Mobilization of this powerful battery of responses against food antigens would be undesirable, partly because it would limit their uptake and metabolic usefulness but more importantly because hypersensitivity to foods can produce intestinal pathology, as typified by celiac disease and other food sensitive enteropathies (FSE).

These conditions are rare, not because intestinal digestion destroys all immunologically relevant food antigens, but because the intestinal immune system can discriminate actively between food antigens and those of pathogenic importance. Contrary to the widespread belief among immunologists, a substantial proportion of ingested protein is absorbed intact in an immunologically relevant form. Thus, each meal results in the absorption of significant amounts of intact protein that certainly are within the range capable of stimulating immune responses if administered by other routes (Swarbrick *et al.*, 1979; Kilshaw and Cant, 1984; Husby *et al.*, 1987; Harmatz *et al.*, 1989). The purpose of this chapter is to review the immunoregulatory mechanisms that prevent the induction of hypersensitivity by this formidable antigenic challenge.

II. IMMUNE RESPONSES TO DIETARY ANTIGENS

The immune system can react in three principal ways when a novel antigen is present in food (Figure 1). First, a local secretory IgA antibody response may occur in the intestine; second, the systemic immune system may be primed, with evidence of serum antibodies and cell mediated immunity (CMI); finally, a state of systemic immunological tolerance may develop, preventing the induction of active immunity when the offending antigen is encountered on subsequent occasions.

Experimental evidence suggests that the production of local IgA antibodies to food antigens may mediate a specific immune exclusion mechanism that, thereafter, prevents the uptake of the appropriate antigen (Swarbrick *et al.*, 1979; Challacombe and Tomasi, 1980). That this mechanism is one means of preventing clinical food hypersensitivity is consistent with the higher frequency of antibodies and hypersensitivity to food proteins that occur in individuals with selective IgA deficiency (Crabbé and Heremans, 1967; Walker, 1987). Nevertheless, most patients with this extremely common form of immune deficiency are entirely normal and have no evidence of food sensitivity. The relative importance of intestinal IgA in the prevention of food sensitivity is challenged further by the fact that stimulating IgA antibodies by immunizing normal animals orally with conventional protein antigens is difficult (Elson and Ealding, 1984; Lycke and Holmgren, 1986; Wilson *et al.*, 1989; van der Heijden *et al.*, 1991; McGhee *et al.*, 1992; Mowat *et al.*, 1993. Further, normal humans have little or no intestinal IgA antibody against food antigens (O'Mahony *et al.*, 1991). Thus, production of secretory IgA antibodies alone is unlikely to account for the absence of hypersensitivity reactions to food antigens, although this mechanism seems likely to provide a useful back-up to other, more potent immunoregulatory mechanisms.

III. ORAL TOLERANCE

Tolerance is a state of specific immunological unresponsiveness to antigens that, under other circumstances, are capable of inducing an active immune response. One of the most reliable means of inducing immunological tolerance in experimental animals is presenting the antigen by the oral route. Tolerance is the usual result of administering a novel antigen to a naive animal by this route. Oral tolerance has been described best in laboratory rodents, but its presence has been implied in many other species including humans (Korenblatt *et al.*, 1968; Lowney, 1968; Walker, 1987), pigs (Miller *et al.*, 1984; Stokes *et al.*, 1987), dogs (Cantor and Dumont, 1967), guinea pigs (Heppell and Kilshaw, 1982), and rabbits (Bhogal *et al.*, 1986). Species differences do occur, however. Inducing oral tolerance in rabbits or guinea pigs (Peri and Rothberg, 1981; Heppell and Kilshaw, 1982) is

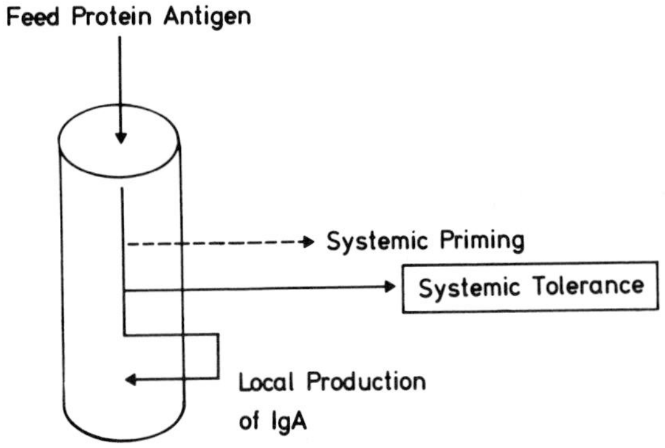

Figure 1 The immunological consequences of feeding antigen. Depending on the antigen, the animal model, and the circumstances involved, oral administration of antigen may stimulate production of secretory IgA antibodies in the intestine, may induce a primary systemic immune response, or may result in systemic unresponsiveness to subsequent challenge with the antigen. In practice, this systemic tolerance is the usual result of feeding a novel protein antigen to a naive mature animal.

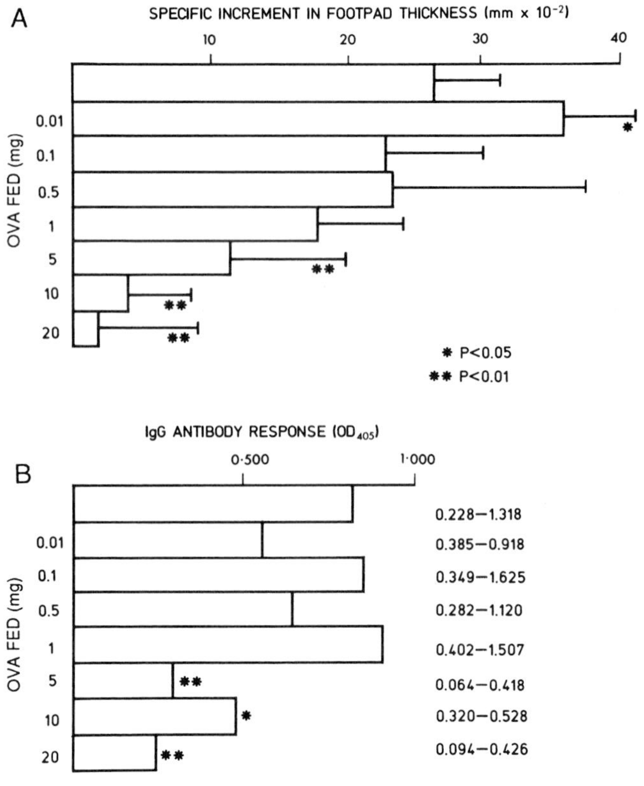

Figure 2 Induction of tolerance by feeding the protein antigen ovalbumin (OVA) to normal adult mice. A dose-dependent suppression of systemic delayed type hypersensitivity (DTH) (A) and IgG antibody (B) responses to subcutaneous challenge with OVA in adjuvant in mice fed OVA. Systemic T cell responses (DTH) are more sensitive to the effects of antigen feeding and also show evidence of priming when the lowest doses of OVA are used.

relatively difficult, whereas ruminants may not develop significant tolerance to dietary materials at all (Stokes, 1984).

The phenomenon is illustrated readily by feeding mice a single dose of a few milligrams of a protein such as ovalbumin (OVA) some time before immunizing the animals with the antigen in adjuvant via an immunogenic route. In most experiments of this type, antigen-fed animals have almost complete suppression of their immune response to the challenge immunization (Figure 2). In this discussion, we focus on oral tolerance to protein antigens and address the hypothesis that this mechanism is the principal means of preventing food hypersensitivity.

A. Background

The possibility that ingestion of antigen might have immunological consequences different from those associated with systemic imunization was raised first in an anecdotal report by Dakin (1829), who described how South American Indians ate poison ivy in an attempt to prevent what we now understand as contact hypersensitivity to the plant (Dakin, 1829). Subsequently, the author and scientist H. G. Wells conducted a large series of experiments that showed that anaphylactic reactions to OVA and other proteins in guinea pigs could be inhibited by prior feeding of the appropriate material (Wells and Osborne, 1911). The immunological nature of the phenomenon first was established by the much later experiments of Chase (1946), using contact sensitizing agents. Exploiting the knowledge that was emerging at that time on cellular immunity and on the induction of tolerance in other systems, Chase's work demonstrated the antigen specificity of oral tolerance and recognized how readily the immune system could be down-regulated by what came to be known as the Sulzberger–Chase phenomenon. Since then, the protocols of inducing oral tolerance and the mechanisms involved have attracted considerable attention, not only from mucosal immunologists but also from individuals interested in using this system as a model of immunoregulation or as a means of artificially inhibiting immune responses to antigens of immunopathological importance.

B. Scope

The induction of systemic tolerance by feeding antigen has been demonstrated with a wide range of nonreplicating antigens. In addition to the many proteins that have been studied, these antigens include contact sensitizing agents (Galister, 1973; Asherson *et al.*, 1977,1979; Newby *et al.*, 1980; Gautam and Battisto, 1985), heterologous red blood cells (Kagnoff, 1978a,1980; Mattingly and Waksman, 1980; Kiyono *et al.*, 1982; MacDonald, 1983), allogeneic leukocytes (Sayegh *et al.*, 1992), and inactivated viruses or bacteria (Stokes *et al.*, 1979; Challacombe and Tomasi, 1980; Rubin *et al.*, 1981). Although the majority of immunological studies have concentrated traditionally on familiar model antigens such as sheep red blood cells (SRBC) and OVA, more recent work also has used proteins of immunopathological importance, including myelin basic protein (MBP), uveal S antigen, and collagen (Nagler-Anderson *et al.*, 1986; Higgins and Weiner, 1988; Lider *et al.*, 1989; Nussenblatt *et al.*, 1990;

Zhang *et al.*, 1990; see Thompson and Staines, 1990, for review). The results obtained using different protein antigens are often similar, indicating the reproducibility of the phenomenon. However, the exact dose required for optimal induction of tolerance may differ, perhaps reflecting size- or charge-related differences in uptake by the intestine as well as inherent differences in immunogenicity.

Virtually all proteins examined have been found to induce oral tolerance, although some controversy exists over whether this also applies to proteins with unusual abilities to bind to and be absorbed by the intestinal mucosa, for example, cholera toxin. Cholera toxin has an almost unique ability to stimulate primary secretory IgA antibody responses after feeding and also has been shown to stimulate systemic antibody and CMI responses by the oral route (Elson and Ealding, 1984; Lycke and Holmgren, 1986; Wilson *et al.*, 1991; McGhee *et al.*, 1992). In addition, cholera toxin acts as an adjuvant for other orally administered proteins, allowing them to provoke both systemic and local immunity rather than the tolerance found after feeding the protein alone. These results suggest that cholera toxin overcomes the immunoregulatory mechanisms that normally produce oral tolerance, but whether this characteristic reflects its ability to bind specifically to enterocytes or its pharmacological effects on cell activation is not clear.

In contrst to the similarities between different proteins, the oral tolerance induced by antigens such as SRBC and contact sensitizing agents may be regulated in quite distinct ways (see subsequent discussion). In the case of SRBCs, this difference may reflect, in part, their particulate nature and the fact that these antigens have a thymus-independent component.

C. Immunological Consequences of Oral Tolerance

All aspects of the immune response can be rendered tolerant by feeding antigen. A single feed of protein antigen will tolerize subsequent systemic IgM, IgG, and IgE antibody responses (Vaz *et al.*, 1977; Ngan and Kind, 1978; Richman *et al.*, 1978; Swarbrick *et al.*, 1979; Challacombe and Tomasi, 1980; Titus and Chiller, 1981; Mowat *et al.*, 1982; Thompson and Staines, 1990), as well as CMI responses measured by lymphocyte proliferation (Challacombe and Tomasi, 1980; Titus and Chiller, 1981; Higgins and Weiner, 1988; Lider *et al.*, 1989), cytokine production (Whitacre *et al.*, 1991), and delayed-type hypersensitivity (DTH) or contact sensitivity *in vivo* (Asherson *et al.*, 1977,1979; Miller and Hanson, 1979; Newby *et al.*, 1980; Titus and Chiller, 1981; Mowat *et al.*, 1982; Gautam and Battisto, 1985; Kay and Ferguson, 1989a,b). CMI responses are much easier to tolerize than are humoral immune responses, requiring less antigen and persisting much longer after feeding (Figure 2; Heppell and Kilshaw, 1982; Mowat *et al.*, 1982; Mowat *et al.*, 1986; Strobel and Ferguson, 1987; Kay and Ferguson, 1989a,b). This finding extends to primed animals, in whom DTH responses can be suppressed fairly readily by feeding OVA after systemic immunization whereas serum antibody repsonses remain relatively unaffected (Lamont *et al.*, 1988a; Peng *et al.*, 1989a). In parallel, oral tolerance to proteins exhibits classical carrier specificity (Hanson *et al.*, 1977; Richman *et al.*, 1978; Titus and Chiller, 1981; Cowdrey and Johlin, 1984) and tolerance of antibody production *in vivo* can be broken if the defective helper T cells are bypassed using an unrelated carrier or are stimulated with lipopolysaccharide (LPS) (Titus and Chiller, 1981; Mowat *et al.*, 1986). When B cells are tolerized by feeding antigen, they recover much more quickly than T cells (Vives *et al.*, 1980).

One exception to the general rule that antibody responses are relatively difficult to tolerize is IgE production, which is remarkably sensitive to inhibition by feeding antigen before or after parenteral immunization (Ngan and Kind, 1978; Jarrett and Hall, 1984; Saklayen *et al.*, 1984). Interestingly, similar findings have been made in the experimental tolerance that can be induced by exposing animals to aerosols of protein antigen (Holt *et al.*, 1981). In conjunction with the fact that IgE and DTH responses are the mechanisms most frequently associated with pathological food hypersensitivity (Mowat, 1993), these results suggest that prevention of food-specific IgE and DTH responses may be the most important biological role of oral tolerance.

The status of mucosal immune responses in orally tolerized animals is less clear. Initial reports suggested that the degree of tolerance of systemic immunity induced by feeding antigen correlated directly with the concomitant development of secretory IgA antibody responses and IgA-mediated immune exclusion (Swarbrick *et al.*, 1979; Challacombe and Tomasi, 1980). In addition, mice fed antigen were reported to have concomitant induction of Peyer's patch T cells that suppressed IgG production but helped the synthesis of IgA antibodies (Richman *et al.*, 1981). However, strain differences in immune exclusion among protein-fed mice do not correlate with their susceptibility to oral tolerance (Stokes *et al.*, 1983a). In addition, several investigators using both protein and nonprotein antigens have shown that intestinal IgA production is tolerized by feeding antigen (Kiyono *et al.*, 1982; MacDonald, 1983). These latter findings are consistent with the apparent absence of IgA antibodies against food antigens in normal individuals and indicate that local IgA production probably is regulated in the same way as systemic immunity in orally tolerant animals.

D. Time Course and Duration of Oral Tolerance

Systemic tolerance can be demonstrated very soon after a single feed of protein. Significantly suppressed responses to systemic challenge with OVA are observed within 2 days of feeding the antigen (Challacombe and Tomasi, 1980). The maximum degree of unresponsiveness then occurs during the first weeks after feeding; in most experimental protocols, a 1- to 2-week gap between feeding and challenge has been found to be the most appropriate. The resulting tolerance is then remarkably persistent, although its exact duration depends on the nature of the systemic immune response under study. Work with OVA has shown that, although tolerance of serum IgG antibody responses had almost disappeared by 6 months after a single feed of OVA, the DTH tolerance remains essentially intact up to at least 18 months (Strobel and Ferguson, 1987). In view of the fact that the average life-span of a laboratory mouse is little more than 2 years, these findings highlight the potency and stability of this immunoregulatory phenomenon. In addition, these data are further evidence that systemic T-cell responses are affected more readily by feeding antigen than is humoral immunity.

Tolerance induced by feeding other antigens such as heterologous red cells may not develop so rapidly, since multiple feeds of SRBCs over a period of >2 weeks often are required for unresponsiveness to be demonstrable. This result may reflect the fact that SRBCs may induce a primary immune response when given orally and that this priming first must be overcome before tolerance ensues (Kagnoff, 1978a,b; David, 1979; Mattingly and Waksman, 1980).

IV. FACTORS THAT INFLUENCE THE INDUCTION AND MAINTENANCE OF ORAL TOLERANCE

A. Nature of Antigen

As we have discussed, a wide range of antigens is capable of inducing oral tolerance. Although differences in dose response, time course, and the exact mechanisms involved may exist, the eventual effects on the systemic immune response are generally similar, irrespective of the antigen. However, certain types of antigen are more likely to provoke active immunity rather than tolerance by the oral route, particularly viable organisms such as viruses and bacteria (Stokes *et al.*, 1979; Rubin *et al.*, 1981). This difference in response is not dependent on the nature of the antigens involved, since the same organisms will induce oral tolerance if killed or inactivated (Rubin *et al.*, 1981). In addition, soluble proteins expressed as gene products in live bacteria are immunogenic when given orally (Dahlgren *et al.*, 1991).

Inducing tolerance by feeding thymus-independent antigens also is generally impossible (Stokes *et al.*, 1979; Titus and Chiller, 1981), even if these are administered in association with a thymus-dependent antigen. Thus, mice fed killed *Escherichia coli* develop tolerance to the thymus-dependent K antigen but acquire local and systemic immunity to the thymus-independent O antigen on the same organism (Stokes *et al.*, 1979). Particulate antigens are also less able than soluble antigens to induce oral tolerance, since OVA coated onto polyglycoside microspheres stimulates active immunity by the oral route (McGhee *et al.*, 1992).

These findings may help explain the ability of the intestinal immune system to discriminate between dietary and pathogenic antigens, since many potentially invasive bacteria will present a large amount of thymus-independent antigen (e.g., LPS) in particulate form and, of course, a large proportion of this material will be viable. How the intestinal immune system can distinguish between immunogenic and tolerogenic materials is not known, but may relate to the ability of viable organisms to provide a persistent stimulus to the immune system or to invade lymphoid tissues beyond the intestinal mucosa. Particulate antigens also may be taken up and processed by the intestine more efficiently, perhaps because such antigens may target M cells in Peyer's patches (Owen, 1977; Pappo and Ermak, 1989), whereas soluble materials may enter diffusely across the villus epithelium.

B. Antigen Dose

A wide range of antigen doses will induce significant oral tolerance; a single feed of a few milligrams of protein is sufficient in mice (Figure 2; Hanson *et al.*, 1977; Mowat *et al.*, 1986). The exact dose required for the optimal effect depends on the protein under study. The different limbs of the systemic immune response are differentially susceptible. Maximal immune suppression after feeding OVA occurs with doses ranging from 1 to 20 mg protein, but DTH responses can be tolerized reproducibly by doses of as little as 100 μg OVA, whereas at least 5–10 mg are necessary to inhibit humoral immunity (Figure 2).

At doses immediately below those that induce tolerance, feeding antigen has no effect on systemic immunity, whereas even lower amounts actually may prime the immune response (Figure 2; Lamont *et al.*, 1989). In mice, systemic priming occurs during doses of 1–50 μg protein and affects T-cell repsonses more than humoral immunity. A similar phenomenon has been noted in piglets, in which large amounts of weaning diet produce tolerance and low amounts prime the animals to develop food sensitivity (Miller *et al.*, 1984). Interestingly, initial exposure to low amounts of food antigens also has been suggested to predispose to eczema in children (Jarrett, 1984).

C. Genetic Background of Host

Since celiac disease is linked closely to the HLA-DQw2 locus of the human major histocompatibility complex (MHC; Howell *et al.*, 1986), determining how genetic factors influence the regulation of immune responses to fed protein antigens under experimental conditions is important. Several early studies noted strain differences in the susceptibility of mouse stains to the induction of oral tolerance by feeding OVA, although these differences were not investigated systematically and their basis was not addressed (Lafont *et al.*, 1982; Stokes *et al.*, 1983a; Tomasi *et al.*, 1983). Similar differences have been observed in the induction of oral tolerance in primed animals (Lafont *et al.*, 1982). In a more detailed analysis of oral tolerance to OVA, we found that the majority of mouse strains was tolerized readily by feeding this antigen (Lamont *et al.*, 1988b). Few consistent genetic influences could be identified, including those encoding the idiotypic regions of immunoglobulins. Interestingly, the susceptibility to induction of oral tolerance did not correlate with differences in tolerance induced by the intravenous route, underscoring the possibility that tolerance to fed antigens involves mechanisms distinct from those that control immunity to parenterally administered antigen (see subsequent text).

One important aspect to emerge from this work was that mice carrying the H-2^d MHC haplotype were particularly susceptible to the induction of tolerance, whereas the H-2^b haplotype frequently was associated with less profound tolerance. Of particular note, BALB/B mice were much more difficult to tolerize than the congenic BALB/c strain (Figure 3; Mowat *et al.*, 1987; Lamont *et al.*, 1988b). Since these mice differ only at the MHC, these data support a possible role for MHC genes in regulating oral tolerance to protein antigens. These strain differences did not reflect differences in the processing of protein in the intestine, but were the result of the inability of the BALB/B immune system to be regulated by tolerogenic protein coming from the intestine (Mowat *et al.*, 1987). The immunological basis of this MHC-linked effect remains to be established. Note that other non-MHC-linked genes have been implicated in oral tolerance, both to OVA and to human γ globulin (Tomasi *et al.*, 1983). These background genes do not appear to operate via the immune exclusion function of secretory IgA antibody, but resistance to tolerance induction correlated with unusually rapid clearance of absorbed antigen from the circulation (Stokes *et al.*, 1983a). Thus, oral tolerance induction may be under the control of several genes that may influence both specific immune responsiveness and nonspecific factors such as protein clearance and catabolism.

One additional level of genetic control that has been noted is that strains of mice with genetically determined systemic lupus erythematosus (SLE)-like autoimmune disease are unusually resistant to the induction of tolerance by feeding certain protein antigens (Cowdrey *et al.*, 1982; Miller *et al.*, 1983; Carr *et al.*, 1985). These well-established experimental models could provide useful means of investigating the immunological basis of antigen-specific regulation of immunity to fed proteins.

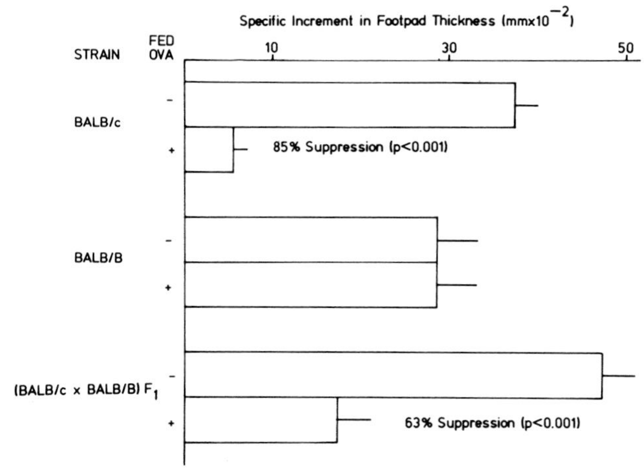

Figure 3 Genetic differences in oral tolerance. BALB/B (H-2^b) mice are resistant to the induction of tolerance by feeding doses of ovalbumin (OVA) that suppress delayed type hypersensitivity (DTH) and antibody responses in congenic BALB/c (H-2^d) mice.

D. Influence of Host Age on Susceptibility to Oral Tolerance

Food hypersensitivities are most common in infants, particularly at or near the time of weaning. Note, therefore, that neonatal and weaning mice exhibit defects in the induction of tolerance by feeding protein antigens. Mice fed OVA on the first day or two of life do not develop the tolerance of systemic immunity found in adults fed the same weight-related dose. Indeed, OVA-fed infant mice show evidence of systemic priming when challenged parenterally as adults, particularly with respect to systemic DTH responses (Hanson, 1981; Strobel and Ferguson, 1984). Similar findings have been reported in neonatal mice exposed early in lactation to gluten present in the milk of mothers fed a gluten-containing diet (Troncone and Ferguson, 1988). In addition, the ability to sensitize calves or piglets by feeding antigen during the preweaning period further supports an age-related defect in oral tolerance at this time (Miller *et al.*, 1984; Stokes, 1984; Barratt *et al.*, 1987; Stokes *et al.*, 1987).

This defect in tolerance does not correlate with differences in the amount of protein absorbed by the neonatal intestine and can be corrected by transfer of mature lymphocytes (Hanson, 1981; Peng *et al.*, 1989a). Thus, the infant response may reflect an inability of the immature immune system to respond appropriately to intestinally derived tolerogen. The adult pattern of susceptibility to tolerance develops after 4 days of age and is established fully around 7 days. However, an additional transient defect in tolerance induction occurs in the days around weaning (Hanson, 1981; Strobel and Ferguson, 1984). This latter phenomenon is not related to the age of the animal, but is influenced by the process of weaning itself and is likely to be determined by the alterations in intestinal microenvironment or in systemic hormone levels associated with weaning.

At the other end of the age spectrum, aging mice have been reported to become increasingly resistant to the induciton of oral tolerance by feeding OVA (S. J. Challacombe, personal communication). Since this observation seems unusual in view of the apparent preservation of the intestinal immune system in aged animals, its significance is unclear.

E. Influence of Intestinal Flora

Evidence from both human and veterinary work suggests that clinical food sensitive enteropathy may develop subsequent to intestinal infection. As we have noted, the changes in gut flora at the time of weaning may be associated with a period of defective oral tolerance. One of several possible explanations for these findings is that bacterial products may influence the regulation of immune responses to dietary antigens.

The immunomodulatory effects of LPS and other bacterial products are well known. Substantial evidence suggests that germ-free mice have defective systemic immune competence (MacDonald and Carter, 1979; Collins and Carter, 1980). That these effects may extend to mucosal immunoregulation was suggested by the fact that germ-free mice cannot be tolerized by feeding SRBC (Wannemuehler *et al.*, 1982b). In addition, inducing tolerance by feeding SRBC to C3H/HeJ mice that have a genetically determined inability to respond to LPS is impossible (Kiyono *et al.*, 1982; Michalek *et al.*, 1982; Mowat *et al.*, 1986; Kitamura *et al.*, 1987). Unlike normal congeneic C3H mice, LPS-unresponsive animals are primed by feeding SRBC and develop systemic antibody and DTH responses as well as local IgA antibodies. These effects were associated with a defect in the induction of suppressor T cells (T_s) and a parallel appearance of contrasuppressor T cells (Suzuki *et al.*, 1986a,b; Kitamura *et al.*, 1987; Fujihashi *et al.*, 1989).

Although these results support an important role for LPS in mucosal immunoregulation, subsequent work by ourselves and others has shown that LPS has no influence on immune responses to fed protein antigens. Oral tolerance to proteins is entirely normal in LPS-unresponsive C3H/HeJ mice, and exogenous LPS has no effect on T-cell tolerance in normal mice fed OVA (Saklayen *et al.*, 1983; Mowat *et al.*, 1986). Thus, bacterial LPS seems unlikely to play an important role in the regulation of immunity to the majority of dietary antigens, which are protein in nature. However, the possibility that other bacterial products may influence these responses cannot be excluded. Clearly, LPS may influence responsiveness to certain antigens, particularly those with a strong thymus-independent component such as SRBCs.

F. Role of Intestinal Absorption and Antigen Uptake

As we shall discuss, oral tolerance to protein antigens reflects the manner in which the protein is processed in the intestine (see subsequent text). Thus, we might predict that any factor that alters either the amount or the chemical nature of the antigen absorbed from the intestine also will influence the immunological consequences of this material. This idea is supported by the high levels of food-specific antibodies that occur in individuals with disorders that cause increased intestinal permeability to macromolecules, for example, Crohn's disease and celiac disease (Cunningham-Rundles, 1987; Walker, 1987). Although increased permeability to antigen may explain in part the absence of tolerance in mice fed OVA incorporated in lipophilic immune stimulating complexes (ISCOM) containing the detergent saponin (Quil A; Figure 4), a firm correlation between antigen uptake and tolerance or priming remains to be established.

G. Nutritional Influences on Oral Tolerance

The function of the immune system is highly dependent on the nutritional status of the host. Several reports have been made that protein-calorie malnutrition compromises the ability of animals to make mucosal immune responses (Chandra *et al.*, 1987). Nutritional deficiencies are most likely to occur in the early neonatal period, when the risk of disordered regulation of immunity to fed antigens is also at its highest. However, little is known of the influence of nutrition on oral tolerance, partly because distinguishing between the effects of malnutrition itself and those that are the result of secondary complications, such as intestinal abnormalities or infection, is frequently difficult. One carefully controlled study has shown that mice on an isocaloric low-protein diet have defective induction of tolerance after feeding OVA and that this defect is related to a primary effect of malnutrition on the immune system (Lamont *et al.*, 1987). If this finding extends to other forms of malnutrition, particularly in developing animals, poor nutritional status could predispose to food hypersensitivity in infancy.

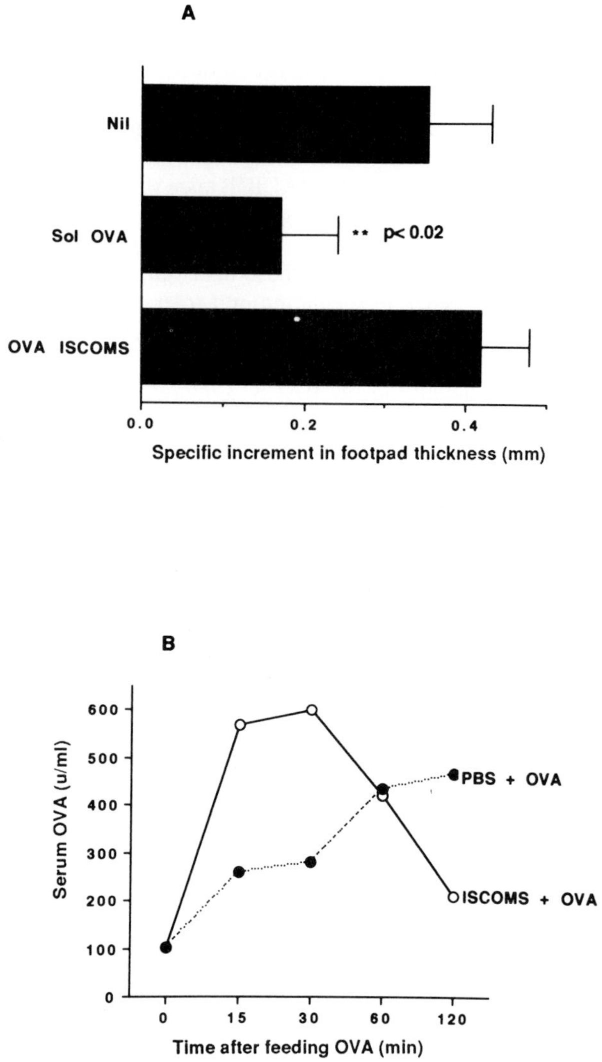

Figure 4 Incorporation in immune stimulating complexes (ISCOMS) prevents the induction of oral tolerance. (A) Mice fed a dose of ovalbumin (OVA), which in soluble form induces tolerance of systemic delayed type hypersensitivity (DTH) responses, are not tolerized if OVA is incorporated into ISCOMS. (B) Feeding ISCOMS increases the speed and amount of OVA uptake into serum after a test feed.

H. Immunological Status of the Host

For many years, researchers have known that inducing systemic tolerance in animals that previously have been primed to the antigen is difficult or impossible. Although initial work suggested that a similar effect of priming extended to oral tolerance (Hanson *et al.*, 1979a), several investigators have since shown that oral tolerance can be induced in parenterally primed mice (Lafont *et al.*, 1982; Higgins and Weiner 1988; Lamont *et al.*, 1988b; Lider *et al.*, 1989; Peng *et al.*, 1989b; Thompson and Staines, 1990). Larger doses of fed antigen or more frequent feeds may be required to obtain degrees of tolerance equivalent to those found in naive animals; also, only a short time window after systemic priming may exist during which oral tolerance is inducible. These findings may help explain why multiple feeds of relatively large amounts of antigen are required to induce tolerance to SRBCs, since these contain antigens to which mice frequently are primed via cross-reacting intestinal flora; a primary immune response can be detected before tolerance ensues (see preceding discussion). As is seen in naive hosts, tolerance to protein antigens in primed animals affects T-cell responses more than humoral immunity (Lamont *et al.*, 1988b; Peng *et al.*, 1989b) and exhibits clear strain differences. However, whether similar immunoregulatory mechanisms govern the tolerance in the two types of host is not clear (see subsequent discussion. Interestingly, studies have shown that feeding specific antigen also can be used to inhibit established autoimmune diseases such as experimental autoimmune encephalomyelitis and collagen-induced arthritis (Higgins and Weiner, 1988; Lider *et al.*, 1989; Thompson and Staines 1990). Thus, the oral route may be potentially useful for immunotherapeutic intervention in antigen-specific immunopathology. The relatively good ability of oral tolerance to overcome systemic priming also may explain the fact that several clinical food sensitivities, including cow milk protein intolerance and eczema, are transient in nature; affected patients apparently acquire specific tolerance.

V. MECHANISMS OF ORAL TOLERANCE

A. Introduction

Most mechanistic studies in oral tolerance were performed during the late 1970s and early 1980s, at a time when the immune system was not understood at the molecular or cellular level. Several different mechanisms were suggested to be responsible for the ability of fed antigen to inhibit immune responsiveness but, as with many other immunoregulatory phenomena, this result usually was seen as a manifestation of T_s activity. Considerable efforts were made to establish the nature and origin of these cells and to understand how fed antigen could induce their activation preferentially. However, T_s have proved resistant to the major advances in molecular and cell biology that have elucidated the basis of most other T cell functions. As a result, researchers now consider T_s unlikely to exist as a discrete population of lymphocytes. The basis of immunoregulation has undergone a period of reexamination. Before reviewing the evidence for T_s and other immunoregulatory mechanisms in oral tolerance, we first discuss briefly how current views have altered our understanding of other forms of tolerance (Table I).

Table I Current Concepts in Systemic Tolerance[a]

Clonal deletion–immature T cells; self-antigens
Clonal anergy–mature T cells; mature/immature B cells
Cytotoxic T cell lysis of APC or of specific B cells
Inhibitory cytokines

[a] Mechanisms that are believed to mediate tolerance to self or parenterally administered antigens.

B. Mechanisms of Peripheral Tolerance and Immunoregulation

Clonal deletion and anergy of antigen-reactive T cells now are believed to be the principal mechanisms responsible for most forms of tolerance induced by parenteral routes (Schwartz, 1989; Holan *et al.*, 1991). Clonal deletion occurs predominantly in the thymus of developing animals, where immature T cells undergo apoptosis after encountering self-antigens on medullary antigen-presenting cells (APC). Clonal deletion also may occur during tolerance induction in the periphery of mature animals, but this event probably reflects a state of specific cellular hyporesponsiveness at the level of antigen-specific T cells. This "anergy" occurs when the molecular signaling events that normally produce T-cell activation after presentation of antigen on APCs are altered and further stimulation by antigen is prevented (Mueller *et al.*, 1989).

Several conditions favor the induction of anergy rather than immune activation, including the amount and nature of the antigen. In addition, growing evidence suggests that clonal anergy is particularly likely when antigen is presented on "nonprofessional" APC which, although expressing appropriate MHC antigens, do not produce the co-stimulatory mediators necessary for T-cell activation (Mueller *et al.*, 1989). APC of this type include a variety of MHC Class II-expressing epithelial cells, indicating the possible importance of this mechanism in regulating immunity in a tissue such as the intestine, where epithelial expression of MHC Class II antigens is a normal event.

Our current understanding of immunoregulation has been increased further in recent years by the discovery that the immune response is controlled by a series of interacting cytokines. Of particular note is the proposal that the outcome of immunization is dependent on the activation of discrete populations of $CD4^+$ helper T cells (T_H), which can be discriminated on the basis of their pattern of cytokine production. T_H1 cells produce interleukin 2 (IL-2), interferon γ (IFNγ), and tumor necrosis factor β (TNFβ; lymphotoxin), and are responsible for DTH responses and cytotoxicity, whereas T_H2 cells produce interleukins 4, 5, 6, 9, and 10 and are classical helper cells for antibody production (Mossmann and Coffman, 1989). The induction of these T-cell subsets by antigen appears to depend on the natue of the APC involved. In addition to playing quite distinct effector roles in the immune system, each of these T-cell subsets can inhibit the functions of the other. The nature of the immune response that eventually occurs reflects the outcome of the interactions between competing cytokines. That production of individual cytokines also can influence whether administration of antigen produces tolerance or immunity is suggested by the findings that antibodies to IFNγ can prevent the induction of tolerance to intravenously administered OVA (Hayglass and Stefura, 1991) as well as the induction of antigen-specific T-cell anergy *in vitro* (Liu and Janeway, 1990). Analogous studies have implicated similar roles for IL4 and transforming growth factor β (TGFβ) in parenterally induced tolerance (Schurmans *et al.*, 1990; Karpus and Swanborg, 1991).

Collectively, these studies indicate that the regulation of immune responses is determined by the way in which antigen is presented to the immune system and that the nature of the eventual response may reflect production of individual cytokines. Ascertaining the relevance of these recent developments to the existing knowledge on oral tolerance discussed in the following sections will be important.

C. Suppressor T Cells and Oral Tolerance

T_s have been implicated in virtually all models of oral tolerance in experimental animals. Early studies in guinea pigs fed contact sensitizing agents noted the presence of an active suppressor mechanism *in vivo* (Chase and Battisto, 1955), and the ability of T cells to transfer tolerance first was reported in 1976 in rats fed bovine serum albumin (BSA; Thomas and Parrott, 1974). Support for a role for T_s came from two approaches. First, the induction of oral tolerance by feeding OVA, cholera toxin, or contact sensitizing agents could be prevented by treating mice with drugs that were believed to be specifically toxic to T_s, for example, cyclophosphamide and 2′-deoxyguanosine (Mowat *et al.*, 1982; Kay and Ferguson, 1989b; Mowat, 1986). By abrogating oral tolerance, cyclophosphamide also allows the development of immune complex glomerulonephritis in mice fed multiple doses of bovine gamma globulin (BGG; Gesualdo *et al.*, 1990). Second, transferable T_s were found after feeding a wide range of experimental antigens, including proteins, contact sensitizing agents, and SRBC as well as several antigens of pathological importance (Ngan and Kind, 1978; Kagnoff, 1978a; Miller and Hanson, 1979; Kiyono *et al.*, 1982; MacDonald, 1983; Gautam and Battisto, 1985; Mowat, 1985,1986; Lider *et al.*, 1989; Nussenblatt *et al.*, 1990; Thompson and Staines, 1990). Interestingly, most evidence showed that T_s could inhibit only systemic T-cell responses in antigen-fed animals, whereas humoral immune responses remained unaffected by T_s activity.

In virtually all cases examined, these suppressor cells were $CD8^+$ T cells that acted in the afferent phase of the immune response. In addition, reports were made of networks in which a number of T_s interacted to produce inhibition of the response (Mattingly and Waksman, 1980; MacDonald, 1982; Gautam and Battisto 1985). As in many other systems, the nature of the T-cell receptor (TcR) expressed on the T_s during oral tolerance has never been elucidated. Nevertheless, one study has proposed that the T_s induced by aerosol exposure of mice to OVA carry the unusual $\gamma\delta$ form of the TcR (McMenamin *et al.*, 1991). In view of the fact that $\gamma\delta^+$ T cells may accumulate in the gut, examining whether these findings extend to oral tolerance would be of interest.

The effector T_s found in antigen-fed animals were believed to originate in the Peyer's patches soon after feeding antigen, before migrating to the mesenteric lymph nodes and then to systemic lymphoid tissues (Asherson *et al.*, 1977,1979; Ngan and Kind, 1978; Mattingly and Waksman, 1978, MacDonald, 1982). This behavior was not shown directly and the site of the interaction between antigen and T_s was never determined. Subsequent studies proposed that the induction of T_s required presentation of fed antigen by specialized APC that differed from conventioanl APC in their expression of molecules thought to be encoded by "I–J" genes found within the MHC Class II locus. *In vivo* treatment with antibodies against I–J molecules prevented the induction of tolerance in mice fed OVA, whereas similar treatment with antibodies against classical MHC Class II antigens had no effect (Mowat *et al.*, 1988). Since the T_s induced by feeding OVA did not themselves express I–J markers, these experiments were interpreted to show that fed antigen associated preferentially with I–J$^+$ APCs that then stimulated T_s. This hypothesis was entirely compatible with contemporary studies in which a network of "I-J-restricted" APCs and T_s appeared to be responsible for a number of other models of tolerance (Green *et al.*, 1983; Granstein and Green, 1985). However, the significance of these findings is now unknown, since the biochemical and genetic nature of the I–J molecule has not been elucidated and its very existence is controversial. Elucidating the molecular basis of the interactions between APCs and regulatory T cells in antigen-fed animals is a major challenge to mucosal immunologists.

An additional layer of complexity in the groups of regulatory T cells found in antigen-fed animals comes from suggestions that, under certain circumstances, a population of "contrasuppressor T cells" (T_{cs}) may counteract the effects of T_s (Suzuki *et al.*, 1986a,b; Kitamura *et al.*, 1987). These T_{cs} first were described as responsible for the lack of oral tolerance in LPS-unresponsive mice fed SRBC and appeared to act by interfering with the ability of T_s to inhibit specific antibody production. Evidence also was presented that the T_{cs} had selective effects on IgA production. More recently, T_{cs} function has been reported to be associated with a small population of spleen and intestinal intraepithelial T lymphocytes (IEL) that express the $\gamma\delta$ TcR (Fujihashi *et al.*, 1989,1990). Although these findings raise many intriguing issues concerning the possible role of mucosal lymphocytes in regulating immunity to dietary antigens, note that the reports of T_{cs} in antigen-fed animals have been made only with SRBC and in an extremely limited number of mouse strains. Further, the existence of these cells is now considered even more unlikely than that of T_s themselves.

D. Other Immunoregulatory Mechanisms

1. Clonal Anergy and Deletion of T Lymphocytes

No studies of clonal deletion or anergy in oral tolerance have been published. However, several workers have reported that T-cell tolerance in antigen-fed mice does not necessarily correlate with the presence of T_s (Titus and Chiller, 1981; Hanson and Miller, 1982; Tomasi *et al.*, 1983). Further, as we have noted, humoral immunity in antigen-fed animals may not be regulated by T_s. Studies using limiting dilution analysis have suggested that individual antigen-specific effector T cells from mice fed MBP are anergic in the absence of T_s (Whitacre *et al.*, 1991). In addition, one report in abstract form has presented evidence for specific absence of T cells expressing the Vβ8.2 TcR in SJL mice fed MBP (Whitacre *et al.*, 1990). Since the immune response to MBP in this strain is dominated by $V\beta8.2^+$ T cells, these results support the possibility that clonal deletion of antigen-specific T cells may occur during oral tolerance. Confirming and extending these findings, perhaps using the superantigen-based approaches that have proved successful in other models of tolerance, is now important.

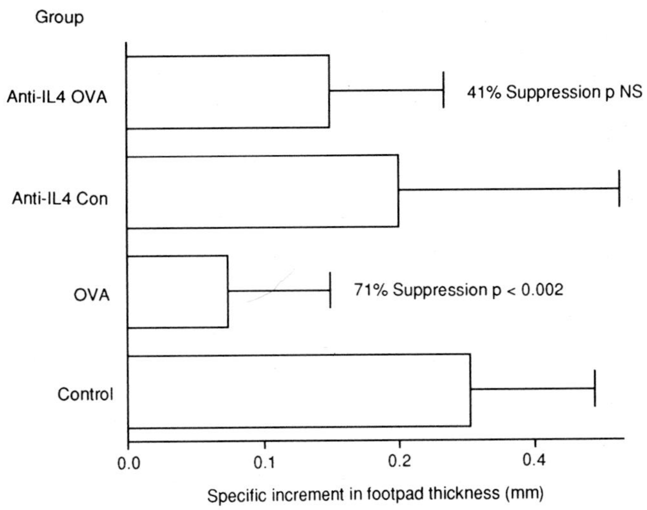

Figure 5 A role for interleukin 4 in oral tolerance. Mice treated with anti-IL4 antibody 1 day before feeding ovalbumin (OVA) do not have the significant tolerance of systemic delayed type hypersensitivity (DTH) responses seen in untreated OVA-fed controls.

2. Role of Cytokines

As we have noted, increasing evidence suggests that preferential induction of individual cytokines may be of critical importance in a number of forms of immunoregulation. That this mechanism may be involved in oral tolerance is suggested by the differential effects of antigen feeding on systemic cellular and humoral immunity, as well as by the possibility that local IgA responses are relatively preserved during oral tolerance. One report has suggested that "T_s" from rats fed MBP can inhibit responses of primed T cells to a third party antigen, a phenomenon that has been ascribed to the involvement of nonspecific soluble mediators released by the T_s after contact with the antigen (Miller *et al.*, 1991a). The cytokines involved have yet to be identified with certainty, but administration of IFNγ interferes with the induction of oral tolerance in mice (Zhang and Michael, 1990), and preliminary studies indicate that *in vivo* depletion of TGFβ (Miller *et al.*, 1991b) or IL-4 (Figure 5) can substantially prevent tolerance in mice fed OVA. These findings indicate the need for more extensive studies of the relationship between cytokine production and oral tolerance.

3. Role of B Lymphocytes and Antibody

Although oral tolerance has been ascribed most frequently to the induction of T_s, several other regulatory mechanisms have been reported. Suppressor B cells have been found in mice fed contact sensitizing agents (Asherson *et al.*, 1977,1979), and oral tolerance to these antigens can be enhanced by administration of polyclonal B cell activators (Newby *et al.*, 1980).

Transferring tolerance using serum-derived material from protein-fed animals is not possible (Hanson *et al.*, 1979b). However, isolated reports suggest that tolerance to SRBCs and certain contact sensitizing agents can be transferred using serum from antigen-fed mice (André *et al.*, 1975; Kagnoff, 1978b; Chalon *et al.*, 1979; Bhogal *et al.*, 1986). The material responsible appears to be IgG and is likely to be an anti-idiotypic antibody rather than an antibody directed at the antigen itself. Regulation of immunity by anti-idiotypic antibody also has been described in mice tolerized by portal vein inoculation of allogeneic lymphocytes (Sato *et al.*, 1988). Although the significance of these findings for more usual forms of oral tolerance has not been established, note that milk from mice tolerized orally or parenterally during pregnancy can induce tolerance in the neonate by transfer of anti-idiotypic antibody (Wannemuehler *et al.*, 1982a; Jarrett and Hall, 1984). Thus, the possibility remains that this mechanism provides a means of conferring tolerance on the neonate at a time when susceptibility to food sensitivity is high.

E. Role of Intestinal Processing in Oral Tolerance

The ability of orally administered antigen to modulate systemic immune responses requires the absorption of small amounts of immunologically intact material from the intestine. Substantial evidence exists that intestinal processing events are critical for oral tolerance to proteins. Serum removed from mice fed OVA 1 hr beforehand induces systemic tolerance when transferred intraperitoneally to naive syngeneic recipients. The tolerance selectively inhibits systemic DTH responses in the recipients and is related to the activation of cyclophosphamide-sensitive T_s by OVA-fed serum (Strobel *et al.*, 1983; Bruce and Ferguson, 1986a,b). Similar findings have been made with other protein antigens (Kay and Ferguson, 1989b; S. Strobel, unpublished observations). The processing event necessary for the generation of the serum tolerogen appears to occur in the intestine itself, since serum taken from mice given equivalent doses of protein by other parenteral routes is never able to reproduce appropriate tolerance in naive recipients (Bruce and Ferguson 1986a). However, the site of this processing is unknown and the relative roles of the intestinal epithelium or local lymphoid cells have not been ascertained. The precise nature of the tolerogen present in OVA-fed serum is also unclear. The tolerogenic material appears in serum within 20–30 min of feeding and therefore is unlikely to involve any immunologically active molecule (Peng *et al.,* 1990). In addition, this result argues against a need for proteolytic digestion. This idea is supported by the fact that the tolerogen reacts with antibodies directed at native OVA (Bruce and Ferguson, 1986b) and elutes on gel filtration columns or high performance liquid chromatography (HPLC) with the native molecule (Bruce and Ferguson, 1986b; H. J. Peng and S. Strobel, personal communication). These findings suggest that a simple filtration mechanism in the intestine may produce deaggregated monomers of protein that are known to be tolerogenic in other systems. However, since the ability of serum to transfer tolerance is not related directly to the absolute amount of protein present (Peng *et al.,* 1990), intestinal processing may cause subtle changes in the charge or conformation of the antigen that influence its immunogenicity.

Proteolytic digestion is unlikely to generate selected peptide fragments containing "suppressor determinants" that can prevent responsiveness to the intact antigen, as suggested in other models (Kölsch, 1984). Feeding artificial peptides usually induces the same degree of tolerance as that found after feeding the intact antigen (Higgins and Weiner, 1988). Rectal administration of proteins also induces tolerance, and *in vivo* inhibition of pancreatic enzyme activity has no effect on induction of oral tolerance (Strobel, 1984). Thus, proteins do not need to undergo proteolysis to induce tolerance by the oral route.

Collectively, these findings support the view that tolerogenic moieties of proteins produced during intestinal processing are responsible for the induction of systemic tolerance, at least for T-cell responses. Since this material has little or no effect on humoral immune responses, however, additional mechanisms must influence the hyporesponsiveness of antibody responses in protein-fed mice.

F. Role of Antigen Presentation in Oral Tolerance

Virtually all immune responses require the activation of T cells by short peptides bound in the surface groove of MHC molecules. Complex nonviable antigens, such as those that induce oral tolerance, first must be taken up by accessory cells in the immune system, processed intracellularly within endosomes, and presented as a complex with MHC Class II antigens. As we have discussed, evidence shows that these APC functions not only control the specificity and level of the resulting immune response but also determine whether active immunity or tolerance occurs after administration of antigen (Mueller *et al.,* 1989).

Therefore, that APC activity appears to be critical in regulating the immunological consequences of feeding antigens is not surprising. This ability first was suggested by the finding that feeding one antigen to naive mice causes transient activation of the reticuloendothelial system (RES) and interferes with the induction of tolerance by feeding a second antigen (Stokes *et al.,* 1983b). Oral tolerance in mice fed OVA also can be prevented by *in vivo* administration of a number of agents that activate the accessory cell functions of the RES, including estrogen, muramyl dipeptide (MDP), and a graft-versus-host reaction (GvHR; Mowat and Parrott, 1983; Strobel *et al.,* 1985; Strobel and Ferguson, 1986). Once again, tolerance of DTH responses was more susceptible to modulation by activating the RES. Further work showed that, although these agents affected many functions of the RES, their effects on oral tolerance correlated specifically with enhanced APC activity in the spleen (Figure 6). In contrast, bacterial LPS, which did not influence DTH tolerance (see preceding discussion), had no ability to enhance antigen presentation. More recently, *in vivo* administration of IFNγ has been shown to prevent the induction of oral tolerance in mice, reinforcing the possible role of agents with the capacity to activate APC (Zhang and Michael, 1990).

The basis of these effects remains to be established, but could include increased expression of MHC Class II antigens, enhanced production of co-stimulatory factors, or alterations in the intracellular processing pathways themselves. The resulting effect may be to alter the balance between distinct populations of APCs so that a larger proportion of fed antigen is presented by APCs with a conventional ability to stimulate T cells, rather than by the putative T_s-activating "I–J$^+$"

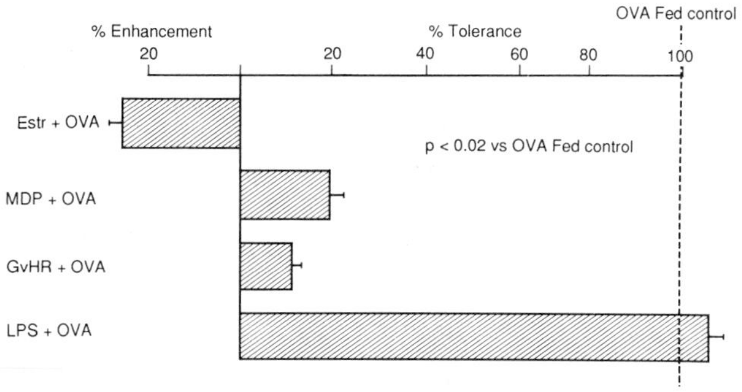

	Prevention of tolerance	Carbon clearance	APC activity	Mucosal DTH
Estradiol	Yes	↑↑	↑	Yes
MDP	Yes	→	↑	Yes
GvHR	Yes	→	↑	Yes (?)
LPS	No	→	↑	(?)

Figure 6 Role of antigen presenting cells in oral tolerance. Treatment of mice with estradiol, muramyl dipeptide (MDP), or a graft versus host reaction (GvHR) prevents the induction of oral tolerance by feeding ovalbumin (OVA) and enhances the ability of splenic adherent cells to present OVA to primed T cells. Bacterial LPS has no effect on oral tolerance to OVA and does not enhance antigen-presenting all (APC) activity *in vivo.*

APCs discussed earlier. Although this hypothesis has yet to be tested in oral tolerance, a differential effect on APC populations of this type may explain the ability of UV light to modulate immune responses *in vivo* (Green *et al.*, 1983).

The influence of the RES on oral tolerance may be of particular relevance in explaining the high incidence of clinical food sensitivity during the period of weaning. As we have discussed, feeding one novel antigen may interfere with tolerance to those encountered subsequently. In addition, a number of products from intestinal flora must have the potential to activate APCs. Thus, modulation of APC function by the rapid exposure to new food antigens and bacterial flora at weaning may help predispose the infant to potentially harmful defects in oral tolerance.

G. Role of the Liver in Oral Tolerance

A large proportion of the antigens absorbed from the intestine will travel directly to the liver via the portal venous system. The liver is the largest tissue of the RES, raising the possibility that this organ may be a major site of the antigen processing events that determine the immunological consequences of antigen feeding.

For many years, researchers have known that administration of antigen directly into the portal system induces a state of tolerance that has many similarities to oral tolerance (Qian *et al.*, 1985; Fujiwara *et al.*, 1986; Sato *et al.*, 1988). An early study in rats indicated that oral tolerance was unaffected when the liver was bypassed by a porto-caval shunt (Thomas *et al.*, 1976), but the many side effects of this surgical maneuver make interpretation of the results difficult. The inability of intravenously injected protein to generate the serum tolerogen found after antigen feeding (Strobel *et al.*, 1983; Bruce and Ferguson, 1986a) also argues against a critical involvement of the liver in oral tolerance, since we might anticipate that intravenously injected antigen also will accumulate rapidly in this organ. Nevertheless, intestinally derived material entering by the portal tracts may be processed by accessory cells distinct from those in contact with the systemic circulation. Thus, a role for the liver in oral tolerance cannot be excluded entirely.

H. Conclusions

Based on the foregoing discussion, clearly multiple mechanisms may be responsible for the induction and maintenance of tolerance to orally administered antigens, presumably reflecting the importance of regulating immune responses to dietary antigens. The role played by individual mechanisms depends on the antigen, the nature of the host animal, and the aspect of the systemic immune response that is under investigation. We have emphasized the view that oral tolerance may be the result of intestinally derived moieties that are presented by specialized APCs to T_s. However, most of the evidence for this mechanism has come from studies of tolerance to protein antigens, and its effects are exerted mainly on systemic cellular immunity. In addition, many of these phenomena have yet to be examined in light of the more recent developments in cellular and molecular immunology. Considerable work remains to be done if the mechanisms regulating immunity to the full range of dietary antigens are to be elucidated.

VI. CLINICAL AND PRACTICAL RELEVANCE OF ORAL TOLERANCE

A. Consequences of Breakdown in Oral Tolerance

We already have discussed the concept that the strength and persistence of oral tolerance indicate its importance in preventing hypersensitivity to food proteins. This idea is based both on the relative infrequency of naturally occurring immunological responsiveness to dietary antigens and on a substantial amount of experimental evidence (Table II).

As we have seen, oral tolerance to proteins in normal mice can be prevented by depleting T_s *in vivo* and by activating APCs. In addition, tolerance does not occur after feeding very low doses of antigen or in animals during the immediate neonatal or weaning periods. In all these cases, subsequent oral challenge of the mice with antigen results in the development of mucosal pathology in the jejunum consisting of crypt hyperplasia, crypt hypertrophy, and increased infiltration of the epithelium by lymphocytes (Mowat and Ferguson, 1981; Mowat and Parrott, 1983; Mowat, 1986; Strobel and Ferguson, 1986; Stokes *et al.*, 1987; Lamont *et al.*, 1988). These features are accompanied by a local cell-mediated immune response in the draining mesenteric lymph nodes (Mowat and Ferguson, 1982; Mowat and Parrott, 1983) and are identical to the early stages of mucosal immunopathology found in other experimental forms of intestinal cell-mediated immunity, including GvHR and allograft rejection (Mowat and Felstein, 1990). Since the intestinal damage in these conditions is caused by the production of T cell-dependent cytokines, a breakdown in oral tolerance is likely to allow the priming of local cytokine-producing T cells that have the capacity to

Table II Factors That Prevent the Induction of Oral Tolerance under Experimental Conditions and Allow the Development of Mucosal Cell-Mediated Immunity and Pathology on Oral Challenge with Antigen[a]

Depletion of T_s
Cyclophosphamide
2′-Deoxyguanosine
Activation of APC
Estradiol
Muramyl dipeptide
Graft-versus-host reaction
Host factors
Immaturity
Low dose of antigen

[a] See text for references.

produce pathology on re-exposure to antigen. Note that the ability of an immunomodulatory agent to allow mucosal DTH is predicted by its effects on tolerance of systemic DTH responses, rather than humoral immunity, thus underlining the importance of preventing T-cell responses to food antigens.

The features of the mucosal immunopathology induced experimentally in the absence of oral tolerance are also qualitatively similar to those found in naturally occurring FSE (Mowat, 1984; Ferguson, 1987). That a defect in oral tolerance may account for the development of FSE under natural conditions is suggested by studies in weaning piglets that have shown that the development of postweaning diarrhea is influenced markedly by the age of introduction of novel antigens and can be prevented by artificially inducing oral tolerance to the antigens to be fed at weaning (Miller *et al.*, 1984; Stokes *et al.*, 1987). Neonatal calves exhibit a similar susceptibility to developing systemic hypersensitivity and enteropathy in response to dietary proteins such as soy protein (Barratt *et al.*, 1987). The mechanisms underlying the naturally occurring conditions have yet to be established, but experimental studies suggest that these may be genetically or maturationally dependent alterations in APCs, intestinal processing, and immunoregulatory T cells.

Table III Use of Oral Tolerance to Prevent Antigen-Specific Immunopathology[a]

Immunopathology	Antigen
Arthritis	Collagen
Encephalomyelitis	Myelin basic protein
Uveoretinitis	Uveal S antigen
Glomerulonephritis	Various proteins
Allograft rejection	Allogeneic leukocytes

[a] Feeding a range of antigens of pathological significance has been found to prevent the induction of associated immunopathological disease. See text for references.

B. Oral Tolerance and Immunotherapy

The oral route offers a convenient and highly acceptable means of administering therapeutic agents. In recent years, interest has developed in the possibility of exploiting oral tolerance to modulate antigen-specific immunopathology (Table III; see Thompson and Staines, 1990, for review). Several experimental immunological diseases can be prevented by prior feeding of appropriate protein antigens, including experimental autoimmune encephalomyelitis (Higgins and Weiner, 1988; Lider *et al.*, 1989; Nussenblatt *et al.*, 1990), collagen-induced arthritis, adjuvant arthritis (Zhang *et al.*, 1990), experimental autoimmune uveoretinitis (Nussenblatt *et al.*, 1990), and immune complex-mediated glomerulonephritis (Devey and Bleasdale, 1984; Gesualdo *et al.*, 1990).

Oral tolerance in these pathological systems shows many phenomenological and mechanistic similarities to that using model protein antigens, affecting T-cell responses predominantly and involving populations of T_s. Encouragingly, in some cases, suppressing established disease by feeding antigen has also proved possible, indicating the possible usefulness of this approach in clinical practice. Although as yet no published reports are available of oral tolerance being exploited for treating clinical disease, a trial of feeding brain-derived material as a means of inhibiting multiple sclerosis is currently underway in the United States (Marx, 1991). Given the increasingly successful identification and purification of autoantigens, similar trials soon could be considered for a variety of organ-specific autoimmune diseases. In addition, feeding allogeneic leukocytes has been reported to suppress specifically the subsequent rejection of cardiac allografts (Sayegh *et al.*, 1992). The possibility of using the oral route to induce specific tolerance to alloantigens in prospective transplant recipients is therefore an attractive, if long-term, proposition. These and other clinical applications of oral tolerance may be helped dramatically by the development of transgenic cattle, whose milk may provide a source of large quantities of specific antigens in an ideal form for oral administration in bulk (Gershon, 1991).

C. Development of Oral Vaccines

A major goal of current vaccine research is the construction of orally active vaccines that contain recombinant proteins or peptides as the immunogen. Such vaccines clearly will be unsuccessful unless the induction of oral tolerance can be overcome. An understanding of the principles involved will assist the design of appropriate vectors. From the foregoing discussion, we can predict that a successful vaccine should be particulate in nature (viable or not) and should contain adjuvant moieties capable of modulating either the uptake of the associated proteins by the intestine or their presentation by APCs within the immune system.

Several approaches that fulfill these conditions have been developed, including attenuated mutant strains of *Salmonella* as vectors for foreign genes and the use of cholera toxin as a mucosal adjuvant (McGhee *et al.*, 1992). Although these vectors have been successful, there are several reasons having nonantigenic vectors that do not themselves induce active immune responses (which could limit the use of multiple immunization). Coating proteins onto polyglycoside microspheres is one possible answer to this problem (McGhee *et al.*, 1992), but these agents have no adjuvant properties. We have shown that incorporation of proteins into ISCOMs containing Quil A (saponin) overcomes the induction of oral tolerance and allows the development of primary immune responses both in the intestine and the systemic immune system (Mowat and Donachie, 1991; Mowat *et al.*, 1991; Mowat, *et al.* 1993). The effectiveness of these small particles (30–40 nm) partly reflects increased uptake of antigen from the intestine, possibly because of the relative stability of ISCOMs in the harsh environment of the gut or because the detergent properties of Quil A potentiate transfer of protein across the epithelium. In addition, Quil A itself is an orally active adjuvant (Chavali and Campbell, 1987) that may enhance APC activity. The success of ISCOMs encourages the belief that continued study of oral tolerance will allow the development of other orally active vaccines.

Acknowledgments

The work of the author discussed in this chapter has been supported by the Medical Research Council (UK) and the Wellcome Trust.

References

André, C., Heremans, J. F., Vaerman, J., and Cambiasco, C. L. (1975). A mechanism for the induction of immunological tolerance by antigen feeding: Antigen–antibody complexes. *J. Exp. Med.* **142,** 1509–1519.

Asherson, G. L., Zembala, M., Perera, M. A. C. C., Mayhew, B., and Thomas, W. R. (1977). Production of immunity and unresponsiveness in the mouse by feeding contact sensitising agents, and the role of suppressor cells in the Peyer's Patches, mesenteric lymph nodes and other lymphoid tissues. *Cell Immunol.* **33,** 145–155.

Asherson, G. L., Perera, M. A. C. C., and Thomas, W. R. (1979). Contact sensitivity and the DNA response in mice to high and low doses of oxazolone: Low dose unresponsiveness following painting and feeding and its prevention by pretreatment with cyclophosphamide. *Immunology* **36,** 449–459.

Barratt, M. E. J., Powell, J. R., Allen, W. D., and Porter, P. (1987). Immunopathology of intestinal disorders in farm animals. *In* "Immunopathology of the Small Intestine" (M. N. Marsh, ed.), pp. 253–258. John Wiley and Sons, Chichester.

Bhogal, B. S., Karkhanis, Y. D., Bell, M. K., Sanchez, P., Zemcik, B., Siskind, G. W., and Thorbecke, G. J. (1986). Production of auto-anti-idiotypic antibody during the normal immune response. XII. Enhanced auto-anti-idiotypic antibody production as a mechanism for apparent B cell tolerance in rabbits after feeding antigens. *Cell. Immunol.* **101,** 93–104.

Bruce, M. G., and Ferguson, A. (1986a). Oral tolerance to ovalbumin in mice: Studies of chemically modified and of "biologically filtered" antigen. *Immunology* **57,** 627–630.

Bruce, M. G., and Ferguson, A. (1986b). The influence of intestinal processing on the immunogenicity and molecular size of absorbed, circulating ovalbumin in mice. *Immunology* **59,** 295–300.

Carr, R. I., Etheridge, P. D., and Tilley, D. (1985). Failure of oral tolerance in NZB/W mice is antigen dependent and parallels antibody patterns in human systemic lupus erythematosus (SLE). *Fed. Proc.* **44,** 1542.

Challacombe, S. J., and Tomasi, T. B. (1980). Systemic tolerance and secretory immunity after oral immunisation. *J. Exp. Med.* **152,** 1459–1472.

Chalon, M-P., Milne, R. W., and Vaerman, J-P. (1979). *In vitro* immunosuppressive effect of serum from orally immunised mice. *Eur. J. Immunol.* **9,** 747–750.

Chandra, R. K., Puri, S., and Vyas, D. (1987). Malnutrition and intestinal immunity. *In* "Immunopathology of the Small Intestine" (M. N. Marsh, ed.), pp. 105–119. John Wiley and Sons, Chichester.

Chase, M. W. (1946). Inhibition of experimental drug allergy by prior feeding of the sensitivity agent. *Proc. Soc. Exp. Biol. Med.* **61,** 257–259.

Chase, M. W., and Battisto, J. R. (1955). The duration of dermal sensitisation following cellular transfer in guinea pigs. *J. Allergy* **26,** 83.

Chavali, S. R., and Campbell, J. B. (1987). Adjuvant effects of orally administered saponins on humoral and cellular immune responses in mice. *Immunobiology* **174,** 347–359.

Collins, F. M., and Carter, P. B. (1980). Development of delayed hypersensitivity in gnotobiotic mice. *Int. Archs. Allergy Appl. Immunol.* **61,** 165–170.

Cowdrey, J. S., and Johlin, B. J. (1984). Regulation of the primary *in vitro* response to TNP-polymerised ovalbumin by T suppressor cells induced by ovalbumin feeding. *J. Immunol.* **132,** 2783–2789.

Cowdrey, J. S., Curtin, M. F., and Steinberg, A. D. (1982). Effect of prior intragastric antigen administration on primary and secondary anti-ovalbumin responses of C57B1/6 and NZB mice. *J. Exp. Med.* **156,** 1256–1261.

Crabbé, P. A., and Heremans, J. F. (1967). Selective IgA deficiency with steatorrhoea. A new syndrome. *Am. J. Med.* **42,** 319.

Cunningham-Rundles, C. (1987). Failure of antigen exclusion. *In* "Food Allergy" (J. Brostoff and S. J. Challacombe, eds.), pp. 223–236. Saunders, Eastbourne.

Dahlgren, U. I. H., Wold, A. E., Hanson, L. A., and Midtvedt, T. (1991). Expression of dietary protein in *E. coli* renders it strongly antigenic to gut lymphoid tissue. *Immunology* **73,** 394–397.

Dakin, R. (1829). Remarks on a cutaneous affection produced by certain poisonous vegetables. *Am. J. Med. Sci.* **4,** 98–100.

David, M. F. (1979). Induction of hyporesponsiveness to particulate antigen by feeding. The sequence of immunologic response to fed antigen. *J. Allergy Clin. Immunol.* **64,** 164–170.

Devey, M. E., and Bleasdale, K. (1984). Antigen feeding modifies the course of antigen-induced immune complex disease. *Clin. Exp. Immunol.* **56,** 637–644.

Elson, C. O., and Ealding, W. (1984). Generalised systemic and mucosal immunity in mice after mucosal stimulation with cholera toxin. *J. Immunol.* **132,** 2736–2741.

Ferguson, A. (1987). Models of immunologically-driven small intestinal damage. *In* "Immunopathology of the Small Intestine" (M. N. Marsh, ed.), pp. 225–252. John Wiley and Sons, Chichester.

Fujihashi, K., Kiyono, H., Aicher, W. K., Green, D. R., Singh, B., Eldridge, J. H., and McGhee, J. R. (1989). Immunoregulatory function of $CD3^+$, $CD4^-$ and $CD8^-$ T cells. $\gamma\delta$ T cell receptor-positive T cells from nude mice abrogate oral tolerance. *J. Immunol.* **143,** 3415–3422.

Fujihashi, K., Taguchi, T., McGhee, J. R., Eldridge, J. H., Bruce, M. G., Green, D. R., Singh, B., and Kiyono, H. (1990). Regulatory function for murine intraepithelial lymphocytes. Two subsets of $CD3^+$, T cell receptor-1^+ intraepithelial lymphocyte T cells abrogate oral tolerance. *J. Immunol.* **145,** 2010–2019.

Fujiwara, H., Qian, J-H., Satoh, S., Kokudo, S., Ikegama, R., and Hamacka, T. (1986). Studies on the induction of tolerance to alloantigens. II. The generation of serum factor(s) able to transfer alloantigen-specific tolerance for delayed-type hypersensitivity by postal venous inoculation with allogeneic cells. *J. Immunol.* **136,** 2763–2768.

Gautam, S. C., and Battisto, J. R. (1985). Orally induced tolerance generates an efferently acting suppressor T cell and an acceptor T cell that together down-regulate contact sensitivity. *J. Immunol.* **135,** 2975–2983.

Gershon, D. (1991). Will milk shake up industry? *Nature* (*London*) **353,** 7.

Gesualdo, L., Lamm, M. E., and Emancipator, S. M. (1990). Defective oral tolerance promotes nephritogenesis in experimental IgA nephropathy induced by oral immunization. *J. Immunol.* **145,** 3684–3691.

Glaister, J. R. (1973). Light, fluorescence and electron microscopic studies of lymphoid cells in the small intestinal epithelium of mice. *Int. Arch. Allergy Appl. Immunol.* **45,** 828.

Granstein, R. D., and Greene, M. I. (1985). Splenic I-J-bearing antigen-presenting cells in activation of suppression: further characterisation. *Cell Immunol.* **91,** 12–20.

Green, D. R., Flood, P. M., and Gershon, R. K. (1983). Immunoregulatory T cell pathways. *Ann. Rev. Immunol.* **1,** 439–464.

Hanson, D. G. (1981). Ontogeny of orally induced tolerance to soluble proteins in mice. I. Priming and tolerance in newborns. *J. Immunol.* **127,** 1518–1522.

Hanson, D. G., and Miller, S. D. (1982). Inhibition of specific immune responses by feeding protein antigens. V. Induction of the tolerant state in the absence of specific suppressor T cells. *J. Immunol.* **128,** 2378–2381.

Hanson, D. G., Vaz, N. M., Maia, L. C. S., Hornbrook, M. M., Lynch, J. M., and Roy, C. A. (1977). Inhibition of specific immune responses by feeding protein Ag's. *Int. Arch. Allergy Appl. Immunol.* **55,** 526–532.

Hanson, D. G., Vaz, N. M., Rawlings, L. A., and Lynch, J. M. (1979a). Inhibition of specific immune responses by feeding protein Ag's. II. Effects of prior passive and active immunisation. *J. Immunol.* **122,** 2261–2266.

Hanson, D. G., Vaz, N. M., Maia, L. C. S., and Lynch, J. M. (1979b). Inhibition of specific immune responses by feeding protein antigens. III. Evidence against maintenance of tolerance to ovalbumin by orally induced antibodies. *J. Immunol.* **123,** 2337–2343.

Harmatz, P. R., Bloch, K. J., Brown, M., Walker, W. A., and Kleinman, R. E. (1989). Intestinal adaptation during lactation in the mouse. I. Enhanced intestinal uptake of dietary protein antigen. *Immunology* **67,** 92–95.

Hayglass, K. T., and Stefura, B. P. (1991). Anti-interferon γ treatment blocks the ability of glutaraldehyde-polymerised allergens to inhibit specific IgE responses. *J. Exp. Med.* **173,** 279–285.

Heppell, L. M., and Kilshaw, P. J. (1982). Immune responses in guinea pigs to dietary protein. I. Induction of tolerance by feeding ovalbumin. *Int. Archs. Allergy Appl. Immunol.* **68,** 54–61.

Higgins, P. J., and Weiner, H. L. (1988). Suppression of experimental autoimmune encephalomyelitis by oral administration of myelin basic protein and its fragments. *J. Immunol.* **140,** 440–445.

Holan, V., Lamb, J. R., and Malkovsky, M. (1991). Immunological tolerance and lymphokines. *Crit. Rev. Immunol.* **10,** 481–493.

Holt, P. G., Batty, J. E., and Turner, K. J. (1981). Inhibition of specific IgE responses in mice by pre-exposure to inhaled antigen. *Immunology* **42,** 409–417.

Howell, M. D., Austin, R. K., Kelleher, D., Nepom, G. T., and Kagnoff, M. F. (1986). An HLA-D region restriction fragment length polymorphism associated with coeliac disease. *J. Exp. Med.* **164,** 333–338.

Husby, S., Foged, N., Host, A., and Svehag, S-E. (1987). Passage of dietary antigens into the blood of children with coeliac disease. Quantification and size distribution of absorbed antigens. *Gut* **28,** 1062–1072.

Jarrett, E. E. (1984). Perinatal influences on IGE responses. *Lancet* **ii,** 797–799.

Jarrett, E. E., and Hall, E. (1984). The development of IgE-suppressive immunocompetence in young animals: Influence of exposure to antigen in the presence or absence of maternal immunity. *Immunology* **53,** 365–373.

Kagnoff, M. F. (1978a). Effects of antigen-feeding on intestinal and systemic immune responses. II. Suppression of delayed type hypersensitivity reactions. *J. Immunol.* **120,** 1509–1513.

Kagnoff, M. F. (1978b). Effects of antigen-feeding on intestinal and systemic immune responses. III. Antigen-specific serum-mediated suppression of humoral antibody responses after antigen-feeding. *Cell. Immunol.* **40,** 186–203.

Kagnoff, M. F. (1980). Effects of antigen-feeding on intestinal and systemic immune responses. IV. Similarity between the suppressor factor in mice after erythrocyte-lysate injection and erythrocyte feeding. *Gastroenterology* **79,** 54–61.

Karpus, W. J., and Swanborg, R. H. (1991). $CD4^+$ suppressor cells inhibit the function of effector cells of experimental autoimmune encephalomyelitis through a mechanism involving transforming growth factor-β. *J. Immunol.* **146,** 1163–1168.

Kay, R., and Ferguson, A. (1989a). The immunological consequences of feeding cholera toxin. I. Feeding cholera toxin suppresses the induction of systemic delayed-type hypersensitivity but not humoral immunity. *Immunology* **66,** 410–415.

Kay, R., and Ferguson A. (1989b). The immunological consequences of feeding cholera toxin. II. Mechanisms responsible for the induction of oral tolerance for DTH. *Immunology* **66,** 416–421.

Kilshaw, P. J., and Cant, A. J. (1984). The passage of maternal dietary proteins into human breast milk. *Int. Arch. Allergy Appl. Immunol.* **75,** 8–15

Kitamura, K., Kiyono, H., Fujihashi, K., Eldridge, J. H., Green, D. R., and McGhee, J. R. (1987). Contrasuppressor cells that break oral tolerance are antigen-specific T cells distinct from T helper ($L3T4^+$), T suppressor ($Lyt2^+$) and B cells. *J. Immunol.* **139,** 3251–3259.

Kiyono, H., McGhee, J. R., Wannemuehler, M. J., and Michalek, S. M. (1982). Lack of oral tolerance in C3H/HeJ mice. *J. Exp. Med.* **155,** 605–610.

Kölsch, E. (1984). Interactions of suppressor and helper antigenic determinants in the dominance of either tolerance or immunity. *Scand. J. Immunol.* **19,** 387–393.

Korenblat, P. E., Rothberg, R. M., Minden, P., and Farr, R. S. (1968). Immune responses of human adults after oral and parenteral exposure to bovine serum albumin. *J. Allergy* **41,** 226–235.

Lafont, S., Andre, C., Andre, F., Gillon, J., and Fargier, M. C. (1982). Abrogation by subsequent feeding of antibody response, including IgE in parenterally immunised mice. *J. Exp. Med.* **155,** 1573–1578.

Lamont, A. G., Gordon, M., and Ferguson, A. (1987). Oral tolerance in protein-deprived mice. I. Profound antibody tolerance but impaired DTH tolerance after antigen feeding. *Immunology* **61,** 333–337.

Lamont, A. G., Bruce, M. G., Watret, K. C., and Ferguson, A. (1988a). Suppression of an established DTH response to ovalbumin in mice by feeding antigen after immunization. *Immunology* **64,** 135–140.

Lamont, A. G., Mowat, A.McI., Browning, M. J., and Parrott, D. M. V. (1988b). Genetic control of oral tolerance to ovalbumin in mice. *Immunology* **63,** 737–739.

Lamont, A. G., Mowat, A. McI., and Parrott, D. M. V. (1989). Priming of systemic and local delayed-type hypersensitivity responses by feeding low doses of ovalbumin to mice. *Immunology* **66,** 595–599.

Lider, O., Santos, L. M. B., Lee, C. S. Y., Higgins, P. J., and Weiner, H. (1989). Suppression of experimental autoimmune encephalomyelitis by oral administration of myelin basic protein. II. Suppression of disease and in vitro immune responses is mediated by antigen-specific $CD8^+$ T lymphocytes. *J. Immunol.* **142,** 748–752.

Liu, Y., and Janeway, C. A. (1990). Interferon γ plays a critical role in induced cell death of effector T cells: A possible third mechanism of self-tolerance. *J. Exp. Med.* **172,** 1735–1739.

Lowney, E. D. (1968). Immunological unresponsiveness to a contact sensitizer in man. *J. Invest. Dermatol.* **512,** 411.

Lycke, N., and Holmgren, J. (1986). Strong adjuvant properties of

cholera toxin on gut mucosal immune responses to orally presented antigens. *Immunology* **59,** 301–308.
MacDonald, T. T. (1982). Immunosuppression caused by antigen feeding. I. Evidence for the activation of a feedback suppressor pathway in the spleen of antigen-fed mice. *Eur. J. Immunol.* **12,** 767–773.
MacDonald, T. T. (1983). Immunosuppression caused by antigen feeding. II. Suppressor T cells mask Peyer's patch B cell priming to orally administered antigen. *Eur. J. Immunol.* **13,** 138–142.
MacDonald, T. T., and Carter, P. B. (1979). Requirement for a bacterial flora before mice generate cells capable of mediating the DTH reaction to sheep red blood cells. *J. Immunol.* **122,** 2624–2629.
McGhee, J. R., Mestecky, J., Dertzbaugh, M. T., Eldridge, J. H., Hirasawa, M., and Kiyono, H. (1992). The mucosal immune system: From fundamental concepts to vaccine development. *Vaccine* **10,** 75–88.
McMenamin, C., Oliver, J., Girn, B., Holt, B. J., Kees, U. R., Thomas, W. R., and Holt, P. G. (1991). Regulation of T-cell sensitization at epithelial surfaces in the respiratory tract: Suppression of IgE responses to inhaled antigens by $CD3^+$ $TcR\alpha^-/\beta^-$ lymphocytes (putative γ/δ T cells). *Immunology* **74,** 234–239.
Marx, J. (1991). Testing of autoimmune therapy begins. *Science* **252,** 27–28.
Mattingly, J. A., and Waksman, B. H. (1978). Immunologic suppression after oral administration of antigen. I. Specific suppressor cells formed in rat Peyer's patches after oral administration of sheep erythrocytes and their systemic migration. *J. Immunol.* **121,** 1878–1883.
Mattingly, J. A., and Waksman, B. H. (1980). Immunologic suppression after oral administration of antigen. II. Antigen specific helper and suppressor factors produced by spleen cells of rats fed sheep erythrocytes. *J. Immunol.* **125,** 1044–1047.
Michalek, S. M., Kiyono, H., Wannemuehler, M. J., Mosteller, L. M., and McGhee, J. R. (1982). Lipopolysaccharide (LPS) regulation of the immune response: LPS influence on oral tolerance induction. *J. Immunol.* **128,** 1992–1998.
Miller, A., Lider, O., and Weiner, H. L. (1991a). Antigen-driven bystander suppression after oral administration of antigens. *J. Exp. Med.* **174,** 791–798.
Miller, A., Roberts, A., Sporn, M., Lider, O., and Weiner, H. L. (1991b). *In vivo* administration of anti-TGFβ antibody increases the severity and duration of experimental allergic encephalomyelitis (EAE) and reverses suppression of EAE by oral tolerance to MBP. *Ann. Neurol.* **30,** 303. (Abstract)
Miller, B. G., Newby, T. J., Stokes, C. R., and, Bourne, F. J. (1984). Influence of diet on postwearing malabsorption and diarrhoea in the pig. *Res. Vet. Sci.* **36,** 187–193.
Miller, M. L., Cowdrey, J. S., and Curtin, M. F. (1983). Gastrointestinal tolerance in autoimmune mice. *Fed. Proc.* **42,** 942.
Miller, S. D., and Hanson, D. G. (1979). Inhibition of specific immune responses by feeding protein antigens. IV. Evidence for tolerance and specific active suppression of cell-mediated immune responses to ovalbumin. *J. Immunol.* **123,** 2344–2350.
Mossmann, T. R., and Coffman, R. L. (1989). T_H1 and T_H2 cells: Different patterns of lymphokine secretion lead to different functional properties. *Ann. Rev. Immunol.* **7,** 145–174.
Mowat, A.McI. (1984). The immunopathogenesis of food sensitive enteropathies. *In* "Local Immune Responses of the Gut" (T. J. Newby and C. R. Stokes, eds.), pp. 199–225. CRC Press, Boca Raton, Florida.
Mowat, A.McI. (1985). The role of antigen recognition and suppressor cells in mice with oral tolerance to ovalbumin. *Immunology* **56,** 253–260.
Mowat, A.McI. (1986). Depletion of suppressor T cells by 2′-deoxyguanosine abrogates tolerance in mice fed ovalbumin and permits the induction of intestinal delayed-type hypersensitivity. *Immunology* **58,** 179–184.
Mowat, A.McI. (1993). The role of the gut-associated lymphoid tissues in food allergy. Proceedings of 4th International Symposium on Clinical Nutrition. (Abstract), in press.
Mowat, A.McI., and Donachie, A. M. (1991). ISCOMS—A novel strategy for mucosal immunization? *Immunol. Today* **12,** 383–385.
Mowat, A.McI., and Felstein, M. V. (1990). Intestinal graft-versus-host reactions in experimental animals. *In* "Graft versus Host Disease" (S. J. Burakoff and J. Ferrara, eds.), pp. 205–244. Marcel Dekker, New York.
Mowat, A.McI., and Ferguson, A. (1981). Hypersensitivity in the small intestinal mucosa. V. Induction of cell mediated immunity to a dietary antigen. *Clin. Exp. Immunol.* **43,** 574–582.
Mowat, A.McI., and Ferguson, A. (1982). Migration inhibition of lymph node lymphocytes as an assay for regional cell-mediated immunity in the intestinal lymphoid tissues of mice immunised orally with ovalbumin. *Immunology* **47,** 365–370.
Mowat, A.McI., and Parrott, D. M. V. (1983). Immunological responses to fed protein antigens in mice. IV. Effects of stimulating the reticuloendothelial system on oral tolerance and intestinal immunity to ovalbumin. *Immunology* **50,** 547–554.
Mowat, A.McI., Strobel, S., Drummond, H. E., and Ferguson, A. (1982). Immunological responses to fed protein antigens in mice. I. Reversal of oral tolerance to ovalbumin by cyclophosphamide. *Immunology* **45,** 104–113.
Mowat, A.McI., Thomas, J. J., and Parrott, D. M. V. (1986). Divergent effects of bacterial lipopolysaccharide on immunity to orally administered protein and particulate antigens in mice. *Immunology* **58,** 677–684.
Mowat, A.McI., Lamont, A. G., and Bruce, M. G. (1987). A genetically determined lack of oral tolerance to ovalbumin is due to failure of the immune system to respond to intestinally derived tolerogen. *Eur. J. Immunol.* **17,** 1673–1676.
Mowat, A.McI., Lamont, A. G., and Parrott, D. M. V. (1988). Suppressor T cells, antigen-presenting cells and the role of I-J restriction in oral tolerance to ovalbumin. *Immunology* **64,** 141–145.
Mowat, A.McI., Donachie, A. M., Reid, G., and Jarrett, O. (1991). Immune stimulating complexes containing Quil A and protein antigen prime class I MHC-restricted T lymphocytes in vivo and are immunogenic by the oral route. *Immunology* **72,** 317–322.
Mowat, A.McI., Maloy, K. J., and, Donachie A. M. (1993). Immune stimulating complexes (ISCOMS) as adjuvants for inducing local and systemic immunity after oral immunization with protein antigens. *Immunology*, in Press.
Mueller, D. L., Jenkins, M. K., and Schwartz, R. H. (1989). Clonal expansion vs functional clonal inactivation. *Ann Rev. Immunol.* **7,** 445–480.
Nagler-Anderson, C., Bober, L. A., Robinson, M. E., Siskind, G. W., and Thorbecke, G. J. (1986). Suppression of type II collagen-induced arthritis by intragastric administration of soluble type II collagen. *Proc. Natl. Acad. Sci. U.S.A.* **83,** 7443–7446.
Newby, T. J., Stokes, C. R., and Bourne, F. J. (1980). Effects of feeding bacterial lipopolysaccharide and dextran sulphate on the development of oral tolerance to contact sensitising agents. *Immunology* **41,** 617–621.
Ngan, J., and Kind, L. S. (1978). Suppressor T-cells for IgE and IgG in Peyer's Patches of mice made tolerant by the oral administration of ovalbumin. *J. Immunol.* **120,** 861–865.
Nussenblatt, R. B., Caspi, R. R., Mahdi, R., Chan, C-C., Roberge, F., Lider, O., and Weiner, H. L. (1990). Inhibition of S-antigen induced experimental autoimmune uveoretinitis by oral induction of tolerance with S-antigen. *J. Immunol.* **144,** 1689–1696.

O'Mahony, S., Arranz, E., Barton, J. R., and Ferguson, A. (1991). Dissociation between systemic and mucosal humoral immune responses in coeliac disease. *Gut* **32,** 29–35.

Owen, R. L. (1977). Sequential uptake of horseradish peroxidase by lymphoid follicle epithelium of Peyer's Patches in the normal unobstructed mouse intestine: An ultra-structural study. *Gastroenterology* **72,** 440–451.

Pappo, J., and Ermak, T. H. (1989). Uptake and translocation of fluorescent latex particles by rabbit Peyer's patch follicle epithelium: A quantitative model for M cell uptake. *Clin. Exp. Immunol.* **76,** 144–148.

Peng, H-J., Turner, M. W., and Strobel, S. (1989a). The kinetics of oral hyposensitization to a protein antigen are determined by immune status and the timing, dose and frequency of antigen administration. *Immunology* **67,** 425–430.

Peng, H-H., Turner, M. W., and Strobel, S. (1989b). Failure to induce tolerance for delayed hypersensitivity to protein antigens in neonatal mice can partially be corrected by spleen cell transfer. *Pediatr. Res.* **26,** 486–471.

Peng, H. J., Turner, M. W., and Strobel, S. (1990). The generation of a tolerogen after a feed of ovalbumin is time dependent and unrelated to the serum level of immunoreactive protein. *Clin. Exp. Immunol.* **81,** 510–515.

Peri, B. A., and Rothberg, R. M. (1981). Circulating antitoxin in rabbits after ingestion of diphtheria toxoid. *Infect. Immun.* **32,** 1148–1154.

Qian, J-H., Hashimoto, T., Fujiwara, H., and Hamaoka, T. (1985). Studies on the induction of tolerance to alloantigens. I. The abrogation of potentials for delayed-type hypersensitivity responses to alloantigens by portal venous inoculation with allogeneic cells. *J. Immunol.* **134,** 3656–3661.

Richman, L. K., Chiller, J. M., Brown, W. R., Hanson, D. G., and Vaz, N. M. (1978). Enterically induced immunologic tolerance. I. Induction of suppressor T lymphocytes by intragastric administration of soluble proteins. *J. Immunol.* **121,** 2429–2434.

Richman, L. K., Graeff, A. S., Yarchoan, R., and Strober, W. (1981). Simultaneous induction of antigen-specific IgA helper T cells and IgG suppressor T cells in the murine Peyer's patch after protein feeding. *J. Immunol.* **126,** 2079.

Rubin, D., Weinder, H. L., Fields, B. N., and Greene, M. I. (1981). Immunologic tolerance after oral administration of reovirus: Requirement for two viral gene products for tolerance induction. *J. Immunol.* **127,** 1697–1701.

Saklayen, M. G., Pesce, A. J., Pollak, V. E., and Michael, J. G. (1983). Induction of oral tolerance in mice unresponsive to bacterial lipopolysaccharide. *Infect. Immun.* **41,** 1383–1385.

Sacklayen, M. G., Pesce, A. J., Pollak, V. E., and Michael, J. G. (1984). Kinetics of oral tolerance: Study of variables affecting tolerance induced by oral administration of antigen. *Int. Arch. Allergy Appl. Immunol.* **73,** 5–9.

Sato, S., Qian, J-H., Kokudo, S., Ikegami, R., Suda, T., Hamaoka, T., and Fujiwara, H. (1988). Studies on the induction of tolerance to alloantigens. III. Induction of antibodies directed against alloantigen-specific delayed-type hypersensitivity T cells by a single injection of allogeneic lymphocytes via portal venous route. *J. Immunol.* **140,** 717–722.

Sayegh, M. H., Zhang, Z. J., Hancock, W. W., Kwok, C. A., Carpenter, C. B., and Wener, H. L. (1992). Down-regulation of the immune response to histocompatibility antigens and prevention of sensitization by skin allografts by orally administered alloantigen. *Transplantation* **53,** 163–166.

Schurmans, S., Heusser, C. H., Qin, H-Y., Merino, J., Brighouse, G., and Lambert, P-H. (1990). *In vivo* effects of anti-IL4 monoclonal antibody on neonatal induction of tolerance and on an associated autoimmune syndrome. *J. Immunol.* **145,** 2465–2473.

Schwartz, R. H. (1989). Self tolerance. *Cell* **57,** 1073–1081.

Stokes, C. R. (1984). Induction and control of intestinal immune responses. (C. R. Stokes and T. J. Newby, eds.), *In* "Local Immune Responses of the Gut." pp. 97–141. CRC Press, Boca Raton, Florida.

Stokes, C. R., Newby, T. J., Huntley, J. H., Patel, D., and Bourne, F. J. (1979). The immune response of mice to bacterial antigens given by mouth. *Immunol.* **38,** 497–502.

Stokes, C. R., Swarbrick, E. T., and Soothill, J. F. (1983a). Genetic differences in immune exclusion and partial tolerance to ingested antigens. *Clin. Exp. Immunol.* **52,** 678–684.

Stokes, C. R., Newby, T. J., and Bourne, F. J. (1983b). The influence of oral immunisation on local and systemic immune responses to heterologous antigens. *Clin. Exp. Immunol.* **52,** 399–406.

Stokes, C. R., Miller, B. G., and Bourne, F. J. (1987). Animal models of food sensitivity. *In* "Food Allergy and Intolerance" (J. Brostoff and S. J. Challacombe, eds.), pp. 286–300. Saunders, Eastbourne.

Strobel, S. (1984). Ph.D. Thesis. Regulation of Intestinal Cell Mediated Immunity. University of Edinburgh, Scotland.

Strobel, S., and Ferguson, A. (1984). Immune responses to fed protein antigens in mice. 3. Systemic tolerance or priming is related to age at which antigen is first encountered. *Pediatr. Res.* **18,** 588.

Strobel, S., and Ferguson, A. (1986). Modulation of intestinal and systemic immune responses to a fed protein antigen, in mice. *Gut* **27,** 829–837.

Strobel, S., and Ferguson, A. (1987). Persistance of oral tolerance in mice fed ovalbumin is different for humoral and cell-mediated immune responses. *Immunology* **60,** 317–318.

Strobel, S., Mowat, A.McI., Drummond, H. E., Pickering, M. G., and Ferguson, A. (1983). Immunological responses to fed protein antigens in mice. 2. Oral tolerance for CMI is due to activation of cyclophosphamide sensitive cells by gut processed antigen. *Immunology* **49,** 451–456.

Strobel, S., Mowat, A.McI., and Ferguson, A. (1985). Prevention of oral tolerance induction to ovalbumin and enhanced antigen presentation during a graft-versus-host reaction in mice. *Immunology* **56,** 57–74.

Suzuki, I., Kitamura, K., Kiyono, H., Kurita, T., Green, D. R., and McGhee, J. R. (1986a). Isotype-specific immunoregulation. Evidence for a distinct subset of T contrasuppressor cells for IgA responses in murine Peyer's patches. *J. Exp. Med.* **164,** 501–516.

Suzuki, I., Kiyono, H., Kitamura, K., Green, D. R., and McGhee, J. R. (1986b). Abrogation of oral tolerance by contrasuppressor T cells suggests the presence of regulatory T cell networks in the mucosal immune system. *Nature (London)* **320,** 451–454.

Swarbrick, E. T., Stokes, C. R., and Soothill, J. F. (1979). Absorption of antigens after oral immunisation and the simultaneous induction of specific systemic tolerance. *Gut* **20,** 121–125.

Thomas, H. C., and Parrott, D. M. V. (1974). Induction of tolerance to a soluble protein antigen by oral administration. *Immunology* **27,** 631–639.

Thomas, H. C., Ryan, C. J., Benjamin, I. S., Blumgart, L. H., and MacSween, R. N. M. (1976). The immune response in cirrhotic rats: The induction of tolerance to orally administered protein antigens. *Gastroenterology* **71,** 114–117.

Thompson, H. S. G., and Staines, N. A. (1990). Could specific oral tolerance by a therapy for autoimmune disease? *Immunol. Today* **11,** 396–399.

Titus, R. G., and Chiller, J. M. (1981). Orally induced tolerance: Definition at the cellular level. *Int. Archs. Allergy Appl. Immunol.* **65,** 323–338.

Tomasi, T. B., Barr, W. G., Challacombe, S. J., and Curran, G. (1983). Oral tolerance and accessory cell function of Peyer's Patches. *Ann. N.Y. Acad. Sci.* **409,** 145–163.

Troncone, R., and Ferguson, A. (1988). In mice, gluten in maternal diet primes systemic immune responses to gliadin in offspring. *Immunology* **64,** 533–537.

Van der Heijden, P. J., Bianchi, A. T. J., Dol, M., Pals, J. W., Stok, W., and Bokhout, B. A. (1991). Manipulation of intestinal immune responses against ovalbumin by cholera toxin and its B subunit in mice. *Immunology* **72,** 89–93.

Vaz, N. M., Maia, L. C. S., Hanson, D. G., and Lynch, J. M. (1977). Inhibition of homocytotropic antibody responses in adult inbred mice by previous feeding of the specific antigen. *J. Allergy Clin. Immunol.* **60,** 110–115.

Vives, J., Parks, D. E., and Weigle, W. O. (1980). Immunologic unresponsiveness after gastric administration of human γ-globulin: Antigen requirements and cellular parameters. *J. Immunol.* **125,** 1811–1816.

Walker, W. A. (1987). Role of the mucosal barrier in antigen handling by Regut. *In* "Food Allergy and Intolerance" (J. Broshoff and S. J. Challacomor, eds.). pp. 209–222. W. B. Saunders, Eastbourne.

Wannemuehler, M. J., Michalek, S. M., and McGhee, J. R. (1982a). Maternal–foetal transfer of suppression to orally administered SRBC. *Fed. Proc.* **41,** 588.

Wannemuehler, M. J., Kiyono, H., Babb, J. L., Michalek, S. M., and McGhee, J. R. (1982b). Lipopolysaccharide (LPS) regulation of the immune response: LPS converts germfree mice to sensitivity to oral tolerance induction. *J. Immunol.* **129,** 959–965.

Wells, H. G., and Osborne, T. B. (1911). The biological reactions of the vegetable proteins. I. Anaphylaxis. *J. Infect. Dis.* **8,** 66–124.

Whitacre, C. C., Gienapp, I. E., Zhang, X., and Heber-Katz, E. (1990). Oral tolerance in experimental autoimmune encephalomyelitis (EAE): A search for the MBP-specific T cell receptor. *FASEB J.* **4,** A1856.

Whitacre, C. C., Gienapp, I. E., Orosz, C. G., and Bitar, D. M. (1991). Oral tolerance in experimental autoimmune encephalomyelitis. III. Evidence for clonal anergy. *J. Immunol.* **147,** 2155–2163.

Wilson, A. D., Stokes, C. R., and Bourne, F. J. (1989). Adjuvant effect of cholera toxin on the mucosal immune response to soluble proteins. Differences between mouse strains and protein antigens. *Scand. J. Immunol.* **29,** 739–745.

Zhang, Z., and Michael, J. G. (1990). Orally inducible immune unresponsiveness is abrogated by IFNγ treatment. *J. Immunol.* **144,** 4163–4165.

Zhang, Z. J., Lee, S. Y., Lider, O., and Weiner, H. L. (1990). Suppression of adjuvant arthritis in Lewis rats by oral administration of type II collagen. *J. Immunol.* **145,** 2489–2493.

17

Functional Aspects of the Peptidergic Circuit in Mucosal Immunity

David W. Pascual · Andrzej M. Stanisz · Kenneth L. Bost

I. INTRODUCTION

When considering the processes of immune protection, we distinguish between those events that govern antigen recognition by lymphoid cells and those that govern nonspecific elimination by macrophages and polymorphonuclear cells. These defense mechanisms are mediated by a cascade of events requiring cell–cell interactions and subsequent release of their soluble products, for example, cytokines, antibodies, and receptor molecules, to regulate these responses. How the nervous system can intervene in such processes, particularly at mucosal sites or mucosa-associated lymphoid tissue (MALT) where these neural mediators have been shown to concentrate, is addressed in this chapter. The contribution of the sensory neurons is examined, particularly the contents of the peripheral nerve fibers (peptidergic fibers) containing the neuropeptides (stored in secretory vesicles) substance P, vasoactive intestinal peptide, somatostatin, gastrin-releasing polypeptide, and calcitonin gene-related peptide.

When considering such cross-communication between the nervous and immune systems, we must examine the intrinsic properties of their mediators. Neuropeptides will, most likely, affect a localized area rather than induce a systemic effect. This property complements the inherent mobility of leukocytes and enhances the opportunity for neural–immune interactions, suggesting that leukocytes may be innervated transiently, especially in light of the ultrastructural studies with rat spleens demonstrating synaptic-like contacts between sympathetic nerve fibers and lymphocytes (Felten and Olschowka, 1987). Further, the close approximation between lymphoid sites and nerve fibers (Felten *et al.*, 1985; Ottaway *et al.*, 1987; Stead *et al.*, 1987b), in particular in mucosal sites of the gut, poses the unique question of whether mediators of one system can induce functional alterations of another system. One manifestation of such neuroimmune communication by which the central nervous system (CNS) can alter the immune system was evident when lesions in the hypothalamus decreased the levels of thymocytes and splenocytes (Roszman *et al.*, 1985). Conversely, an example of immune modification of neural elements is illustrated in the study in which the stimulation of cultured neonatal rat superior cervical ganglion (SCG) with interleukin 1β (IL-1β) resulted in an increase in preprotachykinin (PPT) message with subsequent increase in substance P (SP) production (Jonakait and Schotland, 1990; Hart *et al.*, 1991). Interferon γ (IFNγ) and prostaglandin synthesis inhibitors could reduce both PPT message and SP production induced by IL-1β stimulation. In a similar fashion, when rat SCG were cultured with unstimulated splenocytes (Barbany *et al.*, 1991), tyrosine hydroxylase mRNA diminished by 50% but 400% enhancement of PPT mRNA and 50% enhancement of neuropeptide Y (NPY) were observed. In the presence of concanavalin A (Con A), mitogen-stimulated splenocytes decreased tyrosine hydroxylase mRNA and NPY mRNA expression by 75% and 70%, respectively. PPT mRNA was unaffected by this stimulation. Collectively, these studies suggest that elements from the immune and nervous systems are shared, that is, neurotransmitters, neuropeptides, and neuroendocrine hormones can affect lymphoid function and, conversely, cytokines can affect neural function. Obviously, to grant biological significance to these studies, a mode of uptake of such neuroimmune modifiers by the cells in question must be demonstrated. In this regard, an intriguing aspect of this neuroimmune network is the expression of neuropeptide and neuroendocrine hormone receptors on leukocytes. Over 20 such neuropeptide and neuroendocrine hormone receptors (Bost, 1988) have been identified on normal mononuclear and polymorphonuclear leukocytes and on tumor cell lines (Table I). The expression and regulation of these receptors by leukocytes is energy demanding; therefore, we must assume that their expression is important and not the result of indiscriminate mRNA transcription, that is, these events are regulated. The expression of these receptors by various subpopulations of leukocytes on their cell surfaces provides the means to receive neuronal signals that can alter immune function. Thus, the focus of this chapter is to describe the attributes of the nervous system that contribute to governing the immune surveillance of MALT.

II. MUCOSA-ASSOCIATED LYMPHOID TISSUE NEUROPEPTIDES

A. Substance P and Tachykinins

The CNS-derived 11-amino-acid neuropeptide substance P (SP; Chang and Leeman, 1971) is a product of the sensory

Table I Neuropeptide Receptor Expression by Mononuclear Cells

Neuropeptide receptor[a]	Cell	K_d (n*M*)	Receptor number	Reference
SP-R	Guinea-pig macrophages	19	ND[b]	Hartung *et al.* (1986)
SP-R	IM-9 B lymphoblasts	0.65	22,641	Payan *et al.* (1984a)
SP-R	CH12.LX.C4.4F10 B lymphoma	0.69	632	Pascual *et al.* (1991b)
SP-R	CH12.LX.C4.5F5 B lymphoma	0.69	540	Pascual *et al.* (1991b)
SP-R	BCL_1	0.36	430	Pascual *et al.* (1992)
SP-R	Murine Peyer's patch B cells	0.92	975	Stanisz *et al.* (1987)
SP-R	Murine splenic B cells	0.64	190	Stanisz *et al.* (1987)
SP-R	Murine Peyer's patch T cells	0.50	647	Stanisz *et al.* (1987)
SP-R	Murine splenic T cells	0.62	195	Stanisz *et al.* (1987)
VIP-R	Murine Peyer's patch lymphocytes	0.24	490	Ottaway and Greenberg (1984)
VIP-R	Murine splenic lymphocytes	0.22	880	Ottaway and Greenberg (1984)
VIP-R	Murine lymph node T cells	0.19	3770	Ottaway and Greenberg (1984)
CGRP-R	Murine lymph node T cells	0.35 (high) 48 (low)	265 13,000	Umeda and Arisawa (1989)
VIP-R	Molt 4b T lymphoblasts	7.3	15,000	Beed *et al.* (1983)
VIP-R	U266 IgE myeloma	7.6	41,200	Finch *et al.* (1989)
SOM-R	U266 IgE myeloma	0.005 (high) 100 (low)	1245 $>10^5$	Sreedharan *et al.* (1989a)
SOM-R	Jurkat leukemic T cells	0.003 (high) 66 (low)	150 $>10^5$	Sreedharan *et al.* (1989a)
SOM-R	MOPC 315 myeloma	1.6	40,000	Scicchitano *et al.* (1988b)
CGRP-R	Rat splenic B cells	0.39	745	McGillis *et al.* (1991)
CGRP-R	Rat splenic T cells	0.87	775	McGillis *et al.* (1991)
CGRP-R	$P388D_1$ macrophages	1.8	ND	Abello *et al.* (1991)

[a] SP-R, Substance P receptor; VIP-R, vasoactive intestinal peptide receptor; CGRP-R, calcitonin gene-related peptide receptor; SOM-R, somatostatin receptor.
[b] ND, Not determined.

ganglion cells, and is transported to peripheral sites where it is stored and released on noxious stimulation (Pernow, 1983). Classically, SP is recognized for its ability to contract ileum smooth muscle cells and to act as a pain signal neurotransmitter (Pernow, 1983). The SP amino acid sequence (Table II) is conserved among mammals (bovine, human, and rat sequences) and belongs to a family of related peptides called tachykinins (Erspamer, 1981), each of which bears a common C-terminal amino acid sequence (Phe–X–Gly–Leu–Met–NH_2, where X is a branched aliphatic or aromatic amino acid). An additional feature intrinsic to many of the enteric neuropeptides is the amidation of its C-terminal residue. The two mammalian tachykinin genes encode preprotachykinin A (PPT-A), which generates SP and substance K (SK; neurokinin A), and preprotachykinin B (PPT-B), which produces neurokinin B (neuromedin K). Alternate RNA splicing of the PPT-A gene produces three SP-encoding mRNAs (Nawa *et al.*, 1984; Krause *et al.*, 1987): the α transcript encodes SP only; the β transcript encodes SP, SK, SK(3–10), and neuropeptide K (SK-containing peptide); and the γ transcript encodes SP, SK, SK(3–10), and neuropeptide γ (variant of neuropeptide K). Expression of the different PPT-A mRNAs is both species and tissue dependent (Helke *et al.*, 1990). For instance, in bovine tissues, α-PPT mRNA is predominant in the brain whereas β-PPT mRNA is predominant in the intestine, in contrast to the rat, in which γ- $>\beta$- $>\alpha$-PPT mRNA in all tissues.

Outside the brain, SP is found in greatest concentrations (nanomolar and subnanomolar levels) in the gut (Pernow, 1983). The SP-containing nerve fibers are a major component of the enteric nervous system. Neurons containing SP also innervate lymphoid tissues, that is, spleen and lymph nodes (Felten *et al.*, 1985; Popper *et al.*, 1988; Lorton *et al.*, 1991). Consequently, the presence of SP at nanomolar concentrations is suggestive of an SP contribution to the regulation of immune function in gut-associated lymphoid tissues (GALT). Anatomical data have provided direct evidence for interactions between gut mast cells and nerve fibers containing SP (Stead *et al.*, 1987b). In the Peyer's patches, some evidence suggests that SP-containing nerve fibers infiltrate T-cell zones and associate with macrophages, a result that contrasts with what is observed in the lamina propria. Here, IgA plasma

Table II Sensory Neuropeptide Sequences

Gene	Translated products	Amino acid sequences
Preprotachykinin A	Substance P (SP)	Arg–Pro–Lys–Pro–Gln–Gln–Phe–Phe–Gly–Leu–Met–NH_2
	Substance K (SK)	His–Lys–Thr–Asp–Ser–Phe–Val–Gly–Leu–Met–NH_2
Preprotachykinin B	Neurokinin B (NKB)	Asp–Met–His–Asp–Phe–Phe–Val–Gly–Leu–Met–NH_2
Vasoactive intestinal polypeptide	Vasoactive intestinal peptide (VIP)	His–Ser–Asp–Ala–Val–Phe–Thr–Asp–Asn–Tyr–Thr–Arg–Leu–Arg–Lys–Gln–Met–Ala–Val–Lys–Lys–Tyr–Leu–Asn–Ser–Ile–Leu–Asn–NH_2
	Peptide histidine isoleucine amide (PHI)	His–Ala–Asp–Gly–Val–Phe–Thr–Ser–Asp–Phe–Ser–Arg–Leu–Leu–Gly–Gln–Leu–Ser–Ala–Lys–Lys–Tyr–Leu–Glu–Ser–Leu–Ile–NH_2
	Peptide histidine methionine (PMI)	Positions 1–27 identical with PHI ---------Ser–Leu–Met–NH_2
Somatostatin	Somatostatin	Ala–Gly–Cys–Lys–Asn–Phe–Phe–Trp–Lys–Thr–Phe–Thr–Ser–Cys
Gastrin-releasing polypeptide (humans)	Gastrin-releasing polypeptide (GRP)	Val–Pro–Leu–Pro–Ala–Gly–Gly–Gly–Thr–Val–Leu–Thr–Lys–Met–Tyr–Pro–Arg–Gly–Asn–His–Trp–Ala–Val–Gly–His–Leu–Met–NH_2
Bombesin (frog)	Bombesin	Pyr–Gln–Arg–Leu–Gly–Asn–Gln–Trp–Ala–Val–Gly–His–Leu–Met–NH_2
Calcitonin	Calcitonin	Cys–Gly–Asn–Leu–Ser–Thr–Cys–Met–Leu–Gly–Thr–Tyr–Thr–Gln–Asp–Leu–Asn–Lys–Phe–His–Thr–Phe–Pro–Gln–Thr–Ser–Ile–Gly–Val–Gly–Ala–Pro–NH_2
	Calcitonin gene-related peptide α (CGRP-α)	Ser–Cys–Asn–Thr–Ala–Thr–Cys–Val–Thr–His–Arg–Leu–Ala–Gly–Leu–Leu–Ser–Gly–Gly–Val–Val–Lys–Asp–Asn–Phe–Val–Pro–Thr–Asn–Val–Gly–Ser–Glu–Ala–Phe–NH_2
Calcitonin gene-related peptide β	Calcitonin gene-related peptide β (CGRP-β)	Positions 1–34 identical with CGRP-α ---------Lys–Ala–Phe–NH_2

cells can be found in densely innervated areas, suggesting that these cells may be more likely to be influenced by neuropeptides (Stead *et al.*, 1987a).

Although limited evidence exists demonstrating peptidergic fibers coming into close association with B-cell follicles in mammalian lymphoid tissues, the chicken is potentially the best experimental model to delineate the linkage between the nervous system and B-cell differentiation. The extent of infiltration by peptidergic fibers into the bursa of Fabricius was examined (Zentel and Weihe, 1991). SP, in addition to other enteric neuropeptides—vasoactive intestinal peptide (VIP), calcitonin gene-related peptide (CGRP), and galanin—was found distributed throughout the bursa of Fabricius and bordering B cells in the follicle cortex in three distinct fiber subpopulations: SP-containing, SP + CGRP-containing, and VIP + galanin-containing fibers. VIP-containing fibers were the only such peptidergic fibers that came in contact with some macrophages. However, this association between peptidergic nerve fibers and B cells was not evident with human tonsillar B cells as it was with those B cells in the bursa of Fabricius. SP-containing fibers in human tonsil were seen primarily in the perivascular plexus with low level expression in the interfollicular areas and adjacent to T cells and macrophages (Weihe and Krekel, 1991). In the mesenteric lymph nodes, SP innervation was sparse and was found associated with 5–10% of the arterioles and venules in the medulla adjoining the T-cell region, as well as in the capsule (Popper *et al.*, 1988). In the same study, SP receptor binding sites were examined by quantitative receptor autoradiography. Between 25 and 35% of the germinal centers expressed SP binding sites, whereas limited binding sites were found on arterioles and venules in the T-cell region and internodular region near the capsule. SP-containing fibers also are found in the bronchus-associated lymphoid tissue (BALT). In the rat BALT, SP-containing fibers were localized to the subepithelial zone (Inoue *et al.*, 1990).

To endow biological significance for the expression of SP receptors (SP-R) on lymphocytes and other accessory cells (Bost, 1988; Bost and Pascual, 1992), SP-R expression has been shown by radiolabeled ligand binding studies. Such studies have demonstrated the presence of SP-R on surfaces of B cells and T cells isolated from the spleen and Peyer's patches that have binding characteristics similar to SP-R in neural tissues (Nakata *et al.*, 1988). Evidence to this effect is based on the following observations: (1) similar dissociation constant; (2) similar rank-order displacement by related tachykinins; and (3) identification of 58-kDa protein that binds SP, and (4) the expression of brain SP-R mRNA sequence by $CD4^+$ T lymphocytes isolated from *Schistosomiasis mansoni*-induced granulomas (Elliott *et al.*, 1993). SP-R initially was shown to be expressed by the human B lymphoblastic cell line IM-9 (Payan *et al.*, 1984a); much of our current understanding of the physical characterization of SP-R has been derived from extensive studies of this cell line (Payan *et al.*, 1986). By radiolabel binding studies, these cells have been demonstrated to bind SP with a dissociation constant of 0.65 n*M* and to exhibit a single class of SP-R. IM-9 lymphoblasts preferentially bound SP over other tachykinins via the C terminus since SP fragment (1–4) failed to inhibit radiolabeled SP binding competitively whereas SP fragment (4–11) could compete effectively. Using radiolabeled SP in cross-linking studies (Payan *et al.*, 1986), the SP-R was determined to be a 53,000–58,000 dalton protein. Antireceptor antibodies (Pascual *et al.*, 1989; van Ginkel *et al.*, 1993) have confirmed this finding, which fully supports studies with SP-R in neural tissues. The binding domain for SP-R appears to involve the putative first and third extracellular regions since antibodies directed to peptide sequences to these domains inhibited radiolabeled SP binding to SP-R (van Ginkel *et al.*, 1993). The advent of cloning the rat brain SP-R (Hershey and Krause, 1990) and bovine brain SK-R (Masu *et al.*, 1987) has demonstrated that these receptors belong to G-protein coupled receptor family with seven putative transmembrane spanning regions. This same SP-R exists on lymphocytes as well based on the confirmations by two independent laboratories. Each have shown that murine mononuclear cells express authentic SP-R. A portion of the murine macrophage SP-R was cloned using reverse transcriptase polymerase chain reaction (RT-PCR), and demonstrated complete homology with murine brain SP-R (Bost, 1993). Applying similar strategy, the cDNA for authentic SP-R was cloned and sequenced from liver granulomas isolated from *Schistosomiasis mansoni*-infected mice, and no mRNA for SK-R or neurokinin B could be detected (Elliott *et al.*, 1993). These findings confirm the presence of SP-R on lymphocytes and macrophages, and that the lymphoid SP-R is identical to brain SP-R as opposed to being a separate SP-R isoform.

Functional attributes of SP have been studied best with B lymphocytes and macrophages (Bost and Pascual, 1992; Pascual *et al.*, 1992). Early studies had suggested that SP behaves as a B-cell differentiation factor. When mononuclear fractions from the murine spleen, mesenteric lymph nodes, and Peyer's patches were co-stimulated with 1.0 μg/ml Con A and 10 n*M* SP, IgA production increased by 70, 40, and 300%, respectively (Stanisz *et al.*, 1986). To a lesser extent, IgM levels were altered significantly by 20–40%. Using these culture conditions, no significant increases in IgG secretion by mononuclear cells isolated from these tissues were observed. Consequently, this study does suggest that SP may stimulate IgA secretion preferentially or, alternatively, may indicate that SP is an IgA switching factor (Xu-Amanu *et al.*, 1993). The ramifications of such possibilities are intriguing in light of the abundance of SP-containing neurons in the gut (Hokfelt *et al.*, 1980). Alternatively, SP may stimulate selectively the proliferation of one surface Ig phenotype as opposed to another. Examination of the proliferative effects of SP on these mixed cultures revealed that SP induced 60% increase in the amount of [^{3}H]thymidine incorporated versus cultures treated in the absence of neuropeptide. Although substantial enhancement in IgA production was observed, which mononuclear cell subpopulation or combination was affected most greatly by SP was unclear from this study since each cell subpopulation is known to exhibit SP receptors. Thus, to evaluate SP effects on lymphoid function effectively, SP function had to be assessed with purified lymphoid cell subpopulations.

In an attempt to delineate the mechanisms of how SP behaves as a B-cell differentiation factor (Pascual *et al.*, 1991b,1992; Bost and Pascual, 1992), the direct effect of SP on CD5$^+$ B-lymphoma cell lines CH12.LX.C4.4F10 (an IgA producer) and CH12.LX.C4.5F5 (an IgM producer) was assessed. From radiolabel binding experiments, these CH12LX subclones were shown to bear SP receptors (between 500 and 600 receptors/cell) similar to those levels found on normal B lymphocytes, with binding affinities (K_d ~0.69n*M*) similar to those found on normal B lymphocytes (Stanisz *et al.*, 1987) and IM-9 B lymphoblasts (Payan *et al.*, 1984a) as well. On direct SP stimulation of CH12.LX.C4.4F10 cells, IgA production could be enhanced by 35% at subnanomolar concentrations whereas a similar stimulation on CH12.LX.C4.5F5 cells resulted in no significant change in the amount of IgM produced. SP had no effect on cell proliferation when ascertained by [^{3}H]thymidine uptake. The biological significance for the expression of SP-R on B lymphocytes was enhanced by the observation that SP, in the presence of a secondary signal, could augment immunoglobulin synthesis. The addition of a suboptimal dose of lipopolysaccharide (LPS; 50 ng/ml) with varying concentrations of SP to CH12.LX.C4.5F5 cells resulted in a 172% increase in IgM production at 0.1 n*M* and 1.0 n*M* SP doses. μ Chain message was enhanced only moderately (50–60%) by this mode of stimulation. Modest increases in IgM production also were observed with picomolar concentrations of SP. High doses of SP (100 n*M*) were not as effective in enhancing IgM production as were subnanomolar concentrations of SP suggesting SP-R desensitization at these higher SP concentrations. Moderate increases in IgA production were observed for CH12.LX.C4.4F10 cells stimulated in a similar fashion, as for the IgM-producing CH12 clone. In the presence of suboptimal dose of LPS, again subnanomolar concentrations of SP were most effective in enhancing IgA production by 50%; no differences in α chain message were observed. Further evidence to support that these events are receptor mediated was provided when duplicate cultures were performed in the presence of 1000-fold excess SP antagonist (D-Pro^2-D-Phe^7-D-Trp^9-SP), resulting in the specific inhibition of SP-induced IgM and IgA enhancement and no effect on the enhancement induced by LPS alone. Similar effects mediated by SP also could be shown with purified B cells isolated from the spleen. In one study (Pascual *et al.*, 1991a), >99% sIg$^+$ B lymphocytes isolated from mouse spleens cultured with varying concentrations of SP (0.1 p*M*–100 n*M*) had no effect on Ig production. Again, the presence of a co-stimulating triggering mechanism was required, similar to those required for IL-4 and IL-5 co-stimulation assays. The addition of 10 μg/ml LPS to optimal doses of SP resulted in substantial enhancement of IgM and IgG3 production, as much as 500 and 1000% increase, respectively (Pascual *et al.*, 1991a). Even picomolar concentrations of SP could increase IgM levels significantly. IgA production was enhanced significantly, but only moderately. The significance of this study is twofold. First, SP could stimulate B cells directly in the absence of accessory cells. Second, physiologically relevant concentrations of SP could enhance Ig synthesis by purified B cells. This observation is in agreement with previous reports (Stanisz *et al.*, 1986) about the ability of SP to modify Ig synthesis, although optimal stimulatory concentrations of SP differed. At doses optimal for Ig production, SP in the presence of LPS was antiproliferative for purified B cells, and more inhibitory at higher SP concentrations (Pascual *et al.*, 1991a). An antiproliferative effect of SP also was observed with isolated splenic mononuclear cells treated simultaneously with LPS and SP (Krco *et al.*, 1986); however, the extent of inhibition or the dose effect was not observed. The enhanced antibody production induced by SP in B cells could be explained by the possibility that selected B-cell subpopulations are responsive to SP stimulation. Using the ELISPOT assay, purified splenic B cells subjected to LPS/SP co-stimulation were determined to show increased numbers of spot-forming cells. From these studies analyzing the modulation of Ig synthesis by B cells, we conclude that, despite the differences in the experimental conditions, in each case SP requires a coactivation signal to achieve an augmentation in Ig production. Normal Peyer's patch B lymphocytes are also sensitive to SP stimulation (Pascual *et al.*, 1993). As with splenic B cells, Peyer's patch B cells required a coactivation signal, and in this case, suboptimal dose of recombinant IL-6 was used. Nanomolar concentrations of SP induced 150% increase in IgA, 175% increase in IgG, and 25% increase in IgM. Clearly, these studies suggest differential expression of SP-R on B lymphocyte subpopulations.

Although we have discussed the potential significance of SP as a neuroimmune modulator in various *in vitro* studies, some intriguing aspects to SP *in vivo* function exist. One of the first *in vivo* studies that suggested a possible correlation between SP and Ig production was performed by Helme *et al.* (1987). The premise for this study takes advantage of the selective action of the neurotoxin capsaicin, which destroys unmyelinated sensory neurons present in peripheral tissues when rats are treated neonatally (Buck and Burks, 1986). As a consequence of such treatment, neuropeptides such as SP are depleted from peripheral sites (Nagy *et al.*, 1981,1983; Buck and Burks, 1986). Neonatally capsaicin-treated rats were allowed to mature and were subjected to sheep red blood cells challenge. This treatment resulted in greater than 80% reduction in IgM and IgG plaque-forming cell response by popliteal lymph nodes compared with plaque-forming cell response in SRBC-challenged rats. Clearly, these results denote the significance of neuronal input, particularly the presence of neuropeptides, for the development of antibody responses. This lack of antigen responsiveness or suppression exhibited by capsaicin-pretreated rats was determined to be reversible on coadministration of SP with SRBC. In a subsequent study (Eglezos *et al.*, 1990), a similar magnitude of inhibition in antibody responses was obtained in rats treated with the SP antagonist Spantide during antigen priming. Whereas these studies examined the contribution of SP depletion to antigen challenge, the direct *in vivo* significance of SP for immune function was examined in a study in which the administration of SP via miniosmotic pump for 7 days was examined (Scicchitano *et al.*, 1988a). After a 1-week infusion, lymphocytes from the Peyer's patches were cultured for 7 days in the presence of Con A, and subsequently assessed for Ig production by isotype-specific plaque-forming cell response. A preferential enhancement of IgA-secreting cells (260% increase) in contrast to no significant changes for IgM- and IgG-secreting cells could be demonstrated. When similar analysis was performed with lymphocytes isolated from the spleen, IgA-producing cells were the predominant cell type expressed (~380% increase) although enhancement of IgM-secreting cells also was noted (~190% increase). Enhanced cell-proliferative responses by Peyer's patch and splenic lymphocytes also were observed as a consequence of this *in vivo* SP administration. Similarly, in an antigen-specific system, mice were infused with SP for 1 week via miniosmotic pumps and simultaneously immunized with UV-inactivated rotavirus (Ijaz *et al.*, 1990). Increased levels of antirotavirus antibody in the milk of lactating females as well as in the serum were shown. Using Western blot analysis, increased levels of antibodies to rotaviral antigens VP4, VP6, and VP7 were observed. In summary, *in vivo* infusion of SP stimulates the development of Ig-producing cells whereas *in vivo* SP depletion reduces the number of Ig-producing cells.

In addition to B cells, macrophages have been shown to express receptors for SP and be influenced in their function by SP. Hartung *et al.* (1986) demonstrated the expression of a single class SP-R on guinea pig macrophages with a dissociation constant of 19 n*M*. This binding was mediated via the C terminus. Both human monocytes and guinea pig peritoneal macrophages stimulated with SP at nanomolar concentrations evoked increased chemotaxis (Wiedermann *et al.*, 1989). Further, SP stimulation of monocytes and macrophages enhances the release of cytokines. SP, as well as related tachykinins, induced the release of IL-1-like activity from the mouse macrophage cell line P388D1 in a dose-dependent fashion (Kimball *et al.*, 1988). Human peripheral blood monocytes also could be stimulated by SP to release IL-1, IL-6, and tumor necrosis factor α (TNFα; Lotz *et al.*, 1988). The mode of action in both studies was similar because stimulation was via the SP C terminus, since SP(4–11), SK, and neurokinin A each could induce cytokine release. Whereas these studies show that macrophages are responsive to SP, other studies have found macrophages to be a mobile source of SP, which can be produced by peritoneal macrophages (Pascual and Bost, 1990a) as well as by P388D1 cells (Pascual and Bost, 1990b). Macrophage-derived SP regulates thymocyte proliferation activity, presumably that mediated by IL-1 and IL-6, in an autocrine/paracrine fashion. By culturing P388D1 cells in the presence of a monoclonal anti-SP (N terminus specific) antibody, 40–50% reduction of mouse thymocyte proliferation activity was noted. Peritoneal macrophage-derived SP and its related SP mRNA were later shown to be upregulated by LPS (Bost *et al.*, 1992). An intriguing observation of the relationship between SP and macrophages is that SP can regulate the production and release of cytokines, particularly those responsible either directly or indirectly for IgA production by Peyer's patch lymphocyte cultures. IL-1 (Cowdery *et al.*, 1988) and IL-6 (Beagley *et al.*, 1989) have been shown to promote IgA responses; both of these cytokines are inducible by SP stimulation. In conjunction with anatomical evidence of its vasodilatory properties and histamine releasing abilities, SP at mucosal sites such as gut (Furness and Costa, 1980; Felten *et al.*, 1987; Makhlouf, 1990) and lung (Lundberg and Saria, 1987; Wiederman *et al.*, 1987) represents an additional factor, particularly at localized sites, that can regulate immune function and contribute to inflammation (Payan, 1989). As a result of its association with inflammation and macrophages, SP can be referred to as a pro-inflammatory peptide. Clinical manifestations of SP as a pro-inflammatory peptide are supported by its increased presence at concentrations up to 3 ng/ml in inflammatory exudates (Tissot *et al.*, 1988; Schiogolev *et al.*, 1989). Its presence in synovial fluids isolated from human arthritic patients (Marshall *et al.*, 1990; Argo *et al.*, 1992). Examination of SP-R function from rheumatoid arthritis patients indicates an apparent SP-R desensitization by systemic and synovial fluid lymphocytes. This was evident by the lack in change in SP-mediated lymphocyte proliferation and an associated increase in GM-CSF production (Argo and Stanisz, 1992). With experimental animals, studies (Levine *et al.*, 1984; O'Byrne *et al.*, 1992) suggests that SP contributes to the exacerbation of arthritis. Increased SP and SP receptor expression also has been demonstrated in patients with Crohn's disease and colitis (Koch *et al.*, 1987; Mantyh *et al.*, 1988). In other models of intestinal inflammation, Trichinella-infected rats exhibit increased levels of SP inflamed jejunum (Swain *et al.*, 1992), and treatment with anti-SP antibodies result in reduced gastrointestinal inflammation and restored SP-induced cell proliferation by Con A-stimulated lymphocytes (Argo and Stanisz, 1993).

Limited reports are available of SP modulation of T-cell function. In the one report previously described (Stanisz *et al.*, 1986), Con A stimulation of splenic mononuclear cells suggests that SP may be co-stimulating T cells to release B-cell differentiating cytokines. We have been able to demonstrate that SP promotes Th2-type cytokine production. The addition of SP to Con A-stimulated murine splenic and Peyer's patch $CD4^+$ T cells result in enhanced number of IL-5 producing cells, whereby three- to five-fold increases were noted, while the number of IFN-γ producing cells remain unchanged (D. W. Pascual, submitted). In contrast, SP promotes Th1-type response in murine schistomiasis (Elliott *et al.*, 1993), where increased IFN-γ levels were shown, and no change in IL-5 levels were observed. Obviously, these represent different experimental paradigms, but suggest the influence of SP in T cell-dependent immune responses (Figure 1). In one of the first reports (Payan *et al.*, 1983) describing SP stimulation of lymphocytes, researchers demonstrated that SP behaved as a cell proliferation factor for T cells, yet this proliferation-enhancing ability was not observed with B cells (Pascual *et al.*, 1991a,b). SP co-stimulation of Con A-treated lamina propria lymphocytes (LPL; 64% $CD3^+$ and 11% $CD19^+$) derived from human colon specimens diminished [^{3}H]thymidine incorporation over 50% in a dose-dependent fashion, with maximal effect at nanomolar concentrations (Elitsur and Luk, 1990). Natural killer (NK) activity by murine intestinal intraepithelial leukocytes (IELs) was shown to be enhanced by SP in *in vitro* assays from normal mice as well as in mice infused with SP (Croitoru *et al.*, 1990). As much as a 10-fold increase in NK activity by $Thy1^-$ cells was observed when 10 n*M* SP was incubated with IEL effector cells and Yac-1 target cells.

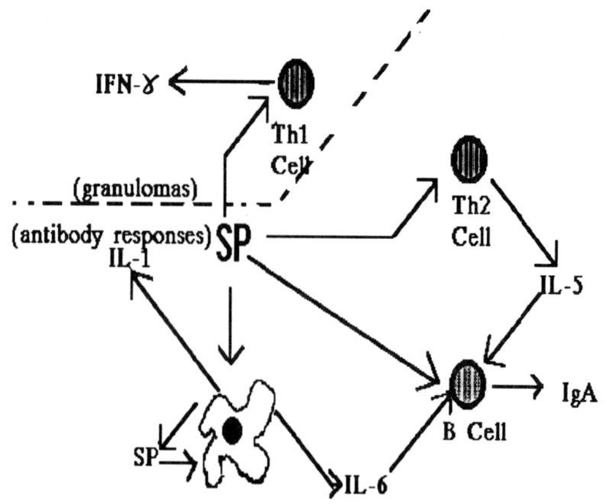

Figure 1 SP participates in the promotion of IgA responses either directly on IgA producing B cells or indirectly on Th2-type cells or macrophages. SP acts as a co-stimulatory signal for B cells activated by antigen or cytokines to elicit an enhanced IgA response, or SP can also provide a co-stimulatory signal to Th2 cells to produce IL-5, an IgA-promoting cytokine. To activated macrophages, SP can induce the production of IL-6, an additional late-acting differentiating factor for IgA and IgG responses. Interestingly, activated macrophages also produce SP, and in an autocrine/paracrine fashion can regulate constitutive IL-1/IL-6 production. Thus, macrophage-produced SP may be important for localized regulation of cytokine-induced inflammation. In addition, SP can also stimulate Th1 cells to produce IFN-γ; however, evidence to this effect has only been shown for schistosomiasis-induced granulomas since no change in the number of IFN-γ-producing cells was observed when normal $CD4^+$ T cells are stimulated with SP and mitogen. Thus, these observations most likely represent separate models of SP induction.

B. Vasoactive Intestinal Peptide

First identified for its potent vasodilatory properties (Said and Mutt, 1970), VIP is a 28-amino-acid peptide with C-terminal amidated asparagine (Table II). No deviation among bovine, rat, human, canine, and porcine sequences was evident, but variations were seen in guinea pig and chicken sequences (McDonald, 1991). VIP is cotranslated from a 1.8- to 2.1-kb mature mRNA that encodes another C-terminal amidated peptide designated PHI (peptide histidine isoleucine amide) and, in humans, PHM (peptide histidine methionine amide) (Gozes *et al.*, 1987; Linder *et al.*, 1987) as the VIP–PHI/PHM preprohormone 170 amino acids in length. The preprohormone is processed into a prohormone of 18 kDa. Further processing generates both VIP and PHI/PHM. Known for its ability to induce vasodilation and act as a potent mediator of smooth muscle relaxation (Said, 1984), VIP is found in the central nervous system as well as in peripheral nerves (Larsson *et al.*, 1976), particularly in the peptidergic nerves (Schultzberg *et al.*, 1980; Ekblad *et al.*, 1987; Makhlouf, 1990). These types of nerve fiber are found abundant in mucosal tissues: gastrointestinal tract, male and female genital tract, upper respiratory and nasal mucosa, and salivary glands (Larsson *et al.*, 1976; Polak and Bloom, 1982). In the gastrointestinal tract, nerve fibers containing VIP are present in both the small and large intestine, with extensive innervation in all layers (Ekblad *et al.*, 1987,1988). VIP also can be found coexisting with SP in similar enteric neurons of the myenteric plexus and submucosal plexus (Makhlouf, 1990). VIP-containing nerve fibers also have been found in lymphoid tissues including the thymus, spleen, and Peyer's patches (Felten *et al.*, 1985; Ottaway *et al.*, 1987).

The presence of VIP receptors (VIP-R) on leukocytes has been determined by radiolabel binding studies (Table I). From these studies and cross-linking experiments, VIP-R has been shown on human MOLT-4b T lymphoblasts (Beed *et al.*, 1983). These cells express a single class VIP-R with an apparent size of 47,000 daltons (Wood and O'Dorisio, 1985), which correlates closely with VIP-R found on liver (Couvineau *et al.*, 1986) and pancreatic acinar cells (McArthur *et al.*, 1987). The VIP-R on the MOLT-4b T cells appears to activate cAMP via a stimulatory guanine nucleotide binding protein (O'Dorisio *et al.*, 1985). Maximum effect was obtained with nonphysiological doses of VIP, but increased cAMP production still was observed at nanomolar concentrations and could synergize with forskolin. The human myeloma cell line U266 also expresses a single class receptor with a K_d of 7.6 nM (Finch *et al.*, 1989), similar to what has been observed with MOLT-4b lymphocytes (K_d = 7.3 nM). Normal mouse lymphocytes also have been shown to express VIP-R. These receptors were found primarily on T cells (Ottaway and Greenberg, 1984). VIP-R density was greatest, in descending order, on lymphocytes isolated from subcutaneous lymph nodes, mesenteric lymph nodes, spleen, and Peyer's patches. In one report (Sreedharan *et al.*, 1991), the authors suggested that they have cloned the human VIP-R gene with libraries derived from the pre-B Nalm 6 cell line, which shares >90% nucleic acid and amino acid sequence homology with the G-protein coupled canine orphan receptor previously cloned by a separate group of investigators (Libert *et al.*, 1989,1990). The deduced sequence of 362 amino acids exhibits a hydropathy profile common to G-protein coupled, seven transmembrane-region type receptors. Cos-6 cells transfected with the cDNA clone for human VIP-R bound radioiodinated VIP with a dissociation constant of 2.5 nM.

The first evidence for VIP mediation of immune function was the finding that polymorphonuclear leukocytes produce VIP (O'Dorisio *et al.*, 1980), but the functional significance of this finding remains to be elucidated. Subsequent studies have shown VIP to inhibit mitogenic-induced proliferation of murine lymphocytes reversibly (Ottaway and Greenberg, 1984; Krco *et al.*, 1986; Stanisz *et al.*, 1986) as a consequence of decreased IL-2 production, but not to affect T suppressor cell activity (Ottaway, 1987; Boudard and Bastide, 1991). Maximum inhibition of mitogen-induced cell proliferation by VIP occurred within the first 24 hr of neuropeptide exposure, and did not appear to be cAMP-dependent (Boudard and Bastide, 1991). Prepro-VIP, synthesized from the preprohormone sequence that encodes three neuropeptides [VIP, PHM (27-mer), and peptide histidine valine (PHV; 42-mer)], also inhibited the proliferation of Con A-stimulated murine lymphoid cells from Peyer's patches, spleen, and mesenteric lymph nodes (Yiangou *et al.*, 1990). Human peripheral blood lymphocytes and human jejunal IEL proliferation responses to Con A were not affected by VIP (Roberts *et al.*, 1991), but LPL proliferation from human colonic specimens was inhibited by nanomolar concentrations of VIP (Elitsur and Luk, 1990).

Short-term (24-hr) Con A stimulation of mesenteric lymphnode cells reduced the number of VIP binding sites (Ottaway, 1987), an indication that VIP receptors on lymphocytes can be regulated. Depletion of L3T4$^+$, but not Lyt2$^+$, mesenteric lymph node cells resulted in diminished radiolabeled VIP binding (Ottaway, 1987), suggesting the preferential expression of VIP receptors on T helper cells. Interestingly, VIP was shown to enhance IgM production (+70%) while preferentially diminishing IgA production (−70%) by Con A-stimulated Peyer's patch mononuclear cells (Stainsz *et al.*, 1986). However, in this study, ascertaining whether VIP was acting directly on VIP-R on B cells (Finch *et al.*, 1989; O'Dorisio *et al.*, 1989) or mediating its effects via VIP-R on T cells and macrophages (Ottaway, 1984; Segura *et al.*, 1991), which in turn stimulated the secretion of cytokines promoting B-cell differentiation, was difficult. VIP-containing neurons have been demonstrated to extend into the T-cell regions of the Peyer's patches (Ottaway *et al.*, 1987), most likely to affect the CD4$^+$ T cells. This population of T cells bears VIP receptors whereas CD8$^+$ cells do not (Ottaway, 1987). Thus, stimulation of CD4$^+$ T cells can modulate Ig synthesis. In this regard, finding that, in the presence of Th2 cells and derived cytokines, VIP could affect B-cell differentiation would not be unexpected. In addition to these activities, VIP has been found to reduce NK cell cytotoxic activity (Rola-Pleszczynski *et al.*, 1985) and to have mast cell secretagogue activity (Piotrowski and Foreman, 1985). VIP can affect lymphocyte migration, since VIP-treated lymphocytes tend to migrate less into mesenteric lymph nodes and Peyer's patches than into spleen, lung, or peripheral blood (Ottaway, 1984). Inhibition of lymphocyte migration out of sheep popliteal lymph nodes also was observed (Moore, 1984). Again, using the murine schistomiasis model, eosinophils in the induced granulomas were found to produce VIP (Mathew *et al.*, 1992), which induces granuloma T cells to generate IL-5. It was also observed that the IL-5-producing T cells were not reactive with soluble ova antigen. Thus, this study suggests that eosinophil-derived VIP can invoke IL-5 release by a T-cell receptor-independent mechanism. In an attempt to understand the endocrine and neuronal contribution to immune protection of the eye, one study (Kelleher *et al.*, 1991) assessed the contribution of various endocrine hormones and neuropeptides to lacrimal secretory component (SC) levels. VIP concentrations of 1.0 μM, but not peptide concentrations from 1.0 nM to 100 nM, were effective in stimulating rat lacrimal gland acinar cells to release SC. This increase in SC output was time dependent, requiring the presence of VIP for 4–7 days, whereas short-term exposure (<24 hr) had no effect.

C. Somatostatin

Widely distributed in the central and peripheral nervous system, the 14-amino-acid peptide somatostatin (growth hormone release-inhibiting hormone; Table II) is present throughout the gastrointestinal tract in nerve cells of the myenteric plexus and submucous plexus (Schultzberg *et al.*,

1980) as well as in endocrine cells (Elde and Hokfelt, 1979; Hokfelt *et al.,* 1980). Its mRNA encodes a preprohormone of 12,800 daltons; after posttranslational processing, somatostatin 14 is generated (Funckes *et al.,* 1983).

The first evidence of lymphocytes expressing somatostatin receptors (Table I) was reported by Bhathena *et al.,* (1981). Somatostatin binding sites were evident on lymphocytes and monocytes, as determined by radiolabel binding studies. Two classes of somatostatin receptors later were identified on human T-cell lines and on an Epstein–Barr virus-transformed B-cell line: high-affinity receptors displayed dissociation constants with picomolar values and low-affinity receptors showed dissociation constants in the nanomolar range (Nakamura *et al.,* 1987). Likewise, examination of the Jurkat human leukemic T-cell line and U266 human IgE myeloma cell line by radiolabel binding studies for the expression of somatostatin receptors showed that these cells exhibited biphasic binding characteristics with high-affinity receptors and K_d values of 3 p*M* (~150 receptors/cell) and 5 p*M* (~1150 receptors/cell), respectively (Sreedharan *et al.,* 1989a). Low-affinity receptors expressed by the Jurkat T cells and U266 myeloma cells displayed binding constants of 66 n*M* and 100 n*M*, respectively. In contrast, only a single class binding receptor for somatostatin was found on the mouse IgA myeloma cells MOPC 315 (Scicchitano *et al.,* 1988b). A dissociation constant of 1.6 n*M* with ~40,000 receptors/cell was obtained. When compared with human lymphoid somatostatin receptors, this evidence suggests that the K_d for this murine somatostatin receptor resembles the low-affinity receptor.

Somatostatin inhibits the release of a variety of hormones including growth hormone, insulin, and VIP (Reichlin, 1986). Similar inhibitory action also is observed in the immune system. Somatostatin at picomolar concentrations inhibited the proliferation of phytohemagglutinin (PHA)-stimulated T lymphocytes and the MOLT-4 T lymphoblasts at the DNA and protein levels (Payan *et al.,* 1984b); nanomolar concentrations were inhibitory for the proliferation of human colonic LPL (Elitsur and Luk, 1990). To obtain similar inhibitory effects, nanomolar (Stanisz *et al.,* 1986) and micromolar (Argo *et al.,* 1991) concentrations of somatostatin were required to inhibit Con A-stimulated murine Peyer's patch and splenic mononuclear cells. However, the *in vivo* administration of somatostatin via miniosmotic pump for constant delivery for 7 days resulted in enhanced suppressive effect with Peyer's patch mononuclear cells were assayed subsequently *in vitro*. A 70% reduction of mitogen-induced cell proliferation was observed with splenocytes from *in vivo*-treated mice, but the addition of somatostatin to these same *in vitro* cultures resulted in greater inhibition, exceeding 90% of cell proliferation. Further examination of the ability of somatostatin to modulate lymphoid function revealed that this neuropeptide exerted an inhibitory effect on IgA (20–50% reduction) and, to lesser degree, on IgM (10–30% reduction) production by murine mononuclear cells from the spleen and Peyer's patches (Stanisz *et al.,* 1986). Similarly, IgA production by MOPC 315 cells was inhibited at nanomolar concentrations of somatostatin by as much as 60% (Scicchitano *et al.,* 1988b). However, at $10^{-12}M$ somatostatin, as much as a 40% increase in IgA production was observed. Further investigation is required to understand the significance of this latter observation.

D. Gastrin-Releasing Polypeptide and Bombesin

The term bombesin refers to a family of peptides that share a conserved 7-amino-acid C terminus (Trp–Ala–Val–Gly–His–Leu–Met–NH_2) that is the minimal fragment required for bombesin-like activity. This tetradecapeptide (Table II) was identified first in frog skin extracts (Anastasi *et al.,* 1971); subsequently, mammalian and avian 27-mer counterparts were identified from gastrointestinal extracts and referred to as gastrin-releasing polypeptide (GRP) (Spindel, 1986). In mammalian gut, GRP is restricted solely to the neurons (Moghimzadeh *et al.,* 1983) and found predominantly in those neurons of the large intestine, whereas fewer neurons are found in the small intestine (Moghimzadeh *et al.,* 1983; Ekblad *et al.,* 1987, 1988). Bombesin/GRP can elicit gastric acid and pancreatic enzyme secretion as well as induce gall bladder and intestinal smooth muscle contraction (Fave *et al.,* 1985; Spindel, 1986). The human GRP gene is 10 kb in length and gives rise to three different mRNA species as a result of alternate splicing. However, the full-sized form is the predominant species (Spindel *et al.,* 1987). The human preprohormone is a 148-amino-acid polypeptide that undergoes posttranslational processing to produce GRP.

Limited reports have been made examining the effects of bombesin/GRP on lymphoid cells. In one study, the proliferative ability of bombesin was assessed and shown to have little or no effect on Con A- or LPS-induced lymphoid cell proliferation (Krco *et al.,* 1986), but was antiproliferative for human colonic LPL (Elitsur and Luk, 1990). However, as an IgA releasing factor, bombesin was shown to enhance effectively the *in situ* release of antigen-specific IgA and IgG antibodies from perfused rat intestine (Jin *et al.,* 1989). The rapid release of these antibodies may be, in part, the result of the evocation of cholecystokinin and gastrin (Freier *et al.,* 1987), which also have been shown to induce the release of IgA and IgG antibodies from the intestine.

E. Calcitonin Gene-Related Peptide

The spontaneous switch in a rat medullary thyroid carcinoma that resulted in diminished calcitonin production led to the discovery of a novel mRNA product that was larger than the calcitonin mRNA (Amara *et al.,* 1982). This new mRNA was shown to result from alternate RNA processing. After posttranslational processing of the 16-kDa prohormone, a novel peptide was generated. This neuropeptide, which was called calcitonin gene-related peptide (CGRP), shared little homology with calcitonin. The alternative gene processing of the calcitonin gene for the production of calcitonin and CGRP appeared to be tissue specific (Rosenfeld *et al.,* 1983). CGRP is a 37-amino-acid peptide (Table II) and shares similar C-terminal amidation with the other sensory neuropeptides. This peptide has the additional feature of a disulfide linkage between cysteine residues at positions 2 and 7. A second CGRP was discovered from a separate gene (Amara *et al.*, 1985) and referred to as β-CGRP, differing from α-CGRP by a conservative amino acid substitution at position 35 (lysine for glutamic acid). CGRP exhibits both potent vasodilatory (Brain *et al.*, 1985) and intestinal smooth muscle relaxant (Barthó *et al.*, 1987) properties. Similar to SP, CGRP is disseminated throughout the central and peripheral nervous systems (Clague *et al.*, 1985; Hanko *et al.*, 1985; Tschopp *et al.*, 1985). During capsaicin treatment, CGRP is co-depleted with SP from unmyelinated sensory neurons (Nagy *et al.*, 1981; Sternini *et al.*, 1987). Immunoreactive nerve fibers containing CGRP have been localized in the medulla and T-cell zone in the mesenteric lymph nodes (Popper *et al.*, 1988). Nerve fibers containing immunoreactive CGRP were detected in arterioles and venules with extensions entering the parenchyma of the mesenteric lymph nodes. By quantitative receptor autoradiography, distinct sites of CGRP binding were determined to be distributed throughout the mesenteric lymph nodes, with the greatest concentration of CGRP binding in −25% of the germinal centers. Binding sites also were observed on 50% of the arterioles and venules in the medulla, T-cell region, and internodular region.

Mouse splenocytes have been shown to express binding sites (Table II) for CGRP. Half-maximal inhibition of radioiodinated CGRP binding to splenocytes was achieved with 0.4 n*M* unlabeled CGRP (Umeda *et al.*, 1988). Subsequent analysis (Umeda and Arisawa, 1989) performed on T cell-enriched fractions (nylon wool nonadherent cells) revealed a biphasic binding curve with a high-affinity binding site (K_d of 0.35 n*M*; 265 sites/cell) and a low-affinity binding site (K_d of 48 n*M*; 13,000 sites/cell). Binding of radiolabeled ligand was unaffected by salmon or human calcitonin. Radioiodinated CGRP binding to T-cell lymphocyte membranes could be dissociated in part by the nucleotide analog Gpp(NH)p, suggesting that the mouse T lymphocyte CGRP receptor may be coupled to the stimulatory guanine nucleotide regulatory binding protein. In contrast to murine lymphocytes, rat lymphocytes (McGillis *et al.*, 1991) demonstrated a single class of high-affinity receptors for radioiodinated CGRP with a dissociation constant of 0.81–0.87 n*M* for splenocytes (970 receptors/cell) and enriched T cells (750 receptors/cell). B cells displayed a similar K_d of 0.39 n*M* and similar numbers of receptors as T cells. Affinity labeling studies cross-linking lymphocytes with radioiodinated CGRP produced three bands when analyzed on SDS–PAGE, all of which could be inhibited specifically with unlabeled CGRP: a high molecular weight form, a 220-kDa protein, and a 75-kDa protein. Macrophages also express CGRP receptors. Plasma membranes prepared from the P388D1 murine macrophage cell line were found to exhibit, minimally, a high-affinity receptor for radiolabeled CGRP with a dissociation constant of 1.8 n*M* (Abello *et al.*, 1991). This CGRP was coupled to adenylate cyclase since nanomolar concentrations of CGRP were effective in stimulating P388D1 adenylate cyclase activity in a dose-dependent fashion.

CGRP inhibited both Con A- and PHA-induced but not LPS-induced proliferation of mouse splenocytes in a dose-dependent fashion, with maximal inhibition seen at a concentration of 10^{-8} *M* (Umeda *et al.*, 1988) within the first 24 hr (Boudard and Bastide, 1991). In contrast to VIP, CGRP had no effect on IL-2 production by Con A-stimulated splenocytes (Boudard and Bastide, 1991), but CGRP increased cAMP levels in enriched murine T cells (Umeda *et al.*, 1988; Boudard and Bastide, 1991). As had been shown with murine T cells, rat lymphocytes stimulated with CGRP also could elicit maximal cAMP production at concentrations near the K_d for the CGRP receptor (McGillis *et al.*, 1991). CGRP also could inhibit macrophage function. Using an ovalbumin-specific T-cell line, CGRP-stimulated peritoneal macrophages inhibited antigen presentation when measured by the decrease in cell proliferation by these T cells (Nong *et al.*, 1989). In the same study, human monocytes pretreated and not co-stimulated with CGRP at nanomolar concentrations could inhibit IFNγ-induced H_2O_2 production effectively. Although the studies examining the immunomodulatory of CGRP are still limited, learning the development of CGRP functional attributes and assessing whether this neuropeptide will enhance or antagonize SP immunostimulatory effects will be interesting since these neuropeptides coexist in peptidergic nerve fibers in lymphoid tissues.

III. PEPTIDERGIC–IMMUNE CIRCUIT

We have provided here the experimental evidence for the existence of the communication system between the nervous and immune systems. Having determined that various neuropeptides do play a role in the modulation of the function of various arms of the cellular and humoral immune network, determining the intracellular mechanisms involved becomes increasingly significant. Further, the shared expression of neuropeptide and cytokine receptors by elements of the immune and nervous systems, as well as the ability to respond to these diametric molecules, supports the existence of such a neural–immune circuit. In view of these observations, efforts were put forth to investigate the possibility that neuropeptides were generated by cells other than those of neuronal origin. Consequently, leukocytes were shown to synthesize SP (Pascual and Bost, 1990b), VIP (Matthew *et al.*, 1992), and somatostatin (Sreedharan *et al.*, 1989b). These findings led some researchers to speculate that the neural–immune network is functionally bidirectional (Spector and Goetzl, 1989). If the neural–immune network is bidirectional as proposed, leukocyte-derived neuropeptides could act at neuronal or endocrine sites, even those at distant sites, in a systemic fashion. However, no *in vivo* evidence exists to support this hypothesis. In fact, even if leukocyte-derived neuropeptides could reach their respective neuronal receptors, the concentrations of leukocyte-derived neuropeptides generally have been found to be 1000-fold less than neuronal concentrations. Thus, at these concentrations, leukocyte-derived neuropeptides seem unlikely to compete effectively with neuronal production and release.

One aspect of the studies addressing leukocyte-derived neuropeptides that has failed to gather consideration is why these neuropeptides are produced by leukocytes. Whereas intricate studies have shown the production of neuropeptides by leukocytes, studies of the purpose of such production have been minimal. One possibility for their production is that low level production of neuropeptides may represent a mechanism for maintaining the expression of their respective receptors on the leukocyte cell surface. In the case of macrophage-derived SP (Pascual and Bost, 1990b), investigators suggested that macrophages produced SP in a paracrine/autocrine fashion to regulate cytokine production. Likewise, eosinophil-derived VIP may be important for nonspecific activation of T cells during schistomiasis. Thus, if leukocyte-synthesized neuropeptides can affect their own function, we must consider them functionally similar to cytokines. It may be important for them not to function at neuronal or endocrine sites; they may, instead, exhibit properties not previously considered. Consequently, leukocyte-derived neuropeptides introduce a novel regulatory circuit to immune regulation. Such an additional regulatory pathway also may have its own mode of neuropeptide release. Previous studies have shown the sensitivity of neural elements to cytokine stimulation to induce the release of neuropeptides (Jonakait and Schotland, 1990; Hart *et al.*, 1991), but these same cytokines may not affect leukocyte-derived neuropeptide release.

Much must still be learned about the mechanisms used by the peptidergic circuit to regulate immune function in MALT. We are beginning to learn about the ability of lymphocytes and macrophages to respond to neuropeptides. Subsequent studies should provide insight into the modulation of neuropeptide receptors on leukocytes, particularly understanding the regulatory mechanisms and events responsible for the expression of neuropeptide receptors. This expression can be especially significant in mucosal tissues, where the presence of neuropeptides is associated greatly with leukocytes. The consequence of understanding the relationship between the nervous system and the immune system will provide a basis for future treatment of mucosal inflammatory diseases, Crohn's disease and colitis, autoimmune diseases, arthritis, and multiple sclerosis (myelin basic protein), as well as for the development of new vaccines to mucosal pathogens. In general, this new field offers additional therapeutic strategies in the manipulation of immunity in various pathological states. Assessing the neuronal component will become more prevalent when addressing immune regulation in MALT. Thus, with the development of cDNA probes and monoclonal antibodies to neuropeptide receptors, the regulation of these receptors on lymphoid cells and macrophages can be addressed readily, providing a functional understanding of the neural–immune network.

References

Abello, J., Kaiserlian, D., Cuber, J. C., Revillard, J. P., and Chayvialle, J. A. (1991). Characterization of calcitonin gene-related peptide receptors and adenylate cyclase response in the murine macrophage cell line P388D1. *Neuropeptides* **19,** 43–49.

Amara, S. G., Jonas, V. J., Rosenfeld, M. G., Ong, E. S., and Evans, R. M. (1982). Alternate RNA processing in calcitonin gene expression generates mRNAs encoding different polypeptide products. *Nature (London)* **298,** 240–244.

Amara, S. G., Arriza, J. L., Leff, S. E., Swanson, L. W., Evans, R. M., and Rosenfeld, M. G. (1985). Expression in brain of a messenger RNA encoding a novel neuropeptide homologous to calcitonin gene-related peptide. *Science* **229,** 1094–1097.

Anastasi, A., Erspamer, V., and Bucci, M. (1971). Isolation and structure of bombesin and alytesin, two alalogous active peptides from the skin of the European amphibians *Bombina* and *Alytes. Experientia* **27,** 166–167.

Argo, A., Padol, I., and Stanisz, A. M. (1991). Immunomodulatory activities of the somatostatin analogue BIM 23014c: Effects on murine lymphocyte proliferation and natural killer activity. *Reg. Peptides* **32,** 129–139.

Argo, A., and Stanisz, A. M. (1992). Are lymphocytes a target for substance P modulation in arthritis? *Seminars Arthritis and Rheumatism* **21,** 252–258.

Argo, A., Stepien, H., and Stanisz, A. M. (1992). Are lymphocytes a target for substance P modulation in arthritis? *Sem. Arthrit. Rheum.* **21,** 1–7.

Argo, A., and Stanisz, A. M. (1993). Inhibition of murine intestinal inflammation by anti-substance P antibody. *Region. Immunol.* **5,** in press.

Barbany, G., Friedman, W. J., and Persson, H. (1991). Lymphocyte-mediated regulation of neurotransmitter gene expression in rat sympathetic ganglia. *J. Neuroimmunol.* **32,** 97–104.

Barthó, L., Lembeck, F., and Holzer, P. (1987). Calcitonin gene-related peptide is a potent relaxant of intestinal muscle. *Eur. J. Pharmacol.* **135,** 449–451.

Beagley, K. W., Eldrige, J. H., Lee, J. H., Kiyono, H., Everson, M. P., Koopman, W. J., Hirano, T., Kishimoto, T., and McGhee, J. R. (1989). Interleukins and IgA synthesis. Human and murine interleukin 6 induce high rate IgA secretion in IgA-committed B cells. *J. Exp. Med.* **169,** 2133–2148.

Beed, E. A., O'Dorisio, M. S., O'Dorisio, T. M., and Gaginella, T. S. (1983). Demonstration of a funtional receptor for vasoactive intestinal polypeptide on MOLT 4b T lymphoblasts. *Reg. Peptides* **6,** 1–12.

Bhathena, S. J., Louie, J., Schechter, G. P., Redman, R. S., Wahl, L., and Recant, L. (1981). Identification of human mononuclear leukocytes bearing receptors for somatostatin and glucagon. *Diabetes* **30,** 127–131.

Bost, K. L. (1988). Hormone and neuropeptide receptors on mononuclear leukocytes. *Prog. Allergy* **43,** 68–83.

Bost, K. L., Breeding, S. A. L., and Pascual, D. W. (1992). Modulation of the mRNAs encoding substance P and its receptor in rat macrophages by LPS. *Region. Immunol.* **4,** 105–112.

Bost, K. L., and Pascual, D. W. (1992). Substance P: A late-acting B lymphocyte differentiation co-factor. *Am. J. Physiol.* **262,** C537–C545.

Boudard, F., and Bastide, M. (1991). Inhibition of mouse T-cell proliferation by CGRP and VIP: Effects of these neuropeptides on IL-2 production and cAMP synthesis. *J. Neurosci. Res.* **29,** 29–41.

Brain, S. D., Williams, T. J., Tippins, J. R., Morris, H. R., and MacIntyre, I. (1985). Calcitonin gene-related peptide is a potent vasodilator. *Nature (London)* **313,** 54–56.

Buck, S. H., and Burks, T. F. (1986). The neuropharmacology of capsaicin: review of some recent observations. *Pharmacol. Rev.* **38,** 179–226.

Chang, M. M., and Leeman, S. E. (1971). Amino acid sequence of substance P. *Nature New Biol.* **232,** 86–87.

Clague, J. R., Sternini, C., and Brecha, N. (1985). Localization of calcitonin gene-related peptide-like immunoreactivity in neurons of the rat gastrointestinal tract. *Neurosci. Lett.* **56,** 63–68.

Couvineau, A., Amiranoff, B., and Laburthe, M. (1986). Solubilization of the liver vasoactive intestinal peptide receptor. Hydrodynamic characterization and evidence for an association with a functional GTP regulatory protein. *J. Biol. Chem.* **261,** 14482–14489.

Cowdery, J. S., Kemp, J. D., Ballas, Z. K., and Weber, S. P. (1988). Interleukin 1 induces T cell mediated differentiation of murine Peyer's patch B cells to IgA secretion. *Reg. Immunol.* **1,** 9–14.

Croitoru, K., Ernst, P. B., Bienenstock, J., Padol, I., and Stanisz, A. M. (1990). Selective modulation of the natural killer activity of murine intestinal intraepithelial leucocytes by the neuropeptide substance P. *Immunology* **71,** 196–201.

Eglezos, A., Andrews, P. V., Boyd, R. L., and Helme, R. D. (1990). Effects of capsaicin treatment on immunoglobulin secretion in the rat: Further evidence for involvement of tachykinin-containing afferent nerves. *J. Neuroimmunol.* **26,** 131–138.

Ekblad, E., Winther, C., Ekman, R., Hakanson, R., and Sundler, F. (1987). Projections of peptide-containing neurons in rat small intestine. *Neuroscience* **20,** 169–188.

Ekblad, E., Ekman, R., Håkanson, R., and Sundler, F. (1988). Projections of peptide-containing neurons in rat colon. *Neuroscience* **27,** 655–674.

Elde, R., and Hokfelt, T. (1979). Localization of hypophysiotropic peptides and other biologically active peptides within the brain. *Ann. Rev. Physiol.* **41,** 587–602.

Elitsur, Y., and Luk, G. D. (1990). Gastrointestinal neuropeptides suppress human colonic lamina propria lymphocyte DNA synthesis. *Peptides* **11,** 879–884.

Elliott, D., Cook, G., Metwali, A., Blum, A. M., Sandor, M., Lynch, R., and Weinstock, J. V. (1993). Molecular characterization and localization of a granuloma T lymphocyte substance P (NK-1) receptor in murine schistosomiasis. *J. Immunol.* 150 (Part II), **#566,** 101A.

Erspamer, V. (1981). The tachykinin peptide family. *Trends Neurosci.* **4,** 267–269.

Fave, G. D., Annibale, B., Magistris, L. D., Severi, C., Bruzzone, R., Puoti, M., Melchiorri, P., Torsoli, A., and Erspamer, V. (1985). Bombesin effects on human GI functions. *Peptides* **6**(Suppl. 3), 113–116.

Felten, D. L., Felten, S. Y., Carlson, S. L., Olschowka, J. A., and Livnat, S. (1985). Noradrenergic and peptidergic innervation of lymphoid tissue. *J. Immunol.* **135,** 755s–765s.

Felten, D. L., Felten, S. Y., Bellinger, D. L., Carlson, S. L., Ackerman, K. D., Madden, K. S., Olschowki, J. A., and Livnat, S. (1987). Noradrenergic sympathetic neural interactions with the immune system: structure and function. *Immunol. Rev.* **100,** 225–260.

Felten, S. Y., and Olschowka, J. (1987). Noradrenergic sympathetic innervation of the spleen: II. Tyrosine hydroxylase (TH)-positive nerve terminals form synapticlike contacts on lymphocytes in the splenic white pulp. *J. Neurosci. Res.* **18,** 37–48.

Finch, R. J., Sreedharan, S. P., and Goetzl, E. J. (1989). High affinity receptors for vasoactive intestinal peptide on human myeloma cells. *J. Immunol.* **142,** 1977–1981.

Freier, S., Eran, M., and Faber, J. (1987). Effect of cholecystokinin and its antagonist, of atropine and of food on the release of immunoglobulin A and immunoglobulin G specific antibodies in the rat intestine. *Gastroenterology* **93,** 1242–1246.

Funckes, C. L., Minth, C. D., Deschenes, R., Magazin, M., Tavianini, M. A., Sheets, M., Collier, K., Weith, H. L., Aron, D. C., Roos, B. A., and Dixon, J. E. (1983). Cloning and characterization of a mRNA-encoding rat preprosomatostatin. *J. Biol. Chem.* **258,** 8771–8787.

Furness, J. B., and Costa, M. (1980). Types of nerves in the enteric nervous system. *Neuroscience* **5,** 1–20.

Gozes, I., Shani, Y., and Rostène, W. H. (1987). Developmental expression of the VIP-gene in brain and intestine. *Brain Res.* **388,** 137–148.

Hanko, J., Hardebo, J. E., Kahrstrom, J., Owman, C., and Sundler, F. (1985). Calcitonin gene-related peptide is present in mammalian cerebrovascular nerve fibers and dilates pial and peripheral arteries. *Neurosci. Lett.* **57,** 91–95.

Hart, R. P., Shadiack, A. M., and Jonakait, G. M. (1991). Substance P gene expression is regulated by interleukin-1 in cultured sympathetic ganglia. *J. Neurosci. Res.* **29,** 282–291.

Hartung, H. P., Wolters, K., and Toyker, K. V. (1986). Substance P: Binding properties and studies on cellular responses in guinea pig macrophages. *J. Immunol.* **136,** 3856–3863.

Helke, C. J., Krause, J. E., Mantyh, P. W., and Bannon, M. J. (1990). Diversity in mammalian tachykinin peptidergic neurons: Multiple peptides, receptors, and regulatory mechanisms. *FASEB J.* **4,** 1606–1615.

Helme, R. D., Eglezos, A., Dandie, G. W., Andrews, P. V., and Boyd, R. L. (1987). The effect of substance P on the regional lymph node antibody response to antigenic stimulation in capsaicin-pretreated rats. *J. Immunol.* **139,** 3470–3473.

Hershey, A. D., and Krause, J. E. (1990). Molecular characterization of a functional cDNA encoding the rat substance P receptor. *Science* **247,** 958–962.

Hokfelt, T., Johansson, O., Ljundahl, A., Lundbent, J. M., and Schultzbert, M. (1980). Peptidergic neurons. *Nature* (*London*) **284,** 515–521.

Ijaz, M. K., Dent, D., and Babiuk, L. A. (1990). Neuroimmunomodulation of *in vivo* anti-rotavirus humoral immune response. *J. Neuroimmunol.* **26,** 159–171.

Inoue, N., Magari, S., and Sakanaka, M. (1990). Distribution of peptidergic nerve fibers in rat bronchus-associated lymphoid tissue:Light microscopic observations. *Lymphology* **23,** 155–160.

Jin, G.-F., Guo, Y.-S., and Houston, C. W. (1989). Bombesin: An activator of specific *Aeromonas* antibody secretion in rat intestine. *Dig. Dis. Sci.* **34,** 1708–1712.

Jonakait, G. M., and Schotland, S. (1990). Conditioned medium from activated splenocytes increases substance P in sympathetic ganglia. *J. Neurosci. Res.* **26,** 24–30.

Kelleher, R. S., Hann, L. E., Edwards, J. A., and Sullivan, D. A. (1991). Endocrine, neural, and immune control of secretory component output by lacrimal gland acinar cells. *J. Immunol.* **146,** 3405–3412.

Kimball, E. S., Persico, F. J., and Vaught, J. L. (1988). Substance P, neurokinin A, and neurokinin B induce generation of IL-1-like activity by P388D1 cells. *J. Immunol.* **141,** 3564–3569.

Koch, T. R., Carney, J. A., and Go, V. W. (1987). Distribution and quantification of gut neuropeptides in normal intestine and inflammatory bowel diseases. *Dig. Dis. Sci.* **32,** 369–376.

Krause, J. E., Chirgwin, J. M., Carter, M. S., Xu, Z. S., and Hershey, A. D. (1987). Three rat preprotachykinin mRNAs encode the neuropeptides substance P and neurokinin A. *Proc. Natl. Acad. Sci. U.S.A.* **84,** 881–885.

Krco, C. J., Gores, A., and Go, V. L. W. (1986). Gastrointestinal regulatory peptides modulate in vitro immune reactions of mouse lymphoid cells. *Clin. Immunol. Immunopathol.* **39,** 308–318.

Larsson, L.-I., Fahrenkrug, J., Schaffalitzsky de Muckadell, O., Sundler, F., Hakanson, R., and Rehfeld, J. (1976). Localization of vasoactive intestinal peptide (VIP) to central and peripheral neurons. *Proc. Natl. Acad. Sci. U.S.A.* **73,** 3197–3200.

Levine, J. D., Clark, R., Devor, M., Helms, C., and Moskowitz, M. A. (1984). Intraneuronal substance P contributes to the severity of experimental arthritis. *Science* **226,** 1218–1221.

Libert, F., Paramentier, M., Lefort, A., Dinsart, C., Van Sande, J., Maenhaut, C., Simons, M.-J., Dumont, J. E., and Vassart, G. (1989). Selective amplification and cloning of four new members of the G protein-coupled receptor family. *Science* **244,** 569–572.

Libert, F., Paramentier, M., Lefort, A., Dumont, J. E., and Vassart,

G. (1990). Complete nucleotide sequence of a putative G protein coupled receptor: RDC1. *Nucleic Acids Res.* **18,** 1917.

Linder, S., Barkhem, T., Norberg, A., Persson, H., Schalling, M., Hökfelt, T., and Magnusson, G. (1987). Structure and expression of the gene encoding the vasoactive intestinal peptide precursor. *Proc. Natl. Acad. Sci. U.S.A.* **84,** 605–609.

Lorton, D., Bellinger, D. L., Felten, S. Y., and Felten, D. L. (1991). Substance P innervation of spleen in rats: Nerve fibers associate with lymphocytes and macrophages in specific compartments of the spleen. *Brain Behav. Immun.* **5,** 29–40.

Lotz, M., Vaughan, J. H., and Carson, D. A. (1988). Effects of neuropeptides on production of inflammatory cytokines by human monocytes. *Science* **241,** 1218–1221.

Lundberg, J. M., and Saria, A. (1987). Polypeptide-containing neurons in airway smooth muscle. *Ann. Rev. Physiol.* **49,** 557–572.

McArthur, K. E., Wood, C. L., O'Dorisio, M. S., Zhou, Z., Gardner, J. D., and Jensen, R. T. (1987). Characterization of receptors for VIP on pancreatic acinar cell plasma membranes using covalent cross-linking. *Am. J. Physiol.* **252,** G404–G412.

McDonald, T. J. (1991). Gastroenteropancreatic regulatory peptide structures: An overview. *In* "Neuropeptide Function in the Gastrointestinal Tract" (E. E. Daniel), pp. 19–86. CRC Press, Boca Raton, Florida.

McGillis, J. P., Humphreys, S., and Reid, S. (1991). Characterization of functional calcitonin gene-related peptide receptors on rat lymphocytes. *J. Immunol.* **147,** 3482–3489.

Makhlouf, G. M. (1990). Neural and hormonal regulation of function in the gut. *Hosp. Prac.* **25,** 79–98.

Mantyh, C. R., Gates, T. S., Zimmerman, R. P., Welton, M. L., Passard, E. P., Vigna, S. R., Maggio, J. E., Kruger, L., and Mantyh, P. W. (1988). Receptor binding sites for substance P, but not substance K or neuromedin K, are expressed in high concentrations by arterioles, venules, and lymph nodules in surgical specimens obtained from patients with ulcerative colitis and Crohn disease. *Proc. Natl. Acad. Sci. U.S.A.* **85,** 3235–3239.

Marshall, K. W., Chiu, B., and Inman, R. D. (1990). Substance P and arthritis analysis of plasma and synovial fluid levels. *Arthritis Rheum.* **33,** 87–90.

Masu, Y., Nakayama, K., Tamaki, H., Harada, Y., Kuno, M., and Nakanishi, S. (1987). cDNA cloning of bovine substance-K receptor through oocyte expression system *Nature* (*London*) **329,** 836–838.

Mathew, R. C., Cook, G. A., Blum, A. M., Metwali, A., Felman, R., and Weinstock, J. V. (1992). Vasoactive intestinal peptide stimulates T lymphocytes to release IL-5 in murine *schistosomiasis mansoni* infection. *J. Immunol.* **148,** 3572–3577.

Moghimzadeh, E., Ekman, R., Håkanson, R., Yanaihara, N., and Sundler, F. (1983). Neuronal gastrin-releasing peptide in the mammalian gut and pancreas. *Neuroscience* **10,** 553–563.

Moore, T. C. (1984). Modification of lymphocyte traffic by vasoactive neurotransmitter substances. *Immunology* **52,** 511–518.

Nagy, J. I., Hunt, S. P., Iversen, L. L., and Emson, P. C. (1981). Biochemical and anatomical observations on the degeneration of peptide containing primary afferent neurons after neonatal capsaicin. *Neuroscience* **6,** 1923–1934.

Nagy, J. I., Iverson, L. L., Goedert, M., Chapman, D., and Hunt, S. D. (1983). Dose dependent effects of capsaicin on primary sensory neurons in the neonatal rat. *J. Neurosci.* **3,** 399–406.

Nakamura, H., Koike, T., Hiruma, T., Sato, T., Tomioka, H., and Yoshida, S., (1987). Identification of lymphoid cell lines bearing receptors for somatostatin. *Immunology* **62,** 655–658.

Nakata, Y., Tanaka, H., Morishima, Y., and Segawa, T. (1988). Solubilization and characterization of substance P binding protein from bovine brainstem. *J. Neurochem.* **50,** 522–527.

Nawa, H., Kotani, H., and Nakanishi, S. (1984). Tissue-specific generation of two preprotachykinin mRNAs from one gene by alternative RNA splicing. *Nature* (*London*) **312,** 729–734.

Nong, Y.-H., Titus, R. G., Ribeiro, J. M. C., and Remold, H. G. (1989). Peptides encoded by the calcitonin gene inhibit macrophage function. *J. Immunol.* **143,** 45–49.

O'Byrne, E. M., Blancuzzi, V., Wilson, D. E., Wong, M., and Jeng, A. Y. (1990). Elevated substance P and accelerated cartilage degradation in rabbit knees injected with interleukin-1 and tumor necrosis factor. *Arthritis Rheum.* **33,** 1023–1028.

O'Dorisio, M. S., O'Dorisio, T. M., Cataland, S., and Balcerzak, S. P. (1980). VIP as a biochemical marker for polymorphonuclear leukocytes. *J. Lab. Clin. Med.* **96,** 666–672.

O'Dorisio, M. S., Wood, C. L., Wenger, G. D., and Vassalo, L. M. (1985). Cyclic AMP-dependent protein kinase in MOLT 4b lymphoblasts: Identification by photoaffinity labeling and activation in intact cells by vasoactive intestinal polypeptide (VIP) and peptide histidine isoleucine (PHI). *J. Immunol.* **134,** 4078–4086.

O'Dorisio, M. S., Shannon, B. T., Fleshman, D. J., and Campolito, L. B. (1989). Identification of high affinity receptors for vasoactive intestinal peptide on human lymphocytes of B cell lineage. *J. Immunol.* **142,** 3533–3536.

Ottaway, C. A. (1984). *In vitro* alteration of receptors for vasoactive intestinal peptide changes in the *in vivo* localization of mouse T cells. *J. Exp. Med.* **160,** 1054–1069.

Ottaway, C. A. (1987). Selective effects of vasoactive intestinal peptide on mitogenic response of murine T cells. *Immunology* **62,** 291–297.

Ottaway, C. A., and Greenberg, F. R. (1984). Interaction of VIP with mouse lymphocytes: Specific binding and the modulation of mitogen responses. *J. Immunol.* **132,** 417–423.

Ottaway, C. A., Lewis, D. L., and Asa, S. L. (1987). Vasoactive intestinal peptide-containing nerves in Peyer's patches. *Brain Behav. Immun.* **1,** 148–158.

Pascual, D. W., and Bost, K. L. (1990a). A monoclonal anti-substance P (SP) antibody recognizes macrophage-generated immunoreactive SP and modulates IL-1 secretion by the same cells. *FASEB J.* **4,** A305 (228).

Pascual, D. W., and Bost, K. L. (1990b). Substance P production by macrophage cell lines: A possible autocrine function for this neuropeptide. *Immunology* **71,** 52–56.

Pascual, D. W., Blalock, J. E., and Bost, K. L. (1989). Anti-peptide antibodies which recognize lymphocyte substance P receptor. *J. Immunol.* **143,** 3697–3702.

Pascual, D. W., McGhee, J. R., Kiyono, H., and Bost, K. L. (1991a). Neuroimmune modulation of lymphocyte function: I. Substance P enhances immunoglobulin synthesis in LPS activated murine splenic B cells. *Int. Immunol.* **3,** 1223–1229.

Pascual, D. W., Xu-Amano, J., Kiyono, H., McGhee, J. R., and Bost, K. L. (1991b). Substance P acts directly upon cloned B lymphoma cells to enhance IgA and IgM production. *J. Immunol.* **146,** 2130–2136.

Pascual, D. W., Bost, K. L., Xu-Amano, J., Kiyono, H., and McGhee, J. R. (1992). The cytokine-like action of substance P upon B cell differentiation. *Regul. Immunol.* **4,** 100–104.

Pascual, D. W., Bost, K. L., Beagley, K. W., Kiyono, H., and McGhee, J. R. (1993). Substance P promotes Peyer's patch and splenic B differentiation. *Adv. Exper. Med. Biol.* in press.

Payan, D. G. (1989). Neuropeptides and inflammation: The role of substance P. *Ann. Rev. Med.* **40,** 341–352.

Payan, D. G., Brewster, D. R., and Goetzl, E. J. (1983). Specific stimulation of human T lymphocytes by substance P. *J. Immunol.* **131,** 1613–1615.

Payan, D. G., Brewster, D. R., and Goetzl, E. J. (1984a). Stereospecific receptors for substance P on cultured IM-9 lymphoblasts. *J. Immunol.* **133,** 3260–3265.

Payan, D. G., Hess, C. A., and Goetzl, E. J. (1984b). Inhibition by somatostatin of the proliferation of T lymphocytes and Molt-4 lymphoblasts. *Cell. Immunol.* **84,** 433–438.

Payan, D. G., McGillis, M. P., and Organist, M. L. (1986). Binding characteristics and affinity labelling of protein constituents of the human IM-9 lymphoblast receptor for substance P. *J. Biol. Chem.* **261,** 14321–14329.

Pernow, B. (1983). Substance P. *Pharmacol. Rev.* **35,** 85–140.

Piotrowski, W., and Foreman, J. C. (1985). On the actions of substance P, somatostatin, and vasoactive intestinal polypeptide on rat peritoneal mast cells and in human skin. *Naunyn-Schmiedebergs Arch. Pharmacol.* **331,** 364–368.

Polak, J. M., and Bloom, S. R. (1982). Distribution and tissue localization of VIP in the central nervous system and seven peripheral organs. *In* "Vasoactive Intestinal Peptide" (S. I. Said), pp. 107–112. Raven Press, New York.

Popper, P., Mantyh, C. R., Vigna, S. R., Maggio, J. E., and Mantyh, P. W. (1988). The localization of sensory nerve fibers and receptor binding sites for sensory neuropeptides in canine mesenteric lymph nodes. *Peptides* **9,** 257–267.

Reichlin, S. (1986). Somatostatin: Historical aspects. *Scand. J. Gastroenterol.* (Suppl.) **119,** 1–10.

Roberts, A. I., Panja, A., Brolin, R. E., and Ebert, E. C. (1991). Human intraepithelial lymphocytes: Immunomodulation and receptor binding of vasoactive intestinal peptide. *Dig. Dis. Sci.* **36,** 341–346.

Rola-Pleszczynski, M., Bulduc, D., and St. Pierre, A. (1985). The effects of VIP on human NK cell function. *J. Immunol.* **135,** 2659–2673.

Rosenfeld, M. G., Mermod, J.-J., Amara, S. G., Swanson, L. W., Sawchenko, P. E., Rivier, J., Vale, W. W., and Evans, R. M. (1983). Production of a novel neuropeptide encoded by the calcitonin gene via tissue-specific RNA processing. *Nature (London)* **304,** 129–135.

Roszman, T. L., Jackson, J. C., Cross, R. J., Titus, M. J., Markesbery, W. R., and Brooks, W. H. (1985). Neuroanatomic and neurotransmitter influences on immune function. *J. Immunol.* **135,** 769s–772s.

Said, S. I. (1984). Vasoactive intestinal polypeptide (VIP): Current status. *Peptides* **5,** 143–150.

Said, S. I., and Mutt, V. (1970). Polypeptide with broad biological activity: Isolation from small intestine. *Science* **169,** 1217–1218.

Schiogolev, S. A., Goetzl, E. J., Urba, W. J. and Longo, D. L. (1989). Appearance of neuropeptides in ascitic fluid after peritoneal therapy with interleukin-2 and lymphokine-activated killer cells for intraabdominal malignancy. *J. Clin. Immunol.* **9,** 169–173.

Schultzberg, M., Hokfelt, T., Nilsson, G., Terenius, L., Rehfeld, J. F., Brown, M., Elde, R., Goldstein, M., and Said, S. (1980). Distribution of peptide- and catecholamine-containing neurons in the gastrointestinal tract of rat and guinea pig: Immunohistochemical studies with antisera to substance P, vasoactive intestinal polypeptide, enkephalins, somatostatin, gastrin/cholecystokinin, neurotension, and dopamine β-hydroxylase. *Nature (London)* **5,** 689–744.

Scicchitano, R., Bienenstock, J., and Stanisz, A. M. (1988a). *In vivo* immunomodulation by the neuropeptide substance P. *Immunology* **63,** 733–735.

Scicchitano, R., Dazin, P., Bienenstock, J., Payan, D. G., and Stanisz, A. M. (1988b). The murine IgA-secreting plasmacytoma MOPC-315 expresses somatostatin receptors. *J. Immunol.* **141,** 937–941.

Segura, J. J., Guerrero, J. M., Goberna, R., and Calvo, J. R. (1991). Characterization of functional receptors for vasoactive intestinal peptide (VIP) in rat peritoneal macrophages. *Reg. Peptides* **33,** 133–143.

Spector, N. H., and Goetzl, E. J. (1989). Preface. *In* "Neuroimmune Networks: Physiology and Diseases" (E. J. Goetzl and N. H. Spector eds.), p. xiii. Liss, New York.

Spindel, E. (1986). Mammalian bombesin-like peptides. *Trends Neurosci.* **9,** 130–133.

Spindel, E. R., Zilberberg, M. D., and Chin, W. W. (1987). Analysis of the gene and multiple messenger ribonucleic acids (mRNAs) encoding human gastrin-releasing peptide: Alternate RNA splicing occurs in neural and endocrine tissue. *Mol. Endocrinol.* **1,** 224–232.

Sreedharan, S. P., Kodama, K. T., Peterson, K. E., and Goetzl, E. J. (1989a). Distinct subsets of somatostatin receptors on cultured human lymphocytes. *J. Biol. Chem.* **264,** 949–952.

Sreedharan, S. P., Peterson, K. E., Kodama, K. T., Finch, R. J., Taraboulos, A., Serwonska, M. H., and Goetzl, E. J. (1989b). Generation and recognition of neuropeptide mediators of cellular communication in immunity and hypersensitivity. *In* "Neuroimmune Networks: Physiology and Diseases" (E. J. Goetzl and N. H. Spector), pp. 113–118. Liss, New York.

Sreedharan, S. P., Robichon, A., Peterson, K. E., and Goetzl, E. J. (1991). Cloning and expression of the human vasoactive intestinal peptide receptor. *Proc. Natl. Acad. Sci. U.S.A.* **88,** 4986–4990.

Stanisz, A. M., Befus, D., and Bienenstock, J. (1986). Differential effects of vasoactive intestinal peptide, substance P, and somatostatin on immunoglobulin synthesis and proliferation by lymphocytes from Peyer's patches, mesenteric lymph nodes, and spleen. *J. Immunol.* **136,** 152–156.

Stanisz, A. M., Scicchitano, R., Dazin, P., Bienenstock, J., and Payan, D. G. (1987). Distribution of substance P receptors on murine spleen and Peyer's patch T and B cells. *J. Immunol.* **139,** 749–754.

Stead, R., Bienenstock, J., and Stanisz, A. M. (1987a). Neuropeptide regulation of mucosal immunity. *Immunol. Rev.* **100,** 333–359.

Stead, R. H., Tomioka, M., Quinonez, G., Simon, G. T., Felten, S. Y., and Bienenstock, J. (1987b). Intestinal mucosal mast cells in normal and nematode-infected rat intestines are in intimate contact with peptidergic nerves. *Proc. Natl. Acad. Sci. U.S.A.* **84,** 2975–2979.

Sternini, C., Reeve, J. R., and Brecha, N. (1987). Distribution and characterization of calcitonin gene-related peptide immunoreactivity in the digestive system of normal and capsaicin-treated rats. *Gastroenterology* **93,** 852–862.

Swain, M. G., Argo, A., Blennerhassett, P., Stainsz, A., and Collins, S. M. (1992). Increased levels of substance P in the myenteric plexus of *Trichinella*-infected rats. *Gastroenterology* **102,** 1913–1919.

Tissot, M., Pradelles, P., and Giroud, J. P. (1988). Substance-P-like levels in inflammatory exudates. *Inflammation* **12,** 25–35.

Tschopp, F. A., Henke, H., Peterman, J. B., Tobler, P. H., Jensen, R., Hokfelt, T., Lundberg, J. H., Cuello, C., and Fischer, J. A. (1985). Calcitonin gene-related peptide and its binding sites in the human central nervous system and pituitary. *Proc. Natl. Acad. Sci. U.S.A.* **82,** 248–252.

Umeda, Y., and Arisawa, M. (1989). Characterization of the calcitonin gene-related peptide receptor in mouse T lymphocytes. *Neuropeptides* **14,** 237–242.

Umeda, Y., Takamiya, M., Yoshizaki, H., and Arisawa, M. (1988). Inhibition of mitogen-stimulated T lymphocyte proliferation by calcitonin gene-related peptide. *Biochem. Biophys. Res. Commun.* **154,** 227–235.

van Ginkel, F. W., Bost, K. L., Kiyono, H., McGhee, J. R., and Pascual, D. W. (1993). Antibodies to rat brain substance P (SP) receptor peptide sequences recognize both brain and lymphoid SP receptors. *J. Immunol.* **150,** (Part II), **#1128,** 198A.

Weihe, E., and Krekel, J. (1991). The neuroimmune connection in human tonsils. *Brain Behav. Immun.* **5,** 41–54.

Wiederman, C. J., Sertl, K., and Pert, C. B. (1987). Neuropeptides and the immune system. Substance P receptors in bronchus-associated lymphoid tissue of rat. *Ann. N.Y. Acad. Sci.* **496,** 205–210.

Wiedermann, C. J., Wiedermann, F. J., Apperl, A., Kieselbach, G., Konwalinka, G., and Braunsteiner, H. (1989). *In vitro* human polymorphonuclear leukocyte chemokinesis and human monocyte chemotaxis are different activities of amino-terminal and carboxyterminal substance P. *Naunyn-Schmiederberg's Arch. Pharmacol.* **340,** 185–190.

Wood, C. L., and O'Dorisio, M. S. (1985). Covalent cross-linking of vasoactive intestinal polypeptide to its receptors on intact human lymphoblasts. *J. Biol. Chem.* **260,** 1243–1247.

Xu-Amano, J., McGhee, J. R., Kiyono, H., Pascual, D. W., and Burrows, P. D. (1993). Effect of substance P (Sub. P) and TGF-β on IgA isotype switching. *J. Immunol.* **150** (Part II), **#975,** 171A.

Yiangou, Y., Serrano, R., Bloom, S. R., Peña, J., and Festenstein, H. (1990). Effects of prepro-vasoactive intestinal peptide-derived peptides on the murine immune response. *J. Neuroimmunol.* **29,** 65–72.

Zentel, H. J., and Weihe, E. (1991). The neuro-B cell link of peptidergic innervation in the Bursa Fabricii. *Brain Behav. Immun.* **5,** 132–147.

18

The Role of B-1 Cells in Mucosal Immune Responses

Frans G. M. Kroese · Aaron B. Kantor · Leonore A. Herzenberg

I. INTRODUCTION

The intestinal lamina propria of the gut contains numerous plasma cells that characteristically secrete IgA. This IgA is transported across the epithelium into the gut lumen to prevent invasion of microorganisms. The high level of IgA in mucosal secretions testifies to its importance as part of the first line of defense of an animal. In fact, approximately 15 million IgA-secreting cells are found in the intestine of the mouse, which is 10 times more than the total number of IgM-secreting cells in lymphoid tissues (Van der Heijden *et al.*, 1987). Given the estimated half-life of 5 days for the vast majority of intestinal IgA plasma cells (Mattioli and Tomasi, 1973), many IgA plasma cells must develop daily from B cells to guarantee a continuous supply of cells. According to the prevailing paradigm, intestinal IgA plasma cells are derived from conventional B cells located mainly in the Peyer's patches of the small intestine (for review, see Phillips-Quagliata and Lamm, 1988; Tseng, 1988).

In this chapter, we review analyses of irradiated and nonirradiated B-cell lineage chimeras and μ,κ transgenic mice from our laboratories that indicate that many intestinal IgA plasma cells arise from Ly-1 B cells that predominate in the peritoneal cavity (Ly-1 B cells are now designated B-1 cells; Kantor *et al.*, 1991). Data from several other laboratories that support this finding are also discussed. Finally, the mucosal IgA plasma cells are considered in the context of the layered immune system (Herzenberg and Herzenberg, 1989).

II. CURRENT VIEW ON THE ORIGIN OF INTESTINAL IgA PLASMA CELLS

Peyer's patches (and appendix) are well known to contain enriched numbers of precursor cells for intestinal IgA plasma cells (Craig and Cebra, 1971,1975; Rudzik *et al.*, 1975; Tseng, 1981,1984). This conclusion was reached mainly after short-term (up to 2 weeks) transfer experiments with various cell populations to X-irradiated animals, and was initiated in the early 1970s by the classic rabbit experiments by Craig and Cebra (1971,1975). Collectively, these (and other) repopulation studies led to the following working model (for reviews, see Phillips-Quagliata and Lamm, 1988; Tseng, 1988). Antigen probably enters the Peyer's patches through specialized epithelial cells (M cells) with short microvilli and an intracellular vesicular transport system, located in the epithelium covering each follicle (Owen, 1977). In the Peyer's patches, antigen is processed by macrophages and presented to T helper cells, leading to the activation of B cells. Committed B cells leave the Peyer's patches, migrate to the mesenteric lymph nodes, and enter the blood circulation by way of the thoracic duct. These cells may expand and differentiate further in the spleen and, after some time, migrate into the gut lamina propria, where they mature to IgA-producing plasma cells. This differentiation process from Peyer's patch precursor B cell to mature IgA-secreting plasma cell in the intestinal lamina propria takes approximately 1 week.

Analysis of the phenotype of the IgA precursor cells located in the murine Peyer's patch shows that the majority of them express sIgM, sIgD, and complement (C3) receptor (Tseng, 1984). Tissue-section staining indicates that these cells are located in the lymphocyte corona of the lymphoid follicle (Butcher *et al.*, 1982). A second but minor population of IgA plasma cell precursors consists of surface/cytoplasmic IgA^+ blastoid cells that are likely to be derived from the IgM^+IgD^+ cells, and are found in the Peyer's patches and, in higher numbers, in the mesenteric lymph nodes and thoracic duct lymph (Guy-Grand *et al.*, 1974; McWilliams *et al.*, 1975; Pierce and Gowans, 1975; Roux *et al.*, 1981). In repopulation studies, this last population of IgA precursors homes immediately after transfer to the gut lamina propria (<24 hr). In Peyer's patches, $sIgA^+$ cells are located almost exclusively in the germinal centers of the lymphoid follicles (Butcher *et al.*, 1982). In the germinal centers, antigen-triggered B cells expand, undergo isotype switching, introduce somatic mutations in their V_H genes, and differentiate into memory cells (for review, see Kroese *et al.*, 1990). Therefore, the (conventional) IgA plasma cell precursors in the Peyer's patches may acquire somatic mutations in their V_H genes, resulting in high affinity antibodies with a narrow specificity.

III. B-1 CELL LINEAGE

B-1 cells (Ly-1 B cells) constitute a small but functionally very important subset of murine B cells that produces much serum immunoglobulin, including autoreactive and antibacterial antibodies. B-1 cells are distinguished from conventional B cells by phenotype, development, anatomical localization, and function (for reviews, see Hardy and Hayakawa, 1986; Herzenberg *et al.*, 1986; Hayakawa and Hardy, 1988; Kipps, 1989; Kantor and Herzenberg, 1993). B-1 cells are virtually absent from lymph nodes and Peyer's patches and are present at low frequency in spleen; however, they constitute a major fraction of the B cells in the peritoneal and pleural cavities. B-1 cells express high levels of sIgM but low levels of sIgD and B220 (RA3-6b2; Coffman and Weissman, 1981). Figure 1 shows the predominance of B-1 cells in the BALB/c peritoneal cavity and the absence of these cells in the Peyer's patches. Conventional B cells, which are dull for IgM and bright for IgD, predominate in Peyer's patches and other secondary lymphoid organs. In the peritoneal and pleural cavities, B-1 cells also express CD11b (Mac-1). B-1 cells can be divided into two independently self-replenishing populations: B-1a cells, which express detectable levels of CD5, and B-1b (formerly called "sister" cells), which do not. Both populations are present in the peritoneal and pleural cavities.

Extensive adoptive transfer studies have shown that B-1 cells and conventional B cells have different developmental pathways and have distinct progenitor cells that develop independently of each other. In essence, B-1 cells arise early during ontogeny from progenitor cells located in the fetal omentum (Solvason *et al.*, 1991) and fetal liver (Solvason *et al.*, 1991; Hardy and Hayakawa, 1992; Kantor *et al.*, 1992). After weaning, B-1 cells maintain themselves by self-replenishment and are independent of the bone marrow. Conventional B cells, in contrast, arise later in ontogeny and are replenished by *de novo* production from adult bone marrow.

Although their overall numbers are low (<5% of the peripheral B cells), B-1 cells produce much of the serum Ig, including half the IgM and IgA in radiation chimeras (Kroese *et al.*, 1989); however, they express a limited repertoire (Förster *et al.*, 1988a; Pennel *et al.*, 1988; Tarlinton *et al.*, 1988) including near exclusive use of V_H11 and V_H12, which are specific for phosphatidylcholine (PtC; Hardy *et al.*, 1989; Pennell *et al.*, 1989; Carmack *et al.*, 1990). B-1 cells produce autoantibodies to Fcγ (rheumatoid factor; Casali *et al.*, 1987; Hardy *et al.*, 1987; Burastero *et al.*, 1988) and thymocytes (Hayakawa *et al.*, 1990), and antibodies that react with microorganismal coat antigen such as α1-3 dextran (Förster and Rajewsky, 1987), PtC, and undefined determinants on *Escherichia coli* (Pennell *et al.*, 1985; Mercolino *et al.*, 1986). These B-1 cell antibodies tend to have low affinity and broad specificity (Lalor and Morahan, 1990). In contrast, B-1 cells respond poorly to commonly used exogenous antigen such as sheep erythrocytes and TNP-KLH; Hayakawa *et al.*, 1984). The majority of B-1 cell antihapten antibodies does not show the high affinity binding or fine specificity of conventional B cells (Lalor and Morahan, 1990). Thus, an apparent dichotomy exists in the expressed repertoire of conventional and B-1 cells. Little is known about the subdivision between B-1a and B-1b cells.

Although mature B-1 cells are only a minor population of B cells, their functional properties suggest that these cells play a crucial role in the first line of protection of the animal against common microorganisms, including those that are ubiquitous in the gut. This hypothesis raises the question of whether B-1 cells could be involved in mucosal IgA immune responses.

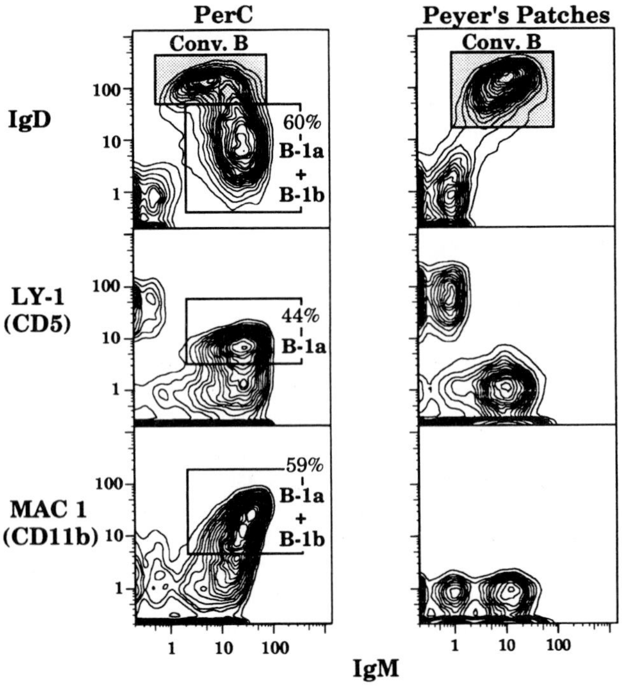

Figure 1 Comparison of Peyer's patch (*right*) and peritoneal cavity (*left*) B cells. Representative plots are shown for untreated Balb/c mice. The FACS phenotype of conventional B, B-1a, and B-1b cells are indicated. Reagents: fluorescein conjugated anti-IgM (DS1); allophycocyanin-conjugated anti-CD5 (53-7); and anti CD11b (M1/70); and biotin-conjugated anti-IgD (AMS9.1) followed by Texas Red–Avidin. The percentages of cells within the boxed populations are given per total number of live lymphocytes after gating on forward and side scatter and propidium iodide. All the plots presented have 5% probability contours.

IV. PERITONEAL RESERVOIR OF PRECURSORS FOR GUT IgA PLASMA CELLS

We examined the possible role of B-1 cells in the mucosal immune response by using stable long-term B lineage chimeras (Kroese *et al.*, 1989,1992). These chimeras exploit the self-replenishing properties of B-1 cells and their poor repopulation by adult bone marrow, especially in the presence of mature B-1 cells. Lethally irradiated mice are reconstituted with syngeneic bone marrow (BM) and peritoneal washout cells (PerC) from immunoglobulin (Ig) allotype (Igh-C) congeneic donors (Figure 2). In these mice, B cells, plasma cells, and serum immunoglobulins derived from either donor population can be distinguished on the basis of the allotype they express.

Multiparameter flow cytometry (fluorescence-activated cell sorting; FACS) analysis of these chimeras (>2 months after transfer) demonstrates that essentially all B cells in Peyer's patch (Figure 3), spleen, and lymph node are conventional B cells derived from the bone marrow donor (b allo-

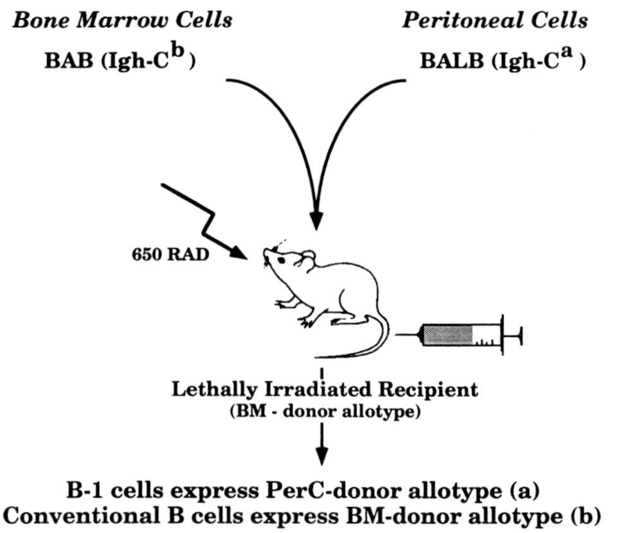

Figure 2 Preparation of radiation chimeras. Recipients [here, b allotype BAB/25 (Igh-C^b)] mice are X-irradiated and reconstituted with peritoneal cells from an a allotype Balbc/Hz and syngeneic (BAB) bone marrow.

type). B cells derived from the PerC donor (a allotype) belong exclusively to the B-1 cell lineage. PerC-derived B-1a and B-1b cells are abundant again in the peritoneal (Figure 3) and pleural cavities of the recipient mouse and are found only at low frequencies in peripheral lymphoid tissues.

Immunohistological analysis of lymphoid organs confirms the FACS data. Specifically, in Peyer's patches only rare surface IgM-, IgD-, or IgA-positive cells of PerC donor allotype are detected in the lymphocyte corona of the lymphoid follicle. However, despite the low overall numbers of PerC-derived B cells in these PerC/BM chimeras, approximately 40% of the IgA plasma cells in the gut lamina propria and half the IgM plasma cells in the spleen are derived from PerC donor cells, even up to 1 year after transfer. Consistently, half the IgA and IgM in the serum are of the PerC donor allotype (Kroese *et al.*, 1989).

Similar data are obtained with nonirradiation B lineage chimeras (Kroese *et al.*, 1989). For example, neonatal chimeras were prepared by transfer of PerC into Igh-C congeneic neonatal homozygotes treated from birth with anti-IgM allotype-specific antibodies (Lalor *et al.*, 1989b). This procedure depletes host B cells but does not affect the injected donor B cells. After stopping the antibody treatment, development of host B-1 cells is suppressed permanently, although host conventional B cells return to normal levels. In these chimeras, B-1 cells are derived exclusively from the PerC donor, and many IgA plasma cells in the gut express the PerC donor Ig allotype (Kroese *et al.*, 1989).

The production of IgA plasma cells from B-1 cells in the nonirradiated chimeras indicates that the repopulation of the lamina propria by PerC-derived cells in the irradiation chimeras is not likely to be the result of nonspecific and immediate homing of cells. Such an aberrant migration pattern could, for example, be induced by the X-irradiation procedure, which may lead to short-term inflammation of the intestine. Immediate nonspecific homing is also unlikely, since PerC-derived IgA plasma cells appear in the intestinal lamina propria of the recipients at least 1–2 weeks after transfer (Kroese *et al.*, 1989).

These findings challenge the prevailing view that the vast majority of IgA plasma cells in the intestinal lamina propria originates from (conventional) B cells located in the Peyer's patches. Instead, the data demonstrate that the murine peritoneal cavity may serve as a huge reservoir of B cells that are capable of differentiating into IgA-secreting plasma cells. Further, given the observation that, even up to 1 year after transfer, PerC-derived IgA plasma cells are seen in the intestinal lamina propria, these PerC-derived plasma cells must be either extremely long-lived (which is rather unlikely; Mattioli and Tomasi, 1973) or derived from self-replenishing precursor cells. Since FACS analysis shows that all PerC-derived $sIgM^+$ cells in these long-term stable chimeras are self-replenishing B-1 cells, the data strongly indicate that B-1 cells present in the peritoneal cavity are responsible for high numbers of intestinal IgA plasma cells.

V. IgA PLASMA CELLS IN μ,κ TRANSGENIC MICE BELONG TO THE B-1 CELL LINEAGE

In a second distinct approach, we examined the lineage origin of intestinal IgA plasma cells in IgM transgenic mice. The introduction of a functionally rearranged immunoglobulin μ heavy-chain transgene interferes with the normal development of the B-cell pool and antibody repertoire (Herzenberg *et al.*, 1987; Herzenberg and Stall, 1989; Müller *et al.*, 1989; Forni, 1990; Grandien *et al.*, 1990; Iacomini *et al.*, 1991). These transgenic mice have severely reduced numbers of B cells. As expected by the principle of allelic exclusion, the rearranged transgene inhibits further endogenous immunoglobulin heavy-chain gene rearrangements and subsequent expression. This inhibition, however, does not occur in all cells. Some B cells express endogenous IgM molecules, often concomitant with the transgenic IgM. FACS analysis and transfer studies with the transgenic mouse lines M54 and M95 have shown that the transgene selectively affects the two B cell lineages: only conventional B cells are depleted in these mice and expression of endogenous immunoglobulins is restricted totally to the B-1 cell lineage (Herzenberg *et al.*, 1987; Herzenberg and Stall, 1989). Endogenous immunoglobulin and transgenic IgM can be distinguished from each other by Igh-C allotype. Despite the loss of endogenous conventional B cells, these mice have almost normal levels of endogenous serum immunoglobulin. Most significantly, serum IgA is near normal in these animals (Grandien *et al.*, 1990).

Similar to the findings with the M54 mice, we have shown that the majority of B cells in the peripheral lymphoid organs of B6-SP6 (μ,κ transgenic) mice expresses only transgenic IgM, whereas many peritoneal B cells express endogenous IgM (either alone or in combination with transgenic IgM; Kroese *et al.*, 1992). These endogenous IgM^+ peritoneal B cells nearly all belong to the B-1 cell lineage as determined by FACS phenotype. Furthermore, transgenic BM poorly

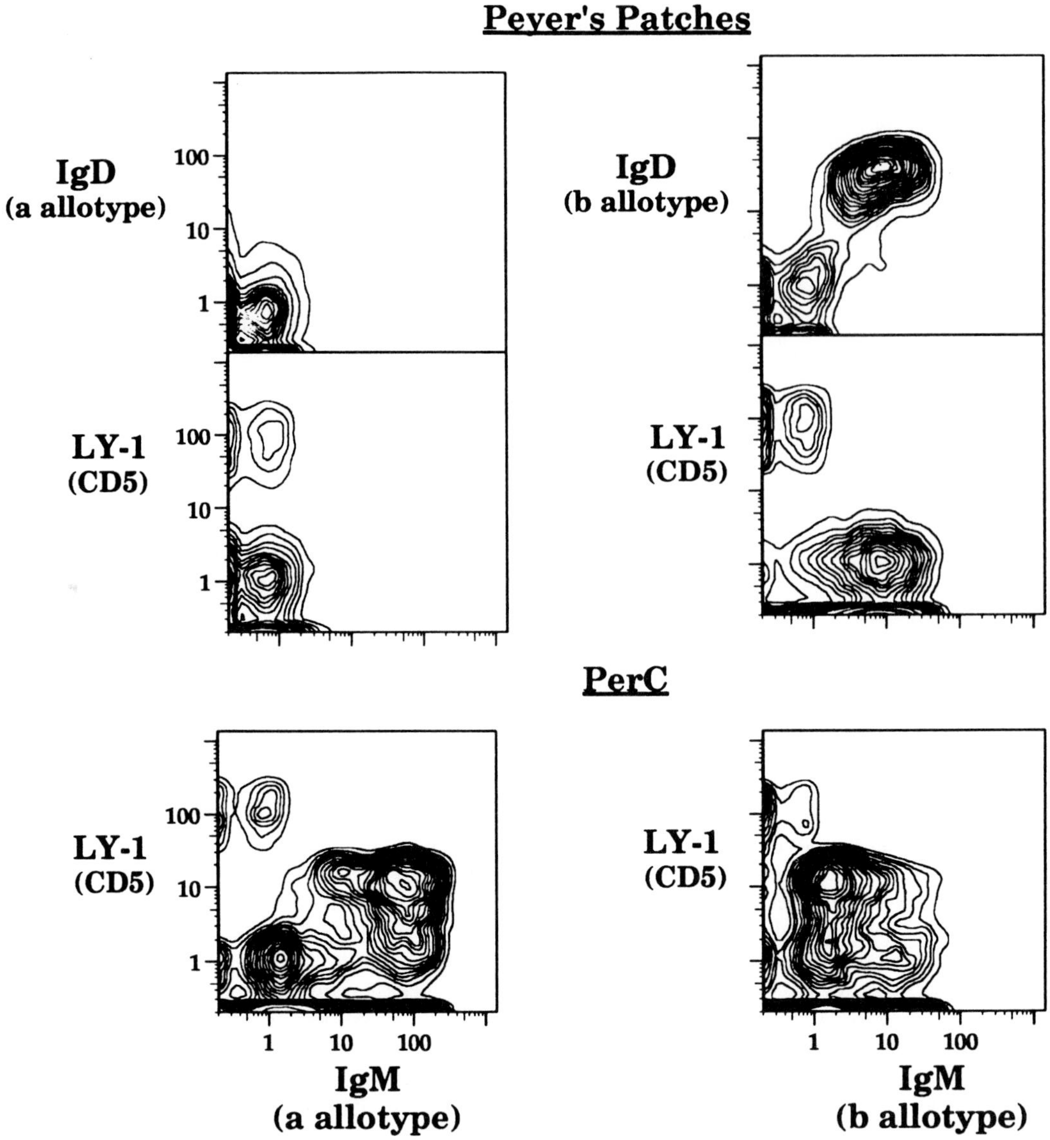

Figure 3 FACS analysis of radiation chimeras. BAB recipients of Balb/c PerC and BAB bone marrow were analyzed 10 wk after transfer. PerC-derived (a allotype) B-1a and B-1b cells are found in the recipient peritoneal cavity (PerC) but not Peyer's patches. Bone marrow-derived (b allotype) conventional B cells predominate in the Peyer's patches and other secondary lymphoid organs. Allotype specific reagents: fluorescein conjugated anti-Igh-6a (IgM of the a allotype, DS1); fluorescein conjugated anti-Igh-6b (IgM of the b allotype, AF6-78); biotin-conjugated anti-Ig5a (IgD of the a allotype, AMS9.1); and biotin-conjugated anti-Ig5b (IgD of the b allotype, AF6-122) (b allotype Mab).

reconstitutes endogenous IgM$^+$ B cells, just as adult BM from normal mice poorly reconstitutes B-1 cells. Most significantly, IgA plasma cells are found in the intestinal lamina propria of these B6-Sp6 mice and approximately 25% of them also contain transgenic IgM in their cytoplasm. Since the constant part of this IgA can be derived only from endogenous heavy-chain genes in these mice and the majority of IgA positive cells do not express the transgenic idiotype, these IgA plasma cells must be the result of an isotype switch from an endogenous IgM-expressing cell. Endogenous IgM is expressed almost exclusively by B-1 cells in these transgenics, suggesting that essentially all IgA plasma cells in the gut lamina propria of these mice belong to the B-1 cell lineage.

VI. ROLE FOR B-1 CELLS IN MUCOSAL IMMUNITY

The two different sets of experiments described earlier (i.e., B lineage chimeras and μ,κ transgenic mice) strongly indicate that B-1 cells generate many IgA plasma cells in the lamina propria. Several other lines of evidence also support our notion that B-1 cells contribute significantly to the gut IgA response. (1) Elegant experiments by Solvason *et al.* (1991) have shown that grafts of fetal omentum into adult severe combined immunodeficiency (SCID) mice reconstitute B-1 cells (both B-1a and B-1b) but not conventional B cells. These grafts also lead to the appearance of IgA plasma cells in the gut and IgM plasma cells in the spleen. (2) Several B-1 cell lymphomas (CH12.LX, CH27, and I.29) preferentially switch *in vitro* from IgM expression to IgA expression (Stavnezer *et al.*, 1985; Arnold *et al.*, 1988; Whitmore *et al.*, 1991). (3) Virtually all B cells in autoimmune viable motheaten mice are B-1 cells; the serum of these mice contains extremely high levels of IgM, IgG3, and IgA (Sidman *et al.*, 1986). (4) CBA/N Xid mice almost completely lack B-1 cells (Herzenberg *et al.*, 1986) and have a defective immune response to certain antigens such as phosphorylcholine and *Salmonella typhimurium* (Mond *et al.*, 1977; O'Brien *et al.*, 1979). However, CBA/N Xid mice populated with B-1 cells from the peritoneum of responsive CBA/CA mice have strong serum and mucosal IgA responses after oral immunization with *S. typhimurium* (Pecquet *et al.*, 1992).

Collectively, these findings are reconciled most easily with the hypothesis that B-1 cells play a significant role in the generation of IgA plasma cells in the intestinal lamina propria. This view is also consistent with the finding that intraperitoneal priming of animals is the most effective route to enhancing mucosal IgA immune responses (Pierce and Gowans, 1975; Pierce and Koster, 1980). In addition, this hypothesis also may explain how surgical removal of Peyer's patches and prolonged thoracic duct cannulation (to deplete Peyer's patch-derived cells) fail to result in a significant drop in numbers IgA plasma cells in the gut lamina propria (Mayrhofer and Fisher, 1979; Heatley *et al.*, 1981; Enders *et al.*, 1988).

Formal proof for a role of B-1 cells in the mucosal immune response requires further study. Rare sIgA$^+$ memory cells in the PerC may be responsible for the repopulation of gut IgA plasma cells after transfer (Kroese *et al.*, 1989). Transfer experiments with sorted B-cell populations into allotype congeneic hosts could clarify this point, as well as distinguish the relative roles of B-1a and B-1b cells.

VII. MUCOSAL IgA RESPONSES AND THE LAYERED IMMUNE SYSTEM

The developmental pattern of the B and T cell lineages can be considered in the context of an evolutionarily layered immune system (Herzenberg and Herzenberg, 1989; Herzenberg *et al.*, 1992; Kantor *et al.*, 1992). In this view, the lymphocyte lineages that develop at different overlapping times during ontogeny of mammals reflect the progressive emergence of layers of hematopoietic progenitor cells during evolution. B-1 cells and some $\gamma\delta$ T cells that arise earliest in ontogeny (Havran and Allison, 1988; Ito *et al.*, 1989) would represent the evolutionarily most primitive layer of the vertebrate immune system. This view is supported by evidence showing that some $\gamma\delta$ T cells (Tonegawa, 1989) and B-1 cells share many characteristics, such as predominant localization outside lymphoid tissues including the mucosal epithelium and restricted repertoires. Conventional B cells and $\alpha\beta$ T cells arise later in ontogeny and are considered more recent evolutionary developments.

Functional considerations indicate that B-1 cells and early $\gamma\delta$ T cells, by nature of their repertoire and anatomical location, may create a first line of defense against invading pathogens. B-1 cells tend to produce a restricted set of low-affinity broad-specificity germ-line antibodies that react with common antigens on ubiquitous microorganisms. In contrast, conventional B cells produce a larger more diverse set of antibodies capable of specific high-affinity interactions with particular pathogens.

The B-1 cell repertoire is established shortly after birth, in part by positive selection, at a time when the animal encounters common exogenous (microorganismal) antigens for the first time. Feedback inhibition from mature B-1 cells (Lalor *et al.*, 1989a,b) and decreased progenitor activity (Hayakawa *et al.*, 1985; Kantor *et al.*, 1992) restrict changes in the B-1 cell antibody repertoire, beginning near adolescence. Thus, the B-1 cell antibody repertoire provides an efficient and early first line of defense against many common bacteria that challenge the animal at birth and throughout life.

Conventional B cells produce a larger more diverse set of antibodies because of continuous generation from stem cells in bone marrow throughout life. These antibodies are capable of specific high-affinity interactions with particular pathogens. The conventional B cell repertoire thus is potentially able to combat any microorganisms, including those that are less common, that escape through the barrier created by the B-1 cell antibodies.

The mucosae are attacked continuously by numerous microorganisms and require a sophisticated immune system that benefits from both layers of the immune system. The importance of a mucosal immune system is indicated by the extremely high numbers of IgA plasma cells in the lamina propria and by the fact that the mucosal immune system is evolutionarily old (Phillips-Quagliata and Lamm, 1988). The layered immune system is clearly evident in the mucosae, as reflected by differentiation into IgA plasma cells from both B-1 cells located in the peritoneal cavity and conventional B cells located in the Peyer's patches. Antigen can be processed by macrophages and presented to T helper cells; the T cells, with antigen, activate the conventional Peyer's patch B cells. These cells leave the patches by way of the mesenteric lymph nodes and thoracic duct into the circulation to migrate back to the gut lamina propria for their final differentiation to IgA-producing plasma cells.

As we have shown in this chapter, some of the gut IgA plasma cells belong to the B-1 cell lineage. B-1 cells reside primarily within the peritoneal and pleural cavities and have not been demonstrated in sizable numbers in the intestinal lamina propria (F. G. M. Kroese, A. B. Kantor, and A. M. Stall, unpublished observations). Where and how these cells receive their initial antigenic stimulus, where these cells switch from IgM expression to IgA expression, and where these cells expand is virtually unknown. Cell kinetics data demonstrate that B-1 cells within the peritoneal cavity do not divide extensively and turn over only approximately 1% per day (Förster *et al.*, 1988b; Deenen and Kroese, 1993). Thus, proliferation of antigen-triggered B-1 cells must take place outside the peritoneal cavity before they differentiate into IgA-secreting cells to give rise to the large number of IgA plasma cells required every day. Perhaps B-1 cells leave the peritoneal cavity through draining lymph nodes or the pleural cavity into the circulation (Kroese *et al.*, 1992).

The relative contribution of the two lineages to the IgA response in normal animals is not known, nor do we know whether both B-1a and B-1b cells could be involved in the production of IgA plasma cells. Importantly, whether the two types of IgA-producing plasma cells exert different functions and have different antibody repertoires remains to be determined. For example, the IgA plasma cells from the B-1 cell lineage might produce low-affinity multireactive IgA to commensal microorganisms and give the animal a baseline level of protection by these antibodies. This IgA might play a role in the maintenance of the gut flora. IgA produced by plasma cells derived from the Peyer's patch, in contrast, could be responsible for producing specific high-affinity antibodies with somatic mutations that are essential to combatting more pathogenic bacteria in the gut. An advanced and layered humoral immune system such as this would be highly practical because it would combine the effective components common to more primitive vertebrates, which are provided by B-1 cells, with the more recently evolved and sophisticated components that are provided by conventional B cells.

Acknowledgments

We thank Willem Ammerlaan and Sharon Adams for their expert technical assistance. This work is supported by NATO collaborative Grant CRG 910195 to F. Kroese and L. A. Herzenberg, by a grant from the Interuniversity Institute for Radiopathology and Radioprotection to F. Kroese, NIH Grant HD-01287 to L. A. Herzenberg, and NIH Grant DK38707 pilot study 1-04 and NRSA award AI-07937 to A. B. Kantor.

References

Arnold, L. W., Grdina, T. A., Whitmore, A. C., and Haughton, G. (1988). Ig isotype switching in B lymphocytes. Isolation and characterization of clonal variants of the murine Ly-1+ B cell lymphoma CH12, expressing isotypes other than IgM. *J. Immunol.* **140,** 4355–4363.

Butcher, E. C., Rouse, R. V., Coffman, R. L., Nottenburg, C. N., Hardy, R. R., and Weissman, I. L. (1981). Surface phenotype of Peyer's patch germinal center cells: implications for the role of germinal centers in B cell differentiation. *J. Immunol.* **129,** 2698–2707.

Carmack, C. E., Shinton, S. A., Hayakawa, K., and Hardy, R. R. (1990). Rearrangement and selection of Vh11 in the Ly-1 B cell lineage. *J. Exp. Med.* **172,** 371–374.

Coffman, R. L., and Weissman, I. L. (1981). B220, a B cell specific member of the T200 glycoprotein family. *Nature (London)* **289,** 681–683.

Craig, S. W., and Cebra, J. J. (1971). Peyer's patches: An enriched source of precursors for IgA-producing immunocytes in the rabbit. *J. Exp. Med.,* **134,** 188–200.

Craig, S. W., and Cebra, J. J. (1975). Rabbit Peyer's patches and popliteal lymph node B lymphocytes: A comparative analysis of their membrane immunoglobulin components and plasma cell precursor potential. *J. Immunol* **114,** 492–502.

Deenen, G. J., and Kroese, F. G. M. (1993) Kinetics of peritoneal B-1a (CD5) B cells in young adult mice. *Eur. J. Immunol.* **23,** 12–16.

Enders, G. A., Balhaus, S., and Brendel, W. (1988). The influence of Peyer's patches on the organ-specific distribution of IgA plasma cells. *Innunology* **63,** 411–414.

Forni, I. (1990). Extensive splenic B cell activation in IgM-transgenic mice. *Eur. J. Immunol.* **20,** 983–989.

Förster, I., Gu., H., and Rajewsky K. (1988a). Germline antibody V regions as determinants of clonal persistence and malignant growth in the B cell compartment. *EMBO J.* **7,** 3693–3703.

Förster, I., and Rajewsky, K. (1987). Expansion and functional activity of Ly-1+ cells upon transfer of peritoneal cells into allotype-congenic newborn mice. *Eur. J. Immunol.* **17,** 521–528.

Förster, I., Vieira, P., and Rajewsky, K. (1988b). Flow cytometric analysis of cell proliferation dynamics in the B cell compartment of the mouse. *Int. Immunol.* **1,** 321–331.

Grandien, A., Coutinho, A., and Andersson, J. (1990). Selective peripheral expansion and activation of B cells expressing endogenous immunoglobulin in μ-transgenic mice. *Eur. J. Immunol.* **20,** 991–998.

Guy-Grand, D. C., Griselli, C., and Vassalli, P. (1974). The gut-associated lymphoid system: Nature and properties of large dividing cells. *Eur. J. Immunol.* **4,** 435–443.

Hardy, R. R., and Hayakawa, K. (1986). Development and physiology of Ly-1 B cells and its human homolog, Leu-1 B. *Immunol. Rev.* **93,** 53–79.

Hardy, R. R., Carmack, C. E., Shinton, S. A., Riblet, R. J., and Hayakawa. (1989). A single V_h gene is utilized predominantly in anti-BrMRBC hybridomas derived from purified Ly-1 B cells. Definition of the V_h11 family. *J. Immunol.* **142,** 3643–3651.

Hardy, R. R., and Hayakawa, K. (1992). Generation of Ly-1 B cells from developmentally distinct precursors: Enrichment by stromal cell culture or cell sorting in CD5 B cells in development and disease. *Ann. N.Y. Acad. Sci.* **651,** 99–111.

Hayakawa, K., and Hardy, R. R. (1988). Normal, autoimmune and malignant CD5+ cells: The LY-1 B lineage. *Ann. Rev. Immunol.* **6,** 197–218.

Hayakawa, K., Hardy, R. R., Honda, M., Herzenberg, L. A., Steinberg, A. D., and Herzenberg, L. A. (1984). Ly-1 B cells: functionally distinct lymphocytes that secrete IgM autoantibodies. *Proc. Natl. Acad. Sci. U.S.A.* **81,** 2494–2498.

Hayakawa, K., Hardy, R. R., Herzenberg, L. A., and Herzenberg, L. A. (1985). Progenitors for Ly-1 B cells are distinct from progenitors for other B cells. *J. Exp. Med.* **161,** 1554–1568.

Hayakawa, K., Carmack, C. E., Hyman, R., and Hardy R. R. (1990). Natural autoantibodies to thymocytes: Origin, VH genes, fine specificities, and the role of Thy-1 glycoprotein. *J. Exp. Med.* **172,** 869–878.

Havran, W. L., and Allison, J. P. (1988). Developmentally ordered appearance of thymocytes expressing different T-cell antigen receptors. *Nature (London)* **335,** 443–445.

Heatley, R. V., Stark, J. M., Horsewood, P., Bandhouvast, E., Cole, F., and Bienenstock, J. (1981). The effects of surgical removal of Peyer's patchers in the rat on systemic antibody responses to intestinal antigen. *Immunology* **44,** 543–548.

Herzenberg, L. A., and Herzenberg, L. A. (1989). Toward a layered immune system. *Cell* **59,** 953–954.

Herzenberg, L. A., and Stall, A. M. (1989). Conventional and Ly-1 B-cell lineages in normal and μ transgenic mice. *Cold Spring Harbor Symp. Quant. Biol.* **54,** 219–225.

Herzenberg, L. A., Stall, A. M., Lalor, P. R., Sidman, C., Moore, W. A., Parks, D. R., and Herzenberg, L. A. (1986). The Ly-1 B cell lineage. *Immunol. Rev.* **93,** 81–102.

Herzenberg, L. A., Stall, A. M., Braun, J., Weaver, D., Baltimore, D., Herzenberg, L. A., and Grosschedl, R. (1987). Depletion of the predominant B-cell population in immunoglobulin μ heavy-chain transgenic mice. *Nature (London)* **329,** 71–73.

Herzenberg, L. A., Kantor, A. B., and Herzenberg, L. A. (1992). Layered evolution in the immune system. A model for the ontogeny and development of multiple lymphocyte lineages. *Ann. N.Y. Acad. Sci.* **651,** 1–9.

Iacomini, J., Yannoutsos, N., Bandyopadhay, S., and Imanishi-kari, T. (1991). Endogenous immunoglobulin expression in mu transgenic mice. *Int. Immunol.* **3,** 185–196.

Ito, K., Bonneville, M., Takagaki, Y., Nakanishi, N., Kanagawa, O., Krecko, E. G., and Tonegawa, S. (1989). Different γδ T-cell receptors are expressed on thymocytes at different stages of development. *Proc. Natl. Acad. Sci. U.S.A.* **86,** 631–635.

Kantor, A. B. and Herzenberg, L. A. (1993). Origin of murine B cell lineages. *Ann. Rev. Immunol.* **11,** 501–538.

Kantor, A. B., *et al.* (1991). A new nomenclature for B cells. *Immunol. Today* **12,** 388.

Kantor, A. B., Stall, A. M., Adams. S., Herzenberg, L. A., and Herzenberg, L. A. (1992). Differential development of progenitor activity for three B cell lineages. *Proc. Natl. Acad. Sci. U.S.A.* **89,** 3320–3324.

Kipps, T. (1989). The CD5 B cell. *Adv. Immunol.* **47,** 117–185.

Kroese, F. G. M., Butcher, E. C., Stall, A. M., Lalor, P. A., Adams, S., and Herzenberg, L. A. (1989). Many of the IgA producing plasma cells in the murine gut are derived from self-replenishing precursors in the peritoneal cavity. *Int. Immunol.* **1,** 75–84.

Kroese, F. G. M., Seijen, H. G., and Nieuwenhuis, P. (1990). Germinal center reaction and B lymphocytes: Morphology and function. *Curr. Top. Pathol.* **84/1,** 103–148.

Kroese, F. G. M., Ammerlaan, W. A. M., and Deenen, G. J. (1992). Location and function of B-cell lineages. *Ann. N.Y. Acad. Sci.* **651,** 44–58.

Lalor, P. A., and Morahan, G. (1990). The peritoneal Ly-1 (CD5) B cell repertoire is unique among murine B cell repertoires. *Eur. J. Immunol.* **20,** 485.

Lalor, P. A., Stall, A. M., Adams, S., and Herzenberg, L. A. (1989a). Permanent alteration of the murine Ly-1 B repertoire due to selective depletion of Ly-1 B cells in neonatal animals. *Eur. J. Immunol.* **19,** 501.

Lalor, P. A., Herzenberg, L. A., Adams, S., and Stall, A. M. (1989b). Feedback regulation of murine Ly-1 B cell development. *Eur. J. Immunol.* **19,** 507–513.

McWilliams, M., Phillips-Quagliata, J. M., and Lamm, M. E. (1975). Characteristics of mesenteric lymph node cells homing to gut-associated lymphoid tissues in syngeneic mice. *J. Immunol.* **115,** 54–58.

Mattioli, C., and Tomasi, T. (1973). The life span of IgA plasma cells from the mouse intestine. *J. Exp. Med.* **138,** 452–460.

Mayrhofer, G., and Fisher, R. (1979). IgA containing plasma cells in the lamina propria of the gut: Failure of the thoracic duct fistula to deplete the numbers in rat small intestine. *Eur. J. Immunol.* **9,** 85–91.

Mercolino, T. J., Arnold, L. W., and Haughton, G. (1986). Phosphatidyl choline is recognized by a series of Ly1+ murine B cell lymphomas specific for erythocyte membranes. *J. Exp. Med.* **163,** 155–165.

Mond, J. R., Lieberman, R., Inman, J., Mosier, D., and Paul, W. (1977). Inability of mice with a defect in B-lymphocyte maturation to respond to phosphorylcholine on immunogenic carriers. *J. Exp. Med.* **146,** 1138–1142.

Müller, W., Rüther, U., Vieira, P., Hombach, J., Reth, M., and Rajewsky, K. (1989). Membrane-bound IgM obstructs B cell development in transgenic mice. *Eur. J. Immunol.* **19,** 923–928.

O'Brien, A. D., Scher, I., Campbell, G. H., MacDermott, R. P., and Formal, S. B. (1979). Susceptibility of CBA/N mice to infection with Salmonella typhimurium: Influence of the X-linked gene controlling B lymphocyte function. *J. Immunol.* **123,** 720–724.

Owen, R. L. (1977). Sequential uptake of horseradish peroxidase by lymphoid follicle epithelium of Peyer's patches in the normal unobstructed mouse intestine; an ultrastructural study. *Gastroenterology* **72,** 440–451.

Pecquet, S. S., Ehrat, C., and Ernst, P. B. (1992). Enhancement of mucosal antibody responses to salmonella typhimurium and the microbial hapten phosphorylcholine in mice with X-linked immunodeficiency by precursors from the peritoneal cavity. *Infect. Immun.* **60,** 503–509.

Pennell, C. A., Arnold, L. W., Lutz, P. M., LoCasio, N. J., Willoughby, P. B., and Haughton, G (1985). Cross-reactive idiotypes and common antigen binding specificities expressed by a series of murine B-cell lymphomas: etiological implications. *Proc. Natl. Acad. Sci. USA* **82,** 3799–3803.

Pennell, C. A., Arnold, L. W., Campbell, G. H., Clarke, S. H., and Haughton, G. (1988). Restricted Ig variable region gene expression among Ly-1+ B cell lymphomas. *J. Immunol.* **141,** 2788–2796.

Pennell, C. A., Mercolino, T. J., Grdina, T. A., Haughton, G., and Clarke, S. H. (1989). Biased immunoglobulin variable region gene expression by Ly-1 B cells is due to clonal selection. *Eur. J. Immunol.* **19,** 1289–1295.

Phillips-Qaugliata, J. M., and Lamm, M. E. (1988). Migration of lymphocytes in the mucosal immune system. *In* "Migration and Homing of Lymphoid Cells" (A. J. Husband, ed.), Vol. II, pp. 53–75. CRC Press, Boca Raton, Florida.

Pierce, N. F., and Gowans, J. L. (1975). Cellular kinetics of the intestinal immune response to cholera toxoid in rats. *J. Exp. Med.* **142,** 1550–1563.

Pierce, N. F., and Koster, F. T. (1980). Priming and suppression of the intestinal response to cholera toxoid/toxin by parenteral toxoid in rats. *J. Immunol.* **124,** 307–311.

Roux, M. E., McWillimas, M., Phillips-Quagliata, J. M., and Lamm, M. E. (1981). Differentiation pathway of Peyer's patch precursors of IgA plasma cells in the secretory immune system. *Cell. Immunol.* **61,** 141–153.

Rudzik, O., Perey, D. Y. E., and Bienenstock, J. (1975). Differential IgA repopulation after transfer of autologous and allogeneic rabbit Peyer's patch cells. *J. Immunol.* **114,** 40–44.

Sidman, C. L., Shultz, L. D., Hardy, R. R., Hayakawa, K., and Herzenberg, L. A. (1986). Production of immunoglobulin isotypes by Ly-1^+ B cells in viable motheaten and normal mice. *Science* **232,** 1423–1425.

Solvason, N., Lehuen, A., and Kearney, J. F. (1991). An embryonic source of Ly1 but not conventional B cells. *Int. Immunol.* **3,** 543–550.

Stavnezer, J., Sirlin, S., and Abbott, J. (1985). Induction of immunoglobulin isotype switching in cultured I.29 B lymphoma cells. Characterization of the accompanying rearrangements of heavy chain genes. *J. Exp. Med.,* **161,** 577–601.

Tarlington, D., Stall, A. M., and Herzenberg, L. A. (1988). Repetitive usage of immunoglobulin V_h and D segemnts in $CD5^+$ Ly-1 B clones from (NZBxNZW)F1 mice. *EMBO J.* **7,** 3705–3710.

Tonegawa, S., Berns, A., Bonneville, M., Farr, A., Ishida, I., Ito, K., Itohara, S., Janeway, C. A., Jr., Kanagawa, O., and Katsuhi, M. (1989). Diversity, development, ligands, and probable functions of $\gamma\delta$ T cells. *Cold Spring Harbor Symp. Quant. Biol.* **LIV,** 31–44.

Tseng, J. (1981). Transfer of lymphocytes of Peyer's patches between immunoglobulin allotype congenic mice: Repopulation of the IgA plasma cells in the gut lamina propria. *J. Immunol.* **127,** 2039–2043.

Tseng, J. (1984). A population of resting IgM-IgD double bearing lymphocytes in Peyer's patches: The major precursor cells for IgA plasma cells in the gut lamina propria. *J. Immunol.* **132,** 2730–2735.

Tseng, J. (1988). Migration and differentiation of IgA precursor cells in the gut-associated lymphoid tissue. *In* "Migration and Homing of Lymphoid Cells" (A. J. Husband, ed.), Vol. II, pp. 77–97. CRC Press, Boca Raton, Florida.

Van der Heijden, P. J., Stok, W., and Bianchi, A. T. J. (1987). Contribution of immunoglobulin-secreting cells in the murine small intestine to the 'background' immunoglobulin production. *Immunology* **62,** 551–555.

Whitmore, A. C., Prowse, D. M., Haughton, G., and Arnold, L. W. (1991). Ig isotype switching in B lymphocytes. The effect of T cell-derived interleukins, cytokines, cholera toxin, and antigen on isotype switch frequency of a cloned B cell lymphoma. *Int. Immunol.* **3,** 95–103.

19

Lymphocyte Homing to Mucosal Effector Sites

Julia M. Phillips-Quagliata • Michael E. Lamm

I. INTRODUCTION

Protection of the mucosae of the gastrointestinal, respiratory, and urogenital tracts, which interface with the environment, is a major preoccupation of the mammalian immune system. The total surface area of these tracts is much greater than that of the skin, and their moist nutrient-rich secretions provide an ideal milieu for the proliferation of many potentially pathogenic microorganisms. The mucosae would continually be infected by viruses, bacteria, and other parasites were they not protected by a variety of competent T cells and natural killer (NK) cells as well as by secretory immunoglobulin (Ig) capable of preventing microbial adhesion. The Ig of major importance in protecting the mucosae is secretory IgA.

II. DISTRIBUTION OF EFFECTOR CELLS IN THE MUCOSA

A. IgA-Producing Plasma Cells

In the gastrointestinal and upper respiratory tracts, nose, middle ear, gall bladder, uterine mucosa, and biliary tree, as well as in the salivary, lactating mammary, prostate, and lacrimal glands, IgA is produced locally (reviewed by Scicchitano *et al.*, 1988). In all these locations, the numbers of plasma cells producing IgA greatly exceed those producing other isotypes, emphasizing the importance of IgA in their defense and, indeed, in the defense of the whole body. Calculations from data of Brandtzaeg *et al.* (1989) indicate that $\sim 5 \times 10^{10}$ IgA-producing immunocytes populate the adult human small bowel alone, compared with a total of approximately 2.5×10^{10} immunocytes producing Ig of all isotypes in the bone marrow, spleen, and lymph nodes. If estimates of the numbers of IgA plasma cells in other mucosal sites are added, approximately 75% of all Ig-producing immunocytes in the body make IgA.

Humans have two subclasses of IgA: IgA1 and IgA2; cells producing these subclasses show regional differences in distribution. For example, IgA1 cells predominate over IgA2 in the spleen, peripheral and mesenteric lymph nodes, tonsils, stomach, and duodenum; the numbers of cells producing the two subclasses are more nearly equivalent in the lacrimal and salivary glands, and IgA2-containing cells predominate in the large intestine (Crago *et al.*, 1984; Kett *et al.*, 1986).

B. T Cells

Although secretory immunoglobulins provide a major protective element, the presence of unique populations of T cells in mucosae such as that of the small intestine strongly suggests that they, too, play an important role in local protection. The two major populations of T cells in the small intestine are intraepithelial T (IEL) and lamina propria T (LPL) lymphocytes.

In mice, IEL consist of a mixed population. About 45% are conventional thymus-processed $Thy1^{+}$T lymphocytes that express T-cell receptor (TCR)$\alpha\beta$. About 10% of these bear CD4 whereas 90% bear classical CD8 molecules, that is, these cells are mostly of the suppressor/cytotoxic phenotype. The other 55% are thymus-independent T cells that arise from bone marrow progenitors migrating directly to the gut. Many of these cells express little or no Thy 1 and bear either TCR$\alpha\beta$ or TCR$\gamma\delta$ and CD8 molecules made only of homodimeric α chains rather than the usual α and β (Lyt 2 and Lyt 3) chains (Parrott *et al.*, 1983; Klein, 1986; Bonneville *et al.*, 1988, 1990; Goodman and Lefrancois, 1988, 1989; Takagaki *et al.*, 1989; De Geus *et al.*, 1990; Guy-Grand *et al.*, 1991a,b; Rocha *et al.*, 1991). These T cells are present in nude and germ-free mice (Guy-Grand *et al.*, 1991a) and do not undergo negative selection against superantigens such as Mls in mouse strains expressing them (Rocha *et al.*, 1991). In all species examined, including humans (Cerf-Bensussan *et al.*, 1985), mice (Guy-Grand *et al.*, 1978), rats (Mayrhofer 1980), and rabbits (Rudzik and Bienenstock, 1974), a high percentage of the IELs contain intracytoplasmic granules with sulfated proteoglycans like those of mucosal mast cells and also contain perforin and the granzymes usually present in cytotoxic T cells. IEL have been shown to be highly cytotoxic in "redirected" cytotoxicity assays involving the TCR–CD3 complex, designed to circumvent the problem of their unknown specificity (Guy-Grand *et al.*, 1991b). The fact that these cells are already cytotoxic, in contrast to peripheral $CD8^{+}$ T cells which must be activated before they will differentiate into cytotoxic cells, implies that inductive stimuli (presumably including bacterial antigens and lymphokines) available in the intestinal microenvironment keep them in a constant state of readiness to kill potential targets. This idea is supported by the finding of Lefrancois and Goodman (1989) that IELs from germ-free mice are not cytolytic but become cytolytic when the mice are adapted to nonsterile conditions. In mice (Wu *et al.*, 1991) and humans (Balk *et al.*, 1991), unusual nonpolymorphic major histocompatibility complex (MHC) Class I antigens QA, TL, and CD1 are present on enterocytes. Evidence suggests that at least some cytotoxic IELs might be restricted by these antigens rather than by conventional Class I antigens. Natural cytotoxicity against classical NK targets also is expressed by intraepithelial cells that contain large granules (Tagliabue *et al.*, 1981, 1982), but whether the cells responsible are genuine NK cells, lacking the TCR, or are members of one of the IEL populations described earlier is controversial. Monoclonal antibodies (MAb) that recognize human (Cerf-Bensussan *et al.*, 1987), mouse (Kilshaw and Murant, 1990), and rat (Cerf-Bensussan *et al.*, 1986) IELs are available. These MAbs stain virtually all IELs and a fraction of LPLs in the appropriate species, but whether the epitopes recognized are involved in migration of the T cells to the intraepithelial site or are induced by some factor(s) produced by or in the vicinity of the intestinal epithelial cells is not clear. Indirect evidence (Kilshaw and Murant, 1990) favors the latter hypothesis, since the determinant recognized on murine IELs is up-regulated by culturing them in the presence of transforming growth factor β (TGFβ). Messenger RNA for TGFβ is known to be present in intestinal epithelial cells, suggesting that they produce this cytokine (Barnard *et al.*, 1989).

T cells and mucosal mast cells, which differ from mast cells in other tissue locations by their lack of serotonin (Enerbäck, 1966), are scattered among the IgA plasma cells in the lamina propria (Guy-Grand *et al.*, 1978). In humans, 95% of LPLs express TCR$\alpha\beta$; approximately 50% are of the helper/inducer phenotype, expressing CD4, and 35% are of the suppressor/cytotoxic phenotype, expressing CD8. Many appear to be memory T cells since they are CD45RO positive (Zeitz *et al.*, 1991). In mice, more than 50% of $CD3^+$ LPLs are $CD4^+$ (Mega *et al.*, 1991). Clear evidence has been presented that human (Kanof *et al.*, 1988) and mouse (Mega *et al.*, 1991) LPLs provide helper function to B cells.

III. IMMUNIZATION OF THE MUCOSA-ASSOCIATED LYMPHOID TISSUES

Because the mucosae interface with the environment and are moist, they are constantly exposed to antigens of microbial origin. In addition, the intestinal mucosa is exposed to antigens derived from food and the respiratory mucosa is exposed to inhaled antigens. During the evolution of the mammalian mucosal immune system, the mucosal lymphoid tissues have become adapted to fulfill several functions necessary for immunological protection: they have developed means of sampling antigens in the environment and of preventing induction of harmful allergic immune responses; they have developed means of optimizing production of protective IgA antibody against pathogens and of passing it into the secretions, where it can act to prevent penetration of mucosae by the pathogens; and they have developed means of distributing effector T and B cells to local and distant mucosal sites.

A. Uptake of Antigen: Role of Epithelial and Dendritic Cells

The apical surfaces of the columnar absorptive cells of the intestinal villus epithelium are bathed in antigen and express MHC Class II antigens. These cells might expected to be capable of taking up antigen and presenting it to local T cells and, indeed, they have been shown, at least *in vitro*, to act as antigen-presenting cells for both murine (Kaiserlian *et al.*, 1989) and human T cells (Mayer and Shlien, 1987). Presentation of antigens by these cells generally, however, leads to the induction of suppressor T cells rather than the T helper cells required for IgA immune responses (Mayer and Shlien, 1987). *In vivo*, these cells may participate in the induction of suppression that often is seen when antigens are delivered by the enteric route (Ngan and Kind, 1978; Richman *et al.*, 1978,1981). Presumably the adaptive advantage of these suppressor mechanisms is to prevent induction of allergy to food proteins and commensal bacteria living within the lumen of the intestine. That immune responses to potential pathogens be actively induced is essential however, to the protection of the mucosae and this induction requires penetration of the mucosae by antigen in a form in which it can stimulate the immune system.

To induce IgA immune responses in the intestinal mucosae, the work of several investigators (Robertson and Cebra, 1976; Cebra *et al.*, 1977; Husband and Gowans, 1978), who have inoculated antigen into sections of small intestine (Thirty–Vella loops) containing or not containing Peyer's patches, demonstrates that antigen must enter the nodular lymphoid tissue of the gut-associated lymphoid tissue (GALT) at some stage of the immunization process. Under physiological conditions, antigen enters these nodules from the lumen of the intestine by way of the specialized epithelium that covers them.

The nodular tissues of GALT and their analogs in bronchus-associated lymphoid tissue (BALT) consist of lymphoid follicles (Figure 1), found singly in the oral mucosa (Nair and Schroeder, 1986), intestine (Burbige and Sobky, 1977; Keren *et al.*, 1978), and bronchi (Racz *et al.*, 1977); van der Brugge-Gamelkoorn *et al.*, 1985) or in clusters in the nose-associated lymphoid tissue of mice and rats (Belal *et al.*, 1977; Spit *et al.*, 1989) and in the tonsils, adenoids, Peyer's patches, and appendix (Bockman and Cooper, 1973; Waksman and Ozer, 1976; Owen and Nemanic, 1978). The follicle-associated epithelium (FAE) is usually quite distinct from the surrounding glandular epithelium and appears to have little glandular or secretory activity (Bockman and Cooper, 1973; Bockman *et al.*, 1983; Owen and Jones, 1974; Owen, 1977), with few goblet cells and few columnar absorptive cells. Within the FAE are cells with short irregular microvilli and many tubules, vesicles, and vacuoles in the cytoplasm; these cells are commonly called M cells. In the small intestine, M cells appear to develop from the same crypt epithelial cell precursors as the villus epithelial cells (Schmidt *et al.*,

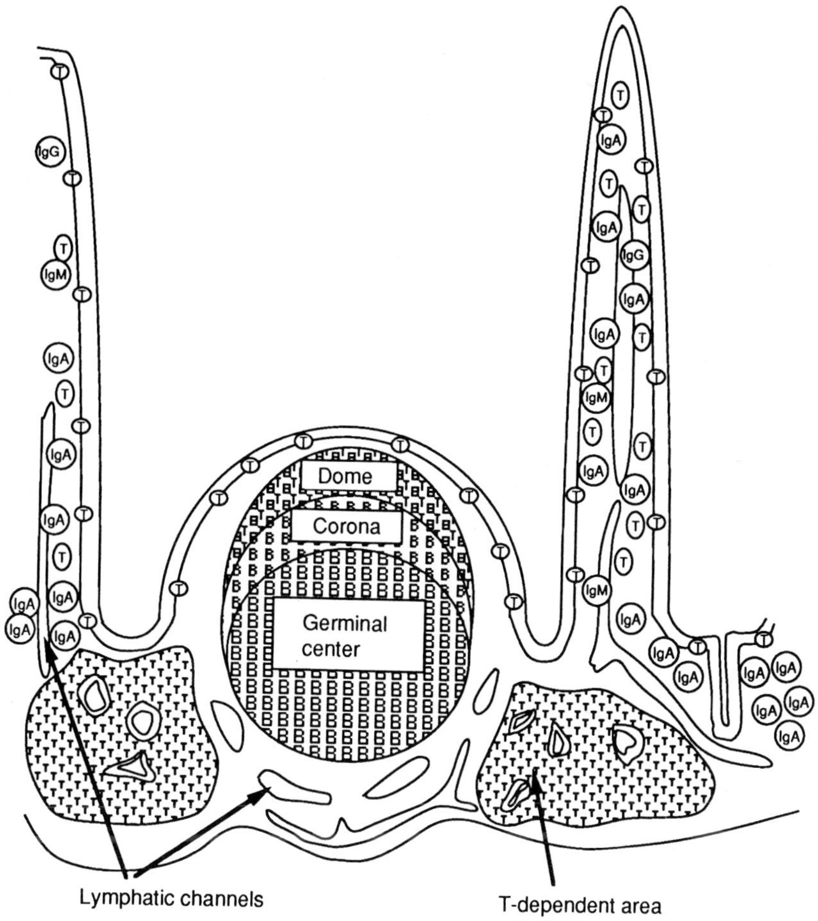

Figure 1 Diagram of MALT nodule with adjacent villi. The numbers of circles representing IgA, IgM, and IgG plasma cells reflect the approximate proportions of these cells in the lamina propria of the small intestine.

1985) but mature more rapidly (Roy, 1987) and bear unique surface antigens (Roy *et al.*, 1987). M cells have been shown to take up and transport various macromolecules intact from the lumen of the intestine (Bockman and Cooper, 1973; Owen and Jones, 1974; Owen, 1977) or bronchi (Richardson *et al.*, 1976; van der Brugge-Gamelkoorn *et al.*, 1985) to the lymphoid cells lying within the "domes" of the nodules immediately beneath them. M cells in the GALT can also transport larger particles such as bacteria (Shimizu and Andrew, 1967; Carter and Collins, 1974) and carbon and latex particles (LeFevre *et al.*, 1978; Owen and Nemanic, 1978), but those in the BALT apparently do not (Bienenstock *et al.*, 1973a,b). GALT M cells also take up and transport immune complexes, using a novel Ig receptor capable of binding either IgA or IgG (Weltzin *et al.*, 1989). A major feature distinguishing molecules capable of inducing strong mucosal immune responses from those that do not is likely to be the presence of an element that promotes binding to GM1 and GM2 gangliosides on the surface of intestinal epithelial cells (Pierce and Koster, 1980; Pierce et al., 1982; Aizpurua and Russell-Jones, 1991), but no clear evidence exists that such gangliosides are restricted to FAE.

Relatively large numbers of $CD4^+$T cells lie in clusters within and immediately beneath the FAE (Bjerke *et al.*, 1988), but that much antigen is presented directly to them by M cells, which are mostly MHC Class II (HLA-DR)-negative, seems unlikely (Hirata *et al.*, 1986; Bjerke *et al.*, 1988). However, many subepithelial DR-positive dendritic cells exist (Brandtzaeg, 1985). Dendritic cells reaching the thoracic duct lymph of mesenteric lymphadenectomized rats have been shown to bear antigens injected into the lumen of the intestine and to present them to primed T cells (Liu and Macpherson, 1991). Presumably such dendritic cells participate in presenting intestinal antigen to GALT T cells, but precisely where presentation takes place is unknown. This event probably occurs within the domes, which contain both B and T cells (Tseng, 1988), and the regional lymph nodes. Dendritic cells have been shown to be extremely supportive of IgA responses in clonal microcultures of primed Peyer's patch B cells and cloned T cells (Schrader *et al.*, 1990). Whether the dendritic cells, macrophages, or even B cells carry antigen down to the B cells in the corona and germinal center is unknown. In GALT nodules, the germinal centers are said to contain macrophages but they lack reticular dendritic cells, which are present in germinal centers in peripheral lymph nodes and spleen (Waksman *et al.,* 1973). Antigen localization in splenic follicles has been shown to be complement dependent (Papamichail *et al.,* 1975; Klaus and Humphrey, 1977), and may require lymphocytes bearing complement receptors (Gray *et al.,* 1984).

B. Lymphatic Drainage

The nodules lack afferent lymphatics. Fluid capable of carrying dissolved antigen and of flushing out unattached cells including dendritic cells and lymphocytes percolates via interstitial spaces across the domes and through the follicle away from the lumen of the mucosal organ. Experiments with dye (Carter and Collins, 1974) have shown that some slight lateral movement of fluid and, presumably, of cells into the lamina propria immediately surrounding the follicle can occur, but is minimized by the pattern of lymphatic drainage of the lymphoid nodules. Most of the fluid is collected into discrete efferent lymph channels that form basket-like structures around the bases of the follicles. From these it passes into the lymphatic network in the wall of the mucosal organ. In this network, the fluid coming from the nodule is mixed with lymph from the surrounding mucosa and drains into the afferent lymphatics of a regional lymph node. In the case of the respiratory mucosae, the regional lymph nodes are the mediastinal (bronchial) lymph nodes; in the case of the small intestine, these are the mesenteric lymph nodes. Lymphocytes in the fluid pass into the regional lymph node where they mature and subsequently are dispersed throughout the body in the blood.

C. Structure–Function Relationships in MALT Nodules

The domes of GALT follicles contain both T lymphocytes and medium-to-large IgM^+IgD^+B lymphocytes and may be equivalent to the marginal zone of the spleen (Nieuwenhuis *et al.,* 1974), whereas the coronas contain mainly small IgM^+IgD^+B lymphocytes and may be equivalent to the mantle zone of the follicles in spleen and lymph nodes (Tseng, 1988). Between the follicles are thymus-dependent areas with many small T cells and conventional high endothelial venules (HEV) through which circulating lymphocytes gain access to the lymphoid nodule.

In the base of the follicle in conventionally reared mammals is always a germinal center containing large DNA-synthesizing B cells that, because they bear on their surface plentiful terminal galactosyl residues, can be stained strongly with fluorescent conjugates of the lectin peanut agglutinin. About 60% of the germinal center cells in GALT express surface IgA (Butcher *et al.,* 1982; Lebman *et al.,* 1987), in contrast to germinal center cells in peripheral lymph nodes, which bear mainly IgM during a primary immune response or IgG during a secondary response (Kraal *et al.,* 1982). Germinal centers in peripheral lymphoid tissue have long been thought to be sites at which B-cell memory and secondary IgG and IgA plasma cell responses are generated (Thorbecke *et al.,* 1974; Klaus and Kunkl, 1981; Nieuwenhuis *et al.,* 1981; Tsiagbe and Thorbecke, 1991); researchers commonly suppose that, in conventional mammals, GALT and BALT germinal centers are maintained by enteric and inhaled antigens respectively. Cebra *et al.* (1991) have discussed the possibility that the precursors of Peyer's patch germinal center cells switch to IgA under the influence of local stimuli, but cannot formally exclude the possibility of selective accumulation of precursors already committed to IgA expression in the germinal centers of Peyer's patches. Studying this problem is difficult because germinal center cells tend to die rapidly in culture and lack "homing" receptors (Reichert *et al.,* 1983), so they cannot reliably be examined by adoptive transfer *in vivo*. The relationship, if any, between the B cells in the domes and the B cells in the coronas and germinal centers of the nodules is unknown. Even with regard to the peripheral lymphoid system, whether primary and memory B cells have the same precursors is still a matter for debate. Some investigators have hypothesized that, when virgin splenic B cells are stimulated with antigen and appropriate T-cell help, they undergo unequal division giving rise both to antibody-forming cells and to secondary or "memory" B cells (Williamson *et al.,* 1976). Work with B cells separated on the basis of their expression of an epitope recognized by the J11d MAb (Bruce *et al.,* 1981) has, instead, indicated that the B cells that give rise to secondary responses may have different precursors from those responsible for primary responses (Linton *et al.,* 1989). Tseng (1988) suggests that the small IgM^+IgD^+B cells in the corona of the Peyer's patch might be virgin B cells that, after encountering their specific antigen, eventually would give rise to IgA plasma cells in the lamina propria at mucosal sites. The B cells in the domes, which are larger than those in the corona and bear the LECAM-1 (MEL 14) antigen (Tseng, 1988) that permits them to migrate through peripheral lymph node HEV (Gallatin *et al.,* 1983), might be memory B cells originally generated in germinal centers and now capable of responding rapidly to a second encounter with specific antigen. However, although MALT nodules clearly are involved in the development of mucosal IgA responses, researchers have not firmly established that this is where priming takes place. In fact, that B cells can be efficiently primed here seems unlikely since very little help (Arny *et al.,* 1984; Dunkley and Husband, 1986) and a great deal of suppression (Ngan and Kind, 1978; Richman *et al.,* 1978,1981) and systemic tolerance induction (Thomas and Parrott, 1974; Hanson *et al.,* 1977; Vaz *et al.,* 1977; Arny *et al.,* 1984; Challacombe and Tomasi, 1987) are the usual responses of Peyer's patch T cells when mice and rats are primed enterically with soluble antigens, although some T-cell help is induced in Peyer's patches by particulate antigens such as sheep erythrocytes (Arny *et al.,* 1984). Inducing an immune response in the mucosa by administering antigen solely via the enteric route is generally difficult, except when viruses (Orgra *et al.,* 1968), cholera toxin (Elson and Ealding, 1984; Lebman *et al.,* 1988; Liang *et al.,* 1988; Chen and Strober, 1990), invasive microorganisms (Carter and Collins, 1974), or repeatedly administered particulate antigens (Crabbé *et al.,* 1969; André *et al.,* 1978; Weisz-Carrington *et al.,* 1979) are used. Immediately after enteric priming, antigen-specific B (Kagnoff, 1977) and T (Kagnoff and Cambell, 1974; Issekutz, 1984) cells usually disappear from the Peyer's patches. Their numbers are then expanded in the regional mesenteric lymph node, suggesting that they actively emigrate, perhaps in association with antigen-coated dendritic cells. Inducing an immune response in the mucosa by first priming via the intraperitoneal route and then boosting with the same antigen via the enteric route is relatively easy (Pierce and Gowans, 1975), that is, the follicles of Peyer's patches may function more as sites of secondary expansion of B cells primed in other lymphoid organs than as sites at which priming occurs. Some antigen injected via the intraperitoneal route might penetrate Peyer's patches from its serosal surface (Dunkley and Husband, 1986), but most of it probably passes into the mediastinal (Carter and Collins, 1974) and perhaps mesenteric lymph nodes, conceivably in conjunction with B cells that are members of the population resident in the peritoneal cavity, as described in a subsequent section. Under natural conditions, T and B cells are likely to be primed in mesenteric lymph nodes by intestinal antigen carried there by macrophages or dendritic cells in the lymph coming from the Peyer's patches. Once primed, the T and B cells can migrate to Peyer's patches and mount secondary responses to antigen retained at that site. Substances such as cholera toxin that act as mucosal adjuvants may not only promote induction of help rather than suppression, but may facilitate penetration of antigen past the Peyer's patch to the mesenteric lymph nodes.

IV. COMMITMENT TO IgA AND MATURATION OF B LYMPHOCYTES IN THE MUCOSAL IMMUNE SYSTEM

A. Factors Affecting Commitment to IgA Production

The mucosal nodules in conventional mammals must have some special characteristic that accounts for the fact that many B cells maturing within them eventually produce IgA. The nature of the special nodular influence is still unclear, although a great deal is now known about cytokines that can influence IgA production. Over the years, most work has been based on the hypothesis that factors available or produced in the mucosal nodules cause preferential switching of immunoglobulin genes downstream from $C\mu$ to $C\alpha$ or proliferation and eventual differentiation of those B cells that do switch to IgA. The prime mover in producing the relevant factors has generally been supposed to be the nodular T cell. Some evidence suggests that T cells derived from Peyer's patches and activated with concanavalin A produce factors that promote greater IgA responses by splenic B cells than do factors produced by similarly activated splenic T cells (Elson *et al.*, 1979; Kawanishi *et al.*, 1982,1983; Arny *et al.*, 1984). Evidence also exists that IgA Fc receptors upregulated on the surface of T helper cells derived from Peyer's patches may help these cells focus on B cells bearing surface IgA (Kiyono *et al.*, 1982,1984). No good evidence exists, however, that recently primed Peyer's patch-derived T cells capable of interacting in a cognate manner with hapten-primed B cells are more likely to contain T-cell clonal precursors capable of helping IgA responses than are similarly primed T cells derived from peripheral lymphoid tissue (Teale, 1983; Arny *et al.*, 1984; Phillips-Quagliata and Al Maghazachi, 1987; Al Maghazachi and Phillips-Quagliata, 1988). In mucosal nodules, cytokines produced by local bystander T cells activated by repeated encounters with environmental antigens or, perhaps, bacterial superantigens (Herman *et al.*, 1991) are likely to help drive B cells toward an almost exclusive commitment to IgA. In agreement with this idea is the observation that interleukin 4 (IL-4) and IL-5, which are of great significance in helping IgA responses, are produced by Th2 rather than Th1 cells (Mosmann *et al.*, 1986) and multiple contacts with antigen are known to be required for generation of Th2 cells (Swain *et al.*, 1988). Peyer's patch and, to a lesser extent, mesenteric lymph node T-cell populations are known to produce much higher ratios of IL-4 to Il-2 than spleen and peripheral lymph node populations (Daynes *et al.*, 1990). Cytokines known to be of importance in promoting IgA responses *in vitro* include TGFβ (Coffman *et al.*, 1989; Sonoda *et al.*, 1989; Kim and Kagnoff, 1990; Lebman *et al.*, 1990a; Kunimoto, 1991), which may promote switching by inducing transcription of the germ-line $C\alpha$ gene (Lebman *et al.*, 1990b; Lin *et al.*, 1991); IL-4 and IL-5 (Coffman *et al.*, 1987; Murray *et al.*, 1987; Beagley *et al.*, 1988; Harriman *et al.*, 1988), which respectively promote activation of B cells potentially able to make IgA as well as differentiation of those that have already switched from surface IgA expression to the secretory state; and IL-6, which promotes high level secretion of IgA (Beagley *et al.*, 1989; Kunimoto *et al.*, 1989). Although these cytokines promote IgA responses, they are not produced solely by mucosal T cells. TGFβ is made by many ubiquitous cell types, so the problem of the uniqueness of mucosal nodules with respect to commitment to IgA production is not solved. Stromal cells unique to the mucosal nodules could be producing crucial factors or the population of B cells on which the factors act could be preselected in some way, so switching to IgA is more likely to occur. The B cells in mucosal nodules are, indeed, selected by virtue of the fact that, to arrive in the mucosal nodule, their precursors must at some time have expressed a surface molecule (Holzmann and Weissman, 1989; Holzmann *et al.*, 1989) necessary for binding to a receptor on the nodular HEV (Streeter *et al.*, 1988). Expression of this molecule may be in some way coupled to the tendency to switch to IgA: For example, the same nuclear factors might be involved.

B. Commitment of Cells to Migration within the Mucosal Immune System

The origins of the effector lymphocytes in the mucosae and the mechanisms by which they arrive there and acquire the properties that distinguish them from cells of the same general type in other locations are under intense investigation. The T-cell pool that contributes to the IELs contains both "conventional" and "unconventional" precursors.

Conventional T-cell precursors include thymus-processed T cells with TCR $\alpha\beta$ and either CD4 or classical CD8 molecules. These cells are derived from cells that encounter antigen in the Peyer's patches and migrate by way of the thoracic duct and blood to colonize the intestinal mucosa (Guy-Grand *et al.*, 1978). Unconventional T cells comprise the cells with TCR$\alpha\beta$ or $\gamma\delta$ that, in mice, lack Thy1 and have homodimeric CD8. Without prior antigenic stimulation, these cells migrate directly from bone marrow to the gut epithelium which, for them, may in some way resemble the thymic epithelium (Guy-Grand *et al.*, 1991a). Conventional and unconventional T cells are likely to use different trafficking signals.

The B-cell pool that contributes to the IgA plasma cells similarly may contain conventional and unconventional B cells. For many years, researchers have known that the lymphoid follicles of both BALT and GALT in mice (Tseng, 1981,1984a) and rabbits (Craig and Cebra, 1971,1975; Rudzik *et al.*, 1975a,b) are highly enriched in precursor B cells that, on intravenous transfer, are capable of replacing the mucosal IgA plasma cell population of recipients after depletion by irradiation. The cells responsible seem to be conventional B cell precursors, now provisionally called B-2 cells (Kantor, 1991a,b). These cells are fetal liver or bone marrow derived, and mature through stages at which they express high levels of surface IgD (Tseng, 1988). Work by Kroese *et al.* (1989) shows, however, that in chimeric mice constructed by reconstituting lethally irradiated mice with mixtures of peritoneal cells and bone marrow cells from congeneic pairs of mice differing in immunoglobulin allotype, 30–40% of the IgA plasma cells appearing in the intestinal lamina propria after about 12 days bear the allotype of the peritoneal cell donor, that is, they appear to be derived from the recycling populations of unconventional B cells, now sometimes called coelomic or B-1 cells (Kantor, 1991a,b), that predominate in the peritoneal and pleural cavities (Hayakawa *et al.*, 1983,1986; Herzenberg *et al.*, 1986) and apparently descend from precursors in the fetal liver and omentum rather than the bone marrow (Solvason *et al.*, 1991). These unconventional B cells express only low levels of IgD and may or may not bear CD5 (Hardy and Hayakawa, 1986; Herzenberg *et al.*, 1986). Very few of the B cells in the Peyer's patches of the recipients of the mixed populations express the allotype of the peritoneal cell donor; these cells seem to be derived mostly from B-2 cells (Kroese *et al.*, 1989). Interpreting the numbers of intestinal IgA plasma cells derived from B-1 rather than B-2 cell populations in the experiments of Kroese *et al.* (1989) is somewhat difficult because when mixed populations of B-1 and B-2 cells are injected into immunodeficient mice, B-1 cells actually seem to suppress the Ig secretory activity of B-2 cells (Riggs *et al.*, 1990). Further, whether the peritoneal precursors of the IgA plasma cells appearing in the lamina propria were unprimed (virgin) cells at the time of transfer, which seems likely from the fact that they take 12 days to appear in lamina propria, or were memory B cells, already primed to intestinal antigens but present for some unknown reason in the peritoneal cavity at the time of transfer, is not certain. In addition, whether the peritoneal IgA plasma cell precursors were or were not contained in the approximately 1% of cells in the population already bearing surface IgA at the time of transfer is unclear. Despite these caveats, the finding is of tremendous interest and potential importance because many B-1 cells make germ-line "natural" antibodies that react both with autoantigens and with common microbial epitopes. Such antibodies are thought to constitute a first line of defense against infection, and a contribution to local immunity in the lamina propria makes good evolutionary sense.

C. Routes of Migration of IgA B Cells

In broad outline, the pattern of immunization, isotype-switching, maturation, and migration of the B cells in the mucosal immune system has, until recently, been thought to be fairly well understood, but the information currently available may be applicable only to conventional B-2 cells. The overall scheme may have to be modified in light of the possibility that the coelomic B-1 cell population contributing to the lamina propria IgA plasma cell population may not pass through MALT nodular lymphoid tissue or lymph nodes.

B-cell proliferation and commitment to IgA production both appear to take place in the lymphoid nodules of BALT and GALT (Jones and Cebra, 1974; Jones *et al.*, 1974; Cebra *et al.*, 1977,1983; Roux *et al.*, 1981; Tseng, 1981,1984a). The cells then leave the lymphoid nodules and pass into the regional lymph nodes, that is, the mesenteric lymph nodes in the case of GALT (Griscelli *et al.*, 1969; Guy-Grand *et al.*, 1974; McWilliams *et al.*, 1975,1977 and the mediastinal lymph nodes in the case of BALT (McDermott and Bienenstock, 1979). In the regional lymph nodes, IgA-committed and mucosa-committed B cells continue to proliferate and mature into blast cells capable of migration. At this stage, they leave the lymph node in its efferent lymph and are transported to the thoracic duct (Gowans and Knight, 1964; Griscelli *et al.*, 1969; Hall *et al.*, 1972; Guy-Grand *et al.*, 1974; Pierce and Gowans, 1975). From the thoracic duct, these cells pass into the blood, which carries them to the lamina propria of various mucosal organs.

In irradiated rabbits, most IgA plasma cells appearing in the spleen 7 days after transfer of Peyer's patch cell populations have been shown to develop from a μ chain-negative population (Jones *et al.*, 1974) that contains α chain-bearing cells (Jones and Cebra, 1974), but no direct evidence exists that the α chain-bearing cells are the precursors. In mice, Peyer's patch cell populations clearly contain two sets of intestinal IgA plasma cell precursors: resting IgM$^+$IgD$^+$ double-bearing, complement receptor-positive cells that give rise to IgA plasma cells in the intestines of irradiated recipients about 12 days after intravenous transfer of normal or lymphoblast-depleted Peyer's patch cell populations (Tseng, 1984a) and DNA-synthesizing surface IgA-bearing B cells that, in double transfer studies done in unirradiated mice, take about 3 days to mature into intestinal IgA plasma cells (Tseng, 1981). The data suggest that the IgM$^+$IgD$^+$ population may represent the corona B cells whereas the DNA-synthesizing IgA-bearing cells may come from germinal centers, but this idea is difficult to prove because germinal center B cells lack surface molecules that would permit them to migrate to lymphoid tissues, and tend to be removed from the circulation in the lungs and liver (Reichert *et al.*, 1983).

Very few cells in radiolabeled Peyer's patch populations have the ability to migrate to lamina propria within 24 hr of intravenous transfer, in contrast to the plentiful numbers of lymphoblasts in mesenteric lymph nodes (Griscelli *et al.*, 1969; Guy-Grand *et al.*, 1974; McWilliams *et al.*, 1975,1977) and thoracic duct lymph (Gowans and Knight, 1964; Hall *et al.*, 1972; Guy-Grand *et al.*, 1974; Pierce and Gowans, 1975; McDermott and Bienenstock, 1979) that do so with alacrity. The Peyer's patch cells that survive intravenous injection seem to require time to mature and develop the surface molecules necessary to allow them to migrate before they can settle in lamina propria. After intravenous injection, these cells generally do so in a nonphysiological site, the spleen (Tseng, 1981); normally, cells leaving the Peyer's patch would be transported by lymph into the regional mesenteric lymph node. After intravenous injection, some radiolabeled DNA-synthesizing Peyer's patch cells can, in fact, cross the walls of blood vessels in the small intestine, reach the intestinal lymph, and be carried into the marginal sinus of the mesenteric node (Roux *et al.*, 1981). Whether they leave from blood vessels in the Peyer's patch or the lamina propria is not known. To study the question, the distribution of IgA-containing radiolabeled Peyer's patch and mesenteric lymph node blasts 30 min after intravenous injection into syngeneic recipients was examined by autoradiography and immunofluorescence in transverse sections of small intestine cut through the center of Peyer's patches (Phillips-Quagliata *et al.*, 1983). More than 90% of the IgA-containing Peyer's patch-derived blasts in each section were located in the Peyer's patch portion of the section, although it only occupied about half the area. The other 10% was found in the lamina propria of the intestine, like the majority of mesenteric lymph node-derived lymphoblasts. The data suggest that Peyer's patch blasts that are sufficiently mature to be capable of migrating to GALT after intravenous injection tend to do so through the HEV of the patch rather than through the walls of vessels in the lamina propria. The ability of mesenteric node versus Peyer's patch IgA-committed blasts to discriminate between the lamina propria and the Peyer's patch strongly suggests that the recognition signals used by B lymphoblasts in these two locations are not the same, although small T lymphocytes may recognize lamina propria vessels by the same molecule used on Peyer's patch HEV (Streeter *et al.*, 1987). Lamina propria IgA-containing B-cell populations have been isolated and shown to be capable of returning to lamina propria after intravenous injection (Tseng, 1984b). The nature of the population with this ability to go back to lamina propria is unclear, but these cells could represent recently arrived mesenteric lymph node blasts that, left undisturbed, would settle down and become plasma cells. Alternatively, these cells could represent a population that actually recirculates through lamina propria. Such a population might be related to the peritoneal B-1 cell population.

Under physiological conditions, maturation of IgA B cells derived from GALT and BALT nodules into blast cells capable of migrating into lamina propria clearly takes place in the draining mesenteric and mediastinal nodes, respectively. Suggested but not proven is the idea that the lymph nodes of the head and neck similarly serve as maturation sites for cells derived from the lymphoid follicles in the lymphoid tissue of the oropharynx (Nair and Schroeder, 1986) and nose (Belal *et al.*, 1977; Spit *et al.*, 1989). By the time they are ready to migrate, the cells are actively synthesizing DNA (Gowans and Knight, 1964; Griscelli *et al.*, 1969; Hall *et al.*, 1972; Guy-Grand *et al.*, 1974; McWilliams *et al.*, 1975,1977; Pierce and Gowans, 1975; McDermott and Bienenstock, 1979), bear surface IgA (Guy-Grand *et al.*, 1974; McWilliams *et al.*, 1975,1977), and lack complement receptors (McWilliams *et al.*, 1975) known to be present on their IgM^+IgD^+ precursors in the Peyer's patch (Tseng, 1984a). Populations of GALT-derived T (Guy-Grand *et al.*, 1974,1978; Parrott and Ferguson, 1974; Rose *et al.*, 1976; Sprent, 1976) and IgG-committed B (McDermott and Bienenstock, 1979) lymphoblasts also follow the same path.

The route by which GALT-derived IgA-committed B cells return to the lamina propria of the gut has been termed the IgA cell cycle (Lamm, 1976). A similarly circular route is apparently followed by BALT-derived IgA-committed B lymphoblasts to the lamina propria in the respiratory tract. Both GALT and BALT nodules, however, contain the precursors of cells eventually capable of migrating to the lamina propria of either the intestine or the respiratory tract (Rudzik *et al.*, 1975a,b). Indeed, the migratory cells derived from GALT and BALT can evidently recognize and settle in both local and distant mucosal sites, leading to the inference that there is a common mucosal immune system with shared endothelial cell markers or chemotactic signals, permitting emigration of the lymphoblasts from the vasculature at several locations. Populations of IgA-committed B lymphoblasts, expanded as a result of immunization in GALT or BALT, are known to be able to settle not only in the intestinal (Guy-Grand *et al.*, 1974; McWilliams *et al.*, 1975, 1977; McDermott and Bienenstock, 1979) and bronchial (McDermott and Bienenstock, 1979) lamina propria but also at sites such as the lactating mammary gland (Roux *et al.*, 1977; McDermott and Bienenstock, 1979), uterine cervix (McDermott and Bienenstock, 1979), and salivary and lacrimal glands (Montgomery *et al.*, 1983). However, a certain regional preference exists, since mesenteric lymph node cells localize much better in the small intestine than in the lungs and the reverse is true of cells from the mediastinal lymph nodes (McDermott and Bienenstock, 1979). Further, intravenously injected labeled cells, taken from the thoracic duct after intraduodenal immunization, lodge preferentially in the jejunum whereas those taken after intracolonic immunization lodge preferentially in the colon (Pierce and Cray, 1982). Cells immunized at proximal rather than distal sites within the small intestine, however, show no preference for localizing at the site of immunization (Husband and Dunkley, 1985). The extent of localization depends on regional blood flow and so can be increased in regions of local inflammation (Rose *et al.*, 1976; Ottaway *et al.*, 1983), but localization is initially independent of local specific antigen, that is, the lymphoblasts are not migrating toward their specific antigen sequestered in lamina propria (Guy-Grand *et al.*, 1974; Parrott and Ferguson, 1974; Hall *et al.*, 1977; Husband, 1982).

The presence of antigen within the lamina propria does, however, influence the outcome of migration: without it, IgA plasma cell precursors that initially localize to lamina propria disappear; with it, they remain (Husband, 1982; Husband and Dunkley, 1985) and proliferate (Husband, 1982; Mayrhofer and Fisher, 1979). The presence of immune T cells is also necessary for optimal localization of these cells (Dunkley and Husband, 1991).

V. MECHANISMS OF MUCOSAL MIGRATION

Compared with our understanding of the pathways of migration of the lymphocyte precursors of mucosal IgA plasma cells, little is known about the underlying mechanisms. For leukocytes in general, including lymphocytes, interactions between reciprocal sets of homing receptors on the circulating cells and so-called vascular addressins on endothelial cells are believed to be critical (Butcher, 1991; Chin *et al.*, 1991; Picker and Butcher, 1992). Some of these sets are expressed constitutively whereas others are induced by local activating signals such as cytokines acting on both circulating and endothelial cells. No individual set by itself is likely to account for a particular regional mode of lymphocyte homing, but the net effect of the expression of multiple interacting sets that individually vary in their binding affinity probably determines the preferential anatomic localization of a particular class of leukocytes.

The best studied vascular addressin relevant to MALT is a receptor on the endothelium of HEV of Peyer's patches and mesenteric lymph nodes and, much less prominently, on the flat-walled venules of mucosal lamina propria (Streeter *et al.*, 1988; Jalkanen *et al.*, 1989; Picker and Butcher, 1992). This addressin, for which a corresponding lymphocyte homing receptor has not yet been identified, is likely to be particularly relevant to the circulation of small lymphocytes through the Peyer's patch and mesenteric lymph node HEV, and possibly through the venules of mucosal lamina propria. Evidence for its role in the highly efficient, directed migration to the lamina propria of the lymphoblasts that are the immediate precursors of mucosal plasma cells is less compelling. For example, the degree of expression of the mucosal addressin is inversely proportional to the homing tendency of mesenteric lymph node-derived IgA plasmablasts, that is, this addressin is expressed much less in lamina propria, to which IgA plasmablasts efficiently home, and much more in Peyer's patches, to which mesenteric node-derived IgA plasmablasts show no directed movement.

In addition to the putative lymphocyte receptor for the mucosal addressin, several other lymphocyte surface moieties have been suggested for accessory roles in homing to MALT, including CD44, integrins, and the high endothelial binding factor for Peyer's patches (Picker and Butcher, 1992). In addition to components of endothelium, local chemoattractants, perhaps including products of the differentiated mucosal epithelium, may play an important role in lymphocyte homing to lamina propria (Czinn and Lamm, 1986). Such a possibility would fit nicely into current multifactorial concepts of cell homing. In turn multifactorial regulation of homing, including local factors, could explain the final localization of B and T lymphoblasts, which segregate themselves after entry into lamina propria. B lymphoblasts initially accumulate around the crypts before distributing themselves in the villi; T lymphoblasts go directly to the lamina propria high in the villi or to the villus epithelium (McDermott *et al.*, 1986). Expression of lymphoblast homing signals is constitutive in the lamina propria of the small intestine, but under hormonal control in the female genital tract (McDermott *et al.*, 1980) and lactating mammary gland (Weisz-Carrington *et al.*, 1978).

We hypothesize (Figure 2) that commitment of the majority of the B cells in MALT both to IgA production and to seeking lamina propria at the plasmablast stage is most likely the end result of antigen- and T cell-driven expansion of B-cell populations initially selected for their ability to cross the endothelium in the MALT nodule or the lamina propria. This ability probably is controlled by different moieties that may or may not, on a stochastic basis, be expressed on cells of the same lineage. Cells that can gain access to the mucosal lymph by extravasating from blood in either the MALT nodule or the lamina propria will eventually arrive via the afferent lymphatics and marginal sinus in the regional lymph node, where they may be primed and expanded in number. Whereas those initially extravasating in the MALT nodule may or may not eventually express lamina propria-seeking tendencies, those extravasating in lamina propria presumably continue to be able to do so after priming and differentiation. After priming and maturation, the cells leave the lymph node in efferent lymph and are carried through the thoracic duct to the blood. Primed B cells that are destined to become plasma cells and fail to express molecules permitting them to cross the endothelium in lamina propria may end up in the spleen or bone marrow. Those cells that express a moiety allowing them to penetrate lamina propria do so and settle there, providing, after the first exposure to a mucosal antigen, an IgM plasma cell response in lamina propria. Primed B memory cell precursors that express the moiety that allows them to cross the HEV of MALT nodules can migrate to these nodules, where they come under the influence of nodular cytokines that drive them toward expansion and the switch to IgA production. Their progeny mature within the draining lymph node into IgA-producing plasmablasts capable of populating the lamina propria. Primed B memory cells derived from lamina propria-seeking precursors that express peripheral lymph node rather than MALT nodule HEV binding moieties may (especially in situations of artificial immunization) encounter their antigen and T-cell help in nonmucosal lymph nodes. If they do, they may give rise to lamina propria IgG rather than IgA plasma cells because only the mucosal nodules contain the T-cell and accessory-cell populations that drive preferential switching to IgA.

Coelomic B-1 cells, which seem not to recirculate through lymph nodes via HEV, may recirculate through lamina propria, reaching regional lymph nodes in the afferent lymph via the marginal sinus. If these cells do not encounter their antigen, they may simply pass through the lymph nodes via their medullary sinuses and return in the efferent lymph to the blood through the thoracic duct. Conceivably, vessels in the peritoneal cavity may share an addressin with lamina

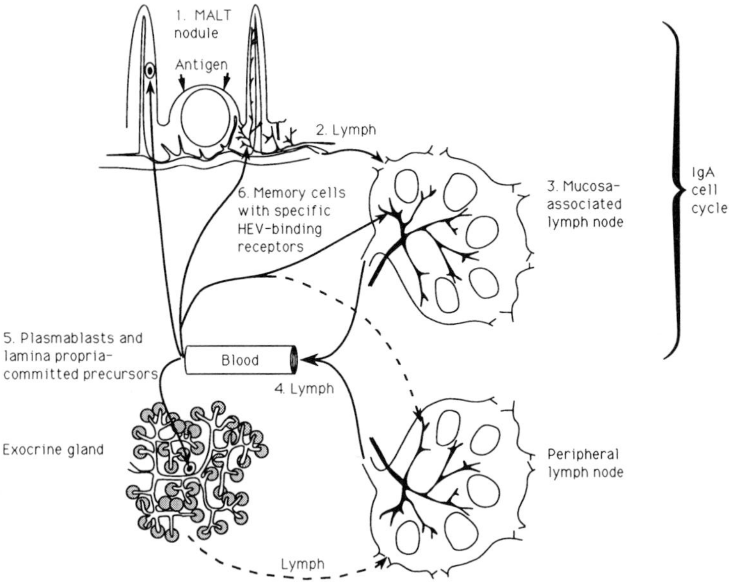

Figure 2 Hypothetical model for the migration of B cells in the mucosal immune system. Open vessels in the MALT nodule and adjacent villi represent lymphatics; solid vessels represent the venous system. (1) Antigen crosses the epithelium of the MALT nodule through the M cells and makes contact with dendritic cells, B cells, and T cells that have entered the nodule through its HEV. Cytokines available in the nodule promote switching to IgA by B cells in the germinal center. (2) A mixed population of cells coming from both the nodule and the lamina propria is carried with antigen in the lymph to the regional mucosa-associated lymph node. (3) In the mucosa-associated lymph node, unprimed B cells are primed and memory B cells are boosted. Some primed B cells mature into IgM-bearing plasmablasts capable of seeding the lamina propria, some into memory B cells capable of recirculating through HEV. B cells derived from memory cells that were boosted by antigen in the MALT nodule mature into IgA plasmablasts. (4) Mature plasmablasts and memory cells leave in efferent lymph and are carried by the blood to the mucosa and exocrine glands as well as to other lymph nodes. (5) Plasmablasts capable of extravasating in lamina propria at mucosal sites and in exocrine glands do so and settle down to become plasma cells, which are mostly IgA producers. Blood-borne unprimed B cells that are capable of extravasating in lamina propria do so; eventually, these cells are transported by lymph to the draining mucosa-associated lymph node, are primed, and so enter the cycle. (6) Memory cells with appropriate HEV-binding receptors enter the MALT nodule or lymph nodes. If they enter the MALT nodule or the mucosa-associated lymph nodes, they encounter their specific antigen again and the population is expanded. Nodular influences that promote IgA production drive the population toward a major commitment to this isotype. If the memory cells enter the peripheral lymph nodes and do not reencounter their antigen, their numbers are not increased. If they do encounter their antigen in peripheral lymph nodes, their numbers are increased but, in the absence of nodular influences that promote IgA responses, they mature into IgG rather than IgA plasma cells.

propria, although not necessarily the same one used by B-2 cell-derived lamina propria plasma cell precursors.

This hypothetical model for the expansion and control of migration of mucosa-seeking B cells admits the possibility of small populations of B-cell precursors with specific ability to seek the lamina propria at sites such as the lactating mammary gland or the proestrous uterus, while avoiding the lamina propria of the intestinal or respiratory tracts. The mammary gland and uterus do not have a nodular lymphoid tissue associated with them and are not generally under intense antigenic bombardment, so these populations generally would not be much expanded. Precursor B cells extravasating from blood in these locations presumably could be immunized by antigens draining into the regional peripheral lymph nodes after experimental immunization, but would be unlikely to become heavily committed to IgA production. Nevertheless, B cells primed in these locations might include a contingent capable of being boosted in BALT or GALT nodules and, subsequently, of populating the mucosae in which they originally extravasated with specific IgA plasma cells, while leaving the respiratory or intestinal tract relatively free of specific IgA plasma cells.

As discussed in more depth elsewhere (Phillips-Quagliata and Lamm, 1988), the evolution of the migratory patterns of IgA B cells in the mucosal immune system probably has a very long history. In modern mammals, the ability of effector cells immunized against pathogens present in the gastrointestinal and respiratory tracts to migrate to other mucosal sites enables them to protect these sites against microbial contamination from the excreta. The delivery of IgA-producing plasmablasts to the lactating mammary gland is of particular significance because it results in transmission in milk of secretory IgA specific for maternal enteric microorganisms to the gastrointestinal tract of the immunologically immature infant. The infant is thus protected against the very microorganisms it is most likely to receive from its mother. The subtle interplay between the cytokines that determine the isotype of the immune response, the homing receptors on the lymphocytes, and the vascular addressins with which they interact, as well as the sex hormones that control expression of the molecules necessary for migration to the lactating mammary gland, is finely tuned and undoubtedly has contributed to the success of mammals in colonizing the earth.

References

Aizpurua, H. J., and Russell-Jones, G. J. (1991). Oral vaccination. Identification of classes of proteins that provoke an immune response upon oral feeding. *J. Exp. Med.* **167,** 440–451.

Al Maghazachi, A., and Phillips-Quagliata, J. M. (1988). Keyhole-limpet hemocyanin-propagated Peyer's patch T cell clones that help IgA responses. *J. Immunol.* **140,** 3380–3388.

André, C., André, F., Druguet, M., and Fargier, M.-C. (1978). Response of anamnestic IgA-producing cells in the mouse gut after repeated intragastric immunization. *In* "Secretory Immunity and Infection" (J. R. McGhee, J. Mestecky, and J. L. Babb, eds.), pp. 583–591. Plenum Press, New York.

Arny, M., Kelly-Hatfield, P., Lamm, M. E., and Phillips-Quagliata, J. M. (1984). T cell help for the IgA response: The function of T cells from different lymphoid organs in regulating the proportions of plasma cells expressing various isotypes. *Cell. Immunol.* **89,** 95–112.

Balk, S. P., Ebert, E., Blumenthal, R. L., McDermott, F. V., Wucherpfenning, K. W., Landau, S. B., and Blumberg, R. S. (1991). Oligoclonal expansion and CD1 recognition by human intestinal epithelial lymphocytes. *Science* **253,** 1411–1415.

Barnard, J. A., Beauchamp, R. D., Coffey, R. J., and Moses, H. L. (1989). Regulation of intestinal epithelial cell growth by transforming growth factor type β. *Proc. Natl. Acad. Sci. U.S.A.* **86,** 1578–1582.

Beagley, K. W., Eldridge, J. H., Kiyono, H., Everson, M. P., Koopman, W. J., Honjo, T., and McGhee, J. R. (1988). Recombinant murine IL-5 induces high rate IgA synthesis in cycling IgA-positive Peyer's patch IgA B cells. *J. Immunol.* **141,** 2035–2042.

Beagley, K. W., Eldridge, J. H., Lee, F., Kiyono, H., Everson, M. P., Koopman, W. J., Hirano, T., Kishimoto, T., and McGhee, J. R. (1989). Interleukins and IgA synthesis: Human and murine IL-6 induce high rate IgA secretion in IgA-committed B cells. *J. Exp. Med.* **169,** 2133–2148.

Belal, A. A., El-Gohery, Y., and Talaat, M. (1977). Nasal and paranasal pathology in experimental bilharziasis. *J. Laryngol. Otol.* **91,** 391–400.

Bienenstock, J., Johnston, N., and Perey, D. Y. E. (1973a). Bronchial lymphoid tissue. I. Morphological characteristics. *Lab. Invest.* **28,** 686–692.

Bienenstock, J., Johnston, N., and Perey, D. Y. E. (1973b). Bronchial lymphoid tissue. II. Functional characteristics. *Lab. Invest.* **28,** 693–698.

Bjerke, K., Brandtzaeg, P., and Fausa, O. (1988). T cell distribution is different in follicle-associated epithelium of human Peyer's patches and villous epithelium. *Clin. Exp. Immunol.* **74,** 270–275.

Bockman, D. E., and Cooper, M. D. (1973). Pinocytosis by epithelium associated with lymphoid follicles in the bursa of Fabricius, appendix and Peyer's patches. An electron microscopic study. *Am. J. Anat.* **136,** 455–478.

Bockman, D. E., Boydston, W. R., and Beezhold, D. H. (1983). The role of epithelial cells in gut-associated immune reactivity. *Ann. N.Y. Acad. Sci.* **409,** 129–143.

Bonneville, M., Janeway, Jr., C. A., Ito, K., Haser, W., Ishida, I., Nakanishi, N., and Tonegawa, S. (1988). Intestinal intraepithelial lymphocytes are a distinct set of $\gamma\delta$ T-cells. Nature (Lond.). **336,** 479–481.

Bonneville, M., Itohara, S., Krecko, E. G., Mombaerts, P., Ishida, I., Katsuki, M., Berns, A., Farr, A. G., Janeway, Jr., C. A., and Tonegawa, S. (1990). Transgenic mice demonstrate that epithelial homing of $\gamma\delta$ T cells is determined by cell lineages independent of T cell receptor specificity. *J. Exp. Med.* **171,** 1015–1026.

Brandtzaeg, P. (1985). Research in gastrointestinal immunology-state of the art. *Scand. J. Gastroenterol.* **20** (Suppl. 114), 137–156.

Brandtzaeg, P., Halstensen, T. S., Kett, K., Krajči, P., Kvale, D., Rognum, T. O., Scott, H., and Sollid, L. M. (1989). Immunobiology and immunopathology of human gut mucosa: humoral immunity and intraepithelial lymphocytes. *Gastroenterology* **97,** 1562–1584.

Bruce, J., Symington, F. W., McKearn, T. J., and Sprent, J. (1981). A monoclonal antibody discriminating between subsets of T and B cells. *J. Immunol.* **127,** 2496–2501.

Burbige, E. J., and Sobky, R. Z. F. (1977). Endoscopic appearance of colonic lymphoid nodules: A normal variant. *Gastroenterology* **72,** 524–526.

Butcher, E. C. (1991). Leukocyte endothelial cell recognition: Three or more steps to specificity and diversity. *Cell* **67,** 1–4.

Butcher, E. C., Rouse, R. V., Coffman, R. L., Nottenburg, C. N., Hardy, R. R., and Weissman, I. L. (1982). Surface phenotype of Peyer's patch germinal center cells: Implications for the role of germinal centers in B cell differentiation. *J. Immunol.* **129,** 2698–2707.

Carter, P. B., and Collins, F. M. (1974). The route of enteric infection in normal mice. *J. Exp. Med.* **139,** 1189–1203.

Cebra, J. J., Kamat, R., Gearhart, P., Robertson, S. M., and Tseng, J. (1977). The secretory IgA system of the gut. *Ciba Found. Symp.* **46,** 5–22.

Cebra, J. J., Cebra, E. R., Clough, E. R., Fuhrman, J. A., Komisar, J. L., Schweitzer, P. A., and Shahin, R. D. (1983). IgA commitment: Models for B-cell differentiation and possible roles for T cells in regulating B-cell development. *Ann. N.Y. Acad. Sci.* **409,** 25–37.

Cebra, J. J., Schrader, C. E., Shroff, K. E., and Weinstein, P. D. (1991). Are Peyer's patch germinal centre reactions different from those occurring in other lymphoid tissues? *Res. Immunol.* **142,** 222–226.

Cerf-Bensussan, N., Guy-Grand, D., and Griscelli, C. (1985). Intraepithelial lymphocytes of human gut: Isolation, characterization and study of natural killer activity. *Gut* **26,** 81–88.

Cerf-Bensussan, N., Guy-Grand, D., Lisowska-Grospierre, B., Griscelli, C., and Bhan, A. K. (1986). A monoclonal antibody specific for rat intestinal lymphocytes. *J. Immunol.* **136,** 76–82.

Cerf-Bensussan, N. Jarry, A., Brousse, N., Lisowska-Grospierre, B., Guy-Grand, D., and Griscelli, C. (1987). A monoclonal antibody (HML-1) defining a novel membrane molecule present on human intestinal lymphocytes. *Eur. J. Immunol.* **17,** 1279–1285.

Challacombe, S. J., and Tomasi, T. B. (1987). Oral tolerance. *In* "Food Allergy and Intolerance" (J. Brostoff and S. J. Challacombe, eds.), pp. 255–268. Baillère Tindall, London.

Chen, K.-S., and Strober, W. (1990). Cholera holotoxin and its B subunit enhance Peyer's patch B cell responses induced by orally administered influenza virus: Disproportionate cholera toxin enhancement of the IgA B cell response. *Eur. J. Immunol.* **20,** 433–436.

Chin, Y.-H., Sackstein, R., and Cai, J.-P. (1991). Lymphocyte-homing receptors and preferential migration pathways. *Proc. Soc. Exp. Biol. Med.* **196,** 374–380.

Coffman, R. L., Shrader, B., Carty, J., Mosmann, T. R., and Bond, M. W. (1987). A mouse T cell product that preferentially enhances IgA production. I. Biologic characterization. *J. Immunol.* **139,** 3685–3690.

Coffman, R. L., Lebman, D. A., and Schrader, B. (1989). Transforming growth factor-β specifically enhances IgA production by lipopolysaccharide-stimulated murine B lymphocytes. *J. Exp. Med.* **170,** 1039–1044.

Crabbé, P. A., Nash, D. R., Bazin, H., Eyssen, H., and Heremans, J. F. (1969). Antibodies of the IgA type in intestinal plasma cells of germ-free mice after oral or parenteral immunization with ferritin. *J. Exp. Med.* **130,** 723–744.

Crago, S. S., Kutteh, W. H., Moro, I., Allansmith, M. R., Radl, J., Haaijman, J. J., and Mestecky, J. (1984). Distribution of IgA1, IgA2 and J-chain-containing cells in human tissues. *J. Immunol.* **132,** 16–18.

Craig, S. W., and Cebra, J. J. (1971). Peyer's patches: An enriched source of precursors for IgA-producing immunocytes in the rabbit. *J. Exp. Med.* **134,** 188–200.

Craig, S. W., and Cebra, J. J. (1975). Rabbit Peyer's patches, appendix and popliteal lymph node B lymphocytes: A comparative analysis of their membrane immunoglobulin components and plasma cell precursor potential. *J. Immunol.* **114,** 492–502.

Czinn, S. J., and Lamm, M. E. (1986). Selective chemotaxis of subsets of B lymphocytes from gut associated lymphoid tissue and its implications for the recruitment of mucosal plasma cells. *J. Immunol.* **136,** 3607–3611.

Daynes, R. A., Araneo, B. A., Dowell, T. A., Huang, K., and Dudley, D. (1990). Regulation of murine lymphokine production *in vivo*. III. The lymphoid tissue microenvironment exerts regulatory influences over T helper cell function. *J. Exp. Med.* **171,** 979–996.

De Geus, B., Van den Enden, M., Coolen, C., Nagelkerken, L., Van der Heijden, P., and Rozin, J. (1990). Phenotype of intraepithelial lymphocytes in euthymic and athymic mice: Implications for differentiation of cells bearing a CD3-associated $\gamma\delta$ T cell receptor. *Eur. J. Immunol.* **20,** 291–298.

Dunkley, M. L., and Husband, A. J. (1986). The induction and migration of antigen-specific helper cells for IgA responses in the intestine. *Immunology* **57,** 379–385.

Dunkley, M. L., and Husband, A. J. (1991). The role of non-B cells in localizing an IgA plasma cell response in the intestine. *Reg. Immunol.* **3,** 336–340.

Elson, C. O., and Ealding, W. (1984). Generalized systemic and mucosal immunity in mice after mucosal stimulation with cholera toxin. *J. Immunol.* **132,** 2736–2741.

Elson, C. O., Heck, J. A., and Strober, W. (1979). T cell regulation of murine IgA synthesis. *J. Exp. Med.* **149,** 632–643.

Enerbäck, E. (1966). Mast cells in rat gastrointestinal mucosa. Monoamine storing capacity. *Acta Pathol. Microbiol. Scand.* **67,** 365–379.

Gallatin, W. M., Weissman, I. L., and Butcher, E. C. (1983). A cell-surface molecule involved in organ-specific homing of lymphocytes. *Nature (London)* **304,** 30–34.

Goodman, T., and Lefrancois, L. (1988). Expression of the γ-δ T-cell receptor on intestinal CD8+ intraepithelial lymphocytes. *Nature (London)* **333,** 855–858.

Goodman, T., and Lefrancois, L. (1989). Intraepithelial lymphocytes. Anatomical site, not T cell receptor form, dictates phenotype and function. *J. Exp. Med.* **170,** 1569–1581.

Gowans, J. L., and Knight, E. J. (1964). The route of recirculation of lymphocytes in the rat. *Proc. R. Soc. London B* **159,** 257–282.

Gray, D., Kumararatne, D. S., Lortan, J., Khan, M., and MacLennan, I. C. M. (1984). Relation of intrasplenic migration of marginal zone B cells to antigen localization on follicular dendritic cells. *Immunology* **52,** 659–669.

Griscelli, C., Vassalli, P., and McCluskey, R. T. (1969). The distribution of large dividing lymph node cells in syngeneic recipient rats after intravenous injection. *J. Exp. Med.* **130,** 1427–1451.

Guy-Grand, D., Griscelli, C., and Vassalli, P. (1974). The gut-associated lymphoid system: nature and properties of the large dividing cells. *Eur. J. Immunol.* **4,** 435–443.

Guy-Grand, D., Griscelli, C., and Vassalli, P. (1978). The mouse gut T lymphocyte, a novel type of T cell. Nature, origin, and traffic in mice in normal and graft-versus host conditions. *J. Exp. Med.* **148,** 1661–1677.

Guy-Grand, D., Cerf-Bensussan, N., Malissen, B., Malassis-Seris, M., Briottet, C., and Vassalli, P. (1991a). Two gut intraepithelial $CD8^+$ lymphocyte populations with different T cell receptors: A role for the gut epithelium in T cell differentiation. *J. Exp. Med.* **174,** 471–481.

Guy-Grand, D., Malassis-Seris, M., Briottet, C., and Vassalli, P. (1991b). Cytotoxic differentiation of mouse gut thymodependent and independent intraepithelial T lymphocytes is induced locally. Correlation between functional assays, presence of perforin and granzyme transcripts, and cytoplasmic granules. *J. Exp. Med.* **173,** 1549–1552.

Hall, J. G., Parry, D. M., and Smith, M. E. (1972). The distribution and differentiation of lymph-borne immunoblasts after intravenous injection into syngeneic recipients. *Cell. Tissue Kinet.* **5,** 269–281.

Hall, J. G., Hopkins, J., and Orlans, E. (1977). Studies on the lymphocytes of sheep. III. Destination of lymph-borne immunoblasts in relation to their tissue of origin. *J. Immunol.* **7,** 30–37.

Hanson, D. G., Vaz, N. M., Maia, L. C., Hornbrook, M. M., Lynch, J. M., and Roy, C. A. (1977). Inhibition of specific immune responses by feeding protein antigens. *Int. Arch. Allergy Appl. Immunol.* **55,** 526–532.

Hardy, R. R., and Hayakawa, K. (1986). Development and physiology of Ly-1 B and its human homolog, Leu-1 B. *Immunol. Rev.* **93,** 53–79.

Harriman, G. R., Kunimoto, D. Y., Elliott, J. F., Paetkau, V., and Strober, W. (1988). The role of IL-5 in IgA B cell differentiation. *J. Immunol.* **140,** 3033–3039.

Hayakawa, K., Hardy, R. R., Honda, M., Herzenberg, L. A., Steinberg, A. D., and Herzenberg, L. A. (1983). The 'Ly 1 B' cell subpopulations in normal, immunodefective and autoimmune mice. *J. Exp. Med.* **157,** 202–218.

Hayakawa, K., Hardy, R. R., and Herzenberg, L. A. (1986). Peritoneal Ly-1 B cells: Genetic control, autoantibody production, increased lambda light chain expression. *Eur. J. Immunol.* **16,** 450–456.

Herman, A., Kappler, J. W., Marrack, P., and Pullen, A. M. (1991). Superantigens: Mechanism of T-cell stimulation and role in immune responses. *Ann. Rev. Immunol.* **9,** 745–772.

Herzenberg, L. A., Stall, A. M., Lalor, P. A., Sidman, C., Moore, W. A., Parks, D. R., and Herzenberg, L. A. (1986). The Ly-1 B cell lineage. *Immunol. Rev.* **93,** 81–102.

Hirata, I., Berrebi, G., Austin, L. L., Keren, D. F., and Dobbins, W. O. (1986). Immunoelectron microscopic localization of HLA-

DR antigen in control small intestine and colon and in inflammatory bowel disease. *Dig. Dis. Sci.* **31,** 1317–1330.

Holzmann, B., and Weissman, I. L. (1989). Peyer's patch-specific lymphocyte homing receptors consist of a VLA-4-like α chain associated with either of two integrin β chains, one of which is novel. *EMBO J.* **8,** 1735–1741.

Holzmann, B., McIntyre, B. W., and Weissman, I. L. (1989). Identification of a murine Peyer's patch specific lymphocyte homing receptor as an integrin molecule with an α chain homologous to human VLA-4a. *Cell* **56,** 37–46.

Husband, A. J. (1982). Kinetics of extravasation and redistribution of IgA-specific antibody-containing cells in the intestine. *J. Immunol.* **128,** 1355–1359.

Husband, A. J., and Dunkley, M. L. (1985). Lack of site of origin effects on distribution of IgA antibody-containing cells. *Immunology* **54,** 215–221.

Husband, A. J., and Dunkley, M. L. (1988). Migration of T effector cells: Role of antigen and tissue specificity. *In* "Migration and Homing of Lymphoid Cells" (A. J. Husband, ed.), Vol. II, pp. 35–52. CRC Press, Boca Raton, Florida.

Husband, A. J., and Gowans, J. L. (1978). The origin and antigen-dependent distribution of IgA-containing cells in the intestine. *J. Exp. Med.* **148,** 1146–1160.

Issekutz, T. B. (1984). The response of gut-associated T lymphocytes to intestinal viral immunization. *J. Immunol.* **133,** 2955–2960.

Jalkanen, S., Nash, G. S., De los Toyos, J., MacDermott, R. P., and Butcher, E. C. (1989). Human lamina propria lymphocytes bear homing receptors and bind selectively to mucosal lymphoid high endothelium. *Eur. J. Immunol.* **19,** 63–68.

Jones, P. P., and Cebra, J. J. (1974). Restriction of gene expression in B lymphocytes and their progeny. III. Endogenous IgA and IgM on the membranes of different plasma cell precursors. *J. Exp. Med.* **140,** 966–976.

Jones, P. P., Craig, S. W., Cebra, J. J., and Herzenberg, L. A. (1974). Restriction of gene expression in B lymphocytes and their progeny. II. Commitment to immunoglobulin heavy chain isotype. *J. Exp. Med.* **140,** 452–469.

Kagnoff, M. (1977). Functional characteristics of Peyer's patch lymphoid cells. IV. Effect of antigen feeding on the frequency of antigen-specific B cells. *J. Immunol.* **118,** 992–997.

Kagnoff, M., and Cambell, S. (1974). Functional characteristics of Peyer's patch lymphoid cells. I. Induction of humoral antibody and cell-mediated allograft reactions. *J. Exp. Med.* **139,** 398–406.

Kaiserlian, D., Vidal, K., and Revillard, J.-P. (1989). Murine enterocytes can present soluble antigen to specific class II-restricted CD4+ T cells. *Eur. J. Immunol.* **19,** 1513–1516.

Kanof, M. E., Strober, W., Fiocchi, C., Zeitz, M., and James, S. P. (1988). CD4 positive Leu-8 negative helper–inducer T cells predominate in the human intestinal lamina propria. *J. Immunol.* **14,** 3029–3036.

Kantor, A. (1991a). A new nomenclature for B cells. *Immunol. Today* **12,** 388.

Kantor, A. (1991b). The development and repertoire of B-1 cells (CD5 B cells). *Immunol. Today* **12,** 389–391.

Kawanishi, H., Salzman, L. E., and Strober, W. (1982). Characteristics and regulatory function of murine Con A-induced cloned T cells obtained from Peyer's patches and spleen: Mechanisms regulating isotype-specific immunoglobulin production by Peyer's patch B cells. *J. Immunol.* **129,** 475–483.

Kawanishi, H., Salzman, L. E., and Strober, W. (1983). Mechanisms regulating IgA class-specific immunoglobulin production in murine gut-associated lymphoid tissues. I. T cells derived from Peyer's patches which switch sIgM B cells to SIgA B cells *in vitro*. *J. Exp. Med.* **157,** 433–450.

Keren, D. F., Holt, P. S., Collins, H. H., Gemski, P., and Formal, S. B. (1978). The role of Peyer's patches in the local immune response to live bacteria. *J. Immunol.* **120,** 1892–1896.

Kett, K., Brandtzaeg, P., Radl, J., and Haaijman, J. (1986). Different subclass distribution of IgA-producing cells in human lymphoid organs and various secretory tissues. *J. Immunol.* **136,** 3631–3635.

Kilshaw, P. J., and Murant, S. J. (1990). A new surface antigen on intraepithelial lymphocytes in the intestine. *Eur. J. Immunol.* **20,** 2201–2207.

Kim, P. H., and Kagnoff, M. F. (1990). Transforming growth factor-β is a co-stimulator for IgA production. *J. Immunol.* **144,** 3411–3416.

Kiyono, H., McGhee, J. R., Mosteller, L. M., Eldridge, J. H., Koopman, W. J., Kearney, J. F., and Michalek, S. M. (1982). Murine Peyer's patch T cell clones. Characterization of antigen-specific helper T cells for immunoglobulin A responses. *J. Exp. Med.* **156,** 1115–1130.

Kiyono, H., Cooper, M. D., Kearney, J. F., Mosteller, L. M., Michalek, S. M., Koopman, W. J., and McGhee, J. R. (1984). Isotype specificity of helper T cell clones. Peyer's patch Th cells preferentially collaborate with mature IgA B cells for IgA responses. *J. Exp. Med.* **159,** 798–811.

Klaus, G. G. B., and Humphrey, J. H. (1977). The generation of memory cells. I. The role of C3 in the generation of B memory cells. *Immunology* **33,** 31–40.

Klaus, G. G. B., and Kunkl, A. (1981). The role of germinal centres in the generation of immunological memory. *Ciba Found. Symp.* **84,** 264–280.

Klein, J. R. (1986). Ontogeny of the Thy-1^-, Lyt-2^+ murine intestinal intraepithelial lymphocyte. Characterization of a unique population of thymus-independent cytotoxic effector cells in the intestinal mucosa. *J. Exp. Med.* **164,** 309–314.

Kraal, G., Weissman, I. L., and Butcher, E. C. (1982). Germinal centre B cells: Antigen specificity and changes in heavy chain class expression. *Nature (London)* **298,** 377–379.

Kroese, H. G. M., Butcher, E. C., Stall, A. M., Lalor, P. A., Adams, S., and Herzenberg, L. A. (1989). Many of the IgA producing plasma cells in murine gut are derived from self-replenishing precursors in the peritoneal cavity. *Int. Immunol.* **1,** 75–84.

Kunimoto, D. Y. (1991). Transforming growth factor-beta in a model of IgA switching. *Immunol. Res.* **10,** 400–403.

Kunimoto, D. Y., Nordan, R. P., and Strober, W. (1989). IL-6 is a potent cofactor of IL-1 in IgM synthesis and of Il-5 in IgA synthesis. *J. Immunol.* **143,** 2230–2235.

Lamm, M. E. (1976). Cellular aspects of immunoglobulin A. *Adv. Immunol.* **22,** 223–290.

Lebman, D. A., and Coffman, R. L. (1988). The effects of Il-4 and IL-5 on the IgA response by murine Peyer's patch B cell subpopulations. *J. Immunol.* **141,** 2050–2056.

Lebman, D. A., Griffin, P. M., and Cebra, J. J. (1987). Relationship between expression of IgA by Peyer's patch cells and functional IgA memory cells. *J. Exp. Med.* **166,** 1405–1418.

Lebman, D. A., Fuhrman, J. A., and Cebra, J. J. (1988). Intraduodenal application of cholera holotoxins increases the potential of clones from Peyer's patch B cells of relevant and unrelated specificities to secrete IgG and IgA. *Reg. Immunol.* **1,** 32–40.

Lebman, D. A., Lee, F. D., and Coffman, R. L. (1990a). Mechanism for transforming growth factor-β and IL-2 enhancement of IgA expression in lipopolysaccharide-stimulated B cell cultures. *J. Immunol.* **144,** 952–959.

Lebman, D. A., Nomura, D. Y., Coffman, R. L., and Lee, F. D. (1990b). Molecular characterization of germ-line immunoglobulin α transcripts produced during transforming growth factor type β-induced isotype switching. *Proc. Natl. Acad. Sci. U.S.A.* **87,** 3962–3966.

Lefevre, M. E., Olivio, R., Vanderhoff, J. W., and Joel, D. D. (1978). Accumulation of latex in Peyer's patches and its subsequent appearance in villi and mesenteric lymph nodes. *Proc. Soc. Exp. Biol. Med.* **159,** 289–302.

Lefrancois, L., and Goodman, T. (1989). *In vivo* modulation of cytolytic activity and Thy-1 expression in TCR-γ/δ^+ intraepithelial lymphocytes. *Science* **243,** 1716–1718.

Liang, X, Lamm, M. E., and Nedrud, J. G. (1988). Oral administration of cholera toxin–Sendai virus conjugate potentiates gut and respiratory immunity against Sendai virus. *J. Immunol.* **141,** 1496–1501.

Lin, Y.-C. A., Shockett, P., and Stavnezer, J. (1991). Regulation of the antibody class switch to IgA. *Immunol. Res.* **10,** 376–380.

Linton, P.-J., Decker, D. J., and Klinman, N. R. (1989). Primary antibody-forming cells and secondary B cells are generated from separate precursor cell populations. *Cell* **59,** 1049–1059.

Liu, L. M., and Macpherson, G. G. (1991). Lymph-borne (veiled) dendritic cells can acquire and present intestinally administered antigens. *Immunology* **73,** 281–286.

McDermott, M. R., and Bienenstock, J. (1979). Evidence for a common mucosal immunologic system. I. Migration of B immunoblasts into intestinal, respiratory and genital tissues. *J. Immunol.* **122,** 1892–1898.

McDermott, M. R., Clark, D. A., and Bienenstock, J. (1980). Evidence for a common mucosal immunologic system. II. Influence of the estrous cycle on B immunoblast migration into genital and intestinal tissues. *J. Immunol.* **124,** 2536–2539.

McDermott, M. R., Horsewood, P., Clark, D. A., and Bienenstock, J. (1986). T lymphocytes in the intestinal epithelium and lamina propria of mice. *Immunology* **57,** 213–218.

McWilliams, M., Phillips-Quagliata, J. M., and Lamm, M. E. (1975). Characteristics of mesenteric lymph node cells homing to gut-associated lymphoid tissue in syngeneic mice. *J. Immunol.* **115,** 54–58.

McWilliams, M., Phillips-Quagliata, J. M., and Lamm, M. E. (1977). Mesenteric lymph node B lymphoblasts which home to the small intestine are precommitted to IgA synthesis. *J. Exp. Med.* **145,** 866–875.

Mayer, L., and Shlien, R. (1987). Evidence for function of Ia molecules on gut epithelial cells in man. *J. Exp. Med.* **166,** 1471–1483.

Mayrhofer, G. (1980). Fixation and staining of granules in mucosal mast cells and intraepithelial lymphocytes in the rat jejunum with special reference to the relationship between the acid glycosaminoglycans in the two cell types. *Histochem. J.* **12,** 513–526.

Mayrhofer, G., and Fisher, R. (1979). IgA-containing cells in the lamina propria of the gut: Failure of a thoracic duct fistula to deplete the numbers in the rat small intestine. *Eur. J. Immunol.* **9,** 85–91.

Mega, J., Bruce, M. G., Beagley, K. W., McGhee, J. R., Taguchi, T., Pitts, A. M., McGhee, M. L., Bucy, R. P., Eldridge, J. H., Mestecky, J., and Kiyono, H. (1991). Regulation of mucosal responses by CD4+ T lymphocytes: Effects of anti-L3T4 treatment on the gastrointestinal immune system. *Int. Immunol.* **3,** 793–805.

Montgomery, P. C., Ayyildiz, A., Lemaître-Coelho, I. M., Vaerman, J.-P., and Rockey, J. H. (1983). Induction and expression of antibodies in secretions: The ocular immune system. *Ann. N.Y. Acad. Sci.* **409,** 428–439.

Mosmann, T. R., Cherwinski, H., Bond, M. W., Giedlin, M. A., and Coffman, R. L. (1986). Two types of murine helper T cell clone I. Definition according to profiles of lymphokine activities and secreted proteins. *J. Immunol.* **136,** 2348–2357.

Murray, P. D., McKenzie, D. T., Swain, S. L., and Kagnoff, M. F. (1987). Interleukin 5 and interleukin 4 produced by Peyer's patch T cells selectively enhance immunoglobulin A expression. *J. Immunol.* **139,** 2669–2674.

Nair, P. N. R., and Schroeder, H. E. (1986). Duct-associated lymphoid tissue (DALT) of minor salivary glands and mucosal immunity. *Immunology* **57,** 171–180.

Ngan, J., and Kind, L. S. (1978). Suppressor T cells for IgE and IgG in Peyer's patches of mice made tolerant by the oral administration of ovalbumin. *J. Immunol.* **120,** 861–865.

Nieuwenhuis, P., van Nouhuijs, C. E., Eggens, J. H., and Keuning, F. J. (1974). Germinal centers and the origin of the B cell system. I. Germinal centers in the rabbit appendix. *Immunology* **26,** 497–507.

Nieuwenhuis, P., Gastkemper, N. A., and Opstelten, D. (1981). Histophysiology of follicular structures and germinal centers in relation to B cell differentiation. *Ciba Found. Symp.* **84,** 246–259.

Ogra, P. L., Karzon, D. T., Righthand, F., and MacGillivray, M. (1968). Immunoglobulin response in serum and secretions after immunization with live and attenuated polio vaccine and natural infection. *N. Engl. J. Med.* **279,** 893–900.

Ottaway, C. A., Bruce, R. G., and Parrott, D. M. V. (1983). The *in vivo* kinetics of lymphoblast localization in the small intestine. *Immunology* **49,** 641–648.

Owen, R. L. (1977). Sequential uptake of horseradish peroxidase by lymphoid follicle epithelium of Peyer's patches in the normal unobstructed mouse intestine: An ultrastructural study. *Gastroenterology* **72,** 440–451.

Owen, R. L., and Jones, A. L. (1974). Epithelial cell specialization within human Peyer's patches: An ultrastructural study of intestinal lymphoid follicles. *Gastroenterology* **66,** 189–203.

Owen, R. L., and Nemanic, P. (1978). Antigen processing structures of the mammalian intestinal tract: An SEM study of lymphoepithelial organs. *Scanning Electron Microsc.* **11,** 367–378.

Papamichail, M., Guttierrez, C., Embling, P., Johnson, P., Holborow, E. J., and Pepys, M. D. (1975). Complement dependency of localization of aggregated IgG in germinal centers. *Scand. J. Immunol.* **4,** 343–347.

Parrott, D. M. V., and Ferguson, A. (1974). Selective migration of lymphocytes within the mouse small intestine. *Immunology* **26,** 571–588.

Parrott, D. M. V., Tait, C., MacKenzie, S., McI. Mowat, A., Davies, M. D. J., and Micklem, H. S. (1983). Analysis of the effector functions of different populations of mucosal lymphocytes. *Ann. N.Y. Acad. Sci.* **409,** 307–319.

Phillips-Quagliata, J. M., and Lamm, M. E. (1988). Migration of lymphocytes in the mucosal immune system. *In* "Migration and Homing of Lymphoid Cells" (A. J. Husband, ed.), Vol. II, pp. 53–76. CRC Press, Boca Raton, Florida.

Phillips-Quagliata, J. M., and Al Maghazachi, A. (1987). T cell clones that help IgA responses. *In* "Recent Advances in Mucosal Immunology" (J. Mestecky, J. R. McGhee, J. Bienenstock, and P. L. Ogra, eds.), Part A, pp. 101–117. Plenum, New York.

Phillips-Quagliata, J. M., Roux, M. E., Arny, M., Kelly-Hatfield, P., McWilliams, M., and Lamm, M. E. (1983). Migration and regulation of B-cells in the mucosal immune system. *Ann. N.Y. Acad. Sci.* **409,** 194–202.

Picker, L. J., and Butcher, E. C. (1992). Physiological and molecular mechanisms of lymphocyte homing. *Ann. Rev. Immunol.* **10,** 561–591.

Pierce, N. F., and Cray, W. C., Jr. (1982). Determinants of the localization and duration of a specific mucosal IgA plasma cell response in enterically immunized animals. *J. Immunol.* **128,** 1311–1315.

Pierce, N. F., and Gowans, J. L. (1975). Cellular kinetics of the intestinal immune response to cholera toxoid in rats. *J. Exp. Med.* **142,** 1550–1563.

Pierce, N. F., and Koster, F. T. (1980). Priming and suppression of the intestinal immune response to cholera toxoid/toxin by parenteral toxoid in rats. *J. Immunol.* **124,** 307–311.

Pierce, N. F., Cray, W. C., and Sacci, J. B. (1982). Oral immunization against experimental cholera: The role of antigen form and antigen combinations in evoking protection. *Ann. N.Y. Acad. Sci.* **409,** 724–732.

Racz, P., Tenner-Racz, K., Myrvik, Q. N., and Fainter, L. K. (1977). Functional architecture of bronchial-associated lymphoid tissue and lymphoepithelium in pulmonary cell-mediated reactions in the rabbit. *J. Reticuloendothel. Soc.* **22,** 59–83.

Reichert, R. A., Gallatin, W. M., Weissman, I. L., and Butcher, E. C. (1983). Germinal center B cells lack homing receptors necessary for normal lymphocyte recirculation. *J. Exp. Med.* **157,** 813–827.

Richardson, J., Bouchard, T., and Ferguson, C. C. (1976). Uptake and transport of exogenous proteins by respiratory epithelium. *Lab. Invest.* **35,** 307–314.

Richman, L. K., Chiller, J. M., Brown, W. R., Hanson, D. G., and Vaz, N. M. (1978). Enterically induced immunological tolerance. I. Induction of suppressor T lymphocytes by intragastric administration of soluble proteins. *J. Immunol.* **121,** 2429–2434.

Richman, L. K., Graeff, A. S., Yarchoan, R., and Strober, W. (1981). Simultaneous induction of antigen-specific IgA helper T cells and IgG suppressor T cells in the murine Peyer's patch after protein feeding. *J. Immunol.* **126,** 2079–2083.

Riggs, J. E., Stowers, R. S., and Mosier, D. E. (1990). The immunoglobulin allotype contributed by peritoneal cavity B cells dominates in SCID mice reconstituted with allotype-disparate mixtures of splenic and peritoneal cavity B cells. *J. Exp. Med.* **172,** 475–484.

Robertson, S. M., and Cebra, J. J. (1976). A model for local immunity. *Ric. Clin. Lab.* **6,** (Suppl. 3), 105–119.

Rocha, B., Vassalli, P., and Guy-Grand, D. (1991). The Vβ repertoire of mouse gut homodimeric α CD8+ intraepithelial T cell receptor α/β+ lymphocytes reveals a major extrathymic pathway of T cell differentiation. *J. Exp. Med.* **173,** 483–486.

Rose, M. L., Parrott, D. M. V., and Bruce, R. G. (1976). Migration of lymphoblasts to the small intestine. II. Divergent migration of mesenteric and peripheral immunoblasts to sites of inflammation in the mouse. *Cell. Immunol.* **27,** 36–46.

Roux, M. E., McWilliams, M., Phillips-Quagliata, J. M., and Lamm, M. E. (1977). Origin of IgA-secreting cells in the mammary gland. *J. Exp. Med.* **146,** 1311–1322.

Roux, M. E., McWilliams, M., Phillips-Quagliata, J. M., and Lamm, M. E. (1981). Differentiation pathway of Peyer's patch precursors of IgA plasma cells in the secretory immune system. *Cell. Immunol.* **61,** 141–153.

Roy, M. J. (1987). Precocious development of lectin (*Ulex europaeus* agglutinin I) receptors in dome epithelium of gut-associated lymphoid tissues. *Cell Tissue Res.* **248,** 483–489.

Roy, M. J., Ruiz, A., and Varvanyis, M. (1987). A novel antigen is common to the dome epithelium of gut and bronchus-associated lymphoid tissues. *Cell Tissue Res.* **248,** 635–644.

Rudzik, O., and Bienenstock, J. (1974). Isolation and characterization of gut mucosal lymphocytes. *Lab. Invest.* **30,** 260–266.

Rudzik, O., Perey, D. Y. E., and Bienenstock, J. (1975a). Differential IgA repopulation after transfer of autologous and allogeneic rabbit Peyer's patch cells. *J. Immunol.* **114,** 40–44.

Rudzik, O., Clancy, R. L., Perey, D. Y. E., Day, R. P., and Bienenstock, J. (1975b). Repopulation with IgA-containing cells of bronchial and intestinal lamina propria after transfer of homologous Peyer's patches and bronchial lymphocytes. *J. Immunol.* **114,** 1599–1604.

Schmidt, G. H., Wilkinson, M. M., and Ponder, B. A. J. (1985). Cell migration pathway in the intestinal epithelium: An *in situ* marker system using mouse aggregation chimeras. *Cell* **40,** 425–429.

Schrader, C. E., George, A., Kerlin, R. L., and Cebra, J. J. (1990). Dendritic cells support production of IgA and other non-IgM isotypes in clonal microculture. *Int. Immunol.* **2,** 563–570.

Scicchitano, R., Stanisz, A., Ernst, P., and J. Bienenstock (1988). A common mucosal immune system revisited. *In* "Migration and Homing of Lymphoid Cells" (A. J. Husband, ed.), Vol. II, pp. 3–34. CRC Press, Boca Raton, Florida.

Shimizu, Y., and Andrew, W. (1967). Studies on the rabbit appendix. I. Lymphocyte-epithelial relations and the transport of bacteria from lumen to lymphoid nodule. *J. Morphol.* **123,** 231–237.

Solvason, N., Lehuen, A., and Kearney, J. F. (1991). An embryonic source of Ly 1 but not conventional B cells. *Int. Immunol.* **3,** 543–550.

Sonoda, E., Matsumoto, R., Hitoshi, Y., Ishii, T., Sugimoto, M., Araki, S., Tominaga, A., Yamaguchi, N., and Takatsu, K. (1989). Transforming growth factor-β induces IgA production and acts additively with interleukin 5 for IgA production. *J. Exp. Med.* **170,** 1415–1420.

Spit, B. J., Hendriksen, E. G. J., Bruijntjes, J. P., and Kuper, C. F. (1989). Nasal lymphoid tissue in the rat. *Cell Tissue Res.* **255,** 193–198.

Sprent, J. (1976). Fate of H-2 activated T lymphocytes in syngeneic hosts. I. Fate in lymphoid tissue and intestines traced with ^{3}H-thymidine, ^{125}I-deoxyuridine, and ^{51}chromium. *Cell. Immunol.* **21,** 278–302.

Streeter, P. R., Berg, E. L., Rouse, B. T. N., Bargatz, R. F., and Butcher, E. C. (1988). A tissue-specific endothelial cell molecule involved in lymphocyte homing. *Nature (London)* **331,** 41–46.

Swain, S. L., McKenzie, D. T., Weinberg, A. D., and Hancock, W. (1988). Characterization of T helper 1 and 2 subsets in normal mice. Helper T cells responsible for IL-4 and IL-5 production are present as precursors that require priming before they develop into lymphokine-secreting cells. *J. Immunol.* **141,** 3445–3455.

Tagliabue, A., Luini, W., Soldateschi, D., and Boraschi, D. (1981). Natural killer activity of gut mucosal lymphoid cells in mice. *Eur. J. Immunol.* **11,** 919–922.

Tagliabue, A., Befus, A. D., Clark, D. A., and Bienenstock, J. (1982). Characteristics of natural killer cells in the murine intestinal epithelium and lamina propria. *J. Exp. Med.* **155,** 1785–1796.

Takagaki, Y., De Cloux, A., Bonneville, M., and Tonegawa, S. (1989). Diversity of $\gamma\delta$ T-cell receptors on murine intestinal intraepithelial lymphocytes. *Nature (London)* **339,** 712–714.

Teale, J. M. (1983). The use of specific helper T cell clones to study the regulation of isotype expression by antigen-stimulated B cell clones. *J. Immunol.* **131,** 2170–2177.

Thomas, H. C., and Parrott, D. M. V. (1974). The induction of tolerance to soluble protein antigens by oral administration. *Immunology* **27,** 631–639.

Thorbecke, G. J., Romano, T. J., and Lerman, S. P. (1974). Regulatory mechanisms in proliferation and differentiation of lymphoid tissue with particular reference to germinal center development. *Prog. Immunol.* **3,** 25–34.

Tseng, J. (1981). Transfer of lymphocytes of Peyer's patches between immunoglobulin allotype congenic mice: Repopulation of the IgA cells in the gut lamina propria. *J. Immunol.* **127,** 2039–2043.

Tseng, J. (1984a). A population of resting IgM-IgD double-bearing lymphocytes in Peyer's patches: The major precursor cells for IgA plasma cells in the gut lamina propria. *J. Immunol.* **132,** 2730–2735.

Tseng, J. (1984b). Repopulation of the gut lamina propria with IgA-containing cells by lymphoid cells isolated from the gut lamina propria. *Eur. J. Immunol.* **14,** 420–425.

Tseng, J. (1988). Migration and differentiation of IgA precursor cells in the gut-associated lymphoid tissue. *In* "Migration and Homing of Lymphoid Cells" (A. J. Husband, ed.), Vol. II, pp. 77–98. CRC Press, Boca Raton, Florida.

Tsiagbe, V. K., and Thorbecke, G. J. (1991). Memory B cells and germinal centres. *Res. Immunol.* **142,** 268–272.

van der Brugge-Gamelkoorn, J., van de Ende, M. B., and Sminia, T. (1985). Nonlymphoid cells of bronchus-associated lymphoid tissue of the rat in situ and in suspension. *Cell Tissue Res.* **239,** 177–182.

Vaz, N. M., Maia, L. C. S., Hanson, D. G., and Lynch, J. M. (1977). Inhibition of homocytotropic antibody responses in adult inbred mice by previous feeding of the specific antigen. *J. Allergy Appl. Immunol.* **60,** 110–115.

Waksman, B. H., and Ozer, H. (1976). Specialized amplification elements in the immune system. *Progr. Allergy* **21,** 1–113.

Waksman, B. H., Ozer, H., and Blythman, H. E. (1973). Appendix and γM-antibody formation. VI. The functional anatomy of the rabbit appendix. *Lab. Invest.* **28,** 614–626.

Weisz-Carrington, P., Roux, M. E., McWilliams, M., Phillips-Quagliata, J. M., and Lamm, M. E. (1978). Hormonal induction of the secretory immune system in the mammary gland. *Proc. Natl. Acad. Sci. U.S.A.* **75,** 2928–2932.

Weisz-Carrington, P., Roux, M. E., McWilliams, M., Phillips-Quagliata, J. M., and Lamm, M. E. (1979). Organ and isotype distribution of plasma cells producing specific antibody after oral immunization: Evidence for a generalized secretory immune system. *J. Immunol.* **123,** 1705–1708.

Weltzin, R., Lucia-Jandris, P., Michetti, P., Fields, B. N., Kraehenbuhl, J. P., and Neutra, M. R. (1989). Binding and transepithelial transport of immunoglobulins by intestinal M cells: Demonstration using monoclonal IgA antibodies against enteric viral proteins. *J. Cell Biol.* **108,** 1673–1685.

Williamson, A. R., Zitron, I. M., and McMichael, A. J. (1976). Clones of B lymphocytes, their natural selection and expansion. *Fed. Proc.* **35,** 2195–2201.

Wu, M., Van Kaer, L., Itohara, S., and Tonegawa, S. (1991). Highly restricted expression of the thymus leukemia antigens on intestinal epithelial cells. *J. Exp. Med.* **174,** 213–218.

Zeitz, M., Scheiferdecker, H. L., Ullrich, R., Jahn, H.-U., James, S. P., and Riecken, E.-O. (1991). Phenotype and function of lamina propria T lymphocytes. *Immunol. Res.* **10,** 199–206.

Section C

Cells, Regulation, and Specificity in the Mucosal Immune System: Effector Sites

Section Editor: Jerry R. McGhee

Part a · The Normal State
(Chapters 20 through 24)

Part b · Mucosal Immunity and Inflammation
(Chapters 25 through 29)

20

Cytokines in the Mucosal Immune System

Deborah A. Lebman • Robert L. Coffman

I. INTRODUCTION

The expression of specific isotypes is regulated by cytokines that act either to mediate heavy-chain class switching or to stimulate the maturation of B cells expressing particular isotypes. The mucosal immune system is distinguished from other secondary lymphoid organs by the predominance of IgA in mucosal secretions. In considering the potential relevance of cytokines in the generation of an IgA response *in vivo,* we must realize that the processes of isotype switching to IgA and maturation of membrane IgA-expressing cells to IgA-secreting cells take place in different anatomical locations. The precursors of IgA-secreting cells are generated primarily in the Peyer's patches (Craig and Cebra, 1971). However, IgA-secreting plasma cells are found in the lamina propria of exocrine tissues (Tomasi, 1983).

Although the actual basis for the preferential generation of an IgA response in mucosal tissues remains unclear, the identification of cytokines that specifically stimulate IgA expression *in vitro* raises the possibility that local production of specific cytokines within mucosal tissues is involved in the establishment of a microenvironment conducive to the generation of a secretory IgA response. Although several cytokines that affect IgA secretion have been described, we must realize that little evidence exists that these cytokines act analogously on IgA secretion *in vivo* and *in vitro*. However, precedence does exist for cytokines that regulate isotype secretion *in vitro* acting similarly *in vivo* (Finkelman *et al.,* 1989). Specifically, interleukin 4 (IL-4), which was shown to mediate isotype switching to IgE *in vitro,* appears to have a similar function *in vivo*. The following sections describe the mechanism of action of different cytokines that influence IgA expression and discuss production of cytokines in mucosal tissues.

II. CYTOKINES THAT INFLUENCE MATURATION OF IgA-EXPRESSING CELLS TO IgA-SECRETING CELLS

A. Interleukin 5

The initial description of a factor in T-cell supernatants that enhanced IgA secretion (IgA-enhancing factor or IL-5) was followed by a series of papers describing its mechanism of action (Coffman *et al.,* 1987; Murray *et al.,* 1987). IL-5 is a dimeric polypeptide with a molecular mass of 45–60 kDa (Bond *et al.,* 1987). The initial reports demonstrated that IL-5 alone caused a four to fivefold enhancement in IgA secretion in cultures of B cells stimulated with the mitogen lipopolysaccharide (LPS). The increase in IgA secretion was augmented further by the addition of a second cytokine, IL-4, which by itself has little effect on IgA secretion. Both cytokines characteristically are produced by a subset of helper T cells—Th2 cells (Mosmann and Coffman, 1989).

The most commonly used culture systems for investigating the effects of cytokines on isotype expression are LPS-stimulated B-cell cultures. The addition of IL-5 to LPS-stimulated cultures of either splenic or Peyer's patch B cells resulted in a comparable three-to-fivefold increase in IgA secretion (Lebman and Coffman, 1988b). To elucidate the mechanism of action of IL-5, Peyer's patches were separated into $mIgA^+$ and $mIgA^-$ populations, which then were stimulated separately with LPS in the presence or absence of IL-5. Interestingly, the results obtained in different laboratories were disparate. Some investigators observed that the majority of IgA was derived from the $mIgA^+$ population and suggested that IL-5 acted to stimulate the maturation of mIgA-expressing cells to IgA-secreting cells (Harriman *et al.,* 1988). However, others observed that the majority of secreted IgA in these cultures was derived from the $mIgA^-$ population (Lebman and Coffman, 1988b). One drawback in using LPS-stimulated cultures to study the effects of cytokines on Peyer's patch populations is the nature of the LPS-responsive population itself. The majority of $mIgA^+$ cells in the Peyer's patch are derived from germinal center cells, which can be distinguished by their ability to bind relatively higher levels of peanut agglutinin (PNA) than non-germinal center cells (Butcher *et al.,* 1982). Peyer's patch cells were separated into PNA^{high} and PNA^{low} populations and stimulated with LPS alone or with IL-5. Not only was the majority of secreted IgA derived from the PNA^{low} population, but the PNA^{high} population was essentially nonresponsive (Lebman and Coffman, 1988b). Thus, a large proportion of $mIgA^+$ cells cannot respond in these cultures.

The mechanism for IL-5-induced enhancement of IgA secretion was resolved using a different culture system. Instead of polyclonally activating B cells with the mitogen LPS, B cells were stimulated with an autoreactive T helper cell (Lebman and Coffman, 1988b), a Th1 cell that secreted neither IL-4 nor IL-5 and, by itself, stimulated substantial proliferation but very little immunoglobulin secretion. In T cell-stimulated cultures, Peyer's patch B cells secreted considerably more IgA than splenic B cells. Further, the majority of secreted IgA in these cultures was derived from the mIgA$^+$ population, suggesting that IL-5 stimulates maturation of IgA-committed precursors and not heavy-chain class switching to IgA.

The previously described studies investigated the effects of IL-5 on B cells that were activated *in vitro*. One of the characteristics of gut-associated lymphoid tissue (GALT) is the presence of chronically active germinal centers in the Peyer's patches. As a consequence, a significant proportion of Peyer's patch mIgA$^+$ cells that are located in the germinal centers are also in cycle, that is, they are activated *in vivo* (Butcher *et al.*, 1982; Lebman *et al.*, 1987). IL-5 induces this *in vivo* activated mIgA$^+$ population to high rate IgA secretion (Beagley *et al.*, 1988). Although the Peyer's patches are the source of precursors of IgA-secreting cells, maturation does not occur within them (Craig and Cebra, 1971; Tomasi, 1983). Thus, if IL-5 acts *in vivo* to stimulate maturation of IgA-expressing cells to IgA-secreting cells, it does not act within the microenvironment of the Peyer's patch. However, evidence suggests that IL-5 can influence IgA secretion *in vivo*. Transgenic mice carrying the IL-5 gene have both elevated levels of serum IL-5 and elevated levels of IgA and IgM (Tominaga *et al.*, 1991).

B. Interleukin 2

In the course of the early studies investigating the IgA-enhancing effects of recombinant cytokines, IL-1, IL-3, granulocyte–macrophage colony stimulating factor (GM-CSF), and interferon γ (IFNγ) were observed not to alter IgA secretion in cultures of LPS-stimulated blasts. However, IL-2 caused a two- to threefold enhancement in IgA secretion in these cultures (Coffman *et al.*, 1987). Additional studies demonstrated that, analogous to IL-5, IL-2 induced a higher level of IgA secretion in T cell-stimulated cultures of Peyer's patch B cells than in similar cultures of splenic B cells (D. A. Lebman and R. L. Coffman, unpublished results). The secreted IgA in these cultures was derived from the mIgA$^+$ population, suggesting that IL-2 can act to cause maturation to IgA secretion (Table I). IL-2 is less effective than the combination of IL-4 and IL-5 in stimulating IgA secretion. However, these data indicate that cytokines characteristic of both Th1 and Th2 cells (cf. Section V; Chapter 20) are capable of playing a role in the terminal differentiation of mIgA-expressing cells.

Table I IgA Secretion in Th-Stimulated Cultures[a]

B cell population[b]	Additions	IgA (ng/ml)
Total PP	Medium	30
	IL-2	60
	IL-4 + IL-5	2000
mIgA$^+$ PP	Medium	130
	IL-2	3000
	IL-4 + IL-5	11800
mIgA$^-$ PP	Medium	<3
	IL-2	20
	IL-4 + IL-5	330

[a] B cells were stimulated with a Th1 helper cell and the indicated additions for 7 days.

[b] T-depleted Peyer's patches (PP) were separated into mIgA$^+$ and mIgA$^-$ populations using flow cytometry.

C. Interleukin 6

IL-6 has a broad range of activities in both lymphoid and nonlymphoid tissues (reviewed by Van Snick, 1990). Historically, the molecule that ultimately was identified as IL-6 was associated with growth and differentiation of B-lineage cells. Accessory cells, particularly macrophages, are a primary source of IL-6 in freshly isolated lymphoid cell cultures (Van Snick, 1990). Consequently, the effect of IL-6 on isotype production in murine lymphocytes was investigated in cultures of purified Peyer's patch B cells in the absence of mitogen (Beagley *et al.*, 1989; Kunimoto *et al.*, 1989). In unfractionated Peyer's patch B cells, IL-6 induced a higher level of IgA secretion than IL-5 (Beagley *et al.*, 1989). Other investigators observed that either IL-5 or IL-6 alone induced a modest increase in IgA secretion in cultures of T cell-depleted Peyer's patch cells, but the combination of the two cytokines greatly increased the level of IgA secretion (Kunimoto *et al.*, 1989). The combination of IL-5 and IL-6 was particularly effective in enhancing IgA secretion. Although IL-6 induced mIgA$^+$ cells that were activated *in vivo* to secrete IgA, it did not increase IgM or IgG secretion in cultures of Peyer's patch B cells. Further, IL-6 did not cause mIgA$^-$ cells to secrete IgA, suggesting that the effect of IL-6 was not stimulation of isotype switching to IgA. Thus, to date, three cytokines—IL-2, IL-5, and IL-6—have been shown to play a role in promoting the maturation of murine mIgA-expressing cells into IgA-secreting cells. However, evidence only exists to substantiate a role *in vivo* for IL-5.

III. CYTOKINES THAT INDUCE ISOTYPE SWITCHING TO IgA

Transforming growth factor β (TGFβ) is a ubiquitous 25-kDa peptide (Sporn *et al.*, 1986) that is pleiotropic in action. TGFβ was characterized initially on the basis of its ability to stimulate anchorage-independent growth of fibroblasts (Assoian *et al.*, 1983). In early studies on its effects on lymphoid populations, TGFβ was shown to inhibit both human T-cell proliferation and immunoglobulin secretion (Kehrl et al., 1986, 1987) and to prevent the maturation of murine pre-B cells to mature B cells (Lee *et al.*, 1987). As a result of these studies, TGFβ was regarded to be immunosuppressive. Since many recombinant cytokines were derived from supernatants of Cos-7 cells, a fibroblast cell line that secretes TGFβ, investigating the effects of TGFβ in B-cell cultures became important. Although Beagley and colleagues did not see any effect of TGFβ on IgA production by unstimulated Peyer's patch B cells (Beagley *et al.*, 1989), Coffman and colleagues (1989a) observed that the addition of TGFβ to LPS-stimulated splenic B cells induced a 5-to 10-fold increase in IgA secretion concomitant with a similar decrease in IgM secretion. Further, the addition of both IL-2 and TGFβ to LPS-stimulated cultures induced an enhancement in IgA secretion that was greater than the combined effects of either cytokine alone, suggesting that IL-2 could synergize with TGFβ in generating an IgA response. The basic finding of this study was confirmed by several other groups of investigators (Sonoda *et al.*, 1989; Chen and Li, 1990; Kim and Kagnoff, 1990a). IL-5 also was observed to synergize with TGFβ to enhance IgA secretion (Sonoda *et al.*, 1989). Interestingly, some variation exists in the ability of TGFβ alone to stimulate IgA secretion. Some investigators have found it necessary to add both TGFβ and IL-2 to cultures to obtain significant enhancement in IgA secretion (Kim and Kagnoff, 1990a).

Studies at the cellular level of the effect of TGFβ on IgA secretion have provided evidence that TGFβ acts to stimulate isotype switching to IgA. In the initial reports on the IgA-enhancing ability of TGFβ, an interesting dichotomy was observed (Coffman *et al.*, 1989a). Although TGFβ enhanced IgA secretion by $mIgA^-$ cells, it inhibited IgA secretion by $mIgA^+$ cells. Nonetheless, TGFβ induced an increase in the proportion of $mIgA^+$ cells (Lebman *et al.*, 1990a). The addition of IL-2 to cultures containing LPS and TGFβ neither caused a further increase in the proportion of $mIgA^+$ cells nor overcame TGFβ-induced inhibition of proliferation, yet the addition of IL-2 to TGFβ-containing cultures caused an additional 10-to 20-fold increase in IgA secretion. The observation that only a small proportion of splenic B cells was induced to express mIgA by TGFβ raised the possibility that expressing mIgA was not necessary to develop into an IgA-secreting cell. To address this issue, splenic B cells were stimulated with LPS in the presence of both TGFβ and IL-2 for 4 days. Subsequently, the $mIgA^+$ and $mIgA^-$ cells were isolated and cultured for an additional 3 days. Virtually all the secreted IgA was derived from cells that were induced to express mIgA. Thus, the combination of TGFβ and IL-2 caused a transition from $mIgA^-$ to $mIgA^+$ to IgA-secreting cells (Lebman *et al.*, 1990a). Additional evidence for the roles of TGFβ and IL-2 in IgA responses was derived from limiting dilution analysis (Kim and Kagnoff, 1990b). TGFβ, but not IL-2, caused approximately a 20-fold increase in the frequency of IgA-secreting cells. Further, the addition of IL-2 to TGFβ-containing cultures increased IgA secretion without increasing the frequency of IgA-secreting cells. Collectively, these studies indicate that TGFβ induces isotype switching to IgA and IL-2 acts to induce terminal differentiation of mIgA-expressing cells.

Molecular analysis of the effects of cytokines on IgA protection has provided additional insights into both the role of cytokines and the specific T helper cell populations in the generation of IgA responses at mucosal sites. Heavy-chain class switching requires a recombination between switch (S) regions located immediately 5′ to each heavy-chain locus (C_H). This recombination juxtaposes a specific variable region (V_H) with a new C_H (Davis *et al.*, 1980). A large body of evidence in normal cells and cell lines demonstrated that this recombination is preceded by the appearance of transcripts containing germ line sequences (Stavnezer *et al.*, 1985, 1988; Lutzker and Alt, 1988; Berton *et al.*,1989; Esser and Radbruch, 1989; Radcliffe *et al.*, 1990). These germline transcipts initiate 5′ to the particular S region to which recombination is targeted and proceed downstream through the constant region. The association of germline transcripts with IgA expression initially was described in the I.29 cell line (Stavnezer *et al.*, 1988). On stimulation with LPS, I.29 cells switch preferentially to either IgA or IgE. However, prior to stimulation, these cells contain germline transcripts consisting of a pseudo-exon 5′ to Sα (Iα) spliced to Cα (Radcliffe *et al.*, 1990). The addition of TGFβ to LPS-stimulated B-cell cultures results in the appearance of similar transcripts (Figure 1; Lebman *et al.*, 1990).

Secreted IgA from cultures stimulated with a Th2 specific for rabbit immunoglobulin is antigen dependent. Further, the secreted IgA in these cultures is derived from $mIgA^+$ cells (D. A. Lebman, unpublished results). In contrast to TGFβ-containing LPS-stimulated cultures, the induction of IgA secretion in Th2 cell-stimulated, antigen-dependent cultures is not accompanied by the appearance of germline α mRNA transcripts (Figure 2). The model proposing that isotype switching is preceded by the appearance of germline transcripts is supported further by the observation that the CH12 lymphoma, which preferentially undergoes isotype switching to IgA, contains germline α mRNA transcripts (Figure 2).

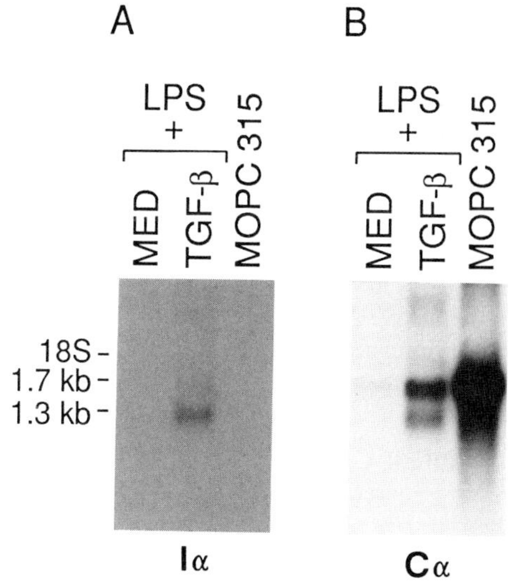

Figure 1 Transforming growth factor β (TGF-β) induces germline α mRNA transcripts. Poly (A)+ RNA was isolated from splenic B cells stimulated for 3 days as indicated. Total mRNA was isolated from the IgA-secreting myeloma MOPC 315. (A) Northern blot was hybridized with a probe specific for germline transcripts (Iα). (B) The same northern blot was hybridized with a constant region probe that would detect both productive and germline α mRNA (Cα). Reprinted with permission from Lebman *et al.* (1990b).

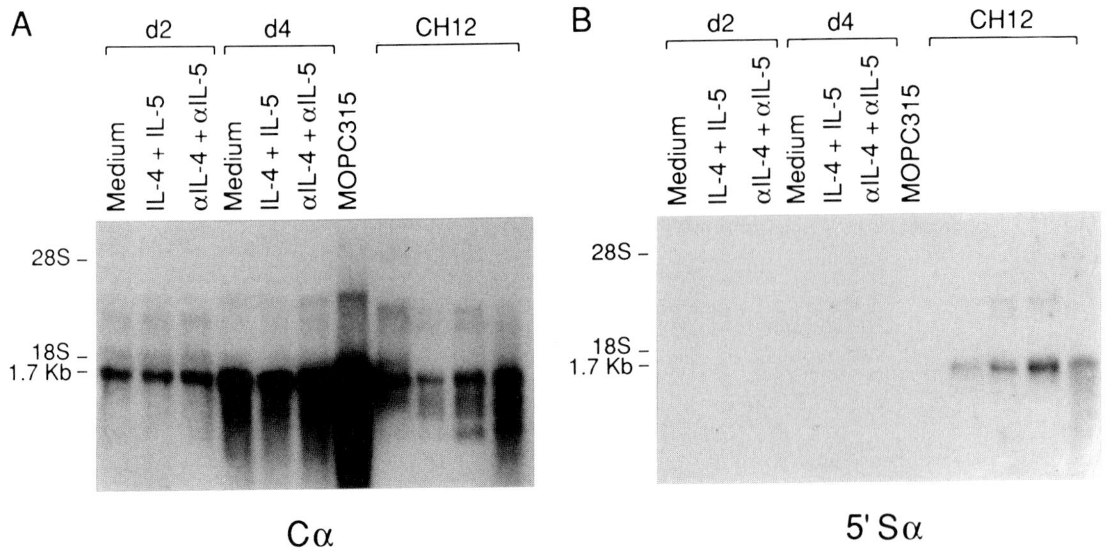

Figure 2 Stimulation with Th2 cells does not induce isotype switching. Peyer's patch B cells were stimulated with a T helper cell specific for rabbit immunoglobulin and rabbit anti-mouse IgA alone or in the presence of cytokines or anti-cytokines, as indicated. (A) Northern blot was hybridized with a Cα probe. (B) Northern blot was hybridized with a probe specific for germline α mRNA (5′Sα).

Thus, studies on the molecular mechanism of isotype switching confirm the functions of TGFβ and Th2 cytokines in isotype switching and maturation of mIgA-expressing cells to IgA-secreting cells, respectively.

IV. CYTOKINES INVOLVED IN IgA EXPRESSION BY HUMAN B CELLS

Several cytokines that act to enhance the maturation of mIgA$^+$ murine B cells to IgA-secreting cells or to induce isotype switching to IgA have been described (Table II). However, the effects of cytokines on isotype secretion by human B cells are not as well documented. The problem in studying the action of cytokines in the human B-cell system appears to stem, in part, from a difficulty in finding methods to stimulate growth and differentiation of human B cells in a way analogous to murine B cell stimulation. However, several groups have approached this problem using different protocols to stimulate B cells. As the results emerge, similarities and differences appear in the response patterns of human and murine B cells. In comparing the results obtained with human B cells to those obtained with murine B cells, note that not only are the stimuli not comparable but the source of cells is also different. The information on murine cells has been gained largely by studying the response of Peyer's patch or splenic B cells whereas, in human studies, the B cells frequently are derived from the tonsils.

Table II Cytokines than Enhance IgA Secretion by Murine B Cells[a]

Isotype switching	Maturation
TGF-β	IL-2
	IL-5
	IL-6

[a] Cytokines are characterized as stimulating heavy chain class switching by mIgA$^-$ cells (isotype switching) or as enhancing secretion by mIgA$^+$ cells (maturation).

Virtually all human B cells can be induced to proliferate by stimulating them for 3 days in the presence of phorbol dibutyrate and ionomycin (Flores-Romo *et al.*, 1990). The addition of either IL-2 or IFNα to these cultures caused enhanced secretion of IgA. In contrast, IL-5 had no effect on IgA secretion in these cultures. A second protocol for inducing human B-cell proliferation is triggering them by cross-linking CD40 antigen (Rousset *et al.*, 1991). To do this, anti-CD40 is presented to B cells on fibroblast cells that stably express FcγRII/CDw32. Since this method of stimulation induces B-cell proliferation in a factor-independent way, it provides a good model system for investigating the effects of cytokines on isotype expression (Rousset *et al.*, 1991). In these cultures, no individual cytokine effectively induces IgA secretion. However, in the presence of IL-4, both IL-2 and IFNγ induce substantial levels of IgA secretion. The combination of IL-4 and IL-5 also increases IgA secretion, albeit not as effectively as the combination of IL-4 and IL-2. The effects of either IL-2 or IFNγ in combination with IL-4 are not limited to IgA. The combination of IL-2 and IL-4 also causes a substantial increase in IgM secretion, whereas IFNγ and IL-4 increase IgG secretion. In contrast, the effect of IL-5 appears to be limited to IgA secretion. No studies are available to indicate whether the increases in isotype expression result from inducing heavy-chain class switching or preferential stimulation of isotype-committed precursors.

On a molecular level, the response of murine and human

B cells to TGFβ is similar. The addition of TGFβ to human splenic B cells stimulated with *Branhamella catarrhalis* results in the induction of germline transcript for both classes of IgA (Islam *et al.*, 1991). The structure of the human germline α mRNA transcripts is analogous to that of the murine transcripts (Nilsson *et al.*, 1991). The genomic sequence of the germline exons for the two human IgA subclasses, as well as the region 5′ to the germline exons, is highly conserved. Further, putative regulatory regions 5′ to the germline exons are conserved between mice and humans. Unfortunately, the signals, if any, that are required to induce these germline α mRNA-producing human B cells to mature to IgA-secreting cells are not established. However, if the molecular mechanisms for isotype switching in human and mouse are similar, TGFβ is likely to induce isotype switching to IgA in both species.

V. CYTOKINE PRODUCTION BY T HELPER SUBSETS

T helper cell subsets have been divided into two distinct classes, Th1 and Th2, on the basis of the pattern of cytokines secreted (Table III; reviewed by Mosmann and Coffman, 1989). Characteristically, Th1 cells secrete IL-2, IFNγ, and lymphotoxin; Th2 cells secrete IL-4, IL-5, and IL-10. Although subsets of Th cells that secrete other patterns of cytokines exist, functionally the Th1 and Th2 subsets are best characterized (Mosmann and Moore, 1991). The relative roles and potential interactions of these subsets in the generation of specific types of immune response can be related to the cytokines they produce. Further, evidence suggests that these subsets play important roles *in vivo* in mice and humans.

Both Th1 and Th2 cells can stimulate B cells to proliferate, undergo clonal expansion, and secrete immunoglobulin (Coffman *et al.*, 1988). B cells can respond to the different helper subsets regardless of their state of activation. However, the Th1 subset of helper cells is less efficient than the Th2 subset in stimulating antibody production by resting B cells. Although growth and maturation per se appear to be relatively independent of the stimulating helper cell, the pattern of isotypes secreted is dependent on the phenotype of the stimulating Th cell (Table IV). Th1 cells are relatively more efficient in stimulating IgG2a responses, whereas Th2 cells are relatively more efficient in stimulating IgE responses. The difference in isotype display potentially is related to the difference in cytokine secretion pattern. Th1 cells secrete IFNγ, which has been shown to be involved in isotype switching to IgG2a (Snapper *et al.*, 1988). On the other hand IL-4, which is a product of Th2 cells, stimulates isotype switching to IgE (Lebman and Coffman, 1988a). Note that the ability of the two helper subsets to stimulate IgA secretion relative to total immunoglobulin secretion is comparable (Table IV).

Table III Cytokine Production by T Helper Subsets[a]

Th1	Th2
IL-2	IL-4
IFNγ	IL-5
Lymphotoxin	IL-6
	IL-10

[a] For each subset the cytokines that are produced uniquely are shown. Data were derived from Mosmann and Moore (1991).

Table IV Patterns of Immunoglobulin Isotype Expression in Th1- and Th2-Stimulated B Cell Cultures[a]

Isotype	Supernatant levels (day 7)[b] (% total response) Th1	Th2
IgA	0.5–1	0.25–1
IgM	50–90	55–90
IgG1	5–20	5–40
IgE	<.01	0.05–2
IgG2a	1–20	0.4–1
IgG2b	0.3–2	0.2–1
IgG3	0.2–1	0.2–0

[a] Cultures of T-depleted spleen cells were stimulated for 7 days with either a Th1 or a Th2 helper cell clone. Th1-stimulated cultures also received anti-IFNγ and IL-2.

[b] Supernatant levels are recorded as percentages of total immunoglobulin secreted.

Th2 cytokines play a significant role in the mediation of allergic responses. IL-4, which stimulates isotype switching to IgE, also has mast cell stimulating activity (Lee *et al.*, 1986). In addition IL-5, whose role in IgA production was discussed in another section (Section II,A), has been shown to enhance eosinophil growth and differentiation both *in vitro* and *in vivo* (Sanderson *et al.*, 1986; Coffman *et al.*, 1989b). IgA can bind to eosinophils and stimulate their degranulation (Abu-Ghazaleh *et al.*, 1989), suggesting a role for IL-5 production in inflammatory bowel disease.

A dichotomy of function between the two predominant helper subsets has been suggested. Th1 cells are associated with delayed-type hypersensitivity whereas Th2 cells are associated with antibody responses (reviewed by Mosmann and Moore, 1991). These two types of response also have been suggested to be mutually exclusive (Parish, 1972). Cytokines produced by the different Th subsets appear to be involved in regulation of the balance of helper subsets. For example, IFNγ inhibits the growth of Th2 cells whereas IL-4 preferentially stimulates their growth (Fernandez-Botran *et al.*, 1988). On the other hand IL-10, which is produced by Th2 cells, inhibits cytokine production by Th1 cells. The interplay of Th cells and cytokines potentially is involved in maintaining the integrity of the mucosal immune system.

VI. CYTOKINE PRODUCTION IN MUCOSAL SITES

The basis for the preferential generation of precursors of IgA-secreting cells in the Peyer's patches remains unclear. Before the cloning of cytokines and the elucidation of their role in regulating isotype expression, investigators had begun to accumulate evidence suggesting that specific T helper populations in the Peyer's patches were involved in the generation of a secretory IgA response (Kawanishi *et al.,* 1983a, b; Kiyono *et al.,* 1984). The discovery that IL-5 enhanced IgA production and was secreted by a specific subset of T helper cells, Th2 cells, provided new impetus for the study of T cells in GALT with an emphasis on cytokine production in mucosal sites. In trying to understand the role of cytokines in the preferential generation of an IgA response in mucosal sites, we must consider the separation of mucosal sites into IgA-inductive and IgA-effector sites. Although the precursors of IgA-secreting cells are generated preferentially in the Peyer's patches, an IgA-inductive site, maturation of these cells to IgA secretion occurs in the lamina propria, an IgA-effector site (Craig and Cebra, 1971; Tomasi, 1983).

Considering the role of IL-5 in IgA secretion, investigators began to look for evidence that IL-5-secreting cells were present in the Peyer's patches (Schoenbeck *et al.,* 1989). Freshly isolated Peyer's patch T cells were separated on the basis of their adherence to *Vicia villosa* agglutinin. On *in vitro* stimulation with a combination of the T-cell mitogen concanavalin A and IL-1, the lectin adherent population secretes IL-5 whereas the lectin nonadherent population secretes IL-2. Interestingly, the supernatants from the adherent but not the nonadherent population supported IgA secretion in cultures of LPS-stimulated splenic B cells. This study provided evidence that Th subsets with both Th1 and Th2 phenotypes were present in an IgA-inductive site.

The ability to assess the actual number of T cells secreting specific cytokines provided a tool for comparing the ratio of Th1 and Th2 subsets in different mucosal sites (Taguchi *et al.,* 1990). Th1 cells were enumerated on the basis of IFN-γ secretion whereas IL-5 secretion was used to define Th2 cells. Although relatively few cytokine-producing cells are found in either freshly isolated spleens or Peyer's patches, the patches contain more cytokine-producing cells, which could reflect the fact that Peyer's patches are a site of chronic antigenic stimulation. On *in vitro* activation, both spleen and Peyer's patch were shown to have relatively equal numbers of IL-5- and IFN-γ-secreting cells. Similarly, relatively equal numbers of IL-5- and IFN -γ -secreting cell are found among intraepithelial lymphocytes (IELs) although, compared with Peyer's patches, IELs have two- to threefold more cytokine-secreting cells. The only mucosal tissue that was enriched for IL-5-secreting cells was the lamina propria, which had a 3 : 1 ratio of IL-5- to IFN-γ-secreting cell (Taguchi *et al.,* 1990). Thus, IgA-effector but not IgA-inductive sites are enriched for Th2 cells. These studies correlate with previous observations (Table III) that both Th1 and Th2 can provide T-cell help for the generation of IgA-producing B cells. Further, they demonstrate that a site that is enriched for IgA-secreting cells, the lamina propria, also is enriched for IL-5-secreting cells, suggesting an *in vivo* role for Th2 cells in the generation of a secretory IgA response.

A great deal of effort has been put forth to correlate $CD4^+$ Th subsets and cytokine production with mucosal immunity, yet freshly isolated IELs also produce cytokines associated with T helper function (Taguchi *et al.,* 1991). However, a major proportion of IELs expresses CD8, and most of these $CD8^+$ cells use $\gamma\delta$ T-cell receptors (TcR; Goodman and Lefrancois, 1988). A considerable proportion of this population expresses both IFN-γ and IL-5 (Taguchi *et al.,* 1991). In fact, in terms of cytokine production, $CD8^+$ $\gamma\delta$ TcR- using cells contain subsets similar to those described for $CD4^+$ Th cells (Taguchi *et al.,* 1991). Although the role of this population is not established, their cytokine production potential raises the possibility that they function at mucosal barriers to regulate immune responses (Taguchi *et al.,* 1990).

VII. CONCLUSIONS

The cloning of cytokines has made it possible to analyze their effects on isotype secretion and to speculate on their role at mucosal surfaces. Although no cytokine appears to be expressed uniquely in a mucosal tissue, the balance of cytokine-expressing cells at mucosal sites may be critical to maintaining the integrity of the mucosal immune system. Thus, the dichotomy of function of Th cells and the role of cytokines in regulating Th balance that has been applied to the study of systemic immunity is equally relevant to mucosal immunity. Although many questions have been answered concerning the *in vitro* actions of cytokines in the regulation of IgA expression, little is known about how these cytokines act *in vivo*.

References

Abu-Ghaazleh, R. I., Fujisawa, T., Mestecky, J., Kyle, R. A., and Gleich, G. J. (1989). IgA induced eosinophil degranulation. *J. Immunol.* **142,** 2393–2400.

Assoian, R. K., Komoriya, A., Meyers, C. A., Miller, D. M., and Sporn, M. B. (1983). Transforming growth factor β in human platelets. Identification of a major storage site, purification, and characterization. *J. Biol. Chem.* **258,** 7155–7160.

Beagley, K. W., Eldridge, J. H., Kiyono, H., Everson, M. P., Koopman, W. J., Honjo, T., and McGhee, J. R. (1988). Recombinant IL-5 induces high rate IgA synthesis in cycling IgA-positive Peyer's patch B cells. *J. Immunol.* **141,** 2035–2042.

Beagley, K. W., Eldridge, J. H., Lee, F., Kiyono, H., Everson, M. P., Koopman, W. J., Hirano, T. J., Kishimoto, T., and McGhee, J. R. (1989). Interleukins and IgA synthesis. Human and murine IL-6 induce high rate IgA secretion in IgA-committed B cells. *J. Exp. Med.* **169,** 2133–2148.

Berton, M. T., Uhr, J. W., and Vitetta, E. S. (1989). Synthesis of germ-line $\gamma 1$ immunoglobulin heavy chain transcripts in resting B cells: Induction by interleukin 4 and inhibition by interferon γ. *Proc. Natl. Acad. Sci. U.S.A.* **86,** 2829–2833.

Bond, M. W., Shrader, B., Mosmann, T. R., and Coffman, R. L. (1987). A mouse T cell product that preferentially enhances IgA production II. Physiochemical characterization. *J. Immunol.* **139,** 3691–3696.

Butcher, E. C., Rouse, R. V., Coffman, R. L., Nottenburg, C. N., Hardy, R. R., and Weissman, I. L. (1982). Surface phenotype of Peyer's patch germinal center cells: Implications for the role of germinal centers in B cell differentiation. *J. Immunol.* **129,** 2698–2707.

Chen, S-S., and Li, Q. (1990). Transforming growth factor β (TGF-β) is a bifunctional immune regulator for mucosal IgA responses. *Cell. Immunol.* **128,** 353–361.

Coffman, R. L., Shrader, B., Carty, J., Mosmann, T. R., and Bond, M. W. (1987). A mouse T cell product that preferentially enhances IgA production. I. Biologic characterization. *J. Immunol.* **139,** 3685–3690.

Coffman, R. L., Seymour, B. H. P., Lebman, D. A., Hiraki, D. D., Christiansen, J. A., Shrader, B., Cherwinski, H. M., Savelkoul, H. F. J., Finkelman, F. D., Bond, M. W., and Mosmann, T. R. (1988). The role of helper T cell products in mouse B cell differentiation and isotype regulation. *Immunol. Rev.* **102,** 5–28.

Coffman, R. L., Lebman, D. A., and Shrader, B. (1989a). Transforming growth factor β specifically enhances IgA production by lipopolysaccharide-stimulated murine B lymphocytes. *J. Exp. Med.* **170,** 1039–1044.

Coffman, R. L., Seymour, B. W., Hudak, S., Jackson, J., and Rennick, D. (1989b). Antibody to interleukin 5 inhibits helminth-induced eosinophilia in mice. *Science* **245,** 308–310.

Craig, S. W., and Cebra, J. J. (1971). Peyer's patches: An enriched source of precursors for IgA- producing immunocytes in the rabbit. *J. Exp. Med.* **134,** 188–200.

Davis, M. M., Calame, K., Early, P. W., Livant, D. L., Joho, R., Weisman, I. L., and Hood, L. (1980). An immunoglobulin heavy-chain gene is formed by at least two recombinational events. *Nature (London)* **283,** 733–739.

Esser, C., and Radbruch, A. (1989). Rapid induction of transcription of unrearranged Sγ1 switch regions in activated murine B cells by interleukin 4. *EMBO J.* **8,** 483–488.

Fernandez-Botran, R., Sanders, V. M., Mosmann, T. R., and Vitetta, E. S. (1988). Lymphokine-mediated regulation of the proliferative response of clones of T helper 1 and T helper 2 cells. *J. Exp. Med.* **168,** 543–558.

Finkelman, F. D., Katona, I. M., Urban, J. F. J., and Paul, W. E. (1989). Control of in vivo IgE production in the mouse by IL-4. *Ciba Found. Symp.* **147,** 3–22.

Flores-Romo, L., Millsum, M. J., Gillis, S., Stubbs, P., Sykes, C., and Gordon, J. (1990). Immunoglobulin isotype production by cycling human B lymphocytes in response to recombinant cytokines and anti-IgM. *Immunology* **69,** 342–347.

Goodman, T., and Lefrancois, L. (1988). Expression of the γ-δ T cell receptor on intestinal $CD8^+$ intraepithelial lymphocytes. *Nature (London)* **333,** 855–858.

Harriman, G. R., Kunimoto, E. Y., Elliot, J. F., Paetkau, V., and Strober, W. (1988). The role of IL-5 in IgA B cell differentiation. *J. Immunol.* **140,** 3033–3039.

Islam, K. B., Nilsson, L., Sideras, P., Hammarstrom, L., and Edvard Smith, C. I. (1991). TGF β1 induces germ-line transcripts of both IgA subclasses in human B lymphocytes. *Int. Immunol.* **3,** 1099–1106.

Kawanishi, H., Saltzman, L. E., and Strober, W. (1983a). Mechanisms regulating IgA class-specific immunoglobulin production in murine gut-associated lymphoid tissues. II. Terminal differentiation of postswitch sIgA-bearing Peyer's patch B cells. *J. Exp. Med.* **158,** 649–668.

Kawanishi, H., Saltzman, L. E., and Strober, W. (1983b). Mechanisms regulating IgA class-specific immunoglobulin production in murine gut associated lymphoid tissues. I. T cells derived from Peyer's patches that switch sIgM B cells to sIgA B cells *in vitro*. *J. Exp. Med.* **157,** 433–450.

Kehrl, J. H., Roberts, A. B., Wakefield, L. M., Jakowlew, S., Sporn, M. B., and Fauci, A. S. (1986). Transforming growth factor β is an important immunomodulatory protein for human B lymphocytes. *J. Immunol.* **137,** 3855–3860.

Kehrl, J. H., Wakefield, L. M., Roberts, A. B., Jakowlew, S., Dernyck, R., Sporn, M. B., and Fauci, A. S. (1987). Production of transforming growth factor β by human T lymphocytes and its potential role in the regulation of T cell growth. *J. Exp. Med.* **163,** 1037–1050.

Kim, P-H., and Kagnoff, M. F. (1990a). Transforming growth factor β1 is a costimulator for IgA production. *J. Immunol.* **144,** 3411–3416.

Kim, P-H., and Kagnoff, M. F. (1990b). Transforming growth factor β 1 increases IgA isotype switching at the clonal level. *J. Immunol.* **145,** 3773–3778.

Kiyono, H., Cooper, M. D., Kearney, J. F., Mosteller, L. M., Michalek, S. M., Koopman, W. J., and McGhee, J. R. (1984). Isotype specificity of helper T cell clones. Peyer's patch Th cells preferentially collaborate with mature IgA B cells for IgA responses. *J. Exp. Med.* **159,** 798–811.

Kunimoto, D. Y., Nordan, R. P., and Strober, W. (1989). IL-6 is a potent cofactor of IL-1 in IgM synthesis and of IL-5 in IgA synthesis. *J. Immunol.* **143,** 2230–2235.

Lebman, D. A., and Coffman, R. L. (1988a). Interleukin 4 causes isotype switching to IgE in T cell-stimulated clonal B cell cultures. *J. Exp. Med.* **168,** 853–862.

Lebman, D. A., and Coffman, R. L. (1988b). The effects of IL-4 and IL-5 on the IgA response by murine Peyer's patch B cell subpopulations. *J. Immunol.* **141,** 2050–2056.

Lebman, D. A., Griffin, P. M., and Cebra, J. J. (1987). Relationship between expression of IgA by Peyer's patch cells and functional IgA memory cells. *J. Exp. Med.* **166,** 1405–1418.

Lebman, D. A., Lee, F. D., and Coffman, R. L. (1990a). Mechanism for transforming growth factor β and IL-2 enhancement of IgA expression in lipopolysaccharide-stimulated B cell cultures. *J. Immunol.* **144,** 952–959.

Lebman, D. A., Nomura, D. Y., Coffman, R. L., and Lee, F. D. (1990b). Molecular characterization of germ-line immunoglobulin A transcripts produced during transforming growth factor type β-induced isotype switching. *Proc. Natl. Acad. Sci. U.S.A.* **87,** 3962–3966.

Lee, F., Yokata, T., Otsuka, T., Meyerson, P., Villaret, D., Coffman, R., Mosmann, T., Renick, D., and Roehm, N. (1986). Isolation and characterization of a mouse interleukin cDNA clone that expresses B cell stimulating factor 1 activities and T cell and mast cell stimulating activities. *Proc. Natl. Acad. Sci. U.S.A.* **83,** 2061–2065.

Lee, G., Ellingsworth, L. R., Gillis, S., Wall, R., and Kincade, P. W. (1987). β transforming growth factors are potential regulators of B lymphopoiesis. *J. Exp. Med.* **166,** 1290–1299.

Lutzker, S., and Alt, F. W. (1988). Structure and expression of germ line immunoglobulin G2b transcripts. *Mol. Cell. Biol.* **8,** 1849–1852.

Mosmann, T. R., and Coffman, R. L. (1989). Th1 and Th2 cells: Different patterns of lymphokine secretion lead to different functional properties. *Annu. Rev. Immunol.* **7,** 145–173.

Mosmann, T. R., and Moore, K. W. (1991). The role of IL-10 in crossregulation of Th1 and Th2 responses. *Immunol. Today* **12,** A49–A53.

Murray, P. D., McKenzie, D. T., Swain, S. L., and Kagnoff, M. F. (1987). Interleukin 5 and interleukin 4 produced by Peyer's patch T cells selectively enhance immunoglobuin A expression. *J. Immunol.* **149,** 2669–2674.

Nilsson, L., Islam, K. B., Olafsson, O., Zalcberg, I., Samakovlis, C., Hammarstrom, L., Edvard Smith, C. I., and Sideras, P. (1991). Structure of TGF-β1 induced human immunoglobulin Cα1 and Cα2 germ-line transcripts. *Int. Immunol.* **3,** 1107–1115.

Parish, C. R. (1972). The relationship between humoral and cell-mediated immunity. *Transplant. Rev.* **13,** 35–66.

Radcliffe, G., Lin, Y-C., Julius, M., Marcu, K. B., and Stavnezer, J. (1990). Structure of germ line immunoglobulin α heavy chain RNA and its location on polysomes. *Mol. Cell. Biol.* **10,** 382–386.

Rousset, F., Garcia, E., and Banchereau, J. (1991). Cytokine-induced proliferation and immunoglobulin production of human B lymphocytes triggered through their CD40 antigen. *J. Exp. Med.* **173,** 705–710.

Sanderson, C. J., O'Garra, A., Warren, D. J., and Klaus, G. G. (1986). Eosinophil differentiation factor also has B cell growth factor activity: Proposed name interleukin 4. *Proc. Natl. Acad. Sci. U.S.A.* **83,** 437–440.

Schoenbeck, S., Hammen, M. J., and Kagnoff, M. F. (1989). *Vicia villosa* agglutinin separates freshly isolated Peyer's patch cells into interleukin 5- or interleukin 2- producing subsets. *J. Exp. Med.* **169,** 1491–1496.

Snapper, C. M., Peschel, C., and Paul, W. E. (1988) IFN-γ stimulates IgG2a secretion by murine B lymphocytes stimulated with bacterial lipopolysaccharide. *J. Immunol.* **140,** 2121–2127.

Sonoda, E., Matsumoto, R., Hitoshi, E., Ishii, T., Sugimoto, M., Araki, S., Toninaga, A., Yamaguchi, N., and Takatsu, K. (1989). Transforming growth factor β induces IgA production and acts additively with interleukin 5 for IgA production. *J. Exp. Med.* **170,** 1415–1420.

Sporn, M. B., Roberts, A. B., Wakefield, L. M., and Assoian, R. K. (1986). Transforming growth factor β: Biological function and chemical structure. *Science* **233,** 532–534.

Stavnezer, J., Sirlin, S., and Abbott, J. (1985). Induction of immunoglobulin isotype switching in cultured I.29 B lymphoma cells: Characterization of the accompanying rearrangements of heavy chain genes. *J. Exp. Med.* **161,** 577–601.

Stavnezer, J., Radcliffe, Y. C., Lin, Y. C., Nietupski, J., Berggren, L., Sitia, R., and Severinson, E. (1988). Immunoglobulin heavy chain switching may be directed by prior induction of transcripts from constant region genes. *Proc. Natl. Acad. Sci. U.S.A.* **85,** 7704–7708.

Taguchi, T., McGhee, J. R., Coffman, R. L., Beagley, K. W., Eldridge, J. H., Takatsu, K., and Kiyono, H. (1990). Analysis of Th1 and Th2 cells in murine gut-associated tissues. Frequencies of $CD4^+$ and $CD8^+$ T cells that secrete IFN-γ and IL-5. *J. Immunol.* **145,** 68–75.

Taguchi, T., Aicher, W., Fujihashi, K., Yamamoto, M., McGhee, J. R., Bluestone, J. A., and Kiyono, H. (1991). Novel function for intestinal intraepithleial lymphocytes. Murine CD3+, γ/δ TCR+ T cells produce IFN-γ and IL-5. *J. Immunol.* **147,** 3736–3744.

Tomasi, T. B., Jr. (1983). Mechanisms of immune regulation at mucosal surfaces. *Rev. Infect. Dis.* **5,** S784–S792.

Tominaga, A., Takaki, S., Koyama, N., Kotah, S., Matsumoto, R., Migita, M., Hitoshi, Y., Hosoya, Y., Yamauchi, S., Kanai, Y., Miyazaki, J-I., Usuku, G., Yamamura, K-I., and Takatsu, K. (1991). Transgenic mice expressing a B cell growth and differentiation factor gene (interleukin 5) develop eosinophilai and autoantibody production. *J. Exp. Med.* **173,** 429–437.

Van Snick, J. (1990). Interleukin 6: An overview. *Annu. Rev. Immunol.* **8,** 253—278.

21

Distribution and Characteristics of Mucosal Immunoglobulin-Producing Cells

Per Brandtzaeg

I. INTRODUCTION

More than two decades ago, the major immunoglobulin (Ig) present in exocrine secretions was shown to be a dimeric IgA covalently bound to an epithelial glycoprotein of about 80 kDa (Tomasi *et al.*, 1965), now called the secretory component (SC). Pentameric IgM likewise is actively enriched in most secretions and is associated with SC, although not in a covalently stabilized complex (Brandtzaeg, 1975). This difference largely explains that secretory IgA (SIgA) survives better than secretory IgM (SIgM) in intestinal fluid (Richman and Brown, 1977). However, a striking heterogeneity exists in SIgA with respect to proteolytic resistance, depending on whether the subclass IgA1 or IgA2 constitutes the Ig moiety (Mestecky and McGhee, 1987).

The secretory immune system is the best defined aspect of mucosal immunity. This adaptive humoral defense mechanism depends on a fascinating cooperation between the local B-cell system and the secretory epithelia. Terminally differentiated B cells, appearing as Ig-producing blasts and plasma cells (collectively called immunocytes) in histologically normal secretory tissues, produce mainly dimers and larger polymers of IgA (Brandtzaeg, 1985). Such polymeric IgA (pIgA) contains a 15-kDa polypeptide called the "joining" or J chain (Mestecky and McGhee, 1987) and therefore can become bound to SC expressed basolaterally on the secretory epithelial cells as a pIg receptor (pIgR; Chapter 10). Pentameric IgM also contains J chain and, hence, can be transported externally by the SC-mediated endocytic mechanism (Brandtzaeg, 1985).

II. NORMAL MUCOSAL STATE

A. Immunoregulatory Mechanisms

Regulation of mucosal immunity is believed to be exerted primarily in organized lymphoepithelial structures such as gut-associated lymphoid tissue (GALT), which includes the Peyer's patches and solitary lymphoid follicles. Additional immune regulation mediating terminal B-cell differentiation, and probably also peripheral tolerance or hyporesponsiveness to nonmicrobial antigens, may involve various cells both in the lamina propria and in the epithelial compartment (Chapters 12, 13 and 16).

B cells that have received their "first signals" of stimulation in GALT migrate with primed T cells through mesenteric lymph nodes to peripheral blood. Both types of memory cells finally are seeded by extravasation into distant gut mucosa and, to some extent, other more remote secretory tissues (Mestecky, 1987; Mestecky and McGhee, 1987; Brandtzaeg and Bjerke, 1990). "Second signals," modulated by various tissue elements expressing HLA Class II determinants and by regulatory T lymphocytes, cause terminal maturation of B cells to Ig-producing immunocytes. Most of these cells apparently belong to clones of an early differentiation stage compatible with gene activation promoting J-chain expression, regardless of concomitant Ig class production (Brandtzaeg, 1974a,1985; Brandtzaeg and Korsrud, 1984; Bjerke and Brandtzaeg, 1990a). The obvious functional goal of this immunoregulatory development is generation of SC-binding pIg locally, where external transport through SC-positive epithelium can take place readily to generate SIgA and SIgM antibodies (Chapter 10).

This brief account of mucosal immune regulation does not give full justice to all the research work that has been performed, mainly in experimental animals. However, how the local inductive and suppressive immunoregulatory mechanisms are achieved is admittedly still obscure (Brandtzaeg *et al.*, 1989). The Peyer's patches have, for the last two decades, been considered the major precursor source of B cells giving rise to the predominant mucosal IgA immunocyte populations (Chapter 13). Particular "switch cells," acting by poorly defined mechanisms on the Ig heavy-chain constant region (C_H) genes to drive the phenotypic expression from IgM directly to IgA, have been postulated in murine Peyer's patches (Kawanishi *et al.*, 1985). Similar cells have been cloned more recently from the human appendix (Benson and Strober, 1988).

The IgA-promoting role of various T cell-derived lymphokines or interleukins (IL) in the mucosal B-cell differentiation process is being subjected to extensive investigation, including studies on IL-2 through IL-12 as well as transforming growth factor β (TGFβ) (Chapter 14). IL-2, IL-5, and perhaps IL-6 are, moreover, involved in the up-regulation of J-chain expression, whereas IL-4 may have an opposing role (Tigges *et al.*, 1989; Takayasu and Brooks, 1991; Randall *et al.*, 1992).

Interestingly, intestinal lamina propria T cells may show particularly high capacity to secrete IL-2 and IL-5 (James, 1991). Further, evidence suggests that J-chain expression can take place independently of Ig production, but the secretion of this peptide depends on its intracellular association with pIgA or pentameric IgM (Brandtzaeg and Berdal, 1975; Kubagawa *et al.*, 1988; Mestecky *et al.*, 1990), perhaps because accessible thiol groups of free J chain prevent its transport from the endoplasmic reticulum (Alberini *et al.*, 1990).

B. Distribution of Ig-Producing Immunocytes in Human Exocrine Tissues

1. Immunohistochemical Methodology for Immunocyte Recording

Specimens of exocrine tissues can be prepared for immunohistochemistry in principally three different ways: as fresh-frozen tissue for cryosections; by a precipitating or coagulative fixative (e.g., ethanol) followed by paraffin wax embedding; or by a cross-linking fixative (e.g., formaldehyde) followed by embedding. Cryosections usually are best suited for membrane-anchored glycoproteins, whereas formaldehyde-fixed tissue is preferred for easily diffusible components of low molecular weight. However, masking of antigenic determinants is a problem in immunohistochemical studies of glycoproteins that have been subjected to cross-linking fixatives, although partial unmasking by enzyme digestion of the tissue sections usually can be achieved, especially when polyclonal antibody reagents are applied (Brandtzaeg, 1982).

For reliable demonstration of interstitial and epithelial Ig distribution, ethanol fixation is undoubtedly the method of choice (Brandtzaeg, 1982). Modification of this approach by including a prefixation tissue washing period is often necessary for visualization of Ig-producing and Ig-bearing cells against a fairly unstained background (Brandtzaeg, 1974b). The antigenic determinants of certain molecules, such as IgA-associated J chain, are masked even in such ethanol-fixed tissue; denaturation of tissue sections in acid urea is therefore necessary for reliable detection of J chain-producing immunocytes of this class (Brandtzaeg, 1983a).

In addition to these important precautions, appropriate morphometric methods must be applied for the quantification of Ig-producing cells to produce meaningful data that can be compared among various laboratories. Immunocyte densities preferably are reported as number of cells/mm^2 of section area or defined tissue compartment. However, in most secretory tissues, the immunocyte density is strikingly heterogeneous so the selection of fields to be evaluated must be performed in a well-defined manner (Korsrud and Brandtzaeg, 1980). Paired staining of two or three Ig isotypes in the same tissue section is always preferable to obtain reliable phenotype ratios (Brandtzaeg 1974b,1982). In the gut lamina propria, reporting the number of immunocytes per length unit of the gut (Figure 1), including the full height of the mucosa (Brandtzaeg and Baklien, 1976), is most representative.

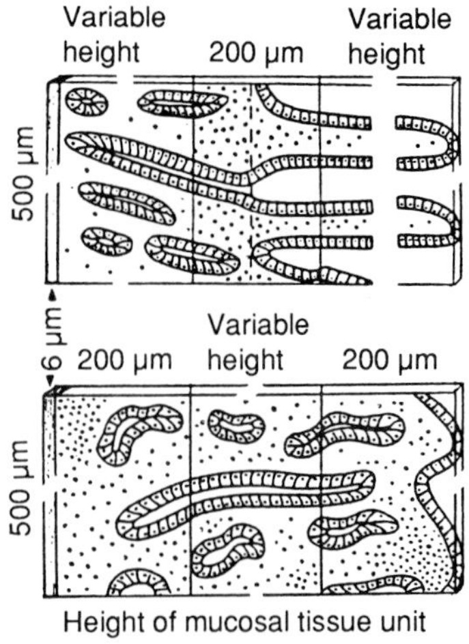

Figure 1 Schematic representation of normal (*top*) and diseased (*bottom*) "tissue unit" defined in a 6-μm thick tissue section (small intestine illustrated). The lamina propria area included varies among different specimens depending on the height of the tissue unit: The total number of Ig-producing immunocytes per unit is determined by this variable as well as by the cell density. The distribution of dots indicates heterogeneity in cell density. The highest density of Ig-producing immunocytes normally is found around the base of the villi in the normal small intestine or close to the lumen in "flat" lesions or normal colonic mucosa. The definition of the corresponding 200-μm zones, which may be used for quantitative comparisons within or between units, is shown by vertical lines. Modified from Brandtzaeg and Baklien (1976).

2. Normal Adult Secretory Tissues

a. Class distribution of Ig-producing cells. Secretory tissues of adults normally contain a remarkable preponderance of IgA-producing immunocytes, including plasma cells and blasts (Figure 2), particularly the intestinal mucosa, as first reported by Crabbé *et al.* (1965) and Rubin *et al.* (1965). We have estimated that almost 10^{10} such cells occur per meter of adult bowel (Brandtzaeg and Baklien, 1976), with a predominance proximally and distally (Figure 3). Absolute figures are difficult to obtain for other secretory tissues in which the cells are distributed much more heterogeneously throughout the stroma than they are in the gastrointestinal lamina propria; however, on the basis of our quantitative data (Figure 4), most gland-associated IgA cells are located in the gut (Brandtzaeg, 1983b). Moreover, the size of this cell population is impressive in view of the comparable figure (2.5×10^{10}) estimated for bone marrow, spleen, and lymph nodes together (Turesson, 1976). Therefore, at least 80% of all Ig-producing immunocytes of the body are located in the gut (Brandtzaeg *et al.*, 1989). A similar estimate has been reported for mice (van der Heijden *et al.*, 1987). Aging does not reduce the remarkable Ig-producing capacity of the intestinal mucosa (Penn *et al.*, 1991).

The large output of IgA in colostrum might imply that lactating mammary glands either harbor a remarkably active secretory immune system or, alternatively, drain pIgA from serum selectively. In fact, human colostrum contains about

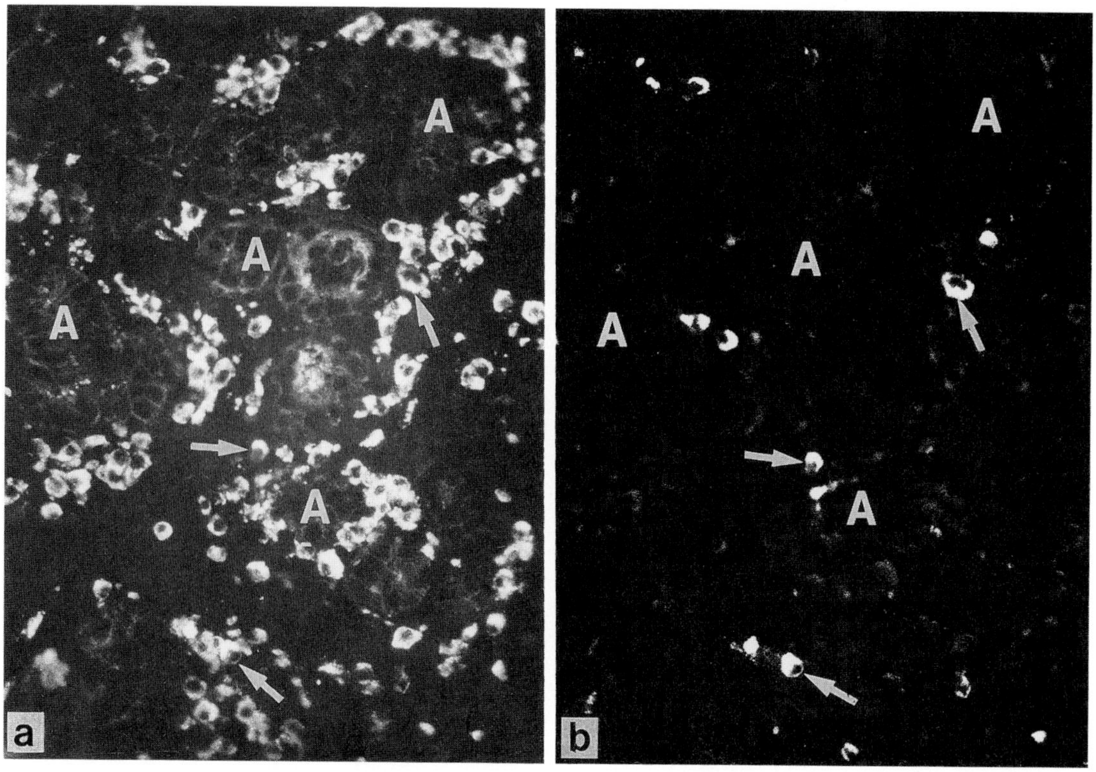

Figure 2 Immunofluorescence staining for IgA (rhodamine) and IgG (fluorescein). (a) Double exposure showing both isotypes. (b) Selective filtration for IgG staining in same field from nasal mucosa. Note relatively few IgG-producing cells (arrows) among densely packed IgA immunocytes adjacent to acini (A), which show selective uptake of IgA. ×190.

300 times more SIgA than stimulated parotid secretion and about 60 times more than normal unstimulated whole saliva (Brandtzaeg, 1983b). However, the density of IgA-producing cells is similar in human salivary and lactating mammary glands, but six to seven times less than in lacrimal glands and colonic mucosa (Figure 4). The daily output of IgA/gm wet weight is, moreover, similar for salivary and lactating mammary glands. Thus a large capacity for storage of IgA in the mammary gland epithelium and the duct system appears to explain the striking output of IgA during feeding. No evidence exists for a selective extracellular accumulation of serum-derived or locally produced pIgA in the glandular stroma (Brandtzaeg, 1983b).

IgM-producing cells normally constitute a substantial but variable fraction of the immunocyte populations in secretory tissues of adults (Figure 5). The reason for the relatively high proportion of this class in the proximal small intestine is unknown (Figure 3). IgG-producing cells constitute 3–5% of the immunocytes in normal intestinal mucosa, but a considerably larger percentage is found in nasal and gastric mucosa (Figure 5). Only occasional IgD and IgE immunocytes are encountered in the gastrointestinal tract, whereas IgD-producing cells constitute a significant fraction (2–10%) of the glandular immunocytes in the upper respiratory tract, including nasal mucosa and salivary and lacrimal glands (Brandtzaeg *et al.*, 1979; Korsrud and Brandtzaeg, 1980; Brandtzaeg, 1984).

We have interpreted this regional difference to suggest that partial sequential downstream switching according to the location of the C_H genes on chromosome 14 (μ–δ–$\gamma3$–$\gamma1$–$\alpha1$–$\gamma2$–$\gamma4$–ε–$\alpha2$) might be a perferential B-cell differentiation pathway in the upper digestive and respiratory tracts, whereas more extensive sequential switching—perhaps combined with direct switching from $C_H\mu$ (IgM) to $C_H\alpha2$ (IgA2)—might be prominent in the distal gut (Brandtzaeg *et al.*, 1986). This notion has been supported by findings in subjects with selective IgA deficiency: The absent IgA immunocytes are replaced largely by the IgM class in gut mucosa but often by J chain-expressing IgD immunocytes in the upper digestive and respiratory tracts (see subsequent discussion).

b. Subclass distribution of Ig-producing cells. Immunohistochemical studies with monoclonal antibodies (MAbs) against the two IgA subclasses have supported further the idea of regional immunoregulatory differences (Kett *et al.*, 1986). Again we found a remarkable disparity between the upper digestive and respiratory tracts compared with the distal gut: IgA1 immunocytes predominated (80–93%) in the former secretory tissues whereas IgA2 immunocytes were usually most frequent (~60%) in the normal large bowel mucosa (Figure 6).

Similar studies with MAbs against the four human IgG subclasses have been difficult to perform because IgG-producing cells are so few in normal gut mucosa. However,

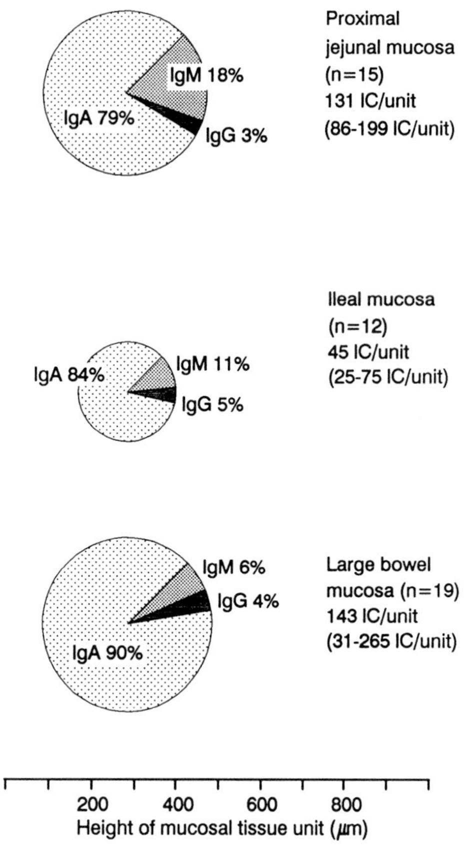

Figure 3 Median numbers (and observed ranges) of Ig-producing immunocytes (IC) per mucosal tissue unit in the normal proximal jejunum, ileum, and large bowel. The median percentage class distributions of the immunocyte populations are given also. All tissue units are 500 μm wide (vertical axis); the median height (horizontal axis) for each specimen category is indicated (n = number of subjects). Data adapted from various immunohistochemical studies reported by the author's laboratory.

we have obtained immunohistochemical results in the large bowel (Nilssen *et al.,* 1991) that, on a relative basis, agree remarkably well with the spontaneous secretion of IgG subclasses observed in cultures of lamina propria lymphoid cells (Scott *et al.,* 1986). Our immunohistochemical studies of IgG-producing cells in upper respiratory tract mucosa (Brandtzaeg *et al.,* 1987), as well as in normal ileal (Bjerke and Brandtzaeg, 1990b) and colonic (Nilssen *et al.,* 1991) mucosa, have shown that IgG1 is the predominating subclass (>55%), which is also the case in normal serum. However, IgG2 cells are generally more frequent (20–35%) than IgG3 cells (4–6%) in the distal intestinal mucosa (Bjerke and Brandtzaeg, 1990b; Nilssen *et al.,* 1991), whereas the reverse is often true in the upper respiratory mucosa (Brandtzaeg *et al.,* 1987).

This IgG subclass disparity also supports the idea that the B-cell switching pathways differ in various regions of the mucosal immune system, as discussed earlier. Although particular T cells or lymphokines that fully explain Ig isotype selection have not been identified, serum IgG subclass responses are well documented to be influenced by the nature of the stimulatory antigen. Many carbohydrate and bacterial antigens preferentially induce an IgG2 response, whereas proteins (which are clearly T cell-dependent antigens) primarily generate a coordinate IgG1 and IgG3 response (Papadea and Check, 1989). Regional environmental factors thus may contribute to the different proportions of IgG subclass-producing cells seen in the upper respiratory and distal gut mucosa. Such environmental influence is likely to explain the disparity observed for the IgA subclass-producing cells as well because proteins stimulate mainly IgA1 whereas carbohydrate antigens, particularly *Escherichia coli* lipopolysaccharide, tend to favor IgA2 responses (Brown and Mestecky, 1985; Mestecky and Russell, 1986; Tarkowski *et al.,* 1990).

The upper respiratory tract microbiota might contribute significantly to B-cell regulation in that region and perhaps explain the prominent local IgD response seen in many IgA-deficient patients (Brandtzaeg *et al.,* 1979,1987; Korsrud and Brandtzaeg, 1980; Brandtzaeg and Korsrud, 1984). Most strains of *Haemophilus influenzae* and *Moraxella (Branhamella) catarrhalis,* which are frequent colonizers of the upper respiratory tract, produce an IgD-binding factor (protein D) and therefore may exert great impact on local B-cell activation by cross-linking surface IgD and HLA Class I determinants (Ruan *et al.,* 1990; Janson *et al.,* 1991). B lymphocytes of the follicular mantle zones in the tonsils are usually strongly positive for both these molecules (Brandtzaeg, 1987), and could be stimulated by protein D to proliferate and differentiate in a polyclonal (antigen-independent) manner. This type of stimulation also might contribute to the fact that, normally, particularly many IgD and IgA1-producing cells exist in the upper digestive and respiratory tracts (Figures 5 and 6). One may speculate that cross-linking of surface IgD favors a sequential differentiation pathway, mainly terminating with IgA1 production, whereas direct switching from IgM to IgA2 predominates in GALT in which lipopolysaccha-

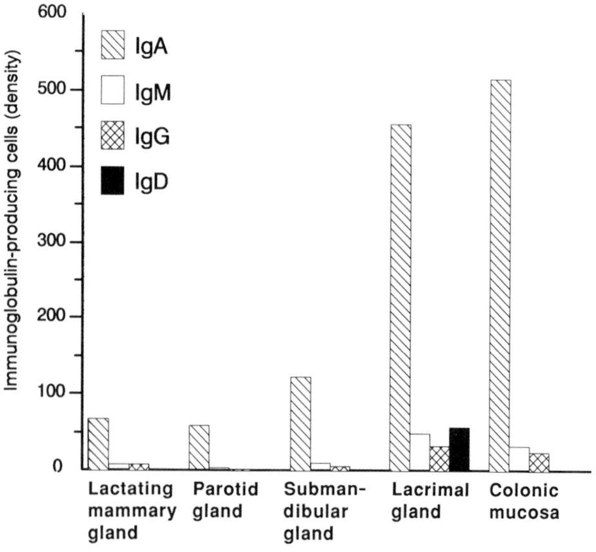

Figure 4 Densities (numbers/mm^2) of immunoglobulin-producing cells of different classes, as indicated, in sections of various normal human secretory tissues. Data adapted from various immunohistochemical studies reported by the author's laboratory.

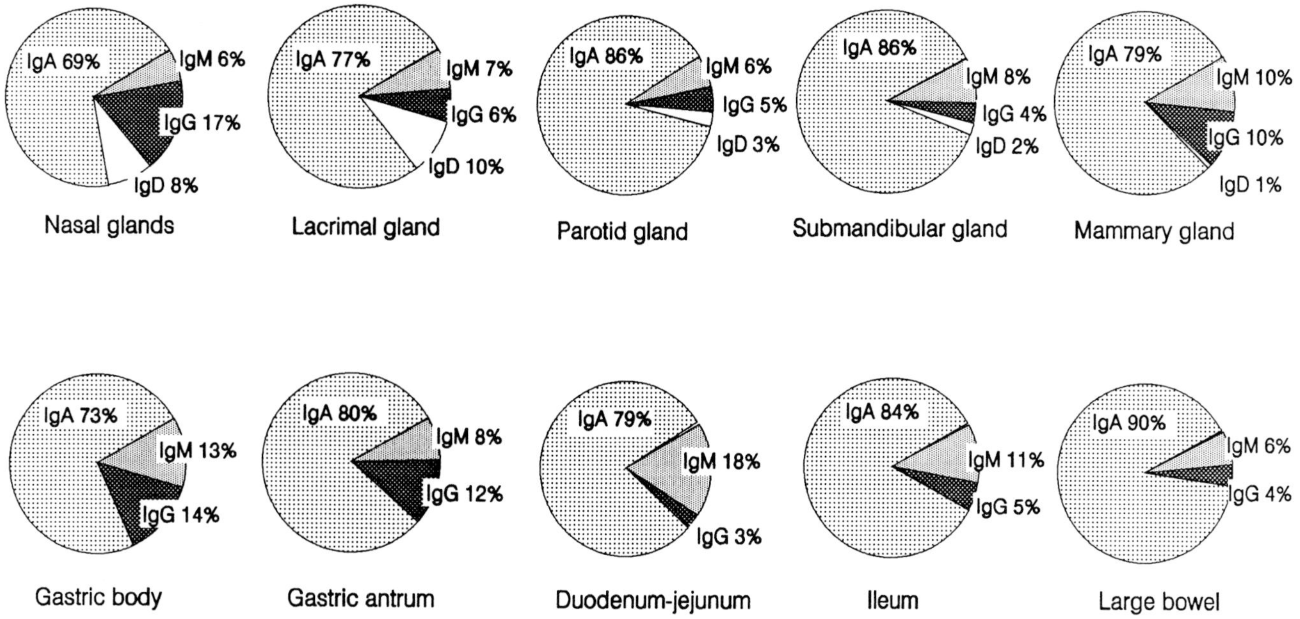

Figure 5 Percentage distribution of IgA-, IgM-, IgG-, and IgD-producing immunocytes in various normal human secretory tissues. Data adapted from various immunohistochemical studies reported by the author's laboratory.

rides could tend to suppress IgD expression (Parkhouse and Cooper, 1977). Perhaps the IgA1 protease-producing bacteria of the upper respiratory tract are equipped with protein D to favor the development of a local secretory immune response that they can evade.

c. J-chain production. Almost 90% of the IgA1 and virtually 100% of the IgA2 immunocytes in normal gut mucosa produce pIgA with associated J chain (Crago *et al.*, 1984; Kett *et al.*, 1988; Bjerke and Brandtzaeg, 1990a). The same is true in other exocrine tissues (Brandtzaeg and Korsrud, 1984). Most of the mucosal IgM immunocytes also produce J chain, which in both classes becomes incorporated into the pIg structure intracellularly (Brandtzaeg, 1983a,1985). However, J-chain incorporation appears not to be necessary for assembly of the polymers and their secretion from the immunocytes (Cattaneo and Neuberger, 1987; Davis and Shulman, 1989), a fact that further attests to the role of this peptide in the generation of the SC binding site of pIgA and pentameric IgM (Brandtzaeg, 1985; Bouvet *et al.*, 1987).

Direct evidence that J chain-positive mucosal IgA immunocytes indeed synthesize a high level of pIgA was obtained first by an SC binding test performed on tissue sections; a striking heterogeneity in the proportion of monomers-to-

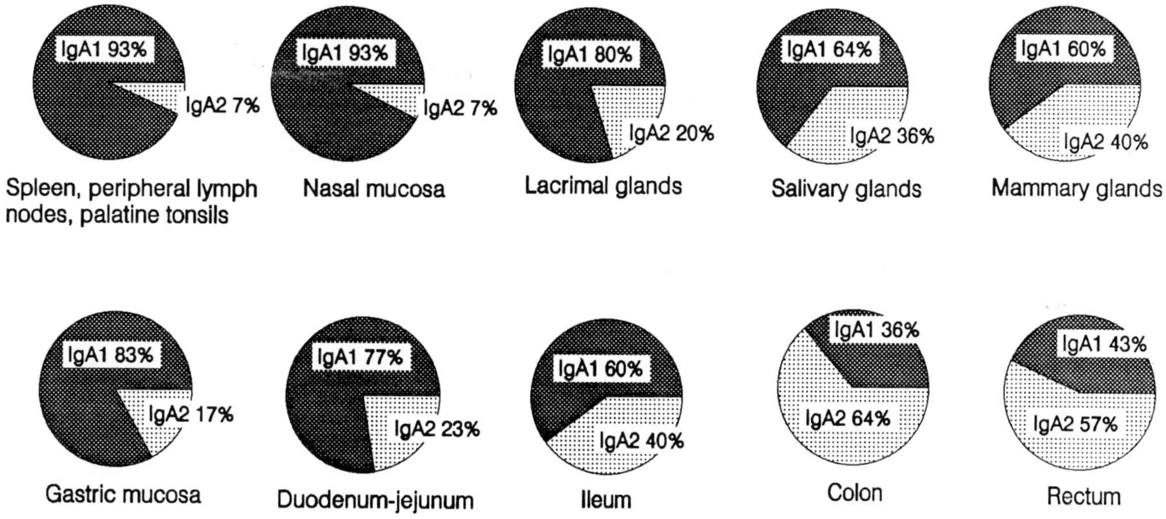

Figure 6 Percentage subclass distribution of IgA-producing immunocytes in various human lymphoid and normal secretory tissues. Based on data from Kett *et al.* (1986).

polymers produced by such immunocytes in lymphoid tissue outside exocrine sites was also suggested (Brandtzaeg, 1973; 1974a) and later confirmed by a spot-ELISA method (Tarkowski *et al.*, 1991). Furthermore, the cytoplasmic affinity for SC shown *in vitro,* as well as the immunohistochemical requirement for unmasking of cytoplasmic J chain (Brandtzaeg, 1983a), support the idea that substantial intracellular polymerization of IgA normally takes place in the J chain-positive immunocytes (Brandtzaeg, 1985). This appears to be different in malignant B-cell lines (Brandtzaeg, 1983a; Moldoveanu *et al.*, 1984), but available methods do not allow accurate determination at the single cell level of the proportion of monomers-to-polymers produced by IgA immunocytes (Tarkowski *et al.*, 1991). Immunoelectron-microscopical localization of J chain in normal intestinal IgA immunocytes suggests that the polymerization process begins in the rough endoplasmic reticulum (Nagura *et al.*, 1979); this notion has been supported by similar studies performed on transformed normal B cells (Moro *et al.*, 1990).

Interestingly, almost 80% of the intestinal IgG-producing cells also normally express cytoplasmic J chain (Brandtzaeg and Korsrud, 1984; Bjerke and Brandtzaeg, 1990a), although this peptide does not become associated with IgG but is degraded intracellularly (Mosmann *et al.*, 1978). Moreover, the J chain is produced by a considerable fraction of IgG cells and most IgD cells in normal nasal mucosa and in salivary, lacrimal, and mammary glands (Brandtzaeg, 1974a; Brandtzaeg *et al.*, 1979; Korsrud and Brandtzaeg, 1980; Brandtzaeg and Korsrud, 1984). When positive for J chain, these mucosal immunocyte classes might be considered terminally differentiated "spin-offs" from early memory clones which, through sequential C_H switching, are on their maturation pathway to pIgA production (Brandtzaeg, 1985).

C. Ontogeny of Mucosal Immunocytes

1. Perinatal Period

Scattered B and T lymphocytes are seen in the human fetal gut lamina propria from 14 weeks gestation (Spencer *et al.*, 1986). A few IgM- and IgG-producing plasma cells have been reported to appear somewhat later and remain in small numbers until birth, whereas IgA immunocytes are either absent or extremely rare (Brandtzaeg *et al.*, 1991). In contrast, human fetal salivary glands sometimes contain additional IgA-producing cells, especially after 30 weeks gestation (Hayashi *et al.*, 1989); most of these immunocytes (~90%) are of the IgA1 subclass and virtually all express J chain (Thrane *et al.*, 1991). This apparent difference in immunological activation between salivary glands and gut mucosa is intriguing (Brandtzaeg *et al.*, 1991). However, fetal GALT is certainly immunocompetent, at least during the final trimester; numerous plasma cells can appear in the intestinal mucosa in response to intrauterine infection (Silverstein and Lukes, 1962).

The postnatal numbers of IgA- and IgM-producing immunocytes in the intestinal lamina propria (including the appendix) and salivary glands start to rise rapidly after 2-4 weeks, the IgA class becoming predominant after 1–2 months (Figure 7). For the first 6 months, moreover, a striking admixture of IgD-producing cells is often seen in the salivary glands (Thrane *et al.*, 1991), which is interesting in relation to terminal B-cell differentiation for this region (see earlier). Also, a considerable proprotion (about 50%) of infants has detectable amounts of IgD in whole saliva during the same time period (Gleeson *et al.*, 1987a). This IgD most likely reaches the secretion by passive diffusion from the local immunocytes because of increased postnatal epithelial permeability.

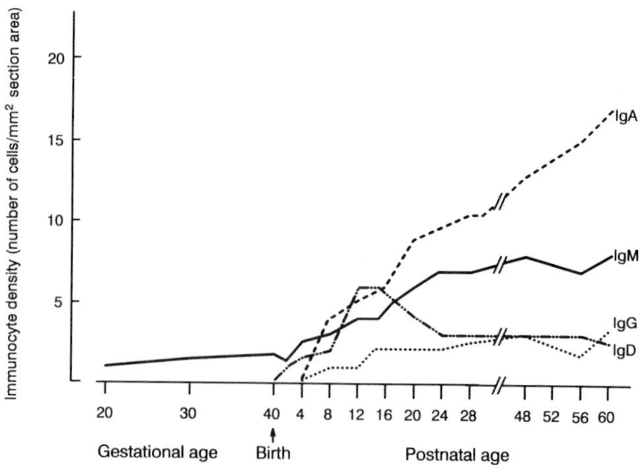

Figure 7 Numeric development of IgA-, IgM-, IgG-, and IgD-producing immunocytes in human parotid glands relative to age in weeks. Based on data from Thrane *et al.* (1991).

During the first 3 months after birth, the IgA1:IgA2 immunocyte ratio observed in salivary glands approaches the normal adult value of approximately 65:35 (Kett *et al.*, 1986), which might reflect an increasing postnatal influx of IgA precursor cells from GALT where the IgA2 isotype normally predominates (Bjerke and Brandtzaeg, 1990b). At the same time, the high level of J-chain expression (94–97%) is maintained for both subclasses (Thrane *et al.*, 1991).

2. Childhood Development

a. Normal state. At an average age of 15 months (Figure 7), the number of IgA immunocytes has approached the lower normal adult range in salivary glands (Korsrud and Brandtzaeg, 1980); the subsequent increase throughout early childhood seems to be small (Hayashi *et al.*, 1989). Blanco *et al.*, (1976) also observed no significant increase of intestinal IgA-producing cells after 1 year, but IgM-producing cells decreased. A similar trend of decreasing intestinal IgM immunocytes with age has been reported by others, although associated with a continuing increase of IgA immunocytes (Savilahti, 1972), even after 2 years (Maffei *et al.*, 1979). In the human appendix, however, no such increase was seen after 5 months (Gebbers and Laissue, 1990).

Cripps *et al.* (1989) reported that almost one-third of infants under 2.5 years of age have only monomeric IgA in saliva, but this finding subsequently was refuted (Smith *et al.*, 1989). The expression of J chain by virtually all salivary IgA immunocytes, both before and after birth (Thrane *et al.*, 1991), strongly suggests that local humoral immunity depends on activation of the secretory immune system in infancy also.

The progressive cellular shift from IgA1 to IgA2 production (Thrane *et al.*, 1991) is reflected in the respective salivary subclass levels (Smith *et al.*, 1989; Müller *et al.*, 1991).

Remarkably, the IgG-producing cell population in the appendix lamina propria becomes substantial after a few months (Gebbers and Laissue, 1990), a feature that can be ascribed to the fact that the 0.1-mm zone adjacent to the numerous lymphoid follicles, and including the domes, contains almost 50% immunocytes of the IgG class (Bjerke *et al.*, 1986). We have suggested that this accumulation reflects local terminal differentiation of B cells belonging to relatively mature memory clones. Generation of such clones in lymphoepithelial structures might reflect the magnitude of topical immunological stimulation and seems to take place increasingly in the order of Peyer's patches (Bjerke and Brandtzaeg, 1986), appendix (Bjerke *et al.*, 1986), and tonsils (Brandtzaeg, 1987). Conversely, dissemination of IgA cell precursors with activated J-chain genes most likely depends on the continuous generation of early memory clones (Brandtzaeg, 1985; Brandtzaeg and Bjerke, 1990). The potency of a lymphoid tissue to function as precursor source for the secretory immune system thus may be related inversely to the local IgG response, in harmony with the major role suggested for Peyer's patches in mucosal IgA responses.

b. Effect of antigenic load. The topical antigenic and mitogenic load seems to be decisive for the postnatal development of mucosal immunity. The indigenous microbial flora is probably of utmost importance, as suggested by the fact that the intestinal IgA system of germ-free or specific pathogen-free mice is normalized after about 4 weeks of conventionalization (Crabbé *et al.*, 1970; Horsfall *et al.*, 1978). *Bacteroides* and *E. coli* strains seem to be particularly stimulative for the development of intestinal IgA immunocytes (Moreau *et al.*, 1978). Artificial colonization of infants with a nonenteropathogenic strain of *E. coli* likewise has resulted in enhanced formation of IgA in the gut (Lodinova *et al.*, 1973). Antigenic constitutents of food probably exert an additional stimulatory effect, as suggested in mice fed hydrolyzed milk proteins (Sagie *et al.*, 1974) and in parenterally fed babies (Knox, 1986). In the latter case, however, a deleterious effect of malnutrition or retarded bacterial colonization cannot be excluded.

Reduced amounts of microbial and dietary antigens apparently explain why the colonic numbers of IgA- and IgM-producing cells are decreased by about 50% after 2–11 months in children who had been subjected to defunctioning colostomies (Wijesinha and Steer, 1982). Postnatal and prolonged observations on defunctioned ileal segments in lambs have revealed even more strikingly a scarcity of immunocytes in the lamina propria. This result was explained by reduced local accumulation of B-cell blasts and might have involved both hampered migration of such precursors into the mucosa and subsequently their decreased local proliferation and differentiation (Reynolds and Morris, 1984).

Geographical variations have a striking impact on the mucosal immune system. In contrast to infants in Sweden, infants in a developing country that are exposed to poliovirus often show substantial levels of salivary SIgA antibodies to poliovirus as early as 1 month after birth and generally approach adult antibody levels by the age of 6 months (Carlsson *et al.*, 1985). Infants heavily exposed to *E. coli* from birth on increase their salivary SIgA antibody levels significantly by 2–3 weeks of age and reach adult levels rapidly (Mellander *et al.*, 1985). In less-exposed infants, such levels are not attained until about 1 year of age, both for total SIgA and for SIgA antibodies to *E. coli* O antigens (Mellander *et al.*, 1984). However, Swedish infants show an indication of enhanced attainment of increased salivary SIgA antibody levels in relation to hospitalization compared with home care, which also often involves more regular breast feeding (Mellander *et al.*, 1984). A striking increase of salivary SIgA in Australian children starting school also has been ascribed to environmental impact, particularly of repeated respiratory tract infections (Gleeson *et al.*, 1987b).

c. Alterations associated with SIDS. The incidence of sudden infant death syndrome (SIDS) is correlated significantly with respiratory viral isolation in the general pediatric population and appears to be increased in cold weather (Milner and Ruggins, 1989). The finding of raised concentrations of IgM and IgA in bronchial lavage fluid, and an increased number of the three major immunocyte classes in interstitial lung tissue, therefore might reflect an intensified local immune response (Forsyth *et al.*, 1989). In keeping with this suggestion, we found significantly elevated numbers of all three major immunocyte classes in the parotid glands on an absolute basis in the order IgA>IgM>IgG (Thrane *et al.*, 1990). The idea of intensified local immunostimulation also was supported strongly by the fact that the parotid glands from the same SIDS victims showed significantly raised numbers of interstitial leukocytes and enhanced epithelial HLA Class II and SC expression (Thrane *et al.*, 1993).

III. MUCOSAL PATHOLOGICAL STATES

Published data on the major Ig-producing immunocyte classes in diseased intestinal mucosae show striking discrepancies (Brandtzaeg and Baklien, 1976; Brandtzaeg *et al.*, 1992; Scott *et al.*, 1992). In addition to general methodological difficulties, as briefly discussed earlier, the selection of tissue samples poses a great problem in infammatory bowel disease, which may show highly varying histopathological features even in the same specimen. Our immunohistochemical results have demonstrated a dramatic and predominant numerical increase of IgG immunocytes, both in ulcerative colitis and in Crohn's disease (Brandtzaeg *et al.*, 1992). Moreover, although the IgA-producing cells remain the overall dominating immunocyte class in the lesion, they are aberrant by showing an increased IgA1 subclass proportion (Kett and Brandtzaeg, 1987) and decreased J-chain expression (Brandtzaeg and Korsrud, 1984; Kett *et al.*, 1988). A significant difference between the mucosal immune response seen in Crohn's disease and ulcerative colitis is the relatively more prominent IgG1 production in the latter disorder (Scott *et al.*, 1986; Kett *et al.*, 1987).

Although much less dramatic, a disproportionate local overproduction of IgG is also a feature of other mucosal inflammatory diseases such as chronic gastritis (Valnes *et al.*, 1986), celiac disease (Scott *et al.*, 1992), chronic rhinitis (Brandtzaeg, 1984), and chronic sialadenitis (Brandtzaeg, 1989). Local defense thus tends to be shifted from immune exclusion mediated by SIgA (and SIgM) to immune elimination through inflammatory and phagocytotic amplification mechanisms induced by IgG antibodies. This shift obviously may be of immunopathological importance for disease activity and persistence (Brandtzaeg *et al.*, 1989,1992).

IV. SELECTIVE IgA DEFICIENCY

A. "Compensatory" Terminal B-Cell Differentiation

The principal finding in gastrointestinal mucosa of subjects with markedly decreased or absent serum IgA is that the IgA-producing immunocytes are reduced in number or completely lacking, whereas IgG- and especially IgM-producing cells are increased substantially (Brandtzaeg *et al.*, 1968,1979; Savilahti, 1973). IgD- and IgE-producing cells are found rarely so the mucosal immunocyte population usually consists of 20–35% IgG and 65–75% IgM (Brandtzaeg *et al.*, 1979; Kanoh *et al.*, 1987; Nilssen *et al.*, 1992). However, the activity of the secretory immune system in IgA deficiency may be quite unpredictable on the basis of the serum level of IgA, although decreased intestinal IgA- to IgM-cell ratio appears to be a good indicator of a significant IgA deficiency after infancy. Thus, the intestinal IgA cell population is commonly intact when serum IgA concentrations are above 18% of the normal average whereas, at values between 18% and 5%, the number of jejunal IgA cells usually is decreased but that of IgM cells is increased (Savilahti, 1974).

Nevertheless, even patients presenting with a truly selective IgA deficiency (serum IgA < 0.05 g/liter) often have a few scattered IgA-producing cells in their intestinal mucosa (McClelland *et al.*, 1976; Scotta *et al.*, 1982); rare cases have indeed been reported to have fairly normal numbers of such immunocytes (Brandtzaeg *et al.*, 1981; Hong and Ammann, 1989; Savilahti and Pelkonen, 1979; Swanson *et al.*, 1968). However, in their jejunal mucosa, the IgM cell population always seems to be expanded aberrantly whereas such expansion is not necessarily seen in their large bowel mucosa (Brandtzaeg *et al.*, 1981; Savilahti and Pelkonen, 1979). IgA immunocytes (and apparently normal secretory immunity) in the gut also has been observed in a patient with severe combined immunodeficiency despite lack of lacrimal, salivary, and serum IgA (Rubinstein *et al.*, 1973). The persistent antigenic and mitogenic load on the intestinal mucosa probably explains these differences. Thus, terminal differentiation to IgA-producing cells takes place when peripheral blood lymphocytes from IgA-deficient patients are infected with Epstein–Barr virus (French and Dawkins, 1990) and sometimes also after mitogen treatment *in vitro* (Conley and Cooper, 1981; Hanson *et al.*, 1983).

As discussed earlier, a striking disparity exists between various exocrine sites in terms of IgD- and IgM-producing cells (Figure 5). These differences are amplified remarkably in IgA-deficient subjects whose glandular tissues from the upper respiratory tract often (but not always) contain an abundance of IgD-producing cells (25–80%) whereas such immunocytes only occasionally amount to 5%, and usually remain below 1%, in the gastrointestinal mucosa (Brandtzaeg *et al.*, 1979,1987; Korsrud and Brandtzaeg, 1980; Kanoh *et al.*, 1987). The compensatory nasal immunocyte population in addition consists of 10–70% IgG cells but only 7–25% IgM cells (Brandtzaeg *et al.*, 1979;1987), whereas the latter immunocytes amount to 65–75% in the gastrointestinal mucosa of IgA-deficient subjects (Brandtzaeg *et al.*, 1979; Kanoh *et al.*, 1987; Nilssen *et al.*, 1992). Notably, compensation with IgD rather than IgM production in respiratory mucosa appears to be associated with reduced resistance to infections (Brandtzaeg *et al.*, 1987).

The IgG1 fraction of the compensatory IgG cell population generally is increased, particularly in the jejunal mucosa where, on average, it represents almost 90% (Nilssen *et al.*, 1992). Interesting in this context is the fact that IgA-deficient subjects often have increased serum levels of IgG1, including casein antibodies belonging to this subclass (Out *et al.*, 1986). In contrast to the normally preferential IgG2 antibody response to polysaccharides, moreover, adults with selective IgA deficiency often show enhanced IgG1 (and IgG3) responses to such antigens, apparently reflecting an immunological maturation delay similar to that seen in early childhood (Roberton *et al.*, 1989).

B. Replacement of J Chain-Positive Immunocytes

When IgA-producing cells appear at secretory sites in IgA deficiency, they show normal or excessive J-chain expression (Brandtzaeg *et al.*, 1979, 1981; Brandtzaeg and Korsrud, 1984). Interestingly, the expanded IgD cell population of the upper respiratory tract also retains its high level (95–100%) of J-chain positivity (Brandtzaeg *et al.*, 1979; Brandtzaeg and Korsrud, 1984), whereas this expression in IgG immunocytes of nasal (~50%) and jejunal (~70%) mucosa is often somewhat reduced compared with normal levels (Brandtzaeg and Korsrud, 1984; Nilssen *et al.*, 1992), perhaps as an effect of inflammatory changes. However, J-chain expression has been reported to be quite high (~90%) for IgG cells in normal rectal mucosa from IgA-deficient subjects (Kanoh *et al.*, 1987).

The total number of Ig-producing immunocytes per defined jejunal mucosal tissue unit (Figure 1) in subjects who completely lacked IgA cells was distributed within a range (40–227) that overlapped with values found for the total immunocyte numbers in normal controls (observed range 86–199) and in adults with treated celiac disease (observed range 144–335) (Brandtzaeg *et al.*, 1979; Nilssen *et al.*, 1992). Also, the total number of Ig-producing cells/mm^2 6-μm thick normal parotid tissue section from an IgA-deficient subject was within the range for normal parotid immunocyte populations (29 compared with 26–98). The immunocyte density (cell number/mm^2) in the lacrimal gland of another IgA-deficient patient likewise was well within the normal range

(432 compared with 307–789). We did not attempt to obtain absolute figures for the nasal immunocyte populations because of the heterogeneous cell distribution within the nasal glands in individual cases, but the impression was that the total number of Ig-producing cells was fairly high in the IgA-deficient specimens compared with normal controls (Brandtzaeg *et al.*, 1987).

These results show that the migration of B cells to secretory sites and their compensatory terminal differentiation are fairly well maintained in IgA deficiency. The prominent J chain-expressing capacity exhibited by the local immunocytes, regardless of the concomitant Ig class produced, probably reflects the fact that these B cells belong to early memory clones whose terminal differentiation pathway to pIgA production has been blocked.

V. SUMMARY

Exocrine tissues contain more than 80% of all Ig-producing cells. The major product of these gland-associated or mucosal immunocytes is pIgA with high affinity for SC expressed by secretory epithelial cells. The SC binding site of poly-IgA and pentameric IgM depends on incorporation of J chain into the polymer structure. The obvious biological significance of the striking J-chain expression shown by immunocytes in secretory tissues is that the locally produced Ig polymers become readily available for external transport through nearby SC-positive epithelium. This important functional goal in terms of clonal differentiation might be sufficient justification for the J chain to be expressed by B cells terminating locally with IgD or IgG production. These immunocytes are probably "spin-offs" from the differentiation process on its way to pIgA production, thus representing a B-cell maturation stage compatible with homing to exocrine tissues. Observations in IgA-deficient individuals suggest that the magnitude of this homing is fairly well maintained, even when the differentiation pathway to pIgA is blocked. Little is known about the immunoregulation underlying the striking disparity of both the class (IgD/IgM) and the subclass (IgA1/IgA2 and IgG2/IgG3) expression patterns shown by gland-associated immunocytes in various regions of the body, but the local microbiota might have a great impact. Whether an inherent disparity exists in imigrating B cells derived from different mucosal precursor sources such as the Peyer's patches and tonsils remains to be shown.

Acknowledgments

Studies in the author's laboratory are supported by the Norwegian Cancer Society, the Norwegian Research Council and Otto Kr. Bruun's Legacy. Hege E. Svendsen is gratefully acknowledged for excellent secretarial assistance.

References

Alberini, C. M., Bet, P., Milstein, C., and Sitia, R. (1990). Secretion of immunoglobulin M assembly intermediates in the presence of reducing agents. *Nature (London)* **347,** 485–487.

Benson, E. B., and Strober, W. (1988). Regulation of IgA secretion by T-cell clones derived from the human gastrointestinal tract. *J. Immunol.* **140,** 1874–1882.

Bjerke, K., and Brandtzaeg, P. (1986). Immunoglobulin- and J chain-producing cells associated with lymphoid follicles in the human appendix, colon and ileum, including Peyer's patches. *Clin. Exp. Immunol.* **64,** 432–441.

Bjerke, K., and Brandtzeg, P. (1990a). Terminally differentiated human intestinal B cells. J chain expression of IgA and IgG subclass-producing immunocytes in the distal ileum compared with mesenteric and peripheral lymph nodes. *Clin. Exp. Immunol.* **82,** 411–415.

Bjerke, K., and Brandtzaeg, P. (1990b). Terminally differentiated human intestinal B cells. IgA and IgG subclass-producing immunocytes in the distal ileum, including Peyer's patches, compared with lymph nodes and palatine tonsils. *Scand. J. Immunol.* **32,** 61–67.

Bjerke, K., Brandtzaeg, P., and Rognum, T. O. (1986). Distribution of immunoglobulin producing cells is different in normal human appendix and colon mucosa. *Gut* **27,** 667–674.

Blanco, A., Linares, P., Andion, R., Alonso, M., and Villares, E. S. (1976). Development of humoral immunity system of the small bowel. *Allerg. Immunopathol.* **4,** 235–240.

Bouvet, J.-P., Pirès, R., Iscaki, S., and Pillot, J. (1987). IgM reassociation in the absence of J-chain. *Immunol. Lett.* **15,** 27–31.

Brandtzaeg, P. (1973). Two types of IgA immunocytes in man. *Nature, (London) New Biol.* **243,**142–143.

Brandtzaeg, P. (1974a). Presence of J chain in human immunocytes containing various immunoglobulin classes. *Nature (London)* **252,** 418–420.

Brandtzaeg, P. (1974b). Mucosal and glandular distribution of immunoglobulin components. Immunohistochemistry with a cold ethanol-fixation technique. *Immunology* **26,** 1101–1114.

Brandtzaeg, P. (1975). Human secretory immunoglobulin M. An immunochemical and immunohistochemical study. *Immunology* **29,** 559–570.

Brandtzaeg, P. (1982). Tissue preparation methods for immunohistochemistry. *In* "Techniques in Immunocytochemistry" (G. R. Bullock and P. Petrusz, eds.), Vol. 1, pp. 1–75. Academic Press, London.

Brandtzaeg, P. (1983a). Immunohistochemical characterization of intracellular J-chain and binding site for secretory component (SC) in human immunoglobulin (Ig)-producing cells. *Mol. Immunol.* **20,** 941–966.

Brandtzaeg, P. (1983b). The secretory immune system of lactating human mammary glands compared with other exocrine organs. *Ann. N.Y. Acad. Sci.* **409,** 353–381.

Brandtzaeg, P. (1984). Immune functions of human nasal mucosa and tonsils in health and disease. *In* "Immunology of the Lung and Upper Respiratory Tract" (J. Bienenstock, Ed.), pp. 28–95. McGraw–Hill, New York.

Brandtzaeg, P. (1985). Role of J chain and secretory component in receptor-mediated glandular and hepatic transport of immunoglobulins in man. *Scand. J. Immunol.* **22,** 111–146.

Brandtzaeg, P. (1987). Immune functions and immunopathology of palatine and nasopharyngeal tonsils. *In* "Immunology of the Ear" (J. M. Bernstein and P. L. Ogra, eds.), pp. 63–106. Raven Press, New York.

Brandtzaeg, P. (1989). Salivary immunoglobulins. *In* "Human Saliva: Clinical Chemistry and Microbiology" (J. O. Tenuvo, ed.), Vol. 2, pp. 1–54. CRC Press, Boca Raton, Florida.

Brandtzaeg, P., and Baklien, K. (1976). Immunohistochemical studies of the formation and epithelial transport of immunoglobulins in normal and diseased human intestinal mucosa. *Scand. J. Gastroenterol.* **11** (Suppl. 36), 1–45.

Brandtzaeg, P., and Berdal, P. (1975). J chain in malignant human IgG immunocytes. *Scand. J. Immunol.* **4,** 403–407.

Brandtzaeg, P., and Bjerke, K. (1990). Immunomorphological characteristics of human Peyer's patches. *Digestion* **46** (Suppl. 2), 262–273.

Brandtzaeg, P., and Korsrud, F. R. (1984). Significance of different J chain profiles in human tissues: Generation of IgA and IgM with binding site for secretory component is related to the J chain expressing capacity of the total local immunocyte population, including IgG and IgD producing cells, and depends on the clinical state of the tissue. *Clin. Exp. Immunol.* **58,** 709–718.

Brandtzaeg, P., Fjellanger, I., and Gjeruldsen, S. T. (1968). Immunoglobulin M: Local synthesis and selective secretion in patients with immunoglobulin A deficiency. *Science* **160,** 789–791.

Brandtzaeg, P., Gjeruldsen, S. T., Korsrud, F., Baklien, K., Berdal, P., and Ek, J. (1979). The human secretory immune system shows striking heterogeneity with regard to involvement of J chain-positive IgD immunocytes. *J. Immunol.* **122,** 503–510.

Brandtzaeg, P., Guy-Grand, D., and Griscelli, C. (1981). Intestinal, salivary, and tonsillar IgA and J-chain production in a patient with severe deficiency of serum IgA. *Scand. J. Immunol.* **13,** 313–325.

Brandtzaeg, P., Kett, K., Rognum, T. O., Söderström, R., Björkander, J., Söderström, T., Petruson, B., and Hanson, L. Å. (1986). Distribution of mucosal IgA and IgG subclass-producing immunocytes and alterations in various disorders. *Monogr. Allergy* **20,** 179–194.

Brandtzaeg, P., Karlsson, G., Hansson, G., Petruson, B., Björkander, J., and Hanson, L. Å. (1987). The clinical condition of IgA-deficient patients is related to the proportion of IgD- and IgM-producing cells in their nasal mucosa. *Clin. Exp. Immunol.* **67,** 626–636.

Brandtzaeg, P., Halstensen, T. S., Kett, K., Krajči, P., Kvale, D., Rognum, T. O., Scott, H., and Sollid, L. M. (1989). Immunobiology and immunopathology of human gut mucosa: Humoral immunity and intraepithelial lymphocytes. *Gastroenterology* **97,** 1562–1584.

Brandtzaeg, P., Nilssen, D. E., Rognum, T. O., and Thrane, P. S. (1991). Ontogeny of the mucosal immune system and IgA deficiency. *Gastroenterol. Clin. North Am.* **20,** 397–439.

Brandtzaeg, P., Halstensen, T. S., and Kett, K. (1992). Immunopathology of inflammatory bowel disease. *In* "Inflammatory Bowel Disease" (R. P. MacDermott and W. F. Stenson, eds.), pp. 95–136. Elsevier, London.

Brown, T. A., and Mestecky, J. (1985). Immunoglobulin A subclass distribution of naturally occurring salivary antibodies to microbial antigens. *Infect. Immun.* **49,** 459–462.

Carlsson, B., Zaman, S., Mellander, L., Jalil, F., and Hanson, L. A. (1985). Secretory and serum immunoglobulin class-specific antibodies to poliovirus after vaccination. *J. Infect. Dis.* **152,** 1238–1244.

Cattaneo, A., and Neuberger, M. S. (1987). Polymeric immunoglobulin M is secreted by transfectants of non-lymphoid cells in the absence of immunoglobulin J chain. *EMBO J.* **6,** 2753–2758.

Conley, M. E., and Cooper, M. D. (1981). Immature IgA B cells in IgA-deficient patients. *N. Engl. J. Med.* **305,** 495–497.

Crabbé, P. A., Carbonara, A. O., and Heremans, J. F. (1965). The normal human intestinal mucosa as a major source of plasma cells containing γA-immunoglobulin. *Lab. Invest.* **14,** 235–248.

Crabbé, P. A., Nash, D. R., Bazin, H., Eyssen, H., and Heremans, J. F. (1970). Immunohistochemical observations on lymphoid tissues from conventional and germ-free mice. *Lab. Invest.* **22,** 448–457.

Crago S. S., Kutteh, W. H., Moro, I., Allansmith, M. R., Radl, J., Haaijman, J. J., and Mestecky, J. (1984). Distribution of IgA1-, IgA2-, and J chain-containing cells in human tissues. *J. Immunol.* **132,** 16–18.

Cripps, A. W., Gleeson, M., and Clancy, R. L. (1989). Molecular characteristics of IgA in infant saliva. *Scand. J. Immunol.* **29,** 317–324.

Davis, A. C., and Shulman, M. J. (1989). IgM—Molecular requirements for its assembly and function. *Immunol. Today* **10,** 118–128.

Forsyth, K. D., Weeks S. C., Koh, L., Skinner, J., and Bradley, J. (1989). Lung immunoglobulins in the sudden infant death syndrome. *Br. Med. J.* **298,** 23–26.

French, M. A. H., and Dawkins, R. L: (1990). Central MHC genes, IgA deficiency and autoimmune disease. *Immunol. Today* **11,** 271–274.

Gebbers, J.-O., and Laissue, J. A. (1990). Postnatal immunomorphology of the gut. *In* "Inflammatory Bowel Disease and Coeliac Disease in Children" (F. Hadziselimovic, B. Herzog, and A. Bürgin-Wolff, eds.), pp. 3–44. Kluwer Academic Publishers, Dordrecht, The Netherlands.

Gleeson, M., Cripps, A. W., Clancy, R. L., Wlodarczyk, J. D., and Hensley, M. J. (1987a). IgD in infant saliva. *Scand. J. Immunol.* **26,** 55–57.

Gleeson, M., Cripps, A. W., Clancy, R. L., Wlodarczyk, J. H., Dobson, A. J., and Hensley, M. J. (1987b). The development of IgA-specific antibodies to *Escherichia coli* O antigen in children. *Scand. J. Immunol.* **26,** 639–643.

Hanson, L., Björkander, J., and Oxelius, V.-A. (1983). Selective IgA deficiency. *In* "Primary and Secondary Immunodeficiency Disorders" (R. K. Chandra, ed.), pp. 62–84. Churchill Livingstone, New York.

Hayashi, Y., Kurashima, C., Takemura, T., and Hirokawa, K. (1989). Ontogenic development of the secretory immune system in human fetal salivary glands. *Pathol. Immunopathol. Res.* **8,** 314–320.

Hong, R., and Ammann, A. J. (1989). Disorders of the IgA system. *In* "Immunologic Disorders in Infants and Children" (E. R. Stiehm ed.), 3 Ed. pp. 329–342. Saunders, Philadelphia.

Horsfall, D. J., Cooper, J. M., and Rowley, D. (1978). Changes in the immunoglobulin levels of the mouse gut and serum during conventionalisation and following administration of *Salmonella typhimurium*. *Aust. J. Exp. Biol. Med. Sci.* **56,** 727–735.

James, S. P. (1991). Mucosal T-cell function. *Gastroenterol. Clin. North Am.* **20,** 597–612.

Janson, H., Hedén, L.-O., Grubb, A., Ruan, M., and Forsgren, A. (1991). Protein D, an immunoglobulin D-binding protein of *Haemophilus influenzae:* Cloning, nucleotide sequence, and expression in *Escherichia coli*. *Infect. Immun.* **59,** 119–125.

Kanoh, T., Nishida, O., Uchino, H., Miyake, T., and Hishitani, Y. (1987). Transport defect of IgM Into luminal space in selective IgA deficiency. *Clin. Immunol. Immunopathol.* **44,** 272–282.

Kawanishi, H., Ozato, K., and Strober, W. (1985). The proliferiative response of cloned Peyer's patch switch T cells to syngenic and allogeneic stimuli. *J. Immunol.* **134,** 3586–3591.

Kett, K., and Brandtzaeg, P. (1987). Local IgA subclass alterations in ulcerative colitis and Crohn's disease of the colon. *Gut* **28,** 1013–1021.

Kett, K., Brandtzaeg, P., Radl, J., and Haaijman, J. F. (1986). Different subclass distribution of IgA-producing cells in human lymphoid organs and various secretory tissues. *J. Immunol.* **136,** 3631–3635.

Kett, K., Rognum, T. O., and Brandtzaeg, P. (1987). Mucosal subclass distribution of immunoglobulin G-producing cells is different in ulcerative colitis and Crohn's disease of the colon. *Gastroenterology* **93,** 919–924.

Kett, K., Brandtzaeg, P., and Fausa, O. (1988). J-chain expression is more prominent in immunoglobulin A2 than in immunoglobulin

A1 colonic immunocytes and is decreased in both subclasses associated with inflammatory bowel disease. *Gastroenterology* **94,** 1419–1425.

Knox, W. F. (1986). Restricted feeding and human intestinal plasma cell development. *Arch. Dis. Child.* **61,** 744–749.

Korsrud, F. R., and Brandtzaeg, P. (1980). Quantitative immunohistochemistry of immunoglobulin- and J-chain-producing cells in human parotid and submandibular glands. *Immunology* **39,** 129–140.

Kubagawa, H., Burrows, P. D., Grossi, C. E., Mestecky, J., and Cooper, M. D. (1988). Precursor B cells transformed by Epstein–Barr virus undergo sterile plasma-cell differentiation: J-chain expression without immunoglobulin. *Proc. Natl. Acad. Sci. U.S.A.* **85,** 875–879.

Lodinova, R., Jouja, V., and Wagner, V. (1973). Serum immunoglobulins and coproantibody formation in infants after artifical intestinal colonization with *Escherichia coli* 083 and oral lysozyme administration. *Pediatr. Res.* **7,** 659–669.

Maffei, H. V. L., Kingston, D., Hill, I. D., and Shiner, M. (1979). Histopathologic changes and the immune response within the jejunal mucosa in infants and children. *Pediatr. Res.* **13,** 733–736.

McClelland, D. B. L., Shearman, D. J. C., and van-Furth, R. (1976). Synthesis of immunoglobulin and secretory component by gastrointestinal mucosa in patients with hypogammaglobulinaemia or IgA deficiency. *Clin. Exp. Immunol.* **25,** 103–111.

Mellander, L., Carlsson, B., and Hanson, L. Å. (1984). Appearance of secretory IgM and IgA antibodies to *Escherichia coli* in saliva during early infancy and childhood. *J. Pediatr.* **104,** 564–568.

Mellander, L., Carlsson, B., Jalil, F., Söderstrom, T., and Hanson, L. Å. (1985). Secretory IgA antibody response against *Escherichia coli* antigens in infants in relation to exposure. *J. Pediatr.* **107,** 430–433.

Mestecky, J. (1987). The common mucosal immune system and current strategies for induction of immune responses in external secretions. *J. Clin. Immunol.* **7,** 265–276.

Mestecky, J., and McGhee, J. R. (1987). Immunoglobulin A (IgA): Molecular and cellular interactions involved in IgA biosynthesis and immune response. *Adv. Immunol.* **40,** 153–245.

Mestecky, J., and Russell, M. W. (1986). IgA subclasses. *Monogr. Allergy* **19,** 277–301.

Mestecky, J., Moldoveanu, Z., Julian, B. A., and Prchal, J. T. (1990). J chain disease: A novel form of plasma cell dyscrasia. *Am. J. Med.* **88,** 411–416.

Milner, A. D., and Ruggins, M. (1989). Sudden infant death syndrome. Recent focus on the respiratory system. *Br. Med. J.* **298,** 689–690.

Moldoveanu, Z., Egan, M. L., and Mestecky, J. (1984). Cellular origins of human polymeric and monomeric IgA: Intracellular and secreted forms of IgA. *J. Immunol.* **133,** 3156–3162.

Moreau, M. C., Ducluzeau, R., Guy-Grand, D., and Muller, M. C. (1978). Increase in the population of duodenal immunoglobulin A plasmocytes in axenic mice associated with different living or dead bacterial strains of intestinal origin. *Infect. Immun.* **121,** 532–539.

Moro, I., Iwase, T., Komiyama, K., Moldoveanu, Z., and Mestecky, J. (1990). Immunoglobulin A (IgA) polymerization sites in human immunocytes: Immunoelectron microscopic study. *Cell Struct. Funct.* **15,** 85–91.

Mosmann, T. R., Gravel, Y., Williamson, A. R., and Baumal, R. (1978). Modification and fate of J chain in myeloma cells in the presence and absence of polymeric immunoglobulin secretion. *Eur. J. Immunol.* **8,** 94–101.

Müller, F., Frøland, S. S., Hvatum, M., Radl, J., and Brandtzaeg, P. (1991). Both IgA subclasses are reduced in parotid saliva from patients with AIDS. *Clin. Exp. Immunol.* **83,** 203–209.

Nagura, H., Brandtzaeg, P., Nakane, P. K., and Brown, W. R. (1979). Ultrastructural localization of J chain in human intestinal mucosa. *J. Immunol.* **23,** 1044–1050.

Nilssen, D. E., Söderström, R., Brandtzaeg, P., Kett, K., Helgeland, L., Karlsson, G., Söderström, T., and Hanson, L. Å. (1991). Isotype distribution of mucosal IgG-producing cells in patients with various IgG-subclass deficiencies. *Clin. Exp. Immunol.* **83,** 17–24.

Nilssen, D. E., Brandtzaeg, P., Frøland, S. S., and Fausa, O. (1992). Subclass composition and J-chain expression of the "compensatory" IgG-cell population in selective IgA deficiency. *Clin. Exp. Immunol.* **87,** 237–245.

Out, T. A., van Munster, P. J. J., De Graeff, P. A., Thé, T. H., Vossen, J. M., and Zegers, B. J. M. (1986). Immunological investigations in individuals with selective IgA deficiency. *Clin. Exp. Immunol.* **64,** 510–517.

Papadea, C., and Check, I. J. (1989). Human immunoglobulin G and immunoglobulin G subclasses: Biochemical, genetic, and clinical aspects. *Crit. Rev. Clin. Lab. Sci.* **27,** 27–58.

Parkhouse, R. M. E., and Cooper, M. D. (1977). A model for the differentiation of B lymphocytes with implications for the biological role of IgD. *Immunol. Rev.* **37,** 105–126.

Penn, N. D., Purkins, L, Kelleher, J., Heatley, R. V., and Mascie-Taylor, B. H. (1991). Ageing and duodenal mucosal immunity. *Age Ageing* **20,** 33–36.

Randall, T. D., Parkhouse, R. M. E., and Corley, R. B. (1992). J chain synthesis and secretion of hexameric IgM is differentially regulated by lipopolysaccharide and interleukin 5. *Proc. Natl. Acad. Sci. U.S.A.* **89,** 962–966.

Reynolds, J. D., and Morris, B. (1984). The effect of antigen on the development of Peyer's patches in sheep. *Eur. J. Immunol.* **14,** 1–6.

Richman, L. K., and Brown, W. R. (1977). Immunochemical characterization of IgM in intestinal fluids. *J. Immunol.* **199,** 1515–1519.

Roberton, D. M., Björkander, J., Henrichsen, J., Söderström, T., and Hanson, L. Å. (1989). Enhanced IgG1 and IgG3 responses to pneumococcal polysaccharides in isolated IgA deficiency. Clin. Exp. Immunol. 75, 201–205.

Ruan, M., Akkoyunlu, M., Grubb, A., and Forsgren., A. (1990). Protein D of *Haemophilus influenzae*. A novel bacterial surface protein with affinity for human IgD. *J. Immunol.***145,** 3379–84.

Rubin, W., Fauci, A. S., Sleisenger, M. H., and Jeffries, G. H. (1965). Immunofluorescent studies in adult celiac disease. *J. Clin. Invest.* **44,** 475–485.

Rubinstein, A., Radl, J., Cottier, H., Rossi, E., and Gugler, E. (1973). Unusual combined immunodeficiency syndrome exhibiting kappa-IgD paraproteinemia, residual gut immunity and graft-versus-host reaction after plasma infusion. *Acta Paediatr. Scand.* **62,** 365–372.

Sagie, E., Tarabulus, J., Maeir, D. M., and Freier, S. (1974). Diet and development of intestinal IgA in the mouse. *Israel J. Med. Sci.* **10,** 532–534.

Savilahti, E. (1972). Immunoglobulin-containing cells in the intestinal mucosa and immunoglobulins in the intestinal juice in children. *Clin. Exp. Immunol.* **11,** 415–425.

Savilahti, E. (1973). IgA deficiency in children. Immunoglobulin-containing cells in the intestinal mucosa, immunoglobulins in secretions and serum IgA levels. *Clin. Exp. Immunol.* **13,** 395–406.

Savilahti, E. (1974). Workshop on secretory immunoglobulins. *In* "Progress in Immunology" (L. Brent and J. Holborow, eds.), pp. 238–243. North Holland, Amsterdam.

Savilahti, E., and Pelkonen, P. (1979). Clinical findings and intestinal immunoglobulins in children with partial IgA deficiency. *Acta Paediatr. Scand.* **68,** 513–519, 1979.

Scott, H., Kett, K., Halstensen, T., Hvatum, M., Rognum, T. O., and Brandtzaeg, P. (1992). The humoral immune system in coeliac disease. *In* "Coeliac Disease" (M. N. Marsh, ed.). pp. 239–282. Blackwell Scientific, Oxford.

Scott, M. G., Nahm, M. H., Macke, K., Nash, G. S., Bertovich, M. J., and MacDermott, R. P. (1986). Spontaneous secretion of IgG subclasses by intestinal mononuclear cells: Differences between ulcerative colitis, Crohn's disease, and controls. *Clin. Exp. Immunol.* **66,** 209–215.

Scotta, M. S., Maggiore, G., Giacomo, C. De., Martini, A., Burgio, V. L., and Ugazio, A. G. (1982). IgA-containing plasma cells in the intestinal mucosa of children with selective IgA deficiency. *J. Clin. Lab. Immunol.* **9,** 173–175.

Silverstein, A. M., and Lukes, R. J. (1962). Fetal response to antigenic stimulus. I. Plasma–cellular and lymphoid reactions in the human fetus to intrauterine infection. *Lab. Invest.* **11,** 918–932.

Smith, D. J., King, W. F., and Taubmann, M. A. (1989). Isotype, subclass, and molecular size of immunoglobulins in salivas from young infants. *Clin. Exp. Immunol.* **76,** 97–102.

Spencer, J., Dillon, S. B., Isaacson, P. G., and MacDonald, T. T. (1986). T cell subclasses in fetal human ileum. *Clin. Exp. Immunol.* **65,** 553–558.

Swanson, W., Dyce, B., Citron, P., Rouleau, C., Feinstein, D., and Haverback, D. J. (1968). Absence of IgA in serum with presence of IgA containing cells in intestinal tract. *Clin. Res.* **16,** 119. (Abstract)

Takayasu, H., and Brooks, K. H. (1991). IL-2 and IL-5 both induce μ_s and J chain mRNA in a clonal B cell line, but differ in their cell-cycle dependency for optimal signaling. *Cell. Immunol.* **136,** 472–485.

Tarkowski, A., Lue, C., Moldoveanu, Z., Kiyono, H., McGhee, J. R., and Mestecky, J. (1990). Immunization of humans with polysaccharide vaccines induces systemic, predominantly polymeric IgA2-subclass antibody responses. *J. Immunol.* **144,** 3770–3778.

Tarkowski, A., Moldoveanu, Z., Koopman, W. J., Radl, J., Haaijman, J. J., and Mestecky, J. (1991). Cellular origins of human polymeric and monomeric IgA: Enumeration of single cells secreting polymeric IgA1 and IgA2 in peripheral blood, bone marrow, spleen, gingiva and synovial tissue. *Clin. Exp. Immunol.* **85,** 341–348.

Thrane, P. S., Rognum, T. O., and Brandtzaeg, P. (1990). Increased immune response in upper respiratory and digestive tracts in SIDS. *Lancet* **335,** 229–230.

Thrane, P. S., Rognum, T. O., and Brandtzaeg, P. (1991). Ontogenesis of the secretory immune system and innate defence factors in human parotid glands. *Clin. Exp. Immunol.* **86,** 342–348.

Thrane, P. S., Rognum, T. O., and Brandtzaeg, P. (1993). Upregulated epithelial expression of HLA-DR and secretory component (SC) in salivary glands: Reflection of mucosal immunostimulation in sudden infant death syndrome (SIDS). *Pediatric Res.* In press.

Tigges, M. A., Casey, L. S., and Koshland, M. E. (1989). Mechanism of interleukin-2 signaling: Mediation of different outcomes by a single receptor and transduction pathway. *Science* **243,** 781–786.

Tomasi, T. B., Tan, E. M., Solomon, A., and Prendergast, R. A. (1965). Characteristics of an immune system common to certain external secretions. *J. Exp. Med.* **121,** 101–124.

Turesson, I. (1976). Distribution of immunoglobulin-containing cells in human bone marrow and lymphoid tissues. *Acta Med. Scand.* **199,** 293–304.

Valnes, K., Brandtzaeg, P., Elgjo, K. and Stave, R. (1986). Quantitative distribution of immunoglobulin-producing cells in gastric mucosa: Relation to chronic gastritis and glandular atrophy. *Gut* **27,** 505–514.

van der Heijden, P. J., Stok, W., and Bianchi, T. J. (1987). Contribution of immunoglobulin-secreting cells in the murine small intestine to the 'background' immunoglobulin production. *Immunology* **62,** 551–55.

Wijesinha, S. S., and Steer, H. W. (1982). Studies of the immunoglobulin-producing cells of the human intestine: The defunctioned bowel. *Gut* **23,** 211–214.

22

T Helper Cells for Mucosal Immune Responses

Hiroshi Kiyono • Jerry R. McGhee

I. INTRODUCTION

The mucosal surfaces in humans are collectively larger than the size of a basketball court and, as such, require an enormous contribution from our immune system for their protection. The humoral immunity for mucosal sites is mediated largely by secretory IgA (SIgA) antibodies, which represent >80% of total Ig in external secretions and are produced as polymeric (usually dimeric) IgA by plasma cells in mucosal effector tissues (see Chapters 7, 11, 21). Most mucosal IgA is produced in the lamina propria of the gastrointestinal tract, where estimates of populations numbering $\sim 1 \times 10^{10}$ plasma cells/m human intestine have been made (Brandtzaeg, 1989). In addition, the bone marrow is a major site for plasma cells that produce monomeric IgA found in serum IgA; these cells constitute the second most dominant isotype in the human circulation. In fact, estimates suggest that approximately two-thirds of the total Ig made in mammals are of the IgA isotype (Solomon, 1980; Conley and Delacroix, 1987). Important questions that arise from these data are: (1) how do we regulate the production of this enormous amount of IgA and (2) why is IgA preferentially produced in mucosal effector sites? As will become clear in this chapter, T cells are of central importance in regulating mucosal immunity, including IgA responses, and T helper (Th) cells constitute the largest cellular component of the mucosal immune system.

We have known for two decades that IgA responses are highly T cell dependent. This knowledge emerged from three separate lines of early work. The first line came from studies of athymic nude mice that were shown to have deficient levels of serum IgA as well as IgG1, IgG2a, and IgG2b whereas IgM levels were normal or even elevated (Crewther and Warner, 1972; Pritchard *et al.,* 1973). Thymic grafting of nude mice restored serum Ig, including IgA, to normal levels (Pritchard *et al.,* 1973). A subsequent study focusing on the serum and plasma cell IgA isotype clearly showed that serum IgA and intestinal IgA plasma cells were deficient in nude mice (Guy-Grand *et al.,* 1975). However, a second study disagreed somewhat with this result and suggested that depressed numbers of IgA plasma cells were found in the lung, parotid, and lactating mammary glands but normal levels were noted in the small intestine (Weisz-Carrington *et al.,* 1979). This discrepancy is most likely explained by age and environmental antigens that impinge on mucosal tissues since aged nude mice showed increases in IgG subclasses and IgA, correlating with increased IgA and IgG plasma cell numbers in bone marrow (Piquet, 1980). Of interest was the finding that deficient numbers of IgA plasma cells also were seen in mucosal tissues of older nude mice, as in younger ones; this study was the first to show that serum IgA originates from bone marrow and not from mucosal sites (Piquet, 1980). These results also suggest that mucosal IgA responses are regulated more tightly by thymus-derived cells than are IgA responses in the bone marrow. A second line of work has shown that neonatal thymectomy results in depressed levels of IgA in serum and external secretions, as well as in diminished SIgA responses (Ebersole *et al.,* 1979; Clough *et al.,* 1971). The final line of evidence stems from studies of patients with immunodeficiencies. For example, patients with ataxia telangiectasia showed complex B and T cell abnormalities with resulting IgA deficiency (Waldmann *et al.,* 1983). Studies also have shown that T-cell abnormalities occur in IgA-deficient subjects (Waldmann *et al.,* 1976); however, this result has not been a universal finding and a deficiency in Th cells alone does not explain IgA deficiency.

To facilitate our discussion of Th cells in IgA responses, we reemphasize that the mucosal immune system can be divided into two separate but interconnected compartments. Mucosal inductive sites include the gut-associated and bronchus-associated lymphoreticular tissues (GALT and BALT) which are placed strategically in the gastrointestinal tract and the upper respiratory tract where they encounter environmental antigens. Several studies have shown that stimulation of Th and IgA precursor B cells in GALT with orally administered antigens leads to the dissemination of B and Th cells to mucosal effector tissues, such as the lamina propria of the gastrointestinal and upper respiratory tracts, and to secretory glands for subsequent antigen-specific SIgA responses (reviewed by McGhee *et al.,* 1989). These mucosal effector tissues have two broad characteristics: (1) they contain Th cells and B cells with enriched numbers of IgA plasma cells, and (2) they are covered by epithelial cells that produce the polymeric Ig receptor (SC) that transports pIgA into the external secretions. The induction of immune B and Th cells in GALT, followed by their exodus to effector sites for the development of mucosal immune responses, is often termed the common mucosal immune system (McGhee *et al.,* 1989; see also Chapters 12, 13, 19, 21, 35, 43). We place a major emphasis on the characteristics of Th cells in GALT and on their function in IgA plasma cell responses in mucosal effector tissues. However, T cells also have been shown to induce B cells to switch from IgM to IgA (and to IgG); this function also receives some attention in this chapter.

II. Th CELLS IN MUCOSAL INDUCTIVE TISSUES

Reviewing certain basic features of Th cell activation and function before discussing Th cell studies in mucosal immune responses may be helpful to the reader. Activation of Th cells by antigen requires processing of the antigen and subsequent reexpression of specific peptide by antigen-presenting cells (APC) in GALT. The APCs in GALT include macrophages, B cells, and dendritic cells that are closely related to the Langerhans cells of skin (reviewed by McGhee *et al.*, 1989). The APCs in GALT process the antigen in endocytic compartments into peptide epitopes that become associated with major histocompatibility complex (MHC) Class II molecules. Th cells are $CD3^+$ $\alpha\beta$ T-cell receptor $(TcR)^+$, and most (but not all) are $CD4^+$; the latter of these cells respond to peptide epitopes associated with MHC Class II in the membrane of the APCs (Marrack and Kappler, 1986; Bierer *et al.*, 1989). Th–APC contact occurs between the $\alpha\beta$ TcR and the presented MHC Class II peptide epitope, forming a ternary complex that is reinforced by reaction of the CD4 molecule with a conserved Class II determinant (Bierer *et al.*, 1989). Other recognition systems also reinforce the Th–APC interaction (Kupfer and Singer, 1989) and contribute to Th-cell activation via the CD3 peptides (Clevers *et al.*, 1988).

Activated Th cells and their derived cytokines are sufficient to induce B cells to enter G_1 phase for completion of the cell cycle and division, as well as for induction of B cells to differentiate terminally into plasma cells. Interestingly, interleukin 4 (IL-4), IL-5, and IL-6, which are tandem products of Th2 cells (see subsequent text), are adept at inducing these three major steps. Nevertheless, the exact requirements for induction of B-cell entry into the cell cycle and subsequent division are not known; however, some studies suggest that Th–B-cell contact is required (Owens, 1988), whereas others suggest that Th cell-derived cytokines (Leclercq *et al.*, 1986) such as IL-2, IL-4, IL-5, and IL-6 are sufficient to stimulate resting B cells and lead to plasma cell induction. As we will see in the discussion that follows, interactions of B cells with Th cells also induce activation of Th cells with subsequent cytokine production and cytokine receptor expression, especially in anamnestic responses in which Th cells have re-entered the quiescent stage (G_0 and G_1) and memory B cells act as APCs for induction of Th cell re-entry into G_1. The subsequent division of and cytokine production by these Th cells may trigger B cells to divide and differentiate into a clonal population of plasma cells. Speculating that the initial induction of Th cells by APCs occurs in GALT, for example, in the Peyer's patches, is tempting; however, memory B cells and Th cells (in G_0) in mucosal effector sites such as the lamina propria of the small intestine may represent the major locale for Th–B-cell interactions resulting in the IgA response.

GALT consists of Peyer's patches, the appendix, and solitary lymphoid nodules, yet most studies, especially in mice, have been done with Peyer's patches (McGhee *et al.*, 1989). The parafollicular regions of Peyer's patches are enriched for T cells and are immediately adjacent to the follicles, or B-cell zones, containing the germinal centers. These T-cell areas possess high endothelial venules (HEV) that are the entry sites for lymphocytes to populate the Peyer's patches continuously. Further, the T-cell zones contain dendritic cells, an important type of APC in GALT for induction of Th cells (Spalding *et al.*, 1983,1984). In GALT, 35–40% of mononuclear cells are $CD3^+$ T cells with a CD4 : CD8 ratio of ~2 : 1 (Table I). The first definitive evidence for functional Th cells in murine Peyer's patches was provided by experiments in which the addition of Peyer's patch T cells to B-cell cultures (from nude mouse Peyer's patches) restored *in vitro* IgM antibody responses to a T cell-dependent antigen (Kagnoff and Campbell, 1974). Further, mice orally primed with heterologous erythrocytes were shown to contain Th cells that supported *in vitro* IgM responses to hapten erythrocyte carrier (Kagnoff, 1975).

Table I Characteristics of Murine T Cell Subsets in Mucosal Inductive and Effector Tissues

Mucosal tissues	Frequency of $CD3^+$ T cells (%)	TcR expression (%) $\alpha\beta$	$\gamma\delta$	Frequency of $CD4^+$ T cells (%)[a]	Ratio of Th1 : Th2	Ratio of CD4 : CD8
Inductive sites						
Peyer's patches	25–35	>90	1–5	60–65	1 : 1	2 : 1
Effector sites						
Lamina propria (GI)	40–60	>95	1–5	55–60	1 : 2–3	2 : 1
Intraepithelium	80–90	35–45	45–65	5–10	1 : 1[b]	1 : 7–8
Salivary glands	40–55	85–95	5–15	40–45	1 : 2	1 : 1

[a] Frequency of $CD4^+$ T cells in $CD3^+$ T cell fraction.
[b] In IELs, $CD8^+$ T cells were separated into IFNγ-producing and IL-5-secreting T cells.

Direct evidence for T-cell regulation of IgA production came from a seminal comparative study with mitogen-activated T cells from Peyer's patches and spleen of mice. Concanavalin A (Con A)-stimulated Peyer's patch T cells selectively induced IgA synthesis in lipopolysaccharide (LPS)-triggered Peyer's patch or spleen B-cell cultures whereas identically treated spleen T cells suppressed IgA, IgG, and IgM production in these cultures (Elson *et al.*, 1979). This work implies that IgA isotype-specific T cells were present in higher frequencies in Peyer's patches and could explain why IgA responses are induced selectively in mucosal tissues. Additional support for this hypothesis was provided in antigen-specific systems in which oral administration of T cell-dependent antigens such as sheep erythrocytes (SRBC), whole bacteria, and soluble proteins induced Th-cell responses in Peyer's patches with resultant IgA responses in spleen and mucosal effector regions (Richman *et al.*, 1981; Kiyono *et al.*, 1983).

A major advance in this area has been the development of an enzymatic dissociation procedure that allows recovery of all lymphoreticular cell subsets from the Peyer's patches (Kiyono *et al.*, 1982b). Cultures from normal mice supported *in vitro* IgM anti-SRBC responses, whereas cells from Peyer's patches of orally immunized mice supported IgA anti-SRBC responses (Kiyono *et al.*, 1982b). Peyer's patch Th cells from the mice given SRBC by the oral route were shown to support IgM and IgA anti-SRBC responses when added to normal B-cell cultures (Kiyono *et al.*, 1982b). Note that this enzyme procedure allows recovery of MHC Class II$^+$ macrophages and dendritic cells (Spalding *et al.*, 1983; Kiyono *et al.*, 1982b) and that Peyer's patch dendritic cells could be induced to form large clusters with CD4$^+$ T cells in the presence of the oxidative mitogen sodium periodate (Spalding *et al.*, 1984). These Peyer's patch dendritic cell–CD4$^+$ T-cell clusters preferentially supported IgA synthesis in either Peyer's patch or spleen B-cell cultures (Spalding *et al.*, 1984).

III. T CELL INDUCTION OF CLASS SWITCHING AND IgA PRODUCTION

Two related developments have helped elucidate how Th cells function to induce and to direct B cells to develop into plasma cells, including those of the IgA isotype. The first was the development of procedures that allow cloning of antigen-specific Th cells and, more recently, analysis of subsets of Th cells that mediate different effector functions (see subsequent discussion). The second was the cloning of cytokines, including IL-1 through IL-13, interferon γ (IFNγ), tumor necrosis factor α and β (TNFα and -β), transforming growth factor β (TGFβ), and others, which has allowed us to determine their roles in the immune response. We will minimize our discussion of cytokines (see Chapter 20 for more details) and mention them only as necessary to understand the function of Th cells in IgA responses.

Two major types of CD4$^+$ T cells have been isolated and cloned from murine Peyer's patches and are separable based on the target B cell affected. These two types of T cells should not be confused with the two Th cell subsets, Th1 and Th2, which are described in more detail in Section IV. One type of T-cell clone induced surface IgM positive (sIgM$^+$) B cells to switch to sIgA expression (Kawanishi *et al.*, 1983a,1985) whereas the second Th cell type preferentially supported antigen-specific IgA responses (Kiyono *et al.*, 1982a,1984,1985). The initial studies with T switch (T_{sw}) cells used T-cell clones derived by mitogen stimulation and IL-2-supported outgrowth that, when added to sIgM$^+$sIgA$^-$ B-cell cultures, resulted in marked increases in sIgA$^+$ cells (Kawanishi *et al.*, 1983a; Figure 1). Peyer's patch T_{sw} cells did not induce IgA secretion, even when incubated with sIgA$^+$ B-cell enriched cultures; however, addition of B-cell growth and differentiation factors readily induced the latter cultures to secrete IgA (Kawanishi *et al.*, 1983b). Specificity studies indicated that T_{sw} cells were autoreactive (Kawanishi *et al.*, 1985), suggesting that the microenvironment of the Peyer's patch was conducive to their induction.

Another population of isotype-specific Th-cell clones derived from Peyer's patches induced the proliferation and differentiation of sIgA$^+$ B cells into IgA-producing plasma cells (Kiyono *et al.*, 1982a,1984; Figure 2). These Peyer's patch Th-cell clones were derived from Peyer's patches of mice fed SRBC (Kiyono *et al.*, 1982a); clones generally were divisible into two groups. One group supported IgM, low IgG, and IgA anti-SRBC responses whereas a second group preferentially supported IgA responses (Kiyono *et al.*, 1982a,1984). These Peyer's patch Th-cell clones expressed Fc receptors for IgA (FcαR; Kiyono *et al.*, 1982a). Hybridomas derived from them secreted IgA binding factors (Kiyono *et al.*, 1985), which helped explain their preferential induction of IgA responses. Further, another study has provided interesting new evidence that the expression of FcαR is always associated with Th2 cells but not Th1 cells (see discussion of Th1 and Th2 cells; Sandor *et al.*, 1990). In this study, large numbers of Th1 and Th2 cell clones were examined for FcαR expression. This receptor was expressed only on Th2 cell clones on stimulation via the TcR–CD3 complex (Sandor *et al.*, 1990). Finally, other investigators also have isolated Th cell clones specific for keyhole limpet hemocyanin (KLH) from mouse Peyer's patches; one of four clones supported antigen-specific IgA responses (Al Maghazachi and Phillips-Quagliata, 1988). Unfortunately, cytokine profiles of T_{sw} cells or cloned Peyer's patch Th cells were not done, so no conclusions could be drawn about the role of cytokines in $\mu \rightarrow \alpha$ switches or in preferential IgA responses. However, in conjunction with current knowledge of Th1 and Th2 cells, as well as their derived cytokines (see Section IV), one could postulate that T cells that are involved in isotype switching might be TGFβ-producing cells whereas FcαR$^+$ Peyer's patch Th cells could be Th2 type cells that preferentially produce IL-5 and IL-6 on antigen stimulation (Figures 1 and 2).

Evidence for T_{sw} cells in human IgA responses also has been presented. Malignant T cells from a patient who suffered from a mycosis fungoides/Sézary-like syndrome (T_{Rac} cells) induced tonsillar sIgM$^+$ B cells to switch to and secrete IgG and IgA (Mayer *et al.*, 1985). Further, T_{Rac} cells, when added to B-cell cultures obtained from patients with hyper-IgM

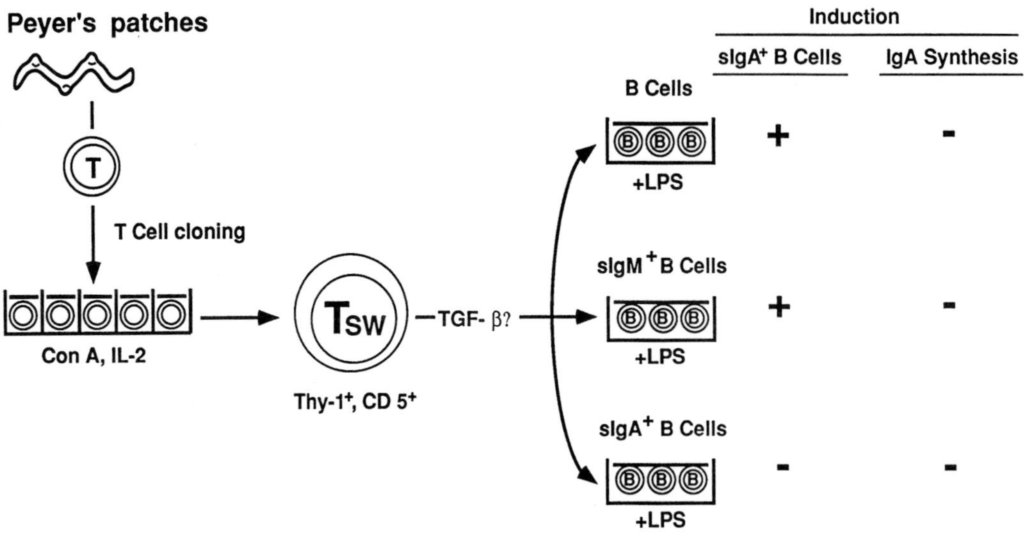

Figure 1 IgA inductive tissue (Peyer's patch) contains switch T cells that induce sIgM$^+$ B cells to become sIgA$^+$ B cells.

immunodeficiency, induced eight of nine cultures to secrete IgG and three of nine to produce IgA (Mayer *et al.*, 1986). T-cell clones also have been obtained from human appendix. These clones, or their derived culture supernatants, provided preferential help for IgA synthesis (Benson and Strober, 1988). Direct evidence was provided that CD3$^+$CD4$^+$CD8$^-$ T-cell clones induced $\mu \rightarrow \alpha$ B-cell switches as well as the terminal differentiation of sIgA$^+$ B cells to IgA-producing plasma cells (Benson and Strober, 1988). Additional studies are needed to determine the mechanism(s) for the observed class switch and the possible contribution of cytokines to this process (see Chapter 20).

The dendritic cells in Peyer's patches, in association with T cells, also have been tested for their potential to induce B-cell and pre-B cell class switching (Spalding and Griffin, 1986). For example, dendritic cell–T cell mixtures from Peyer's patches were shown to induce pre-B cells to undergo $\mu \rightarrow \alpha$ and some $\mu \rightarrow \gamma$ class switches, and to develop into Ig-producing cells of IgA and, to a lesser extent, IgM and IgG isotypes (Spalding and Griffin, 1986). On the other hand, dendritic cell–T cell mixtures from spleen induced pre-B cells to mature and secrete IgM. Further support of a role for dendritic cells and T cells in switching and differentiation comes from experiments that showed that an IL-3-dependent

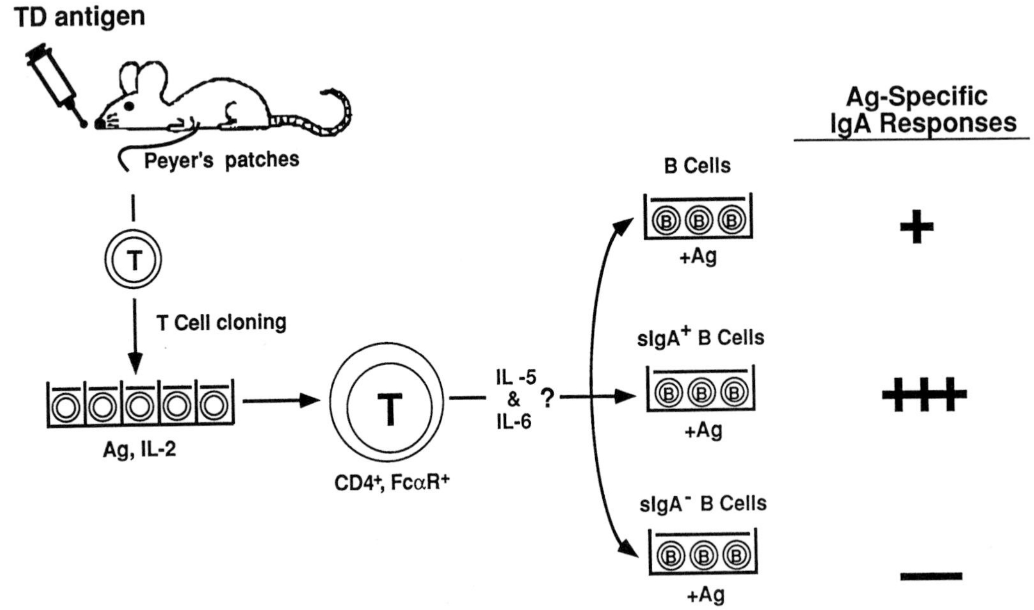

Figure 2 The initial proof for IgA isotype-specific T helper cells that selectively interact with sIgA$^+$ B cells and support IgA responses.

pre-B cell line (LyD9) also could be induced to undergo class switching and maturation (Kinashi *et al.*, 1988). Coculture of LyD9 cells with bone marrow stromal cells or with dendritic cell–T cell mixtures induced *in vitro* maturation and secretion of IgM and IgG (Kinashi *et al.*, 1988). The dendritic cell–T cell mixtures were derived from spleen in this latter study, which may explain the non-IgA isotype profile seen (Kinashi *et al.*, 1988).

IV. ROLE OF Th1 AND Th2 CELLS IN MUCOSAL IMMUNE RESPONSES

A concept of two distinct Th subsets was generated initially based on functional criteria, using uncloned murine Th-cell populations. Th cells were divided into Th1 and Th2 cells according to the difference in their delivery of helper signals to B cells (Tada *et al.*, 1978; Swierkosz *et al.*, 1979; Melchers *et al.*, 1982). The classical Th cells were thought to require cognate interactions between T and B cells to provide helper effects for B cells, in which the former cells responded to carrier antigenic determinants while the latter cells recognized the hapten molecule. This type of Th cell was designated Th1 (Tada *et al.*, 1978; Swierkosz *et al.*, 1979; Melchers *et al.*, 1982; Kim *et al.*, 1985). In contrast to Th1 cells, the other subset of Th cells, known as Th2, did not require a cognate interaction for their helper function, but provided an enhancing signal in a noncognate fashion (Tada *et al.*, 1978; Swierkosz *et al.*, 1979; Melchers *et al.*, 1982; Kim *et al.*, 1985). Th2 type cells also were suggested not to require MHC restriction for their helper activity. Most investigators now agree that Th cells, the majority of which are $CD4^+$, recognize antigen peptide presented by MHC Class II, which is sufficient to induce their activation. Thus, the Th1 and Th2 distinction based on the cognate interaction is less apparent. Further, using the Th1 and Th2 designations in the context described here is more useful.

In early 1986, a completely new concept for Th1 and Th2 cell function was introduced by the analysis of a wide variety of murine Th-cell clones for their profiles of cytokine synthesis (Mosmann *et al.*, 1986). In the original study, a total of 22 different murine Th-cell clones was examined for IL-2, IFNγ, and IL-4 production; approximately half the Th-cell clones produced only IL-2 and IFNγ whereas the other half preferentially secreted IL-4 (Mosmann *et al.*, 1986). Using additional cytokine-specific bioassay and mRNA analysis, a distinct pattern of cytokine production by murine Th1 and Th2 cells was established (Coffman *et al.*, 1988; Mosmann and Coffman, 1989; Mosmann and Moore, 1991; Street and Mosmann, 1991). Th1 cells were capable of producing IL-2, IFNγ, and TNFβ (lymphotoxin) whereas Th2 cells did not produce these cytokines (Table II). On the contrary, Th2 cells exclusively secreted IL-4, IL-5, and IL-6 (and, as later shown IL-10) on antigen or mitogen stimulation (Table II). To date, no specific cell surface molecules that differentiate between Th1 and Th2 cells have been identified. Note that Th1 and Th2 cells can cross-regulate each other via these respective cytokines (Mosmann and Coffman, 1989; Mosmann and Moore, 1991; Street and Mosmann, 1991). IL-2 and IL-4 produced by Th1 and Th2 cells, respectively, are important cytokines for the growth of both types of T cells. IFNγ, a product of Th1 cells, down-regulates Th2 cell function whereas IL-10, secreted by Th2 cells, inhibits Th1 cells (Mosmann and Moore, 1991; Street and Mosmann, 1991).

Table II Th1 and Th2 Cells for the Regulation of IgA Responses

Th subsets	Cytokine produced	Key effect on IgA responses
Th1	IL-2	Augments IgA synthesis; synergizes with IL-5 and TGF-β for enhanced IgA synthesis
	IFNγ	Down-regulate Th1 cells
	TNFβ (LT)	None (? Needs investigation)
	TGFβ(?)	Induces IgA isotype switching
Th2	IL-4	May be involved IgA isotype switching; may augment IL-5 induced IgA synthesis
	IL-5	Induce differentiation of $sIgA^+$ B cells to plasma cells; synergizes with TGF-β to enhance IgA production
	IL-6	Induces maximum IgA synthesis; acts on $sIgA^+$ B cells and induces IgA secreting plasma cells
	IL-10	Down-regulates Th1 cells

The function of Th1 and Th2 cells for B-cell responses has been studied in some detail. Although helper activity can be provided to B cells by both Th-cell subsets, Th2 cells seem to be much more effective (Coffman *et al.*, 1988; Mosmann and Coffman, 1989). This difference could be the result of the profile of cytokines secreted by Th1 and Th2 cells. For example, high doses of IFNγ are immunosuppressive and cause inhibition of B-cell responses (Reynolds *et al.*, 1987; Mosmann and Coffman, 1989). Further, Th1 cells have been shown to kill B cells, directly, probably by production of lymphotoxin and IFNγ (Janeway *et al.*, 1988). Since these two molecules are powerful cytokines for the elimination of intracellularly infected host cells via activation of macrophages and direct cytolytic activity, Th1 cells are perhaps better capable of helping host defenses against intracellular parasites (Mosmann and Coffman, 1989; Mosmann and Moore, 1991; Street and Mosmann, 1991). In addition, Th1 cells have been shown to be involved in the regulation of a Jones–Mote type delayed-type hypersensitivity (DTH) reaction, since co-injection of a Th1 clone and antigen into the footpads of virgin mice led to the induction of antigen-specific and MHC-restricted inflammation (Cher and Mosmann, 1987) whereas Th2 cells did not cause development of any inflammation.

In contrast to Th1 cells and their derived cytokines, cytokines produced by Th2 cells, including IL-4, IL-5, and IL-6, are potent soluble factors for the activation, proliferation, growth, and differentiation of B cells (see more details in Chapter 20). In this regard, Th2-cell clones have been shown to induce growth and differentiation of the majority of B cells in limiting dilution cultures (Lebman and Coffman, 1988). Th2 cells and their secreted cytokines can regulate both resting and large (activated) B-cell populations. In the most cases, resting B cells require direct cell contact with Th2 cells for their activation, growth, and differentiation (Rasmussen *et al.*, 1988). On the other hand, large B cells can proliferate and differentiate in response to culture supernatants from Th2 cells without any physical Th–B-cell linkage (Herron *et al.*, 1988).

Another unique feature of Th1 and Th2 cells is that individual subsets of Th cells can potentiate certain isotypes of B-cell responses because of their secreted cytokines. For example, Th1 cells preferentially support IgG2a synthesis in B-cell cultures (Coffman *et al.*, 1988; Mosmann and Coffman, 1989). IFNγ, a product of Th1 cells, has been shown to be involved in IgG2a isotype switching and to enhance IgG2a synthesis in LPS-stimulated B-cell cultures (Coffman *et al.*, 1988; Snapper *et al.*, 1988). Since IgG2a is a complement-fixing cytotoxic antibody and possesses a high-affinity FcγR on macrophages, this interaction further supports the view that Th1 cells and their secreted cytokines (e.g., IFNγ) are important in host defense against intracellularly infected cells and in DTH responses. Th2 cells, in contrast, support more IgG1, IgE, and IgA responses than Th1 cells (Coffman *et al.*, 1988; Mosmann and Coffman, 1989). Th2-derived IL-4 enhances IgG1 secretion in LPS-triggered B-cell culture via an increase in isotype switching of $sIgG^-$ B cells to $sIgG1^+$ B cells (reviewed by Paul, 1987). However, Th1 cells also can support IgG1 responses (Coffman *et al.*, 1988). Thus, the IgG1 response can be induced in an IL-4-independent manner as well. Several lines of evidence, both *in vivo* and *in vitro,* strongly demonstrated that IL-4 produced by Th2 cells is important for the induction of IgE synthesis (Paul, 1987; Lebman and Coffman, 1988; Finkelman *et al.*, 1990). IL-4 acts directly on $sIgM^+$ B cells and induces them to switch to $sIgE^+$ B cells (Paul, 1987; Lebman and Coffman, 1988). Interestingly, anti-IL-4 or IFNγ treatment shuts down IgE responses both *in vivo* and *in vitro* (Coffman and Carty, 1986; Finkelman *et al.*, 1990). Thus, one can suggest that cross-regulation of Th1 and Th2 cells is important in isotype-specific responses in which IgE responses are Th2 and IL-4 dependent whereas IFNγ produced by Th1 cells down-regulates IL-4-induced IgE responses. Although Ig genes encoding ε and α chains are clustered closely in the 3′ region, IgE responses rarely are seen at normal mucosa. Since relatively high numbers of cytokine-producing Th1 and Th2 cells can be isolated from both IgA inductive and effector sites (Taguchi *et al.*, 1990; Mega *et al.*, 1992), IFNγ produced by Th1 cells may suppress IL-4 production by Th2 cells specifically, whereas the production of other Th2 cytokines (e.g., IL-5 and IL-6) that are essential for IgA synthesis may be maintained.

For IgA responses, clearly Th2 cells regulate the terminal differentiation of $sIgA^+$ B cells to IgA-secreting plasma cells, since the addition of IL-5 or IL-6 to cultures containing either LPS-stimulated splenic B cells or freshly isolated Peyer's patch B cells resulted in the preferential induction of IgA synthesis (see Chapter 20). Th2-like autoreactive Th-cell clones generated from murine Peyer's patches originally were reported to enhance IgA synthesis in LPS-triggered B-cell cultures (Murray *et al.*, 1987). Also, culture supernatants from Th2-cell clones independently were shown to augment IgA production under similar B-cell culture conditions (Coffman *et al.*, 1987). However, when culture supernatants from Th1 clones were tested for IgA-enhancing factor, none of the Th1-cell clone-derived culture supernatants supported IgA responses in LPS-treated B-cell cultures. These findings led to the purification of IgA-enhancing factor; a partial sequence containing 21 amino acids from this factor exactly matched murine IL-5 (Bond *et al.*, 1987). In addition, numerous studies have examined further the molecular aspects of Th2-cell involvement in IgA responses. Researchers now generally accept that Th2-derived IL-5 and IL-6 are essential cytokines for the development of IgA plasma cells (see Chapter 20). However, concluding that only Th2 cells and their secreted IL-5 and IL-6 are important in the regulation of $sIgA^+$ B cell responses would be too simplistic since IL-2, a product of stimulated Th1 cells, has been shown to enhance IgA synthesis in LPS-stimulated B-cell cultures (Coffman *et al.*, 1987). However, the magnitude of IgA enhancement by IL-2 was lower than that of Th2-cell derived cytokines (Coffman *et al.*, 1987). Further, IL-2 synergistically augmented IgA synthesis in TGFβ-treated B-cell cultures in the presence of LPS (Lebman *et al.*, 1990). Therefore, one must emphasize that, although Th2 cells tend to play a major role in the differentiation of $sIgA^+$ B cells to IgA plasma cells, Th1 cells and their cytokines certainly can influence IgA B-cell responses. Thus, an optimal relationship between Th1 and Th2 cells via their respective cytokines is probably essential for the maintenance of appropriate IgA responses in mucosal associated tissues.

To date, most Th1 and Th2 cell studies have been done with cloned T cells. Their natural existence *in vivo* has not been demonstrated directly. However, studies using IFNγ- and IL-5-specific ELISPOT assays and mRNA analysis have revealed that these Th1 and Th2 cells exist *in situ* in both IgA inductive and effector sites (Taguchi *et al.*, 1990; Mega *et al.*, 1992). When freshly isolated $CD3^+CD4^+CD8^-$ T cells from Peyer's patches and lamina propria of intestine were examined for IFNγ-producing Th1 and IL-5-secreting Th2 cells, a distinct pattern of Th1 and Th2 cell distribution was seen (Taguchi *et al.*, 1990). Higher numbers of $CD4^+$ T cells, which were producing IFNγ or IL-5 spontaneously, were always noted in IgA effector tissues compared with IgA inductive sites. In the case of the latter tissue, approximately equal frequencies of IFNγ (Th1)- and IL-5 (Th2)-producing cells were found (Taguchi *et al.*, 1990). Upon T-cell stimulation via the TcR–CD3 complex or lectin receptor, increased numbers of cytokine-producing T cells were evident in both Th1 (IFNγ) and Th2 (IL-5) cell subsets (Taguchi *et al.*, 1990; Xu-Amano *et al.*, 1992). Therefore, an equal appearance of Th1 and Th2 cells in Peyer's patches may represent an appropriate cross-regulation of these two subsets of Th cells that may contribute to the suppression of the $sIgA^+$ B-cell differentiation step. Although Peyer's patches contain significant numbers of $sIgA^+$ B cells, very few IgA plasma cells actually occur in this tissue. In a separate study, using IL-2 and IL-4 as indicators of Th1 and Th2 cells, respectively, Peyer's patches and mesenteric lymph nodes that receive draining lymphocytes from Peyer's patches were suggested to possess both Th1 and Th2 cells (Daynes *et al.,* 1990). Note that cultivation of Peyer's patch T cells with anti-CD3 antibody resulted in the predominant production of IL-4, suggesting that a preferential induction of Th2 cells occurs in IgA inductive sites on stimulation. Collectively, these findings indicated that $CD4^+$ Th cells, which have the potential to become either Th1 or Th2 cells, reside in the IgA inductive sites.

For the induction of Th1 and Th2 responses to antigen-specific IgA responses, one study has provided an important finding that oral administration of T cell-dependent antigen (e.g., SRBC) induced a higher frequency of Th2 (IL-5) cells than of Th1 (IFNγ) cells in T-cell cultures prepared from Peyer's patches and spleen (Xu-Amano *et al.,* 1992). Further, high levels of IL-5-specific mRNA was noted in $CD4^+$ T cells from Peyer's patch T-cell cultures of orally immunized mice. Thus, oral administration of T cell-dependent antigen preferentially induces antigen-specific Th2 cells in IgA inductive sites (Xu-Amano *et al.,* 1992). These antigen-stimulated Th2 cells may leave Peyer's patches and migrate into the IgA effector sites, such as lamina propria of intestine and exocrine glandular tissues, where these cells can provide the necessary cytokines (e.g., IL-5 and IL-6) for $sIgA^+$ B cells to become IgA-secreting plasma cells. In this regard, a higher frequency of Th2 (IL-5) cells than IFNγ-producing Th1 cells was seen in IgA effector sites (Taguchi *et al.,* 1990; Mega *et al.,* 1992; see Section V).

Several studies have provided strong evidence that human Th cells also can be separated into Th1 and Th2 cells according to their cytokine profile (reviewed by Romagnani, 1991). *Mycobacterium tuberculosis*-specific $CD4^+$ Th-cell clones generated from healthy donors were categorized as Th1 type cells, since these clones produced IFNγ and IL-2 (Del Prete *et al.,* 1991). On the other hand, *Toxocara canis*-specific $CD4^+$ Th-cell clones secreted Th2 cytokines, including IL-4 and IL-5. In addition, allergen-specific $CD4^+$ Th-cell clones from atopic disease patients were preferentially grouped as Th2 cells (Parronchi *et al.,* 1991). Therefore, clearly Th1 and Th2 cells exist in both murine and human systems. The cross-regulation of Th1 and Th2 cells via respective cytokines thus can influence the outcome of isotype-specific responses. Further, the nature of antigen and its presentation to Th cells will affect the induction of Th1 and Th2 cells. Since both IgA inductive and effector sites possess several immunologically unique features and are exposed continuously to a wide variety of environmental antigens, considering $CD4^+$ Th cells in mucosal associated tissues to have novel interaction pathways between Th1 and Th2 cells to regulate mucosal IgA immune responses is logical (Figure 3).

V. Th CELLS IN MUCOSAL EFFECTOR TISSUES

Antigen uptake via M cells or follicle-associated epithelial (FAE) cells into mucosal associated lymphoreticular tissues (including GALT and BALT) results in antigen stimulation of B and T lymphocytes that leave IgA inductive tissues via the efferent lymphatics. These lymphocytes then home to the effector sites, including the lamina propria of the upper respiratory and gastrointestinal tracts, the reproductive tract, and exocrine glandular tissues through the common mucosal immune pathway.

The lamina propria of the gastrointestinal tract has been characterized as an example of a major mucosal effector site (reviewed by Brandtzaeg, 1984; Brandtzaeg *et al.,* 1985). Note that, in contrast to IgA inductive sites, major studies for the characterization of lamina propria T cells have been done in the human system. The intestinal lamina propria contains primarily B cells (including plasma cells), T cells, and macrophages. In addition, mucosal inflammatory cells such as eosinophils and mast cells are also present in lamina propria. Among B-lineage cells, which represent 20–40% of lamina propria cells, approximately 80% of the plasma cells in the small intestine produce antibodies of the IgA isotype (Brandtzaeg, 1984; Brandtzaeg *et al.,* 1985), as reflected by an abundant production of IgA in external secretions of mucosal effector tissues. Substantial numbers of T cells are also present in this tissue; approximately 50% of lamina propria lymphocytes are $CD3^+$ T cells (Brandtzaeg, 1984; Brandtzaeg *et al.,* 1985; Mega *et al.,* 1992; Table I). The majority of $CD3^+$ T cells is $CD4^+CD8^-$ (~40–60% of $CD3^+$ T cells) and the ratio of CD4 to CD8 is ~2–3 : 1 (Brandtzaeg, 1984;

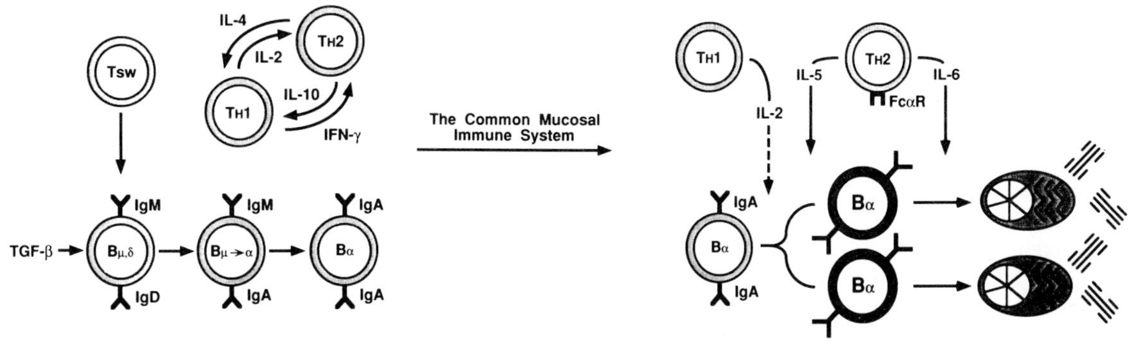

Figure 3 Current concepts for T cell and cytokine regulation of IgA responses in IgA inductive (*left*) and effector (*right*) sites.

Brandtzaeg *et al.*, 1985; Mega *et al.*, 1992). These $CD4^+$ T cells have been shown to exert helper effects on Ig secretion, including the IgA isotype in B-cell cultures prepared from the lamina propria and the peripheral blood (Clancy *et al.*, 1984; Elson *et al.*, 1985). In addition, when $CD4^+$ T cells isolated from human mesenteric lymph nodes, a population of T lymphocytes that is presumably on its way to lamina propria regions, were cultured with B cells, elevated IgA secretion compared with IgG and IgM was noted (Pang *et al.*, 1986). This helper function for the IgA isotype was higher with mesenteric lymph node $CD4^+$ T cells than with peripheral blood $CD4^+$ T cells. These findings provide evidence that $CD4^+$ T cells in IgA effector tissues such as intestinal lamina propria can provide helper functions for IgA B cell responses.

The $CD4^+$ Th cells in intestinal lamina propria can be separated further into helper–inducer (Leu 8^- and $2H4^-$) and suppressor–inducer (Leu 8^+ and $2H4^+$) phenotypes based on their immunological function as well as Leu 8 and 2H4 expression (James *et al.*, 1986; Kanof *et al.*, 1988). Lamina propria $CD4^+$ Th cells possessed higher numbers of cells with a phenotype associated with helper–inducers and a corresponding decrease in the proportion of suppressor–inducer type $CD4^+$ T cells compared with their systemic counterparts (e.g., peripheral blood; James *et al.*, 1986). $CD4^+$ T cells that coexpress Leu 8 suppress Ig synthesis. On the other hand, Leu 8^- and $CD4^+$ T cells isolated from lamina propria support both IgA and IgG synthesis in pokeweed mitogen (PWM)-stimulated peripheral blood B-cell cultures (Kanof *et al.*, 1988). In another study, the possible existence of preactivated IgA isotype-specific Th cells in normal human lamina propria was suggested (Smart *et al.*, 1988). When the T cell-enriched fraction from the human colonic mucosa, which contained a 3 : 1 ratio of CD4 : CD8, was tested for enhancing function, maximum enhancing activity was seen for the IgA isotype with increasing numbers of T cells. Further, cocultivation with PWM in this system had no significant effect on IgA synthesis, suggesting that lamina propria Th cells were activated *in situ* (Smart *et al.*, 1988). Further, normal lamina propria T cells were shown to possess higher gene expression associated with cell activation compared with T cells in systemic tissues (Zeitz *et al.*, 1988). $CD4^+$ T cells isolated from normal nonhuman primates had high percentages of IL-2 receptor (IL-2R)-positive cells that contained increased mRNA levels for this receptor. Collectively, these findings indicate that intestinal lamina propria contains significant numbers of activated $CD4^+$ Th cells that are capable of providing helper signals for the enhancement of IgA responses.

Since the concomitant appearance of activated $CD4^+$ Th cells and high numbers of IgA plasma cells are always seen in IgA effector sites such as the intestinal lamina propria, an interesting possibility was raised that Th2 cells may occur in high frequency in these tissues (Taguchi *et al.*, 1990). When $CD4^+$ T cells were isolated from normal murine lamina propria and tested for IFNγ-producing Th1 and IL-5-secreting Th2 cells by respective cytokine-specific ELISPOT assays, although significant numbers of Th1 cells were seen in lamina propria, the frequency of Th2 cells was always higher (Th1 : Th2 = 1 : 3). Thus, greater numbers of IL-5-producing Th2 cells were present in IgA effector sites at which Th cells were activated *in vivo* in response to environmental antigens (Taguchi *et al.*, 1990). Further, Northern blot analysis of mRNA from lamina propria T cells of normal nonhuman primates revealed that higher message levels for IL-4 and IL-5 were seen compared with T-cell fractions from systemic tissues, including peripheral lymph nodes and spleen (James *et al.*, 1990). In addition to the Th2 cytokines, mRNA levels for IL-2 and IFNγ (Th1 cytokines) also were increased in lamina propria T cells (James *et al.*, 1990). Based on these observations, one can envision that higher numbers of Th2 cells than Th1 cells reside in lamina propria; however, both subsets of $CD4^+$ Th cells are activated and are producing their respective cytokines for the regulation of the IgA response.

The occurrence of activated $CD4^+$ Th cells with a higher frequency of Th2 cells at IgA effector sites seems to provide an appropriate environment for IgA B-cell responses. However, one must always remember that Th2 cells also play an important role in classical allergic responses in which IgE synthesis and the numbers of eosinophils and mast cells are increased. The intestinal mucosa has a significant number of mast cell precursors that is higher than elsewhere in the body (Crapper and Schrader, 1983). Thus, IL-3 produced by both Th1 and Th2 cells in intestinal lamina propria could induce these precursors to become mature mast cells. $CD4^+$ T cells isolated from mesenteric lymph nodes of *Nippostrongylus brasiliensis*-infected rats were shown to produce IL-3, which can induce mucosal mast cells from bone marrow cultures (McMenamin *et al.*, 1985). In other studies, $CD4^+$ Th cells from the thoracic duct of *Trichinella spiralis*-infected rats were separated into two subsets according to OX22 expression (Wang *et al.*, 1990). When $OX22^+$ $CD4^+$ Th cells were transferred adoptively to naive rats and then challenged with *T. spiralis*, this subset of $CD4^+$ Th cells substantially enhanced the number of mucosal mast cells. In contrast, $OX22^-CD4^+$ Th cells increased the number of resident eosinophils in the intestine (Wang *et al.*, 1990). Further, this latter $CD4^+$ Th-cell subset provided helper activity for B cells and conferred protection against *T. spiralis*. Thus, the models of mucosal regulation by $CD4^+$ Th1 and Th2 cells are complex. One must always envision the importance of $CD4^+$ Th cells in regulation of mucosal associated responses other than the IgA B-cell responses.

In addition to lamina propria T cells, large numbers of T cells also are found in the intraepithelial compartment of the intestine. Intraepithelial lymphocytes (IELs) possess several unique features in terms of their TcR expression, T-cell subsets, and immunological functions (see Chapter 24). One of the novel characteristics of murine IELs is that IEL preparations contain $CD8^+$ T cells that produce Th1 and Th2 cytokines spontaneously (Taguchi *et al.*, 1990,1991). Approximately equal numbers of IFNγ- and IL-5-secreting $CD8^+$ T cells that express either TcR $\alpha\beta$ or TcR $\gamma\delta$ were seen in isolated IELs (Taguchi *et al.*, 1991). The immunological role of these cytokine-producing TcR $\alpha\beta^+$ and TcR $\gamma\delta^+$ $CD8^+$ T-cell subsets in mucosal immune responses remains to be elucidated. In addition to their cytokine production capability, most studies have provided evidence that a distinct subset of IEL T cells can provide an immunoregulatory function for IgA responses (Fujihashi *et al.*, 1990,1992). When TcR $\gamma\delta^+$ T cells from IELs of mice orally immunized with T cell-dependent antigen were transferred adoptively to mice orally tolerized with the same antigen, the oral tolerance was converted to antigen-specific immune responses including those of the IgA isotype (Fujihashi *et al.*, 1990,1992). On the other hand, TcR $\alpha\beta^+$ T cells from IELs of the same mice provided helper function for IgA responses (Fujihashi *et al.*, 1992). Thus, subsets of IEL T cells also could be important in regulating the IgA response, that is, TcR $\gamma\delta^+$ Th cells could provide protection or augmentation of TcR $\alpha\beta^+$ Th cells in the presence of oral tolerance to maintain appropriate IgA responses at the mucosal barrier.

In addition to the lamina propria regions of the gastrointestinal tract, another important IgA effector site is represented by exocrine glandular tissues. In this regard, saliva has been extensively used as a convenient secretion to analyze induction of antigen-specific SIgA responses. Further, salivary glands contain high numbers of IgA-producing cells (Mega *et al.*, 1992; see Chapter 15). The lymphocytes from murine submandibular glands contain approximately 40–55% CD3$^+$ T cells with a CD4:CD8 ratio of 1.0 (Mega *et al.*, 1992) (Table I). A similar finding also was observed in rats, in which the lymphocytes were shown to contain approximately 60% W3/13$^+$ T cells with a CD4:CD8 ratio of 1.3 (Pappo *et al.*, 1988). When the frequency of Th1 and Th2 cells was examined in CD4$^+$ T cells isolated from murine salivary glands, IL-5-producing Th2 cells were always more abundant than IFNγ-secreting Th1 cells (Mega *et al.*, 1992). This finding was in complete agreement with other studies in which the intestinal lamina propria region was shown to contain cytokine-producing CD4$^+$ Th cells with a preference for Th2 cells (Taguchi *et al.*, 1990).

VI. SUMMARY: OVERVIEW OF Th CELL REGULATION OF MUCOSAL IMMUNE RESPONSES

IgA inductive tissues (e.g., GALT or Peyer's patches) and IgA effector sites such as intestinal lamina propria and salivary glands contain several distinct T-cell subsets that possess unique biological characteristics for the induction and regulation of IgA immune responses. In GALT, two major subsets of T cells are present that are capable of regulating IgA isotype switching and terminal differentiation of post-switched sIgA$^+$ B cells to become IgA plasma cells (Figures 1 and 2). The T_{sw} cells act on sIgM$^+$ B cells in Peyer's patches and induce them to switch sIgA$^+$ B cells. Whether T_{sw} cells produce TGFβ for the induction of IgA isotype switching still is not known. Further, testing whether T_{sw} cells can be categorized into a family of Th1 or Th2 cells is important. The other subset of T cells is composed of helper T cells that possess the capability to interact preferentially with sIgA$^+$ B cells and induce them to become IgA-secreting plasma cells. This type of Th cell tends to fall in the category of Th2 cells, which can produce IL-5 and IL-6 for the differentiation of sIgA$^+$ B cells to high IgA-secreting plasma cells (Figures 2 and 3). The exact immunological mechanism for this selective interaction between Th2 cells and sIgA$^+$ B cells remains to be elucidated.

GALT has been shown to contain CD4$^+$ Th cells that can become either Th1 or Th2 cells. Both Th1 and Th2 cells are essential for the regulation of IgA B-cell responses since IL-2 and IL-5 and IL-6 (and perhaps others) produced by Th1 and Th2 cells, respectively, are important cytokines for the enhancement of IgA responses. Oral administration of T cell-dependent antigens induces antigen-specific Th1 and Th2 cells, with preferential induction of IL-5-producing Th2 cells. Thus, stimulation of Th cells and IgA precursor B cells in GALT via the oral route is an important consideration for the induction of appropriate antigen-specific IgA responses in distant mucosal effector sites.

In IgA effector sites, CD4$^+$ Th cells that can augment IgA B-cell responses are present in intestinal lamina propria. As one might expect, because of the unique immunological and physiological characteristics of the gut in which lymphocytes are exposed continuously to environmental antigens, CD4$^+$ Th cells are activated *in situ* and produce immunoregulatory cytokines. IFNγ- and IL-2-producing Th1 and IL-5- and IL-6-secreting Th2 CD4$^+$ Th cells are found in this tissue. The ratio of Th1 to Th2 cells is approximately 1:2–3, which provides an appropriate environment for sIgA$^+$ B cells to become IgA plasma cells since Th2 cells secrete essential cytokines (IL-5 and IL-6) for these B cells. A similar situation also occurs in other IgA effector tissues such as the salivary glands, a major IgA source for the oral cavity. The salivary glands contain cytokine-producing CD4$^+$ Th cells with a high frequency of Th2 cells. Note that Th1 and Th2 cells are important in the induction and regulation of IgA responses because of cross-regulation of Th1 and Th2 cells via respective cytokines. Further, cytokines (e.g., IL-2, IL-5, and IL-6) produced by these two subsets of CD4$^+$ T cells are essential for mucosal IgA immune responses. In addition to these CD4$^+$ Th cells that reside in IgA effector tissue (e.g., intestinal lamina propria), T cells reside in the epithelium itself (IELs) and also can be important regulatory cells for mucosal IgA responses.

Clearly T cells, especially CD4$^+$ Th cells, are an essential element in the induction and maintenance of appropriate IgA responses in mucosal associated tissues. This view has been demonstrated convincingly *in vivo*. Chronic treatment of mice with monoclonal anti-CD4 antibody dramatically reduced the numbers of IgA plasma cells in intestinal lamina propria (Mega *et al.*, 1991). In addition to IgA effector sites, IgA inductive sites such as the Peyer's patches also are affected by chronic CD4$^+$ Th cell deficiency. The size of Peyer's patches, especially the germinal centers where induction of IgA precursor B cells occurs, was reduced significantly (Mega *et al.*, 1991). A subset of T cells, $V_{\beta1}{}^+$ T cells elegantly were shown to be essential to the IgA response in chickens (Cihak *et al.*, 1991). Multiple injections of anti-TcR2 ($V_{\beta1}$-specific antibody) in embryonic life followed by thymectomy after hatching deleted $V_{\beta1}{}^+$ T cells in young birds. In these birds, IgA antibody production was impaired completely, whereas other types of antibody production were maintained

(Cihak *et al.*, 1991). Further, antigen-specific secretory IgA antibodies were not induced in response to mucosal immunization with tetanus vaccine. These *in vivo* studies further emphasize that IgA responses are CD4$^+$ Th cell dependent. The last study provided additional evidence that a subset of CD4$^+$ Th cells plays an important role in the induction and regulation of mucosal IgA responses. The concept of IgA-specific Th cells remains an important and essential part of our understanding of the precise regulatory mechanisms of the mucosal IgA response.

Acknowledgments

H. Kiyono and J. R. McGhee are supported in part by U. S. Public Health Service Grants AI 18958, AI 19674, AI 30366, DE 08228, DE 09837, DK 44240, and DE 04217 and NIAID Contract AI 15128. H. Kiyono is a recipient of NIH RCDA DE 00237. We are indebted to Drs. Dennis McGee, Katherine Merrill, Kohtaro Fujihashi, and Masafumi Yamamoto (University of Alabama at Birmingham) for their helpful suggestions. We thank Ms. Sheila Weatherspoon for the preparation of this manuscript.

References

AI Maghazachi, A., and Phillips-Quagliata, J. M. (1988). Keyhole limpet hemocyanin-propagated Peyer's patch T cell clones that help IgA responses. *J. Immunol.* **140,** 3380–3388.

Benson, E. B., and Strober, W. (1988). Regulation of IgA secretion by T cell clones derived from the human gastrointestinal tract. *J. Immunol.* **140,** 1874–1882.

Bierer, B. E., Sleckman, B. P., Ratnofsky, S. E., and Burakoff, S. J. (1989). The biologic roles of CD2, CD4 and CD8 in T-cell activation *Annu. Rev. Immunol.* **7,** 579–599.

Bond, M. W., Shrader, B., Mosmann, T. R., and Coffman, R. L. (1987). A mouse T cell product that preferentially enhances IgA production. II. Physiochemical characterization. *J. Immunol.* **139,** 3691–3696.

Brandtzaeg, P. (1985). Research in gastrointestinal immunology. State of arts. *Scand. J. Gastroenterol.* **20** (Suppl. 114)**,** 137–156.

Brandtzaeg, P. (1989). Overview of the mucosal immune system. *Curr. Top. Microbiol. Immunol.* **146,** 13–25.

Brandtzaeg, P., Valnes, K., Scott, H., Rognum, T. O., Bjerke, K., and Baklien, K. (1985). The human gastrointestinal secretory immune system in health and disease. *Scand. J. Gastroenterol.* **20** (Suppl. 114)**,** 17–38.

Cher, D. J., and Mosmann, T. R. (1987). Two types of murine helper T cell clone. II. Delayed-type hypersensitivity is mediated by Th1 clones. *J. Immunol.* **138,** 3688–3694.

Cihak, J., Hoffman-Fezer, G., Ziegler-Heibrock, H. W. L., Stein, H., Kaspers, B., Chen, C. H., Cooper, M. D., and Lösch, U. (1991). T cells expressing the $V_{\beta 1}$ T-cell receptor are required for IgA production in the chicken. *Proc. Natl. Acad. Sci. U.S.A.* **88,** 10951–10955.

Clancy, R., Cripps, A., and Chipchase, H. (1984). Regulation of human gut B lymphocytes by T lymphocytes. *Gut* **25,** 47–51.

Clevers, H., Alarcon, B., Wileman, T., and Terhorst, C. (1988). The T cell receptor/CD3 complex: A dynamic protein ensemble. *Annu. Rev. Immunol.* **6,** 629–662.

Clough, J. D., Mims, L. H., and Strober, W. (1971). Deficient IgA antibody responses to arsanilic acid bovine serum albumin (BSA) in neonatally thymectomized rabbits. *J. Immunol.* **106,** 1624–1629.

Coffman, R. L., and Carty, J. (1986). A T cell activity that enhances polyclonal IgE production and its inhibition by interferon-γ. *J. Immunol.* **136,** 949–954.

Coffman, R. L., Shrader, B., Carty, J., Mosmann, T. R., and Bond, M. W. (1987). A mouse T cell product that preferentially enhances IgA production. I. Biologic characterization. *J. Immunol.* **139,** 3685–3690.

Coffman, R. L., Seymour, B. W., Lebman, D. A., Hiraki, D. D., Christiansen, J. A., Shrader, B., Cherwinski, H. M., Savelkoul, H. F., Finkelman, F. D., Bond, M. W., and Mosmann, T. R. (1988). The role of helper T cell products in mouse B cell differentiation and isotype regulation. *Immunol. Rev.* **102,** 5–28.

Conley, M. E., and Delacroix, D. L. (1987). Intravascular and mucosal immunoglobulin A: Two separate but related systems of immune defense? *Ann. Intern. Med.* **106,** 892–899.

Crapper, R. M., and Schrader, J. W. (1983). Frequency of mast cell precursors in normal tissues determined by an *in vitro* assay: Antigen induces parallel increase in the frequency of P cell precursors and mast cells. *J. Immunol.* **131,** 923–928.

Crewther, P., and Warner, N. L. (1972). Serum immunoglobulins and antibodies in congenitally athymic (nude) mice. *Austr. J. Exp. Biol. Med. Sci.* **50,** 625–635.

Daynes, R. A., Araneo, B. A., Dowell, T. A., Huang, K., and Dudley, D. (1990). Regulation of murine lymphokine production *in vivo*. III. The lymphoid tissue microenvironment exerts regulatory influences over T helper cell function. *J. Exp. Med.* **171,** 979–996.

Del Prete, G. F., De Carli, M., Mastromauro, C., Biagiotti, R., Macchia, D., Falagiani, P., Ricci, M., and Romagnani, S. (1991). Purified protein derivative of *Mycobacterium tuberculosis* and excretory-secretory antigen(s) of *Toxocara canis* expand *in vitro* human T cells with stable and opposite (type 1 T helper or type 2 T helper) profile of cytokine production. *J. Clin. Invest.* **88,** 346–350.

Ebersole, J. L., Taubman, M. A., and Smith, D. J. (1979). The effect of neonatal thymectomy on the level of salivary and serum immunoglobulins in rats. *Immunology* **36,** 649–657.

Elson, C. O., Heck, J. A., and Strober, W. (1979). T-cell regulation of murine IgA synthesis. *J. Exp. Med.* **149,** 632–643.

Elson, C. O., Machelski, E., and Weiserbs, D. B. (1985). T cell-B cell regulation in the intestinal lamina propria in Crohn's disease. *Gastroenterology* **89,** 321–327.

Finkelman, F. D., Holmes, J., Katona, I. M., Urban, J. F., Jr., Beckman, M. P., Park, L. S., Schooley, K. A., Coffman, R. L., Mosmann, T. R., and Paul, W. E. (1990). Lymphokine control of *in vivo* immunoglobulin isotype selection. *Annu. Rev. Immunol.* **8,** 303–333.

Fujihashi, K., Taguchi, T., McGhee, J. R., Eldridge, J. H., Bruce, M. G., Green, D. R., Singh, B., and Kiyono, H. (1990). Regulatory function for murine intraepithelial lymphocytes. Two subsets of CD3$^+$, T cell receptor-1$^+$, intraepithelial lymphocytes T cells abrogate oral tolerance. *J. Immunol.* **145,** 2010–2019.

Fujihashi, K., Taguchi, T., Aicher, W. K., McGhee, J. R., Bluestone, J. A., Eldridge, J. H. and Kiyono, H. (1992). Immunoregulatory functions for murine intraepithelial lymphocytes: γ/δ TCR$^+$ T cells abrogate oral tolerance, while α/β TCR$^+$ T cells provide B cell help. *J. Exp. Med.* **175,** 695–707.

Guy-Grand, D., Griscelli, C., and Vassalli, P. (1975). Peyer's patches, gut IgA plasma cells and thymic function: Study in nude mice bearing thymic grafts. *J. Immunol.* **115,** 361–364.

Herron, L. R., Coffman, R. L., Bond, M. W., and Kotzin, B. L. (1988). Increase autoantibody production by NZB/NZW B cells in response to interleukin 5. *J. Immunol.* **141,** 842–848.

James, S. P., Fiocchi, C., Graeff, A. S., and Strober, W. (1986). Phenotypic analysis of lamina propria lymphocytes. Predominance of helper-inducer and cytolytic T-cell phenotype and deficiency of suppressor-inducer phenotypes in Crohn's disease and control patients. *Gastroenterology* **91,** 1483–1489.

James, S. P., Kwan, W. C., and Sneller, M. C. (1990). T cells in inductive and effector compartments of the intestinal mucosal immune system of nonhuman primates differ in lymphokine mRNA expression, lymphokine utilization and regulatory function. *J. Immunol.* **144,** 1251–1256.

Janeway, C. A., Jr. Carding, S., Jones, B., Murray, J., Portoles, P., Rasmussen, R., Rojo, J., Saizawa, K., West, J., and Bottomly, K. (1988). CD4$^+$ T cells: Specificity and function. *Immunol. Rev.* **101.** 39–80.

Kagnoff, M. F. (1975). Functional characteristics of Peyer's patch cells. III. Carrier priming of T cells by antigen feeding. *J. Exp. Med.* **142,** 1425–1435.

Kagnoff, M. F., and Campbell, S. (1974). Functional characteristics of Peyer's patch lymphoid cells. I. Induction of humoral antibody and cell-mediated allograft reactions. *J. Exp. Med.* **139,** 398–406.

Kanof, M. E., Strober, W., Fiocchi, C., Zeitz, M., and James, S. P. (1988). CD4 positive Leu-8 negative helper-inducer T cells predominate in the human intestinal lamina propria. *J. Immunol.* **141,** 3029–3036.

Kawanishi, H., Saltzman, L., and Strober, W. (1983a). Mechanisms regulating IgA class-specific immunoglobulin production in murine gut-associated lymphoid tissues. I. T cells derived from Peyer's patches that switch SIgM B cells to SIgA cells *in vitro*. *J. Exp. Med.* **157,** 433–450.

Kawanishi, H., Saltzman, L., and Strober, W. (1983b). Mechanisms regulating IgA class-specific immunoglobulin production in murine gut-associated lymphoid tissues. II. Terminal differentiation of postswitch SIgA-bearing Peyer's patch B cells. *J. Exp. Med.* **158,** 649–669.

Kawanishi, H., Ozato, K., and Strober, W. (1985). The proliferative response of cloned Peyer's patch switch T-cells to syngeneic and allogeneic stimuli. *J. Immunol.* **134,** 3586–3591.

Kim, J., Woods, A., Becker-Dunn, E., and Bottomly, K. (1985). Distinct functional phenotypes of cloned Ia- restricted helper T cells. *J. Exp. Med.* **162,** 188–201.

Kinashi, T., Inaba, K., Tsubata, T., Tashiro, K., Palacios, R., and Honjo, T. (1988). Differentiation of an interleukin 3-dependent precursor B-cell clone into immunoglobulin-producing cells *in vitro*. *Proc. Natl. Acad. Sci. U.S.A.* **85,** 4473–4477.

Kiyono, H., McGhee, J. R., Mosteller, L. M., Eldridge, J. H., Koopman, W. J., Kearney, J. F., and Michalek, S. M. (1982a). Murine Peyer's patch T-cell clones: Characterization of antigen-specific helper T cells for immunoglobulin A responses. *J. Exp. Med.* **156,** 1115–1130.

Kiyono, H., McGhee, J. R., Wannemuehler, M. J., Frangakis, M. V., Spalding, D. M., Michalek, S. M., and Koopman, W. J. (1982b). *In vitro* immune responses to a T cell-dependent antigen by cultures of disassociated murine Peyer's patch. *Proc. Natl. Acad. Sci. U.S.A.* **79,** 596–600.

Kiyono, H., Mosteller, L. M., Eldridge, J. H., Michalek, S. M., and McGhee, J. R. (1983). IgA responses in *xid* mice: Oral antigen primes Peyer's patch cells for *in vitro* immune responses and secretory antibody production. *J. Immunol.* **131,** 2616–2622.

Kiyono, H., Cooper, M. D., Kearney, J. F., Mosteller, L. M., Michalek, S. M., Koopman, W. J., and McGhee, J. R. (1984). Isotype-specificity of helper T cell clones. Peyer's patch Th cells preferentially collaborate with mature IgA B cells for IgA responses. *J. Exp. Med.* **159,** 798–811.

Kiyono, H., Mosteller-Barnum, L. M., Pitts, A. M., Williamson, S. I., Michalek, S. M., and McGhee, J. R. (1985). Isotype-specific immunoregulation: IgA binding factors produced by Fcα receptor$^+$ T cell hybridomas regulate IgA responses. *J. Exp. Med.* **161,** 731–747.

Kupfer, A., and Singer, S. J. (1989). Cell biology of cytotoxic and helper T-cell functions: Immunofluorescence microscopic studies of single cells and cell couples. *Annu. Rev. Immunol.* **7,** 309–337.

Lebman, D. A., and Coffman, R. L. (1988). Interleukin 4 causes isotype switching to IgE in T cell-stimulated clonal B cell cultures. *J. Exp. Med.* **168,** 853–862.

Lebman, D. A., Lee, F. D., and Coffman, R. L. (1990). Mechanism for transforming growth factor β and IL-2 enhancement of IgA expression in lipopolysaccharide-stimulated B cell cultures. *J. Immunol.* **144,** 952–959.

Leclercq, L., Cambier, J. C., Mishal, Z., Julius, M. H., and Theze, J. (1986). Supernatant from a cloned helper T cell stimulates most small resting B cells to undergo increased I-A expresion, blastogenesis and progression through cell cycle. *J. Immunol.* **136,** 539–545.

McGhee, J. R., Mestecky, J., Elson, C. O., and Kiyono, H. (1989). Regulation of IgA synthesis and immune response by T cells and interleukins. *J. Clin. Immunol.* **9,** 175–199.

McMenamin, C., Jarrett, E. E. E., and Sanderson, A. (1985). Surface phenotype of T cells producing growth of mucosal mast cells in normal rat bone marrow culture. *Immunology* **55,** 399–403.

Marrack, P., and Kappler, J. (1986). The antigen-specific, major histocompatibility comlex-restricted receptor on T cells. *Adv. Immunol.* **38,** 1–30.

Mayer, L., Posnett, D. N., and Kunkel, H. G. (1985). Human-malignant T-cells capable of inducing an immunoglobulin class switch. *J. Exp. Med.* **161,** 134–144.

Mayer, L., Kwan, S. P., Thompson, C., Ko, H. S., Chiorazzi, N., Waldmann, T., and Rosen, F. (1986). Evidence for a defect in "switch" T cells in patients with immunodeficiency and hyperimmunoglobulin M. *N. Engl. J. Med.* **314,** 409–413.

Mega, J., Bruce, M. G., Beagley, K. W., McGhee, J. R., Tagucht, T., Pitts, A. M., McGhee, M. L., Blicy, P. R., Eldridge, J. H., Mestecky, J., and Kiyono, H. (1991). Regulation of mucosal responses by CD4$^+$ T lymphocytes: Effect of anti-L324 treatment on the gastrointestinal immune system. *Int. Immunol.* **3,** 793–805.

Mega, J., McGhee, J. R., and Kiyono, H. (1992). Cytokine and Ig producing cells in mucosal effector tissues: Analysis of IL-5 and IFN-γ producing T cells, TCR expression and IgA plasma cells from mouse salivary gland associated tissues. *J. Immunol.* **148,** 2030–2039.

Melchers, I., Fey, K., and Eichmann, K. (1982). Quantitative studies on T cell diversity. III. Limiting dilution analysis of precursor cells for T helper cells reactive to xenogeneic erythrocytes. *J. Exp. Med.* **156,** 1587–1603.

Mosmann, T. R., and Coffman, R. L. (1989). Thl and Th2 cells: Different patterns of lymphokine secretion lead to different functional properties. *Annu. Rev. Immunol.* **7,** 145–173.

Mosmann, T. R., and Moore, K. W. (1991). The role of IL-10 in cross regulation of Thl and Th2 responses. *Immunol. Today* **12,** A49–A53.

Mosmann, T. R., Cherwinsky, H., Bond, M. W., Giedlin, M. A., and Coffman, R. L., (1986). Two types of murine helper T cell clone. I. Definition according to profiles of lymphokine activities and secreted proteins. *J. Immunol.* **136,** 2348–2357.

Murray, P. D., McKenzie, D. T., Swain, S. L., and Kagnoff, M. F. (1987). Interleukin 5 and interleukin 4 produced by Peyer's patch T cells selectively enhance immunoglobulin A expression. *J. Immunol.* **139,** 2669–2674.

Owens, T. (1988). A noncognate interaction with anti-receptor antibody-activated helper T cells induces small resting murine B cells to proliferate and to secrete antibody. *Eur. J. Immunol.* **18,** 395–401.

Pang, G., Yeung, S., Clancy, R. L., Cripps, A. W., Hennessy, E. J., and Santhanam, A. N. (1986). Regulation of IgA secretion in polyclonally induced *in vitro* human lymphocyte cultures: The function of T and B cells from mesenteric lymph node and peripheral blood. *Clin. Exp. Immunol.* **64,** 158–165.

Pappo, J., Ebersole, J. L., and Taubman, M. A. (1988). Phenotype of mononuclear leucocytes resident in rat major salivary and lacrimal glands. *Immunology* **64,** 295–300.

Parronchi, P., Macchia, D., Piccinni, M. P., Biswas, P., Simonelli, C., Maggi, E., Ricci, M., Ansari, A. A., and Romagnani, S. (1991). Allergen-and bacterial antigen-specific T-cell clones established from atopic donors show a different profile of cytokine production. *Proc. Natl. Acad. Sci. U.S.A.* **88,** 4538–4542.

Paul, W. E. (1987). Interleukin 4/B cell stimulatory factor 1: One lymphokine, many functions. *FASEB J.* **1,** 456–461.

Piquet, P.-F. (1980). Change in the humoral response of athymic nude mice with aging. *Scand. J. Immunol.* **12,** 233–238.

Pritchard, H., Riddaway, J., and Micklem, H. S. (1973). Immune responses in congenitally thymus-less mice. II. Quantitative studies of serum immunoglobulins, the antibody response to sheep erythrocytes, and the effect of thymus allografting. *Clin. Exp. Immunol.* **13,** 125–138.

Rasmussen, R., Takatsu, K., Harada, N., Takahashi, T., and Bottomly, K. (1988). T cell-dependent hapten-specific and polyclonal B cell responses require release of interleukin 5. *J. Immunol.* **140,** 705–712.

Reynolds, D. S., Boom, W. H., and Abbas, A. K. (1987). Inhibition of B lymphocyte activation of interferon-γ. *J. Immunol.* **139,** 767–773.

Richman, L. K., Graeff, A. S., Yarchoan, R., and Strober, W. (1981). Simultaneous induction of antigen-specific IgA helper T cells and IgG suppressor T cells in the murine Peyer's patch after protein feeding. *J. Immunol.* **126,** 2079–2083.

Romagnani, S. (1991). Human Th1 and Th2 subsets: Doubt no more. *Immunol. Today* **12,** 256–257.

Sandor, M., Gajewski, T., Thorson, J., Kemp, J. D., Fitch, F. W., and Hoover, R. G., (1990). $CD4^+$ murine T cell clones that express high levels of immunoglobulin binding belong to the interleukin 4-producing T helper cell type 2 subset. *J. Exp. Med.* **171,** 2171–2176.

Smart, C. J., Trejdosiewicz, L. K., Badr-El-Din, S., and Heatley, R. V. (1988). T lymphocytes of the human colonic mucosa: Functional and phenotypic analysis. *Clin. Exp. Immunol.* **73,** 63–69.

Snapper, C. M., Peschel, C., and Paul, W. E. (1988). IFN-γ stimulates IgG2a secretion by murine B cells stimulated with bacterial lipopolysaccharide. *J. Immunol.* **140,** 2121–2127.

Solomon, A. (1980). Monoclonal immunoglobulins as biomarkers of cancer. *In* "Cancer Markers" (S. Sell, ed.), pp. 57–87. Humana Press, Clifton, New Jersey.

Spalding, D. M., and Griffin, J. A. (1986). Different pathways of differentiation of pre-B cell lines are induced by dendritic cells and T cells from different lymphoid tissues. *Cell* **44,** 507–515.

Spalding, D. M., Koopman, W. J. Eldridge, J. H., McGhee, J. R., and Steinman, R. M. (1983). Accessory cells in murine Peyer's patch. I. Identification and enrichment of functional dendritic cells. *J. Exp. Med.* **157,** 1646–1959.

Spalding, D. M., Williamson, S. I., Koopman, W. J., and McGhee, J. R. (1984). Preferential induction of polyclonal IgA secretion by murine Peyer's patch dendritic cell-T cell mixtures. *J. Exp. Med.* **160,** 941–946.

Street, N. E., and Mosmann, T. R. (1991). Functional diversity of T lymphocytes due to secretion of different cytokine patterns. *FASEB J.* **5,** 171–177.

Swierkosz, J. E., Marrack, P., and Kappler, J. (1979). Functional analysis of T cells expressing Ia antigens. I. Demonstration of helper T-cell heterogeneity. *J. Exp. Med.* **150,** 1293–1309.

Tada, T., Takemori, T., Okumura, K., Nonaka, M., and Tokuhisa, T. (1978). Two distinct types of helper T cells involved in the secondary antibody response: Independent and synergistic effects of Ia^- and Ia^+ helper T cells. *J. Exp. Med.* **147,** 446–458.

Taguchi, T., McGhee, J. R., Coffman, R. L., Beagley, K. W., Eldridge, J. H., Takatsu, K., and Kiyono, H. (1990). Analysis of Th1 and Th2 cells in murine gut-associated tissues. Frequencies of $CD4^+$ and $CD8^+$ T cells that secrete IFN-γ and IL-5. *J. Immunol.* **145,** 68–77.

Taguchi, T., Aicher, W. K., Fujihashi, K., Yamamoto, M., McGhee, J. R., Bluestone, J. A., and Kiyono, H. (1991). Novel function for intestinal intraepithelial lymphocytes. Murine $CD3^+$, γ/δ TCR^+ T cells produce IFN-γ and IL-5. *J. Immunol.* **147,** 3736–3744.

Waldmann, T. A., Broder, S., Krakauer, R., Durm, M., Meade, B., and Goldman, C. (1976). Defects in IgA secretion and in IgA specific suppressor cells in patients with selective IgA deficiency. *Trans. Assoc. Am. Phys.* **89,** 215–223.

Waldmann, T. A., Broder, S., Goldman, C. K., Frost, K., Korsmeyer, S. J., and Medici, M. A. (1983). Disorders of B cells and helper T cells in the pathogenesis of the immunoglobulin deficiency of patients with ataxia teleangiectasia. *J. Clin. Invest.* **71,** 282–295.

Wang, C. H., Korenaga, M., Greenwood, A., and Bell, R. G. (1990). T-helper subset function in the gut of rats: Differential stimulation of eosinophils, mucosal mast cells and antibody-forming cells by $0X8^-$ $0X22^-$ and $Ox8^-$ $0X22^+$ cells. *Immunology* **71,** 166–175.

Weisz-Carrington, P., Schrater, A. F., Lamm, M. E., and Thorbecke, G. J. (1979). Immunoglobulin isotypes in plasma cells of normal and athymic mice. *Cell. Immunol.* **44,** 343–351.

Xu-Amano, J., Aicher, W. K., Taguchi, T., Kiyono, H., and McGhee, J. R. (1992). Selective induction of Th2 cells in murine Peyer's patches by oral immunization. *Int. Immunol.* **4,** 433–445.

Zeitz, M., Greene, W. C., Peffer, N. J., and James, S. P. (1988). Lymphocytes isolated from the intestinal lamina propria of normal nonhuman primates have increased expression of genes associated with T cell activation. *Gastroenterology* **94,** 647–655.

23

Human Gastrointestinal Mucosal T Cells

Stephen P. James • Martin Zeitz

I. INTRODUCTION

T cells in the gastrointestinal (GI) tract are thought to play a central role in GI host defense and in regulation of GI function. Cells present in organized lymphoid sites such as the Peyer's patches, mesenteric lymph nodes, and appendix are thought to carry out specialized tasks necessary for initiating responses to antigens present in the intestinal lumen. After activation, cells leave these sites and recirculate in the systemic circulation, from which they enter the diffuse lamina propria compartment of the mucosa. The intestinal lamina propria and epithelium constitute the largest single T-cell site in humans. Peyer's patches are much less prominent in humans than in rodents. In addition, the lamina propria of the colon of humans normally contains large numbers of lymphocytes, whereas that of rodents contains few lymphocytes. Substantial evidence suggests that T lymphocytes associated with the human GI tract have unique characteristics that reflect their specialized roles in host defense in the mucosa (Table I). In this chapter, the phenotypic and functional characteristics of human and nonhuman primate GI T cells are reviewed. By necessity, the ability to manipulate mucosal T cells in humans experimentally is, for the most part, limited to *in vitro* studies of isolated cells or tissue explants. Despite these limitations, considerable information is available concerning the function of human GI T cells. Further, this information serves as the foundation for the study of diseases of the human GI tract.

II. PHENOTYPIC CHARACTERISTICS

A. Lymphocyte Subpopulations

Many of the characteristics of mucosal lymphocytes are probably the result of prior activation in response to antigens and mitogens present in the GI lumen. Lymphocytes in the intestinal mucosa first interact with antigens in the organized lymphoid tissues (Peyer's patches and lymphoid follicles in the colon) and further differentiate and mature in the germinal centers of the lymphoid follicles. Thereafter, they rapidly leave the mucosa and migrate through the mesenteric lymph nodes and the thoracic duct to reach the systemic circulation. From the blood, these antigen-activated lymphocytes migrate back to the mucosa and extravasate preferentially into the lamina propria, becoming lamina propria lymphocytes (LPL), and the intraepithelial compartment above the basement membrane, becoming intraepithelial lymphocytes (IEL). Thus, most of the lymphocytes that enter the diffuse compartments of the GI tract (LPL, IEL) are likely to have had prior antigen activation and are likely to be memory cells.

Memory T cells are, by definition, cells that already have been in contact with antigens; they are adapted to their new tasks by the expression of various surface antigens that are absent from or expressed to a lesser degree on naive cells, by an altered pattern of lymphokine secretion, by different functional capacities, and by changes in their proliferative responses to different stimuli (Sanders *et al.*, 1988b). Previously, *in vitro* activation of CD45RA-positive,CD29-negative peripheral blood T lymphocytes by antigen has been shown to lead to a transition to CD45RA-negative,CD29-positive T cells (Akbar *et al.*, 1988; Clement *et al.*, 1988). This finding and functional studies have led to the conclusion that naive (or virgin) T cells can be distinguished from memory T cells by their expression of different antigen specificities of the CD45 cell-surface glycoprotein complex or CD29, the β1 chain of the integrin family (Sanders *et al.*, 1988a). The transition from naive to memory T-cell function is accompanied by a shift from the 205/220-kDa determinant (recognized by 2H4 monoclonal antibody) to the 180-kDa form (recognized by UCHL1 monoclonal antibody) of the CD45 cell-surface glycoprotein complex. These different molecules represent cell-type specific alternative splicing from a common precursor gene (Streuli *et al.*, 1987; Akbar *et al.*, 1988). Other markers have been described that are coexpressed with CD45 or CD29 after the transition from naive to memory T cells (Sanders *et al.*, 1988a). Naive T cells can be characterized as CD45RA-high, LFA-3-low, CD2-low, LFA-1-low, CD45R0-low, and CD29-low; memory T cells represent the reciprocal subset.

CD4- and CD8-positive T cells are present in the lamina propria in similar proportions compared with the peripheral blood (Selby *et al.*, 1983; James *et al.*, 1986; Schieferdecker *et al.*, 1990). Thus, regarding the major T-cell subpopulations, peripheral blood T cells and lamina propria T cells do not appear to be different. However, further investigations showed that only few lamina propria lymphocytes express CD45RA (recognized by 2H4) and the vast majority of cells are CD45R0 positive (recognized by UCHL1) (Schieferdecker *et al.*, 1990; Figure 1). In contrast, in peripheral blood, approximately 30% of T cells are CD45RA positive and

Table I Evidence for Specialized T Cell Function in the Mucosal Immune System[a]

	Mesenteric node	Lamina propria	Peripheral blood
Proliferation			
Specific antigen	+ +	−	+ + +
Mitogens	+ + + +	+ + +	+ + + +
Anti-CD3	N.D.[b]	+	+ + + +
Anti-CD2	N.D.	+ + +	+ + +
Surface glycoproteins			
CD45R		10%	33%
CD45R0	N.D.	93%	41%
CD29	N.D.	47%	60%
HML-1	N.D.	32%	2%
Leu-8	N.D.	11%	56%
Activation			
IL-2Ra	<5%	15–20%	<5%
Lymphokine production			
IL-2	+ +	+ + + +	N.D.
IFN-γ	+ +	+ + + +	N.D.
IL-4	+ + + +	+ + + +	N.D.
IL-5	+ + + +	+ + + +	N.D.
Lymphokine utilization			
IL-2	+ + +	+ + + +	+ +
IL-4	+ + + +	+/−	+ +
Regulatory function			
Helper activity	+ +	+ + + +	+ + + +
CD4 suppressor activity	N.D.	+/−	+ + + +

[a] Based on a compilation of studies from humans and nonhuman primates.
[b] N.D., Not determined.

30–50% are CD45R0 positive. Thus, the CD45 phenotype of LPLs resembles that of memory T cells. However, expression of another marker of memory T cells, CD29 (β1 integrin), is not increased in the lamina propria compared with peripheral blood. The phenotype of lamina propria T lymphocytes therefore only partially corresponds to that of memory T cells as defined by *in vitro* studies with peripheral blood lymphocytes. These phenotypic studies are an indication that T cells in the human intestinal lamina propria are a specialized memory T-cell subset.

B. Receptors Controlling Lymphocyte Migration

Naive and memory T cells are likely to have specific migration pathways throughout the body that enable antigen-specific immune responses to be concentrated at specific sites. Directed migration into normal or inflamed tissues probably is controlled by expression of a distinct pattern of specific adhesion molecules on the cell surface. The best studied "homing" receptor is the L-Selectin (LAM-1, LECAM-1, Leu-8, MEL 14) molecule. The L-Selectin antigen is expressed on neutrophils and monocytes and on subpopulations of T and B cells (Gatenby *et al.*, 1982; Kansas *et al.*, 1985a,b), but is not expressed on platelets. On circulating cells, 60–70% of T cells are L-Selectin positive, including both $CD4^+$ and $CD8^+$ cells. Although most L-Selectin-positive T cells are CD45RA positive, L-Selectin-positive T cells are found in both the naive (CD45RA-positive) and memory (CD29-positive) T-cell subsets. The latter observation is substantiated by the finding that some L-Selectin positive lymphocytes can respond to recall antigens (Bookman *et al.*, 1986). About half the circulating B cells are L-Selectin positive; evidence is presented in this chapter that these subpopulations differ in function. L-Selectin is expressed weakly on natural killer (NK) cells. Although L-Selectin expression is modulated rapidly by activation (Kanof and James, 1988), it is expressed stably in high levels on some T-cell lines (Bookman *et al.*, 1986) and clones and on some B-cell lines.

Few lymphocytes in the human or primate intestinal lamina propria are L-Selectin positive, whereas the majority of cells in mesenteric lymph nodes, which presumably drain the Peyer's patches, are L-Selectin positive (James *et al.*, 1986, 1987a; Figure 2). Several explanations for this observation are apparent. One explanation is based on the observation that substantial activation of lymphocytes occurs in the intestinal lamina propria (Zeitz *et al.*, 1988a; see subsequent dis-

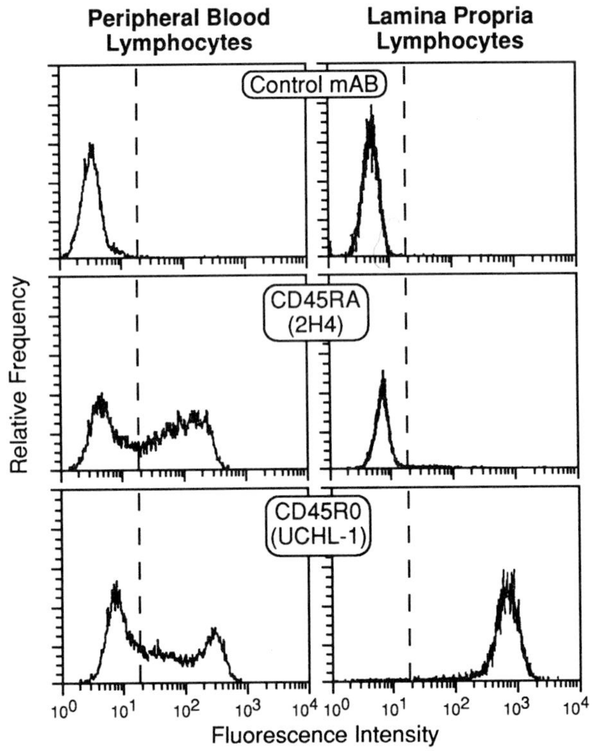

Figure 1 Expression of CD45RA and CD45R0 on human peripheral blood (PBL; *left*) and intestinal lamina propria lymphocytes (LPL; *right*). PBL and LPL were isolated from macroscopically normal small intestine and were stained with monoclonal antibodies 2H4 (CD45RA) or UCHL-1 (CD45R0) and analyzed by flow cytometry. LPL are nearly devoid of CD45RA-positive cells and express a high percentage of CD45R0-positive cells.

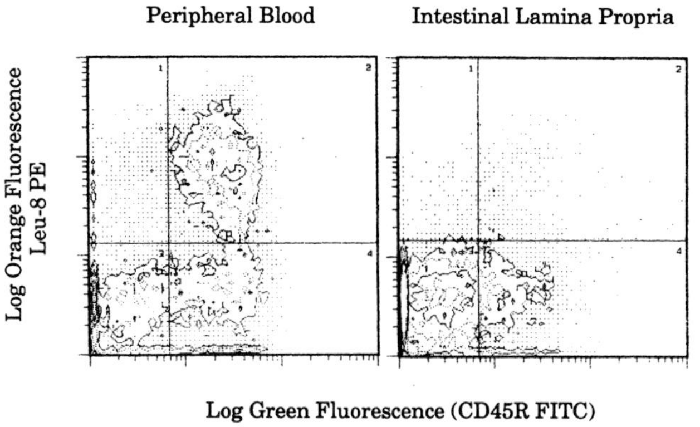

Figure 2 Expression of Leu-8/MEL14 lymph node homing receptor on intestinal lymphocytes. Peripheral blood (*left*) and intestinal lamina propria (*right*) lymphocytes from a normal nonhuman primate were stained with anti-CD45RA FITC and anti-Leu-8-PE and analyzed by dual fluorescence flow cytometry. Few lymphocytes in the lamina propria express the peripheral lymph node homing receptor or CD45RA.

cussion). Therefore, cells in the lamina propria might not express L-Selectin because they are in an activated state associated with low L-Selectin expression. However, this explanation is unlikely to be complete. First, when lamina propria lymphocytes are isolated and cultured in the absence of any stimulus, they do not re-express L-Selectin (Berg *et al.*, 1991). Further, intestinal lamina propria lymphocytes have little if any mRNA for L-Selectin following activation with potent inducers of L-Selectin mRNA, such as phorbol 12-myristute 13-acetate (PMA), these cells continue to lack L-Selectin mRNA (Berg *et al.*, 1991). Finally, only a proportion of L-Selectin-negative cells in the intestinal lamina propria actually are activated and express interleukin 2 (IL-2) receptors. L-Selectin-negative lymphocytes in the intestinal lamina propria share some characteristics with L-Selectin-negative lymphocytes in the circulation. The latter do not have evidence of activation, do not express L-Selectin mRNA and are not able to express L-Selectin after induction with PMA. Further, L-Selectin-negative cells isolated from the intestinal lamina propria and circulating L-Selectin-negative lymphocytes both have a similar high level of helper activity in pokeweed mitogen (PWM)-stimulated cultures. Based on these findings, L-Selectin-negative cells in the circulation are actually likely to arise from L-Selectin-positive precursors by a process of differentiation that remains to be defined. Further, these data suggest that L-Selectin-negative cells preferentially enter the intestinal lamina propria. The mechanism by which this occurs is as yet unknown, but may involve increased expression of other adhesion molecules that are known to be present on memory lymphocytes (Sanders *et al.*, 1988a) or other as yet undefined adhesion molecules. Finally, lymphocytes that enter the lamina propria are likely to acquire additional characteristics that may be unique to their microenvironment, for example, expression of HML-1 (see subsequent discussion).

Since lymphoid cells in the intestinal lamina propria have the phenotypic and functional characteristics of "memory" lymphocytes, including low expression of CD45RA (James *et al.*, 1986, 1987a) and high expression of CD45R0 (Schieferdecker *et al.*, 1991), glycoproteins expressed on memory lymphocytes may be important in localization of cells to the intestinal lamina propria. In addition to increased expression of the CD45R0 glycoprotein, circulating memory lymphocytes have been shown to have increased expression of a number of molecules that have been implicated in cell adhesion and cellular interactions, including CD2, LFA-1, LFA-3, CD29, and CD44 (Sanders *et al.*, 1988a). As indicated earlier, both CD29 (β chain (β_1 chain of integrins) and CD44 may play a role in localization of lymphoid cells to mucosal endothelium; therefore CD29 and CD44 may be important in intestinal homing.

Although lymphocytes in the intestinal lamina propria have almost exclusively the surface glycoprotein characteristics of memory lymphocytes, this alone does not account for mucosal lymphocyte localization for several reasons. First, cells with the memory phenotype are heterogeneous for the L-Selectin phenotype, that is, CD45RA-negative lymphocytes can be L-Selectin positive or negative. In addition, both L-Selectin positive and L-Selectin-negative $CD4^+$ T cells are able to respond to the recall antigen purified protein derivative (PPD) (Takada *et al.*, 1989), indicating that the presence or absence of the L-Selectin antigen is not a marker of immunological memory. Similarly, long-term memory B cells have been shown to be L-Selectin positive (Kraal *et al.*, 1988). Finally, although human intestinal lamina propria lymphocytes do not bind to peripheral lymph nodes, they do bind to human appendix or murine Peyer's patch lymph nodes; however, they have no increased binding to mucosal tissue in comparison with peripheral blood lymphocytes (Jalkanen *et al.*, 1989). In contrast, lamina propria lymphoblasts have greatly increased binding to mucosal tissues. Therefore, the exclusive localization of L-Selectin-negative lymphocytes to the lamina propria is not solely the result of the presence of memory cells in this subset. These observations suggest that newly expressed molecules or a change in density of surface molecules such as CD44 on activated lymphocytes (Willerford *et al.*, 1989) may be a critical determinant of localization of lymphocytes in the intestinal mucosa.

C. Mucosal T-Cell Specific Antigens

Monoclonal antibodies have been developed for rats (RGL1; Cerf-Bensussan *et al.*,1986), mice (M290; Kilshaw and Murant, 1990) and humans (HML-; Cerf-Bensussan, 1987; Ber-Act8; Kruschwitz *et al.*,1991) that recognize lymphocyte surface antigens that are expressed nearly exclusively in the mucosal immune system. By immunohistology and flow cytometry, approximately 40% of lamina propria lymphocytes and nearly all IELs in humans were shown to express the surface antigen recognized by HML-1 (Cerf-Bensussan *et al.*, 1987; Schieferdecker *et al.*, 1990; Ullrich *et al.*, 1990a). Reactivity also is seen in a few cells in the extrafollicular areas of lymph nodes and tonsils, as well as in splenic red pulp (Kruschwitz *et al.*, 1991).

Immunoprecipitation and polyacrylamide gel electrophoresis (PAGE) have shown that the HML-1 antigen is a heterodimer comprising a 150-kDa α chain and a 120-kDa β chain (Cerf-Bensussan *et al.*, 1992). Using monoclonal antibody Ber-Act8, which recognizes a different epitope of the same antigen, a trimeric structure also has been described (150; 125; and 105-kDa subunits; Kruschwitz *et al.*, 1991). Both the α and the β chain of HML-1 are glycosylated. Pulse–chase experiments indicate that precursor forms exist for both subunits; the larger α chain precursor (160 kDa) is reduced in size by posttranslational cleavage of a 10-kDa peptide and the smaller β chain precursor is increased in size by modification of the *N*-glycans (Cerf-Bensussan *et al.*, 1992).

Dual color cytofluorometry has shown that HML-1 is expressed preferentially on $CD8^+$ T cells; however, a significant proportion of $CD4^+$ lamina propria T cells also expresses HML-1 (Schieferdecker *et al.*, 1990; Figure 3). The low number of CD45RA-positive cells in the human intestinal lamina propria is almost exclusively HML-1 negative. Therefore, HML-1 has been hypothesized to be a tissue-specific memory T-cell marker exclusively expressed in the environment of the gut (Schieferdecker *et al.*, 1991). However, only a partial overlap in expression of CD29 and HML-1 is seen. In one study, the differential expression of homing-associated adhesion molecules on human peripheral blood T cells was investigated (Pricker *et al.*, 1990). The small proportion of circulating human T cells expressing the mucosal lymphocyte-associated antigen recognized by the monoclonal antibody Ber-Act8 (identifying the same antigen as HML-1) was shown also to have the CD29-low phenotype. These results are in agreement with the finding of an intermediate expression of CD29 on lamina propria T cells and further

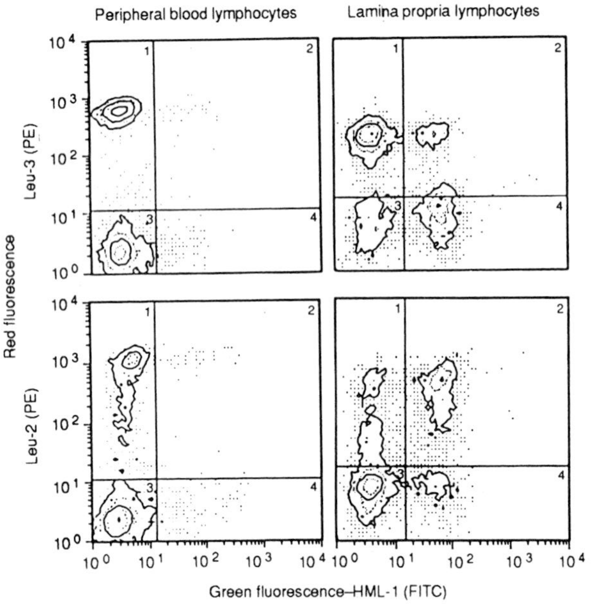

Figure 3 HML-1 antigen is expressed on both CD4 and CD8 positive lamina propria lymphocytes. Dual color flow cytometry analysis of human peripheral blood (*left*) and intestinal lamina propria (*right*) lymphocytes that were stained with anti-CD4 PE or anti-CD8 PE and HML-1 plus FITC anti-mouse IgG. HML-1 is nearly absent on peripheral blood lymphocytes. More CD8 than CD4 lamina propria lymphocytes express HML-1.

support the hypothesis of a tissue-specific modulation of memory or homing-associated T-cell surface antigens.

Expression of HML-1 is induced on HML-1-negative peripheral blood lymphocytes by *in vitro* activation using various stimuli (Schieferdecker *et al.*, 1990). However, certain differences are seen in the kinetics of expression of HML-1 when compared with the established T-cell activation antigen CD25. CD25 can be detected very early after mitogenic stimulation (within the first 24 hr), maximal expression is on day 1 or 2, and the number of positive cells decreases rapidly during the following days. In contrast, HML-1 is expressed later, maximal expression is on day 5–7, and only a slight decrease occurs up to day 10. In addition, whereas nearly 100% of activated T cells become CD25 positive, HML-1 expression in mitogen-stimulated cultures does not exceed 50% (Schieferdecker *et al.*, 1990). HML-1 therefore can be defined as an activation marker with characteristics shared by T-cell differentiation antigens used for the definition of memory T cells, that is expressed *in vivo* only in the environment of the intestine.

The function of the antigen recognized by HML-1 is not completely understood. The phenotypic data mentioned earlier and the kinetics of expression after activation are indications that this antigen may define a subset of memory T cells located in the intestinal immune system. In one study, tryptic peptides cleaved from purified β chain of HML-1 were sequenced and the amino acid sequence was compared with a protein data bank, revealing strong homology with the integrin β chains (Cerf-Bensussan *et al.*, 1992). Although the primary structure of the α chain of HML-1 has not been determined, these data indicate that HML-1 may be a novel human integrin. Integrins mediate cell–cell adhesion and binding to extracellular matrix components and, therefore, play important roles in lymphocyte homing, differentiation, and activation. Preliminary evidence suggests that triggering HML-1 with monoclonal antibody was co-stimulatory activity on human intestinal and peripheral T cells (Sarnacki *et al.*, 1991; H. Schieferdecker and M. Zeitz, unpublished results). Although the natural ligand of HML-1 is not known, HML-1 might be an important surface molecule in the regulation of the local immune response in the intestine.

D. T-Cell Receptor Expression in the Intestinal Mucosa

More than 95% of the normal intestinal lamina propria T cells express the $\alpha\beta$ T-cell receptor (TcR) heterodimer (Ullrich *et al.*, 1990a). Although T cells are found in the human epithelium (IEL) as in the mouse, in humans only about 10% of small bowel IELs (range: 5–20%) express this receptor. In the colon, a much higher proportion of IELs expresses $\gamma\delta$ receptors (Deusch *et al.*, 1991; Porcelli *et al.*, 1991). Thus, in humans the majority of T cells in the mucosa express the $\alpha\beta$ TcR that predominates in the periphery. Using polymerase chain reaction (PCR) amplification for different specific Vβ families, only a few Vβ families have been shown to predominate in human IELs (Balk *et al.*, 1991; VanKerckhove *et al.*, 1992). Further, sequences of VDJC showed evidence of oligoclonality of T-cell clones from human IELs.

Results for lamina propria T lymphocytes also showed skewing toward particular families, however, the level of heterogeneity was intermediate between peripheral blood and IELs. These interesting results suggest that factors may exist in the intestinal epithelium, for example, exogenous antigens or superantigens perhaps in combination with unique major histocompatibility complex (MHC) determinants expressed in the epithelium, that drive selective expansion of specific families of T cells.

III. ACTIVATION OF LAMINA PROPRIA T CELLS

T-cell activation is followed by an early expression of the IL-2 receptor on the cell surface. The interaction of the IL-2 receptor with IL-2 is a critical event in T-cell proliferation, differentiation, and function (Greene *et al.,* 1986). Intestinal T cells are in close proximity to a large number of antigens and substances with mitogenic properties. Therefore, the question arises whether lamina propria T cells differ in their state of activation from T cells in other sites of the immune system. Using Northern blot analysis in nonhuman primates to study the transcription of the gene for the IL-2 receptor α chain (CD25), mRNA for the IL-2 receptor α chain has been shown to be clearly detectable in freshly isolated lymphocytes from the intestinal lamina propria whereas, in the other populations from the spleen, mesenteric lymph nodes, or the peripheral blood, IL-2 receptor mRNA is found only after activation *in vitro* (Zeitz *et al.,* 1988a; Figure 4).

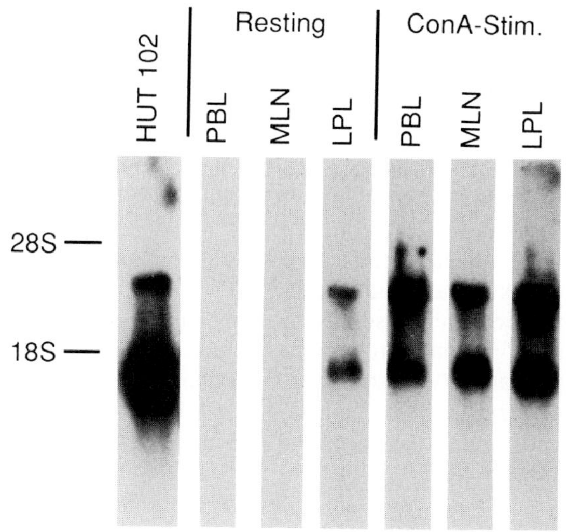

Figure 4 IL-2 receptor alpha chain mRNA is present in freshly isolated lamina propria lymphocytes. RNA was isolated from HUT 102 cell line (positive control), resting peripheral blood lymphocytes (PBL), mesenteric lymph nodes (MLN), or lamina propria lymphocytes (LPL) of a normal nonhuman primate. RNA was also isolated from lymphocytes that were activated with concanavalin A (Con A) *in vitro*. Northern blot of total cellular RNA was hybridized with probe specific for IL-2 receptor alpha chain. 10μg of RNA was loaded per lane.

Correspondingly, by flow cytometry, 15% (range; 6–29%) of freshly isolated intestinal lamina propria lymphocytes have been shown to be CD25 positive, but less than 3% of the other lymphocyte populations have that phenotype. $CD4^+$ and $CD8^+$ T cells express CD25 to a similar extent. The increased CD25 expression of lamina propria lymphocytes is correlated with a high proliferative response to low doses of IL-2, indicating that the IL-2 receptors are able to transduce the signal after IL-2 binding. In agreement with an increased state of activation of lamina propria T cells, these cells are able to synthesize high amounts of IL-2 after activation (Zeitz *et al.,* 1988a). Lamina propria lymphocytes also express MHC Class II antigens (Zeitz *et al.,* 1988a) and other T-cell activation markers (Peters *et al.,* 1986). Expression of CD25 in the lamina propria has been confirmed in humans by immunohistology of frozen tissue sections (Ullrich *et al.,* 1990b) and flow cytometry (Schieferdecker *et al.,* 1990). The finding that the mucosal T-cell associated antigen recognized by HML-1 is an antigen that can be induced by activation further supports the concept of an increased activation of lamina propria T cells. The increased state of activation of lamina propria T cells may be the result of the continuous exposure to antigens and mitogens from the gut lumen. The increased state of activation of lamina propria T cells and their unique phenotype are accompanied by characteristic functional changes after stimulation with antigens in comparison with cells from other compartments of the immune system.

IV. LYMPHOKINE PRODUCTION AND UTILIZATION BY INTESTINAL T CELLS

Many of the functions carried out by T cells in the GI immune system are thought to be mediated, at least in part, by their secreted lymphokines. Therefore, a detailed understanding of the lymphokines produced by mucosal T cells is necessary to understand their function. Further, alterations in the patterns of cytokines produced by mucosal cells may be important in the pathogenesis of intestinal disease. Experiments have been carried out to determine whether differences exist in the steady-state levels of lymphokine mRNA after activation of lymphocytes isolated from different sites of normal nonhuman primates (James *et al.,* 1990). Using conventional Northern blots, no specific hybridization with different lymphokine probes was detected in unactivated lymphocytes obtained from any site. When lymphocytes from different sites were activated with a combination of ionomycin and PMA, both mesenteric lymph node and lamina propria T cells were found to express high levels of mRNA for IL-4 and IL-5, in comparison with cells from peripheral blood, spleen, or peripheral lymph nodes (Figure 5). Lamina propria lymphocytes also had the highest levels of IL-2 mRNA, whereas mesenteric lymph node IL-2 mRNA was lower. In contrast, interferon γ (IFNγ) mRNA was low in mesenteric lymph nodes compared with all other sites. Thus, intestinal lamina propria lymphocytes have high capacity to express IL-2, IFNγ, IL-4, and IL-5 mRNA whereas mesen-

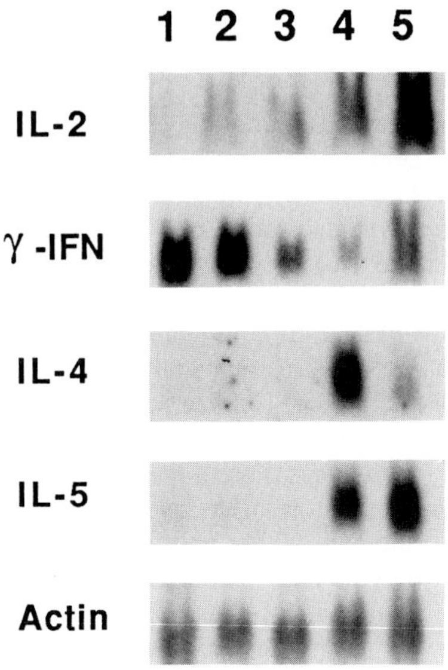

Figure 5 Northern blot for lymphokine mRNA in intestinal lymphocytes. Lymphocytes were obtained from different sites in a normal nonhuman primate (1, peripheral blood; 2, spleen; 3, peripheral node; 4, mesenteric node; 5, lamina propria) and were activated with ionomycin and PMA. Total cellular RNA was hybridized with probes for IL-2, IFN gamma, IL-4, IL-5, and actin. Activated intestinal lymphocytes have high expression of IL-4 and IL-5 mRNA.

teric lymph node cells have much lower capacity to express IL-2 and IFNγ but have a high capacity to express IL-4 and IL-5 mRNA after activation. The higher potential for expression of IL-2 was confirmed at the level of secreted proteins in studies of isolated primate lamina propria lymphocytes, in which activated intestinal T cells were demonstrated to have high production of IL-2 bioactivity (Zeitz *et al.*, 1988a). These studies indicate that mucosal T cells may be substantially different from T cells in other sites with respect to their potential for modulating immune responses; additional evidence that this is the case is described subsequently.

The ability of human IELs to produce lymphokines also has been examined. IELs isolated from surgically resected specimens have an ability similar to that of peripheral blood lymphocytes to produce IL-2 and IFNγ in response to stimulation with phytohemagglutinin (PHA; Ebert, 1990). Previously human IELs were shown to proliferate poorly in response to mitogens, but the addition of sheep erythrocytes or anti-CD2 monoclonal antibodies greatly enhances their proliferative responses. Similarly, addition of sheep erythrocytes greatly enhances lymphokine production by human IELs. These preliminary results indicate that human IELs, like murine IELs, have substantial potential for production of lymphokines. However, the extent to which lymphokines are produced *in vivo* and their physiological effects in the human GI epithelium are unclear.

Studies also have been carried out to examine the capacity of intestinal T-cell populations to use IL-2 or IL-4 as a growth factor. The proliferative responses of T cells isolated from either mesenteric lymph node or lamina propria were compared with those of T cells from peripheral blood or spleen of normal nonhuman primates (James *et al.*, 1990). Background proliferative responses and responses induced by concanavalin A (Con A) were not significantly different among the different cell populations. Human recombinant IL-2 induced dose-dependent proliferative responses of nonhuman primate T cells that were highest in T cells isolated from the intestinal lamina propria. In contrast, when T cells were cultured with recombinant human IL-4 alone, significant dose-dependent proliferative responses were not observed in T cells isolated from any site. When T cells from peripheral blood, spleen, or mesenteric lymph node were cultured with IL-4 and PMA, dose-dependent proliferative responses were observed; responses were highest in T cells isolated from the mesenteric lymph node. In contrast, T cells from the lamina propria did not exhibit a significant proliferative response to IL-4 + PMA at any dose, although these cells showed a high response to Con A and had the highest responses to IL-2 alone. These findings suggest that T cells in inductive and effector compartments of the mucosal immune system may differ in important ways in their responses to lymphokines. In particular, IL-4 may be an important autocrine factor in the mesenteric lymph nodes for T-cell growth and differentiation, whereas IL-2 may be the critical autocrine factor for growth and differentiation of T cells in the lamina propria.

V. IMMUNOREGULATORY FUNCTION OF INTESTINAL T CELLS

As indicated in the introduction the GI immune system is confronted with the necessity of responding to or being tolerant of various pathogens and antigens in the GI tract. One of the ways in which this response is accomplished is through regulation of immune responses by T cells. T cells exert their regulatory influence (help, suppression) on immunoglobulin synthesis, which is the major focus of this section, but also exert regulatory influences on other lymphoid and nonlymphoid cells. These regulatory influences probably are mediated in part by the secreted products of T cells and, as discussed earlier, evidence suggests that mucosal T cells may be characterized by the high potential for production of certain cytokines after activation.

In earlier studies, isolated human lamina propria cells were found to be similar to peripheral blood cells in the capacity to regulate PWM-stimulated immunoglobulin synthesis (James *et al.*, 1985). Lamina propria T cells had a similar capacity to provide help, and did not appear to have any increased suppressor function in comparison to peripheral blood lymphocytes. When lamina propria $CD4^+$ T cells were discovered to differ phenotypically from peripheral blood T cells (see previous discussion), the helper function of lamina propria T cells was re-examined in several ways. For some time, researchers have known that immunoglobulin synthesis is suppressed in PWM-stimulated cultures at high CD4/B cell ratios. This phenomenon is caused by the fact that the $CD4^+$ population is heterogeneous, that is, that the $CD4^+LAM\text{-}1^-$ population has high helper activity and the $CD4^+LAM\text{-}1^+$ subpopulation, which represents about 60% of $CD4^+$ T cells, suppresses immunoglobulin synthesis (Kanof *et al.,* 1987). The *in vitro* variation of the inhibitory function of $CD4^+$LAM-1^+ T cells with changes in the T cell/B cell ratio may be caused by the requirement of the inhibitory effect of these cells for direct contact between T and B cells. Further, the LAM-1 molecule may be involved in the function of these cells since, when the $CD4^+$LAM-1^+ subpopulation is treated with anti-LAM-1 under conditions that cross-link the monoclonal antibody, the suppressor function of these cells is enhanced. When $CD4^+$ T cells from the lamina propria were studied using similar methods, lamina propria $CD4^+$ cells did not suppress immunoglobulin synthesis at high T cell/B cell ratios. The ability of these cells to inhibit immunoglobulin synthesis was not enhanced by treatment with anti-LAM-1 (Kanof *et al.,* 1988; Figure 6). The helper and suppressor capacity of the $CD4^+$LAM-1^- and the $CD4^+$LAM-1^+ subpopulations does not appear to be inherently different in the lamina propria, since highly purified preparations of these two cell types have identical function, whether isolated from the lamina propria or peripheral blood (Kanof et al, 1988b). Thus, these studies confirm the fact that the predominance of $CD4^+$LAM-1^- cells in the intestinal lamina propria indicates that their net functional capacity is shifted significantly toward helper function in comparison with T cells in the peripheral blood.

The suppressor function of $CD8^+$ lamina propria T cells has been studied also. The proportion of $CD8^+$ cells in the lamina propria is similar to that in peripheral blood. In PWM-stimulated cultures, these cells have a similar ability to inhibit immunoglobulin synthesis (James *et al.,* 1985). However,

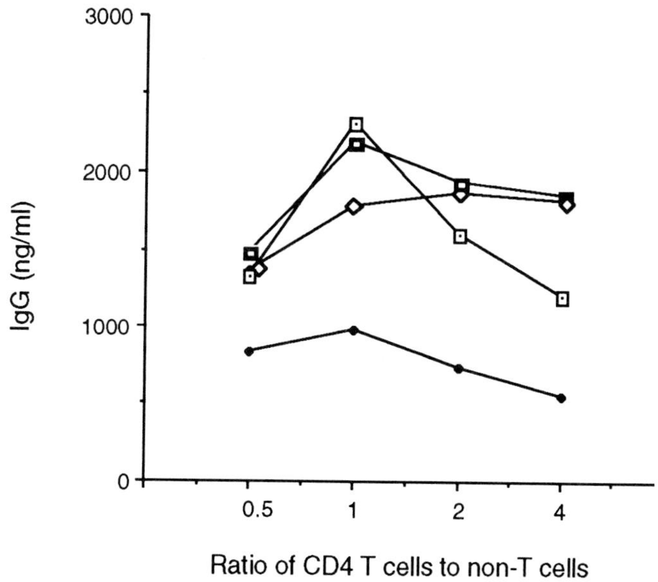

Figure 6 Regulatory function of intestinal lamina propria CD4 T cells. CD4 T cells from human peripheral blood (□, ◆) or intestinal lamina propria (◘, ◇) were cultured with non-T cells and pokeweed mitogen (PWM) for 10 days in presence (◆, ◇) or absence (□, ◘) of anti-Leu-8 monoclonal antibody. IgG in culture supernatants was determined by ELISA. Lamina propria CD4 T cells do not inhibit IgG synthesis at high T/B ratios.

only modest suppressor activity is found unless the cells are activated by exposure to a mitogen such as Con A. Currently, whether the suppressor function of lamina propria T cells differs from that of peripheral blood cells is unclear; however, as noted earlier, an increased proportion of $CD8^+$ cells from the intestinal lamina propria expresses IL-2 receptors, indicating that these cells are in a more activated state. The function of lamina propria $CD8^+$ cells also may differ from that of peripheral blood but, as for the studies of $CD4^+$ cells, these differences may not become apparent until new and more specific methods are identified to study subpopulations of suppressor lymphocytes.

In the studies described in this section using human lamina propria $CD4^+$ T cells, no IgA isotype specificity was observed, that is, no evidence was found that lamina propria T cells preferentially augment IgA synthesis rather than IgG or IgM (James *et al.,* 1985). This result might seem surprising in view of the evidence presented earlier that mucosal T cells have high potential for expression of lymphokines such as IL-5 that enhance IgA B-cell differentiation (Murray *et al.,* 1987; Yokota *et al.,* 1987; Harriman *et al.,* 1988). However, the evidence suggests that, within the intestinal lamina propria, the great preponderance of IgA-secreting cells is not determined by preferential production of IgA-specific helper factors but that the B cells that enter and undergo differentiation in the lamina propria already are committed to IgA production.

Since the studies discussed already indicated significant differences in the production and utilization of lymphokines by mesenteric lymph node and lamina propria T cells, studies were carried out to determine whether these differences might result in differences in the regulatory function of these T-cell populations (James *et al.,* 1990). First, to evaluate this question, the effect of exogenous (recombinant, r) lymphokines on the capacity of PWM stimulated human lymphocytes to produce immunoglobulin was determined. Both rIL-2 and rIFNγ enhanced immunoglobulin synthesis in a dose-dependent fashion. In related studies, IL-2 was demonstrated to enhance the helper activity of mucosal T cells for immunoglobulin synthesis (James and Graeff, 1987). In contrast, as previously described (Jelinek and Lipsky, 1988), recombinant human IL-4 caused a dose-dependent inhibition of immunoglobulin synthesis. This inhibitory effect was reversed by addition of recombinant human IFNγ. The reversal of the IL-4 inhibitory effect by IFNγ was observed only at low doses of IL-4, and was not observed at high doses of IL-4 (1000 U/ml).

These results suggested that lamina propria T cells, which express higher levels of IL-2 and IFNγ mRNA, would have greater helper function for immunoglobulin synthesis than mesenteric lymph node T cells. In other studies, nonhuman primate mesenteric lymph node and lamina propria T cells were cultured with autologous spleen B cells, alone or in the presence of increasing doses of recombinant human IL-4. Significantly more immunoglobulin was produced in cultures containing lamina propria T cells than mesenteric lymph node T cells, and the helper effect of lamina propria T cells was less inhibitable by exogenous IL-4 (James *et al.,* 1990). In summary, these studies of the immunoregulatory potential of lamina propria T cells *in vitro* indicate that such cells have high potential for helper activity, consistent with their phenotypic characteristics and potential for lymphokine gene expression discussed previously.

VI. T CELL ANTIGEN–RECEPTOR TRIGGERED FUNCTION OF INTESTINAL LYMPHOCYTES

Many of the functional studies described so far have relied on the activation of lymphoid cells using mitogens to study their function. This approach to the study of lymphocytes might not necessarily be representative of the outcome of exposure of lamina propria lymphocytes to specific antigens or pathogens. Therefore an animal model was established to examine this question in more detail. The function of lymphocytes isolated from the intestinal lamina propria of nonhuman primates with rectal infection with *Chlamydia trachomatis* (Serovar L2; lymphogranuloma venereum) was studied (James *et al.*, 1987b; Zeitz *et al.*, 1988b). This infectious model is of particular interest because the histopathological features of lymphogranuloma venereum bear a striking resemblance to those of Crohn's disease of the colon. As expected, T cells from peripheral blood, spleen, mesenteric lymph nodes, and particularly draining lymph nodes had a significant proliferative response when exposed to *C. trachomatis* antigens. However, T cells isolated from either the involved rectum or distant sites in the lamina propria did not exhibit a proliferative response when challenged with chlamydial antigens, although they did proliferate in response to mitogens such as Con A (Figure 7). This failure of lamina propria T cells to exhibit antigen-specific proliferative responses in lymphogranuloma venereum is not because of the absence of functional antigen-presenting cells or the presence of suppressor cells. Further, this finding may be a more general aspect of T-cell function in the lamina propria, since similar results were obtained in studies of animals rectally immunized with *Bacillus* Calmette-Guérin (BCG). Other lines of evidence also indicate that TcR-triggered activation of lamina propria lymphocytes may differ from that of circulating T cells. Anti-CD3-mediated activation of lamina propria lymphocytes is markedly lower than that of peripheral blood lymphocytes, but activation through the CD2 alternative pathway is normal in lamina propria lymphocytes (Qiao *et al.*, 1991). The most interesting aspect of these studies was that, although T cells from the lamina propria were unable to proliferate in response to antigens, antigen-specific T cells are present in this site, as was shown by experiments in which lamina propria T cells exposed to specific antigens could provide help for immunoglobulin synthesis (Figure 7). Thus, antigen-specific T cells are present in the intestinal lamina propria but, at least in certain circumstances, they have lost the capacity for proliferation while retaining the capacity to mediate helper function on antigen stimulation. An important implication of this study is that T-cell proliferation may not be a suitable test for the presence of antigen-specific T cells in sites of active mucosal inflammation, and tests of T-cell function may be required to demonstrate the presence of antigen-specific T cells.

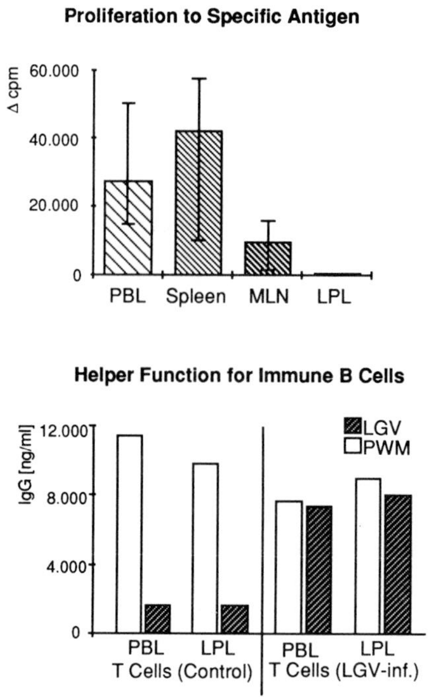

Figure 7 Antigen-specific proliferation of intestinal lamina propria lymphocytes (LPL) and antigen-induced production of helper factors by lamina propria T cells. Lymphocytes from the peripheral blood (PBL), the spleen, mesenteric lymph nodes (MLN), or the intestinal lamina propria (LPL) were isolated from nonhuman primates infected with *Chlamydia trachomatis*. Cell populations were stimulated with chlamydial antigens *in vitro*, and proliferation was measured by [^{3}H]thymidine incorporation (delta cpm; *left*). Spleen B cells from infected animals were cocultured with T cells from uninfected animals (control) or infected animals (LGV-inf) and cultures were stimulated either with pokeweed mitogen (PWM) or with chlamydial antigens (LGV). IgG production was measured in culture supernatants (*right*). Lamina propria T cells from immune animals do not proliferate but do provide help for Ig synthesis in the presence of chlamydial antigens.

VII. CYTOTOXIC FUNCTION OF INTESTINAL LYMPHOCYTES

Cytotoxic lymphocytes might play an important role in the function of the intestinal immune system and in the pathogenesis of intestinal disease in several different ways (James and Strober, 1986). First, cytolytic cells might play a role in injuring, either directly or indirectly via a bystander effect, any of the following cells: infectious organisms, neoplastic cells, infected cells, normal epithelial cells, altered epithelial cells, or stromal cells of the intestine. Second, the absence or inhibition of function of cytolytic cells might have a negative role in a disease state, because absence or a deficiency of activity might cause a local immunodeficiency state. Third, cytolytic cells might have indirect effects through their interactions with other cells of the GI immune system. Several different lymphocyte-mediated cytotoxic mechanisms might be active in the intestine, including NK cell cytotoxicity, antibody-dependent cellular cytotoxicity, T-cell mediated cytotoxicity, and, finally, lymphokine activated killer cell cytotoxicity. Both phenotypic and functional studies are consistent with the conclusion that the effector cells of NK and antibody-dependent all cytotoxicity activity are infrequent in the intestinal lamina propria (James and Graeff, 1985). On the other hand, evidence suggests that T-cell cytotoxicity plays an important role in immune function in the intestine. T-cell cytotoxicity is typified by the classical cytotoxic T lymphocyte (CTL) assay, in which the cytolytic effector cell specifically recognizes specific antigen in the context of HLA Class I determinants. Based on discussion of lymphocyte phenotypes in the intestine, clearly T cells are present with the typical markers of cytolytic T cells. However, showing experimentally that functional cytolytic T cells are present in this site has been much more problematic. To demonstrate this function, one must not only obtain functional mucosal lymphocytes, but also have an assay system that utilizes a target cell with the appropriate antigenic and HLA determinants, a requirement that is usually not possible in human experiments. In animal modes, demonstrating the presence of antigen-specific cytolytic T cells during viral infection (Issekutz *et al.,* 1984) and in animals immunized with alloantigens (Klein and Kagnoff, 1987) has been possible. To date, however, no convincing demonstration has been made of antigen-specific cytolytic T-cell function in humans. However, progress in our understanding of cytolytic T-cell function may allow for the study of these cells without actually knowing the antigen or MHC specificity of the effector cell. When cytolytic T cells are exposed to monoclonal anti-CD3 antibodies and target cells that are capable of binding the monoclonal antibody via Fc receptors, the effector cell is triggered to lyse the target cell without a requirement for MHC or antigenic specificity (Phillips and Lanier, 1986). Similarly, lectins such as PHA can trigger the same process, although this triggering is not limited to that of cytolytic T cells. Thus, the previous demonstration that the intestinal mucosa contains cells capable of mediating lectin-dependent cytotoxicity is indirect evidence that the intestinal mucosa contains cytolytic T cells (MacDermott *et al.,* 1980). These observations have been extended further by the demonstration of anti-CD3-triggered cytotoxicity mediated by intestinal lymphocytes (Shanahan *et al.,* 1988). Interestingly, peripheral blood $CD8^+$ lymphocytes that mediate CD3- or lectin-triggered cytotoxicity are primarily Leu-7 positive, whereas this phenotypic marker is infrequent on intestinal lymphocytes, suggesting that the frequency of this cytolytic T-cell type is very low in the lamina propria or, more likely, that in the intestine cytolytic T cells may not express this antigen. The physiological significance of these findings is uncertain at present, since the *in vitro* experiments only indicate that cells with potential for cytolytic function are present in the intestine. Whether these cells are triggered normally or during disease processes remains to be shown. Speculating that this form of non-antigen-specific killing may be important is interesting; for example, bacterial products might trigger killing of innocent bystander cells under certain conditions.

VIII. SUMMARY

The findings presented in this chapter provide substantial evidence that lymphocytes in the intestinal lamina propria differ from lymphocyte populations in the circulation or in other tissue sites in a number of ways. First, lamina propria lymphocytes are phenotypically distinct because few of these cells normally express the LAM-1 or CD45RA antigens. The presence of these molecules on $CD4^+$ T cells correlates with suppressor and suppressor–inducer function. Therefore the majority of $CD4^+$ T cells in the intestinal lamina propria has the phenotype associated with high helper activity. A substantial proportion of lamina propria lymphocytes also shows evidence of activation, based on expression of the IL-2 receptor α chain and HLA-DR molecules. Lymphocytes in the intestinal lamina propria are different in their potential for expression of lymphokine gene products, since activated cells from the lamina propria have high expression of mRNA for IL-2, IL-4, IL-5, and IFN γ in comparison with circulating lymphocytes. Mesenteric lymph node T cells also differ from circulating lymphocytes in their high expression of IL-4 and IL-5 mRNA. An additional difference between mesenteric lymph node and lamina propria T cells is that the former are capable of proliferating in response to IL-4, whereas the latter are not. These phenotypic and mRNA differences of lamina propria lymphocytes also correlate well with their high helper activity for immunoglobulin synthesis *in vitro* in the PWM system. T cells with the potential for cytolytic activity are present in the intestinal lamina propria, although as yet no definitive evidence exists that they are cytolytically active under physiological or pathological conditions. Finally, in a model system of intestinal inflammation (lymphogranuloma venereum in nonhuman primates), lamina propria T cells at the site of inflammation were unable to respond to specific antigens with proliferation but did respond with high helper activity. These observations are all consistent with the conclusion that T cells in the lamina propria are pleomorphic, but are highly enriched for subpopulations of activated memory cells that are geared for effector functions such as helper and cytolytic functions. These functions are likely to be critical in maintaining normal host defense in the mucosal environment.

References

Akbar, A. N., Terry, L., Timms, A., Beverley, P. C., and Janossy, G. (1988). Loss of CD45R and gain of UCHL1 reactivity is a feature of primed T cells. *J. Immunol.* **140,** 2171–2178.

Balk, S. P., Ebert, E. C., Blumenthal, R. L., McDermott, F. V., Wucherpfennig, K. W., Lanndau, S. B., and Blumberg, R. S. (1991). Oligoclonal expansion and CD1 recognition by human intestinal intraepithelial lymphocytes. *Science* **253,** 1411–1415.

Berg, M., Murakawa, Y., Camerini, D., and James, S. P. (1991). Lamina propria lymphocytes are derived from circulating cells that lack the Leu-8 lymph node homing receptor. *Gastroenterology* **101,** 90–99.

Bookman, M. A., Groves, E. S., and Matis, L. A. (1986). Expression of MEL-14 is not an absolute requirement for dissemination to lymph nodes after adoptive transfer of murine T lymphocyte clones. *J. Immunol.* **137,** 2107–2114.

Cerf-Bensussan, N., Guy-Grand, D., Lisowska-Grospierre, B., Griscelli, C., and Bhan, A. K. (1986). A monoclonal antibody specific for rat intestinal lymphocytes. *J. Immunol.* **136,** 76–82.

Cerf-Bensussan, N., Jarry, A., Brousse, N., Liskowska-Grospierre, B., Guy-Grand, D., and Griscelli, C. (1987). A monoclonal antibody (HML-1) defining a novel membrane molecule present on human intestinal lymphocytes. *Eur. J. Immunol.* **17,** 1270–1286.

Cerf-Bensussan, N., Begue, B., Gagnon J., and Meo, T. (1992). The human intraepithelial lymphocyte marker HML 1 is an integrin consisting of a beta-7 subunit associated with a distinctive alpha chain. *Eur. J. Immunol.* **22,** 273–277.

Clement, L. T., Yamashita, N., and Martin, A. M. (1988). The functionally distinct subpopulations of human CD4+ helper/inducer T lymphocytes defined by anti-CD45R antibodies derive sequentially from a differentiation pathway that is regulated by activation-dependent post-thymic differentiation. *J. Immunol.* **141,** 1464–1470.

Deusch, K., Luling, F., Reich, K., Classen, M., Wagner, H., and Pfeffer, K. (1991). A major fraction of human intraepithelial lymphocytes simultaneously expresses the T cell receptor, the CD8 accessory molecule and preferentially uses the V 1 gene segment. *Eur. J. Immunol.* **21,** 1053–1059.

Ebert, E. C. (1990). Intraepithelial lymphocytes: Interferon-gamma production and suppressor/cytotoxic activities. *Clin. Exp. Immunol.* **32,** 81–85.

Gatenby, P. A., Kansas, G. S., Xian, C. Y., Evans, R. L., and Engleman, E. G. (1982). Dissection of immunoregulatory subpopulations of T lymphocytes within the helper and suppressor sublineages in man. *J. Immunol.* **129,** 1997–2000.

Greene, W. C., Leonard, W. J., and Depper, J. M. (1986). Growth of human T lymphocytes: An analysis of interleukin 2 and its cellular receptor. *Prog. Hematol.* **14,** 283–301.

Harriman, G. R., Kunimoto, D. Y., Elliott, J. F., Paetkau, V., and Strober, W. (1988). The role of IL-5 in IgA B cell differentiation. *J. Immunol.* **140,** 3033–3039.

Issekutz, T. B. (1984). The response of gut-associated T lymphocytes to intestinal viral immunization. *J. Immunol.* **133,** 2955–2960.

Jalkanen, S., Nash, G. S., De los Toyos, J., MacDermott, R. P., and Butcher, E. C. (1989). Human lamina propria lymphocytes bear homing receptors and bind selectively to mucosal lymphoid high endothelium. *Eur. J. Immunol.* **19,** 63–68.

James, S. P., and Graeff, A. S. (1985). Spontaneous and lymphokine induced cytotoxic activity of monkey intestinal lymphocytes. *Cell. Immunol.* **93,** 387–397.

James, S. P., and Graeff, A. S. (1987). Effect of IL-2 on immunoregulatory function of intestinal lamina propria T cells in normal nonhuman primates. *Clin. Exp. Immunol.* **70,** 3394–3402.

James, S. P., and Strober, W. (1986). Cytotoxic lymphocytes and intestinal disease. *Gastroenterology* **90,** 235–240.

James, S. P., Fiocchi, C., Graeff, A. S., and Strober, W. (1985). Immunoregulatory function of lamina propria T cells in Crohn's disease. *Gastroenterology* **88,** 1143–1150.

James, S. P., Fiocchi, C., Graeff, A. S., and Strober, W. (1986). Phenotypic analysis of lamina propria lymphocytes: Predominance of helper-inducer and cytolytic T cell phenotypes and deficiency of suppressor–inducer phenotypes in Crohn's disease and control patients. *Gastroenterology* **91,** 1483–1489.

James, S. P., Graeff, A. S., and Zeitz, M. (1987a). Predominance of helper-induced T cells in mesenteric lymph nodes and intestinal lamina propria of normal non-human primates. *Cell. Immunol.* **107,** 372–383.

James, S. P., Graeff, A. S., Zeitz, M., Kappus, E., and Quinn, T. C. (1987b). Cytotoxic and immunoregulatory function of intestinal lymphocytes in LGV proctitis of non-human primates. *Infect. Immun.* **55,** 1137–1143.

James, S. P., Kwan, W. C., and Sneller, M. C. (1990). T cells in inductive and effector compartments of the intestinal mucosal immune system of nonhuman primates differ in lymphokine mRNA expression, lymphokine utilization, and regulatory function. *J. Immunol.* **144,** 1251–1256.

Jelinek, D. F., and Lipsky, P. E. (1988). Inhibitory influence of IL-4 on human B cell responsiveness. *J. Immunol.* **141,** 164–173.

Kanof, M. E., and James, S. P. (1988). Leu-8 antigen expression is diminished during cell activation but does not correlate with effector function of activated T lymphocytes. *J. Immunol.* **140,** 3701–3706.

Kanof, M. E., Strober, W., and James, S. P. (1987). Induction of CD4 suppressor T cells with anti-Leu-8 antibody. *J. Immunol.* **139,** 49–54.

Kanof, M. E., Strober, W., Fiocchi, C., Zeitz, M., and James, S. P. (1988). CD4 positive Leu-8 negative helper-inducer T cells predominate in the human intestinal lamina propria. *J. Immunol.* **141,** 3029–3036.

Kansas, G. S., Wood, G. S., Fishwild, D. M., and Engleman, E. G. (1985a). Functional characterization of human T lymphocyte subsets distinguished by monoclonal anti-Leu-8. *J. Immunol.* **134,** 2995–3002.

Kansas, G. S., Wood, G. S., and Engleman, E. G. (1985b). Maturational and functional diversity of human B lymphocytes delineated with anti-Leu-8. *J. Immunol.* **134,** 3003–3006.

Kilshaw, P., and Murant, S. (1990). A new surface antigen on intraepithelial lymphocytes in the intestine. *Eur. J. Immunol.* **20,** 2201–2207.

Klein, J. R., and Kagnoff, M. F. (1987). Spontaneous in vitro evolution of lytic specificity of cytotoxic T lymphocyte clones isolated from murine intestinal epithelium. *J. Immunol.* **138,** 58–62.

Kraal, G., Weissman, I. L., and Butcher, E. C. (1988). Memory B cells express a phenotype consistent with migratory competence after secondary but not short-term primary immunization. *Cell. Immunol.* **115,** 78–87.

Kruschwitz, M., Fritsche, G., Schwarting, R., Micklem, K., Mason, D. Y., Falini, B., and Stein, H. (1991). Ber-ACT8: A new monoclonal antibody to the mucosa lymphocyte antigen. *J. Clin. Pathol.* **44,** 636–645.

MacDermott, R. P., Franklin, G. O., Jenkins, K. M., Kodner, I. J., Nash, G. S., and Weinrieb, I. J. (1980). Human intestinal mononuclear cells. 1. Investigation of antibody-dependent, lectin-induced, and spontaneous cell-mediated cytotoxic capabilities. *Gastroenterology* **78,** 47–56.

Murray, P. D., McKenzie, D. T., Swain, S. L., and Kagnoff, M. F. (1987). Interleukin 5 and interleukin 4 produced by Peyer's patch T cells selectively enhance immunoglobin A expression. *J. Immunol.* **139,** 2669–2674.

Peters, M., Secrist, H., Anders, K. R., Nash, G. S., Schloemann, S., and MacDermott, R. P. (1986). Increased expression of cell surface activation markers by intestinal mononuclear cells. *Clin. Res.* **35,** 462.

Phillips, J. H., and Lanier, L. L. (1986). Lectin-dependent and anti-CD3 induced cytotoxicity are preferentially mediated by peripheral blood cytotoxic T lymphocytes expressing Leu-8 antigen. *J. Immunol.* **136,** 1579–1585.

Picker, L. J., Terstappen, L. W. M. M., Rott, L. S., Streeter,

P. R., Stein, H., and Butcher, E. C. (1990). Differential expression of homing-associated adhesion molecules by T cell subsets in man. *J. Immunol.* **145,** 3247–3255.

Porcelli, S., Brenner, M. B., and Band, H. (1991). Biology of human T cell receptor. *Immunol. Rev.* **120,** 137–183.

Qiao, L., Schürman G., Betzler M., and Meuer S. C. (1991). Functional properties of human lamina propria T lymphocytes assessed with mitogenic monoclonal antibodies. *Immunol. Res.* **10,** 218–225.

Sanders, M. E., Makgoba, M. W., Sharrow, S. O., Stephany, D., Springer, T. A., Young, H. A., and Shaw, S. (1988a). Human memory T lymphocytes express increased levels of three cell adhesion molecules (LFA-3, CD2, and LFA-1) and three other molecules (UCHL1, CDw29, and Pgp-1) and have enhanced IFN-gamma production. *J. Immunol.* **140,** 1401–1407.

Sanders, M. E., Malegapuru, W., Makgoba, M., W., and Shaw, S. (1988b). Human naive and memory T cells: reinterpretation of helper induced and suppressor-inducer subsets. *Immunol. Today* **9,** 195–199.

Sarnacki, S., Begue, B., Jarry, A., and Cerf-Bensussan, N. (1991). Human intestinal intraepithelial lymphocytes, a distinct population of activated T cells. *Immunol. Res.* **10,** 302–305.

Schieferdecker, H. L., Ullrich, R., WeiB-Breckwoldt, A. N., Schwarting, R., Stein, H., Riecken, and E. O., Zeitz, M. (1990). The HML-1 antigen of intestinal lymphocytes is an activation antigen. *J. Immunol.* **144,** 2511–2519.

Schieferdecker, H. L., Ullrich, R., and Zeitz, M. (1991). Phenotype of HML-1-positive T cells in the human intestinal lamina propria. *Immunol. Res.* **10,** 207–210.

Selby, H. L., Janossy, G., Bofill, M., and Jewell, D. P. (1983). Lymphocyte subpopulations in the human small intestine. The findings in normal mucosa and in the mucosa of patients with adult coeliac disease. *Clin. Exp. Immunol.* **52,** 219–228.

Shanahan, F., Deem, R., Nayersina, R., Leman, B., and Targan, S. (1988). Human mucosal T-cell cytotoxicity. *Gastroenterology* **94,** 960–967.

Streuli, M., Hall, L. R., Saga, Y., Schlossman, S. F., and Saito, H. (1987). Differential usage of three exons generate at least five different mRNAs encoding human leukocyte common antigens. *J. Exp. Med.* **166,** 1548–1566.

Takada, S., Koide, J., and Engleman, E. G. (1989). Differences in surface phenotype between cytolytic and non-cytolytic CD4+ T cells. MHC class II-specific cytotoxic T lymphocytes lack Leu 8 antigen and express CD2 in high density. *J. Immunol.* **142,** 3038–3044.

Ullrich, R., Schieferdecker, H. L., Ziegler, K., Riecken, E. O., and Zeitz, M. (1990a). CD8 T cells in the human intestine express surface markers of activation and are preferentially located in the epithelium. *Cell. Immunol.* **128,** 619–627.

Ullrich, R., Zeitz, M., Heise W., L'age, M., Ziegler, K., Bergs, C., and Riecken, E. O. (1990b). Mucosal atrophy is associated with loss of activated T cells in the duodenal mucosa of human immunodeficiency virus (HIV)-infected patients. *Digestion* **46,** (Suppl. 2), 302–307.

Van Kerckhove, C., Russell, G. J., Deusch, K., Reich, K., Bhan, A. K., DerSimonian, H., and Brenner, M. B. (1992). Oligoclonality of human intestinal intraepithelial T cells. *J. Exp. Med.* **175,** 57–63.

Willerford, D. M., Hoffman, P. A., and Gallatin, W. M. (1989). Expression of lyphocyte adhesion receptors for high endothelium in primates. Anatomic partitioning and linkage to activation. *J. Immunol.* **142,** 3416–3422.

Yokota, T, Coffman, R. L., Hagiwara, H., Rennick, D. M., Takebe, Y., Yokota, K., Gemmell, L., Shrader, B., Yang, G., Meyerson, P., Luh, J., Hoy, P., Pene, J., Briere, F., Spits, H., Banchereau, J., De Vries, J., Lee, F. D., Arai, N., and Arai, K. -I. (1987). Isolation and characterization of lymphokine cDNA clones encoding mouse and human IgA-enhancing factor and eosinophil colony-stimulating factor activities: Relationship to interleukin 5. *Proc. Natl. Acad. Sci. U.S.A.* **84,** 7388–7392.

Zeitz, M., Green, W. C., Peffer, N. J., and James, S. P. (1988a). Lymphocytes isolated from the intestinal lamina propria of normal non-human primates have increased expression of genes associated with T cell activation. *Gastroenterology* **94,** 647–655.

Zeitz, M., Quinn, T. C., Graeff, A. S., and James, S. P. (1988b). Mucosal T cells provide helper function but do not proliferate when stimulated by specific antigen in Lymphogranuloma venereum proctitis in non-human primates. *Gastroenterology* **94,** 353–366.

24

Basic Aspects of Intraepithelial Lymphocyte Immunobiology

Leo Lefrancois

I. INTRODUCTION

Intraepithelial lymphocytes (IELs) constitute the first immune cell line of defense in the intestine, that is, IgA in the intestinal lumen is likely to represent the first immunological defense encountered by an intestinal pathogen, followed by the anti-invasive glycocalyx of the intestinal mucosa. Any organism that was able to traverse these barriers could encounter IELs, which are interspersed between the columnar epithelial cells of the villi in the small and large intestine (Figure 1). Thus, infection of the epithelium with the subsequent expression of peptidic foreign antigen associated with major histocompatibility complex (MHC) molecules could result in IELs mounting an immune response. Alternatively, IELs could respond directly to foreign antigens such as intact bacteria. However, the precise *in vivo* function of IELs remains elusive. This chapter highlights the most recent findings in this area and presents the current questions being addressed in IEL research.

II. PHENOTYPE OF INTRAEPITHELIAL LYMPHOCYTES

A. T-Cell Receptor Expression

As can other T cells, IELs can be subdivided into two classes based on T-cell receptor (TcR) type: those expressing $\alpha\beta$ TcRs and those expressing $\gamma\delta$ TcRs. However, mouse small intestinal IELs (Bonneville *et al.*, 1988; Goodman and Lefrancois, 1988) and human large intestinal IELs (Deusch *et al.*, 1991) contain much higher percentages of $\gamma\delta$ T cells than do other lymphoid sites. Mouse IEL populations can contain 20–80% $\gamma\delta$ T cells and human large intestinal IEL isolates contain, on average, 37% (range: 13–87%) $\gamma\delta$ T cells. Human small intestinal IELs are composed of ~10% $\gamma\delta$ T cells (mean 13% of 28 samples; Jarry *et al.*, 1990), but this percentage is considerably higher than that observed in lamina propria (<1–5%), indicating that $\gamma\delta$ T cells exhibit a predilection for the intestinal mucosa, regardless of their location along the intestinal tract. Although a monoclonal antibody (MAb) specific for the rat $\gamma\delta$ TcR has not yet been described, studies using anti-CD3 and anti-$\alpha\beta$ TcR MAbs suggest that $\gamma\delta$ T cells constitute 10–50% of rat small intestinal IELs (Viney *et al.*, 1989/1990; Vaage *et al.*, 1990; Fangmann *et al.*, 1991). In addition, $\gamma\delta$ T cells constitute a large percentage of IELs in the chicken (Bucy *et al.*, 1988) and in ruminants (Hein and MacKay, 1991). The factors controlling IEL subset ratios in the various species are not known. The demonstration that human large intestine contains significantly higher percentages of $\gamma\delta$ T cells than human small intestine (although these values were not obtained from the same donors) suggests species-specific as well as organ-specific factor involvement in the control of IEL subpopulations.

B. CD4 and CD8 Expression

An interesting characteristic of IELs is their predominant expression of CD8. In the mouse >90% of IELs are CD8$^+$, irrespective of TcR expression (Parrot *et al.*, 1983; Goodman and Lefrancois, 1989). Human TcR $\alpha\beta$ IELs are primarily CD8$^+$ but CD4$^+$CD8$^-$ and CD4$^-$CD8$^-$ TcR $\gamma\delta$ IELs can be detected. Human peripheral blood $\gamma\delta$ T cells are ~25% CD8$^+$ whereas human $\gamma\delta$ IELs are 50–80% CD8$^+$ (Trejdosiewicz *et al.*, 1989; Jarry *et al.*, 1990; Deusch *et al.*, 1991). Predominant CD8 expression implies that IELs will react with antigen in a class I MHC-restricted fashion, which has been demonstrated for some $\alpha\beta$ IELs but not for $\gamma\delta$ IELs (see subsequent discussion).

Although most IELs are CD8$^+$, a significant percentage expresses CD4 and CD8 (double positives, DPs). DPs have been noted for mouse (Mosley *et al.*, 1990a; Lefrancois, 1991) and rat IELs (Fangmann *et al.*, 1991). In the latter, 30% of the IELs are CD4$^+$CD8$^+$. In the mouse, ~10% of $\alpha\beta$ IELs are CD4$^+$CD8$^+$, but in some experiments >80% of $\alpha\beta$ IELs are CD4$^+$CD8$^+$ (Lefrancois, 1991a; Table I). Outside the thymus, the gut is the only site in which substantial numbers of CD4$^+$CD8$^+$ T cells can be found. In contrast to the majority of thymic DPs, intestinal DPs express high levels of TcR. Moreover, intestinal DPs lack the CD8 β chian (Ly3), which further distinguishes them from their thymic CD8β^+ counterparts (Lefrancois, 1991a). Double-positive IELs are constitutively cytolytic but do not proliferate in response to anti-TcR MAb stimulation (Gramzinski *et al.*, 1993). Thus, CD4$^+$CD8$^+$ IELs appear functionally mature in some respects. Determining whether intestinal DPs serve as develop-

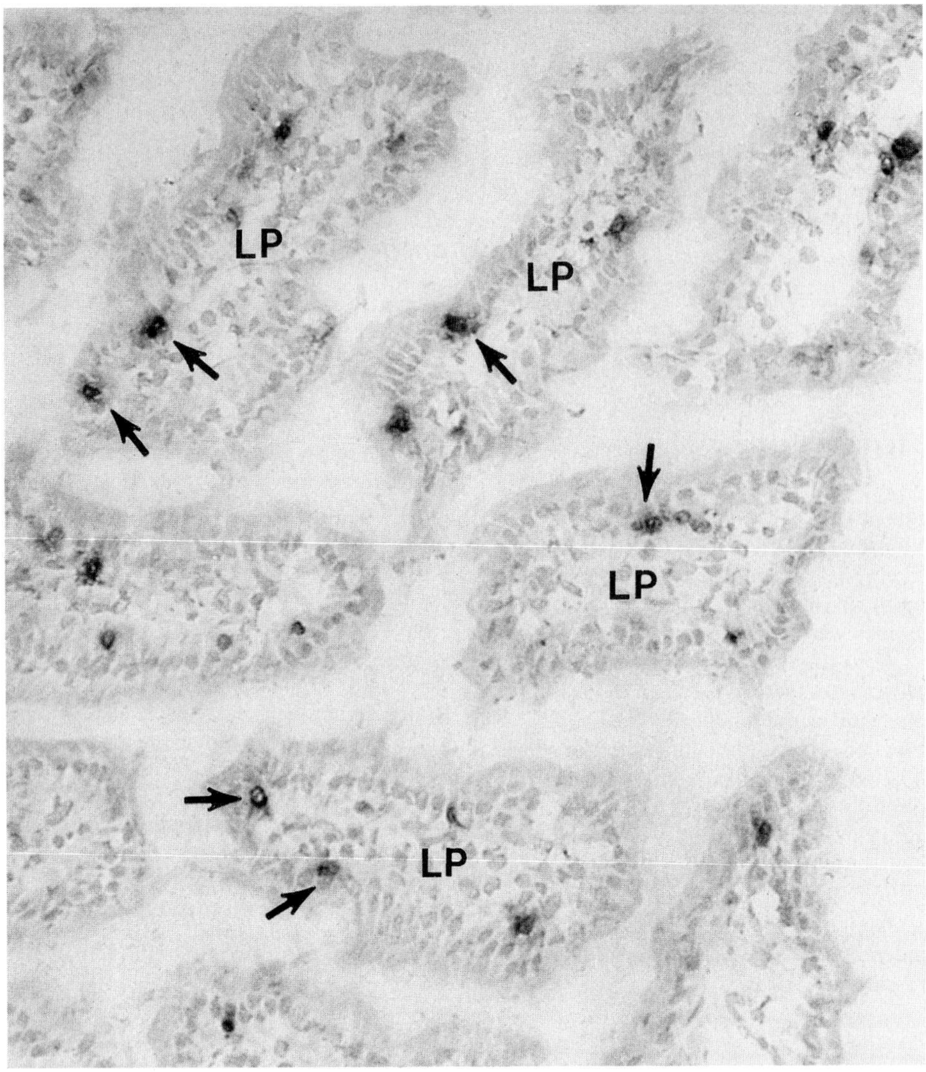

Figure 1 Localization of $\gamma\delta$ intraepithelial lymphocytes (IELs). Frozen sections of mouse small intestine were reacted with the GL3 MAb followed by incubation with a peroxidase-labeled anti-hamster Ig reagent and development with DAB. Arrows indicate IELs. LP, lamina propria.

mental intermediates during IEL differentiation is an area of current study.

C. T-Cell Differentiation Antigens; A Partial List

1. Thy1

In contrast to the vast majority of other mouse peripheral T cells, a substantial proportion of IELs lacks Thy1 (Parrot *et al.*, 1983). Roughly 20% of $\alpha\beta$ IELs and 70% of $\gamma\delta$ IELs are Thy1$^-$ (Table I). Freshly isolated IELs are constitutively cytolytic, as measured by a redirected lysis assay (Goodman and Lefrancois, 1989). The majority of such cytolytic activity is confined to the Thy1$^+$ subset of either $\gamma\delta$ or $\alpha\beta$ IELs, although some controversy exists over this point (Viney *et al.*, 1989/1990; Guy-Grand *et al.*, 1991a). In our hands, Thy1$^+$ IELs exhibit at least 100-fold greater cytolytic activity than Thy1$^-$ IELs. The IEL population of germ-free mice is composed primarily of $\gamma\delta$ T cells that are Thy1$^-$ and weakly or non-cytolytic. After introduction of these animals into non-germ-free conditions, IELs begin to express Thy1 and, simultaneously, become cytolytically active (Lefrancois and Goodman, 1989). Additionally, substantial numbers of $\alpha\beta$ IELs infiltrate the epithelium and the number of $\gamma\delta$ IELs increases (Bandeira *et al.*, 1990b; T. Goodman and L. Lefrancois, unpublished results). These results suggest that Thy1 expression and cytolytic activity of IELs are inducible by environmental antigens, likely to be derived from bacteria colonizing the gut. Moreover, gut colonization results in the expansion or the recruitment of $\alpha\beta$ IELs. Whether these effects are the result of direct activation of IELs via antigen–TcR interactions remains to be demonstrated.

Table I Relative Frequencies of Intraepithelial Lymphocyte Subpopulations[a]

TcR $\gamma\delta$ IEL subset	(%)	TcR $\alpha\beta$ IEL subset	(%)
Thy1$^+$ CD4$^-$8$^+$ Ly3$^-$ CD5$^-$	26 ± 5	Thy1$^+$ CD4$^-$8$^+$ Ly3$^+$ CD5$^+$	50 ± 17
Thy1$^-$ CD4$^-$8$^+$ Ly3$^-$ CD5$^-$	74 ± 5	Thy1$^+$ CD4$^-$8$^+$ Ly3$^-$ CD5$^-$	33 ± 19
		Thy1$^-$ CD4$^-$8$^+$ Ly3$^-$ CD5$^-$	14 ± 3
		Thy1$^-$ CD4$^-$8$^+$ Ly3$^+$ CD5$^-$	4 ± 3
		Thy1$^+$ CD4$^+$8$^+$ Ly3$^-$ CD5$^+$	9 ± 8

[a] IELs from a minimum of eight experiments using at least three mouse strains were analyzed for the expression of the indicated determinants by two- and three-color fluorescence flow cytometry.

We have attempted to duplicate this differentiation scheme *in vitro*. Thy1$^-$ IELs were purified by fluorescence activated cell sorting (FACS) and stimulated *in vitro* with anti-TcR MAb. In response to anti-CD3 stimulation in the presence of interleukin 2 (IL-2), Thy1$^-$ noncytolytic IELs proliferated, acquired cytolytic activity, and began to express Thy1 (Figure 2; Gramzinski *et al.*, 1993). However, CD5 and CD8β were not induced by activation. The *in vitro* differentiated population therefore phenotypically resembled the Thy1$^+$ CD8β^-CD5$^-$ IEL subset expressing either TcR subtype (Table I). *In vivo* reconstitution experiments using highly purified IEL subsets will be required to determine whether these results represent an *in vitro* correlate to IEL differentiation *in vivo*.

2. CD8β

The absence of CD8β (Ly3) on subsets of IELs has been known for some time (Parrot *et al.*, 1983). Multicolor fluorescence analysis has been employed to demonstrate that all $\gamma\delta$ IELs and ~50% of $\alpha\beta$ IELs are CD8β^- (Table I; Lefrancois, 1991a). Human CD8$^+$ $\gamma\delta$ IELs are also predominantly CD8β^- (Jarry *et al.*, 1990). Interestingly, those CD4$^-$CD8$^-$ $\gamma\delta$ T cells from thymus or spleen that are induced to express CD8 are also CD8β^-, suggesting that $\gamma\delta$ T cells in general are unable to synthesize or express CD8β (Cron *et al.*, 1989; MacDonald *et al.*, 1990a).

CD8 exists as a cell-surface complex, usually dimers, of β chains associated with α or α' chains (Ledbetter and Seaman, 1982). The α' chain lacks a portion of the cytoplasmic tail that the α chain contains, but is otherwise identical to the α chain. The α but not the α' chain is sufficient to allow signal transduction via CD8 (Zamoyska *et al.*, 1989). Since many IELs are CD8β^-, we determined which α chain type was expressed by these cells. IELs expressed CD8α but little CD8α' compared with thymocytes, which expressed roughly equivalent quantitites of α and α' (Figure 3; CD8β is difficult to label). These results are worth considering in light of the finding that anti-CD8 MAbs greatly inhibit anti-TcR MAb-triggered CD8$^+$ lymph node T-cell proliferation, but only marginally inhibit Thy1$^-$ IELs and do not inhibit Thy1$^+$ IEL proliferation (see subsequent discussion). This apparent lack of signal transduction does not appear to be the result of the predominant use of α' chains by IELs or the lack of association of IEL CD8 with the *src*-like kinase p56^{lck} that is involved in TcR–CD8 signal transduction (Gramzinski and Lefrançois, unpublished observations).

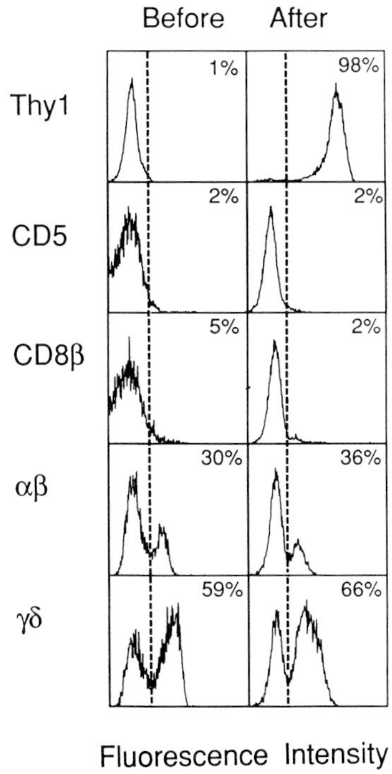

Figure 2 *In vitro* differentiation of Thy1$^-$ intraepithelial lymphocytes (IELs). Thy1$^-$ IELs were purified by removal of Thy1$^+$ cells by fluorescence-activated cell sorting. Thy1$^-$ IELs were stimulated *in vitro* with immobilized anti-CD3 in the presence of IL-2 for 5 days. The cells were analyzed for the indicated determinants before and after culture.

3. CD5

Whereas virtually all peripheral T cells and thymocytes express CD5 to some degree, certain IEL subsets do not. Mouse (Lefrancois, 1991a) and human $\gamma\delta$ IELs lack CD5 (Trejdosiewicz *et al.*, 1989; Jarry *et al.*, 1990), in contrast to peripheral $\gamma\delta$ T cells. Further, approximately 50% of mouse, rat (Fangmann *et al.*, 1991), and human $\alpha\beta$ IELs are CD5$^-$ (Table I). CD5 expression does not appear to correlate with Thy1 or CD8β expression. The functional significance of the absence of CD5 is unknown. However, a ligand for CD5 has been identified as the CD72/Lyb-2 B-cell surface protein (Van de Velde *et al.*, 1991). Perhaps the lack of IEL CD5 expression reflects the lack of a necessity for IEL–B cell interactions. Alternatively, other IEL-specific interaction molecules may be present but remain unidentified.

4. CD45

The CD45 antigens are a family of high molecular weight glycoproteins (170–260 kDa) that are expressed exclusively

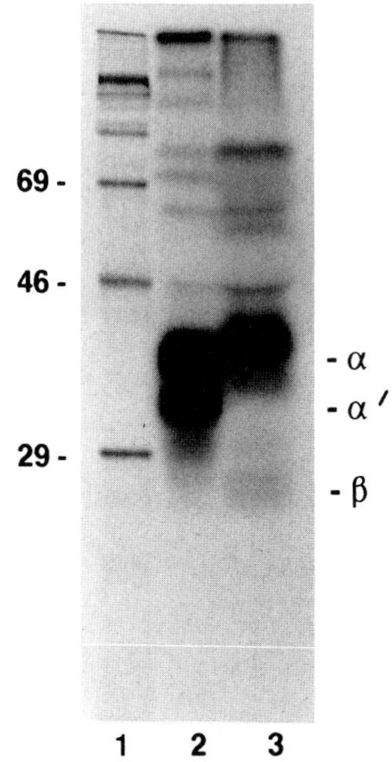

Figure 3 Biochemical analysis of intraepithelial lymphocyte (IEL) CD8. CD8 was immunoprecipitated from surface-labeled thymocytes (lane 2) or IELs (lane 3) and analyzed by SDS–PAGE.

by hematopoietic cells. The intracytoplasmic domain of CD45 is a tyrosine phosphatase thought to play a role in a signal transduction cascade involving CD4/CD8, $p56^{lck}$, and TcR (Clark and Ledbetter, 1989). The function of the CD45 extracellular domain is not known, but the B lymphocyte adhesion molecule CD22 has been shown to interact with T-cell CD45 (Stamenkovic *et al.*, 1991). Eight CD45 isoforms are possible that are generated by alternative mRNA splicing of three exons (4,5, and 6) near the 5′ end of the CD45 gene (Thomas and Lefrancois, 1988). Antigenic determinants encoded by these exons or expressed on subsets of CD45 molecules (e.g., carbohydrate antigens) are termed CD45-restricted determinants (CD45R). Distinct CD45 isoforms are expressed in a developmentally regulated fashion during T-cell differentiation. $CD8^+$ peripheral T cells can be distinguished from $CD4^+$ T cells by CD45 isoform type; the $CD4^+$ subset can be subdivided further by CD45 isoform expression (Lefrancois and Goodman, 1987; Bottomly *et al.*, 1989). In addition to isoforms generated via mRNA splicing, other modifications of CD45 occur that can be detected by MAbs or biochemical analysis. Examples of these modifications are the CT1 and M371 determinants, which are carbohydrate-dependent CD45 epitopes (Lefrancois, 1987; Kilshaw and Baker, 1989). CT1 is expressed by early fetal thymocytes and by activated $CD8^+$ cytotoxic T lymphocyte (CTL) clones *in vitro*. Interestingly, CT1 is expressed at high levels by a subset of $Thy1^-$ IELs of either TcR type (Goodman and Lefrancois, 1989). Thus, the only *in vivo* sites of CT1 expression are the fetal thymus and the gut. One could speculate that a functional link exists between CT1 expression in these sites, since T-cell differentiation occurs in the fetal thymus and is likely to occur in the intestinal mucosa (see subsequent discussion).

CD45 isoform expression by human and mouse IELs has been analyzed using MAbs and molecular techniques. Mouse IELs express a 260-kDa isoform that is not generated by mRNA splicing but appears to be the result of hyperglycosylation of the molecule (Goodman *et al.*, 1990). This form is not present in significant quantities on other T cells. The polymerase chain reaction (PCR) and restriction mapping of the resulting products were used to analyze mouse IEL CD45 alternative exon usage. Three mRNA isoforms were detected: one utilizing a single variable exon (exon 5) and two containing two variable exons (exons 4 and 5 or exons 5 and 6). In addition, MAbs specific for exon 4-encoded determinants (generally B-cell specific) react with a subset of IELs.

Human IELs have been shown to express CD45 determinants that generally are associated with activated T cells. The majority of human IELs are CD45RO (no expression of alternative exons) and $CD45RA^-$, in contrast to peripheral T cells which are ~50% CD45RO and ~50% $CD45RA^+$ (Halstensen *et al.*, 1990). $CD45RA^+$ T cells are thought to be naive whereas CD45RO cells are memory or activated cells. These results agree with those demonstrating that fresh mouse IELs are constitutively cytolytic, implying that they are activated *in situ*. The antigens involved in this activation process have not been identified.

5. IEL-Specific Integrin Expression

The MAb M290 stains ~90% of mouse IELs and ~20% of $CD8^+$ lymph node T cells, although to a much lower intensity than that obtained with IELs (Kilshaw and Murant, 1990). M290 does not react with significant numbers of $CD4^+$ lymph node T cells or with B cells. M290 immunoprecipitates from IELs a complex of 3–4 proteins with apparent molecular weights similar to those of previously described integrins. N-Terminal sequences of the mouse M290 120-kDa β subunit and the β_7 integrin chain have been shown to be identical (Yuan *et al.*, 1991). However, β_7 mRNA expression does not correlate with M290 expression, since B cells and spleen cells have high levels of β_7 mRNA. The β_7 subunit is likely to be utilized by lymphocytes other than IELs and the M290 MAb is likely to react with the α subunit of the IEL integrin (Yuan *et al.*, 1991).

Human and rat IELs appear to express a molecular complex similar or identical to that recognized by the M290 MAb. In the human, the HML-1 antigen is expressed by ~90% of IELs but also is found on ~40% of lamina propria T cells, primarily of the $CD8^+$ subset (Cerf-Bensussan *et al.*, 1987). Outside the intestine, HML-1 is expressed on few lymphoid cells. However, HML-1 is inducible on peripheral blood T cells by mitogen or antigen activation (Schieferdecker *et al.*, 1990). HML-1 has been shown to recognize an antigen identical to that recognized by the MAbs B-ly7, Ber-Act8, and LF61. B-ly7 was generated against a hairy cell leukemia cell line (HCL); all these MAbs react with the majority of HCL lines (Kruschwitz *et al.*, 1991). The MAbs immunoprecipitate a trimeric 150/125/105~kDa complex similar to that immunoprecipitated by M290 from mouse IELs, although M290 also precipitated several proteins of lower M_r. In the rat, the cellular distribution and biochemical characteristics of the antigens recognized by the RGL-1 MAb are similar to those of the HML-1 and M290 antigens (Cerf-Bensussan *et al.*, 1986). Interestingly, RGL-1 reacted with a high percentage of rapidly dividing cells in the mesenteric lymph node and the thoracic duct. These cells are thought to be immediate precursors of IELs (probably of the $\alpha\beta$ TcR type) and other intestinal T cells. Overall, the results indicate that IELs are likely to use adhesion structures that share common subunits with other lymphocyte integrins but also contain subunits restricted in expression to IELs and their precursors. These complexes may be involved in homing of IELs to the gut mucosa or may play a role in IEL adherence to the basement membrane during residence in the gut. Since IELs turn over much less rapidly than the villous epithelial cells that are sloughed into the intestinal lumen every few days, IELs require a specific mechanism to remain in the villi as the epithelium migrates "over" them. Histological analysis generally shows IELs to be closely apposed to the basement membrane, where they may interact specifically with components of that structure.

III. MATURATION AND SELECTION OF INTRAEPITHELIAL LYMPHOCYTES

A. $\gamma\delta$ T Cells

1. Origin

Studies using nude mice and thymectomized bone marrow or fetal liver irradiation chimeras have demonstrated that a significant proportion of mouse $\gamma\delta$ IELs is extrathymically derived (Bonneville *et al.*, 1990; DeGeus *et al.*, 1990; Lefrancois *et al.*, 1990; Mosley *et al.*, 1990b; Bandeira *et al.*, 1990a; Guy-Grand *et al.*, 1990a). In our hands, Thy1$^+$ and Thy1$^-$ $\gamma\delta$ IEls are generated in ATXBM mice. Thy1$^+$ $\gamma\delta$ IELs can be found in some but not all nude mice. These results indicate that Thy1 expression is not necessarily linked to thymic derivation. Prior to T cell colonization of the thymus at 11 days of mouse fetal ontogeny, Vγ5 rearrangements (the predominant Vγ region utilized by IELs) can be detected in fetal gut and liver, indicating that extrathymic γ TcR rearrangement can occur (Carding *et al.*, 1990). In addition, the recombination activating gene 1 is expressed by IELs (subset analysis was not performed), albeit at much lower levels than in thymocytes (Guy-Grand *et al.*, 1991b). Thus, significant extrathymic maturation of $\gamma\delta$ IELs occurs in the mouse intestine. Studies of rat IELs have demonstrated that the majority are thymus-derived and express the $\alpha\beta$ TcR (Viney *et al.*, 1989/1990; Vaage *et al.*, 1990; Fangmann *et al.*, 1991). However, a thorough analysis of $\gamma\delta$ IEL maturation in the rat has not been performed, in part because of the lack of an anti-$\gamma\delta$ TcR MAb. Whether $\gamma\delta$ IELs mature before or after arrival in the intestine and what other cell types are involved in the maturation (e.g., intestinal epithelial cells) is currently being studied.

2. TcR V Region Expression

Mouse $\gamma\delta$ IELs express a restricted set of Vγ and Vδ regions. Vγ5 is expressed by 50–80% of $\gamma\delta$ IELs as detected by MAb binding. The MAb GL5 is Vγ5 specific and reacts with IELs from all mouse strains except four that contain a polymorphism in the Vγ5 region that results in a single amino acid change (Goodman *et al.*, 1992). A small percentage of IELs, ~5%, expresses Vγ2 whereas Vγ3 expression cannot be detected by a Vγ3-specific MAb. PCR analysis and DNA sequencing revealed that significant numbers of in-frame Vγ4 mRNAs were present in IELs (Asarnow *et al.*, 1989; Takagaki *et al.*, 1989). for the most part, other Vγ regions do not appear to be utilized by IELs.

The expression of Vδ regions is somewhat more extensive than that of Vγ regions. Using the MAb GL2, which is Vδ4-specific, we have shown that Vδ4 is expressed by 15–60% of $\gamma\delta$ IELs, depending on the mouse strain (see subsequent discussion). Two-color analysis using the GL5 and GL2 MAbs indicates that virtually all the Vδ4$^+$ subset is contained in the Vγ5$^+$ population, whereas significant numbers of Vγ5$^+$/Vδ4$^-$ IELs are observed (L. Lefrancois and T. Goodman, unpublished results). Other Vδ-specific MAbs are not available at this time. However, Northern blot and PCR analysis reveals that Vδ6 is used frequently whereas Vδ5 and Vδ7 are utilized at lower frequencies. Vδ1, 2, and 3 are not expressed in significant quantities.

Unlike the $\gamma\delta$ TcRs expressed by dendritic epidermal cells of the skin and the reproductive tract, IEL TcR sequences contain significant junctional diversity. Non-germ-line encoded (NGE) nucleotides and shortened V and J ends are present in the rearranged γ gene sequences, resulting in a great deal of junctional diversity (Asarnow *et al.*, 1989; Takagaki *et al.*,1989). The various mechanisms for generating junctional diversity are used extensively in δ gene rearrangements, including use of multiple D and different J segments, insertion of NGE nucleotides, and imprecise joining. Thus, $\gamma\delta$ IELs have the potential to react with a large array of antigens, which may be required to respond to the bacteriological load of the intestine.

The genetics of human $\gamma\delta$ IELs has not been extensively studied. One report claimed that the relative percentages of Vγ9$^+$ and Vγ2$^+$ (these chains preferentially associate) IELs from the small intestine are similar to those present in peripheral blood $\gamma\delta$ cells (Jarry *et al.*, 1990). Also, $\gamma\delta$ IELs utilize primarily the non-disulfide-linked form of the TcR, in contrast to peripheral $\gamma\delta$ cells which use the disulfide-linked form (Spencer *et al.*, 1989). In the colon, an average of 70% of $\gamma\delta$ IELs uses the Vδ1 gene segment, compared with 40% of $\gamma\delta$ peripheral blood T cells (Deusch *et al.*, 1991). Moreover, whereas ~60% of $\gamma\delta$ peripheral blood T cells uses Vγ9 and Vδ2, only ~20% of colonic IELs expresses these V regions. The J region usage of the Vδ2$^+$ IELs was also distinct from that of peripheral $\gamma\delta$ T cells; the Jδ1 segment was used much less frequently by IELs than by peripheral $\gamma\delta$ T cells. The junctional diversity of colonic $\gamma\delta$ TcRs has not been analyzed.

In sum, $\gamma\delta$ IELs utilize a restricted subset of V regions and, on rearrangement, significant junctional diversity is generated. Further diversity is produced by differing combinations (e.g., Vδ4-Vγ5; Vδ6-Vγ5). The results from the genetic analysis of human and mouse $\gamma\delta$ IELs further strengthen the likelihood that a distinct $\gamma\delta$ lineage exists that preferentially localizes to the intestinal mucosa.

3. $\gamma\delta$ TcR Selection

Although the preferential use of V regions suggests an ongoing selection process, such a mechanism has not been demonstrated. However, in the case of V$\delta4^+$ mouse IELs, extrathymic positive or negative selection can occur (Lefrancois *et al.*, 1990). Using recombinant inbred and congeneic mouse strains we demonstrated that positive selection of V$\delta4^+$ IELs is dependent on the presence of Class II MHC I–E moelcules, particularly I–E^k. V$\delta4^+$ IELs increase from ~30% in I–E strains to ~60% of total $\gamma\delta$ IELs in I–E^k strains. However, IELs from AKR/J mice (also I–E^k) are of the V$\delta4^{low}$ phenotype. We have shown that this phenotype is the result of an active negative selection of V$\delta4^+$ IELs in this strain (L. Lefrancois, unpublished results). Non-MHC antigens appear to be involved in V$\delta4^+$ IEL selection, but these antigens have not been identified. Many instances of I-E-dependent selection of T cells expesing various Vβ regions have been reported; in many cases, retroviral superantigens derived from mouse mammary tumor virus are responsible for the selection (reviewed by Acha-Orbea and Palmer, 1991). Perhaps viral or bacterial superantigens are involved in $\gamma\delta$ IEL selection as well.

An interesting aspect of V$\delta4^+$ IEL selection is the fact that the selection requires Class II MHC expression but the selected IELs are CD8$^+$. Although CD8$^+$ IELs might be expected to be Class I MHC restricted, selection by Mls (i.e., viral superantigens) also has been shown for peripheral CD8$^+$ $\alpha\beta$ T cells to be Class II I–E dependent (MacDonald *et al.*, 1990b). Thus, superantigen selection appears to bypass the normal accessory molecule restriction of a particular T cell subset, yet data obtained from mice lacking Class I MHC because of disruption of the β-2 microglobulin gene also should be considered. IELs from these animals contain apparently normal numbers of CD8$^+$ $\gamma\delta$ T cells, whereas CD8$^+$ $\alpha\beta$ IELs are essentially absent (Raulet *et al.*, 1991). Moreover, IELs from these mice express their normal complement of TcR V regions. Thus, Class I MHC does not appear to be involved in the generation of $\gamma\delta$ IELs, but this finding does not preclude the possibility that $\gamma\delta$ IELs react with antigens in the context of Class I MHC. Since these cells do not mature in the thymus where most Class I MHC-based selection occurs, alternative selection mechansims are likely to be in place for $\gamma\delta$ IELs.

The latter possibility is strengthened by studies of IELs in mice expressing an alloantigen-specific transgenic $\gamma\delta$ TcR (Barrett *et al.*, 1992). In mice expressing this transgene and the selecting alloantigen, $\gamma\delta$ T cells are deleted in the thymus and spleen. However, IELs with normal receptor levels are present in these animals that are unresponsive to activation. As the mice age, these anergic self-reactive IELs gradually diminish in number. Thus, selection of $\gamma\delta$ T cells in epithelial tissue appears to be dependent on induction of clonal anergy with eventual deletion.

B. $\alpha\beta$ T Cells

1. Origin

In contrast to $\gamma\delta$ IELs, most $\alpha\beta$ IELs require the thymus for maturation. However, some variable extrathymic production of $\alpha\beta$ IELs appears to occur. In thymectomized irradiated bone marrow chimeras, significant numbers of donor-derived $\alpha\beta$ IELs were detected in some animals but not in others. In nude mice, $\alpha\beta$ IELs are found rarely (Bandeira *et al.*, 1990b; Bonneville *et al.*, 1990; DeGeus *et al.*, 1990) although an occasional preparation can contain large numbers of these cells (L. Lefrancois, unpublished results).

A putative "thymoindependent" $\alpha\beta$ population has been proposed to exist in the gut (Murosaki *et al.*, 1991; Rocha *et al.*, 1991). This contention is based on the finding that certain Vβ regions that are not found on peripheral T cells are expressed by a subset of IELs (reviewed by Lefrancois, 1991c). Lack of deletion in the IEL compartment was considered evidence that these cells do not mature in the thymus. The forbidden V regions are expressed by CD8β^- IELs but not by CD8β^+ IELs supporting the concept that the CD8β^- $\alpha\beta$ TcR subset is derived extrathymically. However, the data from nude mice and thymectomized chimeras must be considered. Since few $\alpha\beta$ T cells generally are found in nude mice, the CD8β^- subset may be more likely to require some thymic influence, perhaps via interaction with thymus-derived CD8$\beta^+\alpha\beta$ IELs or other T cells. Alternatively, these forbidden clones could traffic through the thumus and escape deletion only to be tolerized in the periphery. In this regard, whether IELs expressing forbidden V regions are functional has not been shown. Further studies of this intriguing subset are required to understand their origin and function.

2. $\alpha\beta$ TcR Selection

As just discussed, Vβ selection in the gut does not necessarily occur as predicted by the selection patterns of other peripheral T cells. To understand in more detail the relationship between CD8β expression and V region selection, we analyzed CD4$^+$CD8$^+$ IELs that are CD8β^-. Table II shows the results of analysis of Vβ6 and Vβ14 expression in CD4$^-$CD8$^+$ and CD4$^+$CD8$^+$ IELs compared with lymph node T cells. The interesting result is that, although Vβ6 was expressed in CD4$^-$CD8$^+$ IELs, it was deleted from lymph node T cells as well as from CD4$^+$CD8$^+$ IELs. Most V$\beta6^+$ IELs were found in the CD8β^- subset (data not shown). Vβ14 was expressed in all lymph node and IEL subsets. These results indicate that CD8β expression (or lack of it) is not sufficient to explain the expression of forbidden V regions. A thorough analysis of several Vβ regions in various mouse strains confirmed these findings and also demonstrated other nonpredicted selection patterns (Badiner *et al.*, 1993).

Data from studies of human $\alpha\beta$ IELs indicate that a restricted subset of V regions is expressed by IELs compared with peripheral blood T cells (Balk *et al.*, 1991; Van Kerckhove *et al.*, 1991). In two independent studies, V region analysis demonstrated that IELs were oligoclonal, expressing predominant V regions, some of which were shared among IELs of different individuals. In one study, an oligoclonal T-cell line and a clone expressing a dominant V region were shown to react with CD1, a nonpolymorphic Class I-like molecule (see subsequent discussion). Oligoclonal expansion was proposed to occur in response to a restricted set of antigens, some of which may be nonpolymorphic.

Table II TcR Vβ Expression in Intraepithelial Lymphocytes and Lymph Node Subsets[a]

	% Positive			
	Lymph node subset		IEL subset	
Vβ	CD4	CD8	$CD4^-8^+$	$CD4^+8^+$
6	0.5 ± 0.4	0.5 ± 0.2	4.7 ± 2.5	0.5 ± 0.4
14	9.5 ± 0.4	18.6 ± 4.9	10.6 ± 5.7	6.9 ± 2.5

[a] AKR/J IELs were isolated and expression of the indicated antigens was tested by three-color fluorescence flow cytometry.

C. Epithelial Cell Involvement

Since most γδ IELs and perhaps a subset of αβ IELs (at least in the mouse) mature outside the thymus, several investigators have proposed the involvement of the intestinal epithelium in IEL differentiation. Thymic and gut epithelium are endoderm derivatives and have several similar characteristics. Villous epithelium constitutively expresses MHC Class II molecules; this expression can be up-regulated by lymphokines such as interferon γ (IFNγ; reviewed by Bland, 1988). Intestinal epithelial cells are able to process and present antigen to Class II-restricted T cells, although whether IELs respond to epithelium-presented antigen is not known.

Several studies have suggested that γδ T cells in general may react with nonpolymorphic antigens such as heat-shock proteins or Class I-like molecules such as CD1 or TLA. The demonstration that TLA in the mouse and CD1 in the mouse and the human are expressed prominently by intestinal epithelial cells supports this theory (Bleicher *et al.*, 1990; Hershberg *et al.*, 1990). TLA also is expressed by ~50% of αβ IELs and ~25% of γδ IELs and is predominantly expressed by the $Thy1^-$ subset (Hershberg *et al.*, 1990). TLA and CD1 exhibit restricted expression patterns, with predominant expression in the intestine, suggesting an important role for these molecules in intestinal immunity. Although αβ IEL reactivity to CD1 has been demonstrated, as discussed earlier, γδ IEL reactivity to nonclassical MHC molecules has not been reported.

IV. FUNCTIONAL PROPERTIES

A. Cytolytic Activity

Freshly isolated $CD8^+$ mouse IELs are constitutively cytolytic but do not possess natural killer activity. This activity is confined largely to the $Thy1^+$ subset; γδ and αβ IELs are cytolytic. The cytolytic activity is measured using a redirected lysis assay in which IELs are reacted with an anti-TcR MAb followed by incubation with a radiolabeled target cell that expresses an Ig Fc receptor. In this way, a measure of total cytolytic capability is obtained irrespective of the specificity of the effector cell. Since $CD8^+$ lymph node T cells are negative in this assay, IELs are assumed to be activated *in situ* by the supposed constant antigenic bombardment of the intestinal mucosa. This theory is supported by the finding that colonization of the gut induces Thy1 expression and cytolytic activity in IELs. However, a specific target cell for IEL cytolytic activity has not been found. IELs did not lyse a panel of tumor target cells and also did not lyse antigen-presenting cells (not derived from gut) that were preincubated with bacterial lysates (T. Goodman and L. Lefrancois, unpublished results). Thus, either the correct antigenic moiety has not been tested or the antigen-presenting cell employed was lacking in a necessary component. "Preactivated" IELs may recognize antigen only as presented by intestinal epithelium. Purified $CD8^+$ IELs do not exhibit natural killer activity.

TcR αβ IELs can be primed against alloantigen or viral antigen (Ernst *et al.*, 1986; London *et al.*, 1989; Offit and Dudzik, 1989; Lefrancois, 1991b). Reovirus infection results in the generation of MHC-restricted virus-specific cytolytic $Thy1^+$ TcR αβ IELs. TcR γδ IELs do not respond to reovirus antigens. However, whether resident αβ IELs respond to viral challenge or whether other T cells infiltrate the mucosa after infection is not clear. A cytolytic CD1-specific human IEL line has been produced by stimulation of jejunal IELs with phytohemagglutinin (PHA), lymphokines, and allogeneic peripheral blood lymphocytes (Balk *et al.*, 1991). Thus, at least some αβ IELs have characteristics of classical cytotoxic T lymphocytes. The specificity of γδ IELs remains unknown.

B. Proliferative Capacity

Several reports indicate that IELs respond poorly or not at all to proliferative signals including mitogens, phorbol esters, or anit-TcR MAb (Ebert, 1989; Mowat *et al.*, 1989; Mosley *et al.*, 1991). However, we routinely maintain IELs in culture for several weeks after stimulation with anti-TcR MAb. In our hands, culture of $Thy1^+$ IELs with immobilized anti-CD3 or anti-γδ/αβ MAb results in significant proliferation (Gramzinski *et al.*, 1993). Proliferation is the result of an IL-2–IL-2 receptor autocrine pathway, yet the maximum proliferation of IELs is 10–20% of that obtained with $CD8^+$ lymph node cells (Figure 4). $Thy1^-$ IELs proliferated significantly less than $Thy1^+$ IELs in response to anti-TcR stimulation, but proliferation was enhanced by the addition of IL-2 to the cultures (Figure 4). Interestingly, the addition of anti-CD8 MAbs to the cutlures strongly inhibits $CD8^+$ lymph node T-cell proliferation but only marginally affects IEL proliferation (Gramzinski *et al.*, 1993). This result suggests that IEL CD8 is functionally distinct or that the IEL CD8 signal transduction pathway differs from that of peripheral T cell CD8. Overall, the results indicate that IELs are able to respond to proliferative signals but to a reduced level compared with lymph node T cells. This phenomenon could be the result of down-regulation of proliferative pathways by continuous antigenic stimulation or the result of our lack of knowledge of the growth requirements of IELs.

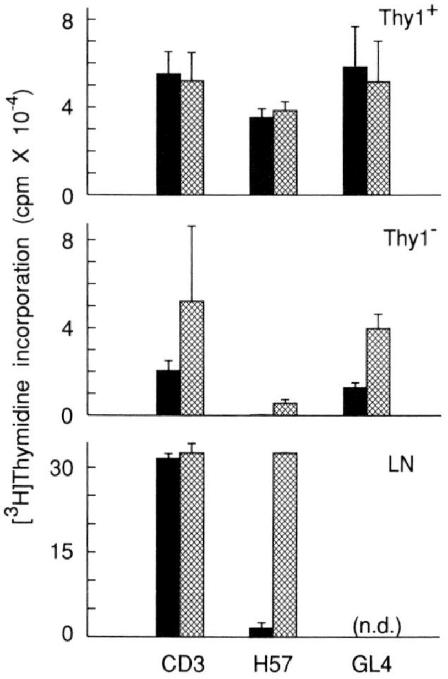

Figure 4 Proliferative capacity of intraepithelial lymphocytes (IELS). Thy1$^+$ (*top*) or Thy1$^-$ (*middle*) CD4$^-$CD8$^+$ IELs or CD4$^-$CD8$^+$ lymph node (*bottom*) T cells were stimulated *in vitro* for 3 days with immobilized anti-CD3, anti-$\alpha\beta$ TcR (H57), or anti-$\gamma\delta$ TcR (GL4) MAb in the absence (solid bars) or presence (hatched bars) of recombinant IL-2. Cells were pulsed with [^{3}H]thymidine for the final 24 hr of culture followed by harvesting and scintillation counting. n.d., Not done.

C. Lymphokine Production

IELs produce an array of lymphokines similar to those produced by other CD8$^+$ T cells. *In situ* analysis demonstrates that IELs produce IFNγ and IL-5 (Taguchi *et al.*, 1990). Analysis of culture supernatants from anti-TcR MAb-activated $\gamma\delta$ or $\alpha\beta$ IELs indicates that both subsets produce IL-2, IFNγ and transforming growth factor β (TGFβ) but do not produce IL-4 (Barrett *et al.*, 1990). The role of IEL lymphokine production in intestinal immune responses remains to be elucidated.

D. Regulatory Role for $\gamma\delta$ IEL?

Some intriguing data have been reported suggesting that $\gamma\delta$ T cells, including IELs, may function as regulatory cells (Fujihashi *et al.*, 1989,1990). Using a system of oral tolerance to sheep red blood cells (SRBC), these authors demonstrated that transfer of antigen-primed CD4$^-$CD8$^-$ splenic $\gamma\delta$ T cells from nude mice or $\gamma\delta$ IELs from normal mice can reverse oral tolerance. This function was attributed to Thy1$^-$ $\gamma\delta$ IELs of either CD4$^-$CD8^{+-} or CD4$^-$CD8$^-$ phenotype. This phenomenon has not been reported for other antigens, and whether the antigen-primed $\gamma\delta$ T cells can respond to SRBCs has not been shown. Significant efforts should be applied to determining whether this function is generalized and to analyzing the specificity of such regulatory cells.

V. SUMMARY

The complexity of the IEL compartment rivals that found in the thymus. Indeed, mounting evidence suggests that the intestine may be a lymphocyte generative organ analogous in some ways to the thymus. In the case of $\gamma\delta$ IELs, clearly extrathymic maturation occurs. Although this pathway has not been proven to exist in humans, it seems likely based on the phenotypic similarities between mouse and human $\gamma\delta$ IELs that distinguish them from peripheral $\gamma\delta$ T cells. Restricted V gene usage by IELs suggests that their surveillance capabilities are skewed toward a discrete set of antigens that is likely to be tissue specific. The TcRs expressed appear to be polyclonal, based on junctional sequences.

TcR $\alpha\beta$ IELs also appear to express a restricted set of V regions preferentially. However, skewing toward particular V region usage appears to be the result of oligoclonal expansion of certain IEL clones, perhaps in response to a limited array of antigens. For a subset of $\alpha\beta$ IELs that expresses forbidden V regions, the TcR selection process is distinct from that of conventional CD8$^+$ T cells, including other IELs. Whereas most $\alpha\beta$ IELs are thymus derived, the role of the thymus in the production of forbidden $\alpha\beta$ IEL clones is unclear.

Although much progress has been made in the areas of IEL phenotypic characterization, *in vitro* functional assays, and TcR expression, the specificity and function of IELs *in vivo* remains obscure. At least some $\alpha\beta$ IELs can respond to antigens such as viral proteins in a conventional MHC-restricted cytotoxic T-lymphocyte response. The function of the $\alpha\beta$ T-cell subsets that are unique to the IEL compartment, for example, the CD4$^+$CD8$^+$ IELs, remains to be determined. With respect to $\gamma\delta$ IELs, no defined "conventional" responses for $\gamma\delta$ T cells are known. We are hard-pressed to define specific functions at this time. Except for assumptions concerning function made based on phenotype and anatomical location, little substantive progress has been made. The development of novel *in vivo* and *in vitro* assays may be required before a breakthrough is realized in the area of IEL function.

Acknowledgments

I would like to thank Gloria Badiner, Tom Goodman, Rozenne LeCorre, and Robert Gramzinski for their perseverance in generating much of the data presented from our laboratory. I also thank Earl Adams for his expert assistance with flow cytometry.

References

Acha-Orbea, H., and Palmer, E. (1991). MLS—A retrovirus exploits the immune system. *Immunol. Today* **12**, 356–361.

Asarnow, D. M., Goodman, T., Lefrancois, L., and Allison, J. P. (1989). Distinct antigen receptor repertoires of two classes of murine epithelium-associated T cells. *Nature* (*London*) **341**, 60–62.

Badiner, G., Goodman, T. G., and Lefrancois, L. (1993). Selection of intestinal intraepithelial lymphocyte T-cell receptors—evidence for a dynamic tissue-specific process. *Int. Immunol.* **5,** 223–226.

Balk, S. P., Ebert, E. C., Blumenthal, R. L., McDermott, F. V., Wucherpfennig, K. W., Landau, S. B., and Blumberg, R. S. (1991). Oligoclonal expansion and CD1 recognition by human intestinal intraepithelial lymphocytes. *Science* **253,** 1411–1415.

Bandeira, A., Itohara, S., Bonneville, M., Burlen-Defranoux, O., Mota-Santos, T., Coutinho, A., and Tonegawa, S. (1990a). Extrathymic origin of intestinal intraepithelial lymphocytes bearing T-cell antigen receptor $\gamma\delta$. *Proc. Natl. Acad. Sci. U.S.A.* **88,** 43–47.

Bandeira, A., Mota-Santos, T., Itohara, S., Degermann, S., Heusser, C., Tonegawa, S., and Coutinho, A. (1990b). Localization of γ/δ T cells to the intestinal epithelium is independent of normal microbial colonization. *J. Exp. Med.* **172,** 239–244.

Barrett, T., Gajewski, T., Lee, N., Widacki, S. M., Chang, E. B., Lefrancois, L., and Bluestone, J. A. (1990). Localization and functional characterization of intra-epithelial lymphocyte subsets activated with anti-α/β and γ/δ T cell receptor antibodies. *FASEB J.* **4,** 1864.

Barrett, T. A., Delvy, M. L., Kennedy, D. M., Lefrancois, L., Matis, L. A., Dent, A. L., Hedrick, S. M., and Bluestone, J. A. (1992). Mechanism of self-tolerance of γ/δ T cells in epithelial tissue. *J. Exp. Med.* **175,** 65–70.

Bland, P. (1988). MHC class II expression by the gut epithelium. *Immunol. Today* **9,** 174–178.

Bleicher, P., Balk, S. P., Hagen, S. J., Blumberg, R. S., Flotte, T. J., and Terhorst, C. (1990). Expression of murine CD1 on gastrointestinal epithelium. *Science* **250,** 679–682.

Bonneville, M., Janeway, C. A., Ito, N., Haser, W., Ishida, I., Nakanishi, N., and Tonegawa, S. (1988) Intestinal intraepithelial lymphocytes are a distinct set of $\gamma\delta$ T cells. *Nature (London)* **336,** 479–481.

Bonneville, M., Itohara, S., Krecko, E. G., Mombaerts, P., Ishida, I., Katsuki, M., Berns, A., Farr, A. G., Janeway, C. A., and Tonegawa, S. (1990). Transgenic mice demonstrate that epithelial homing of γ/δ T cells is determined by cell lineages independent of T cell receptor specificity. *J. Exp. Med.* **171,** 1015–1026.

Bottomly, K., Luqman, M., Greenbaum, L., Carding, S., West, J., Pasqualini, T., and Murphy, D. B. (1989). A monoclonal antibody to murine CD45R distinguishes CD4 T cell populations that produce different cytokines. *Eur. J. Immunol.* **19,** 617–623.

Bucy, R. P., Chen, C-. L. H., Cihak, J., Losch, U., and Cooper, M. D. (1988). Avian T cells expressing γ/δ receptors localize in the splenic sinusoids and the intestinal epithelium. *J. Immunol.* **141,** 2200–2205.

Carding, S. R., Kyes, S. Jenkinson, E. J., Kingston, R., Bottomly, K., Owen, J. J. T., and Hayday, A. (1990). Developmentally regulated fetal thymic and extrathymic T-cell receptor $\gamma\delta$ gene expression. *Genes Dev.* **4,** 1304–1315.

Cerf-Bensussan, N., Guy-Grand, D., Lisowska-Grospierre, B., Griscelli, C., and Bhan, A. K. (1986). A monoclonal antibody specific for rat intestinal lymphocytes. *J. Immunol.* **136,** 76–82.

Cerf-Bensussan, N., Jarry, A., Brousse, N., Lisowska-Grospierre, B., Guy-Grand, D., and Griscelli, C. (1987). A monoclonal antibody (HML-1) defining a novel membrane molecule present on human intestinal lymphocytes. *Eur. J. Immunol.* **17,** 1279–1285.

Clark, E. A., and Ledbetter, J. A. (1989). Leukocyte cell surface enzymology: CD45 (LCA, T200) is a protein tyrosine phosphatase. *Immunol. Today* **10,** 225–228.

Cron, R. Q., Gajewski, T., Sharrow, S. O., Fitch, F. W., Matis, L. A., and Bluestone, J. A. (1989). Phenotypic and functional analysis of murine $CD3^+$, $CD4^-$, $CD8^-$ TCR-$\gamma\delta$-expressing peripheral T cells. *J. Immunol.* **142,** 3754–3762.

De Geus, B., Van den Enden, M., Coolen, C., Nagelkerken, L., Van der Heijden, P., and Rozing, J. (1990). Phenotype of intraepithelial lymphocytes in euthymic and athymic mice: Implications for differentiation of cells bearing a CD3-associated $\gamma\delta$ T cell receptor. *Eur. J. Immunol.* **20,** 291–298.

Deusch, K., Luling, F., Reich, K., Classen, M., Wagner, H., and Pfeffer, K. (1991). A major function of human intraepithelial lymphocytes expresses the γ/δ T cell receptor, the CD8 accessory molecule and perferentially uses the Vδ1 gene segment. *Eur. J. Immunol.* **21,** 1053–1059.

Ebert, E. C. (1989). Proliferative responses of human intraepithelial lymphocytes to various T cell stimuli. *Gastroenterology* **97,** 1372–1381.

Ernst, P. B., Clark, D. A., Rosenthal, K. L., Befus, A. D., and Bienenstock, J. (1986). Detection and characterization of cytotoxic T lymphocyte precursors in the murine intestinal intraepithelial leukocyte population. *J. Immunol.* **136,** 2121–2126.

Fangmann, J., Schwinzer, R., and Wonigeit, K. (1991). Unusual phenotype of intestinal intraepithelial lymphocytes in the rat: predominance of T cell receptor $\alpha/\beta^+/CD2^-$ cells and high expression of the RT6 alloantigen. *Eur. J. Immunol.* **21,** 753–760.

Fujihashi, K., Kiyono, H., Aicher, W. K., Green, D. R., Singh, B., Eldridge, J. H., and McGhee, J. R. (1989). Immunoregulatory function of $CD3^+$, $CD4^-$, and $CD8^-$ T cells. $\gamma\delta$ T cell receptor-positive T cells from nude mice abrogate oral tolerance. *J. Immunol.* **143,** 3415–3422.

Fujihashi, K., Taguchi, T., McGhee, J. R., Eldridge, J. H., Bruce, M. G., Green, D. R., Singh, B., and Kiyono, H. (1990). Regulatory function for murine intraepithelial lymphocytes. Two subsets of $CD3^+$, T cell receptor-1^+ intraepithelial lymphocyte T cells abrogate oral tolerance. *J. Immunol.* **145,** 2010–2019.

Goodman, T., and Lefrancois, L. (1988). Expression of the $\gamma\delta$ T cell receptor on intestinal $CD8^+$ intraepithelial lymphocytes. *Nature (London)* **333,** 855–858.

Goodman, T., and Lefrancois, L. (1989). Intraepithelial lymphocytes. Anatomical site, not T cell receptor form, dictates phenotype and function. *J. Exp. Med.* **170,** 1569–1581.

Goodman, T. G., Chang, H.-L., Esselman, W. J., LeCorre, R., and Lefrancois, L. (1990). Characterization of the CD45 molecule on murine intestinal intraepithelial lymphocytes. *J. Immunol.* **145,** 2959–2966.

Goodman, T., LeCorre, R., and Lefrancois, L. (1992). A T-cell receptor $\gamma\delta$-specific monoclonal antibody detects a Vγ5 region polymorphism. *Immunogenetics* **35,** 65–68.

Gramzinski, R. A., Adams, E., Gross, J. A., Goodman, T. G., Allison, J. P., and Lefrancois, L. (1993). T-cell receptor-triggered activation of intraepithelial lymphocytes *in vitro*. *Int. Immunol.* **5,** 145–153.

Guy-Grand, D., Malassis-Seris, M., Briottet, C., and Vassalli, P. (1991a). Cytotoxic differentiation of mouse gut thymodependent and independent intraepithelial lymphocytes is induced locally. Correlation between functional assays, presence of perforin and granzyme transcripts, and cytoplasmic granules. *J. Exp. Med.* **173,** 1549–1552.

Guy-Grand, D., Cerf-Bensussan, N., Malissen, B., Malassis-Seris, M., Briottet, C., and Vassalli, P. (1991b). Two gut intraepithelial $CD8^+$ lymphocyte populations with different T cell receptors: A role for the gut epithelium in T cell differentiation. *J. Exp. Med.* **173,** 471–481.

Halstensen, T., Scott, H., and Brandtzaeg, P. (1990). Human $CD8^+$ intraepithelial T lymphocytes are mainly $CD45RA^-RB^+$ and show increased co-expression of CD45R0 in celiac disease. *Eur. J. Immunol.* **20,** 1825–1830.

Hein, W. R., and Mackay, C. R. (1991). Prominence of $\gamma\delta$ T cells in the ruminant immune system. *Immunol. Today* **12,** 30–34.

Hershberg, R., Eghtesady, P., Sydora, B., Brorson, K., Cheroutre,

H., Modlin, R., and Kronenberg, M. (1990). Expression of the thymus leukemia antigen in mouse intestinal epithelium. *Proc. Natl. Acad. Sci. U.S.A.* **87,** 9727–9731.

Jarry, A., Cerf-Bensussan, N., Brousse, N., Selz, F., and Guy-Grand, D. (1990). Subsets of $CD3^+$ (T cell receptor α/β or γ/δ) and $CD3^-$ lymphocytes isolated from normal human gut epithelium display phenotypical features different from their counterparts in peripheral blood. *Eur. J. Immunol.* **20,** 1097–1103.

Kilshaw, P. J., and Baker, K. C. (1989). A new antigenic determinant on intraepithelial lymphocytes and its association with CD45. *Immunology* **67,** 160–166.

Kilshaw, P. J., and Murant, S. J. (1990). A new surface antigen on intraepithelial lymphocytes in the intestine. *Eur. J. Immunol.* **20,** 2201–2207.

Kruschwitz, M., Fritzsche, G., Schwarting, R., Micklem, K., Mason, D. Y., Falini, B., and Stein, H. (1991). Ber-ACT8: New monoclonal antibody to the mucosa lymphocyte antigen. *J. Clin. Pathol.* **44,** 636–645.

Ledbetter, J. A., and Seaman, W. E. (1982). The Lyt-2, Lyt-3 macromolecules: Structural and functional studies. *Immunol. Rev.* **68,** 197–218.

Lefrancois, L. (1987). Expression of carbohydrate differentiation antigens during ontogeny of the murine thymus. *J. Immunol.* **139,** 2220–2229.

Lefrancois, L. (1991a). Phenotypic complexity of intraepithelial lymphocytes of the small intestine. *J. Immunol.* **147,** 1746–1751.

Lefrancois, L. (1991b). Intraepithelial lymphocytes of the intestinal mucosa: Curiouser and curiouser. *Sem. Immunol.* **3,** 99–108.

Lefrancois, L. (1991c). Extrathymic differentiation of intraepithelial lymphocytes: Generation of a separate and unequal T-cell repertoire? *Immunol. Today* **12,** 436–438.

Lefrancois, L. and Goodman, T. (1987). Developmental sequence of T200 antigen modifications in murine T cells. J. Immunol. **139,** 3718–3724.

Lefrancois, L., and Goodman, T. (1989). *In vivo* modulation of cytolytic activity and Thy-1 expression in TCR-$\gamma\delta^+$ intraepithelial lymphocytes. *Science* **243,** 1716–1718.

Lefrancois, L., LeCorre, R., Mayo, J., Bluestone, J. A., and Goodman, T. (1990). Extrathymic selection of TCR $\gamma\delta^+$ T cells by class II major histocompatibility molecules. *Cell* **63,** 333–340.

London, S. D., Cebra, J. J., and Rubin, D. H. (1989). Intraepithelial lymphocytes contain virus-specific, MHC-restricted cytotoxic T cell precursors after gut mucosal immunization with reovirus serotype 1/Lang. *Reg. Immunol.* **2,** 98–102.

MacDonald, H. R., Schreyer, M., Howe, R. C., and Bron, C. (1990a). Selective expression of CD8α (Ly-2) subunit on activated thymic γ/δ cells. *Eur. J. Immunol.* **20,** 927–930.

MacDonald, H. R., Lees, R. K., and Chvatchko, Y., (1990b). $CD8^+$ T cells respond clonally to Mls-1^a-encoded determinants. *J. Exp. Med.* **171,** 1381–1386.

Mosley, R. L., Styre, D., and Klein, J. R. (1990a) CD4+ CD8+ murine intestinal intraepithelial lymphocytes. *Int. Immunol.* **2,** 361–365.

Mosley, R. L., Styre, D., and Klein, J. R. (1990b). Differentiation and functional maturation of bone marrow-derived intestinal epithelial T cells expressing membrane T cell receptor in athymic radiation chimeras. *J. Immunol.* **145,** 1369–1375.

Mosley, R. L., Whetsell, M., and Klein, J. R. (1991). Proliferative properties of murine intestinal intraepithelial lymphocytes (IEL): IEL expressing TCR$\alpha\beta$ or TCR$\gamma\delta$ are largely unresponsive to proliferative signals mediated via conventional stimulation of the CD3-TCR complex. *Int. Immunol.* **3,** 563–569.

Mowat, A. M. I., McInnes, I. B., and Parrott, D. M. V. (1989). Functional properties of intra-epithelial lymphocytes from mouse small intestine. IV. Investigation of the proliferative capacity of IEL using phorbol ester and calcium ionophore. *Immunology* **66,** 398–403.

Murosaki, S., Yoshikai, Y., Ishida, A., Nakamura, T., Matsuzaki, G., Takimoto, H., Yuuki, H., and Nomoto, K. (1991). Failure of T cell receptor Vβ negative selection in murine intestinal intraepithelial lymphocytes. *Int. Immunol.* **3,** 1005–1013.

Offit, P. A. and Dudzik, K. I. (1989). Rotavirus-specific cytotoxic T lymphocytes appear at the intestinal mucosal surface after rotavirus infection. *J. Virol.* **63,** 3507–3512.

Parrott, D. M. V., Tait, C., MacKenzie, S., Mowat, A. M., Davies, M. D. J., and Micklem, H. S. (1983). Analysis of the effector functions of different populations of mucosal lymphocytes. *Ann. N.Y. Acad. Sci.* **409,** 307–320.

Raulet, D. H., Spencer, D. M., Hsiang, Y-H., Goldman, J. P., Bix, M., Liao, N.-S., Zijlstra, M., Jaenisch, R., and Correa, I. (1991). Control of $\gamma\delta$ T-cell development. *Immunol. Rev.* **120,** 185–204.

Rocha, B., Vassalli, P., and Guy-Grand, D. (1991). The Vβ repertoire of mouse gut homodimeric α $CD8^+$ intraepithelial T cell receptor α/β^+ lymphocytes reveals a major extrathymic pathway of T cell differentiation. *J. Exp. Med.* **173,** 483–486.

Schieferdecker, H. L., Ullrich, R., Weiss-Breckwoldt, A. N., Schwarting, R., Stein, H., Riecken, E. O., and Zeitz, M. (1990). The HML-1 antigen of intestinal lymphocytes is an activation antigen. *J. Immunol.* **144,** 2541–2549.

Spencer, J., Isaacson, P. G., Diss, T. C., and MacDonald, T. T. (1989). Expression of disulfide-linked and non-disulfide-linked forms of the T cell receptor $\gamma\delta$ heterodimer in human intestinal intraepithelial lymphocytes. *Eur. J. Immunol.* **19,** 1335–1338.

Stamenkovic, I., Sgroi, D., Aruffo, A., Sy, M. S., and Anderson, T. (1991). The B lymphocyte adhesion molecule CD22 interacts with leukocyte common antigen CD45R0 on T cells and α2-6 sialyltransferase, CD75, on B cells. *Cell* **66,** 1133–1144.

Taguchi, T., McGhee, J. R., Coffman, R. L., Beagley, K. W., Eldridge, J. H., Takatsu, K., and Kiyono, H. (1990). Analysis of Th1 and Th2 cells in murine gut-associated tissues. Frequencies of $CD4^+$ and $CD8^+$ T cells that secrete IFN-γ and IL-5. *J. Immunol.* **145,** 68–77.

Takagaki, Y., DeCloux, A., Bonneville, M., and Tonegawa, S. (1989). Diversity of $\gamma\delta$ T-cell receptors on murine intestinal intraepithelial lymphocytes. *Nature (London)* **339,** 712–714.

Thomas, M., and Lefrancois, L. (1988). Differential expression of the leucocyte common antigen family. *Immunol. Today* **9,** 321–326.

Trejdosiewicz, L. K., Smart, C. J., Oakes, D. J., Howdle, P. D., Malizia, G., Camapana, D., and Boylston, A. W. (1989). Expression of T-cell receptors Tcr1 (γ/δ) and Tcr2 (α/β) in the human intestinal mucosa. *Immunology* **68,** 7–12.

Vaage, J. T., Dissen, E., Ager, A., Roberts, I., Fossum, S., and Rolstad, B. (1990). T cell receptor-bearing cells among rat intestinal intraepithelial lymphocytes are mainly α/β^+ and are thymus dependent. *Eur. J. Immunol.* **20,** 1193–1196.

Van de Velde, H., von Hoegen, I., Luo, W., Parnes, J. R., and Thielemans, K. (1991). The B-cell surface protein CD72/Lyb-2 is the ligand for CD5. *Nature (London)* **351,** 662–665.

Van Kerckhove, C., Russell, G. J., Deusch, K., Reich, K., Bhan, A. K., DerSimonian, H., and Brenner, M. B. (1991). Oligoclonality of human intestinal intraepithelial T cells. *J. Exp. Med.* **175,** 57–63.

Viney, J. L., MacDonald, T. T., and Kilshaw, P. J. (1989/1990). $\alpha\beta$ T cell receptor expression in rat intestinal epithelium. *Immunol. Lett.* **3,** 49–54.

Viney, J. L., Kilshaw, P. J., and MacDonald, T. T. (1990). Cytotoxic α/β^+ and γ/δ^+ T cells in murine intestinal epithelium. *Eur. J. Immunol.* **20,** 1623–1626.

Yuan, Q., Jiang, W. M., Hollander, D., Leung, E., Watson, J. D., and Krissansen, G. W. (1991). Identity between the novel integrin β_7 subunit and an antigen found highly expressed on intraepithelial lymphocytes in the small intestine. *Biochem. Biophys. Res. Commun.* **176,** 1443–1449.

Zamoyska, R., Derham, P., Gorman, S. D., von Hoegen, P., Bolen, J. B., Veillette, A., and Parnes, J. R. (1989). Inability of CD8α' polypeptides to associate with p56^{lck} correlates with impaired function *in vitro* and lack of expression *in vivo*. *Nature (London)* **342,** 278–281.

25

IgE-Mediated Responses in the Mucosal Immune System

Kimishige Ishizaka

I. INTRODUCTION

IgE is the least component of immunoglobulins. The concentration of IgE in the serum of normal individuals is on the order of 100–300 ng/ml. However, IgE antibodies have unique biological activities. The antibodies sensitize mast cells and basophilic granulocytes of homologous species; the reaction of antigen to cell-bound IgE antibodies induces the release of various mediators that cause allergic reactions. Under normal circumstances, allergic diseases are induced by exposure to extrinsic antigens such as allergens. Therefore, IgE-mediated allergic diseases are induced most frequently in the respiratory tract, gastrointestinal tract, and skin. Since the IgE antibody response also is induced by allergens, conceivably IgE antibodies formed in mucosal lymphoid tissues may play important roles in allergic diseases. Indeed, IgE-producing cells are detected more frequently in mucosal lymphoid tissues than in the major lymphoid organs such as spleen and peripheral lymph nodes (Tada and Ishizaka, 1970). High frequency of IgE-producing cells in mucosal lymphoid tissues appears to be the result of local immune response to extrinsic antigens. Different from IgA, IgE in secretions does not contain secretory component (SC) and has the same physicochemical properties as IgE present in the serum (Newcomb and Ishizaka, 1970). To date, mechanisms of the IgE antibody response and IgE-mediated hypersensitivity reactions have been studied in experimental models using splenic lymphocytes, peritoneal or bone marrow-derived mast cells, and peripheral blood basophilic granulocytes. In this chapter, the fundamental mechanisms of IgE-mediated responses, which were elucidated using these systems, are summarized briefly with some attention to mucosal immune systems.

II. BASIC MECHANISMS INVOLVED IN THE IgE ANTIBODY RESPONSE

A. Dissociation between the IgE and IgG Antibody Response

In atopic patients, IgE antibody levels in serum do not show much fluctuation. Considering that the half-life of IgE in normal individuals is 2–3 days, formation of IgE antibodies appears to be persistent in these patients. Although the quantity of allergen inhaled by the patients during a pollen season is on the order of micrograms, the IgE and IgG antibody levels in their serum increase after the season and the antibody levels are well maintained during the remainder of the year (Ishizaka, 1976). Another unique characteristic of atopic patients is a relatively high concentration of IgE antibodies among various isotypes. Unless the patients receive immunotherapy, the concentration of IgE antibodies against allergen in their serum is comparable to that of IgG antibodies and usually higher than that of IgA antibodies. Considering that the concentration of total serum IgE is less then 1/10,000 of the concentration of total IgG, the immune response of atopic patients to allergens includes some conditions favorable for the IgE isotype.

A series of experiments in inbred strains of mice revealed that persistent IgE antibody formation was obtained only when genetically high responder strains were immunized with a minute dose of a potent immunogen and an appropriate adjuvant (Ishizaka, 1976). An increase in the dose of the immunogen resulted in an increase in the magnitude of IgG antibody response, but made the IgE antibody response transient and caused dissociation of the IgE antibody response and IgG antibody response.

As expected, the IgE antibody response appears to be controlled by immune response (Ir) genes that are linked to the major histocompatibility complex (MHC). However, an entirely different type of genetic control was found in the mouse that uniquely controls the IgE isotype. For example, SJL and AKR mice showed a poor IgE antibody response to various protein antigens despite a substantial IgG antibody response to the same antigen (Levine, 1971). This genetic control provides another restriction for the persistent IgE antibody formation and causes dissociation of IgE antibody response and IgG antibody response.

B. Role of IL-4 in IgE Synthesis

The IgE antibody response is highly T cell dependent, suggesting that T cell-derived lymphokines are involved in the differentiation of B cells to IgE-forming cells. Indeed, results of experiments by several groups of investigators revealed that interleukin 4 (IL-4) from helper T cells is essential to IgE production. That stimulation of mouse B cells with lipopolysaccharide (LPS) results in the differentiation of B cells and the formation of a variety of Ig isotypes except IgE is well known. However, culture of the same B cells with LPS and 300–1000 units/ml recombinant IL-4 results in the formation of IgE and selective enhancement of IgG1 formation, accompanied by decreases in IgG2b and IgG3 formation (Coffman *et al.*, 1986). The concentration of IL-4 required for switching of B cells for IgE synthesis was much higher than the physiological concentration. However, addition of IL-5 with IL-4 diminished the minimum concentration of IL-4 required for IgE synthesis to 5–10 units/ml.

The effect of IL-4 on IgE synthesis also was demonstrated in *in vitro* immunoglobulin formation by human peripheral blood mononuclear cells (PBMC) (Pene *et al.*, 1988). Culture of normal human PBMCs with 100 units/ml human IL-4 resulted in the formation of IgE. IL-4 also induced IgG4 synthesis. For the formation of IgE by normal human B cells, however, both T cells and monocytes are required (Pene *et al.*, 1988). Additional studies have shown that interaction of B cells with T cells is required for IL-4-induced IgE synthesis by normal B cells (Vercelli *et al.*, 1989; Parronchi *et al.*, 1990).

The major effect of IL-4 on IgE synthesis is switching of resting B cells to the precursors of IgE-forming cells that bear surface IgE. Culture of pure murine B cells with LPS and IL-4 resulted in the appearance of IgE-bearing B cells and IgG1-bearing B cells; depletion of $sIgE^+$ B cells developed in the culture abolished IgE formation in the system (Snapper *et al.*, 1988). The mechanism for isotype switching is the deletion of immunoglobulin gene segments. Yoshida *et al.*, (1990) characterized immunoglobulin switch circular DNA present in lymph nodes of mice infected with the nematode *Nippostrongylus brasiliensis* and in normal splenic lymphocytes cultured with LPS and IL-4, and identified two kinds of circular DNA as excision products of switch recombination of immunoglobulin heavy-chain constant region genes. One of them was a recombinant between $C\mu$ and $C\gamma1$, and the other was a recombinant between $C\gamma1$ and $C\varepsilon$ (Figure 1). Such circular DNA was not detected when spleen cells were cultured with LPS alone. Further, no ε circles were identified for the switch from $C\mu$ to $C\varepsilon$. Thus, in the IL-4-mediated class switch, switch recombination appears to occur in a successive manner, first from $C\mu$ to $C\gamma1$ and then from $C\gamma1$ to $C\varepsilon$. Detection of switch circular DNAs supports the notion that IL-4 triggers the switch recombination rather than selects the preswitched cells for ε. Indeed, IL-4 induces germ-line ε chain transcription in normal B cells (Geronclakis, 1990); however, IL-4 alone is not sufficient for the formation of switch circular DNA. More recently, similar findings were obtained in human lymphocyte systems. Induction of ε switching occurs through a recombination deletion event. In the human system, however, switching might occur in successive steps from IgM to IgG4 and IgG4 to IgE (Gascan *et al.*, 1991). Not only IL-4 but also T cell–B cell interaction is required for switching (Vercelli *et al.*, 1987). The relative contributions of IL-4 and $CD4^+$ T cells to the switching remain to be determined. However, direct T cell–B cell interactions were reported to provide the first signal, which is required for initiating B cells to respond to IL-4, and IL-4 was reported to direct switching to IgG4 and IgE (Vercelli *et al.*, 1989).

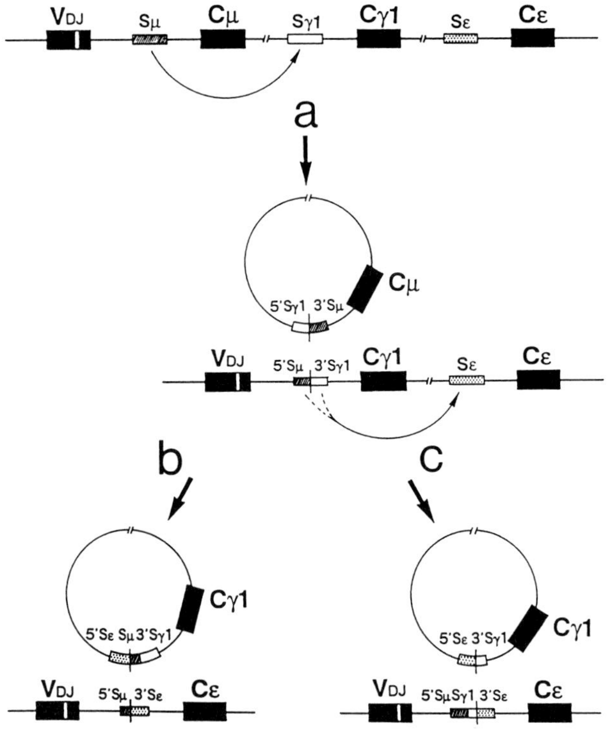

Figure 1 Successive switch recombination from μ to $\gamma1$ (a), and then from $\gamma1$ to ε (b or c). Two kinds of switch circular DNAs are detected; one is from the recombination between $C\mu$ and $C\gamma1$; the other is between $C\gamma1$ and $C\varepsilon$. In some ε switch circles (b), $S\mu$ sequence is inserted between $S\varepsilon$ and $S\gamma1$, indicating that the $S\mu$ sequences in the $\gamma1$ gene were used for recombination with $S\varepsilon$. In the other ε circle, no $S\mu$ sequence was retained on the excision product (c). Reprinted with permission from Yoshida *et al.* (1990).

C. Suppression of IgE Synthesis by Antagonists to IL-4

The effect of IL-4 on B cells has been shown to be counteracted by interferon γ (IFNγ). This cytokine inhibits not only the IL-4-induced increase in Ia expression and FcεRII expression on resting B cells, but also the formation of IgE and IgG1 by B cells stimulated with LPS plus IL-4 (Coffman and Carty, 1986). The IL-4-induced formation of IgE by human PBMC also was inhibited by IFNγ or IFNα (Pene *et al.*, 1988). These findings suggest that the proportion among various cytokines in the environment of B cells may affect the distribution of antibodies among various isotypes.

As expected, *in vitro* IgE synthesis by murine B cells stimulated by IL-4 and LPS could be inhibited by monoclonal anti-IL-4. Suppressive effects of the monoclonal antibody or IFNγ suggested the possibility that anti-IL-4 or IFNγ might be effective in suppressing *in vivo* IgE synthesis. Indeed, an intraperitoneal injection of 20 mg monoclonal anti-IL-4 into BALB/c mice resulted in suppression of IgE synthesis induced by infection of *Nippostrongylus brasiliensis* (Finkelman *et al.,* 1986). Similarly, an intravenous iv injection of anti-IL-4 suppressed the secondary IgE antibody response of mice to a protein antigen as well as the on-going IgE antibody formation. The results support the concept that IL-4 is required for the IgE antibody response. However, that an injection of 1–2 mg anti-IL-4 into mice failed to affect the IgE synthesis is rather surprising. Results of an attempt to suppress *in vivo* IgE synthesis with IFNγ were also discouraging. In the experiment carried out by Finkelman *et al.* (1988), enhanced IgE and IgG1 formation was induced by injecting goat antimouse IgD antibodies; the anti-IgD-treated mice received intraperitoneal injections of 12,500–50,000 u IFNγ twice daily for 3 days. The results showed that the treatment with 25,000 u or more of IFNγ per injection reduced both IgE and IgG1 levels to one-fifth to one-tenth; however, 6250 u of IFNγ per injection did not have a significant effect on IgE and IgG1 synthesis. The quantities of IFNγ required to regulate the IgE synthesis appear to be too much for clinical purposes. Indeed, clinical application of IFNγ for the treatment of hay fever was unsuccessful. Li *et al.* (1990) injected up to 0.2 mg recombinant IFNγ 3 times a week to rhinitis patients who were allergic to ragweed. After 4 weeks of treatment, however, no effect was observed in weekly symptom score or serum IgE antibody titer. Another course of the same treatment was given to the same patients prior to ragweed season; however, the treatment gave no significant effect on the IgE antibody titer and failed to suppress the secondary IgE antibody response observed after the ragweed season.

D. Requirement of IL-4-Producing Helper T cells for IgE Synthesis

As described earlier, the persistent IgE antibody response is obtained only when high responder mice were immunized with a minute dose of a potent immunogen. Since this dose of antigen with antigen-presenting cells is not sufficient to stimulate helper T cells for IL-4 or Il-2 production, one may speculate that differentiation of B cells to IgE-forming plasma cells is triggered by cognate interaction between antigen-specific helper T cells and B cells rather than by bystander effects of IL-4. If cognate interaction is the mechanism, anti-IL-4 or IFNγ has much less chance of preventing the effect of helper T cells.

Mosmann *et al.* (1986) described that mouse helper T-cell clones can be classified into two subtypes, Th1 and Th2, that produce different interleukins on antigenic stimulation. Both subtypes express Lyt 1 and L3T4; however, Th1 produces IL-2, IFNγ, and lymphotoxin whereas Th2 produces IL-4 and IL-5. Coffman *et al.* (1988) found that both Th1 and Th2 clones can provide help to B cells under appropriate conditions; however, important differences are seen in the Ig isotypes produced by B cells in response to the different T-cell subsets. These investigators employed rabbit IgG-specific helper T-cell clones, and induced polyclonal activation of normal B cells by coculture of the B cells and the Th clone with rabbit antimouse Ig antibodies. As shown in Table I, these researchers found that the Th2 clone gave much better help than the Th1 clone for the production of Ig. The major Ig produced by the B cells with the Th2 clone were IgM and IgG1, but a substantial quantity of IgE also was produced in the culture. In contrast, the same B cells failed to form IgE when they were cultured with the Th1 clone. Since IFNγ suppresses Ig formation, these investigators added anti-IFNγ antibody and supplemented the Th1 system with IL-2. Under these conditions, substantial amounts of IgM, IgG1, and IgG2a were produced, but IgE was not detected in the culture supernatant (c.f. Table I). However, the addition of IL-4 to the Th1 system resulted in the formation of IgE. These results show that Th2 cells, which form IL-4, are essential for IgE synthesis. Accumulated evidence suggests that the Th1 and Th2 subsets do not represent distinct lineages, and a single helper T cell can develop into either Th1 or Th2 (Swain *et al.,* 1990). For example, Gajewski *et al.* (1989) have shown that Th1 clones developed when antigen-primed lymph node cells were activated by antigen and then propagated in the presence of IFNγ, whereas propagation of the same antigen-activated lymph node cells by recombinant IL-2 alone resulted in preferential development of Th2 clones. Also, the presence of IL-4 during the propagation of antigen-activated cells facilitated the development of Th2 clones (Fernandez-Botran *et al.,* 1988).

Table I Isotype Distribution of Polyclonal Response of Normal B Cells to RGG-Specific Helper T Cell Clones[a]

Isotype	Th2 (ng/ml)	Th1 (ng/ml)	Th1 +IL-2 + anti-IFNγ (ng/ml)
IgM	98,000	248	65,000
IgE	187	<1	<1
IgA	487	<1	825
IgG_1	21,600	<8	5280
IgG_{2a}	39	14	2760
IgG_{2b}	189	<8	135
IgG_3	354	<8	474

[a] Reprinted with permission from Coffman *et al.* (1988).

In contrast to the murine system, human helper T-cell clones cannot be classified into Th1 and Th2 subtypes (Paliard *et al.,* 1988). Some helper cell clones form IL-2, IL-4, and IFNγ. Romagnani *et al.* (1989) reported that the frequency of IL-4-producing Th clones is higher in atopic patients than in nonatopic individuals. More recently, however, the same investigators found that the frequency of IL-4-producing Th clones also depends on the immunogen (Parronchi *et al.,* 1991). These investigators have isolated Th clones specific for allergen, and those specific for the other immunogens such as tetanus toxoid or purified protein derivative (PPD) of tubercle bacilli, from peripheral blood of the same atopic patients and have examined profiles of interleukin production by each clone. The researchers found that the majority of Th clones specific for allergen produced IL-4 alone or IL-4 with a limited amount of IFNγ, whereas essentially all T-cell clones specific for bacterial antigen produced both IL-4 and IFNγ. When the T-cell clones were cultured with autologous B cells and respective antigen, IgE synthesis was observed only with Th clones that can produce IL-4 alone or IL-4 with a limited amount of IFNγ. The reasons for the differences in the profiles of interleukin production among allergen-specific Th cells and bacterial antigen-specific Th cells are not known. However, the results indicate that repeated natural exposures to an allergen provide favorable conditions for the development of Th2-like helper cells or that mucosal tissues provide a favorable environment for the development of IL-4-producing helper T cells (see Chapters 19 and 20).

III. IgE-MEDIATED ALLERGIC REACTIONS

A. Structural Basis of Sensitization of Mast Cells with IgE Antibodies

The most important immunological property of IgE antibody is the ability to sensitize homologous tissues for reaginic hypersensitivity reactions. This ability is a common property for IgE for all mammalian species in which this immunoglobulin isotype has been described. Sensitization of homologous tissues with IgE is the result of its binding to mast cells and basophils. Indeed, IgE binds to normal basophils and mast cells with high affinity. As shown in Table II, the number of receptors (FcεRI) per mast cell and basophil granulocyte is 2–3 × 10^5 per cell. The forward rate constant (k_1) and dissociation constant (k_{-1}) for the binding of IgE to the receptors are on the order of 1–2 × 10^5 M^{-1} sec^{-1} and 2–10 × 10^{-5} sec^{-1}, respectively. Thus, the equilibrium constant (K_A) between IgE and the receptors is on the order of 10^9 to 10^{10} M^{-1} (Ishizaka, 1985). As shown in Table II, these values are comparable for human and rodent IgE. It is well known that an optimal latent period for skin sensitization by IgE antibodies is 1 to 3 days and that the sensitization with IgE antibodies persists for a long period of time. High affinity of IgE for FcεRI and a low dissociation constant between IgE and the receptors on mast cells explains why a minute dose of IgE antibodies can sensitize homologous tissues and why the sensitization with the antibodies is so persistent.

IgE binds to mast cells and basophils through the Fc portion of the molecule. The affinity of the Fc fragments of E myeloma protein for FcεRI was comparable to that of native IgE molecules. Application of recombinant gene technology led to cloning of the human ε chain gene. Recombinant Fcε chain fragments blocked passive sensitization of human skin to Prausnitz–Küstner reactions and could sensitize cultured human basophils for anti-IgE-induced histamine release (Ishizaka *et al.*, 1986). Indeed, recombinant Fcε peptide, in the dimeric form, and native IgE had comparable affinity for FcεRI on human basophils.

Helm *et al.* (1988,1989) prepared a series of overlapping recombinant Fcε gene products that represent smaller fragments of Fcε and found that the peptide representing amino acid sequence 301–376 in the ε chain could block the *in vivo* passive sensitization of human skin mast cells and the *in vitro* sensitization of human basophils with human IgE antibodies (c.f. Figure 2). However, approximately 10-fold higher molar concentrations of the recombinant peptide than E myeloma protein were required for 50% inhibition of Prausnitz–Küstner reaction or histamine release (Helm *et al.*, 1989). Thus, the recombinant peptides that represent the C-terminal 30 amino acids of Cε2 and the N-terminal half (46 amino acids) of the Cε3 domain appear to contain the structures involved in the binding of IgE to FcεRI.

The precise regions involved in the binding of FcεRI were identified by expressing chimeric ε heavy-chain genes composed of a mouse Vh domain and human Cε in which various domains were replaced by their murine counterparts. This approach was based on the fact that human IgE binds to FcεRI on human mast cells but not to FcεRI on mouse mast cells, whereas mouse IgE can bind to FcεRI on mast cells from both species (Conrad *et al.*, 1983). Nissin *et al.* (1991) found that all the chimeric IgE molecules that contain the murine Cε3 domain bound equally to both the rodent and the human FcεRI, whereas replacement of the mouse second constant region domain (Cε2) with human Cε2 did not affect the binding capacity of the mutated IgE to murine mast cells nor its ability to mediate degranulation. These findings show

Table II Affinity of IgE for IgE Receptors on Mast Cells and Basophils of Homologous Species

Cells	Number of receptors/cells ($\times 10^{-5}$)	k_1 ($\times 10^{-5}$ M^{-1} sec^{-1})	k_{-1} ($\times 10^5$ sec^{-1})	K_A ($\times 10^{-9}$ M^{-1})
Rat basophilic leukemia cells	3.55 ± 0.67	149 ± 0.19	1.85 ± 0.07	7.84
Normal rat mast cells	3.08 + 0.49	1.65 ± 0.42	2.05 ± 0.21	8.05
Normal mouse mast cells[a]	2.30 + 0.59 (3.21 + 0.73)	1.94 + 0.16 (2.23)	11.07 + 0.23 (6.24)	1.75 (3.57)
Cultured human basophils	3.06 + 0.28	1.88 + 0.32	9.94 + 0.36	2.75

[a] Peritoneal mast cells from BALB/c mice; numbers in parentheses are obtained with mast cells form CBA mice.

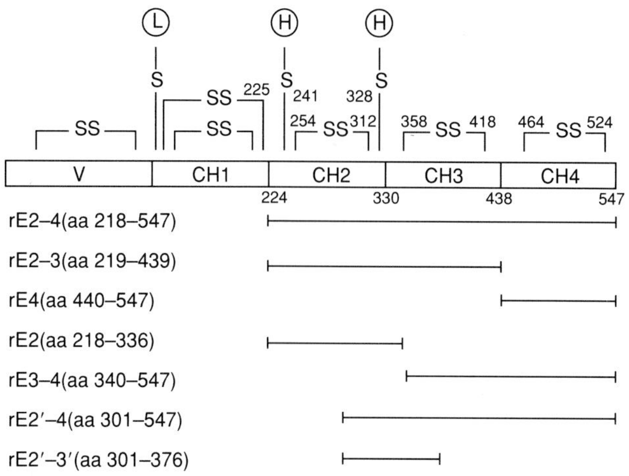

Figure 2 ε chain fragments having affinity for FcεRI. (*Top*) Covalent structure of the human ε chain, indicating the positions of the intra-chain disulfide bonds (SS), the interheavy (S-H) and heavy–light (S-L) chain disulfide bonds, and the boundaries of the five structural domains, that is, variable (v) and constant (c) regions. (*Bottom*) Peptides synthesized by *E. coli* expression of gene fragments encoding the indicated protein sequences. Among the peptides rE 2-4, rE 2-3, rE 2′-4, and rE 2′-3′ could block passive sensitization of human skin with IgE antibodies. Reprinted with permission from Helm *et al.* (1988).

that the Cε3 domain is involved in the binding of FcεRI. The C-terminal half of the Cε2 domain, which is essential for peptide 301–376 to bind to FcεRI, appears to play an important role in the stabilization of the conformation of the binding site.

The FcεRI on rodent mast cells consist of three different polypeptide chains that is, α, β, and γ; the gene encoding each polypeptide chain was cloned (Kinet *et al.*, 1987,1988; Blank *et al.*, 1989). The binding site for IgE is known to be present on the α chain; however, precise structures involved in the high affinity binding are not known.

B. Immunological and Biochemical Mechanisms for Mediator Release

Mast cells and basophils are triggered for mediator release when cell-bound IgE antibody molecules are cross-linked by multivalent antigen. Experiments have shown that direct cross-linking of FcεRI by divalent antireceptor antibodies resulted in the release of mediators and degranulation (Ishizaka and Ishizaka, 1978). In this artificial system, IgE is not involved in triggering mediator release. Under physiological conditions, however, IgE antibodies are anchored to FcεRI. Thus, cross-linking of IgE by multivalent antigen mediates the bridging of receptor molecules, which in turn triggers activation of mast cells. FcεRI is suspected to be one of the few membrane components through which mediator release can be triggered. Since no immunoglobulin other than IgE will bind to FcεRI with high affinity, triggering of mediator release through FcεRI can be mediated only by IgE antibodies.

Cross-linking of cell-bound IgE on FcεRI on mast cells results in activation of various membrane-associated enzymes, which leads to the release of vasoactive amines such as histamine and derivatives of arachidonic acid (c.f. Figure 3). The major biochemical pathway for mediator release is not known. However, researchers generally believe that the activation of phospholipase C (PLC) may play a key role in the early stage of the biochemical process for mediator release. The activation of this enzyme results in the cleavage of phosphatidylinositol 4,5-diphosphate to form inositol 1,4,5-triphosphate (IP_3) and diacylglycerol (DAG). IP_3 in turn induces intracellular mobilization of Ca^{2+} from endoplasmic reticulum, whereas DAG activates protein kinase C. An increase in intracellular Ca^{2+} in mast cells is well known to result in histamine release.

Phospholipase A_2 in mast cells is activated by cross-linking of FcεRI. This enzyme is involved in the release of both histamine and arachidonate (Nakamura *et al.*, 1991). Particularly, this enzyme appears to be important for the formation of arachidonic acid, which would be the source of prostaglandins and leukotrienes. Arachidonic acid could be formed by hydrolysis of DAG by DAG lipase and of monoacylglycerol by MAG lipase (c.f. Figure 3). However, experiments on bone marrow-derived murine mast cells indicated that the major pathway for the formation of arachidonate is hydrolysis of phospholipids by phospholipase A_2 (PLA_2) (Nakamura *et al.*, 1991).

Arachidonic acid is converted to prostaglandins through cyclooxygenase pathways and to leukotrienes through lipoxygenase pathways (Holgate *et al.*, 1988). PLA_2 also may be involved in the formation of platelet activating factor (PAF). These derivatives appear to be involved in causing immediate allergic reactions and participate in inducing allergic inflammation.

In addition to histamine and vasoactive amines described earlier, mast cells release several chemotatic factors and granule-associated proteolytic enzymes. Further, studies indicate that cross-linking of cell-bound IgE on mouse mast cells by multivalent antigen induces synthesis and release of various interleukins such as IL-1, IL-3, IL-4, IL-6, granulocyte–macrophage colchy stimulating factor (GM-CSF), and tumernecrosis factor (TNFα) (Burd *et al.*, 1989; Gurish *et al.*, 1991). IgE-dependent stimulation of IL-3-dependent mouse mast cell lines resulted in the formation of IL-3, IL-4, IL-5, and IL-6 (Plaut *et al.*, 1989). These findings suggest that the cytokines may be involved in causing allergic inflammation. Several lines of evidence have been accumulated that TNFα from mast cells recruits leukocytes and contributes to IgE-dependent inflammation. An important question that remains to be answered is whether cross-linking of FcεRI on human mast cells may induce the formation of such cytokines. If this is the case, cytokines such as TFNα from lung mast cells may contribute to late phase reactions expressed in human lung.

C. Role of IgE Antibodies in Allergic Disease and Mucosal Immunity

Allergic rhinitis or pollinosis is well established to be caused by IgE antibodies to which the patients are sensitive.

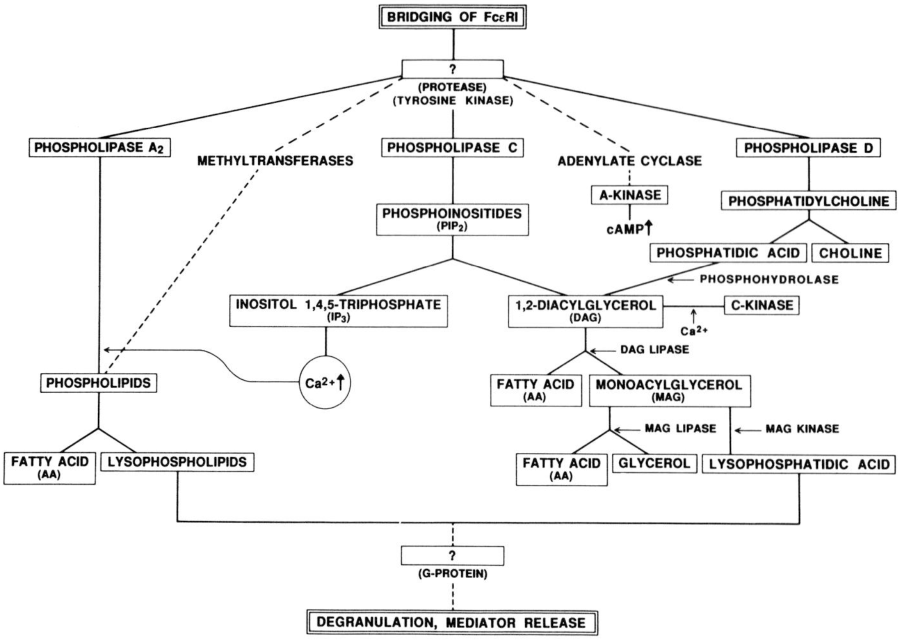

Figure 3 Schematic model of biochemical events in mast cells induced by cross-linking of cell-bound IgE antibodies by multivalent antigen. How triggering signals from FcεRI are transmitted to enzymes such as phospholipase C and phospholipase A_2 is not known but possible participation of protein tyrosine kinase or GTP-binding protein is predicted. An increase in intracellular Ca^{2+} is sufficient to induce mediator release. Under physiological conditions, both mobilization of intracellular Ca^{2+} and Ca^{2+} influx contribute to the increase in intracellular Ca^{2+}.

In allergic patients who have not received immunotherapy, a statistical correlation is seen between the concentration of IgE antibodies in the serum and their symptom score during the season (Lichtenstein *et al.,* 1973). Many of their symptoms can be explained by the release of vasoactive amines from mast cells, which cause an increase in vascular permeability and contraction of smooth muscles. On the other hand, asthma represents an inflammatory disease of the bronchi and has not been considered an IgE-mediated allergic disease. However, in extrinsic asthma, inhaling allergen can induce both immediate (20 min) and late phase (4–12 hr) increase in airway resistance. Inhaling allergen also can produce a prolonged increase in nonspecific bronchial reactivity, one of the characteristic symptoms in asthma. The immediate response is caused by IgE-dependent mediator release from mast cells whereas late phase response is caused by inflammation. Dolovich *et al.* (1973) demonstrated that allergic inflammation in human skin can be induced by anti-IgE, suggesting that the inflammation was the consequence of mediator release from mast cells that was induced by allergen–IgE antibody reactions at the early stage. Proving a casual relationship between chronic (not seasonal) exposure to an allergen such as dermatophagoides and a chronic disease such as asthma is very difficult. However, evidence has been presented that IgE antibodies to dust mite, cat, and cockroach allergens are each significantly correlated with asthma (Pollart *et al.,* 1989). Thus, epidemiolgical studies indicate that IgE antibodies against allergens play an essential role not only in hay fever but also in chronic asthma.

Accumulated evidence indicates that IgE antibodies play an important role in immunity against some parasites (Capron *et al.,* 1987). Another possible role of IgE antibodies would be increasing vascular permeability, resulting in an increase in local concentration of antibodies of the other isotypes (Steinberg *et al.,* 1974). Since IgE-mediated reaction occurs immediately after antigen exposure. IgG antibodies accumulated into the site effectively participate in immunity. Mucosal tissues are rich in mast cells, which should have been sensitized with IgE antibodies formed in mucosal lymphoid tissues. One may expect that the role IgE antibodies play as "gate keepers" may be important in local immunity in mucosal tissues.

References

Blank, U., Ra, C., Miller, L., White, K., Metzger, H., and Kinet, J-P. (1989) Complete structure and expression in transfected cells of high affinity IgE receptor. *Nature* (*London*) **337,** 187–189.

Burd, P. R., Rogers, H. W., Gordon, J. R., Martin, C. A., Jayaraman, S., Wilson, S. D., Dvorak, A. M., Galli, S. J., and Dorf, M. E. (1989). Interleukin 3-dependent and independent mast cells stimulated with IgE and antigen express multiple cytokines. *J. Exp. Med.* **170,** 245–257.

Capron, A., Dessaiut, J. P., Capron, M., Ouma, J. H., and Butterworth, A. (1987). Immunity to schistosomes; Progress toward vaccine. *Science* **238,** 1065–1072.

Coffman, R. L., and Carty, J. (1986). A T cell activity that enhances polyclonal IgE production and its inhibition by interferon γ. *J. Immunol.* **136,** 949–954.

Coffman, T., Ohara, J., Bond, M., Carty, J., Zlotnik, A., and Paul, W. E. (1986). B cell stimulatory factor-1 enhances the IgE response of lipopolysaccharide activated B cells. *J. Immunol.* **136,** 4538–4541.

Coffman, R. L., Seymour, B. W. P., Liebman, D. A., Hitaki, D. D., Christensen, J. A., Shrader, B., Cherwinski, H. M., Savelkaul, H. F., Finkelman, F. D., Bond, M. W., and Mosmann, T. T. (1988). The role of helper T cell products in mouse B cell differentiation and isotype regulation. *Immunol. Rev.* **102,** 5–28.

Conrad, D. H., Wingard, J. R., and Ishizaka, T. (1983). The interaction of human and rodent IgE with the human basophil IgE receptor. *J. Immunol.* **130,** 327–333.

Dolovich, J., Hargreave, F. E., Chalmers, R., Shire, K. J., Gouldie, J., and Bienenstock, J. (1973). Late cutaneous allergic response in isolated IgE-dependent reaction. *J. Allergy Clin. Immunol.* **52,** 38–46.

Fernandez-Botran, R., Sanders, V. M., Mosmann, T. R., and Vitella, E. S. (1988). Lymphokine-mediated regulation of the proliferative response of clones of T helper 1 and T helper 2 cells. *J. Exp. Med.* **168,** 543–558.

Finkelman, F. D., Katona, I. M., Urban, J. F., Jr., Snapper, G. M., Ohara, J., and Paul, W. E. (1986). Suppression of *in vivo* polyclonal IgE responses by monoclonal antibody to the lymphokine, BSF1. *Proc. Natl. Acad. Sci. U.S.A.* **83,** 9675–9678.

Finkelman, F. D., Katona, I. M., Mossman, T. R., and Coffman, R. L. (1988). IFNγ regulates the isotypes of Ig secreted during *in vivo* humoral immune response. *J. Immunol.* **140,** 1022–1027.

Gajewski, T. F., Joyce, J., and Fitch, F. W. (1989). Antiproliferative effect of IFNγ in immune regulation. III. Differential selection of TH1 and TH2 murine helper T lymphocyte cones using recombinant IL-2 and recombinant IFNγ. *J. Immunol.* **143,** 15–22.

Gascan, Gauchat, J.-F., Rocarolo, M. G., Yssel, H., Spits, H., and deVries, J. E. (1991). Human B cell clones can be induced to proliferate and to switch to IgE and IgG4 synthesis by interleukin 4 and a signal provided by activated $CD4^+$ T cell clones. *J. Exp. Med.* **173,** 747–750.

Gerondakis, S. (1990). Structure and expression of murine germ-line immunoglobulin ε heavy chain transcripts induced by interleukin 4. *Proc. Natl. Acad. Sci. U.S.A.* **83,** 1581–1585.

Gurish, M. F., Ghildyal, N., Arm, J., Austen, K. F., Avraham, S., Reynolds, D., and Stevens, R. L. (1991). Cytokine mRNA are preferentially increased relative to secretary granule protein mRNA in mouse bone marrow-derived mast cells that have undergone IgE-mediated activation and degranulation. *J. Immunol.* **146,** 1527–1533.

Helm, B., Marsh, P., Vercelli, D., Padlan, E., Gould, H., and Geha, R. (1988). The mast cell binding site on human immunoglobulin E. *Nature* (*London*) **331,** 180–183.

Helm, B., Kebo, D., Vercelli, D., Glovsky, M. M., Gould, H., Ishizaka, K., Geha, R., and Ishizaka, T. (1989). Blocking of passive sensitization of human mast cells and basophils granulocytes with IgE antibodies by a recombinant human ε chain fragment of 76 amino acids. *Proc. Natl. Acad. Sci. U.S.A.* **86,** 9465–9469.

Holgate, S. T., Robinson, C., and Church, M. K. (1988). Mediator of immediate hypersensitivity. *In* "Allergy, Principles and Practice" (E. Middleton, C. E. Reed, E. F. Ellis, N. F. Adkinson, and J. W. Yunginger, eds.), Vol. 1, pp. 235–263. Mosby, St. Louis, Missouri.

Ishizaka, K. (1976). Cellular event in the IgE antibody response. *Adv. Immunol.* **23,** 1–75.

Ishizaka, K. (1985). Immunoglobulin E. *Meth. Enzymol.* **116,** 76–94.

Ishizaka, T., and Ishizaka, K. (1978). Triggering of histamine release from rat mast cells by divalent antibodies against IgE receptors. *J. Immunol.* **120,** 800–805.

Ishizaka, T., Helm, B., Hakimi, J., Niebyl, J., and Ishizaka, K. (1986). Biological properties of a recombinant human immunoglobulin ε chain fragment. *Proc. Natl. Acad. Sci. U.S.A.* **83,** 8323–8327.

Kinet, J-P, Metzger, H., Hakimi, J., and Kochan, J. (1987). A cDNA presumptively coding for the α subunit of the receptor with high affinity for immunoglobulin ε. *Biochemistry* **26,** 4605–4610.

Kinet, J.-P., Blank, U., Ra, C., White, K., Metzger, H., and Kochan, J. (1988). Isolation and characterization of cDNAs coding for the β subunit of the high affinity receptor for immunoglobulin E. *Proc. Natl. Acad. Sci. U.S.A.* **85,** 6483–6487.

Levine, B. B. (1971). Genetic factors in reagin production in mice. *In* "Biochemistry of the acute Allergic Reactions" (K. F. Austen and E. L. Becker eds.), pp. 1–11. Blackwell, Oxford.

Li, J. T. C., Yunginger, J. W., Reed, C. E., Jaffe, H. S., Nelson, D. R., and Gleich, G. L. (1990). Lack of suppression of IgE production by recombinant interferon gamma. A controlled trial in patients with allergic rhinitis. *J. Allergy Clin. Immunol.* **85,** 934–940.

Lichtenstein, L. M., Ishizaka, K., Norman, P. S., Sobotka, A. K., and Hill, B. M. (1973). IgE antibody measurement in ragweed hay fever. Relationship of clinical severity and the results of immunotherapy. *J. Clin. Invest.* **52,** 472–482.

Mossman, T. R. Cherwinki, H., Bond, M. W., Giedlin, M. A., and Coffman, R. L. (1986). Two type of murine helper T cell clone I. Definition according to profiles of lymphokine activities and secreted proteins. *J. Immunol.* **136,** 2348–2357.

Nakamura, T., Fonteh, A. N., Hubband, W. C., Triggiani, M., Inagaki, N., Ishizaka, T., and Chilton, F. H. (1991). Arachidonic acid metabolism during antigen and ionophore activation of the mouse bone marrow-derived mast cells. *Biochim. Biophys. Acta* **1085,** 191–200.

Newcomb, R. W., and Ishizaka, K. (1970). Physiocochemical and antigenic studies on human γE in respiratory fluid. *J. Immunol.* **105,** 85–89.

Nissin, A., Jouvin, M. H., and Eschar, Z. (1991). Mapping of the high affinity Fcε receptor binding site to the third constant region domain of IgE. *EMBO J.* **10,** 101–107.

Paliard, X., Malefijt, R. D., Yssel, H., Blauchard, D., Chreiten, I., Adams, J., deVries, J., and Spits, H. (1988). Simultaneous production of IL-2, IL-4 and IFNγ by activated human $CD4^+$ and $CD8^+$ T cell clones. *J. Immunol.* **141,** 849–855.

Parronchi, P., Tiri, A., Macchia, D., de Carli, M., Biswas, P., Simonelli, C., Maggi, E., Del Prete, G., Ricci, M., and Romagnani, S. (1990). Noncognate contact-dependent B cell activation can promote IL-4 dependent *in vitro* human IgE synthesis. *J. Immunol.* **144,** 2102–2108.

Parronchi, P., Macchia, D., Piccini, M-P, Blowas, P., Simonelli, C., Maggi, E., Ricci, M., Ansari, A. A., and Romagnani, S. (1991). Allergen and bacterial antigen-specific T cell clones established from atopic donors show a different profile of cytokine production. *Proc. Natl. Acad. Sci. U.S.A.* **88,** 4538–4542.

Pene, J., Rousset, F., Briere, F., Chretien, I., Bonnefoy, J. Y., Spits, H., Yokota, T., Arai, N., Arai, K., Banchereau, J., and deVries, J. E. (1988). IgE production by human B cells is induced by IL-4 and suppressed by interferons, γ, α and prostaglandin E2. *Proc. Natl. Acad. Sci. U.S.A.* **85,** 6880–6884.

Plaut, M., Pierce, J. H., Watson, C. J., Hanley-Hyde, J., Nordan, R. P., and Paul, W. E. (1989). Mast cell lines produce lymphokine in response to cross-linkage of FcεRI or to calcium ionophores. *Nature* (*London*) **339,** 64–67.

Pollart, S. M., Chapman, M. D., Fiocco, G. P., Rose, G., and Platts-Mills, T. A. E. (1989). Epidemiology of acute asthma: IgE antibodies to common inhalent allergens as a risk factor for emergency room visits. *J. Allergy Clin. Immunol.* **83,** 875–882.

Romagnani, S., Del Prete, G. F., Maggi, E., Parronchi, P., Tiri, A., Macchia, D., Guidizi, M. G., Almerigogna, F., and Ricci, M. (1989). Role of interleukins in induction and regulation of human IgE synthesis. *Clin. Immunol. Immunopathol.* **50,** 513–523.

Snapper, C. M., Finkelman, F. D., and Paul, W. E. (1988). Regulation of IgG1 and IgE production by interleukin 4. *Immunol. Rev.* **102,** 51–75.

Steinberg, P., Ishizaka, K., and Norman, P. S. (1974). Possible role of IgE-mediated reaction in immunity. *J. Allergy Clin. Immunol.* **54,** 359–366.

Swain, S. L., Weinberg, A. D., and English, M. (1990). $CD4^+$ T cell subsets. Lymphokine secretion of memory cells and of effector cells that develop from precursors in vitro. *J. Immunol.* **144,** 1788–1799.

Tada, T., and Ishizaka, K. (1970). Distribution of γE-forming cells in lymphoid tissues of the human and monkey. *J. Immunol.* **104,** 377–387.

Vercelli, D., Jabara, H. H., Arai, K., and Geha, R. S. (1989). Induction of human IgE synthesis requires interleukin 4 and T/B cell interactions involving the T cell receptor/CD3 complex and MHC. Class II antigens. *J. Exp. Med.* **169,** 1295–1307.

Yoshida, K., Matsuoka, M., Usuda, S., Mori, A., Ishizaka, K., and Sakano, H. (1990). Immunoglobulin switch circular DNA in the mouse infected with *Nippostrongylus brasiliensis:* Evidence for successive class switching from μ to ε via $\gamma 1$. *Proc. Natl. Acad. Sci. U.S.A.* **87,** 7829–7833.

26

Inflammation: Mast Cells

A. D. Befus

I. INTRODUCTION

One hallmark of the virtually ubiquitous mast cell is that it bears thousands of high affinity receptors for IgE. When IgE antibodies occupying these receptors are cross-linked by specific antigens, the cell is activated and releases, in an explosive or more slowly timed manner, a myriad of stored or newly synthesized inflammatory mediators. Such allergic reactions which may have both immediate and late phases are prominent at mucosal surfaces presumably because of the pronounced antigenic exposures at these sites and the positive, but poorly understood, relationship between IgE production and mucosal surfaces. In addition, the presence and abundance of mast cells at mucosal surfaces, at times in the epithelium but normally in the underlying lamina propria and associated musculature, contributes to hypersensitivity reactions at these sites.

However, not only the clinical significance of mast cells in mucosal allergic responses such as extrinsic asthma (see Chapter 44) and food allergies (see Chapter 40), but evidence that these cells are willing participants in normal physiological events and in many, if not most, non-IgE-mediated inflammatory reactions throughout the body has spawned extensive investigations. Moreover, in rodents and in humans, abundant evidence suggests that mast cell populations at mucosal surfaces can be distinguished by the high proportion of cells with a characteristic "mucosal" phenotype.

Although some of the information is sparse and often restricted to studies in only a single species or with *in vitro* approximations of *in vivo* populations, cells of this "mucosal" phenotype are distinct from mast cells elsewhere. They differ in their protein composition and arsenal of mediators, their discriminating responsiveness to certain secretagogues that activate mast cells from other, largely connective tissue sites, and their restricted responsiveness to the fleet of anti-allergic and anti-inflammatory drugs (see Befus, 1989).

This chapter provides a summary of the general properties of mast cells; their ontogeny, mediator repertoire, responsiveness to activating, and regulatory stimuli; and their spectrum of functions. However, a primary focus is on the distinctive qualities of mast cells at mucosal surfaces that may uncover functions specific to these locations. Given the breadth of this volume and the limitations that it poses on each chapter, readers who seek more extensive information are referred to several reviews of mast cells and their heterogeneity and function (Bienenstock, 1988; Befus, 1989; Benyon *et al.*, 1989; Galli, 1990; Gordon *et al.*, 1990; Schwartz, 1990; Miller, 1992).

II. STRATEGIES TO EXPLORE MAST CELL HETEROGENEITY AND FUNCTION

In 1966, Enerback clarified some confusing literature and established that mast cell populations in the gastrointestinal tract of the rat were morphologically, histochemically, and functionally distinct from more widely studied mast cells in the peritoneal cavity and connective tissues (see Enerback, 1987; Galli, 1990). These two cell populations have become known as intestinal mucosal mast cells (IMMC) and connective tissue mast cells (CTMC), of which the peritoneal mast cell (PMC) has been studied most widely because of the ease of its isolation and purification. Numerous reviews are available of the details of the distinctions between these two mast cell types, so this information will not be repeated in a comprehensive manner. However, a brief description of the evolution of the field may help the reader place specific information in the appropriate context.

In mice, the dramatic increase in the numbers of IMMCs that follows intestinal helminth infection is dependent on an intact thymus. In contrast, in many situations increases in the numbers of CTMCs are not thymus dependent. This thymus dependency of intestinal mastocytosis is based on the requirement for interleukin 3 (IL-3); repetitive administration of IL-3 reconstitutes the ability of athymic mice to express hyperplasia of IMMCs (Abe and Nawa, 1988). However, this explanation may be an oversimplification since other T cell-derived cytokines, including IL-4 (see Galli, 1990) and IL-10 (Thompson-Snipes *et al.*, 1991), are also cofactors for mast cell development.

To characterize IMMCs more fully and compare them with CTMCs, structural, histochemical, and immunohistochemical analyses have been conducted on the cells *in situ*. For example, characteristics of their proteoglycan content and expression of certain serine proteases have been evaluated with such approaches. In addition, procedures were developed to disperse mast cells from the intestine and other tissues enzymatically and mechanically. Mast cell-specific components were studied in such cell mixtures and strategies were developed to enrich and purify the cells or some of their components for further analyses.

In the rat, purifying PMCs and IMMCs from their respective sources is possible but, in the mouse, although PMCs can be purified, the isolation and purification of IMMCs has been an insurmountable challenge. Similarly, mast cells from the human intestine have been impossible to purify, although dispersed mixtures of intestinal cells containing up to 30% mast cells have been studied (Befus *et al.*, 1987). These dispersed cell populations from the human intestine, and from lung as well (Schulman, 1990), contain two distinct populations of mast cells, histochemically analogous to PMCs and IMMCs of rats. These and other histochemical studies of mast cells from human tissues (e.g., Enerback, 1987) have established that these two histochemically distinct populations are found in virtually all sites investigated to date, although their relative abundance varies. Whether these populations are functionally distinct as in the rat remains to be confirmed. Schwartz and colleagues provided compelling evidence that the cell populations differ in protease content; the cell type histochemically analogous to the PMC expresses both chymase and tryptase (MC^{TC}) in considerable abundance, whereas the IMMC-like mast cell expresses only tryptase (MC^{T}) in abundance (Irani *et al.*, 1986).

In vitro culture also has been a powerful tool with which to investigate mast cells and their phenotypic heterogeneity. Since the original observations by several investigators of mast cell development and persistence in IL-3-containing cultures of murine bone marrow or lymphoid tissues, such systems have been employed to investigate mast cell ontogeny and phenotype. Much has been learned from these cultures. The development of clonal populations or populations "frozen" in a particular phenotype by viral transformation (Reynolds *et al.*, 1988) has aided greatly in dissecting very complicated issues of phenotypic diversity. Galli (1990) identified the benefits of these approaches and appropriately expressed caution about the relationship of these cultured cells to *in vivo* populations or to their development.

The bases for mast cell heterogeneity are complex (e.g., Befus, 1989; Kitamura, 1989) and have been expressed thoughtfully by Galli (1990). Although two easily distinguished populations (CTMC and IMMC) can be identified in rodents, whether or not these are the only two populations distinct in so many ways is unclear. Other equally distinct populations may exist in different tissues or in other species, or perhaps only minor variations of these two themes exist. As new information has been uncovered, mast cell populations from various sources have been shown to differ in a number of characteristics. However, the information is not of sufficient quantity or clarity to allow useful definition of cell subsets beyond their location, perhaps because the bases for heterogeneity are diverse and may include distinct mast cell lineages (irreversible commitment to a particular phenotype at some phase in development), processes of cell maturation and differentiation in response to selected microenvironmental stimuli, renewal after activation and mediator depletion or synthesis, and acquistion of components produced by other cell types (Galli, 1990).

In recent years, a powerful tool with which to study mast cell heterogeneity and function has been the use of mice of the W/W^{v} or Sl/Sl^{d} genotypes. Although both these strains of mice are congenitally mast cell deficient, the natures of their deficiencies are distinct. W/W^{v} mice are deficient in the stem cells of the mast cell lineage. Their mast cell deficiency can be reconstituted with normal bone marrow, and they are capable of producing mast cell growth factors. Sl/Sl^{d} mice have a deficit in the tissue microenvironment that induces mast cell development, but possess mast cell precursors. Kitamura and colleagues (Kitamura, 1989) used these mice to explore the defects and the ontogeny and function of mast cells. Alone and in collaboration with Kitamura, Galli and co-workers have defined these experimental approaches carefully and presented an algorithm for their use (Galli, 1990).

III. ONTOGENY

Mast cells can be detected in many tissues before birth, but their numbers are generally low (Watkins *et al.*, 1976). In sites such as the peritoneal cavity and intestine, mast cells do not approach normal adult levels until 2–3 months of age (Watkins *et al.*, 1976; Woodbury *et al.*, 1978). As indicated earlier, mastocytosis in selected tissues such as the intestine can occur in response to certain stimuli; in some cases, as in the intestinal mucosa in response to helminthic infection, this activation is thymus dependent, but in other cases it is not.

Mast cell precursors are derived from pleuripotent hemopoietic stem cells; in humans, these cells express CD34 (Kirshenbaum *et al.*, 1991). During their development, and under the influence of IL-3 and IgE, mast cell precursors become committed to the mast cell lineage that, in some tissues such as mesenteric lymph nodes of helminth-infected mice, can be identified as a mast cell committed precursor (MCCP) line by the ability to develop into granulated mast cells in fibroblast-conditioned medium and in the absence of exogenous IL-3 (perhaps an autocrine pathway of IL-3 production; Ashman *et al.*, 1991; Figure 1). This fibroblast-conditioned medium is a rich source of stem cell factor (SCF, c-*kit* ligand; Williams *et al.*, 1990), a multipotent growth factor with mast cell growth activity. W/W^{v} mice are deficient in MCCP but produce SCF, whereas Sl/Sl^{d} mice generate MCCP but are deficient in SCF (Jarboe and Huff, 1989).

Several environmental factors have the potential to impinge on this stem cell and committed precursor to facilitate differentiation and subsequent maturation. These factors include SCF (c-*kit* ligand; Tsai *et al.*, 1991), CD45 ligand (Broxmeyer *et al.*, 1991), IL-3 (Ashman *et al.*, 1991), IL-4 (Hamaguchi *et al.*, 1987), IL-10 (Thompson-Snipes *et al.*, 1991), and nerve growth factor (NGF; Matsuda *et al.*, 1991; Figure 1). Both IL-4 and NGF appear to facilitate development of CTMC-like MCs (Hamaguchi *et al.*, 1987; Matsuda *et al.*, 1991). To date, no information is available on the microenvironmental factors that selectively induce or enhance the development of IMMC-like MCs. Granulocyte–macrophage colony stimulating factor (GM-CSF) (Bressler *et al.*, 1989), interferon γ (IFNγ; Nafziger *et al.*, 1990), transforming growth factor β (TGF_{β}; Broide *et al.*, 1989), and even hista-

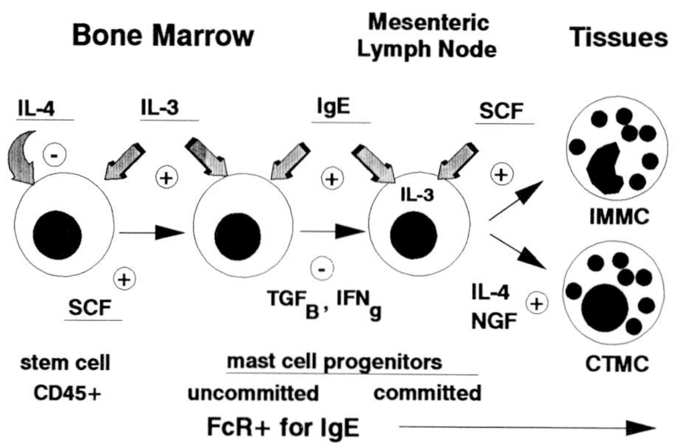

Figure 1 Factors that regulate the ontogeny of mast cells during the course of their development from stem cells to mature tissue-dwelling subpopulations (abbreviations in text).

mine (Schneider *et al.*, 1990) may down-regulate these developmental processes (Figure 1).

The commitment to CTMC or IMMC characteristics appears not to be irreversible, that is, the cells of one or the other phenotype are capable of changing into cells of the other phenotype, a process referred to by Kitamura and colleagues as transdifferentiation. The experimental approaches employed and evidence for this phenomenon have been reviewed by Kitamura (1989) and Galli (1990), although the extent to which transdifferentiation might occur *in vivo* and the signaling systems involved have not been explored.

IV. REPERTOIRE OF MEDIATORS

Mast cells throughout the body have the potential to produce a spectrum of powerful mediators (Table I), many of which are pro-inflammatory, especially when large quantities are released in an explosive manner. Some of the best known mediators are produced in advance, for example, histamine, proteases, and other enzymes, and are stored in cytoplasmic granules in association with the proteoglycan matrix. When the cell is activated, exocytosis of granule contents occurs, in turn initiating a complex of cascading events with short-term or more prolonged time courses. In addition, activation induces the synthesis of lipid and other mediators that are released immediately into the local milieu, including prostaglandins, leukotrienes, platelet activating factor-acether (PAF-acether), and nitric oxide (Table I).

Considerable excitement has surrounded observations that mast cells constitutively express certain cytokines (Table I) and, when activated, rapidly produce mRNA for an impressive array of cytokines. However, much of this information on cytokines has been established with cell lines, and some studies have been restricted to measuring mRNA rather than the protein products. Thus, the extent to which mast cells are an important source of cytokines *in vivo* requires considerable investigation. That rodent and human mast cells are a prominent source of the multifunctional mediator tumor necrosis factor α (TNFα; Bissonnette and Befus, 1990; Gor-

Table I Distribution of Mediators in Mast Cell Types[a]

	Cell type				
	Rodent			Human	
Mediator	CTMC	IMMC	BMMC	SKIN[b]	UC[b]
Preformed					
Amines					
Histamine	+	+	+	+	+
Serotonin	+	+	+	−?	−?
Chemotactic peptides					
ECF	+			+?	+?
NCF	+			+?	+?
Enzymes					
Chymase	RMCPI	RMCPII	+	+	−
Cathepsin G				+	−
Tryptase	+	+	+	+	+
Carboxypeptidase	+		+	+	+
Lysosomal	+	+?	+	+	+
Proteoglycans					
Heparin	+	−	−	+	
Chrondroitin sulfates					
diB		+			
E		+	+	−	+
Newly synthesized					
PAF	+	+	+	+	+
Nitric oxide	+	+			
Arachidonic acid metabolites					
PGD_2	+	+	+	+	+
LTB_4	−	+	+		
LTC_4 (and metabolites)	−	+	+	+	+
Cytokines					
TNFα (stored and newly made)	+	+	+	+ (little stored)	+
IL-1,3,4,6	+		+		
IL-10,IFNγ, etc.			+		
Acquired from other cells					
Eosinophil					
Peroxidase			+		
Major basic protein				+	

[a] Abbreviations: ECF/NCF, eosinophil/neutrophil chemotactic factors; RMCP, rat mast cell protease; PAF, platelet activating factor-acether; PGD_2 prostaglandin D_2; LT, leukotriene; TNF, tumor necrosis factor; IL, interleukin; IFNγ, gamma interferon.

[b] The evaluation of mediator distribution in human mast cells is based on the most abundant mast cell type in the named tissue, recognizing that histochemically and protease content-distinct populations are mixed in all tissues.

don and Galli, 1991; Benyon *et al.*, 1991a) and that important effects emanate from its release from mast cells (Klein *et al.*, 1989; Gordon and Galli, 1991) has been well established. However, factors other than IgE that dictate whether or not mast cells, macrophages, or other cells are the immediate source of TNFα in an inflammatory event remain to be clarified.

Unfortunately, given the heterogeneity of mast cells, the mosaic of information that one draws on to present a summary of their mediators (Table I) comes from studies with mast cells from different species and collected from different tissue sites by a profusion of techniques. Thus, one must be cautious when making generalizations and be careful to establish that the mediator repertoire of mast cells in a particular site does or does not follow closely the pattern of the "generalized" mast cell. Equal caution must be taken when discussing the functions of these mediators; some may have functions that can be generalized easily in different species or tissues, for example, well-known actions of histamine on the vasculature or the substrate specificities of selected enzymes. However, other mediators may express site-specific functions dictated by conditions in the local microenvironment. For example, the overall actions of histamine in a tissue may vary from those in another tissue or at another time in the same tissue. Such distinct responses could depend on the abundance and competence of selected cell populations designated to respond to this mediator, because of their expression of H1, H2, or H3 histamine receptors or because of alterations in the catabolism or activity of the mediator itself.

Finally, although in our efforts to understand cascading networks of biological responses we use reductionist approaches, mast cells release a spectrum of mediators at one time and no mediator can be viewed in isolation. Moreover, depending on the stimulus applied, mast cells may release mediators in a differential fashion. For example, histamine can be released in preference to 5-hydroxytryptamine (5HT) and vice versa by murine skin mast cells (e.g., Meade *et al.*, 1988). For human skin mast cells, although the magnitude of histamine release is similar with both secretagogues, an IgE-dependent stimulus releases 10- to 20-fold more prostaglandin D_2 (PGD_2) and leukotriene C_4 (LTC_4) than the neuropeptide substance P (see Benyon *et al.*, 1989). Few of these types of issues have been analyzed with the care needed to provide more than a "generalized" view of mast cells.

V. MODULATION OF MAST CELL FUNCTION

A. Activation

Until recently, studies of the factors that stimulate mast cells have focused largely on secretagogues for histamine or other mediators such as 5HT, arachidonic acid metabolities, proteases, or lysosomal enzymes. The list of such secretagogues is long (Figure 2), yet unlikely to be complete. For example, although rodent IMMCs are unique in many ways and one might speculate that they are responsive to signals specific for the intestinal or other mucosal environments, no secretagogues have been identified that stimulate IMMCs but fail to stimulate CTMCs. In contrast, numerous secretagogues such as certain neuropeptides and endorphins activate CTMCs but not IMMCs (e.g., Bienenstock, 1988).

In addition to the classical antigen-specific IgE-dependent sensitization of mast cells, antigen-specific sensitization has been attributed also to a T cell-derived factor not cross-reactive with IgE (e.g., Meade *et al.*, 1988). However, progress in the characterization of this factor has been slow and its potential relevance for mast cells other than in murine skin requires additional study. Other mast cell activating factors are not known to be linked to antigen in a specific manner, although after antigen challenge the cascade of events may lead to continued mast cell activation, perhaps in a mediator-specific fashion, insuring the continued participation of these cells in the ongoing immune and inflammatory responses.

For example, complement-derived anaphylatoxins, certain neuropeptides, endogenous opiates, rat mast cell protease I (RMCP I), or relatively poorly known factors from a variety of cell types collectively called HRFs (histamine releasing factors) may be important in different pathological states. HRFs include connective tissue activating peptide II (CTAP

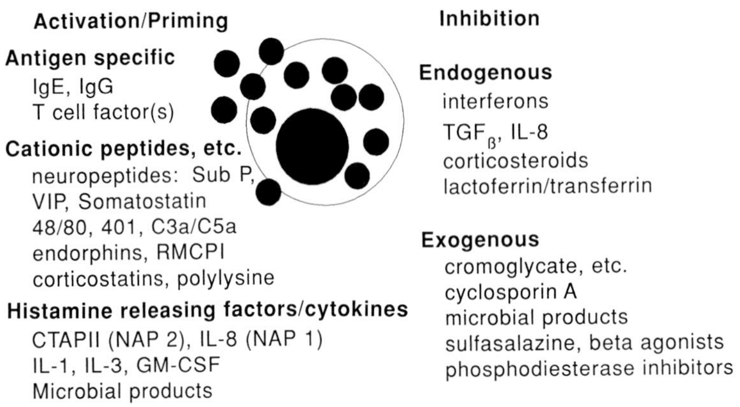

Figure 2 Factors that activate, prime or inhibit mast cell functions (abbreviations in text).

II), the closely related cleavage product, neutrophil-activating peptide (NAP 2) (Baeza *et al.*, 1990), or, in the hands of some authors, neutrophil activating peptide 1 (NAP 1) (Dahinden *et al.*, 1989), now recognized as IL-8. In addition to these HRFs, at least one other HRF activity with an apparent molecular mass of 40–41 kDa remains to be fully characterized (Baeza *et al.*, 1990). The elucidation of the different uses of and cascades of responses to these pathways of mast cell activation will contribute much to our understanding of the functions of these cells.

Perhaps more complex than the cytokine network in modulating mast cell function is the interaction between mast cells and the nervous system. The close anatomical association of mast cells and nerves in the mucosa (Stead *et al.*, 1987), the role of substance P and mast cell activation in wheal and flare reactions (see Stead *et al.*, 1990), the differential activation of mast cell subpopulations by neuropeptides and endorphins (e.g., Shanahan *et al.*, 1985), and even the classical Pavlovian conditioning of mast cell secretion (MacQueen *et al.*, 1989) disclose the breadth of the spectrum of nervous control of mast cell function. Moreover, this interaction is bidirectional; mast cell activation, in turn, regulates nervous system function through mediators such as PDG_2 (e.g., Undem and Weinreich, 1989).Given the elaborate, partially autonomous enteric nervous system, in studies of the physiology of the intestinal mucosa or other mucosal sites an understanding of normal mast cell–nerve interactions and of their alterations in inflammatory states clearly will be beneficial.

The intestinal mucosa may be a rich source of other factors that stimulate mast cell secretion, such as hitherto poorly studied endogenous components or exogenous factors derived from infectious agents or foodstuffs. For example, several studies have established that members of the defensin/corticostatin family of polypeptides derived from neutrophils and other cell types (Lehrer *et al.*, 1991) are potent stimulators of histamine secretion from mast cells (A. Bateman, C. Mowat, D. Befus, and S. Solomon, unpublished results). One member of this family, cryptdin, appears to be derived from Paneth cells in the intestinal crypt as well as from other intestinal leukocytes (e.g., Ouellette and Lualdi, 1990). Determining whether or not this member of the family has specificity for the activation of IMMCs or for differential mediator release, as opposed to other members of the family that might activate CTMCs, will be interesting.

A similar specificity of activation, differential mediator release, or inhibition may exist for other endogenous intestinal components or for toxins or other metabolic products of the intestinal flora. Lipophilic but not hydrophilic bile acids have been shown to induce cytotoxic release of histamine from CTMCs as well as from cultured mast cells with some properties of IMMCs (Quist *et al.*, 1991). Clearly evidence exists for activation (Konig *et al.*, 1989) and inhibition (Nakagomi *et al.*, 1990) of CTMCs by bacterial products, but to date no studies of differential activation, mediator secretion, or inhibition of IMMCs have been conducted. As such investigations are done in the near future, exploring markers of mast cell function other than simply histamine secretion will be important. For example, cytokine production, protein biosynthesis, and other metabolic activities associated with growth, differentiation, and maturation must become more widely used in assaying mast cell involvement in these and other physiological and pathophysiological pathways.

B. Inhibition

Although much effort has been invested in the search for drugs that inhibit the activation of mast cells (Figure 2) or antagonize selected mediators such as histamine or arachidonic acid metabolites, no fully satisfactory or specific drugs have been discovered. For a review of many drugs that inhibit the actions of mast cells, including corticosteroids, disodium cromoglycate, sulfasalazine, cyclosporin A, and antihistamines, see Benyon *et al.*, (1991b). Certain drugs appear to affect mast cells in multiple sites (e.g., corticosteroids), whereas others inhibit CTMCs but appear to be without effect on IMMCs in rodents (e.g., disodium cromoglycate). The actions of these drugs may be diverse, in part depending on site and duration of use. For example, the observations that dexamethasone appears to induce ingestion of IMMCs by macrophages (Soda *et al.*, 1991) requires careful investigation.

Unfortunately, the information from human mast cells is confusing because all populations of human mast cells are mixed (as discussed earlier). Whether or not a partial response to the drug (e.g., 30–70% inhibition) reflects a limited responsiveness by all cells in the mixed population or a marked response by some cells and no response by others is unclear.

In the future, more emphasis will be placed on studies of endogenous inhibitors of mast cell activation (Figure 2) and development. This area of research has been neglected to date, yet many pathways for the regulation of mast cell function must exist *in vivo*. For example, we have established that interferons inhibit histamine and TNFα release from CTMCs and IMMCs in rats (Bissonnette and Befus, 1990). We have shown that, after preincubation of rat CTMCs with TGFβ, the release of TNFα and histamine is inhibited (E.Y. Bissonnette and A. D. Befus, unpublished observations). Others have shown that IL-8 (Grant *et al.*, 1991) and lactoferrin (Theobald *et al.*, 1987) inhibit histamine secretion.

VI. PLETHORA OF FUNCTIONS

Given the tremendous spectrum of mediators stored and secreted by mast cells, or newly synthesized and released when the cell is activated, concisely listing the specific functions of the mast cell is difficult. In a broad biological sense, mast cells have been shown to be involved in responses ranging from elicitation of cardiopulmonary responses in anaphylaxis (Takeishi *et al.*, 1991), experimental allergic encephalomyelitis (Dietsch and Hinrichs, 1989), and host defenses (Matsuda *et al.*, 1987; Abe and Nawa, 1988) to immune complex- (Ramos *et al.*, 1990) and substance P-induced inflammation (Yano *et al.*, 1989). Accordingly, in this chapter a more generalized conceptualization of mast cell function will be outlined (Figure 3).

The targets of mediators secreted by mast cells may include almost any cell in the body: connective tissue cells, endothelium, epithelium, cells of the immune system, and cells of the nervous system, as well as smooth muscle. These targets may respond to interaction with mast cell mediators in a number of ways, including alterations in their survival; short term secretory, contractile, migratory, or other functional responses; competency, proliferation, differentiation, or maturation; and overall tissue or organ physiology or pathophysiology. Many of these responses are associated with inflammation, its associated tissue damage, and subsequent repair processes.

In addition to the knowledge of mast cell mediators that have been studied for many years, for example, histamine and certain arachidonic acid metabolites, priorities for investigation in the next few years will lie in evaluating the production and roles of mast cell-derived cytokines in inflammatory conditions of differing etiology. For example, when are mast cells a prominent source of TNFα (e.g., Gordon and Galli, 1991) in comparison with other cell sources of this potent cytokine? Another emphasis will be on elucidating the *in vivo* substrates and functional activities of the multiple serine and other proteases in the mast cell (Schwartz, 1990). For example, the catalytic site of mast cell tryptase appears to be critical in tryptase augmentation of histamine-induced smooth muscle contraction in dog bronchi (see Caughey, 1990), tryptase mitogenic activity for fibroblasts (Ruoss *et al.*, 1991), and degradation of bronchodilatory neuropeptides such as VIP (vasoactive intestinal polypeptide) and PHM (peptide histidine-methionine) (Caughey, 1990). Understanding the orchestration of release of proteases and their activities in inflammatory sites promises to clarify many aspects of mast cell function *in vivo*.

Postulating that this variety of functions of proteases and other mast cell-derived mediators is not restricted to pronounced inflammatory reactions, but is ongoing during the course of normal physiological homeostasis, albeit in subtle unobtrusive ways, is reasonable. Such subtle and ongoing mast cell function, perhaps driven by both the endocrine (Befus, 1990) and the nervous (Stead *et al.*, 1990) system, is likely to be difficult to measure, given our emphasis to date on assay systems in which explosive degranulation events have been evaluated. Innovative approaches are required to begin to address this hypothesis and to address specifically its implications in the context of the homeostasis of mucosal function in health and disease.

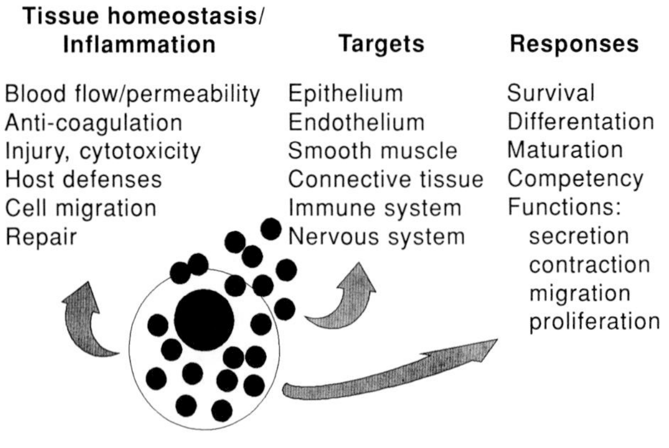

Figure 3 Physiology and pathophysiology of mast cell activation in the maintenance of tissue homeostasis.

References

Abe, T., and Nawa, Y. (1988). Worm expulsion and mucosal mast cell response induced by repetitive IL-3 administration in *Strongyloides ratti*-infected nude mice. *Immunology* **63,** 181–185.

Ashman, R. I., Jarboe, D. L., Conrad, D. H., and Huff, T. F. (1991). The mast cell-committed progenitor. *In vitro* generation of committed progenitors from bone marrow. *J. Immunol.* **146,** 211–216.

Baeza, M. L., Reddigari, S. R., Kornfeld, D., Ramani, N., Smith, E. M., Hossler, P. A., Fischer, T., Castor, C. W., Gorevic, P. G., and Kaplan, A. P. (1990). Relationship of one form of human histamine-releasing factor to connective tissue activating peptide-II. *J. Clin. Invest.* **85,** 1516–1521.

Befus, A. D. (1989). Mast cells are that polymorphic! *Reg. Immunol.* **2,** 176–187.

Befus. A. D. (1990). Reciprocal interactions between mast cells and the endocrine system. *In* "The Neuroendocrine–Immune Network" (S. Freier, ed.), pp. 39–52. CRC Press, Boca Raton, Florida.

Befus, A. D., Dyck, N., Goodacre, R., and Bienenstock, J. (1987). Mast cells from the human intestinal lamina propria. Isolation, histochemical subtypes, and functional characterization. *J. Immunol.* **138,** 2604–2610.

Benyon, R. C., Lowman, M. A., Ress, P. H., Holgate, S. T., and Church, M. K. (1989). Mast cell heterogeneity. *In* "Asthma Reviews" (J. Morley, ed.), Vol. 2, pp. 151–189. Academic Press, London.

Benyon, R. C., Bissonnette, E. Y., and Befus, A. D. (1991a). Tumor necrosis factor-alpha dependent cytotoxicity of human skin mast cells is enhanced by anti-IgE antibodies. *J. Immunol.* **147,** 2253–2258.

Benyon, R. C., Bissonnette, E. Y., and Befus, A. D. (1991b). Intestinal mast cells in IBD: pathogenesis and therapeutic implications. *In* "Current Topics in Gastroenterology. Inflammatory Bowel Disease" (R. MacDermott and W. Stenson, eds.). pp. 189–199. Elsevier, New York.

Bienenstock, J. (1988). An update on mast cell heterogeneity. *J. Allergy Clin. Immunol.* **81,** 763–769.

Bissonnette, E. Y., and Befus, A. (1990). Inhibition of mast cell-mediated cytotoxicity by interferons alpha/beta, and gamma. *J. Immunol.* **145,** 3385–3390.

Bressler, R. B., Thompson, H. L., Keefer, J. M., and Metcalfe, D. D. (1989). Inhibition of the growth of IL-3-dependent mast cells from murine bone marrow by recombinant granulocyte–macrophage colony-stimulating factor. *J. Immunol.* **143,** 135–139.

Broide, D. H., Wasserman, S. I., Alvaro-Garcia, J., Zvaifler, N. J., and Firestein, G. A. (1989). Transforming growth factor-β selectively inhibits IL-3 dependent mast cell proliferation without affecting mast cell function or differentiation. *J. Immunol.* **143,** 1591–1597.

Broxmeyer, H. E., Lu, L., Hangoc, G., Cooper, S., Hendrie, P. C., Ledbetter, J. A., Xiao, M., Williams, D. E., and Shen, F.-W. (1991). CD45 cell surface antigens are linked to stimulation of early human myeloid progenitor cells by interleukin 3 (IL-3), granulocyte/macrophage colony-stimulating factor (GM-CSF), a GM-CSF/IL-3 fusion protein, and mast cell growth factor (a c-*kit* ligand). *J. Exp. Med.* **174,** 447–458.

Caughey, G. H. (1990). Tryptase and chymase in dog mast cells. *In* "Neutral Proteases of Mast Cells" (L. B. Schwartz, ed.), pp. 67–89. Karger, Basel.

Dahinden, C. A., Kurimoto, Y., de Weck, A. L., Lindley, I., Dewald, B., and Baggiolini, M. (1989). The neutrophil-activating peptide NAF/NAP-1 induces histamine and leukotriene release by interleukin 3-primed basophils. *J. Exp. Med.* **170,** 1787–1792.

Dietsch, G. N., and Hinrichs, D. J. (1989). The role of mast cells in the elicitation of experimental allergic encephalomyelitis. *J. Immunol.* **142,** 1476–1481.

Enerback, L. (1987). Mucosal mast cells in the rat and in man. *Int. Arch. Allergy Appl. Immunol.* **82,** 249–255.

Galli, S. J. (1990). New insights into "the riddle of the mast cells:" Microenvironmental regulation of mast cell development and phenotypic heterogeneity. *Lab. Invest.* **62,** 5–33.

Gordon, J. R., and Galli, S. J. (1991). Release of both preformed and newly synthesized tumor necrosis factor α (TNFα)/cachectin by mouse mast cells stimulated via the Fc_ERI. A mechanism for the sustained action of mast cell-derived TNFα during IgE-dependent biological responses. *J. Exp. Med.* **174,** 103–107.

Gordon, J. R., Burd, P. R., and Galli, S. J. (1990). Mast cells as a source of multifunctional cytokines. *Immunol. Today* **11,** 458–464.

Grant, J. A., Alam, R., and Lett-Brown, M. A. (1991). Histamine-releasing factors and inhibitory factors. *Int. Arch. Allergy Appl. Immunol.* **94,** 141–143.

Hamaguchi, Y., Kanakura, Y., Fujita, J., Takeda, S., Nakano, T., Tarui, S., Honjo, T., and Kitamura, Y. (1987). Interleukin 4 as an essential factor for in vitro clonal growth of murine connective tissue type mast cells. *J. Exp. Med.* **165,** 268–273.

Irani, A. A., Schechter, N. M., Craig, S. S., DeBlois, G., and Schwartz, L. B. (1986). Two types of human mast cells that have distinct neutral protease compositions. *Proc. Natl. Acad. Sci. U.S.A.* **83,** 4464–4448.

Jarboe, D. L., and Huff, T. F. (1989). The mast cell-committed progenitor. II. W/W^v mice do not make mast cell-committed progenitors and Sl/Sl^d fibroblasts do not support development of normal mast cell-committed progenitors. *J. Immunol.* **142,** 2418–2423.

Kirshenbaum, A. S., Kessler, S. W., Goff, J. P., and Metcalfe, D. D. (1991). Demonstration of the origin of human mast cells from CD34+ bone marrow progenitor cells. *J. Immunol.* **146,** 1410–1415.

Kitamura, Y. (1989). Heterogeneity of mast cells and phenotypic change between subpopulations. *Ann. Rev. Immunol.* **7,** 59–76.

Klein, L. M., Lavker, R. M., Matis, W. L., and Murphy, G. F. (1989). Degranulation of human mast cells induces an endothelial antigen central to leukocyte adhesion. *Proc. Natl. Acad. Sci. U.S.A.* **86,** 8972–8976.

Konig, W., Konig, B., Scheffer, J., Hacker, J., and Goebel, W. (1989). Role of cloned virulence factors (mannose-resistant haemagglutination, mannose-resistant adhesions) from uropathogenic *Escherichia coli* strains in the release of inflammatory mediators from neutrophils and mast cells. *Immunology* **67,** 401–407.

Lehrer, R. I., Ganz, T., and Selsted, M. E. (1991). Defensins: Endogenous antibiotic peptides of animal cells. *Cell* **64,** 229–230.

MacQueen, G., Marshall, J., Perdue, M., Siegel, S., and Bienenstock, J. (1989). Pavlovian conditioning of rat mucosal mast cells to secrete rat mast cell protease II. *Science* **243,** 83–85.

Matsuda, H., Nakano, T., Kiso, Y., and Kitamura, Y. (1987). Normalization of anti-tick response of mast cell-deficient W/W^v mice by intracutaneous injection of cultured mast cells. *J. Parasitol.* **73,** 155–160.

Matsuda, H., Kannan, Y., Ushio, H., Kiso, Y., Kanemoto, T., Suzuki, H., and Kitamura, Y. (1991). Nerve growth factor induces development of connective tissue-type mast cells *in vitro* from murine bone marrow cells. *J. Exp. Med.* **174,** 7–14.

Meade, R., Van Loveren, H., Parmentier, H., Iverson, G. M., and Askenase, P. W. (1988). The antigen-binding T cell factor Pcl-F sensitizes mast cells for *in vitro* release of serotonin. *J. Immunol.* **141,** 2704–2713.

Miller, H. R. P. (1992). Mast cells: Their function and heterogeneity. *In* "Allergy and Immunity to Helminths: Common Mechanisms or Divergent Pathways?" (R. Moqbel, ed.). pp. 228–248. Taylor and Francis, London and Washington, DC. ■.

Nafziger, J., Arock, M., Guilloson, J-J., and Wietzerbin, J. (1990). Specific high-affinity receptors for interferon-γ on mast cell precursors. *Eur. J. Immunol.* **20,** 113–117.

Nakagomi, K., Takeuchi, M., Tanaka, H., and Tomizuka, N. (1990). Studies on inhibitors of rat mast cell degranulation produced by microorganisms. I. Screening of microorganisms, and isolation and physico-chemical properties of eurocidins C, D and E. *J. Antibiot.* **43,** 462–469.

Ouellette, A. J., and Lualdi, J. C. (1990). A novel mouse gene family coding for cationic, cysteine-rich peptides. *J. Biol. Chem.* **265,** 9831–9837.

Quist, R. G., Ton-nu, H-T., Lillienau, J., Hofmann, A. F., and Barrett, K. E. (1991). Activation of mast cells by bile acids. *Gastroenterology* **101,** 446–456.

Ramos, B. F., Qureshi, R., Olsen, K. M., and Jakschik, B. A. (1990). The importance of mast cells for the neutrophil influx in immune complex-induced peritonitis in mice. *J. Immunol.* **145,** 1868–1873.

Reynolds, D. S., Serafin, W. E., Faller, D. V., Dvorak, A. M., Austen, K. F., and Stevens, R. L. (1988). Immortalization of murine connective tissue-type mast cells at multiple stages of their differentiation by coculture of splenocytes with fibroblasts that produce Kirsten sarcoma virus. *J. Biol. Chem.* **263,** 12783–12791.

Ruoss, S. J., Hartmann, T., and Caughey, G. H. (1991). Mast cell tryptase is a mitogen for cultured fibroblasts. *J. Clin. Invest.* **88,** 493–499.

Schneider, E., Piquet-Pellorce, C., and Dy, M. (1990). New role for histamine in interleukin-3-induced proliferation of haematopoietic stem cells. *J. Cell Physiol.* **143,** 337–343.

Schulman, E. S., Pollack, R. B., Post, T. J., and Peters, S. P. (1990). Histochemical heterogeneity of dispersed human lung mast cells. *J. Immunol.* **144,** 4195–4201.

Schwartz, L. B. (1990). Neutral proteases of mast cells. *Monogr. Allergy* **27,** 1–165.

Shanahan, F. L., Denburg, J. A., Fox, J., Bienenstock, J., and Befus, A. D. (1985). Mast cell heterogeneity. Effects of neuroenteric peptides on histamine release. *J. Immunol.* **135,** 1331–1337.

Soda, K., Kawabori, S., Perdue, M. H., and Bienenstock, J. (1991). Macrophage engulfment of mucosal mast cells in rats treated with dexamethasone. *Gastroenterology* **101,** 929–937.

Stead, R. H., Tomioka, M., Quinonez, G., Simon, G. T., Felten, S. Y., and Bienenstock, J. (1987). Intestinal mucosal mast cells in normal and nematode-infected rat intestines are in intimate contact with peptidergic nerves. *Proc. Natl. Acad. Sci. U.S.A.* **84,** 2975–2979.

Stead, R. H., Perdue, M. H., Blennerhassett, M. G., Kakuta, Y, Sestini, P., and Bienenstock, J. (1990). The innervation of mast cells. *In* "The Neuroendocrine–Immune Network" (S. Freier, ed.), pp. 19–37. CRC Press, Boca Raton, Forida.

Takeishi, T., Martin, T. R., Katona, I. M., Finkelman, F. D., and Galli, S. J. (1991). Differences in the expression of the cardiopulmonary alterations associated with anti-immunoglobulin E-induced or active anaphylaxis in mast cell-deficient and normal mice. Mast cells are not required for the cardiopulmonary changes associated with certain fatal anaphylactic responses. *J. Clin. Invest.* **88,** 598–608.

Theobald, K., Grob-Weege, W., Keymling, J., and Konig, W. (1987). Inhibition of histamine release in vitro by a blocking factor from human serum: Comparison with the iron binding proteins transferrin and lactoferrin. *Agents Act.* **20,** 10–16.

Thompson-Snipes, L., Dhar, V., Bond, M. W., Mosmann, T. R., Moore, K. W., and Rennick, D. (1991). Interleukin-10: A novel stimulatory factor for mast cells and their progenitors. *J. Exp. Med.* **173,** 507–510.

Tsai, B. M., Shih, L-S., Newlands, G. F. J., Takeishi, T., Langley, K. E., Zsebo, K. M., Miller, H. R. P., Geissler, E. N., and Galli, S. J. (1991). The rat c-*kit* ligand, stem cell factor, induces the development of connective tissue-type and mucosal mast cells in vivo. Analysis by anatomical distribution, histochemistry, and protease phenotype. *J. Exp. Med.* **174,** 125–131.

Undem, B. J., and Weinreich, D. (1989). Functional interactions between mast cells and peripheral neurons. *In* "Neuroimmune Networks: Physiology and Disease" (E. J. Goetzl and N. H. Spector, eds.), pp. 155–162. Liss, New York.

Watkins, S. G., Dearin, J. L., Yong, L. C., and Wilhelm, D. L. (1976). Association of mastopoiesis with haemopoietic tissues in the neonatal rat. *Experientia* **32,** 1339–1340.

Williams, D. E., Eisenman, J., Baird, A., Rauch, C., Van Ness, K., March, C. J., Park, L. S., Martin, U., Mochizuki, D. Y., Boswell, H. S., Burgess, G. S., Cosman, D., and Lyman, S. D. (1990). Identification of a ligand for the c-*kit* protooncogene. *Cell* **63,** 167–174.

Woodbury, R. G., and Neurath, H. (1978). Purification of an atypical mast cell protease and its levels in developing rats. *Biochemistry* **7,** 4298–4304.

Yano, H., Wershil, B. K., Arizono, N., and Galli, S. J. (1989). Substance P-induced augmentation of cutaneous vascular permeability and granulocyte infiltration in mice is mast cell dependent. *J. Clin. Invest.* **84,** 1276–1286.

27

Cytokines in the Liver and Gastrointestinal Tract

Fernando Anaya-Velazquez • Graham D. F. Jackson • Peter B. Ernst • Brian J. Underdown • Jack Gauldie

I. INTRODUCTION

Although immunological interactions between the liver and the intestine have been described for years, the liver often is perceived to function primarily as a "scavenger" within the reticuloendothelial system. The broader contributions of the liver can be appreciated if one considers that this organ can function in lymphopoiesis (particularly in neonates), clearance of immune complexes, antigen presentation, acute inflammation, IgA transport, local synthesis of immunoglobulin, cell-mediated cytotoxicity, and immune regulation through the production of regulatory cells and cytokines.

The liver and intestine exchange immunological information via the portal vein and bile. Since some immunological responses in the liver are associated with pathological conditions in the intestine, both organs are likely to act in concert to coordinate some of their immune responses. In this chapter, we describe the production and function of cytokines in the liver and intestine using the paradigm of parasitic infestations to illustrate the dynamic immunological interventions between these tissues.

II. OVERVIEW OF CYTOKINE PRODUCTION

Cytokines are soluble small-to-intermediate sized proteins produced by a variety of cells in response to injury, infection, or antigenic challenges. These molecules can function in an autocrine, paracrine, or endocrine fashion, the latter being relevant to the communication between the gut and the liver. Their functions are diverse and include the regulation of growth, differentiation, and function of a variety of immune cells (Arai *et al.*, 1990; Finkelman *et al.*, 1991). Cytokines also help orchestrate numerous interactions between the immune system and physiological processes by altering the microenvironment and biomatrix surrounding these cells. Most of what we know about the effects of cytokines is related to inflammatory events, whereas relatively little is known about the function of these molecules under physiological conditions (Arai *et al.*, 1990).

The number of well-characterized cytokines has grown tremendously during the last 5 years. Two important developments that have helped elucidate the role of these factors in the immune response are the availability of recombinant cytokines and neutralizing antibodies. Among the best characterized cytokines are interferon (IFNα, β, γ), tumor necrosis factor (TNF), lymphotoxin (LT), interleukins (IL) 1–12, and growth factors including epidermal growth factor (EGF), platelet-derived growth factor (PDGF), and transforming growth factors (TGF), as well as granulocyte–macrophage (GM-CSF), granulocyte (G-CSF), and macrophage (M-CSF) colony stimulating factors (reviewed by (Arai *et al.*, 1990; Finkelman *et al.*, 1991; Mosmann and Moore, 1991). In addition to these mediators, an entirely new class of cytokine has been discovered and characterized, describing a group of small secreted chemotactic factors referred to as the platelet factor 4 (PF4) superfamily (Schall, 1991). All these molecules share a similar primary structure and have a four-cysteine motif. The superfamily has two major subclasses: those with a "Cys–X–Cys" structure include PF4 and IL-8 and those with a "Cys–Cys" structure including the RANTES/SIS cytokines. These cytokines act on a wide range of cells and collaborate in a cytokine network with neuroendocrine factors, adhesion molecules, and nonpeptide factors to influence the function of cells bearing the appropriate receptors and to modify the inflammatory or immune responses in tissues.

The complexities of the cytokine network, including the cascades of events that lead to the indirect effects of a cytokine, are sometimes difficult to dissect and evaluate. This complexity can be illustrated by cytokine production by monocytes, T cells, and mast cells in the intestine and liver. Using the tools at hand, a framework that describes the source and effects of many cytokines can be drawn and the link between the gut and liver can be exposed.

III. INITIATION OF CYTOKINE PRODUCTION: INTERACTIONS AMONG CELLS AND ANTIGEN

Cells in the intestine are involved in the absorption of nutrients, motility, and immune functions; all these functions are coordinated by nerves, hormones, cytokines, or other factors (Marshall *et al.*, 1989; Kiyono *et al.*, 1991; Strober *et al.*, 1991). To develop a model of cytokine function in the gut and liver, we first consider the distribution of monocytes, T cells, and mast cells; their response to nematode infestation; the progressive increase in cytokine synthesis; and their effects.

The primary immune inductive sites in the intestine are aggregates of lymphocytes and antigen-presenting cells and include the Peyer's patches. Other antigen presenting cells, lymphoid cells, and leukocytes (including mast cells or their precursors) are scattered diffusely throughout the lamina propria and epithelium (effector sites).

Although the liver is composed largely of parenchymal cells, an enormous complement of immune or inflammatory cells is also present. The major antigen-presenting cell is believed to be the Kupffer cell. T and B lymphocytes, natural killer cells, and other inflammatory cells including the occasional mast cell are also found. Lymphocytes and other inflammatory cells are found primarily in the portal triads, adjacent to the biliary tracts and throughout the parenchyma (Jones and Altorfer, 1988). Plasma cells also are found near biliary spaces, but this observation is relatively rare under normal circumstances. One question that arises is whether hepatic lymphocytes are trapped from peripheral and portal blood or whether the liver has its own endogenous population of lymphoid cells. The enrichment for B and T cell precursors in the liver, particularly in infancy, suggests that the liver is not merely a sink for trapped lymphocytes from the blood, but does actively accumulate cells with a particular function. Further, this organ contains a proportionally larger number of B cells than blood or spleen (Manning *et al.*, 1984). Collectively, these observations suggest that the liver has the cellular capacity to respond to antigens and cytokines by mediating cytotoxic activity, antibody production, and the release of cytokines.

Stimulation of the intestinal cells by luminal antigen is believed to occur primarily in the inductive sites (Ernst *et al.*, 1988). These aggregates lie below specialized epithelial cells (M cells) that act as preferential sampling sites of luminal antigen (Owen and Jones, 1974; Neutra *et al.*, 1987; Pappo *et al.*, 1988). Some antigen also crosses intact or disrupted epithelium and contributes to the stimulation of naive or sensitized cells in the epithelium or the underlying lamina propria (Bland and Warren, 1986; Mayer *et al.*, 1991). Antigen-stimulated lymphocytes or cytokines reach the portal circulation and traffic to the liver. Alternatively, this immunological information may enter the lymph or blood and eventually reach the liver via the hepatic artery. In either case, substantial communication occurs between the intestine and the liver after antigenic stimulation.

An interesting consequence of the response of the liver to luminal antigens is the induction of oral tolerance, which is a state of reduced responsiveness (Ernst *et al.*, 1988) that is believed to be beneficial to the host by limiting immune responses to the myriad of enteric antigens. The role of the liver in this process has been implicated by experiments in which the portal circulation was made to bypass the liver prior to oral immunization (Cantor and Dumont, 1967). Moreover, immunization with alloantigens into the portal vein inhibits subsequent graft rejection (Qian *et al.*, 1987). Thus, by dealing with the immunogenicity of luminal antigens, the liver is linked quite closely to the intestine. Although cellular studies have verified these results, little information is available on the factors or cytokines that may be mediating this process.

IV. INITIATION OF CYTOKINE PRODUCTION: ACUTE INFLAMMATION

In response to parasitic or other infections and injuries, the host responds initially with an acute inflammatory response (Fey and Gauldie, 1990; Heinrich *et al.*, 1990; Stadnyk and Gauldie, 1991). The acute inflammatory response may be divided into the local inflammatory response—coagulation, kinin generation, phospholipid metabolism with vasodilation and cellular emigration—and the systemic acute phase response—fever, leukocytosis, changes in the concentrations of plasma heavy metals, and increased plasma levels of a number of hepatocyte-derived proteins (Gauldie *et al.*, 1989; Heinrich *et al.*, 1990; Stadnyk and Gauldie, 1991). These two responses are not clearly separable since many of the systemic changes seen during local inflammation are the result of the production of mediators at the primary site of inflammation. The systemic component of acute inflammation, that is, increases in the plasma "acute phase reactants" (APR), has received considerable attention as a marker for the detection of inflammation.

Corticosteroids have a direct effect on the regulation of many genes in the liver, but may make a greater contribution by enhancing the effects of other factors such as IL-6 (Baumann and Gauldie, 1990). IL-1 and TNF also have the ability to regulate APR; however, neither could regulate the full response *in vitro,* even in the presence of corticosteroids. IL-6 (also referred to as hepatocyte stimulating factor) acts via a heterodimeric receptor to activate nuclear factors that regulate the expression of acute phase protein genes (Gauldie *et al.*, 1989; Heinrich *et al.*, 1990; Richards *et al.*, 1991). This activity of IL-6 is mimicked by leukemia inhibitory factor (LIF), IL-11, and oncostatin M (OM), which also can synergize with IL-1 or TNF and corticosteroids. IL-1, IL-6, LIF, OM, and IL-11 all act through separate receptors, meaning a broad range of factors can contribute independently in response to inflammation regardless of the tissue affected and differences in local cytokine responses.

The hepatocytes respond to these factors in a specific manner as a result of direct, additive, synergistic, or inhibitory actions of the cytokines (Stadnyk and Gauldie, 1991). Type I acute phase proteins include opsonins, complement components, and transport proteins and are stimulated by combinations of cytokines such as IL-1 and IL-6. Type II proteins include fibrinogen, haptoglobin, and all the antiproteases and are stimulated only by IL-6 or IL-6-like cytokines. Other cytokines, including IFNγ and TGF modulate the hepatic response (Zuraw and Lotz, 1990). The complexity of the interactions is illustrated further by the fact that IL-1 can inhibit the effect of IL-6 induction on some type II proteins. Thus, in predicting the response of hepatocytes, one must consider which factors are released at the site of inflammation as well as their sequence of release, which contribute to the network of signals that reach the liver.

The cells producing cytokines that regulate gene expression in the liver are quite diverse (Andus *et al.*, 1991; Stadnyk and Gauldie 1991). Macrophages, both resident tissue and circulating (monocytes), provide a link between the inflammatory response and immune system by antigen presentation and activation of lymphocytes. Through the secretion of cytokines, especially IL-1 and TNF, macrophages communicate with other tissues to elicit systemic inflammatory changes (Andus *et al.*, 1991). Other cells involved at the site of inflammation also may participate in the acute phase response through the release of cytokines. These cells include lymphocytes, neutrophils, and platelets; stromal cells such as fibroblasts, endothelial cells, and smooth muscle cells; and epithelial cells such as keratinocytes.

V. CYTOKINE PRODUCTION IN RESPONSE TO INFECTION WITH NEMATODES

Several parasitic infections cause intestinal inflammation and permit studies on the impact of cytokine production during inflammation. Two nematode infections of the rodent with similar but distinct life cycles are *Nippostrongylus brasiliensis* and *Trichinella spiralis*. Subcutaneously administered infectious L3 stage larvae of *N. brasiliensis* have an obligatory host lung stage before they arrive as L4 stage larvae in the small intestine. In that site, the worms mature to adults and live in the proximal jejunum where they mate and secrete eggs prior to expulsion. In contrast, infective larvae (L4) of *T. spiralis* recovered from skeletal muscle of mammals are ingested, allowing them to undergo rapid molts in the proximal jejunum. Subsequently, the worms mature and mate; newborn larvae (L1) arise few a days later. L1 larvae migrate via the portal vein to skeletal muscle throughout the host, where they encyst. The adults of the two species occupy a different niche within the host intestine: *N. brasiliensis* remains in the intestinal lumen, usually at the base of the villi, whereas *T. spiralis* lives within the epithelium (Stadnyk and Gauldie, 1991).

During infection with *N. brasiliensis,* alveolar macrophages become activated and spontaneously secrete IL-1 and IL-6 during the passage of the larvae through the host lungs. These cells continue to secrete increased amounts of these cytokines while the parasite inhabits the intestine (Stadnyk and Gauldie, 1991), leading to changes in serum APR. IL-1 and IL-6 were detected in the supernatants of cultures of isolated intestinal cells from normal animals, and levels were increased in cultures from rats infected with *N. brasiliensis*. In contrast, no APR changes occur and neither alveolar nor peritoneal macrophages from *T. spiralis*-infected rats secrete greater than normal amounts of IL-1 or IL-6, whereas the intestinal cell cytokine levels from animals infected with *T. spiralis* were reduced compared with normal levels. However, cells in the infected intestine are capable of producing IL-1 nd IL-6 (and other cytokines) *in vitro* but do not appear to be activated *in vivo* during intestinal pathology caused by *T. spiralis* or, most significantly, during the inflammation induced by direct intestinal infection with the L4 stage of *N. brasiliensis*. These observations suggest that tissue activation and cytokine secretion occur because of the effects of parasite migration through the lung and that the inflamed intestine does not generate an acute phase response to nematode infection, as might have been predicted.

Other cells also may produce cytokines during nematode infections. Intraepithelial lymphocytes (IEL), found at the basolateral surfaces of epithelial cells, have been shown to produce several different cytokines including IL-2, IL-3, IL-5, IL-6, IFNγ, TNFα, and TGFβ in the absence of parasitic infection (Dillon *et al.*, 1987; Barrett *et al.*, 1990; Taguchi *et al.*, 1990). The epithelium itself also has been shown to produce EGF/urogastrone in humans (Wright *et al.*, 1990) and IL-6 in freshly isolated cell preparations (K. Beagley, personal communication). Although these cytokines and their potential effects are impressive, few studies have evaluated this condition *in situ*. Part of this response may reflect the effects of cell isolation and manipulation *in vitro*.

IEL deserve special attention since they have interesting cytoplasmic granules, appear to be thymus independent, and express novel surface antigens including T-cell repertoires that are not found elsewhere in the body (Lefrancois, 1991). The large population of Thy1$^-$CD8$^+$ IEL has been shown to mediate antibody enhancement in orally tolerized animals, but IEL-derived cytokines have not been implicated directly (Fujihashi *et al.*, 1990). IFNγ (Zhang and Michael, 1990) and TGFβ (L. Zettel and P. Ernst, unpublished observations) have been shown to prevent or reverse tolerance, since both these cytokines are produced by IEL they may contribute to the enhancement of antibody responses. Since IELs are mostly CD8$^+$, their ability to produce so many cytokines may compensate for the absence of CD4 helper T cells (Th) in this compartment. Since nematodes and other pathogens are found in close association with the epithelium, the IEL may have evolved an important role in the host response to infections through cytokine generation and other functions.

Most analyses of T-cell function in parasitized animals have focused on cytokine production by Th cells from the spleen or mesenteric lymph node, providing an interesting model of Th cell heterogeneity and its implications for function. Studies have shown that Th cells segregate into subsets based on their cytokine profile (Mosmann and Coffman, 1987). Thus, Th1 cells are a source of IL-2, IL-3, IFNγ, LT, GM-CSF, and TNF-β. In turn, Th2 cells produce IL-3, IL-4, IL-5, IL-6, IL-10, GM-CSF, and TNF (Mosmann and Moore, 1991). Interestingly IL-10, which is produced by Th2 but not Th1 cells, leads to the inhibition of Th1 cell development but not that of Th2 cells (Mosmann and Moore, 1991). During infection with *N. brasiliensis* or *T. spiralis,* mice mount a strong Th2 cell-like response in their spleen or mesenteric lymph nodes, including the ability to synthesize more IL-4 and IL-5 while producing less IFNγ and IL-2 (Pond *et al.*, 1989; Street *et al.*, 1990; Mosmann and Moore, 1991).

VI. EFFECTS OF CYTOKINE PRODUCTION DURING INFECTION WITH NEMATODES

The characteristics of Th2 stimulation during nematode infection include elevated IgE antibody production, eosinophilia, and mastocytosis (Finkelman *et al.*, 1988,1991; Coffman *et al.*, 1989; Wang *et al.*, 1989; Madden *et al.*, 1991; Urban *et al.*, 1991). These immunological manifestations are explained by the production of IL-3, IL-4, and IL-5, which can contribute to these changes. Evidence implicating cytokine control of the immune response *in vivo* in some nematode infections comes from experiments in which various neutralizing antibodies have been injected into an animal. Several studies have shown that either anti-IL-4 or anti-IL-3 antibody can inhibit partially the induction of mucosal mastocytosis in *N. brasiliensis*-infected mice, and that a combination of these two antibodies blocks the *N. brasiliensis*-induced increase in mucosal mast cell number by approximately 90% (Finkelman *et al.*, 1991). The injection of anti-IL-4 and anti-IL-4 receptor monoclonal antibodies into mice infected with *N. brasiliensis* or *H. polygyrus* totally blocks the IgE responses to both primary and secondary inoculations. Likewise, a neutralizing anti-IL-5 monoclonal antibody has been shown to block peripheral blood and tissue eosinophilia completely in mice infected with *N. brasiliensis* (Coffman *et al.*, 1989). Remarkably, treatment with anti-IL-5 antibodies does not block expulsion of *N. brasiliensis;* however, the expulsion is inhibited completely by an anti-CD4 antibody (Katona *et al.*, 1988). The cytokine IFNα appears to inhibit the development of blood and solid tissue eosinophilia, at least in *N. brasiliensis*-infected mice (Finkelman *et al.*, 1991). Thus, $CD4^+$ T cells, by some mechanism other than the induction of eosinophil, mast cell, or IgE responses, make an essential contribution to protective immunity in *N. brasiliensis*-infected mice. Interestingly, clearance of *H. polygyrus* is blocked by anti-IL-4 antibody (Urban *et al.*, 1991), showing that mechanisms of protection differ.

IL-3 production by IELs also may lead to local mast cell hyperplasia induced by these infections. Mast cells also produce a range of cytokines (Gordon *et al.*, 1990) and, since the IELs contain a vast number of mast cell precursors that are able to differentiate during nematode infestations (Crapper and Schrader, 1983; Guy-Grand *et al.*, 1984), they also may contribute to additional cytokine production.

In addition to the alterations in the immune and inflammatory response, infection with intestinal nematodes has been shown to affect intestinal physiology. Changes observed in association with musocal inflammation are consistent with the prediction that lymphocytes or mast cells in the epithelium and lamina propria may modulate epithelial proliferation, differentiation, and function. This hypothesis is supported by studies showing altered epithelial structure and function after challenge with antigen in sensitized animals (King and Miller, 1984; Harari *et al.*, 1987; Patrick *et al.*, 1988; Crowe *et al.*, 1990), as well as by reports that cytokines or mast cell mediators modulate the expression of secretory component and major histocompatibility (MHC) Class II molecules on enterocytes (Sollid *et al.*, 1987; Kvale *et al.*, 1988; Phillips *et al.*, 1990) and enterocyte function (Barrett, 1991).

Complementing these responses to antigen in the epithelium, smooth muscle contractility also is altered by antigen in sensitized animals (Palmer and Castro, 1986). This altered contractility may involve the effects of mast cells or T cells (Vermillion *et al.*, 1989,1991) on sodium pump activity (Muller *et al.*, 1989) or impaired neurotransmitter release (Collins et al., 1991). At least some of these changes do not require contact with the parasite, since uninfected segments of intestine experience similar alterations in physiological function (Marzio *et al.*, 1990). These observations suggest that inflammatory mediators or cytokines from mast cells or T cells may act as hormones and modulate distant tissues. A coordinated physiological response mediated by the immune system during infection with intestinal nematodes could assist in the catharsis associated with the expulsion of these parasites.

VII. EXTENSION TO THE LIVER

Two reviews (Andus *et al.*, 1991; Richards *et al.*, 1991) have summarized the effects of a number of cytokines on the liver (see Table I). These authors have emphasized three aspects about the interactions between the liver and cytokines, including (1) cytokines as signal molecules reaching the liver from extraheptaic inflammatory sites and leading to changes in hepatocyte metabolism, including the acute phase response; (2) the role of the liver as a source and scavenger of cytokines; and (3) the role of cytokines during diseases of the liver itself.

The liver responds quite dramatically to intestinal infection with nematodes. For example, mast cells are increased in the portal areas of the liver of rats infected with *N. brasiliensis* (Figure 1) or *Taenia taeniaeformis* (Ishiwata *et al.*, 1991). As noted earlier, mast cells rarely are seen in the normal liver, either as young mast cells in the space of Disse (Balabaud *et al.*, 1988) or as mature mast cells in the perisinusoidal space (Jezequel *et al.*, 1986). Our studies suggest that some of these mast cells in normal or parasitized animals may arise from hepatic precursors in response to an increase in mast cell growth factors emanating from the intestine or hepatic T cells (see Table II).

The function of hepatic mast cells is unclear, although their presence during nematode infection reflects the ability of the liver to respond to intestinal sensitization. After the administration of 48/80, histamine is released by hepatic mast cells into the bile. Using a more physiological stimulus, feeding ovalbumin to sensitized animals also causes an increase in biliary histamine (G. D. F. Jackson *et al.*, unpublished observations). Presumably, histamine and other mediators from mast cells contribute to changes in the liver including altered blood flow, the accumulation of inflammatory cells, and possibly chronic changes such as fibrosis through the production of TNF or TGFβ by mast cells. Since significant synthesis and transport of IgA also occurs in the liver of rodents (Manning *et al.*, 1984), the exchange of immunological information between the liver and intestine via the portal circulation and the bile may play a role in host resistance.

Table I Cytokines Affecting the Liver[a]

Cytokine	Main source
IL-1	Monocytes, endothelium, smooth muscle, keratinocytes
IL-2	Lymphocytes
IL-6	Monocytes, lymphocytes, fibroblasts, endothelium, smooth muscle, keratinocytes
TNFα	Monocytes
LIF/HSF III	Tumor cells
IL-11	Stromal cells, T cells, monocytes
Oncostatin M	Stromal cells, T cells, monocytes
IFNα/β	Mononuclear cells
IFNγ	T lymphocytes
EGF	Gastrointestinal glands
TGFα	Fibroblasts, embryonic cells, keratinocytes, monocytes
TGFβ	Monocytes, platelets, hemopoietic cells, lymphocytes, placenta, keratinocytes, kidney, fibroblasts, bone
FGF	Endothelial cells, pituitary cells
PDGF	Platelets, monocytes
IGF-1	Hepatocytes, tumor cells
IGF-2	Liver, yolk sac

[a] Modified with permission from Andus *et al.*, (1991).

In some other parasitic diseases, cytokines produced in the liver may act directly to clear the liver of parasites. IL-1, IL-6, IFNγ, and TNF directly or indirectly interfere with the development of malaria parasites in the liver via an L-arginine-dependent effector mechanism (Nussler *et al.*, 1991). Similarly, both the sporozoites and the erythrocytic stages of malaria parasites have been established to modulate the hepatic phase of malaria by cytokines (notably IFNγ, TNFα, and IL-6), either directly or as a result of a cascade of events (Mazier *et al.*, 1990). Th2 cytokines have been suggested to be selectively induced during infection with *Schistosoma mansoni* (Pearce *et al.*, 1991) and IL-5 production is associated with the eosinophilia. However, anti-IL-5 antibody *in vivo* can decrease the number of eosinophils but has no other effect on the appearance of the hepatic granulomas.

Table II Frequency of Mast Cell Precursors in Mononuclear Cells from Liver and Peripheral Blood of Normal CBA Mice[a]

Origin of cells	Frequency/10^6 cells (95% confidence interval)
Perfused liver	148 (107–189)
Nonperfused liver	357 (289–425)
Peripheral blood	115 (94–137)

[a] Purified mononuclear cells from normal spleen were cultured in the presence of interleukin 3 (WEHI-conditioned media) using limiting dilution as described elsewhere (Crapper and Schrader, 1983). Based on the presence of colonies of mast cells individual wells were scored and the frequency of mast cell precursors was calculated.

Additional evidence suggests that cytokines can be produced in the liver and modulate other functions in this site. After immunization of rats, the number of cells expressing CD25 (IL-2 receptor) increases from 10 to 24% (G. D. F. Jackson *et al.*, unpublished observations). This increase is associated mainly with CD8$^+$ cells in the portal region. This evidence of activation again suggests that local cytokine production by immune or inflammatory cells or other nonparenchymal cells occurs in the liver, in agreement with the observations that cytokines such as TNFα, IL-1, and IL-6 are produced by hepatic mononuclear cells (Decker, 1990), whereas parenchymal and fat-storing cells may produce these as well as fibroblast growth factor (FGF), TGFα, and IFNα (Northemann *et al.*, 1990). In turn, perisinusoidal cells are the major source of circulating insulin-like (IGF-1) (Murphy *et al*, 1987) and also can express TGFβ1 (Nakatsukkasa *et al.*, 1990). Hepatic sinusoidal endothelial cells produce cytokines such as a basic FGF-like molecule (Rosenbaum *et al.*, 1989). liver parenchymal cells also have been shown to express IL-8 genes *in vitro*, implying that the liver may participate in inflammatory processes by the production of leukocyte chemotactic factors. From these reports, we can see that antigen or inflammatory signals emanating from the gut via the portal circulation clearly stimulate host of cytokine responses in the liver.

Cytokines affect many metabolic functions of the liver including its amino acid, protein, lipid, and carbohydrate metabolism. Mineral metabolism, detoxification, and bile excretion also may be influenced by certain cytokines. Carbohydrate metabolism is increased by several cytokines including IGF-1, IL-6, EGF, and IGF-2 (Andus *et al.*, 1991). In particular, IL-6 can stimulate hepatic glucose release from prelabeled glycogen pools *in vitro;* likewise, antisera to this cytokine significantly decrease monocyte-derived glucose-releasing factor (GFR) activity, implicating IL-6 as a glucoregulatory factor that acts by inhibiting glycogen synthase (Ritchie, 1990). In addition, lipid metabolism is raised by IL-1, IFNα, TNFα/β, and IFNγ. TNF increases serum triglyceride levels *in vivo* by stimulating hepatic lipogenesis and very low density lipoprotein (VLDL) production. However, IL-4 has been found to block the effect of TNF, IL-1, and IL-6 on lipogenesis but to have no effect on the ability of IFNγ to stimulate this response (Endo, 1991; Grunfeld *et al.*, 1991). Thus, the liver can respond in a number of ways to cytokines produced in response to local or intestinal inflammation by altering its immunological characteristics, inflammatory response, and metabolic processes.

VIII. SUMMARY

Infection with intestinal nematodes has been a useful tool in exploring the peculiarities of cytokine production and func-

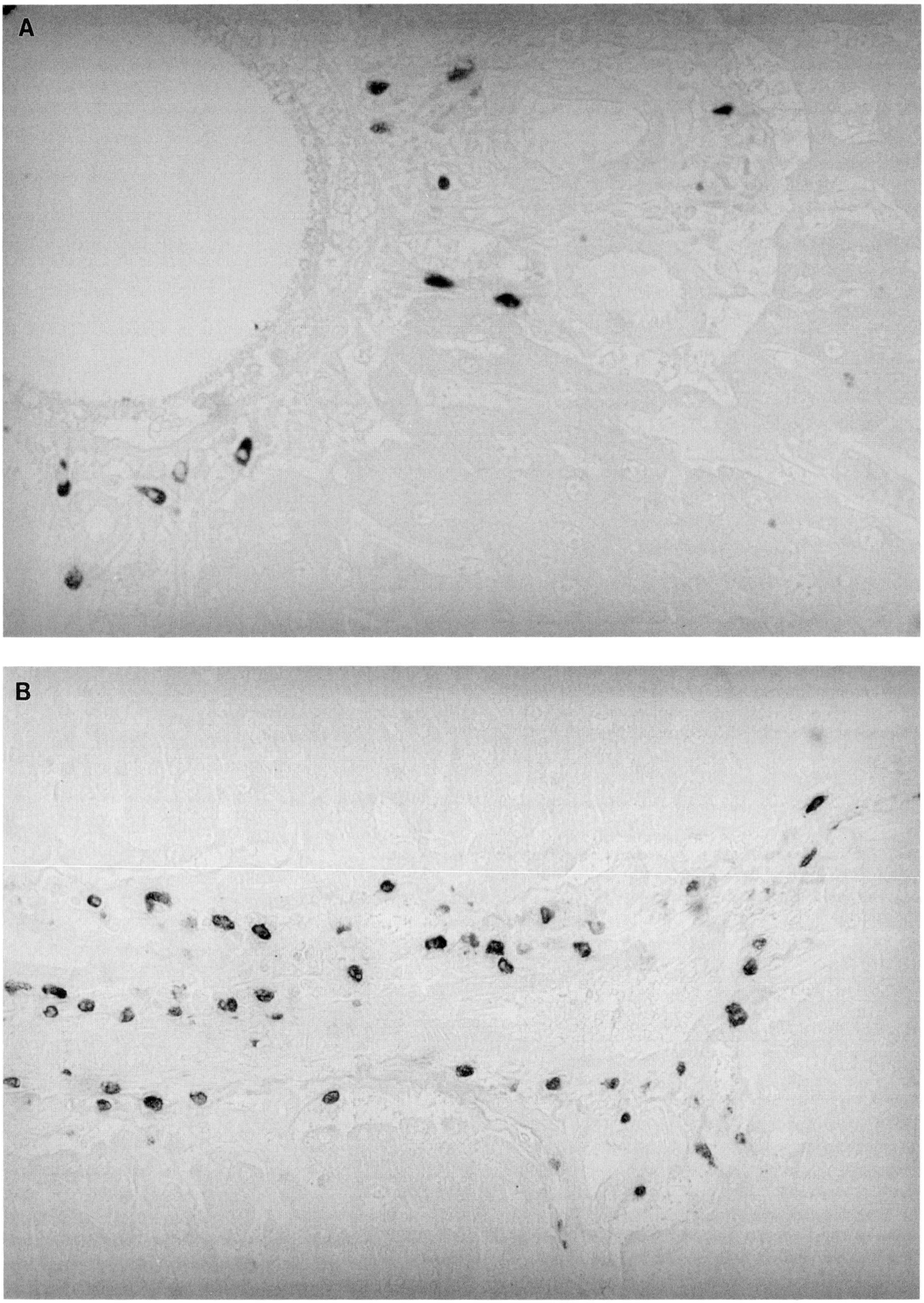

Figure 1 Hepatic mast cell response during intestinal inflammation. Histological sections of liver from mice infected with *N. brasiliensis* were prepared and stained with toluidine blue. A marked increase in mast cells was observed, particularly close to the portal triad as seen in cross (A) or longitudinal (B) sections. Mast cells rarely are seen in uninfected mice.

tion. Although the acute inflammatory response may not be invoked during the intestinal phase of a nematode infection, a significant activation of Th2 cells appears to occur that could account for the characteristic changes in the intestinal mucosa and possibly the mastocytosis in the liver. Interestingly, Th2 cells also are believed to enhance IgA responses through the production of IL-4, IL-5, and IL-6; however, the immunological picture observed during a mucosal IgA response and nematode infestation could not be more different. Clearly, a significant gap exists in our current understanding of the control of mucosal immunity. Cytokines produced in the intestine and liver are quite pleiotropic and the discrete expression of genes encoding cytokines or their receptors may combine with tolerogenic mechanisms involving the liver to focus a response toward the desired end point. In view of the protective responses governed by cytokines, a better understanding of cytokine regulation and the manner in which their pleiotropic effects are prevented certainly will be a key issue for future research.

Studies of the local and systemic effects of intestinal nematodes constitute a useful approach to demonstrating the immunologial link between the intestine and the liver. The nature of the interaction can include an exchange of antigen, hematopoietic precursors, immune cells, or potent intercellular messengers such as cytokines. Additional knowledge about the intestinal–hepatic axis could facilitate the successful development of oral vaccines and intestinal transplantation.

Acknowledgments

The studies summarized in this chapter were supported in part by the Medical Research Council of Canada.

References

Andus, T., Bauer, J., and Gerok, W. (1991). Effects of cytokines on the liver. *Hepatology* **13,** 354–375.

Arai, K., Lee, F., Miyajima, A., Miyatake, S., Arai, N., and Yokota, T. (1990). Cytokines: Coordinators of immune and inflammatory responses. *Ann. Rev. Biochem.* **59,** 783–836.

Balabaud, C., Boulard, A., Quinton, A., Saric, J., Bedin, C., Boussarie, L., and Bioulac-Sage. P. (1988). Light and transmission electron microscopy of sinusoids in human liver. *In* "Sinusoids in Human Liver" (P. Bioulac-Sage and C. Balabaud, eds.), pp. 87–110. Kupffer Cell Foundation, Rijswijk, Iceland.

Barrett, K. E. (1991). Immune-related intestinal chloride secretion. III. Acute and chronic effects of mast cell mediators on chloride secretion by a human colonic epithelial cell line. *J. Immunol.* **147,** 959–964.

Barrett, T., Gajewski, T., Lee, N., Widacki, S. M., Chang, E. B., Lefrancois, L. and Bluestone, J. A. (1990). Localization and functional characterization of intraepithelial lymphocyte subsets activated with anti-$\alpha\beta$ and $\gamma\delta$ T cell receptor antibodies. *FASEB J.* **4,** A1864.(Abstract)

Baumann, H., and Gauldie, J. (1990). Regulation of hepatic acute phase plasma protein genes by hepatocyte stimulating factors and other mediators of inflammation. *Mol. Biol. Med.* **7,** 147–159.

Bland, P. W., and Warren, L. G. (1986). Antigen presentation by epithelial cells of the rat small intestine I. Kinetics, antigen specificity and blocking by anti-Ia antisera. *Immunology* **58,** 1–7.

Cantor, H. M., and Dumont, A. E. (1967). Hepatic suppression of sensitization to antigen absorbed into the portal system. *Nature (London)* **215,** 744–745.

Coffman, R. L., Seymour, B. W. P., Hudak, S., Jackson, J., and Rennick, D. (1989). Antibody to interleukin-5 inhibits helminth-induced eosinophilia in mice. *Science* **245,** 308–310.

Collins, S. M., Blennerhasett, P., Vermillion, D. L., Davis, K., Langer, J., and Ernst, P. B. (1992). On the mechanism of impaired acetylcholine release in the inflamed rat intestine. *Am. J. Physiol. Gastrointest. Liver Physiol.* **263,** G198–G204.

Crapper, R. M., and Schrader, J. W. (1983). Frequency of mast cell precursors in normal tissues determined by an in vitro assay: Antigen induces parallel increase in the frequency of P cell precursors and mast cells. *J. Immunol.* **131,** 923–928.

Crowe, S. E., Sestini, P., and Perdue, M. H. (1990). Allergic reactions of rat jejunal mucosa. Ion transport responses to luminal antigen and inflammatory mediators. *Gastroenterology* **99,** 74–82.

Decker, K. (1990). Biologically active products of stimulated liver macrophages (Kupffer cells). *Eur. J. Biochem.* **192,** 245–261.

Dillon, S. B., Dalton, B. J., and MacDonald, T. T. (1987). Lymphokine production by mitogen and antigen activated mouse intraepithelial lymphocytes. *Cell. Immunol.* **103,** 326–338.

Endo, Y. (1991). Parallel relationship between the increase in serotonin in the liver and the hypoglycaemia induced in mice by interleukin-1 and tumour necrosis factor. *Immunol. Lett.* **27,** 75–79.

Ernst, P. B., Scicchitano, R., Underdown, B. J., and Bienenstock, J. (1988). Oral immunization and tolerance. *In* "Immunology of the Gastrointestinal Tract and Liver" (M. F. Heyworth and A. L. Jones, eds.), pp. 125–144. Raven Press, New York.

Fey, G., and Gauldie, J. (1990). The acute phase response of the liver in inflammation. *In* "Progress in Liver Diseases" (H. Popper and F. Schaffner, eds.), pp. 89–116. Saunders, Philadelphia.

Finkelman, F. D., Katona, I. M., Urban, J. F., Jr., Holmes, J., Ohara, J., Tung, A. S., Sample, J. V. G., and Paul, W. E. (1988). IL-4 is required to generate and sustain in vivo IgE repsonses. *J. Immunol.* **141,** 2335–2341.

Finkelman, F. D., Pearce, E. J., Urban, J. F., and Sher, A. (1991). Regulation and biological function of helminth-induced cytokine responses. *Immunol. Today* **12,** A62–A66.

Fujihashi, K., Taguchi, T., McGhee, J. R., Eldridge, J. H., Bruce, M. G., Green, D. R., Singh, B., and Kiyono, H. (1990). Regulatory function for murine intraepithelial lymphocytes: Two subsets of CD3+, T cell receptor-1+ intraepithelial lymphocyte T cells abrogate oral tolerance. *J. Immunol.* **145,** 2010–2019.

Gauldie, J., Richards, C., Northemann, W., Fey, G., and Baumann, H. (1989). IFN-β2/BSF2/IL-6 is the monocyte-derived HSF that regulates receptor-specific acute phase gene regulation in hepatocytes. *Ann. N.Y. Acad. Sci.* **557,** 46–59.

Gordon, J. R., Burd, P. R., and Galli, S. J. (1990). Mast cells as a source of multifunctional cytokines. *Immunol. Today* **11,** 458–464.

Grunfeld, C., Soued, M., Adi, S., Moser, A. H., Fiers, W., Dinarello, C. A., and Reingold, K. R. (1991). Interleukin 4 inhibits stimulation of hepatic lipogenesis by tumor necrosis factor, interleukin 1 and interleukin 6 but not by interferon-α. *Cancer Res.* **51,** 2803–2807.

Guy-Grand, D., Dy, M., Luffau, G., and Vassalli, P. (1984). Gut mucosal mast cells. Origin, traffic, and differentiation, *J. Exp. Med.* **160,** 12–28.

Harari, Y., Russell, D. A., and Castro, G. A. (1987). Anaphylaxis-mediated epithelial Cl-secretion and parasite rejection in rat intestine. *J. Immunol.* **138,** 1250–1255.

Heinrich, P. C., Castell, J. B., and Andus, T. (1990). Interleukin-6 and the acute phase response. *Biochem. J.* **265,** 621–636.

Ishiwata, K., Oku, Y., Kamiya, M., and Ohbayashi, M. (1991). Phenotypic changes in hepatic mast cells accumulating around the metacestodes of *Taenia taeniaeformis* in rats, *Acta Pathol. Microbiol. Immunol. Scand.* **99,** 179–186.

Jezequel, A. M., Macari, G., Brunelli, E., and Orlandi, F. (1986). A hitherto undescribed component of the perisinusoidal space in normal human liver: The mast cell. *In* "Frontiers of Gastrointestinal Research", (P. Rozen, ed.), pp. 126–131. Karger, Basel.

Jones, A. L., and Altorfer, J. (1988). Immunological functions of the liver. *In* "Immunology of the Gastrointestinal Tract and Liver," M. F. Heyworth and A. L. Jones, eds.), pp. 159–171. Raven Press, New York.

Katona, I. M., Urban, J. F., and Finkelman, F. D. (1988). The role of L3T4+ and Lyt 2+ T cells in the IgE response and immunity to *Nippostongylus brasiliensis. J. Immunol.* **140,** 3206–3211.

King, S. J., and Miller, H. R. P. (1984). Anaphylactic release of mucosal mast cell protease and its relationship to gut permeability in *Nippostrongylus*-primed rats. *Immunology* **51,** 653–660.

Kiyono, H., Fujihashi, K., Taguchi, T., Aicher, W. K., and McGhee, J. R. (1991). Regulatory functions for murine intraepithelial lymphocytes in mucosal responses. *Immunol. Res.* **10,** 324–330.

Kvale, D., Lovhaug, D., Sollid, L. M., and Brandtzaeg, P. (1988). Tumor necrosis factor-α upregulates expression of secretory component, the epithelial receptor for polymeric Ig, *J. Immunol.* **140,** 3086–3089.

Lefrancois, L. (1991). Extrathymic differentiation of intraepithelial lymphocytes: Generation of a separate and unequal T cell repertoire. *Immunol. Today* **12,** 436–438.

Madden, K. B., Urban, J. F., Jr., Ziltener, H. J., Schrader, J. W., Finkelman, F. D., and Katona, I. M. (1991). Antibodies to IL-3 and IL-4 suppress helminth-induced intestinal mastocytosis. *J. Immunol.* **147,** 1387–1391.

Manning, R. J., Walker, P. G., Carter, L., Barrington, P. J., and Jackson, G. D. F. (1984). Studies on the origins of biliary immunoglobulins in rats. *Gastroenterology* **87,** 173–179.

Marshall, J. S., Bienenstock, J., Perdue, M. H., Stanisz, A. M., Stead, R. H., and Ernst, P. B. (1989). Novel cellular interactions and networks involving the intestinal immune system and its microenvironment. *Acta Pathol. Microbiol. Immunol. Scand.* **97,** 383–394.

Marzio, L., Blennerhassett, P., Chiverton, S., Vermillion, D. L., Langer, J., and Collins, S. M. (1990). Altered smooth muscle function in worm-free gut regions of *Trichinella*-infected rats. *Am. J. Physiol. Gastrointest. Liver Physiol.* **259,** G306–G313.

Mayer, L., Panja, A., and Li, Y. (1991). Antigen recognition in the gastrointestinal tract: Death to the dogma. *Immunol. Res.* **10,** 356–359.

Mazier, D., Renia, L., Nussler, A., Pied, S., Marussig, M., Goma, J., Grillot, D., Miltgen, F., Drapier, J. C., Corradin, G., Del Giudice, G., and Grau, G. E. (1990). A crucial role for liver nonparenchymal cells. *Immunol. Lett.* **25,** 65–70.

Mosmann, T. R., and Coffman, R. L. (1987). Two types of mouse helper T-cell clone. Implications for immune regulation. *Immunol. Today* **8,** 223–227.

Mosmann, T. R., and Moore, K. W. (1991). The role of IL-10 in crossregulation of T_H1 and T_H2 responses. *Immunol. Today* **12,** A49–A53.

Muller, M. J., Huizinga, J. D., and Collins, S. M. (1989). Altered smooth muscle contraction and sodium pump activity in the inflamed rat intestine. *Am. J. Physiol.* **257,** G570–G577.

Murphy, L. J., Bell, J. I., and Friesen, H. G. (1987). Tissue distribution of insulin-like growth factor I and II messenger ribonucleic acid in the adult rat. *Endocrinology* **120,** 1279–1282.

Nakatsukkasa, H., Nagy, P., Evarts, R. P., Hsia, C. C., Marsden, E., and Thorgeirsson, S. S. (1990). Cellular distribution of transforming growth factor-β1 and procollagen types I,II, and IV transcripts in carbon tetrachloride-induced rat liver fibrosis. *J. Clin. Invest.* **85,** 1833–1843.

Neutra, M. R., Phillips, T. L., Mayer, E. L., and Fishkind, D. J. (1987). Transport of membrane-bound macromolecules by M-cells in follicle associated epithelium of rabbit Peyer's patch. *Cell Tissue Res.* **247,** 537–546.

Northemann, W., Hattori, M., Baffet, G., Braciak, T. A., Fletcher, F. G., Abrahams, L. H., Gauldie, J., Baumann, M., and Fey, G. H. (1990). Production of interleukin-6 by hepatoma cells. *Mol. Biol. Med.* **7,** 273–285.

Nussler, A., Drapier, J. C., Renia, L., Pied, S., Miltgen, F., Gentilini, M., and Mazier, D. (1991). L-Arginine-dependent destruction of intrahepatic malaria parasites in response to tumor necrosis factor and/or interleukin-6 stimulation. *Eur. J. Immunol.* **21,** 227–230.

Owen, R. L., and Jones, A. L. (1974). Epithelial cell specialization within human Peyer's patches: An ultrastructural study of intestinal lymphoid follicles. *Gastroenterology* **66,** 189–203.

Palmer, J. M., and Castro, G. A. (1986). Anamnestic stimulus-specific myoelectrical responses associated with intestinal immunity in the rat. *Am. J. Physiol.* **250,** G266–G273.

Pappo, J., Steger, H. J., and Owen, R. L. (1988). Differential adherence of epithelium overlying gut-associated lymphoid tissue. An ultrastuctural study. *Lab. Invest.* **58,** 692–697.

Patrick, M. K., Dunn, T. J., Buret, A., Miller, H. R. P., Huntley, J. F., Gibson, S., and Gall, D. G. (1988). Mast cell protease release and mucosal ultrastructure during intestinal anaphylaxis in the rat. *Gastroenterology* **94,** 1–9.

Pearce, E. J., Caspar, P., Grzych, J.-M., Lewis, F. A., and Sher, A. (1991). Downregulation of Th1 cytokine production accompanies induction of Th2 responses by a parasitic helminth *Schistosoma mansoni. J. Exp. Med.* **173,** 159–166.

Phillips, J. O., Everson, M. P., Moldoveanu, Z., Lue, C., and Mestecky, J. (1990). Synergistic effect of IL-4 and IFN-gamma on the expression of polymeric Ig receptor (secretory component) and IgA binding by human epithelial cells. *J. Immunol.* **145,** 1740–1744.

Pond, L., Wassom, D. L., and Hayes, C. E. (1989). Evidence for differential induction of helper T cell subsets during *Trichinella spiralis* infection. *J. Immunol.* **143,** 4232–4237.

Qian, J. H., Hashimoto, T., Fujiwara, J., and Hamaoka, T. (1987). Studies on the induction of tolerance to alloantigens. I. The abrogation of potentials for delayed-type-hypersensitivity response to alloantigens by portal venous inoculation with allogeneic cells. *J. Immunol.* **134,** 3656–3661.

Richards, C., Gauldie, J., and Baumann, H. (1991). Cytokine control of acute phase protein expression. *Eur. Cytokine Net.* **2,** 89–98.

Ritchie, D. G. (1990). Interleukin-6 stimulates hepatic glucose release from prelabeled glycogen pools. *Am. J. Physiol.* **258,** E57–E64.

Rosenbaum, J., Mavier, P., Preaux, A. M., and Dhumeaux, D. (1989). Demonstration of a basic fibroblast growth factor-like molecule in mouse hepatic endothelial cells. *Biochem. Biophys. Res. Commun.* **164,** 1099–1104.

Schall, T. J. (1991). Biology of the RANTES/SIS cytokine family. *Cytokine* **3,** 165–183.

Sollid, L. M., Kvale, D., Brandtzaeg, P., Markussen, G., and Thorsby, E. (1987). Interferon gamma enhances expression of secretory component, the epithelial receptor for polymeric immunoglobulins. *J. Immunol.* **138,** 4303–4306.

Stadnyk, A. W., and Gauldie, J. (1991). The acute phase protein response during parasitic infection. *Immunoparasitology* **12,** A7–A12.

Street, N. E., Schumacher, J. H., Fong, T. A. T., Bass, H., Fiorentino, D. F., Leverah, J. A., and Mosmann, T. R. (1990). Heterogeneity of mouse helper T cells. Evidence from bulk cultures and limiting dilution cloning for precursors of Th1 and Th2 cells. *J. Immunol.* **144,** 1629–1639.

Strober, W., Harriman, G. R., and Kunimoto, D. R. (1991). Early steps of IgA B cell differentiation. *Immunol. Res.* **10,** 386–388.

Taguchi, T., McGhee, J. R., Coffman, R. L., Beagley, K. W., Eldridge, J. H., Takatsu, K., and Kiyono, H. (1990). Analysis of Th1 and Th2 cells in murine gut-associated tissues. Frequencies of CD4+ and CD8+ cells that secrete IFN gamma and IL-5. *J. Immunol.* **145,** 68–77.

Urban, J. F., Jr., Katona, I. M., Paul, W. E., and Finkelman, F. D. (1991). Interleukin 4 is important in protective immunity to a gastrointestinal nematode infection in mice. *Proc. Natl. Acad. Sci. U.S.A.* **88,** 5513–5517.

Vermillion, D. L., Ernst, P. B., Scicchitano, R., and Collins, S. M. (1989). Antigen-induced contraction of jejunal smooth muscle in the sensitized rat. *Am. J. Physiol.* **255,** G701–G708.

Vermillion, D., Ernst, P. B., and Collins, S. M. (1991). T lymphocyte modulation of intestinal muscle function in the *Trichinella* infected rat. *Am. J. Physiol. Gastrointest. Liver Physiol.* **101,** G701–G708.

Wang, J. M., Rambaldi, A., Biondi, A., Chen, Z. G., Sanderson, C. J., and Mantovani, A. (1989). Recombinant human interleukin 5 is a selective eosinophil chemoattractant. *Eur. J. Immunol.* **19,** 701–705.

Wright, N. A., Pike, C., and Elia, G. (1990). Induction of a novel epidermal growth factor-secreting cell lineage by mucosal ulceration in human gastrointestinal stem cells, *Nature (London)* **343,** 82–85.

Zhang, Z., and Michael, J. G. (1990). Orally inducible immune unresponsiveness is abrogated by IFN-γ treatment. *J. Immunol.* **144,** 4163–4165.

Zuraw, B. L., and Lotz, M. (1990). Regulation of the hepatic synthesis of C1 inhibitor by the hepatocyte stimulating factors interleukin-6 and interferon-γ. *J. Biol. Chem.* **265,** 12664–12670.

28

Cytotoxic Lymphocytes in Mucosal Effector Sites

Steven D. London

I. INTRODUCTION

Lymphocytes that express cytotoxic function are a major component of the immune system. Cytotoxic lymphocytes can be classified broadly into two groups based on their antigenic specificity. The first group is antigen specific and is thought to be involved in the rejection of tissues expressing nonself major histocompatability complex (MHC) antigens (alloantigens). Antigen-specific cytotoxic cells also are thought to be important in the elimination of cells infected with a wide number of intracellular pathogens via recognition of pathogen-specific antigens (nominal antigens) complexed with self MHC molecules. Antigen-specific cytotoxic T lymphocytes (CTL) are T-cell receptor bearing $CD3^+$ T lymphocytes. These cells are usually $CD8^+$ and are restricted by MHC Class I molecules. However, $CD4^+$ MHC Class II-restricted CTLs also have been found to exist as a subpopulation of CTLs. The second group of cytotoxic effector cells includes a variety of cell types that are not antigen or MHC restricted and often exist in the absence of specific infections or diseased states. In this chapter, I review the cytotoxic lymphocyte compartment of mucosal tissues with emphasis on antigen-specific cytotoxic cells. Although the primary focus of this review is the CTLs, a description of nonspecific cytotoxic cells in mucosal tissues is also included. The presence of nonspecific cytotoxic cells in mucosal tissues may indicate that they play a functional role in protection of mucosal areas. In addition, their presence should be appreciated since they can complicate the detection of specific cytotoxic effector cells in specific CTL assays.

II. NONSPECIFIC CYTOTOXIC CELLS IN GUT MUCOSAL TISSUES

Several different types of nonspecific cytotoxic cell have been described based on target preference, surface phenotype, and responsiveness to various biological factors. Natural killer cells (NK) lyse Yac-1 targets and express asialo-GM1, NK-1 antigen, and low levels of Thy 1 antigen. These cells are responsive to interferon and interleukin 2 (IL-2) *in vitro* (Welsh, 1984; Brooks and Henney, 1985). Natural cytotoxic cells (NC) lyse WEHI-164 targets, are negative for the NK cell markers, and are responsive to IL-2 and IL-3 *in vitro* (Stutman *et al.*, 1978; Lattime *et al.*, 1983). Spontaneously cytotoxic T lymphocytes (SC) were described initially as arising from splenocytes cultured in the absence of mitogen, antigen, or interleukins. These cells bear high levels of Thy 1 and lyse P-815 cells (Ching *et al.*, 1977). The origin of and interrelationship among these cytotoxic cells is not clear, and is complicated by observations of the breakdown in specificity of cultured antigen-specific CTLs (Wilson and Shortman, 1984). The levels of these types of nonspecific cytotoxic activity have been analyzed in various mucosal lymphoid populations. Peyer's patch lymphocytes obtained from conventionally reared mice have been shown to contain undetectable levels of cytotoxic activity to the NK-sensitive target Yac-1 in 4-hr (Tagliabue *et al.*, 1981,1983/1984) or 16-hr (Tagliabue *et al.*, 1983/1984) ^{51}Cr release assays. NK activity was not induced by a 24-hr incubation of Peyer's patch lymphocytes with a source of IL-2 or IL-3 (Tagliabue *et al.*, 1983/1984). However, the incubation of Peyer's patch lymphocytes with irradiated peritoneal exudate cells and 10% concanavalin A (Con A)-conditioned medium has been shown to result in the generation of cytotoxic activity to Yac-1 target cells (London *et al.*, 1986). These results may be analogous to the observation that Peyer's patches lack terminally differentiated B cells (plasma cells) although they are capable of generating antibody secreting cells in *in vitro* cultures (Kiyono *et al.*, 1982). In contrast to NK cytotoxicity, normal Peyer's patch lymphocytes lyse the NC-sensitive target WEHI-164 in 16-hr ^{51}Cr release assays. Peyer's patch lymphocytes have higher levels of NC activity than either spleen or peripheral lymph node lymphocytes (Tagliabue *et al.*, 1983/1984). Peyer's patch lymphocytes obtained from conventionally reared mice also were found to contain a population of novel naturally cytotoxic effector cells that have been termed natural cytotoxic T cells (NCTC) (Gautam *et al.*, 1986). NCTC effector cells were able to lyse a wide variety of syngeneic and allogeneic tumor cell lines as well as syngeneic or allogeneic Con A-induced T lymphoblasts. These cells are characterized as plastic nonadherent, nylon wool adherent Thy 1^+ Ia^+ asialo-$GM1^+$ T cells (Gautam *et al.*, 1986) and have been identified in several inbred strains of mice. Of all lymphoid tissues tested, only Peyer's patch lymphocytes were found to contain NCTC activity.

In addition to Peyer's patch lymphocytes, intraepithelial lymphocytes (IEL) have been analyzed for the presence of naturally occurring cytotoxic cells. NC (Tagliabue *et al.*, 1983/1984) activity has been observed in purified populations of unprimed IELs. Whereas IELs of normal mice do not express cytotoxicity toward the SC target P-815 (Goodman and Lefrancois, 1988), such cytotoxicity can be elicited *in vitro* by culturing IELs in the presence of Con A-conditioned medium (Ernst *et al.*, 1985) or *in vivo* after immunization by the combined feeding and parenteral inoculation of allogeneic splenocytes or tumor cells (Klein and Kagnoff, 1984). The literature regarding the presence of NK cytotoxicity among IELs is more complex, with some reports of this activity in normal mice (Petit *et al.*, 1985; Tagliabue *et al.*, 1981,1982, 1983/1984; Klein, 1986) and some reports of this activity only in mice experimentally stimulated with allogeneic splenocytes or tumor cells (Klein and Kagnoff, 1984; Carman *et al.*, 1986; Goodman and Lefrancois, 1988). The inconsistent finding of NK activity in isolated IELs may be related to differences in environmental conditions. For example, specific pathogen-free mice and germ-free mice, compared with conventionally reared mice, have lower numbers of IELs and phenotypically altered IEL populations (Carman *et al.*, 1986; Lefrancois and Goodman, 1989; Guy-Grand *et al.*, 1991a). Utilizing an antigen nonspecific "redirected" cytotoxicity assay, some investigators have reported that the cytotoxic potential of IELs is unrelated to gut antigen stimulation (Guy-Grand *et al.*, 1991b) whereas others have shown a striking environmental influence on the cytotoxic potential of particular IEL subpopulations (Lefrancois and Goodman, 1989). The redirected cytotoxicity assay has demonstrated clearly that IELs from conventionally reared mice are constitutively lytic (Lefrancois and Goodman, 1989; Viney *et al.*, 1990; Guy-Grand *et al.*, 1991b). Thus, environmental factors may have a strong influence on the nature and immune potential of IELs, so these factors should be considered in the planning and interpretation of experiments involving IELs. In addition, these results suggest that the activation of nonspecific cytotoxic effector populations that occurs during an antigen-specific response may be a nonspecific defense mechanism that is important for the protection of the gut mucosa from infection with environmental pathogens.

The cytotoxic lymphocyte response to gut mucosal infection with an enteric murine coronavirus, mouse hepatitis virus (MHV), has been analyzed. Although an antigen-specific CTL response was not detected, a novel non-MHC-restricted cytotoxic IEL effector cell population has been identified that is highly cytotoxic to target cells infected with this virus (Carman *et al.*, 1986). These predominantly asialo-GM1$^+$ Thy 1$^-$ Lyt 1$^-$ Lyt 2$^-$ cytotoxic effector cells were present in immune and normal mice. Elimination of asialo-GM1$^+$ cells *in vivo* resulted in an increased persistence of virus in gut tissues as well as decreased cytotoxic activity of isolated IELs to MHV infection *in vitro* (Carman *et al.*, 1986). Although MHV-specific CTLs have been difficult to demonstrate and MHV-specific CTL clones have been obtained only recently (Yamaguchi *et al.*, 1988), antibody-independent B lymphocyte-mediated lysis of MHV-infected cells has been shown to occur (Wysocka *et al.*, 1989). This lysis is likely to be mediated by selective fusion of B lymphocytes and MHV-infected cells, facilitated by the neutral pH membrane-fusing activity of MHV E2 protein. Note that a similar mechanism of nonspecific cytolysis may control MHV infection at mucosal surfaces and that this activity is carried out by a unique cell population present only in the intestinal epithelium.

III. GUT MUCOSAL CYTOTOXIC T LYMPHOCYTES

A. Allospecific Cytotoxic T Lymphocytes

Kagnoff and Campbell (1974) were the first to demonstrate that Peyer's patch lymphocytes express CTL activity by generating allogeneic specific CTLs in secondary mixed lymphocyte reaction (MLR) of cultured Peyer's patch lymphocytes from normal mice. The precursor CTLs were identified as T cells by pretreatment with anti-theta serum and complement (Kagnoff and Campbell, 1974). Intraperitoneal injection or chronic feeding of MHC disparate tumor cells (EL-4 cells into BALB/c mice) was found to increase the level of allogeneic cytotoxicity developed in secondary MLR cultures of primed rather than normal Peyer's patch lymphocytes, suggesting that the gut mucosal application of stimulator cells results in an increase in precursor frequency (Kagnoff, 1978). In contrast to tumor cells bearing major MHC differences, tumor cells bearing minor MHC differences induced a CTL response in Peyer's patches after intrapeitonael priming but not after chronic feeding (Kagnoff, 1978).

The intraperitoneal injection of allogeneic tumor cells has been shown to generate allogeneic specific CTLs recoverable from IELs and lamina propria lymphocytes (LPL) 6–11 days after immunization (Davies and Parrott, 1980,1981; Parrott *et al.*, 1983). This cytotoxic activity was observed without re-stimulation of isolated effector cells in an *in vitro* MLR. Control mice do not respond to allogeneic targets, and the subcutaneous route of immunization does not generate high levels of CTL activity in the gut mucosa (Davies and Parrott, 1981; Parrott *et al.*, 1983). LPLs contained the highest levels of cytotoxic activity of all tissues tested after intraperitoneal immunization; this cytotoxicity lasted for prolonged periods (>40 days; Parrott *et al.*, 1983). The phenotype of both alloantigen-specific effectors and precursor CTLs (pCTLs) generated *in vitro* in primary isolated IEL MLR cultures was shown to be Thy 1$^+$ Lyt 2$^+$ (Ernst *et al.*, 1986). The frequency of alloantigen-specific pCTLs was found to be approximately threefold higher among unfractionated splenocytes than in isolated IELs (Ernst *et al.*, 1986).

Alloantigen-specific CTL clones have been obtained from isolated IELs derived from BALB/c mice that were immunized twice, intragastrically and intraperitoneally, with allogeneic tumor cells (EL-4) (Klein *et al.*, 1985; Klein and Kagnoff, 1987). Two types of effector clone were generated: (1) clones that were antigen specific with respect to proliferation and cytolytic activity and (2) clones that were antigen specific for proliferation but were not cytolytic when maintained in 4% Con A-conditioned medium. When cultured in the presence of 25% Con A-conditioned medium for 4 days, these clones exhibited broad lytic potential and were cytotoxic for EL-4 cells, P-815 cells (SC), and Yac-1 cells (NK), as well as for syngeneic and allogeneic lipopolysaccharide

(LPS) blasts. Although one clone (D3) was reported lytic for syngeneic LPS blasts, it does not lyse itself when ^{51}Cr-labeled D3 cells are used as targets. The phenotype of both types of clones was Thy 1$^+$ Lyt 2$^+$ (Klein *et al.*, 1985; Klein and Kagnoff, 1987). These broadly cytotoxic clones may be an *in vitro* counterpart of the broadly cytotoxic NCTC cells observed in normal Peyer's patches. The presence of broadly cytotoxic cells in gut mucosal tissues might be one mechanism by which mucosal tissues are protected from infection with particular intracellular pathogens.

B. Vaccinia Virus-Specific Cytotoxic T Lymphocytes

Although early studies have indicated that gut mucosal tissues have the capability to contain CTLs, whether mucosal application of antigen is a necessary prerequisite for the generation of CTL activity in these tissues is not clear. Further, the generation of allospecific CTLs with precursors that are present at an extremely high frequency (Lindahl and Wilson, 1977) may not be a good indication of the potential of Peyer's patches to generate CTL activity directed to nominal antigens associated with environmentally encountered pathogens. Gut mucosal infection with vaccinia virus has provided direct evidence that some gut associated tissue contains virus-specific CTLs. After enteric injection, mesenteric lymph node lymphocytes had a strong vaccinia-specific T helper cell and CTL response (Issekutz, 1984). Vaccinia-specific T helper cell and CTL responses were not observed in Peyer's patches. Since Peyer's patches are one source of lymphocytes that migrate to the mesenteric lymph nodes, one interpretation of these results is that Peyer's patches are an inductive site from which virus-specific Th cells and CTLs were stimulated. In this scenario, the absence of detection of these cells in Peyer's patches is a consequence of their rapid migration to mesenteric lymph nodes.

C. Reovirus-Specific Cytotoxic T Lymphocytes

Reovirus serotype 1, strain Lang (reovirus 1/L), is a naturally occurring enteric virus that is stable within the gastrointestinal tract (Sabin, 1959; Rubin and Fields, 1980). The observation that reovirus 1/L preferentially binds to and is transported from the intestinal lumen into Peyer's patches through microfold (M) cells (Wolf *et al.*, 1981,1983) and its ability to stimulate the appearance of IgA-committed memory cells in Peyer's patches and distal lymphoid tissues after intraduodenal immunization (London *et al.*, 1986) suggest that reovirus 1/L is an effective mucosal immunogen. Further, the marked expansion of cells expressing the GCT antigen (an antigen present on subpopulations of CD8$^+$ T and germinal center B cells) after a single intraduodenal application of reovirus 1/L provides additional evidence of the ability of reovirus 1/L to stimulate Peyer's patch T and B cell subpopulations acutely (London *et al.*, 1990).

In studies aimed at analyzing the potential of gut mucosal tissues to generate virus-specific CTLs, researchers found that a single intraduodenal application of reovirus 1/L generates the appearance of detectable levels of virus-specific cytotoxicity in Peyer's patch and mesenteric lymph node lymphocytes on *in vitro* re-stimulation (London *et al.*, 1986). Although this was the first demonstration of virus-specific pCTLs in Peyer's patches, these results confirm those found with vaccinia virus infection and offer further support that the CTL response observed in mesenteric lymph nodes in both systems may have originated from migrating Peyer's patch lymphocytes. Peyer's patch effectors show the surface phenotype of CTLs (Thy 1$^+$ Lyt 2$^+$), are MHC restricted, and are virus-specific (London *et al.*, 1986). In addition, the phenotype of the pCTLs prior to their *in vitro* stimulation also was shown to be Thy 1$^+$ Lyt 2$^+$ (London *et al.*, 1990). Although the virus-specific cytotoxic cells derived from Peyer's patches were found not to be selective for the immunizing serotype of reovirus, as was reported previously for nonmucosal lymphocytes (Finberg *et al.*, 1979), they were not cross-reactive with unrelated virus antigens (London *et al.*, 1986). The lack of serotype specificity was found not to be unique to Peyer's patch-derived lymphocytes but also was displayed by intraperitoneally primed splenocytes (London *et al.*, 1986,1989a) and is similar to the CTL response observed with a number of other viruses, including two other members of the Reoviridae family of viruses: blue-tongue virus (Jeggo and Wardley, 1982) and Group A rotavirus (Offit and Dudzik, 1988) (see subsequent discussion).

Since reovirus-specific pCTLs have been demonstrated in Peyer's patches, determining whether they were generated locally or whether they represent a population of lymphocytes stimulated elsewhere that have localized preferentially in the patch was of interest. Two observations suggest that the former possibility occurs: (1) Peyer's patches contain virus-specific helper activity that has been shown to be required for the generation of effector CTLs on *in vitro* re-stimulation in the reovirus system (London *et al.*, 1986) and (2) significantly higher levels of virus-specific cytotoxicity are generated from cultures of Peyer's patches than from peripheral lymph nodes 2–6 days after intraduodenal immunization (London *et al.*, 1986). The frequency of reovirus-specific pCTLs in these tissues was confirmed directly. A 100-fold difference in frequency (1675/10^6 CD8$^+$ Peyer's patch lymphocytes vs. 17/10^6 peripheral lymph node CD8$^+$ lymphocytes) was found 6 days after enteric immunization. In addition, the gradient of pCTLs that initially was established early after infection was found to exist for a prolonged period after the single intraduodenal injection of reovirus 1/L. The frequency of pCTLs was an order of magnitude greater in Peyer's patches than in peripheral lymph nodes (14.5-fold higher; 1235/10^6 CD8$^+$ vs. 85/10^6 CD8$^+$) 6 months after reovirus infection (London *et al.*, 1986).

In addition to the pCTLs in Peyer's patches, virus-specific pCTLs also occur as a component of the IEL compartment. MHC Class I antigen-restricted reovirus-specific effector CTLs are generated from *in vitro* cultured IELs 1 week after the intraduodenal application of reovirus 1/L (London *et al.*, 1989b). IEL effectors have been shown to be Thy 1$^+$ CD8$^+$ lymphocytes, and reovirus-specific IEL pCTLs also are likely to express the Thy 1 antigen (C. Cuff, D. H. Rubin, and J. J. Cebra, unpublished observation). The frequencies of pCTLs in the epithelial and Peyer's patch lymphoid compartments are similar (100–300/10^6 $CD8^+$ Peyer's patch lymphocytes vs. 50–200/10^6 $CD8^+$ IEL lymphocytes) 1 week after intraduodenal immunization (Cebra *et al.*, 1991). IEL pCTLs have been observed to persist for up to 4 weeks (Cebra *et al.*, 1991; C. Cuff, D. H. Rubin, and J. J. Cebra, unpublished observation). Since IELs are an enriched source of $\gamma\delta$ T-cell receptor (TcR)-bearing lymphocytes, determining whether IEL reovirus-specific effector or precursor CTLs expressed this or the more common $\alpha\beta$ TcR was of interest. Collectively, the following observations strongly suggest the latter: (1) >90% of TcR^+ cells express the $\alpha\beta$ TcR in *in vitro* cultured IEL preparations that also have been shown to contain reovirus-specific cytotoxic activity; (2) oral infection of germ-free mice with reovirus 1/L results in a marked increase of $\alpha\beta$-expressing lymphocytes in the epithelium that can be stimulated *in vitro* to generate reovirus-specific CTLs; and (3) adoptive transfer of normal Peyer's patch lymphocytes to mice that harbor the severe combined immunodeficiency defect (SCID), followed by oral reovirus infection 2 days later, results in an increase in the number of IELs, many of which express the $\alpha\beta$ TcR (Cebra *et al.*, 1991; C. Cuff, D. H. Rubin, and J. J. Cebra, unpublished observation).

The ability of adoptively transferred Peyer's patch lymphocytes to respond to reovirus infection and repopulate the gut epithelium of SCID mice confirms studies suggesting that Peyer's patch lymphocytes are able to populate the gut epithelium with thymodependent lymphocytes (Guy-Grand *et al.*, 1991a, and references therein). In addition, the adoptive transfer of reovirus-immune Peyer's patch lymphocytes into SCID mice prevents the establishment of a disseminated infection in these immunodeficient mice (George *et al.*, 1990). The transfer of $CD8^+$ GCT^+ reovirus-immune Peyer's patch lymphocytes, but not naive lymphocytes or B cells, contains disseminated reovirus infection in SCID mice 1 week after challenge (A. George, D. H. Rubin, and J. J. Cebra, unpublished observation). Thus, this cell population, which has been shown to include both reovirus-specific precursor and effector CTLs (London *et al.*, 1990), contains virus-specific effector cells that are functionally relevant and important in the containment of virus infections *in vivo*. Similarly, the adoptive transfer of reovirus-immune Thy 1^+ $CD8^+$ IELs confers protection on neonatal mice when challenged with a lethal neurotropic strain of reovirus (Cuff *et al.*, 1991).

The presence of precursors for virus-specific CTLs, diffusely scattered in the intestinal epithelium, and the ability of enterically applied reovirus 1/L to generate a CTL response in Peyer's patches that can persist for many months demonstrates that a CTL response exists among the repertoire of immune responses that can occur in Peyer's patches and the gut epithelium. For viruses that initially impinge on the wet epithelium, the presence of virus-specific CTLs and natural effector (i.e., NK) cells at this location could result in the local containment, limitation, and resolution of the infectious agent rather than its dissemination. The ability to mount a mucosal CTL response may be advantageous to the host, because local containment could prevent sequelae associated with infection at distal sites.

D. Rotavirus-Specific Cytotoxic T Lymphocytes

Gut mucosal infection with rotavirus provides another informative viral stimulus for the study of gut mucosal immunity. Rotaviruses, like reoviruses, are members of the Reoviridae family of nonenveloped doubled-stranded RNA viruses. These viruses share similar structural features and replicative strategies, yet their interaction with the gut mucosa is strikingly different. Whereas reovirus infection of the gut mucosa is a potent stimulator of virus-specific and nonspecific responses, the virus infection is subclinical and is resolved in the gut within 10–12 days (Cebra *et al.*, 1991). In contrast, gut mucosal infection with rotavirus results in a generalized infection of small intestinal villous epithelial cells and can cause acute viral gastroenteritis in humans and animals (Offit and Dudzik, 1989a, and references therein).

Infection of mice with several strains of rotavirus is a potent inducer of virus-specific CTLs. Rotavirus infection by either oral or parenteral route elicits effector CTLs in multiple lymphoid tissues that can be detected without *in vitro* amplification (Offit and Dudzik, 1988,1989b; Offit and Svoboda, 1989; Offit *et al.*, 1991b). Effector and precursor CTLs are serotype nonspecific Thy 1^+ $CD8^+$ lymphocytes (Offit and Dudzik, 1988,1989b; Offit and Svoboda, 1989; Dharakul *et al.*, 1991; Offit *et al.*, 1991a). Although these effectors usually are elicited by infection with replicating virus, inoculation with noninfectious virus has been shown to be capable of eliciting rotavirus-specific CTLs (Offit and Dudzik, 1989a).

The tissue distribution of rotavirus-specific CTLs has been analyzed after various routes of immunization. The salient observations from these studies follow: (1) Six days after oral immunization, effector CTLs were detected among Peyer's patch, mesenteric lymph node, LPL, spleen, and IEL lymphocyte populations (Offit and Dudzik, 1989b; Offit *et al.*, 1991b). (2) Six days after intraperitoneal or subcutaneous immunization, effector CTLs were detected among Peyer's patch, mesenteric lymph node, LPL, spleen, and peripheral lymph node lymphocytes. Effector CTLs were observed in IELs after intraperitoneal but not subcutaneous immunization (Offit and Dudzik, 1989b; Offit *et al.*,1991b). (3) Four weeks after oral, intraperitoneal, or subcutaneous immunization, pCTLs (as assayed by *in vitro* culture) were detected in Peyer's patch, mesenteric lymph node, LPL, spleen, and peripheral lymph node but not IEL lymphocyte populations (Offit and Dudzik, 1989b; Offit *et al.*, 1991b). (4) IEL effector CTLs obtained from orally infected mice were shown to be $CD3^+$ and express the $\alpha\beta$ form of the TcR (Offit *et al.*, 1991b). (5) When the frequency of pCTLs was analyzed 3, 6, and 21 days after immunization, the site of rotavirus infection determined that pCTL first appeared in Peyer's patch and mesenteric lymph nodes three days after oral infection. Three days after footpad infection, pCTLs were detected first in the inguinal peripheral lymph node. At six days, pCTLs were 30-fold higher in Peyer's patches after oral infection and ~7-fold higher in inginual peripheral lymph node after footpad infection. However, by 21 days, pCTLs were distributed uniformly throughout the lymphoid system (with the exception of IEL), regardless of the route of immunization (Offit and Dudzik, 1988; Offit *et al.*, 1991b). Thus, in contrast to results obtained with gut mucosal reovirus infection, which suggested that the route of immunization may be important for the generation and maintenance of a gut mucosal CTL response, the route of immunization with rotavirus does not appear to be as important for the generation of disseminated gut mucosal responses. The lack of persistence of rotavirus-specific pCTLs in the epithelium also contrasts with results obtained with gut mucosal reovirus infection. These discrepancies are likely to be the results of differences in virus dissemination and interaction with the immune system, and suggest that different strategies for particular mucosal pathogens may be devised that elicit protective T-cell immunity at mucosal surfaces.

The potential functional relevance of rotavirus-specific CTLs has been demonstrated in two animal model systems. In the first example, Thy 1^+ $CD8^+$ splenocytes obtained from intraperitoneally immunized mice passively protect suckling mice against diarrhea induced by rotavirus challenge (Offit and Dudzik, 1990). In the second, rotavirus infection was cleared in SCID mice after the transfer of immune $CD8^+$ splenic lymphocytes from intraperitoneally immunized histocompatible mice (Dharakul *et al.*, 1990,1991). Interestingly, $CD8^+$ immune splenocytes or Thy 1^+ $CD8^+$ IELs obtained from orally immunized mice only temporarily cleared rotavirus infection of SCID mice (Dharakul *et al.*, 1990,1991). Whether the suboptimal ability of orally immunized spleen and IELs to contain rotavirus infection in SCID mice is a result of intrinsic differences in cell population after oral or intraperitoneal immunization or is simply a technical problem remains to be resolved.

IV. PULMONARY CYTOTOXIC CELLS

The lung is another mucosal site that has been shown to contain nonspecific and specific cytotoxic effector cells. Natural killer cell activity is normally present in the lung and is enhanced after influenza infection in mice (Wyde *et al.*, 1977). Seven days after infection with influenza virus, $\gamma\delta$ TcR-expressing cells are found to predominate in the lungs of mice (Carding *et al.*, 1990). Although these cells are not constitutively cytotoxic when recovered directly from the respiratory tract, cytotoxic function can be induced by culturing them in the presence of monoclonal antibody to CD3 and low concentrations of IL-2 (Eichelberger *et al.*, 1991a). Although the function of these $\gamma\delta$ TcR-expressing cells remains an enigma, they may have a role in the containment and resolution of infections in the lung by either cytolytic or noncytolytic (i.e., secretion of cytokines) mechanisms.

Antigen-specific CTLs also have been shown to be a component of the immune repertoire of the lung. Immunization with allogeneic tumor cells by both the intratrachial and the intraperitoneal route have resulted in the accumulation of alloantigen-specific CTLs in the lung and spleen (Liu *et al.*, 1982, and references therein). Viral-specific CTLs also are generated after pulmonary infection with several viruses that replicate in the respiratory epithelium. For example, influenza virus-specific precursor and effector CTLs are found in the lung shortly after intratrachial infection (Bennink *et al.*, 1978; Ennis *et al.*, 1978; Yap *et al.*, 1978a; Allan *et al.*, 1990). The ability of adoptively transferred influenza virus-specific CTLs to limit viral replication in the pulmonary tract has been shown (Yap *et al.*, 1978b; Lukacher *et al.*, 1984; Taylor and Askonas, 1986). However, recent data suggest that CTLs are not the sole effectors capable of terminating influenza infection. For example, adoptive transfer of influenza virus-specific MHC Class II-restricted Th clones allows athymic mice to recover from pulmonary influenza virus infection in the absence of MHC Class I-restricted CTLs (Scherle *et al.*, 1992). Clearance of influenza virus infection also has been reported in normal mice depleted of $CD8^+$ T cells *in vivo* and in transgenic mice, homozygous for a β_2-microglobulin gene disruption, that lack functional Class I MHC glycoproteins and $CD8^+$ $\alpha\beta^+$ T cells (Eichelberger *et al.*, 1991b). Pulmonary infection with respiratory syncytial virus (RSV) also has been shown to elicit the generation of precursor and effector CTLs in the lungs and spleen of mice (Bangham *et al.*, 1985; Taylor *et al.*, 1985; Gupta *et al.*,1990). The appearance of $CD8^+$ lymphocytes in the lungs of RSV-infected mice correlates with the elimination of infectious virus from the pulmonary tract (Kimpen *et al.*, 1991). *In vivo* depletion of $CD8^+$ T cells suggests that their presence is important for the cessation of viral replication in the lung (Graham *et al.*, 1991). In a number of studies, the transfer of RSV-specific CTLs has been shown to be capable of clearing virus from the lungs of mice (Cannon *et al.*, 1987; Munoz *et al.*, 1991; Nicholas *et al.*, 1991; Trudel *et al.*, 1991). Although transferred CTLs limit viral replication in the pulmonary tract, some studies have correlated their transfer with increased pulmonary disease (Cannon *et al.*, 1988; Graham *et al.*, 1991).

V. CONCLUSIONS

The idea that both antigen-specific and nonspecific cytotoxic cells are an integral component of mucosal tissues is becoming increasingly evident. Although much research has focused on the gastrointestinal and respiratory tracts, cytotoxic cells are likely to be components of the immune repertoire of other mucosal tissues. The specifics of the cytotoxic response are likely to vary depending on the nature and location of the immune stimulus. For example, studies of the eye have revealed site-specific immunoregulation of CTL development and have demonstrated the presence of the less commonly observed $CD4^+$ MHC Class II-restricted CTLs in mucosal tissues. In the eye, the placement of tumor cells in two anatomically distinct regions (anterior chamber and subconjunctiva) elicits tumor-specific pCTLs (Ksander and Streilein, 1990, and references therein). However, the pCTLs differentiate into cytotoxic effector CTLs only in the subconjunctiva, thereby allowing tumor rejection to occur only in this site. Recurrent herpes simplex virus-1 (HSV-1) infection of the corneal stroma of the eye often results in stromal pathology and, ultimately, in vision impairment. HSV-1-specific MHC Class II-restricted CD4$^+$ CTLs have been implicated as constituting one of the mechanisms leading to stromal immunopathology in herpetic infections (Doymaz *et al.*, 1991).

A better understanding of how to stimulate cytotoxic cells in mucosal tissues, their recirculation pathways between mucosal and systemic tissues, and their function in mucosal sites is warranted since these cells may limit pathogens or may be involved in pathogenesis at mucosal sites. The series of observations that CTLs are elicited in response to a number of nonviral intracellular pathogens suggests that such cells might be a more generalized component of the immune system. CTL responses have been identified for the protozoan parasites *Leishmania* (Smith *et al.*, 1991) and *Toxoplasma gondii* (Hakim *et al.*, 1991; Khan *et al.*, 1991), for malaria *Plasmodium berghei* circumsporozoite protein (Aggarwal *et al.*, 1990, and references therein), and for the gram-positive bacterium *Listeria monocytogenes* (Pamer *et al.*, 1991). In studies of immunity to malaria, researchers found that oral immunization with attenuated *Salmonella typhimurium* recombinants containing the full-length *P. bergehei* circumsporozoite gene induces protective immunity against intravenous sporozoite challenge in the absence of antibodies. Immunity was found to be mediated through the induction of circumsporozoite-specific CD8$^+$ CTLs (Aggarwal *et al.*, 1990). Thus, the mucosal application of *S. typhimurium,* a bacterium known to interact with Peyer's patches, is capable of inducing a systemic CTL response that can control heterologous infections. This elegant study suggests that oral *Salmonella* vectors may be useful for the generation of specific CTL responses, which may be useful for the containment of viral or nonviral infections of mucosal or systemic tissues.

Acknowledgments

The author would like to thank Drs. John J. Cebra, Donald H. Rubin, Christopher F. Cuff, and Anna George for providing unpublished data for this chapter.

References

Aggarwal, A., Kumar, S., Jaffe, R., Hone, D., Gross, M., and Sadoff, J. (1990). Oral *Salmonella:* Malaria circumsporozoite recombinants induce specific CD8$^+$ cytotoxic T cells. *J. Exp. Med.* **172,** 1083–1090.

Allan, W., Tabi, Z., Cleary, A., and Doherty, P. C. (1990). Cellular events in the lymph node and lung of mice with influenza. Consequences of depleting CD4$^+$ T cells. *J. Immunol.* **144,** 3980–3986.

Bangham, C. R. M., Cannon, M. J., Karzon, D. T., and Askonas, B. A. (1985). Cytotoxic T-cell response to respiratory syncytial virus in mice. *J. Virol.* **56,** 55–59.

Bennink, J., Effros, R. B., and Doherty, P. C. (1978). Influenza pneumonia: Early appearance of cross reactive T cells in lungs of mice primed with heterologous type A viruses. *Immunology* **35,** 503–509.

Brooks, C. G., and Henney, C. S. (1985). Interleukin-2 and the regulation of natural killer activity in cultured cell populations. *Contemp. Top. Mol. Immunol.* **10,** 63–92.

Cannon, M. J., Stott, E. J., Taylor, G., and Askonas, B. A. (1987). Clearance of persistent respiratory syncytial virus infections in immunodeficient mice following transfer of primed T cells. *Immunology* **62,** 133–138.

Cannon, M. J., Openshaw, P. J. M., and Askonas, B. A. (1988). Cytotoxic T cells clear virus but augment lung pathology in mice infected with respiratory syncytial virus. *J. Exp. Med.* **168,** 1163–1168.

Carding, S. R., Allan, W., Kyes, S., Hayday, A., Bottomly, K., and Doherty, P. C. (1990). Late dominance of the inflammatory process in murine influenza by $\gamma/\delta+$ T cells. *J. Exp. Med.* **172,** 1225–1231.

Carman, P. S., Ernst, P. B., Rosenthal, K. L., Clark, D. A., Befus, A. D., and Bienenstock, J. (1986). Intraepithelial leukocytes contain a unique subpopulation of NK-like cytotoxic cells active in the defense of gut epithelium to enteric murine coronavirus. *J. Immunol.* **136,** 1548–1553.

Cebra, J. J., Cuff, C. F., and Rubin, D. H. (1991). Relationship between alpha/beta T cell receptor/CD8$^+$ precursors for cytotoxic T lymphocytes in the murine Peyer's patches and the intraepithelial compartment probed by oral infection with reovirus. *Immunol. Res.* **10,** 321–323.

Ching, L. M., Marbrook, J., and Walker, K. Z. (1977). Spontaneous clones of cytotoxic T cells in culture. I. Characteristics of the response. *Cell. Immunol.* **31,** 284–292.

Cuff, C. F., Cebra, C. K., Lavi, E., Molowitz, E. H., Rubin, D. H., and Cebra, J. J. (1991). Protection of neonatal mice from fatal reovirus infection by immune serum and gut derived lymphocytes. *In* "Immunology of Milk and the Neonate" (J. Mestecky, C. Blair, and P. L. Ogra, eds.), pp. 307–315. Plenum Press, New York.

Davies, M. D. J., and Parrott, D. M. V. (1980). The early appearance of specific cytotoxic T cells in murine gut mucosa. *Clin. Exp. Immunol.* **42,** 273–279.

Davies, M. D. J., and Parrott, D. M. V. (1981). Cytotoxic T cells in small intestine epithelial, lamina propria and lung lymphocytes. *Immunology* **44,** 367–371.

Dharakul, T., Rott, L., and Greenberg, H. B. (1990). Recovery from chronic rotavirus infection in mice with severe combined immunodeficiency: Virus clearance mediated by adoptive transfer of immune CD8$^+$ T lymphocytes. *J. Virol.* **64,** 4375–4382.

Dharakul, T., Labbe, M., Cohen, J., Bellamy, A. R., Street, J. E., Mackow, E. R., Fiore, L., Rott, L., and Greenberg, H. B. (1991). Immunization with baculovirus-expressed recombinant rotavirus proteins VP1, VP4, VP6, and VP7 induces CD8$^+$ T lymphocytes that mediate clearance of chronic rotavirus infection in SCID mice. *J. Virol.* **65,** 5928–5932.

Doymaz, M. Z., Foster, C. M., Destephano, D., and Rouse, B. T. (1991). MHC II-restricted, CD4$^+$ cytotoxic T lymphocytes specific for herpes simplex virus-1: Implications for the development of herpetic stromal keratitis in mice. *Clin. Immunol. Immunopathol.* **61,** 398–409.

Eichelberger, M., Allan, W., Carding, S. R., Bottomly, K., and Doherty, P. C. (1991a). Activation status of the CD4$^-$8$^-$ $\gamma\delta$-T cells recovered from mice with influenza pneumonia. *J. Immunol.* **147,** 2069–2074.

Eichelberger, M., Allan, W., Zijlstra, M., Jaenisch, R., and Doherty, P. C. (1991b). Clearance of influenza virus respiratory infection in mice lacking Class I major histocompatibility compelx-restricted CD8$^+$ T cells. *J. Exp. Med.* **174,** 875–880.

Ennis, F. A., Wells, M. A., Butchko, G. M., and Albrecht, P. (1978). Evidence that cytotoxic T cells are part of the host's response to influenza penumonia. *J. Exp. Med.* **148,** 1241–1250.

Ernst, P. B., Petit, A., Befus, A. D. Clark, D. A. Rosenthal, K. L., Ishizaka, T., and Bienenstock, J. (1985). Murine intestinal intraepithelial lymphocytes II. Comparison of freshly isolated and cultured intraepithelial lymphocytes. *Eur. J. Immunol.* **15,** 216–221.

Ernst, P. B., Clark, D. A., Rosenthal, K. L., Befus, A. D., and Bienenstock, J. (1986). Detection and characterization of cytotoxic T lymphocyte precursors in the murine intestinal intraepithelial leukocyte population. *J. Immunol.* **136,** 2121–2126.

Finberg, R., Weiner, H. L., Fields, B. N., Benacerraf, B., and Burakoff, S. J. (1979). Generation of cytolytic T lymphocytes after reovirus infection: Role of S1 gene. *Proc. Natl. Acad. Sci U.S.A.* **76,** 442–446.

Gautam, S. C., Beckman, K., and Batisto, J. R. (1986). Natural cytotoxic T cells (NCTC) that differ from natural killer (NK) and natural cytotoxic (NC) cells are present in Peyer's patches of mice. *Cell. Immunol.* **101,** 463–475.

George, A., Kost, S. I., Witzleben, C. L., Cebra, J. J., and Rubin, D. H. (1990). Reovirus-induced liver disease in severe combined immunodeficient (SCID) Mice. A model for the study of viral infection, pathogenesis, and clearance, *J. Exp. Med.* **171,** 929–934.

Goodman, T., and LeFrancois, L. (1988). Expression of the γ-δ T-cell receptor on intestinal $CD8^+$ intraepithelial lymphocytes. *Nature (London)* **333,** 855–858.

Graham, B. S., Bunton, L. A., Wright, P. F., and Karzon, D. T. (1991). Role of T lymphocyte subsets in the pathogenesis of primary infection and rechallenge with respiratory syncytial virus in mice. *J. Clin. Invest.* **88,** 1026–1033.

Gupta, R., Yewdell, J. W., Olmsted, R. A., Collins, P. L., and Bennink, J. R. (1990). Primary pulmonary murine cytotoxic T lymphocyte specificity in respiratory syncytial virus pneumonia. *Microb. Pathogen.* **9,** 13–18.

Guy-Grand, D., Cerf-Bensussan, N., Malissen, B., Malassis-Seris, M., Briottet, C., and Vassalli, P. (1991a). Two gut intraepithelial $CD8^+$ lymphocyte populations with different T cell receptors; A role for the gut epithelium in T cell differentiation. *J. Exp. Med.* **173,** 471–481.

Guy-Grand, D., Malassis-Seris, M., Briottet, C., and Vassalli, P. (1991b). Cytotoxic differentiation of mouse gut thymodependent and independent intraepithelial T lymphocytes is induced locally. Correlation between functional assays, presence of perforin and granzyme transcripts, and cytoplasmic granules. *J. Exp. Med.* **173,** 1549–1552.

Hakim, F. T., Gazzinelli, R. T., Denkers, E., Hieny, S., Shearer, G. M., and Sher, A. (1991). $CD8^+$ T cells from mice vaccinated against *Toxoplasma gondii* are cytotoxic for parasite-infected or antigen-pulsed host cells. *J. Immunol.* **147,** 2310–2316.

Issekutz, T. B. (1984). The response of gut-associated T lymphocytes to intestinal viral immunization. *J. Immunol.* **133,** 2955–2960.

Jeggo, M. H., and Wardley, R. C. (1982). Generation of cross-reactive cytotoxic T lymphocytes following immunization of mice with various blue-tongue virus types. *Immunology* **45,** 629–635.

Kagnoff, M. F. (1978). Effect of antigen-feeding on intestinal and systemic immune responses. I. Priming of precursor cytotoxic T cells by antigen feeding. *J. Immunol.* **120,** 395–399.

Kagnoff, M. F., and Campbell, S. (1974). Functional characteristics of Peyer's patch lymphoid cells I. Induction of humoral antibody and cell-mediated allograft reactions. *J. Exp. Med.* **139,** 398–406.

Khan, I. A., Ely, K. H., and Kasper, L. H. (1991). A purified parasite antigen (p30) mediates $CD8^+$ T cell immunity against fatal *Toxoplasma gondii* infection in mice. *J. Immunol.* **147,** 3501–3506.

Kimpen, J. L. L., Richy, G. A., and Ogra, P. L. (1991). Development of mucosal T cell immunity to respiratory syncytial virus (RSV): Role in clearance pulmonary infection *Pediatr. Res.* 29, 176A (Abstract).

Kiyono, H., McGhee, J. R., Wannemuehler, M. J., Frangakis, M. V., Spalding, D. M., Michalek, S. M., and Koopman, W. J. (1982). *In vitro* immune responses to a T cell-dependent antigen by cultures of disassociated murine Peyer's patch. *Proc. Natl. Acad. Sci. U.S.A.* **79,** 596–600.

Klein, J. R. (1986). Ontogeny of the $Thy1^-$, $Lyt2^+$ murine intestinal intraepithelial lymphocyte: characterization of a unique population of thymus-independent cytotoxic effector cells in the intestinal mucosa. *J. Exp. Med.* **164,** 309–314.

Klein, J. R., and Kagnoff, M. F. (1984). Nonspecific recruitment of cytotoxic effector cells in the intestinal mucosa of antigen-primed mice. *J. Exp. Med.* **160,** 1931–1936.

Klein, J. R., and Kagnoff, M. F. (1987) Spontaneous *in vitro* evolution of lytic specificity of cytotoxic T lymphocyte clones isolated from murine intestinal epithelium. *J. Immunol.* **138,** 63–69.

Klein, J. R., Lefrancois, L., and Kagnoff, M. F. (1985). A murine cytotoxic T lymphocyte clone from the intestinal mucosa that is antigen specific for proliferation and displays broadly reactive inducible cytotoxic activity. *J. Immunol.* **135,** 3697–3703

Ksander, B. R., and Streilein, J. W. (1990). Failure of infiltrating precursor cytotoxic T cells to acquire direct cytotoxic function in immunologically privileged sites. *J. Immunol.* **145,** 2057–2063.

Lattime, E. C., Pecoraro, G. A., Cuttito, M. J., and Stutman, O. (1983). Murine non-lymphoid tumors are lysed by a combination of NK and NC cells. *Int. J. Cancer.* **32,** 523–528.

Lefrancois, L., and Goodman, T. (1989). *In vivo* modulation of cytolytic activity and Thy-1 expression in TCR-$\gamma\delta^+$ intraepithelial lymphocytes. *Science* **243,** 1716–1718.

Lindahl, K. F., and Wilson, D. B. (1977). Histocompatability antigen-activated cytotoxic T lymphocytes. I. Estimates of the absolute frequency of killer cells generated *in vitro*. *J. Exp. Med.* **145,** 500–507.

Liu, M. C., Ishizaka, K., and Plaut, M (1982). T lymphocyte responses of murine lung: immunization with alloantigen induces accumulation of cytotoxic and other T lymphocytes in the lung. *J. Immunol.* **129,** 2653–2661.

London, S. D., Rubin, D. H., and Cebra, J. J. (1986). Gut mucosal immunization with reovirus serotype 1/L stimulates virus-specific cytotoxic T cell precursors as well as IgA memory cells in Peyer's patches. *J. Exp. Med.* **165,** 830–847.

London, S. D., Cebra, J. J., and Rubin, D. H. (1989a). The reovirus-specific cytotoxic T cell response is not restricted to serotypically unique epitopes associated with the virus hemagglutinin. *Microb. Pathogen.* **6,** 43–50.

London, S. D., Cebra, J. J., and Rubin, D. H. (1989b). Intraepithelial lymphocytes contain virus-specific, MHC-restricted cytotoxic cell precursors after gut mucosal immunization with reovirus serotype 1/Lang. *Reg. Immunol.* **2,** 98–102.

London, S. D., Cebra-Thomas, J. A., Rubin, D. H., and Cebra, J. J. (1990). CD8 lymphocyte subpopulations in Peyer's patches induced by reovirus serotype 1 infection. *J. Immunol.* **144,** 3187–3194.

Lukacher, A. E., Braciale, V. L., and Braciale T. J. (1984). *In vivo* effector function of influenza virus-specific cytotoxic T lymphocyte clones is highly specific. *J. Exp. Med.* **160,** 814–826.

Munoz, J. L., McCarthy, C. A., Clark, M. E., and Hall, C. B. (1991). Respiratory syncytial virus infection in C57BL/6 mice: clearance of virus from the lungs with virus-specific cytotoxic T cells. *J. Virol.* **65,** 4494–4497.

Nicholas, J. A., Rubino, K. L., Levely, M. E., Meyer, A. L., and Collins, P. L. (1991). Cytotoxic T cell activity against the 22-kDa protein of human respiratory syncytial virus (RSV) is associated with a significant reduction in pulmonary RSV replication. *Virology* **182,** 664–672.

Offit, P. A., and Dudzik, K. I. (1988). Rotavirus-specific cytotoxic T lymphocytes cross-react with target cells infected with different rotavirus serotypes. *J. Virol.* **62,** 127–131.

Offit, P. A., and Dudzik, K. I. (1989a). Noninfectious rotavirus strain RRV induces an immune response in mice which protects against rotavirus challenge. *J. Clin. Microbiol.* **27,** 885–888.

Offit, P. A., and Dudzik, K. I. (1989b). Rotavirus-specific cytotoxic T lymphocytes appear at the intestinal mucosal surface after rotavirus infection. *J. Virol.* **63,** 3507–3512.

Offit, P. A., and Dudzik, K. I. (1990). Rotavirus-specific cytotoxic T lymphocytes passively protect against gastroenteritis in suckling mice. *J. Virol.* **64,** 6325–6328.

Offit, P. A., and Svoboda, Y. M. (1989). Rotavirus-specific cytotoxic T lymphocyte response of mice after oral inoculation with candidate rotavirus vaccine strains RRV or WC3. *J. Inf. Dis.* **160,** 783–788.

Offit, P. A., Boyle, D. B., Both, G. W., Hill, N. L., Svoboda, Y. M., Cunningham, S. L., Jenkins, R. J., and McCrae, M. A. (1991a). Outer capsid glycoprotein vp7 is recognized by cross-reactive, rotavirus-specific, cytotoxic T lymphocytes. *Virology* **184,** 563–568.

Offit, P. A., Cunningham, S. L., and Dudzik, K. I. (1991b). Memory and distribution of virus-specific cytotoxic T lymphocytes (CTL) and CTL precursors after rotavirus infection. *J. Virol.* **65,** 1318–1324.

Pamer, E. G., Harty, J. T., and Bevan, M. J. (1991). Precise prediction of a dominant class I MHC-restricted epitope of *Listeria monocytogenes*. *Nature* (*London*) **353,** 852–855.

Parrott, D. M. V., Tait, C., MacKenzie, S., Mowat, A. McI., Davies, M. D. J., and Micklem, H. S. (1983). Analysis of the effector functions of different populations of mucosal lymphocytes. *Ann. N.Y. Acad. Sci.* **409,** 307–320.

Petit, A., Ernst, P. B., Befus, A. D., Clark, D. A., Rosenthal, K. L., Ishizaka, T., and Bienenstock, J. (1985). Murine intestinal intraepithelial lymphocytes. I. Relationship of a novel Thy-1^-, Lyt-1^-, Lyt-2^+, granulated subpopulation to natural killer cells and mast cells. *Eur. J. Immunol.* **15,** 211–215.

Rubin, D. H., and Fields, B. N. (1980). Molecular basis of reovirus virulence: Role of the M2 gene. *J. Exp. Med.* **152,** 853–868.

Sabin, A. B. (1959). Reoviruses; A new group of respiratory and enteric viruses formerly classified as Echo-type 10 is described. *Science* **130,** 1387–1389.

Scherle, P., Palladino, G., and Gerhard, W. (1992). Mice can recover from pulmonary influenza virus infection in the absence of class I-restricted cytotoxic T cells. *J. Immunol.* **148,** 212–217.

Smith, L. E., Rodrigues, M., and Russell, D. G. (1991). The interaction between $CD8^+$ cytotoxic T cells and *Leishmania*-infected macrophages. *J. Exp. Med.* **174,** 499–505.

Stutman, O., Paige, C., and Figarella, E. F. (1978). Natural cytotoxic cells against solid tumors in mice. I. Strain and age distribution and target cell susceptibility. *J. Immunol.* **121,** 1819–1826.

Tagliabue, A., Luini, W., Soldateschi, D., and Boraschi, D. (1981). Natural killer activity of gut mucosal lymphoid cells in mice. *Eur. J. Immunol.* **11,** 919–922.

Tagliabue, A., Befus, A. D., Clark, D. A., and Bienenstock, J. (1982). Characterization of NK cells in the murine intestinal epithelium and lamina propria. *J. Exp. Med.* **155,** 1785–1796.

Tagliabue, A., Villa, L., Scapigliati, G., and Boraschi, D. (1983/1984). Peyer's patch lymphocytes express natural cytotoxicity but not natural killer activity. *Nat. Immunol. Cell Growth Regul.* **3,** 95–101.

Taylor, G., Scott, E. J., and Hayle, A. J. (1985). Cytotoxic lymphocytes in the lungs of mice infected with respiratory syncytial virus. *J. Gen. Virol.* **66,** 2533–2538.

Taylor, P. M., and Askonas, B. A. (1986). Influenza nucleoprotein-specific cytotoxic T-cell clones are protective *in vivo*. *Immunology* **58,** 417–420.

Trudel, M., Seguin, N. C., and Binz, H. (1991). Protection of Balb/c mice from respiratory syncytial virus infection by immunization with a synthetic peptide derived from the G glycoprotein. *Virology* **185,** 749–757.

Viney, J. L., Kilshaw, P. J., and MacDonald, T. T. (1990). Cytotoxic α/β^+ and γ/δ^+ T cells in murine intestinal epithelium. *Eur. J. Immunol.* **20,** 1623–1626.

Welsh, R. M. (1984). Natural killer cells and interferon. *CRC Crit. Rev. Immunol.* **5,** 55–93.

Wilson, A., and Shortman, K. (1984). Degradation of specificity in cytolytic T lymphocyte clones; Mouse strain dependence and interstrain transfer of nonspecific cytolysis. *Eur. J. Immunol.* **14,** 951–956.

Wolf, J. L., Rubin, D. H., Finberg, R, Kauffman, R. S., Sharpe, A. H., Trier, J. S., and Fields, B. N. (1981). Intestinal M cells: A pathway for entry of reovirus into the host. *Science* **212,** 471–472.

Wolf, J. L., Kauffman, R. S., Finberg, R., Dambrauskas, R., Fields, B. N., and Trier, J. S. (1983). Determinants of reovirus interaction with the intestinal M cells and absorptive cells of murine intestine. *Gastroenterology* **85,** 291–300.

Wyde, P. R., Couch, R. B., Mackler, B. F., Cate, T. R., and Levy, B. M. (1977). Effects of low and high passage influenza virus infection in normal and nude mice. *Infect. Immun.* **15,** 221–229.

Wysocka, M., Korngold, R., Yewdell, J., and Bennink, J. (1989). Target and effector cell fusion accounts for B lymphocyte-mediated lysis of mouse hepatitis virus-infected cells. *J. Gen. Virol.* **70,** 1465–1472.

Yamaguchi, K., Kyuwa, S., Nakanaga, K., and Hayami, M. (1988). Establishment of cytotoxic T-cell clones specific for cells infected with mouse hepatitis virus. *J. Virol.* **62,** 2505–2507.

Yap, K. L., and Ada, G. L. (1978a). Cytotoxic T cells in the lungs of mice infected with an influenza A virus. *Scand. J. Immunol.* **7,** 73–80.

Yap, K. L., Ada, G. L., and McKenzie, I. F. C. (1978b). Transfer of specific cytotoxic T lymphocytes protects mice inoculated with influenza virus. *Nature* (*London*) **273,** 238–239.

29

Mucosal Immunity to Viruses

Brian R. Murphy

The mucosal surfaces of the body, including primarily the respiratory and gastrointestinal tracts, are infected readily with a wide variety of DNA and RNA viruses. Important viral pathogens of mucosal surfaces such as paramyxoviruses and rotaviruses cause serious disease on first infection. In contrast to the lifelong immunity induced by viruses such as measles virus and polioviruses that cause systemic disease, mucosal immunity is usually more transient, so reinfection by mucosal pathogens is common. Disease often occurs during reinfection but is usually less severe than that experienced during first infection. Several general observations of the effectiveness of the mucosal immune system in altering the course of viral infection follow: (1) In the absence of antibody, severe disease can occur. (2) In the presence of low to moderate levels of antibody, infection results in a milder illness. (3) In the presence of intermediate levels of antibody, an asymptomatic infection occurs. (4) In the presence of high levels of antibody, infection can be prevented (Ogra and Karzon, 1969b). Because of the difficulty in maintaining a very high level of mucosal immunity, the major function of the mucosal immune system appears to be that of converting a severe infection into a mild or asymptomatic one. The high volume, rapid transit time, and hostile environment of the respiratory and gastrointestinal tracts most likely contribute to the inability to maintain high levels of mucosal antibodies.

In this quantitative balance between virus and host, the host calls on the cellular and humoral immune systems to limit the extent of virus replication, to clear virus, and to prevent reinfection. Although the secretory IgA system has evolved specifically to protect mucosal surfaces, significant contributions to mucosal immunity are made by the cellular arm of the immune system and by the transudation of antiviral IgG antibodies onto mucosal surfaces.

I. CELLULAR ANTIVIRAL IMMUNE MECHANISMS OPERATIVE ON MUCOSAL SURFACES

Natural killer (NK) cells, major histocompatibility complex (MHC) Class I-restricted $CD8^+$ cytotoxic T cells (Tc) and MHC Class II-restricted $CD4^+$ helper T cells (Th) each can function as antiviral effector cells against viruses that infect mucosal surfaces.

A. NK cells

Humans with an inherited deficiency of NK cells experience more severe herpes virus infections than normal individuals (Biron *et al.*, 1989). The infected individuals eventually clear the virus infection in a fashion comparable to that of immunocompetent hosts. These observations suggest that NK cells, which do not exhibit virus-specific antiviral activity, can play an important early role in limiting the extent of certain mucosal viral infections.

B. Tc Cells

Tc cells appear to be the major T cell effector with antiviral activity (Yap *et al.*, 1978; Kast *et al.*, 1986; Taylor and Askonas, 1986; Dharakul *et al.*, 1990; Offit and Dudzik, 1990; Munoz *et al.*, 1991). The Tc cell receptor recognizes a short peptide derived from an endogenously produced viral protein in the context of the MHC Class I β_2-microglobulin heterodimer expressed on the surface of an infected cell (Madden *et al.*, 1991). Since the MHC Class I restriction elements are present on almost all cells except neurons, Tc cells can exert their antiviral effects against almost all infected cells of mucosal surfaces. Since viral infection of a cell generally is required for antigen presentation by the MHC Class I β_2-microglobulin heterodimer, clearly Tc cells cannot function to prevent infection, but must function to eliminate cells already infected or, alternatively, to restrict virus replication in cells already infected. The net effect of Tc cell activity is preventing further spread of virus and terminating infection in cells already infected. Passive transfer of Tc-cell clones to animals results in restriction of virus replication in mucosal epithelial cells, demonstrating the functional capabilities of this T-cell subset (McDermott *et al.*, 1987; Cannon *et al.*, 1988; Mackenzie *et al.*, 1989; Munoz *et al.*, 1991). Tc cell antiviral activity generally is associated with the clearance of virus and the reduction of virus-associated pathology (Lukacher *et al.*, 1984; Mackenzie *et al.*, 1989; Munoz *et al.*, 1991). However, disease enhancement was seen in one viral infection after passive transfer of large numbers of respiratory syncytial virus-specific cloned Tc cells that were capable of clearing virus infection (Cannon *et al.*, 1988).

The time course of Tc-cell activation during viral infection is consistent with this predominant role in clearance of virus infection. Primary (also called direct) Tc cell cytotoxic activity of pulmonary lymphocytes peaks early during paramyxovirus (respiratory syncytial virus) infection (day 7) and declines to barely detectable levels by day 12 (Anderson *et al.*, 1990). Thus, restriction of virus replication in mucosal tissues mediated by Tc cells is active early during the acute stage of the virus infection, but this activity wanes rapidly by day 28 (Connors *et al.*, 1991). These observations suggest that the Tc-cell component of the immune response is operative primarily during the early phase of infection from the time just before peak titers of virus are reached to the time virus-infected cells are cleared, and later exists in an inactive (or memory) state (Connors *et al.*, 1991; Nicholas *et al.*, 1991). For viruses that replicate rapidly at mucosal surfaces, such as influenza viruses and parmyxoviruses, the proliferation of memory Tc cells is unlikely to be sufficiently rapid to alter significantly the peak titer of virus achieved in the respiratory tract (McMichael *et al.*, 1983; Endo *et al.*, 1991; Webster *et al.*, 1991). However, Tc cells actively generated from memory cells may reach levels that accelerate viral clearance (McMichael *et al.*, 1983). Since disease is experienced when peak titers of viruses are attained, immunization with antigens that induce predominantly Tc activity in the absence of antibody is, not surprisingly, much less successful in restricting replication of challenge virus and preventing illness than immunization that induces a sustained antibody response (Andrew *et al.*, 1987; Endo *et al.*, 1991; Webster *et al.*, 1991).

C. Th Cells

Although Th cells are known to provide help to B cells, thereby augmenting antibody response, Th cells themselves have been shown to have direct antiviral activities *in vivo* (McDermott *et al.*, 1987; Taylor *et al.*, 1990). The contribution made by the direct antiviral activity of the Th response to the overall immunity that is induced appears to be of lower magnitude than that of the Tc cells consistent with the more limited distribution of its restricting element, the MHC Class II α,β heterodimer, which is present predominantly on B lymphocytes and antigen-presenting cells such as macrophages and dendritic cells. In addition to having antiviral activity, Th cells also can mediate immunopathology (Leung and Ada, 1980; Taylor *et al.*, 1990).

Animals depleted of either Th or Tc cells prior to infection with influenza A viruses can, however, clear virus at rates similar to those of fully immunocompetent animals (Lightman *et al.*, 1987; Eichelberger *et al.*, 1991a,b), indicating that the immune system is functionally redundant; multiple components from both the humoral and the cellular immune systems contribute to clearance of infection.

II. IgG ANTIBODIES ON MUCOSAL SURFACES

IgG antibodies present in the blood can gain access to mucosal surfaces by passive diffusion and can exert antiviral activity. Much of the IgG antibody present at mucosal surfaces is derived from serum, as indicated by the following observations: (1) A linear relationship exists between titer of serum and nasal wash IgG influenza virus antibodies (Wagner *et al.*, 1987). (2) The ratio of IgG1/IgG3 influenza virus-specific antibody is similar in serum and nasal washes (Wagner *et al.*, 1987). (3) The active transport of IgG antiviral antibodies across mucosal surfaces occurs infrequently, if at all, whereas transport of IgA and IgM antibodies is the rule (Murphy *et al.*, 1982). Although most of the IgG present in mucosal secretions is derived by transudation from serum, virus-specific IgG antibodies produced by the mucosa also can contribute to total antiviral activity in mucosal secretions (Ogra *et al.*, 1974; Johnson *et al.*, 1986; McBride and Ward, 1987). Further, in IgA-deficient patients, mucosal production and secretion of IgG and IgM antiviral antibodies can compensate for the deficiency of production and secretion of IgA antibodies (Ogra *et al.*, 1974).

The antiviral activity of IgG antibodies against viruses that replicate on mucosal surfaces has been documented following transudation of antibodies that are derived from three different sources: (1) antibodies produced by the host (Clements *et al.*, 1986); (2) maternally derived antibodies (Lepow *et al.*, 1961; Puck *et al.*, 1980; Reuman *et al.*, 1983,1987); and (3) passively transferred polyclonal or monoclonal antibodies (Bodian and Nathanson, 1960; Ramphal *et al.*, 1979; Prince *et al.*, 1985; Offit *et al.*, 1986; Besser *et al.*, 1988). The IgG antiviral antibodies can prevent infection (Lepow *et al.*, 1961), decrease virus replication (Bodian and Nathanson, 1960; Lepow *et al.*, 1961; Prince *et al.*, 1985; Clements *et al.*, 1986), and eliminate or lessen the severity of disease (Puck *et al.*, 1980). In the case of respiratory viruses, serum IgG antibodies restrict virus replication in the lung more effectively than in the trachea or nose (Ramphal *et al.*, 1979; Prince *et al.*, 1985). Further, passively transferred IgG antibodies restrict the replication of poliovirus to a greater extent in the throat than in the lower intestinal tract (Bodian and Nathanson, 1960). These data suggest that a gradient exists regarding the ability of serum IgG derived antibodies to restrict virus replication on mucosal surfaces; this gradient is lung > nasopharynx > lower intestinal tract (Sabin *et al.*, 1963a,b; Reuman *et al.*, 1983; Murphy *et al.*, 1986a,b,1988,1989; Kimman *et al.*, 1987,1989; Johnson *et al.*, 1988). One possible explanation for this gradient is that serum antibodies can diffuse more readily across alveolar walls than across the mucosa of the upper respiratory tract and that the hostile environment of the gastrointestinal tract and the dilution of the IgG antibodies with the intestinal secretions further limit the effectiveness of passively derived IgG antibodies at this site. The mechanism of the antiviral activity of IgG antibodies *in vivo* is related to direct neutralization of virus infectivity, as evidenced by the restriction of respiratory syncytial virus replication in the lungs of passively immunized rodents depleted of complement, and by the finding that $F(ab)_2$ fragments of IgG can restrict pulmonary virus replication as effectively as whole IgG molecules. Thus, complement-dependent immune cytolysis and antibody-dependent cell cytotoxicity are not required for the antiviral activity of IgG antibodies (Prince *et al.*, 1990). However, complement appears to be necessary for the efficient clearance of influenza A virus infection in mice (Hicks *et al.*, 1978).

Many viruses infect mucosal surfaces during the first 6 months of life when maternal IgG antibodies are present. In addition, immunizing infants with live poliovirus vaccine when passively acquired maternal antibodies are present is routine. For these reasons, interest has arisen in studying the effect of passively derived IgG antibodies on the development of immunity to viral infections. Such antibodies clearly can significantly modify the immune response to viruses that replicate on mucosal surfaces. The magnitude of the mucosal and systemic antibody response to a viral infection that takes place in the presence of passively acquired IgG antibody can be reduced significantly despite a high level of virus replication (Sabin *et al.*, 1963a; Murphy *et al.*, 1986a; Kimman *et al.*, 1987). However, a secondary IgG antibody response is seen in subjects immunosuppressed by passively transferred IgG antibodies on rechallenge with virus or antigen, even in subjects who failed to mount a detectable primary antibody response (Sabin *et al.*, 1963b; Reuman *et al.*, 1983). Despite the reduction in magnitude of the primary antibody response to initial infection in such subjects, partial resistance to subsequent challenge is evident (Sabin *et al.*, 1963a; Reuman *et al.*, 1983; Murphy *et al.*, 1989). The suppressive effect of passively acquired IgG antibody on the induction of resistance to challenge is greatest when viral antigen is administered parenterally rather than mucosally (Murphy *et al.*, 1989). A secretory IgA response still can develop in individuals whose IgG antibody response is suppressed by passively derived IgG, suggesting that the mucosal IgA antibody response is suppressed less easily by passive IgG antibody than is the systemic IgG response (Jayashree *et al.*, 1988; Kimman and Westenbrink, 1990). This finding provides a partial explanation for the development of mucosal resistance to infection in the presence of maternally derived antibodies.

A second way in which passively derived IgG can modify the antibody response to virus is altering the functional activity (i.e., quality) of the antiviral antibodies that are induced (Murphy *et al.*, 1988). The neutralizing activity of a given amount of virus antigen-specific antibody is decreased markedly when the viral infection occurs in the presence of passively derived IgG antibodies (Murphy *et al.*, 1988). The mechanisms by which passively acquired IgG antibodies mediate their effects on the magnitude and quality of the antibody response remain to be defined.

III. MUCOSAL IgA ANTIBODY RESPONSE

Although passively transferred IgG antibodies and Th and Tc effector cells contribute to mucosal immunity, the major mediators of resistance to viral infection on mucosal surfaces are IgA antibodies. IgA antiviral antibodies are likely to play major roles in clearance of viral infections, modification of the severity of disease on reinfection, and prevention of infection on reexposure to virus.

A. Viral Antigens Recognized by IgA Antibodies

The major viral antigens that induce a protective antibody response are the surface glycoproteins of viruses that contain lipid envelopes or the proteins present on the surface of icosahedral viruses. IgA antibodies recognize the same viral antigens as IgG antibodies; evidence is accumulating that they also recognize the same epitopes on these glycoproteins. For instance, polyclonal IgA antibodies, like polyclonal IgG antibodies, recognize the hemagglutinin of influenza virus (Murphy *et al.*, 1982; Clements *et al.*, 1986); the gp70 (fusion) and gp90 (attachment) glycoproteins of respiratory syncytial virus (Murphy *et al.*, 1986b); the gp340 of Epstein–Barr virus (Yao *et al.*, 1991); the VP1, VP2, and VP3 of polioviruses (Zhaori *et al.*, 1989); and the VP4 of VP7 of rotaviruses (Conner *et al.*, 1991; Shaw *et al.*, 1991; Richardson and Bishop, 1990). In general, the specificity of the neutralizing activity of IgA and IgG antibodies for antigenically related variant viruses appears to be similar (Buscho *et al.*, 1972; Richman *et al.*, 1974), that is, the mucosal IgA antibody response does not appear to be more broad than the systemic IgG antibody response. However, the antigens of viruses that replicate on mucosal surfaces can be modified by intestinal enzymes to expose new epitopes on the surface proteins of such viruses. Thus, the immunogenicity of a virus that replicates in the intestinal tract can differ from that of a parenterally administered inactivated vaccine produced from tissue-culture grown virus. For example, the mucosal IgA response to the poliovirus VP3 protein—which is cleaved by intestinal enzymes following oral administration of live virus, thereby exposing unique epitopes on the protein—is greater than that following immunization with inactivated virus given parenterally (Zhaori *et al.*, 1989), despite the finding that the mucosal IgA responses to VP1 and VP2 are comparable for the two conditions.

The IgA antibody response to the attachment and fusion glycoprotein antigens on respiratory syncytial virus is depressed during infection of infants that have maternal antibodies. Further, the age of the subject correlates with the response to the fusion protein, and the level of maternally derived antibodies is related inversely to the response to the G glycoprotein (Murphy *et al.*, 1986a). Thus, factors influencing IgA responses to viral glycoproteins are complex; protein structure, age of host, and presence of passively acquired IgG antibody all contribute to the magnitude and quality of the response.

IgA monoclonal antibodies to viruses that infect mucosal surfaces have been produced to define further the antigens and epitopes seen by IgA antibodies (Maoliang, 1986; Weltzin *et al.*, 1989; Lyn *et al.*, 1991). The same antigens and epitopes appear to be recognized by IgG and IgA monoclonal antibodies. Variants selected with neutralizing IgA and IgG monoclonal antibodies have been shown to have identical reactivity patterns against a panel of monoclonal antibodies (Maoliang, 1986) or to have identical amino acid substitutions (Lyn *et al.*, 1991). Some epitopes of the HN glycoprotein of Sendai virus are recognized by IgA antibodies but not by IgG antibodies; however, a large panel of IgG and IgA monoclonal antibodies must be analyzed to determine whether any epitopes or antigenic sites on viral proteins are seen exclusively by IgA antibodies (Lyn *et al.*, 1991). The mechanism of heavy chain switching, in which the antibody binding regions are maintained but constant regions of the heavy chains are exchanged, is compatible with the observations just outlined, namely, that IgG and IgA in general have similar specificities for viral antigens and their epitopes.

B. Time Course of the Mucosal IgA Response to Viral Infection

The mucosal IgA response to viral infection is rapid after first infection and can be detected as early as day 3 following infection (Blandford and Heath, 1972; Rubin *et al.*, 1983). The time course for an idealized mucosal IgA response is given in Figure 1. The primary response peaks within the first 6 weeks and can decrease to a low, often barely detectable, level by 3 months (Buscho *et al.*, 1972; (Sonza and Holmes, 1980; Kaul *et al.*, 1981; Friedman, 1982; Friedman *et al.*, 1989; Bishop *et al.*, 1990; Coulson *et al.*, 1990; Nishio *et al.*, 1990). This short duration of the primary mucosal antibody response is compatible with the susceptibility to reinfection that is common for viruses that infect mucosal surfaces. Reinfection results in a secondary antibody response, indicating immunological memory characterized by a rapid rise in IgA antibody titer, a rise to a higher peak titer, and maintenance of detectable levels of antibody over a longer period of time (Buscho *et al.*, 1972; Kaul *et al.*, 1981; Wright *et al.*, 1983; Merriman *et al.*, 1984; Yamaguchi *et al.*, 1985; Bishop *et al.*, 1990; Coulson *et al.*, 1990).

In addition to a mucosal IgA response, a serum IgA response occurs after mucosal viral infection. The latter appears to be more sustained than the mucosal response (Friedman *et al.*, 1989). A correlation between the magnitude of the serum and mucosal IgA antiviral antibody responses has been observed in some instances, suggesting that some of the serum IgA antibody is a spill-over from mucosal sites (Burlington *et al.*, 1983). The polymeric structure of postinfection antiviral serum IgA antibodies is consistent with a mucosal origin of B cells that secrete IgA antibody into the systemic circulation since serum IgA antibodies are generally monomeric (Brown *et al.*, 1985; Ponzi *et al.*, 1985). However, polymeric IgA serum antibodies can be induced by parenteral immunization of immune individuals with inactivated influenza virus vaccine (Brown *et al.*, 1987), suggesting that memory IgA cells of mucosal origin might seed systemic sites after infection and that antigenic stimulation of such cells yields IgA antibodies with a polymeric nature and subclass that are characteristic of mucosal IgA antibodies. The detection of IgA-producing B lymphocytes in the peripheral blood or spleen after mucosal viral infection or immunization with inactivated antigen is compatible with this suggestion (Yarchoan *et al.*, 1981; Czerkinsky *et al.*, 1987; London *et al.*, 1987). The number of these B cells peaks early within the first 2 weeks after antigenic stimulation and decreases rapidly thereafter. These circulating cells could seed not only systemic sites but also mucosal sites at locations other than the site of antigenic stimulation (Czerkinsky *et al.*, 1987).

The number of virus-specific IgG-, IgA-, or IgM-secreting B cells at mucosal sites of virus replication has been studied in both the lungs and the small intestine, and differences were noted. An IgG B-cell response predominated in the lungs (Jones and Ada, 1986) whereas an IgA B-cell response predominated in the intestine (Merchant *et al.*, 1991).

C. Local Nature of the Mucosal IgA Antibody Response

Evidence for the existence of a common mucosal immune system comes from the observation that immunization of a mucosal site often leads to detectable immune responses at distant mucosal sites (Mestecky, 1987). This seeding of distal mucosal sites is likely to be the result of trafficking of locally stimulated mucosal B lymphocytes to distince sites, where they reside as IgA plasma cells actively producing antibody or as memory B cells (Rudzik *et al.*, 1975; Czerkinsky *et al.*, 1987; Mestecky, 1987). Such trafficking of antiviral IgA-producing cells can occur from the gastrointestinal tract mucosa to the respiratory tract mucosa and perhaps vice versa (Waldman *et al.*, 1986; Chen *et al.*, 1987; Hirabayashi *et al.*, 1990). Although this common mucosal system exists, it appears to be relatively inefficient at protecting sites not directly stimulated with antigen (Ogra *et al.*, 1969b; Smith *et al.*, 1970; Nedrud *et al.*, 1987). Oral immunization with live adenovirus vaccine in enteric coated capsules selectively

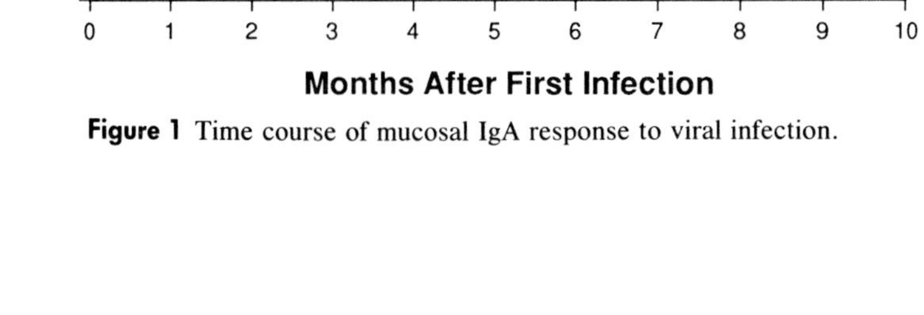

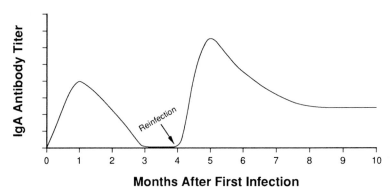

Figure 1 Time course of mucosal IgA response to viral infection.

infects the lower intestinal tract and induces a fecal IgA and serum IgG antiviral antibody response, but fails to induce a detectable nasal wash IgA antibody response (Smith *et al.*, 1970; Scott *et al.*, 1972). In contrast, live adenovirus vaccine administered to the upper respiratory tract induces a vigorous nasal wash antibody response (Smith *et al.*, 1970). In a similar study with live poliovirus virus vaccine in infants, selective infection of the colon via a colostomy orifice resulted in a vigorous neutralizing IgA antibody response in the colon, but not in the nasopharynx (Ogra *et al.*, 1969b). When the upper respiratory tract of these infants was challenged with poliovirus vaccine, vaccine virus replicated to high titer in the pharynx but the colon was resistant to replication to vaccine virus, as indicated by absence of virus shedding from the lower gastrointestinal tract (Ogra *et al.*, 1969b). Similar studies with rotavirus infection in infants and children demonstrated that the IgA antiviral response in the duodenum, which is the major site of viral replication, was greater than that in saliva, a distant mucosal site not known to support rotavirus replication (Grimwood *et al.*, 1988). In experimental studies in rodents, immunization of the gut with inactivated parainfluenza virus vaccine plus adjuvant was less protective than intranasally administered vaccine (Nedrud *et al.*, 1987). However, a protective response to influenza virus infection in the lung was observed after oral immunization of mice (Chen *et al.*, 1987). These studies in humans and animals suggest that induction of protective mucosal IgA responses at distant mucosal sites is likely to be difficult to achieve and that augmentation of the distant IgA response by immunological adjuvants is likely to be required.

The local nature of the mucosal antibody response, even within the respiratory tract, was observed in two studies. In the first study, the quantity of mucosal antibody in sputum or nasal secretions of volunteers given an inactivated influenza A virus vaccine by aerosol was a function of the size of the aerosolized particles (Waldman *et al.*, 1970). The subjects vaccinated with an aerosol containing small particles that are deposited predominantly in the lung had high sputum but low nasal secretion antibody titers, whereas individuals immunized with large particles that are deposited predominantly in the nose had high nasal but low sputum antibody titers. In the second study, intranasal administration of inactivated influenza A virus vaccine induced a greater nasal wash neutralizing antibody response than salivary antibody response, indicating that the site of antigenic stimulation, that is, the nasal passages, had a greater mucosal response than the distant site, that is, the salivary glands (Waldman *et al.*, 1968). These observations demonstrate that mucosal antibody responses are more localized than systemic antibody responses, which are disseminated via the circulatory system. A partial explanation for the local nature of the mucosal responses comes from the finding that the concentration of virus-specific IgA-producing B cells at the site of antigenic stimulation is much higher than that at more distant sites (Dharakul *et al.*, 1988). Although trafficking of B cells between mucosal sites occurs, the level of antiviral antibody and resistance to infection achieved at distant sites appears to be much less than at sites of direct antigenic stimulation. Mucosal immunization thus is achieved most successfully by antigenic stimulation of sites directly involved in viral replication.

D. Mechanism of Antiviral Activities of IgA Antibodies

The mechanism of neutralization of the infectivity of animal viruses by immunoglobulins is complex; a variety of mechanisms contribute to loss of viral infectivity (Outlaw and Dimmock, 1991). IgA antibodies are able to neutralize the infectivity of viruses efficiently and more closely resemble IgG antibodies in their efficiency of neutralization than do IgM antibodies, which have a lower overall activity (Nguyen *et al.*, 1986; Mazanec *et al.*, 1987; Outlaw and Dimmock, 1991; Renegar and Small, 1991a). IgA antibodies are able to neutralize the infectivity of viruses by several different mechanisms. First, aggregation of virus by IgA antibodies is associated with a decrease in virus infectivity, a finding that contrasts with that for IgM (Outlaw and Dimmock, 1990). Second, IgA antibodies to influenza appear to be more efficient than IgG antibodies in preventing attachment of virus to infected cells by being able to block 70–90% of virus particles from attaching to cell receptors (Outlaw and Dimmock, 1991). The polymeric nature of the IgA molecule is thought to contribute in part to this difference. Third, IgA antibodies can prevent the penetration of attached virus into the infected cell (Nguyen *et al.*, 1986; Outlaw and Dimmock, 1991). Fourth, IgA antibodies, like IgG antibodies, also act to neutralize viruses after penetration of the host cell (Outlaw and Dimmock, 1991). Thus, IgA antibodies appear similar to IgG in their efficiency of neutralization *in vitro*, but because of their polymeric nature appear to be more efficient at preventing attachment of certain viruses to susceptible cells.

IgA antibodies can have other effects on the immune system such as promoting uptake of viral antigens via immunoglobulin receptors present on the specialized absorptive epithelial cells called M cells (Weltzin *et al.*, 1989). Thus, virus neutralized by IgA antibodies whose attachment to specific cell receptors for virus has been blocked still can bind to M cells and be transported to the subepithelial macrophages that are in proximity to M cells. In this manner, viral antigen–IgA immume complexes destined for excretion in stools can gain access to antigen-presenting cells and thereby promote the overall immune response. Thus, IgA antibodies have direct (neutralization) and indirect means of preventing diseases caused by viruses that replicate on mucosal surfaces.

Few studies have compared IgG and IgA antibodies for their efficacy *in vivo*. However, with the availability of neutralizing monoclonal IgA and IgG antibodies directed to the attachment glycoprotein of Sendai virus, researchers have been able to compare the *in vivo* efficacies of IgA and IgG antibodies that have specificity for the same viral glycoprotein (Mazanac *et al.*, 1992). Mice passively immunized intranasally with IgG or IgA antibodies, either before or up to 24 hr after intranasal challenge with Sendai virus, were protected equally against pulmonary virus replication. Monomeric and polymeric IgA antibodies were equally efficacious. These data are consistent with the similarities of IgG and IgA antibodies in their *in vitro* neutralizing activities and their similar abilities to recognize the same antigenic sites and epitopes on viral antigens. In a separate study, a neutralizing polymeric monoclonal IgA anti-influenza A virus hemagglutinin antibody, administered systemically, was able to restrict the replication of influenza virus in the upper respiratory tract of the mouse (Renegar and Small, 1991a). However, a similar effect was not observed when a comparable amount of IgG monoclonal antibody of the same specificity was administered. Thus, the main advantage of IgA antibodies in protecting mucosal surfaces of the respiratory tract appears to be their ability to be transported selectively across mucosal surfaces, not an inherently greater antiviral activity.

E. IgA Antibodies Are Associated with the Clearance of Infectious Virus from Mucosal Surfaces

The appearance of IgA antibodies in mucosal secretions correlates with the cessation of virus excretion during mucosal viral infections in animals and humans in both the respiratory and gastrointestinal tracts (Figure 2; McIntosh *et al.*, 1978,1979; Keller and Dwyer, 1968; Ogra, 1970; Corthier and Vannier, 1983). This suggests that the IgA antibodies neutralize the infectivity of viruses present in mucosal secretions and are partially responsible for clearance of infectious virus from such secretions is reasonable. The appearance of virus–IgA or virus–IgM immune complexes at the time of virus clearance is consistent with the role of IgA in resolution of virus infection (Corthier and Vannier, 1983). Whether antibodies produced during the course of viral infection can clear virus-infected cells from mucosal surfaces in the absence of T cells remains to be determined, but antibodies alone can clear systemic viral infections (Levine *et al.*, 1991). As mentioned earlier, animals rendered deficient in Tc or Th cell responses are able to clear virus infection in a manner similar to their fully immunocompetent counterparts (Lightman *et al.*, 1987; Eichelberger *et al.*, 1991a,b), suggesting that antibodies can participate in clearance of virus-infected cells from mucosal surfaces and that they might be sufficient in this regard. However, the relative roles of IgG and IgA antibodies in such processes remain to be defined. Passive transfer studies of both polyclonal IgA and IgG antiviral antibodies or antibody-producing cells in T-cell deficient animals will be needed to address the question of the role of antibodies in viral clearance.

F. IgA Antibodies Are the Major Mediators of Mucosal Immunity

Researchers long have recognized that immunization of the mouse by a mucosal route could, under certain circumstances, induce greater resistance to virus infection than systemic immunization and that resistance correlated with the level of mucosal antibodies (de St. Groth and Donnelly, 1950). Since that time, a large body of literature has emerged that associates the level of mucosal antibodies, either neutralizing or IgA antibodies, with resistance to a variety of viral infections in humans and animals (Table I). The resistance associated with IgA antibodies is manifested by prevention of infection or by decreasing the severity of infection. A quantitative relationship exists between the level of mucosal IgA antibodies and the extent of virus replication (Ogra and Karzon, 1969b). This association provides compelling, but not definitive, evidence that IgA antibodies are the primary mediators of mucosal resistance to viral infection. One study even demonstrated that local IgA memory in the absence of detectable IgA antibodies was associated with resistance to viral infection (Kimman *et al.*, 1989). In this instance, a local IgA response to reinfection appeared to be sufficiently rapid to limit the extent of virus replication or, alternatively, undetectable levels of antibody were present that modified the infection.

Definitive proof that IgA antibodies are the mediators of mucosal immunity has been forthcoming. Four studies demonstrate that passively transferred IgA antibodies are associated with resistance to virus infection on mucosal surfaces. (1) Neutralizing monoclonal IgA antibodies to the HN glycoprotein of Sendai virus (a murine parainfluenza virus) could protect against virus infection when administered intranasally

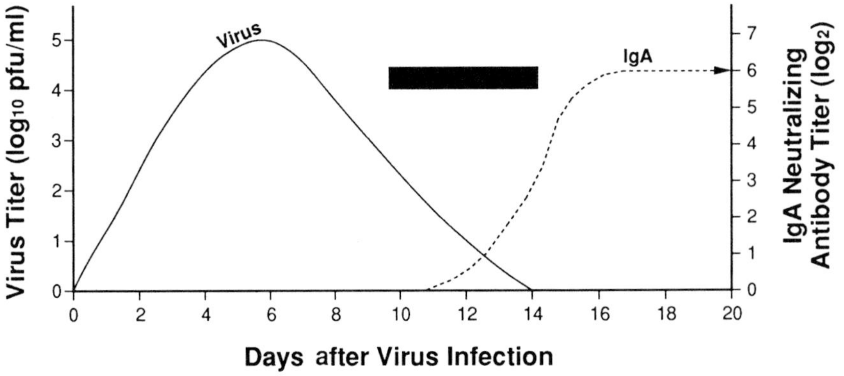

Figure 2 An idealized viral infection of a mucosal surface in which clearance of infectious virus is associated with the appearance of neutralizing IgA antibodies. The black bar indicates the time when IgA–virus immune complexes are likely to be present.

Table I Association of Mucosal Antibodies with Resistance to Viral Infections

Studies in humans or animals	Virus	Resistance observed[a]: Modified infection or disease	Resistance observed[a]: Prevented infection	References
Humans				
	Respiratory syncytial virus	+		Mills *et al.* (1971)
	Respiratory syncytial virus	+		Watt *et al.* (1990)
	Parainfluenza virus		+	Smith *et al.* (1966)
	Influenza A virus	+		Clements *et al.* (1986)
	Influenza A virus		+	Clements *et al.* (1983)
	Influenza A virus		+	Johnson *et al.* (1986)
	Influenza A virus	+	+	Murphy *et al.* (1973)
	Influenza A virus	+		Reuman *et al.* (1990)
	Rhinovirus		+	Perkins *et al.* (1969)
	Rotavirus[b]	+		Hjelt *et al.* (1987)
	Rotavirus	+		Ward *et al.* (1989)
	Rotavirus	+	+	Ward *et al.* (1990)
	Poliovirus	+		Onorato *et al.* (1991)
	Poliovirus	+		Ogra and Karzon (1969a)
	Poliovirus	+	+	Ogra and Karzon (1969b)
Animals				
Mice	Influenza virus	+	+	de St. Groth and Donnelly (1950)
Mice	Influenza virus		+	Liew *et al.* (1984)
Mice	Parainfluenza virus	+		Nadrud *et al.* (1987); Liang *et al.*, (1988)
Hamsters	Parainfluenza virus	+	+	Ray *et al.* (1988)
Bovine	Respiratory syncytial virus	+		Kimman and Westenbrink (1990)

[a] Best estimate based on data presented.
[b] Serum IgA but not IgG was associated with milder illness.

before virus infection (Mazanec *et al.*, 1987). (2) Intranasally administered polymeric anti-influenza virus IgA antibodies that had been purified from mucosal secretions provided passive protection against virus infection when administered before virus challenge (Tamura *et al.*, 1990). (3) Systemically administered monoclonal polymeric IgA but not monoclonal IgG antibodies against influenza virus passively protected the respiratory tract of the mouse against influenza virus challenge (Renegar and Small, 1991a). (4) Inoculation of hybridoma cells secreting nonneutralizing polymeric IgA antibodies against a reovirus surface protein provided resistance to reovirus replication in the gastrointestinal tract (M. Neutra, personal communication). These studies clearly demonstrate that antiviral IgA antibodies are capable of mediating resistance to mucosal virus infection. Using a different approach, another study demonstrated that the mucosal immunity induced by infection with influenza virus is abrogated by instillation of anti-IgA antibody into the respiratory tract prior to virus challenge (Renegar and Small, 1991b). These data provides convincing evidence that the IgA antibodies induced by prior virus infection are the mediators of resistance to reinfection and that other mediators of antiviral activity such as Tc or Th cells or IgG antibodies make little contribution to resistance. Thus, three major lines of evidence, namely, the consistent association of the level of IgA antibodies with the extent of resistance to virus infection, the mediation of mucosal resistance to virus infection by passive transfer of IgA antibodies, and the abrogation of infection-induced resistance to virus challenge by anti-IgA antibody treatment of the upper respiratory tract, clearly demonstrate that IgA antibodies are the major mediators of mucosal resistance to viral infections.

In conclusion, both cellular and humoral immune systems participate actively in the resolution of viral infections from mucosal surfaces, including the elimination of virus-infected cells, but T cells are likely to make a greater contribution in this phase of infection. In contrast, IgA antibodies play the major role in resistance to reinfection with a relatively minor direct role contributed by Tc and Th cells and IgG antibodies.

References

Anderson, J. J., Norden, J., Saunders, D., Toms, G. L., and Scott, R. (1990). Analysis of the local and systemic immune responses induced in BALB/c mice by experimental respiratory syncytial virus infection. *J. Gen. Virol.* **71,** 1561–1570.

Andrew, M. E., Coupar, B. E. H., Boyle, D. B., and Ada, G. L. (1987). The roles of influenza virus haemagglutinin and nucleoprotein in protection: Analysis using vaccinia virus recombinants. *Scand. J. Immunol.* **25,** 21–28.

Besser, T. E., Gay, C. C., McGuire, T. C., and Evermann, J. F. (1988). Passive immunity to bovine rotavirus infection associated with transfer of serum antibody into the intestinal lumen. *J. Virol.* **62,** 2238–2242.

Biron, C. A., Byron, K. S., and Sullivan, J. L. (1989). Severe herpesvirus infections in an adolescent without natural killer cells. *N. Engl. J. Med.* **320,** 1731–1735.

Bishop, R., Lund, J., Cipriani, E., Unicomb, L., and Barnes, G. (1990). Clinical serological and intestinal immune responses to rotavirus infection of humans. *In* "Medical Virology 9" (L. M. de la Maza, and E. M. Peterson, eds.), pp. 85–110. Plenum Press, New York.

Blandford, G., and Heath, R. B. (1972). Studies on the immune response and pathogenesis of Sendai virus infection of mice. I. The fate of viral antigens. *Immunology* **22,** 637–649.

Bodian, D., and Nathanson, N. (1960). Inhibitory effects of passive antibody on virulent poliovirus excretion and on immune response in chimpanzees. *Bull. Johns Hopkins Hosp.* **107,** 143–162.

Brown, T. A., Murphy, B. R., Radl, J., Haaijman, J. J., and Mestecky, J. (1985). Subclass distribution and molecular form of immunoglobulin A hemagglutinin antibodies in sera and nasal secretions after experimental secondary infection with influenza A virus in humans. *J. Clin. Microbiol.* **22,** 259–264.

Brown, T. A., Clements, M. L., Murphy, B. R., Radl, J., Haaijam, J. J., and Mestecky, J. (1987). Molecular form and subclass distribution of IgA antibodies after immunization with live and inactivated influenza A vaccines. *In* "Recent Advances in Mucosal Immunology" (J. Mestecky, J. R. McGhee, J. Bienenstock, and P. L. Ogra, eds.), Part B, pp. 1691–1700. Plenum, New York.

Burlington, D. B., Clements, M. L., Meiklejohn, G., Phelan, M., and Murphy, B. R. (1983). Hemagglutinin specific antibody responses in the IgG, IgA and IgM isotypes as measured by ELISA after primary or secondary infection of man with influenza A virus. *Infect. Immun.* **41,** 540–545.

Buscho, R. F., Perkins, J. C., Knopf, H. L. S., Kapikian, A. Z., and Chanock, R. M. (1972). Further characterization of the local respiratory tract antibody response induced by intranasal instillation of inactivated rhinovirus 13 vaccine. *J. Immunol.* **108,** 169–177.

Cannon, M. J., Openshaw, P. J. M., and Askonas, B. A. (1988). Cytotoxic T cells clear virus but augment lung pathology in mice infected with respiratory syncytial virus. *J. Exp. Med.* **168,** 1163–1168.

Chen, K.-S., Burlington, D. B., and Quinnan, G. V. (1987). Active synthesis of hemagglutinin-specific immunoglobuling A by lung cells of mice that were immunized intragastrically with inactivated influenza virus vaccine. *J. Virol.* **61,** 2150–2154.

Clements, M. L., O'Donnell, S., Levine, M. M., Chanock, R. M., and Murphy, B. R. (1983). Dose response of A/Alaska/6/77 (H3N2) cold-adapted reassortant vaccine virus in adult volunteers: Role of local antibody in resistance to infection with vaccine virus. *Infect. Immun.* **40,** 1044–1051.

Clements, M. L., Betts, R. F., Tierney, E. L., and Murphy, B. R. (1986). Serum and nasal wash antibodies associated with resistance to experimental challenge with influenza A wild-type virus. *J. Clin. Microbiol.* **24,** 157–160.

Conner, M. E., Gilger, M. A., Estes, M. K., and Graham, D. Y. (1991). Serologic and mucosal immune response to rotavirus infection in the rabbit model. *J. Virol.* **65,** 2562–2571.

Connors, M., Collins, P. L., Firestone, C.-Y., and Murphy, B. R. (1991). Respiratory syncytial virus (RSV) F, G, M2 (22K), and N proteins each induce resistance to RSV challenge, but resistance induced by M2 and N proteins is relatively short-lived. *J. Virol.* **65,** 1634–1637.

Corthier, G., and Vannier, P. (1983). Production of coproantibodies and immune complexes in piglets infected with rotavirus. *J. Infect. Dis.* **147,** 293–296.

Coulson, B. S., Grimwood, K., Masendycz, P. J., Lund, J. S., Mermelstein, N., Bishop, R. F., and Barnes, G. L. (1990). Comparison of rotavirus immunoglobulin A coproconversion with other indices of rotavirus infection in a longitudinal study in childhood. *J. Clin. Microbiol.* **28,** 1367–1374.

Czerkinsky, C., Prince, S. J., Michalek, S. M., Jackson, S., Russell, M. W., Moldoveanu, Z., McGhee, J. R., and Mestecky, J. (1987). IgA antibody-producing cells in peripheral blood after antigen ingestion: Evidence for a common mucosal immune system in humans. *Proc. Natl. Acad. Sci. U.S.A.* **84,** 2449–2453.

De St. Groth, S. F., and Donnelley, M. (1950). Studies in experimental immunology of influenza. IV. The protective value of active immunization. *Aust. J. Exp. Biol. Med. Sci.* **28,** 61–75.

Dharakul, T., Riepenhoff-Talty, M., Albini, B., and Ogra, P. L. (1988). Distribution of rotavirus antigen in intestinal lymphoid tissues: Potential role in development of the mucosal immune response to rotavirus. *Clin. Exp. Immunol.* **74,** 14–19.

Dharakul, T., Rott, L., and Greenberg, H. B. (1990). Recovery from chronic rotavirus infection in mice with severe combined immunodeficiency: Virus clearance mediated by adoptive transfer of immune $CD8^+$ T lymphocytes. *J. Virol.* **64,** 4375–4382.

Eichelberger, M., Allan, W., Zijlstra, M., Jaenisch, R., and Doherty, P. C. (1991a). Clearance of influenza virus respiratory infection in mice lacking class I major histocompatibility complex-restricted $CD8^+$ T cells. *J. Exp. Med.* **174,** 875–880.

Eichelberger, M. C., Wang, M., Allan, W., Webster, R. G., and Doherty, P. C. (1991b). Influenza virus RNA in the lung and lymphoid tissue of immunologically intact and CD4-depleted mice. *J. Gen. Virol.* **72,** 1695–1698.

Endo, A., Itamura, S., Iinuma, H., Funahashi, S.-I., Shida, H., Koide, F., Nerome, K., and Oya, A. (1991). Homotypic and heterotypic protection against influenza virus infection in mice by recombinant vaccinia virus expressing the haemagglutinin or nucleoprotein gene of influenza virus. *J. Gen. Virol.* **72,** 699–703.

Friedman, M. G. (1982). Radioimmunoassay for the detection of virus-specific IgA antibodies in saliva. *J. Immunol. Meth.* **54,** 203–211.

Friedman, M. G., Phillip, M., and Dagan, R. (1989). Virus-specific IgA in serum, saliva, and tears of children with measles. *Clin. Exp. Immunol.* **75,** 58–63.

Grimwood, K., Lund, J. C. S., Coulson, B. S., Hudson, I. L., Bishop, R. F., and Barnes, G. L. (1988). Comparison of serum and mucosal antibody responses following severe acute rotavirus gastroenteritis in young children. *J. Clin. Microbiol.* **26,** 732–738.

Hicks, J. T., Ennis, F. A., Kim, E., and Verbonitz, M. (1978). The importance of an intact complement pathway in recovery from a primary viral infection: Influenza in decomplemented and in C5-deficient mice. *J. Immunol.* **121,** 1437–1445.

Hirabayashi, Y., Kurata, H., Funato, H., Nagamine, T., Aizawa, C., Tamura, S.-I., Shimada, K., and Kurata, T. (1990). Comparison of intranasal inoculation of influenza HA vaccine combined with cholera toxin B subunit with oral or parenteral vaccination. *Vaccine* **8,** 243–249.

Hjelt, K., Grauballe, P. C., Paerregaard, A., Nielsen, O. H., and Krasilnikoff, P. A. (1987). Protective effect of preexisting rotavirus-specific immunoglobulin A against naturally acquired rotavirus infection in children. *J. Med. Virol.* **21,** 39–47.

Jayashree, S., Bhan, M. K., Kumar, R., Raj, P., Glass, R., and Bhandari, N. (1988). Serum and salivary antibodies as indicators of rotavirus infection in neonates. *J. Infect. Dis.* **158,** 1117–1119.

Johnson, M. P., Meitin, C. A., Bender, B. S., and Small, P. A. (1988). Passive immune serum inhibits antibody response to recombinant vaccinia virus. *In* "Vaccines 88: Modern Approaches to New Vaccines Including Prevention of AIDS" (R. M. Chanock, R. A. Lerner, F. Brown, and H. Ginsberg, eds.), pp. 189–192. Cold Spring Harbor Laboratory Press, Cold Spring Harbor, New York.

Johnson, P. R., Feldman, S., Thompson, J. M., Mahoney, J. D., and Wright, P. E. (1986). Immunity to influenza A virus infection in young children. A comparison of natural infection, live cold-adapted vaccine, and inactivated vaccine. *J. Infect. Dis.* **154,** 121–127.

Jones, P. D., and Ada, G. L. (1986). Influenza virus-specific antibody-secreting cells in the murine lung during primary influenza virus infection. *J. Virol.* **60,** 614–619.

Kast, W. M., Bronkhorst, A. M., de Waal, L. P., and Melief, C. J. M. (1986). Cooperation between cytotoxic and helper T lymphocytes in protection against lethal Sendai virus infection. *J. Exp. Med.* **164,** 723–738.

Kaul, T. N., Welliver, R. C., Wong, D. T., Udwadia, R. A., Riddlesberger, K., and Ogra, P. L. (1981). Secretory antibody response to respiratory syncytial virus infection. *Am. J. Dis. Child* **135,** 1013–1016.

Keller, R., and Dwyer, J. E. (1968). Neutralization of poliovirus by IgA coproantibodies. *J. Immunol.* **101,** 192–202.

Kimman, T. G., and Westenbrink, F. (1990). Immunity to human and bovine respiratory syncytial virus. *Arch. Virol.* **112,** 1–25.

Kimman, T. G., Westenbrink, F., Schreuder, B. E. C., and Straver, P. J. (1987). Local and systemic antibody response to bovine respiratory syncytial virus infection and reinfection in calves with and without maternal antibodies. *J. Clin. Microbiol.* **25,** 1097–1106.

Kimman, T. G., Westenbrink, R., and Straver, P. J. (1989). Priming for local and systemic antibody memory responses to bovine respiratory syncytial virus: Effect of amount of virus, virus replication, route of administration and maternal antibodies. *Vet. Immunol. Immunopathol.* **22,** 145–160.

Lepow, M. L., Warren, R. J., Gray, N., Ingram, V. G., and Robbins, F. C. (1961). Effect of Sabin type 1 poliomyelitis vaccine administered by mouth to newborn infants. *N. Engl. J. Med.* **264,** 1071–1078.

Leung, K. N., and Ada, G. L. (1980). Cells mediating delayed-type hypersensitivity in the lungs of mice infected with an influenza A virus. *Scand J. Immunol.* **12,** 393–400.

Levine, B., Hardwick J. M., Trapp, B. D., Crawford, T. O., Bollinger, R. C., and Griffin, D. E. (1991). Antibody-mediated clearance of alphavirus infection from neurons. *Science* **254,** 856–860.

Liang, X., Lamm, M. E., and Nedrud, J. G. (1988). Oral administration of cholera toxin-Sendai virus conjugate potentiates gut and respiratory immunity against Sendai virus. *J. Immunol.* **141,** 1495–1501.

Liew, F. Y., Russell, S. M., Appleyard, G., Brand, C. M., and Beale, J. (1984). Cross-protection in mice infected with influenza A virus by the respiratory route is correlated with local IgA antibody rather than serum antibody or cytotoxic T cell reactivity. *Eur. J. Immunol.* **14,** 350–356.

Lightman, S., Cobbold, S., Waldmann, H., and Askonas, B. A. (1987). Do L3T4$^+$ cells act as effector cells in protection against influenza virus infection? *Immunology* **62,** 139–144.

London, S. D., Rubin, D. H., and Cebra, J. J. (1987). Gut mucosal immunization with reovirus serotype 1/L stimulates virus-specific cytotoxic T cell precursors as well as IgA memory cells in Peyer's patches. *J. Exp. Med.* **165,** 830–847.

Lukacher, A. E., Braciale, V. L., and Braciale, T. J. (1984). *In vivo* effector function of influenza virus-specific cytotoxic T lymphocyte clones is highly specific. *J. Exp. Med.* **160,** 814–826.

Lyn, D., Mazanec, M. B., Nedrud, J. G., and Portner, A. (1991). Location of amino acid residues important for the structure and biological function of the haemagglutinin-neuraminidase glycoprotein of Sendai virus by analysis of escape mutants. *J. Gen. Virol.* **72,** 817–824.

McBride, B. W., and Ward, K. A. (1987). Herpes simplex-specific IgG subclass response in herpetic keratitis. *J. Med. Virol.* **21,** 179–189.

McDermott, M. R., Lukacher, A. E., Braciale, V. L., Braciale, T. J., and Bienenstock, J. (1987). Characterization and *in vivo* distribution of influenza-virus-specific T-lymphocytes in the murine respiratory tract. *Am. Rev. Respir. Dis.* **135,** 245–249.

McIntosh, K., Masters, H. B., Orr, I., Chao, R. K., and Barkin, R. M. (1978). The immunologic response to infection with respiratory syncytial virus in infants. *J. Infect. Dis.* **138,** 24–32.

McIntosh, K., McQuillin, J., and Gardner, P. S. (1979). Cell-free and cell-bound antibody in nasal secretions from infants with respiratory syncytial virus infection. *Infect. Immun.* **23,** 276–281.

Mackenzie, C. D., Taylor, P. M., and Askonas, B. A. (1989). Rapid recovery of lung histology correlates with clearance of influenza virus by specific CD8$^+$ cytotoxic T cells. *Immunology* **67,** 375–381.

McMichael, A. J., Gotch, F. M., Noble, G. R., and Beare, P. A. S. (1983). Cytotoxic T-cell immunity to influenza. *N. Engl. J. Med.* **309,** 13–17.

Madden, D. R., Gorga, J. C., Strominger, J. L., and Wiley, D. C. (1991). The structure of HLA-B27 reveals nonamer self-peptides bound in an extended conformation. *Nature (London)* **353,** 321–325.

Maoliang, W. (1986). Production of IgA monoclonal antibodies against influenza A virus. *J. Virol. Meth.* **13,** 21–26.

Mazanec, M. B., Lamm, M. E., Lyn, D., Portner, A., and Nedrud, J. G. (1992). Comparison of IgA versus IgG monoclonal antibodies for passive immunization of the murine respiratory tract. *Virus Res.* **23,** 7–12.

Mazanec, M. B., Nedrud, J. G., and Lamm, M. E. (1987). Immunoglobulin A monoclonal antibodies protect against Sendai virus. *J. Viol.* **61,** 2624–2626.

Merchant, A. A., Groene, W. S., Cheng, E. H., and Shaw, R. D. (1991). Murine intestinal antibody response to heterologous rotavirus infection. *J. Clin. Microbiol.* **29,** 1693–1701.

Merriman, H., Woods, S., Winter, C., Fahnlander, A., and Corey, L. (1984). Secretory IgA antibody in cervicovaginal secretions from women with genital infection due to herpes simplex virus. *J. Infect. Dis.* **149,** 505–510.

Mestecky, J. (1987). The common mucosal immune system and current strategies for induction of immune responses in external secretions. *J. Clin. Immunol.* **7,** 265–276.

Mills, J., van Kirk, J. E., Wright, P. F., and Chanock, R. M. (1971). Experimental respiratory syncytial virus infection of adults. *J. Immunol.* **107,** 123–130.

Munoz, J. L., McCarthy, C. A., Clark, M. E., and Hall, C. B. (1991). Respiratory syncytial virus infection in C57BL/6 mice: Clearance of virus from the lungs with virus-specific cytotoxic T cells. *J. Virol.* **65,** 4494–4497.

Murphy, B. R., Chalhub, E. G., Nusinoff, S. R., Kasel, J., and Chanock, R. M. (1973). Temperature-sensitive mutants of influenza virus. III. Further characterization of the *ts*-1[E] influenza A recombinant (H_3N_2) virus in man. *J. Infect. Dis.* **128,** 479–487.

Murphy, B. R., Nelson, D. L., Wright, P. F., Tierney, E. L., Phelan, M. A., and Chanock, R. M. (1982). Secretory and systemic immunological response in children infected with live attenuated influenza A virus vaccines. *Infect. Immun.* **36,** 1102–1108.

Murphy, B. R., Alling, D. W., Snyder, M. H., Walsh, E. E., Prince, G. A., Chanock, R. M., Hemming, V. G., Rodriguez, W. J., Kim, H. W., Graham, B. S., and Wright, P. F. (1986a). Effect of age and preexisting antibody on serum antibody response of infants and children to the F and G glycoproteins during respiratory syncytial virus infection. *J. Clin. Microbiol.* **24,** 894–898.

Murphy, B. R., Graham, B. S., Prince, G. A., Walsh, E. E., Chanoch, R. M., Karzon, D. T., and Wright, P. F. (1986b). Serum and nasal-wash immunoglobulin G and A antibody response of infants and children to respiratory syncytial virus F and G glycoproteins following primary infection. *J. Clin. Microbiol.* **23,** 1009–1014.

Murphy, B. R., Olmstead, R. A., Collins, P. L., Chanock, R. M., and Prince, G. A. (1988). Passive transfer of respiratory syncytial virus (RSV) antiserum suppresses the immune response to the RSV fusion (F) and large (G) glycoproteins expressed by recombinant vaccinia viruses. *J. Virol.* **62,** 3907–3910.

Murphy, B. R., Collins, P. L., Lawrence, L., Zubak, J., Chanock, R. M., and Prince, G. A. (1989). Immunosuppression of the antibody response to respiratory syncytial virus (RSV) by preexisting serum antibodies: Partial prevention by topical infection of the respiratory tract with vaccinia virus-RSV recombinants. *J. Gen. Virol.* **70,** 2185–2190.

Nedrud, J. G., Liang, X., Hague, N., and Lamm, M. E. (1987). Combined oral/nasal immunization protects mice from Sendai virus infection. *J. Immunol.* **139,** 3484–3492.

Nguyen, T. D., Bottreau, E., Bernard, S., Lantier, I., and Aynaud, J. M. (1986). Neutralizing secretory IgA and IgG do not inhibit attachment of transmissible gastroenteritis virus. *J. Gen. Virol.* **67,** 939–943.

Nicholas, J. A., Rubino, K. L., Levely, M. E., Meyer, A. L., and Collins, P. L. (1991). Cytotoxic T cell activity against the 22-kDa protein of human respiratory syncytial virus (RSV) is associated with a significant reduction in pulmonary RSV replication. *Virology* **182,** 664–672.

Nishio, O., Sumi, J., Sakae, K., Ishihara, Y., Isomura, S., and Inouye, S. (1990). Fecal IgA antibody responses after oral poliovirus vaccination in infants and elder children. *Microbiol. Immunol.* **34,** 683–689.

Offit, P. A., and Dudzik, K. I. (1990). Rotavirus-specific cytotoxic T lymphocytes passively protect against gastroenteritis in suckling mice. *J. Virol.* **64,** 6325–6328.

Offit, P. A., Shaw, R. D., and Greenberg, H. B. (1986). Passive protection against rotavirus-induced diarrhea by monoclonal antibodies to surface proteins vp3 and vp7. *J. Virol.* **58,** 700–703.

Ogra, P. L. (1970). Distribution of echovirus antibody in serum, nasopharynx, rectum, and spinal fluid after natural infection with echovirus type 6. *Infect. Immun.* **2,** 150–155.

Ogra, P. L., and Karzon, D. T. (1969a). Poliovirus antibody response in serum and nasal secretions following intranasal inoculation with inactivated poliovaccine. *J. Immunol.* **102,** 15–23.

Ogra, P. L., and Karzon, D. T. (1969b). Distribution of poliovirus antibody in serum, nasopharynx and alimentary tract following segmental immunization of lower alimentary tract with poliovaccine. *J. Immunol.* **102,** 1423–1430.

Ogra, P. L., Coppola, P. R., MacGillivray, M. H., and Dzierba, J. L. (1974). Mechanism of mucosal immunity to viral infections in γA immunoglobulin-deficiency syndromes. *Proc. Soc. Exp. Biol. Med.* **145,** 811–816.

Onorato, I. M., Modlin, J. F., McBean, A. M., Thomas, M. L., Losonsky, G. A., and Bernier, R. H. (1991). Mucosal immunity induced by enhanced-potency inactivated and oral polio vaccines. *J. Infect. Dis.* **163,** 1–6.

Outlaw, M. C., and Dimmock, N. J. (1990). Mechanisms of neutralization of influenza virus on mouse tracheal epithelial cells by mouse monoclonal polymeric IgA and polyclonal IgM directed against the viral haemagglutinin. *J. Gen. Virol.* **71,** 69–76.

Outlaw, M. C., and Dimmock, N. J. (1991). Insights into neutralization of animal viruses gained from study of influenza virus. *Epidemiol. Infect.* **106,** 205–220.

Perkins, J. C., Tucker, D. N., Knopf, H. L. S., Wenzel, R. P., Kapikian, A. Z., and Chanock, R. M. (1969). Comparison of protective effect of neutralizing antibody in serum and nasal secretions in experimental rhinovirus type 13 illness. *Am. J. Epidemiol.* **90,** 519–526.

Ponzi, A. N., Merlino, C., Angeretti, A., and Penna, R. (1985). Virus-specific polymeric immunoglobulin A antibodies in serum from patients with rubella, measles, varicella, and herpes zoster virus infections. *J. Clin. Microbiol.* **22,** 505–509.

Prince, G. A., Horswood, R. L., and Chanock, R. M. (1985). Quantitative aspects of passive immunity to respiratory syncytial virus infection in infant cotton rats. *J. Virol.* **55,** 517–520.

Prince, G. A., Hemming, V. G., Horswood, R. L., Baron, P. A., Murphy, B. R., and Chanock, R. M. (1990). Mechanism of antibody-mediated viral clearance in immunotherapy of respiratory syncytial virus infection of cotton rats. *J. Virol.* **64,** 3091–3092.

Puck, J. M., Glezen, W. P., Frank, A. L., and Six, H. R. (1980). Protection of infants from infection with influenza A virus by transplacentally acquired antibody. *J. Infect, Dis.* **142,** 844–849.

Ramphal, R., Cogliano, R. C., Shands, J. W., and Small, P. A. (1979). Serum antibody prevents lethal murine influenza pneumonitis but not tracheitis. *Infect. Immun.* **25,** 992–997.

Ray, R., Glaze, B. J., Moldoveanu, Z., and Compans, R. W. (1988). Intranasal immunization of hamsters with envelope glycoproteins of human parainfluenza virus type 3. *J. Infect, Dis.* **157,** 648–654.

Renegar, K. B., and Small, P. A. (1991a). Passive transfer of local immunity to influenza virus infection by IgA antibody. *J. Immunol.* **146,** 1972–1978.

Renegar, K. B., and Small, P. A. (1991b). Immunoglobulin A mediation of murine nasal anti-influenza virus immunity. *J. Virol.* **65,** 2146–2148.

Reuman, P. D., Paganini, C. M. A., Ayoub, E. M., and Small, P. A. (1983). Maternal–infant transfer of influenza-specific immunity in the mouse. *J. Immunol.* **130,** 932–936.

Reuman, P. D., Ayoub, E. M., and Small, P. A. (1987). Effect of passive maternal antibody on influenza illness in children: A prospective study of influenza A in mother–infant pairs. *Pediatr. Infect. Dis. J.* **6,** 398–403.

Reuman, P. D., Bernstein, D. I., Keely, S. P., Sherwood, J. R., Young, E. C., and Schiff, G. M. (1990). Influenza-specific ELISA IgA and IgG predict severity of influenza disease in subjects prescreened with hemagglutination inhibition. *Antiviral Res.* **13,** 103–110.

Richardson, S. C., and Bishop, R. F. (1990). Homotypic serum antibody responses to rotavirus proteins following primary infection of young children with serotype 1 rotavirus. *J. Clin. Microbiol.* **28,** 1891–1897.

Richman, D. D., Murphy, B. R., Tierney, E. L., and Chanock, R. M. (1974). Specificity of the local secretory antibody to influenza A virus infection. *J. Immunol.* **113,** 1654–1656.

Rubin, D. H., Anderson, A. O., and Lucis, D. (1983). Potentiation of the secretory IgA response by oral and enteric administration of CP 20,961. *Ann. N.Y. Acad. Sci.* **409,** 866–870.

Rudzik, R., Clancy, R. L., Perey, D. Y. E., Day, R. P., and Bienenstock, J. (1975). Repopulation with IgA-containing cells of bronchial and intestinal lamina propria after transfer of homologous Peyer's patch and bronchial lymphocytes. *J. Immunol.* **114,** 1599–1604.

Sabin, A. B., Michaels, R. H., Krugman, S., Eiger, M. E., Berman, P. H., and Warren, J. (1963a). Effect of oral poliovirus vaccine in newborn children. I. Excretion of virus after ingestion of large doses of type I or of mixture of all three types, in relation to level of placentally transmitted antibody. *Pediatrics* **31,** 623–640.

Sabin, A. B., Michaels, R. H., Ziring, P., Krugman, S., and Warren, J. (1963b). Effect of oral poliovirus vaccine in newborn children. II. Intestinal resistance and antibody response at 6 months in children fed type I vaccine at birth. *Pediatrics* **31,** 641–654.

Scott, R. M., Dudding, B. A., Romano, S. V., and Russell, P. K.

(1972). Enteric immunization with live adenovirus type 21 vaccine. II. Systemic and local immune responses following immunization. *Infect. Immun.* **5,** 300–304.

Shaw, R. D., Groene, W. S., Mackow, E. R., Merchant, A. A., and Cheng, E. H. (1991). VP4-specific intestinal antibody response to rotavirus in a murine model of heterotypic infection. *J. Virol.* **65,** 3052–3059.

Smith, C. B., Purcell, R. H., Bellanti, J. A., and Chanock, R. M. (1966). Protective effect of antibody to parainfluenza type 1 virus. *N. Engl. J. Med.* **275,** 1145–1152.

Smith, T. J., Buescher, E. L., Top, F. H., Altemeier, W. A., and McCown, J. M. (1970). Experimental respiratory infection with type 4 adenovirus vaccine in volunteers: Clinical and immunological responses. *J. Infect. Dis.* **122,** 239–248.

Sonza, S., and Holmes, I. H. (1980). Coproantibody response to rotavirus infection. *Med. J. Aust.* **2,** 496–499.

Tamura, S.-I., Funato, H., Hirabayashi, Y., Kikuta, K., Suzuki, Y., Nagamine, T., Aizawa, C., Nakagawa, M., and Kurata, T. (1990). Functional role of respiratory tract haemagglutinin-specific IgA antibodies in protection against influenza. *Vaccine* **8,** 479–485.

Taylor, P. M., and Askonas, B. A. (1986). Influenza nucleoprotein-specific cytotoxic T-cell clones are protective *in vivo*. *Immunol.* **58,** 417–420.

Taylor, P. M., Esquivel, F., and Askonas, B. A. (1990). Murine $CD4^+$ T cell clones vary in function *in vitro* and in influenza infection *in vivo*. *Int. Immunol.* **2,** 323–328.

Wagner, D. K., Clements, M. L., Reimer, C. B., Snyder, M. H., Nelson, D. L., and Murphy, B. R. (1987). Analysis of IgG antibody responses after live and inactivated influenza A vaccine indicate that nasal wash IgG is a transudate from serum. *J. Clin. Microbiol.* **25,** 559–562.

Waldman, R. H., Kasel, J. A., Fulk, R. V., Togo, Y., Hornick, R. B., Heiner, G. G., Dawkins, A. T., and Mann, J. J. (1968). Influenza antibody in human respiratory secretions after subcutaneous or respiratory immunization with inactivated virus. *Nature (London)* **218,** 594–595.

Waldman, R. H., Wood, S. H., Torres, E. J., and Small, P. A. (1970). Influenza antibody response following aerosol administration of inactivated virus. *Am. J. Epidemiol.* **91,** 575–584.

Waldman, R. H., Stone, J., Bergmann, K. C., Khakoo, R., Lazzell, V., Jacknowitz, A., Waldman, E. R., and Howard, S. (1986). Secretory antibody following oral influenza immunization. *Am. J. Med. Sci.* **292,** 367–371.

Ward, R. L., Bernstein, D. I., Shukla, R., Young, E. C., Sherwood, J. R., McNeal, M. M., Walker, M. C., and Schiff, G. M. (1989). Effects of antibody to rotavirus on protection of adults challenged with a human rotavirus. *J. Infect. Dis.* **159,** 79–88.

Ward, R. L., Bernstein, D. I., Shukla, R., McNeal, M. M., Sherwood, J. R., Young, E. C., and Schiff, G. M. (1990). Protection of adults rechallenged with a human rotavirus. *J. Infect. Dis.* **161,** 440–445.

Watt, P. J., Robinson, B. S., Pringle, C. R., and Tyrrell, D. A. J. (1990). Determinants of susceptibility to challenge and the antibody response of adult volunteers given experimental respiratory syncytial virus vaccines. *Vaccine* **8,** 231–236.

Webster, R. G., Kawaoka, Y., Taylor, J., Weinberg, R., and Paoletti, E. (1991). Efficacy of nucleoprotein and haemagglutinin antigens expressed in fowlpox virus as vaccine for influenza in chickens. *Vaccine* **9,** 303–308.

Weltzin, R., Lucia-Jandris, P., Michetti, P., Fields, B. N., Kraehenbuhl, J. P., and Neutra, M. R. (1989). Binding and transepithelial transport of immunoglobulins by intestinal M cells: Demonstration using monoclonal IgA antibodies against enteric viral proteins. *J. Cell Biol.* **108,** 1673–1685.

Wright, P. F., Murphy, B. R., Kervina, M., Lawrence, E. M., Phelan, M. A., and Karzon, D. T. (1983). Secretory immunological response after intranasal inactivated influenza A virus vaccinations: Evidence for immunoglobulin A memory. *Infect. Immun.* **40,** 1092–1095.

Yamaguchi, H., Inouye, S., Yamauchi, M., Morishima, T., Matsuno, S., Isomura, S., and Suzuki, S. (1985). Anamnestic response in fecal IgA antibody production after rotaviral infection of infants. *J. Infect. Dis.* **152,** 398–400.

Yao, Q. Y., Rowe, M., Morgan, A. J., Sam, C. K., Prasad, U., Dang, H., Zeng, Y., and Rickinson, A. B. (1991). Salivary and serum IgA antibodies to the Epstein–Barr virus glycoprotein gp340: Incidence and potential for virus neutralization. *Int. J. Cancer* **48,** 45–50.

Yap, K. L., Ada, G. L., and McKensie, I. F. C. (1978). Transfer of specific cytoxic T lymphocytes protects mice inoculated with influenza virus. *Nature (London)* **273,** 238–239.

Yarchoan, R., Murphy, B. R., Strober, W. Schnieder, H. S., and Nelson, D. L. (1981). Specific anti-influenza virus antibody production *in vitro* by human peripheral blood mononuclear cells. *J. Immunol.* **127,** 2588–2594.

Zhaori, G., Sun, M., Faden, H. S., and Ogra, P. L. (1989). Nasopharyngeal secretory antibody response to poliovirus type 3 virion proteins exhibit different specificities after immunization with live or inactivated poliovirus vaccines. *J. Infect. Dis.* **159,** 1018–1024.

Section D

Mucosal Immunization and Vaccines

Section Editor: Pearay L. Ogra

(Chapters 30 through 34)

30

Passive Immunization: Systemic and Mucosal

Kathryn B. Renegar • Parker A. Small, Jr.

The passive transfer of maternal immunity is responsible for keeping all mammalian species alive. The process of evolution developed effective mechanisms for the passive transfer of both systemic and mucosal immunity from the mother to her offspirng. Experimental passive transfer of systemic immunity via serum antibody is well established, but the experimental passive transfer of mucosal immunity has been accomplished only recently. This chapter addresses the contributions of both natural and experimental mechanisms to the study of passive immunization.

I. NATURAL PASSIVE IMMUNIZATION

A. Systemic Immunity

The transfer of systemic immunity (IgG) from mother to offspring occurs prenatally via the placenta or yolk sac and after birth via the colostrum. Species vary in the contribution each route makes to the transfer of immunity (Waldman and Strober, 1969) and can be grouped into three categories (Table I) based on this variation.

1. Prenatal Transfer Only

The first group, using prenatal transfer only, includes primates, rabbits, and guinea pigs. Transport of IgG in primates occurs almost exclusively through the placenta. IgG transfer occurs via receptor-mediated transcytosis across the syncytiotrophoblast and transcellular transport through the fetal endothelium (Leach *et al.*, 1990). Human placental transfer of protective IgG antibodies against a number of pathogens including rotavirus (Hjelt *et al.*, 1985), hepatitis B (Hockel and Kaufman, 1986), measles (Lennon and Black, 1986), and group B streptococcus (Baker *et al.*, 1988) has been reported. Prenatal transfer of IgG in the rabbit occurs via the yolk sac and in the guinea pig via both the yolk sac and the fetal gut (Waldman and Strober, 1969).

2. Combined Prenatal and Postnatal Transfer

The group using combined prenatal and postnatal transfer includes rats, mice, cats, and dogs. Prenatal transmission occurs via the yolk sac/placenta and the fetal gut in the rat (Waldman and Strober, 1969). IgG is bound rapidly to receptors on the surface of the yolk sac membrane (Mucchielli *et al.*, 1983), endocytosed in clathrin-coated vesicles, and, early in gestation, is stored in subapical vacuoles. By late gestation, the antibody has been hydrolyzed or transferred to fetal capillaries (Jollie, 1985). Prenatal transmission in mice occurs by a similar mechanism (Gardner, 1976).

Although placental transfer occurs, studies in rodents have shown that most transport of antibody occurs postnatally from colostrum or milk (Nejamkis *et al.*, 1975; Oda *et al.*, 1983; Kohl and Loo, 1984; Arango-Jaramillo *et al.*, 1988; Barthold *et al.*, 1988; Heiman and Weisman, 1989). Postnatal transmission of systemic immunity from colostrum and milk occurs over a period of 10–21 days, depending on the species, with a gradual decrease in transmission over the last 3 days of the period (Waldman and Strober, 1969), and is limited to antibodies of the IgG class (Hammerberg *et al.*, 1977; Appleby and Catty, 1983). Transport is a receptor-mediated process (Simister and Rees, 1983). In rats, the receptor is found in enterocytes of the proximal intestine during the early postnatal period but is absent after weaning (Jakoi *et al.*, 1985). The receptor is specific for IgG and its Fc fragment and consists of two similar polypeptides of 48,000–52,000 daltons (p51) in association with β_2-microglobulin (Jakoi *et al.*, 1985; Simister and Mostov, 1989). The Fc binding subunit (p51) has three extracellular domains and a transmembane region, all of which are homologous to the corresponding domains of Class I major histocompatibility complex (MHC) antigens (Simister and Mostov, 1989).

3. Postnatal Transfer Only

Ruminants (cattle, sheep, goats), horses, and pigs (reviewed by Tizzard, 1987) use only postnatal transfer. Transport of colostral proteins from the lumen of the ileum in ruminants is largely nonspecific but, in the horse and pig, IgG and IgM are absorbed preferentially. Proteins are taken up actively by epithelial cells through pinocytosis and passed through these cells into the lacteals and intestinal capillaries (Tizzard, 1987). Intestinal absorption occurs for only the first 24–48 hours after birth, then the "open gut" closes down and no further transfer from milk or colostrum occurs (Waldman and Strober, 1969; Francis and Black, 1984; Ellis *et al.*, 1986; Tizzard, 1987). Newborn piglets have also been shown to absorb colostral lymphoid cells during this time period (Tuboly *et al.*, 1988).

Absorption of colostral immunoglobulin is normally extremely effective, supplying the newborn with serum immunoglobulin (particularly IgG) at a level approaching that found in adults (Tizzard, 1987); however, failure of passive transfer

Table I Transfer of Immunity to Offspring

Prenatal transfer	
	Primates
	Rabbit
	Guinea Pig
Combined prenatal and postnatal transfer	
	Rat
	Mouse
	Cat
	Dog
Postnatal transfer	
	Ruminants
	Horse
	Pig

(FPT) can occur and, when it does, can pose a considerable problem in animal husbandry. About 25% of newborn foals fail to obtain sufficient quantities of immunoglobulin (McGuire *et al.*, 1975; Tizzard, 1987). In the McGuire study (1975), 2 of 9 FPT foals died of infections within a few days of birth and 5 of the remaining 7 developed nonfatal respiratory infections between 2 and 5 weeks of age. McGuire *et al.* (1976) also reported FPT in calves, finding that 85% of calves less than 3 weeks old dying from infectious diseases had significant hypogammaglobulinemia. Although adequate methods to diagnose and treat FPT are available (Tizzard, 1987; Bertone *et al.*, 1988), the phenomenon remains a significant veterinary problem.

B. Mucosal Immunity

Mother's milk provides passive protection of the mucosal surfaces it contacts. This protection may be mediated by nonspecific factors found in milk, for example, lactoferrin, lysozyme, fatty acids, and complement, or by specific antibody (reviewed by Goldman *et al.*, 1985). The antibody composition of milk differs from that of colostrum (Tizzard, 1987) and the class of protective antibody in milk varies with the species and the route of immunization of the mother. With the exception of IgG in rodents, these protective antibodies are not absorbed systemically by the suckling offspring but exert their protective effect locally by neutralizing viruses or virulence factors and by binding to microbial pathogens to prevent their attachment to the mucosal surface (Goldman *et al.*, 1985). Secretory IgA is especially suited to this protective role since secretory component enhances its resistance to proteolytic enzymes and gastric acid (Kenny *et al.*, 1967; Tomasi, 1970; Zikan *et al.*, 1972; Lindh, 1975) providing extra antibody stability in mucosal secretions.

1. Milk Antibody in Rodents

Rodents have been a popular model for the study of passive transfer of maternal immunity via milk; however, this group of animals has a major drawback as a model for passive mucosal immunity. Rats and mice can actively transport IgG from the gut into the serum for approximately 2 weeks (Section I,A,2). Thus, observed protection could be the result of antibody in the milk bathing the mucosal surfaces or of maternal antibody being transported into the serum and secretions of the offspring. This caveat should be kept in mind during the evaluation of the many reports of milk-borne protection in these species. Three rodent models in which protection of mucosal surfaces is due to milk-borne, not serum-derived, antibody are described here.

The predominant immunoglobulin in mouse milk is IgG, although significant levels of IgA can also be present (Ijaz *et al.*, 1987). Protection of infant mice from colonization with *Campylobacter jejuni* can be achieved by the consumption of immune milk at and after the time of bacterial challenge. The milk in this study contained high concentrations of specific IgG antibodies and very little specific IgA antibody; infant mice were not protected by prior consumption of colostrum. Milk antibody was required in the gut lumen for protection to be observed (Abimiku and Dolby, 1987). A similar requirement for antibodies active at the intestinal cell surface in murine immunity to primate rotavirus SA-11 was reported by Offit *et al.* (1984).

In rats, protection against dental caries by milk can be due to IgG or SIgA antibodies, depending on the route of maternal immunization. Rat dams immunized intravenously with heat-killed *Streptococcus mutans* developed IgG antibodies in their colostrum, milk, and serum. Their offspring demonstrated significant protection against *S. mutans*-induced caries formation. Rat dams locally injected in the region of the mammary gland with heat-killed *S. mutans* or fed formalin-killed *S. mutans* developed SIgA antibodies in their colostrum and milk. Their offspring were also protected against caries formation (Michalek and McGhee, 1977). Caries protection in suckling rats theoretically could be due to either bathing mucosal surfaces or antibody leakage into the saliva from the serum. Nonimmune adult rats can be protected from *S. mutans*-induced caries by feeding on lyophilized immune bovine milk or on immune bovine whey containing specific IgG (Michalek *et al.*, 1978a,1987). Since adult rats are unable to transport orally administered IgG into their serum, protection is from milk-derived antibodies bathing the oral cavity.

2. Milk Antibody in Ungulates

In ruminants (sheep, cattle, goats), the predominant antibody in both colostrum and milk is IgG_1. The predominant antibody in the colostrum of pigs and horses is also IgG but, as lactation progresses and colostrum becomes milk, IgA predominates (Tizzard, 1987). Protection can be mediated by either antibody class. Whereas bathing of the mucosal surfaces by milk-derived antibodies can provide passive immunity to some pathogens, the high rate of infections in FPT foals and calves shows that milk (mucosal immunity) alone cannot provide complete protection to neonates.

In cattle and pigs, passive immunity against enteric infections with viruses such as rotaviruses and coronaviruses [transmissible gastroenteritis (TGE)] is dependent on the continual presence in the gut lumen of a protective level of specific antibodies (Crouch, 1985). In swine, passive immunity against intestinal infection with the TGE virus is generally more complete in piglets ingesting IgA antibodies than in those ingesting IgG antibodies, although both classes of antibody are protective. The class of antibody present in sow milk depends on the route of immunization (Bohl and Saif, 1975). In cattle, passive immunity in calf scours (neonatal bovine colibacillosis caused by *Escherichia coli*) correlates with the level of specific IgA antibody in milk (Wilson and Jutila, 1976).

3. Milk Antibody in Primates

In primates, IgA is the predominant immunoglobulin in both colostrum and milk (Tizzard, 1987). Both lysozyme and SIgA in human milk remain bioavailable in the digestive tract of the early infant (Eschenburg *et al.*, 1990). Human milk has been shown to contain SIgA antibodies against at least five viruses and nine bacterial pathogens, as well as against fungi, parasites, and food antigens (Goldman *et al.*, 1985). Mucosal immunity to rotavirus, for example, was shown to be transferred to the infant by the SIgA in milk. A positive correlation was found between titers of secretory component in mother's milk and infant feces, and virus-specific IgA was found in infant fecal samples (Rahman *et al.*, 1987). In addition to providing passive mucosal immunity, human breast milk also stimulates the early local production of SIgA in the urinary and gastrointestinal tracts, thus accelerating the development of an active local host defense system in the infant (Prentice, 1987; Koutras and Vigorita, 1989).

II. EXPERIMENTAL PASSIVE IMMUNIZATION

Since the first transfer of immunity by the injection of serum (von Behring and Kitasato, 1890), passive transfer of humoral immunity has been investigated intensively. The use of specific serum antibody (IgG) to transfer protection to nonimmune individuals has become so routine that it is now common medical practice in, for example, the postexposure prophylaxis of rabies and tetanus and the treatment of snakebite (Arnold, 1982; Centers for Disease Control, 1991a,b).

Local immunity has been correlated with the level of IgA in various secretions (Table II). However, direct demonstration of the mediation of local immunity by injected IgA could not occur until specific transport of passively administered IgA had been confirmed.

Table II Correlation of IgA with Local Immunity

Anatomical site	Agent	Reference
Eye/tears	Newcastle disease virus	Katz and Kohn (1976)
	Shigella	Levenson *et al.* (1988)
	Staphylococcus aureus	Mondino *et al.* (1987)
Mouth/saliva	*Streptococcus mutans*	Michalek *et al.* (1978b,1983a,b); Morisaki *et al.* (1983); Russell and Mestecky (1986)
Gastrointestinal tract	Campylobacter jejuni	Burr *et al.* (1988)
	Canine parvovirus	Nara *et al.* (1983)
	Escherichia coli	Porter *et al.* (1977); Chidlow and Porter (1979); Evans *et al.* (1988)
	Giardia	Kaplan *et al.* (1985)
	Poliovirus	Fox (1984)
	Shigella flexneri	Keren *et al.* (1988,1989)
	Transmissible gastroenteritis virus of swine	DeBuysscher and Berman (1980)
	Vibrio cholerae	Svennerholm *et al.* (1978); Jertborn *et al.* (1986)
Respiratory tract (nose and/or trachea)	*Hemophilus influenzae*	Clancy *et al.* (1983)
	Influenza virus	Bergman and Waldman (1988); Brown *et al.* (1988); Hirabayashi *et al.* (1990); Meitin *et al.* (1991)
	Parainfluenza, type 1	Smith *et al.* (1966)
	Penumococcal polysaccharide	Lue *et al.* (1988)
	Sendai virus	Nedrud *et al.* (1987)
	Streptococcal M protein	Kurono and Mogi (1987); Poirier *et al.* (1988)
Urinary tract	*Escherichia coli*	Layton and Smithyman (1983)
	Ovalbumin	Husband and Clifton (1989)
Reproductive tract	*Chlamydia*	Lamont *et al.* (1978); Brunham *et al.* (1983); Ogra *et al.* (1989)
Skin	Miscellaneous bacteria and fungi	Metze *et al.* (1991)

A. Transport of Passively Administered IgA to Mucosal Surfaces

1. Gastrointestinal Tract

In rabbits, rats, and mice, polymeric IgA can be and is transported efficiently from the circulation into the bile via the liver (Orlans *et al.*, 1978,1983; Delacroix *et al.*, 1982; Koertge and Butler, 1986a; Mestecky and McGhee, 1987). These species express secretory component on their hepatocytes (Socken *et al.*, 1979) and, in addition, have polymeric IgA as the primary molecular form in their serum (Vaerman, 1973; Heremans, 1974). Serum IgA is also transported efficiently into bile in cattle (Butler *et al.*, 1986). In fact, most IgA in ruminant bile may be of serum origin.

Transport of serum IgA into bile in humans has been reported (Delacroix *et al.*, 1982; Dooley *et al.*, 1982), although IgA transport is about 50-fold less efficient than in rats and rabbits. The human biliary IgA level is approximately 20% of the human serum IgA level and, under physiologic conditions, only 50% of human biliary IgA is derived from the serum (Vaerman and Delacroix, 1984). Although transport is possible, passively administered IgA does not reach high levels in human bile. In one study, less than 3% of intravenously injected radiolabeled polymeric IgA was found in human bile after 24 hr (Vaerman and Delacroix, 1984). This subject is reviewed in Chapter 10.

2. Saliva

Serum polymeric IgA can be transported into saliva in dogs (Montgomery *et al.*, 1977), monkeys (Challacombe *et al.*, 1978), and humans (Delacroix *et al.*, 1982; Kubagawa *et al.*, 1987). In humans, the amount of IgA acquired from the serum is low (only 2% from the serum) compared with the amount acquired from local production (Delacroix *et al.*, 1982). Transfer of polymeric IgA from serum into canine saliva is a selective process requiring secretory component (Montgomery *et al.*, 1977), whereas transport into oral fluids in monkeys appears to be by leakage from the plasma into the crevicular spaces surrounding the deciduous molars (Challacombe *et al.*, 1978).

3. Milk

In sheep, active transport of IgA from the circulation into milk seems likely (Sheldrake *et al.*, 1984); however, studies on the transport of IgA into murine milk have produced conflicting results. Using radiolabeled IgA, Halsey *et al.* (1983) demonstrated in the mouse that IgA can be transported from the circulation into milk during early lactation. Other investigators (Russell *et al.*, 1982; Koertge and Butler, 1986b), using assays based on antibody-binding activity, were unable to show transport of IgA into murine milk. Using radiolabeled IgA, Koertge and Butler (1986b) were able to show that the IgA present in milk was degraded and suggested that the previous study (Halsey *et al.*, 1983) detected only IgA fragments that had been transudated into the milk from the serum and not specifically transported IgA. Passively administered IgA is not transported into the milk of rats (Dahlgren *et al.*, 1981; Koertge and Butler, 1986b).

4. Respiratory Tract

Only a limited number of studies on the transport of antibodies into respiratory secretions have been reported, but the results have shown that selective transport of passively administered serum IgA into the respiratory tract is possible in sheep and mice. Because of their importance as background information for the experiments demonstrating the passive transfer of local immunity by IgA, these respiratory transport studies will be addressed in more detail.

a. Sheep. Using the intravenous (iv) injection of radioiodinated ovine immunoglobulin, Scicchitano *et al.* (1984) showed that 35% of the IgA in the mediastinal lymph of sheep is plasma derived. These investigators further demonstrated (Scicchitano *et al.*, 1986), by the simultaneous injection of radiolabeled IgA and radiolabeled IgG_1 or IgG_2, that IgA is transported selectively into ovine respiratory secretions. Transport of IgA, calculated 24 hr postinjection, was approximately 4.5 times greater than transport of IgG, and the transported IgA was intact in the secretions. Biologic activity of transported IgA was not determined.

b. Mice. Mazanec *et al.* (1989) found that, 4–5 hr after the iv injection of radiolabeled monomeric or polymeric IgA anti-Sendai virus monoclonal antibodies into mice, transport of polymeric IgA into nasal secretions was 3–7 times more efficient than transport of monomeric IgA whereas polymeric IgA transport into bronchioalveolar lavages was only 1–3 times more efficient. This difference probably reflects an increased contribution of serum antibody to bronchioalveolar secretions because of the transudation of IgG into alevolar fluids. Transport of polymeric IgA into the gut was 4–5 times more efficient than the transport of monomeric IgA, as expected. The agreement of the nasal secretion and gut transport indices suggests that transport could occur by a similar mechanism. The investigators were unable to demonstrate the presence of functionally intact polymeric IgA in the upper respiratory tract.

The polymeric IgA transported into murine nasal secretions in the studies reported by Renegar and Small (1991a) was, in contrast, functionally intact. To avoid problems associated with the quantitation of intact compared with degraded radiolabeled IgA in secretions (described by Koertge and Butler, 1986b), this study used an anti-influenza enzyme-linked immunosorbent assay (ELISA) to evaluate the transport of monomeric or polymeric IgA or IgG_1 monoclonal anti-influenza antibodies into the nasal secretions of mice. Any antibodies detected by this assay were, of necessity, functional. Nonimmune mice were injected intravenously with influenza-specific monomeric or polymeric IgA or IgG_1 and sacrificed at varying times between 2 and 24 hr postinjection. Nasal wash, serum, and bile samples were collected and assayed by ELISA for anti-influenza antibody. The peak nasal wash polymeric IgA titer was reached 4 hr after antibody injection and was approximately 35 times greater than the nasal wash titer of either monomeric immunoglobulin.

To determine whether polymeric IgA was transported selectively relative to IgG_1, the investigators injected a mixture of the two monoclonal antibodies intravenously into nonimmune mice and calculated a selective transport index (STI) for nasal antibody for each mouse. An STI greater than 1 indicates that polymeric IgA was transported specifically relative to IgG_1 whereas a value of 1 indicates that the same extent of transport, leakage, or transudation of both polymeric IgA and IgG_1 occurred in that animal. Of the 31 mice studied, 29 showed an STI greater than 1 (average STI at 4 hr was 36 ± 19) demonstrating the selective transport of polymeric IgA relative to IgG_1. Selective transport of polymeric IgA relative to monomeric IgA was also demonstrated.

Thus, transport of serum IgA into nasal secretions is possible in some species. The relevance of this transport to the passive transfer of local immunity will be addressed in Section II,B,2,a.

B. Protection of Mucosal Surfaces by Passively Administered Antibodies

Studies on the passive transfer of local immunity can be classified into two categories. In the first category are studies in which the antibody is introduced into the local secretions exogenously or mixed with the target pathogen prior to host challenge. The second category includes those studies in which systemically administered polymeric IgA must be transported physiologically (i.e., by secretory component-mediated mechanisms) to its site of activity.

1. Exogenously Administered Antibody

The studies in this category have investigated the role of IgA in mucosal immunity by feeding antibody or instilling it intranasally, then challenging, or by administering antibody–pathogen mixtures intranasally.

a. Oral antibody. Offit *et al.* (1984) demonstrated the ability of milk-derived IgG and IgA to protect the murine intestine from infection with primate rotavirus SA-11. Suckling mice were protected by milk from dams that had been immunized orally with SA-11 virus. This protective activity was detected in both the IgG and IgA fractions, but the IgA fraction was more potent *in vivo* than the IgG fraction. In newborn mice from immune dams foster-nursed on seronegative dams, the presence of circulating systemic antirotavirus antibodies in high titer did not protect against SA-11 viral infection. Thus, the specific antibody had to be present in the gut lumen to protect the intestinal cell surface from viral infection, and SIgA could mediate this protection.

b. Intranasal antibody. Three studies have shown that exogenously administered IgA can protect against intranasal challenge with a pathogen. Bessen and Fischetti (1988) showed that SIgA given by the intranasal route protected mice against streptococcal infection. Live streptococci were mixed with affinity-purified human salivary SIgA or serum IgG antibodies directed toward the streptococcal M6 protein. The mixture was administered intranasally to mice. The SIgA antibody protected against streptococcal infection whereas the serum antibody had no effect. This study suggested that SIgA alone is capable of protecting the mucosa against bacterial invasion.

Mazanec *et al.* (1987) demonstrated that IgA can protect mucosal surfaces against viral infection. Ascites fluid containing IgA anti-Sendai virus monoclonal antibody was administered intranasally to lightly anesthetized mice before and after the mice were challenged intranasally with live virus. Mice were sacrificed 3 days later and lung viral titers were determined. Animals treated with the specific monoclonal antibody were protected against viral infection. Additional work from the same laboratory showed that local immunity to Sendai virus also can be mediated by intranasal IgG (Mazanec *et al.* (1992). Tamura *et al.* (1991) purified anti-influenza SIgA antibodies from the respiratory tracts of mice immunized with influenza hemagglutinin molecules. This IgA, when given intranasally, protected nonimmune mice from influenza infection. Protection, which was observed up to 3 days after antibody administration, was proportional to the amount of IgA administered and was observed at IgA doses equivalent to naturally occurring antibody titers.

These studies show that local IgA or IgG can protect against viral or bacterial infection of the mucosa. They do not show that physiologically transported (secretory) IgA or serum-derived IgG actually does so. For that demonstration, antibody must be administered parenterally and transported into the mucosal secretions by a physiologic mechanism. The studies presented in the next section satisfy that criterion.

2. Systemically Administered Antibody

The definitive studies in this category have involved the respiratory and gastrointestinal tracts, although passive transfer of uterine immunity by polymeric IgA also has been observed (K. B. Renegar, A. C. Menge, P. A. Small, Jr., and J. Mestecky, unpublished results). Work with the respiratory and gastrointestinal tracts will be presented in more detail.

a. Respiratory tract. Numerous studies have shown that passively administered serum anti-influenza antibody (IgG) can prevent lethal viral pneumonia (Loosli *et al.*, 1953; Barber and Small, 1978; Ramphal *et al.*, 1979; Kris *et al.*, 1988). Serum antibody, however, does not prevent influenza infection of the upper respiratory tract (Barber and Small, 1978; Ramphal *et al.*, 1979; Kris *et al.*, 1988). Protection of the nose correlates with an increased nasal secretion IgA antibody level (Table II), making influenza an excellent model in which to investigate the hypothesis that nasal immunity is mediated by SIgA.

The first demonstration of the passive transfer of local immunity by physiologically transported SIgA was reported by Renegar and Small (1991a) in the murine influenza model. These researchers showed, as described in Section II,A,4,b, that intravenously administered polymeric IgA is transported into nasal secretions in a physiologic manner. To determine whether intravenously administered polymeric IgA anti-influenza monoclonal antibody could mediate protection against local influenza virus challenge, passively immunized mice were challenged intranasally while awake with influenza virus. The mice were sacrificed 24 hr later and the amount of virus shed in their nasal secretions was determined. Of the 24 saline-injected control mice, 23 shed virus into the nasal secretions whereas only 5 of the 25 polymeric IgA-injected mice shed virus; those 5 that did shed virus had a low viral titer. The observed protection was significant ($p < 0.001$). Passive immunization with influenza-specific polymeric IgA, therefore, conferred complete protection against viral infection in 80% of the mice and partial protection in the remaining 20%.

To determine whether serum IgG_1 also could confer local protection to influenza challenge, the relative abilities of equivalent virus-neutralizing doses of influenza-specific polymeric IgA or IgG_1 to protect against influenza challenge were compared. Intravenous polymeric IgA significantly reduced viral shedding compared with either intravenous saline or intravenous IgG_1. Intravenous IgG_1 also reduced viral shedding ($p < 0.02$); however, the protection against infection was not significant ($p = 0.5$), since viral shedding was prevented in only 1 of 8 mice injected. Additional studies (K. B. Renegar and P. A. Small, Jr., unpublished results) have shown that IgG_1 can also mediate local protection against influenza infection, but 10 times the polymeric IgA protective dose is required to produce this protection.

The passive protection studies showed that IgA *can* mediate local immunity. To confirm that IgA *is* the mediator of local immunity, a method to abolish IgA-mediated protection was needed. Mice passively immunized with polymeric IgA were given nose drops of anti-IgA antibody 10 min before and 6 hr after they were challenged intranasally with influenza virus suspended in anti-IgA antiserum. Anti-IgA treatment abrogated IgA-mediated protection in the passively immunized mice (Renegar and Small, 1991a). To show that passive transfer of local immunity by IgA was a reflection of the natural situation, the abrogation technique was extended to mice convalescent from influenza infection (Renegar and Small, 1991b). Nonimmune mice and convalescent mice, that is, mice that had recovered from an influenza virus infection 4–6 weeks earlier and were therefore naturally immune, were treated intranasally with antiserum to IgA or IgG or with a mixture of antisera to IgG and IgM, then challenged while awake with influenza virus mixed with antiserum. Intranasal administration of antiserum was continued at intervals for 24 hr. Mice were killed 1 day after viral challenge, and their nasal washes were assayed for virus shedding (Figure 1). Nonimmune mice all became infected, regardless of whether the virus was administered in saline, normal rabbit serum, or anti-immunoglobulin antiserum. Convalescent mice, as expected, were protected from viral infection. Administration of influenza virus in either anti-IgG or a mixture of anti-IgG and anti-IgM antisera did not affect protection, that is, the convalescent mice were still immune. Administration of virus in anti-IgA antiserum, however, abrogated convalescent immunity. These results show that IgA is the major (if not the sole) mediator of mucosal immunity to influenza virus in the murine nose and suggest that passive immunization mimics the role SIgA plays in natural immunity.

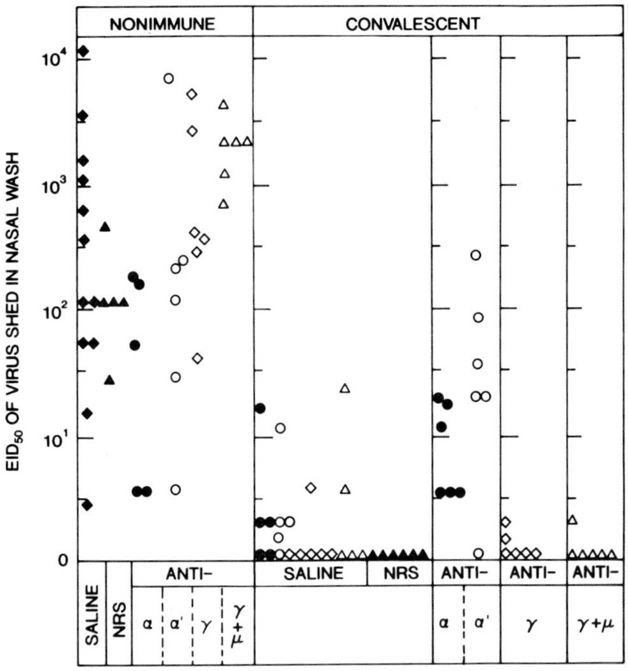

Figure 1 Effect of intranasal installation of anti-IgA, anti-IgG, anti-IgM, or NRS on nasal immunity of convalescent mice. Virus shedding from 12 nonimmune saline-treated mice (◆) is shown in the left column. Experiment 1 (●): nonimmune and convalescent mice were treated intranasally with 10 μl anti-IgA (anti-α) and challenged with influenza virus in anti-IgA. Convalescent control mice were treated similarly, except saline was substituted for anti-IgA. Experiment 2 (○): nonimmune and convalescent mice were treated with 20 μl anti-IgA (anti-α). Convalescent control mice were treated similarly with saline. Experiment 3 (▲): nonimmune and convalescent mice were treated with 20 μl NRS. Experiment 4 (◇): nonimmune and convalescent mice were treated with 20 μl anti-IgG (anti-γ). Convalescent control mice were treated with saline. Experiment 5 (△): nonimmune and convalescent mice were treated with 20 μl anti-IgG and anti-IgM (anti-γ + μ). Convalescent control mice were treated with saline. EID_{50}, 50% egg infective dose. Reprinted with permission from Renegar and Small (1991b).

b. Gastrointestinal tract. Additional evidence that secretory IgA is the mediator of local immunity comes from studies of the gastrointestinal tract. Polymeric IgA hybridomas against *Vibrio cholerae* were generated and the resulting monoclonal antibodies used to determine whether IgA can mediate immunity toward a bacterial pathogen in the gut (Winner *et al.*, 1991). The investigators selected a clone that produced dimeric monoclonal IgA antibodies directed against an Ogawa-specific lipopolysaccharide carbohydrate antigen exposed on the bacterial surface. These antibodies were able to cross-link bacterial organisms *in vitro*, suggesting that they might be effective in preventing mucosal colonization by the pathogen *in vivo*. To provide continuous physiologic (i.e., secretory component-mediated) transport of specific antibody into the gut, hybridoma cells were injected subcutaneously into the backs of adult BALB/c mice. These "backpack" tumors released monoclonal IgA into the circulation and the serum IgA was transported into the gut lumen. Neonatal mice bearing these backpack tumors survived challenge with *V. cholerae* whereas neonatal mice bearing backpack tumors of unrelated IgA hybridomas and non-tumor-bearing neonatal mice died. This ingenious model provides the first evidence that secretory IgA alone can mediate mucosal immunity to a bacterial pathogen and serves as the second example of the passive transfer of local immunity by IgA.

3. Implications for Passive Immunization

The general approach of passive parenteral transfer of mucosal immunity should be a useful research tool for determining the role of SIgA in protection against other pathogens and at other mucosal surfaces. The possibility of therapy by passively administered IgA antibody is more problematic. Generation of gastrointestinal protection by feeding specific antibodies is certainly possible and already has been reported in cattle (Tsunemitsu *et al.*, 1989). Passive protection by injection is, however, highly speculative because of the questionable efficiency of transport to the targeted mucosal surface and the potential adverse effects of intravenous IgA antibody. Serum IgA has been associated with both decreased complement activation (Russell *et al.*, 1989) and decreased immune lysis (Griffiss and Goroff, 1983). Systemically administered polymeric IgA may also be highly suppressive of both specific humoral and cellular responses (K. B. Renegar, S. Taylor, and P. A. Small, Jr., unpublished observations). A more thorough knowledge of the role IgA can play in regulating the immune response is needed before passive mucosal immunization via parenteral antibody administration can become an acceptable means of therapy in humans.

References

Abimiku, A. G., and Dolby, J. M. (1987). The mechanism of protection of infant mice from intestinal colonisation with *Campylobacter jejuni*. *J. Med. Microbiol.* **23,** 339–344.

Appleby, P., and Catty, D. (1983). Transmission of immunoglobulin to foetal and neonatal mice. *J. Reprod. Immunol.* **5,** 203–213.

Arango-Jaramillo, S., Wisseman, C. L., Jr., and Azad, A. F. (1988). Newborn rats in the murine typhus enzootic infection cycle: Studies on transplacental infection and passively acquired maternal antirickettsial antibodies. *Am. J. Trop. Med. Hyg.* **39,** 391–397.

Arnold, R. E. (1982). Treatment of rattlesnake bites. *In* "Rattlesnake Venoms; Their Actions and Treatment" (A. T. Tu, ed.), pp. 315–338. Marcel Dekker, New York.

Baker, C. J., Rench, M. A., Edwards, M. S., Carpenter, R. J., Hays, B. M., and Kasper, D. L. (1988). Immunization of pregnant women with a polysaccharide vaccine of group B streptococcus. *N. Engl. J. Med.* **319,** 1180–1185.

Barber, W. H., and Small, P. A., Jr. (1978). Local and systemic immunity to influenza infections in ferrets. *Infect. Immun.* **21,** 221–228.

Barthold, S. W., Beck, D. S., and Smith, A. L. (1988). Mouse hepatitis virus and host determinants of vertical transmission and maternally-derived passive immunity in mice. *Arch. Virol.* **100,** 171–183.

Bergman, K.-C., and Waldman, R. H. (1988). Enhanced murine respiratory tract IgA antibody respone to oral influenza vaccine when combined with a lipoidal amine (avridine). *Int. Arch. Allergy Appl. Immunol.* **87,** 334–335.

Bertone, J. J., Jones, R. L., and Curtis, C. R. (1988). Evaluation of a test kit for determination of serum immunoglobulin G concentration in foals. *J. Vet. Intern. Med.* **2,** 181–183.

Bessen, D., and Fischetti, V. A. (1988). Passive acquired mucosal immunity to group A streptococci by secretory immunoglobulin A. *J. Exp. Med.* **167,** 1945–1950.

Bohl, E. H., and Saif, L. J. (1975). Passive immunity in transmissible gastroenteritis of swine: Immunoglobulin characteristics of antibodies in milk after inoculationg virus by different routes. *Infect. Immun.* **11,** 23–32.

Brown, T. A., Murphy, B. R., Radl, R., Haaijman, J. J., and Mestecky, J. (1988). Subclass distribution and molecular form of immunoglobulin A hemagglutinin antibodies in sera and nasal secretions after experimental secondary infection with influenza A virus in humans. *J. Clin. Microbiol.* **22,** 259–264.

Brunham, R. C., Kuo, C.-C., Cles, L., and Holmes, K. K. (1983). Correlation of host immune response with quantitative recovery of *Chlamydia trachomatis* from the human endocervix. *Infect. Immun.* **39,** 1491–1494.

Burr, D. H., Caldwell, M. B., Bourgeois, A. L., Morgan, H. R. Wistar, R., Jr., and Walker, R. I. (1988). Mucosal and systemic immunity to *Campylobacter jejuni* in rabbits after gastric inoculation. *Infect. Immun.* **56,** 99–105.

Butler, J. E., Frenyo, V. L., Whipp, S. C., Wilson, R. A., and Koertge, T. E. (1986). The metabolism and transport of bovine serum SIgA. *Comp. Immunol. Microbiol. Infect. Dis.* **9,** 303–315.

Centers for Disease Control (1991a). Rabies prevention—United States: Recommendations of the Immunization Practices Advisory Committee (ACIP). *Morbid. Mortal. Wkly. Rep.* **40 (RR-3),** 7–8.

Centers for Disease Control (1991b). Diptheria, tetanus, and pertussis: Recommendations for vaccine use and other preventative measures: recommendations of the Immunization Practices Advisory Committee (ACIP). *Morbid. Mortal. Wkly. Rep.* **40 (RR-10),** 21–22.

Challacombe, S. J., Russell, M. W., Hawkes, J. E., Bergmeier, L. A., and Lehner, T. (1978). Passage of immunoglobulins from plasma to the oral cavity in rhesus monkeys. *Immunology* **35,** 923–931.

Chidlow, J. W., and Porter, P. (1979). Intestinal defense of the neonatal pig; Interrelationship of gut and mammary function providing surface immunity against colibacillosis. *Vet. Rec.* **104,** 496–500.

Clancy, R. L., Cripps, A. W., Husband, A. J., and Buckley, D. (1983). Specific immune response in the respiratory tract after administration of an oral polyvalent bacterial vaccine. *Infect. Immun.* **39,** 491–496.

Crouch, C. F. (1985). Vaccination against enteric rota and coronaviruses in cattle and pigs: Enhancement of lactogenic immunity. *Vaccine* **3,** 284–291.

Dahlgren, U., Ahlstedt, S., Hedman, L., Wadsworth, C., and Hanson, L. Å. (1981). Dimeric IgA in the rat is transferred from serum into bile but not into milk *Scand. J. Immunol.* **14,** 95–98.

DeBuysscher, E. V., and Berman, D. T. (1980). Secretory immune response in intestinal mucosa and salivary gland after experimental infection of pigs with transmissible gastroenteritis virus. *Am. J. Vet. Res.* **41,** 1214–1220.

Delacroix, D. L., Hodgson, H. J., McPherson, A., Dive, C., and Vaerman, J. P. (1982). Selective transport of polymeric immunoglobulin A in bile. Quantitative relationships of monomeric and polymeric immunoglobulin A, immunoglobulin M, and other proteins in serum, bile, and saliva. *J. Clin. Invest.* **70,** 230–241.

Delacroix, D. L., Malburny, G. N., and Vaerman, J. P. (1985). Hepatobiliary transport of plasma IgA in the mouse: contribution to the clearance of intravascular IgA. *Eur. J. Immunol.* **15,** 893–899.

Dooley, J. S., Potter, B. J., Thomas, H. C., and Sherlock, S. (1982). A comparative study of the biliary secretion of human dimeric and monomeric IgA in the rat and in man. *Hepatology* **2,** 323–327.

Ellis, T. M., Carman, H., Robinson, W. F., and Wilcox, G. E. (1986). The effect of colostrum-derived antibody on neonatal transmission of caprine arthritis–encephalitis virus infection. *Aust. Vet. J.* **63,** 242–245.

Eschenburg, G., Heine, W., and Peters, E. (1990). [Fecal SIgA and lysozyme excretion in breast feeding and formula feeding.] *Kinderarztl. Prax.* **58,** 255–260. (in German)

Evans, D. G., Evans, D. J., Jr., Opekun, A. R., and Graham, D. Y. (1988). Nonreplicating oral whole cell vaccine protective against enterotoxigenic *Escherichia coli* (ETEC) diarrhea: Stimulation of anit-CFA (CFA/I) and anti-enterotoxin (anti-LT) intestinal IgA and protection against challenge with ETEC belonging to heterologous serotypes. *FEMS Microbiol. Immunol.* **1,** 117–125.

Fox, J. P. (1984). Modes of action of poliovirus vaccines and relation to resulting immunity. *Rev. Infect. Dis.* **6,** S352–S355.

Francis, M. J., and Black, L. (1984). The effect of vaccination regimen on the transfer of foot and mouth disease antibodies from the sow to her piglets. *J. Hyg. Lond.* **93,** 123–131.

Gardner, M. M. (1976). Localization of rabbit gamma globulins in the mouse visceral yolk sac placenta. *Anat. Rec.* **184,** 665–677.

Goldman, A. S., Ham-Pong, A. J., and Goldblum, R. M. (1985). Host defenses: Development and maternal contributions. *Adv. Pediatr.* **32,** 71–100.

Griffiss, J. M., and Goroff, D. K. (1983). IgA blocks IgM and IgG-initiated immune lysis by separate molecular mechanism. *J. Immunol.* **130,** 2882–2885.

Halsey, J. F., Mitchell, C. S., and McKenzie, S. J. (1983). The origin of secretory IgA in milk: A shift during lactation from a serum origin to local synthesis in the mammary gland. *Ann. N.Y. Acad. Sci.* **409,** 452–459.

Hammerberg, B., Musoke, A. J., Williams, J. F., and Leid, R. W. (1977). Uptake of colostral immunoglobulins by the suckling rat. *Lab. Anim. Sci.* **27,** 50–53.

Heiman, H. S., and Weisman, L. E. (1989). Transplacental or enteral transfer of maternal immunization-induced antibody protects suckling rats from type III group B streptococcal infection. *Pediatr. Res.* **26,** 629–632.

Heremans, J. F. (1974). Immunoglobulin A. *In* "The Antigens, Vol. 2". (M. Sela, ed), pp. 365–522. Academic Press, New York.

Hirabayashi, Y., Kurata, H., Funato, H., Nagamine, T., Aizawa, C., Tamura, S., Shimada, K., and Kurata, T. (1990). Comparison of intranasal inoculation of influenza HA vaccine combined with cholera toxin B subunit with oral or parenteral vaccination. *Vaccine* **8,** 243–248.

Hjelt, K., Grauballe, P. C., Nielsen, O. H., Schiotz, P. O., and Krasilnikoff, P. A. (1985). Rotavirus antibodies in the mother and her breast-fed infant. *J. Pediatr. Gastroenterol. Nutr.* **4,** 414–420.

Hockel, M., and Kaufmann, R. (1986). Placental transfer of class G immunoglobulins treated with beta-propiolactone (beta-PL) for intravenous application—A case report. *J. Perinat. Med.* **14,** 205–208.

Husband, A. J., and Clifton, V. L. (1989). Role of intestinal immunization in urinary tract defense. *Immunol. Cell Biol.* **67,** 371–376.

Ijaz, M. K., Sabara, M. I., Frenchick, P. J., and Babiuk, L. A. (1987). Effect of different routes of immunization with bovine rotavirus on lactogenic antibody response in mice. *Antiviral Res.* **8,** 283–297.

Jakoi, E. R., Cambier, J., and Saslow, S. (1985). Transepithelial transport of maternal antibody: Purification of IgG receptor from newborn rat intestine. *J. Immunol.* **135,** 3360–3364.

Jertborn, M., Svennerholm, A. M., and Holmgren, J. (1986). Saliva, breast milk, and serum antibody responses as indirect measures of intestinal immunity after oral cholera vaccination or natural disease. *J. Clin. Microbiol.* **24,** 203–209.

Jollie, W. P. (1985). Immunocytochemical localization of antibody during placental transmission of immunity in rats. *J. Reprod. Immunol.* **7,** 261–274.

Kaplan, B. S., Uni, S., Aikawa, M., and Mahmoud, A. A. (1985). Effector mechanism of host resistance in murine giardiasis: Specific IgG and IgA cell-mediated toxicity. *J. Immunol.* **134,** 1975–1981.

Katz, D., and Kohn, A. (1976). Antibodies in blood and secretions of chickens immunized parenterally and locally with killed Newcastle disease virus vaccine. *Dev. Biol. Stand.* **33,** 290–296.

Kenny, J. F., Boesman, M. I., and Michaels, R. H. (1967). Bacterial and viral coproantibodies in breast-fed infants. *Pediatrics* **39,** 202–213.

Keren, D. F., McDonald, R. A., and Carey, J. L. (1988). Combined parenteral and oral immunization results in an enhanced mucosal immunoglobulin A response to *Shigella flexneri. Infect. Immun.* **56,** 910–915.

Keren, D. F., McDonald, R. A., Wassef, J. S., Armstrong, L. R., and Brown, J. E. (1989). The enteric immune response to Shigella antigens. *Curr. Top. Microbiol. Immunol.* **146,** 213–223.

Koertge, T. E., and Butler, J. E. (1986a). Dimeric mouse IgA is transported into rat bile five times more rapidly than into mouse bile. *Scand. J. Immunol.* **24,** 567–574.

Koertge, T. E., and Butler, J. E. (1986b). Dimeric M315 is transported into mouse and rat milk in a degraded form. *Mol. Immunol.* **23,** 839–845.

Kohl, S., and Loo, L. S. (1984). The relative role of transplacental and milk immune transfer in protection against lethal neonatal herpes simplex virus infection in mice. *J. Infect. Dis.* **149,** 38–42.

Koutras, A. K., and Vigorita, V. J. (1989). Fecal secretory immunoglobulin A in breast milk versus formula feeding in early infancy. *J. Pediatr. Gastroenterol. Nutr.* **9,** 58–61.

Kris, R. M., Yetter, R. A., Cogliano, R., Ramphal, R., and Small, P. A., Jr. (1988). Passive serum antibody causes temporary recovery from influenza virus infection of the nose, trachea, and lung of nude mice. *Immunology* **63,** 349–353.

Kubagawa, H., Bertoli, L. F., Barton, J. C., Koopman, W. J., Mestecky, J., and Cooper, M. D. (1987). Analysis of paraprotein transport into the saliva by using anti-idiotype antibodies. *J. Immunol.* **138,** 435–439.

Kurono, K., and Mogi, G. (1987). Secretory IgA and serum type IgA in nasal secretions and antibody activity against the M protein. *Ann. Otol. Rhinol. Laryngol.* **96,** 419–424.

Lamont, H. C., Semine, D. Z., Leveille, C., and Nichols, R. L. (1978). Immunity to vaginal reinfection in female guinea pigs infected sexually with *Chylamydia* of guinea pig inclusion conjunctivitis. *Infect. Immun.* **19,** 807–813.

Layton, G. T., and Smithyman, A. M. (1983). The effects of oral and combined parenteral/oral immunization against an experimental *Escherichia coli* urinary tract infection in mice. *Clin. Exp. Immunol.* **54,** 305–312.

Leach, L., Eaton, B. M., Firth, J. A., and Contractor, S. F. (1990). Uptake and intracellular routing of peroxidase-conjugated immunoglobulin-G by the perfused human placenta. *Cell Tisue Res.* **261,** 383–388.

Lennon, J. L., and Black, F. L. (1986). Maternally derived measles immunity in era of vaccine-protected mothers. *J. Pediatr.* **108,** 671–676.

Levenson, V. I., Chernokhvostova, E. V., Lyubinskaya, M. M., Salamatova, S. A., Dzhikidze, E. K., and Stasilevitch, Z. K. (1988). Parenteral immunization with Shigella ribosomal vaccine elicits local IgA. *Int. Arch. Allergy Appl. Immunol.* **87,** 25–31.

Lindh, E. (1975). Increased resistance of immunoglobulin dimers to proteolytic degradation after binding of secretory component. *J. Immunol.* **114,** 284–286.

Loosli, C. G., Hamre, D., and Berlin, B. S. (1953). Airborne influenza virus A infection in immunized animals. *Trans. Assoc. Am. Phys.* **66,** 222–230.

Lue, C., Tarkowski, A., and Mestecky, J. (1988). Systemic immunization with pneumoccocal polysaccharide vaccine induces predominantly IgA_2 response of peripheral blood lymphocytes and increases both serum and secretory antipneumococcal antibodies. *J. Immunol.* **140,** 3793–3800.

McGuire, T. C., Poppie, M. J., and Banks, K. L. (1975). Hypogammaglobulinemia predisposing to infection in foals. *J. Am. Vet. Med. Assoc.* **166,** 71–75.

McGuire, T. C., Pfeiffer, N. E., Weikel, J. M., and Bartsch, R. C. (1976). Failure of colostral immunoglobulin transfer in calves dying from infectious disease. *J. Am. Vet. Med. Assoc.* **169,** 713–718.

Mazanec, M. B., Nedrud, J. G., and Lamm, M. E. (1987). Immunoglobulin A monoclonal antibodies protect against Sendai virus. *J. Virol.* **61,** 2624–2626.

Mazanec, M. B., Nedrud, J. G., Liang, X., and Lamm, M. E. (1989). Transport of serum IgA into murine respiratory secretions and its implications for immunization strategies. *J. Immunol.* **142,** 4275–4281.

Mazanec, M. B., Lamm, M. E., Lyn, D., Portner, A., and Nedrud, J. G. (1992). Comparison of IgA versus IgG monoclonal antibodies for passive immunization of the murine respiratory tract. *Virus Res.* **23,** 1–12.

Meitin, C. A., Bender, B. S., and Small, P. A., Jr. (1991). Influenza immunization: Intranasal live vaccinia recombinant contrasted with parenteral inactivated vaccine. *Vaccine* **9,** 751–756.

Mestecky, J., and McGhee, J. R. (1987). Immunoglobulin A (IgA): Molecular and cellular interactions involved in IgA biosynthesis and immune response. *Adv. Immunol.* **40,** 153–245.

Metze, D., Kersten, A., Jurecka, W., and Gebhart, W. (1991). Immunoglobulins coat microorganisms of skin surface: a comparative immunohistochemical and ultrastructural study of cutaneous and oral microbial symbionts. *J. Invest. Dermatol.* **96,** 439–445.

Michalek, S. M., and McGhee, J. R. (1977). Effective immunity to dental caries: passive transfer to rats of antibodies to *Streptococcus mutans* elicits protection. *Infect. Immun.* **17,** 644–650.

Michalek, S. M., McGhee, J. R., Arnold, R. R., and Mestecky, J. (1978a). Effective immunity to dental caries: Selective induction of secretory immunity by oral administration of *Streptococcus mutans* in rodents. *Adv. Exp. Med. Biol.* **107,** 261–269.

Michalek, S. M., McGhee, J. R., and Babb, J. L. (1978b). Effective immunity to dental caries: Dose-dependent studies of secretory immunity by oral administration of *Streptococcus mutans* to rats. *Infect. Immun.* **19,** 217–224.

Michalek, S. M., Morisaki, I., Gregory, R. L., Kiyono, H., Hamada, S., and McGhee, J. R. (1983a). Oral adjuvants enhance IgA responses to *Streptococcus mutans*. *Mol. Immunol.* **20,** 1009–1018.

Michalek, S. M., Morisaki, I., Harmon, C. C., Hamada, S., and McGhee, J. R. (1983b). Effective immunity to dental caries: Gastric intubation of *Streptococcus mutans* whole cells or cell walls induces protective immunity in gnotobiotic rats. *Infect. Immun.* **39,** 645–654.

Michalek, S. M., Gregory, R. L., Harmon, C. C., Katz, J., Richardson, G. J., Hilton, T., Filler, S. J., and McGhee, J. R. (1987). Protection of gnotobiotic rats against dental caries by passive immunization with bovine milk antibodies to *Streptococcus mutans*. *Infect. Immun.* **55,** 2341–2347.

Mondino, B. J., Laheji, A. K., and Adamu, S. A. (1987). Ocular immunity to *Staphylococcus aureus*. *Invest. Ophthalmol. Vis. Sci.* **28,** 560–564.

Montgomery, P. C., Khaleel, S. A., Goudswaard, J., and Virella, G. (1977). Selective transport of an oligomeric IgA into canine saliva. *Immunol. Commun.* **6,** 633–642.

Morisaki, I., Michalek, S. M., Harmon, C. C., Torii, M., Hamada, S., and McGhee, J. R. (1983). Effective immunity to dental caries: enhancement of salivary anti-*Streptococcus mutans* antibody responses with oral adjuvants. *Infect. Immun.* **40,** 577–591.

Mucchielli, A., Laliberte, F., and Laliberte, M. F. (1983). A new experimental method for the dynamic study of the antibody transfer mechanism from mother to fetus in the rat. *Placenta* **4,** 175–183.

Nara, P. L., Winters, K., Rice, J. B., Olsen, R. G., and Krakowka, S. (1983). Systemic and local intestinal antibody response in dogs given both infective and inactivated canine parvovirus. *Am. J. Vet. Res.* **44,** 1989–1995.

Nedrud, J. G., Liang, X., Hague, N., and Lamm, M. E. (1987). Combined oral/nasal immunization protects mice from Sendai virus infection. *J. Immunol.* **139,** 3484–3492.

Nejamkis, M. R., Nota, N. R., Weissenbacher, M. C., Guerrero, L. B., and Giovanniello, O. A. (1975). Passive immunity against Junin virus in mice. *Acta Virol. Praha.* **19,** 237–244.

Oda, M., Izumiya, K., Sato, Y., and Hirayama, M. (1983). Transplacental and transcolostral immunity to pertussis in a mouse model using acellular pertussis vaccine. *J. Infect. Dis.* **148,** 138–145.

Offit, P. A., Clark, H. F., Kornstein, M. J., and Plotkin, S. A. (1984). A murine model of oral infection with a primate rotavirus (simian SA-11). *J. Virol.* **51,** 233–236.

Ogra, P. L., Okamoto, Y., Freihorst, J., La Scolea, L. J., Jr., and Merrick, J. M. (1989). Immunization of the gastrointestinal tract with bacterial and viral antigens: Implications in mucosal immunity. *Immunol. Invest.* **18,** 559–570.

Orlans, E., Peppard, J., Reynolds, J., and Hall, J. (1978). Rapid active transport of immunoglobulin A from blood to bile. *J. Exp. Med.* **147,** 588–592.

Orlans, E., Peppard, J. V., Payne, A. W., Fitzharris, B. M., Mullock, B. M., Hinton, R. H., and Hall, J. G. (1983). Comparative aspects of the hepatobiliary transport of IgA. *Ann. N.Y. Acad. Sci.* **409,** 411–427.

Poirier, T. P., Kehoe, M. A., and Beachey, E. H. (1988). Protective immunity evoked by oral administration of attenuated aroA *Salmonella typhimurium* expressing cloned streptococcal M protein. *J. Exp. Med.* **168,** 25–32.

Porter, P., Parry, S. H., and Allen, W. D. (1977). Significance of immune mechanisms in relation to enteric infections of the gastrointestinal tract in animals. *Ciba Found. Symp.* **46,** 55–75.

Prentice, A. (1987). Breast feeding increases concentrations of IgA in infants' urine. *Arch. Dis. Child.* **62,** 792–795.

Rahman, M. M., Yamauchi, M., Hanada, N., Nishikawa, K., and Morishima, T. (1987). Local production of rotavirus specific IgA in breast tissue and transfer to neonates. *Arch. Dis. Child.* **62,** 401–405.

Ramphal, R., Cogliano, R. C., Shands, J. W., Jr., and Small, P. A., Jr., (1979). Serum antibody prevents lethal murine influenza penumonitis but not tracheitis. *Infect. Immun.* **25,** 992–997.

Renegar, K. B., and Small, P. A., Jr. (1991a). Passive transfer of local immunity to influenza virus infection by IgA antibody. *J. Immunol.* **146,** 1972–1978.

Renegar, K. B., and Small, P. A., Jr. (1991b). Immunoglobulin A mediation of murine nasal anti-influenza virus immunity. *J. Virol.* **65,** 2146–2148.

Russell, M. W., and Mestecky, J. (1986). Potential for immunological intervention against dental caries. *J. Biol. Buccale* **14,** 159–175.

Russell, M. W., Brown, T. A., and Mestecky, J. (1982). Preferential transport of IgA and IgA-immune complexes into bile compared with other external secretions. *Mol. Immunol.* **19,** 677–682.

Russell, M. W., Reinholdt, J., and Kilian, M. (1989). Anti-inflammatory activity of human IgA antibodies and their Fab alpha fragments: Inhibition of IgG-mediated complement activation. *Eur. J. Immunol.* **19,** 2243–2249.

Scicchitano, R., Husband A. J., and Cripps, A. W. (1984). Immunoglobulin-containing cells and the origin of immunoglobulins in the respiratory tract of sheep. *Immunol.* **52,** 529–537.

Scicchitano, R., Sheldrake R. F., and Husband, A. J. (1986). Origin of immunoglobulins in respiratory tract secretion and saliva of sheep. *Immunol.* **58,** 315–321.

Sheldrake, R. F., Husband, A. J., Watson, D. L., and Cripps, A. W. (1984). Selective transport of serum-derived IgA into mucosal secretions. *J. Immunol.* **132,** 363–368.

Simister, N. E., and Mostov, K. E. (1989). An Fc receptor structurally related to MHC class I antigens. *Nature (London)* **337,** 184–187.

Simister, N., and Rees, A. R. (1983). Properties of immunoglobulin G-Fc receptors from neonatal rat intestinal brush borders. *Ciba Found. Symp.* **95,** 273–286.

Smith, C. B., Purcell, R. H., Bellanti, J. A., and Chanock, R. M. (1966). Protective effect of antibody to parainfluenza type 1 virus. *N. Engl. J. Med.* **275,** 1145–1152.

Socken, D. J., Jeejeebhoy K. N., Bazin H., and Underdown, B. J. (1979). Identification of secretory component as an IgA receptor on rat hepatocytes. *J. Exp. Med.* **150,** 1538–1548.

Svennerholm, A., Lange, S., and Holmgren, J. (1978). Correlation between intestinal synthesis of specific immunoglobulin A and protection against experimental cholera in mice. *Infect. Immun.* **21,** 1–6.

Tamura, S., Funato, H., Hirabayashi, Y., Suzuki, Y., Nagamine, T., Aizawa, C., and Kurata, T. (1991). Cross-protection against influenza A virus infection by passively transferred respiratory tract IgA antibodies to different hemagglutinin molecules. *Eur. J. Immunol.* **21,** 1337–1344.

Tizzard, I. (1987). Immunity in the fetus and newborn. *In* "Veterinary Immunology—An Introduction" (I. Tizzard, ed), 3d Ed., pp. 171–184. Saunders, Philadelphia.

Tomasi, T. B., Jr. (1970). The structure and function of mucosal antibodies. *Ann. Rev. Med.* **21,** 281–298.

Tsunemitsu, H., Shimizu, M., Hirai, T., Yonemichi, H., Kudo, T., Mori, K., and Onoe, S. (1989). Protection against bovine rotaviruses in newborn calves by continuous feeding of immune colostrum. *Nippon Juigaku Zasshi* **51,** 300–308.

Tuboly, S., Bernath, S., Glavits, R., and Medveczky, I. (1988). Intestinal absorption of colostral lymphoid cells in newborn piglets. *Vet. Immunol. Immunopathol.* **20,** 75–85.

Vaerman, J. P. (1973). Comparative immunochemistry of IgA. *Res. Immunochem. Immunobiol.* **3,** 91.

Vaerman, J. P., and Delacroix, D. L. (1984). Role of the liver in the immunobiology of IgA in animals and humans. *Contrib. Nephrol.* **40,** 17–31.

von Behring, E., and Kitasato, S. (1890). On the acquisition of immunity against diphtheria and tetanus in animals. *Deutsch. Med. Wochenschr.* **16,** 1113–1114. (German)

Waldman, T. A., and Strober, W. (1969). Metabolism of immunoglobulins. *Progr. Allergy* **13,** 1–110.

Wilson, R. A., and Jutila, J. W. (1976). Experimental neonatal colibacillosis in cows: Immunoglobulin classes involved in protection. *Infect. Immun.* **13,** 100–107.

Winner, L., III, Mack, J., Weltzin, R., Mekalanos, J. J., Kraehenbuhl, J.-P., and Neutra, M. R. (1991). New model for analysis of mucosal immunity: Intestinal secretion of specific monoclonal immunoglobulin A from hybridoma tumors protects against Vibrio cholerae infection. *Infect. Immun.* **59,** 977–982.

Zikan, J., Mestecky, J., Schrohenloher, R. E., Tomana, M., and Kulhavy, R. (1972). Studies on human secretory immunoglobulin A. V. Trypsin hydrolysis at elevated temperatures. *Immunochemistry* **9,** 1185–1193.

31

Common Mucosal Immune System and Strategies for the Development of Vaccines Effective at the Mucosal Surfaces

Jiri Mestecky · Rebecca Abraham · Pearay L. Ogra

I. INTRODUCTION

Mucosal tissues constitute an enormous surface area and serve as primary portals of entry for most infectious agents. The immune response generated as a result of such host–pathogen interactions are targeted primarily to prevent local or systemic disease. That mucosal surfaces constitute an elaborate system of defense mechanisms including the mucosa-associated lymphoid tissue (MALT) is not surprising (Hanson and Brandtzaeg, 1989). However, the impact of the mucosal lymphoid tissues relative to the mechanisms of host–pathogen interaction has been recognized only in the last two decades. Current interest in mucosal vaccines stems, to a large extent, from our new understanding of mucosal immunity (Ogra *et al.*, 1980; Mestecky and McGhee, 1987; McGhee and Mestecky, 1990).

The concept of a common mucosal system has been elaborated by a number of prominent workers (for reviews, see McDermott and Bienenstock, 1979; Phillips-Quagliata and Lamm, 1988; Scicchitano *et al.*, 1988) and has gained wide acceptance in relation to mucosal immunity (Tomasi *et al.*, 1965). This concept refers to a specific defense system that operates at external mucosal surfaces and functions somewhat independently of the immunological reactivity in the systemic sites and the bloodstream. This system includes the inductive sites of the gut-associated lymphoid tissue (GALT), the bronchus-associated lymphoid tissue (BALT), and the immunocompetent elements in the effector sites in the genital mucosa, salivary glands, respiratory tract, pharynx, and mammary glands. The predominant immunoglobulin present in mucous secretions is secretory IgA (SIgA). Other elements of immunity are also present in varying amounts, for example, IgA (serum type), IgG, IgM, T lymphocytes, and components of cell-mediated immunity (Tomasi *et al.*, 1965).

II. ORIGIN OF MUCOSAL ANTIBODIES

Early studies concerning the origin of IgA antibodies in secretions considered the possibility that they are transferred from the circulatory pool (for reviews, see Brandtzaeg, 1985a; Mestecky *et al.*, 1991a). Infusion of 1–2 liters of plasma into immunodeficient patients resulted in the appearance of immunochemically detectable IgA in the saliva of a few patients (South *et al.*, 1966). Further, finding monoclonal IgA in the saliva of patients with IgA myeloma (Coelho *et al.*, 1974) gave support to the original proposal that mIgA from plasma is polymerized during the secretory component (SC)-mediated transport through the epithelial cells (Tomasi *et al.*, 1965). However, many subsequent studies performed in animal models and in humans clearly have shown that, in most species, plasma-derived IgA contributes only small amounts of IgA to external secretions, except in rabbits, rats, and mice, in which plasma-derived polymeric IgA is transported effectively by hepatocytes that express SC into the bile and ultimately into the intestine (Brown and Kloppel, 1989; Mestecky *et al.*, 1991a). Radiolabeled human IgA injected intravenously into humans appeared in only very small quantities in human nasal secretions, saliva, intestinal fluid, and bile (Delacroix *et al.*, 1982; Jonard *et al.*, 1984; Mestecky *et al.*, 1991a). Even in IgA myeloma patients, whose plasma contained extremely high levels of pIgA, salivary IgA was not elevated and monoclonal IgA detected by anti-idiotypic antibodies constituted only 0.4–3.9% of the total salivary IgA (Kubagawa *et al.*, 1987).

Immunochemical and immunohistochemical studies of SIgA and of mucosal tissues and glands convincingly established that almost all IgA found in external secretions originates from the locally assembled pIgA produced by plasma cells found in abundance in mucosal tissues and secretory glands and is transported selectively (Lawton and Mage, 1969; Bienenstock and Strauss, 1970; Brandtzaeg, 1985a; Mestecky *et al.*, 1991a). However, locally produced pIgA may compete successfully with the plasma-derived pIgA for the epithelial receptor SC. Nevertheless, additional studies of the transport of intravenously injected purified pIgA into IgA-deficient patients should be performed to solve this problem. In normal individuals, such passive immunizations with intravenously administered pIgA appear to be unlikely to provide immunity on mucosal surfaces.

In animals, the transport of plasma-derived pIgA into external secretions is rather controversial. Some investigators (Halsey *et al.*, 1983) demonstrated the transport of pIgA in external secretions whereas others (Russell *et al.*, 1982; Koertge and Butler, 1986) found that such transport is rather limited.

The importance of local mucosal antigenic stimulation in the respiratory and intestinal tracts has been demonstrated by the observation that the titer of specific IgA antibody to poliovirus is highest in intestinal sites that have direct contact with the poliovirus antigen after segmental colonic immunization of subjects with double-barreled colostomies (Ogra and Karzon, 1971). In other studies, intranasal immunization with inactivated poliovaccine induced a specific nasopharyngeal IgA antibody response, often in the absence of any detectable response in the serum (Ogra and Karzon, 1971). The lack of mucosal antibody-producing plasma cells in germ-free animals and in human neonates is another example of the role of local antigenic exposure in the development of mucosal immunity, since such situations are associated with a significantly reduced mass of microbial and dietary antigens in the respiratory and enteric membranes (Tomasi, 1976).

Sufficient information is not available about the development of other immunoglobulins in the mucosal surface. However, a significant amount of the IgG and IgM antibodies in external secretions of the nasopharynx and intestine appears to be synthesized locally. Some evidence suggests that compensation for IgA antibody in patients with a selective absence or deficiency of IgA is effected largely by the increased local synthesis of IgM and, to some extent, IgG in the secretory sites (Ogra *et al.*, 1974). T lymphocytes and cell-mediated immune responses in the mucosal surfaces also may be local phenomena (Waldman and Ganguly, 1974); they depend on local exposure to antigen, migration recirculation, and homing to other mucosal surfaces after initial antigenic stimulation, a sequence of events that appears to be remarkably similar to that described for IgA antibody (Tomasi, 1976).

III. COMMON MUCOSAL IMMUNE SYSTEM

The presence of large numbers of Ig-producing cells, mostly of the IgA isotype, in lamina propria of the gastrointestinal and respiratory tracts and in secretory glands was described during the early 1960s (for review, see Heremans, 1974; Lamm, 1976). However, studies of the origin of their precursors, the migratory pathways, and the regulation of local differentiation in IgA-producing plasma cells were initiated in the early 1970s in several laboratories. In both humans and animals, mucosal IgA plasma cells were found to be derived from precursors localized in the IgA-inductive sites, primarily in GALT (Bienenstock, 1985; Phillips-Quagliata and Lamm, 1988; Scicchitano *et al.*, 1988). Further, exposure of such IgA precursor cells to environmental antigens and their subsequent migration to remote mucosal tissues and glands results in dissemination of SIgA-mediated specific immune responses. The physiological importance of these findings is considerable. Stimulation at an IgA-inductive site (e.g., GALT) is likely to lead to the generalized protection of remote sites such as nasopharynx and genital tract; SIgA antibodies in milk of orally immunized mothers may protect the gastrointestinal and possibly upper respiratory tract of breast-fed neonates (Mestecky, 1987; Mestecky *et al.*, 1991b). Further, the existence of this common mucosal immune system can be exploited in the design of novel types of vaccines that, for example, given orally result in protection at mucosal surfaces and glands (e.g., mammary gland) that are less accessible to local immunization. The site of stimulation and type and delivery of antigen play important roles in the extent of dissemination of SIgA-mediated immune responses and must be given special consideration in design of vaccines effective in the protection of mucosal surfaces (McGhee and Mestecky, 1990).

A. Evidence in Animals

In many experimental models, local antigenic stimulation of mucosal surfaces and secretory glands has been demonstrated to result in the production of specific antibodies, not only at the site of stimulation but also in the circulation and in remote external secretions (for reviews see Mestecky, 1987; Phillips-Quagliata and Lamm, 1988; Scicchitano *et al.*, 1988). Heremans and Bazin (1971) showed that the IgA-producing cells in orally immunized germ-free mice are found in the intestinal as well as the extraintestinal lymphoid organs, including mesenteric lymph nodes and spleen, and, in other experiments (Alley *et al.*, 1986), bone marrow. Jacobson *et al.* (1961) noted the ability of Peyer's patches to repopulate other tissues and restore their immunological capacities: mice subjected to total body irradiation, but with shielded Peyer's patches, retained their immune functions. This finding was interpreted as evidence of migration of lymphocytes from Peyer's patches to peripheral organs. However, Craig and Cebra (1971) clearly demonstrated for the first time that Peyer's patches are also an enriched source of precursors of mucosal IgA plasma cells. Adoptive transfer of lymphocytes from Peyer's patches but not peripheral lymph nodes from a donor rabbit into an irradiated recipient resulted in repopulation of the recipient intestine by IgA plasma cells of donor allotype. A host of subsequent studies (for reviews, see Lamm, 1976; Phillips-Quagliata and Lamm, 1988; Scicchitano *et al.*, 1988) convincingly established that—in rabbits, mice, and rats—GALT (with adjacent mesenteric lymph nodes), and in some experiments, BALT (Bienenstock, 1985) contains precursors of IgA plasma cells capable of repopulating intestines, respiratory tract, and salivary, lacrimal, mammary, and cervical glands of the uterus with IgA plasma cells. When peripheral lymph nodes and spleen were used as sources of lymphocytes in these adoptive transfer experiment, few IgA-producing cells were seen in these mucosal tissues and glands. Lymphoblasts displayed a more pronounced homing capacity than unstimulated small lymphocytes, which may explain why mesenteric lymph nodes are often a better source of cells for repopulation studies than Peyer's patches (Lamm, 1976). The local presence of an antigen on mucosal surfaces leads to an additional increase of IgA plasma cells secreting corresponding specific antibodies, apparently because of the local clonal expansion of antigen-specific lymphoblasts arriving to these locales rather than their antigen-driven increased immigration (Husband and

Gowans, 1978). In some experiments, mucosal tissues of orally immunized animals contained IgA cells secreting antibodies specific for the ingested antigen. Transfer of lymphocytes from mesenteric lymph nodes of orally immunized donors into naive recipients yielded similar results (De Buysscher and Dubois, 1978; Weisz-Carrington *et al.*, 1979).

These studies provided a cellular basis for the earlier experiments of Montgomery *et al.* (1974), who stimulated great interest by their demonstration of specific antibodies to dinitrophenylated *Pneumococcus* in milk of lactating rabbits fed this conjugated antigen. Numerous subsequent studies (for reviews, see Mestecky, 1987; Mestecky and McGhee, 1987; Russell and Mestecky, 1988; McGhee and Mestecky, 1992) with oral administration of various particulate and soluble antigens to experimental animals fully confirmed Montgomery's observations and extended them to other external secretions. Elegant experiments from Montgomery's laboratory excluded the possibility that free antigens absorbed from mucosal sites, rather than committed lymphocytes, are carried by the circulation to mucosal sites to initiate local IgA responses (Montgomery *et al.*, 1976). Direct evidence for the importance of Peyer's patch-derived IgA plasma cell precursors in dissemination of SIgA-mediated immune response specific to bacterial antigen was provided by Robertson and Cebra (1976). Two isolated ileal loops—one with and the other without a Peyer's patch—were constructed without the interruption of the flow of blood and lymph. After the introduction of antigens [dinitrophenylated keyhole limpet hemocyanin (KLH) and *Salmonella typhimurium*] into the loop that contained the Peyer's patch, an SIgA response was detected in both loops whereas these antigens introduced into a loop devoid of Peyer's patches did not induce an immune response. These observations directly implicated Peyer's patches as the sources of precursor cells that are capable of undergoing direct antigen-driven stimulation to proliferate, migrate, differentiate, and repopulate the intestinal lamina propria with cells that secrete *specific* IgA antibodies. Further, IgA from several secretions of a *single* animal orally immunized with the dinitrophenyl hapten on a carrier displayed, on isoelectric focusing, identical spectrotypes, suggesting that IgA cells that populate various exocrine tissues are derived from a common clone (Montgomery *et al.*, 1983). As summarized in several review articles (Lamm 1976; Mestecky, 1987; Mestecky and McGhee, 1987; Phillips-Quagliata and Lamm, 1988; Scicchitano *et al.*, 1988), the concept of a common mucosal immune system was proposed which, in a simplified form, is shown in Figure 1.

B. Evidence in Humans

Because of ethical and biological limitations, the adoptive transfer of IgA-precursor cells is impossible to perform in humans. Thus, the evidence for the existence of the common mucosal immune system is inevitably indirect. Nevertheless,

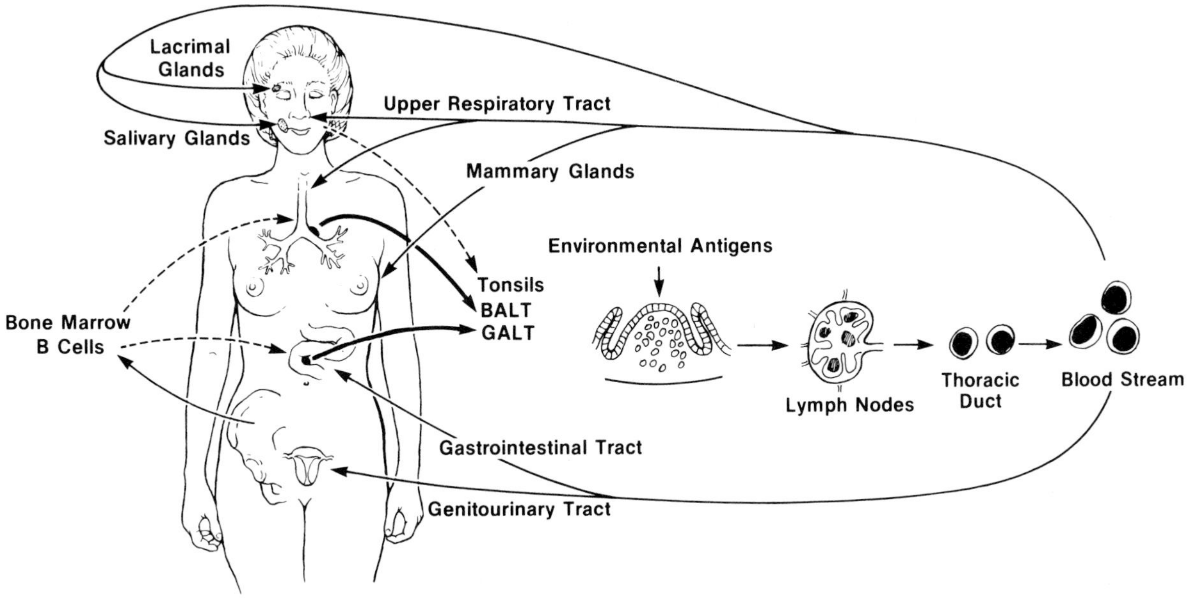

Figure 1 Hypothetical diagram of the common mucosal immune system in humans. Lymphoid cells, presumably from the bone marrow, enter the Peyer's patches (PP) and probably other gut-associated lymphoid tissues (GALT) through high endothelial venules. Under the local influence of T cells and accessory cells, the arriving B cells express surface IgA. Environmental antigens enter Peyer's patches through pinocytotic and phagocytic M cells and interact with resident accessory, T, and B cells. IgA-committed and antigen-sensitized B cells and lymphoblasts leave and enter the regional lymph nodes, then the lymph and circulation. Finally, such cells populate various exocrine glands and mucosa-associated tissues, where terminal differentiation into IgA-secreting plasma cells occurs. In animals, bronchus-associated lymphoid tissues (BALT) apparently play a role analogous to that of GALT.

data accumulated during the last decade lend strong credence to this contention.

External secretions of glands that are remote from the site of antigen stimulation contain natural SIgA antibodies to such antigens. For example, colostrum and milk as well as tears contain high levels of antibodies to an oral bacterium, *Streptococcus mutans* (Arnold *et al.*, 1976; Allansmith *et al.*, 1982). This bacterium colonizes the oral cavity of children only after the eruption of the primary definition; thus, local stimulation of the immune apparatus of the mammary gland during breastfeeding is unlikely to play a role in the induction of such antibodies. The fact has been well established (Ogra *et al.*, 1983; Ladjeva *et al.*, 1989) that human milk contains SIgA antibodies against a broad spectrum of food and microbial antigens that are encountered by inhalation and ingestion. Thus, in the absence, or presence in low titers, of corresponding antibodies in serum, the most probable explanation for the presence of specific SIgA antibodies in these external secretions would consider the dissemination and lodging of antigen-sensitized IgA-committed antibody-forming cells to mucosal tissues and glands.

Evidence for this hypothesis was strengthened further by a number of oral immunization studies (for reviews, see Mestecky, 1987; Mestecky and McGhee, 1987,1989; McGhee and Mestecky, 1992). Live or killed microorganisms or their antigenic products given by the oral route induced specific SIgA antibodies in milk, tears, saliva, and nasal secretions (Goldblum *et al.*, 1975; Mestecky *et al.*, 1978; Czerkinsky *et al.*, 1987). Such antibodies appeared in parallel in all external secretions examined; corresponding pre-existing serum antibodies usually were not elevated as a consequence of oral immunization (Mestecky *et al.*, 1978; Clancy *et al.*, 1983; Bergmann *et al.*, 1986; Czerkinsky *et al.*, 1987). Further, subsequent oral boosting with the same antigen led to higher levels of SIgA in these secretions, compared with the levels induced by the first ingestion.

Antigens used for such immunizations included whole bacteria [e.g., *S. mutans* (Mestecky *et al.*, 1978; Czerkinsky *et al.*, 1987; Taubman and Smith, 1989), *Haemophilus influenzae* (Clancy *et al.*, 1983)] and their products [e.g., glucosyltransferase (Taubman and Smith, 1989) or carbohydrate antigens (Taubman and Smith, 1989) of *S. mutans*] and live or killed viruses [e.g., poliovirus (Ogra and Karzon, 1969), influenza virus (Waldmann *et al.*, 1986; Bergmann *et al.*, 1986)] as well as their modified antigens (Waldmann *et al.*, 1986). Generally, particulate antigens induce higher responses than corresponding soluble ones probable because of better uptake and limited digestion.

Because cells from human lymphoid tissues are not easily obtainable, cellular studies have been limited to the examination of lymphocytes from the peripheral blood. However, in the IgA cell cycle described earlier IgA-committed cells specific for ingested antigens should be present in the peripheral blood before their emigration to and lodging in the mucosal tissues and glands. This is indeed the case and has been demonstrated in several studies (Czerkinsky *et al.*, 1987, 1991; Kantele, 1990; Quiding *et al.*, 1991).

First, mitogen-stimulated peripheral blood lymphocytes have been shown to secrete predominantly pIgA; the intracellular distribution of IgA subclasses resembles that in secretory tissues (Kutteh *et al.*, 1980). Based on these results, researchers proposed that a large proportion of such cells is composed of precursors of IgA-producing plasma cells that populate mucosal tissues. Therefore, these studies complemented and extended earlier observations of Friedman *et al.* (1975), in which extracorporeal cesium irradiation of peripheral blood of leukemic patients resulted in a decrease in salivary but not serum IgA levels.

Commitment of peripheral blood lymphocytes to secrete IgA antibodies specific for ingested antigen became obvious from several independent experiments. Peripheral blood lymphocytes from volunteers orally immunized with a single dose of combined cholera B-subunit/whole-cell vaccine secreted IgA antibodies to the ingested antigen into tissue culture supernatants (Lycke *et al.*, 1985). When examined on a single-cell level, peripheral blood lymphocytes that secreted specific IgA antibodies were detected in 4 of 6 volunteers who had been immunized orally with enterically coated capsules containing *S. mutans* (Czerkinsky *et al.*, 1987). These cells are detectable in peripheral blood before the appearance of specific SIgA antibodies in external secretions that included saliva and tears. Interestingly, one of the volunteers was IgA deficient, so peripheral blood lymphocytes produced and external secretions contained specific IgM antibodies. Peroral immunization of volunteers with *Salmonella typhi* also led to the transient presence of predominantly IgA-secreting cells in the peripheral blood, but secretory and serum IgA antibodies were absent (Kantele *et al.*, 1986).

In the most recent study (Czerkinsky *et al.*, 1991), specific antibody-secreting cells were detected in cell suspensions of minor salivary glands surgically removed after ingestion of *Vibrio cholerae* vaccine by human volunteers. Sequential experiments revealed that specific IgA antibody-producing cells appear first in the peripheral blood and then in minor salivary glands; corresponding antibodies appeared later in saliva.

Collectively, these experiments strongly suggest that the stimulation of GALT by oral immunization can be exploited for the induction of a secretory immune response to several additional microbial agents that infect mucosal surfaces distant from the gastrointestinal tract.

C. How "Common" Is the Common Mucosal Immune System?

In the original concept of the common mucosal immune system, GALT and BALT served as sources of precursors of the IgA plasma cells from all mucosal tissues and glands. However, several studies have considered the possibility that additional lymphoid tissues may fulfill this function. Surgical removal of visible GALT and extended drainage of the thoracic duct resulted in approximately 50% reduction in the number of IgA plasma cells in the intestinal lamina propria (Heatley *et al.*, 1981). Thus, other sources seem to contribute to the pool of IgA precursor cells (Figure 2).

1. Tonsils

The tonsils at the top of the digestive and respiratory tracts are exposed continually to antigens in inhaled air and ingested

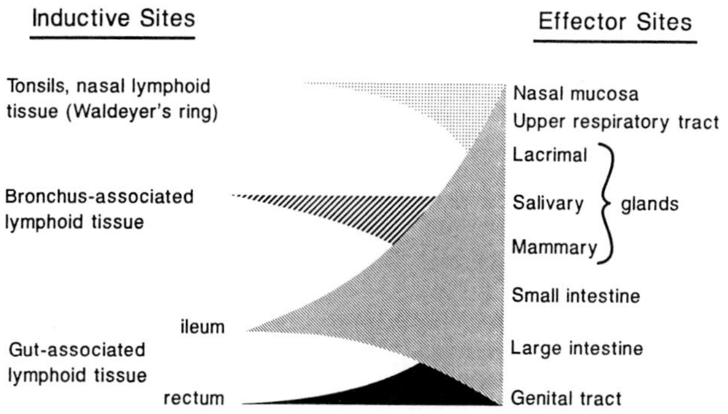

Figure 2 Subcompartmentalization in the common mucosal immune system. In addition to gut- and bronchus-associated lymphoid tissues, IgA-inductive sites in the Waldeyers ring of oropharyngeal lymphoid tissue (nasal, palatinal, and lingual tonsils) or rectum also may contribute to the pool of precursor cells that preferentially populate upper respiratory or lower-intestinal and genital tract.

food. They display a unique architecture similar to that of lymph nodes (cell types, development of germinal centers on exposure to antigens; Brandtzaeg, 1985b) and have deep, partly branched crypts that increase their surface area enormously and trap environmental materials. Antigen-processing and-presenting cells as well as T and B cells are represented abundantly in specific tonsillar tissue compartments (Brandtzaeg, 1987). Human tonsillar germinal center cells reveal IgM as the prominent surface isotype, followed by IgA, IgG, and IgD (Tsunoda *et al.*, 1980). Cells from palatine and nasopharyngeal tonsils have been proposed to contribute to the population of cells that supplies distant mucosal sites with IgA precursors, particularly the upper respiratory and digestive tracts (Brandtzaeg, 1987). Supporting circumstantial evidence is based on (1) the expression of intracellular J chain, a probable marker of pIgA synthesis by cultured tonsillar cells (Brandtzaeg, 1987), and the secretion of pIgA into supernatants and (2) the distribution of IgA subclasses with a predominance of IgA1, typical of the upper respiratory and digestive tracts (Brandtzaeg, 1987). In addition, reduced nasopharyngal antibody response to orally administered live poliovirus was demonstrated in tonsillectomized children (Ogra and Karzon, 1971). Before tonsillectomy, poliovirus IgA antibody was present in appreciable titers in the nasopharynx of all children previously immunized with live attenuated poliovirus vaccine. Significantly, however, after tonsillectomy the pre-existing IgA poliovirus antibody levels in the nasopharynx sharply declined in all the patients studied. Mean antibody titers decreased 3- to 4-fold. Individual titers in several children declined 4- to 8-fold (Ogra and Karzon, 1971).

Note that tonsils are absent from commonly used animals (except rabbits). Although rats have been shown to possess nasal associated lymphoid tissue, which might be an equivalent structure (Evans *et al.*, 1985), intranasal immunization of rats or mice does not result in disseminated antibody response in other mucosal tissues, although responses in the posterior cervical lymph nodes and serum can be demonstrated (Evans *et al.*, 1983; Dunn *et al.*, 1990). The human nasal mucosa also contains T lymphocytes (Chin *et al.*, 1969; Kapikian *et al.*, 1969; Ogra *et al.*, 1991), HLA-DR expressing dendritic and epithelial cells (Kim *et al.*, 1969), and abundant IgA-secreting plasma cells (predominantly IgA1), which may originate in BALT or tonsillar tissue (Buynak *et al.*, 1979; Belshe *et al.*, 1982). Intranasal immunization in humans has been used particularly against respiratory pathogens (e.g., influenza, parainfluenza viruses) but the responses have been analyzed only in the nasal secretions and serum (Kim *et al.*, 1971; Richardson *et al.*, 1978). We do not know whether the intranasal route of immunization, which most likely involves the nasopharyngeal tonsils, generates antibodies of other mucosal sites. It is possible that specific antibodies induced by intranasal immunization will be restricted primarily to the upper respiratory tract.

2. Rectal Lymphoid Tissues

Although Peyer's patches are found primarily in the lower segments of the small intestine, similar structures also occur in the large intestine, especially in the rectum (Strindel, 1935). Such lymphoid follicles, called lymphoglandular complexes, are found in the large intestine with a frequency that increases from colon to rectum. B and T lymphocytes have been detected and IgA-producing plasma cells are quite numerous in the lamina propria (Kett *et al.*, 1986). Interestingly, the distribution of IgA1- and IgA2-producing cells in the colorectum (Crago *et al.*, 1984; Kett *et al.*, 1986) is remarkably similar to that of the female genital tract (Kutteh *et al.*, 1988). Further, the rectum and genital tract have common lymphoid drainage, and venous blood from these tissues avoids the portal vein and, thus, the liver. The rectal route of immunization has been considered in only a few human and animal studies (Forrest *et al.*, 1990; Lehner *et al.*, 1992a,b). When examined (Forrest *et al.*, 1990), external secretions (intestinal juice and saliva) contained antibodies specific for rectally administered antigens. Additional experiments will be necessary to evaluate fully the efficacy of rectal immunization for the induction of specific antibodies in remote external secretions (e.g., tears, milk, and saliva) and in genital secretions. Limited results (Lehner *et al.*, 1992a,b) suggest that this route of immunization may be effective for the induction of virus-specific mucosal antibodies, especially in the female genital tract of monkeys.

D. Peritoneal Cavity

Results concerning the properties and repopulation potential of Ly-1^+ ($CD5^+$, B-1) B cells from the peritoneal cavity of mice have provided new insights into the origin and precursors of IgA plasma cells in mucosal tissues. As many as half the IgA plasma cells found in the murine intestinal wall were derived from a distinct lineage of self-replenishing and long-living peritoneal lymphoid cells (Kroese *et al.*, 1988,1989). Interestingly, $sIgA^+$ cells constitute no more than 1% of total peritoneal cells; thus, a considerable proportion of IgA plasma cells in the murine gut originating from peritoneal Ly-1^+ B cells is derived from the $sIgA^-$ population. Subsequently, Solvason *et al.* (1991) demonstrated convincingly that the transfer of omental and peritoneal cells (which did not contain antibody-forming cells) or fetal omental graft from C57BL/

6 × BALB/c mice under the kidney capsule of severely compromised immunodeficient (SCID) mice resulted in the population of the gut with numerous IgA-producing plasma cells. Co-staining with anti-allotypic reagents clearly confirmed their donor origin. Pecquet *et al.* (1992) have reconstituted irradiated Xid mice that are nonresponsive to *S. typhimurium* with peritoneal $CD5^+$ B cells from responsive CBA/Ca donors and observed a strong mucosal IgA and IgG response to oral immunization with this antigen; such responses were not observed in animals reconstituted with $CD5^-$ B cells from the bone marrow. An identical pattern of immune responses was observed when phosphorylcholine–bovine serum albumin (BSA) conjugates were used. The authors concluded that the mucosal IgA responses to certain antigens are dependent on the presence of peritoneal $CD5^+$ cells. Further, intraperitoneal (ip) immunization of animals has been used (Beh *et al.*, 1975; Pierce and Gowans, 1975; Dunkley and Husband, 1990; Thapar *et al.*, 1990) as an extremely effective route of immunization for the induction of both systemic and mucosal immune responses. A vigorous IgA antibody response was promoted by ip priming when the same antigen was given subsequently enterically or systemically. In contrast, primary intraduodenal immunization was substantially less effective. All investigators generally agree that the IgA-secreting plasma cells found in mucosal tissues of animals are derived from two relatively independent sources, Peyer's patches and peritoneum. Although both sources contain precursors of plasma cells that are committed, to a large degree, to synthesis of IgA, their surface phenotypes, maturation pattern, specific antibody repertoires, and stimulation routes are quite different.

The precursors of mucosal IgA plasma cells in humans have been assumed also to originate from Peyer's patches. The possibility that such cells may be derived from the peritoneum has not been considered. Studies of the human mucosal immune system, as related to the IgA plasma cells and $CD5^+$ cells in individual compartments, are limited. Solvason and Kearney (1992) demonstrated the presence of pro/pre-B cells in fetal omentum and liver as early as 8 weeks gestation; 40% of B cells found in the omentum were $CD5^+$. Histochemical examination revealed that the human fetal omentum contains more $CD5^+$ cells than the liver; the authors (Solvason and Kearney, 1992) propose that this tissue should be considered a primary lymphoid organ and a site of B-cell generation, in addition to the fetal liver and bone marrow. Because Peyer's patches in newborns are not well developed, apparently because of lack of stimulation with luminal antigens, such cells are not likely to be derived from Peyer's patches and must originate elsewhere, perhaps in the peritoneum. Analyses of intestinal B cells from normal adults revealed that 55% of B cell-enriched populations were $CD5^+$ (Peters *et al.*, 1989). When examined for Ig secretion, the $CD5^+$ B-cell population contained 4 times the number of IgA-secreting cells than the $CD5^-$ population. In sum, the evidence derived from studies of the ontogeny of the immune system in humans and animals, the phenotypes of B cells in different lymphoid compartments, immune responses generated by various routes of immunization, and adoptive transfer of B cells obtained from the peritoneum into immunodeficient mice favor the possibility that IgA-secreting plasma cells in mucosal tissue are derived not only from the Peyer's patches but also from the peritoneum.

IV. VACCINES BASED ON THE COMMON MUCOSAL SYSTEM

A. Viral Vaccines

An increased understanding of the general principles of mucosal immunity have led to an exponential expansion in investigative efforts to develop mucosal vaccines (for reviews, see Mestecky, 1987; McGhee and Mestecky, 1990, McGhee *et al.*, 1992). Throughout the last century, many microorganisms and their products have been given by the oral route as potential vaccines (Mestecky and McGhee, 1989; Gilligan and Li Wan Po, 1991). Currently, the vaccines approved for human use contain live adeno and polioviruses, whereas other vaccines such as those against influenza, rabies, hepatitis, respiratory syncytical, rota, and cytomegaloviruses are under investigation (Mestecky and McGhee, 1989; McGhee and Mestecky, 1990; Gilligan and Li Wan Po, 1991; O'Hagan, 1992). Developments with available vaccines and relevant information concerning experimental vaccines are summarized here.

1. Poliovirus

Poliovirus causes an acute infectious disease that, in its serious form, affects the central nervous system causing flaccid paralysis. The introduction of inactivated (Salk) polio vaccine (IPV) in 1955, followed by the trivalent oral (Sabin) poliovirus vaccine (OPV) in 1963, has resulted since 1979 in the elimination of endogenously transmitted paralytic disease caused by wild poliovirus in the United States and in many other parts of the world. However, 5–10 cases of vaccine-associated poliomyelitis occur every year in the United States after immunization with OPV (Ogra and Faden, 1986).

Numerous epidemiological and clinical studies have demonstrated that the extent and nature of circulating antibody responses following parenteral administration of IPV are similar to those following successful immunization with orally ingested OPV (Ogra *et al.*, 1980). The response is characterized by the appearance of serum IgM and IgG in a predictable sequence. IgA is detectable in serum at a later stage and may remain at low levels. OPV induces a state of local resistance in the alimentary tract to subsequent viral reinfection. However, the alimentary immunity after naturally acquired wild virus infection is more profound than after immunization with OPV (Ogra, 1984). In contrast, parenteral administration of IPV affords very little alimentary immunity (Ogra *et al.*, 1980). Experimental studies with OPV and IPV administered to children have shown that OPV elicits development of SIgA antibody to poliovirus in the nasopharynx and intestine 1–3 weeks after immunization, that persist over a period of as long as 5–6 years. Immunization with IPV fails to induce a secretory antibody response in the nasopharynx or intestines. Administration of a large dose of IPV into the nasopharynx or intestine elicits a local SIgA response without an associated SIgA response in the serum (Ogra *et al.*, 1980). Subsequent studies have demonstrated that reimmunization with IPV–Salk in individuals previously primed with parenterally administered IPV–Salk resulted in a booster effect and modest secretory antibody response. However, reimmunization of IPV–Salk vaccinated subjects with a single booster dose of OPV resulted in a marked enhancement of SIgA antibody response (Ogra, 1984).

Early studies therefore demonstrated the advantages of Sabin OPV administered orally to Salk IPV administered parenterally in inducing an efficient mucosal response. Despite the infrequent use of IPV–Salk in the United States, several European and Scandinavian countries and certain provinces of Canada have relied successfully on the parenteral administration of IPV. In the late 1970s, an enhanced potency preparation of IPV (IPV-EP) was introduced in the United States. Comparative studies have shown that routine parenteral immunization with three doses of the vaccine induces serum antibody responses similar to those after immunization with OPV. Virus-specific neutralizing and enzyme-linked immunosorbent assay (ELISA) antibody activity in nasopharyngeal secretions (NPS) was observed in about 56 and 82% of subjects who received IPV-EP and in 56 and 82% of subjects who received OPV, respectively (Zhaori *et al.*, 1988). In contrast, only 15–20% of IPV–Salk immunized subjects exhibited a neutralizing antibody response, demonstrating the superiority of IPV–EP to IPV–Salk in inducing neutralizing and ELISA secretory antibody responses (Zhaori *et al.*, 1988; Onorato *et al.*, 1991). Elegant studies carried out with OPV or IPV-EP poliovaccines have suggested that other host factors in the mucosa, such as the enzymatic environment, could play an important role in the development of immune response (Roivainen and Hovi, 1988).

During its replication in the gut, OPV as well as naturally acquired wild poliovirus is cleaved by proteolytic enzymes. Such cleavage has been shown experimentally to alter the antigenic nature of the virus (Roivainen and Hovi, 1988). The effects of such interaction and the development of secretory antibody response to poliovirus virion proteins against intact or trypsin-treated poliovirus type 3 have been studied in the nasopharyngeal samples of four groups of infants immunized with OPV, IPV-EP, or a combined vaccination of IPV-EP followed by OPV (Zhaori *et al.*, 1989; Ogra and Garofalo, 1990). ELISA SIgA and, less frequently, neutralizing antibody activity were detected in the NPS in IPV-EP and IPV–Salk vaccinated subjects when tested against the whole virus, compared with a decline in secretory antibody activity when tested against cleaved virus. On the other hand, the secretory antibody activity in NPS samples from OPV vaccinees exhibited a significant increase in neutralizing and ELISA activity against cleaved virus compared with intact virus. These observations suggest that antigenic sites are exposed by trypsin cleavage, in case of live oral vaccine, and elicit a mucosal secretory antibody response. This response is not possible for inactivated vaccines administered parenterally.

The virion proteins of poliovirus also have been characterized and the neutralization antigenic site determined (Emini *et al.*, 1982). The major antigenic site for virus neutralization appears to be on the capsid protein VP1 of poliovirus type 3. The antibody response in the serum and SIgA to different virion proteins with OPV or IPV or a combination of the two vaccines was studied (Zhaori *et al.* 1989; Ogra and Garofalo, 1990). Infants in both OPV and IPV-EP vaccinated groups developed similar SIgA antibody responses to VP1 and VP2 in the NPS. VP3-specific response was observed in 75% of subjects immunized with OPV. The IPV-immunized subjects exhibited poor VP3 response. Therefore, in addition to VP1 neutralization association, sites associated with VP3 also play an important role in the magnitude and quality of the immune response elicited by immunization with OPV.

Vaccine-associated poliomyelitis is a major drawback of OPV. Several studies (Faden *et al.*, 1990) show that the incorporation of at least one dose of IPV at the start of the immunization schedule could reduce the risk of vaccine-associated poliomyelitis and increase systemic as well as local antibody production. However, the long-term immunity to poliovirus provided by such a combined vaccination schedule has yet to be determined (Faden *et al.*, 1990). In addition, repeated contact with circulating vaccine virus may be important in causing intestinal reinfection and boosting local and humoral immunity, as is possible with such combined vaccines.

Another major concern with OPV is the formation of neurovirulent mutants (revertant virus) as it replicates in the gut. Sabin type 2 and 3 vaccine viruses have been reported to revert to neurovirulent phenotypes (Burke *et al.*, 1988). The types of potential sites of mutations associated with virulence are complex. These sites may include single base substitutions at either the 5′ or the 3′ noncoding regions of the viral genome (Evans *et al.*, 1985) or changes in the amino acid sequence of capsid proteins (Evans *et al.*, 1983). Prolonged fecal virus shedding has been proposed to be a function of development of revertants (Dunn *et al.*, 1990). However, the frequency of such reversion after different vaccination schedules has not been well defined. Studies carried out in our laboratory (Ogra *et al.*, 1991) have demonstrated that fecal shedding of nonvaccine type poliovirus revertants is not uncommon after immunization with OPV, regardless of prior immunization status. The nature of the virus shed in four groups of infants immunized with OPV, IPV-EP, or a combined vaccination of OPV and IPV-EP were analyzed. In group 1 receiving only one OPV dose, two of three (67%) isolates were nonrevertants. In group 2 receiving two doses of OPV, 11 of 12 (67%) isolates were found to be revertants. In groups 3 and 4, receiving doses of IPV-EP followed by OPV, over 90% of isolates were of the reverted virus types. On examining the frequency of reversion for different serotypes, evidently all type 2 poliovirus isolates tested were revertant types, irrespective of the immunization group. Significantly, all poliovirus type 3 revertants were observed in subjects previously primed with IPV-EP. In addition, nasopharyngeal antibody response was observed more significantly in subjects shedding revertants in the feces, irrespective of prior immunization with OPV or IPV-EP. Therefore, wild (virulent) virus or development of reversion during replication of OPV in the gut may provide a more potent stimulus for induction of mucosal immune response than attenuated parent strains of vaccine viruses. Although combined immunization with IPV-EP followed by OPV is effective in inducing both systemic and secretory antibody responses, it affords no protection against generation of nonattenuated virulent revertants in vaccinees (Ogra *et al.*, 1991).

2. Respiratory Syncytial Virus

Respiratory syncytial virus (RSV) is a major viral respiratory pathogen causing severe lower respiratory tract infection in early childhood. Despite the wide prevalence of RSV disease and a high rate of morbidity and mortality among children, no vaccine is currently available for prevention of this respiratory disease.

The earliest attempt to develop an effective vaccine occurred in the mid-1960s using a formalin-inactivated whole virus vaccine (Chin *et al.*, 1969). The vaccine, when evaluated in field trials, did not elicit any SIgA response nor did it show any immediate untoward effects. Subsequently, however, a number of vaccinees developed an exaggerated form of acute lower respiratory illness following natural exposure to the virus (Kapikian *et al.*, 1969; Kim *et al.*, 1969). Several other attempts were made to develop inactivated or attenuated vaccine, none of which have been successful (Buynak *et al.*, 1979; Belshe *et al.*, 1982). Investigative efforts also were directed at the use of low temperature adapted virus (Kim *et al.*, 1971) or other temperature sensitive mutants of the virus (TS1 and TS2). However, such vaccine candidates also showed poor infectivity and immunogenicity (Wright *et al.*, 1971; Richardson *et al.*, 1978).

RSV encodes for two major glycoproteins: G (G-Gp), which facilitates attachment of virus to the host cell, and F (F-Gp), which mediates spread of infection via cell-to-cell fusion. More recent studies by different workers have shown that these glycoproteins can induce protective immunity against infection with RSV (Routledge *et al.*, 1988). Monoclonal antibodies prepared against either glycoprotein, when passively administered to cotton rats and mice, were found to generate pulmonary resistance to subsequent intranasal challenge with the virus (Walsh *et al.*, 1987). Intranasal immunization with viral proteins was found to induce higher antibody titers in lungs than immunization by the intraperitoneal route. With refinements of molecular techniques, cDNA copies of the mRNAs for both glycoproteins have been cloned and live recombinant vaccinia viruses have been constructed that express RSV F or G glycoproteins. Experimental studies on rodents and monkey produced high titer antibody response to RSV F and G glycoprotein and showed significant resistance to intranasal challenge with RSV (Elango *et al.*, 1986; Stott *et al.*, 1987). However, immunization of chimpanzees with such recombinant viruses failed to induce a high level of RSV-specific antibody and resistance to RSV challenge (Collins *et al.*, 1990).

Experimental immunization of cotton rats with RSV or a live recombinant vaccinia virus expressing the RSV F-Gp via intranasal, parenteral, or enteric routes uniformly resulted in the development of RSV antibody in the serum and respiratory tract that was increased significantly after subsequent intranasal challenge with RSV (Kanesaki *et al.*, 1991). The IgA antibody response in bronchoalveolar fluid was two- to threefold higher after intranasal or enteric immunization than after intradermal immunization. The IgA antibody response in nasal wash was not significantly different among the three immunization groups, although the mean antibody titer was highest in the intranasal immunization group (Kanesaki *et al.*, 1991). Complete resistance to replication of RSV challenge was observed in lungs of cotton rats immunized by intranasal or enteric routes, compared with those immunized intradermally. Enteric or intradermal immunization conferred partial protection on the upper respiratory tract but complete protection was observed after intranasal administration. These studies indicate that although enteric immunization is quite effective in inducing antibody responses in the respiratory tract, intransal immunization is superior. A combined immunization with both enteric and intranasal routes could, however, afford better antiviral immunity. These findings highlight the importance of immunization or infection of the respiratory tract itself to provide complete immunity (Ogra and Karzon, 1969). Several experimental studies on cotton rats (Wathen *et al.*, 1991), BALB/c mice (Connors *et al.*, 1991), and humans (Hall *et al.*, 1991) also have demonstrated the importance of F and G glycoproteins as protective antigens. In addition to live or inactivated vaccines, subunit vaccines prepared from fusion proteins are also under development (Murphy *et al.*, 1988). Immunostimulating complex (ISCOM) vaccine (Morien *et al.*, 1984), made from fusion protein and nucleoprotein of human RSV, also has been found to induce circulating neutralizing antibody when given by the mucosal intranasal route (Truedel *et al.*, 1990). Intranasal vaccination with ISCOM induced eightfold higher neutralizing antibody titers than live virus vaccine or subunit vaccine with adjuvant (Truedel *et al.*, 1990).

3. Rotavirus

Rotavirus is the leading cause of diarrhea in infants and young children worldwide, and represents the single most important cause of morbidity and mortality in children and infants in developing countries (Kapikian *et al.*, 1969). No vaccine has been approved for human use to date.

Rotavirus is a segmented double-stranded RNA virus capable of genetic reassortment, with the potential for antigenic changes. The major inner capsid polypeptide VP6 and, possibly contains the domain for the common group antigen shared by most human and animal rotavirus. Neutralizing antibody responses have been associated with outer capsid polypeptides VP7 and VP3, and hemagglutinin activity with VP3 (Greenberg *et al.*, 1988).

Based on earlier observation (Wyatt *et al.*, 1979), a "Jennerian" approach has been applied to the development of a vaccine for human rotavirus. This approach was possible because human and animal rotaviruses share a common group antigen VP6. A number of candidate vaccines have undergone clinical trials with limited success, including RIT 4374, WC3, MMU 18006, and SA-11. RIT 4374 derived from bovine rotavirus (strain NCDV) provided a high level of protection (88%) against clinically significant diarrhea in children ages 6–12 months (Vesikari *et al.*, 1986). However, the vaccine later failed to provide protection to children under 6 months of age (DeMol *et al.*, 1986). Similar results were obtained with rhesus rotavirus strain (RRV) MMU 18006 (Christy *et al.*, 1988). The bovine rotavirus vaccine WC3 provided protection against moderate to severe diarrhea in children 3–12 months of age (Clark *et al.*, 1988). Purified empty capsids of vervel monkey rotavirus (SA-11) have been evaluated in mice, but no data are available concerning their use in humans. Reassortant vaccines derived from rhesus virus and human rotavirus serotypes 1, 2, and 4 have been tested in adults and infants (Halsey *et al.*, 1988). Oral administration of reassortant vaccines has been found to be effective in inducing antibody seroconversion in over 70% of vaccinees, often associated with significant viral replication and shedding in the feces. The vaccine appears to be tolerated well by both adults and children. A safety tested strain of human rotavirus (CJN) appears to be distinct from other candidate vaccines (Ward *et al.*, 1986). Molecular approaches to vaccine development are also underway. A recombinantly expressed VP4 protein may be considered a viable candidate for rotavirus vaccine in the future (Mackow *et al.* 1990).

The role of SIgA antibody in protection against natural or vaccine-induced rotavirus infection remains controversial (Glass *et al.*, 1986). Several studies have demonstrated the presence of rotavirus-specific SIgA activity in breast milk and significant protection against rotavirus enteritis in breastfed infants (Sheridan *et al.*, 1984). However, a positive relationship between the levels of fecal SIgA and protection from infection has not been observed consistently (Glass *et al.*, 1986).

4. Adenovirus

Inactivated vaccines against adenoviruses were licensed initially for parenteral use more than 20 years ago. However, the detection of a living monkey virus (SV40) in such inactivated vaccine preparations and the consistency in their protective efficacy against acute respiratory illness necessitated their withdrawal from the civilian market in the 1960s. Subsequently, live mucosal vaccines were developed against several adenovirus serotypes (types 4, 7, and 21), but the use of these vaccines has been restricted largely to military populations in whom these serotypes cause a large share of acute respiratory disease (Top *et al.*, 1971). Mucosal immunization with enteric-coated live adenovirus preparations has been highly effective against acute respiratory disease caused by adenoviruses in military recruits (Dudding *et al.*, 1973). After oral immunization with type 21 vaccine and after natural infection with virus of type 1, 4, 6, or 7, the characteristics of the serum antibody response appear to be similar to those of the responses to other mucosal viral infections, particularly with respect to the development of IgM and IgG antibody responses. The SIgA and, frequently, the secretory IgG antibody responses have been observed regularly in the nasal secretions after natural infection (Ogra *et al.*, 1980). After immunization with enteric-coated vaccines, SIgA antibody is detected regularly in feces; however, nasal secretions do not manifest significant adenovirus-specific SIgA antibody activity. The adenoviruses types 1, 2, and 5 that are associated with childhood illnesses have been shown to be safe and immunogenic when administered to adult volunteers using the same technique of enteric immunization (Steinhoff, 1991). However, the approach of enteric immunization has not been used in children.

The precise role of serum rather than secretory nasopharyngeal antibody in adenovirus-induced respiratory disease remains to be defined. After natural infection, homotypic reinfection is a rare phenomenon. On the other hand, after enteric immunization, homotypic reinfection occurs frequently in association with shedding of virus in the respiratory tract, although clinical illness is rare. These observations suggest that other mechanisms, such as serum antibody or T cell-mediated immunity, also may play a role in the mechanisms of mucosal defense in adenovirus infections. Unfortunately, no information is available about the development and function of adenovirus-specific cell-mediated immune response after natural infection in humans.

5. Rabies Vaccine

Animal rabies is endemic in virtually all parts of the world. Human infection continues to be a uniformly fatal disease. Attempts at reducing the animal reservoir of the disease have been frustrated by the multiplicity of animal species in which the virus replicates (Baer, 1988). Vaccinia virus recombinants expressing rabies virus glycoproteins have been utilized as a replicating vaccine, administered orally in wild animals. Immunization with one such glycoprotein vaccine in raccoons induced specific neutralizing antibody to rabies virus in serum (Rupprecht *et al.*, 1986). The animals resisted rabies virus challenge 28 and 205 days after immunization. Significantly, however, oral immunization with other attenuated antigenic variants of rabies virus (strain CVS-11 or ERA) failed to induce significant seroconversion (Rupprecht *et al.*, 1986). Although oral immunization with recombinant rabies vaccine appears to be highly successful in such experimental settings, information concerning the development of SIgA antibody response is not available at this time.

6. Simian and Human Immune Deficiency Viruses

Although on a world-wide scale more than 70% of AIDS cases are acquired by the heterosexual route of transmission (Padian, 1987; Johnson 1988; Piot *et al.*, 1988; Alexander, 1990; Naz and Ellaurie, 1990), the role of mucosal immunity and development of vaccines that may be effective in the prevention of sexually acquired disease have not received due attention (McGhee and Mestecky, 1990,1992). However, an animal model has clearly demonstrated that systemically immunized rhesus macaques that are protected against systemic challenge with simian immunodeficiency virus (SIV) develop infection when the virus is introduced in the vagina or urethra (Miller *et al.*, 1989). In view of the relative independence of systemic and mucosal immune compartments, future immunization efforts should be aimed at inducing protective immunity in both compartments. Whether SIgA anti-SIV- or anti-HIV-specific antibodies neutralize corresponding viruses before they infect susceptible cells in the genital tract (T cells, macrophages, Langerhans cells, and probably epithelial cells) or also neutralize virus intracellularly has not been established. Further, the role of mucosal cytotoxic T cells in the prevention of spreading of infection by eliminating infected cells has not been established.

Exploration of immunization routes that lead to the preferential induction of immune responses in genital tract secretions and tissues should receive further attention. In macaques, combination of oral–vaginal and rectal immunizations has yielded promising results (Lehner *et al.*, 1992a,b).

B. Influenza Virus

Several studies performed in animal models indicate that mucosal antibodies, especially SIgA, play a prominent role in the prevention of influenza virus infection of the upper respiratory tract (Shvartsman and Zykov, 1976; Liew *et al.*, 1984; Small, 1990; Renegar and Small, 1991a,b); systemic antibodies and cell-mediated immunity are apparently more important in the recovery phase from the infection and in prevention of viral pneumonia (Liew *et al.*, 1984). Antibodies against both hemagglutinin (HA) and neuraminidase (NA) of influenza protect mice from experimental infection. Antibodies against HA are thought to neutralize viruses whereas anti-NA is thought to prevent release of viruses from infected cells (Askonas *et al.*, 1982).

Oral administration of live virus or inactivated vaccine (Bergmann and Waldman, 1989) to mice results in HA virus-specific antibodies in lung lavage fluids. Since influenza vaccine is only moderately immunogenic, mucosal adjuvants such as cholera toxin (Chen and Quinnan, 1989) have been used in oral immunization protocols. In one study (Moldoveanu *et al.*, 1993), the use of microencapsulated influenza vaccine in mice preserved immunogenicity of vaccine given orally or by the systemic route and also resulted in higher serum and secretory antibody levels, which persisted longer than when an unencapsulated vaccine was used.

Humans orally immunized with inactivated influenza vaccine exhibited an SIgA antibody response in nasal and other external secretions (Bergmann *et al.*, 1986; Waldmann *et al.*, 1986; Bergmann and Waldman, 1989). Higher oral doses induced better responses in the age groups most commonly afflicted, that is, the elderly and children with chronic bronchitis, both of which responded well to the oral vaccine (Bergmann and Waldman, 1989). Several studies also have been performed of aerosol immunization with attenuated virus, a procedure that presumably immunizes via BALT. Nasal washes of these vaccinees contain high titers of SIgA and anti-HA and lesser amounts of IgM and IgG (Murphy *et al.*, 1982; Murphy and Clements, 1989). Individuals who developed nasal SIgA anti-HA also developed serum IgA and anti-HA responses (Brown *et al.*, 1985).

In summary, ample evidence supports the conclusion that oral immunization with killed virus, intranasal (BALT) immunization with attenuated strains, or perhaps combinations of the two, should provide SIgA immunity in the upper respiratory tract.

C. Bacterial Vaccines

Mucosal immunizations with numerous bacterial species and their products have been explored in humans and in animals for more than 100 years (for reviews, see Gay, 1924; Besredka, 1927; Mestecky and McGhee, 1989). Although the list of bacterial species used for mucosal immunization includes some 17 important mucosal and systemic pathogens, we discuss only those that have been used in human orally delivered vaccines.

1. *Salmonella*

Salmonellae effectively colonize the gastrointestinal tract in a species-specific fashion, for example, *S. typhi* affects humans whereas *S. typhimurium* causes mouse typhoid (Curtiss *et al.*, 1989). Further, these bacteria can penetrate into the Peyer's patches and can reach systemic tissues via the mesenteric lymph nodes and the bloodstream. The advantages of using *Salmonella* in antigen delivery is reviewed elsewhere (Curtiss *et al.*, 1989; Cardenas and Clements, 1992). Thus, vaccines for immunity to typhoid have been developed and, in some instances, have been given by the oral route (Kantele *et al.*, 1986). The avirulent galactose epimeraseless (*gal E*) *S. typhi* Ty21a was field tested extensively and shown to be safe and to induce immunity when given systemically (Levine *et al.*, 1986). However, when Ty21a was given by the oral route, it was less effective; multiple oral doses were required. Nevertheless, a number of attenuated *Salmonella* strains and mutants are being tested and hold promise for use as oral vaccines (Curtiss *et al.*, 1989).

2. Cholera

A major cause of severe diarrheal disease in developing countries is cholera, which is produced by the enterotoxigenic strains of *V. cholerae*. Partially protective SIgA antibodies are found in the intestine of those who recover and may work synergistically with antibodies to cholera toxin and to surface antigens to provide protection (Holmgren *et al.*, 1989). Two types of oral cholera vaccines currently are being tested: mutant cholera strains that colonize the gut and induce a local antibody response (Levine *et al.*, 1983) and a combined vaccine consisting of killed cholera vibrios and purified B toxin subunit (Clemens *et al.*, 1988). The latter vaccine has been field tested extensively in cholera endemic areas, and has been shown to give rise to a long-lasting protective immunity (Holmgren *et al.*, 1989).

3. Shigellosis

The *Shigellae* are gram-negative pathogens that penetrate through the epithelial cells in the large intestine and induce bacillary dysentery. Most efforts toward development of immunity have involved attenuated oral vaccines (Hale and Formal, 1989). The bacterium contains a large (120–140 mDa) plasmid that encodes invasion plasmid antigens (*ipa*), permitting the construction of enteroinvasive vaccines using *Esche-*

richia coli and *Salmonella* as recipients. The plasmid has been transferred to *E. coli* K-12, and conjugal transfer of *His* and *Pro* markers from *Shigella flexneri* into the *E. coli* yielded a vaccine strain (EC104) that expressed *Shigella* antigens (Hale and Formal, 1989). This strain has been used to immunize monkeys orally, but resulted in a high incidence of diarrhea when tested in humans. The Ty21a *gal E* mutant of *S. typhi* has been used as a recipient of a 120-mDa plasmid of *Shigella sonnei,* which encodes the O-polysaccharide side chain of the somatic antigen. This oral vaccine provided 40% protection from challenge by virulent *S. sonnei*. Thus, oral vaccines with recombinant bacteria containing *Shigella* plasmids are promising and ultimately may induce protection from bacterial dysentery.

4. *Haemophilus influenzae*

Haemophilus influenzae [nontypable (NTHI)] has been used as a component of oral vaccine given to human volunteers as a protective measure against acute bronchitis (Clancy *et al.,* 1989). Killed NTHI vaccine was given 3 times in tablets. Previous studies (Clancy *et al.,* 1983) from the same group of investigators revealed that oral immunization induces haemophilus-specific SIgA in saliva of vaccinees. However, no difference in NTHI colonization of throats of orally immunized or placebo-administered individuals were noted (Clancy *et al.,* 1989).

5. *Streptococcus mutans*

Mutants streptococci are involved in the development of dental caries. Numerous studies performed in the last 20 years have shown that oral immunization of human volunteers with formalin-killed *S. mutans* and with certain bacterial products such as enzyme glucosyltransferase induces enzyme-neutralizing antibodies in saliva and reduces *S. mutans* counts in dental plague (Russell and Mestecky, 1986; Taubman and Smith, 1989; Michalek and Childers, 1990; Russell, 1992). Further, *S. mutans*-specific SIgA antibodies were detected in tears, colostrum, and milk as well as parotid, submandibular, and submaxillar saliva of vaccinees (Mestecky *et al.,* 1978; Gregory *et al.,* 1985; Czerkinsky *et al.,* 1987). Although the mechanisms involved in the protection against dental caries have not been established convincingly, antibodies apparently play a dominant role.

V. SUMMARY

The selective induction of humoral and cellular immune responses in mucosal tissues is desirable for the prevention of various systemic as well as predominantly mucosa-restricted infections. The enormous surface area of mucosal membranes is protected primarily by antibodies produced locally by large numbers of plasma cells distributed in the subepithelial spaces of mucosal membranes and in the stroma of secretory glands. In contrast to the large variety of currently available injectable vaccines that stimulate systemic immunity, vaccines administered nonparenterally to stimulate mucosal immunity preferentially are used infrequently.

Current knowledge of the origins and migratory pathways of B and T lymphocytes destined for mucosal tissues indicates that the development and application of vaccines to exploit the remarkable principles of the common mucosal immune system will achieve the ultimate goal—protection of mucosal membranes.

References

Alexander, N. J. (1990). Sexual transmission of human immunodeficiency virus: Virus entry into the male and female genital tract. *Fertil. Steril.* **54,** 1–18.

Allansmith, M. R., Burns, C. A., and Arnold, R. R. (1982). Comparison of agglutinin titers to *Streptococcus mutans* in tears, saliva, and serum. *Infect. Immun.* **35,** 202–205.

Alley, C. D., Kiyono, H., and McGhee, J. R. (1986). Murine bone marrow IgA responses to orally administered sheep erythrocytes. *J. Immunol.* **136,** 4414–4419.

Arnold, R. R., Mestecky, J., and McGhee, J. R. (1976). Naturally occurring secretory immunoglobulin A antibodies to *Streptococcus mutans* in human colostrum and saliva. *Infect. Immun.* **14,** 355–362.

Askonas, B. A., McMichael, A. J., and Webster, R. G. (1982). The immune response to influenza viruses and the problem of protection against infection. *In* "Basic and Applied Influenza Research" (A. S. Beare, ed.), p. 159. CRC Press, Boca Raton, Florida.

Baer, G. M. (1988). Oral rabies vaccination. An overview. *Rev. Infect. Dis.* **10S,** 644–648.

Beh, K. J., Husband, A. J., and Lascelles, A. K. (1975). Intestinal response of sheep to intraperitoneal immunization. *Immunology* **37,** 385–388.

Belshe, R. B., Van Voris, L. P., and Mufson, M. A. (1982). Parenteral administration of live respiratory syncytial virus vaccine: Results of a field trial. *J. Infect. Dis.* **145,** 311–319.

Bergmann, K.-C., and Waldman, R. H. (1989). Oral immunization with influenza virus: Experimental and clinical studies. *Curr. Top. Microbiol. Immunol.* **146,** 83–89.

Bergmann, K. C., Waldmann, R. H., Tischner, H., Pohl, W.-D. (1986). Antibody in tears, saliva and nasal secretions following oral immunization of humans with inactivated influenza virus vaccine. *Int. Arch. Allergy Appl. Immunol.* **80,** 107–109.

Besredka, A. (1927). "Local Immunization." Williams and Wilkins, Baltimore.

Bienenstock, J. (1985). Bronchus associated lymphoid tissue. *Int. Arch. Allergy Appl. Immunol.* **76,** 62–69.

Bienenstock, J., and Strauss, H. (1970). Evidence for synthesis of human colostral γA as 11S dimer. *J. Immunol.* **105,** 274–277.

Brandtzaeg, P. (1985a). The role of J chain and secretory component in receptor-mediated glandular and hepatic transport of immunoglobulins in man. *Scand. J. Immunol.* **22,** 111–146.

Brandtzaeg, P. (1985b). Research in gastrointestinal immunology-state of the art. *Scand. J. Gastroenterol.* **20** (Suppl. 114), 137–156.

Brandtzaeg, P. (1987). Immune functions and immunopathology of palatine and nasopharyngeal tonsils. *In* "Immunology of the Ear" (J. M. Bernstein and P. L. Ogra, eds.), pp. 63–106. Raven Press, New York.

Brown, T. A., Murphy, B. R., Radl, J., Haaijman, J. J., and Mestecky, J. (1985). Subclass distribution and molecular form of immunoglobulin A hemagglutinin antibodies in sera and nasal secretions after experimental secondary infection with influenza A virus in humans. *J. Clin. Microbiol.* **22,** 259–264.

Brown, W. R., and Kloppel, T. M. (1989). The liver and IgA: Immunological, cell biological and clinical implications. *Hepatology* **9,** 763–784.

Burke, K. L., Dunn, G., Ferguson, M., Minor, P. D., and Almond, J. W. (1988). Antigen chimeras of poliovirus as potential new vaccines. *Nature (London)* **332,** 81–82.

Buynak, E. B., Weibel, R. E., Carlson, A. J., McLean, A. A., and Hilleman, M. R. (1979). Further investigations of virus administered parenterally. *Proc. Soc. Exp. Biol. Med.* **160,** 272–277.

Cardenas, L., and Clements, J. D. (1992). Oral immunization using live attenuated *Salmonella* spp. as carriers of foreign antigens. *Clin. Microbiol. Rev.* **5,** 328–342.

Chen, K.-S., and Quinnan, G. V., Jr. (1989). Efficacy of inactivated influenza vaccine delivered by oral administration. *Curr. Top. Microbiol. Immunol.* **146,** 101–106.

Chin, J., Magoffin, R. L., Shearer, L. A., Schieble, J. H., and Lennette, E. H. (1969). Field evaluation of a respiratory syncytial virus vaccine and a trivalent parainfluenza virus vaccine in a pediatric population. *Am. J. Epidemiol.* **89,** 449–463.

Christy, C., Madore, H. P., Pichichero, M., E. Gala, C., Pincus, P., Vosefski, D., Hoshino, Y., Kapikian, A., and Dolin, R. (1988). Field trial of rhesus rotavirus vaccine in infants. *Pediatrics* **7,** 645–650.

Clancy, R. L., Cripps, A. W., Husband, A. J., and Buckley, D. (1983). Specific immune response in the respiratory tract after administration of an oral polyvalent bacterial vaccine. *Infect. Immun.* **39,** 491–496.

Clancy, R. L., Wallace, F. J., Cripps, A. W., and Pang, G. T. (1989). Protection induced against acute bronchitis—The use of human and rat models to determine mechanisms of action of oral immunization with *Haemophilus influenza. Curr. Top. Microbiol. Immunol.* **146,** 181–185.

Clark, H. F., Bonian, F. E., Bell, L. M., Modesto, K., Gouvea, V., and Plotkin, S. A. (1988). Protective effects of WC3 vaccine against rotavirus diarrhea in infants during a predominantly serotype 1 rotavirus season. *J. Infect. Dis.* **158,** 570–587.

Clemens, J. D., Harris, J. R., Sack, D. A., Chakraborty, J., Ahmed, F., Stanton, B. F., Khan, M. U., Kay, B. A., Huda, N., Khan, M. R., Yunus, M., Raghava Rao, M., Svennerholm, A. -M., and Holmgren, J. (1988). Field trial of oral cholera vaccines in Bangladesh: Results of a one year of followup. *J. Infect. Dis.* **158,** 60–69.

Coelho, I. M., Pereira, M. T., and Virella, G. (1974). Analytical study of salivary immunoglobulins in multiple myeloma. *Clin. Exp. Immunol.* **17,** 417–426.

Collins, P. L., Purcell, R. H., London, W. T., Lawrence, L. A., Chanock, R. M., and Murphy, B. R. (1990). Evaluation in chimpanzees of vaccinia virus recombinants that express the surface glycoproteins of human respiratory syncytial virus. *Vaccine* **8,** 164–168.

Connors, M., Collins, P. L., Firestone, C. Y., and Murphy, B. R. (1991). Respiratory syncytial virus (RSV) F, G, M2 (22K), and N proteins each induce resistance to RSV challenge, but resistance induced by M2 and N proteins is relatively short-lived. *J. Virol.* **65,** 1634–1637.

Crago, S. S., Kutteh, W. H., Moro, I., Allansmith, M. R., Radl, J., Haaijman, J. J., and Mestecky, J. (1984). Distribution of IgA1-, IgA2-, and J chain-containing cells in human tissues. *J. Immunol.* **132,** 16–18.

Craig, S. W., and Cebra, J. J. (1971). Peyer's patches: An enriched source of precursors for IgA-producing immunocytes in the rabbit. *J. Exp. Med.* **134,** 188–200.

Curtiss, R., III, Kelly, S. M., Gulig, P. A., and Nakayama, K. (1989). Selective delivery of antigens by recombinant bacteria. *Curr. Top. Microbiol. Immunol.* **146,** 35–49.

Czerkinsky, C., Prince, S. J., Michalek, S. M., Jackson, S., Russell, M. W., Moldoveanu, Z., McGhee, J. R., and Mestecky, J. (1987). IgA antibody producing cells in peripheral blood after antigen ingestion: Evidence for a common mucosal immune system in humans. *Proc. Natl. Acad. Sci. U.S.A.* **84,** 2449–2453.

Czerkinsky, C., Svennerholm, A.-M., Quiding, M., Jonsson, R., and Holmgren, J. (1991). Antibody-producing cells in peripheral blood and salivary glands after oral cholera vaccination of humans. *Infect. Immun.* **59,** 996–1001.

De Buysscher, E. V., and Dubois, P. R. (1978). Detection of IgA anti-*Escherichia coli* plasma cells in the intestine and salivary glands of pigs orally and locally infected with *E. coli. Adv. Exp. Med. Biol.* **107,** 593–600.

Delacroix, D. L., Hodgson, H. J. F., McPherson, A., Dive, C., and Vaerman, J.-P. (1982). Selective transport of polymeric IgA in bile: Quantitative relationships of monomeric and polymeric IgA, IgM, and other proteins in serum, bile, and saliva. *J. Clin. Invest.* **70,** 230–241.

DeMol, P., Zissis, G., Butzler, J. P., Mutwewingabo, A., and Andre, F. E. (1986). Failure of live, attenuated oral rotavirus vaccine. *Lancet* **2,** 108.

Dudding, B. A., Top, F. H., Jr. Winter, P. E., Buescher, E. L., Lamson, T. H., and Leibovitz, A. (1973). Acute respiratory disease in military trainees: The adenovirus surveillance program 1966–1971. *Am. J. Epidemiol.* **97,** 187–98.

Dunkley, M. L., and Husband, A. J. (1990). Routes of priming and challenge for IgA antibody-containing cell responses in the intestine. *Immunol. Lett.* **26,** 165–170.

Dunn, G., Begg, N. T., Cammack, N., and Minor, P. D. (1990). Virus excretion and mutation by infants following primary vaccination with live oral poliovaccine from two sources. *J. Med. Virol.* **32,** 92–95.

Elango, N., Prince, G. A., Murphy, B. R., VenKatesan, S., Chanock, R. M., and Moss, B. (1986). Resistance to human respiratory syncytial virus (RSV) infection induced by immunization of cotton rats with a recombinant vaccinia virus expressing RSV G glycoprotein. *Proc. Natl. Acad. Sci. U.S.A.* **83,** 1906–1910.

Emini, E. A., Jameson, B. A., Lewis, A. J., Larsen, G. R., and Wimmer, E. (1982). Poliovirus neutralization epitopes: Analysis and localization with neutralizing monoclonal antibodies. *J. Virol.* **43,** 997–1005.

Evans, D. M. A., Minor, P. D., Schild, G. C., and Almond, J. W. (1983). Critical role of an eight amino acid sequence of VP1 in neutralization of poliovirus type 3. *Nature (London)* **304,** 459–462.

Evans, D. M., Dunn, G., Minor, P. D., Schild, G. C., Cann, A. J., Stanway, G., Almond, J. W., Currey, K., and Maizel, J. V., Jr. (1985). Increased neurovirulence is associated with a single nucleotide change in noncoding region of Sabin type 3 poliovaccine. *Nature* **314,** 548–550.

Faden, H., Modlin, J. F., Thoms, M. L., McBean, A. M., Ferdon, M. B., and Ogra, P. L. (1990). Comparative evaluation of immunization with live attenuated and enhanced-potency inactivated trivalent poliovirus vaccines in childhood: Systemic and local immune response. *J. Infect. Dis.* **162,** 1291–1297.

Forrest, B. D., Shearman, D. J. C., and LaBrooy, J. T. (1990). Specific immune response in humans following rectal delivery of live typhoid vaccine. *Vaccine* **8,** 209–212.

Friedman, B. K., Greenberg, B., and McNamara, T. F. (1975). Effect of extracorporeal cesium irradiation on secretory and serum immunoglobulins. *J. Dent. Res.* **54,** 96. (Abstract)

Gay, F. P. (1924). Local resistance and local immunity to bacteria. *Physiol. Rev.* **4,** 191–214.

Gilligan, C. A., and Li Wan Po, A. (1991). Oral vaccines: Design and delivery. *Int. J. Pharm.* **73,** 1–24.

Glass, R. I., Stoll, B. J., Wyatt, R. G., Hoshino, Y., Banu, H., and Kapikian, A. Z. (1986). Observations questioning a protective role for breast feeding in severe rotavirus diarrhea. *Acta Pediatr. Scand.* **75,** 713–718.

Goldblum, R. M., Ahlstedt, S., Carlsson, B., Hanson, L. Å., Jodal, U., Lidin-Janson, G., and Sohl-Ackerlund, A. (1975). Antibody-forming cells in human colostrum after oral immunization. *Nature (London)* **257,** 797–799.

Greenberg, H. B., Offit, P. A., and Shaw, R. D. (1988). Neutralization of rotaviruses *in vitro* and *in vivo:* Molecular determinants of protection and role of local Immunity. *In* "Mucosal Immunity and Infections at Mucosal Surfaces" (W. Strober, M. Lamm, and J. R. McGhee, eds.), pp. 325–329. Oxford University Press, New York.

Gregory, R. L., Schöller, M., Filler, S. J., Crago, S. S., Prince, S. J., Allansmith, M. R., Michalek, S. M., Mestecky, J., and McGhee, J. R. (1985). IgA antibodies to oral and ocular bacteria in human external secretions. *Protides Biol. Fluids* **32,** 53–56.

Hale, T. L., and Formal, S. B. (1989). Oral shigella vaccines. *Curr. Top. Microbiol. Immunol.* **146,** 205–211.

Hall, C. B., Walsh, E. E., Long, C. E., and Schnabel, K. C. (1991). Immunity to and frequency of reinfection with respiratory syncytial virus. *J. Infect. Dis.* **63,** 693–698.

Halsey, J. F., Mitchell, C. S., and McKenzie, S. J. (1983). The origin of secretory IgA in milk: A shift during lactation from a serum origin to local synthesis in the mammary gland. *Ann. N.Y. Acad. Sci.* **409,** 452–459.

Halsey, N. A., Anderson, E. L., Sears, S. D., Steinhoff, M., Wilson, M., Belshe, R. B., Midthun, K., Kapikian, A. Z., Chanock, R. M., Samorodin, R., Burns, B., and Clements, M. L. (1988). Human rhesus reassortant rotavirus vaccines. Safety and immunogenecity in adults, infants, and children. *J. Infect. Dis.* **158,** 1261–1267.

Hanson, L. Å., and Brandtzaeg, P. (1980). The mucosal defense system. *In* "Immunological Disorders in Infants and Children" (E. R. Steihm, and V. A. Fulginiti, eds.). pp. 137–164. Saunders, Philadelphia.

Heatley, R. V., Stark, J. M., Horsewood, P., Bandouvas, E., Cole, F., and Bienenstock, J. (1981). The effects of surgical removal of Peyer's patches in the rat on systemic antibody responses to intestinal antigen. *Immunology* **44,** 543–548.

Heremans, J. F. (1974). Immunoglobulin A. *In* "The Antigens" (M. Sela, ed.), Vol. II, pp. 365–522. Academic Press, New York.

Heremans, J. F., and Bazin, H. (1971). Antibodies induced by local antigenic stimulation of mucosal surfaces. *Ann. N.Y. Acad. Sci.* **190,** 268–274.

Holmgren, J., Clemens, J., Sack, D. A., Sanchez, J., and Svennerholm, A.-M. (1989). Oral immunization against cholera. *Curr. Top. Microbiol. Immunol.* **146,** 197–204.

Husband, A. J., and Gowans, J. L. (1978). The origin and antigen-dependent distribution of IgA-containing cells in the intestine. *J. Exp. Med.* **148,** 1146–1160.

Jacobson, L. O., Marks, E. K., Simmons, E. L., and Gaston, E. O. (1961). Immune response in irradiated mice with Peyer's patch shielding. *Proc. Soc. Exp. Biol. Med.* **108,** 487–493.

Johnson, A. M. (1988). Heterosexual transmission of human immunodeficiency virus. *Brit. Med. J.* **296,** 1017–1020.

Jonard, P. P., Rambaud, J. C., Dive, C., Vaerman, J.-P., Galian, A., and Delacroix, D. L. (1984). Secretion of immunoglobulins and plasma proteins from the jejunal mucosa: Transport data and origin of polymeric immunoglobulin A. *J. Clin. Invest.* **74,** 525–535.

Kanesaki, T., Murphy, B. R., and Collins, P. L., and Ogra, P. L. (1991). Effectiveness of enteric immunization in the development of secretory immunoglobulin A response and the outcome of infection with respiratory syncytial virus. *J. Virol.* **65,** 657–663.

Kantele, A. (1990). Antibody secreting cells in the evaluation of the immunogenicity of an oral vaccine. *Vaccine* **8,** 321–326.

Kantele, A., Avrilommi, M., and Jokinen, I. (1986). Specific immunoglobulin-secreting human blood cells after peroral vaccination against *Salmonella typhi. J. Infect. Dis.* **153,** 1126–1131.

Kapikian, A., and Chanock, R. M. (1990). Rotaviruses. *In* "Virology" (B. N. Fields, D. M. Knipe, R. M. Chanock, M. S. Hirsh, J. L. Melnick, and T. P. Morath, eds.), 2d Ed., Vol. 2, pp. 1335–1404. Raven Press, New York.

Kapikian, A. Z., Mitchell, R. H., Chanock, R. M., Shvedoff, R. A., and Stewart, C. E. (1969). An epidemiologic study of altered clinical reactivity to respiratory syncytial (RS) virus infection in children previously vaccinated with an inactivated RS virus vaccine. *Am. J. Epidemiol.* **89,** 405–421.

Kett, K., Brandtzaeg, P., Radl, J., and Haaijman, J. J. (1986). Different subclass distribution of IgA producing cells in human lymphoid organs and various secretory tissues. *J. Immunol.* **136,** 3631–3635.

Kim, H. W., Canchola, J. G., and Brandt, C. D., Pyles, G., Chanock, R. M., Jensen, K., and Parrott, R. H. (1969). Respiratory syncytial virus disease in infants despite prior administration of antigenic inactivated vaccine. *Am. J. Epidemiol.* **89,** 422–434.

Kim, H. W., Arrobio, J. O., Pyles, G., Brandt, C. D., Camargo, E., Chanock, R. M., and Parrott, R. H. (1971). Clinical and immunological response of infants and children to administration of low temperature adapted respiratory syncytial virus. *Pediatrics* **48,** 745–755.

Koertge, T. E., and Butler, J. E. (1986). Dimeric M315 is transported into mouse and rat milk in degraded form. *Mol. Immunol.* **23,** 839–845.

Kroese, F. G. M., Butcher, E. C., Stall, A. M., Lalor, P. A., Adams, S., and Herzenberg, L. (1988). Many of the IgA plasma cells in the murine gut are derived from self replenishing precursors in the peritoneal cavity. *Int. Immunol.* **1,** 75–84.

Kroese, F. G. M., Butcher, E. C., Stall, A. M., and Herzenberg, L. A. (1989). A major peritoneal reservoir of precursors for intestinal IgA plasma cells. *Immunol. Invest.* **18,** 47–58.

Kubagawa, H., Bertoli, L. F., Barton, J. C., Koopman, W. J., Mestecky, J., and Cooper, M. D. (1987). Analysis of paraprotein transport into the saliva by using anti-idiotype antibodies. *J. Immunol.* **138,** 435–439.

Kutteh, W. H., Koopman, W. J., Conley, M. E., Egan, M. L., and Mestecky, J. (1980). Production of predominantly polymeric IgA by human peripheral blood lymphocytres stimulated *in vitro* with mitogens. *J. Exp. Med.* **152,** 1424–1429.

Kutteh, W. H., Hatch, K. D., Blackwell, R. E., and Mestecky, J. (1988). Secretory immune system of the female reproductive tract. I. Immunoglobulin and secretory component-containing cells. *Obstet. Gynecol.* **71,** 56–60.

Ladjeva, I., Peterman, J. H., and Mestecky, J. (1989). IgA subclasses of human colostral antibodies specific for microbial and food antigens. *Clin. Exp. Immunol.* **78,** 85–90.

Lamm, M. E. (1976). Cellular aspects of immunoglobulin A. *Adv. Immunol.* **22,** 223–290.

Lawton, A. R., and Mage, R. G. (1969). The synthesis of secretory IgA in the rabbit. I. Evidence for synthesis of an 11S dimer. *J. Immunol.* **102,** 693–697.

Lehner, T., Bergmeier, L. A., Panagiotidi, C., Brookes, R., Tao, L., Gearing, A. J. H., and Adams, S. (1992a). A primate model of immunization inducing mucosal and systemic immunity to SIV antigens. 7th International Conference on Mucosal Immunology, Prague.

Lehner, T., Bergmeier, L. A., Panagiotidi, C., Tao, L., Brookes,

R., Klavinskis, L. S., Walker, P., Walker, J. Ward, R. G., Hussain, L., Gearing, A. J. H., and Adams, S. E. (1992). Induction of mucosal and systemic immunity to recombinant simian immunodeficiency viral protein. *Science* **258,** 1365–1369.

Levine, M. M., Kaper, J. B., Black, R. E. (1983). New knowledge on pathogenesis of bacterial enteric infections as applied to vaccine development. *Microbiol. Rev.* **47,** 510–550.

Levine, M. M., Black, R. E., Ferreccio, C., Clements, M. L., Lanata, C., Rooney, J., and Germanier, R. (1986). The efficacy of attenuated *Salmonella typhi* oral vaccine strain Ty21a evaluated in controlled field trials. *In* "Development of Vaccines and Drugs against Diarrhea" (J. Holmgren, A. Lindberg, and R. Möllby, eds.), pp. 90–101. Studentilitteratur, Lund, Sweden.

Liew, F. Y., Russell, S. M., Appleyard, G., Brand, C. M., and Beale, J. (1984). Cross-protection in mice infected with influenza A virus by the respiratory route is correlated with local IgA antibody rather than serum antibody or cytotoxic T cell reactivity. *Eur. J. Immunol.* **14,** 350–356.

Lycke, N., Lindholm, L., and Holmgren, J. (1985). Cholera antibody production *in vitro* by peripheral blood lymphocytes following oral immunization of humans and mice. *Clin. Exp. Immunol.* **62,** 39–47.

Mackow, E. R., Vo, P. T., Broome, R., Bass, D., and Greenberg, H. B. (1990). Immunization with poliovirus expressed VP4 protein passively protects against simian and murine rotavirus challenge. *J. Virol.* **64,** 1698–1703.

McDermott, M. R., and Bienenstock, J. (1979). Evidence for a common mucosal immunologic system: I. Migration of B immunoblasts into intestinal, respiratory, and genital tissues. *J. Immunol.* **122,** 1892–1898.

McGhee, J. R., and Mestecky, J. (1990). In defense of mucosal surfaces. Development of novel vaccines for IgA responses protective at the portals of entry of microbial pathogens. *Infect. Dis. Clin. North Am.* **4,** 315–341.

McGhee, J. R., and Mestecky, J. (1992). The mucosal immune system in HIV infection and prospects for mucosal immunity to AIDS. *AIDS Res. Rev.* **2,** 289–312.

McGhee, J. R., Mestecky, J., Dertzbaugh, M. T., Eldridge, J. H., Hirasawa, M., and Kiyono, H. (1992). The mucosal immune system: From fundamental concepts to vaccine development. *Vaccine* **10,** 75–88.

Mestecky, J. (1987). The common mucosal immune and current strategies for induction of immune response in external secretions. *J. Clin. Immunol.* **7,** 265–276.

Mestecky, J., and McGhee, J. R. (1987). Immunoglobulin A (IgA): Molecular and cellular interactions involved in IgA biosynthesis and immune response. *Adv. Immunol.* **40,** 153–245.

Mestecky, J., and McGhee, J. R. (eds.) (1989). New strategies for oral immunization. Proceedings of the international symposium. *Curr. Top. Microbiol. Immunol.* **146.**

Mestecky, J., McGhee, J. R., Arnold, R. R., Michalek, S. M., Prince, S. J., and Babb, J. L. (1978). Selective induction of an immune response in human external secretions by ingestion of bacterial antigen. *J. Clin. Invest.* **61,** 731–737.

Mestecky, J., Lue, C., and Russell, M. W. (1991a). Selective transport of IgA. Cellular and molecular aspects. *Gastroenterol. Clin. North Am.* **20,** 441–471.

Mestecky, J., Blair, C., and Ogra, P. L. (eds.) (1991b). Immunology of milk and the neonate. Proceedings of the international symposium. *Adv. Exp. Med. Biol.* **310.**

Michalek, S. M., and Childers, N. K. (1990). Development and outlook for a caries vaccine. *Crit. Rev. Oral Biol. Med.* **1,** 37–54.

Miller, C. J., Alexander, N. J., Sutjipto, S., Lackner, A. A., Gettie, A., Lowenstine, L. J., Jennings, M., and Marx, P. A. (1989). Genital mucosal transmission of simian immunodeficiency virus: Animal model for heterosexual transmission of human immunodeficiency virus. *J. Virol.* **63,** 4277–4284.

Moldoveanu, A., Novak, M., Huang, W.-Q., Gilley, R. M., Staas, J. K., Schafer, D., Compans, R. W., and Mestecky, J. (1993). Oral immunization with influenza virus in biodegradable microspheres. *J. Infect. Dis.* **167,** 84–90.

Montgomery, P. C., Cohen, J., and Lally, E. T. (1974). The induction and characterization of secretory IgA antibodies. *Adv. Exp. Med. Biol.* **45,** 453–462.

Montgomery, P. C., Lemaitre-Coelho, I., and Lally, E. T. (1976). The effect of circulating antibodies on secretory IgA antibody induction following oral immunization with dinitrophenylated *Pneumococcus. Ric. Clin. Lab.* **6** (Suppl. 3), 93–99.

Montgomery, P. C., Ayyildiz, A., Lemaitre-Coelho, I. M., Vaerman, J.-P., and Rocky, J. H. (1983). Induction and expression of antibodies in secretions: The ocular immune system. *Ann. N.Y. Acad. Sci.* **409,** 429–439.

Morein, B., Sundquist, B., Hogland, S., Da Isgaard, K., and Osterhaus, A. (1984). ISCOM, a novel structure for antigenic presentation of membrane proteins from enveloped viruses. *Nature (London)* **308,** 457–460.

Murphy, B. R., and Clements, M. L. (1989). The systemic and mucosal immune response of humans to influenza A virus. *Curr. Top. Microbiol. Immunol.* **146,** 107–116.

Murphy, B. R., Nelson, D. L., Wright, P. F., Tierney, E. L., Phelan, M. A., and Chanock, R. M. (1982). Secretory and systemic immunological response in children infected with live attenuated influenza A virus vaccines. *Infect. Immun.* **36,** 1102–1008.

Murphy, B. R., Prince, G. A., Collins, P. L., Van Wyke Coelingh, K., Olmsted, R. A., Spriggs, M. K., Parrott, R. H., Kim, H. W., Brandt, C. D., and Chanock, R. M. (1988). Current approaches to the development of vaccines effective against parainfluenza and respiratory syncytial virus. *Virus Res.* **11,** 1–15.

Naz, R. K., and Ellaurie, M. (1990). Reproductive immunology of human immunodeficiency virus (HIV-1) infection. *Am. J. Reprod. Immunol.* **23,** 107–114.

Ogra, P. L. (1984). Mucosal immune response to poliovirus vaccines in childhood. *Rev. Infect. Dis.* **6** (Suppl. 2), 361–368.

Ogra, P. L., and Faden, H. S. (1986). Poliovirus vaccines live or dead. *J. Pediatr.* **108,** 1031–1033.

Ogra, P. L., and Garofalo, R. (1990). Secretory antibody response to viral vaccines. *Prog. Med. Virol.* **37,** 156–189.

Ogra, P. L., and Karzon, D. T. (1971). Formation and function of poliovirus antibody in different tissues. *Prog. Med. Virol.* **13,** 156–193.

Ogra, P. L., and Karzon, D. T. (1969). Distribution of poliovirus antibody in serum, nasopharynx, and alimentary tract following segmental immunization of lower alimentary tract with poliovaccine. *J. Immunol.* **102,** 1423–1430.

Ogra, P. L., Coppola, P. R., MacGillivray, M. H., and Dzierba, J. L. (1974). Mechanism of mucosal immunity to viral infections in gamma A immunoglobulin-deficiency syndromes. *Proc. Soc. Exp. Biol. Med.* **145,(3),** 811–816.

Ogra, P. L., Fishaut, M., and Gallagher, M. R. (1980). Viral vaccination via the mucosal route. *Rev. Infect. Dis.* **2,** 352–369.

Ogra, P. L., Losonsky, G. A., and Fishaut, M. (1983). Colostrum-derived immunity and maternal–neonatal interactions. *Ann. N.Y. Acad. Sci.* **409,** 82–93.

Ogra, P. L., Faden, H. S., Abraham, R., Duffy, L. C., Sun, M., and Minor, P. D. *et al.* (1991). Effect of prior immunity on the shedding of virulent revertant virus in feces after oral immunization with live attenuated poliovirus vaccines. *J. Infect. Dis.* **164,** 191–194.

O'Hagan, D. T. (1992). Oral delivery of vaccines. Formulation and clinical pharmacokinetic considerations. *Clin. Pharmacokinet.* **22,** 1–10.

Onorato, I. M., Modlin, J. F., McBean, A. M., Thoms, M. L., Losonsky, G. A., and Bernier, R. H. (1991). Mucosal immunity induced by enhanced potency inactivated and oral polio vaccines. *J. Infect. Dis.* **163,** 1–6.

Padian, N. S. (1987). Heterosexual transmission of acquired immune deficiency syndrome: International perspectives and national projections. *Rev. Infect. Dis.* **9,** 947–960.

Pecquet, S. S., Ehrat, C., and Ernst, P. B. (1992). Enhancement of mucosal antibody responses to *Salmonella typhimurium* and microbial hapten phosphorylcholine in mice with X-linked immunodeficiency by B-cell precursors from the peritoneal cavity. *Infect. Immun.* **60,** 503–509.

Peters, M. G., Secrist, H., Anders, K. R., Nash, G. S., Rich, S. R., and MacDermott, R. P. (1989). Normal human intestinal B lymphocytes. Increased activation compared with peripheral blood. *J. Clin. Invest.* **83,** 1827–1833.

Phillips-Quagliata, J. M., and Lamm, M. E. (1988). Migration of lymphocytes in the mucosal immune system. *In* "Migration and Homing of Lymphoid Cells" (A. J. Husband, ed.), Vol. II, pp. 53–75. CRC Press, Boca Raton, Florida.

Pierce, N. F., and Gowans, J. L. (1975). Cellular kinetics of the intestinal immune response to cholera toxoid in rats. *J. Exp. Med.* **142,** 1550–1563.

Piot, P., Plummer, F. A., Mhalu, F. S., Lamboray, J.-L., Chin, J., and Mann, J. M. (1988). AIDS: An international perspective. *Science* **239,** 573–579.

Quiding, M., Nordström, I., Kilander, A., Anderson, G., Hanson, L. Å., Holmgren, J., and Czerkinsky, C. (1991). Intestinal immune responses in humans. Oral cholera vaccination induces strong intestinal antibody responses and interferon-γ production and evokes local immunological memory. *J. Clin. Invest.* **88,** 143–148.

Renegar, K. B., and Small, P. A., Jr. (1991a). Passive transfer of local immunity to influenza virus infection by IgA antibody. *J. Immunol.* **146,** 1972–1978.

Renegar, K. B., and Small, P. A., Jr. (1991b). Immunoglobulin A mediation of murine nasal anti-influenza virus immunity. *J. Virol.* **65,** 2146–2148.

Richardson, L. S., Belshe, R. B., London, W. T., Sly, D. L., Prevar, D. A., Camargo, E., and Chanock, R. M. (1978). Evaluation of five temperature sensitive mutants of respiratory syncytial virus in primate. I. Viral shedding, immunologic response and associated illness. *Med. Virol.* **3,** 91–100.

Robertson, S. M., and Cebra, J. J. (1976). A model for local immunity. *Ric. Clin. Lab.* **6** (Suppl. 3), 105–119.

Roivainen, M., and Hovi, T. (1988). Cleavage of VP1 and modification of antigenic site 1 of type 2 polioviruses by intestinal trypsin. *J. Virol.* **62,** 3536–3539.

Routledge, E. G., Willcocks, M. M., Samson, A. C., Morgan, L., Scott, R., Anderson, J. J., and Toms, G. L. (1988). The purification of four respiratory syncytial virus proteins and their evaluation as protective agents against experimental infection in BALB/c mice. *J. Gen. Virol.* **69,** 293–303.

Rupprecht, C. E., Wiktor, T. J., Johnston, D. H., Hamir, A. N., and Dietzschold, B., Wunner, W. H., Glickman, L. T., and Koprowski, H. (1986). Oral immunization and protection of raccoons (*Procyon totor*) with a vaccinia rabies glycoprotein recombinant virus vaccine. *Proc. Natl. Acad. Sci. U.S.A.* **83,** 7947–7950.

Russell, M. W. (1992). Immunization against dental caries. *Curr. Opin. Dent.* **2,** 72–80.

Russell, M. W., and Mestecky, J. (1986). Potential for Immunological Intervention Against Dental Caries. *J. Biol. Buccale* **14,** 159–175.

Russell, M. W., and Mestecky, J. (1988). Induction of the mucosal immune response. *Rev. Infect. Dis.* **10,** S440–S446.

Russell, M. W., Brown, T. A., and Mestecky, J. (1982). Preferential transport of IgA and IgA immune complexes to bile compared with other secretions. *Mol. Immunol.* **19,** 677–682.

Scicchitano, R., Stanisz, A., Ernst, P., and Bienenstock, J. (1988). A Common Mucosal Immune System Revisited. *In* "Migration and Homing of Lymphoid Cells" (A. J. Husband, ed.), Vol. II, pp. 1–34. CRC Press, Boca Raton, Florida.

Sheridan, J. F., Smith, C. C., Manak, M. M., and Aurelian, L. (1984). Prevention of rotavirus induced diarrhea in neonatal mice born to dams immunized with empty capsid of simian rotavirus SA-11. *J. Infect. Dis.* **149,** 434–438.

Shvartsman, Y. S., and Zykov, M. P. (1976). Secretory anti-influenza immunity. *Adv. Immunol.* **22,** 291–330.

Small, P. A., Jr. (1990). Influenza: Pathogenesis and host defense. *Hosp. Prac.* **25,** 51–62.

Solvason, N., and Kearney, J. F. (1992). The human fetal omentum: A site of B cell generation. *J. Exp. Med.* **175,** 397–404.

Solvason, N., Lehuen, A., and Kearney, J. F. (1991). An embryonic source of Ly1 but not conventional B cells. *Int. Immunol.* **3,** 543–550.

South, M. A., Cooper, M. D., Wollheim, F. A., Hong, R., and Good, R. A. (1966). The IgA system. I. Studies of the transport and immunochemistry of IgA in saliva. *J. Exp. Med.* **123,** 615–627.

Stienhoff, M. C. (1991). Viral vaccines for the prevention of childhood pneumonia in developing nations. Priorities and prospects. *Rev. Infect. Dis.* **13,** S562–70.

Stott, E. J., Taylor, G., Ball, L. A., Anderson, K., Young, K. K., King, A. M., and Wertz, G. W. (1987). Immune and histopathological response in animals vaccinated with recombinant vaccinia viruses that express individual genes of human respiratory syncytial virus. *J. Virol.* **61,** 3855–3861.

Strindel, H. (1935). Bartel's Tonsille des Mastdarmes und ihre Stellung in der Pathologie des lymphatischen Apparates des Mastdarme. *Zbl. Chirurgie* **62,** 2594.

Taubman, M. A., and Smith, D. J. (1989). Oral immunization for the prevention of dental disease. *Curr. Top. Microbiol. Immunol.* **146,** 187–195.

Thapar, M. A., Parr, E. L., and Parr, M. B. (1990). Secretory immune response in the mouse vaginal fluid after pelvic, parenteral or vaginal immunization. *Immunology* **70,** 121–125.

Tomasi, T. B. (1976). "The Immune System of Secretions." Prentice-Hall, Englewood Cliffs, New Jersey.

Tomasi, T. B., Jr., Tan, E. M., Solomon, A., and Prendergast, R. A. (1965). Characteristics of an immune system common to certain external secretions. *J. Exp. Med.* **121,** 101–124.

Top, F. H., Jr., Buescher, E. L., Bancroft, W. H., and Russell, P. K. (1971). Immunization with live types 7 and 4 adenovirus vaccines. II. Antibody response and protective effect against acute respiratory disease due to adenovirus type 7. *J. Infect. Dis.* **124,** 155–160.

Truedel, M., Nadon, F., Seguin, C. (1990). Efficient intranasal vaccination of mice against human respiratory syncytial virus with an experimental iscoms subunit vaccine. *In* "Advances in Mucosal Immunology" (S. Challacombe, P. W. Bland, C. R. Stokes, R. V. Heatley, and A. McMowat, eds.), pp. 379. Kluwer Academic Publishers, Boston.

Tsunoda, R., Yaginuma, Y., and Kojima, M. (1980). Immunocytological studies on the constituent cells of the secondary modules in human tonsil. *Acta Pathol. Jpn.* **30,** 33–57.

Vesikari, T., Kapikian, A. Z., Delem, A., and Zissis, G. (1986). A comparative trial of rhesus monkey (RRV-1) and bovine (RIT 4237) oral rotavirus vaccines in young children. *J. Infect. Dis.* **153,** 832–839.

Waldman, R. H., and Ganguly, R. (1974). Immunity to infections on secretory surfaces. *J. Infect. Dis.* **130,** 419–440.

Waldmann, R. H., Stone, J., Bergmann, K.-Ch., Khakoo, R., Lazzell, V., Jacknowitz, A., Waldman, E. R., and Howard, S. (1986). Secretory antibody following oral influenza immunization. *Am. J. Med. Sci.* **292,** 367–371.

Walsh, E. E., Hall, C. B., Briselli, M., Brandriss, M. W., and Schlesinger, J. J. (1987). Immunization with glycoprotein subunits of respiratory syncytial virus to protect cotton rats against viral infection. *J. Infect. Dis.* **155,** 1198–1204.

Ward, R. L., Bernstein, D. I., Young, E. C., Sherwood, J. R., Knowlton, D. R., and Schiff, G. M. (1986). Human rotavirus studies in volunteers: Determination of infectious dose and serological response to infection. *J. Infect. Dis.* **154,** 871–880.

Wathen, M. W., Kakuk, T. J., Brideau, R. J., Hausknecht, E. C., Cole, S. L., and Zaga, R. M. (1991). Vaccination of cotton rats with a chimeric FG glycoprotein of human respiratory syncytial virus induces minimal pulmonary pathology on challenge. *J. Infect. Dis.* **163,** 477–482.

Weisz-Carrington, P., Roux, M. E., McWilliams, M., Phillips-Quagliata, J. M., and Lamm, M. E. (1979). Organ and isotype distribution of plasma cells producing specific antibody after oral immunization: Evidence for a generalized secretory immune system. *J. Immunol.* **123,** 1705–1708.

Wright, P. F., Mills, J. V., and Chanock, R. M. (1971). Evaluation of a temperature-sensitive mutant of respiratory syncytial virus in adults. *J. Infect. Dis.* **124,** 505–511.

Wyatt, R. G., Mebus, C. A., Yolken, R. H., Kalica, A. R., James, H. D., Jr., Kapikian, A. Z., and Chanock, R. M. (1979). Rotavirus immunity in gnotobiotic calves: Heterologous resistance to human virus induced by bovine virus. *Science* **203,** 548–550.

Zhaori, G., Sun, M., and Ogra, P. L. (1988). Characteristics of the immune response to poliovirus virion polypeptides after immunization with live or inactivated polio vaccines. *J. Infect. Dis.* **158,** 160–165.

Zhaori, G., Sun, M., Faden, H. S., and Ogra, P. L. (1989). Nasopharyngeal secretory antibody response to poliovirus type 3 virion proteins exhibit different specificities after immunization with live or inactivated poliovirus vaccines. *J. Infect. Dis.* **159,** 1018–1024.

32

Antigen Delivery Systems: New Approaches to Mucosal Immunization

Suzanne M. Michalek • John H. Eldridge • Roy Curtiss III • Kenneth L. Rosenthal

I. INTRODUCTION

The concept of vaccination as a means to eradicate disease began almost 200 years ago when Jenner showed that inoculation of a child with cow pox provided protection from a lethal small pox infection. Progress in this area moved slowly for many years. In fact, only during the past few decades have notable advances been made in the development of vaccines, that is, in the formulation of new ones and the improvement of existing ones, through the application of modern technology. In designing a vaccine, several aspects that need to be considered are its safety for use in animals (including humans), the convenience and cost of reproducibly generating the vaccine in large quantities, and its effectiveness in inducing the desired host response. Another important consideration is the route of immunization. Most infectious diseases involve colonization of or invasion through mucosal surfaces by the pathogen; therefore, developing methods for the induction of mucosal immune responses that will serve as a first line of defense is important. Oral administration of antigen has been shown to result in the induction of mucosal IgA antibodies in our external secretions (Mestecky, 1987; McGhee and Mestecky, 1990). This route of immunization has advantages over other means because the vaccines can be administered easily and have, potentially, no side effects. However, major limitations are the acidic pH and the presence of degradative enzymes in the gastrointestinal tract, which can break down the immunogens prior to antigen uptake and presentation to lymphoid cells in IgA inductive sites, for example, the gut-associated lymphoid tissue (GALT). Perhaps for these reasons, particulate antigens, especially when presented as viable organisms, are effective in inducing local and generalized secretory and systemic immune responses. At least three possible reasons exist to explain why particulate antigens are more effective oral immunogens than soluble antigens. First, the size of these macromolecular complexes may allow them to survive more effectively in low pH, bile salts, and proteolytic enzymes of the stomach and gastrointestinal tract. Second, at least some particulates are adsorbed through the M cells into the Peyer's patches with greater efficiency than soluble molecules, thus providing a higher local antigen concentration within this mucosal immune inductive site. Third, the major portion of an ingested soluble protein antigen will cross the epithelial barrier of the gut in the form of amino acids and low molecular weight peptides. The recognition of these peptides by gut lymphoid cells at sites other than the inductive environment of the Peyer's patches has been proposed as the stimulus initiating systemic tolerance after antigen feeding (Bland and Warren, 1986), and may provide a negative signal to the mucosal immune system as well. This information and the availability of modern technology have facilitated the development of antigen delivery systems with immunopotentiating activity for the induction of protective mucosal and systemic immune responses against microbial pathogens. Antigen delivery systems that have received considerable attention for their use in vaccine development are liposomes, biodegradable microspheres, and recombinant *Salmonella* and viral vectors.

II. LIPOSOMES AS VACCINE DELIVERY SYSTEMS

A. Introduction

Since the discovery by Bangham and co-workers (1965) that the addition of water to a flask containing a film of phospholipids resulted in the appearance of microscopic closed vesicles, liposomes have been studied extensively for use in targeted drug delivery and more recently as vaccine delivery systems. A number of aspects pertaining to the usefulness of liposomes as vaccine delivery systems are listed in Table I; several of these are discussed further in a subsequent section. Briefly, liposomes can act as immunoadjuvants in potentiating immune responses. Therefore, the amounts of antigen needed to induce a response are smaller when incorporated into liposomes than when given alone. Liposomes also can convert nonimmunogenic substances into immunogenic forms, for example, by rendering soluble substances particulate in nature. A variety of substances can be incorporated into liposomes including multiple antigens, adjuvants, and substances such as antibodies to cell-surface antigens for targeted delivery. Liposomes are taken up by macrophages and by M cells (specialized epithelial cells covering Peyer's patches) for antigen processing or presentation to other lymphoid cells for the induction of immune responses. Liposome also can present antigens to lymphoid cells directly

Table I Usefulness of Liposomes as a Delivery System and Immunoadjuvant for Vaccine Development

1. Small amounts of antigen may be suitable as immunogen
2. Nonimmunogenic substances may be converted to immunogenic forms (e.g., soluble antigens can be rendered "particulate" in form)
3. Adjuvants can be incorporated into the aqueous phase or membrane of liposomes containing antigens
4. Targeting agents can be incorporated into liposomes for delivery to specific host cells
5. Can be administered safely by oral or systemic routes for the induction of antibody responses to the incorporated antigen in external secretions or serum, respectively
6. Are taken up by macrophages and M cells and can substitute for antigen-presenting cells
7. Can mediate DNA or RNA transfection of cells

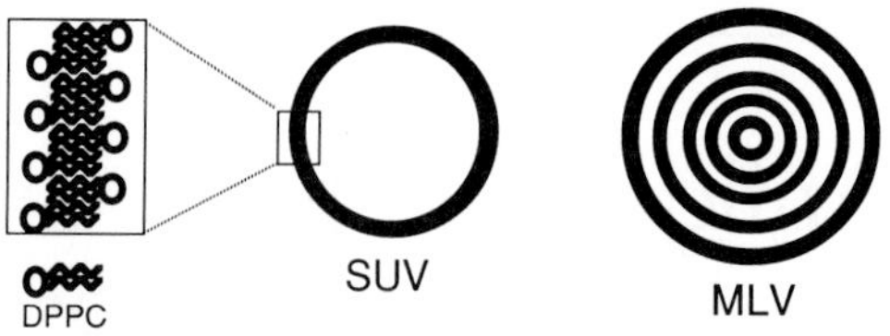

Figure 1 Schematic depiction of the two basic forms of liposomes. The small unilamellar vesicle (SUV) illustrates the bilayered membrane composed of dipalmitoyl phosphatidylcholine (DPPC) surrounding an aqueous core. The multilamellar vesicle (MLV) is characterized by several lipid bilayers separated by thin aqueous phases.

for the induction of immune responses. Since liposomes can be composed of substances (e.g., phospholipids) that constitute host cells, they should represent nontoxic, safe, and efficacious vaccine delivery systems for use in animals, including humans. Liposomes also have been shown to mediate DNA or RNA transfection of cells and may represent a useful means of transfer of genetic material encoding vaccine antigens. For more detailed discussion of this subject, the reader is referred to extensive reviews by others (Felgner *et al.*, 1987; Ostro, 1987; Swenson *et al.*, 1988; Gregoriadis, 1990; New, 1990; van Rooijen, 1990; Alving, 1991).

B. Properties of Liposomes

Liposomes are composed of a bilayered (bimolecular sheet) phospholipid membrane (lamella) forming vesicles enclosing and surrounded by an aqueous solution (Figure 1). The amphipathic nature of phospholipid molecules accounts for the spontaneous formation of vesicles, with the hydrophilic (water-soluble or polar) head portion oriented toward the aqueous phase and the hydrophobic (water-insoluble) tail pointing into the bilayer. Thus, in preparing liposome vaccines, water-soluble substances can be incorporated into the enclosed aqueous space whereas lipid-soluble molecules can be added to the solvent during vesicle formation and incorporated into the lipid bilayer. Almost any substance, regardless of its solubility, size, shape, or electric charge, can be incorporated into liposomes as long as it does not interfere with vesicle formation.

Depending on conditions used for production, liposomes can vary in size from 0.01 μm (Cornell *et al.*, 1982) to 150 μm (Pagano and Weinstein, 1978) (red blood cells are ~10 μm in diameter), as well as in form. The two standard forms of liposomes are multilamellar and unilamellar (Figure 1). Multilamellar vesicles (MLV) have several lipid bilayers separated by thin aqueous phases. Unilamellar vesicles have a single bilayer membrane surrounding an aqueous core and are characterized as being small (SUV) or large (LUV). Liposomes can be prepared to vary in their membrane stability, fluidity, and permeability depending on their lipid content (e.g., ratio of phospholipid to cholesterol). The incorporation of charged amphiphiles renders the liposomal surface positively or negatively charged. Each of these properties influences how effective a liposome preparation will be as a delivery system.

Several procedures for producing liposomes have been described (reviewed in Bangham *et al.*, 1974; Pagano and Weinstein, 1978; Kirby and Gregoriadis, 1984; New, 1990); however, a commonly used method involves sonication of the aqueous phospholipid suspension. The liposomes generated by this method are heterogeneous in size and form. For vaccine delivery systems, techniques must be used that reproducibly generate liposome preparations of controlled size and composition. Microemulsification of liposome suspensions is one technique that reproducibly results in homogeneous liposomes. The lipsomes are produced in a pressurized chamber and, by controlling the pressure and cycling time, small unilamellar liposomes of the desired diameter are generated (Mayhew *et al.*, 1984; Childers *et al.*, 1989). This procedure has been used extensively to generate liposomes containing antigens, especially mutans streptococcal antigens, for use as oral vaccines (reviewed by Michalek *et al.*, 1989; Michalek and Childers, 1990). Another method for preparing liposomes involves the generation of dehydrated–rehydrated vesicles (Gregoriadis *et al.*, 1990; reviewed by Gregoriadis, 1990). This procedure has been shown to result in high-yield entrapment of drugs and has been used to incorporate reproducibly various substances such as tetanus toxoid, influenza virus subunit peptides, recombinant hepatitis B surface antigen, *Leishmania major,* antigens and poliovirus. A direct comparison of the various liposome preparations for their effective use as vaccine delivery systems for the induction of protective immune response remains to be done.

C. Processing of Liposome Vaccines

Several explanations have been proposed for how liposomes can be effective delivery systems and adjuvants for the induction of immune responses (reviewed by Gregoriadis, 1990; van Rooijen, 1990; Alving, 1991). Liposomes, regardless of their composition and size, can adsorb to most cells and release their incorporated substances, which then can act on the cell. Liposomes also can be taken up by macrophages and other phagocytic cells in the blood, lymph, and various tissues (e.g., lymph nodes, liver, and spleen) with the subsequent release of antigen. The liver and spleen take up nearly all liposomes given by the intravenous route, whereas most liposomes injected via the subcutaneous or intramuscular route are retained at the site of injection and are taken up by infiltrating macrophages. The ability of antigen presenting cells to take up and process antigens associated with liposomes more efficiently for enhanced immune responses is another explanation for the immunoadjuvant property of liposomes. The liposomes also have been suggested to act directly in presenting antigen to lymphoid cells for the induction of responses. Further studies are necessary, however, to better define the mechanism(s) involved in the adjuvanticity of liposomes.

Although the fate of liposomes given orally remains controversial, vesicles composed of cholesterol and phospholipids are resistant to detergents or phospholipases and are also more resistant to degradation by enzymes in the gastrointestinal tract. In extensive studies in an experimental rat model (Childers *et al.*, 1990), liposomes have been shown to be taken up by M cells present in the epithelium covering the Peyer's patches (Figure 2). The liposomes are detected in endosomes in the M cells and appear to be transversing the cell, moving toward the underlying lymphoid cells. The presentation of antigen within liposomes to lymphoid cells in this IgA-inductive tissue can result in a mucosal immune response as manifested by the appearance of IgA antibodies in external secretions.

D. Liposome Vaccines in Vivo

During the past decade, numerous studies have been performed to establish the usefulness of the liposome vaccine delivery system in inducing protective immune responses against various infectious diseases. Although studies frequently have involved systemic routes of administration, evidence is accumulating that demonstrates that liposomes can serve as carriers of antigens and as adjuvants for inducing enhanced mucosal immune responses when given as an oral vaccine. Table II lists several, but not all, studies that have used liposomes as vaccine delivery systems. In the oral immunization studies, mucosal IgA immune responses were

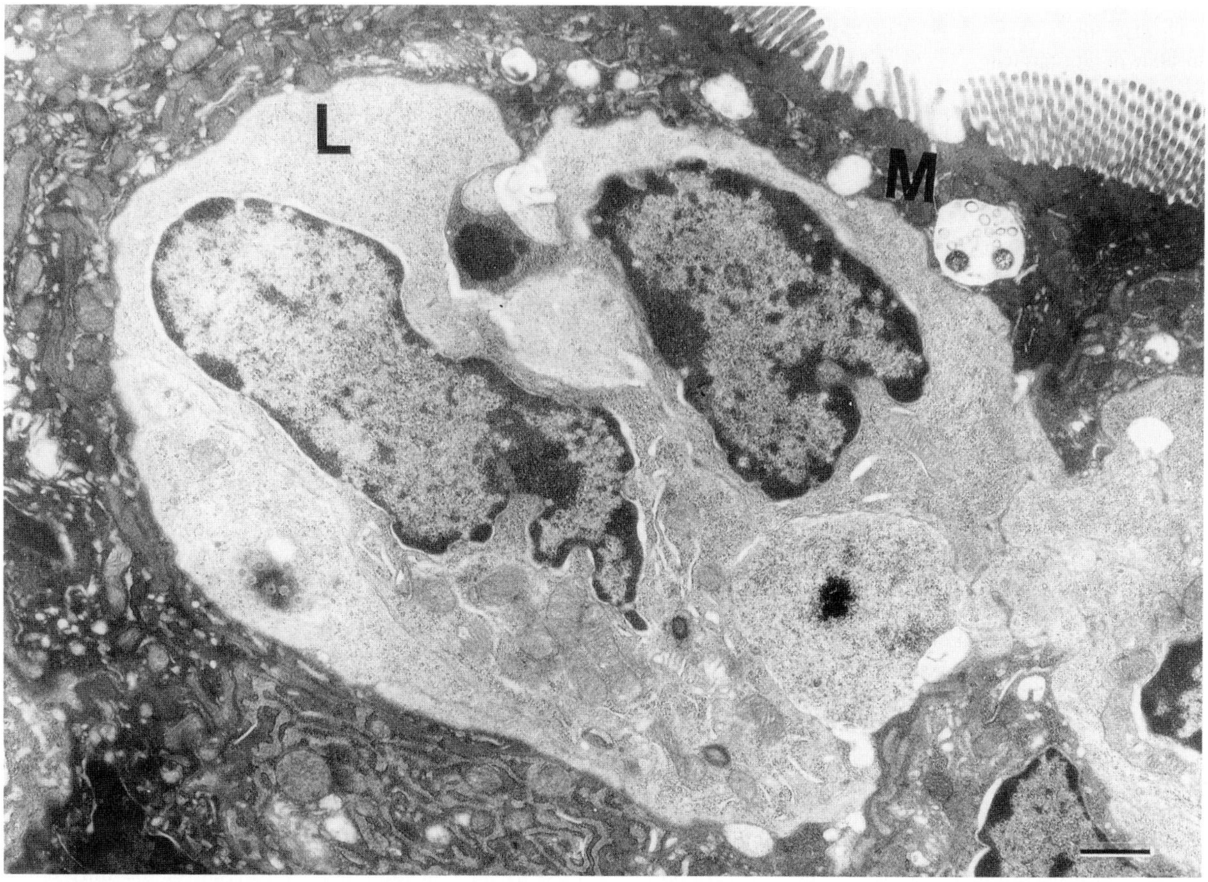

Figure 2 Electron micrograph of a section of rat Peyer's patch tissue from a ligated intestinal segment exposed to a suspension of liposomes (SUV) for 2 hr. Illustrated is an M cell (M) with an endocytic vesicle containing liposomes and a closely associated lymphoid cell (L). Bar: 1.0 μm. Reprinted with permission from Childers *et al.* (1990 and John Wiley & Sons, Inc. Copyright 1990).

Table II Immunization Studies with Liposomal Vaccine Delivery Systems[a]

Antigen/adjuvant	Liposome composition	Route of administration	Host	Major findings	References
Cholera toxin/lipoidal amine/ lipid A	DPPC, Chol, DP (M L V)	po	Rats	Enhanced intestinal IgA response	Pierce and Sacci (1984); Pierce *et al.* (1984)
mutans streptococcal anti-idiotypic antibodies carbohydrate/lipophilic MDP peptide-CTB protein-CTB proteins ribosomes	DPPC, Chol, DP (S U V)	po	Rats	Adjuvant effect—induction of salivary IgA antibodies; reduced infection by mutans streptococci	Gregory *et al.* (1986); Michalek *et al.* (1989,1990,1992); Jackson *et al.* (1990); Childers *et al.* (1991)
mutans streptococcal carbohydrate–protein conjugate		po	Rats	Adjuvant effect—induction of serum and salivary antibodies	Wachsmann *et al.* (1985, 1986)
Streptococcus mutans carbohydrate	DPPC, Chol, DP	po	Humans	Adjuvant effect—induction of salivary and serum IgA antibodies	Childers *et al.* (1991)
Bacteroides gingivalis fimbriae/L18-MDP or GM-53-MDP	DPPC, Chol	po or sc	Mice	Adjuvant effect—enhanced by GM-53-MDP > L18-MDP (salivary and serum antibodies)	Ogawa *et al.* (1989)
Plasmodium falciparum recombinant protein/lipid A/alum	DMPC, DMPG, Chol	im	Monkey	Adjuvant effect—enhanced by alum and lipid A (serum antibody)	Richards *et al.* (1989)
Herpes simplex virus acylpeptide of glycoprotein D/MLA/MTP-PE	PC, Chol, PS (M L V)	ip	Mice	Adjuvant effect enhanced by acylpeptide and further enhanced by MLA or MTP-PE (serum antibody); protected against lethal challenge	Brynestad *et al.* (1990)
Influenza virus hemagglutinin and neuraminidase/B30-MDP/ L18-MDP	MDP-virosomes ± Chol	ip	Mice Guinea pigs	Adjuvant effect enhanced by chol (stabilized) and B30 MDP (serum antibody and cellular immune response)	Nerome *et al.* (1990)

[a] Abbreviations: PC, phosphatidylcholine; DMPC, dimyristoyl phosphatidylcholine; DPPC, dipalmitoyl phosphatidylcholine; DP, diacetyl phosphate; Chol, cholesterol; MDP, *N*-acetyl muramyl-L-threonyl-D-isoglutamine; MLA, monophosphoryl lipid A; MTP-PE, muramyl tripeptide phosphatidylethanolamine; CTB, cholera toxin B subunit; SUV, small unilamellar vesicles; MLV, multilamellar vesicles, im, intramuscular; ip, intraperitoneal; sc, subcutaneous; po, per os (oral).

induced; in some cases the induction of the response correlated with protection against disease. In these studies and in those involving systemic routes of liposome vaccine administration, the spatial arrangement of the antigens within liposomes and the characteristics of the vesicles such as size and number of lamellae were not actually determined. Researchers generally accept that a physical association between the liposome membrane and antigen (as opposed to their simple mixing) is an important consideration in formulating a delivery system for inducing immune responses. Antigen can be incorporated into the aqueous phase of the vesicles, adsorbed onto their surface, partitioned into the bilayers (hydrophobic antigens), or covalently coupled to a membrane component. The specific formulation of liposome delivery systems may differ for the development of vaccines that are effective in inducing protective immunity against different infectious organisms. Further studies will be required to resolve this issue.

III. BIODEGRADABLE MICROSPHERES

A. Introduction

As first suggested by Strannegard and Yurchinson (1969), the particulate form of an antigen may enhance its effectiveness as an oral immunogen. Currently, the only approved method to adjuvant vaccines for human use is to adsorb protein antigens onto aluminum salts to create a particulate. These particulates potentiate the antibody response after systemic administration through the creation of an antigen depot, the induction of inflammation at the site of injection, and the directed delivery of the particulate antigen into the draining lymph nodes. However, the size and properties of aluminum compounds are sensitive to slight changes in the conditions of their preparation and their age (Nail *et al.*, 1976a,b), and they are not effective carriers for mucosal immunization. Among the approaches under investigation to improve vaccine delivery to systemic and mucosal lymphoid cells is the generation of polymeric particulate adjuvants.

Litwin and Singer (1965) demonstrated a modest enhancement in the circulating antibody response to human gamma globulin adsorbed onto polystyrene latex particles that had been administered intravenously to rabbits. This adjuvant activity was shown to be dependent on the adsorption of the antigen to the particles, was most apparent at limiting antigen doses, and was equivalent when particles of various diameters from 0.05 to 1.3 μm were tested. In contrast, Kreuter *et al.* (1986, 1988) reported that subcutaneous injection of mice with bovine serum albumin (BSA) adsorbed to either poly(methylmethacrylate) or polystyrene particles potentiated the anti-BSA response to a greater extent than adsorption to aluminum hydroxide. The possibility of using polymeric particles coated with antigen for the induction of a mucosal antibody response was reported by Cox and Taubman (1984), who stated that the oral administration of dinitrophenyl–bovine gamma globulin (DNP–BGG) on 1- to 3-μm glutaraldehyde-activated polyacrylamide beads was generally more effective in eliciting a salivary IgA anti-DNP response than was an equivalent dose of the soluble DNP–BGG. However, no supporting data were provided in this communication, so determining the degree to which the mucosal response was potentiated is impossible. More recently, O'Hagan *et al.* (1989a) tested 0.1- and 3-μm poly (butyl-2-cyanoacrylate) particles with adsorbed ovalbumin (OVA) as carriers for mucosal immunization. When orally administered on 4 consecutive days to primed rats, both the 0.1- and the 3-μm OVA-coated particles induced the appearance of specific IgA antibodies in saliva; the 0.1-μm particles also induced a serum IgG response. In contrast, oral boosting with soluble OVA was without effect.

B. Immunization Studies with Antigens Incorporated within Polymeric Particulates

Although clearly synthetic polymeric particulates with antigen adsorbed to their surface can serve as adjuvants that may enhance systemic or mucosal immune responses, many antigens will not adsorb effectively to their surface. Further, the exposed antigen is subject to elution or degradation after *in vivo* administration, an especially important consideration in the case of oral immunization. Incorporation of the vaccine within the polymer can allow virtually any antigen to be used, providing protection from degradation and control over the time of release. Several antigen-containing polymer systems have been investigated, some of which are listed in Table III with the conditions used to evaluate their effectiveness and the major experimental findings.

1. Antigens Incorporated within Polymeric Agglomerates and Implantable Pellets

Methylmethacrylate was polymerized by gamma irradiation in the presence of whole formalin-inactivated influenza virions (Kreuter and Speiser, 1976) or split influenza vaccine (Kreuter *et al.*, 1976) to yield agglomerates of poly(methylmethacrylate). After subcutaneous administration to guinea pigs or intraperitoneal administration to mice, the vaccine–polymer agglomerates were shown to elicit serum hemagglutination inhibition titers that exceeded those induced by equivalent doses of the free or aluminum hydroxide adjuvanted vaccines. Incorporation of the vaccines into the polymer by this approach was suggested because the adsorption of antigens to the agglomerate after polymerization provided less adjuvant activity. The vaccine-containing agglomerates exhibited a delay in the time of the antibody response relative to the other vaccine forms.

Preis and Langer (1979) used a solvent casting process to produce 0.3-mm pellets of ethylene-vinyl acetate copolymer, each of which contained 100 μg BSA. Subcutaneous implantation of one pellet per mouse was shown to elicit a circulating anti-BSA response, as measured by indirect hemagglutination, which was equivalent to that stimulated by two injections, each of which contained 50 μg BSA emulsified in complete Freund's adjuvant (CFA). The authors proposed that the immunopotentiation afforded by this delivery system resulted from prevention of antigen degradation and sustained release by diffusion through the copolymer. In a subsequent modification of this approach, BSA-containing pellets were prepared with a novel biodegradable polymer, CTTH-iminocarbonate, formed by linking tyrosine dipeptide units together through hydrolytically labile bonds between the tyrosine side-chain groups (Kohn *et al.*, 1986). This polymer was chosen for evaluation because the degradation products include derivatives of L-tyrosine, which have been reported to exhibit adjuvant activity. Following implantation, the BSA-containing CTTH-iminocarbonate pellets were shown to induce substantially enhanced antibody responses relative to the same dose of free BSA. Although the CTTH-iminocarbonate pellets did not potentiate the humoral response to the same extent as the previously described BSA-containing ethylene-vinyl acetate pellets (Preis and Langer, 1979), their *in vivo* biodegradation obviated the need for surgical removal.

2. Antigens Incorporated within Polymeric Microspheres

Incorporation of vaccines within polymeric microspheres can provide a system combining the advantages of a particulate adjuvant, which protects and controls the release of the antigen, with ease of administration by injection or mucosal application. Microencapsulation involves the coating of a bioactive agent, such as a vaccine, in a protective wall material that is generally polymeric in nature. The microsphere product is a free-flowing powder of spherical particles that can be produced across a size range from <1 μm to as large as 3 mm in diameter. The systems that have been investigated for vaccine delivery include microspheres formed by cross-

Table III Immunization Studies with Antigens Incorporated in Polymeric Delivery Systems[a]

Polymer/form	Antigen	Route of administration	Host	Major findings	References
Polmethylmethacrylate Agglomerate	Influenza virus	sc, ip	Guinea pigs, mice	Adjuvant effect—enhanced serum HAI titer	Kreuter and Speiser (1976)
Polyethylene-vinyl acetate Pellets	OVA	sc implant	Mice	Adjuvant effect—enhanced serum indirect HA titer equivalent to FCA	Preis and Langer (1979)
Poly(CTTH-iminocarbonate) Pellets	BSA	sc implant	Mice	Adjuvant effect—enhanced serum indirect HA titer exceeded two doses of free BSA	Kohn *et al.* (1986)
Polyacryl-starch Microspheres (0.5–2.0 μm)	HSA	im, iv	Mice	Adjuvant effect—enhanced serum ELISA titer anti-matrix response induced	Artursson *et al.* (1986)
Polymerized RSA Microspheres (100–200 μm)	Nodamura virus	im	Rabbits	Adjuvant effect—equivalent to FIA, antibody response to glutaraldehyde polymerized RSA induced	Martin *et al.* (1988)
Polyacrylamide Microspheres (2.5 μm)	OVA	po	Rats	Adjuvant effect—induction of salivary IgA in ip-primed host	O'Hagan *et al.* (1989b)
Poly(lactide-co-glycolide) Microspheres (100 μm)	p72:TT	sc, im	Mice	Weak primary response, effective booster	Altman and Dixon (1989)
Poly(lactide-co-glycolide) Microspheres (1–10 μm)	SEB toxoid	sc, im, ip, it, po	Mice, rhesus macaques	Adjuvant effect—plasma IgG equivalent to FCA after im; pulsed release; plasma, salivary, bronchial, gut IgA after or it	Eldridge *et al.* (1989,1990a,b,1991a,b,1992)
Poly(lactide-co-glycolide) Microspheres (1–10 μm)	Influenza virus	sc, ip, po	Mice	Adjuvant effect—oral booster induced salivary IgA, enhanced serum HAI titer and protection	Moldoveanu *et al.* (1989,1992)
Poly(lactide-co-glycolide) Microspheres (1–10 μm)	SIV	sc, ip	Mice rhesus macaques	Adjuvant effect—enhanced serum IgG response	Eldridge *et al.* (1992)
Poly(lactide-co-glycolide) Microspheres (5 μm)	OVA	sc, ip	Mice, Rats	Adjuvant effect—enhanced serum IgG response significantly greater than FCA in mice	O'Hagan *et al.* (1991a,b)

[a] Abbreviations: OVA, ovalbumin; BSA, bovine serum albumin; HSA, human serum albumin; SEB, staphylococcal enterotoxin B; p72:TT, 28-amino-acid peptide from the surface glycoprotein of hepatitis B virus conjugated to tetanous toxoid; SIV, simian immunodeficiency virus; sc, subcutaneous; ip, intraperitoneal; im, intramuscular; iv, intravenous; it, intratracheal; po, per os; HAI, hemagglutination inhibition; HA, hemagglutination; FIA, Freund's incomplete adjuvant; FCA, Freund's complete adjuvant.

linking natural substances such as starch or albumin and synthetic polymers.

In an attempt to produce a biocompatible microsphere antigen delivery system from a natural substance, Artursson *et al.* (1986) formulated 0.5 to 2.0-μm microspheres containing human serum albumin (HSA) from acryl starch activated with ammonium peroxydisulfate and cross-linked with *N,N,N′,N′*-tetramethylethylenediamine. When administered to mice by intramuscular or intravenous injection, the HSA–polyacryl starch microspheres stimulated a circulating anti-HSA antibody response that reached and remained for >200 days at approximately 500-fold the peak level induced by the injection of free HSA. However, an antibody response to the cross-linked starch was demonstrated in inhibition of antibody binding studies. In another approach that investigated the use of a natural substance under conditions under which it is normally nonimmunogenic, Martin *et al.* (1988) intramuscularly immunized rabbits with 100- to 200-μm microspheres containing Nodamura virus, that were formed by glutaraldehyde cross-linking of autologous rabbit serum albumin (RSA). In this system, the circulating antivirus antibody response was low and responses also were detected to glutaraldehyde cross-linked RSA. Thus, although the number of studies examining cross-linked natural substances to formulate vaccine-containing microspheres has been limited, the induction of antibody responses to the microsphere matrix is a problem that appears to preclude their application in human immunization.

O'Hagan *et al.* (1989b) examined the ability of antigen-containing synthetic polymer microspheres to potentiate salivary and plasma antibody responses. Oral administration of 1 mg OVA entrapped in polyacrylamide microspheres on each of 4 consecutive days to rats that had been primed previously by intraperitoneal injection of OVA in saline generated a statistically significant salivary IgA response, in the absence of a rise in circulating antibodies, 65 days following oral boosting. These microspheres were macroporous particles of 2.55-μm mean diameter with the OVA partially exposed on their surface. Control animals that received soluble OVA as the oral booster did not respond. These authors did not report on the adjuvant activity or tissue reactivity after systemic injection of these polyacrylamide microspheres, but the known neurotoxicity of polyacrylamide bars this formulation from all but experimental applications.

More recently, considerable effort has been placed in the evaluation of microspheres formulated from poly(DL-lactide-co-glycolide) (DL-PLG) for the parenteral and enteral delivery of vaccines because of the proven biocompatibility and biodegradability of this copolymer. DL-PLG is in the class of copolymers from which resorbable sutures, resorbable surgical clips, and controlled-release drug implants and microspheres are made (Redding *et al.*, 1984). These polyesters are approved for and have a 30-year history of safe use in humans. After introduction into the body, DL-PLG induces only a minimal inflammatory response and biodegrades through hydrolysis of ester linkages to yield the normal body constituents lactic and glycolic acids (Tice and Cowsar, 1984; Visscher *et al.*, 1987; Figure 3). Further, the rate at which DL-PLG biodegrades is a function of the ratio of lactide to glycolide in the copolymer (Miller *et al.*, 1977), thus determining the time after administration when release initiates as well as the subsequent rate of release.

Altman and Dixon (1989) examined the immune response induced by immunization with peptide 72 (p72), a 28-amino-acid peptide from the surface glycoprotein of hepatitis B virus, conjugated to tetanus toxoid (p72 : TT). Subcutaneous injection of mice with p72 : TT incorporated into 50- to 100-μm DL-PLG microspheres that were designed to release the antigen at a uniform rate over a period of 1–12 months resulted in a very weak primary antibody response. However, the microencapsulated p72 : TT retained antigenicity, as judged by the ability to prime for an anamnestic secondary response. Further, if the microencapsulated p72 : TT was injected in an inflammatory vehicle such as incomplete Freund's adjuvant (IFA), a high primary antibody response was induced, suggesting that the difference seen between these noninflammatory controlled release DL-PLG microspheres and the previously described pellets (Preis and Langer, 1979; Kohn *et al.*, 1986) may be related to inflammation induced by the implants.

In contrast to the results obtained with the relatively large DL-PLG microspheres investigated by Altman and Dixon (1989), the systemic administration of staphylococcal enterotoxin B (SEB) (Eldridge *et al.*, 1989,1990a,b,1991a,b,1992), influenza vaccine (Moldoveanu *et al.*, 1989,1992), simian immunodeficiency virus (SIV; Marx *et al.*, 1993), and OVA (O'Hagan *et al.*, 1991a,b) in 1- to 10-μm DL-PLG microspheres resulted in strongly potentiated primary antibody

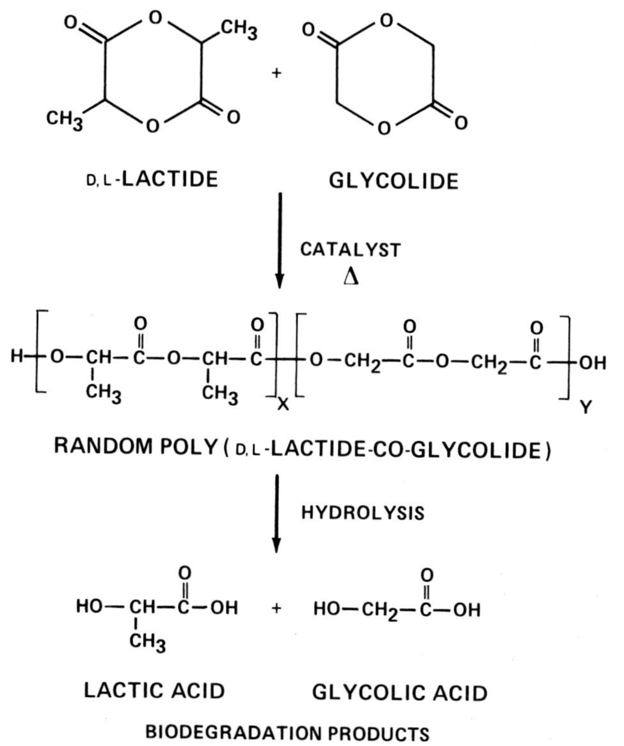

Figure 3 Synthesis, structure, and biodegradation products of poly(D,L-lactide-co-glycolide) (DL-PLG). Polymerization of D,L-lactide and glycolide, the respective cyclic dimers of lactic and glycolic acids, into the high molecular weight DL-PLG through ionic, ring opening, addition polymerization. On exposure to water, this aliphatic polyester degrades through hydrolysis of ester linkages to yield the biocompatible products lactic and glycolic acids.

responses without the need for an additional vehicles. In the case of SEB toxoid, mice immunized with 50 μg vaccine in 1- to 10-μm DL-PLG microspheres mounted a neutralizing plasma antitoxin response that was equivalent in level and duration to that induced by the same dose of toxoid emulsified in CFA without a significant inflammatory response (Eldridge *et al.*, 1991b). This antibody level was 512-fold and 64-fold that induced by soluble and alum-precipitated toxoid, respectively. Similar immunopotentiation was obtained in rhesus macaques immunized by the intramuscular injection of microencapsulated SEB toxoid or whole formalin-inactivated SIV (Marx *et al.*, 1993). Direct comparison of the antibody responses elicited by subcutaneous immunization with 1- to 10-μm versus 10- to 110-μm microspheres, formulated from the same lot of DL-PLG and containing the same percentage of SEB toxoid by weight, demonstrated that the 1- to 10-μm microspheres provided approximately 20-fold greater immune enhancement (Eldridge *et al.*, 1991b). This enhanced potentiation by the <10-μm microspheres correlated with the phagocytosis and transportation of a large number of these particles, but not those >10 μm, to the lymph nodes draining the injection site. These data suggest that the efficient delivery of vaccine by the <10-μm microspheres into antigen-presenting cells, which then carry it to an immune inductive environment, is a more effective approach to the enhancement of antibody responses than the depot release of free antigen provided by larger microspheres, and a probable explanation for the poor adjuvancy observed in the studies by Altman and Dixon (1989).

An additional difference in the behavior of <10-μm versus >10-μm microspheres noted in the studies by Eldridge *et al.* (1991b) was an accelerated rate of antigen release by the smaller microspheres after *in vivo* administration, presumably as a result of phagocytosis. This difference formed the basis for the design of a single-injection multiple-release microsphere formulation consisting of a mixture of 1- to 10-μm and 20- to 50-μm microspheres containing SEB toxoid (Eldridge *et al.,* 1991a). Mice injected with this mixture of microspheres mounted a biphasic antitoxin response in which the first phase of antibody increase corresponded to the release of vaccine from the 1- to 10-μm component. The second phase corresponded to the release of vaccine from the 20- to 50-μm microspheres and stimulated an anamnestic secondary rise in antitoxin levels. These results indicate that blends of DL-PLG microspheres differing in their size or lactide-to-glycolide ratio are capable of functioning as adjuvant systems with the ability to provide one or more discrete booster releases of antigen after a single administration.

To evaluate the possibility of using DL-PLG microspheres as vehicles for oral immunization, the adsorption of fluorochrome-containing microspheres was studied in mice (Eldridge *et al.,* 1989,1990a). At various times after oral administration, the gut and other lymphoid tissues were serial frozen sectioned and the microspheres within tissue were observed by fluorescence microscopy. At early time points, tissue penetration in the gut was restricted to the Peyer's patches (Figure 4), only microspheres ≤ 10 μm in diameter were adsorbed, and the adsorbed microspheres were within Peyer's patch macrophages. With increasing time after administration, the number of microspheres in the Peyer's patches fell and they were observed sequentially in the mesenteric lymph nodes and spleen, suggesting that orally delivered microspheres could be capable of delivering vaccine antigens to both mucosal and systemic immune inductive tissues. When mice were given three oral administrations, at 30-day intervals, of SEB toxoid in 1- to 10-μm DL-PLG microspheres, they exhibited a steady rise in their plasma levels of IgG antitoxin and significant levels of SIgA antitoxin in saliva, gut fluids, and bronchial-alveolar fluids 20 days after the third dose (Eldridge *et al.,* 1989,1991a). In contrast, mice orally immunized with nonencapsulated SEB toxoid mounted only a weak IgM response in plasma and none in mucosal secretions. In similar experiments, Moldoveanu *et al.* (1989,1992) have examined the immune response to influenza virus vaccine encapsulated in 1- to 10-μm DL-PLG microspheres. Their studies have shown that systemic immunization with microencapsulated influenza potentiates the plasma hemagglutination inhibition titer, that encapsulation protects influenza vaccine from acid degradation, and that oral boosting with encapsulated vaccine is particularly effective in the induction of salivary IgA anti-influenza antibodies.

To date, the studies with DL-PLG microspheres have served to illustrate the potential of this approach to mucosal immunization with nonliving vaccine antigens. Current studies in this area are being directed toward microsphere adsorption from the gut, a process that is enhanced by increased microsphere hydrophobicity (Eldridge *et al.,* 1990a); alternative routes of mucosal administration such as respiratory tissues (Eldridge *et al.,* 1991a); and multirelease formulations for mucosal immunization.

IV. AVIRULENT *SALMONELLA* STRAINS AS LIVE VECTOR ANTIGEN DELIVERY SYSTEMS

A. Introduction

The concept of using avirulent *Salmonella* mutants as oral vaccine delivery systems began almost a decade ago (Formal *et al.,* 1981; Curtiss *et al.,* 1983; Curtiss, 1986; reviewed by Curtiss, 1990; Hackett, 1990). This idea was based on separate and yet interrelated areas of research. *Salmonella typhi* and *S. typhimurium* are pathogenic bacteria in humans and mice, respectively. Virulent strains of *Salmonella* colonize in the intestine and then migrate to deeper tissues, especially the spleen and liver, which can lead to a bacteremia and subsequent death (Collins and Carter, 1972). The findings of Carter and Collins (1974) demonstrated the initial site of *S. typhimurium* infection is the GALT, which is also a major IgA inductive site. This identification and the ability to attenuate *Salmonella,* in conjunction with the development of genetic techniques to incorporate recombinant DNA into these *Salmonella* mutants, prompted the use of avirulent *Salmonella* strains as potential live vectors for expression of cloned genes specifying colonization or virulence antigens of other pathogens. These antigen delivery systems could be administered orally to induce mucosal IgA responses locally in the intestine and in other secretions, as well as systemic humoral and cellular immune responses.

For the development of an oral *Salmonella* vaccine, several facts must be considered. Oral vaccines consisting of killed *Salmonella* are poor immunogens, whereas the live organism is very effective in inducing mucosal immune responses, presumably because of their ability to colonize in the gastrointestinal tract. However, the systemic dissemination of *Salmonella* organisms can result in death as a result of the effects of the endotoxin load. Therefore, a live vaccine strain must be completely avirulent to the host and yet highly immunogenic for the induction of the desired immune responses. For safety of the vaccine strain, it should have two or more attenuating deletion mutations to preclude loss of the avirulence phenotype by reversion or gene transfer. The vaccine vector–carrier strain should be effective in expressing, in the animal host, cloned genes encoding virulence factors of other pathogens at adequate levels and in appropriate form for the induction of immune responses that render the host protected against infection and disease.

The following sections discuss characteristics of several avirulent *Salmonella* mutants and the effectiveness of recombinant avirulent *Salmonella* strains as bivalent vaccine delivery systems for the induction of immune responses protective against various pathogens. The reader is referred to a review

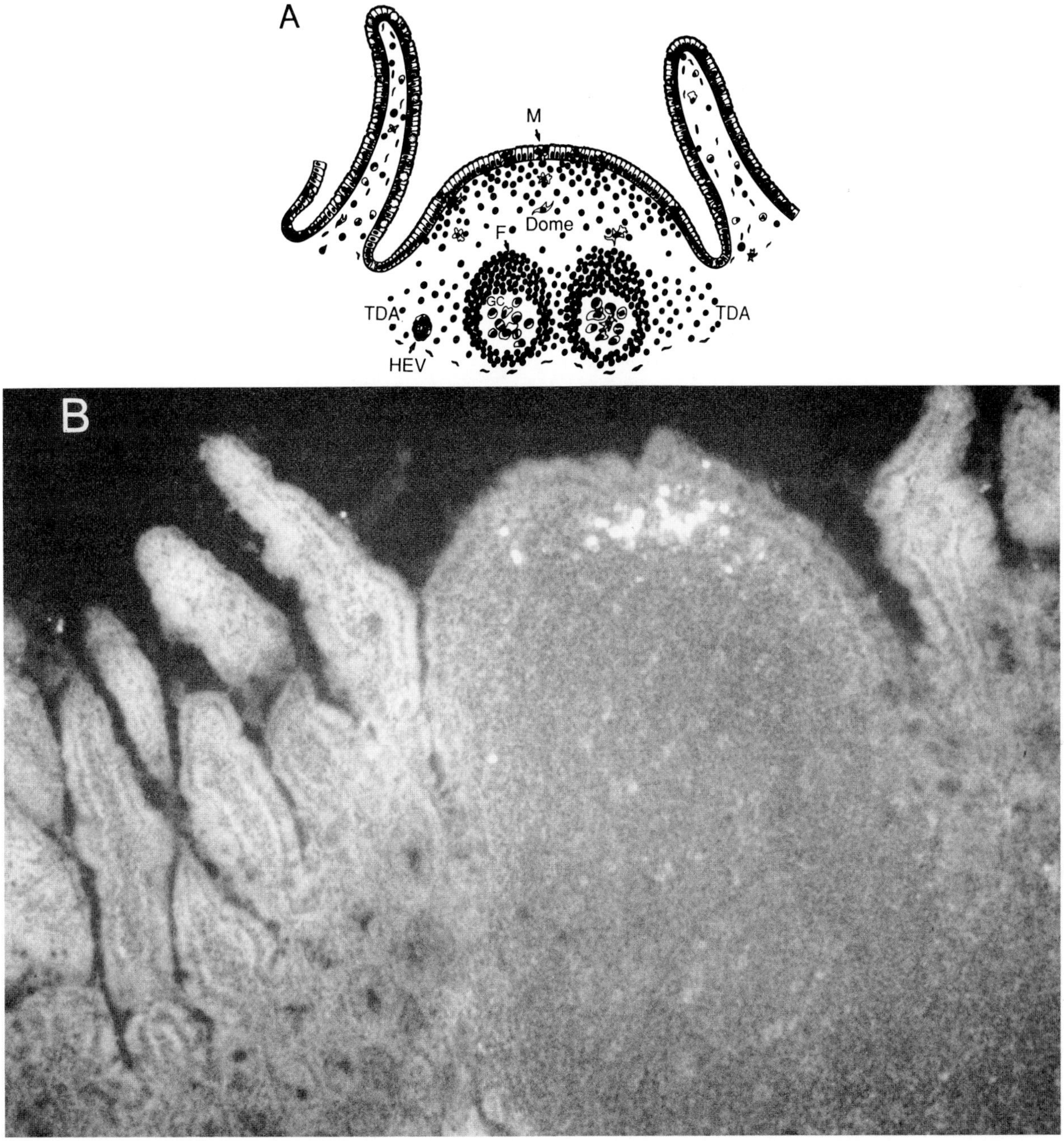

Figure 4 Adsorption of coumarin-containing DL-PLG microspheres into the Peyer's patches. (A) Schematic showing the cellular organization of a Peyer's patch. M, M cell; F, follicle; GC, germinal center; TDA, T cell-dependent area; HEV, high endothelial venule; dome, macrophage-containing dome region. (B) Coumarin-containing DL-PLG microspheres visualized by fluorescene microscopy in the M cells and dome region macrophages in a 6-μm frozen section of duodenum obtained from a mouse 24 hr after oral administration of a suspension of 1- to 10-μm microspheres in water.

by Curtiss (1990) for a more comprehensive coverage of this area.

B. Avirulent Salmonella *Mutants*

Several avirulent mutants of the human pathogen *S. typhi* and of the murine pathogens *S. typhimurium* and *S. cholerae-suis* have been derived and characterized for their potential usefulness as vaccine delivery systems (Table IV). The *galE* mutants of *Salmonella* are unable to synthesize the enzyme UDP-galactose epimerase. These mutants are defective in lipopolysaccharide (LPS) biosynthesis (rough) when grown in the absence of galactose, but synthesize a complete LPS (smooth) when grown in the presence of galactose. *Salmonella typhimurium galE* mutants are avirulent and retain their

Table IV Characteristics of Selected Avirulent *Salmonella* Mutants[a]

		Colonizes		Attenuates/Immunogenic		
Mutation	Phenotype	Guy	Spleen	*S. typhimurium*	*S. choleraesuis*	*S. typhi*
galE	UDP-galactose epimerase; reversibly rough	?	?	Y/Y	N/N	N/?
Δ*aro*	Requires *p*-aminobenzoic acid	Y	Fair	Y/Y	Y/±	±/±
Δ*cya*	Adenylate cyclase;					
Δ*crp*	cAMP receptor protein; slow growth	Y	Poor	Y/Y	Y/Y	±/±
ˇPla⁻	No virulence plasmid	Y	Poor	±/Y	?/?	NA
Δ*cdt*	Defective in colonizing deep tissues	Y	Poor	Y/Y	Y/Y	Y/±[b]
Δ*phoP*	Macrophage sensitive	Poor	No	Y/Y	?/?	?/?
phoP[c]	Constitutive expression of some virulence antigens	?	?	±/Y	?/?	?/?
ompR	Positive activator of outer membrane protein genes	Y	Y	Y/Y	?/?	?/?

[a] ?, Unknown; Y, yes; N, no; ±, partial effect; NA, not applicable.
[b] When combined with Δcya and Δcrp mutations.

immunogenicity, as exemplified by their ability to induce responses protective against challenge with virulent *Salmonella* strains (Germanier, 1972; Germanier and Furer, 1971; Hone *et al.*, 1987). However, the *S. typhi* Ty21 a *galE* vaccine strain (Germanier and Furer, 1975) is undoubtedly avirulent and immunogenic because of mutations in addition to *gal E,* since *S. typhi galE* generated by recombinant methods causes typhoid fever in human volunteers (Hone *et al.*, 1988). Also the *galE* mutants of *S. choleraesuis* are virulent, probably because of their requirement for only low amounts of galactose for complete LPS synthesis (Nnalue and Stocker, 1986). Little information is available regarding the ability of *galE* mutants to colonize the gut or deeper tissues such as the spleen.

The Δ*aroA* mutants of *S. typhimurium* (Hoiseth and Stocker, 1981) are avirulent primarily because of their requirement for *p*-aminobenzoic acid (PABA) which is not provided by the animal host. These mutants can colonize the gut and the spleen, and have been shown to be immunogenic. A Δ*aroA* mutation also has been shown to be attenuating for *S. choleraesuis* in mice (Nnalue and Stocker, 1987). The addition of the Δ*purE* mutation to a Δ*aroA S. typhi* strain leads to hyperattenuation with very low immunogenicity (Levine *et al.*, 1987). *Salmonella typhi* strains with Δ*aroC* and Δ*aroD* mutations are avirulent and immunogenic in humans, but nevertheless are capable of causing fever and adverse reactions when given at high doses (Tacket *et al.*, 1992).

During the past several years, mutants defective in global gene regulation have been evaluated for influencing colonization and virulence (reviewed by Curtiss, 1990), leading to the discovery that Δ*cya* Δ*crp S. typhimurium* mutants unable to synthesize cyclic AMP (cAMP) and the cAMP receptor protein (CRP) (Pastan and Adhya, 1976) are highly attenuated for infection in mice and induce a protective response against challenge with a virulent strain when fed orally to mice (Curtiss and Kelly, 1987; Curtiss *et al.*, 1988). These mutants grow slowly *in vitro* and *in vivo,* which may contribute to their attenuation. A Δ*cya* Δ*crp S. typhi* mutant is both avirulent and immunogenic in human volunteers (Tacket *et al.*, 1992) but, unlike the Δ*aroC* Δ*aroD S. typhi* strains, causes symptoms in some volunteers and is not as immunogenic at the dose given as would be desirable (Tacket *et al.*, 1992). An additional mutation that diminishes the ability of *Salmonella* to colonize deep tissues (*cdt*) completely eliminates any adverse reactions without diminishing immunogenicity S. M. Kelly and R. Curtiss III, unpublished observations).

Salmonella typhimurium phoP mutants, prepared to eliminate nonspecific acid phosphatases in strains to use for transposon Tn*phoA* mutagenesis, are avirulent when administered to mice by oral or intraperitoneal routes (Galan and Curtiss, 1989), which may be the result of an inability to multiply in macrophages (Fields *et al.*, 1986). These mutants can induce an immune response that is protective against challenge by virulent *Salmonella* (Galan and Curtiss, 1989). Mutants that constitutively express the *phoP* gene lead to the complete activation of some *Salmonella* genes and the complete shut down of others (Miller and Mekalanos, 1990). These *phoP*^{C} mutants are totally avirulent and highly immunogenic for mice; however, these mutants revert at high frequency to a form that is virulent (Miller and Mekalanos, 1990).

Dorman *et al.* (1989) have demonstrated that *S. typhimurium* mutants with mutations in the *ompR* gene are avirulent and highly immunogenic. The *ompR* gene product is part of a two-component regulatory system that affects the regulation of genes for a number of outer membrane proteins (*ompC* and *ompF*), as well as influencing expression of other genes whose expression is dependent on changes in osmolarity.

C. *Bivalent* Salmonella *Vaccine Strains*

Several attenuated *Salmonella* mutant strains have been shown to be effective as live antigen delivery systems for potential vaccine development (Table V). These mutants can be detected in GALT following oral administration to the

Table V Recombinant Avirulent *Salmonella:* Selected Immunization Studies

Salmonella mutant	Foreign antigen expressed	Major finding	References
S. typhimurium Δ*aroA*	*Streptococcus pyogenes* M protein (cytoplasmic)	Induction of salivary and serum antibodies in mice; protected against challenge by virulent *S. typhimurium* or M5 streptococci	Poirier *et al.* (1988)
	E. coli K88 fimbrial antigen (surface)	Induction of serum anti-K88 antibodies	Dougan *et al.* (1986)
	B subunit of *E. coli* enterotoxin	Induction of secretory (gut) and serum antibody	Dougan *et al.* (1987); Maskell *et al.* (1987)
	Leishmania major gp63 antigen	Induction of serum antibodies and antigen -specific Th1 cells in mice; protected against challenge with *L. major*	Yang *et al.* (1990)
S. typhimurium Δ*thyA* Δ*asd* and Δ*aroA*	*Streptococcus sobrinus* SpaA and, *Streptococcus mutans* glucosyltransferase	Induction of salivary and serum antibodies	Katz *et al.* (1987)
S. typhimurium Δ*cya* Δ*crp* Δ*asd*	*Streptococcus sobrinus* SpaA (cytoplasmic)	Induction of salivary and serum antibody responses	T. Doggett (personal communication)
	Francisella tularensis 17-kDa membrane protein	Protection against *F. tularensis* challenge	Sjostedt *et al.* (1990)
	Bordetella pertussis FHA	Serum antibody responses	Parker *et al.* (1990)
S. typhi Ty21a *galE*	*Shigella flexneri* 2a O antigen	Induction of humoral response	Baron *et al.* (1987)
	Shigella sonnei form 1 antigen	Induction of serum antibodies in humans; protected against challenge with virulent *S. sonnei*	Black *et al.* (1987)

host, but do not cause systemic disease. In several of these studies, mucosal immune responses as well as serum antibody and cell-mediated immune responses have been induced that were specific for the *Salmonella* and the foreign antigen(s) expressed by the carrier strain. However, several questions remain unanswered regarding the usefulness of this antigen delivery system in animals, including humans. Whether the amount, form, or location (e.g., cytoplasmic, periplasmic, or surface) of the heterologous virulence antigen(s) expressed by the *Salmonella* vector will influence the nature or magnitude of the immune response is still unknown. The mutation(s) induced to render the *Salmonella* safe for vaccine use may limit the expression of the cloned virulence antigen or the ability of the expressed antigen to induce a protective immune response. Further information is needed on the nature of the antigen and the use of adjuvants in these delivery systems for optimal immunization. In this regard, through immunological and molecular biological techniques, we can define T- and B-cell epitopes of the antigen involved in the induction of mucosal responses and can incorporate the gene encoding these regions into the *Salmonella* vector. Also, genetic fusion of the gene encoding the antigen to the gene encoding the B subunit of cholera toxin or *Escherichic coli* enterotoxin may result in an enhanced specific immune response (adjuvant effect). Further studies will be required to define the feasibility, safety, and effectiveness of these approaches in inducing the desired host response. Also determining whether *Salmonella* vaccine strains can induce tolerance or suppress the induction of a response based on host susceptibility to components of the vector, such as LPS, or to the expressed cloned antigen(s) will be important. The effect of the host immune response to the *Salmonella* vector and the expressed cloned antigen on subsequent immunizations with *Salmonella* and the same or different expressed cloned antigens or adjuvants will require further investigation to define strategies for developing live vaccine delivery systems for optimal induction of protective host responses to microbial pathogens.

V. USE OF RECOMBINANT VIRAL VECTORS FOR MUCOSAL IMMUNIZATION

A. Introduction

Advances in molecular biology and the development of genetic engineering techniques allow the insertion of genes encoding immunologically important antigens into viruses. Such recombinant viral vectors should function as live subunit vaccines and should share the advantages of live attenuated viral vaccines without the possibility of reversion. Recombinant viral vaccines have the advantage of being inexpensive to produce and deliver and have the important property of being able to induce high levels of humoral and cell-mediated immunity. Indeed, inserted viral gene products will be synthesized endogenously and processed in cells infected with a live recombinant vector, thus resulting in antigen presentation to T cells in the same fashion as natural infection. An ideal virus vector should readily admit insertion of foreign DNA sequences, be nonpathogenic, and be capable of eliciting protective immunity to foreign antigens or pathogens in the host. Viral vectors that have been well studied include vaccinia virus (Mackett *et al.*, 1982) and adenovirus (Graham, 1990). Vaccinia virus vectors capable of expressing as many as four distinct antigens at the same time have been constructed (Moss and Flexner, 1987), including information encoding antigens from pathogenic organisms as well as immunomodulatory molecuels such as cytokines (Ramshaw *et al.*, 1987). The tremendous potential of vaccinia virus as a single-inoculation multivalent vaccine is attractive. Although limited in the amount of foreign genetic information that can be inserted, adenoviruses have the same advantages and can be used as oral vaccines (Graham, 1990).

The study and application of live recombinant viral vectors as mucosal vaccines is in its infancy. Indeed, although many studies have been performed that test the efficacy of recombinant viral vaccines to protect animals after mucosal immunization, these studies have not critically examined the induction of mucosal immune responses or the mechanisms of protection (Ogra *et al.*, 1989).

Our intention here is not to comprehensively list all studies that have examined the use of recombinant viruses after mucosal vaccination. Rather, we highlight some of the systems that are providing the major impetus for further investigations concerning the use of recombinant viruses in eliciting mucosal immunity.

B. Recombinant Rabies Virus Vectors: Bait to Prevent the Bite

Rabies remains a major public health problem in many parts of the world, including Europe and North America, where infected wild animals constitute a significant reservoir for the virus. Experience has shown that control of rabies in wildlife cannot be achieved by reducing the reservoir species through hunting, poisoning or gassing. Instead, immunization of wild reservoir animals offers an alternative approach (Steck *et al.*, 1982). Clearly, the only realistic route for the vaccination of large numbers of wild animals is oral administration of vaccine, which was first attempted by Baer *et al.* (1971) in North America and by Mayr *et al.* (1972) in Europe. Oral vaccination is achieved by placing vaccine in sponge baits that are coated with wax containing beef tallow or fish oil and tetracycline as a biomarker. The tetracycline allows identification of animals that have ingested the bait by fluorescence of their teeth. Using this method, acceptance rates of bait ingestion of about 70% have been achieved in a number of wild animal populations (Johnston *et al.*, 1988). In small-scale field trials, live attenuated rabies virus vaccine introduced in baits was used successfully to vaccinate foxes in Europe (Steck *et al.*, 1982; Schneider and Cox, 1983; Pastoret *et al.*, 1987; Brochier *et al.*, 1988). Unfortunately, other mammalian species such as the skunk and raccoon, which are major rabies virus vectors in North America, have been refractory to efficient oral immunization against rabies (Rupprecht *et al.*, 1986). Additionally, the stability of attenuated rabies virus is poor, attenuated virus remains pathogenic to some rodents, and reversion to virulence occurs at a significant frequency (Kieny *et al.*, 1988). Finally, inactivated rabies virus has been shown to be ineffective when administered orally (Kieny *et al.*, 1988).

To improve the safety, stability, and efficacy of the vaccine used in the field, several recombinant viruses containing the rabies virus glycoprotein gene have been constructed (Kieny *et al.*, 1984). Initial studies demonstrated that intradermal or footpad inoculation of rabbits and mice with a vaccinia–rabies glycoprotein (VRG) recombinant virus resulted in high concentrations of rabies virus neutralizing antibodies (Wiktor *et al.*, 1984). Subsequently, administration of 10^8 plaque-forming units (pfu) of VRG subcutaneously, intradermally, or orally to foxes was shown to elicit the production of titers of rabies neutralizing antibodies equal or superior to those obtained with conventional vaccine, and was shown to confer complete protection to severe intracerebral challenge with street rabies virus (Blancou *et al.*, 1986). More recently, virus isolation, immunofluorescence, and polymerase chain reaction (PCR) were used to show that VRG could be detected in the buccal mucosa and tonsils of foxes for only 48 hr following oral immunization (Thomas *et al.*, 1990), thus minimizing the risk of additional spread or recombination with other orthopoxviruses.

Rupprecht *et al.* (1986,1988) demonstrated that raccoons, a major rabies virus vector in North America, fed bait containing VRG developed rabies neutralizing antibodies and resisted street rabies virus infection for up to 6 months after feeding. This observation was important, since live attenuated rabies vaccine administered orally failed to immunize raccoons. This study also demonstrated that a minimum virus-neutralizing antibody titer may not be applicable as an indication of adequate animal vaccination. Clearly, virus-neutralizing antibody alone is unsuitable as the sole criterion of successful rabies immunization in all species. Further studies have shown that cats, dogs, skunks, and badgers also can be immunized effectively against rabies with VRG by the oral route (Tolson *et al.*, 1987; Koprowski, 1989). However, higher doses of VRG ($10^{9.6}$ pfu) appeared to be required to generate antibodies in dogs and badgers (Koprowski, 1989).

In addition to recombinant vaccinia virus, other recombinant vectors capable of expressing rabies glycoprotein have been developed, including recombinant human adenovirus type 5 (Prevec *et al.*, 1990) and raccoon poxvirus vectors (Esposito *et al.*, 1988). Recombinant adeno–rabies virus has been shown to elicit neutralizing antibodies and protection against rabies virus challenge following oronasal immunization in mice, dogs, skunks, foxes, and raccoons (Prevec *et al.*, 1990). Similarly, raccoons fed sponge baits loaded with raccoon poxvirus recombinants expressing rabies glycoprotein developed high levels of neutralizing antibodies and were protected from lethal street rabies virus challenge (Esposito *et al.*, 1988). Thus, a vast number of species have been shown to be immunized effectively and protected against rabies following oral administration of live recombinant viral vaccines.

C. Recombinant Adenovirus Vaccines: A Natural Mucosal Immunogen

The use of vaccinia virus vectors is well advanced and their efficacy as recombinant vaccines has been demonstrated in numerous systems. Nevertheless, problems of toxicity may limit their acceptance for widespread use. Further, distinct viral vectors may be required for different pathogens and multiple vectors may be necessary to boost immunized individuals. The approach that we are investigating involves the use of recombinant human adenoviruses as potential vaccines. We have focused on the use of human adenovirus type 5 (Ad5). Ad5 is a nononcogenic virus that causes mild respiratory illness in humans (Rubin and Rorke, 1988). Human adenoviruses have been well characterized both genetically and biochemically, and methods to construct recombinant vectors are well established (Graham and Prevec, 1990). One advantage to adenoviruses as vaccines is the fact that they may be administered orally, a vaccination route that may be critical in generating immunity to viruses that are transmitted mucosally (Couch *et al.*, 1963). Indeed, a single oral administration of live adenovirus type 4 and 7 vaccine in enteric-coated capsules was shown to be safe and effective in suppressing adenovirus-induced acute respiratory disease in millions of United States military recruits without evidence of adverse reactions (Top *et al.*, 1971a,b). From these studies we conclude a benign gut infection with adenovirus types 4 and 7 induced neutralizing antibodies and protection of the lungs from infection with these viruses, thus supporting the concept of the common mucosal immune system (McDermott and Bienenstock, 1979). These results suggest that oral immunization with adenovirus recombinants may induce mucosal immunity at distant mucosal sites such as the respiratory and genital tracts.

Respiratory syncytial virus (RSV) is one of the leading causes of pediatric viral respiratory tract disease worldwide (McIntosh and Chanock, 1985; Murphy *et al.*, 1988). Conventional approaches to RSV vaccine development have not been successful. For example, developing attenuated RSV strains for vaccination has not been possible and parenteral administration of formalin-inactivated RSV was associated paradoxically with enhanced disease after subsequent natural infection. Therefore, live recombinant vaccinia and adenoviruses that express the glycoproteins of RSV were constructed. After intranasal inoculation of mice, vaccinia recombinants expressing the G protein of RSV generated antibody against RSV and protection against intranasal challenge (Stott *et al.*, 1986). Intranasal administration to cotton rats of Ad5 recombinants capable of expressing RSV F glycoprotein (Ad5-F) was shown to be three- to fourfold more immunogenic than Ad5-F administered intraduodenally (Collins *et al.*, 1990). Interestingly, although administration of Ad5-F by either route did not induce detectable levels of RSV neutralizing antibodies, intranasal administration provided complete protection, whereas immunization by the intraduodental route conferred incomplete but significant resistance. Additional studies (Hsu *et al.*, 1991) demonstrated that recombinant adenovirus types 4 and 7 of RSV F glycoprotein protected dogs from challenge after intratracheal inoculation. Ferrets immunized intranasally with these vectors also showed an 80–100% reduction in challenge virus titer, despite the fact that neutralizing antibodies to RSV were not detected (Hsu *et al.*, 1991).

After intranasal administration, recombinant adenovirus capable of expressing vesicular stomatitis virus (VSV) glycoprotein was shown to immunize and protect a number of animal species, including mice, dogs, calves, and piglets, from challenge with wild-type rhabdovirus (Prevec *et al.*, 1989). Moreover, oral hepatitis B virus (HBV) vaccines based on live recombinant adenovirus types 4 and 7 have been developed and shown to protect hamsters (Morin *et al.*, 1987) and chimpanzees (Lubeck *et al.*, 1989) from acute clinical disease following HBV challenge.

Most of the studies concerning mucosal vaccination with recombinant viral vectors have focused on the generation of serum neutralizing antibodies and protection against challenge. Few studies have focused on the generation of mucosal IgA or on the generation of antiviral cytotoxic T lymphocytes (CTLs) after mucosal vaccination. McDermott *et al.* (1989b) have shown that recombinant adenovirus containing the glycoprotein B gene of herpes simplex virus (HSV) was able to protect mice from a lethal challenge with HSV-2. This protection appeared to be primarily T-cell mediated (McDermott *et al.*, 1989a). We used the same vector (AdHSVgB) to demonstrate that intranasal inoculation primed mice for the generation of anti-HSV CTLs. This anti-HSV CTL activity was detected in both the spleens and local lymph nodes of recombinant adenovirus-immunized mice (Gallichan *et al.*, in press). Thus, we have shown that mucosal vaccination with a recombinant adenovirus vector primes mice for both a systemic and local T cell-mediated immune response. The stability of adenoviruses, as well as their ease of propagation and administration, holds promise that they may be highly suitable for widespread vaccination programs against mucosal infections.

D. AIDS and STDs: The Challenge of Mucosal Immunity

The World Health Organization has estimated that 80% of human immunodeficiency virus (HIV) transmission worldwide is heterosexual. Heterosexual transmission is becoming increasingly important in developed countries as the epidemic progresses (Forrest, 1991). Most of the efforts on candidate HIV vaccines have concentrated on the systemic route of vaccination. However, since systemic and mucosal immune systems are compartmentalized, parenterally administered vaccines do not consistently induce mucosal immunity and are poorly effective against mucosal pathogens. This conclusion was confirmed by the observation that rhesus macaque monkeys immunized with whole inactivated SIV vaccines, which provide protection against low-dose intravenous challenge with cell-free SIV, did not protect against low-dose intravaginal challenge (Sutjipto *et al.*, 1990).

These results suggest that oral or locally administered vaccines may be necessary to induce effective immunity against these sexually transmitted viruses, perhaps because of the common mucosal immune system that permits the generation of immune responses to mucosally presented antigens at distant mucosal surfaces (McDermott and Bienenstock, 1979). Initial studies have shown no signficant mucosal antibody response in gastrointestinal, salivary, or genital secretions of rhesus monkeys given microencapsulated inactivated whole SIV orally (Miller and Gardner, 1991). Interestingly, however, mice inoculated intravaginally with live virulence-attenuated HSV generated intravaginal anti-HSV IgA and CTLs and were protected against intravaginal challenge with wild-type HSV-2 (McDermott *et al.,* 1984). These studies suggest that live virus vectors that infect and replicate within the mucosa, particularly the genital mucosa, may induce strong local immune responses.

Clearly, the ability of recombinant viral vaccines able to express SIV and HIV gene products after mucosal immunization should be evaluated to determine whether genital mucosal immunity and protection against genital mucosal infection can be elicited (Miller and Gardner, 1991). In particular, examination of adenovirus recombinants, which are known to induce strong mucosal protective immunity in the lung after oral administration, or recombinants of HSV should be examined. Recombinant adeno–HIV (Prevec *et al.,* 1991) and adeno–SIV have been produced. We demonstrated that adeno–HIV was able to induce a humoral immune response to HIV core proteins in mice and rhesus macaque monkeys (Prevec *et al.,* 1991). We intend to utilize adeno–SIV recombinants in studies concerning the generation of mucosal immunity and protection from mucosal SIV challenge. The urgency of our need for a vaccine against AIDS should serve as a major impetus for studies concerning the use of live recombinant viral vectors to generate mucosal immunity.

Acknowledgments

The studies on liposome, biodegradable microspheres, and *Salmonella* vaccine delivery systems were supported in part by U.S. Public Health Service Grants DE 08182, DE 09081, DE 08228, DE 00232, AI 28147, DE 06669, and DE 04217 from the National Institutes of Health and Contract DAMD17-86-6162 from the U.S. Army Medical Research Acquisition Activity. The authors thank Noel Childers and Jenny Katz for their critical assessment of this review and Vickie Barron and Amie Stoppelbein for secretarial support.

References

Altman, A., and Dixon, F. (1989). Immunomodifiers in vaccines. *Adv. Vet. Sci. Comp. Med.* **33,** 301–343.

Alving, C. R. (1991). Liposomes as carriers of antigens and adjuvants. *J. Immunol. Meth.* **140,** 1–13.

Artursson, P., Martensson, I.-L., and Sjoholm, I. (1986). Biodegradable microspheres III: Some immunological properties of polyacryl starch microparticles. *J. Pharmaceut. Sci.* **75,** 697–701.

Baer, G. M., Abelseth, M. K., and Debbie, J. G. (1971). Oral vaccination of foxes against rabies. *Am. J. Epidemiol.* **93,** 487–490.

Bangham, A. D., Standish, M. M., and Watkins, J. C. (1965). Diffusion of univalent ions across the lamellae of swollen phospholipids. *J. Mol. Biol.* **13,** 238–252.

Bangham, A. D., Hill, M. W., and Miller, N. G. A. (1974). Preparation and use of liposomes as models of biological membranes. *In* "Methods in Membrane Biology" (E. D. Korn, ed.), pp. 1–68. Plenum Press, New York.

Baron, L. S., Kopecko, D. J., Formal, S. B., Seid, R., Guerry, P., and Powell, C. (1987). Introduction of *Shigella flexneri* 2a type and group antigen genes into oral typhoid vaccine strain *Salmonella typhi* Ty21a. *Infect. Immun.* **55,** 2797–2801.

Black, R. E., Levine, M. M., Clements, M. L., Losonsky, G., Herrington, D., Berman, S., and Formal, S. B. (1987). Prevention of shigellosis by a *Salmonella typhi–Shigella sonnei* bivalent vaccine. *J. Infect. Dis.* **155,** 1260–1265.

Blancou, J., Kieny, M. P., Lathe, R., Lecocq, J. P., Pastoret, P. P., Soulebot, J. P., and Desmettre, P. (1986). Oral vaccination of the fox against rabies using a live recombinant vaccinia virus. *Nature (London)* **322,** 373–375.

Bland, P. W., and Warren, L. G. (1986). Antigen presentation by epithelial cells of the rat small intestine. *Immunology* **58,** 9–14.

Brochier, B. M., Thomas, I., Ioken, A., Ginter, A., Kalpers, J., Paquot, A., Lostly, F., and Pastoret, P.-P. (1988). A field trial in Belgium to control for fox rabies by oral immunization. *Vet. Rec.* **123,** 618–621.

Brynestad, K., Babbitt, B., Huang, L., and Rouse, B. T. (1990). Influence of peptide acylation, liposome incorporation, and synthetic immunomodulators on the immunogenicity of a 1-23 peptide of glycoprotein D of Herpes Simplex Virus: Implications for subunit vaccines. *J. Virol.* **64,** 680–685.

Carter, P. B., and Collins, F. M. (1974). The route of enteric infection in normal mice. *J. Exp. Med.* **139,** 1189–1203.

Childers, N. K., Michalek, S. M., Eldridge, J. H., Denys, F. R., Berry, A. K., and McGhee, J. R. (1989). Characterization of liposomes suspensions by flow cytometry. *J. Immunol. Meth.* **119,** 135–143.

Childers, N. K., Denys, F. R., McGee, N. F., and Michalek, S. M. (1990). Ultrastructural study of liposome uptake by M cells of rat Peyer's patch: An oral vaccine system for delivery of purified antigen. *Reg. Immunol.* **3,** 8–16.

Childers, N. K., Michalek, S. M., Pritchard, D. G., and McGhee, J. R. (1991). Mucosal and systemic responses to an oral liposome–*Streptococcus mutans* carbohydrate vaccine in humans. *Reg. Immunol.* **3,** 289–296.

Collins, F. M., and Carter, P. B. (1972). Comparative immunogenicity of heat-killed and living oral *Salmonella* vaccines. *Infect. Immun.* **6,** 451–458.

Collins, P. L., Prince, G. A., Camargo, E., Purcell, R. H., Chancock, R. M., Murphy, B. R., Davis, A. R., Lubeck, M. D., Mizutani, S., and Hung, P. P. (1990). Evaluation of the protective efficacy of recombinant vaccinia viruses and adenoviruses that express respiratory syncytial virus glycoproteins. *In* "Vaccines '90" (F. Brown, R. M. Chanock, H. S. Ginsberg, and R. A. Lerner, eds.), pp. 79–84. Cold Spring Harbor Laboratory Press, Cold Spring Harbor, New York.

Cornell, B. A., Fletcher, G. C., Middleburst, J., and Separovic, F. (1982). The lower limits to the size of small sonicated vesicles. *Biochim. Biophys. Acta* **690,** 15–19.

Couch, R. B., Chanock, R. M., Cate, T. R., Lang, D. J., Knight, V., and Huebner, R. J. (1963). Immunization with types 4 and 7 adenovirus by selective infection of the intestinal tract. *Am. Rev. Respir. Dis.* **88,** 394–403.

Cox, D. S., and Taubman, M. A. (1984). Oral induction of the secretory antibody response by soluble and particulate antigens. *Int. Arch. Appl. Immunol.* **75,** 126–131.

Curtiss, R., III (1986). Genetic analysis of *Streptococcus mutans* virulence and prospects for an anticaries vaccine. *J. Dent. Res.* **65,** 1034–1045.

Curtiss, R., III (1990). Attenuated *Salmonella* strains as live vectors for the expression of foreign antigens. *In* "New Generation Vaccines" (G. C. Woodrow and M. M. Levine, eds.), pp. 161–188. Marcel Dekker, New York.

Curtiss, R., III, and Kelly, S. M. (1987). *Salmonella typhimurium* deletion mutations lacking adenylate cyclase and cyclic AMP receptor protein are avirulent and immunogenic. *Infect. Immun.* **55,** 3035–3043.

Curtiss, R., III, Holt, R. G., Barletta, R., Robeson, J. P., and Saito, S. (1983). *Escherichia coli* strains producing *Streptococcus mutans* proteins responsible for colonization and virulence. *Ann. N.Y. Acad. Sci.* **409,** 688–695.

Curtiss, R., III, Goldschmidt, R. M., Fletchall, N. B., and Kelly, S. M. (1988). Avirulent *Salmonella typhimurium* Δ*cya* Δ*crp* oral vaccine strains expressing a streptococcal colonization and virulence antigen. *Vaccine* **6,** 155–160.

Dorman, C., Chatfield, S., Higgins, C., Hayward, C., and Dougan, G. (1989). Characterization of porin and *ompR* mutants of a virulent strain of *Salmonella typhimurium: ompR* mutants are attenuated in vivo. *Infect. Immun.* **57,** 2136–2140.

Dougan, G., Sellwood, R., Maskell, D., Sweeney, K., Liew, F. Y., Beesley, J., and Hormaeche, C. (1986). *In vivo* properties of a cloned K88 adherence antigen determinant. *Infect. Immun.* **52,** 344–347.

Dougan, G., Hormaeche, C. E., and Maskell, D. J. (1987). Live oral *Salmonella* vaccines: Potential use of attenuated strains as carriers of heterologous antigens to the immune system. *Parasite Immunol.* **9,** 151–160.

Eldridge, J. H., Gilley, R. M., Staas, J. K., Moldoveanu, Z., Meulbroek, J. A., and Tice, T. R. (1989). Biodegradable microspheres: vaccine delivery system for oral immunization. *Curr. Top. Microbiol. Immunol.* **146,** 59–66.

Eldridge, J. H., Hammond, C. J., Meulbroek, J. A., Staas, J. K., Gilley, R. M., and Tice, T. R. (1990a). Controlled vaccine release in the gut-associated lymphoid tissues. I. Orally administered biodegradable microspheres target the peyer's patches. *J. Controlled Release* **11,** 205–214.

Eldridge, J. H., Staas, J. K., Meulbroek, J. A., McGhee, J. R., Tice, T. R., and Gilley, R. M. (1990b). Disseminated mucosal antitoxin antibody responses induced through oral or intratracheal immunization with toxoid containing biodegradable microspheres. *In* "Advances in Mucosal Immunology" (T. T. MacDonald, S. J. Challacombe, D. W. Bland, C. R. Stokes, R. V. Heatley, and A. McL. Mowat, ed.), pp. 375–378. Kluwer Academic Publishers, London.

Eldridge, J. H., Staas, J. K., Meulbroek, J. A., McGhee, J. R., Tice, T. R., and Gilley, R. M. (1991a). Biodegradable microspheres as a vaccine delivery system. *Mol. Immunol.* **28,** 287–294.

Eldridge, J. H., Staas, J. K., Meulbroek, J. A., McGhee, J. R., Tice, T. R., and Gilley, R. M. (1991b). Biodegradable and biocompatible poly(DL-lactide-co-glycolide) microspheres as an adjuvant for staphylococcal enterotoxin B toxoid which enhance the level of toxin-neutralizing antibodies. *Infect. Immun.* **59,** 2978–2985.

Esposito, J. J., Knight, J. C., Shaddock, J. H., November, F. J., and Baer, G. M. (1988). Successful oral rabies vaccination of raccoons with raccoon poxvirus recombinants expressing rabies virus glycoprotein. *Virology* **165,** 313–316.

Felgner, P. L., Gadek, T. R., Holm, M., Roman, R., Chan, H. W., Wenz, M., Northrop, J. P., Ringold, G. M., and Danielsen, M. (1987). Lipofection: A highly efficient, lipid-mediated DNA-transfection procedure. *Proc. Natl. Acad. Sci. U.S.A.* **84,** 7413–7417.

Fields, P. I., Swanson, R. V., Haidaris, C. G., and Heffron, F. (1986). Mutants of *Salmonella typhimurium* that cannot survive within the macrophage are avirulent. *Proc. Natl. Acad. Sci. U.S.A.* **83,** 5189–5193.

Formal, S. B., Baron, L. S., Kopecko, D. J., Powell, C., and Life, C. A. (1981). Construction of a potential bivalent vaccine strain: introduction of *S. sonnei* form I antigen genes into the *galE Salmonella typhi* Ty21a typhoid vaccine strain. *Infect. Immun.* **34,** 746–750.

Forrest, B. D. (1991). Women, HIV, and mucosal immunity. *Lancet* **337,** 835–836.

Galan, J., and Curtiss, R. (1989). Virulence and vaccine potential of *phoP* mutants of *Salmonella typhimurium. Microb. Pathogen.* **6,** 433–443.

Gallichan, W. S., Johnson, D. C., Graham, F. L., and Rosenthal, K. L. (1993). Mucosal immunity and protection following intranasal immunization with recombinant adenovirus expressing herpes simplex virus glycoprotein B. *J. Inf. Dis.*, in press.

Germanier, R. (1972). Immunity in experimental salmonellosis. III. Comparative immunization with viable and heat-inactivated cells of *Salmonella typhimurium. Infect. Immun.* **5,** 792–797.

Germanier, R., and Furer, E. (1971). Immunity in experimental salmonellosis. II. Basics for the avirulence and protective capacity of *galE* mutants of *Salmonella typhimurium. Infect. Immun.* **4,** 663–673.

Germanier, R., and Furer, E. (1975). Isolation and characterization of *Gal E* mutant Ty 21A of *Salmonella typhi:* A candidate strain for a live, oral typhoid vaccine. *J. Infect. Dis.* **131,** 553–558.

Graham, F. L. (1990). Adenoviruses as expression vectors and recombinant vaccines. *Trends Biotech.* **8,** 85–87.

Graham, F., and Prevec, L. (1990). Manipulation of adenovirus vectors. *In* "Methods in Molecular Biology" (E. J. Murray and J. M. Walker, eds.), Vol. 7, pp. 1–19. Humana Press, Clifton, New Jersey.

Gregoriadis, G. (1990). Immunological adjuvants: A role for liposomes. *Immunol. Today* **11,** 89–97.

Gregoriadis, G., daSilva, H., and Florence, A. T. (1990). A procedure for the efficient entrapment of drugs in dehydration–rehydration liposomes (DRVs). *Int. J. Pharmaceut.* **65,** 235–242.

Gregory, R. L., Michalek, S. M., Richardson, G., Harmon, C., Hilton, T., and McGhee, J. R. (1986). Characterization of immune response to oral administration to *Streptococcus sobrinus* ribosomal preparation in liposomes. *Infect. Immun.* **54,** 780–786.

Hackett, J. (1990). *Salmonella*-based vaccines. *Vaccine* **8,** 5–11.

Hoiseth, S. K., and Stocker, B.A.D. (1981). Aromatic-dependent *Salmonella typhimurium* are non-virulent and effective as live vaccines. *Nature (London)* **291,** 238–239.

Hone, D., Marona, R., Attridge, S., and Hackett, J. (1987). Construction of defined *galE* mutants of *Salmonella* for use as vaccines. *J. Infect. Dis.* **156,** 167–174.

Hone, D., Attridge, S., Forrest, B., Morona, R., Daniels, D., LaBrooy, J., Bartholomeusz, R., Shearman, D., and Hackett, J. (1988). A *galE via* (vi antigen-negative) mutant of *Salmonella typhi* Ty2 retains virulence in humans. *Infect. Immun.* **56,** 1326–1333.

Hsu, K-H. L., Lubeck, M. D., Davies, A. R., Bhat, R. A., Selling, B. H., Bhat, B. M., Mizutani, S., Hung, P. P., Murphy, B. R., Collins, P. L., and Chanock, R. M. (1991). Immunogenicity and protective efficacy of adenovirus vectored respiratory syncytial virus vaccine. *In* "Vaccines '91" (R. M. Chanock, H. S. Ginsberg, F. Brown, and R. A. Lerner, eds.), pp. 293–297. Cold Spring Harbor Laboratory Press, Cold Spring Harbor, New York.

Jackson, S., Mestecky, J., Childers, N. K., and Michalek, S. M. (1990). Liposomes containing anti-idiotypic antibodies: an oral vaccine to induce protective secretory immune responses specific for pathogens of mucosal surfaces. *Infect. Immun.* **58,** 1932–1936.

Johnston, D. H., Voigt, D. R., MacInnes, C. D., Bachmann, P.,

Lawson, K. F., and Rupprecht, C. E. (1988). An aerial baiting system for the distribution of attenuated or recombinant rabies vaccines for foxes, raccoons, and skunks. *Rev. Infect. Dis.* **10,** Suppl. 4, 660–664.

Katz, J., Michalek, S. M., Curtiss, R., III, Harmon, C., Richardson, G., and Mestecky, J. (1987). Novel oral vaccines: The effectiveness of cloned gene products on inducing secretory immune responses. *Rec. Adv. Mucosal Immunol.* **216B,** 1741–1747.

Kieny, M. P., Lathe, R., Drillen, R., Spehner, D., Skory, S., Schmitt, D., Wiktor, T., Koprowski, H., and Lecocq, J.-P. (1984). Expression of rabies virus glycoprotein from a recombinant virus. *Nature (London)* **312,** 163–166.

Kieny, M. P., Blancou, J., Lathe, R., Pastoret, P.-P., Soulebot, J.-P., Desmettre, P., and Lecocq, J.-P. (1988). Development of animal recombinant DNA vaccine and its efficacy in foxes. *Rev. Infect. Dis.* **10,** Suppl. 4, 799–802.

Kirby, C. F., and Gregoriadis, G. (1984). A simple procedure for preparing liposomes capable of high encapsulation efficiency under mild conditions. *In* "CRC Liposomes Technology," (G. Gregoriadis, ed.), Vol. 1, pp. 19–27. CRC Press, Boca Raton, Florida.

Kohn, J., Niemi, S. M., Albert, E. C., Murphy, J. C., Langer, R., and Fox, J. G. (1986). Single-step immunization using a controlled release biodegradable polymer with sustained adjuvant activity. *J. Immunol.* **95,** 31–38.

Koprowski, H. (1989). Rabies oral immunization. *Curr. Top. Microbiol. Immunol.* **146,** 137–151.

Kreuter, J., and Speiser, P. P. (1976). New adjuvants on a polymethylmethacrylate base. *Infect. Immun.* **13,** 204–210.

Kreuter, J., Mauler, R., Gruschkau, H., and Speiser, P. P. (1976). The use of new polymethylmethacrylate adjuvants for split influenza vaccines. *Exp. Cell Biol.* **44,** 12–19.

Kreuter, J., Berg, U., Liehl, E., Soliva, M., and Speiser, P. P. (1986). Influence of particle size on the adjuvant effect of particulate polymeric adjuvants. *Vaccine* **4,** 125–129.

Krueter, J., Liehl, E., Berg, U., Soliva, M., and Speiser, P. P. (1988). Influence of hydrophobicity on the adjuvant effect of particulate polymeric adjuvants. *Vaccine* **6,** 253–256.

Levine, M. M., Herrington, D., Murphy, J., Morris, J., Losonsky, G., Tall, B., Lindberg, A., Svenson, S., Baqar, S., Edwards, M., and Stocker, B. (1987). Safety, infectivity, immunogenicity, and *in vivo* stability of two attenuated auxotrophic mutant strains of *Salmonella typhi,* 541Ty and 543Ty, as live oral vaccines in man. *J. Clin. Invest.* **79,** 888–902.

Litwin, S. D., and Singer, J. M. (1965). The adjuvant action of latex particulate carriers. *J. Immunol.* **95,** 1147–1152.

Lubeck, M. D., Davis, A. R., Chengalvala, M., Natuk, R. J., Morin, J. E., Molnar-Kimber, K., Mason, B. B., Bhat, B. M., Mizutani, S., Hung, P. P., and Purcell, R. H. (1989). Immunogenicity and efficacy testing in chimpanzees of an oral hepatitis B vaccine based on live recombinant adenovirus. *Proc. Natl. Acad. Sci. U.S.A.* **86,** 6763–6767.

McDermott, M. R., and Bienenstock, J. B. (1979). Evidence for a common mucosal immunologic system. I. Migration of B immunoblasts into intestinal, respiratory and genital tissues. *J. Immunol.* **122,** 1892–1898.

McDermott, M. R., Smiley, J. R., Brais, P. L. J., Rudzroga, H. E., and Bienenstock, J. B. (1984). Immunity in the female genital tract after intravaginal vaccination of mice with an attenuated strain of herpes simples virus type 2. *J. Virol.* **51,** 747–753.

McDermott, M. R., Goldsmith, C. A., Rosenthal, K. L., and Brais, P. L. J. (1989a). T lymphocytes in the genital lymph nodes protect mice from intravaginal infection with herpes simplex virus type 2. *J. Infect. Dis.* **159,** 460–466.

McDermott, M. R., Graham, F. L., Hanke, T., and Johnson, D. C. (1989b). Protection of mice against lethal challenge with herpes simplex virus by vaccination with an adenovirus vector expressing HSV glycoprotein B. *Virology* **169,** 244–247.

McGhee, J. R., and Mestecky, J. (1990). In defense of mucosal surfaces. Development of novel vaccines for IgA responses protective at the portal of entry of microbial pathogens. *Infect. Dis. Clin. North. Am.* **4,** 315–341.

McIntosh, K., and Chanock, R. M. (1985). Respiratory syncytial virus. *In* "Virology" (B. N. Fields, ed.), pp. 1285–1304. Raven Press, New York.

Mackett, M., Smith, G. L., and Moss, B. (1982). Vaccinia virus: A suitable eukaryotic cloning and expression vector. *Proc. Natl. Acad. Sci. U.S.A.* **79,** 7415–7419.

Martin, M. E. D., Dewar, J. B., and Newman, J. F. E. (1988). Polymerized serum albumin beads possessing slow release properties for use in vaccines. *Vaccine* **6,** 33–38.

Marx, P. A., Compans, R. W., Gettie, A., Staas, J. K., Gilley, R. M., Mulligan, M. J., Yamshchikov, G. V., Chen, D., and Eldridge, J. H. (1993). Protection against vaginal SIV transmission with microencapsulated vaccine. *Science* **260,** 1323–1327.

Maskell, D. J., Sweeney, K. J., O'Callaghan, D., Hormaeche, C. E., Liew, F. Y., and Dougan, G. (1987). *Salmonella typhimurium aroA* mutants as carriers of the *Escherichia coli* heat-labile enterotoxin B subunit to the murine secretory and systemic immune system. *Microb. Pathogen.* **2,** 211–221.

Mayhew, E., Lazo, R., Vail, W. J., King, J., and Green, A. M. (1984). Characterization of liposomes prepared using a microemulsifier. *Biochim. Biophys. Acta* **775,** 169–174.

Mayr, A., Kraft, H., Jaeger, O., and Haacke, H. (1972). Oral Immunisierrung von Füchsen gegen Tollwut. *Zentralbl. Veterinar. Med.[B]* **19,** 615–625.

Mestecky, J. (1987). The common mucosal immune system and current strategies for induction of immune responses in external secretions. *J. Clin. Immunol.* **7,** 265–276.

Michalek, S. M., and Childers, N. K. (1990). Development and outlook for a caries vaccine. *Crit. Rev. Oral Biol. Med.* **1,** 37–54.

Michalek, S. M., Childers, N. K., Katz, J., Denys, F. R., Berry, A. K., Eldridge, J. H., McGhee, J. R., and Curtiss, R., III (1989). Liposomes as oral adjuvants. *Curr. Top. Microbiol. Immunol.* **146,** 51–58.

Michalek, S. M., Childers, N. K., Katz, J., Dertzbaugh, M., Zhang, S., Russell, M. W., Macrina, F. L., Jackson, S., and Mestecky, J. (1992). Liposomes and conjugate vaccines for antigen delivery and induction of mucosal immune responses. *In* "Genetically Engineered Vaccines: Prospects for Oral Disease Prevention" (J. Ciardi, J. R. McGhee and J. Keith, eds.). Plenum, New York. *Adv. Exp. Med. Biol.* **327,** 191–198.

Miller, C., and Gardner, M. B. (1991). AIDS and mucosal immunity: Usefulness of the SIV macaque model of genital mucosal transmission. *J. Acq. Immune Def. Syn.* **4,** 1169–1172.

Miller, R. A., Brady, J. M., and Cutwright, D. E. (1977). Degradation rates of resorbable implants (polylactates and polyglycolates): Rate modification with changes in PLA/PGA copolymer ratios. *J. Biomed. Mater. Res.* **11,** 711–719.

Miller, S., and Mekalanos, J. (1990). Constitutive expression of the PhoP regulon attenuates *Salmonella* virulence and survival within macrophages. *J. Bacteriol.* **172,** 2485–2490.

Moldoveanu, Z., Novak, M., Huang, W.-Q., Gilley, R. M., Staas, J. K., Schafer, D., Compans, R. W., and Mestecky, J. (1993). Oral immunization with influenza virus in microspheres. *J. Infect. Dis.* **167,** 84–90.

Moldoveanu, Z., Staas, J. K., Gilley, R. M., Ray, R., Compans, R. W., Eldridge, J. H., Tice, T. R., and Mestecky, J. (1989). Immune responses to influenza virus in orally and systemically immunized mice. *Curr. Top. Microbiol. Immunol.* **146,** 91–99.

Morin, J. E., Lubeck, M. D., Barton, J. E., Conley, A. J., Davis,

A. R., and Hung, P. P. (1987). Recombinant adenovirus induces antibody response to hepatitis B virus surface antigen in hamsters. *Proc. Natl. Acad. Sci. U.S.A.* **84,** 4626–4630.

Moss, B., and Flexner, C. (1987). Vaccinia virus expression vectors. *Ann. Rev. Immunol.* **5,** 305–324.

Murphy, B. R., Prince, G. A., Collins, P. L., Coelingh, K. V. W., Olmstead, R. A., Spriggs, M. K., Parrott, R. H., Kim, H.-W., Brandt, C. D., and Chanock, R. M. (1988). Current approaches to the development of vaccines against parainfluenza and respiratory syncytial viruses. *Virus Res.* **11,** 1–15.

Nail, S. L., White, J. L., and Hem, S. L. (1976a). Structure of aluminum hydroxide gel. I. Initial precipitate. *J. Pharm. Sci.* **65,** 1188–1191.

Nail, S. L., White, J. L., and Hem, S. L. (1976b). Structure of aluminum hydroxide gel. II. Aging mechanism. *J. Pharm. Sci.* **65,** 1192–1195.

Nerome, K., Yoshioka, Y., Ishida, M., Okuma, K., Oka, T., Kataoka, T., Inoue, A., and Oya, A. (1990). Development of a new type of influenza subunit vaccine made by muramyldipeptide-liposomes: Enhancement of humoral and cellular immune responses. *Vaccine* **8,** 503–509.

New, R. R. C. (1990). "Liposomes: A Practical Approach." Oxford University Press, New York.

Nnalue, N. A., and Stocker, B. A. D. (1986). Some *galE* mutants of *Salmonella choleraesuis* retain virulence. *Infect. Immun.* **54,** 635–640.

Nnalue, N. A., and Stocker, B. A. D. (1987). Test of the virulence and live-vaccine efficacy of auxotrophic and *galE* derivatives of *Salmonella choleraesuis. Infect. Immun.* **55,** 955–962.

Ogawa, T., Shimairchi, H., and Hamada, S. (1989). Mucosal and systemic immune responses in BALB/c mice to *Bacteroides gingivalis* fimbriae administered orally. *Infect. Immun.* **57,** 3466–3471.

Ogra, P. L., Leibovitz, E. E., and Zhao-Ri, G. (1989). Oral immunization and secretory immunity to viruses. *Curr. Top. Microbiol. Immunol.* **146,** 73–81.

O'Hagan, D. T., Palin, K., Davis, S. S., Artursson, P., and Sjoholm, I. (1989b). Microparticles as potentially orally active immunological adjuvants. *Vaccine* **7,** 421–424.

O'Hagan, D. T., Palin, K. J., and Davis, S. S. (1989a). Poly(butyl-2-cyanoacrylate) particles as adjuvants for oral immunization. *Vaccine* **7,** 213–216.

O'Hagan, D. T., Jeffery, H., Roberts, M. J. J., McGee, J. P., and Davis, S. S. (1991a). Controlled release microparticles for vaccine development. *Vaccine* **9,** 768–771.

O'Hagan, D. T., Rahman, D., McGee, J. P., Jeffery, H., Davies, M. C., Williams, P., and Davis, S. S. (1991b). Biodegradable microparticles as controlled release antigen delivery systems. *Immunology* **73,** 239–242.

Ostro, M. J. (1987). Liposomes. *Sci. Amer.* **256,** 102–111.

Pagano, R. E., and Weinstein, J. N. (1978). Interactions of liposomes with mammalian cells. *Ann. Rev. Biophys. Bioeng.* **7,** 435–468.

Parker, C., Molina, N., Kelly, S., Curtiss, R., and Yu, J. (1990). Live oral attenuated *Salmonella typhimurium* vaccine vectors which induce formation of antibody to *Bordetella pertussis. In* "Proceedings of the Sixth International Symposium on Pertussis" (C. R. Manclark, ed.), pp. 189–195. DHHS Publication No. (FDA) 90-1664. Department of Health and Human Service, Bethesda, Maryland.

Pastan, I., and Adhya, S. (1976). Cyclic adenosine 5′-monophosphate in *Escherichia coli. Bacteriol. Rev.* **40,** 527–551.

Pastoret, P.-P., Frisch, R., Blancou, J., Brochier, B., Wolff, F., Roboly, O., and Schneider, L. G. (1987). Campagne internationale de vaccination antirabique du renard par voie orale menée au grandduché du Luxembourg, en Belgique et an France. *Ann. Méd. Vét.* **131,** 441–447.

Pierce, N. F., and Sacci, J. B., Jr. (1984). Enhanced mucosal priming by cholera toxin and procholeragenoid with a lipoidal amine adjuvant (avridine) delivered in liposomes. *Infect. Immun.* **44,** 469–473.

Pierce, N. F., Sacci, J. B., Jr., Alving, C. R., and Richardson, E. C. (1984). Enhancement by lipid A of mucosal immunogenicity of liposome-associated cholera toxin. *Rev. Infect. Dis.* **6,** 563–566.

Poirier, T. P., Kehoe, M. A., and Beachey, E. H. (1988). Protective immunity evoked by oral administration of attenuated *aroA Salmonella typhimurium* expressing cloned streptococcal M protein. *J. Exp. Med.* **168,** 25–32.

Preis, I., and Langer, R. (1979). A single-step immunization by sustained antigen release. *J. Immunol.* **28,** 193–197.

Prevec, L., Schneider, M., Rosenthal, K. L., Belbeck, L. W., Derbyshire, J. B., and Graham, F. L. (1989). Use of human adenovirus-based vectors for antigen expression in animals. *J. Gen. Virol.* **70,** 429–434.

Prevec, L., Campbell, J. B., Christie, B. S., Belbeck, L., and Graham, F. L., (1990). A recombinant human adenovirus vaccine against rabies. *J. Infect. Dis.* **161,** 27–30.

Prevec, L., Christie, B. S., Laurie, K. E., (Smith) Bailey, M. M., Graham, F. L., and Rosenthal, K. L. (1991). Immune response to HIV-1 gag antigens induced by recombinant adenovirus vectors in mice and rhesus macaque monkeys. *J. Acq. Immune Def. Syn.* **4,** 568–576.

Ramshaw, I. A., Andrew, M. E., Phillips, S. M., Boyl, D. B., and Couper, B. E. (1987). Recovery of immunodeficient mice from a vaccinia virus IL-2 recombinant infection. *Nature (London)* **329,** 545–546.

Redding, T. W., Schally, A. V., Tice, T. R., and Meyers, W. E. (1984). Long acting delivery systems for peptides: inhibition of rat prostate tumors by controlled-release of D-Trp^6-LH-RH from injectable microcapsules. *Proc. Natl. Acad. Sci. U.S.A.* **81,** 5845–5851.

Richards, R. L., Swartz, G. M., Jr., Schultz, C., Hayre, M. D., Ward, G. S., Ballou, W. R., Chulay, J. D., Hockmeyer, W. T., Berman, S. L., and Alving, C. R. (1989). Immunogenicity of liposomal malaria sporozoite antigen in monkeys: Adjuvant effects of aluminum hydroxide and non-pyrogenic liposomal lipid A. *Vaccine* **7,** 506–512.

Rubin, B. A., and Rorke, L. B. (1988). Adenovirus vaccines. *In* "Vaccines" (S. A. Plotkin and E. A. Mortimer, Jr., eds.), pp. 492–512. Saunders, Toronto.

Rupprecht, C. E., Wiktor, T. J., Johnston, D. H., Hamir, A. N., Dietzschold, B., Wunner, W. H., Glickman, L. T., and Koprowski, H. (1986). Oral immunization and protection of raccoons (*Procyon lotor*) with a vaccinia-rabies glycoprotein recombinant virus vaccine. *Proc. Natl. Acad. Sci. U.S.A.* **83,** 7946–7950.

Rupprecht, C. E., Hamir, A. N., Johnston, D. H., and Koprowski, H. (1988). Efficacy of a vaccinia-rabies glycoprotein recombinant virus vaccine in raccoons (*Procyon lotor*). *Rev. Infect. Dis.* **10,** Suppl. 4, 803–809.

Schneider, L. G., and Cox, J. H. (1983). Ein Feldversuch zur oralen Immunisierung von Füchsen gegen die Tollwut in der Bundesrepublik Deutschland. I. Unschädlichkeit, Wirksamkeit und Stabilität der Vakzine SAD B19. *Tierärztl. Umsch.* **38,** 315–324.

Sjostedt, A., Sandstrom, G., and Tarnvik, A. (1990). Immunization of mice with an attenuated *Salmonella typhimurium* strain expressing a membrane protein of *Francisella tularensis.* A model for identification of bacterial determinants relevant to the host defense against tularemia. *Res. Microbiol.* **141,** 887–891.

Steck, F., Wandeler, A., Bichsel, P., Capt, S., Hafliger, U., and Schneider, L. (1982). Oral immunization of foxes against rabies: Laboratory and field studies. *Comp. Immunol. Microbiol. Infect. Dis.* **5,** 165–171.

Stott, E. J., Ball, L. A., Young, K. K., Furze, J., and Wertz, G. W. (1986). Human respiratory syncytial virus glycoprotein G expressed from a recombinant vaccinia virus vector protects mice against live-virus challenge. *J. Virol.* **60,** 607–613.

Strannegard, O., and Yurchison, A. (1969). Formation of agglutinating and reaginic antibodies in rabbits following oral administration of soluble and particulate antigens. *Int. Arch. Allergy Appl. Immunol.* **35,** 579–590.

Sutjipto, S., Pedersen, N. C., Miller, C. J., Gardner, M. B., Hanson, C. V., Gettie, A., Jennings, M., Higgins, J., and Marx, P. A. (1990). Inactivated simian immunodeficiency virus vaccine failed to protect rhesus macaques from intravenous or genital mucosal infection but delayed disease in intravenously exposed animals. *J. Virol.* **64,** 2290–2297.

Swenson, C. E., Popescu, M. C., and Ginsberg, R. S. (1988). Preparation and use of liposomes in the treatment of microbial infections. *Crit. Rev. Microbiol.* **15,** S1–S31.

Tacket, C., Hone, D., Curtiss, R., Kelly, S. M., Losonsky, G., Guers, L., Harris, A., Edelman, R., and Levine, M. (1992). Comparison of the safety and immunogenicity of Δ*aroC* Δ*aro*D and Δ*cya* Δ*crp Salmonella typhi* strains in adult volunteers. *Infect. Immun.* **60,** 536–541.

Thomas, I., Brochier, B., Languet, B., Blancou, J., Peharpre, D., Kieny, M. P., Desmettre, P., Chappuis, G., and Pastoret, P.-P. (1990). Primary multiplication site of the vaccinia–rabies glycoprotein recombinant virus administered to foxes by the oral route. *J. Gen. Virol.* **71,** 37–42.

Tice, T. R., and Cowsar, D. R. (1984). Biodegradable controlled release parenteral systems. *Pharmacol. Technol. J.* **8,** 26–31.

Tolson, N. D., Charlton, K. M., Stewart, R. B., Campbell, J. B., and Wiktor, T. J. (1987). Immune response in skunks to a vaccinia virus recombinant expressing the rabies virus glycoprotein. *Can. J. Vet. Res.* **51,** 363–366.

Top, F. H., Grossman, R. A., Bartelloni, P. J., Segal, H. E., Dudding, B. A., Russell, P. K., and Buescher, E. L. (1971a). Immunization with live types 7 and 4 adenovirus vaccines. I. Safety, infectivity, antigenicity, and potency of adenovirus type 7 vaccine in humans. *J. Infect. Dis.* **124,** 148–154.

Top, F. H., Buescher, E. L., Bancroft, W. H., and Russell, P. K. (1971b). Immunization with live type 7 and 4 adenovirus vaccines. II. Antibody response and protective effect against acute respiratory disease due to adenovirus type 7. *J. Infect. Dis.* **124,** 155–160.

van Rooijen, N. (1990). Liposomes as carrier and immunoadjuvant of vaccine antigens. *In* "Bacterial Vaccines" (A. Mizrahi, ed.), pp. 255–279. Liss, New York.

Visscher, G. E., Robison, R. L., and Argentieri, G. I. (1987). Tissue response to biodegradable injectable microcapsules. *J. Biomater. Appl.* **2,** 118–131.

Wachsmann, D., Klein, J. P., Scholler, M., and Frank, R. M. (1985). Local and systemic immune response to orally administered liposome-associated soluble *S. mutans* cell wall antigen. *Immunology* **54,** 189–194.

Wachsmann, D., Klein, J. P., Scholler, M., Ogier, J., Ackerman, F., and Frank, R. M. (1986). Serum and salivary antibody responses in rats orally immunized with *Streptococcus mutans* carbohydrate protein conjugate associated with liposomes. *Infect. Immun.* **52,** 408–413.

Wiktor, T. J., Macfarlan, R. I., Reagan, K. J., Dietzschold, B., Curtis, P. J., Wunner, W. H., Kieny, M.-P., Lathe, R., Lecocq, J.-P., Mackett, M., Moss, B., and Koprowski, H. (1984). Protection from rabies by a vaccinia virus recombinant containing the rabies virus glycoprotein gene. *Proc. Natl. Acad. Sci. U.S.A.* **81,** 7194–7198.

Yang, D. M., Fairweather, N., Button, L. L., McMaster, W. R., Kahl, L. P., and Liew, F. Y. (1990). Oral *Salmonella typhimurium* ($AroA^-$) vaccine expressing a major Leishmanial surface protein (gp63) preferentially induces T helper 1 cells and protective immunity against leishmaniasis. *J. Immunol.* **145,** 2281–2285.

33

Mucosal Adjuvants

Charles O. Elson • Mark T. Dertzbaugh

I. INTRODUCTION

Adjuvants are agents that enhance immune responses. Adjuvants stimulate an immune response that is of greater magnitude than the response that occurs when the antigen is given alone. Many if not most antigens yield only weak or poor immune responses when given by themselves. The need for strong and reliable adjuvants has been accentuated by modern molecular techniques that generate weakly immunogenic recombinant proteins or peptides from pathogens for use in vaccines, leading to a renewed interest in vaccine adjuvants, particularly those that can be used in humans (Hooper, 1991). Adjuvants have been shown to affect virtually every measurable aspect of antibody response, including the kinetics, duration, quantity, isotype, and avidity as well as the generation of neutralization or protection. Adjuvants have been shown to affect specificity of antibody responses as well, that is, they alter the selection of epitopes of complex antigens to which antibody will be directed (Hui *et al.*, 1991). Adjuvants also can enhance the development of cell-mediated immunity, both delayed hypersensitivity mediated by CD4 cells and cytotoxic lymphocyte responses mediated by CD8 cells. However, the number of adjuvants that stimulate cell-mediated immune responses tends to be smaller than the number of those that stimulate antibody formation.

Although adjuvants have been used empirically by immunologists for many years, the mechanisms by which they act are not well understood. Part of the problem has been that the adjuvants themselves have been very complex, making the evaluation of mechanisms difficult (Waksman, 1979). More highly purified molecules have been isolated from traditional adjuvants, for example, muramyl dipeptide from mycobacteria and monophosphoryl lipid A from endotoxin, simplifying the dissection of their effects and making elucidation of the mechanisms more probable. The reader is referred to several reviews on adjuvants (White, 1967; Waksman, 1979; Warren *et al.*, 1986; Spriggs and Koff, 1991) for a detailed discussion, but a number of themes or concepts have emerged that will be addressed here. Waksman (1979) has made the point that one must define the target cell on which the adjuvant acts, the distribution of the adjuvant in relation to the location of those target cells, the function of the target cell affected by the adjuvant, and the cellular and molecular mode of action of the adjuvant on the target cell. This information is either rudimentary or nonexistent for most adjuvants. Clearly the best understood adjuvants have a multiplicity of effects on immune cells and different adjuvants can have very divergent effects on the same cells. Potential mechanisms of adjuvant activity after systemic administration are shown in Table I. The possible effects of a given adjuvant are complex, may overlap, and are likely to be multiple. Many adjuvants are surface active agents or surfactants, but how this characteristic translates into these cellular and molecular mechanism is unclear.

Although many if not all of these mechanisms are likely to apply to mucosal adjuvants as well, there is a profound dearth of data and information on agents with mucosal adjuvanticity. This is not because such agents are not needed, because it is remarkably difficult to deliberately immunize for mucosal responses. However, many pathogens either invade through or cause disease at mucosal surfaces. Aside from ease of administration by the mucosal route, mucosal immunization has a distinct advantage. Unlike injectable forms of antigen, which confer primarily systemic immunity, mucosal immunization confers two types of immunity: systemic and mucosal. Mucosal immunity is responsible for protecting the mucosal surface of the host from pathogens and toxins, primarily through the production of secretory IgA. This antibody is elicited only by direct stimulation of mucosal lymphoid tissue.

Most protein antigens are not only poor immunogens when given mucosally but, in fact, induce tolerance instead. Mucosal adjuvants must overcome this potential outcome of mucosal antigen exposure. (The reader is referred to other chapters in this volume that discuss in detail the mucosal immune system, oral immunization, and oral tolerance.) An important concept for this discussion is that of the common mucosal immune system, in which immunization of one mucosal surface also sensitizes other mucosal surfaces at remote sites. This paradigm has formed the basis for a strategy of oral immunization in which the antigen is delivered into the intestine, which has the greatest amount of mucosal lymphoid tissue, to prime the entire mucosal immune system. Such priming is followed by local mucosal or systemic boosting. The intestine is a very harsh environment for most antigens because of its intrinsic properties as a digestive organ. An antigen must survive luminal enzymes, bile salts, trapping by mucus, and propulsion by intestinal motility to be taken up by M cells in the follicle-associated epithelium and be delivered to the gut-associated lymphoid tissue (GALT). Antigen delivery systems and adjuvants are considered in separate chapters of this volume, but this separation may not

Table I General Mechanisms of Adjuvant Action[a]

Prolonged release of antigen over weeks, months
Generation of inflammation, that is, macrophage (APC) activation
Selective antigen localization in thymic dependent areas
Increased uptake and presentation of antigen by accessory cells
Alteration of antigen processing pathway; class I vs class II
Stimulation of T helper cells, nonspecific or specific, Th1 of Th2
Stimulation of increased cytokine production
Stimulation of B cell isotype switching, proliferation, differentiation
Enhanced maturation of T and B cell precursors
Elimination of suppressor cells

[a] Adapted from Waksman (1979).

reflect reality. Injections of antigen into Peyer's patches can generate IgA responses (Andrew and Hall, 1982), so simple delivery of antigen into GALT may be sufficient to generate mucosal responses to some antigens. In addition, lipopolysaccharide (LPS) present in the gut lumen in large quantities may serve as an adjuvant locally in GALT. Once in GALT, antigens must undergo the various processing and presentation steps by accessory cells, presentation to helper T cells, stimulation of specific B cells, and so on. Each of these steps could potentially be affected by mucosal adjuvants. Different mucosal surfaces have different microenvironments, so mucosal adjuvants may have different effects at different mucosal sites.

The remainder of this chapter reviews current knowledge about mucosal adjuvants. The relatively sparse number of agents that are discussed and the relative paucity of information about them illustrates how much need and opportunity exists for more work in this area.

II. CHOLERA TOXIN AND *ESCHERICHIA COLI* HEAT-LABILE TOXIN

Cholera toxin (CT) has been shown to enhance the immunogenicity of relatively poor mucosal immunogens when mixed or conjugated together with them and given orally. Thus, CT and its B subunit (CTB) have generated a great deal of interest as potential adjuvants for oral vaccines (Dertzbaugh and Elson, 1991). CT is one of the most potent mucosal immunogens yet identified. Its immunogenic properties (Pierce and Gowans, 1975; Pierce and Cray, 1982; Elson and Ealding, 1984a,b, 1985,1987), including prolonged mucosal memory (Lycke and Holmgren, 1986a), are exactly those desired for an effective oral vaccine. Whether these properties extend to the antigens for which CT acts as an adjuvant is unknown, but early data suggest that this does occur.

The molecular structure of CT has been characterized extensively (Betley *et al.*, 1986). This toxin is composed of A and B subunits. The toxigenic A subunit (28 kDa) is involved in the ADP-ribosylation of the adenylate cyclase regulatory protein Gs. The A subunit (CTA) is cleaved posttranslationally into the A1 and A2 peptides, the former of which is toxigenic. Crystallographic data on the closely reatled *E. coli* heat-labile toxin indicate that the A2 peptide mediates the association of the A1 peptide with the binding subunits (Sixma *et al.*, 1991). CTB is a homopentamer of five identical noncovalently associated subunits (11.6 kDa) that serve as the carrier for the A subunit. The CTB pentamer binds to the monosialoganglioside GM1 (Cuatrecasas, 1973) that is present on all nucleated cells, including intestinal epithelial cells. Such membrane binding may induce a conformational change that allows the A1 peptide to penetrate the cell (Cuatrecasas, 1973). The exact mechanism of entry is unknown, but may involve endocytosis and transcytosis in endosomes (Lencer *et al.*, 1992).

Enterotoxigenic strains of *E. coli* produce several types of heat-labile enterotoxin (LTs), some of which are highly homologous to CT and others that differ in their protein sequence and carbohydrate-binding specificities (Fukuta *et al.*, 1988). LT-I toxin of *E. coli*, which is highly homologous to CT, has been used with success as an adjuvant (Clements *et al.*, 1988). Although these two toxins will be discussed together and are assumed to be equivalent in this section, the protein sequence of LT-I B subunit does differ by 20% from CTB (Dallas and Falkow, 1980). Thus, the two proteins may have some different properties as mucosal adjuvants. Another toxin of interest is Shiga toxin, which has been demonstrated to elicit potent SIgA responses when administered to the intestine and may show promise as yet another oral adjuvant (Keren *et al.*, 1989).

A. Cholera Toxin as a Mucosal Adjuvant: General Characteristics

The initial demonstration of the adjuvant effects of CT was in studies on whether the feeding of CT resulted in oral tolerance. CT was fed to mice either alone or with the unrelated protein antigen keyhole limpet hemocyanin (KLH). CT did not induce oral tolerance to itself and, when both proteins were fed together, abrogated tolerance to KLH (Elson and Ealding, 1984a). At the same time, CT also induced an intestinal SIgA response to KLH that did not occur when KLH was fed alone. The ability of CT to act as a mucosal adjuvant has been confirmed since by a number of other investigators with a variety of antigens (Table II).

The ability of CT to act as a mucosal adjuvant depends on a number of parameters. To induce immunity to the target antigen, CT must be administered simultaneously with the antigen (Lycke and Holmgren, 1986b). In addition, both the antigen and CT must be administered by the same route, that is, mucosally. Giving CT and the antigen by different routes is not effective, suggesting that CT alters the mucosal lymphoid tissue in a manner that favors responsiveness to the antigens presented to it. Given orally, CT may provide the necessary signals that alter the regulatory environment of GALT from one of suppression to one of responsiveness. The dose of CT required for the adjuvant effect is not clearly defined, and may vary depending on the antigen involved. Although very small amounts of CT suffice to potentiate the immune response to CTB, much larger amounts have been used to enhance mucosal responses to viruses. Because CT induces long-term immunological memory as an antigen (Lycke and Holmgren, 1986a), one might expect memory to be generated when CT is used as an adjuvant and recent data indicates that this is the case (Vajdy and Lycke, 1992). The adjuvant effect observed for CT also probably depends on the type of antigen administered. CT has been used with success orally with proteins and viruses, and parenterally as a vaccine carrier for polysaccharides (Robbins *et al.*, 1989). Despite these successes, we and others have been unable to stimulate SIgA responses to ovalbumin when it is mixed and given orally with CT (Wilson *et al.*, 1990; C. O. Elson, unpublished observation), so the adjuvanticity of CT may not apply to all antigens. The suitability of a given antigen for this method will probably have to be determined empirically. The adjuvanticity of CT may be related to and dependent on its immunogenicity: the response of mice to KLH given with CT orally was significantly higher in H-2 congeneic mouse strains, which are high responders to CT, than in strains that are low responders to CT (Elson, 1992). The LPS gene locus also seems to influence CT adjuvanticity (Elson, 1992).

CT possesses the B- and T-cell epitopes required to elicit systemic immunity; as such, it has been used effectively as a carrier for several parenterally administered experimental vaccines (Que *et al.*, 1988; Szu *et al.*, 1989; Cryz *et al.*, 1990). Clearly CT generates a strong mucosal and systemic response to itself when coadministered as an adjuvant. Whether the strong immunogenicity of CT will limit its effectiveness as an adjuvant has yet to be determined.

B. Role of Cholera Toxin Subunits in Mucosal Adjuvanticity

Although CT has definite mucosal adjuvanticity in mice, whether similar effects would occur in humans is not known. However, from a practical perspective, the use of holotoxin is not feasible in humans because of its toxicity (Levine *et al.*, 1983). One approach being explored to resolve this problem is the use of nontoxic B subunit instead. McKenzie and Halsey (1984) were the first to report that horseradish peroxidase (HRP) chemically conjugated to CTB elicited higher antibody levels in the gut and serum than were observed after feeding either HRP alone or an unconjugated mixture of HRP and

Table II Use of Cholera Toxin as a Mucosal Vaccine Adjuvant

Antigen[a]	Route[b]	Form of CT[c]	Conjugation method[d]	Result	Reference
KLH	po	CT	None	+	Elson and Ealding (1984a)
KLH	po	CT	None	+	Lycke and Holmgren (1986b)
		CT-B	None	−	
HRP	po	CT-B	Glutar	+ +	McKenzie and Halsey (1984)
			None	+	
HA	in	CT-B	None	+	Tamura *et al.* (1988)
HA	po	CT	None	+	Chen and Quinnan (1989)
FLU	po	CT	None	+	
OVA	po	LT	None	+	Clements *et al.* (1988)
		LT-B	None	−	
OVA	po	CT	Glutar	+ +	Van der Heijden *et al.* (1991)
		CT-B	Glutar	+	
M	in	CT-B	SPDP	+	Bessen and Fischetti (1988)
I/II	po	CT-B	SPDP	−	Czerkinsky *et al.* (1989)
		CT	None	+	
SV	po/in virus	CT	None	+	Nedrud *et al.* (1987)
SV	po/in virus	CT-B	Glutar	−	Liang *et al.* (1988)
SV	po	CT	Glutar	+	Liang *et al.* (1989b)
H. pylori	po	CT	None	+	Czinn and Nedrud (1991)
PAc	in	CT-B	None	+	Takahashi *et al.* (1990)

[a] FLU, Whole influenza virus; KLH, keyhole limpet hemocyanin; OVA, ovalbumin; HRP, horseradish peroxidase; HA, hemagglutinin of influenza virus; I/II, surface antigen of *S. mutans;* M, conserved M protein epitope of group A streptococci; PAc, protein antigen of serotype c *Streptococcus mutans;* SV, Sendai virus.
[b] Route of immunization: in, intranasally; po, per os.
[c] CT, Cholera toxin; CT-B, B subunit of cholera toxin; LT, heat-labile enterotoxin of *E. coli;* LT-B, B subunit of LT.
[d] None, mixed only; glutar, glutaraldehyde; SPDP, *n*-succimidyl-3,2-pyridyl dithiopropionate.

CTB. Since then, the use of CTB as a vaccine adjuvant has been examined by others with mixed success. In one report, mixtures of KLH and CTB were unable to stimulate immunity to KLH unless very small doses (<50 ng) of holotoxin were added (Lycke and Holmgren, 1986b); however, KLH conjugated to CTB was not tested. The use of CTB conjugates has been reported to be effective in some cases (Bessen and Fischetti, 1988; Tamura *et al.*, 1988), but not in others (Liang *et al.*, 1988; Czerkinsky *et al.*, 1989). The poor responses that have been observed with CTB conjugates in some cases may be the result of the coupling procedure. The degree of cross-linking and the coupling procedure used can affect the immunogenicity of protein conjugates significantly (Verheul *et al.*, 1989). Genetic fusion of peptides to CTB has been accomplished, generating chimeric neoantigens (Sanchez *et al.*, 1988; Schodel and Will, 1989) that are immunogenic when fed to mice (Dertzbaugh *et al.*, 1990).

Few data are available to date on the role of the A subunit. In mice, the holotoxin is consistently more potent than the B subunit, both for immunogenicity and adjuvanticity. Liang *et al.* (1989a) concluded that GM1 binding but not toxic activity was necessary for the mucosal adjuvanticity of CT–Sendai virus conjugates. Conversely, Lycke *et al.* (1992) found that E coli LT with a single amino acid mutation in the A subunit ($112^{Glu \rightarrow Lys}$) was unable to act as an adjuvant. This question remains to be answered. Further work is necessary to determine whether CTB can replace holotoxin as an adjuvant and to define the role of the A subunit.

C. Site of Adjuvant Activity

The requirement for CT to be given at the same time and by the same route as antigen indicates that its adjuvant effect is exerted at the mucosal surface, but the exact site is unknown. As discussed earlier, our current understanding is that the induction of mucosal immune responses occurs in GALT and requires the transport of antigen by specialized M cells into the underlying lymphoid follicles, where antigen processing and presentation to antigen-specific T cells and B cells presumably occurs. We assume that the adjuvant effect of CT is exerted in these lymphoid follicles, but we acknowledge that no direct evidence for this assumption exists. Gut epithelial cells can act as antigen-presenting cells (APCs) *in vitro,* although the functional effect of that presentation has been suppression (Bland and Warren, 1986; Mayer and Schlien, 1987). Gut epithelial cells bind the great majority of CT and, in an immunohistochemical light microscopic study, CT was present within epithelial cells as well as within mononuclear cells in the underlying lamina propria (Hansson *et al.*, 1984). In addition, CT has been reported to increase intestinal permeability to luminal antigens (Lycke *et al.*, 1991). Thus, the epithelium and the lamina propria are both possible sites for CT adjuvanticity.

D. Antigen Uptake into Follicles

One reason proposed for the effectiveness of CT and CTB as oral immunogens is their ability to bind to epithelial cells and thus persist at mucosal surfaces; the same may be true for their adjuvant function. Increased uptake into intestinal follicles may be an important mechanism by which CT potentiates the immune response to particulate antigens to which it is conjugated. Colloidal gold particles 8–12 nm in size to which CT had been conjugated selectively localized to the M cells of the follicle-associated epithelium after being administered into the murine intestine (M. Neutra, personal communication), whereas soluble CT was bound diffusely to the microvillous surface of all enterocytes. This result suggests that CTB bound to particles does not bind efficiently to GM1 ganglioside in the enterocyte brush border, perhaps because the particles do not efficiently penetrate the mucus coat (which is sparse over the follicle-associated epithelium) or because the GM1 ganglioside of M cells, with their less developed glycocalyx, may be more available to the particles than the GM1 ganglioside of the epithelial cell microvilli. This observation may pertain to the results of Liang *et al.*, who found that GM1 binding but not toxic activity was necessary for the mucosal adjuvanticity of CT–Sendai virus conjugates, and indicates that the mechanism of CT adjuvanticity for particulate antigens may be different from that for soluble antigens.

E. Cellular Targets of Adjuvanticity

1. Antigen-Presenting Cells

Little is known about the mechanism of antigen processing in GALT. Mucosal antigens must be presented to T cells in the context of the appropriate major histocompatibility complex (MHC) Class II molecules (Elson and Ealding, 1985). CT and CTB do not alter macrophage APC antigen uptake or processing *in vitro* (Woogen *et al.*, 1987) or MHC Class II expression (Bromander *et al.*, 1991). However, CT has been shown to stimulate the production of interleukin 1 (IL-1) *in vitro,* an effect that may enhance antigen presentation (Lycke *et al.*, 1989). Bromander *et al.* (1991) have presented evidence that part of CT adjuvanticity is the result of its potentiation of antigen presentation by enhanced IL-1 production. Stimulation of APCs may be a major mechanism of CT adjuvanticity; however, the results obtained *in vitro* may not correspond with events *in vivo* with chronically stimulated APCs.

2. T Cells

After an exogenous antigen is taken up and processed by APCs, it is re-expressed on the cell surface as peptide fragments in association with MHC Class II molecules. The peptide fragments lie in a cleft in the MHC Class II molecule and the T-cell receptor recognizes both the foreign peptide and adjacent facets of the self MHC Class II molecule (Unanue and Cerottini, 1989). Such triggering of T cells is a critical step in the induction of immune response because T cells play an important regulatory role, both positive and negative, the outcome of which determines whether a response occurs and, if so, how large it will be. The experimental basis for these statements rests on work done with systemic lymphoid tissue, but the same also appears to hold true for immune responses in mucosal tissues. Not only is the response to CT itself T cell dependent (Lycke *et al.*, 1987), but it is also genetically restricted by MHC Class II molecules (Elson and Ealding, 1985; Elson and Solomon, 1990). The same rules are likely to apply also to protein antigens for which CT is acting as a mucosal adjuvant.

Mucosal lymphoid follicles contain both CD4 helper cells and CD8 cytotoxic suppressor cells. Murine CD4 helper T cells have been subdivided further into Th1 and Th2 subtypes based on the pattern of cytokines that they secrete (Mosmann and Coffman, 1989). The Th1 helper cells secrete IL-2 and interferon γ (IFNγ) whereas Th2 cells produce IL-4 and IL-5. The latter cytokines have been shown to be important in generating IgA responses *in vitro* (Murray *et al.*, 1987); interestingly, this Th2 subtype may be expressed preferentially in mucosal follicles such as Peyer's patches. Whether one or the other of these subtypes is stimulated preferentially by CT as an immunogen or as an adjuvant is currently unknown and awaits study. CT appears to be able to stimulate the Th2 helper cell subtype *in vivo* because CT given orally stimulates not only a secretory IgA response but also an equally strong plasma IgG1 anti-CT response, which are associated with the Th2 function (Elson *et al.*, 1988).

Feeding CT to mice induced oral tolerance to DTH, but not for antibody responses to CT (Kay and Ferguson, 1989), suggesting that mucosal CT may inhibit the Th1 cells but not Th2 cells. CT does inhibit Th1 clones preferentially *in vitro* (Gajewski *et al.*, 1990). However, as an adjuvant CT seems able to boost either Th1 or Th2 responses. Xu Amano *et al.* (1993) found that CT augmented a predominant Th2 response when tetanus toxoid (TT) was given mucosally but also augmented Th1 responses when TT and CT were given together parenterally. Much needs to be learned about the effect of CT and CTB on cytokine expression by both CD4 and CD8 T cells, effects that are likely to be extremely important in the net effect of these molecules in GALT.

One hypothesis for the mucosal adjuvanticity of CT is that it may alter the T-cell regulatory environment within mucosal lymphoid follicles, for example, the inhibition of suppressor cells. The addition of both CT and CTB to lymphocytes *in vitro* is quite inhibitory (Woogen *et al.*, 1987) and preferentially inhibits the $CD8^+$ T-cell subset (Elson *et al.*, 1990). Some *in vivo* evidence in a graft vs. host system suggests that CT inhibits suppressor cells (Lange *et al.*, 1978). Consistent with this finding, we have found, in an adoptive transfer system, that feeding of KLH to mice generates suppressor T cells that inhibit both a secretory IgA and a plasma IgG response to KLH but that feeding of both KLH and CT eliminates this suppression (C. O. Elson, S. P. Holland, M. Dertzbaugh, C. Cuff, and A. Anderson, unpublished data). The *in vitro* inhibition of T-cell activation by CTB has features that suggest that similar inhibition may occur *in vivo* because it can be accomplished with brief pulses lasting only minutes and the concentrations required should be achievable *in vivo*. These data collectively support the notion that regulatory inhibition of T-cell subsets is an important feature in both the mucosal immunogenicity and the adjuvanticity of CT.

Most of the work done with CT has focused on the antibody response. Little is known about the delayed hypersensitivity (DTH) response to CT. In other systems, DTH responses are regulated independently of humoral responses, so one cannot extrapolate results with antibody responses to DTH. Supporting this point are data of Kay and Ferguson (1989a,b), mentioned earlier who found that feeding CT or its toxoid prior to systemic immunization induced oral tolerance for the DTH response but not for the antibody response to CT. Experiments with cell transfer indicated that this oral tolerance for DTH involved the induction of suppressor cells. Interestingly, the T cells that suppress DTH reactions are $CD4^+$ whereas the T cells that suppress antibody responses are $CD8^+$. Whether CT would have similar effects as a mucosal adjuvant, that is, induction of antibody but not cellular responses to a second antigen, is unknown. This attribute may be desirable for some vaccine candidates and undesirable for others, such as those for intracellular pathogens. This question will need to be addressed in each system to determine how DTH responses are affected by CT.

3. B Cells

Many stages of B-cell development must be traversed before reaching the antibody-secreting plasma cell. The major steps of B-cell development, including isotype commitment or switching, clonal expansion, and terminal differentiation are all dependent on and regulated by various cytokines that act on B cells at defined stages of development (Tesch *et al.*, 1986). For example, IgE and IgG1 isotype production is enhanced preferentially by IL-4 (Snapper and Paul, 1987) and IgA isotype is enhanced by IL-5 (Murray *et al.*, 1987) and by TGFβ (Coffman *et al.*, 1989). CT could affect any one or more of these steps. Precisely how CT interaacts with B cells or with the critical cytokines that regulate them has only just begun to be examined.

CT may possess some pharmacological activity that drives B cells toward IgA-committed precursors. Lebman *et al.* (1988) have shown that CT given intraduodenally can change the isotype pattern displayed by Peyer's patch B cells primed for an unrelated hapten from IgM to IgG and IgA after antigen-dependent clonal expansion *in vitro*. CT appears to alter nonspecifically the responsiveness of Peyer's patch B cells to isotype switching signals present in the *in vitro* cultures, perhaps by a direct effect on B cells or by the effect of CT on cytokine-mediated signals within the Peyer's patch. Lycke and Strober (1989) have shown that CT enhances the effect of both IL-4 and IL-5 on purified B cells stimulated by LPS *in vitro*. In the presence of CT, IL-4 enhanced IgG1-producing B cells 3- to 4-fold; IL-5 had a similar effect on IgA-producing B cells. These results suggest that CT promotes isotype switching of surface IgM^+ B cells in synergy with interleukins, at least to a moderate extent, but determining the exact molecular mechanism involved awaits molecular genetic analysis. The interaction of CT and interleukins on B cells of GALT *in vivo* must be explored further to understand the process that drives B cells to commit to a predominantly IgA isotype expression.

Little information is available concerning the effects of CT on B-cell clonal expansion. Woogen et al. (1987), found that CT inhibited proliferation of purified B cells *in vitro* when they were stimulated polyclonally by either anti-IgM or LPS;

CTB inhibited B cells stimulated by anti-IgM but not by LPS. Lycke *et al.* (1989) also found that CT inhibited the B-cell proliferative response to LPS, but observed a mild stimulatory effect on B-cell proliferation relative to the control if the culture period was prolonged to 6 days and low doses of CT were used. The effects of CT on B-cell proliferation *in vivo*, particularly after the brief exposures expected there, remains to be determined. Certainly the large numbers of plasma cells producing anti-CT in the lamina propria after oral immunization with CT, which has been estimated at up to 5% of the total at the peak of the response, indicates that clonal expansion occurs and is vigorous *in vivo*. The effect of CT on terminal differentiation of B cells has yet to be examined.

F. Summary

Much remains to be learned about the mechanisms of CT immunogenicity and adjuvanticity, including the relative contributions of the two subunits. The dose, timing, route, antigen type, and genetic background of the host are all important variables. Indications are that the mechanism of CT adjuvanticity involves multiple aspects of immune induction in the mucosa, including increased uptake of antigen; enhancement of IL-1 production by APCs; altered regulation by T cells, especially inhibition of CD8 suppressor cells; stimulation of B-cell switching to IgA and IgG; and possibly, enhancement of B-cell clonal expansion. Different components of these multiple effects may be of more importance for some antigens than for others.

III. IMMUNOSTIMULATING COMPLEXES

Immunostimulating complex (ISCOM) is a term coined by Morein to describe 40-nm cage-like particles that form spontaneously on mixing cholesterol with the saponin, Quil A (Morein, 1987). Protein antigens can be incorporated in such particles, and the Quil A serves as a built-in adjuvant. The incorporation of the protein into ISCOMs is via hydrophobic interactions; however, a wide variety of proteins can be incorporated by palmitification of the protein before incorporation, or acidification to expose hydrophobic groups in conjunction with the addition of phosphatidyl choline (Morein *et al.*, 1990; Mowat and Donachie, 1991). Much smaller amounts of antigen are effective in ISCOMs that are needed for oil adjuvants (Nagy *et al.*, 1990). ISCOMs have been used effectively parenterally in a variety of species including mice, cats, sheep, cattle, and monkeys (Morein, 1990).

ISCOMs stimulate a strong antibody response in all immunoglobulin classes (Lovgren, 1988). They also strongly stimulate cell-mediated immunity, as measured by proliferative T-cell responses and delayed hypersensitivity (Fossum *et al.*, 1990). Perhaps a unique feature of ISCOMs is their ability to induce $CD8^+$ cytolytic T lymphocyte (CTL) responses. Thus, a single subcutaneous immunization of mice with ISCOMs containing either purified human immunodeficiency virus (HIV) gp160 or influenza hemagglutinin resulted in priming of HIV-specific or influenza-specific $CD8^+$ MHC Class I-restricted CTLs (Takahashi *et al.*, 1990a). This result indicates that ISCOMs somehow cause exogenous proteins to enter the endogenous pathway of antigen processing. The Quil A component appears to be essential for this effect because it does not occur with simple liposomes or with free palmitified antigen (Mowat and Donachie, 1991). The ability of ISCOMs to stimulate cytolytic T cells may be unique among adjuvants and has generated much interest in this adjuvant system, particularly for vaccination against viral pathogens.

Mucosal adjuvanticity of ISCOMs also has been demonstrated, although in a limited number of studies to date. An experimental influenza virus vaccine administered intranasally on two occasions generated high levels of antibody and protection against challenge infection that was equivalent to that after subcutaneous immunization (Lovgren *et al.*, 1990). Mowat and colleagues have reported that administration of ovalbumin (OVA) in ISCOMs converts the response from the oral tolerance that is seen when OVA is fed alone to a state of antibody and cell-mediated immunity and, after repeated feeding, the generation of OVA-specific CTLs. After several administrations orally, strong secretory IgA antibody responses to OVA could be detected in intestinal washings. Thus, the oral administration of OVA in ISCOMs generated a wide spectrum of humoral and cellular immune responses (Mowat and Donachie, 1991; Mowat *et al.*, 1991). Finally, parenteral immunization in the pelvic presacral space with sheep erythrocyte membrane proteins in ISCOMs generated significant IgA titers in vaginal fluid against this antigen in mice (Thapar *et al.*, 1991). Thus, ISCOMs may be useful at a number of mucosal surfaces, and the mucosal route may help avoid the toxicity that has been observed after the parenteral use of these particulates in small animals. Such toxicity may limit the usefulness of this adjuvant. However, immunostimulatory but nontoxic fractions of Quil A have been identified that may reduce or eliminate this potential problem (Kensil *et al.*, 1991). These early studies suggest that ISCOMs may be a very useful adjuvant system for generating mucosal responses.

IV. BACTERIAL LIPOPOLYSACCHARIDE AND LIPID A

The adjuvant activity of LPS was demonstrated first by Johnson *et al.* (1956). An unusual feature of its adjuvanticity relative to other agents is that it can be delivered at a site and a time different from antigen (Ulrich *et al.*, 1991). LPS has multiple effects on the immune system, including the stimulation of macrophages and their production of cytokines such as IL-1 and colony stimulating factor (CSF), mitogenicity for B cells, alteration of MHC Class II expression on APCs, the stimulation of IFNγ production, and the stimulation of delayed hypersensitivity (Ohta *et al.*, 1982; Warren *et al.*, 1986). Despite its potent adjuvant effects, LPS has been used as an adjuvant only experimentally because of its toxicity. The lipid A component of LPS is its active moiety, that is, the administration of purified lipid A can reproduce all the toxic and biological effects of LPS (Chiller *et al.*, 1973).

Many studies have been done on chemical modifications of lipid A in an effort to find a less toxic but still immunostimulatory compound (Takayama *et al.*, 1981; Takada and Kotani, 1989). Multiple such forms of lipid A have been produced and some have undergone fairly extensive testing as nontoxic but effective immunological adjuvants. One of these, monophosphoryl lipid A, has been shown to have many of the adjuvant effects of lipid A or LPS itself, that is, it stimulates macrophages to release IL-1, tumor necrosis factor α (TNFα), and CSF, increases production of IFNγ *in vivo*, and can increase the nonspecific resistance of mice to bacterial infection (Ulrich *et al.*, 1991). This material can be combined with other adjuvants and has been given safely to humans.

Relatively little work has been done to test such lipid A derivatives as mucosal adjuvants. LPS increased serum antibody against inhaled bovine serum albumin (BSA) or OVA when it was included in the inhalant (Mizoguchi *et al.*, 1986), and enhanced the anti-BSA response after oral administration of BSA in liposomes (Ogawa *et al.*, 1986). These studies suggest that monophosphoryl lipid A may be an effective adjuvant at mucosal surfaces; however, its effects appear complex. Studies in rodents suggest that LPS depresses the response to certain antigens such as sheep red blood cells (SRBC) given orally; the administration of LPS to germ-free mice causes oral tolerance to SRBC when these were fed subsequently to the same mice (Michalek *et al.*, 1983a). In addition, the IgA immune responses in LPS-resistant C3H/HeJ mice are greater than the responses of their LPS-responsive C3H/HeN counterpart, suggesting that LPS induces mucosal hyporesponsiveness in the latter (Babb and McGhee, 1980; Kiyono *et al.*, 1980,1982). Coadministration of LPS or lipid A orally with myelin basic protein (MBP) to rats enhanced the generation of oral tolerance to this antigen; in contrast, LPS given subcutaneously at the time of antigen feeding abrogated oral tolerance to MBP (Khoury *et al.*, 1990). Other investigators have reported that administration of LPS intravenously to mice abrogates humoral (IgG) but not cellular (DTH) oral tolerance to OVA (Mowat *et al.*, 1986). These studies illustrate that the effects of LPS or lipid A at mucosal surfaces are complex and require further study. The effect of LPS or lipid A on different forms of antigen and at various mucosal surfaces, including those that are not normally bathed in bacterial endotoxin, need to be defined. Because antigen and LPS or lipid A do not need to be given by the same route, combined parenteral and mucosal administration may be effective in stimulating mucosal responses, as has been found in studies with *Shigella* LPS (Keren *et al.*, 1988). Finally, lipid A derivatives can be combined with other adjuvants. Such combinations may have much greater efficacy than lipid A alone. The availability of the nontoxic lipid A derivatives for use in humans makes a reexamination of their mucosal adjuvant effects a high priority.

V. *BORDETELLA PERTUSSIS* PERTUSSIGEN

Bordetella pertussis whole cell bacteria have been used parenterally as a vaccine against pertussis and as an adjuvant for other antigens. Obviously this material is a complex mixture, including LPS as well as variable amounts of pertussis toxin. Pertussis toxin (pertussigen) has been crystallized (Munoz *et al.*, 1981) and its gene cloned (Locht *et al.*, 1986). This substance has many biological effects, probably related to its ability to bind to signal transducing G proteins in a diverse number of cell types. Pertussigen has been tested in purified form and was found to have adjuvant activity. Pertussigen particularly enhances the cell-mediated immune response as measured by increased delayed skin responses to soluble antigens and increased inflammatory responses such as footpad swelling after injection of Freund's complete adjuvant. These effects of pertussigen appear to be mediated through T cells because footpad swelling does not occur in athymic nude mice. *Bordetella* and pertussigen both increase IgG and IgE responses to antigens and have been reported to be able to abrogate humoral (Herzenberg and Tokuhisa, 1982) and cell-mediated (Tamura *et al.*, 1985) tolerance to antigens in some systems, an effect of some interest for mucosal immunity because of the propensity for tolerance induction by antigen feeding. Similar to LPS or lipid A, pertussigen can be given by a different route and at a different time than antigen and still exert its adjuvant effects.

The data on its mucosal adjuvanticity are sparse. One can induce IgE antibody responses to OVA in rats by feeding OVA and administering pertussigen either intradermally, intraperitoneally, or orally (Bazin and Platteau, 1976; Jarrett *et al.*, 1976). The IgE isotype is not one that vaccines usually are intended to induce, so the value of this ability of pertussigen is questionable. Perhaps related to its ability to induce IgE responses or, alternatively, to induce DTH, immunization with nematode worm antigens plus pertussigen stimulated resistance to two different intestinal nematodes in rodents (Murray et al., 1979; Mitchell and Munoz, 1983). When SRBC antigen plus pertussigen was delivered to nasal mucosa, a strong respiratory immunization in mice was induced (Birnabaum and Pinto, 1976).

The propensity for this agent to produce adverse effects is a real concern. *Bordetella pertussis* vaccine has been associated with severe reactions in humans, including encephalopathy (Cavanagh *et al.*, 1981). These potential toxicities may be lessened by administration via a mucosal route; however, in the intestine, pertussigen has induced hypersecretory responses to some inflammatory mediators and neurotransmitters and this responsiveness may be prolonged (Crowe *et al.*, 1990). These and other potential adverse reactions with pertussigen are likely to limit its usefulness as an adjuvant even by mucosal routes, except for experimental use.

VI. AVRIDINE

Avridine [*N*,*N*-dioctadecyl *N*′,*N*′-bis(2-hydroxyethyl)propanediamine] is a synthetic lipoidal amine developed as an inducer of interferon production. However, this molecule subsequently was found to possess properties that made it potentially useful as a vaccine adjuvant, especially as a mucosal adjuvant. Its adjuvant activity probably is related to its ability to stimulate interferon production and thus up-regulate antigen presentation by macrophages.

When administered intraduodenally, avridine has been shown to enhance the uptake, localization, and retention of antigen in Peyer's patches (Anderson *et al.*, 1985). One of the ways in which avridine may exert this effect is by slowing the rate of degradation of antigen, as has been observed for microcapsules.

Avridine has been used to protect mice against aerosol challenge with Rift Valley Fever virus (Anderson *et al.*, 1987). Formalin-inactivated virus was combined with avridine and administered either subcutaneously (sc) or intraduodenally (id). The use of avridine was found to stimulate production of both secretory IgA and serum IgG. The response elicited by id administration was found to protect the mucosa from aerosol challenge, but also increased the predilection of the mice to develop encephalitis on parenteral challenge. Further, the survival rate was only 62% for mice immunized id compared with a survival rate of 100% for mice immunized sc. The reason for this effect is not clear, but it suggests that mucosal vaccination can have both positive and negative consequences, depending on the agent and the adjuvant being used for vaccination.

The effectiveness of avridine as an adjuvant reportedly is increased by incorporating it into liposomes (Pierce and Sacci, 1984). When avridine-containing liposomes were coadministered with cholera toxin, the efficiency of priming for an anamnestic response increased 5- to 7-fold. No such adjuvant effect was observed for the liposomes alone. Interestingly, cholera toxin did not have to be incorporated into the liposomes for this effect to occur. However, neither avridine nor the liposomes had any effect on the strength of the immune response to either primary or secondary exposure to cholera toxin. In general, most antigens have been found to elicit better immunity in GALT when packaged in liposomes. However, as described earlier, cholera toxin is a unique antigen with respect to mucosal immunity, and is not representative of most antigens administered orally.

Somewhat surprising was the reported effectiveness of avridine as an adjuvant for influenza virus (Bergmann and Waldman, 1988). Coadministration of killed virus with avridine-containing liposomes orally was reported to enhance the IgA response in the respiratory tract. However, no antibody response was detected in the serum. This observation is unusual, since most mucosally administered vaccines elicit both secretory and systemic immunity. Further, most orally administered vaccines require boosting locally to stimulate appreciable secretory immunity in remote mucosal sites.

An interesting study examined the effectiveness of avridine as an adjuvant for eliciting secretory immunity in tears (Peppard *et al.*, 1988). Dinitrophenyl (DNP)-*Pneumococcus* was coadministered with or without avridine-containing liposomes by ocular-topical (ot) or oral routes. When DNP-*Pneumococcus* was administered without avridine-containing liposomes, whether administered to the eye or orally, IgA responses were detected in tears. However, the antibody response in tears was always greater by the ot route. In contrast to the results observed for respiratory IgA, the use of avridine-containing liposomes reduced the IgA antibody response found in tears, compared with antigen alone, when administered either ot or orally. However, the serum IgG response was increased slightly when avridine was coadministered with the antigen.

In summary, avridine has shown some promise as a vaccine adjuvant, and currently is being used as an adjuvant for parenterally administered veterinary vaccines. Although avridine clearly is able to stimulate mucosal immunity at some sites, its ability to stimulate systemic immunity via mucosal immunization is less clear.

VII. MURAMYL DIPEPTIDE

Muramyl dipeptide (MDP; *N*-acetyl muramyl-L-alanyl-D-isoglutamine) is derived from the cell wall of mycobacteria, is the smallest structural component of the cell wall that still retains adjuvant activity, and is one of the active components contained in Freund's complete adjuvant. The effectiveness of Freund's as an adjuvant for parenterally administered vaccines is well documented. Freund's has been used extensively for experimental vaccines and immunotherapy. Although several reports are available on the use of MDP as a mucosal adjuvant, the literature is not nearly as extensive as it is for parenterally administered vaccines.

In several instances, oral administration of MDP has been used to stimulate nonspecific immunity to bacteria and to tumor cells. Oral administration of MDP to mice protected them against challenge with *Klebsiella pneumoniae* (Parant *et al.*, 1978) and increased cytolytic activity after intravenous challenge with tumor cells (Okutomi *et al.*, 1990). In both cases, the increase in nonspecific immunity was probably the result of induction of cytokines. MDP is known to be a potent inducer of IL-1, which can up-regulate macrophages and T cells. Although not directly relevant to mucosal immunity, these results do show that MDP is absorbed by the gut and suggest that it can affect the immunoregulatory environment of the mucosa-associated lymphoid tissue.

MDP has been used as an adjuvant for intravaginal immunization in mice (Thapar *et al.*, 1990a). Multiple large doses of horse ferritin were combined with aluminum hydroxide, muramyl dipeptide, monophosphoryl lipid A, or cholera toxin. Although MDP was not the most effective adjuvant for this route, it was shown to potentiate the secretory immune response to horse ferritin. Depending on the route of immunization chosen, the level and isotype of antibody to horse ferritin varied (Thapar *et al.*, 1990b). Pelvic immunization induced greater IgA and IgG responses in the vagina than did intravaginal immunization. Although IgG responses were elevated only slightly relative to sc-immunized mice, the IgA response was elevated dramatically by pelvic immunization.

MDP also has been used as an adjuvant for oral immunization (Michalek *et al.*, 1983b). Trinitrophenyl (TNP)-haptenated whole cells or cell wall from the cariogenic bacterium

Streptococcus mutans combined with MDP was administered intragastrically to mice. MDP boosted anti-TNP IgA responses in LPS-responsive C3H/HeN mice, but not in LPS-unresponsive C3H/HeJ mice. The salivary immune response to *S. mutans* whole cells or cell walls in gnotobiotic rats was augmented more than 2-fold when coadministered orally with MDP. The use of MDP in combination with *S. mutans* resulted in a significant reduction in bacterial colonization of the tooth surface and number of carious lesions produced (Morasaki *et al.*, 1983). MDP augmented the mucosal immune response to *Neisseria gonorrhoeae* major outer membrane protein when given into the intestine or injected directly into Peyer's patches (Jeurissen *et al.*, 1987). Lipophilic derivatives of MDP have been synthesized and tested for their mucosal adjuvanticity. Some enhanced the mucosal response of rats to the soluble protein BSA when coadministered in saline; others were active only when incorporated with antigen in liposomes (Ogawa *et al.*, 1986).

The observations just discussed suggest that MDP can be taken up by mucosal surfaces and can stimulate both secretory and systemic immunity to antigens coadministered with it. The mechanism of action at these sites is unknown, but is probably due, at least in part, to the ability of MDP to induce IL-1 production and increase processing and presentation of antigen by macrophages.

VIII. MISCELLANEOUS ADJUVANTS

Many different compounds have been examined for their potential to act as adjuvants. In general, the literature on the use of these compounds as mucosal adjuvants is sparse. Items included on this list are nonionic block copolymers, vitamin A, synthetic double-stranded polyribonucleotide complexes such as poly I : C (an interferon inducer), polyacrylic compounds, glucan analogs, pyran copolymers, and proteosomes (peptide–multimeric protein complexes). The utility of these compounds has yet to be established, although these and a number of others appear interesting.

References

Anderson, A. O., MacDonald, T. T., and Rubin, D. H. (1985). Effect of orally administered avridine on enteric antigen uptake and mucosal immunity. *Int. J. Immunother.* **1**, 107–115.

Anderson, A. O., Wood, O. L., King, A. D., and Stephenson, E. H. (1987). Studies on anti-viral mucoal immunity with the lipoidal amine adjuvant. *In* "Recent Advances in Mucosal Immunology" (J. Mestecky, J. R. McGhee, J. Bienenstock, and P. L. Ogra, ed.), pp. 1781–1790. Plenum, New York.

Andrew, E., and Hall, J. G. (1982). IgA antibodies in the bile of rats. I. Some characteristics of the primary response. *Immunology* **45**, 169–175.

Babb, J. L., and McGhee, J. R. (1980). Mice refractory to lipopolysaccharide manifest high immunoglobulin A responses to orally administered antigen. *Infect. Immun.* **29**, 322–328.

Bazin, H., and Platteau, B. (1976). Production of circulating reaginic (IgE) antibodies by oral administration of ovalbumin to rats. *Immunology* **30**, 679–684.

Bergmann, K. C., and Waldman, R. H. (1988). Enhanced murine respiratory tract IgA antibody response to oral influenza vaccine when combined with a lipoidal amine (avridine). *Int. Arch. Allergy Appl. Immunol.* **87**, 334–335.

Bessen, D., and Fischetti, V. A. (1988). Influence of intranasal immunization with synthetic peptides corresponding to conserved epitopes of M protein on mucosal colonization by group A streptococci. *Infect. Immun.* **56**, 2666–2672.

Betley, M., Miller, V., and Mekalanos, J. (1986). Genetics of bacterial enterotoxins. *Ann. Rev. Microbiol.* **40**, 577–605.

Birnabaum, S., and Pinto, M. (1976). Local and systemic opsonic adherent, hemagglutinating and rosette forming activity in mice induced by respiratory immunization with sheep red blood cells. *Z. Immunitätsforsch.* **151**, 69–77.

Bland, P. W., and Warren, L. G. (1986). Antigen presentation by epithelial cells of the rat small intestine. 1. Kinetics, antigen specificity and blocking by anti-Ia antisera. *Immunology* **58**, 8–16.

Bromander, A., Holmgren, J., and Lycke, N. (1991). Cholera toxin stimulates IL-1 production and enhances antigen presentation by macrophages *in vitro*. *J. Immunol.* **146**, 2908–2014.

Cavanagh, N. P., Brett, E. M., Marshall, W. C., and Wilson, J. (1981). The possible adjuvant role of *Bordetella pertussis* and pertussis vaccine in causing severe encephalopathic illness: A presentation of three case histories. *Neuropediatr.* **12**, 374–381.

Chen, K. S., and Quinnan, G. V. (1989). Efficacy of inactivated influenza vaccine delivered by oral administration. *Curr. Top. Microbiol. Immunol.* **146**, 101–106.

Chiller, J. M., Skidmore, B. J., Morrison, D. C., and Weigle, W. O. (1973). Relationship of the structure of bacterial lipopolysaccharides to its function in mitogenesis and adjuvanticity. *Proc. Natl. Acad. Sci. U.S.A.* **70**, 2129–2132.

Clements, J. D., Hartzog, N. M., and Lyon, F. L. (1988). Adjuvant activity of *Escherichia coli* heat-labile enterotoxin and effect on the induction of oral tolerance in mice to unrelated protein antigens. *Vaccine* **6**, 269–277.

Coffman, R. L., Lebman, D. A., and Shrader, B. (1989). Transforming growth factor beta specifically enhances IgA production by lipopolysaccharide-stimulated murine B lymphocytes. *J. Exp. Med.* **170**, 1039–1044.

Crowe, S. E., Sestini, P., and Perdue, M. H. (1990). Allergic reactions of rat jejunal mucosa. Ion transport responses to luminal antigen and inflammatory mediators. *Gastroenterology* **99**, 74–82.

Cryz, S. J., Cross, A. S., Sadoff, J. C., and Furer, E. (1990). Synthesis and characterization of *Escherichia coli* O18 O-polysaccharide conjugate vaccines. *Infect. Immun.* **58**, 373–377.

Cuatrecasas, P. (1973). Gangliosides and membrane receptors for cholera toxin. *Biochemistry* **12**, 3558–3566.

Czerkinsky, C., Russell, M. W., Lycke, N., Lindblad, M., and Holmgren, J. (1989). Oral administration of a streptococcal antigen coupled to cholera toxin B subunit evokes strong antibody responses in salivary glands and extramucosa tissues. *Infect. Immun.* **57**, 1072–1077.

Czinn, S. J., and Nedrud, J. G. (1991). Oral immunization against *Heliobacter pylori*. *Infect. Immun.* **59**, 2359–2363.

Dallas, W. S., and Falkow, S. (1980). Amino acid sequence homology between cholera toxin and *Escherichia coli* heat-labile toxin. *Nature (London)* **288**, 499–501.

Dertzbaugh, M. T., and Elson, C. O. (1991). Cholera toxin as a mucosal adjuvant. *In* "Topics in Vaccine Adjuvant Research" (D. Spriggs and W. Koff, ed.), pp. 119–132. CRC Press, Boca Raton, Florida.

Dertzbaugh, M. T., Peterson, D. L., and Macrina, F. L. (1990). Cholera toxin B-subunit gene fusion: Structural and functional analysis of the chimeric protein. *Infect. Immun.* **58**, 70–79.

Elson, C. O. (1992). Cholera toxin as a mucosal adjuvant: Effects of H-2 major histocompatibility complex and *lps* genes. *Infect. Immun.* **60,** 2874–2879.

Elson, C. O., and Ealding, W. (1984a). Cholera toxin feeding did not induce oral tolerance in mice and abrogated oral tolerance to an unrelated protein antigen. *J. Immunol.* **133,** 2892–2897.

Elson, C. O., and Ealding, W. (1984b). Generalized systemic and mucosal immunity in mice after mucosal stimulation with cholera toxin. *J. Immunol.* **132,** 2736–2741.

Elson, C. O., and Ealding, W. (1985). Genetic control of the murine immune response to cholera toxin. *J. Immunol.* **135,** 930–932.

Elson, C. O., and Ealding, W. (1987). Ir gene control of the murine secretory IgA response to cholera toxin. *Eur. J. Immunol.* **17,** 425–428.

Elson, C. O., and Solomon, S. (1990). Activation of cholera toxin specific T cells in vitro. *Infect. Immun.* **58,** 3711–3716.

Elson, C. O., Ealding, W., Woogen, S., and Gaspari, M. (1988). Some new perspectives on IgA immunization and oral tolerance derived from the unusual properties of cholera toxin as a mucosal immunogen. *In* "Mucosal Immunity and Infections at Mucosal Surfaces" (W. Strober, M. E. Lamm, J. R. McGhee, and S. P. James, ed.), pp. 392–400. Oxford University Press, New York.

Elson, C. O., Holland, S., and Woogen, S. (1990). Preferential inhibition of the CD8+ T cell subset by cholera toxin (CT) and its B subunit (CT-B). *FASEB J.* **4,** A1864.

Fossum, C., Bergstrom, M., Lovgren, K., Watson, D. L., and Morein, B. (1990). Effect of iscoms and their adjuvant moiety (matrix) on the initial proliferation and IL-2 responses: Comparison of spleen cells from mice inoculated with iscoms and/or matrix. *Cell. Immunol.* **129,** 414–425.

Fukuta, S., Magnani, J. L., Twiddy, E. M., Holmes, R. K., and Ginsburg, V. (1988). Comparison of the carbohydrate-binding specificities of cholera toxin and *Escherichia coli* heat-labile enteroxins LTh-I, LTh-IIa, and LTh-IIb. *Infect. Immun.* **56,** 1748–1756.

Gajewski, T. F., Schell, S. R., and Fitch, F. W. (1990). Evidence implicating utilization of different T cell receptor-associated signaling pathways by TH1 and TH2 clones. *J. Immunol.* **144,** 4110–4120.

Hansson, H. A., Lange, S., and Lonnroth, I., (1984). Internalization in vivo of cholera toxin in the small intestinal epithelium of the rat. *Acta Pathol. Microbiol. Immunol. Scand.* **92,** 15–21.

Herzenberg, L. A., and Tokuhisa, T. (1982). Epitope-specific regulation I. Carrier-specific induction of suppression for IgG antihapten antibody responses. *J. Exp. Med.* **155,** 1730–1740.

Hooper, C. (1991). The new age of vaccine adjuvants. *J. NIH Res.* **3,** 21–23.

Hui, G. S. N., Chang, S. P., Gibson, H., Hashimoto, A., Hashiro, C., Barr, P. J., and Kotani, S. (1991). Influence of adjuvants on the antibody specificity to the *Plasmodium falciparum* major merozoite surface protein, gp195. *J. Immunol.* **147,** 3935–3941.

Jarrett, E. E., Haig, D. M., McDougall, W., and McNulty, E. (1976). Rat IgE production. II. Primary and booster reaginic antibody responses following intradermal or oral immunization. *Immunology* **30,** 671–677.

Jeurissen, S. H., Sminia, T., and Beuvery, E. C. (1987). Induction of mucosal immunoglobulin A immune response by preparations of *Neisseria gonorrhoeae* porin proteins. *Infect. Immun.* **55,** 253–257.

Johnson, A. J., Gaines, S., and Landy, M. (1956). Studies on the O antigen of *Salmonella typhosa*. V. Enhancement of the antibody response to protein antigens by the purified lipopolysaccharide. *J. Exp. Med.* **103,** 225–233.

Kay, R. A., and Ferguson, A. (1989a). The immunological consequences of feeding cholera toxin. I. Feeding cholera toxin suppresses the induction of systemic delayed-type hypersensitivity but not humoral immunity. *Immunology* **66,** 410–415.

Kay, R. A., and Ferguson, A. (1989b). The immunological consequences of feeding cholera toxin. II. Mechanisms responsible for the induction of oral tolerance for DTH. *Immunology* **66,** 416–421.

Kensil, C. R., Patel, U., Lennick, M., and Marciani, D. (1991). Separation and characterization of saponins with adjuvant activity from *Quillaja saponaria* Molina cortex. *J. Immunol.* **146,** 431–437.

Keren, D. F., McDonald, R. A., and Carey, J. L. (1988). Combined parenteral and oral immunization results in an enhanced mucosal immunoglobulin. A response to *Shigella flexneri*. *Infect. Immun.* **56,** 910–915.

Keren, D. F., Brown, J. E., McDonald, R. A., and Wassef, J. S. (1989). Secretory immunoglobulin A response to shiga toxin in rabbits: Kinetics of the initial mucosal immune response and inhibition of toxicity *in vitro* and *in vivo*. *Infect. Immun.* **57,** 1885–1889.

Khoury, S. J., Lider, O., Al-Sabbagh, A., and Weiner, H. L. (1990). Suppression of experimental autoimmune encephalomyelitis by oral administration of myelin basic protein. III. Synergistic effect of lipopolysaccharide. *Cell. Immunol.* **131,** 302–310.

Kiyono, H., Babb, J. L., Michalek, S. M., and McGhee, J. R. (1980). Cellular basis for elevated IgA responses in C3H/HeJ mice. *J. Immunol.* **125,** 732–737.

Kiyono, H., McGhee, J. R., Wannemeuhler, M. J., and Michalek, S. M. (1982). Lack of oral tolerance in C3H/HeJ mice. *J. Exp. Med.* **155,** 605–610.

Lange, S., Lindholm, L., and Holmgren, J. (1978). Interaction of cholera toxin and toxin derivatives with lymphocytes. III. Modulating effects in vivo by cholera toxin on the graft-vs-host reactivity of lymphoid cells: Suggested inhibition of suppressor cells. *Int. Arch. Allegy Appl. Immunol.* **57,** 364–374.

Lebman, D. A., Fuhrman, J. A., and Cebra, J. J. (1988). Intraduodenal application of cholera holotoxin increases the potential of clones from Peyer's patch B cells of relevant and unrelated specificities to secrete IgG and IgA. *Reg. Immunol.* **1,** 32–40.

Lencer, W. I., Delp, C., Neutra, M. R., and Madara, J. L. (1992). Mechanism of cholera toxin action on a polarized human intestinal epithelial cell line: role of vesicular traffic. *J. Cell Biol.* **117,** 1197–1209.

Levine, M. M., Kaper, J. B., Black, R. E., and Clements, M. L. (1983). New knowledge on pathogensis of bacterial enteric infections as applied to vaccine development. *Microbiol. Rev.* **47,** 510–550.

Liang, X. P., Lamm, M. E., and Nedrud, J. G. (1988). Oral administration of cholera toxin–Sendai virus conjugate potentiates gut and respiratory immunity against Sendai virus. *J. Immunol.* **141,** 1495–1501.

Liang, X., Lamm, M. E., and Nedrud, J. G. (1989a). Cholera toxin as a mucosal adjuvant: Glutaraldehyde treatment dissociates adjuvanticity from toxicity. *J. Immunol.* **143,** 484–490.

Liang, X. P., Lamm, M. E., and Nedrud, J. G. (1989b). Cholera toxin as a mucosal adjuvant for respiratory antibody responses in mice. *Reg. Immunol.* **2,** 244–248.

Locht, C., Barstad, P. A., Coligan, J. E., Mayer, L., Munoz, J. J., Smith, S. G., and Keith, J. M. (1986). Molecular cloning of pertussis toxin genes. *Nucleic Acids Res.* **14,** 3251–3261.

Lovgren, K. (1988). The serum antibody response distributed in subclasses and isotypes after intranasal and subcutaneous immunization with influenza virus immunostimulating complexes. *Scand. J. Immunol.* **27,** 241–245.

Lovgren, K., Kaberg, H., and Morein, B. (1990). An experimental influenza subunit vaccine (iscom): Induction of protective immunity to challenge infection in mice after intranasal or subcutaneous administration. *Clin. Exp. Immunol.* **82,** 435–439.

Lycke, N., and Holmgren, J. (1986a). Intestinal mucosal memory and presence of memory cells in lamina propria and Peyer's patches in mice 2 years after oral immunization with cholera toxin. *Scand. J. Immunol.* **23,** 611–616.

Lycke, N., and Holmgren, J. (1986b). Strong adjuvant properties of cholera toxin on gut mucosal immune responses to orally presented antigens. *Immunology* **59,** 301–308.

Lycke, N., and Strober, W. (1989). Cholera toxin promotes B cell isotype differentiation. *J. Immunol.* **142,** 3781–3787.

Lycke, N., Erikson, L., and Holmgren, J. (1987). Protection against cholera toxin after oral immunization is thymus-dependent and associated with intestinal production of neutralizing IgA antitoxin. *Scand. J. Immunol.* **25,** 413–419.

Lycke, N., Bromander, A. K., Ekman, L., Karlsson, U., and Holmgren, J. (1989). Cellular basis of immunomodulation by cholera toxin *in vitro* with possible association to the adjuvant function in vivo. *J. Immunol.* **142,** 20–27.

Lycke, N., Karlsson, U., Sjolander, A., and Magnusson, K. E. (1991). The adjuvant action of cholera toxin is associated with an increased intestinal permeability for luminal antigens. *Scand. J. Immunol.* **33,** 691–698.

Lycke, N., Tsuji, T., and Holmgren, J. (1992). The adjuvant effect of Vibrio cholerae and Escherichia coli heat-labile enterotoxins is linked to their ADP-ribosyltransferase activity. *Eur. J. Immunol.* **22,** 2277–2281.

McKenzie, S. J., and Halsey, J. F. (1984). Cholera toxin B subunit as a carrier protein to stimulate a mucosal immune response. *J. Immunol.* **133,** 1818–1824.

Mayer, L., and Schlien, R. (1987). Evidence for function of Ia molecules on gut epithelial cells in man. *J. Exp. Med.* **166,** 1471–1483.

Michalek, S. M., McGhee, J. R., Kiyono, H., Colwell, D. E., Eldridge, J. H., Wannemuehler, M. J., and Koopman, W. J. (1983a). The IgA response: Inductive aspects, regulatory cells, and effector functions. *Ann. N.Y. Acad. Sci.* **409,** 48–69.

Michalek, S. M., Morisaki, I., Gregory, R. L., Kiyono, H., Hamada, S., and McGhee, J. R. (1983b). Oral adjuvants enhance IgA responses to *Streptococcus mutans*. *Mol. Immunol.* **20,** 1009–1018.

Mitchell, G. F., and Munoz, J. J. (1983). Vaccination of genetically susceptible mice against chronic infection with *Nematospiroides dubius* using pertussigen as adjuvant. *Aust. J. Exp. Biol. Med. Sci.* **61,** 425–434.

Mizoguchi, K., Nakashima, I., Hasegawa, Y., Isobe, K., Nagase, F., Kawashima, K., Shimokata, K., and Kato, N. (1986). Augmentation of antibody responses of mice to inhaled protein antigens by simultaneously inhaled bacterial lipopolysaccharides. *Immunobiology* **173,** 63–71.

Morasaki, I., Michalek, S. M., Harmon, C. C., Torii, M., Hamada, S., and McGhee, J. R. (1983). Effective immunity to dental caries: Enhancement of salivary anti-*Streptococcus mutans* antibody responses with oral adjuvants. *Infect. Immun.* **40,** 577–591.

Morein, B. (1987). Potentiation of the immune response by immunization with antigens in defined multimeric physical forms. *Vet. Immunol. Immunopathol.* **17,** 153–159.

Morein, B. (1990). The iscom: An immunostimulating system. *Immunol. Lett.* **25,** 281–283.

Morein, B., Ekstrom, J., and Lovgren, K. (1990). Increased immunogenicity of a nonamphipathic protein (BSA) after inclusion into iscoms. *J. Immunol. Meth.* **128,** 177–181.

Mosmann, T. R., and Coffman, R. L. (1989). Th1 and Th2 cells: Different patterns of lymphokine secretion lead to different functional properties. *Ann. Rev. Immunol.* **7,** 145–174.

Mowat, A. M., and Donachie, A. M. (1991). ISCOMS–A novel strategy for mucosal immunization? *Immunol. Today* **12,** 383–385.

Mowat, A. M., Thomas, M. J., MacKenzie, S., and Parrott, D. M. V. (1986). Divergent effects of bacterial lipopolysaccharide on immunity to orally administered protein and particulate antigens in mice. *Immunology* **58,** 677–684.

Mowat, A. M., Donachie, A. M., Reid, G., and Jarrett, O. (1991). Immune-stimulating complexes containing Quil A and protein antigen prime class I MHC-restricted T lymphocytes *in vivo* and are immunogenic by the oral route. *Immunology* **72,** 317–322.

Munoz, J. J., Arai, H., Bergman, R. K., and Sadowski, P. L. (1981). Biological activities of crystalline pertussigen from *Bordetella pertussis*. *Infect. Immun.* **33,** 820–826.

Murray, M., Robinson, P. B., Grierson, C., and Crawford, R. A. (1979). Immunization against *Nippostrongylus brasiliensis* in the rat. A study on the use of antigen extracted from adult parasites and the parameters which influence the level of protection. *Acta Trop. (Basel)* **36,** 297–322.

Murray, P. D., McKenzie, D. T., Swain, S. L., and Kagnoff, M. F. (1987) Interleukin 5 and interleukin 4 produced by Peyer's patch T cells selectively enhance immunoglobulin A expression. *J. Immunol.* **139,** 2669–2674.

Nagy, B., Hoglund, S., and Morein, B. (1990). Iscom (immunostimulating complex) vaccines containing mono- or polyvalent pili of enterotoxigenic *E. coli;* immune response of rabbit and swine. *Zentralbl. Veterinärmed.* **37,** 728–738.

Nedrud, J. G., Liang, X. P., Hague, N., and Lamm, M. E. (1987). Combined oral/nasal immunization protects mice from Sendai virus infection. *J. Immunol.* **139,** 3484–3492.

Ogawa, T., Kotani, S., and Shimauchi, H. (1986). Enhancement of serum antibody production in mice by oral administration of lipophilic derivatives of muramylpeptides and bacterial lipopolysaccharides with bovine serum albumin. *Methods Find. Exp. Clin. Pharmacol.* **8,** 19–26.

Ohta, M., Nakashima, I., and Kato, N. (1982). Adjuvant action of bacterial lipopolysaccharide in induction of delayed-type hypersensitivity to protein antigens. II. Relationships of intensity of the action to that of other immunological activities. *Immunobiology* **163,** 460–466.

Okutomi, T., Inagawa, H., Nishizawa, T., Oshima, H., Soma, G., and Mizuno, D. (1990). Priming effect of orally administered muramyl dipeptide on induction of exogenous tumor necrosis factor. *J. Biol. Resp. Mod.* **9,** 564–569.

Parant, M., Parant, F., and Chedid, L. (1978). Enhancement of the neonate's nonspecific immunity to *Klebsiella* infection by muramyl dipeptide, a synthetic immunoadjuvant. *Proc. Natl. Acad. Sci. U.S.A.* **75,** 3395–3399.

Peppard, J. V., Mann, R. V., and Montgomery, P. C. (1988). Antibody production in rats following ocular-topical or gastrointestinal immunization: Kinetics of local and systemic antibody production. *Curr. Eye Res.* **7,** 471–481.

Pierce, N. F., and Cray, W. C. (1982). Determinants of the localization, magnitude, and duration of a specific mucosal IgA plasma cell response in enterically immunized rats. *J. Immunol.* **128,** 1311–1315.

Pierce, N. F., and Gowans, J. L. (1975). Cellular kinetics of the intestinal immune response to cholera toxoid in rats. *J. Exp. Med.* **142,** 1550–1563.

Pierce, N. F., and Sacci, J. B. J. (1984). Enhanced mucosal priming by cholera toxin and procholeragenoid with a lipoidal amine adjuvant (avridine) delivered in liposomes. *Infect. Immun.* **44,** 469–473.

Que, J. U., Cryz, S. J., Ballou, R., Furer, E., Gross, M., Young, J., Wasserman, G. J., Loomis, L. A., and Sadoff, J. C. (1988). Effect of carrier selection on immunogenicity of protein conjugate vaccines against *Plasmodium falciparum* circumsporozoites. *Infect. Immun.* **56,** 2645–2649.

Robbins, J., Schneerson, R., Szu, S. C., Fattom, A., Yang, Y., Lagergard, T., Chu, C., and Sorensen, U. S. (1989). Prevention of invasive bacterial diseases by immunization with polysaccharide-protein conjugates. *In* "New Strategies for Oral Immunization" (J. Mestecky and J. R. McGhee, ed.), pp. 169–180. Springer-Verlag, New York.

Sanchez, J., Svennerhom, A. M., and Holmgren, J. (1988). Genetic fusion of a nontoxic heat-stable enterotoxin-related decapeptide-antigen to cholera toxin B subunit. *FEBS Lett.* **241,** 110–114.

Schodel, F., and Will, H. (1989). Construction of a plasmid for expression of foreign epitopes as fusion proteins with subunit B of *Escherichia coli* heat-labile enterotoxin. *Infect. Immun.* **57,** 1347–1350.

Sixma, T. K., Pronk, S. E., Kalk, K. H., Wartna, E. S., van Zanten, B. A. M., Witholt, B., and Hol, W. G. (1991). Crystal structure of a cholera toxin-related heat-labile enterotoxin from *E. coli. Nature (London)* **351,** 371–377.

Snapper, C. M., and Paul, W. E. (1987). Interferon-gamma and B cell stimulatory factor-1 reciprocally regulate Ig isotype production. *Science* **236,** 944–947.

Spriggs, D. R., and Koff, W. C., eds. (1991). "Topics in Vaccine Adjuvant Research." CRC Press, Boca Raton, Florida.

Szu, S. C., Li, X., Schneerson, R., Vickers, J. H., Bryla, D., and Robbins, J. B. (1989). Comparative immunogenicities of Vi polysaccharide-protein conjugates composed of cholera toxin or its B subunit as a carrier bound to high- or lower-molecular weight Vi. *Infect. Immun.* **57,** 3823–3827.

Takada, H., and Kotani, S. (1989). Structural requirements of lipid A for endotoxicity and other biological activities. *Crit. Rev. Microbiol.* **16,** 477–523.

Takahashi, H., Takeshita, T., Morein, B., Putney, S., Germain, R. N., and Berzofsky, J. A. (1990). Induction of CD8+ cytotoxic T cells by immunization with purified HIV-1 envelope protein in ISCOMs. *Nature (London)* **344,** 873–875.

Takahashi, I., Okahashi, N., Kanamoto, T., Asakawa, H., and Koga, T. (1990). Intranasal immunization of mice with recombinant protein antigen of serotype c *Streptococcus mutans* and cholera toxin B subunit. *Arch. Oral Biol.* **35,** 475–477.

Takayama, K., Ribi, E., and Cantrell, J. L. (1981). Isolation of a nontoxic lipid A fraction containing tumor regression activity. *Cancer Res.* **41,** 2654–2660.

Tamura, S. I., Tanaka, H., Takayama, R., Sato, H., Sato, Y., and Uchida, N. (1985). Break of unresponsiveness of delayed-type-hypersensitivity to sheep red blood cells by pertussis toxin. *Cell. Immunol.* **92,** 376–382.

Tamura, S., Samegai, Y., Kurata, H., Nagamine, T., Aizawa, C., and Kurata, T. (1988). Protection against influenza virus infection by vaccine inoculated intranasally with cholera toxin B subunit. *Vaccine* **6,** 409–413.

Tesch, H., Muller, W., and Rajewsky, K. (1986). Lymphokines regulate immunoglobulin isotype expression in an antigen-specific immune response. *J. Immunol.* **136,** 2892–2895.

Thapar, M. A., Parr, E. L., and Parr, M. B. (1990a). The effect of adjuvants on antibody titers in mouse vaginal fluid after intravaginal immunization. *J. Reprod. Immunol.* **17,** 207–216.

Thapar, M. A., Parr, E. L., and Parr, M. B. (1990b). Secretory immune responses in mouse vaginal fluid after pelvic, parenteral, or vaginal immunization. *Immunology* **70,** 121–125.

Thapar, M. A., Parr, E. L., Bozzola, J. J., and Parr, M. B. (1991). Secretory immune responses in the mouse vagina after parenteral or intravaginal immunization with an immunostimulating complex (ISCOM). *Vaccine* **9,** 129–133.

Ulrich, J. T., Cantrell, J. L., Gustafson, G. L., Myers, K. R., Rudbach, J. A., and Hiernaux, J. R. (1991). The adjuvant activity of monophosphoryl lipid A. *In* "Topics in Vaccine Adjuvant Research" (D. R. Spriggs and W. C. Koff, ed.), pp. 133–143. CRC Press, Boca Raton, Florida.

Unanue, E. R., and Cerottini, J. C. (1989). Antigen presentation. *FASEB J.* **3,** 2496–2502.

Van der Heijden, P. J., Bianchi, A. T., Dol, M., Pals, J. W., Stok, W., and Bokhout, B. A. (1991). Manipulation of intestinal immune responses against ovalbumin by cholera toxin and its B subunit in mice. *Immunology* **72,** 89–93.

Vajdy, M., and Lycke, N. Y. (1992). Cholera toxin adjuvant promotes long-term immunological memory in the gut mucosa to unrelated immunogens after oral immunization. *Immunology* **75,** 488–492.

Verheul, A. F. M., Versteeg, A., DeReuver, M. J., Jansze, M., and Snippe, H. (1989). Modulation of the immune response to pneumococcal type 14 capsular polysaccharide-protein conjugates by the adjuvant quil A depends on the properties of the conjugates. *Infect. Immun.* **57,** 1078–1083.

Waksman, B. H. (1979). Adjuvants and immune regulation by lymphoid cells. *Springer Sem. Immunopathol.* **2,** 5–33.

Warren, H. S., Vogel, F. R., and Chedid, L. A. (1986). Current status of immunological adjuvants. *Ann. Rev. Immunol.* **4,** 369–388.

White, R. G. (1967). Concepts relating to the mode of action of adjuvants. *In* "International Symposium on Adjuvants of Immunity" (R. H. Regamey, W. Hennessen, D. Ikic, and J. Ungar, ed.), pp. 3–12. Karger, Basel.

Wilson, A. D., Clarke, C. J., and Stokes, C. R. (1990). Whole cholera toxin and B subunit act synergistically as an adjuvant for the mucosal immune response of mice to keyhole limpet haemocyanin. *Scand. J. Immunol.* **31,** 443–451.

Woogen, S. D., Ealding, W., and Elson, C. O. (1987). Inhibition of murine lymphocyte proliferation by th B subunit of cholera toxin. *J. Immunol.* **139,** 3764–3770.

Xu-Amano, J., Jackson, R. J., Staats, H. F., Fujihashi, K., Kiyono, H., Burrows, P. D., Elson, C. O., Pillai, S., and McGhee, J. R. (1993). Helper T cell subsets for IgA responses. Oral immunization with tetanus toxoid and cholera toxin as adjuvant selectively induces Th2 cells in mucosa-associated tissues. *J. Exp. Med.,* in press.

34

Monoclonal Secretory IgA for Protection of the Intestinal Mucosa against Viral and Bacterial Pathogens

Jean-Pierre Kraehenbuhl • Marian R. Neutra

I. ROLE OF SECRETORY IgA IN INTESTINAL PROTECTION: UNRESOLVED ISSUES

A. Current Views of the Role of IgA

Secretory IgA is the major class of immunoglobulin found in the secretions bathing mucosal surfaces in the normal gastrointestinal tract, in part because immunoglobulin transport across epithelial surfaces into secretions is a receptor-mediated process requiring specific interaction of polymeric immunoglobulins (primarily dimeric IgA) with the polymeric immunoglobulin receptor (Kraehenbuhl and Neutra, 1992a; Mostov *et al.,* 1980,1984). In addition, monomeric IgG that enters secretions through fluid-phase transport or paracellular leakage is degraded readily by proteases in the intestine, whereas dimeric or polymeric SIgA resists hydrolysis (Lindh, 1975). Since SIgA has at least four antigen binding sites, it should be more effective than IgG in forming microbe–antibody complexes and aggregating intestinal pathogens. Whether the polymeric nature of sIgA is essential to its protective function, however, has not been proven.

The mechanisms by which IgA may prevent epithelial contact and mucosal disease are discussed in detail in Chapter 11 but are summarized here to provide background for specific studies using monoclonal IgAs. Bacteria aggregated by IgA may be unable to exploit motility and chemotactic mechanisms to move through mucus and toward epithelial targets (McCormick *et al.,* 1988). Aggregates of bacteria, viruses and macromolecules would be cleared efficiently from the lumen by peristalsis, and clearance is thought to be enhanced by entrapment of IgA–microbe complexes in the interstices of the mucus gel (Neutra and Forstner, 1987). Although a specific interaction of IgA and mucus glycoproteins has been proposed (Creeth, 1978), it has not been confirmed in studies using highly purified mucins (Crowther *et al.,* 1985). Evidence also suggests that IgA can protect epithelial surfaces by specifically blocking the microbial adhesins required for attachment (Williams and Gibbons, 1972). This hypothesis has been difficult to test, however, since most bacteria can use multiple adhesion mechanisms, and polyclonal SIgAs in secretions are directed against multiple antigens and epitopes. This idea is difficult to prove even with monoclonal IgAs, because the large size of dimeric or polymeric immunoglobulins may sterically hinder microbial binding sites even when directed against a nonadhesive component.

Secretory IgA has been found, in most studies, to lack complement-fixing, opsonizing, and direct bacteriocidal activity (Mestecky, 1988; Childers *et al.,* 1989; Kerr, 1990). These characteristics are consistent with its function in the external milieu, usually in the absence of serum proteins and macrophages. On the other hand, SIgA in the lumen may interact with molecules in milk such as lactoferrin and lactoperoxidase and enhance their bacteriocidal activities (Arnold *et al.,* 1980; Tenovuo *et al.,* 1982). In addition, evidence suggests that SIgA can enhance antibody-dependent cytotoxicity by mucosal lymphocytes, and has been suggested to somehow "arm" lymphocytes in the lumen and thus promote direct killing of bacteria (Tagliabue *et al.,* 1985).

B. Importance of Specific IgAs in Protection

Testing of these ideas has been hampered by the limited availability of specific dimeric IgAs in quantities sufficient for *in vivo* and *in vitro* experimentation. Monoclonal IgA antibodies were generated against viral pathogens that colonize and invade mucosal surfaces of the respiratory system (see Chapters 29 and 30). These reagents were used to show that IgAs can indeed provide protection against airway infection and subsequent pulmonary disease, whether applied passively to mucosal surfaces (Mazanec *et al.,* 1987) or secreted actively into the airways after intravenous injection (Renegar and Small, 1991). Passive application of corresponding monoclonal IgGs also was protective, however, suggesting that the dimeric nature of IgA may be important only in insuring transepithelial delivery and increasing protease resistance. On the other hand, precisely measuring local concentrations of secreted immunoglobulins in the microenvironment of epithelial surfaces and within the mucus coat requires special techniques (Haneberg *et al.,* in press). Experiments often involve application of large amounts of exogenous antibodies to the luminal side of the mucus blanket.

In the intestine, abundant evidence is found that SIgA in secretions is associated with protection against enterotoxigenic and invasive enteric pathogens (Levine *et al.*, 1983,1988), but whether SIgA alone can provide such protection has not been clear. Transport of enteric bacteria and viruses by M cells and subsequent "sampling" by cells in organized mucosal lymphoid tissues generally results in production of both IgG- and IgA-producing cells, and in some cases also induces cell-mediated immunity. After oral immunization or natural disease, the presence of all these types of immune protection, as well as nonimmune protection mechanisms, complicates the analysis of IgA action. In addition, the SIgA response *in vivo* is polyclonal and, although the antigen specificities have been documented partially, in some cases (Sears *et al.*, 1984; Svennerholm *et al.*, 1984; Cancellieri and Fara, 1985; Tacket *et al.*, 1990), little information is available concerning the exact epitopes that are present after intestinal passage and M cell transport and that are most immunogenic in the mucosa (for review, see Kraehenbuhl and Neutra, 1992b; Neutra and Kraehenbuhl, 1992). Finally, the relative protective capacities of individual SIgAs have not been tested systematically or compared in the intestinal system. These issues must be addressed for each of the many bacterial, viral, protozoal, and parasitic pathogens that colonize the intestinal lumen, infect the intestinal mucosa, or use the intestinal epithelium as an invasion route.

C. Role of IgA in Modulating the Mucosal Immune Response

Secretory IgA antibodies in mucosal or glandular secretions are able to bind to the apical membranes of M cells in follicle-associated epithelia and enter organized mucosal lymphoid tissue from the lumen by M-cell transepithelial transport (Roy and Varvayanis, 1987; Weltzin *et al.*, 1989). This transport allows secretory IgA and sIgA–antigen complexes to interact with lymphocytes and antigen-presenting cells that express IgA binding sites. IgA binding sites (FcA receptors) on T- and B-cell subsets have been detected in peripheral and mucosal lymphoid tissue from several species (Kerr, 1990). Once transported into organized mucosal lymphoid tissue, IgA antibodies (associated or not with antigen) could mediate several functions. First, they may modulate the immune response in the organized mucosal lymphoid tissue: polymeric but not monomeric IgA is known to upregulate FcA receptors on cloned T cells (Kiyono and McGhee, 1987). Some of the T cells in Peyer's patches expressing FcA receptors are able to function as helper cells, increasing the number of IgA-positive B cells (Kiyono *et al.*, 1984). Pre-incubation of these T helper cells with IgA, however, blocks this response (Kiyono *et al.*, 1985). Second, since antigen–SIgA complexes are transported across M cells into the underlying lymphoid tissue (Weltzin *et al.*, 1989), FcA receptors on antigen-presenting cells (B cells and macrophages) may facilitate uptake and processing of antigens. In this way, re-uptake of secreted IgA may constitute an amplification loop, enhancing the immune response and contributing to secondary responses. Finally, IgA re-uptake by M cells may regulate an immune response through the idiotypic network. Anti-idiotypic IgA antibodies in glandular and mucosal secretions could follow the M-cell uptake pathway to prime the mucosal immune system actively. Such a mechanism has been proposed to explain why breast-fed infants that acquire the IgA repertoire of their mothers via milk respond to parenteral or peroral vaccines (Hanson *et al.*, 1990). Whether the anti-idiotypic network can be used in mucosal vaccine strategies remains to be established.

II. GENERATION AND ANALYSIS OF MONOCLONAL IgA

A. Development of Methods for Production of IgA Hybridomas

Conventional systemic immunization methods followed by fusion of spleen cells with myeloma cells yields IgA hybridomas only rarely. We now recognize that mucosal immunization, and the isotype switch that occurs under the influence of specific cytokines in the organized mucosal lymphoid tissue, is a prerequisite for generation of IgA-committed lymphoblasts (Kiyono *et al.*, 1984; McGhee *et al.*, 1989). These lymphoblasts are known to migrate from inductive sites in the mucosa to regional mesenteric lymph nodes, to proliferate and there to return via the bloodstream to mucosal effector sites (Craig and Cebra, 1971). Several investigators have exploited this migration phenomenon to obtain IgA hybridomas. For example, IgA hybridomas were generated by fusion of spleen cells from mucosally immunized mice (Colwell *et al*, 1986; Mazanec *et al.*, 1987). Fusion of cells from mesenteric lymph nodes and thoracic duct lymph (Styles *et al.*, 1984; Rits *et al.*, 1986) or a mixture of cells from mesenteric lymph nodes and Peyer's patches (Komisar *et al.*, 1982) also yielded significant numbers of IgA hybridomas. We have found that fusion of Peyer's patch cells alone provides a very efficient means of generating IgA hybridomas, and that immunization by gastric intubation or intraluminal injection alone, without intraperitoneal priming, is effective (Weltzin *et al.*, 1989; Winner *et al.*, 1991; Michetti *et al.*, 1992; Apter *et al.*, 1993a). In our experience, direct injection into Peyer's patch tissue is less effective, presumably because the immune response is most efficient when M cells deliver the immunogens directly to organized assemblies of antigen-processing and presenting cells (Ermak *et al.*, 1990). Cells are isolated 5 days after the last peroral immunization by excision of Peyer's patch mucosa and digestion in collagenase, followed by maceration of the tissue. Released cells are fused with mouse myeloma cells using standard procedures. In our hands, at least 50% of the pathogen- or antigen-specific hybridomas generated by this method are of the IgA type. When *Salmonella typhimurium* was used as mucosal immunogen, all 48 stable anti-*Salmonella* hybridomas obtained produced IgA antibodies (Michetti *et al.*, 1992).

B. *Evaluation of Monoclonal IgAs*

The antigen specificities of mucosally derived IgA antibodies are determined using standard immunochemical assays such as enzyme-linked immunosorbent assay (ELISA), Western immunoblot, and immunoprecipitation. Before evaluating their function in protection, however, these antibodies must be shown to be structurally and functionally analogous to the IgAs produced by normal subepithelial plasma cells. To verify the molecular forms of IgA produced, antibodies concentrated from IgA hybridoma supernatants are separated by gradient SDS–PAGE under nonreducing conditions and visualized by immunoblot analysis (Weltzin *et al.*, 1989; Winner *et al.*, 1991). We have found that almost all IgA hybridomas derived from Peyer's patch cells produce IgA primarily in dimeric form, with some monomers and higher polymers. IgAs metabolically labeled in hybridoma culture, when injected intravenously into rats, were transported efficiently into bile and recovered as dimers and polymers with molecular weights that increased by an amount consistent with the addition of secretory component (SC) during transport across hepatocytes (Weltzin *et al.*, 1989). This result confirms that the monoclonal IgAs are recognized by polymeric immunoglobulin receptors and can be transported into secretions, either by hepatocytes and epithelial cells *in vivo* or by epithelial cells in culture, as described subsequently.

III. EXPERIMENTAL METHODS FOR TESTING PROTECTIVE FUNCTIONS OF MONOCLONAL IgA

A. *Passive Oral Administration* in Vivo

SIgA functions on mucosal surfaces. Passive application of monoclonal IgA or IgG antibodies to respiratory mucosa provides protection against viral infection. Thus, assuming that oral ingestion of specific IgAs might protect against enteric infections seems reasonable. The environment of the gastrointestinal tract lacks the specific IgA proteases produced by certain *respiratory* pathogens, but is extremely rich in digestive proteases that readily degrade IgG and monomeric IgA (Brown *et al.*, 1970; Underdown and Dorrington, 1974; Lindh, 1975). Secretory polymeric IgA is relatively resistant to these enzymes; secretory IgA of human milk can survive the stomach and intestine since it can be recovered from feces (Cancellieri and Fara, 1985; Hanson *et al.*, 1990). Ingestion of human milk from orally immunized mothers that contained natural polyclonal secretory IgA against *Vibrio cholerae* lipopolysaccharide (LPS) has been shown to protect infants against cholera (Glass *et al.*, 1983).

Monoclonal IgA lacks secretory component, however, and would be degraded more readily in the gastrointestinal tract (Underdown and Dorrington, 1974; Lindh, 1975). Although dimeric IgA is more stable than monomeric IgG, the exact survival time of dimeric monoclonal IgA without SC in the human stomach and intestine is not known. A more difficult problem is that of achieving effective predictable antibody distribution over the lining of the entire 4.5 m of human intestine after an oral dose, and correctly timing the oral IgA to coincide with local microbial challenge. Whereas normally secreted IgA antibodies are delivered into intestinal crypts and directly onto epithelial surfaces, orally administered IgA might never reach these sites. Despite these concerns, evidence suggests that oral monoclonal IgA can protect the intestinal mucosa passively. For example, studies in our laboratories showed that, in suckling mice (in which protease activity is low), a single oral dose of monoclonal IgA provided passive protection against viral and bacterial challenge for up to 3 hr. Further, human serum immunoglobulins (primarily IgG), fed with infant formula, appeared to prevent intestinal disease in high risk infants (Eibl *et al.*, 1988).

B. *Hybridoma "Backpack" Tumor Method*

To achieve continuous widespread delivery of monoclonal IgA into secretions, we took advantage of the facts that hybridoma cells can form immunoglobulin-producing tumors *in vivo* (Harris *et al.*, 1982) and that circulating dimeric IgA binds to epithelial pIg receptors and is transported into secretions (Jackson *et al.*, 1977). Serum antibodies can diffuse readily to IgA-transporting epithelial cells in the liver and intestine because capillaries in these tissues are fenestrated (with the exception of Peyer's patches; Allen and Trier, 1991). When IgA-producing hybridoma cells are injected subcutaneously on the upper backs of adult BALB/c mice, well-organized tumors with blood and lymphatic vessels form within 1–2 weeks. In newborns, the cells grow in a more dispersed fashion under the loose dorsal skin. In adult mice, increasing levels of specific monoclonal IgA in serum were shown to be accompanied by increasing levels in secretions (Winner *et al.*, 1991). In contrast, antibodies from IgG-producing hybridoma tumors enter secretions in low amounts despite very high blood levels. Thus, with the IgA hybridoma backpack tumor method, monoclonal IgA can be delivered continually into secretions via the physiological route, with addition of secretory component. Mice bearing hybridoma tumors are not strictly analogous to normal immunized mice secreting endogenous IgA, however. In a normal mucosal immune response, dimeric IgA is produced locally by subepithelial plasma cells and blood levels of IgA are relatively low (Mestecky, 1988) whereas, in "backpack" mice, blood and tissue levels of monoclonal antibody may be very high (Winner *et al.*, 1991). This method nevertheless allows for assessment of the protective capacities of specific SIgA antibodies in the absence of other immune protection mechanisms, and has been applied in studies of several pathogens that can colonize or invade the mouse intestine.

C. *Epithelial Monolayers* in Vitro

The development of improved epithelial cell culture systems and the availability of well-characterized lines of human intestinal epithelial cells have opened the way for new *in vitro* approaches to analysis of mucosal immune protection. Certain cell lines and subclones derived from human colon carcinomas form confluent polarized monolayers in culture that display many of the features of the normal differentiated intestinal epithelium (Rousset, 1986; Huet *et al.*, 1987; Madara *et al.*, 1987; Neutra and Louvard, 1989). Although these cell lines do not strictly replicate normal cell phenotypes and do not reproduce the complex microenvironment of mucosal surfaces, they provide valuable models in which to test the interactions of microbial pathogens and toxins with epithelial cells and the ability of IgA to prevent these interactions.

Confluent MDCK (Madin-Darby canine kidney) cells and Caco-2 (human colon carcinoma) cells have been used to evaluate *Salmonella* factors involved in attachment and invasion (Finlay *et al.*, 1988; Finlay and Falkow, 1990; Lee and Falkow, 1990). Studies in our laboratories have shown that monolayers of subcloned HT29 cells, representing either absorptive cell or goblet cell phenotypes in various stages of differentiation, also can be infected by *S. typhimurium*. The presence in the apical medium of specific monoclonal IgAs directed against a surface component of *S. typhimurium* significantly reduced epithelial infection in both MDCK and HT29 cells. Relatively high concentrations of antibody were required, however, perhaps because the nonimmune protection mechanisms such as peristalsis and clearance that operate in concert with IgA *in vivo* are not present *in vitro*.

In other studies, monoclonal IgA directed against the B subunit of cholera toxin protected confluent polarized T84 cell monolayers against toxin binding, and thus also prevented the toxin-induced chloride secretory response (Apter *et al.*, 1991). Some epithelial cell lines or clones express endogenous polymeric immunoglobulin receptors and are capable of vectorial IgA transport (Roa *et al.*, 1987); others can be transfected with receptor cDNA to induce receptor expression (Hirt *et al.*, 1992). This approach allowed testing of epithelial protection during active IgA secretion *in vitro* (Mazanec *et al.*, 1992). In addition, this model has been used to demonstrate transport of IgA immune complexes from the basolateral to the apical compartment, suggesting that IgA secretion may serve to clear antigens or pathogens from the interstitial compartment (Kaetzel *et al.*, 1991).

IV. EVALUATION OF IgA PROTECTION AGAINST ENTERIC PATHOGENS

A. Vibrio cholerae

Vibrio cholerae causes disease by colonizing the epithelial surface of the intestinal mucosa and secreting cholera toxin that binds with high affinity to a specific ganglioside, GM1, in cell membranes. Entry of vibrios into the luminal microenvironment is associated with expression of the *ToxR* gene product, which in turn regulates several other genes including those involved in adherence, colony formation, and toxin production (Taylor *et al.*, 1987; Miller *et al.*, 1989). *Vibrio cholerae* infection or immunization with bacterial cells and toxin evokes SIgA directed against both toxin and bacterial surface components including LPS. SIgA secretion is associated with protection against subsequent challenge (Cash *et al.*, 1974; Levine *et al.*, 1983; Svennerholm *et al.*, 1984). The relative importance of specific IgAs in protection, however, was not established. Both cholera toxin and *V. cholerae* bind to M cells and are transported efficiently into Peyer's patch mucosa, so both would be expected to evoke specific IgA lymphoblasts. We used such cells to generate hybridomas that produce monoclonal IgAs directed against a strain-specific carbohydrate epitope of bacterial LPS that is exposed on the bacterial surface (Winner *et al.*, 1991), and against the binding subunit of cholera toxin (CTB) (Apter *et al.*, 1991). We then tested the protective capacities of these IgAs against virulent organisms and toxin *in vivo* and *in vitro* (Apter *et al.*, 1991).

Using the hybridoma backpack tumor system in suckling mice, we showed that secretion of monoclonal SIgA directed against a single Ogawa strain-specific LPS epitope protected mice against oral challenge with 100 times the LD_{50} of virulent Ogawa organisms (Winner *et al.*, 1991). Protection was specific, since mice were not protected by secretion of irrelevant IgAs and anti-LPS tumors failed to protect against virulent *V. cholerae* of the Inaba strain (Winner *et al.*, 1991). Secretion of anti-CTB IgA from hybridoma tumors, in contrast, failed to protect against the same challenge (Apter *et al.*, 1991), presumably because anti-LPS IgA effectively aggregates vibrios in the lumen and prevents colonization (Manning, 1987) whereas antitoxin IgA permits colonization. Once colonies are established, the secreted antitoxin IgA may not be of sufficient concentration or affinity to intercept toxin secreted directly into the enterocyte glycocalyx on the mucosal surface. In addition, SIgA may not diffuse readily into the extracellular pilus-rich matrix of established bacterial colonies.

The same monoclonal IgAs were tested for their ability to provide passive oral protection against live organisms or purified toxin. Oral administration of a single dose of as little as 5 μg anti-LPS IgA prevented *V. cholerae*-induced diarrheal disease, but only when the bacterial challenge was given within 3 hr of the IgA (Apter *et al.*, 1991), confirming the need for repeated administration or continuous secretion of IgA to compensate for peristalsis and clearance. Oral delivery of up to 80 μg antitoxin IgA failed to protect against live vibrios, but did provide some protection against oral challenge with the ED_{50} (5 μg) of toxin alone. Collectively, these studies indicate that anti-LPS SIgA is much more efficient than antitoxin SIgA in providing protection against virulent *V. cholerae*. This result is consistent with evidence from oral cholera vaccine trials in which antibodies against the bacterial cells were found to be an important component in protection (Levine *et al.*, 1988; Holmgren *et al.*, 1989; Kaper, 1989).

B. Salmonella typhimurium

Salmonella typhimurium infection in mice is analogous to *Salmonella typhi* infection (typhoid fever) in humans. Both cause lethal systemic disease by invading the intestinal mucosa via the M cells of Peyer's patches and also via enterocytes (Takeuchi, 1975; Hohmann *et al.*, 1978; Kohbata, 1986) and then spreading via the bloodstream to the liver, spleen, and other organs. We used this model to test whether secretory IgA alone can prevent infection of the mucosa by an invasive organism and hence prevent systemic disease (Michetti *et al.*, 1992). Hybridomas were generated after oral immunization of BALB/c mice with attenuated mutant strains of *S. typhimurium* and 48 stable IgA-producing cell lines were obtained. One of these, called Sal 4, produced monoclonal dimeric IgA directed against a surface carbohydrate epitope present on wild-type organisms.

Sal 4 IgA was tested for protection in adult mice using the hybridoma backpack tumor method (Michetti *et al.*, 1992). As control, a *S. typhimurium* mutant was identified and characterized that lacked the epitope and "escaped" IgA-mediated aggregation *in vitro*, but was nevertheless fully virulent. Backpack tumor-bearing mice challenged with wild-type organisms were protected against systemic disease, whereas those challenged with the "escape" mutant were infected consistently. When using this method with invasive organisms, however, recall that abnormally high levels of specific IgA are present in the blood and tissues of tumor-bearing mice that might provide protection after invasion has occurred. Mice with Sal 4 tumors, however, were not protected against intraperitoneal challenge with *S. typhimurium*. Further, tumor-bearing mice showed a dramatic decrease in *S. typhimurium* recovered from Peyer's patch mucosa. Thus, secreted monoclonal IgA, not the circulating antibody, provided the protection observed. These experiments confirm that SIgA protects by preventing access of organisms to the mucosal surface.

C. Quantitative Aspects of IgA Protection

New approaches such as monoclonal IgA antibodies *in vitro* and a novel "wick" method for sampling of undiluted fluids from mucosal surfaces (Haneberg *et al.*, in press) can now be used to estimate the concentrations of IgA required to protect mucosal surfaces *in vivo*. For example, 4-5 dimeric IgA molecules per cholera holotoxin, or one antibody dimer per B subunit, were required to protect cultured monolayers of T84 enterocytes against toxin-induced chloride secretion (Apter *et al.*, 1991). However, approximately 500,000 specific monoclonal IgA molecules per bacterium were required to protect MDCK cell monolayers against *Salmonella typhimurium* (Michetti *et al.*, 1992). Specific IgA concentrations attained *in vivo* may also be in the μg range. Undiluted mucous secretions harvested by wicks directly from the surface of the small intestinal mucosa of cholera toxin-immunized adult mice contained up to 80 μg/ml of specific anti-cholera toxin IgA. In mice bearing IgA hybridoma tumors, 10 to 15 μg/ml of monoclonal IgA antibody was measured in the same secretions. Lower IgA concentrations could be protective *in vivo* when nonspecific protection mechanisms such as mucus and peristaltic clearance are also at play.

V. STRATEGIES FOR PRODUCTION OF ENGINEERED SECRETORY IgA

In the studies described earlier, monoclonal IgA was administered passively to mucosal surfaces or delivered into secretions of BALB/c mice from hybridoma backpack tumors. The tumor method allows identification of protective antibodies that might be used for passive protection in other species. If IgA antibodies are to be used for this purpose, they should be most effective if secretory component is attached to the antibody, to confer protease resistance.

A. Cloning of the Polymeric Immunoglobulin Receptor and Secretory Component

During normal secretion of dimeric or polymeric IgA, SC is added during receptor-mediated transepithelial transport across mucosal and glandular tissue (Kraehenbuhl and Neutra, 1992a). SC corresponds to the five immunoglobulin-like domains of the polymeric immunoglobulin receptor, and is generated by proteolytic cleavage of the receptor either during transport or at the luminal epithelial cell surface (Mostov *et al.*, 1984; Schaerer *et al.*, 1990). This receptor has been cloned and its primary sequence established in rabbit (Mostov *et al.*, 1984; Schaerer *et al.*, 1990), rat (Banting *et al.*, 1989), and human (Krajči *et al.*, 1989). IgA binds to the outermost Ig-like domain of the receptor (Frutiger *et al.*, 1986). After cleavage of the receptor, a disulfide bond is formed between cysteine residues on the fifth domain of SC and on the Fc portion of one of the IgA monomers. Domains 2, 3, and 4 of SC do not participate in binding but are required to position the cysteine residues involved in disulfide bonds (Solari *et al.*, 1985). A three-dimensional molecular model of the Ig-like domains of SC has been derived from the SC sequence, and from the crystal structure of the immunoglobulin Vκ light chain and the first immunoglobulin-like domain of CD4. The IgA binding site is situated on the first 30 amino acids of domain 1, and corresponds to the first β strand and the loop situated between the first and second β strands (Bakos *et al.*, 1991). In CD4, the analogous loop is involved both in major histocompatibility complex (MHC) Class II interaction and in binding of HIV gp120.

Transfection of several cell types with the cDNA encoding the pIg receptor has resulted in production of membrane-bound receptor and cleaved free SC that can recognize dimeric IgA. These cells include fibroblasts (Dietcher *et al.*, 1986), myeloma cells (P. Michetti and J. P. Kraehenbuhl, unpublished results), epithelial cells including MDCK (Casanova *et al.*, 1990; Hirt *et al.*, 1992,1993), and mammary epithelial cells (Schaerer *et al.*, 1990). In all cases, the receptor was cleaved to produce SC that was released into the medium; in the case of epithelial cells, cleavage and release was polarized as in normal epithelia.

B. Methods for Addition of SC to Monoclonal IgA

Three approaches have been developed in our laboratories to generate complexes of recombinant SC and monoclonal

IgA: coculture of epithelial monolayers and IgA hybridoma cells, transfection of hybridoma cells with cDNA encoding SC, and mixing of recombinant SC with IgA *in vitro*. All three strategies require the insertion of SC cDNA into efficient expression vectors.

The coculture method essentially replicates normal epithelial transport *in vivo*. Epithelial cells such as MDCK cells have been transfected by us and others with rabbit or human pIg receptor cDNA (Casanova *et al.,* 1990). We used an inducible expression vector that contains a kidney-specific MTV promoter and a glucocorticoid-responsive element (Hirt *et al.,* 1992). Stable transfected epithelial cells were grown on permeable substrates (Transwell fiter units) to confluency, and pIg receptor expression was induced. We and others have shown that trafficking of the receptor in the MDCK cell system reflects the behavior observed in normal intestinal epithelial cells (Casanova *et al.,* 1990). When these epithelial monolayers were cultured with IgA-producing hybridoma cells embedded in a collagen gel in the lower chamber of the Transwell device, IgA antibodies were transported efficiently and recovered on the apical side, associated both covalently and noncovalently with SC (Hirt *et al.,* 1993). Although this system produced only 0.1–0.2 μg SIgA per 5 $\times 10^6$ MDCK cells per 24 hr, it provided a source of pure monoclonal SIgA assembled in the normal physiological manner for the first time.

We also have shown that SC cDNA can be introduced into myeloma cells and expressed under the influence of a μ enhancer. This result led to a second approach for production of engineered SIgA in which IgA-producing hybridoma cells were transfected with the cDNA encoding SC. In this case, the cDNA was inserted into vector containing a μ enhancer element and an SV40 promoter. Although one might expect that expression of recombinant SC in hybridoma cells might impair normal IgA assembly, in fact large amounts of complexes containing both SC and IgA were produced by the transfected cells. Preliminary experiments indicate that these molecules exhibit higher resistance to proteases *in vitro* than does IgA produced by nontransfected hybridoma cells. This system might prove to be a valid one for production of engineered SIgA, but whether the assembly of SC and IgA is exactly analogous to that of normal SIgA produced *in vivo* remains to be established.

The third approach may prove to be less complex and more practical, and involves *in vitro* assembly of recombinant SC and monoclonal IgA dimers produced separately by hybridoma cells and one of several transfected cell lines. Although transfected myeloma cells and other cell types can produce free SC, we have attempted to increase the efficiency of SC production by inserting cDNA into the vaccinia virus genome using, as vector, a plasmid containing an efficient vaccinia promoter flanked by thymidine kinase sequences required for homologous recombination. Significant amounts of SC were recovered in the supernatant of infected HeLa cells in suspension and in CV-1 anchorage-dependent cells. Recombinant SC produced in this system binds noncovalently to monoclonal IgA dimers produced by hybridoma cells. The engineered SIgA molecules produced through these three procedures now must be tested *in vivo* and *in vitro* to assess their stability as well as their protective properties.

VI. CONCLUSIONS

Monoclonal IgA antibodies may be used in the future to passively protect immunologically naive children and immunocompromised individuals against mucosal infections. The monoclonal antibody technology reviewed in this chapter could also contribute important information for the design of novel mucosal vaccines. Protective epitopes on pathogenic microorganisms identified using monoclonal IgA antibodies could be subsequently inserted into vaccine vehicles that are transported into organized mucosal lymphoid tissues. In addition, the use of monoclonal IgAs *in vitro* as well as *in vivo* will serve to better define the role(s) of secretory antibodies in preventing adherence and invasion of mucosal tissues by pathogens.

Acknowledgments

We thank the current and former members of our laboratory who contributed to the work discussed here: R. Weltzin, L. Winner, J. Mack, P. Michetti, H. Amerongen, W. Lencer, F. Apter, R. Hirt, and E. Schaerer. The collaboration of J. Mekalanos, M. Mahan, and J. Slauch is gratefully acknowledged.

References

Allan, C. H., and Trier, J. S. (1991). Structure and permeability differ in subepithelial villus and Peyer's patch follicle capillaries. *Gastroenterology* **100,** 1172–1179.

Apter, F. M., Lencer, W. I., Mekalanos, J. J., and Neutra, M. R. (1991). Analysis of epithelial protection by monoclonal IgA antibodies directed against cholera toxin B subunit *in vivo* and *in vitro*. *J. Cell Biol.* **115,** 399a.

Arnold, R. R., Brewer, M., and Gauthier, J. J. (1980). Bacterial activity of human lactoferrin: Sensitivity of a variety of microorganisms. *Infect. Immun.* **28,** 893–898.

Bakos, M. A., Kurosky, A., and Goldblum, R. M. (1991). Characterization of a critical binding site for human polymeric Ig on secretory component. *J. Immunol.* **147,** 3419–3426.

Banting, G., Brake, B., Braghetta, P., Luzio, J. P., and Stanley, K. K. (1989). Intracellular targeting signals of polymeric immunoglobulin receptors are highly conserved between species. *FEBS Lett.* **254,** 177–183.

Brown, W. R., Newcomb, R. W., and Ishizaka, I. K. (1970). Proteolytic degradation of exocrine and serum immunoglobulins. *J. Clin. Invest.* **49,** 1374–1380.

Cancellieri, V., and Fara, G. M. (1985). Demonstration of specific IgA in human feces after immunization with live Ty21a *Salmonella typhi* vaccine. *J. Infect. Dis.* **151,** 482–484.

Casanova, J. E., Breitfeld, P. P., Ross, S. A., and Mostov, K. E. (1990). Phosphorylation of the polymeric immunoglobulin receptor required for its efficient transcytosis. *Science* **248,** 742–745.

Cash, R. A., Music, S. I., Libonati, J. P., Craig, J. P., Pierce, N. F., and Hornick, R. B. (1974). Response of man to infection with *Vibrio cholerae*. II. Protection from illness afforded by previous disease and vaccine. *J. Infect. Dis.* **130,** 325–333.

Childers, N. K., Bruce, M. G., and McGhee, J. R. (1989). Molecular mechanisms of immunoglobulin A defense. *Annu. Rev. Microbiol.* **43,** 503–536.

Colwell, D. E., Michalek, S. M., and McGhee, J. R. (1986). Method for generating a high frequency of hybridomas producing monoclonal IgA antibodies. *Meth. Enzymol.* **121,** 42–51.

Craig, S. W., and Cebra, J. J. (1971). Peyer's patches: An enriched source of precursors for IgA-producing immunocytes in the rabbit. *J. Exp. Med.* **134,** 188–200.

Creeth, J. M. (1978). Constituents of mucus and their separation. *Br. Med. Bull.* **34,** 17–24.

Crowther, R., Lichtman, S., Forstner, J., and Forster, G. (1985). Failure to show secretory IgA binding by rat intestinal mucin. *Fed. Proc.* **44,** 691.

Czerkinsky, C., Russell, M. W., Lycke, N., Lindblad, M., and Holmgren, J. (1989). Oral administration of a streptococcal antigen coupled to cholera toxin B subunit evokes strong antibody responses in salivary glands and extramucosal tissues. *Infect. Immun.* **57,** 1072–1077.

Deitcher, D. L., Neutra, M. R., and Mostov, K. E. (1986). Functional expression of the polymeric immunoglobulin receptor from cloned DNA in fibroblasts. *J. Cell Biol.* **102,** 911–919.

Eibl, M. M., Wolf, H. M., Furnkranz, H., and Rosenkranz, A. (1988). Prevention of necrotizing enterocolitis in low birth weight infants by IgA-IgG feeding. *N. Engl. J. Med.* **319,** 1–17.

Ermak, T. H., Steger, H. J., and Pappo, J. (1990). Phenotypically distinct subpopulations of T cells in domes and M cell pockets of rabbit gut-associated lymphoid tissues. *Immunology* **71,** 530–537.

Finlay, B. B., and Falkow, S. (1990). *Salmonella* interactions with polarized human Caco-2 epithelial cells. *J. Infect. Dis.* **162,** 1096–1106.

Finlay, B. B., Gumbiner, B., and Falkow, S. (1988). Penetration of *Salmonella typhimurium* through a polarized Madin–Darby canine kidney monolayer. *J. Cell Biol.* **107,** 221–230.

Frutiger, S., Hughes, G. J., Hanly, W. C., Kingzette, M., and Jaton, J. C. (1986). The amino-terminal domain of rabbit secretory component is responsible for noncovalent binding to immunoglobulin A dimers. *J. Biol. Chem.* **261,** 16673–16681.

Glass, R. I, Svennerholm, A.-M., Stoll, B. J., Khan, M. R., Hossain, K. M. B., Huq, I. M., and Holmgren, J. (1983). Protection against cholera in breast-fed children by antibodies in breast milk. *New Engl. J. Med.* **308,** 1389–1392.

Haneberg, B., Kendall, D., Amerongen, H. M., Apter, F. M., Kraehenbuhl, J. P., and Neutra, M. R. (1993). Induction of specific secretory IgA responses in small intestine, colon-rectum, and vagina measured with a new method for collection of secretions from local mucosal surfaces. *Infect. Immun.,* in press.

Hanson, L. A., Adlerberth, I., Carlsson, B., Zaman, S., Hahn Zoric, M., and Jalil, F. (1990). Antibody-mediated immunity in the neonate. *Pediatr. Pathol.* **25,** 371–376.

Harris, M. C., Douglas, S. D., Kolski, G. B., and Polin, R. A. (1982). Functional properties of anti-group B streptococcal monoclonal antibodies. *Clin. Immunol. Immunopathol.* **24,** 342–350.

Hirt, R. P., Hughes, G. J., Frutiger, S., Michetti, P., Perregaux, C., Jeanguenat, N., Neutra, M. R., and Kraehenbuhl, J.-P. (1993). Transcytosis of the polymeric immunoglobulin receptor requires phosphorylation of serine 664 in the absence but not in the presence of dimeric IgA. *Cell* **74,** 245–255.

Hirt, R., Poulain-Godefroy, O., Billotte, J., Kraehenbuhl, J. P., and Fasel, N. (1992). Highly inducible synthesis of heterologous proteins in epithelial cells carrying a glucocorticoid-responsive vector. *Gene* **111,** 199–206.

Hohmann, A. W., Schmidt, G., and Rowley, D. (1978). Intestinal colonization and virulence of *Salmonella* in mice. *Infect. Immun.* **22,** 763–770.

Holmgren, J., Clemens, J., Sack, D. A., and Svennerholm, A. M. (1989). New cholera vaccines. *Vaccine* **7,** 94–96.

Huet, C., Sahuquillo-Merino, C., Coudrier, E., and Louvard, D. (1987). Absorptive and mucus-secreting subclones isolated from multipotent intestinal cell line (HT-29) provide new models for cell polarity and terminal differentiation. *J. Cell Biol.* **105,** 345–357.

Jackson, G. D. F., Lemaitre-Coelho, I., and Vaerman, J. P. (1977). Transfer of MOPC-315 IgA to secretions in MOPC-315 tumor-bearing and normal BALB/c mice. *In* "Protides of the Biological Fluids" (H. Peters, ed.), pp. 919–922. Pergamon Press, New York.

Kaetzel, C. S., Robinson, J. K., Chintalacharuvu, K. R., Vaerman, J.-P., and Lamm, M. E. (1991). The polymeric immunoglobulin receptor (secretory component) mediates transport of immune complexes across epithelial cells: A local defense function for IgA. *Proc. Natl. Acad. Sci. USA* **88,** 8796–8800.

Kaper, J. B. (1989). *Vibrio cholerae* vaccines. *Rev. Infect. Dis.* **11** (Suppl. 3), 5568–5573.

Kerr, M. A. (1990). The structure and function of human IgA. *Biochem. J.* **271,** 285–296.

Kiyono, H., and McGhee, J. R. (1987). Mucosal T cell networks: Role of Fc alpha R + T cells and Ig BF alpha in the regulation of the IgA response. *Int. Rev. Immunol.* **2,** 157–182.

Kiyono, H., Cooper, M. D., Kearney, J. F., Mosteller, L. M., Michalek, S. M., Koopman, W. J., and McGhee, J. R. (1984). Isotype specificity of helper T cell clones. Peyer's patch T cells preferentially collaborate with mature IgA B cells for IgA responses. *J. Exp. Med.* **159,** 798–811.

Kiyono, H., Mosteller-Barnum, L. M., Pitts, A. M., Williamson, S. I., and McGhee, J. R. (1985). Isotype-specific immunoregulation. IgA-binding factors produced by Fc alpha receptor positive cell hybridomas regulate IgA responses. *J. Exp. Med.* **161,** 731–747.

Kohbata, S., Yokobata, H., and Yabuuchi, E. (1986). Cytopathogenic effect of *Salmonella typhi* GIFU 10007 on M cells of murine ileal Peyer's patches in ligated ileal loops: An ultrastructural study. *Microbiol. Immunol.* **30,** 1225–1237.

Komisar, J. L., Fuhrman, J. A., and Cebra, J. J. (1982). IgA-producing hybridomas are readily derived from gut-associated lymphoid tissue. *J. Immunol.* **128,** 2376–2378.

Kraehenbuhl, J. P., and Neutra, M. R. (1992a). Transepithelial transport and mucosal defense. II. Secretion of IgA. *Trends Cell Biol.* **2,** 2:134–138.

Kraehenbuhl, J. P., and Neutra, M. R. (1992b). Molecular and cellular basis of immune protection of mucosal surfaces. *Physiol. Rev.* **72,** 853–879.

Krajči, P., Solberg, R., Sandberg, M., Oyen, O., Jahnsen, T., and Brandtzaeg, P. (1989). Molecular cloning of the human transmembrane secretory component (poly-Ig-receptor) and its mRNA expression in human tissues. *Biochem. Biophys. Res. Commun.* **158,** 783–789.

Lee, C. A., and Falkow, S. (1990). The ability of *Salmonella* to enter mammalian cells is affected by bacterial growth state. *Proc. Natl. Acad. Sci. U.S.A.* **87,** 4304–4308.

Levine, M. M., Kaper, J. B., Black, R. E., and Clements, M. L. (1983). New knowledge on pathogenesis of bacterial enteric infections as applied to vaccine development. *Microbiol. Rev.* **47,** 510–550.

Levine, M. M., Herrington, D., Losonsky, G., Tall, B., Kaper, J. B., Ketley, J., Tacket, C. O., and Cryz, S. (1988). Safety, immunogenicity, and efficacy of recombinant live oral cholera vaccines, CVD 103 and CVD 103-HgR. *Lancet* **ii,** 467–470.

Lindh, E. (1975). Increased resistance of immunoglobulin A dimers to proteolytic degradation after binding of secretory component. *J. Immunol.* **14,** 284–286.

McCormick, B. A., Stocker, B. A. D., Laux, D. C., and Cohen, P. S. (1988). Roles of motility, chematoxis and penetration through and growth in intestinal mucus in the ability of a virulent strain of *S. typhimurium* to colonize the large intestine of the streptomycin-treated mouse. *Infect. Immun.* **50,** 2209–2217.

McGhee, J. R., Mestecky, J., Elson, C. O., and Kiyono, H. (1989). Regulation of IgA synthesis and immune response by T cells and interleukins. *J. Clin. Immunol.* **9,** 175–199.

Madara, J. L., Stafford, J., Dharmsathaphorn, K., and Carlson, S. (1987). Structural analysis of a human intestinal epithelial cell line. *Gastroenterology* **92,** 1133–1145.

Manning, P. A. (1987). Involvement of cell envelope components in the pathogenesis of *Vibrio cholerae:* Targets for cholera vaccine development. *Vaccine* **5,** 83–87.

Mazanec, M. B., Kaetzel, C. S., Lamm, M. E., Fletcher, D., and Nedrud, J. G. (1992). Intracellular neutralization of virus by immunoglobulin A antibodies. *Proc. Natl. Acad. Sci. USA* **89,** 6901–6905.

Mazanec, M. B., Nedrud, J. G., and Lamm, M. E. (1987). Immunoglobulin A monoclonal antibodies protect against Sendai virus. *J. Virol.* **61,** 2624–2626.

Mestecky, J. (1988). Immunobiology of IgA. *Am. J. Kidney Dis.* **12,** 378–383.

Michetti, P., Mahan, M. J., Slauch, J. M., Mekalanos, J. J., and Neutra, M. R. (1992). Monoclonal secretory IgA protects against oral challenge with the invasive pathogen *Salmonella typhimurium. Infect. Immun.* **60,** 1786–1792.

Miller, J. F., Mekalanos, J. J., and Falkow, S. (1989). Coordinate regulation and sensory transduction in the control of bacterial virulence. *Science* **243,** 916–922.

Mostov, K. E., Kraehenbuhl, J. P., and Blobel, G. (1980). Receptor mediated transcellular transport of immunoglobulins: Synthesis of secretory component as multiple and larger transmembrane forms. *Proc. Natl. Acad. Sci. U.S.A.* **77,** 7257–7261.

Mostov, K. E., Friedlander, M., and Blobel, G. (1984). The receptor for transepithelial transport of IgA and IgM contains multiple immunoglobulin-like domains. *Nature* (*London*) **308,** 37–43.

Neutra, M. R., and Forstner, J. F. (1987). Gastrointestinal mucus: synthesis, secretion and function. *In* "Physiology of the Gastrointestinal Tract," Vol. 2. (L. R. Johnson, ed.). pp. 975–1009. Raven Press, New York.

Neutra, M. R., and Kraehenbuhl, J. P. (1992). Transepithelial transport and mucosal defense. *I.* The role of M cells. *Trends Cell Biol.* **2,** 134–138.

Neutra, M. R., and Louvard, D. (1989). Differentiation of intestinal cells *in vitro. In* "Functional Epithelial Cells in Culture" (K. S. Matlin and J. D. Valentich, eds.), pp. 363–398. Alan R. Liss, Inc., New York.

Renegar, K. B., and Small, P. A. J. (1991). Passive transfer of local immunity to influenza virus infection by IgA antibody. *J. Immunol.* **146,** 1972–1978.

Rits, M., Cormont, F., Bazin, H., Maykens, R., and Vaerman, J. P. (1986). Rat monoclonal antibodies VI. Production of IgA secreting hybridomas with specificity for the 2,4-dinitrophenyl (DNP) hapten. *J. Immunol. Meth.* **89,** 81–87.

Roa, R. C., Kaetzel, C. S., and Lamm, M. E. (1987). Induction of secretory component synthesis in colonic epithelial cells. *Adv. Exp. Biol. Med.* **216B,** 1071–1077.

Rousset, M. (1986). The human colon carcinoma cell lines HT-29 and Caco-2: Two *in vitro* models for the study of intestinal differentiation. *Biochimie* **68,** 1035–1040.

Roy, M. J., and Varvayanis, M. (1987). Development of dome epithelium in gut-associated lymphoid tissues: Association of IgA with M cells. *Cell Tissue Res.* **248,** 645–651.

Schaerer, E., Verrey, F., Racine, L., Tallichet, C., Rheinhardt, M., and Kraehenbuhl, J. P. (1990). Polarized transport of the polymeric immunoglobulin receptor in transfected rabbit mammary epithelial cells. *J. Cell Biol.* **110,** 987–998.

Sears, S. D., Richardson, K., Young, C., Parker, C. D., and Levine, M. M. (1984). Evaluation of the human immune response to outer membrane proteins of *Vibrio cholerae. Infect. Immun.* **44,** 439–444.

Solari, R., and Kraehenbuhl, J. P. (1987). Receptor-mediated transepithelial transport of polymeric immunoglobulins. *In* "The Mammary Gland. Development, Regulation and Function" (M. C. Neville and C. W. Daniel, eds.), pp. 269–298. Plenum Press, New York.

Solari, R., Kuhn, L. C., and Kraehenbuhl, J. P. (1985). Antibodies recognizing different domains of the polymeric immunoglobulin receptor. *J. Biol. Chem.* **260,** 1141–1145.

Styles, J. M., Dean, C. J., Gyure, L. A., Hobbs, S. M., and Hall, J. G. (1984). The production of hybridomas from the gut-associated lymphoid tissue of tumor-bearing rats. II. Peripheral intestinal lymph as a source of IgA producing cells. *Clin. Exp. Immunol.* **57,** 365–370.

Svennerholm, A. M., Jertborn, M., Gothefors, L., Karim, A. M. M. M., Sack, D. A., and Holmgren, J. (1984). Mucosal antitoxic and antibacterial immunity after cholera disease and after immunization with a combined B subunit-whole cell vaccine. *J. Infect. Dis.* **149,** 884–893.

Tacket, C. O., Forrest, B., Morona, R., Attridge, S. R., LaBrooy, J., Tall, B. D., Reymann, M., Rowely, D., and Levine, M. M. (1990). Safety, immunogenicity, and efficacy against cholera challenge in humans of a typhoid-cholera hybrid vaccine derived from *Salmonella typhi* Ty21a. *Infect. Immun.* **58,** 1620–1627.

Tagliabue, A., Villa, L., Boraschi, D., Peri, G., DeGori, V., and Nencioni, L. (1985). Natural anti-bacterial activity against *Salmonella typhi* by human T4+ lymphocytes armed with IgA antibodies. *J. Immunol.* **135,** 4178–4182.

Takeuchi, A. (1975). Electron microscope observations on penetration of the gut epithelial barrier by *Salmonella typhimurium. Microbiol.* 174–181.

Taylor, R. K., Miller, V. L., Furlong, D. B., and Mekalanos, J. J. (1987). Use of phoA gene fusions to identify a pilus colonization factor coordinately regulated with cholera toxin. *Proc. Natl. Acad. Sci. U.S.A.* **84,** 2833–2837.

Tenovuo, J., Moldoveanu, Z., Mestecky, J., Pruitt, K. M., and Rahemtulla, B. M. (1982). Interaction of specific and innate factors of immunity: IgA enhances the antimicrobial effect of the lactoperoxidase system against *Streptococcus mutans. J. Immunol.* **128,** 726–730.

Underdown, B. J., and Dorrington, K. J. (1974). Studies on the structural and conformational basis for the relative resistance of serum and secretory immunoglobulin A to proteolysis. *J. Immunol.* **112,** 949–959.

Weltzin, R. A., Lucia-Jandris, P., Michetti, P., Fields, B. N., Kraehenbuhl, J. P., and Neutra, M. R. (1989). Binding and transepithelial transport of immunoglobulins by intestinal M cells: Demonstration using monoclonal IgA antibodies against enteric viral proteins. *J. Cell Biol.* **108,** 1673–1685.

Williams, R. C., and Gibbons, R. J. (1972). Inhibition of bacterial adherence by secretory immunoglobulin A: A mechanism of antigen disposal. *Science* **177,** 697–699.

Winner, L. S., III, Weltzin, R. A., Mekalanos, J. J., Kraehenbuhl, J. P., and Neutra, M. R. (1991). New model for analysis of mucosal immunity: Intestinal secretion of specific monoclonal immunoglobulin A from hybridoma tumors protects against *Vibrio cholerae* infection. *Infect. Immun.* **59,** 977–982.

PART II

Mucosal Diseases

Section E

Stomach, Intestine, and Liver

Section Editor: Pearay L. Ogra

(Chapters 35 through 42)

35

Gut-Associated Lymphoid Tissue

Thomas T. MacDonald • Jo Spencer

I. INTRODUCTION

The mucosal immune system consists of a series of coordinated and specialized lymphoid tissues with the complex task of protecting the most vulnerable of the surfaces of the body that interact with the external environment. The gut associated tissues (Peyer's patches, appendix, colonic and cecal patches, isolated lymphoid aggregates) in conjunction with mesenteric lymph nodes and the lymphoid elements of gut epithelium and lamina propria account for the bulk of the body's lymphoid mass. In comparison, the contribution of other secondary lymphoid organs such as the spleen and other lymph nodes is minor.

The organized lymphoid structures of the gastrointestinal tract have anatomical features in common that distinguish them from other secondary lymphoid tissues. The most obvious of these common features is the lack of a defined capsule or afferent lymphatics and the presence of a specialized covering epithelium (follicle-associated epithelium, FAE) which facilitates the transmission of antigen from the gut lumen. In this chapter, the term gut-associated lymphoid tissue (GALT) is used to describe any organized aggregate of lymphoid tissue with a specialized FAE. Large numbers of lymphoid/myeloid cells are also present in the mucosa between the follicular structures in the epithelium and lamina propria; these are considered independently. The possible role of the epithelium itself in mucosal immunology is discussed as well.

II. STRUCTURE AND CELLULAR COMPOSITION OF ORGANIZED GUT-ASSOCIATED LYMPHOID TISSUE IN HUMANS

A. Stomach

The normal stomach mucosa is devoid of organized lymphoid tissue and lymphoid/myeloid cells are sparse in the lamina propria. A scattering of T cells is seen in the lamina propria; a few are found in the epithelium. In the lamina propria, IgA plasma cells predominate over IgM and IgG cells. In chronic gastritis, plasma cells of all isotypes increase, but the increase in IgG cells is especially profound (Brandtzaeg, 1987). An increase in epithelial T cells is seen also (Kazi *et al.*, 1989). A striking feature of the stomach is the acquisition of organized lymphoid aggregates in association with *Helicobacter pylori* infection (Figure 1). In children, this aggregation is especially striking and leads to antral nodularity that is visible at gastroscopy (Wyatt and Rathbone, 1988; Hassall and Dimmick, 1991).Whether this acquired lymphoid tissue functionally resembles Peyer's patches, has an M-cell containing FAE, and is capable of generating a secretory IgA response to gastric antigens remains to be established. B cells have been identified in the gastric epithelium close to follicles in *H. pylori* gastritis (Wotherspoon *et al.*, 1991).

B. Peyer's Patches

The organized lymphoid tissue of the small intestine was described first by de Peyer in 1667. Structurally, Peyer's patches are organized areas of lymphoid tissue in the mucosa of the small bowel. These patches usually contain follicle centers and well-defined cellular zonation (Figure 2). These areas are overlain by a specialized lymphoepithelium without crypts or villi.

The epithelial cells overlying the follicle are derived from crypts of Lieberkuhn adjacent to the follicles. Follicle-associated eptiehlium is different from columnar villus epithelium because it is cuboidal, contains few goblet cells, and does not contain secretory component (Bjerke and Brandtzaeg, 1988). In addition, specialized "M" cells, also derived from adjacent crypts (Bye *et al.*, 1984), so called because they have microfolds rather than microvilli on their surface, are found (Owen and Jones, 1974). M cells have a number of morphological and functional specializations—attenuated processes to adjacent cells and very close association with lymphocytes. Clusters of $CD3^+$ T cells lie next to M cells in the epithelium, which can be identified by their lack of brush border alkaline phosphatase (Bjerke *et al.*, 1988). Significant numbers of $CD4^+$ T cells are found in follicle epithelium compared with villus epithelium. M cells are deficient in cytoplasmic acid phosphatase and microvillus-associated alkaline phosphatase (Owen *et al.*, 1986). These cells are also probably HLA-DR^- (Bjerke and Brandtzaeg, 1988), so they are unlikely to play a role in antigen presentation but are more likely a portal of entry for some types of antigen into the dome area of the follicle. This role has been clearly shown for reovirus in mice, which only adheres to and penetrates

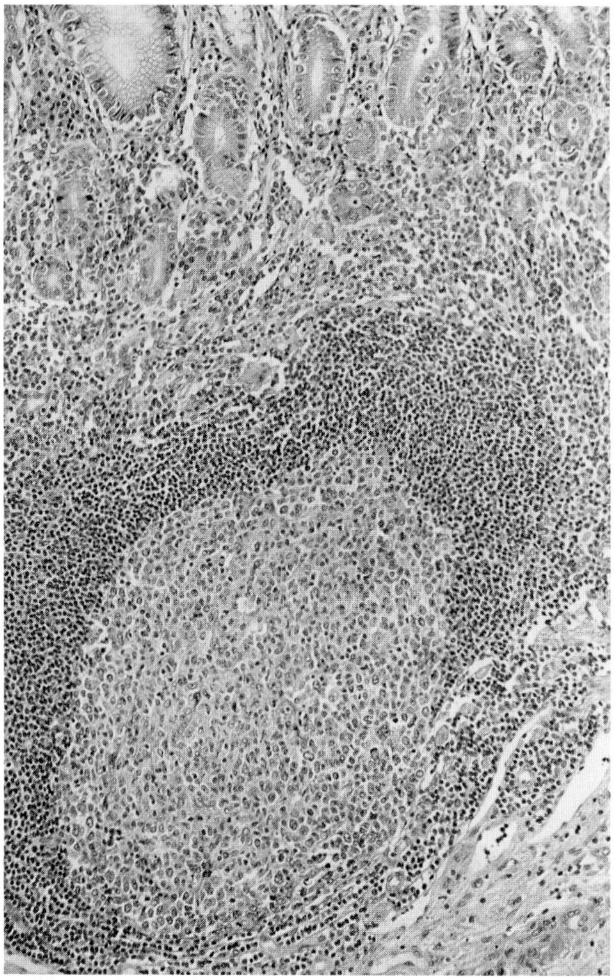

Figure 1 Acquired lymphoid tissue in the stomach of a patient with *Helicobacter pylori* gastritis. Note the large reactive follicle center. Hematorylin and eosin stain (H&E), ×100.

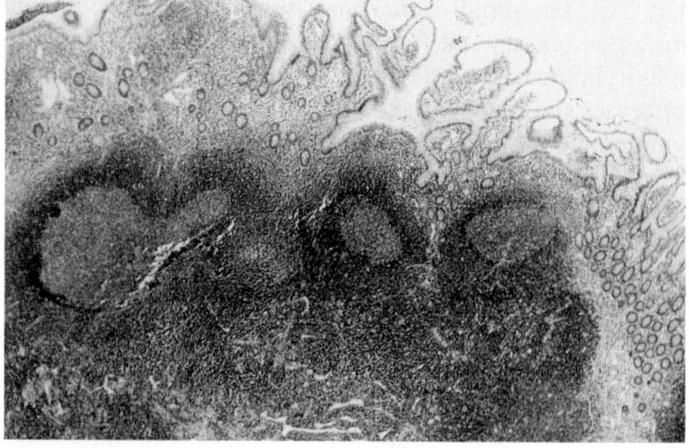

Figure 2 Histological appearance of Peyer's patch in human terminal ileum. H&E, ×27.

the M cells of the FAE (Wolf *et al.*, 1981); poliovirus (Sicinski *et al.*, 1990); and horseradish peroxidase, which also is taken up preferentially by M cells (Owen, 1977).

At birth, approximately 100 Peyer's patches with five follicles or more exist in human small intestine; the majority of these Peyer's patches are found in the distal small intestine (Cornes, 1965a). The number of Peyer's patches increases to 225–300 in the whole small intestine by late adolescence and then decreases with increasing age, so the small intestine from 90-yr-old individuals has roughly the same number of Peyer's patches as at birth (Cornes, 1965b). The assumption by Cornes that five or more follicles are necessary before a lymphoepithelial structure can be called a Peyer's patch is arbitrary; to categorize even a single nodule as a Peyer's patch is reasonable provided FAE is present. In normal intestine, all organized mucosal follicles can be shown to have FAE, if the tissue is properly oriented for sectioning. Many Peyer's patches with one to four follicles are evident in small intestine, both macroscopically and microscopically; Cornes' estimates, although useful for comparative studies, seriously underestimate the amount of organized lymphoid tissue in the human gut.

1. Morphological and Immunohistochemical Characteristics of Human Peyer's Patches

The most prominent feature of Peyer's patches is the follicle center, containing centrocytes and centroblasts. The follicle center is surrounded by a mantle of small lymphocytes that merge into the mixed-cell zone of the dome. The dome area also contains plasma cells, dendritic cells, macrophages, and small cells with cleaved nuclei (centrocyte-like cells) that infiltrate the overlying epithelium. These centrocyte-like cells can be identified immunohistochemically as B cells in frozen sections (Spencer *et al.*, 1986b). B cells are rarely seen in villus or crypt epithelium, if at all.

2. T-Cell Populations in Peyer's Patches

Immunohistochemical staining of Peyer's patches with anti-CD3 monoclonal antibodies shows T cells to be present in the greatest density in the areas surrounding the high endothelial venules (HEV; Figure 3). Interleukin 2 (IL-2) receptor positive T cells are also present in this area. T cells are also present surrounding the follicle, in the mixed-cell zone in the dome, and in the lymphoepithelium (Spencer *et al.*, 1986b). In humans, in contrast to mice, the T-cell zone extends between the follicle center and the muscularis mucosa. Occasional T cells are seen in the follicle center. Most of the T cells are $CD4^{+}$.

3. B Cells and Plasma Cells in Peyer's Patches

Human Peyer's patches contain large numbers of B cells (Figure 4). The narrow mantle zone surrounding the follicle center is composed of cells expressing surface IgM or IgD (Figure 5). The B cells that surround the mantle zone, are present in the mixed-cell zone of the dome, and infiltrate the epithelium, do not express IgD but do express sIgM or sIgA (Spencer *et al.*, 1986b). A major difference between rodent and human Peyer's patches is that, in humans, cells with

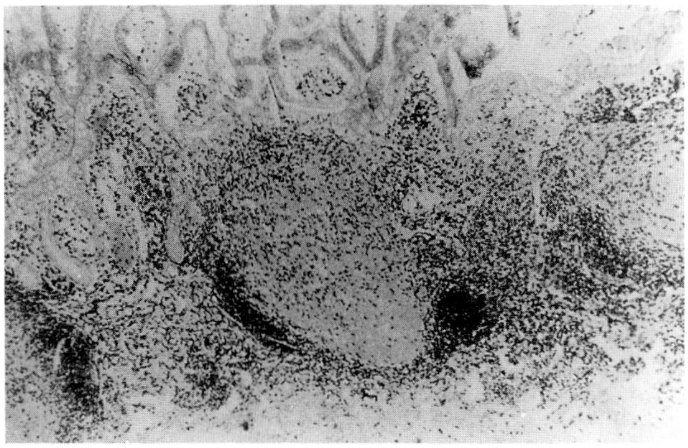

Figure 3 Immunohistochemical localization of $CD3^+$ cells in human Peyer's patch. Most T cells are in the interfollicular zones. Immunoperoxidase, ×26.

surface IgD are restricted to a narrow zone around the follicle center whereas, in rats, the majority of the B cells surrounding the follicle centers, including those in the dome and dome epithelium, express sIgM and sIgD (Spencer *et al.*, 1986c). Germinal center formation is not seen in Peyer's patches of the fetus and only occurs after antigenic exposure at birth (Bridges *et al.*, 1959).

Most of the cells with abundant cytoplasmic immunoglobulin are in the dome area in human Peyer's patches. Most contain IgA with fewer cIgM cells (Spencer *et al.*, 1986b). Some workers have reported that cIgG plasma cells are as abundant as cIgA cells in the dome (Bjerke and Brandtzaeg, 1986). Cells with cIgA also exist in the T-cell zone surrounding the HEV, but the dense accumulation of IgA-containing immunoblasts around the HEV in rodents is not seen in humans (Spencer *et al.*, 1986c).

4. Macrophages and Accessory Cells in Peyer's Patches

In humans, B cells, activated T cells, dendritic cells, follicular dendritic cells, and macrophages express Class II molecules necessary for antigen presentation to $CD4^+$ T cells. All these cell types are present in normal Peyer's patches. Numerous nonlymphoid HLA-DR^+ cells with cytoplasmic processes are present in the dome area of human Peyer's patches and in the T-cell zones. The HLA-DR^+ cells in the dome do not stain with antimacrophage markers such as RFD7 or lysozyme (although these cells are abundant in adjacent lamina propria), but do stain with S-100 (Spencer *et al.*, 1986b). These cells are probably dendritic cells but the HLA-DR^+ cells between the follicles in the T-cell zones are probably interdigitating cells. The dome epithelium itself is also HLA-DR^+ (Spencer *et al.*, 1986a) and also may be capable of presenting antigen to the numerous lymphoid cells in the epithelium. The presence of dendritic cells in the mixed-cell zone of the dome, immediately underlying the M cells, which are Class II^-, suggests that in Peyer's patches most antigen presentation takes place in the dome region.

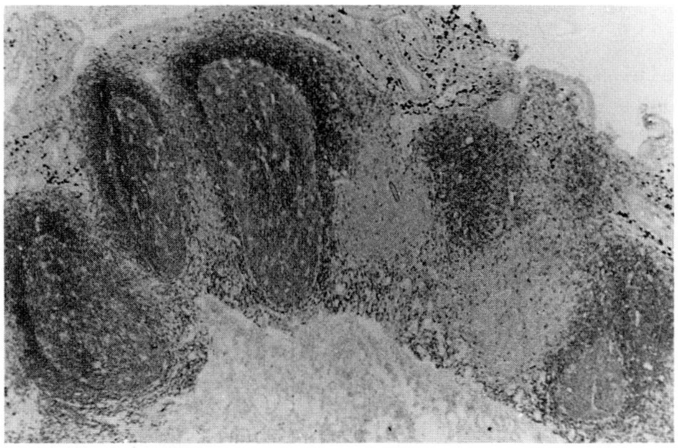

Figure 4 Immunohistochemical localization of B cells ($CD20^+$) in human Peyer's patch. Immunoperoxidase, ×25.

C. Organized Lymphoid Tissue of the Colon

Organized lymphoid tissue in human colon was described first by Dukes and Bussey (1926), who counted the number of single lymphoid follicles in human colon of different ages. These investigators showed in children, eight follicles per square centimeter of colonic mucosa, which decrease to three per square centimeter in older persons. Aggregates of follicles akin to those seen in the multifollicular Peyer's patches in the small bowel are not seen in human colon. The bulk of the lymphoid tissue in colonic lymphoid follicles lies below the muscularis mucosa, the follicles producing points of discontinuity in the latter (O'Leary and Sweeney, 1986). Unless colonic lymphoid tissue is oriented properly, it may appear as though it has no FAE. Serial sections, however, of reoriented blocks invariably reveals FAE (Figure 6). Normally, only about 1% of colonic follicles contain a germinal center, but a characteristic of Crohn's disease of the colon is that the percentage of lymphoid follicles containing a germinal center is increased dramatically (O'Leary and Sweeney, 1986). In addition, numerous ectopic lymphoid follicles occur within the inflamed mucosa. Aphthous ulceration overlying colonic lymphoid follicles is the earliest sign of Crohn's disease of the colon (Rickert and Carter, 1980). Colonic lymphoid follicles also have a dome epithelium with M cells, similar in many regards to the specialized lymphoepithelium overlying Peyer's patches, although, in proportion to the mass of lymphoid tissue, colonic FAE is less than that of Peyer's patches (Jacob *et al.*, 1987). The number of follicles is greater in the rectum than in the colon, and FAE of rectal follicles contains more M cells than FAE in the proximal colon.

D. Appendix

The human appendix is a blind sac, 5–8 cm long, extending from the cecum near the ileocecal junction. The most striking feature of the appendix is the presence of numerous lymphoid nodules separated by regions of lamina propria, into which the glandular crypts penetrate. The types of cells and the zonal arrangement are very similar to those of human Peyer's

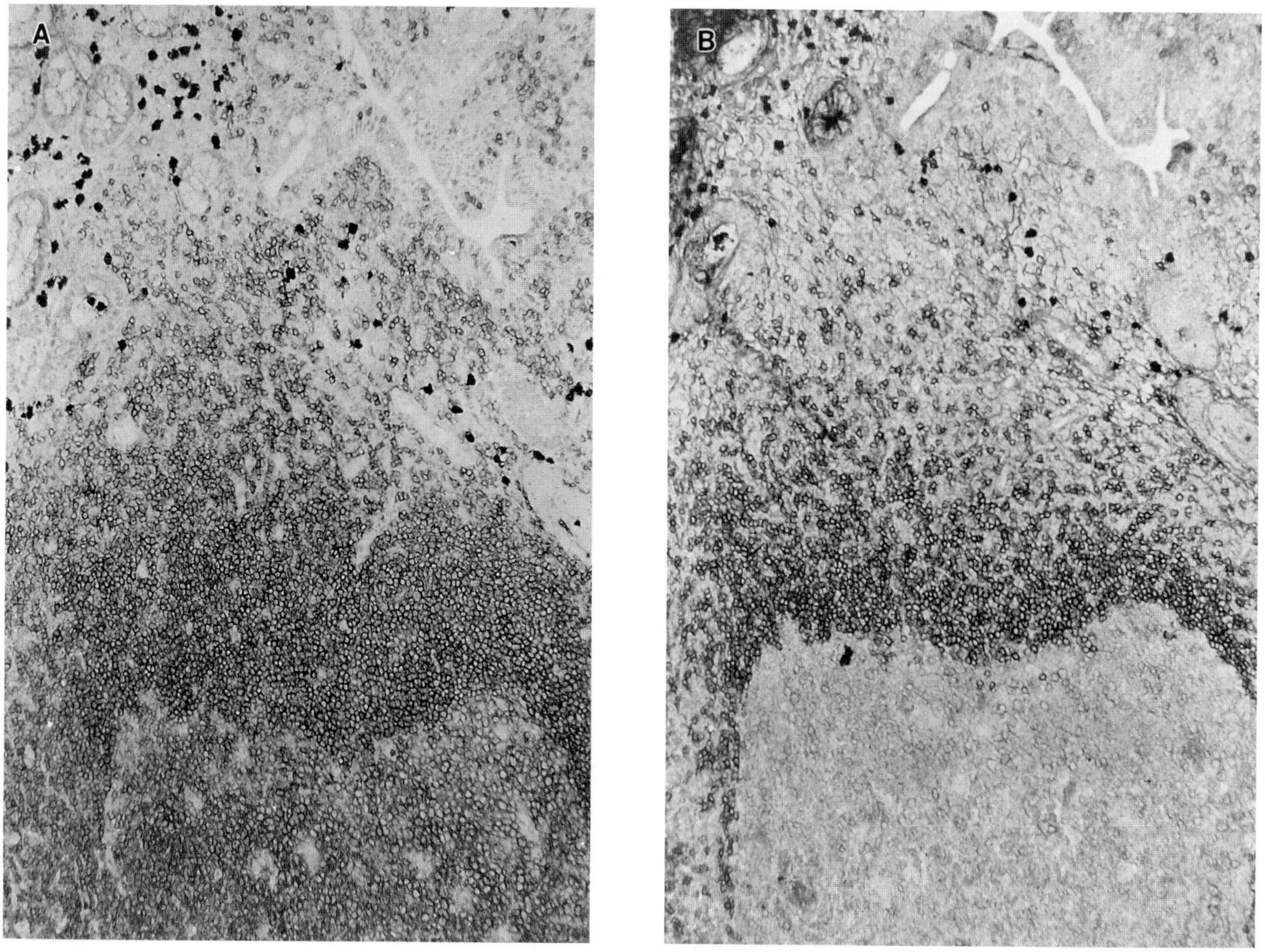

Figure 5 Mantle and dome regions of a human Peyer's patch. (A) Stained with CD20, B cells are seen in the follicle, mantle zone, and extending into the dome epithelium. (B) Stained with anti-IgD, the mantle zone is seen to be strongly IgD^+, but the follicle center cells and most of those in the dome are IgD^-. Immunoperoxidase, ×100.

patches. The most prominent feature of the lymphoid nodules is the reactive follicle center, surrounded by a narrow mantle of cells that merges with the mixed-cell zone below the epithelium. The mantle and mixed-cell zone contain $CD4^+$ T cells but are mostly IgM^+IgD^- B cells (Spencer *et al.*, 1985). The FAE that contains T and B cells is often $HLA\text{-}DR^+$. The T-cell zone lies mostly between the follicle center and the muscularis mucosa (Figure 7). Lysozyme-containing macrophages are uncommon in the dome region; most of the $HLA\text{-}DR^+$ cells with cytoplasmic processes stain with S-100 and are probably dendritic cells (Spencer *et al.*, 1985). $S\text{-}100^+$ cells occasionally can be seen in the epithelium.

IgG-producing plasma cells predominate in the region immediately adjacent to the follicles and in the dome, but the majority of plasma cells in the lamina propria between the follicles are IgA producing (Bjerke *et al.*, 1986).

III. INTESTINAL MUCOSA

A. Gut Epithelium as a Lymphoid Organ

The mucosa between the follicles makes up most of the mass of the intestine. Extensive lymphoid/myeloid elements are found in the connective tissue of the lamina propria; numerous lymphocytes (mostly T cells but never B cells, macrophages, or plasma cells) are found in the gut epithelium. Small bowel villus enterocytes also express HLA-DR (Scott *et al.*, 1980). Thus, both the gut epithelium and the lamina propria may be sites at which mucosal immune responses may be initiated.

1. Class II Gene Expression in the Epithelium

The expression of Class II major histocompatibility complex (MHC) products on gut epithelium was seen first in the

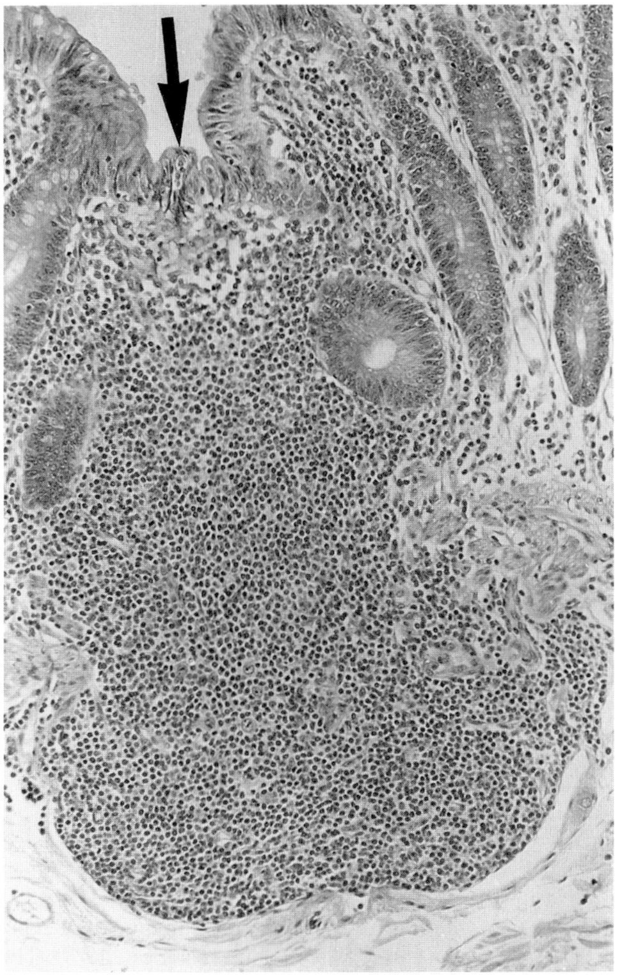

Figure 6 Colonic lymphoid follicle. Arrow shows the small follicle-associated epithelium (FAE). H&E, ×100.

guinea pig (Wiman *et al.*, 1978) and later in human small intestine (Figure 8; Scott *et al.*, 1980). In humans, normal large intestine and stomach epithelium are HLA-DR$^-$ (Selby *et al.*, 1983b; Spencer *et al.*, 1986d), as are crypt epithelial cells. Peyer's patch epithelium is also HLA-DR$^+$ (Spencer *et al.*, 1986a), although in the rat it appears to be HLA-DR$^-$ (Mayrhofer *et al.*, 1983). HLA-DR expression in the human fetal gut epithelium first appears at 19–20 weeks gestation (MacDonald *et al.*, 1988). In humans, normal small intestinal epithelial cells are HLA-DP$^-$ and -DQ$^-$ (Scott *et al.*, 1987).

Epithelial HLA-DR expression in humans is increased in chronic inflammatory bowel disease (Selby *et al.*, 1983b), celiac disease (Arato *et al.*, 1987), gastritis (Spencer *et al.*, 1986d), and autoimmune enteropathy (Mirakian *et al.*, 1986). In untreated celiac disease expression of HLA-DP and -DQ on the surface epithelial cells is also common in some patients (Scott *et al.*, 1987). In patients with ulcerative colitis in whom intestinal inflammation has been reduced by steroids, the epithelium becomes HLA-DR$^-$ (Poulsen *et al.*, 1986). Similar changes in Class II expression are seen in rat intestinal epithelium during small intestinal inflammation caused by *Trichinella spiralis* infection and graft-versus-host disease (Mason *et al.*, 1981; Barclay and Mason, 1982).

Interferon gamma (IFNγ) can increase HLA-DR expression on human transformed intestinal epithelial cell lines and on rat epithelial cell lines (Cerf-Bensussan *et al.*, 1984; Sollid *et al.*, 1987). Activation of lamina propria T cells in explants of human small intestine with mitogens *in vitro* results in IFNγ production and an increase in HLA-DR expression by crypt epithelial cells (MacDonald *et al.*, 1988). Thus good, but circumstantial, evidence exists that increased epithelial HLA-DR expression during inflammation is caused by local production of IFNγ by activated mucosal T cells. Whether the increased HLA-DR expression is of any pathogenic significance or is merely an epiphenomenon is unknown. Indeed, we know very little about the control of gene expression in intestinal epithelial cells in normal and pathological conditions. The increased HLA-DR expression by enterocytes in

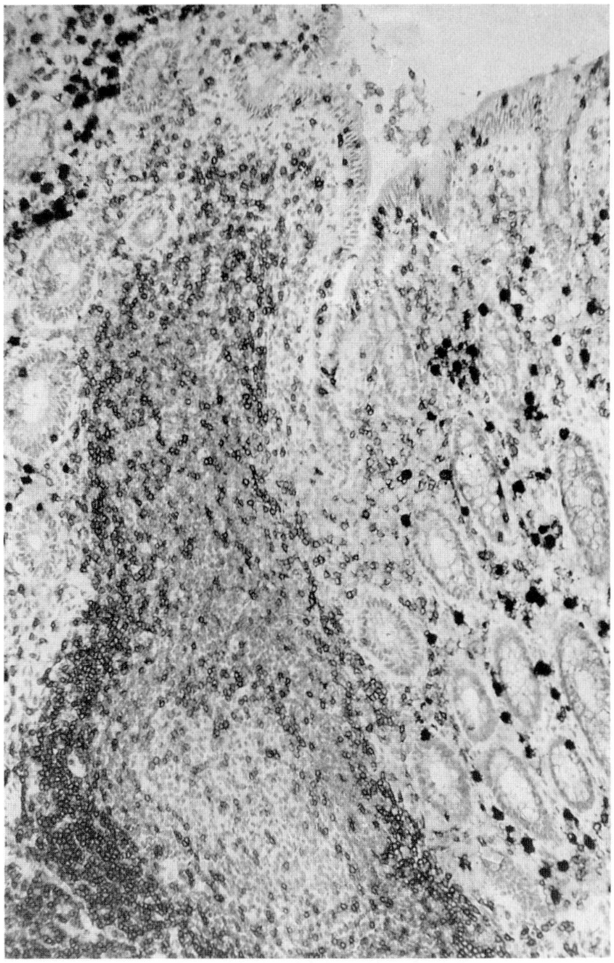

Figure 7 T cells in human appendix. Immunoperoxidase with anti-CD3, ×100.

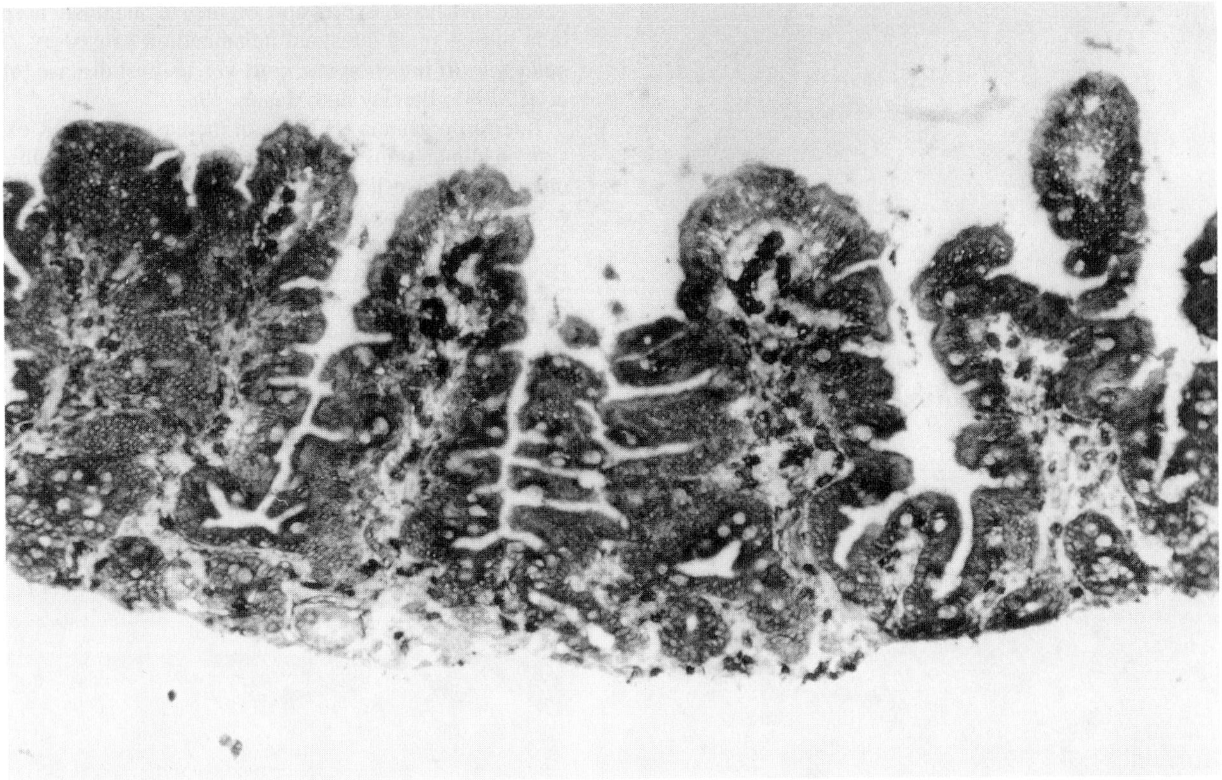

Figure 8 HLA-DR expression in normal human small intestine. The epithelium is strongly positive, as are many cells in the lamina propria. Immunoperoxidase, ×100.

inflammation is not the only change, since increased expression of secretory component on villus cells also occurs in celiac disease (Scott *et al.*, 1981).

2. T-Cell Populations of the Gut Epithelium—Intraepithelial Lymphocytes

If epithelial cells can present enteric antigens, the most likely cells to be stimulated will be intraepithelial lymphocytes (IEL), situated basally above the basement membrane (Figure 9). The majority of IELs in humans use the $\alpha\beta$ T cell receptor (TcR) (Brandtzaeg *et al.*, 1989). These cells are unusual because oligoclonal expansion of certain Vβ genes appears to occur in healthy individuals (Balk *et al.*, 1991; Spencer *et al.*, 1991b). Only about 10% of IELs in healthy individuals use the $\gamma\delta$ TcR (Groh *et al.*, 1989; Jarry *et al.*, 1990), and the function of these cells in humans is still unclear. An important difference between blood $\gamma\delta$ TcR$^+$ T cells and those in the gut epithelium is that, whereas most of these cells in the blood use the Vδ2 gene product, those in the gut use the Vδ1 gene product (Spencer *et al.*, 1989; Halstensen *et al.*, 1989). Differences also exist in CD45 expression between epithelial $\alpha\beta$ TcR$^+$ and $\gamma\delta$ TcR$^+$ T cells. Only about half the $\alpha\beta$ TcR$^+$ IELs are CD45R0$^+$, whereas the majority of the $\gamma\delta$ TcR$^+$ IELs are CD45R0$^+$ (Halstensen *et al.*, 1990).

The distribution of cells expressing different forms of the TcR has been examined in disease states. $\gamma\delta$ TcR$^+$ IELs are not increased in inflammatory bowel disease (Fukushima *et al.*, 1991), but are increased dramatically in untreated celiac disease (Spencer *et al.*, 1989; Halstensen *et al.*, 1989). This increase, however, is not specific for celiac disease since, in severe cases of cow milk sensitive enteropathy, the most important differential diagnosis of celiac disease in children, $\gamma\delta$ TcR$^+$ T cells also are raised in number in the epithelium (Spencer *et al.*, 1991a).

In untreated celiac disease, the number of $\alpha\beta$ TcR$^+$ IELs coexpressing CD45R0 increases to 75%, whereas the number

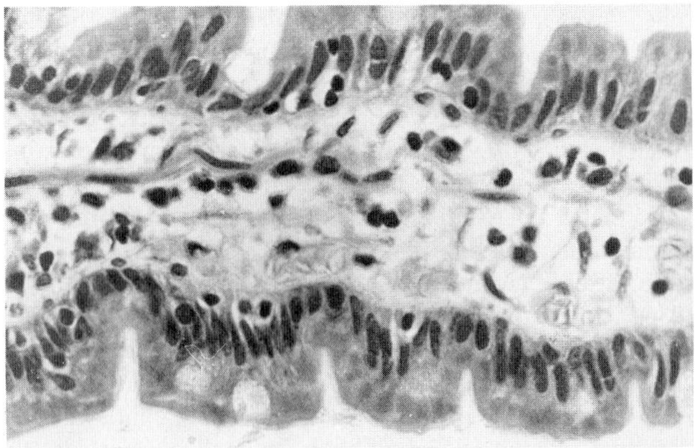

Figure 9 Intraepithelial lymphocytes in human small intestine. Most lie basally within the epithelium. H & E, ×64.

of $\gamma\delta$ TcR^+ IELs coexpressing CD45R0 actually decreases to 59% (Halstensen *et al.*, 1990).

3. Function of Class II Molecules on Epithelial Cells

That normal small intestinal enterocytes could present nominal antigen (ovalbumin) to antigen-primed T cells was demonstrated first in the rat (Bland and Warren, 1986a). Somewhat surprisingly, the cells induced to proliferate were $CD8^+$ and were capable of antigen-specific suppressor activity (Bland and Warren, 1986b). In humans, isolated intestinal epithelial cells can act as stimulators in the mixed lymphocyte reaction (MLR) and also can present the antigen tetanus toxoid to syngeneic peripheral blood T cells (Mayer and Schlien, 1987). The cells responding to allo-determinants on epithelial cells in the MLR were $CD8^+$, which classically would be expected to respond to Class I MHC differences. However the proliferation of $CD8^+$ cells in the MLR was inhibited by anti-Class II antisera. $CD8^+$ cells activated by epithelial cells in the MLR were potent suppressors of polyclonal B-cell proliferation. To our knowledge, no data are currently available on antigen presentation by enterocytes to IELs, so these cells may respond differently.

The functional consequences of increased epithelial Class II expression for mucosal immunity are unclear. In humans, enterocytes from patients with inflammatory bowel disease (IBD) preferentially activate allogeneic $CD4^+$ lymphocytes with profound helper activity, whereas enterocytes from control patients activate allogeneic $CD8^+$ lymphocytes with suppressor activity (Mayer and Eisenhardt, 1990). Puzzlingly, enterocytes from patients with IBD have this property regardless of whether or not the bowel is inflamed, indicating that an inherent function of their epithelial cells rather than increased Class II expression is responsible for this phenomenon. In mice, increased epithelial Class II expression (induced by systemic administration of IFNγ) increases the antigen-presenting capacity of enterocytes and also renders mice less susceptible to oral tolerance (Zhang and Michael, 1990). These data might suggest that increased epithelial Class II expression leads to sensitization to enteric antigens and therefore might play a role in intestinal inflammation. The nature of the restriction element for T cells in the gut epithelium, and the role of MHC products in antigen presentation in the gut, is an area of great interest since gut epithelium in humans is among the few sites at which the nonclassical MHC molecule CD1d (Blumberg *et al.*, 1991) is expressed.

B. Intestinal Lamina Propria

The lamina propria is the layer of connective tissue between the epithelium and the muscularis mucosa. This layer is made up of smooth muscle cells, fibroblasts, lymphatics, and blood vessels, and makes up the villus core over which the absorptive epithelial cells migrate from the crypts to the villus tips. The most striking feature of adult human large and small intestinal lamina propria is the infiltrate of lymphoid/myeloid cells. The large numbers of macrophages, dendritic cells, and T cells in the lamina propria make it likely that antigen crossing the epithelium may be processed and presented to lamina propria $CD4^+$ T cells. These cells could provide B cell help, as well as function in mucosal cell-mediated immunity.

1. Plasma Cells in the Lamina Propria

As first observed almost 25 years ago, the major plasma cell isotype and, hence, the major immunoglobulin isotype in the intestinal secretions is IgA (Tomasi *et al.*, 1965; Crabbe and Heremans, 1966). IgA plasma cells make up 30–40% of the mononuclear cells in human intestinal lamina propria and small B cells make up 15–45% of the cells (MacDonald *et al.*, 1987). In the jejunum, around 80% of the total plasma cells secrete IgA, around 18% secrete IgM, and only 3% secrete IgG (Crabbe and Heremans, 1966; Brandtzaeg, 1987). These same relative proportions are seen also in the ileum and the colon, although fewer IgM plasma cells exist there than in the proximal small intestine. In addition, immediately adjacent to lymphoid follicles throughout the gut is an increase in IgG plasma cells (Bjerke and Brandtzaeg, 1986). IgD and IgE plasma cells are very uncommon. Most of the plasma cells, regardless of isotype, are found in the region around the crypts. Slightly more than half the IgA plasma cells in the gut secrete IgA2 (Crago *et al.*, 1984), in contrast to tonsils and lymph nodes in which most IgA is IgA1. In addition, the majority of IgA secreted by the plasma cells is dimeric IgA; 100% of IgA2 immunocytes are J-chain positive and 88% of IgA1 immunocytes are J-chain positive (Kett *et al.*, 1988). Dimeric IgA binds specifically via a J-chain–secretory component interaction to the basolateral aspect of crypt epithelial cells and is actively transported into the lumen.

No plasma cells exist in the lamina propria at birth (Perkkio and Savilahti, 1980) although a rapid expansion occurs after birth. Also, a dramatic reduction in IgA plasma cells occurs in the lamina propria of children with defunctioned colostomies (Wijesinha and Steer, 1982).

2. T Cells in the Lamina Propria

Immunohistochemical staining reveals that most of the T cells in the lamina propria are $CD4^+$ (Janossy *et al.*, 1980). Lamina propria $CD4^+$ T cells differ from blood $CD4^+$ T cells because the former do not bear the human homology of the murine lymph node homing receptor, Leu8 (Berg *et al.*, 1991). By immunohistochemistry, virtually no lamina propria T cells in normal bowel are $CD25^+$ (Choy *et al.*, 1990); however, by fluorescence activated cell sorting (FACS) analysis on isolated cells, about 10% are $CD25^+$ (Schreiber *et al.*, 1991). Equal numbers are $CD45RA^+$ and $CD45RO^+$, indicating that some may be memory cells (Halstensen *et al.*, 1990). Many studies have been done in which functional aspects of lamina propria T cells have been examined. All these studies, however, have utilized a technique in which the final cell preparation is virtually all small mononuclear cells with no plasma cells (Bull and Bookman, 1977). Since cells isolated from the lamina propria would be expected to contain many plasma cells, the so-called lamina propria T cells used in all these studies may, in fact, be derived from blood in the tissues, from the lymphatics, which are filled with lymphocytes in diseased bowel, or from Peyer's patches. The presence of T cells in the lamina propria is not totally dependent on luminal antigen, since they are present in the fetus (Spencer *et al.*, 1986e,f), but their numbers do increase after birth. The presence of plasma cells in the lamina propria, however, is antigen dependent.

3. Macrophages and Dendritic Cells in the Lamina Propria

Most of the HLA-DR$^+$ cells in the lamina propria of the large and small intestine are macrophages and dendritic cells (Selby *et al.*, 1983a). Note, however, that the distinction between these two cell types in the lamina propria is vague and controversial. Isolating these cells in any great number is virtually impossible, so most studies have used immunohistological or immunochemical techniques to characterize these cells. HLA-DR$^+$ antigen-presenting cells such as skin Langerhans cells, veiled cells, and interdigitating cells can be recognized by their long cytoplasmic protrusions, few lysosomes, strong presence of membrane ATPase, and weak or absent acid phosphatase activity. Cells with these characteristics cannot be isolated from normal human colon or ileum but can be isolated readily from Crohn's disease tissue (Wilders *et al.*, 1984).

The relative proportions of dendritic type cells to phagocytic type cells in human gut is unclear. Wilders *et al.* (1984) showed that, at the tops of the villi in normal intestine, a population of HLA-DR$^+$, strongly acid phosphatase positive cells exists. These cells are probably phagocytic macrophages identical to the population of 25F9$^+$ cells (a marker of mature macrophages) also identified in human small intestine (Hume *et al.*, 1987). Wilders *et al.* (1984) also reported that HLA-DR$^+$, weakly acid phosphatase-positive cells were sparse in normal intestine but were more abundant in Crohn's bowel, throughout the full mucosal thickness. In contrast, Selby *et al.* (1983a) reported that, in the normal human small intestine, 80–90% of the HLA-DR$^+$ histiocytes were weakly acid phosphatase-positive, weakly nonspecific esterase-positive, and strongly membrane ATPase-positive, suggesting that these cells are dendritic cells. In normal colon, Selby also reported that most of the HLA-DR$^+$ cells were strongly acid phosphatase- and esterase-positive and were weakly ATPase-positive. This work indicates that, in the small bowel, most of the HLA-DR$^+$ accessory cells are antigen-presenting cells, whereas in the large bowel most are phagocytic.

4. Changes in Lamina Propria Cell Populations in Disease States

Many studies have been done on the changes in the lamina propria cellular infiltrate in disease states. Reviewing these studies in detail is beyond the scope of this chapter. In general, these studies have been uninformative with respect to understanding gastrointestinal disease. In the food-sensitive enteropathies and inflammatory bowel diseases, an increase in lamina propria T cells occurs and CD4$^+$ cells still predominate. In inflammatory bowel disease, lamina propria CD4$^+$ cells show increased levels of activation antigens (Choy *et al.*, 1990; Schreiber *et al.*, 1991), and show increased reactivity to recall microbial antigens (Pirzer *et al.*, 1991). Lamina propria plasma cells of all isotypes also are increased in celiac disease, Crohn's disease, ulcerative colitis, and in the stomach in gastritis (Brandtzaeg, 1987). Several striking features of this condition are worth noting. Adjacent to fissures in Crohn's disease is a dramatic increase in IgG plasma cells (Brandtzaeg, 1987) and, in both ulcerative colitis and Crohn's disease, increased proportions of IgA1 plasma cells are seen (Kett and Brandtzaeg, 1987).

References

Arato, A., Savilahti, E., Taenio, V.-M., Verkasalo, M., and Klemola, T. (1987). HLA-DR expression, natural killer cells and IgE containing cells in the jejunal mucosa of coeliac children. *Gut* **28,** 988–994.

Balk, S. P., Ebert, E. C., Blumenthal, R. L., McDermott, F. V., Wucherpfennig, K. W., Landau, S. B., and Blumberg, R. S. (1991). Oligoclonal expansion and CD1 recognition by human intestinal intraepithelial lymphocytes. *Science* **253,** 1411–1415.

Barclay, A. N., and Mason, D. W. (1982). Induction of Ia antigen in rat epidermal cells and gut epithelium by immunologic stimuli. *J. Exp. Med.* **156,** 1665–1676.

Berg, M., Murakawa, Y., Camerini, D., and James, S. P. (1991). Lamina propria lymphocytes are derived from circulating cells that lack the Leu-8 lymph node homing receptor. *Gastroenterology* **101,** 90–99.

Bjerke, K., and Brandtzaeg, P. (1986). Immunoglobulin- and J chain-producing cells associated with lymphoid follicles in the human appendix, colon, and ileum, including Peyer's patches. *Clin. Exp. Immunol.* **64,** 432–441.

Bjerke, K., and Brandtzaeg, P. (1988). Lack of relation between expression of HLA-DR and secretory component (SC) in follicle-associated epithelium of human Peyer's patches. *Clin. Exp. Immunol.* **71,** 502–507.

Bjerke, K., Brandtzaeg, P., and Rognum, T. O. (1986). Distribution of immunoglobulin producing cells is different in normal human appendix and colon mucosa. *Gut* **27,** 667–674.

Bjerke, K., Brandtzaeg, P., and Fausa, O. (1988). T cell distribution is different in follicle-associated epithelium of human Peyer's patches and villous epithelium. *Clin. Exp. Immunol.* **74,** 270–275.

Bland, P. W., and Warren, L. G. (1986a). Antigen presentation by epithelial cells of the rat small intestine. 1. Kinetics, antigen specificity and blocking by anti-Ia antisera. *Immunology* **58,** 1–7.

Bland, P. W., and Warren, L. G. (1986b). Antigen presentation by epithelial cells of the rat small intestine. 2. Selective induction of suppressor T cells. *Immunology* **58,** 9–14.

Blumberg, R. S., Terhorst, C., Bleicher, P., McDermott, F. V., Allan, C. H., Landau, S. B., Trier, J. S., and Balk, S. P. (1991). Expression of a nonpolymorphic MHC Class 1-like molecule, CD1D, by human intestinal epithelial cells. *J. Immunol.* **147,** 2518–2524.

Brandtzaeg, P. (1987). The B cell system. *In* "Food Allergy and Intolerance" (J. Brostoff and S. B. Challacombe, eds.), pp. 118–155. Bailliere Tindall, London.

Brandtzaeg, P., Bosnes, V., Halstensen, T. S., Scott, H., Sollid, L. M., and Valnes, K. N. (1989). T lymphocytes in human gut epithelium express preferentially the α/β antigen receptor and are often CD45/UCHL1-positive. *Scand. J. Immunol.* **30,** 123–128.

Bridges, R. A., Condie, R. M., Zak, S. J., and Good, R. A. (1959). The morphologic basis of antibody formation development during the neonatal period. *J. Lab. Clin. Med.* **53,** 331–359.

Bull, D. M., and Bookman, M. A. (1977). Isolation and functional characterization of human intestinal mucosal lymphoid cells. *J. Clin. Invest.* **59,** 966–974.

Bye, W. A., Allan, C. H., and Trier, J. S. (1984). Structure, distribution, and origin of M cells in Peyer's patches of mouse ileum. *Gastroenterology* **86,** 789–801.

Cerf-Bensussan, N., Quaroni, A., Kurnick, J. T., and Bhan, A. K. (1984). Intraepithelial lymphocytes modulate Ia expression by intestinal epithelial cells. *J. Immunol.* **132,** 2244–2252.

Choy, M-Y., Richman, P. I., Walker-Smith, J. A., and MacDonald, T. T. (1990). Differential expression of CD25 on lamina propria T cells and macrophages in the intestinal lesions in Crohn's disease and ulcerative colitis. *Gut* **31,** 1365–1370.

Cornes, J. S. (1965a). Number, size, and distribution of Peyer's patches in the human small intestine. Part 1. The development of Peyer's patches. *Gut* **6,** 225–229.

Cornes, J. S. (1965b). Number, size, and distribution of Peyer's patches in the human small intestine. Part 2. The effect of age on Peyer's patches. *Gut* **6,** 230–233.

Crabbe, P. A., and Heremans, J. F. (1966). The distribution of immunoglobulin containing cells along the human gastrointestinal tract. *Gastroenterology* **51,** 305–316.

Crago, S. S., Kutteh, W. H., Moro, I., Allansmith, M. R., Radl, J., Haaijman, J. J., and Mestecky, J. (1984). Distribution of IgA1^{-}, IgA2^{-}, and J chain-containing cells in human tissues. *J. Immunol.* **132,** 16–18.

Dukes, C., and Bussey, H. J. R. (1926). The number of lymphoid follicles of the human large intestine. *J. Pathol. Bacteriol.* **29,** 111–116.

Fukushima, K., Masuda, T., Ohtani, H., Sasaki, I., Funayama, Y., Matsuno, S., and Nagura, H. (1991). Immunohistochemical characterization, distribution, and ultrastructure of lymphocytes bearing T-cell receptor $\gamma\delta$ in inflammatory bowel disease. *Gastroenterology* **101,** 670–678.

Groh, V., Porcelli, S., Fabbi, M., Lanier, L., Picker, L. J., Anderson, T., Warnke, R. A., Bhan, A. K., Strominger, J. L., and Brenner, M. B. (1989). Human lymphocytes bearing the T cell receptor γ/δ are phenotypically diverse and evenly distributed throughout the lymphoid system. *J. Exp. Med.* **169,** 1277–1294.

Halstensen, T. S., Scott, H., and Brandtzaeg, P. (1989). Intraepithelial T cells of the TcR$\gamma/\delta+$ CD8$-$ and Vδ1/Jδ1+ phenotypes are increased in coeliac disease. *Scand. J. Gastroenterol.* **30,** 665–672.

Halstensen, T. S., Farstad, I. N., Scott, H., Fausa, O., and Brandtzaeg, P. (1990). Intraepithelial TcR $\alpha/\beta+$ lymphocytes express CD45RO more often than the TcR $\gamma\delta+$ counterparts in coeliac disease. *Immunology* **71,** 460–466.

Hassall, E., and Dimmick, J. E. (1991). Unique features of Helicobacter pylori disease in children. *Dig. Dis. Sci.* **36,** 417–423.

Hume, D. A., Allan, W., Hogan, P. G., and Doe, W. F. (1987). Immunohistochemical characterization of macrophages in human liver and gastrointestinal tract. Expression of CD4, HLA-DR, OKM1, and the mature macrophage marker 25F9 in normal and diseased tissue. *J. Leukocyte Biol.* **42,** 474–484.

Jacob, E., Baker, S. J., and Swaminathan, S. P. (1987). "M" cells in the follicle-associated epithelium of the human colon. *Histopathology* **11,** 941–952.

Janossy, G., Tidman, N., Selby, W. S., Thomas, J. A., Granger, S., Kung, P. C., and Goldstein, G. (1980). Human T lymphocytes of inducer and suppressor type occupy different microenvironments. *Nature (London)* **288,** 81–84.

Jarry, A., Cerf-Bensussan, N., Brousse, N., Selz, F., and Guy-Grand, D. (1990). Subsets of CD3+ T cell receptor ($\alpha\beta$ or $\gamma\delta$) and CD3$-$ lymphocytes isolated from normal human gut epithelium display phenotypical features different from their counterparts in peripheral blood. *Eur. J. Immunol.* **20,** 1097–1104.

Kazi, J. I., Sinniah, R., Jaffrey, N. A., Alam, S. M., Zaman, V., Zuberi, S. J., and Kazi, A. M. (1989). Cellular and humoral immune responses in *Campylobacter pylori*-associated chronic gastritis. *J. Pathol.* **159,** 231–237.

Kett, K., and Brandtzaeg, P. (1987). Local IgA subclass alterations in ulcerative colitis and Crohn's disease of the colon. *Gut* **28,** 1013–1021.

Kett, K., Brandtzaeg, P., and Fausa, O. (1988). J-chain expression is more prominent in immunoglobulin A2 than in immunoglobulin A1 colonic immunocytes and is decreased in both subclasses associated with inflammatory bowel disease. *Gastroenterology* **94,** 1419–1425.

MacDonald, T. T., Spencer, J., Viney, J. L., Williams, C. B., and Walker-Smith, J. A. (1987). Selective biopsy of Peyer's patches during ileal endoscopy. *Gastroenterology* **93,** 1356–1362.

MacDonald, T. T., Weinel, A., and Spencer, J. M. (1988). HLA-DR expression in human fetal intestinal epithelium. *Gut* **29,** 1342–1348.

Mason, D. W., Dallman, M., and Barclay, A. N. (1981). Graft-versus-host disease induces expression of Ia antigen in rat epidermal cells and gut epithelium. *Nature (London)* **293,** 150–151.

Mayer, L., and Eisenhardt, D. (1990). Lack of induction of suppressor T cells by intestinal epithelial cells from patients with inflammatory bowel disease. *J. Clin. Invest.* **86,** 1255–1260.

Mayer, L., and Shlien, R. (1987). Evidence for function of Ia molecules on gut epithelial cells in man. *J. Exp. Med.* **166,** 1471–1483.

Mayrhofer, G., Pugh, C. W., and Barclay, A. N. (1983). The distribution, ontogeny and origin in the rat of Ia-positive cells with dendritic morphology and of Ia antigen in epithelia, with special reference to the intestine. *Eur. J. Immunol.* **13,** 112–122.

Mirakian, R., Richardson, A., Milla, P. J., Walker-Smith, J. A., Unsworth, J., Savage, M. O., and Bottazzo, G. F. (1986). Protracted diarrhoea of infancy, evidence in support of an autoimmune variant. *Br. Med. J.* **293,** 1132–1136.

O'Leary, A. D., and Sweeney, E. C. (1986). Lymphoglandular complexes of the colon, structure and distribution. *Histopathology* **10,** 267–283.

Owen, R. L. (1977). Sequential uptake of horseradish peroxidase by lymphoid follicle epithelium of Peyer's patches in normal unobstructed mouse intestine. An ultrastructural study. *Gastroenterology* **72,** 440–451.

Owen, R. L., and Jones, A. L. (1974). Epithelial cell specialization within human Peyer's patches, an ultrastructural study of intestinal lymphoid follicles. *Gastroenterology* **66,** 189–203.

Owen, R. L., Apple, R. T., and Bhalla, D. K. (1986). Morphometric and cytochemical analysis of lysosomes in rat Peyer's patch follicle epithelium, their reduction in volume fraction and acid phosphatase content in M cells compared to adjacent enterocytes. *Anat. Rec.* **216,** 521–527.

Perkkio, M., and Savilahti, E. (1980). Time of appearance of immunoglobulin-containing cells in the mucosa of the neonatal intestine. *Pediatr. Res.* **14,** 953–955.

Pirzer, U., Schönhaar, A., Fleischer, B., Hermann, E., Meyer zum Büschenfelde, K-H. (1991). Reactivity of infiltrating T lymphocytes with microbial antigens in Crohn's disease. *Lancet* **338,** 1238–1239.

Poulsen, L. O., Elling, P., Sorensen, F. B., and Hoedt-Rasmussen, K. (1986). HLA-DR expression and disease activity in ulcerative colitis. *Scand. J. Gastroenterol.* **21,** 364–368.

Rickert, R. R., and Carter, H. W. (1980). The "early" ulcerative lesion of Crohn's disease, correlative light- and scanning electron-microscopic studies. *J. Clin. Gastroenterol.* **2,** 11–19.

Schreiber, S., MacDermott, R. P., Raedler, A., Pinnau, R., Bertovich, M. J., and Nash, G. S. (1991). Increased activation of isolated intestinal lamina propria mononuclear cells in inflammatory bowel disease. *Gastroenterology* **101,** 1020–1030.

Scott, H., Solheim, B. G., Brandtzaeg, P., and Thorsby, E. (1980). HLA-DR-like antigens in the epithelium of the human small intestine. *Scand. J. Immunol.* **12,** 77–82.

Scott, H., Brandtzaeg, P., Solheim, B. G., and Thorsby, E. (1981). Relation between HLA-DR-like antigens and secretory component (SC) in jejunal epithelium of patients with coeliac disease or dermatitis herpetiformis. *Clin. Exp. Immunol.* **44,** 233–238.

Scott, H., Sollid, L. M., Fausa, O., and Brandtzaeg, P. (1987). Expression of major histocompatability Class 11 subregion products by jejunal epithelium in histocompatability Class 11 subregion products by jejunal epithelium in patients with coeliac disease. *Scand. J. Immunol.* **26,** 563–571.

Selby, W. S., Poulter, L. W., Hobbs, S., Jewell, D. P., and Janossy, G. (1983a). Heterogeneity of HLA-DR-positive histiocytes in human intestinal lamina propria, a combined histochemical and immunohistological analysis. *J. Clin. Pathol.* **36,** 379–384.

Selby, W. S., Janossy, G., Mason, D. Y., and Jewell, D. P. (1983b). Expression of HLA-DR antigens by colonic epithelium in inflammatory bowel disease. *Clin. Exp. Immunol.* **53,** 614–618.

Sicinski, P., Rowinski, J., Warchol, J. B., Jarzabek, Z., Gut, W., Szczygiel, B., Bielecki, K., and Koch, K. (1990). Poliovirus type 1 enters the human host through intestinal M cells. *Gastroenterology* **98,** 56–58.

Sollid, L. M., Kvale, D., Brandtzaeg, P., Markussen, G., and Thorsby, E. (1987). Interferon-γ enhances expression of secretory component, the epithelial receptor for polymeric immunoglobulins. *J. Immunol.* **138,** 4303–4306.

Spencer, J., Finn, T., and Isaacson, P. G. (1985). Gut associated lymphoid tissue. A morphological and immunocytochemical study of the human appendix. *Gut* **26,** 672–679.

Spencer, J., Finn, T., and Isaacson, P. G. (1986a). Expression of HLA-DR antigens on epithelium associated with lymphoid tissue in the human gastrointestinal tract. *Gut* **27,** 153–157.

Spencer, J., Finn, T., and Isaacson, P. G. (1986b). Human Peyer's patches. An immunohistochemical study. *Gut* **27,** 405–410.

Spencer, J., Finn, T., and Isaacson, P. G. (1986c). A comparative study of the gut-associated lymphoid tissue of primates and rodents. *Virchows Arch. Cell Pathol.* **51,** 509–519.

Spencer, J., Pugh, S., and Isaacson, P. G. (1986d). HLA-D region antigen expression on stomach epithelium in absence of autoantibodies. *Lancet* **2,** 983.

Spencer, J. M., Dillon, S. B., Isaacson, P. G., and MacDonald, T. T. (1986e). T cell subclasses in human fetal ileum. *Clin. Exp. Immunol.* **65,** 553–558.

Spencer, J. M., MacDonald, T. T., Finn, T. T., and Isaacson, P. G. (1986f). Development of Peyer's patches in human fetal terminal ileum. *Clin. Exp. Immunol.* **64,** 536–543.

Spencer, J., Isaacson, P. G., Diss, T. C., and MacDonald, T. T. (1989). Expression of disulphide linked and non-disulphide linked forms of the T cell receptor gamma/delta heterodimer in human intestinal intraepithelial lymphocytes. *Eur. J. Immunol.* **19,** 1335–1339.

Spencer, J., Isaacson, P., MacDonald, T. T., Thomas, A. J., and Walker-Smith, J. A. (1991a). Gamma/delta T cells and the diagnosis of coeliac disease. *Clin. Exp. Immunol.* **85,** 109–113.

Spencer, J., Choy, M.-Y., and MacDonald, T. T. (1991b). T cell receptor expression in normal and diseased human intestine. *J. Clin. Pathol.* **44,** 915–918.

Tomasi, T. B., Tan, E. M., Soloman, E. A., and Prendergast, R. A. (1965). Characterization of an immune system common to certain external secretions. *J. Exp. Med.* **121,** 101–124.

Wilders, M. M., Drexhage, H. A., Kokje, M., Verspaget, H., and Meuwissen, G. M. (1984). Veiled cells in chronic idiopathic inflammatory bowel disease. *Clin. Exp. Immunol.* **55,** 377–387.

Wijesinha, S. S., and Steer, H. W. (1982). Studies of the immunoglobulin-producing cells of the human intestine, the defunctioned bowel. *Gut* **23,** 211–214.

Wiman, K., Curman, B., Forsum, U., Klareskog, L., Malmnas-Tjernlund, U., Rask, L., Tragardh, L., and Peterson, P. A. (1978). Occurrence of Ia antigens on tissues of non-lymphoid origin. *Nature (London)* **276,** 711–713.

Wolf, J. L., Rubin, D. H., Finberg, R., Kauffman, R. S., Sharpe, A. H., Trier, J. S., and Fields, B. N. (1981). Intestinal M cells, A pathway for entry of reovirus into host. *Science* **212,** 471–472.

Wotherspoon, A. C., Ortiz-Hitalgo, C., Falzon, M. R., and Isaacson, P. G. (1991). *Helicobacter pylori*-associated gastritis and primary B cell lymphoma. *Lancet* **338,** 1175–1176.

Wyatt, J. I., and Rathbone, B. J. (1988). Immune response of the gastric mucosa to *Campylobacter pylori*. *Scand. J. Gastroenterol.* **23** (Suppl 142), 44–49.

Zhang, Z., and Michael, J. G. (1990). Orally inducible immune unresponsiveness is abrogated by IFN-γ treatment. *J. Immunol.* **144,** 4163–4165.

36

Alpha Chain Disease and Related Lymphoproliferative Disorders

Jean-Claude Rambaud • Jean-Claude Brouet • Maxime Seligmann

I. ALPHA CHAIN DISEASE

Heavy chain diseases (HCD) are lymphoproliferative disorders of B cells that are characterized by the production of immunoglobulin (Ig) molecules consisting of incomplete heavy chains devoid of light chains.

Alpha chain disease (αHCD; Seligmann *et al.*, 1968) is by far the most frequent type of HCD. αHCD involves primarily the IgA secretory system. The vast majority of patients is affected with the digestive form of αHCD, which primarily involves the small intestine and the mesenteric lymph nodes.

A. Pathology

The pathological features of αHCD are, in most cases, in accordance with their initial description (Rambaud *et al.*, 1968; Galian *et al.*, 1977). Apart from a few cases described in this chapter, αHCD involves the whole length of the small intestine, except sometimes the terminal ileum, without intervening normal mucosa. Three grades of increasing malignancy can be recognized. At stage A, the cellular infiltrate is localized mainly to the mucosa, with occasional limited infiltration of adjacent submucosa. Villi are more or less shortened and widened; crypts are sparse and atrophic; and lamina propria is infiltrated massively by mature and occasional younger plasma cells (Figure 1). Stage C corresponds to an immunoblastic lymphoma with plasmacytoid features (Figure 2), either forming discrete ulcerated tumor(s) or extensively infiltrating long segments of the small intestine (Figure 3). Stage B is intermediate between A and C. The infiltrate largely invades at least the submucosa; plasma cells are frankly dystrophic and some large immunoblastic or centroblastic-like cells are observed, usually located in the deeper area of the infiltrate and sometimes clustering in small nodules. Occasionally numerous reactive follicles may be observed within mucosa or submucosa at stages A and B (Isaacson *et al.*, 1989; Price, 1990).

Mesenteric lymph nodes usually (but not always at stage A) are involved in the pathological process. According to the cell type of the infiltrate and to the degree of architectural disorganization, three histological stages (A, B, and C) equivalent to those described in the small intestine can be identified. Spreading to other lymph nodes (retroperitoneal, mediastinal, and peripheral lymph nodes), other parts of the digestive tract (stomach, colon, Waldeyer's ring), and other organs such as liver, spleen, bone marrow, pleura, or central nervous system initially was considered to be very rare, except when enteric lesions were at stage C (Seligmann *et al.*, 1969; Rambaud and Matuchansky, 1973; Reyes *et al.*, 1985; Kumar *et al.*, 1988).

Histological lesions may progress at a given site from stage A to B or from stage B to C, but of utmost importance for proper pretherapeutic staging is the fact that different stages can be found at the same time in different organs or lymph nodes or even at different sites within the same organ.

This overview of αHCD pathology requires some additions. In very few patients, intestinal lesions apparently spare the duodenum or even the jejunum or, in contrast, are limited to a short segment of the latter (Nemes *et al.*, 1981). Spread of the disease in the digestive tract outside the enteromesenteric area is not so uncommon, even at stage A. This spread usually concerns gastric or colorectal mucosa; in some cases the disease is confined to these organs, sparing the small bowel (Rambaud and Halphen, 1989). In stomach, numerous signet-ring cells can be admixed with plasma cells (Tungekar, 1986). Other rare primary localizations of αHCD are the respiratory tract (Seligmann and Rambaud, 1978) and the thyroid (Tracy *et al.*, 1984). In a single case, the disease appeared to involve peripheral non-mucosa-associated lymphoid tissue only (Takahashi *et al.*, 1988).

In a few instances, plasma cells synthesizing the αHCD protein were limited to a continuous band in the superficial part of the intestinal mucosa. The deeper zone was infiltrated by centrocytic-like cells forming lymphoepithelial lesions; the immunohistological study of these cells showed their common clonal origin with plasma cells. In addition, multiple reactive nonneoplastic follicles were present in the mucosa and submucosa. These follicles tended to be more or less penetrated by the centrocytic-like cell infiltrate. This peculiar pattern of αHCD pathological lesions was observed initially by Galian *et al.* (1977) and Nemes *et al.* (1981), but was reemphasized and better characterized by Isaacson *et al.* (1989). For these authors, these peculiar forms of αHCD merely reflect the similarity between αHCD and the Western gastrointestinal lymphomas of the mucosa-associated lymphoid tissue (MALT) type. Indeed, Isaacson *et al.* (1989) and Price (1990) reported the presence, in usual pathological forms of αHCD at stages A and B, of well-demarcated foci

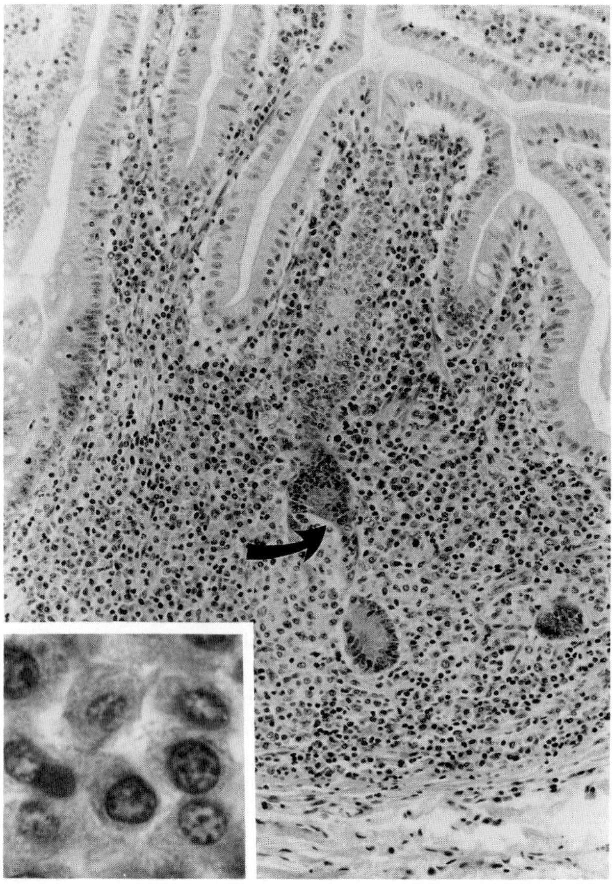

Figure 1 Alpha chain disease at stage A. Histological pattern of the jejunal mucosa. A lymphoepithelial lesion is indicated by the arrow. Hematoxylin and eosin (H&E), ×115. *Inset:* Detail of the plasma cell infiltrate. H & E, ×950.

of centrocytic-like cells centered around crypts and forming characteristic lymphoepithelial lesions (Figure 1).

Few cytogenetic studies have been performed; karyotypic abnormalities involving chromosome 14 have been observed (Gafter *et al.*, 1980), including rearrangements of 14q32 (Berger *et al.*, 1986).

B. Epidemiology

The age distribution of αHCD is in sharp contrast with that of multiple myeloma as well as that of intestinal lymphomas occurring in western Europe. The great majority of patients is between 15 and 35 years old, with a slight preponderance in males. The geographical origin of the patients is very peculiar. Table I shows the geographical distribution of 130 cases that had been reported, or diagnosed in our laboratory, prior to 1978. Since then, several hundred cases have been recorded in the same and other countries from Africa, Central and South America, the Indian subcontinent, the Middle East, the Far East, and southern and eastern Europe. Obviously a wide spectrum of racial and ethnic origin exists. Most patients originated from and had been living in areas with a high degree of infestation by intestinal microorganisms. In

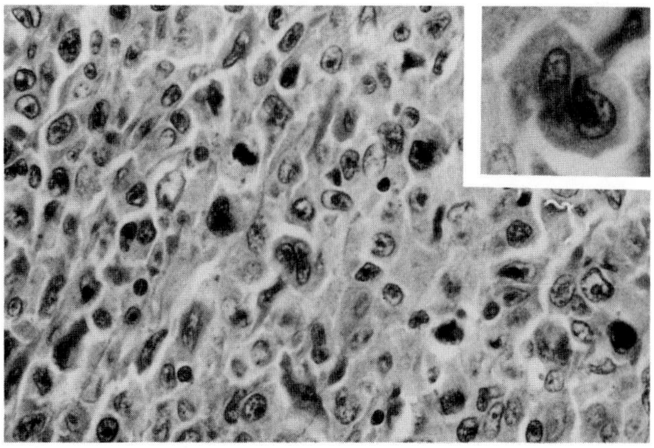

Figure 2 Alpha chain disease at stage C. Histological pattern of the jejunal cellular infiltrate (immunoblastic lymphoma). H & E, ×840. *Inset:* Malignant immunoblast. H & E, ×744. Reprinted with permission from Navab *et al.* (1978).

addition, many of these patients were of low socioeconomic background and were exposed to conditions of poor hygiene.

These epidemiologic features and the complete remissions achieved at the early stage of the disease by antibiotic treatment alone strongly suggest that environmental factors, providing local and protracted antigenic stimulation, play an important role in the pathogenesis of αHCD. No specific microorganisms could be found by bacterological, virological, or parasitological studies (Harzic *et al.*, 1985). The postulated antigenic stimulation by such agent(s) may have occurred many years before the disease became clinically manifest, particularly during infancy. The absence of the Fab region in the αHCD protein precludes its use for identifying

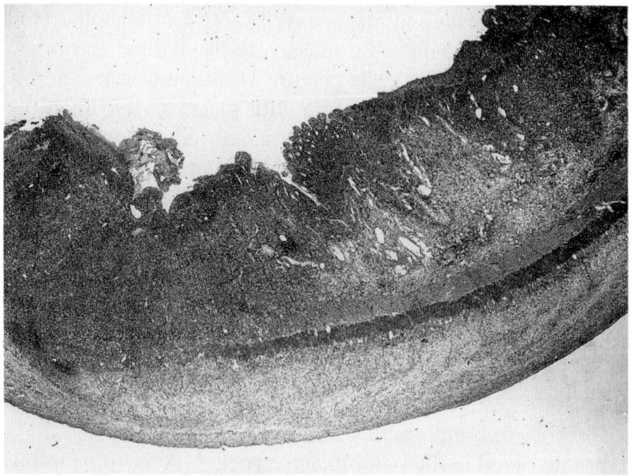

Figure 3 Alpha chain disease at stage C. Histological pattern of the jejunal wall obtained during staging laparotomy. Note the invasion of submucosa and muscularis propria by the tumeral process and the ulceration of the left part of the mucosa. H & E, ×9. Reprinted with permission from Galian *et al.* (1977).

Table I Geographical Origin of the First 130 Patients with αHCD[a]

Africa		Far East	
Tunisia	25	Pakistan	2
Algeria	21	Cambodia	1
Morocco	3	India	1
South Africa	3	Europe	
Nigeria	2	Spain	10
Zaire	1	Turkey	9
Mali	1	South Italy	6
		Yugoslavia	2
Middle East		Greece	2
Iran	13	Finland	1
Israel	10	Portugal	2
Lebanon	2	Netherlands	1[b]
Egypt	2	Great Britain	1[b]
Syria	1	The Americas	
Saudi Arabia	1	United States	1[b]
Libya	1	Columbia	1
Kuwait	1	Mexico	1
Iraq	1	Argentina	1

[a] Reprinted with permission from Seligmann *et al.* (1979).
[b] Respiratory form of the disease.

putative antigenic stimuli. The environmental factors could trigger the clonal proliferation directly or, alternatively, could represent only predisposing factors. In either case, that the plasma cell proliferation resulting from this postulated antigenic stimulation appears to lead, in these patients to the production of an HCD protein rather than of a whole myeloma globulin is remarkable. Indeed, we know of only two patients with the typical clinicopathological pattern of αHCD in whom a complete monoclonal IgA was found in serum (Chantar *et al.*, 1974; Tangun *et al.*, 1975) whereas, in another patient with the same features, a γHCD protein was demonstrated in the serum and intestinal cells (Bender *et al.*, 1978). In a few other patients with similar features, the massive small intestinal plasma cell infiltrate was polyclonal with high plasma levels of polymeric IgA (Brandtzaeg and Baklien, 1977; Gilinsky *et al.*, 1985; Colombel *et al.*, 1988).

The association with an underlying immunodeficiency that could be the result of malnutrition, especially in early infancy (Dutz *et al.*, 1971), or of genetic factors is not ruled out. In fact, the role of environmental factors does not exclude the possibility of predisposing genetic factors, although no familial cases have been reported and although the search in Tunisia by the Tufrali Group for serum Ig abnormalities in the patient's relatives has been negative, as have HLA typing studies.

C. Laboratory Diagnosis

1. Serum and Other Fluids

The demonstration, by immunochemical methods, of the presence of Ig α heavy chains devoid of light chains in the serum (or jejunal fluid) is mandatory for the diagnosis of αHCD.

The abnormal Ig chains are not evidenced by serum electrophoresis in nearly half the cases (Seligmann *et al.*, 1979). When detectable by this procedure, the pathological protein rarely, if ever, shows the discrete narrow spike suggestive of a monoclonal Ig abnormality. Instead, α chains feature a broad band that may extend from the α2 to the β2 region. This remarkable electrophoretic behavior of αHCD may be related to the tendency of these chains to polymerize or to their high carbohydrate content (Seligmann *et al.*, 1979).

The identification of the αHCD proteins therefore relies on serum immunoelectrophoresis, immunoselection, or immunofixation. The pathological protein may escape detection by the first method when its serum concentration is low. Moreover, lack of precipitation of the abnormal protein with anti-light chain antisera may be observed for some monoclonal IgA myeloma proteins (Seligmann *et al.*, 1969). Immunoselection combined with immunoelectrophoresis allows the detection of αHCD proteins in most cases (Doe *et al.*, 1979). This technique, however, requires rather large amounts of highly selected antisera to κ and λ light chains, capable of precipitating completely all monoclonal and polyclonal Ig molecules. Finally, immunofixation (O'Reilly *et al.*, 1981) is easier to perform, is sensitive, and allows the detection of αHCD when the level of polyclonal IgA is low or when the migration of the pathological protein extends beyond the β region. All αHCD proteins appear to belong to the α1 subclass; no α2 HCD protein has been found in over 100 studied cases (Seligmann, 1977). Since one-third of the normal secretory IgA molecules belong to the α2 subclass, this finding is obviously significant, although it remains unexplained.

Of note, other serum Ig abnormalities may be found in αHCD. Serum levels of normal polyclonal Ig molecules of all classes may be reduced independent of the protein-losing enteropathy. In addition, serum monoclonal IgG were disclosed in four cases of αHCD.

The αHCD protein, bound to the secretory piece, is present in significant amounts in the jejunal fluid of patients with the digestive form of αHCD (Seligmann *et al.*, 1969). The immunochemical techniques used for the detection of αHCD protein are the same as for serum; however, jejunal fluid must be collected carefully and concentrated to avoid protein degradation. In some patients with the clinicopathological features of αHCD, the pathological protein can be found in the jejunal fluid but cannot be detected in the serum (Rambaud *et al.*, 1983).

In almost all instances of αHCD, only minimal amounts of HCD are present in the urine and monoclonal light chains are always absent.

2. Cellular Studies

The study of proliferating plasma cells or immunoblasts by conventional immunofluorescence or immunoperoxidase techniques, on cell suspensions (from lymph nodes or bone marrow) or histological sections, demonstrates the presence of intracytoplasmic α heavy chains in the absence of light chains in most cases (Preud'homme *et al.*, 1979). However, exceptions to this pattern do exist since κ light chains were found in the cytoplasm or at the surface of the proliferating plasma cells in three cases of αHCD (Preud'homme *et al.*, 1979). Immunochemical studies permit the detection of the rare cases of nonsecretory αHCD, in patients with the characteristic clinicopathological pattern but without detectable αHCD protein in the serum or jejunal fluid (Rambaud *et al.*,1983; Matuchansky *et al.*, 1989). In one such case, molecular studies identified the mechanism responsible for the absence of secretion (Cogné and Preud'homme, 1990): a deletion had occurred of the polyadenylation site for secretory α1 chain mRNA; however, the membrane form of the abnormally short α heavy chain was produced.

D. Structure of the αHCD Protein and Productive α Genes

Most HCD proteins consist primarily of the Fc region and have a normal carboxyl terminal. The missing portion of the heavy chain therefore usually is located within the Fd fragment (Seligmann *et al.*, 1979). Indeed, most αHCD proteins lack the variable and first constant domains. In four of five αHCD proteins studied in our laboratory (Seligmann *et al.*, 1979), the sequence started with a valine residue corresponding to position 222 of the α1 heavy chain, that is, the first amino acid of the hinge region. In the fifth case, the normal hinge region sequence was preceded by a short stretch of amino acids whose sequence did not belong obviously to Ig-related sequences (Wolfenstein-Todel *et al.*, 1974). Sub amino-terminal sequences of unknown origin also have been found in some cases of γ- and μHCD (Franklin and Frangione, 1975; Seligmann *et al.*, 1979; Barnikol-Watanabe *et al.*, 1984).

Of note, the sequence of αHCD proteins was difficult to assess because of technical difficulties in the isolation of the pathological protein or because of the existence of a heterogenous amino-terminal sequence most likely created by limited proteolytic cleavage of the amino-terminal end of the hinge region (Seligmann, 1977). Biosynthesis experiments indicated that HCD proteins are not a mere degradation product of a normal chain, but that truly short heavy chains are synthesized by the cells (Buxbaum and Preud'homme, 1972).

The latter results were confirmed by the nucleotide sequence analysis of the α mRNA and of the rearranged productive α1 genes from invaded mesenteric lymph nodes. In three reported cases (Bentaboulet *et al.*, 1989; Tsapis *et al.*, 1989; Cogné and Preud'homme, 1990) as well as in eight additional patients (Fakhfakh *et al.*, 1992), the α mRNA was short, lacking the whole V_H and C_H1 segments. A striking additional feature of these α mRNAs was the presence, at their 5′ ends, of a 20- to 80-nucleotide stretch that had no homology with Ig or non-Ig sequences stored in data banks. This sequence of unknown origin was in frame with that of the hinge, C_H2, and C_H3 α domains. Therefore, a proteolytic cleavage must take place within the cell since the serum protein usually is devoid of an abnormal amino-terminal sequence. However, such inserted sequences might account for those rare proteins with such an unusual amino-terminal end (see previous discussion). Biosynthesis studies in one case showed two different α chains of slightly different molecular masses, which may correspond to the two species of α chains (Tsapis *et al.*, 1989). Of note, no homology existed between the inserted sequences from different patients (which might have provided a clue about the pathogenesis of αHCD).

Analysis of the sequence of the productive α1 chain genes in three cases indicated that these non-Ig sequences arise by various mechanisms. In two cases, the extra sequence found in the mRNA originated from part of a very long sequence (289 and 360 bp) that replaced the V_H gene (Tsapis *et al.*, 1989; Cogné and Preud'homme, 1990). In the other case (Bentaboulet *et al.*, 1989), the mRNA insert corresponded to two composite exons from the J_H region, including a 62-nucleotide insertion of unknown origin. Again, analysis of the inserted sequences at the DNA level yielded no indication of their possible derivation. The lack of a C_H1 domain was related to a deletion event affecting the whole C_H1 exon in two cases and the 5′ end of the C_H exon in the third case. Analysis of the flanking sequences of these deletions provided no clue about the mechanism underlying this event. Another remarkable feature of these altered α1 genes was a high degree of mutation affecting primarily the J_H region, which retains a low homology (66–90%) with its germ-line counterpart. These alterations within the J_H region appear to be a common feature of sequenced γ- and αHCD productive genes (Cogné *et al.*, 1989); these changes result in an unusual splicing, using alternative splice sites and eliminating a large part of the remnant V_H and J_H segments. In addition, we sequenced a nonfunctional α1 gene implicated in a t(9,14) translocation and found strikingly similar abnormalities, including a high number of mutations and a deletion of the 3′ end of a V_H rearranged gene (Pellet *et al.*, 1990).

Interestingly, the single nucleotide sequence established for a rearranged κ light chain gene in cells from a patient with γHCD exhibited similar features (Cogné *et al.*, 1988a), indicating that these unusual genetic alterations took place in different genetic loci located on different chromosomes. With respect to αHCD we observed, in all eight cases studied, the presence of rearranged κ genes and of nonproductive κ mRNA (Fakhfakh *et al.*, 1992).

Overall, the study of nucleic acids in αHCD as well as in other varieties of HCD has not yet generated comprehensive insights into the pathogenesis of these disorders. The abnormalities are distinct from those of mouse plasmocytoma and bear some similarities to those of cells from some nonsecreting lymphoma cell lines that produce truncated μ chains in the absence of light chains (Cogné *et al.*, 1988b).

E. Clinical Features

The usual presentation of αHCD is remarkably uniform; its pattern has not been modified noticeably since its early description (Rambaud *et al.*, 1968; Rambaud and Seligmann, 1976; Gargouri and Amor, 1982). The onset is usually gradual, but may be abrupt. The time from appearance of the first symptom to diagnosis ranges from 1 month to 6 years; an intermittent clinical course is not rare. Table II gives the frequency of presenting symptoms and signs in two series of patients. In fact, two clinical patterns can be distinguished.

In the majority of patients diagnosed in developed countries of western Europe, the clinical presentation is chronic diarrhea with evidence of malabsorption. However, a profuse watery diarrhea may be observed; water and electrolyte imbalance may result in atypical presentations, such as nephrogenic diabetes insipidus (Economidou *et al.*,1976). Apart from signs of protein-caloric malnutrition and specific deficiencies, finger clubbing is the single frequent physical finding, present more often than in any other enteric disease.

The second presentation pattern usually follows the neglected or misdiagnosed preceding one, but in rare cases may occur first. This presentation is the result of the occurrence, usually at stage C, of digestive tract tumors or of voluminous abdominal adenomegalies and their complications. Abdominal examination often finds abdominal masses; surgical emergencies may be due to intestinal intussusception or perforation of ulcerated lesions, but rarely to digestive hemorrhage. Pains may simulate acute appendicitis or pancreatitis and are related to lymph node necrosis. Chronic obstruction as a result of stenosing infiltration or masses has been also observed. Pathological study of surgical resection or biopsy is essential for diagnosis.

Some patients, often with this "tumoral" syndrome and usually at stage C, may present with signs of tumoral dissemination to liver, spleen, Waldeyer's ring, peripheral lymph nodes, or bone marrow. The rare isolated gastric localizations of αHCD are revealed by epigastric pain, vomiting, and often weight loss.

F. Digestive Investigations

Usual biological investigations confirm the malabsorption syndrome and protein-losing enteropathy (Table III). The frequent increase in alkaline phosphatase initially was considered of intestinal origin, but this symptom later proved to be rare; the source of the enzyme is mainly hepatic. Owing to the proposed etiopathogenesis of αHCD, results of parasitological (Table III), bacteriological, and virological studies are interesting, although rather disappointing (Harzic *et al.*, 1985). Bacterial colonization of the jejunal lumen is found in the majority of patients, but usually is moderate and anaerobes are absent. D-Glucose and [^{14}C]glycyl-cholyl breath test are negative. *Giardia lamblia* and isolated cases of infestation by various parasites are present in one-third of patients (Rambaud and Seligmann, 1976). Nevertheless, clinical symptoms and laboratory evidence of malabsorption and plasma protein digestive loss usually improve strikingly after a short course of antibiotic and antiparasitic treatment, without or before any apparent change in the small bowel mucosal lesions (Rambaud *et al.*, 1978). This amelioration must be kept in mind for patient follow-up.

Small intestinal radiographs usually show enlarged duodenal and jejunal folds and a polypoid pattern, with diffusion of lesions to the whole small bowel length. Radiographs also may show stenosis caused by lymph nodes compression or

Table II Clinical Presentation of αHCD

Symptoms and signs	Prevalence[a] (%)	
Chronic diarrhea	100	89
with overt steatorrhea	47	
watery appearance	14	
uncertain type	29	
Abdominal pain	93	100
Vomiting	41	?
Tetany	38	?
Fever	21	37
Loss of weight	97	87
Finger blubbing	47	39
Abdominal mass(es)	24	39
Ascites	12	8.5
Edema	24	?
Peripheral nodes	0	30

[a] Figures are percentages of the total number of patients in a series of 34 patients diagnosed in Western Europe (Rambaud and Seligmann, 1976; left column) and a series of 51 patients diagnosed in Tunisia (Gargouri and Amor, 1982; right column).

Table III Main Laboratory Findings Related to Intestinal Involvement in 34 Cases of αHCD[a]

Laboratory data	Prevalence (%)
Hemoglobin <13 g/dl	68
Serum potassium <3.5 m*M*	55
Serum albumin	
2.4–35 g/liter	46
<2.5 g/liter	46
Serum cholesterol <0.15 g/liter	89
Serum calcium <9.0 mg/dl	71
Absorption serum tests	
Fecal fats <6 g/24 hr	5
6–15 g/24 hr	45
>15 g/24 hr	50
Abnormal D-xylose test	83
Abnormal Schilling test	56
Protein-losing enteropathy[b]	71

[a] Data from Rambaud and Seligmann (1976).
[b] Nearly constant with the sensitive α1-antitrypsin clearance test.

infiltrating lesions, ulcerations or defects, or internal fistulas (Navab *et al.*, 1978; Matsumoti *et al.*, 1990).

Since αHCD nearly always affects the duodenum and jejunum, endoscopy with biopsies, using a long-ending view instrument and immunohistochemistry, is a major tool for its diagnosis. In the experience of the Tunisian–French Lymphoma Study Group Tufrali (Halphen *et al.*, 1986), the sensitivity of this method for diagnosis was 0.92, with no false positives. Among the macroscopic patterns, the infiltrative one was the most sensitive (0.8) and specific (0.96) in differentiating so-called Mediterranean lymphoma (see subsequent text) from other small intestinal lesions, but was unable to distinguish between αHCD and other diseases covered by this imprecise denomination. Ileocoloscopy with systematic biopsies, even in the absence of macroscopic abnormalities, is necessary to ascertain the extent of the disease, even at stage A. Such biopsies are also required for careful stomach examination during upper endoscopy. In the pure gastric localizations of αHCD, thick, rugae, erosive "gastritis," and some ulcers localized in the antrum have been described (references in Rambaud and Halphen, 1989).

G. Course and Treatment

The spontaneous course of αHCD may be relentless or interrupted by periods of clinical improvement often induced by blind antibiotic treatment. The length of the delay between the first symptom and diagnosis does not correlate with the pathological stage of the disease at the time of diagnosis (Rambaud and Halphen, 1989). Death may occur at any stage because of complications (infections, hypoglycemia, surgical emergency) or because of cachexia due to malabsorption and tumor growth. A single case of spontaneous, apparently complete remission, without control small intestinal biopsy, was reported after withdrawal from an unfavorable environment (Sala *et al.*, 1983).

Treatment may prevent the often fatal outcome. The modalities of treatment depend on a precise knowledge of the extent and histological stage of the disease. Because of the frequent asynchrony of the histological lesions between sites, laparotomy according to a precise protocol (Tabbane *et al.*, 1988) is necessary, except in patients displaying stage C peripheral lesions. The follow-up should include a periodic search for αHCD protein in serum and urine, intestinal absorption tests, small intestinal X-rays, upper esophagogastroduodenojejunal endoscopy, and ileocoloscopy with multilevel biopsies studied by immunohistochemical techniques.

Our present therapeutic guidelines, drawn from a personal series of 19 patients, Tufrali Group experience (Ben-Ayed *et al.*, 1989), the series of 20 patients published by Martinez and Chantar (1983) and a pool of 40 individual well-studied cases from the literature references in Rambaud and Halphen, 1989) are described here.

Patients with stage A lesions limited to the gut and to mesenteric lymph nodes should be treated first by oral antibiotics, including metronidazole, which also eradicates the frequent infestation by *Giardia lamblia.* Any other parasite should be eradicted as well. Of 28 patients, 39% achieved a complete clinical, histological, and immunological remission with antibiotic therapy alone, including a case treated without tetracycline. Antibiotics usually have a dramatic effect on the malabsorption syndrome, whether or not a true remission of the disease will be obtained.

The duration of treatment before complete remission was assessed varied from 5 to 36 months; the actual delay for obtaining the remission could have been shorter. Invasion of the submucosa by the plasma cell infiltrate, involvement of mesenteric lymph nodes or other parts of the digestive tract, and the presence of cellular atypias at histological or electron microscope examination do not preclude the efficacy of oral antibiotics. In view of the possible and unpredictable evolution of stage A lesions to overt malignancy, chemotherapy should not be instituted too late in unresponsive patients. When a complete remission of the disease is obtained, maintenance antibiotic therapy does not seem necessary.

At stages B and C, antiparasitic and antibiotic treatments are also useful since they may improve the malabsorption syndrome. Patients with stage B lesions, or with stage A lesions without marked improvement after a 6-month course of antibiotic treatment or a complete remission within 12 months, should be given combination chemotherapy. Again, some patients will not improve, even after salvage chemotherapy. Some of these patients progress to stage C lesions and die, whereas others apparently remain at stage A and remain asymptomatic for long periods of time on tetracycline treatment.

At stage C, patients with disseminated immunoblastic lesions of the small intestine require an intensive chemotherapy regimen to the extent allowed by their nutritional state. When a focal tumor is found, its surgical resection followed by combination chemotherapy including an anthracycline may induce a complete and prolonged remission.

The overall complete remission rate in all Tunisian patients was 52% (64.3% for stages B and C), with a median survival of 67% at 3 years. Relapses, sometimes after a long disease-free interval, may occur after treatment at any stage of the disease. Since most patients are young, those with disseminated stage C lesions that show a good response after four cycles of conventional or salvage chemotherapy could be submitted to autologous bone marrow transplantation (Perrot *et al.*, 1988).

Supportive therapy by intravenous infusion of water, electrolytes, calcium and magnesium salts, blood, or albumin and, in some cases, enteral or total parenteral nutrition is often necessary before laparotomy and during the early period of treatment.

II. RELATIONSHIP BETWEEN ALPHA CHAIN DISEASE, IMMUNOPROLIFERATIVE SMALL INTESTINAL DISEASE, AND "MEDITERRANEAN" LYMPHOMA

Since the first publications on αHCD (Rambaud *et al.*, 1968; Seligmann and Rambaud, 1969), the similarity of its epidemiology and clinical pattern with those of "Mediterranean'' lymphoma described previously in Israel (Ramot *et al.*, 1965; Eidelman *et al.*, 1966) was stressed; most of these lymphomas were suggested, to be in fact, αHCD (Seligmann and Rambaud, 1969; Rambaud and Matuchansky, 1973). Because of the frequent absence of adequate immunochemical studies, a World Health Organization (1976) memorandum stated that all ''Mediterranean'' lymphomas the pathology of which was identical to that of αHCD, whether or not αHCD protein was synthesized by proliferating cells, should be named Immunoproliferative Small Intestinal Disease (IPSID). Further experience revealed that most cases of IPSID were, in fact, αHCD, including rare cases in which the abnormal protein was absent from serum but detected in the gastric (Coulbois *et al.*, 1986) or jejunal (Rambaud *et al.*, 1983) juice or only at a cellular level (Rambaud *et al.*, 1983; Matuchansky *et al.*, 1989). However, in a few similar patients, proliferating cells synthesized other monoclonal Igs or polyclonal IgA (Rambaud and Halphen, 1989).

Does IPSID include all the previously described ''Mediterranean'' lymphomas? Rambaud *et al.* (1982) reported four young patients, born in countries in which IPSID is observed, with a clinical history and presentation identical to those of this syndrome. However, the pathological lesions, consisting of extensive follicular lymphoid hyperplasia of the small intestine associated in one case with multicentric follicular center cell (or centrocytic-like?) lymphoma, were quite different from those of αHCD. Immunological studies were unable to disclose αHCD protein synthesis or primary Ig deficiency. Review of the literature revealed that previously reported cases of this disorder, which should not be confused with multiple lymphomatous polyposis of the gut, had been observed primarily in the same epidemiological context as IPSID.

Thus, one of the goals of the Tunisian–French Intestinal Lymphoma Study Group was to reevaluate prospectively in Tunisia the nosology of Mediterranean lymphoma. All subsequent patients referred to the group with the suspicion of intestinal lymphoma, from 1981 to 1985, were investigated thoroughly. All those who proved to suffer from a small intestinal lymphoma were submitted to detailed immunological investigations, and all but one had a laparotomy. Among the 55 patients, 39% had IPSID and in all of them αHCD protein synthesis was demonstrated; 46% showed an extensive cellular proliferation infiltrating all or the proximal half of the small intestinal mucosa and submucosa, consisting of benign-appearing follicular lymphoid structures surrounded and more-or-less destroyed by a low-grade malignant lymphoid proliferation consisting of small cleaved cells (Cammoun *et al.*, 1989). Gross tumor foci of usually higher malignancy than the diffuse lesions were found in association with the latter proliferation in nearly 50% of cases (Figure 4). No evidence of production of αHCD protein was observed in any of these patients. A provisional denomination of ''non-IPSID extensive small intestinal lymphoma'' (ESIL) was proposed (Rambaud and Halphen, 1989). Finally, 15% patients had a Western type, that is, localized small intestinal lymphoma, associated in three cases with extensive villous atrophy of the mucosa. Note that Tunisian patients with IPSID and those with non-IPSID extensive small intestinal lymphoma originated from different parts of the country.

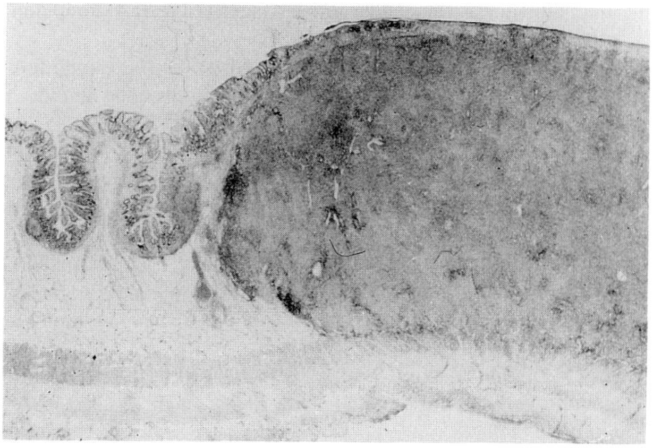

Figure 4 Non-IPSID extensive small intestinal lymphoma. Histological pattern of jejunal resection. Note, on the left, the multiple hyperplastic follicles and the lymphomatous band and, on the right, a tumoral mass. H & E, ×8.

Acknowledgments

We are grateful to Annie Galian for kindly providing the photographs of the figures.

References

Barnikol-Watanabe, S., Milhaesco, E., Mihaesco, C., Barnikol, K. U., and Hilschmann, N. (1984). Primary structure of μ chain disease protein BOT. *Hoppe Seyler's Z. Physiol. Chem.* **365,** 105–110.

Ben-Ayed, F., Halphen, M., and Najjar, T. (1989). Treatment of alpha chain disease. Results of a prospective study in 21 Tunisian patients by the Tunisian–French Intestinal Lymphoma Study Group. *Cancer* **63,** 1251–1256.

Bender, S. W., Danon, F., Preud'homme J. L., Posselt, H. G., Toettger, P., and Seligmann, M. (1978). Gamma heavy chain disease simulating alpha chain disease. *Gut* **19,** 1148–1152.

Bentaboulet, M., Mihaesco, E., Gendron, M. C., Brouet, J. C. and Tsapis, A. (1989). Genomic alterations in a case of alpha heavy chain disease leading to the generation of composite exons from the JH region. *Eur. J. Immunol.* **19,** 2093–2098.

Berger, R., Bernheim, A., Tsapis, A., Brouet, J. C., and Seligmann, M. (1986). Cytogenetic studies in four cases of alpha chain disease. *Cancer Genet. Cytogenet.* **22,** 219–223.

Brandtzaeg, P., and Baklien, K. (1977). Characterization of the IgA immunocyte population and its product in a patient with excessive intestinal formation of IgA. *Clin. Exp. Immunol.* **30,** 77–88.

Buxbaum, J. N., and Preud'homme, J. L. (1972). Alpha and gamma heavy chain diseases in man: Intracellular origin of the aberrant polypeptides. *J. Immunol.* **109,** 1131–1137.

Cammoun, M., Jaafoura, H., Tabbane, F., Halphen, M., and Group Tufrali (1989). Immunoproliferative small intestinal disease without alpha chain disease: A pathological study. *Gastroenterology* **96,** 750–763.

Chantar, C., Escartin, P., Plaza, A. G., Corugedo, A. F., Arenas J. I., and Sanz, E. (1974). Diffuse plasma cell infiltration of the small intestine with malabsorption associated to IgA monoclonal gammopathy. *Cancer* **34,** 1620–1630.

Cogné, M., and Preud'homme, J. L. (1990). Gene deletions force nonsecretory a-chain disease plasma cells to produce membrane form α-chain only. *J. Immunol.* **145,** 2455–2458.

Cogné, M., Bakshshi, A., Korsmeyer, S. J., and Guglielmi, P. (1988a). Gene mutations and alternate RNA splicing result in truncated Ig L chains in human αH chain disease. *J. Immunol.* **141,** 1738–1744.

Cogné, M., Mounir, S., Preud'homme, J. L., Nau, F., and Guglielmi, P. (1988b). Burkitt's lymphoma cell lines producing truncated μ immunoglobulin chains lacking part of the variable region. *Eur. J. Immunol.* **18,** 1485–1489.

Cogné, M., Preud'homme, J. L., and Guglielmi, P. (1989). Immunoglobulin gene alterations in human heavy chain diseases. *Res. Immunol.* **140,** 487–502.

Colombel, J. F., Rambaud, J. C., and Vaerman, J. P. (1988). Massive plasma cell infiltration of the digestive tract. Secretory component as the rate-limiting factor of immunoglobulin secretion in external fluids. *Gastroenterology* **95,** 1106–1113.

Coulbois, J., Galian, P., Galian, A., Couteaux, B., Danon, F., and Rambaud, J. C. (1986). Gastric form of alpha chain disease. *Gut* **27,** 719–725.

Doe, W. F., Danon, F., and Seligmann, M. (1979). Immunodiagnosis of alpha chain disease. *Clin. Exp. Immunol.* **36,** 189–197.

Dutz, W., Asvadi, S., Sadri, S., and Kohout, E. (1971). Intestinal lymphoma and sprue: a systematic approach. *Gut* **12,** 804–810.

Economidou, J. C., Manousos, O. N., and Katsaros, D. (1976). Alpha chain disease causing kaliopenic nephropathy and fatal intestinal perforations. *Am. J. Dig. Dis.* **21,** 577–585.

Eidelman, S., Parkins, R. A., and Rubin, C. E. (1966). Abdominal lymphoma presenting as malabsorption. A clinico-pathologic study of nine cases in Israel and review of the literature. *Medicine* **45,** 111–117.

Fakhfakh, F., Dellagi, K., Ayadi, H., Bouguerra, A., Fourati, R., Ben-Ayed, F., Brouet, J. C., and Tsapis, A. (1992). α-Heavy chain disease α mRNA contain nucleotide sequences of unknown origins. *Eur. J. Immunol.* **22,** 3037–3040.

Franklin, E. C., and Frangione, B. (1975). Structural variants of human immunoglobulins. *Contemp. Top. Mol. Immunol.* **4,** 89–125.

Gafter, U., Kesler, E., Shabtay, F., Shaked, P., and Djaldetti, M. (1980). Abnormal chromosome marker (D14 q+) in a patient with alpha heavy chain disease. *J. Clin. Pathol.* **33,** 136–144.

Galian, A., Lecestre, M.-J., Scotto, J., Bognel, C., Matuchansky, C., and Rambaud, J. C. (1977). Pathological study of alpha-chain disease, with special emphasis on evolution. *Cancer* **39,** 2981–2101.

Gargouri, M., and Amor, N. B. (1982). La maladie des chaînes lourdes alpha en Tunisie en 1981. *Med. Chir. Dig.* **11,** 163–167.

Gilinsky, N. H., Mee, A. S., and Beatty, D. W., (1985). Plasma cell infiltration of the small bowel: Lack of evidence for a nonsecretory form of alpha-heavy chain disease. *Gut* **26,** 928–934.

Halphen, M., Najjar, T., Jaafoura, H., Cammoun, M., and Group Tufrali (1986). Diagnostic value of upper intestinal fiber endoscopy in primary small intestinal lymphoma. A prospective study by the Tunisian–French Intestinal Lymphoma Group. *Cancer* **58,** 2140–2145.

Harzic, M., Girard-Pipau, F., Halphen, M., Ferchal, F., Pérol, Y., and Rambaud, J.-C. (1985). Etude bactériologique, parasitologique et virologique de la flore digestive dans la maladie des chaînes alpha. *Gastroenterol. Clin. Biol.* **9,** 472–479.

Isaacson, P. G., Dogan, A., Stephen Pice, S. K., and Spencer, J. (1989). Immunoproliferative small intestinal disease. An immunohistochemical study. *Am. J. Surg. Pathol.* **13,** 1023–1033.

Kumar, P. V., Esfahani, F. N., Tabei, S. Z., and Malek-Zadeh, R. (1988). Cytopathology of alpha chain disease involving the central nervous system and pleura. *Acta Cytol.* **32,** 902–907.

Martinez, J., and Chantar, C. (1983). Tratamiento del linfoma primitivo intestinal. *In* "Linfoma Primitivo Intestinal" (C. Chantar, ed.), pp. 151–160. Laboratorios Robert, Madrid.

Matsumoto, T., Iada, M., Matsui, T., Tanaka, H., and Fujushima, M. (1990). The value of double-contrast study of the small intestine in immunoproliferative small intestinal disease. *Gastrointest. Radiol.* **15,** 159–163.

Matuchansky, C., Cogné, M., Lemaire, M., Babin, P., Touchard, G., Chamaret, S., and Preud'homme, J. L. (1989). Nonsecretory alpha chain disease with immunoproliferative small-intestinal disease. *N. Engl. J. Med.* **320,** 1534–1539.

Navab, F., Mobarhan, S., Banisadre, M., Rambaud, J. C., and Mojtabai, A. (1978). The evolution of alpha-chain disease. *Gastroenterol. Clin. Biol.* **2,** 983–988.

Nemes, Z., Thomazy, V., and Szeifert, G. V. (1981). Follicular centre cell lymphoma with alpha heavy chain disease. *Virch. Arch. Pathol. Anat.* **394,** 119–132.

O'Reilly, D. S., Adjukiewicz, A., and Whicher, J. T. (1981). Biochemical findings in a case of mu chain disease. *Clin. Chem.* **27,** 331–333.

Pellet, P., Tsapis, A., and Brouet, J. C. (1990). Alpha heavy chain disease of patient MAL: Structure of the non-functional rearranged gene translocated on chromosome 9. *Eur. J. Immunol.* **20,** 2731–2735.

Perrot, S., Delchier, J. C., Farcet, J. P., Kuentz, M., Haioun, C., and Soule, J. C. (1988). Maladie des chaînes lourdes alpha (MCLα) disséminée: Résultats préliminaires d'un traitement par chimiothérapie intensive et autogreffe de moelle. *Gastroenterol. Clin. Biol.* **12,** 98. (Abstract)

Preud'homme, J. L., Brouet, J. C., and Seligmann, M. (1979). Cellular immunoglobulins in human gamma and alpha heavy chain diseases. *Clin. Exp. Immunol.* **37,** 283–291.

Price, S. K. (1990). Immunoproliferative small intestinal disease: A study of 13 cases with alpha heavy chain disease. *Histopathology* **17,** 7–17.

Rambaud, J. C., and Halphen, M. (1989). Immunoproliferative small intestinal disease (IPSID): Relationship with alpha-chain disease and "Mediterranean" lymphomas. *Gastroenterol. Int.* **2,** 33–41.

Rambaud, J. C., and Matuchansky, C. (1973). Alpha-chain disease. Pathogenesis and relation to Mediterranean lymphoma. *Lancet* **1,** 1430–1432.

Rambaud, J. C., and Seligmann, M. (1976). Alpha-chain disease. *Clin. Gastroenterol.* **5,** 341–358.

Rambaud, J. C., Bognel, C., Prost, A., Bernier, J. J., Le Quintrec, Y. Lambling, A., Danon, F., Hurez, D., and Seligmann, M. (1968). Clinico-pathological study of a patient with "Mediterranean" type of abdominal lymphoma and a new type of IgA abnormality ("Alpha chain disease"). *Digestion* **1,** 321–336.

Rambaud, J. C., Piel, J. L., Galian, A., Leclerc, J. P., Danon, F., Girard-Pipau, F., Modigliani, R., and Illoul, G. (1978). Rémission complète clinique, histologique et immunologique d'un cas de maladie des chaînes alpha traitée par antibiothérapie orale. *Gastroenterol. Clin. Biol.* **2,** 49–62.

Rambaud, J. C., de Saint-Louvent, P., Marti, R., Galian, A., Mason, D. Y., Wassef, M., Licht, H., Valleur, P., and Bernier, J. J. (1982). Diffuse follicular lymphoid hyperplasia of the small intestine without primary immunoglobulin deficiency. *Am. J. Med.* **73,** 125–132.

Rambaud, J. C., Galian, A., Danon, F., Preud'homme, J. L., Brandtzaeg, P., Wassef, R. G., Le Carrer, M., Mehaut, M. A., Voinchet, O. L., Pérol, R. G., and Chapman, A. (1983). Alpha-chain disease without qualitative serum IgA abnormality. Report of two cases, including a "nonsecretory" form. *Cancer* **51,** 686–693.

Ramot, B., Shanin, N., and Bubis, J. J. (1965). Malabsorption syndrome in lymphoma of small intestine. *Isr. J. Med. Sci.* **2,** 221–226.

Reyes, F., Piquet, J., Gourdin, M. F., and Haioun, C., Intrator, L., Tulliez, M. K., Roberti, A., and Rambaud, J. C. (1985). Immunoblastic lymphoma involving the bone marrow in a patient with alpha-chain disease. Clinical and immunoelectron microscopic study. *Cancer* **55,** 1007–1014.

Sala, P., Tonutti, E., Mazzolini, S., Antonutto, G., and Bamezza, M. (1983). Alpha-heavy chain disease. Report of a case with spontaneous regression. *Scand. J. Haematol.* **31,** 149–154.

Seligmann, M., and Rambaud, J. C. (1978). Alpha chain disease, a possible model for the pathogenesis of human lymphomas. *In* Immunopathology of Lymphoreticular Neoplasms (R. A. Good and J. J. Twomey, eds.), pp. 425–447. Plenum Press, New York.

Seligmann, M. (1977). Immunobiology and pathogenesis of alpha chain disease. *Ciba Found. Symp.* **46,** 263–281.

Seligmann, M., and Rambaud, J. C. (1969). IgA abnormalities in abdominal lymphoma (alpha chain disease). *Isr. J. Med. Sci.* **5,** 151–157.

Seligmann, M., Danon, F., Hurez, D., Mihaesco, E., and Preud'homme, J. L. (1968). Alpha chain disease: A new immunoglobulin abnormality. *Science* **162,** 1396–1397.

Seligmann, M., Mihaesco, E., Hurez, D., Mihaesco, C., Preud'homme, J. L., and Rambaud, J. C. (1969). Immunochemical studies in four cases of alpha chain disease. *J. Clin. Invest.* **48,** 2374–2389.

Seligmann, M., Mihaesco, E., Preud'homme, J. L., Danon, F., and Brouet, J. C. (1979). Heavy chain diseases: Current findings and concepts. *Immunol. Rev.* **48,** 145–167.

Tabbane, F., Mourali, N., Cammoun, M., and Najjar, T. (1988). Results of laparotomy in immuno-proliferative small intestinal disease. *Cancer* **61,** 1699–1706.

Takahashi, K., Naito, M., Matsuoka, Y., and Takatsuki, K. (1988). A new form of alpha-chain disease with generalized lymph node involvement. *Pathol. Res. Pract.* **183,** 717–723.

Tangun, Y., Saracbasi, Z., Inceman, S., Danon, F., and Seligmann, M. (1975). IgA myeloma globulin and Bence Jones proteinuria in a diffuse plasmacytoma of the small intestine simulating alpha chain disease. *Ann. Int. Med.* **83,** 673.

Tracy, R. P., Kyle, R. A., and Leitch, J. M. (1984). Alpha heavy-chain disease presenting as goiter. *Am. J. Clin. Pathol.* **82,** 336–339.

Tsapis, A., Bentaboulet, M., Pellet, P., Mihaesco, E., Thierry, D., Seligmann, M., and Brouet, J. C. (1989). The productive gene for alpha-H chain disease protein MAL is highly modified by insertion-deletion processes. *J. Immunol.* **143,** 3821–3827.

Tungekar, M. F. (1986). Gastric signet-ring cell lymphoma with alpha heavy chains. *Histopathology* **10,** 725–733.

Wolfenstein-Todel, C., Mihaesco, E., and Frangione, B. (1974). "Alpha chain disease" protein DEF: Internal deletion of a human immunoglobulin A heavy chain. *Proc. Natl. Acad. Sci. U.S.A.* **71,** 974–978.

World Health Organization (1976) WHO Meeting Report. Alpha-chain disease and related lymphomas. *Arch. Fr. Mal. App. Dig.* **54,** 615–624.

37

Gastritis and Peptic Ulcer

Bertil Kaijser

I. INTRODUCTION

Tlhe idea that bacteria or immunological factors might play an important role in the pathogenesis of gastritis and ulcus duodeni or ventriculi has attracted researchers for many years. Autoimmunity has been studied, as has the role of eosinophilia. Little attention has been paid to early descriptions of spiral bacteria in human biopsy specimens from gastric mucosa (Freedberg *et al.*, 1940). In 1982, a gram-negative microaerophilic curved rod was cultured successfully by Robert Warren in Perth, Australia, in biopsy specimens from patients with histological signs of gastritis (Warren, 1983). This event was the start of the new perspective of the pathogenesis of gastritis and ulcus, in which bacteria have been accepted to play an important role. The first report was followed by a number of publications confirming the idea.

II. MICROBIOLOGY

The curved rod that was isolated originally was named *Campylobacter pylori*. Intense scrutiny of its taxonomic features compared with other *Campylobacter* species showed major differences between *C. pylori* and true *Campylobacter* with respect to ultrastructure, cellular fatty acid composition, respiratory quinones, growth characteristics, RNA sequencing, and enzymes. Distinct from most other bacteria and especially other *Campylobacter, C. pylori* possesses a potent urease activity, a property that also might have important pathogenic implications. This cell surface enzyme is composed of two subunits of approximately 30 and 60 kDa; the genes that encode this enzyme have been sequenced (Clayton *et al.*, 1990; Dunn *et al.*, 1990). The unique characteristics of the bacterium has motivated formation a new genus; the organism is now called *Helicobacter pylori* (Goodwin *et al.*, 1989).

Bacteria closely related to *H. pylori* have been found in the stomach of primates (Baskerville and Newell, 1988), whereas other *Helicobacter* species such as *H. mustelae* have been isolated in the stomach of ferrets; *H. felis* has been isolated from cats (Lee *et al.*, 1988; Fox *et al.*, 1990).

Curved rods other than *H. pylori* have been found in a few humans with gastritis, but the significance of this result is not clear (Dye *et al.*, 1989).

III. EPIDEMIOLOGY

Several investigations have shown a relationship between age and prevalence of *H. pylori* in healthy individuals (Dooley *et al.*, 1989). In the age group under 30 years, prevalence is not higher than 10% whereas, in the age group of 50–60 years and older, corresponding figures are more than 60%. Race and socioeconomic circumstances influence the prevalence also (Megraud *et al.*, 1989). In several publications, persons with duodenal ulcer (prevalence of *H. pylori* close to 100%) or gastric ulcer (prevalence of *H. pylori* approximately 80%) clearly have been shown to harbor *H. pylori* significantly more often than age-matched healthy controls (Wyatt, 1989).

The mode of transmission of *H. pylori* is known not in detail. Person-to-person transmission seems likely, since clustering of cases has been reported in families or nursing homes (Drumm *et al.*, 1990). Infection from environmental sources is also possible. The bacteria have not, however, been isolated in environmental sources such as water, food, or domestic animals. They have not been found in stools of humans. Transmission via endoscopes has been suggested, and gastroenteroscopists have been shown to have a higher prevalence than corresponding control individuals (Mitchell *et al.*, 1989).

IV. PATHOGENESIS

Helicobacter pylori clusters around the junctions between cells and never penetrates the cells. The bacteria also may harbor in metaplastic gastric epithelium of the esophagus or duodenum (Steer, 1975; Talley *et al.*, 1988). They are never found in the blood and rarely are found in other parts of the body (de Cothi *et al.*, 1989; Dye *et al.*, 1989). *Helicobacter pylori* has been reported to induce intense inflammatory reaction with dominating neutrophils in the antrum and in the body of the stomach, sometimes followed by hypochlorhydria. *Helicobacter pylori* also has been suggested to produce a protein capable of inhibiting parietal cell function (Cave and Vargas, 1989). Biopsy specimens from gastritis patients with *H. pylori* show focal epithelial cell damage and inflammatory response in the lamina propria consisting of mononucler cells and granulocytes. A marked systemic IgG and IgA response accompanies the inflammatory reaction to *H.*

pylori, including T lymphocyte and plasma cell proliferation (Perez-Perez *et al.*, 1988; Evans *et al.*, 1989).

The capacity of *H. pylori* to escape the bactericidal activity of gastric acid juices, and to colonize the epithelium and thereby damage epithelial cells and induce an inflammatory reaction has attracted the interest of many researchers. Possible virulence factors such as urease, adhesins, proteases, phospholipases, and cytotoxins have been suggested. The production of a very potent urease might protect the bacteria against the gastric acid. Patients with active duodenal ulcers and *H. pylori* have been reported to secrete more acid and release more gastrin (Levi *et al.*, 1989).

V. DIAGNOSIS

The most reliable procedure for diagnosis is the isolation of *H. pylori* from biopsy specimens taken from the relevant epithelium. The clinical drawback is that biopsies are required; no other specimens are adequate. A less sensitive and specific procedure is the biopsy-urease test (McNulty *et al.*, 1989). A medium containing urea with pH-sensitive dye is inoculated with the mucosal biopsy specimen. Urease in a positive specimen splits the urea and causes raised pH via production of ammonia. A color indicator reacts to the increased pH. Another noninvasive test is the urea breath test (Graham *et al.*, 1987). ^{14}C-Labeled urea is given perorally with liquid. If urease activity is in the stomach, labeled CO_2 is split off and expired in the breath, from which it can be recorded with a mass spectrometer. A third noninvasive method, reliable and increasingly used, is the antibody determination (see subsequent section).

VI. IMMUNOLOGY

Serum antibody response against *H. pylori* antigen has been measured using several different antibody techniques such as agglutination, complement fixation, enzyme-linked immunosorbent assays (ELISA), and immunoblotting (Jones *et al.*, 1986; Bolton and Hutchison, 1989; Kosunen *et al.*, 1989; Reiff *et al.*, 1989). Different antigen preparations have been used, for example, whole cell antigens, glycine extracts, urease antigen, 120-kDa protein, and sonicated bacteria (Hirschl *et al.*, 1988; Bolton and Hutchinson, 1989). Crude antigens often have shown cross reactions with other bacteria.

IgG antibodies have been shown to be recorded significantly more often in patients with active chronic gastritis than in patients with normal morphology. The antibodies, furthermore, appear significantly more often in patients with *H. pylori* than in bacteria-negative patients (Perez-Perez *et al.*, 1988; Evans *et al.*, 1989). An increased level of IgA antibodies often is seen simultaneously with IgG antibodies. High levels of IgM antibodies are less common, which might indicate that the infection is a chronic one in most cases. A certain overlap of increased antibody titers is found in diseased and healthy persons, complicating the predictive value of the antibody test.

After treatment of patients with antimicrobial drugs the increased antibody levels, mainly IgG and IgA antibodies, decrease in 1–2 months (Vaira *et al.*, 1988; van Bohemen *et al.*, 1989). The patients who become free of *Helicobacter* as a consequence of antimicrobial treatment are expected to show even lower antibody level within the next 6 months. In patients in whom the bacteria remain, a new antibody increase might be expected (Oderda *et al.*, 1989). Immunological methods, that is, antibody determination, rather than cumbersome endoscopic methods can be used to screen the pertinent patient group with gastroenterological disease. This technique is especially valuable in younger patients, in whom the finding of low antibody level is a satisfactory result and need not be followed by endoscopy with biopsy to rule out malignancies. Follow-up of patients treated with antimicrobial drugs also can be performed very well by antibody determination.

Why the local immune response of the mucous membrane cannot clear the gastrointestinal tract of *H. pylori* without antimicrobial treatment is still unclear. *Helicobacter pylori* gastritis is apparently an immunopathological disease. Most of the morphological and histological changes can be accounted for by most immune response mechanisms. Activation of the inflammatory reaction and self-damaging mediators such as complement factors, interleukin 6, and so on are important. An autoimmune component seems probable.

In all discussions of "new" infectious diseases, the question is raised whether or not a protective immunity is possible. In terms of cost–benefit, considerations of this kind are most relevant. The induction of prophylactic immunity against *H. pylori* seems unlikely. Urease was suggested as a vaccine candidate (Pallen and Clayton, 1990). However, animal experiments with other urease-producing *Helicobacter* species have shown that urease-producing microorganisms have no marked toxic effect on the mucous membrane.

An induction of immune response to *H. pylori* already has been shown and has no influence on the eradication of the bacteria—they are already there. Furthermore, the bacteria apparently induce an inflammatory reaction with immunopathological effects. If vaccination were possible, it would have to be done in young individuals with no *H. pylori* present.

VII. TREATMENT

Helicobacter pylori bacteria are sensitive *in vitro* to most commonly used antimicrobial drugs such as ampicillin, cefalosporins, erythromycin, penicillin, quinolones, and tetracyclines (Goodwin *et al.*, 1986). They are resistant to nalidixic acid, trimethoprim, sulfonamides, and vancomycin.

Despite the good *in vitro* results, the treatment *in vivo* does not always eradicate the bacteria. Reasons for failure might be development of resistance or loss of activity in the presence of acid. Better results have been obtained with combinations of drugs such as bismuth salts and amoxycillin or tinidazole or amoxycillin and tinidazole (Marshall *et al.*, 1988; Rauws *et al.*, 1988; Oderda *et al.*, 1989). Even greater effectiveness has been achieved using triple therapy of bismuth salts, amoxycillin or tetracycline, and metronidazole. In 90% or more cases, the patient was cleared after treatment (Borody *et al.*, 1988; Börsch *et al.*, 1988). Another very promising therapy study combining omeprazole and amoxycillin showed a marked effect on eradication and ulcer relapse during a 6-month follow-up (Unge *et al.*, 1991).

VIII. CONCLUSION

Based on extensive studies since the first report in 1983, *H. pylori* evidently play an important role in the etiology of gastritis and peptic ulcer. *Helicobacter pylori* is found in the mucous membrane of the stomach or duodenum in patients with gastritis or peptic ulcer more commonly than in healthy people. The prevalence increases with age and is high in some ethnic groups. *Helicobacter pylori* induce an inflammatory reaction with immunopathological effects. An increased antibody level, mainly IgG and IgA, is seen in the serum of the patients. This antibody response has an important diagnostic value. However, the immune response does not eradicate *H. pylori*. Treatment of patients has been discussed extensively. A combination of bismuth and one or two antimicrobial drugs, preferably metronidazole and amoxycillin or omeprazole in combination with amoxycillin, has been suggested.

References

Baskerville, A., and Newell, D. G. (1988). Naturally occurring chronic gastritis and *C. pylori* infection in the rhesus monkey: A potential model for gastritis in man. *Gut* **19,** 465–472.

Bolton, F. J., and Hutchinson, D. N. (1989). Evaluation of three *Campylobacter pylori* antigen preparations for screening sera from patients undergoing endoscopy. *J. Clin. Pathol.* **42,** 723–726.

Borody, T., Cole, P., Noonan, S., Morgan, A., Ossip, G., Maysey, J., and Brandl, S. (1988). Long-term *Campylobacter pylori* recurrence post-eradication. *Gastroenterology* **94,** A43.

Börsch, G., Mai, U., and Opferkuch, W. (1988). Oral triple therapy (OTT) may effectively eradicate *Campylobacter pylori* (*C.p.*) in man: A pilot study. *Gastroenterology* **94,** A44.

Cave, D. R., and Vargas, M. (1989). Effect of a *Campylobacter pylori* protein on acid secretion by parietal cells. *Lancet* **2,** 187–189.

Clayton, C. L., Pallen, M. J., Kleanthous, H., Wren, B. W., and Tabaqchali, S (1990). Nucleotide sequence of two genes from *Helicobacter pylori* encoding for urease subunits. *Nucleic Acids Res.* **18,** 362.

de Cothi, G. A., Newbold, K. M., and O'Connor, H. J. (1989). *Campylobacter*-like organisms and heterotopic gastric mucosa in Meckel's diverticula. *J. Clin. Pathol.* **42,** 132–134.

Dooley, C. P., Cohen, H., Fitzgibbons, P. L., Bauer, M., Appleman, M. D., Perez-Perez, G. I., and Blaser, M. J. (1989). Prevalence of *Helicobacter pylori* infection and histologic gastritis in asymptomatic persons. *N. Engl. J. Med.* **121,** 1562–1566.

Drumm, B., Perez-Perez, G. I., Blaser, M. J., and Sherman, P. M. (1990). Intrafamilial clustering of *Helicobacter pylori* infection. *N. Engl. J. Med.* **322,** 359–363.

Dunn, B. E., Campbell, G. P., Perez-Perez, G. I., and Blaser, M. J. (1990). Purification and characterization of urease from *Helicobacter pylori. J. Biol. Chem.* **265,** 9494–9499.

Dye, K. R., Marshall, B. J., Frierson, H. F., Jr., Guerrant, R. L., and McCallum, R. W. (1989). Ultra-structure of another spiral organism associated with human gastritis. *Dig. Dis. Sci.* **34,** 1787–1791.

Evans, D. J., Jr., Evans, D. G., Graham, D. Y., and Klein, P. H. (1989). A sensitive and specific serologic test for detection of *Campylobacter pylori* infection. *Gastroenterology* **96,** 1004–1008.

Fox, J. G., Correa, P., Taylor, N. S., Lee, A., Otto, G., Murphy, J. C., and Rose, R. (1990). *Helicobacter mustelae*-associated gastritis in ferrets: An animal model of *Helicobacter pylori* gastritis in humans. *Gastroenterology* **99,** 352–361.

Freedberg, A. S., and Barron, L. E. (1940). The presence of spirochetes in human gastric mucosa. *Am. J. Dig. Dis.* **7,** 443–445.

Goodwin, C. S., Blake, P., and Blincow, E. (1986). The minimum inhibitory and bactericidal concentrations of antibiotics and antiulcer agents against *Campylobacter pyloridis. J. Antimicrob. Chemother.* **17,** 309–314.

Goodwin, C. S., Armstrong, J. A., Chilvers, T., Peters, M., Collins, M. D., Sly, L., and McConnell, W., and Harper, W. E. S. (1989). Transfer of *Campylobacter pylori* and *Campylobacter mustelae* to *Helicobacter* gen. nov. as *Helicobacter pylori* comb. nov. and *Helicobacter mustelae* comb. nov. respectively. *Int. J. Syst. Bact.* **39,** 397–405.

Graham, D. Y., Klein, P. D., Evans, D. R., Jr., Evans, D. G., Alpert, L. C., Opekun, A. R., and Boutton, T. W. (1987). *Campylobacter pylori* detected noninvasively by the ^{13}C-urea breath test. *Lancet* **1,** 1174–1177.

Hirschl, A. M., Pletschette, M., Hirschl, M. H., Berger, J., Stanek, G., and Rotter, M. L. (1988). Comparison of different antigen preparations in an evaluation of the immune response to *Campylobacter pylori. Eur. J. Clin. Microbiol. Infect. Dis.* **7,** 570–575.

Jones, D. M., Eldridge, J., Fox, A. J., Sethi, P., and Whorwell, P. J. (1986). Antibody to the gastric *Campylobacter*-like organism ("*Campylobacter pyloridis*")—Clinical correlations and distribution in the normal population. *J. Med. Microbiol.* **22,** 57–62.

Kosunen, T. U., Höök, J., Rautelin, H. I., and Myllylä, G. (1989). Age-dependent increase of *Campylobacter pylori* antibodies in blood donors. *Scand. J. Gastroenterol.* **24,** 110–114.

Lee, A., Hazell, S. L., O'Rourke, J., and Kouprach, S. (1988). Isolation of a spiral-shaped bacterium from the cat stomach. *Infect. Immun.* **56,** 2843–2850.

Levi, S., Beardshall, K., Swift, I., Foulkes, W., Playford, R., Ghosh, P., and Calam, J. (1989). Antral *Helicobacter pylori*, hypergastrinaemia, and duodenal ulcers. Effect of eradicating the organism. *Br. Med. J.* **299,** 1504–1505.

McNulty, C. A. M., Dent, J. C., Uff, J. S., Gear, M. W. L., and Wilkinsson, S. P. (1989). Detection of *Campylobacter pylori* by the biopsy urease test: An assessment in 1445 patients. *Gut* **30,** 1058–1062.

Marshall, B. J., Goodwin, C. S., Warren, J. R., Murray, R., Blincow, E. D., Blackbourn, S. J., Phillips, M., Waters, T. E., and Sanderson, C. R. (1988). Prospective double-blind trial of duodenal ulcer relapse after eradication of *Campylobacter pylori. Lancet* **ii,** 1437–1441.

Megraud, F., Brassens-Rabbe, M. P., Denis, F., Belbouri, A., and Hoa, D. Q. (1989). Seroepidemiology of *Campylobacter pylori* infection in various populations. *J. Clin. Microbiol.* **27,** 1870–1873.

Mitchell, H. M., Lee, A., and Carrick, J. (1989). Increased incidence of *Campylobacter pylori* infection in gastroenterologists: Further evidence to support person-to-person transmission of *C. pylori. Scand. J. Gastroenterol.* **24,** 396–400.

Oderda, G., Vaira, D., Holton, J., Ainley, C., Altare, F., and Ansaldi, N. (1989). Amoxycillin plus tinidazole for *Campylobacter pylori* gastritis in children: Assessment by serum IgG antibody, pepsinogen I, and gastrin levels. *Lancet* **i,** 690–692.

Pallen, M. J., and Clayton, C. L. (1990). Vaccination against *Helicobacter pylori* urease. *Lancet* **336,** 186–187.

Perez-Perez, G. I., Dworkin, B. M., Chodods, J. E., and Blaser, M. J. (1988). *Campylobacter pylori* antibodies in humans. *Ann. Intern. Med.* **109,** 11–17.

Rauws, E. A. J., Langenberg, W., Houthoff, H. J., Zanen, H. C., and Tytgat, G. N. J. (1988). *Campylobacter pyloridis*-associated chronic active antral gastritis. A prospective study of its prevalence and the effects of antibacterial and antiulcer treatment. *Gastroenterology* **94,** 33–40.

Reiff, A., Jacobs, E., and Kist, M. (1989). Seroepidemiological study of the immune response to *Campylobacter pylori* in potential risk groups. *Eur. J. Clin. Microbiol. Infect. Dis.* **8,** 592–596.

Steer, H. W. (1975). Ultrastructure of cell migration through the gastric epithelium and its relationship to bacteria. *J. Clin. Pathol.* **28,** 639–646.

Talley, N. J., Cameron, A. J., Shorter, R. G., Zinsmeister, A. R., and Phillips, S. F. (1988). *Campylobacter pylori* and Barrett's esophagus. *Mayo Clin. Proc.* **63,** 1176–1180.

Unge, P., Eriksson, K., Bergman, B., Carling, L., Ekström, P., Gad, A., Glise, H., Gnarpe, H., Jansson, R., Lindholmer, C., Sandzen, B., Strandberg, L., and Stubberod, A. (1991). Omeprazole and amoxycillin in patients with duodenal ulcer: Effect on *Helicobacter pylori* eradication and ulcer relapse during a 6-month follow-up. Sixth International Workshop on *Campylobacter, Helicobacter,* and Related Organisms, Sydney, Australia. (Abstract)

Vaira, D., Holton, J., Cairns, S. R., Falzon, M., Polydorou, A., Dowsett, J. F., and Salmon, P. R. (1988). Antibody titres to *Campylobacter pylori* after treatment for gastritis. *Br. Med. J.* **297,** 397.

van Bohemen, C. G., Langenberg, M. L., Rauws, E. A. J., Oudbier, J., Weterings, E., and Zanen, H. C. (1989). Rapidly decreased serum IgG to *Campylobacter pylori* following elimination of *Campylobacter* in histological chronic biopsy *Campylobacter*-positive gastritis. *Immunol. Lett.* **20,** 59–62.

Warren, J. R. (1983). Unidentified curved bacilli on gastric epithelium in active chronic gastritis. *Lancet* **1,** 1273.

Wyatt, J. I. (1989). *Campylobacter pylori,* duodenitis, and duodenal ulceration. *In* "Campylobacter pylori, and Gastroduodenal Disease" (B. J. Rathbone and R. V. Heathley, eds.) pp. 117–124. Blackwell Scientific, Oxford.

38

The Role of the Mucosal Immune System in Ulcerative Colitis and Crohn's Disease

Hans-Christian Reinecker • Stefan Schreiber • William F. Stenson • Richard P. MacDermott

I. INTRODUCTION

Because of the continuous exposure of the intestine to a wide variety of bacterial, viral, and dietary antigens, host defense mechanisms are constantly necessary and depend on essential functions mediated by the intestinal mucosal immune system. The mucosal immune system has developed a unique set of immunological protective mechanisms and effector capabilities that normally prevent damage to the intestine but, in the case of inflammatory bowel disease (IBD), may perpetuate and exacerbate intestinal injury. In healthy individuals, nutrients must be allowed to cross the interface of the external environment (the gut lumen) and the intestinal mucosa while injurious agents must be prevented from entering effectively and specifically (Tomasi *et al.*, 1965; Mestecky and McGhee, 1987; Brandtzaeg *et al.*, 1988). Thus, a critical function of the normal mucosal immune system is to recognize and neutralize specifically infectious agents and potentially injurious toxins or antigens (Hanson *et al.*, 1980; Underdown and Schiff, 1986). Discrimination between self and nonself is vital so host tissues are not damaged while host protective defense mechanisms are being employed. In ulcerative colitis and Crohn's disease, the normally protective inflammatory response is not down-regulated and the highly activated effector cells produce prolonged and intense damage of the intestine. Advances in our understanding of normal immune and inflammatory processes in the intestinal mucosa have provided new insights into the immunopathogenic mechanisms involved in autoimmune and chronic inflammatory gastrointestinal diseases such as ulcerative colitis and Crohn's disease (MacDermott and Stenson, 1988a,b).

An effective immune response begins with the specific processing of antigens by monocytes and macrophages, which endocytose large molecules and infectious organisms such as bacteria and viruses (Unanue and Allen, 1987). After lysosomal processing, smaller fragments are generated that interact with major histocompatibility complex (MHC) Class II or Class I determinants. Antigen recognition events by lymphocytes involve the antigen-specific T-cell receptor–CD2 complex. The T-cell receptor complex specifically recognizes Class II cell surface determinants in conjunction with antigen fragments on the macrophage surface. Other cell types, in addition to the macrophage, now are known to have Class II antigens on their surfaces and to be capable of antigen presentation. The gastrointestinal tract in particular is populated by many potential antigen-presenting cells, including epithelial cells and endothelial cells as well as dendritic cells and macrophages. The presence of a variety of antigen-presenting cells further enhances the ability of the intestine to mount specific mucosal immune responses against the many different luminal antigens to which it is exposed (Bland and Warren, 1986a,b). Specific antigen recognition is pivotal to the normal function of T cells, which both regulate immune responses through T helper cell function and serve as effector cells by carrying out T cell-mediated cytotoxicity.

Cytokines are produced by macrophages (Dinarello, 1988) and T cells induce B cells to mature into plasma cells and to secrete immunoglobulins. Presentation of antigens to B cells initiates an orderly and precise sequence of events during which genes that encode for variable regions are joined with genes that encode the constant regions of heavy and light chains of immunoglobulins. This rearrangement of genes results in the formation of specific DNA that produces a specific messenger RNA that allows a B cell to secrete an isotype- and subclass-defined antibody that is specific to the initiating antigen. The normal gastrointestinal immune system has unique mechanisms that allow mucosal B cells to "switch" from predominantly IgM production to IgA production (Kawanishi *et al.*, 1983a,b). A series of cell- and cytokine-mediated regulatory events is involved in the production of IgA, which is the major mucosal protective immunoglobulin. Within normal human mucosal lymphoid follicles, T-cell subsets produce specific B-cell switch, differentiation, and growth factors that regulate IgA production by B cells (Coffman *et al.*, 1987).

T-cell recognition functions are controlled by the formation of a T-cell receptor complex with two polypeptide chains (alpha and beta) that have variable regions. Sensitized T cells recognize specific antigens in conjunction with MHC Class II molecules. Helper T lymphocytes then are stimulated by interleukin 1 (IL-1) released from antigen-activated macrophages (Dinarello, 1988). Increased production of IL-2 by T cells further stimulates helper T cells to undergo cell cycle progression and clonal expansion (Smith, 1988). Specific helper T cells lead to enhanced production of immunoglobulins. Therefore, carefully regulated expansion of immunoglobulin-producing B cells in the mucosa by T cell-derived cytokines (Strickland *et al.*, 1974) normally occurs in response to specific infectious agents or stimulating antigens to provide a protective immune response.

In ulcerative colitis and Crohn's disease, the normal sequence of T-cell and B-cell regulating events is altered so an up-regulated immune and highly activated chronic inflammatory response ensues.

Although the specific and effective protection provided by the normal immune response in the intestine does not lead to injury to the surrounding tissue in ulcerative colitis and Crohn's disease, the continuous production of chemotactic cytokines, pro-inflammatory cytokines, inflammatory mediators, and other injurious molecules leads to damaging rather than healing processes. The normal protective mucosal immune response should be down-regulated when it is no longer needed, but in IBD the continuous up-regulation of the immune response results in highly activated specific and nonspecific damage to the surrounding intestinal tissue. In the remaining sections of this chapter, we discuss recent progress that has been made in our understanding of the role of the mucosal immune system in ulcerative colitis and Crohn's disease.

II. PERIPHERAL BLOOD LYMPHOCYTE ACTIVATION

Initial descriptions of immunological alterations in IBD focused on peripheral blood lymphocyte function (Strickland *et al.*, 1974; Thayer *et al.*, 1976; Auer *et al.*, 1978,1979). Auer and co-workers (Auer *et al.*, 1978,1979) demonstrated that, in patients with long-term steroid-treated Crohn's disease, lymphocytopenia and a decrease in T cells occurred that was dependent on disease duration whereas, in new-onset untreated Crohn's disease patients, no alterations were found. More recent studies (Selby and Jewell, 1983; Yuan *et al.*, 1983) using monoclonal antibodies against T lymphocytes and their subsets have not demonstrated any differences between IBD patients and controls. Therefore, attention now has turned to the concept that, although the absolute number of certain types of lymphocytes may not differ from normal in IBD, the functional state and degree of activation may be altered (Figure 1).

Raedler and co-workers (Raedler *et al.*, 1985a,b,1986,1988; Schreiber *et al.*, 1991) and Pallone and co-workers (Fais *et al.*, 1987; Pallone *et al.*, 1987) have demonstrated the increased state of activation of peripheral blood T cells in IBD. Using the T9 antigen, which is identical to the transferrin receptor and is expressed during early lymphocyte activation, Raedler and colleagues observed that 24% of active Crohn's disease peripheral blood T lymphocytes express early activation markers (Raedler *et al.*, 1985b). The extent of peripheral blood T-lymphocyte activation was dependent on disease activity; only 10% of T cells expressed the T9 antigen in inactive Crohn's disease (Raedler *et al.*, 1985b; Schreiber *et al.*, 1991). Peripheral blood T-cell activation was not specific for IBD, but was observed also in a variety of autoimmune diseases including systemic lupus erythematosus, rheumatoid arthritis, and Behcet's disease. In contrast, peripheral blood T-cell activation was not increased in bacterial or viral colitis (Raedler *et al.*, 1985a). Interestingly, in IBD, a high percentage of activated T9 antigen-positive T cells coexpressed Fc receptors for polymeric IgA (Fcα receptor), which was not observed in the autoimmune disorders that also exhibited increased peripheral blood T-cell activation (Raedler *et al.*, 1985a,1986,1988; Schreiber *et al.*, 1991).

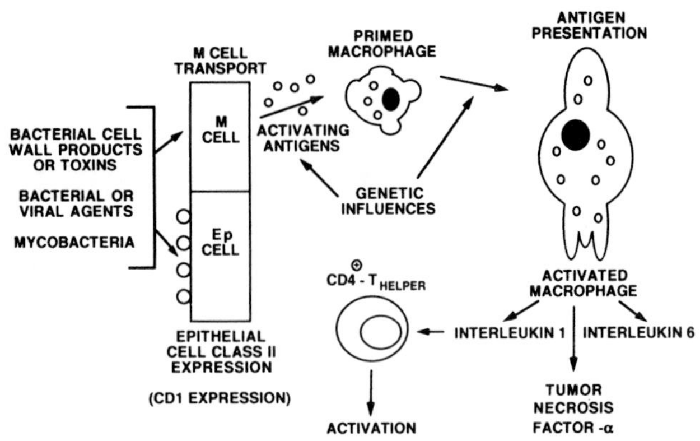

Figure 1 Activating events in IBD. Bacterial cell wall products, infectious agents, and/or toxins can be transported across M cells or presented by class II antigens on epithelial cells to prime and activate macrophages. After antigen presentation, the primed and activated macrophages synthesize and secrete a variety of molecules, including pro-inflammatory cytokines such as interleukin 1, interleukin 6, and tumor necrosis factor α. The pro-inflammatory cytokines in turn activate a number of important cell-mediated events and processes, including $CD4^+$ T helper cells in the intestine. In IBD, therefore, macrophages and lymphocytes are in a highly activated and up-regulated state with the resultant secretion of numerous pro-inflammatory and immunoregulatory molecules.

The work of Pallone and co-workers (Fais *et al.*, 1987; Pallone *et al.*, 1987) demonstrated that, in Crohn's disease, the T9 antigen in conjunction with other early lymphocyte-activation markers is expressed in increased proportions on both peripheral blood mononuclear cells and isolated intestinal lamina propria mononuclear cells. This work indicated that heightened cellular activation processes in IBD may be important in the intestine. The observation that a high percentage of activated peripheral blood T cells expresses Fcα receptors and exhibits the functional capability of up-regulating IgA secretion *in vitro* provides intriguing evidence that either particular subpopulations in the peripheral blood are activated or activated intestinal lymphocyte populations can migrate from inflamed intestine into the peripheral blood compartment during IBD.

Mueller *et al.* (1990) demonstrated increased serum levels of soluble IL-2 receptor in Crohn's disease patients (Figure 2). Soluble IL-2 receptor can be shed from the surface of T cells or macrophages during cellular activation. The authors also observed an enhanced capacity of Crohn's disease peripheral blood mononuclear cells to secrete soluble IL-2 receptor *in vitro,* both spontaneously and after stimulation with phytohemagglutinin (PHA). Moreover, Crabtree and co-workers found that increased serum levels of soluble IL-2

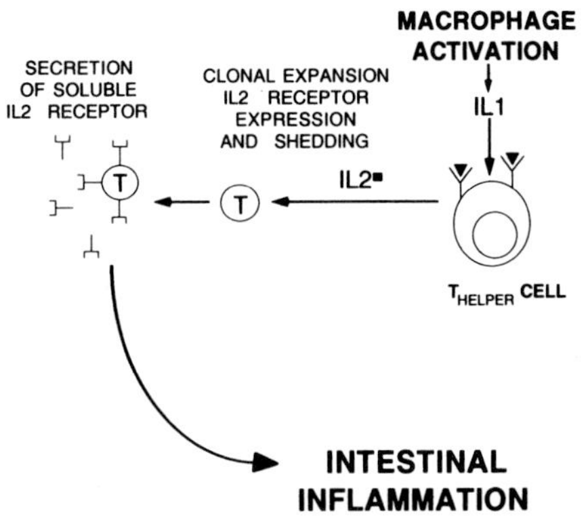

Figure 2 T cell-mediated immunity in IBD. With macrophage activation and the subsequent secretion of pro-inflammatory cytokines such as interleukin 1 (IL1), intestinal T helper cells are highly activated. The increased state of activation of intestinal T cells can be determined by demonstrating activation antigen markers on the cell surface. Subsequently, clonal expansion occurs because of the increased production of interleukin 2 (IL2) and interleukin 2 receptors on intestinal lymphocytes. With activation and expansion of the intestinal T cell repertoire, soluble interleukin 2 receptors are secreted and shed from T cells so they circulate in the serum. The expression and secretion of soluble interleukin 2 receptors as well as TNF-γ and IL-6 may provide a convenient and reliable immunologic marker of intestinal inflammation in ulcerative colitis and Crohn's disease patients in the future.

receptor correlated with the inflammatory activity in Crohn's disease patients (Crabtree *et al.*, 1990). This work indicates that activated lymphocytes in IBD may be able to modulate the immune response by the synthesis and secretion and/or shedding of biologically active molecules. Moreover, measurement of these molecules, such as soluble IL-2 receptor or cytokines produced by activated mononuclear cells, ultimately may provide useful serum markers to correlate the level of tissue inflammation with an ongoing active disease state.

We have demonstrated (Schreiber *et al.*, 1992) an enhanced capacity of isolated IBD intestinal lamina propria mononuclear cells to release soluble IL-2 receptor spontaneously. Enhanced secretion of soluble IL-2 receptors by intestinal mononuclear cells is not specific to either ulcerative colitis or Crohn's disease, but also can be observed in colonic diverticulitis. These studies suggest that activation events observed in the peripheral blood may be related to ongoing inflammatory events in the diseased intestine. This hypothesis also is supported by *in vivo* studies by Mahida *et al.* (1990), who demonstrated that soluble IL-2 receptor is secreted from the inflamed intestine into portal vein blood in Crohn's disease patients.

III. INTESTINAL LYMPHOCYTE ACTIVATION

Immunohistological studies have characterized the numbers and types of inflammatory cells in diseased IBD mucosa (Selby *et al.*, 1984; Fais *et al.*, 1987; Kontinen *et al.*, 1987; MacDonald *et al.*, 1990a), but have yielded conflicting results regarding intestinal lymphocyte activation in Crohn's disease and ulcerative colitis (Figure 1). Although a number of groups have described the increased expression of lymphocyte activation antigens (including 4F2, transferrin receptor, IL-2 receptor, and HLA-DR; Pallone *et al.*, 1987; Allison *et al.*, 1990a; MacDonald *et al.*, 1990), other observations have not demonstrated a rise in activated mucosal lymphocytes (Selby *et al.*, 1984). Allison *et al.* (1990) observed increased T-cell activation in IBD mucosa as demonstrated by the appearance of CD7 but, in contrast, increased IL-2 receptor expression was not seen. Fais and Pallone (1989) noted that intestinal epithelial cells may be capable of expressing activation antigens such as 4F2 and transferrin receptor during active IBD.

We have used flow cytometric analysis of isolated colonic lamina propria mononuclear cells to demonstrate that lymphocyte activation antigens including the IL-2 receptor, the transferrin receptor, and the 4F2 antigen are expressed in increased percentages of intestinal B cells and T cells, as well as in $CD4^+$ and $CD8^+$ T lymphocyte subpopulations, in both active ulcerative colitis and Crohn's disease (Schreiber *et al.*, 1991a). Moreover, 5-aminosalicylic acid (5-ASA), which can be used successfully in the treatment of intestinal inflammation in IBD, inhibits lymphocyte activation and antibody secretion by mitogen-stimulated peripheral blood cells (MacDermott *et al.*, 1989; Schreiber *et al.*, 1991b). Collectively, these studies provide evidence that activation of B- and T-cell populations occurs in the intestine as well as in the peripheral blood of patients with IBD. James and co-workers reported elevated levels of IL-2 mRNA in the mucosa of Crohn's disease patients (Figure 2), but not in that of patients with ulcerative colitis (James *et al.*, 1991).

James and co-workers (Kansas *et al.*, 1985; James *et al.*, 1986; Kanof *et al.*, 1988; James, 1991) have demonstrated that, in contrast to peripheral blood, only a small number of normal lamina propria T cells expresses the Leu8 molecule. Most lymphocytes within the intestine, therefore, are of the $Leu8^-$ $CD4^+$ phenotype and, thus, may be able to enhance B-cell activation and immunoglobulin secretion (Kansas *et al.*, 1985; James *et al.*, 1986; Kanof *et al.*, 1988; James, 1991). This result may help explain the heightened state of intestinal B-cell activation and differentiation in normal human intestine. Moreover, the functional capabilities of $CD4^+Leu8^-$ T cells in IBD intestinal mucosa constitute an important area for future studies.

IV. HOMING OF LYMPHOBLASTS

Follicle-associated epithelium contains microfold (M) cells that are derived directly from undifferentiated immature epithelial stem cells in the crypts that surround Peyer's patches. M cells cover the lymphoid follicles in the gastrointestinal tract and provide a site for the selective sampling of intraluminal antigens (Owen and Jones, 1974), which then are transcytosed into the underlying lymphoid tissues of Peyer's patches (Wolf *et al.*, 1981). Among the characteristic morphological features that distinguish M cells from absorptive epithelial cells is the presence of fewer, shorter, and wider microvilli (Owen and Nemanic, 1978). Vesicles in the M-cell cytoplasm transport antigens through the cell. The antigens then come into contact with lymphocytes and macrophages that have migrated into an intercellular space or central hollow that indents into the M cell (Bockman and Cooper, 1973). M cells themselves do not have Class II antigens on their surfaces and do not process or present antigens. M cells, thus, primarily perform a transport function by moving selected antigens from the lumen into the mucosa, so subsequent macrophage processing and antigen presentation in the intestinal lymphoid follicles will initiate a specific mucosal immune response. Among the infectious agents known to be transcytosed by M cells are reoviruses, *Vibrio cholerae,* and mycobacteria. Similarly, large molecules, including horseradish peroxidase, ferritin, and certain lectins, also are transcytosed by M cells.

Antigen-stimulated lymphocytes from intestinal lymphoid follicles then begin a "maturational journey," in which they leave the intestinal tract and migrate into afferent lymphatics that drain into mesenteric lymph nodes (Bienenstock *et al.*, 1978; Dunkley and Husband, 1987). Lymphocytes then enter efferent lymphatics and pass through the thoracic duct into the peripheral blood. During this process, the lymphoctyes mature into T-cell and B-cell lymphoblasts. B lymphocytes become surface IgA-bearing lymphoblasts after being promoted to switch their immunoglobulin isotype by regulatory ("switch") T cells within the Peyer's patch (Kawanishi *et al.*, 1983a,b; Cebra *et al.*, 1984). B lymphoblasts mature into IgA-secreting plasma cells after homing to mucosal sites. The homing of lymphoblasts results in mature B cells arriving at a variety of secretory sites (Bienenstock *et al.*, 1978; Mestecky, 1987) by interactions between specific "homing antigens" (Jalkanen *et al.*, 1986,1988) on the surfaces of the lymphoblasts and "addressins" (Streeter *et al.*, 1988), specific receptors on the surfaces of high endothelial venules. Thus, a selective recognition of lymphocyte-specific proteins by intergrin family adhesion molecules found on endothelial cells in specific organs regulates the distribution of lymphoid effector cells to the intestine and other mucosal secretory sites. Lymphoblasts recirculate or "home" to the sites of the original antigenic stimulation as well as to other mucosal secretory sites. In humans, the cell interaction, adherence, and extravasation process is mediated by an 85- to 95-kDa class of lymphocyte surface glycoprotein that defines "homing receptors" for high endothelial venules and is present on normal human mucosal lamina propria lymphocyte populations (Jalkanen *et al.*, 1986,1988; Hamann *et al.*, 1988). IgA B cells preferentially migrate to mucosal secretory lymphoid sites, whereas T cells primarily home to peripheral lymph nodes. These differences in migration between B cells and T cells, as well as differences in the migration of lymphoblasts based on their tissue of origin, are due to cell surface homing receptor interactions with high endothelial venules (Streeter *et al.*, 1988).

Antigenic stimulation and chronic inflammation result in a rapid increase in the number of high endothelial venules (identified morphologically by their typical cuboidal, plump appearance). Increase in the number of high endothelial venules is caused by both enhanced differentiation and stimulation of proliferation (Jalkanen *et al.*, 1986,1988). Cytokines, including IL-1, interferon gamma (IFNγ), and tumor necrosis factor (TNF-α), increase lymphoblast adherence to endothelial cells, trigger the development of endothelial cell differentiation markers, and enhance the expression of endothelial adhesion molecules. Increased expression of adhesion molecules on endothelial cells allows an increase in the influx of antigen-specific sensitized lymphocytes, as well as monocytes and granulocytes, into areas of chronic inflammation or areas in which cell-mediated host defense processes are needed. High endothelial venules increase in number in areas that are in close proximity to developing granulomas. The presence of high endothelial venules thus is associated closely with dense lymphocytic infiltrates, particularly when the mononuclear cell-mediated processes are persistent. Although most studies to date have focused on the maturation and homing events related to lymphocytes (Jalkanen *et al.*, 1986,1988; Hamann *et al.*, 1988; Streeter *et al.*, 1988), the migration of granulocytes and macrophages into tissue sites also is regulated by interactions with similar endothelial cell adhesion molecules. Therefore, different cell surface receptors now are known to be involved in determining which lymphocytes become localized to both normal and inflamed intestine.

After antigenic stimulation in the gastrointestinal tract, IgA lymphoblasts also circulate to a number of other mucosal secretory sites including breast, lung, and eye, where antigen-specific antibodies are secreted (Bienenstock *et al.*, 1978; Mestecky, 1987). Homing of stimulated lymphoblasts to mucosal secretory sites allows the secretion of protective antibodies directed against antigens within the gastrointestinal lumen into lung, breast, and eye fluids. Once lymphoblasts have "homed" to the gastrointestinal mucosa and have matured into effector cells, they provide protective immunity within the lamina propria. The appearance of Fcα receptor-expressing activated T cells in the peripheral blood of IBD patients, as well as the enhanced IgA secretion by peripheral blood B cells during active disease, may be related to the outpouring of activated lymphoblasts from involved intestine and their participation in the homing process in active IBD (MacDermott *et al.*, 1981,1983; Raedler *et al.*, 1985a,1986,1988; MacDermott, 1988; MacDermott and Stenson, 1988b; Schreiber *et al.*, 1991). Further, we have observed in collaborative studies with the Jalkanen laboratory that activated lymphoblasts from the intestine also will adhere to human synovial tissue, raising the possibility that altered cell homing to the synovium could lead to the joint manifestations (arthralgias) observed in active IBD.

V. ALTERATIONS IN IMMUNOGLOBULIN SYNTHESIS AND SECRETION

Long-standing IBD is characterized by a mixed cellular infiltrate composed predominantly of B cells and T cells. The B cells normally are arrayed in areas subjacent to ulcerations in IBD, whereas T cells are found around granulomas and in submucosal areas of Crohn's disease lesions. In the normal intestine, IgA-positive B cells predominate. In IBD, however, IgG-containing cells are increased more than other plasma cell types and are present in deeper tissue layers (Brandtzaeg *et al.*, 1988). The intestinal lumen contains numerous immunogenic molecules that physiologically stimulate the normal mucosal immune system, which reacts by mounting a protective immune response. The normal protective mucosal immune response is characterized by a number of features: It is effective, selective, controlled, and localized. These properties are, in part, mediated by IgA, the major immunoglobulin in the normal intestine. IgA protects passively by aggregation and immune exclusion rather than by activation of the complement cascade or induction of an intense inflammatory response, which could cause localized tissue damage.

In IBD, on the other hand, the mucosal immune system exhibits a markedly heightened IgG immune response because of defective or altered immunoregulation. Our studies have provided evidence for the presence of highly activated T cells and B cells, as evidenced by the heightened spontaneous immunoglobulin secretion observed from intestinal and peripheral blood mononuclear cells, particularly of IgG and IgG subclasses (MacDermott *et al.*, 1981; MacDermott, 1988; MacDermott and Stenson, 1988b). We have observed that peripheral blood mononuclear cells (PBMNs) from patients with new-onset untreated IBD display a strikingly high level of spontaneous IgG, IgA, and IgM secretion compared with PBMNs from normal individuals, which demonstrate little spontaneous secretion of antibodies (MacDermott *et al.*, 1981,1983; MacDermott, 1988; MacDermott and Stenson, 1988b). The pattern of markedly elevated spontaneous immunoglobulin secretion is not unique to IBD PBMNs, since we have observed the same secretion pattern from normal human rib bone marrow mononuclear cells, as well as from PBMNs obtained from patients with systemic lupus erythematosus and Henoch–Schoenlein purpura (Alley *et al.*, 1982; Beale *et al.*, 1982; MacDermott *et al.*, 1983). Raedler *et al.* (1985a,1988) reported increased numbers of Fcα receptor-bearing activated T lymphocytes in the blood of IBD patients. The increased numbers of Fcα receptor-positive activated T cells in IBD may contribute to the enhanced secretion of IgA (Raedler *et al.*, 1985a,1988).

Intestinal mononuclear cells have unique capabilities and differ in their functional characteristics from PBMNs (MacDermott *et al.*, 1981;1983;1986;1987; MacDermott, 1988; Scott *et al.*, 1986). Intestinal mononuclear cells from normal mucosa spontaneously secrete enormous amounts of IgA (MacDermott *et al.*, 1983,1986). Both phenotypic and functional parameters indicate an increased state of activation of normal lamina propria T and B cells, which may be induced through continous antigenic stimulation by luminal antigens (Peters *et al.*, 1989). This hypothesis is supported by the demonstration of a higher degree of activation antigen expression (IL-2 receptor and transferrin receptor) on normal colonic lamina propria lymphocytes compared with lymphocytes from the normal small intestine. The enhanced *in vivo* activation of normal intestinal B lymphocytes in comparison to PBMNs may lead to heightened spontaneous *in vitro* immunoglobulin secretion (Schreiber *et al.*, 1991). IBD intestinal monuclear cells exhibit decreased spontaneous IgA secretion (MacDermott *et al.*, 1983;1986) but exhibit instead markedly increased IgG secretion compared with control intestinal mononuclear cells (Scott *et al.*, 1986; MacDermott and Nahm, 1987).

Changes in IgA subclass secretion in IBD are consistent with the migration of monomeric IgA- and IgA1-secreting cells from peripheral blood into the diseased intestine and could represent a normal mucosal response to intestinal antigens or pathogens related to IBD (MacDermott *et al.*, 1986). The integrity and function of the mucosal immune system is critically dependent on complex regulatory events that sustain a continuous IgA-mediated immune response. The decrease in dimeric IgA and IgA2 in IBD could lead to less effective antigen exclusion and decreased host protection by the mucosal immune response (MacDermott *et al.*, 1986). The overall decreased IgA production (MacDermott *et al.*, 1983;1986), coupled with a shift leading to an increase in the percentage of monomeric IgA and IgA1, results in a local dimeric IgA and IgA2 deficiency in IBD (MacDermott and Nahm, 1987) that could lead to an impairment of critical mucosal immune defense mechanisms.

When compared with normal control intestinal mononuclear cells, IBD mononuclear cells show a marked increase in spontaneous secretion of IgG (Scott *et al.*, 1986). The greatest increase in spontaneous IgG secretion is seen in ulcerative colitis intestinal mononuclear cells because of the secretion of large amounts of IgG1 with a concomitant increase in IgG3 secretion. Crohn's disease intestinal mononuclear cells exhibit increased IgG secretion, primarily because of IgG1 and IgG2 (Scott *et al.*, 1986). We have observed similar alterations in IgG subclass concentrations in the sera of active untreated IBD patients, thus underscoring the *in vivo* relevance of our *in vitro* findings (MacDermott *et al.*, 1988).

Increased total IgG and IgG subclass secretion by isolated IBD intestinal mononuclear cells *in vitro* is most likely the result of increased numbers and altered ratios of intestinal plasma cell populations in IBD. The total lymphocyte number has been observed to be four times greater than normal in intestinal specimens from patients with both ulcerative colitis and Crohn's disease (Brandtzaeg *et al.*, 1974; Baklien and Brandtzaeg, 1975; Rosedrans *et al.*, 1980; Scott *et al.*, 1983; Keren *et al.*, 1984; Van Spreeuwel *et al.*, 1985); the major increase occurs in IgG-containing cells. Compared with control specimens, the numbers of IgG-containing cells were 30 times greater whereas numbers of IgA-containing cells were 2 times greater and those of IgM-containing cells 5 times greater than normal. The increased *in vitro* secretion of total IgG and IgG subclasses from IBD intestinal mononuclear cells most likely is related to the increased percentage of IgG-containing cells present *in vivo* in inflamed mucosa. Kett *et al.* (1987) have observed increased IgG1-containing cells in ulcerative colitis patients and increased IgG2-containing cells in Crohn's disease patients. Finally, Badr-el-Din *et al.* (1988) have provided evidence for defective IgA production in ulcerative colitis. Disease specificity control studies by Van Spreeuwel *et al.* (1985) have revealed that, in comparison with IBD biopsies, significantly fewer IgG-containing cells were found in biopsies of patients with acute infectious colitis.

The analysis of immunoglobulin isotype regulation may provide important clues for the delineation of new pathophysiological principles in IBD. Traditionally, IgA has been viewed as the major protective mucosal immunoglobulin of the intestine. Now, in IBD, IgG and its subclasses appear to play a very important role in injurious pathophysiological processes. The study by Kaulfersche *et al.* (1988) assessed lamina propria mononuclear cell heterogeneity and demonstrated that T- and B-cell populations in IBD lamina propria appear to be polyclonal in nature. The question that remains, therefore, is whether or not IgG secretion in IBD might be restricted clonally and, thus, represent a defined response against a group of specific antigens or might be a markedly up-regulated nonspecific response to common luminal agents that are potent inducers of inflammation.

Intriguing questions regarding the pathophysiology of IBD are raised by the observation that IgG subclasses represent discrete and specific immune responses. Different antigens and mitogens induce antibody responses restricted to particular IgG subclasses in both murine and human systems (Gronowicz and Couthino, 1976; Skakib and Stanworth, 1980; Slack *et al.*, 1980; McKearn *et al.*, 1982; Scott and Nahm, 1984). IgG1 and IgG3 antibodies account for the predominant IgG response to proteins and T-cell dependent antigens (Skakib and Stanworth, 1980; Heiner, 1984; Oxelius, 1984). Both IgG1 and IgG3 are better complement pathway activators and opsonins than IgG2 and IgG4 (Skakib and Stanworth, 1980; Waldmann *et al.*, 1983; Heiner, 1984; Oxelius, 1984). IgG2 provides the predominant IgG response to carbohydrates and many bacterial antigens. IgG2 and IgG4 deficiencies therefore are associated with recurrent bacterial infections (e.g., otitis media, pneumococcal respiratory tract infections, pericarditis, meningococcal infections) and with some rare inherited immunodeficiency disorders (such as ataxia telangiectasia and Wiskott–Aldrich syndrome). The increased production of IgG2 in Crohn's disease therefore may represent an inappropriate immune response that could partially contain, but not eradicate, a chronic infectious process (MacDermott and Nahm, 1987). Delineation of the stimuli and antigens that induce increased secretion of IgG subclasses in intestinal mucosa may provide valuable insights into possible etiologic and immunopathogenic aspects of IBD (MacDermott and Nahm, 1987).

We now know that (1)intestinal mononuclear cells in health and disease constitute a unique immunological compartment with distinct functional capabilities; (2) major alterations occur with respect to spontaneous antibody secretion in IBD, thereby demonstrating potential regulatory defects in the mucosal immune system in IBD; (3) within the intestine involved with disease itself, major alterations in antibody secretion occur, particularly with respect to IgA and IgG subclasses; and (4) further research addressing the specificity and function of IgG antibodies secreted in IBD may delineate important effector mechanisms.

VI. COMPLEMENT PATHWAY ACTIVATION IN INFLAMMATORY BOWEL DISEASE

Complement pathway activation, by either the classical or the alternative pathway, leads to the generation of products that not only maintain normal host defense integrity, but also result in inflammation and tissue destruction. Products of the complement activation pathway include large fragments of C_3 (i.e., C_3b, C3bi) that have considerable opsonic activity and small, low molecular weight fragments (from both C3 and C5) that can stimulate leukocytes directly and possess chemotactic activity. Human C3a, C4a, and C5 can activate smooth muscle cells, small blood vessels, mast cells, and basophils directly, whereas phagocytes respond only to C5a via specific receptors (Stoughton, 1972; Petersson *et al.*, 1975; Grant *et al.*, 1976; Siraganian and Hook, 1976; Hartman and Glovsky, 1981; Stimler *et al.*, 1981,1983; Yancey *et al.*, 1985). Investigators have proposed pathogenic roles for complement system molecules in IBD, but the nature and extent of their involvement in the immunopathophysiology of IBD is still undefined. Some of the clinical findings and histological changes that occur in IBD are consistent with the biological activities of C3a, C4a, C5a, and C3b. Phagocytosis of bacteria and cellular debris occurs at an accelerated rate during intestinal inflammation, in part because of opsonization by complement components, as well as increased priming and activation of monocytes and macrophages. Synergism of IFNγ and C5a also may be of great importance in IBD with respect to the induction of leukotriene release (Nielson *et al.*, 1988). Moreover, C5a, like LTB4, is a potent chemotactic agent for neutrophils and increases vascular permeability (Wilkinson, 1982; Charo *et al.*, 1986). Neutrophils demonstrate distinct polarization and enhanced aggregation as well as increased adherence after activation by C5a (Ward and Newman, 1969; Craddock *et al.*, 1977,1978; Fernandez *et al.*, 1978; Smith *et al.*, 1979; Hammerschmidt *et al.*, 1980; Perez *et al.*, 1980; Tonnesen *et al.*, 1984; Charo *et al.*, 1986), a mechanism that may contribute to the large number of neutrophils present in IBD mucosa. Thus, the pathophysiological and histological changes seen in IBD may be caused, in part, by the biological activities of C3b and C5a coupled with other potent inflammatory mediators such as leukotriene B4 (LTB4) released in response to bacterial cell wall components.

Several studies have found normal levels of C3 and C4 in the peripheral blood of IBD patients. The state of activation of the alternative pathway in IBD has been reported in different studies to be decreased, normal, or increased (Lake *et al.*, 1979; D'Amelio *et al.*, 1983; Elmgreen, et al.). In support of decreased activation of the alternative pathway is a study that observed the depression of properidin and properidin convertase, in addition to diminished consumption of C3–C9 after incubation with cobra venom of sera from patients with Crohn's disease and ulcerative colitis (Lake *et al.*, 1979;

D'Amelio *et al.*, 1983). C5a activity was reported to be diminished in Crohn's sera; decreased consumption of the major complement component C3 was noted; and, finally, a reduced generation of C5a after stimulation was seen (D'Amelio *et al.*, 1983). In other studies, an increased level of activation of complement pathways in IBD (Hodgson *et al.*, 1977; Elmgreen *et al.*, 1983; Simonsen and Elmgreen, 1985; Peterson *et al.*, 1988) was demonstrated. After radioiodinated C3 was injected intravenously, both the synthesis and the catabolism of C3 were found to be increased in patients with Crohn's disease and ulcerative colitis, suggesting an increased state of complement pathway activation (Hodgson *et al.*, 1977; Simonsen and Elmgreen, 1985). The levels of C3c in Crohn's disease patients were 10-fold greater than those in healthy persons or ulcerative colitis patients (Elmgreen *et al.*, 1983). C3c levels did not correlate with disease activity in Crohn's disease. In another study, levels of C3d were elevated in 6 of 20 patients with Crohn's disease, as were those of C4 in 9 of 20 cases (Peterson *et al.*, 1988). Moreover, levels of C3d correlated with C4d concentrations in patient sera. Elevated levels of C3c in Crohn's disease suggest hypercatabolism of C3 and activation of the complement cascade in IBD. Elevated levels of C3d and C4d underscore activation of the classical pathway in Crohn's disease.

Studies by Halstensen *et al.* (1990) have demonstrated the possible direct role of complement in tissue destruction in ulcerative colitis. The authors used monoclonal antibodies against a neoepitope, only expressed by activated C3b and the cytolytically active terminal complement complex, to identify potential complement-induced damage in tissue sections from inflamed IBD intestine. Of 11 patients with ulcerative colitis, 9 showed activated C3b deposited apically on the surface epithelium of involved mucosa, whereas no deposits were seen in 31 matched noninflamed specimens or in 16 of 17 healthy controls. Moreover, a striking colocalization of IgG1, activated C3b, and terminal complement complex was observed in 4 of the 11 ulcerative colitis patients. Thus, IgG1, secreted into the lumen during ulcerative colitis, may provide a mechanism for contiguous bowel involvement seen via complement activation. Further, an increased vascular deposition of terminal complement complex in both ulcerative colitis and Crohn's disease (Halstensen *et al.*, 1989a) could be demonstrated. Interestingly, 5 of 10 ulcerative colitis specimens and 1 of 5 Crohn's disease samples contained terminal complement complex located outside the blood vessels in the mucosa or the submucosa. In IBD, significantly more C3c reactivity was associated with terminal complement complex deposition, thus indicating continuous complement activation and deposition within the blood vessel wall (Halstensen *et al.*, 1989b). These findings are consistent with the *in vivo* studies by Ahrenstedt *et al.* (1990), who found that both C3 and C4 levels in jejunal perfusates of Crohn's disease patients were increased compared with healthy controls (Ahrenstedt *et al.*, 1990). A major role for complement activation in IBD, therefore, could be participation in the acute effector events of tissue destruction. In addition, complement as part of immune complexes could lead to enhanced phagocytosis and could participate in the *in vitro* release of potent mediators such as LTB_4 by neutrophils (Nielson *et al.*, 1986).

VII. GRANULOCYTE AND MACROPHAGE FUNCTION

During active ulcerative colitis and Crohn's disease, large numbers of neutrophils and monocytes leave the bloodstream and migrate into the inflamed mucosa and submucosa (Figure 3). These cells carry out a series of destructive effector events, and continue to migrate on through the bowel wall into the intestinal lumen. The biological events that occur during inflammation are the result of a multiplicity of interacting mediators and autacoids (auto-pharmacological substances that exert a potent local activity). The regulatory events that control the level of inflammation can be divided into three areas (Figure 3): (1) the process of adhesion and migration through the intestinal mucosa, (2) the secretion of cytokines by lymphocytes, monocytes, and macrophages, and (3) the pro-inflammatory role of lipid mediators such as leukotrienes, prostaglandins, and platelet activating factor (PAF).

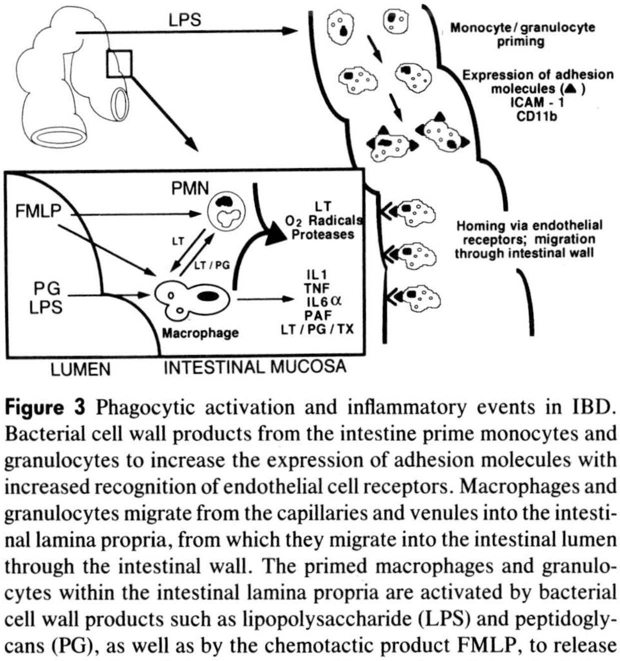

Figure 3 Phagocytic activation and inflammatory events in IBD. Bacterial cell wall products from the intestine prime monocytes and granulocytes to increase the expression of adhesion molecules with increased recognition of endothelial cell receptors. Macrophages and granulocytes migrate from the capillaries and venules into the intestinal lamina propria, from which they migrate into the intestinal lumen through the intestinal wall. The primed macrophages and granulocytes within the intestinal lamina propria are activated by bacterial cell wall products such as lipopolysaccharide (LPS) and peptidoglycans (PG), as well as by the chemotactic product FMLP, to release a variety of pro-inflammatory cytokines and mediators including interleukin 1 (IL1) tumor necrosis factor (TNF), interleukin 6 (IL6), platelet activating factor (PAF), leukotrienes (LT), and prostaglandins (PG/TX). In addition, destructive molecules such as oxygen radicals and proteases are produced. The involvement of granulocytes and macrophages in inflammatory bowel disease adds an acute inflammatory component to the chronic cell-mediated intestinal injurious processes involved in IBD.

Polymorphonuclear leukocyte (PMN) function initially was evaluated in IBD by assessing migration, chemotaxis, adherence, and phagocytosis. Studies by Rhodes and co-workers suggested intrinsic abnormalities of PMN function in IBD, and also revealed that inhibitors of chemotactic factor activity are present in the sera of Crohn's disease and ulcerative colitis patients (Rhodes *et al.*, 1981; Wandall and Binder, 1982). Interestingly, no functional difference between PMNs from normal controls and those from IBD patients were observed with respect to phagocytic capacity or chemotaxis induced by zymosan-activated serum or casein (Morain *et al.*, 1981).

Saverymuttu *et al.* (1985a,b) subsequently carried out a series of pivotal functional studies in which peripheral blood phagocytes (granulocytes and monocytes) were isolated, labeled *in vitro* with ^{111}indium-labeled tropolonate, and reinjected into the patient. The migration of the labeled cells was assessed with time, using a whole body gamma-radiation camera. In 20 of 22 patients with Crohn's disease, over 90% of radiolabeled phagocytes accumulated rapidly in the inflamed intestine (Saverymuttu *et al.*, 1985a). A similar study conducted in 15 ulcerative colitis patients showed enhanced migration into areas of inflamed bowel (Saverymuttu *et al.*, 1985b). These studies established the greatly increased migration of monocytes, macrophages, and PMNs into the intestine, which occurs in IBD, and showed that monitoring phagocytic cell movement could be of potential value in the clinical assessment of IBD patients (Saverymuttu *et al.*, 1985a,b). These findings also indicated the likely central importance of granulocytes and macrophages in mediating inflammation in IBD (Saverymuttu *et al.*, 1985a,b). The introduction of ^{99m}technetium-labeled hexamethyl propylene amine oxine as a leukocyte label in Crohn's disease by Schoelmerich *et al.* (1988) refined the technique and further eased the assessment of phagocytic cell migration in IBD. The selective labeling of mononuclear phagocytes (monocytes) by ^{99m}T-labeled stannous colloid likewise has improved our understanding of macrophage migration in IBD (Pullman *et al.*, 1988).

The binding of phagocytes to blood vessel endothelial cells, followed by migration into the diseased bowel, is mediated through well-characterized adhesion molecules (Figure 3) including LFA-1 (lymphocyte function-associated antigen 1; CD11a) which binds to ICAM-1 (intercellular adhesion molecule 1; CD54). Although great advances have been made regarding our understanding of the integrin family of cell surface molecules, their participation in intestinal inflammation is only now being examined. Studies by Malizia *et al.* (1991) have demonstrated that, during IBD, the expression of ICAM-1 on endothelial cells increases dramatically and is accompanied by an increase of CD11a on mononuclear phagocytes. This study demonstrated the potential importance of adhesion molecules in mediating granulocyte and monocyte influx into the diseased intestine, which promises to be one of the central areas for future investigation of the immunopathogenesis of IBD, as well as for the development of new treatment strategies.

VIII. PRO-INFLAMMATORY CYTOKINES

Lymphocytes and macrophages synthesize and secrete a number of potent pro-inflammatory mediators (Figure 1) after stimulation and activation by molecules that are present in large amounts in the intestinal lumen, such as bacterial cell wall products (Fiocchi, 1989). Inflammatory events are mediated in part by the multitude of effects and actions of IL-1 (IL-1α and IL-1β), IL-6, and TNFα (cachectin). When the two forms of IL-1 (α and β) are compared, they exert very similar functions despite their different sources and their structural dissimilarities. The best known activities of IL-1 include the induction of fever ("endogenous pyrogen"), the stimulation of acute-phase protein synthesis, and the initiation of critical lymphocyte activation events. TNF, which shares only 3% homology with IL-1, is identical to "cachectin," which causes hemodynamic shock and cachexia associated with various disease states.

Human T-cell activation requires both a cross-linking mechanism for the T-cell antigen–receptor complex and the presence of IL-1 which, under physiological conditions, are both provided by the macrophage. In addition to macrophages, B cells, astrocytes, mesangial cells, keratinocytes, and endothelial cells also can act as accessory cells by producing or expressing membrane-bound IL-1. IL-1 also promotes B-cell activation and differentiation, particularly when acting in synergism with IL-4. Moreover, IL-1 can induce other B cell-regulating factors such as IFN-γ and IL-2 as well as IL-6. Finally, IL-1 will act in an autocrine loop on the macrophage itself, and will stimulate further IL-1 production as well as induce prostaglandin E_2 (PGE_2) and granulocyte–macrophage colony stimulating factor (GM-CSF) secretion.

Work by Isaacs and co-workers (Isaacs *et al.*, 1990) as well as by Rachmilewitz and co-workers (1991; Ligumsky *et al.*, 1990) has focused on cytokines involved in the initiation of intestinal lymphocyte activation. Ligumsky and co-workers (1990) detected increased levels of IL-1 in inflamed mucosa from patients with both Crohn's disease and ulcerative colitis. Moreover, *in vitro*, increased amounts were synthesized in cultured biopsies as well, indicating that mucosa-resident cells secrete IL-1. Isaacs and co-workers (1990) as well as Stevens and co-workers (1990) demonstrated that IL-1 mRNA was present in the mucosa of a majority of IBD patients. Increasing interest therefore has focused on the role of pro-inflammatory cytokines in the initiation and enhancement of intestinal inflammatory processes.

In IBD intestinal mucosa, increased quantities of IL-1β mRNA have been detected, presumably produced by mononuclear phagocytes (Ligumsky *et al.*, 1990). Mahida and co-workers (1989) studied IL-1β release from isolated intestinal lamina propria mononuclear cells and observed enhanced spontaneous secretion by monocytes from IBD patients, compared with normal controls. Lipopolysaccharide (LPS) further enhanced IL-1β production by IBD lamina propria mononuclear cells but not by those from normal controls (Mahida *et al.*, 1989). Moreover, depletion of macrophages abolished IL-1β secretion (Mahida *et al.*, 1989). Satsangi and co-workers (1987) demonstrated that PBMNs from Crohn's disease patients secrete increased amounts of IL-1, both spontaneously as well as after being stimulated with LPS, compared with normal controls. Cominelli and co-workers demonstrated that increased IL-1 concentrations play a key role in the pathogenesis of rabbit immune complex colitis and that tissue levels of IL-1 correlate with the severity of inflammation (Cominelli and Dinarello, 1989; Cominelli *et al.*, 1990). IL-1 mRNA was detectable as early as 4 hr after induction of colitis, indicating that IL-1 gene expression occurs as a very early event in experimental immune complex colitis (Cominelli *et al.*, 1990). The rise in IL-1 preceded the increase of PGE_2 and LTB_4. Moreover, treatment with IL-1 receptor antagonist (IL-1ra) reduced the extent and severity of the inflammatory response associated with immune complex colitis in rabbits (Cominelli *et al.*, 1990).

Studies by Isaacs *et al.* (1992) using the polymerase chain reaction (PCR) to detect cytokines in intestinal lamina propria showed a more frequent presence of IL-1, IL-6, and TNFα in Crohn's disease and ulcerative colitis patients compared with normal patients. We have observed that lamina propria monunuclear cells isolated from endoscopic biopsies from patients with active IBD spontaneously secreted high amounts of IL-1β (Reinecker *et al.*, 1993).

MacDonald and co-workers (1990b) investigated the secretion of TNFα in IBD using a spot enzyme-linked immunosorbent assay (ELISA) technique. In Crohn's disease and in a subgroup of ulcerative colitis patients, TNFα-screting intestinal mononuclear cells were increased in frequency in comparison with normal controls. We have found very low spontaneous *in vitro* release of TNFα from lamina propria mononuclear cells isolated from endoscopic biopsies from normal donors and IBD patients (Reinecker *et al.*, 1993). However, stimulation of lamina propria mononuclear cells with pokeweed mitogen (PWM) induced an enhancement of TNFα release that was significantly higher in IBD than in normal controls (Reinecker *et al.*, 1993).

IL-6 also can be released by monocytes as one of the proinflammatory cytokines, and is involved in regulating the final maturation of B cells into antibody-forming plasma cells (Hilbert, 1989). IL-6 shares a number of characteristics with granulocyte colony stimulating factor (G-CSF) and can be induced *in vitro* by IL-1β (Yasukawa *et al.*, 1987). Shirota and co-workers (1990) reported that normal epithelium can express IL-6 as well as its receptor, a finding that may be of importance in IBD. Moreover, Mitsuymama *et al.* (1991) reported increased serum levels of IL-6, in Crohn's disease and ulcerative colitis patients, that decline with treatment of the patients. Increased levels of IL-6, spontaneously secreted by lamina propria mononuclear cells from ulcerative colitis patients, were observed by Kusagami *et al.* (1991). We have observed an enhancement of IL-6 secretion by lamina propria mononuclear cells in ulcerative colitis but not in Crohn's disease patients or normal controls (Reinecker *et al.*, 1993).

Intriguingly, many of the biological activities of IL-1, IL-6, and TNFα overlap, particularly those leading to amplification of immunological and inflammatory processes. TNFα and IL-6 share many of the systemic properties and functions of IL-1, including the enhancement of cellular catabolism, induction of acute phase proteins, and pyrogenic activity. TNFα activates endothelial cells and can induce IL-1 and IL-6. Both IL-1 and TNFα stimulate PGI_2, PGE_2, and PAF secretion by cultured endothelial cells. Therefore, sustained inflammation leading to tissue destruction in IBD could be mediated to a significant extent by the potent biological activities of IL-1, IL-6, and TNFα

IX. PROSTAGLANDINS

Mucosal hyperemia, increased microvascular permeability, and edema are typical changes seen in a variety of intestinal inflammatory states, independent of the cause. Soluble lipid mediators released during the process of inflammation (Figure 4) can induce inflammatory tissue damage *in vivo*. These molecules cause tissue edema by increasing vascular (postcapillary venule) permeability to albumin and other macromolecules and cause hyperemia by inducing vasodilation. Other functional changes (including diminished salt and water absorption) that are characteristic of intestinal inflammation also may be related to soluble mediators, but their pathogenesis is less clear.

Arachidonic acid is liberated from the second carbon in phospholipids by a specific enzyme, phospholipase A_2. Whereas the remaining lysophosphatide can undergo further degradation or subsequently can be acetylated to form PAF, arachidonic acid can enter two principal metabolic pathways, the cyclooxygenase and the lipoxygenase pathways (Bach, 1982; Parker, 1984). The pathway leading to prostaglandin synthesis is initiated by the enzyme cyclooxygenase, which

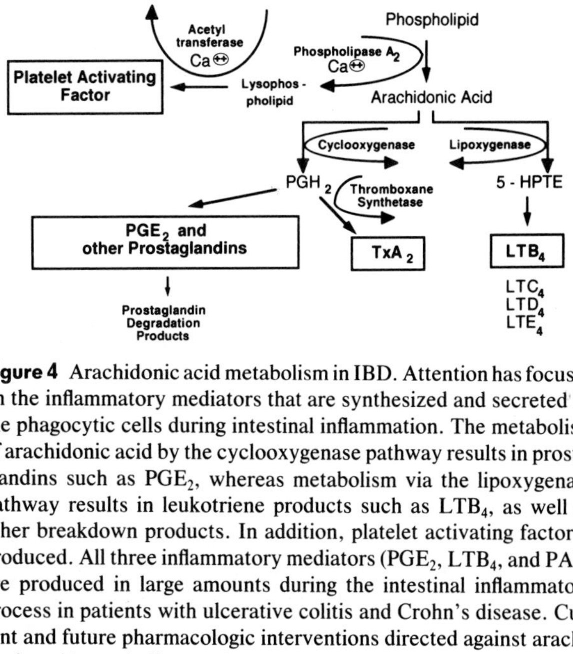

Figure 4 Arachidonic acid metabolism in IBD. Attention has focused on the inflammatory mediators that are synthesized and secreted by the phagocytic cells during intestinal inflammation. The metabolism of arachidonic acid by the cyclooxygenase pathway results in prostaglandins such as PGE_2, whereas metabolism via the lipoxygenase pathway results in leukotriene products such as LTB_4, as well as other breakdown products. In addition, platelet activating factor is produced. All three inflammatory mediators (PGE_2, LTB_4, and PAF) are produced in large amounts during the intestinal inflammatory process in patients with ulcerative colitis and Crohn's disease. Current and future pharmacologic interventions directed against arachidonic acid metabolism pathways are being developed.

catalyzes the transformation of arachidonic acid into unstable endoperoxides and then into prostaglandin G_2 (PGG_2) and prostaglandin H_2 (PGH_2), from which PGE_2, PGD_2, PGF_{2a}, PGI_2, and thromboxane A_2 (TxA_2) are derived (Bach, 1982; Parker, 1984). Almost all mammalian cells, including intestinal epithelium and cells associated with inflammatory events (i.e., macrophages, platelets, endothelial cells, mast cells), are capable of producing prostaglandins (Bach, 1982; Parker, 1984).

An alternative metabolic pathway for arachidonic acid is provided by the enzyme 5-lipoxygenase. The first product of the action of 5-lipoxygenase on arachidonic acid is a short-lived hydroperoxide metabolite, which again is transformed by 5-lipoxygenase to the epoxide leukotriene A_4 (LTA_4). Subsequent reaction products include LTB_4 and a series of metabolites (Figure 4)—LTC_4, LTD_4, and LTE_4 (Bach, 1982; Lewis and Austen, 1984; Parker, 1984; MacGlashin *et al.*, 1986). On release into the extracellular space, these leukotrienes can be oxidized (i.e., by interaction with myeloperoxidase and H_2O_2) to sulfoxide metabolites. However, 5-lipoxygenase and subsequent enzymes of this pathway have been shown to exist definitely only in a small number of cell types, including neutrophils, eosinophils, basophils, monocytes, macrophages, and mast cells (Lewis and Austen, 1984; MacGlashin *et al.*, 1986). Moreover, the key enzyme, 5-lipoxygenase, can utilize other unsaturated fatty acids in addition to arachidonic acid, thus leading to different products.

Eicosanoids, including dietary compounds such as the omega-3 unsaturated fatty acids contained in fish oil, have unique biological properties: They are not stored in tissues but are synthesized *de novo* in response to stimulation (Douglas, 1985). Furthermore, cell–cell interactions involving products of the eicosanoid pathway are of increasing interest. Some cells will synthesize *de novo* their own eicosanoid precursors from arachidonic acid, others will acquire precursors from neighboring cells in close physical proximity, thus leading to different final products (Douglas, 1986). The pattern of eicosanoid production is tissue specific and most of these short-lived mediators exert their action only in the immediate microenvironment of the secreting cell. In most cases, eicosanoids are not the sole mediators of a certain function, but act in synergy with other regulatory mechanisms (Bach, 1982; Lewis and Austen, 1984; Parker, 1984; MacGlashin *et al.*, 1986; Douglas, 1985).

Prostaglandins, in particular those of the E series, have biological properties that can induce some of the morphological changes observed in inflamed tissue, for example, enhanced microvascular permeability and subsequent edema, vasodilation, and induction of pain (Bach, 1982; Parker, 1984). Physiological concentrations of PGE_2 have little effect, whereas pharmacological concentrations may impair electrolyte and water transport.

Clearly IBD is associated with increased levels of prostaglandin production. Elevated levels of prostaglandins (primarily PGE_2) are found in the stool, venous blood, and rectal mucosa in IBD, and elevated levels of metabolites are found in urine (Sharon *et al.*, 1978; Gould, 1981; Gould *et al.*, 1981). When incubated *in vitro*, biopsies of rectal mucosa from patients with ulcerative colitis contain increased amounts of PGE_2 and TxB_2 (Sharon *et al.*, 1978). An *in vivo* estimate of prostaglandin synthesis by rectal mucosa is achieved using a dialysis bag that is filled with buffer and placed into the patient's rectum (Lauritsen *et al.*, 1985). Prostaglandin levels in IBD, whether in mucosa, serum, or rectal dialysate, correlate with disease activity; successful medical management results in a reduction in prostaglandin levels (Rampton *et al.*, 1980; Lauritsen *et al.*, 1985).

The source of the prostaglandins in colonic mucosa in IBD is not well defined; epithelial cells, endothelial cells, fibroblasts, and mononuclear inflammatory cells all can produce prostaglandins. From isolation studies, intestinal mononuclear cells appear to be responsible for as much as or more prostaglandin synthesis than intestinal epithelial cells (Zifroni *et al.*, 1983). This finding is consistent with studies of inflammatory cells in other organ systems in which mononuclear cells were found to be the major source of prostaglandin synthesis (Bach, 1982; Parker 1984).

However, evidence against a significant primary role for prostaglandins as pro-inflammatory mediators in IBD also exists. Clinical evidence comes from a few small studies of nonsteroidal anti-inflammatory drugs (NSAIDs), particularly indomethacin, in IBD (Levy and Gaspar, 1975; Gilat *et al.*, 1979; Campieri *et al.*, 1980; Gould *et al.*, 1981). Indomethacin and other NSAIDs are potent inhibitors of cyclooxygenase but not lipoxygenase (Vane, 1971). Use of these drugs in rheumatoid arthritis and other inflammatory diseases results in both decreased prostaglandin synthesis and clinical improvement, effects that helped establish a role for prostaglandins as important mediators of inflammation. In contrast to their usefulness in rheumatoid arthritis, NSAIDs have no role in the medical management of IBD. Small trials of indomethacin administered orally (Lauritsen *et al.*, 1985) and rectally (Levy and Gaspar, 1975; Sharon *et al.*, 1978; Flower and Blackwell, 1979; Gilat *et al.*, 1979; Campieri *et al.*, 1980; Rampton and Sladen, 1981; Hawkey, 1982; Terano *et al.*, 1984) revealed no improvement in ulcerative colitis. Moreover, some reports have suggested that both indomethacin and flubiprofen, another NSAID, may cause clinical deterioration in ulcerative colitis, despite the decrease in prostaglandin production (Campieri *et al.*, 1980; Gould *et al.*, 1981; Rampton and Sladen, 1981,1984). The failure of NSAIDs to induce clinical improvement in IBD, despite their inhibition of prostaglandin production, suggests that prostaglandins and other inflammatory mediators such as PAF and leukotrienes may all need to be inhibited to reduce tissue injury.

These clinical observations are also compatible with reports characterizing PGE_2 as an anti-inflammatory agent in the regulation of mononuclear cell activation. PGE_2, as well as glucocorticoids or α-fetoprotein, down-regulates HLA Class II expression on activated macrophages and thus impairs their ability to present antigen (Hokland *et al.*, 1981; Madsen *et al.*, 1981; Snyder *et al.*, 1982). PGE_2 inhibits the release of inflammatory mediators from stimulated leukocytes via induction of cAMP (Zurier *et al.*, 1974). Prostaglandins of the E series, as well as prostacyclin (PGI_2), inhibit leukocyte chemotaxis (Gallin *et al.*, 1985), adherence to various substrates including endothelium (Boxer *et al.*, 1980), phagocytosis (Cox and Karnovsky, 1973), and generation of toxic oxygen radicals (Lehmeyer and Johnston, 1978). Proliferative responses of human lymphocytes to mitogens, lymphocyte-mediated cytotoxicity, and antibody production are all inhibited by PGE_2 (Goldyne and Stobo, 1981). Moreover, anti-inflammatory effects of PGE_2 can be confirmed *in vivo*: PGE_2 compounds suppress adjuvant arthritis (Aspinall and Cammarata, 1969; Glenn and Rohloff, 1971; Zurier *et al.*, 1973), carrageenan-induced inflammation (Glenn and Rohloff, 1971; Zurier *et al.*, 1973), and immune complex-induced inflammation (Kunkel *et al.*, 1979). An anti-inflammatory effect produced by PGE_2 may be of importance in spontaneous remissions in IBD. PGE decreases the affinity of neutrophil formyl methionyl-leucyl-phenylalanine (FMLP)-receptors (Fantone *et al.*, 1983), resulting in decreased neutrophil degranulation (Fantone *et al.*, 1981), which may be another role for anti-inflammatory actions of prostaglandins of the E series in IBD.

X. LEUKOTRIENES

Whereas the cyclooxygenase pathway is present in almost all mammalian cells, the 5-lipoxygenase pathway is found primarily in cells of bone marrow origin involved in the inflammatory process (i.e., mast cells, neutrophils, monocytes, and macrophages; Borgeat and Samuelsson, 1979; Stenson and Parker, 1984). The major products of the 5-lipoxygenase pathway (Figure 4) are 5-hydroxy-6,8,11,14-eicosatetraenoic acid (5-HETE) and LTB_4, LTC_4, LTD_4, and LTE_4. LTB_4 and, to a lesser extent, 5-HETE exert potent chemotactic activities on neutrophils. LTB_4, in the presence of neutrophils, also induces enhanced vascular permeability. The sulfidoleukotrienes induce smooth muscle contraction in the lung, blood vessels, and gastrointestinal tract (Buckell *et al.*, 1978; Stenson and Parker, 1984).

Incubation of IBD mucosa with radiolabeled arachidonic acid results in the synthesis of large quantities of LTB_4 and 5-HETE and smaller quantities of PGE_2 and TxB_2 (Sharon and Stenson, 1984). IBD mucosa produces larger quantities of lipoxygenase and cyclooxygenase products than does normal mucosa. Patterns of arachidonate lipoxygenase metabolism are similar for ulcerative colitis and Crohn's disease. Lipid extracts of IBD mucosa contain large amounts of LTB_4, up to 50-fold as much as normal mucosa (Rampton and Sladen, 1984). A concentration of 250 ng LTB_4/g, as typically found in IBD mucosa, is equivalent of a concentration of 5×10^{-7} *M*, which is well within the range of biological activity of LTB_4. Levels of both PGE_2 and LTB_4 were markedly higher in rectal dialysates from ulcerative colitis patients and declined to normal levels after treatment with a short course of prednisolone (Lauritsen *et al.*, 1985).

The presence of large numbers of neutrophils and mononuclear phagocytes in IBD mucosa suggests that a chemotactic factor (or factors) is present in IBD mucosa that induces neutrophils to migrate out of the circulation and into the tissue. LTB_4 is a potent chemoattractant for human neutrophils (Ford-Hutchinson *et al.*, 1984); however, other chemotactic compounds (IL-8, MCP-1) are present in IBD mucosa. In an attempt to sort out the contributions of various chemotactic factors for neutrophil infiltration in IBD, a study was done using homogenized IBD mucosa as the chemotactic stimulus for ^{51}Cr-labeled neutrophils in a Boyden chamber, revealing that most of the chemotactic activity is lipophilic and coelutes with LTB_4 standards in reverse-phase high performance liquid chromatography (HPLC) (Stenson, 1988). If the findings using the *in vitro* assay for neutrophil chemotaxis in the Boyden chamber can be extrapolated to the *in vivo* situation, one could argue that LTB_4 is the chemotactic mediator that, in addition to adhesion molecules, is primarily responsible for neutrophils leaving the circulation and entering the intestinal tissue in IBD. The generation of LTB_4 is certainly not the initiating event in IBD, nor is it specific to IBD.

Although the role of LTB_4 in IBD has been studied most extensively, preliminary reports are available of a possible role for the sulfidoleukotrienes (LTC_4, LTD_4, LTE_4; Peskar *et al.*, 1985). Crohn's colitis mucosa produced 3-fold more sulfidoleukotrienes than normal mucosa produced under both stimulated and unstimulated conditions (Peskar *et al.*, 1985). The predominant sulfidoleukotriene found was LTE_4, suggesting that released LTC_4 is degraded rapidly by peptidases.

XI. PLATELET ACTIVATING FACTOR

The ability to induce platelet aggregation and granulocyte activation by PAF led to its recognition as a potent inflammatory mediator. The primary pathway of PAF biosynthesis is by reacetylation at the 2 position of the lysophosphatide produced by phospholipase A_2. Degradation of PAF occurs via deacetylation by acetylhydrolase.

PAF can be synthesized by a variety of cell types including PMNs, macrophages, mast cells, eosinophils, basophils, endothelial cells, and platelets. PAF actually consists of multiple species, including saturated homologs and unsaturated analogs, as well as derivatives from lysophosphatides with polar head groups other than choline (Mueller *et al.*, 1984; Ludwig and Pinckard, 1987; Oda *et al.*, 1985; Weintraub *et al.*, 1985; Satouchi *et al.*, 1985; Ramesha and Pickett, 1987). Some of the pro-inflammatory activities of PAF include induction of aggregation, chemotaxis, and chemokinesis of PMNs (McManus *et al.*, 1980; Pinckard *et al.*, 1980; Shaw *et al.*, 1981); monocyte aggregation and initiation of superoxide secretion (Ingraham *et al.*, 1982; Yasaka *et al.*, 1982; Hartung, 1983; Hartung *et al.*, 1983; Gay *et al.*, 1986); and the induction of prostaglandin and leukotriene release by eosinophils, neutrophils platelets, endothelial cells, moncytes, and epithelial cells (Lin *et al.*, 1982; O'Flaherty *et al.*, 1984; Bussolino *et al.*, 1985; O'Flaherty, 1985; Brock and Gimbrone, 1986; Brunynzeel *et al.*, 1986). Direct contraction of vascular smooth muscle also can be induced, as can enhanced vascular permeability and intestinal edema (Sanchez-Crespo *et al.*, 1982; Hartung *et al.*, 1983). Some of these effects may involve cyclooxygenase-derived arachidonic acid products or histamine as secondary mediators (Humphrey *et al.*, 1982; Archer *et al.*, 1985; Hwang *et al.*, 1985).

The role of PAF in IBD is just beginning to be studied

(Figure 4). The studies by Eliakim *et al.* (1988) suggest the involvement of PAF as a pro-inflammatory mediator in IBD, which can be reduced in activity by steroids and 5-ASA. Thus, the role of PAF in IBD deserves intensive future investigation, particularly with respect to the different derivatives of PAF. PAF activity may contribute significantly to the inflammatory changes seen in IBD. The biological function of PAF is related closely to the prostaglandins and leukotrienes, which can be induced by PAF and can induce PAF synthesis as well (Shaw *et al.*, 1981; O'Flaherty *et al.*, 1984; O'Flaherty, 1985; Sun and Hsueh, 1988). Little is known currently about the mechanisms that may regulate PAF synthesis and degradation in IBD. The use of specific PAF antagonists in the treatment of IBD patients constitutes an important area for future clinical investigation.

XII. CONCLUSION

Within the gastrointestinal tract, many different cell types contribute to the development of a successful mucosal immune response. M cells within the follicle-associated epithelium overlie Peyer's patches and can mediate the transcytosis of antigens and infectious agents to the underlying cells of the mucosal immune system. Immature cells within Peyer's patches (lymphoid follicles) are stimulated to recognize specific antigens but, instead of migrating directly to adjacent lamina propria, these cells migrate out of the gastrointestinal tract. Maturation and activation occurs while the cells are traversing through the lymphatic system. After subsequent circulation of stimulated lymphoblasts in the peripheral blood, mature activated T and B cells "home" to the intestine as specific effector cells.

In addition to producing specific cytokines that regulate cell function, lamina propria and intraepithelial T cells also secrete nonspecific inflammatory mediators, such as IFNγ, that enhance antigen-presenting capabilities through the increased expression of Class II MHC determinants on epithelial cells and other cell types.

The intestine is fully capable of mounting an intense protective inflammatory reaction in response to infectious agents or injurious substances. Antigen presentation by intestinal macrophages triggers the production of cytokines and inflammatory mediators. Antibodies leading to complement pathway activation produce chemotactic factors and activate macrophages and granulocytes to produce pro-inflammatory cytokines and other destructive molecules. Eosinophils and mast cells are also important cell types in the intestinal immune response. The final manifestations of intestinal inflammation are, in large part, the result of the production of a wide variety of pro-inflammatory cytokines, chemotactic cytokines, and inflammatory mediators such as prostaglandins, leukotrienes, and PAF.

Intestinal inflammation in IBD is characterized by the increased activation of B and T lymphocytes in both peripheral blood and intestinal lamina propria. Activation events lead to the secretion of soluble IL-2 receptors, TNF-α, and IL-6, which can be detected in diseased intestine and peripheral blood and may serve as important markers of disease activity.

During active IBD, the homing to mucosal sites of lymphoblasts involved in the regulation and production of IgA is altered. Not only can increased spontaneous secretion of IgA by peripheral blood mononuclear cells be found, but IgA synthesis by intestinal lamina propria mononuclear cells is decreased in favor of immunoglobulins of the IgG-isotype. Whereas in Crohn's disease the enhancement of IgG secretion is mostly in the form of IgG_2 and IgG_1, in ulcerative colitis a particular increase of IgG_1 and IgG_3 is observed. Through activation of complement components, the dramatic increase in IgG may contribute to the tissue destruction seen in IBD.

Monocytes and granulocytes appear to cause pivotal initiating events and enact specific effector mechanisms by migrating in large numbers into the intestinal mucosa during chronic inflammation. Because macrophages and granulocytes secrete large amounts of pro-inflammatory cytokines, lipid autacoids, and toxic metabolites, they contribute significantly to the heightened state of activation of the mucosal immune system in IBD. The investigation of important new areas, including the mechanisms leading to activation and amplification of inflammatory events as well as to the down-regulation of mucosal immune responses, will provide novel therapeutic approaches in the future.

References

Ahrenstedt, O., Knutson, L., Nilsson, B., Nilson-Ekdahl K., Odlind B., and Hallgren R. (1990). Enhanced local production of complement components in the small intestines of patients with Crohn's disease *N. Engl. J. Med.* **322,** 1345–1349.

Alley, C. D., Nash, G. S., and MacDermott, R. P. (1982). Marked *in vitro* spontaneous secretion of AIgA by human rib bone marrow mononuclear cells. *J. Immunol.* **128,** 2804–2808.

Allison, M. C., Poulter, L. W., Dhillon, A. P., and Pounder, R. E. (1990). Immunohistological studies of surface antigen on colonic lymphoid cells in normal and inflamed mucosa. *Gastroenterology* **99,** 421–430.

Archer, C. B., MacDonald, D. M., Morley, J., Page C. P., Paul W., and Sanjar, S. (1985). Effects of serum albumin, indomethacin and histamine H_1-antagonists on PAF-acether-induced inflammatory responses in the skin of experimental animals and man. *Br. J. Pharmacol.* **85,** 109–113.

Aspinall, R. L., and Cammarata, P. S. (1969). Effect of prostaglandin E_2 on aduvant arthritis. *Nature (London)* **224,** 1320–1321.

Auer, I.O., Wechsler, W., Ziemer, E., Malchow, H., and Sommer, H. (1978). Immune status in Crohn's disease. 1. Leukocyte and lymphocyte subpopulations in peripheral blood. *Scand. J. Gastroenterol.* **13,** 561–571.

Auer, I. O., Gotz, S., Ziemer, E., Malchow, H., and Ehms, H. (1979). Immune status in Crohn's disease, 3. Peripheral blood lymphocytes, enumerated by means of F(ab) 2-antibody fragments, null and T lymphocytes. *Gut* **20,** 261–268.

Bach, M. K. (1982). Mediators of anaphylaxis and inflammation. *Ann. Rev. Microbiol.* **36,** 371–413.

Badr-El-Din, S., Trejdosiewicz, L. K., Heatley, R. V., and Losowsky, M. S.. (1988). Local immunity in ulcerative colitis: Evidence for defective secretory IgA production. *Gut* **29,** 1070–1075.

Baklien, K., Brandtzaeg, P. (1975). Comparative mapping of the local distribution of immunoglobulin containing cells in ulcerative colitis and Crohn's disease of the colon. *Clin. Exp. Immunol.* **22,** 197–209.

Beale, M. G., Nash, G. S., Bertovich, M. J., and MacDermott, R. P. (1982). Similar disturbances in B-cell activity and regulatory T-cell function in Henoch–Schonlein purpura and systematic lupus erythematosus. *J. Immunol.* **128,** 486–491.

Bland, P. W., and Warren, L. G. (1986a). Antigen presentation by epithelial cells of the rat small intestine. I. Kinetics, antigen specificity and blocking by anti-1a antisera. *Immunology* **58,** 1–7.

Bland, P. W., and Warren, L. G. (1986b). Antigen presentation by epithelial cells of the rat small intestine. II. Selective induction of suppressor T cells. *Immunology* **58,** 9–14.

Bienenstock, J., McDermott, M., Befus, D., and O'Neill, M. (1978). A common mucosal immunologic system involving the bronchus, breast and bowel. *Adv. Exp. Med. Biol.* **107,** 53–59.

Bockman, E. E., and Cooper, M. D. (1973). Pinocytosis by epithelium associated with lymphoid follicles in the Bursa of Fabricius, appendix, and Peyer's patches: An electron microscopic study. *Am. J. Anat.* **136,** 455–461.

Borgeat, P., and Samuelsson, B. (1979). Transformation of arachidonic acid by rabbit polymorphonuclear leukocytes. *J. Biol. Chem.* **254,** 2643–2646.

Boxer, L. A., Allen, J. M., Schmidt, M., Yoder, M., and Baehner, R. L. (1980). Inhibition of polymorphonuclear leukocyte adhesion by prostacyclin. *J. Lab. Clin. Med.* **95,** 672–678.

Brandtzaeg, P., Baklien, K., Fausa, O., and Hoel, P. S. (1974). Immunohistologic characterization of local immunoglobulin formation in ulcerative colitis. *Gastroenterology* **66,** 1123–1136.

Brandtzaeg, P., Sollid, L. M., Thrane, P. S., Kvale, P. S., Bjerke K., Scott, H., Kett, K., and Rognum, T. O. (1988). Lymphoepithelial interactions in the human mucosal immune system. *Gut* **29,** 1116–1130.

Brock, T. A., and Gimbrone, M. A., Jr. (1986). Platelet activating factor alters calcium homeostasis in cultured vascular endothelial cells. *Am. J. Physiol.* **252,** H1086–H1092.

Brunynzeel, P. L. B., Koenderman, L., Kok, P. T., Hameling, M. L., and Verhagen, J. (1986). Platelet activating factor (PAF-acether)-induced leukotriene C_4 formation and luminol-dependent chemiluminescence by uman eosinophils. *Pharmacol. Res. Commun.* **18,** 61–69.

Buckell, N. A., Gould, S. R., Day, D. W., and Lennard Jones, J. E. (1978). Controlled trial of sodium cromoglycate in chronic persistent ulcerative colitis. *Gut* **19,** 1140–1143.

Bussolino, F., Aglietta, M., Sanavio, F., Stacchini, A., Lauri, D., and Camussi, G. (1985). Alkylether phosphoglycerides influence calcium into human endothelial cells. *J. Immunol.* **135,** 2748–2753.

Campieri, M., Lanfranchi, G. A., Bazzochi, G., Brignola, C., Benatti, A., Boccia, S., and Labo, G. (1980). Prostaglandins, indomethacin and ulcerative colitis. *Gastroenterology* **78,** 193.

Cebra, J. J., Komisar, J. L., and Schweitzer, P. A. (1984). ^{C}H isotype "switching" during normal B-lymphocyte development. *Ann. Rev. Immunol.* **2,** 493–548.

Charo, I. F., Yuen, C., Perez, H. D., and Goldstein, I. M., (1986). Chemotactic peptides modulate adherence of human polymorphonuclear leukocytes to monolayers of cultured endothelial cells. *J. Immunol.* **136,** 3412–3419.

Coffman, R. L., Shrader, B., Carty, J., Mosmann, T. R., and Bond, M. W. (1987). A mouse T cell product that preferentially enhances IgA production, I. Biologic characterization. *J. Immunol.* **139,** 3685–3690.

Cominelli, F., and Dinarello, C. A. (1989). Interleukin-1 in the pathogenesis of and protection from inflammatory bowel disease. *Biotherapy* **1(4),** 369–375.

Cominelli, F., Nast, C.C., Clark, B. D., Schindler, R., Lierena, R., Eysselein, V. E., Tompson, R. C., and Dinarello, C. A.. (1990). Interleukin-1 (IL-1) gene expression, synthesis and effect of specific IL-1 receptor blockade in rabbit immune complex colitis. *J. Clin. Invest.* **86(3)** 972–980.

Cox, J. P., and Karnovsky, M. L. (1973). The depression of phagocytosis by exogenous cyclic nucleotides, prostaglandins and theophylline. *J. Cell Biol.* **59,** 480–490.

Crabtree, J. E., Juby, L. D., Heatley, R. V., Lobo, A. J., Bullimore, D. W., and Axon, A. T. R. (1990). Soluble interleukin-2 receptor in Crohn's disease: Relation of serum concentrations to disease activity. *Gut* **31,** 1033–1036.

Craddock, P. R., Hammerschidt, D., White, J. G., Dalmosso, A. P., and Jacob, H. S. (1977). Complement (C5a)-induced granulocyte aggregation *in vitro*: A possible mechanism of complement-mediated leukostasis and leukopenia. *J. Clin. Invest.* **60,** 260–264.

Craddock, P. R., White, J. G., and Jacob, H. S. (1978). Potentiation of complement (C5a)-induced granulocyte aggregation by cytochalasin B. *J. Lab. Clin. Med.* **91,** 490–499.

Dinarello, C. A. (1988). Biology of interleukin-1. *FASEB* **2,** 108–115.

D'Amelio, R. Rosi, P., and Le Moli, S. (1983). *In vitro* studies on cellular and humoral chemotaxis in Crohn's disease using the under agarose gel technique. *Gut* **24,** 525–531.

Douglas, W. W. (1985). Autocoids. *In:* "Goodman and Gilman's The pharmacological basis of therapeutics" (A. G. Gilman, and L. S. Goodman, eds.), pp. 604–659. Macmillan, New York.

Dunkley, M. L., and Husband, A. J. (1987). Distribution and functional characteristics of antigen-specific helper T cells arising after Peyer's patch immunization. *Immunology* **61,** 475–482.

Eliakim, R., Karmeli, F., Razin, E., and Rachmilewitz, D. (1988). Role of platelet-activating factor in ulcerative colitis: Enhanced production during active disease and inhibition by sulfasalazine and prednisone. *Gastroenterology* **95,** 1167–1172.

Fais, S., and Pallone, F. (1989). Ability of human colonic epithelium to express the 4F2 antigen, the common acute lymphoblastic leukemia antigen and the transferrin receptor. *Gastroenterology* **97,** 1435–1441.

Fais, S., Pallone, F., Squarcia, O., Biancone, L., Paoluzi, P., and Biorivant, M. (1987). HLA-DR antigens on colonic epithelial cells in inflammatory bowel disease, I. Relation to the state of activation of lamina propria lymphocytes and to the epithelial expression of other surface markers. *Clin. Exp. Immunol.* **68,** 605–612.

Fantone, J. C., Kunkel, S. L., and Ward, P. A. (1981). Suppression of human polymorphonuclear function after intravenous infusion of prostaglandin E1. *Prostaglandins Med.* **7,** 195–198.

Fantone, J. C., Marasco, W. A., Elgas, L. J., and Ward, P. A. (1983). Anti-inflammatory effects of prostaglandin E_1: *In vivo* modulation of the formyl peptide chemotactic receptor on the rat neutrophil. *J. Immunol.* **130,** 1495–1497.

Fernandez, H. N., Henson, P. M., Otani, A., and Hugli, T. E. (1978). Chemotactic response to human C3a and C5a anaphylatoxins, I. Evaluation of C3a and C5a leukotaxis *in vitro* and under simulated *in vivo* conditions. *J. Immunol.* **120,** 109–115.

Fiocchi, C. (1989). Lymphokines and the intestinal immune response. Role in inflammatory bowel disease. *Immunol. Invest.* **18,** 91–102.

Flower, R. J., and Blackwell, G. J. (1979). Anti-inflammatory steroids induce biosynthesis of a phospholipase A2 inhibitor which prevents prostaglandin generation. *Nature (London)* **278,** 456–459.

Ford-Hutchinson, W. W., Bray, M. A., and Doig, M. V. (1984). Leukotriene B, a potent chemotactic and aggregating substance released from polymorphonuclear leukocytes. *Nature (London)* **266,** 264–265.

Gallin, J. I., Sandler, J. A., and Clyman, R. J. (1985). Agents that increase cyclic AMP inhibit accumulation of cGMP and depress human monocyte locomotion. *J. Immunol.* **120,** 492–496.

Gay, J. C., Beckman, J. K., Zaboy, K. A., and Lukens, J. N. (1986).

Modulation of neutrophil oxidative responses to soluble stimuli by platelet-activating factor. *Blood* **67,** 931–936.

Gilat, T., Ratan, J., Rosen, P., and Peled, Y. (1979). Prostaglandins and ulcerative colitis. *Gastroenterology* **77,** 1083.

Glenn, E. M., and Rohloff, N. (1971). Anti-arthritic and anti-inflammatory effects of certain prostaglandins. *Proc. Soc. Exp. Biol. Med.* **139,** 290–294.

Goldyne, M. E., and Stobo, J. D. (1981). Immunoregulatory role of prostaglandins and related lipids. *Crit. Rev. Immunol.* **2,** 189–223.

Gould, S. R. (1981). Assay of prostaglandin-like substances in feces and their measurement in ulcerative colitis. *Prostaglandins* **11,** 489–497.

Gould, S. R., Brash, A. R., Conolly, M. E., and Lennard-Jones, J. E. (1981). Studies of prostaglandins and sulphasalazine in ulcerative colitis. *Prostaglandins Leukotrienes Med.* **6,** 165–182.

Grant, J. A., Dupree, E., and Thueson, D. O. (1977). Complement-mediated release of histamine from human basophils. III. Possible regulatory role of microtubules and microfilaments. *J. Allergy Clin Immunol.* **60,** 306–311.

Gronowicz, E., and Couthino, A. (1976). Heterogeneity of B cells: Direct evidence of selective triggering of distinct subpopulations by polyclonal activators. *Scand. J. Immunol.* **5,** 55.

Halstensen T. S., Mollnes T. E., Fausa O, and Brandtzaeg P. (1989a). Deposits of terminal complement complex (TCC) in muscular mucosae and submucosal vessels in ulcerative colitis and Crohn's disease of the colon. *Gut.* **30,** 361–366.

Halstensen T. S., Mollnes T. E., and Brandtzaeg P. (1989b). Persistent complement activation in submucosal blood vessels of active inflammatory bowel disease: Immunohisto chemical evidence Gastroenterology. **97(1):** 10–19.

Halstensen, T. S., Mollnes, T. E., Garred, P., Fausa, O., Brandtzaeg, P. (1990). Epithelial deposition of immunoglobulin G1 and activated complement (C3b and terminal complement complex) in ulcerative colitis. *Gastroenterology* **98,** 1264–1271.

Hamann, A., Jablonski-Westrich, D., Scholz, K. U., Duijvestijn, A., Butcher, E. C., and Thiele, H. G. (1988). Regulation of lymphocyte homing I. Alterations in homing receptor expression and organ-specific high endothelial venule binding of lymphocytes upon activation. *J. Immunol.* **140,** 737–743.

Hammerschmidt, D. E., Bowers, T. K., Lammi-Keefe, C. J., Jacob, H. S., and Craddock, P. R. (1980). Granulocyte aggregometry: A sensitive technique for the detection of C5a and complement activation. *Blood* **55,** 898–902.

Hanson, L. A., Ahlstedt, S., Anderson, B., Carlsson, B., Dahlgren, U., Lidin-Janson, G., Mattsby Baltzer I., and Svanborg Eden, C. (1980). *J. Reticuloendothel. Soc.* **28** (suppl.), 1s–9s.

Hartman, C. T., Fr., and Glovsky, M. M. (1981). Complement activation requirements for histamine release from human leukocytes: Influence of purified $C3a_{hu}$ and $C5a_{hu}$ on histamine release. *Int. Arch. Allergy Appl. Immunol.* **66,** 274–281.

Hartung, H. P. (1983). Acetyl glyceryl ether phosphorylcholine (platelet activating factor) mediates heightened metabolic activity in macrophages. *Int. J. Immunopharmacol.* **5,** 115–121.

Hartung, H. P., Parnham, M. J., Winkelmann, J., Englberger, W., and Hadding, U. (1983). Platelet activating factor (PAF) induces the oxidative burst in macrophages. *Int. J. Immunopharmacol.* **5,** 115–121.

Hawkey, C. J. (1982). Evidence that prednisolone is inhibitory to the cyclooxygenase activity of human rectal mucosa. *Prostaglandins* **23,** 397–409.

Hawthorne, A. B., Daneshmend, T. K., and Hawkey, C. J. (1990). Fish oil in ulcerative colitis: Final results of a controlled clinical trial. *Gastroenterology* **99,** A174.

Heiner, D. C. (1984). Significance of immunoglobulin G (IgG) subclasses, *Am. J. Med.* **76,** 1.

Hodgson, H. J. F., Potter, B. J., and Jewell, D. P. (1977). C3 metabolism in ulcerative colitis and Crohn's disease. *Clin. Exp. Immunol.* **28,** 490–495.

Hokland, M., Larsen, B., Heron, I., and Plesner, T. (1981). Corticosteroids decrease the expression of beta-2 microglobulin and histocompatibility antigens on human peripheral blood lymphocytes *in vitro*. *Clin. Exp. Immunol.* **44,** 239–246.

Humphrey, D. M., McManus, L. M., Satouchi, K., Hanahan, D. J., and Pinkard, R. N. (1982). Vasoactive properties of acetyl glyceryl ether phosphorylcholine (AGEPC) and AGEPC analogues. *Lab. Invest.* **46,** 422–427.

Hwang, S. B., Chang-Ling, L, Lam, M H, and Shen, T. Y. (1985). Characterization of cutaneous vascular permeability induced by platelet activating factor (PAF) in guinea pigs and rats and its inhibition by a PAF receptor antagonist. *Lab. Invest.* **52,** 617–630.

Ingraham, L. M., Coates, T. D., Allen, J. M., Higgins, C. P., Baehner, R. L, and Boxer, L. A. (1982). Metabolic, membrane and functional responses of human polymorphonuclear leukocytes to platelet-activating factor. *Blood* **59,** 1259–1266.

Isaacs, K. L., Sartor, R. B., and Haeskil, J. S. (1992). Cytokine messenger RNA profiles in inflammatory bowel disease mucosa detected by polymerase chain reaction amplification. *Gastroenterology* **103,** 1587–1595.

Jalkanen, S., Reichert, R. A.,Gallatin, W. M., Bargatze, R. F., Weissman, I. L., and Butcher, E. C. (1986). Homing receptors and the control of lymphocyte migration. *Immunol. Rev.* **91,** 39–60.

Jalkanen, S., Streeter, P., Lakey, E., Bargatze, R., and Butcher, E. C. (1988). Lymphocytic and endothelial cell recognition elements that control lymphocyte traffic to mucosa-associated lymphatic tissues. *Monogr. Allergy* **24,** 144–149.

James, S. P. (1991). Mucosal T cell function. *In* "Mucosal Immunology. Gastroenterology Clinics of North America" (R. P. MacDermott and C. O. Elson, eds.), pp. 567–612. W. B. Saunders, Philadelphia.

James, S. P., Fiocchi, C., Graeff, A. S., and Strober, W. (1986). Phenotypic analysis of lamina propria lymphocytes: Predominance of helper-inducer and cytolytic T-cell phenotypes and deficiency of suppressor-inducer phenotypes in Crohn's disease and control patients. *Gastroenterology* **91,** 1483–1492.

James, S. P., Murakawa, Y., and Kanof, M. E. (1991). Role of intestinal T-cells and intestinal lymphokine production in inflammatory bowel disease. *In* "Frontiers of Mucosal Immunology" (M. Tsuchiya, ed.), pp. 727–731. Elsevier, Amsterdam.

Kanof, M. E., Strober, W., Fiocchi, C., Zeitz, M., and James, S. P. (1988). CD4 positive leu-8 negative helper-inducer T cells predominate in the human intestinal lamina propria. *J. Immunol.* **141,** 3036–3041.

Kansas, G. S., Wood, G. S.,Fishwild, D. M., and Engleman, E. G. (1985). Functional characterization of human T-lymphocyte subsets distinguished by monoclonal anti-leu-8. *J. Immunol.* **134,** 2995–3000.

Kaulfersch, W., Fiocchi, C., and Waldmann, T. H. (1988). Polyclonal nature of the intestinal mucosal lymphocyte populations in inflammatory bowel disease. *Gastroenterology* **95,** 364–370.

Kawanishi, H., Saltzman, L. E., and Strober, W. (1983a). Mechanisms regulating IgA class-specific immunoglobulin production in murine gut-associated lymphoid tissues, I. T cells derived from Peyer's patches that switch sIgM B cells *in vitro*. *J. Exp. Med.* **157,** 433–450.

Kawanishi, H., Saltzman, L., and Strober, W. (1983b). Mechanisms regulating IgA class-specific immunoglobulin production in murine gut-associated lymphoid tissues, II. Terminal differentiation of postswitch SIgA-bearing Peyer's patch B cells. *J. Exp. Med.* **158,** 649–669.

Keren, D. F., Appelman, H. D., Dobbins, W. O., Wells, J. J.,

Whisenant, B., Foley, J., Diererle, R., and Geisinger, K. (1984). Correlation of histopathologic evidence of disease activity with the presence of immunoglobulin-containing cells in the colon of patients with inflammatory bowel disease. *Human Pathol.* **15,** 757–763.

Kett, K., Rognum, T. O., and Brandtzaeg, P. Mucosal subclass distribution of IgG-producing cells is different in ulcerative colitis and Crohn's disease of the colon. *Gastroenterology* **94,** 1419–1425.

Hilbert, D. M., Cancro, M. P., Scherle, P. A., Nordan, R. P., Van Snick, J., Gerhard, and W., Rudikoff, S. T. (1989). Cell derived IL-6 is differentially required for antigen-specific antibody secretion by primary and secondary B cells *J. Immunol.* **143,** 4019–4024.

Kotinen, Y. T., Bergroth, V., Nordstroem, D., Segerberg-Konttinen, M., Seppala, K., and Salaspuro, M. (1987). Lymphocyte activation *in vivo* in the intestinal mucosa of patients with Crohn's disease. *J. Clin. Lab. Immunol.* **22,** 59–63.

Kunkel, S. L., Thrall, R. T., Kunkel, R. G., McCormick, J. R., Ward, P. A., and Zurier, R. B. (1979). Suppression of immune complex vasculitis in rats by prostaglandin. *J. Clin. Invest.* **64,** 1525–1528.

Kusagami, K., Kuroiwa, A., and Haruta, J. (1991). Interleukin-6 activities in lamina propria mononuclear cells from patients with ulcerative colitis. *Gastroenterology* **100,** 5, A591.

Lake, A. M., Stitzel, A. E., Urmson, J. R., Walker, W. A., and Spitzer, R. E. (1979). Complement alteration in inflammatory bowel disease. *Gastroenterology* **76,** 1374–1379.

Lauristen, K., Laursen, L. S., Bukhave, K., and Rachmilewitz, D. (1985). Effects of systemic prednisolone on arachidonic acid metabolites determined by equilibirum *in vivo* dialysis of rectum in severe relapsing ulcerative colitis (Abstr.). *Gastroenterology* **88,** 1466.

Lehmeyer, J. E., and Johnston, R. B. (1978). Effect of anti-inflammatory drugs and agents that elevate intracellular levels of cyclic AMP on the release of toxic oxygen metabolites by phagocytes: Studies in a model of tissue bound IgG. *Clin. Immunol. Immunopathol.* **9,** 482–490.

Levy, N., and Gaspar, E. (1975). Rectal bleeding and indomethacin suppositories. *Lancet* **1,** 577.

Lewis, R. A., and Austen, K. F. (1984). The biologically active leukotrienes: Biosynthesis, metabolism, receptors, functions and pharmacology. *J. Clin. Invest.* **73,** 889–897.

Ligumsky, M., Simon, P. L., Kameli, F., and Rachmilewitz D. (1990). Role of interleukin-1 in inflammatory bowel disease: Enhanced production during active disease. *Gut* **31,** 686–689.

Lin, A. H., Morton, D. R., and Gorman, R. R. (1982). Acetyl glyceryl ether phosphorylcholine stimulates leukotriene B_4 synthesis in human polymorphonuclear leukocytes. *J. Clin. Invest.* **70,** 1058–1065.

Ludwig, J. C., and Pinckard, R. N. (1987). Diversity in the chemical structures of neutrophil-derived platelet activating factors. *In* "New Horizons in Platelet Activating Factor Research" (C. M. Winslow and J. L. Lee, eds.), pp. 59–71. John Wiley & Sons, New York.

MacDermott, R. P. (1988). Altered secretion patterns of IgA and IgG subclasses by IBD intestinal mononuclear cells. *In* "Inflammatory Bowel Diseases—Basic Resarch and Clinical Implications" (H. Goebell, B. M. Peskar, H. Malchow eds.), pp. 105–111. MTP Press, Flacon House, Lancaster, England.

MacDermott, R. P., and Nahm, M. H. (1987). Expression of human immunoglobulin G subclassed in inflammatory bowel disease. *Gastroenterology* **93,** 1127.

MacDermott, R. P., and Stenson, W. F. (1988a). Alterations of the immune system in ulcerative colitis and Crohn's disease. *Adv. Immunol.* **42,** 285–323.

MacDermott, R. P., and Stenson, W. F. (1988b). The role of the immune system in Inflammatory Bowel Disease. *Immunol. Allerg. Clin. N. Am.* **8,** 521–542.

MacDermott, R. P., Nash, G. S., Bertovich, M. J., Seiden, M. V., Bragdon, M. J., and Beale, M. G. (1981). Alterations of IgA, IgM, and IgG by peripheral blood mononuclear cells, and by human bone marrow mononuclear cells from patients with ulcerative colitis and Crohn's disease. *Gastroenterology* **81,** 844–852.

MacDermott, R. P., Beale, M. G., Alley, C. D., Nash, G. S., Bertovich, M. J., and Bragdon, M. J. (1983). Synthesis and secretion of IgA, IgM, and IgG by peripheral blood mononuclear cells in human disease states, by isolated human intestinal mononuclear cells, and by human bone marrow mononuclear cells from ribs. *In* "The Secretory Immune System" (McGhee, J. R. and Mestecky, J., eds.), *NY Acad. Sci.* **409,** 498.

MacDermott, R. P., Delacroix, D. L., Nash, G. S., Bertovich, M. J., Mohrman, R. F., and Vaerman, J. P. Altered patterns of secretion of monomeric IgA and IgA subclass 1 (IgA1) by peripheral blood and intestinal mononuclear cells in inflammatory bowel disease. (1986). *Gastroenterology* **91,** 379–385.

MacDermott, R. P., Nash, G. S., Auer, I. O., Schlien, R., Lewis, B. S., Madassery, J., and Nahm, M. H (1988). Alterations in serum IgG subclasses in patients with ulcerative colitis and Crohn's disease. *Gastroenterology* **94,** A275.

MacDermott, R. P., Schloemann, S. R., Bertovich, M. J., Nash, G. S., Peters, M., and Stenson, W. F. (1989). Inhibition of antibody synthesis by 5-aminosalicylic acid. *Gastroenterology* **96,** 442–448.

MacDonald, T. T., Choy, M. Y., Hutchings, P., and Cooke, A. (1990a) Activated T cells in macrophages in the intestinal mucosa of children with inflammatory bowel disease. *In:* "Advances in Mucosal Immunology" (T. T. MacDonald, S. J. Challacombe, P. W. Bland, C. R. Stokes, R. V. Heatly, A. McI Movat, eds.), pp. 683–690. Kluwer, Boston.

MacDonald, T. T., Hutchings, P., Choy, M. Y., Murch, S., and Cooke, A. (1990b). Tumour necrosis factor-alpha and interferon-gamma production measured at the single-cell level in normal and inflamed human intestine. *Clin. Exp. Immunol.* **81(2),** 301–305.

MacGlashin, D. W., Peters, S. P., Warner, J., and Lichtenstein, L. M. (1986). Characteristics of human basophil sulfidopeptide leukotriene release: Releasability defined as the ability of the basophil to respond to dimeric cross-links. *J. Immunol.* **136,** 2231–2239.

McKearn, J. P., Paslay, J. W., Slack, J. H., Baum, C., and Davie, J. M. (1982). B cell subsets and differential responses to mitogens. *Immunol. Rev.* **64,** 10.

MacManus, L. M., Hanahan, D. J., Demopoulos, C. A., and Pinckard, R. N. (1980). Pathobiology of the intravenous infusion of acetyl glyceryl ether phosphorylcholine (AGPEC), a synthetic platelet activating factor (PAF), in the rabbit. *J. Immunol.* **124,** 2919–2924.

Madsen, M., Kissmeyer-Nielson, F., and Rasmussen, P. (1981). Decreased expression of HLA-DR antigens on peripheral blood B lymphocytes during glucocorticoid treatment. *Tissue Antigens* **17,** 195–204.

Mahida, Y. R., Wu, K., and Jewell, D. P. (1989). Enhanced production of interleukin-1-beta by mononuclear cells isolated from mucosa with active ulcerative colitis or Crohn's disease. *Gut* **30(6),** 835–838.

Mahida, Y. R., Gallagher, A., Kurlak, L., and Hawkey, C. J. (1990). Plasma and tissue interleukin-2 receptor levels in inflammatory bowel disease. *Clin. Exp. Immunol.* **82,** 75–80.

Malizia, G., Calabrese, A., Cottone, M, Raimondo, M., Trejdosiewicz, L. K., Smart, C. J., Olivia, L., and Pagliaro, L. (1991). Expression of leukocyte adhesion molecules by mucosal mononuclear phagocytes in inflammatory bowel disease. *Gastroenterology* **100,** 150–159.

Mestecky, J. (1987). The common mucosal immune system and current strategies for induction of immune responses in external secretions. *J. Clin. Immunol.* **7,** 265–276.

Mestecky, J., and McGhee, J. R. (1987). Immunoglobulin A (IgA): Molecular and cellular interactions involved in IgA biosynthesis and immune response. *Adv. Immunol.* **40,** 153–245.

Mitsuymama, K., Sada, M., and Tanikawa, K. (1991). Significance of interleukin 6 in patients with inflammatory bowel disease. Gastroenterologia japonica. **26,** 20–28.

Morain, C. O., Segal, A. A., Walker, D., and Levi, A. J. (1981) Abnormalities of neutrophil function do not cause the migration defect in Crohn's disease. *Gut* **22,** 817–822.

Mueller, C. H., Knoflach, P., and Zielinski, C. C. (1990). T cell activation in Crohn's disease. Intestinal levels of soluble interleukin-2 receptor in serum and in supernatants of stimulated peripheral blood mononuclear cells. *Gastroenterology* **98,** 639–646.

Mueller, H. W., O'Flaherty, J. T., and Wykle, R. L. (1984). The molecular species distribution of platelet-activating factor synthesized by rabbit and human neutrophils. *J. Biol. Chem.* **259,** 14554–14559.

Nielson, O. H., Elmgreen, J., Thomsen, B. S., Ahnfelt-Ronne, I., and Wiik, A. (1986). Release of leukotriene B4 and 5- hydoxyeicosatetraenoic acid during phagocytosis of artificial immune complexes by peripheral neutrophils in chronic inflammatory bowel disease. *Clin. Exp. Immunol.* **65,** 465–471.

Nielson, O. H., Elmgreen, J. and Ahnfelt, R. I. (1988). Serum interferon activity in inflammatory bowel disease. Arachidonic acid release and lipoxygenation activated by alpha-class interferon in human neutrophils. *Inflammation* **12(2),** 169–179.

Oda, M., Satouchi, K, Yasunaga, K., and Saito, K. (1985). Molecular species of platelet-activating factor generated by human neutrophils challenged with ionophore A23187. *J. Immunol.* 134, 1090–1093.

O'Flaherty, J. T. (1985). Neutrophil degranulation: Evidence pertaining to its mediation by the combined effects of leukotriene B_4, platelet-activating factor and 5-HETE. *J. Cell Physiol.* **122,** 229–239.

O'Flaherty, J. T., Wykle, R. L., Thomas, M. J., *et al.* (1984). Neutrophil degranulation responses to combinations of arachidonate metabolites and platelet-activating factor. *Res. Commun. Chem. Pathol. Pharmacol.* **43,** 3–23.

Owen, R. L., and Jones, A. L. (1974). Epithelial cell specialization within human Peyer's patches: An ultrastructural study of intestinal lymphoid follicles. *Gastroenterology* **66,** 189–203.

Owen, R. L., and Nemanic, P. (1978). Antigen processing structures of the mammalian intestinal tract: An SEM study of lymphoepithelial organs. "Scanning Elec. Microsc., **II,** 367–378. IL.

Oxelius, V. A. (1984). Immunoglobulin G (IgG) subclasses and human disease. *Am. J. Med.* **76,** 7–18.

Pallone, F., Fais, S., Squarcia, O., Biancone, L., Pozzilli, P., and Boirivant, M. (1987). Activation of peripheral blood and intestinal lamina propria lymphocytes in Crohn's disease: *In vivo* state of activation and *in vitro* response to stimulation as defined by the expression of early activation antigens. *Gut* **28,** 745–753.

Parker, C. W. (1984). Mediators: Release and function. *In* "Fundamental Immunology" (W. E. Paul, ed), pp. 697–750. Raven Press, New York.

Perez, H. D., Goldstein, I. M., Webster, R. O., and Henson, P. M. (1981). Enhancement of the chemotactic activity of human C5 des Arg by an anionic polypeptide ("cochemotaxin") in normal serum and plasma. *J. Immunol.* **126,** 800–804.

Peskar, B. M., Dreyling, K. W., and Hoppe, U. (1985). Formation of sulfidopeptide- leukotrienes (SP-LT) in normal human colonic tissue, colonic carcinoma and Crohn's disease (Abstr.). *Gastroenterology* **88,** 1537.

Peters, M. G., Secrist, H., Anders, K. A., Nash, G. S., Rich, S. R., and MacDermott, R. P. (1989). Normal human intestinal B lymphocytes: Increased activation compared to peripheral blood. *J. Clin. Invest.* **83,** 1827–1833.

Peterson, N. E., Elmgreen, J., Teisner, B., and Svehag, S. E. (1988). Activation of classical pathway complement in chronic inflammation: Elevated levels of circulating C3d and C4d split products in rheumatoid arthritis and Crohn's disease. *Acta Med. Scand.* **223,** 557–560.

Petersson, B. A., Nilsson, A., and Stalenheim, G. (1975). Induction of histamine release and desensitization in human leukocytes: Effect of anaphylatoxin. *J. Immunol.* **114,** 1581–1584.

Pinckard, R. N., McManus, L. M., Demopoulos, C. A., Halonen, M., Clarck, P. O. Shaw, J. O., Kniker, W. T., and Hanahan, D. J. (1980). Moelcular pathobiology of acetyl glyceryl ether phosphorylcholine (AGEPC): Evidence for the structural identity with platelet activating factor (PAF). *J. Reticuloendothel. Soc.* **28,** 95s–103s.

Pullman, W. E., Sullivan, P. J., Barratt, P. J., Lising, J., Booth, J. A., and Doe, W. F. (1988). Assessment of inflammatory bowel disease activity by technetium 99m phagocyte scanning. *Gastroenterology* **95,** 989–996.

Rachmilewitz, D., Eliakim, R., and Simon, P., et al. (1991). Role of cytokines and platelet activating factor in the pathogenesis of inflammatory bowel disease. *In* "Falk Symposium 60: Inflammatory Bowel Disease: Progress in Basic Research and Clinical Implications" (H. Goebell, K. Ewe, H. Malchow, and Ch. Koelbel, eds.), pp. 153–159. Kluwer Academic Publishers, Lancaster, London.

Raedler, A., Fraenkel, S., Klose, G., and Thiele, H. G. (1985a). Elevated numbers of peripheral T cells in inflammatory bowel diseases displaying T9 antigen and Fc alpha receptors. *Clin. Exp. Immunol.* **60,** 518–524.

Raedler, A., Fraenkel, S., Klose, G., Seyfarth, K., and Thiele, H. G. (1985b). Involvement of the immune system in the pathogenesis of Crohn's disease: Expression of the T9 antigen on peripheral immunocytes correlated with the severity of the disease. *Gastroenterology* **88,** 978–983.

Raedler, A., Bredow, G., Kirch, W., Thiele, H. G., Gtreten, H. (1986). *In vivo* activated T cells in autoimmune disease. *J. Clin. Lab. Immunol.* **19,** 181–186.

Raedler, A., Schreiber, S., Schulz, K. H., Peters, S., Greten, H., and Thiele, H. G. (1988). Activated Fc-alpha T-cells in Crohn's disease are involved in regulation of IgA. *Adv. Exp. Med. Biol.* **237,** 665–673.

Ramesha, C. S., and Pickett, W. C. (1987). Species-specific variations in the molecular heterogeneity of the platelet activating factor. *J. Immunol.* **138,** 1559–1563.

Rampton, D. S., Sladen, G. E., and Youlten, L. Y. (1980). Rectal mucosal prostaglandin E2 release and its relation to disease activity; Electrical potential differences and treatment in ulcerative colitis. *Gut* **21,** 591–596.

Rampton, D. S., and Sladen, G. E. (1981). Prostaglandin synthesis inhibitors in ulcerative colitis: Flurbiprofen compared with conventional treatment. *Prostaglandins* **21,** 417–425.

Rampton, D. S., and Sladen, G. E. (1984). The relationship between rectal mucosa prostaglandin production and water and electrolyte transport in ulcerative colitis. *Digestion Intern.* **30,** 13–22.

Reinecker, H-C., Steffen, M., Witthoeft, T., Pflueger, I., Schreiber, S., MacDermott, R. P., and Raedler, A. (1993). Enhanced secretion of TNF-α, IL-6, and IL-1β by isolated lamina propria mononuclear cells from patients with ulcerative colitis and Crohn's disease. *Clin. Exp. Immunol.* **94,** in press.

Rhodes, J. M., Bartholomew, T. C., and Jewell, D. P. (1981). Inhibition of leukocyte motility by drugs used in ulcerative colitis. *Gut* **22,** 642–647.

Rosedrans, P. M. C., Meijer, C. J. L. M., and van der Wal, A. M. (1980). Immunoglobulin-containing cells in inflammatory bowel disease of the colon: A morphometrica and immunohistochemical study. *Gut* **21,** 941–947.

Sanchez-Crespo, M., Alonso, F., Inarrea, P, Alvaarez, V., and Egido, J. (1982). Vascular actions of synthetic PAF-acether (a synthetic platelet activating factor) in the rat: Evidence for a platelet independent mechanism. *Immunopharmacol.* **4,** 173–185.

Satouchi, K., Oda, M., Yasunaga, K., and Saito, K. (1985). Evidence for the production of 1-acyl-2-acetyl-sn-glyceryl-3-phosphorylcholine concomitantly with platelet activating factor. *Biochem. Biophys. Res. Commun.* **128,** 1409–1417.

Satsangi, J., Wolstencroft, R. A., and Cason, J. (1987). Interleukin-1 in Crohn's disease. *Clin. Exp. Immunol.* **67(3),** 594–605.

Saverymuttu, S. H., Chadwick, V. S., and Hodgson, H. J. (1985a). Granulocyte migration in ulcerative colitis. *Eur. J. Clin Invest.* **15,** 60–68.

Saverymuttu, S. H., Peters, A. M., Lavender, J. P., Chadwick, V. S., and Hodgson, H. J. (1985b). *In vivo* assessment of granulocyte migration to diseased bowel in Crohn's disease. *Gut* **26,** 378–383.

Schoelmerich, J., Schmidt, E., Shumichen, C., Bilmann, P., Schmidt, H., and Gerok, W. (1988). Scintigraphic assessment of bowel involvement and disease activity in Crohn's disease using technetium 99m hexamethyl propylene amine oxine as leukocyte labei. *Gastroenterology* **95,** 1287–1293.

Schreiber, S., MacDermott, R. P., Raedler, A., *et al.* (1992). Increased *in vitro* release of soluble interleukin-2 receptor by colonic lamina propria mononuclear cells in inflammatory bowel disease. *Gut* **33,** 236–241.

Schreiber, S., MacDermott, R. P., Raedler, A., Pinnau, R., Bertovich, M. J., and Nash, G. S. (1991a). Increased activation of isolated intestinal lamina propria mononuclear cells in inflammatory bowel disease. *Gastroenterology* **101,** 1020–1030.

Schreiber, S., Nash, G. S., Raedler, A., Conn, A. R., Rombeau, J. L., and MacDermott, R. P. (1991). Human lamina propria mononuclear cells are activated in inflammatory bowel disease. *In:* "Frontiers of Mucosal Immunology" (Tsuchiya M. ed.), pp. 749–753, Elsevier, Amsterdam.

Scott, B. B., Goodall, A., Stephenson, R., and Jenkins, D. (1983). Rectal mucosa plasma cells in inflammatory bowel disease. *Gut* **21,** 519–524.

Scott, M. G., and Nahm, M. H. (1984). Mitogen induced IgG subclass expression. *J. Immunol.* **135,** 1454–1460.

Scott, M. G., Nahm, M. H., Macke, K., Nash, G. S., Bertovich, M. J., and MacDermott, R. P. (1986). Spontaneous secretion of IgG subclasses by intestinal mononuclear cells: Differences between ulcerative colitis, Crohn's disease and controls. *Clin. Exp. Immunol.* **66,** 209–215.

Selby, W. S., and Jewell, D. P. (1983). T lymphocyte subsets in inflammatory bowel disease: Peripheral blood. *Gut* **24,** 99–105.

Selby, W. S., Janossy, G., Bofill, M., and Jewell, D. P. (1984). Intestinal lymphocyte subpopulations in inflammatory bowel disease: An analysis by immunohistological and cell isolation techniques. *Gut* **25,** 32–40.

Sharon, P., Ligumsky, M., Rachmilewitz, D., and Zor, U. (1978). Role of prostaglandins in ulcerative colitis; Enhanced production during active disease and inhibition by sulfasalazine. *Gastroenterology* **75,** 638–640.

Sharon, P., and Stenson, W. F. (1984). Enhanced synthesis of leukotriene B4 by colonic mucosa in inflammatory bowel disease. *Gastroenterology* **86,** 453–360.

Shaw, J. O., Pinckard, R. N., Ferrigni, K. S., McManus, L. M., and Hanahan, D. J. (1981). Activation of human neutrophils with 1-O-hexadecyl/oxtadecyl-2-acetyl-sn-glyceryl-3-phosphorylcholine (platelet activating factor). *J. Immunol.* **127,** 1250–1255.

Shirota, K, LeDuy, L., Yuan, S., and Jothy, S. (1990). Interleukin-6 and its receptor are expressed in human intestinal epithelial cells. *Virchows Archiv B Cell Pathol.* **58,** 303–308.

Simonsen, T., and Elmgreen, J. (1985). Defective modulation of complement in Crohn's disease. *Scand. J. Gastroenterol.* **20,** 883–886.

Siraganian, R. P., and Hook, W. A. (1976). Complement-induced histamine release from human basophils, II. Mechanism of the histamine release reaction. *J. Immunol.* **116,** 639–646.

Skakib, F., and Stanworth, D. R. (1980). Human IgG subclasses in health and disease: A review, part II. *Ricerca Clin. Lab.* **10,** 561.

Smith, C. W., Hollers, J. C., and Patrick, R. A. (1979). Motility and adhesiveness in human neutrophils: Effects of chemotactic factors. *J. Clin. Invest.* **63,** 221–229.

Smith, K. A. (1988). The interleukin 2 receptor. *Adv. Immunol.* **42,** 165–179.

Snyder, D. S., Beller, D. I., and Unanue, E. R. (1982). Prostaglandins modulate macrophage Ia expression. *Nature (London)* **299,** 163–165.

Stenson, W. F., and Parker, C. W. (1984). Leukotrienes. *Adv. Intern. Med.* **30,** 175–199.

Stevens, C., Walz, G., and Zanker, B (1990). Interleukin-6, interleukin-1-beta and tumor necrosis factor: Expression in inflammatory bowel disease. *Gastroenterology* **98,** A475.

Stimler, N. P., Brocklehurst, W. E., Bloor, C. M., and Hugli, T. E. (1981). Anaphylatoxin-mediated contraction of guinea pig lung strips: A nonhistamine tissue response. *J. Immunol.* **126,** 2258–2261.

Stenson, W. (1988). Luecotriene B4 in inflammatory bowel disease. *In* "Inflammatory Bowel Diseases—Basic Resarch and Clinical Implications" (H. Goebell, B. M. Peskar, and H. Malchow, eds.), pp. 143–159. MTP Press, Flacon House, Lancaster, England.

Stimler, N. P., Bloor, C. M., and Hugli, T. E. (1983). C3a-induced contraction of guinea-pig lung parenchyma: Role of cyclooxygenase metabolites. *Immunopharmacology* **5,** 251–257.

Stoughton, R. B. (1972). Cutaneous responses to human C3 anaphylatoxin in man. *Clin. Exp. Immunol.* **11,** 13–20.

Streeter, P. R., Berg, E. L., Rouse, B. T. Bargatze, R. F., and Butcher, E. C. (1988). A tissue-specific endothelial cell molecule involved in lymphocyte homing. *Nature (London)* **331,** 441–446.

Strickland, R. G., Korsmeyer, S., Soltis, R. D., Wilson, I. D., and Williams, R. C. Jr. (1974). Peripheral blood T and B cells in chronic inflammatory bowel disease. *Gastroenterology* **67,** 569–577.

Sun, S., and Hsueh, W. (1988). Bowel necrosis induced by tumor necrosis factor in rats is mediated by platelet-activating factor. *J. Clin. Invest.* **81,** 1328–1331.

Terano, T., Salmon, J. A., and Moncada, S. (1984). Biosynthesis and biological activity of leukotriene B5. *Prostaglandins* **27,** 217–232.

Thayer, W. R., Charland, C., and Field, C. E. (1976). The subpopulations of circulating white blood cells in inflammatory bowel disease. *Gastroenterology* **71,** 379–384.

Tomasi, T. B., Tan, E. M., Solomon, A., *et al.* (1965). Characteristics of an immune system common to certain external secretions. *J. Exp. Med.* **121**; 101–124.

Tonnesen, M. G., Smedly, L. A., and Henson, P. M. (1984). Neutrophil-endothelial cell interactions: Modulation of neutrophil adhesiveness induced by complement fragments C5a and C5a des Arg and formyl, methionyl-leucly-phenylalanine. *J. Clin. Invest.* **74,** 1581–1592.

Underdown, B. J., and Schiff, J. M. (1986). Immunoglobulin A; Strategic defense initiative at the mucosal surface. *Ann. Rev. Immunol.* **4,** 389–417.

Unanue, E. R., and Allen, P. M. (1987). The basis for the immunoregulatory role of macrophages and other accessory cells. *Science* **236,** 551–557.

Van Spreeuwel, J. P., Lindeman, J., and Meijer, A.C.J.L.M. (1985). A quantitative study of immunoglobulin-containing cells in the differential diagnosis of acute colitis. *J. Clin. Pathol.* **38,** 774–777.

Vane, J. R. (1971). Inhibition of prostaglandin synthesis as a mechanism of action for aspirin-like drugs. *Nature New Biol.* **231,** 232–235.

Waldmann, T. A., Broder, S., Goldman, C. K., Frost, K., Korsmeyer, S. J., and Medici, M. A. (1983). Disorders of B cells and helper T cells in the pathogeneiss of the immunoglobulin deficiency of patients with ataxia telangiectasia. *J. Clin. Invest.* **71,** 282–295.

Wandall, J. H., and Binder, V. (1982). Leukocyte function in ulcerative colitis. *Gut* **23,** 758–765.

Ward, P. A., and Newman, L. J. (1969). A neutrophil chemotactic factor from human C'5. *J. Immunol.* **102,** 93–99.

Weintraub, S. T., Ludwig, J. C., and Mott, G. E. (1985). Fast atom bombardment-mass spectrometric identification of molecular species of platelet-activating factor produced by stimulated human polymorphonuclear leukocytes. *Biochem. Biophys. Res. Commun.* **129,** 868–876.

Wilkinson, P. C. (1982). Chemotaxis and Inflammation, 2nd ed., p. 93. Churchill Livingstone, Edinburgh.

Wolf, J. L., Rubin, D. H., Finberg, R., Kauffman, R. S., Sharpe, A. H., Trier, J. S., and Fields, B. N. (1981). Intestinal M cells: A pathway for entry of reovirus into the host. *Science* **212,** 471–472.

Yancey, K. B., Hammer, C. H., Harvath, L., Renfer, L., Frank, M. M., and Lawley, T. J. (1985). Studies of human C5a as a mediator of inflammation in normal human skin. *J. Clin. Invest.* **75,** 486–495.

Yasaka, T., Boxer, L. A., and Baehner, R. L. (1982). Monocyte aggregation and superoxide anion release in response to formyl-methionyl-leucyl-phenylalanine (FMLP) and platelet-activating factor (PAF). *J. Immunol.* **128,** 1939–1944.

Yasukawa, K, Hirano, T., Watanabe, Y., Muratani, K., Matsuda, T., Nakai, S., and Kishimoto, T. (1987). Structure and expression of human B cell stimulatory factor-2 (BSF-2/IL-6) gene. *EMBO. J.* **6(10),** 2929–2945.

Yuan, S. Z., Hanauer, S. B., Kluskens, L. F., and Kraft, S. C. (1983). Circulating lymphocyte subpopulations in Crohn's disease. *Gastroenterology* **85,** 1313–1318.

Zifroni, A., Treves, A. J., Sachar, D. B., and Rachmilewitz, D. (1983). Prostanoid synthesis by cultured intestinal epithelial and mononuclear cells in inflammatory bowel disease. *Gut* **24,** 659–664.

Zurier, R. B., Hoffstein, S., and Weissmann, G. (1973). Suppression of acute and chronic inflammation in adrenalectomized rats by pharmacologic amounts of prostaglandins. *Arthritis Rheum.* **16,** 606–618.

Zurier, R. B., Weissmann, G., and Hoffstein, S. (1974). Mechanisms of lysosomal enzyme release from human leukocytes, II. Effects of cAMP and cGMP, autonomic agonists and agents which affect microtubule function. *J. Clin. Invest.* **53,** 297–309.

39

Malabsorption Syndromes and Intestinal Protein Loss

D. Nadal • C. P. Braegger • P. Knoflach • B. Albini

I. INTRODUCTION

Absorption of nutrients and the permeability of the intestines are affected by a variety of disorders involving the immune system (Doe and Hapel, 1983; Kalser, 1985b; Wright and Heyworth, 1989). Conversely, malabsorption and malnutrition may impact the status of the immune system and, thus, the gut-associated lymphoid tissue (GALT) (Doe and Hapel, 1983; Chandra and Wadhwa, 1989). Further, increased permeability of the intestines to microbial and nutrient antigens can lead to enhanced and abnormal immune responses (King and Toskes, 1985; Cunningham-Rundles, 1987). In this chapter, we discuss malabsorption, immunologically mediated diseases leading to malabsorption, intestinal protein loss, and the effects of malabsoprtion and increased leakiness of the intestines on the immune system.

Malabsorption syndromes are defined by the failure of the patient to absorb ingested nutrients appropriately. Inappropriate absorption can occur in a wide variety of conditions with a broad spectrum of pathogenic mechanisms (Doe and Hapel, 1983; Kalser, 1985b; Wright and Heyworth, 1989). Malabsorption, on the other hand, may result in a gamut of effects, ranging from isolated deficiencies, such as occult anemia, to life-threatening conditions. Most severe malabsorption syndromes are characterized clinically by abdominal distention, diarrhea, progressive loss of weight, malaise, borborygmi, and, in children, failure to thrive (Frazer, 1956). Passage of abnormal stools is important diagnostically for many of the syndromes; the characteristics of the stools reflect the nature of the unabsorbed foodstuff. The stools often are bulky, yellow to grey, greasy, and soft. Bowel movements tend to be frequent.

Lymphoid cells represent one-fourth of all cells of the mucosa (Kagnoff, 1981). Therefore, that GALT is integrated closely in the homeostasis of the gastrointestinal tract and that it is involved in the pathogenesis of a large number of gastrointestinal diseases is not surprising. Malnutrition, on the other hand, can lead to a dysregulation of the immune response and, thus, to a dysfunction of GALT (Doe and Hapel, 1983; Chandra and Walhwa, 1989). A brief look at some salient features of nutrient uptake by the gut should provide a starting point for the discussion of malabsorption syndromes.

A. Absorption of Nutrients

The primary function of the gut to assimilate nutrients is accomplished in two stages, digestion and absorption (Kalser, 1985a). In the first "intraluminal" stage, ingested food is broken down into smaller molecules. In the second "intestinal" stage, the foodstuff thus prepared reaches the body fluids by passage across the intestinal mucosal epithelium and subsequently is removed from the intestines via capillaries and lymphatics to reach blood circulation. The passage across enterocytes may be effected passively by diffusion or actively by transport mechanisms. Although absorption occurs preferentially in the small intestines, many cells and tissues of the gut and of other organ systems contribute to the assimilation process. Thus, fat assimilation requires integration of the functions of the liver and the biliary tract, the pancreas, the jejunum, and the ileum. Integration and regulation of these diverse activities involves hormonal networks and neural interactions; these two systems affect the immune system and thus also GALT. Immune effectors may be involved in the triggering of other components of the gastrointestinal tissue; thus, release of mucus from goblet cells may be induced by immune complexes (Walker *et al.*, 1977) or via anaphylactic responses (Lake *et al.*, 1980).

In the stomach, ingested fat is emulsified, hypertonic nutrients are diluted, protein digestion is initiated by pepsin, and intrinsic factor, necessary for the absorption of vitamin B_{12} in the small intestine, is produced. Arrival of food in the duodenum triggers release of gut hormones, which coordinate output of pancreatic enzymes and bile and may increase secretion of immunoglobulins by GALT (Freier *et al.*, 1989). The multitiered regulation of digestion and absorption is illustrated vividly by the interaction of enterocyte peptidases and pancreatic proenzymes. The brush border-associated enteropeptidase is necessary to activate trypsin (Rinderknecht, 1986). Therefore, impaired protein digestion may reflect a variety of defects: injury to enterocyte brush border, genetically determined enteropeptidase deficiency of enterocytes, as well as disorders of the exocrine pancreas.

Enterocyte brush border membranes contain a number of peptidases that brake down both large proteins and oligopeptides (Erickson and Kim, 1990). Peptidases are also present in the enterocyte cytoplasm.

Carrier-mediated transport through enterocytes is available for single amino acids and for an as yet unknown number of small peptides (Erickson and Kim, 1990). Patients with defects in transport systems for single amino acids (e.g., cystin) still can absorp the amino acid as component of oligopeptides (Steinhardt and Adibi, 1986). Iron and calcium are absorbed most efficiently in the most proximal portion of the intestines. Most other nutrients, water, and solutes are taken up with highest efficiency in the jejunum. The ileum is the primary site of absorption of vitamin B_{12} and of bile salts. The colon is a relatively impermeable barrier for most nutrients. However, sodium and organic acids can be absorbed, and protons can be secreted into the lumen (Kalser, 1985a,c).

Appropriate absorption of food components depends (1) on their adequate preparation, that is, digestion or conjugation with appropriate factors in the intestinal lumen; (2) on the structural and functional integrity of the mucosal epithelium; and (3) on the removal of absorbed moieties by body fluids, predominantly via lymphatics. Absorption may be accomplished by diffusion or solvent drag, occurring preferentially along intercellular spaces, or by active transport employing carrier molecules and occurring across intestinal epithelial cells. For each component of food, that is, fat, protein, carbohydrate, solutes, and water, a well-defined and, in general, distinct pathway for assimilation exists. However, absorption of one food component may influence uptake of other nutrients; in this way, fat-soluble vitamin uptake is determined by the efficiency of fat absorption.

B. Absorption of Nutrients and Immunity

In addition to absorption, the gastrointestinal tract also has other functions, prominent among which is the elimination of environmental noxae and parasites (Hanauer and Kraft, 1985; Kagnoff, 1989a).

The gastrointestinal tract can be envisioned as an invagination of the environment into the host's body. The gut mucosa indeed is the largest host interphase with the outside world. This interphase has two functions: (1) it is a barrier to deleterious outside stimuli and (2) it is the site of active exchange. Since molecules have to pass through the mucosal epithelium, this area lacks the mechanical protection that the multilayered and keratinized epithelium of the skin can provide, which may explain the accumulation of a variety of nonspecific host defense mechanisms in the gut, as well as the tremendous accumulation of immunologically reactive cells. Saliva, mucus, gastric juice, and bile salts, in conjunction with peristalsis, epithelial cell turnover, and low phagocytic potential of epithelial cells, are well designed to prevent foreign particulate matter and macromolecules from entering the mucosa. Obviously, GALT, divided into its two compartments, the intraepithelial lymphocytes (IEL) and the lamina propria lymphocytes (LPL), contributes a stacked specific defense mechanism encompassing humoral and cellular immunity (see Sections A–C of this handbook).

Some of the immune effectors may play a direct role in assimilating nutrients. Thus, macromolecules, on complexing with IgA, are impaired in their adherence to intestinal epithelial cells. At the same time, complexing with IgA may enhance the intraluminal digestion of nutrients (Walker and Bloch, 1983), and binding of antigens by SIgA will reduce the potential to initiate IgG responses. Secretory antibodies and IEL may be essential to reducing systemic immunization to the contents of the intestines. IgA present in milk may play an important role for the immunoregulation of the newborn. (Ahlstedt *et al.*, 1977; Crago and Mestecky, 1985).

C. Immunity and Malabsorption

The immune system can be involved in the pathogenesis of malabsorption syndromes (1) by interfering with digestion (e.g., antibodies to the intrinsic factor in pernicious anemia); (2) by mediating epithelial cell damage; (3) by interfering with the removal of absorbed food-derived moieties; and (4) by allowing microbial overgrowth. Mechanisms of malabsorption also may facilitate the entry of antigenic material into the mucosa and thus induce overstimulation of the immune system. Finally, malabsorption leading to malnutrition may interfere with the normal life cycle and responsiveness of immunologically reactive cells of GALT and of the immune reactivity in general.

Clinically, malabsorption may be defined as the presence of unabsorbed food components in the stool, accompanied by weight loss or failure to gain weight on an appropriate diet (Kalser, 1985b; Wright and Heyworth, 1989). Sometimes gastrointestinal manifestations are lacking or remain subclinical. Depending on the site of involvement along the digestive tract and on the extent of the damage, malabsorption may involve one or more of the constituents of food: carbohydrates, proteins, fats, small organic compounds such as vitamins, and minerals. Exquisitely "specific" malabsorption is exemplified by vitamin B_{12} deficiency leading to pernicious anemia. On the other hand, panmalabsorption encompasses all foodstuffs to a lesser or greater degree. Diverse etiologies and pathogenic pathways may result in the same or similar nutrient deficiencies; one disease may express, in various patients and at different times, various degrees and types of malabsorption, as seen, for example, in celiac disease.

The traditional pathophysiological classification of malabsorption syndromes is based on the stage of nutrient uptake affected (Kalser, 1985b; Wright and Heyworth, 1989). The intraluminal stage may be affected either in its digestive phase or by decreased availability of ingested nutrients (Wright and Heyworth, 1989). Similarly, the intestinal stage may be deranged, by interference either with digestion at the level of the epithelial cells or with movement across the epithelium. Finally, the transport stage may be affected, most frequently, via lymphatics. However, several malabsorption syndromes exist in which a clear-cut assignment to one of these groups is not possible and in which additional as-yet-unknown factors may be involved (Kalser, 1985b; Wright and Heyworth, 1989).

Diseases evolving from disorders affecting the intraluminal stage have been reviewed extensively elsewhere and will not be discussed further. In this chapter, delineating selected aspects of malabsorption confined to the intestinal stage and to lymphatic transport (Table I) seems appropriate. Malabsorption at the intestinal stage often involves deficient carbohydrate digestion at the brush border of epithelial cells or impaired transport of fat or proteins through these cells. The impairment of transport mechanisms may be restricted to a single substance. Finally, transfer of fat and proteins from the mucosa to other organ systems for metabolism or storage may be hampered by obstruction of capillaries or intestinal lymphatic vessels.

II. MALABSORPTION SYNDROMES

In an attempt to classify malabsorption syndromes involving immune mechanisms from the perspective of pathogenesis, the syndromes may be categorized as (1) diseases definitively associated with infectious agents; (2) syndromes possibly associated with microbes; and (3) disorders not associated with infectious agents (Table II).

A. *Malabsorption Syndromes Associated with Infectious Agents*

Chronic infection of the small intestine is the leading cause of malabsorption. Malabsorption after infection is found in apparently immunocompetent as well as in immunocompromised hosts. Malabsorption in immunodeficient hosts indeed results most often from the increased susceptibility to infection and the direct action of the microorganisms on the small intestines. However, this does not always seem to be the case; malabsorption without demonstrable infection has been reported repeatedly in various immunodeficiency syndromes (Doe, 1983; Brown and Strober, 1988). The epidemic of acquired immunodeficiency syndrome (AIDS; for review, see Kotler, 1991a) has increased the number of patients suffering from malnutrition dramatically. Since this latter topic is of great importance and rather new, it will be discussed in some detail. The outcome of malabsorption may be complicated by the complex metabolic changes induced by the reactions of the host to infectious agents (Beisel, 1987). Changes occur in the hormonal homeostasis, carbohydrate metabolism, and nitrogen balance. Other than the mildest infections usually entail anorexia, and, with fever, increased oxygen consumption (~ 13% increase per 1°C). In recurrent or chronic infectious diseases, both the host defense and general nutritional status may be critically reduced, especially in children and adolescents.

1. Gastroenteritis in the Immunocompetent Host

With fully functioning specific and nonspecific host defense, acute gastroenteritis is a self-limited disease of short duration. Malabsorption usually does not develop in such patients. Long-lasting, chronic, or recurrent infections, on the other hand, can lead to malabsorption, especially in children (Owen, 1989). Pathogenic determinants that lead to protracted diarrhea are not fully understood. Protein-calorie mal-

Table I Classification of Malabsorption Syndromes[a]

Stage of absorption	Defects	Prototype diseases
Maldigestion	Pancreatic secretions	Chronic pancreatitis, pancreatic neoplasm, cystic fibrosis
	Mechanical/microclimate derangements	Postgastrectomy syndrome, enzyme inactivation, Zollinger–Ellison syndrome, congenital enterokinase deficiency
	Brush border enzymes	Disaccharidase deficiencies, lactase, sucrase-isomaltase, trehalase deficiency peptidase deficiencies
Malabsorption: Intestinal Stage	Intraluminal derangements	Bacterial overgrowth, ileal dysfunction, hepatocellular disease, cholestasis
	Mucosal cells	Gluten-induced enteropathy, tropical sprue, short bowel syndrome, endocrinopathies, drug-induced disease (Neomycin, Colchicine), acute bacterial enteritis, Crohn's disease, Mediterranean lymphoma, Kaposi sarcoma, adenocarcinomas, dermatitis herpetiformis, psoriasis, Köhler-Dager syndrome
	Vasculature	Radiation enteritis, chronic mesenteric vascular insufficiency
	Food allergy	Milk allergy, protein-losing enteropathy with allergy
	Systemic diseases	Dysgammaglobulinemias, alpha heavy chain disease, systemic lupus erythematosus, scleroderma, autoimmune and immune complex vasculitides, mastocytosis, amyloidosis, malnutrition (exogenous)
	Genetic disorders (single enzymes)	Hartnup disease, cystinuria, vitamin D, magnesium deficiencies, chloridorrhea, vitamin B_{12} malabsorption, abetalipoproteinemia, glucose–galactose malabsorption
	Unclassified	Whipple's disease, congenital malrotation of intestines, idiopathic steatorrhea
Transport Stage	Lymphatic obstruction	Retroperitoneal malignancy, intestinal lymphangiectasia, heart insufficiency, sarcoidosis

[a] Syndromes discussed in this chapter are underlined.

Table II Malabsorption Syndromes with Known or Likely Links to the Immune System

Category	Syndrome	Histopathology	Distribution
Associated with infectious agents	Infections in immunocompetent host	Variable villous flattening, inflammation, usually few microbes	Localized, patchy
	Infections in immunodeficient host (including AIDS)	Variable villous flattening, epithelial defects, weak inflammatory response, few plasma cells. Lymphocytes; no granulomata, usually many microbes	Patchy–diffuse
Presumably associated with infectious agents	Tropical sprue	Shortened and thickened villi, plasma cells in LP increased in numbers	Diffuse, proximal jejunum
	Whipple's disease	Numerous PAS-positive foamy macrophages	Patchy
	Sarcoidosis	Lymphatics obstructed, lymph node involvement	Patchy
No association with infectious agents	Gluten-induced enteropathy (including dermatitis herpetiformis)	Flat mucosa, crypt hyperplasia, increased IEL, increased plasma cells in LP	Diffuse–patchy, proximal jejunum
	Cow's milk intolerance	Similar to above	Similar to above
	Crohn's disease	Noncaseating granulomas with giant cells; epithelial disruption; T cells predominate surrounding ulcera	Patchy, small intestines
	Immunoproliferative small intestinal diseases	Thick, indurated segments of small intestines; extensive infiltrates with lymphocytes, immunoblasts, plasma cells; reduced crypts and villi, sometimes flat mucosa, ulcera	
	Eosinophilic gastroenteritis	Eosinophil granulocytes in lamina propria	Patchy
	Connective tissue diseases	Collagen accumulation in lamina propria	Patchy–diffuse
	Pernicious anemia	None in small intestinal mucosa	

nutrition seems to predispose to chronic diarrhea by inducing changes in the intestinal mucosa (Gracey, 1981). There is thinning of the gut wall, flattening of villi, and a cuboidal to squamous "metaplasia" of enterocytes. Inflammatory infiltrates in the *lamina propria* also are seen frequently in children with protein-calorie malnutrition, suggesting decreased host-defense. In severe protein-calorie defects, cell-mediated immunity (Seth *et al.*, 1982) is more likely to be affected than humoral immunity. It seems, therefore, that malnourishment is a primary factor predisposing to chronic diarrhea, both by direct effects on the intestinal mucosa and by impairment of host defense. The spiral of deficiency of nutrients leading to chronic diarrhea, which results in malabsorption, which aggravates the malnutrition, is a major killer of children in the developing countries of this world. Children with persistent diarrhea and malnutrition have recently been shown to be frequently infected with *Giardia lamblia*. Of interest are reports that children with giardiasis of short duration had IgG and IgA antibodies to a 57 kDa Giardia heat shock protein (HSP), whereas patients with chronic infections lacked the IgA response to this antigen (Char *et al.*, 1993). Since IgM class antibodies to this moiety were abundant in these patients, the authors of this report suggest a derranged switch from IgM to IgG and IgA in these subjects; this defect must be antigen specific, however, since total immunoglobulin isotypes were elevated in these children. Minute and very specific immunodeficiencies thus may exist in patients that are routinely declared "immunocompetent."

In *Giardia lamblia* infestation, diarrhea results from disruption of the brush border of epithelial cells and disaccharidase (Veghelyi, 1939; Cortner, 1959; Meyer and Radulescu, 1979). In some studies, these parasites also have been found within the intestinal mucosa (Brandborg *et al.*, 1967; Hoskins *et al.*, 1967; Morecki and Parker, 1967). Yeast infection and bacterial overgrowth may coexist with *G. lamblia* infestation. Co-infections as well as creation of mechanical barriers to absorption (Erlandsen and Chase, 1974; Poley and Rosenfield, 1981), competition for nutrients (Yardley and Bayless, 1967; Cowen and Campbell, 1973), and alteration of intestinal motility (Castro *et al.*, 1976) have been proposed as pathogenic mechanisms leading to malabsorption in these patients. In this infestation, IELs seem to be increased in density (Dobbins, 1986), suggesting a contribution of the immune system to the pathogenesis of malabsorption or to its perpetuation.

Extensive involvement of the small intestines in gastrointestinal tuberculosis may cause steatorrhea and other manifestations of malabsorption (Shin *et al.*, 1988) as a consequence of impaired lymphatic transport from the gut, especially when the mesenteric lymphatic system is involved ("tabes mesenterica"; Gorbach, 1989). In addition, intestinal luminal obstruction may lead to bacterial overgrowth (King and Toskes, 1985). Although many patients with gastrointestinal tuberculosis have no symptoms, the increasing incidence of tuberculosis in the United States (Bloom and Murray, 1992) may enhance the relevance of this condition for medical professionals in the near future. Overgrowth of bacteria that occurs in surgical patients with blind loops or short bowel may lead to malabsorption (Weser, 1976). However, note that malabsorption is seen only infrequently in infections or infestations of immunocompetent, well-nourished hosts.

2. Gastroenteritis in the Immunocompromised Host

The immunocompromised host is susceptible to a wider range of microorganisms than the immunocompetent individual; the infections in patients with immunodeficiencies tend to be protracted, recurrent, or chronic. Usually, these infections do not resolve completely even with aggressive antimicrobial treatment. The spectrum of potential pathogens obviously depends on the nature of the underlying immune defects (Doe, 1983; Doe and Hapel, 1983; Brown and Strober, 1988; Kagnoff, 1989a).

a. Primary immunodeficiencies. Many of the congenital deficiencies of the host defense system may lead to malabsorption (Demarchi *et al.*, 1983; Kagnoff, 1989a). The importance of an intact immune system is demonstrated by the high prevalence of gastrointestinal disease in patients with immunodeficiency, even when nonspecific defense mechanisms are functioning (Brown and Strober, 1988). Incidence and frequency of malabsorption varies among the distinct entities. Immunodeficiencies of B cells and immunoglobulins are more common than deficiencies of the T-cell system (Figure 1; Stiehm, 1990). Malabsorption deficiency occurs less frequently in patients with isolated immunoglobulin deficiencies than in children with severe combined immunodeficiency.

In general, the severity of the intestinal involvement correlates well with the extent of the immunodeficiency. However, severe immunodeficiencies may not be associated with intestinal disease, suggesting that local immune responses may be dissociated from systemic immunity; this option has been shown convincingly in the case of IgA. Patients with reduced serum IgA concentrations may have normal secretory IgA, and individuals with reduced secretory IgA may show normal serum IgA concentrations (Strober *et al.*, 1976). Thus, evaluation of the local status of GALT often is necessary to understand the underlying defect of the immune system.

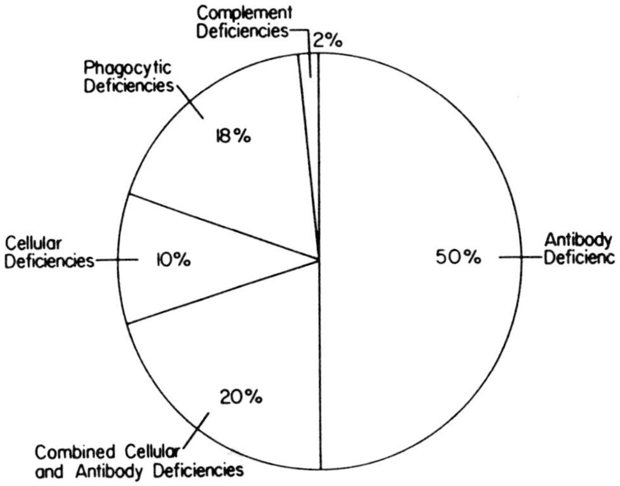

Figure 1 The frequency of primary immunodeficiencies categorized according to the host defense mechanisms. (Reproduced with kind permission of the author and publisher from Stiehm, 1990.)

IgA deficiencies, in Caucasians the most common (1 : 500) and fortunately usually the most benign of primary immunodeficiencies (among Japanese, the incidence is much lower; Kanoh, 1991), only seldom lead to gastrointestinal disease (Fisher *et al.*, 1982; Kagnoff, 1989a). However, IgA deficiencies may be associated with nodular lymphoid hyperplasia of the intestines (Brown and Strober, 1988), inflammatory bowel disease (IBD; Hodgson and Jewell, 1977; Doe and Hapel, 1983), and disaccharidase deficiencies (Dubois *et al.*, 1970). Patients with IgA deficiency also may have a propensity for infestation with *G. lamblia*. Although isolated deficiency of the secretory piece has been described (Strober *et al.*, 1976), the patient developed diarrhea and intestinal candidiasis but not malabsorption. Ample evidence exists for "immune exclusion breakdown" in IgA-deficient patients (Soothill *et al.*, 1976; Cunningham-Rundles *et al.*, 1979; Cunningham-Rundles, 1987). However, conclusive demonstration of a direct relationship between IgA deficiency and immune exclusion breakdown still is lacking (Brown and Strober, 1988). Similarly, the increased incidence of food allergies in IgA-deficient patients requires further analysis to understand the mechanism linking the two pnenomena (Cunningham-Rundles *et al.*, 1979).

In patients with X-linked hypogammaglobulinemia, described by Bruton (1952) and characterized by Good and his collaborators (Peterson *et al.*, 1965), gastrointestinal disorders become seldom manifest. In a few patients, inflammation of the colonic mucosa, acute or chronic rotavirus infection (Saulsbury *et al.*, 1980), infestation with *G. lamblia*, bacterial overgrowth (Ament *et al.*, 1973), or lactase deficiency (Dubois *et al.*, 1970) is apparent.

Much more frequent are gastrointestinal disorders in patients with common variable hypogammaglobulinemia (CVH). In a study of 50 patients with this primary immunodeficiency, 60% had diarrhea and 40% had malabsorption (Hermans *et al.*, 1976). In CVH, the lamina propria of the intestine usually shows a reduction in numbers of plasma cells of all isotypes (Brown *et al.*, 1972a,b). There may be a partial villous atrophy, which does not improve with gluten restriction (Brown *et al.*, 1972a). IBD may occur in patients with CVH more frequently than in immunocompetent individuals (Kagnoff, 1989a). Bacterial overgrowth is documented in CVH patients (Brown *et al.*, 1972b; Hermans *et al.*, 1976), and infections with *Heliobacter jejuni* may resemble IBD when lasting over prolonged periods of time (Ahnen and Brown, 1982). In CVH, *Shigella* and *Salmonella* also may be seen (Hermans *et al.*, 1976; Ahnen and Brown, 1982). Over 65% of patients with CVH have an infestation with *G. lamblia;* this protozoan causes extensive tissue damage in some of these patients (Brown *et al.*, 1972b; Ament *et al.*,

1973; Hermans *et al.*, 1976). In addition, cryptosporidiosis (Current *et al.*, 1983) and strongyloidiasis (Brandt de Oliveira *et al.*, 1981) have been reported in CVH patients.

Interestingly, pernicious anemia and atrophy of the entire stomach mucosa, associated with normal gastrin levels, occurs frequently in CVH patients (Twomey *et al.*, 1969; Brown *et al.*, 1972a). CVH patients may show intestinal nodular lymphoid hyperplasia (Hermans *et al.*, 1976). The nodules contain many IgA-bearing B cells but few mature IgA-producing plasma cells. The striking difference in the frequency and severity of gastrointestinal symptoms and malabsorption between CVH and X-linked hypogammaglobulinemia is still puzzling, but may find an explanation in the concomitant T-cell derangements of CVH.

Congenital thymic aplasia, described by DiGeorge (1968), sometimes manifests with malabsorption as well as other gastrointestinal symptoms (Cleveland, 1975). Similarly, chronic mucocutaneous candidiasis may lead to carbohydrate intolerance, iron deficiency, and diarrhea (Asquith, 1979; Brown and Strober, 1988).

Combined B- and T-cell defects lead in many patients to severe gastrointestinal disorders, including severe malabsorption. Jejunal villi may be shortened and the mucosa may show appreciably increased numbers of vacuolated macrophages and tissue edema (Brown and Strober, 1988; Kagnoff, 1989a). Some patients with Nezelof's syndrome, a T-cell deficiency associated with variable B-cell defects (Stiehm, 1990), have malabsorption (Ament, 1975). Ataxia telangiectasia, a T-cell deficiency often combined with IgA deficiency, may develop mild malabsorption (Ament *et al.*, 1973). Steatorrhea and vitamin B_{12} deficiency have been described in the Wiskott–Aldrich syndrome, encompassing a T-cell defect and decreased IgM synthesis (Ament *et al.*, 1973).

In chronic granulomatous disease, phagocyte deficiency in which the oxidative metabolism is disturbed in neutrophilic granulocytes (Stiehm *et al.*, 1989a), steatorrhea and panmalabsorption have been seen (Ament and Ochs, 1973). Lipid-filled pigmented macrophages similar to those observed in Whipple's disease appear sometimes in the mucosa. Some patients with this disorder may have lesions resembling those of Crohn's disease (Werlin *et al.*, 1982).

Whereas in most primary immunodeficiency patients with gastrointestinal symptoms, intestinal infections are the likely causes of malabsorption, others have malabsorption without any such apparent infection. The pathogenic mechanisms involved in the latter conditions are not known.

Since mucosal lesions in primary immunodeficiency syndromes often are patchy and therefore can be missed easily, several biopsies should be taken of the same patient. *In situ* hybridization techniques may be useful for the identification of infectious agents in tissue samples. Correction of the immunodeficiency, for example, replacement of immunoglobulin, often reverses malabsorption and histological changes.

b. Secondary immunodeficiencies. Secondary or acquired immunodeficiencies develop in the wake of a host of infections and other diseases. In the following section, malabsorption associated with AIDS and with some neoplasms will be discussed. Malabsorption and intestinal protein loss as causes of impaired immune responsiveness are covered in Section IV of this chapter.

i. The acquired immunodeficiency syndrome (AIDS). AIDS increasingly has gained in importance among secondary immunodeficiencies. AIDS patients often have involvement of the gastrointestinal system (Friedman-Kien, 1981; Gottlieb *et al.*, 1981; Fischel *et al.*, 1990; Kotler, 1991a). The spread of AIDS during recent years has contributed appreciably to the number of individuals suffering from chronic diarrhea and malabsorption syndromes. Whereas AIDS was defined originally in developed countries by Kaposi sarcoma and *Pneumocystis carinii* pneumonia, in Africa and Caribbean countries, AIDS is most impressively defined by the "enteropathic" variant, consisting of chronic diarrhea (more than 30 days of diarrhea over a 2 month period), wasting, and fever (Keusch *et al.*, 1992).

Studies performed in industrialized as well as developing countries have documented gastrointestinal dysfunction in 50–90% of individuals testing positive for antibodies to the human immunodeficiency virus (HIV) (Malenbranche *et al.*, 1983; Budhraja *et al.*, 1985; Friedman and Owen, 1989). and 30–60% have malabsorption (Brasitus and Sitrin, 1990). Several mechanisms have been postulated in attempts to explain the high rate of intestinal dysfunction in this immunodeficiency. The gut is a major route of infection in AIDS, which has been considered one of the factors leading to the high incidence of intestinal derangements in this disease (Kagnoff *et al.*, 1991). Nevertheless, in patients with blood-borne HIV infection, for example, hemophiliacs, intestinal involvement is high also (Okubo and Yasunaga, 1991). Table III lists the main pathogens responsible for gastrointestinal morbidity in AIDS, as well as the currently available methods for their detection and the therapy regimens—in part still experimental—for their eradication. A depletion of helper T cells in the mucosa was hypothesized to lead to impaired immune responses to antigenic moieties and mitogens. This immunodeficiency could render the patients susceptible to infection with opportunistic and nonopportunistic intestinal pathogens (Brown and Strober, 1988). These pathogens then could lead to debilitating diarrhea and malabsorption. Alternatively, HIV infection of small intestinal mucosal cells could be responsible for malabsorption directly (Nelson *et al.*, 1988; Fox *et al.*, 1989; Ullrich *et al.*, 1989; Yolken *et al.*, 1991). AIDS patients also have anorexia, resulting in severe malnutrition in conjunction with malabsorption. Diarhea and loss of body weight are the most common clinical manifestations of gastrointestinal AIDS; in Africa, AIDS often is called "Slim's disease" (Greene, 1988).

The ratio of $CD4^+$ to $CD8^+$ cells, which is decreased severely in the blood of AIDS patients, has been reported to be decreased (Rodgers *et al.*, 1986) or increased (Kotler *et al.*, 1986) in the intestinal mucosa. In another study (Riecken *et al.*, 1991), a decrease of $CD4^+$ LPLs has been demonstrated in patients with AIDS, but this decrease was much smaller than that seen for blood lymphocytes. At the same time, a significant increase of $CD8^+$ cells was seen (Riecken *et al.*, 1991). Interestingly, the activation marker

Table III Diagnosis and Treatment of Intestinal Infections in Patients with AIDS

Organism	Diagnosis	Treatment
Fungi		
Candida sp.	SS: gram, culture	Nystatin, Amphotericin B, Fluconazole, Clotrimazole
Protozoa		
Cryptosporidium	SS or DA: Ziehl–Neelson, monoclonal antibody; SBB with histology	Experimental: Spiramycin, Transfer Factor, Hyperimmune Bovine Serum and Colostrum, Monoclonal Antibodies, Somatostatin
Isospora belli	SS or DA: Ziehl–Neelson, modified acid-fast	Trimethoprim-Sulfamethoxazole
Microsporidia	SS or DA: Chromotropy; SBB	None proven
Giardia lamblia	SS or DA: microscopy or ELISA	Metronidazole, Quinacrine-HCl, Furazolidone
Strongyloides stercoralis	SS or DA for rhabditiform larvae; SBB	Thiabendazole
Viruses		
Cytomegalovirus	SBB	Gancyclovir, Foscarnet
Herpes simplex		Acyclovir
Bacteria		
Mycobacterium Avium-intracellulare	SS or DA: Ziehl–Neelson, culture or genome detection	Rifampin or Rifabutin + Clofasimine, Ethambutol, Ethionamide, Streptomycin and Clarythromycin
Mycobacterium tuberculosis	SS or DA: Ziehl–Neelson, culture or genome detection	Isoniazid, Rifampin, Pyrazinamide, Streptomycin
Salmonella typhimurium	SS: gram, culture	Antibiotics
Shigella	SS: gram, culture	Antibiotics

DA, duodenal aspirate; SBB, small bowel biopsy; SS, stool smear.

CD25 is expressed on fewer T cells in the mucosa of AIDS patients than in that of healthy subjects (Riecken *et al.*, 1991). The same authors suggested that $CD4^+$ cells in the mucosa may be less susceptible to HIV-induced cell death, but may respond to HIV infection by improper activity.

The number of IgA-producing intestinal plasma cells has been found to be decreased (Kotler *et al.*, 1987) or normal (Rodgers and Kagnoff, 1987) in AIDS patients compared with normal individuals. A study of the parotid glands of AIDS patients suggests that IgA production may be reduced severely; Muller *et al.* (1991) have found a decrease of both IgA1 and IgA2 concentrations in the secretion of this gland. This local mucosal reduction of IgA was accompanied by a significant increase of serum IgA, but correlated well with decreased CD4 : CD8 ratios for blood T cells (Muller *et al.*, 1991). Immune complexes, predominantly consisting of IgA1 (Jackson *et al.*, 1988), have been demonstrated in some AIDS patients. The impact of circulating immune complexes on tissue lesions and immunoregulation in AIDS is not yet understood.

A direct pathogenic effect of HIV on gastrointestinal tract cells in AIDS patients has not yet been demonstrated convincingly, albeit several findings do suggest such an effect (Kotler *et al.*, 1984; Rodgers *et al.*, 1986; Brown and Strober, 1988). Intestinal disease has been shown to occur often in patients with AIDS who do not have other intestinal infections (Kotler *et al.*, 1984). However, inability to demonstrate infectious agents may not be equated with absence of the infectious agents.

Genetic material of HIV has been reported in the intestinal epithelium of AIDS patients (Mathjis *et al.*, 1988; Nelson *et al.*, 1988), and HIV core antigen (p24) has been found in various cell types of the intestinal mucosa (René *et al.*, 1988; Reka *et al.*, 1989; Ullrich *et al.*, 1989). Scientists generally agree that 20–40% of patients with AIDS have HIV-infected mononuclear cells in the lamina propria of the intestines (Fox *et al.*, 1989), even early in the disease. Some colonic epithelial cell lines can be infected with HIV (Kagnoff *et al.*, 1991). HIV seems to attach to some cell lines via CD4. HIV infection of the line HT29, however, cannot be inhibited by antibodies to CD4 (Kagnoff *et al.*, 1991). Whether infection of epithelial cells with HIV is important in the pathogenesis of intestinal disorders of AIDS patients is not known, since the consequences of infection of mucosal cells with HIV are not understood as well as those of infection of systemic lymphocytes and macrophages (Kotler, 1991b). Recently, no significant difference in D-xylose uptake could be detected in patients with or without HIV gp41 in their duodenal mucosa (Ehrenpreis *et al.*, 1992). In this study, HIV was present only in *lamina propria* mononuclear cells, and not in neuroendocrine cells or enterocytes. Presence of HIV in enterocytes was associated with the most severe malabsorption in another group of AIDS patients (Heise *et al.*, 1991); localization of HIV in enterocyte, however, seems to be a rare event, since four out of five patients with HIV in the small intestine had the viral antigens only in infiltrating mononuclear cells. Heise *et al.* (1991) conclude that infection of the intestines with HIV is an early event and that infection of enterocytes alters their differentiation and function, which leads to malabsorption.

The histopathology of HIV-associated intestinal disorders may suggest a difference between directly HIV-induced tissue lesions and those mediated by secondary intestinal infections. Partial villous atrophy combined with crypt hyperplasia seems characteristic in patients with the latter, whereas patients without detectable secondary infections seem to show minimal villous atrophy and reduced mitotic figures in the crypt. Kotler *et al.*, (1984) have shown extensive degeneration of intestinal crypt cells among patients with AIDS, with a presentation reminiscent of graft-versus-host reactions (Sapin *et al.*, 1977). Lactase and β-glucosidase, as well as alkaline phosphatase, deficiencies in intestinal epithelium of AIDS patients suggest delay of intestinal epithelial cell maturation. In six AIDS patients with fat malabsorption, only the two patients infected with opportunistic enteropathogens (*Cryptosporidium* spp. and *Isospora belli*) had abnormal ileal absorptive functions (Kapembwa *et al.*, 1990). These data suggest that in nonsuperinfected AIDS gastroenteritis, only the upper jejunum is involved in malabsorption, whereas superinfection extends the involvement to the ileum.

Among the most frequently diagnosed intestinal parasites of AIDS patients are *Cryptosporidium, Isospora belli, Microsporidium* (Levine, 1980), *G. lamblia,* and *Strongyloides stercoralis* (René *et al.*, 1991). The relative importance of other agents such as *Blastocystis hominis, Dientamoeba fragilis, Balantidium coli,* and nonpathogenic *Entamoeba* strains has not yet been clarified. In immunocompetent patients, infestation with these pathogens usually responds well to therapy and is of short duration; in AIDS patients, the course is protracted and severe.

Cryptosporidium, known prior to 1982 almost exclusively as an animal pathogen (Current *et al.*, 1983; Navin and Juranek, 1984), increasingly causes disease in immunocompetent and immunocompromised humans (René *et al.*, 1991). In immunologically competent patients, this parasite causes mild diarrhea, nausea, abdominal cramps, anorexia, and low grade fever. In immunodeficient hosts, the organism often leads to a devastating disease manifesting with protracted diarrhea and malabsorption (Soave *et al.*, 1984; Navin and Juranek, 1984; René *et al.*, 1989,1991); up to 25 bowel movements per day have been reported in *Cryptosporidium*-infested AIDS patients (Whiteside *et al.*, 1984). The diarrhea most likely is of the enterotoxin-induced secretory type (Friedman and Owen, 1989; René *et al.*, 1991); however, enterotoxin secretion by *Cryptosporidium* has not yet been shown conclusively. Note that immunocompetent individuals infested with *Cryptosporidium* report a history of contacts with animals; such an association is lacking in AIDS patients. Cryptosporidiosis in AIDS patients is unremitting and, in general, refractory to therapy.

Isospora belli, rare in immunocompetent individuals, causes chronic profuse watery diarrhea in AIDS patients, resulting in dehydration, weight loss, and steatorrhea (DeHovitz *et al.*, 1986), especially in patients in developing countries (DeHovitz *et al.*, 1986; Sevankambo *et al.*, 1987). *Microsporidium* has been reported to play a pathogenic role in malabsorption syndromes of AIDS (Desportes *et al.*, 1985; Dobbins and Weinstein, 1985; Orenstein *et al.*, 1990). On the other hand, *G. lamblia* and *Entamoeba histolytica* do not show a more severe progression in AIDS patients than in immunocompetent hosts (René *et al.*, 1991), a puzzling finding.

One of the first clinical manifestations of the decay of immune functions in HIV-infected patients is the colonization of the gastrointestinal tract by *Candida* species (René *et al.*, 1991). Most commonly, *Candida* is found in the oral cavity and in the esophagus, the latter causing odynophagia and dysphagia (Klein *et al.*, 1984; René *et al.*, 1991). Ulcers in the mouth and the esophagus rarely spread to the submucosa or to distant organs. The normal function of neutrophilic granulocytes in AIDS patients may explain the relatively successful containment of *Candida*. Although the gastrointestinal tract cannot be cleared completely of this yeast, response to treatment often is good. *Candida* has not been shown to cause severe malabsorption.

Salmonella typhimurium and *Shigella flexneri* have been demonstrated in the feces and blood of patients with AIDS (Soave *et al.*, 1984; Dobbins and Weinstein, 1985; Glaser *et al.*, 1985; Jacobs *et al.*, 1985; Whimbey *et al.*, 1986; Baskin *et al.*, 1987). Antibiotic-resistant *Heliobacter jejuni* has been seen to persist in a patient with AIDS (Dworkin *et al.*, 1986; Whimbey *et al.*, 1986; Laughon *et al.*, 1988). Rather frequently, patients with bacterial intestinal infections and AIDS have atypical mycobacteria (Damsker and Bottone, 1985; Roth *et al.*, 1985), most common among which is *Mycobacterium avium-intracellulare; Mycobacterium malmoense* and, most recently described, *Mycobacterium ganavense* may be involved more often than yet recognized. These microorganisms are found in lymph nodes, bone marrow, spleen, liver, and the stool of some AIDS patients. Clinically, intestinal mycobacterial infection in AIDS is characterized by diarrhea. Despite large numbers of acid-fast microorganisms, a striking absence of granulomatous tissue lesions can occur in this syndrome (Shin *et al.*, 1988) *Mycobacterium tuberculosis* has joined HIV in a diabolic marriage, causing outbreaks of multidrug-resistant tuberculosis in HIV-positive patients (Chaisson, 1993). The rapid progression of *M. tuberculosis* infections in immunodeficient patients enhances propensity for development of multidrug resistance. Most recently, the mutual enhancement of *M. tuberculosis* and HIV infections has become better understood. Wallis *et al.* (1993) have obtained elegant data suggesting that PPD stimulates peripheral blood mononuclear cells to produce large amounts of tumor necrosis factor-α (TNF-α); TNF-α up-regulates HIV expression *in vitro,* and it can be hypothesized that co-infection with *M. tuberculosis* thus may enhance HIV-disease progression. On the other hand, Forte *et al.* (1992) showed that T-cell mediated destruction of macrophages harboring mycobacteria was significantly impaired in patients infected with HIV. *M. tuberculosis* in AIDS most commonly involves the lungs, but extrapulmonary involvement is not unusual.

Cytomegalovirus (CMV) is by far the most frequent opportunistic virus in gastrointestinal disorders of AIDS (Figure 2; Welch *et al.*, 1984). Severe CMV disease occurs virtually only in severely immunocompromised hosts. The gastrointestinal disease may involve the stomach, duodenum, and colon and, most frequently, the rectosigmoid (Centers for Disease Control, 1982; Frank and Raicht, 1984; Meiselman *et al.*, 1985). Histological findings include isolated viral inclusion bodies, vasculitis, and inflammatory cell infiltrates as well as ischemic and gangrenous lesions (Clayton, 1991). The clinical

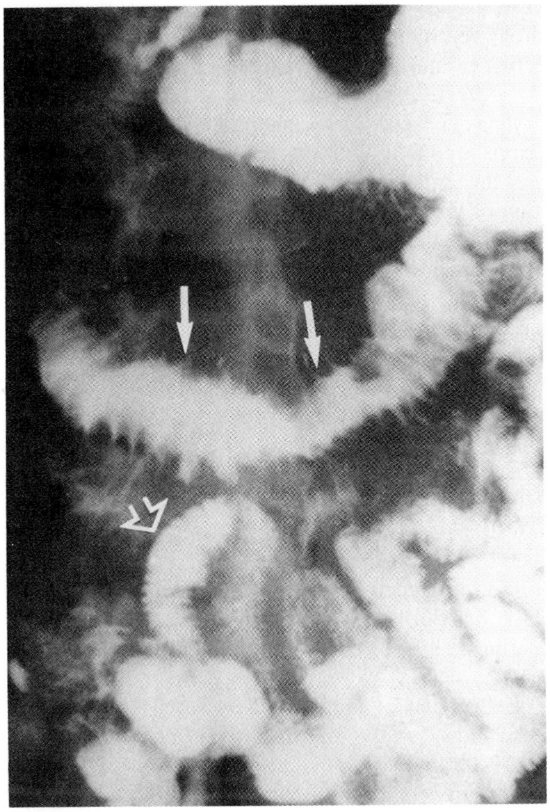

Figure 2 CMV enteritis. A 45-year-old male with 3 weeks of malaise, diarrhea, and weight loss. The X-ray shows dilatation, fluid retention, and marked edema of the jejunum (arrow) with only mild fold prominence in the ileum (open arrow). [Reproduced from Baer, J. and Hilton, S. (1991). Radiologic changes in AIDS. *In* "Gastrointestinal and Nutritional Manifestations of the Acquired Immunodeficiency Syndrome" (D. P. Kotler, ed.). Raven Press, New York, with the kind permission of the authors and the publisher.]

presentation varies from asymptomatic infection to debilitating enteritis, colitis, or even perforation of the bowel (Foucar *et al.*, 1981; Frank and Raicht, 1984). Sometimes the CMV infection mimics IBD (Brown and Strober, 1988). Bacteremia with enteric organisms may accompany CMV enteritis and colitis. The diagnosis relies on virus culture from biopsy material and demonstration of inclusion bodies in tissue sections (René *et al.*, 1991). Blood culture is not useful, since many patients have CMV in the blood without any disease (Masur and Fauci, 1989). For treatment, 9(1,3-dihydroxy-2-proepoxymethyl)guanine (DHPG, Ganciclovir; Koretz *et al.*, 1986) and phosphoformate (Foscarnet) are used (Weber *et al.*, 1987). Life-long suppression of the virus may be necessary.

Herpes simplex virus infects perioral and perianal regions, the rectum, the oropharynx, and the esophagus of patients with AIDS (Siegal *et al.*, 1981; Goodell *et al.*, 1983; René *et al.*, 1991). Lesions are hemorrhagic, ulcerative, or necrotic. Acyclovir-resistant herpes simplex virus infections usually can be treated with foscarnet or vidarabine (Safrin *et al.*, 1991).

In patients with Kaposi's sarcoma (Kaposi, 1872) of the gastrointestinal tract, malabsorption has been described (Bryk *et al.*, 1978), as has protein-losing enteropathy (Perrone *et al.*, 1981; Laine *et al.*, 1987) and intestinal perforation (Mitchell and Feder, 1949) or obstruction (White and King, 1964). Non-Hodgkin's lymphomas, a rather common and often fatal complication of AIDS, involve the gastrointestinal tract in up to 25% of cases (Ziegler *et al.*, 1984; Ioachim *et al.*, 1985). These lymphomas are usually of the B-cell type, show a translocation between chromosomes 8 and 14 (Peterson *et al.*, 1985; Berheim and Berger, 1988), and may arise from polyclonal B-cell stimulation by Epstein–Barr virus (EBV) and other viral agents (Knowles *et al.*, 1989). The intestinal lesions may lead to bleeding, perforation, and retroperitoneal lymphadenopathy (Potter *et al.*, 1984; Subar *et al.*, 1991).

Since Zidovudine (AZT) is associated with hematologic toxicity, it is likely that this drug also interferes with the rapidly proliferating intestinal epithelium. Fortunately, however, clinical trials have not documented any significant adverse intestinal reactions to AZT therapy (e.g., Volberding *et al.*, 1990), and Ullrich *et al.* (1992) report even trends of morphologic and functional normalization of small intestines in HIV-antibody positive patients with gastrointestinal involvement without secondary enteric infections, when treated with AZT. This data would be in good agreement with reports on weight gains in AIDS patients upon AZT treatment (Yarchoan *et al.*, 1986); they are, however, statistically not significant and have to be interpreted with caution.

ii. Neoplastic diseases not associated with AIDS. Some patients with lymphomas, lymphosarcomas, thymomas, or chronic lymphatic leukemia may lose their ability to synthesize one or more classes of immunoglobulins (Brown and Strober, 1988). The resulting hypoglobulinemia may increase their susceptibility to intestinal infections and lead to malabsorption. Increased immunoglobulin catabolism, sometimes seen in patients with severe burns, nephrotic syndrome, or protein-losing enteropathy, may initiate the same chain of events.

B. Malabsorption Syndromes Possibly Associated with Infectious Agents

The syndromes discussed in the following section—tropical sprue, Whipple's disease, and sarcoidosis—long have been considered potentially related to infections. Definitive demonstration of such an association, however, has not yet been accomplished, with the possible exception of Whipple's disease.

1. Tropical Sprue

Within weeks, months, or, more commonly, 1–2 yr of arrival, visitors to the tropics may develop tropical sprue (Sheehy, 1985; Klipstein, 1989). The illness is characterized by acute onset with an episode of explosive diarrhea that resolves within a week into chronic gastrointestinal symptoms, including abdominal distension and cramps. Many patients develop milk intolerance because of lactase deficiency

(Klipstein, 1989); some individuals manifest alcohol intolerance (Klipstein, 1989). After 1–3 months, the folate stores of the body are depleted. Anorexia, malabsorption, and progressive weight loss follow. Glossitis and, eventually, symptoms of anemia occur 1–3 months later (Gardner, 1958). Adults are affected more often than children. The disease may occur as a single case, or in epidemics (O'Brien and England, 1971; Jones *et al.*, 1972). Formerly, the condition was believed to develop exclusively in European travelers or immigrants, but now the disease is recognized to affect native populations of the endemic, (i.e., tropical) areas even more often (Thomas and Clain, 1976).

The epidemiological aspects of tropical sprue strongly suggest an infectious cause. However, no single specific infectious agent has been isolated to date (Sheehy 1985;Klipstein, 1989). Contamination of the small intestines by coliform bacteria including *Klebsiella pneumoniae, Eschericia coli,* and *Enterobacter cloacae* (Gorbach *et al.*, 1969) has been considered to play a role in the pathogenesis of tropical sprue because these bacteria synthesize enterotoxins and ethanol, which are able to damage intestinal mucosa (Klipstein *et al.*, 1973,1978). Also, a not-yet-identified virus may be associated with this disease. Dietary lipids may have some relevance for the pathogenesis. Secondary folic acid deficiency seems to play a perpetuating role, since treatment with folic acid may lead to resolution of the disease (Chuttani *et al.*, 1968).

Pathophysiologically, tropical sprue is characterized by impaired production of intrinsic factor and hydrochloric acid by the stomach and net secretion of water and electrolytes by the jejunum (Corcino *et al.*, 1983). Malabsorption of carbohydrates, amino acids, fat, fat-soluble vitamins, vitamin B_{12}, and bile salts occurs (Klipstein, 1989). In chronic disease, megaloblastic anemia develops because of deficiency of folic acid and vitamin B_{12}. In 50% of the patients, hypoalbuminemia and decreased serum concentrations of cholesterol are seen; one-third of patients present with a mild hypocalcemia.

Diagnosis of tropical sprue is based on the exclusion of other pathognomonic entities such as intestinal infestation by parasites and small intestinal contamination with coliform bacteria. The mucosa shows lengthening of the crypts, broadening and shortening of the villi (which are usually thickened and coalesce to form leaves), and infiltration by cells characteristic of chronic inflammation. These changes are seen already early in disease. Less than 10% of the patients have a classical "flat mucosa". Jejunal biopsy allows differentiation from gluten enteropathy (flat villi), infiltrative disorder (lymphoma), and Whipple's disease. The optimal treatment consists of oral folic acid (5 mg/day for 6 months), tetracycline (250 mg qid for 1 month, followed by 250 mg bid for 5 months), and 1000 μg vitamin B_{12} several times initially and then at monthly intervals (Klipstein, 1989). Clinical improvement with the appropriate treatment gives final evidence for the correctness of the diagnosis.

2. Whipple's Disease

Recently, the etiologic agent of Whipple's disease or intestinal lypodystrophy, first described in 1907 (Whipple, 1907), has been tentatively identified as *Tropheryma wippelii*. The disease has not been reproduced in animals; clinically, the disorder commonly is defined as a systemic bacterial illness affecting primarily middle-aged Caucasian males (Dobbins, 1985). Affected individuals have a history of intermittent arthralgia in several joints, lasting for years. The actual illness develops gradually with diarrhea turning into steatorrhea in 93% of the patients, with subsequent weight loss and a deterioration of the patients' general status. Normocytic and normochromic anemia is noted in 90% of the patients. Half the patient population demonstrates hypotension and hyperpigmentation. Other clinical manifestations include low grade fever, peripheral lymphadenopathy, and neurological abnormalities. A few patients have Whipple's disease without gastrointestinal involvement (Mansbach *et al.*, 1978). Most frequently, such extragastrointestinal Whipple's disease seems to involve neural tissue (Feurle *et al.*, 1979; Brown *et al.*, 1990; Wroe *et al.*, 1991; Amarenco *et al.*, 1991). In some cases, diagnosis may be delayed when gastrointestinal involvement occurs only after many years. Thus, IgA nephropathy and hypercalcemia have been reported to preceed gastrointestinal symptoms of Whipple's disease by 2 to 5 years (Stoll *et al.*, 1993), and chronic polyarthritis by 16 years in one patient (Scheib and Quinet, 1990).

The diagnosis is established by small bowel biopsy; the disease shows, in the proximal small intestine, typical club-shaped villi and a lamina propria replete of macrophages loaded with sickle-form particles (SPC cells) intensively stained by periodate–Schiff reagent (PAS) (Sieracki and Fine, 1959). Such SPC cells are found in virtually all organs, but most prominently in the lamina propria of the small intestine and its lymphatic drainage, the heart valves, and the central nervous system.

Electronmicroscopically, the Whipple organism resembles structurally intact or degenerating bacteria (Dobbins and Kawanishi, 1981). The bacillus is gram positive, and is present not only in macrophages but also in intestinal epithelial cells, lymphatic and capillary endothelial cells, smooth muscle cells, polymorphonuclear leucocytes, plasma cells, mast cells, and IELs. The nucleotide sequence of bacterial 16 S ribosomal DNA from the intestinal biopsy of a patient with Whipple's disease was shown to have close relation to *Rhodococcus, Streptomyces,* and *Actinobacter* genera, and weaker homology with mycobacteria (Wilson *et al.*, 1991). One year later, Relman *et al.* (1992) reported on a 1321-base-long bacterial 16S rRNA sequence amplified by PCR from duodenal tissue of a patient with Whipple's disease. Subsequently, it was shown that the same sequence was present in intestinal tissue of all five patients studied with Whipple's disease, but in none of the 10 patients with other diseases. Phylogenetic analysis suggested that the bacterium is a gram-positive actinomycete, unrelated to any of the known genera. This bacterium (as yet uncultured) was named *Tropheryma whippelii.*

Most patients respond to treatment with antibiotics. Currently, the recommended regimen is penicillin G (1.2 million Units/day) and streptomycin (1.0 g/day) for 10–14 days, followed by trimethoprim/sulfamethoxazole for 1 yr (Trier, 1989a).

3. Sarcoidosis

Sarcoidosis may involve, among other organs, the gastrointestinal tract (Fick and Hunninghake, 1988); the stomach is the most common gastrointestinal site. However, small intestinal involvement also has been described and may cause malabsorption and protein-losing enteropathy (Sterling, 1951). Differential diagnosis includes Crohn's disease. Colonic sarcoidosis is seen only infrequently. The words of Longcope and Freiman (1952), that "the etiology of sarcoidosis still is obscure," remain valid. Within lesional tissue, acid-fast coccobacillary microorganisms have been seen (Canturee, 1982). These findings are compatible with the presence of wall-deficient bacteria, most likely related to mycobacteria or non-diphtheria *Corynebacterium* species. However, mycobacteria, especially atypical mycobacteria, have been associated most frequently with sarcoidosis (Vanek and Schwarz, 1970; Mitchell *et al.,* 1992; Saboor *et al.,* 1992). Nevertheless, convincing evidence for a pathogenic role of these microorganisms has never been established. Twenty years ago, combined infection with mycobacteria and viruses has been suggested to explain the pathogenesis of sarcoidosis (Hanngren *et al.,* 1974). *Bacillus* Calmette–Guerin (BCG) vaccination in individuals with virus-induced T-cell impairment has been proposed to lead to sarcoidosis. In addition to microbial agents, chemicals and drugs have been discussed in the framework of a pathogenesis for sarcoidosis, as have allergy and autoimmunity (Fick and Hunninghake, 1988). Sarcoidosis occurs in a familial pattern (Prendville *et al.,* 1982) and some clinical manifestations have been associated with HLA-encoded antigens.

The granulomatous lesions of sarcoidosis are characterized by large numbers of T cells. These T cells are predominantly carrying α/β TcR on their surface, as do the T cells in granulomata of tuberculosis (Tazi *et al.,* 1991), and they show signs of recent antigenic stimulation (Du Bois *et al.,* 1992). As in many other inflammatory conditions, increased expression of adhesion molecules is seen in sarcoidosis, where it may contribute to extravasation, aggregation in tissue and granuloma formation (Shakoor and Hamblin, 1992). Similarly most likely reflecting inflammation, alveolar macrophages in sarcoidosis have been shown to release spontaneously tumor necrosis factor-α (TNF-α), interleukin 1(IL-1) (Strausz *et al.,* 1991), and prostaglandin E2 (PGE2); however, there was no correlation between the amount of inflammatory mediators released and clinical status of disease or steroid usage (Pueringer *et al.,* 1993). Of more potential interest for the understanding of the pathogenesis of tissue lesions in sarcoidosis is a report on a defect at the level of G-proteins in peripheral blood lymphocytes of patients with sarcoidosis (Nemoz *et al.,* 1993). These authors hypothesize that a defect in the negative control of adenylate cyclase, mediated by the inhibitory G-protein Gi, prevents the lowering of cAMP necessary for normal mitogenic responses of blood lymphocytes. In addition, both cAMP and cGMP phosphodiesterase activities were found decreased in blood lymphocytes of sarcoidosis patients.

The small intestine malabsorption in this disease arises indirectly, through lymphatic obstruction following mesenteric lymph node enlargement. Dilated lacteals can be seen in patient intestinal biopsies (Sprague *et al.,* 1984).

C. Malabsorption Syndromes Not Associated with Infectious Agents

Several malabsorption syndromes are not related to infectious agents but are associated with immune responses and heightened activity of GALT. These conditions comprise a heterogeneous group of diseases, usually with poorly understood pathogenesis, and present with a gamut of tissue lesions (Table II). In some of these syndromes, immunoreactive cells could be the primary mediators of the pathogenesis; in others, exogenous noxae, primarily extraintestinal diseases, and inborn errors of metabolism may be of etiological importance.

1. Gluten-Induced Enteropathy

The first description of "sprue" is attributed to Areteus of Cappadocia (1856), who lived in the second century of our era. Nevertheless, the formal definition of gluten-induced enteropathy (GIE; synonyms: celiac disease, celiac sprue) still is not fully satisfactory and its causes are poorly understood. Gee (1888) described the clinical manifestations of GIE in pediatric patients; Thaysen (1932) gave the classical description of this syndrome in adults. In the early 1950s, Dicke (1950) established the association between the clinical syndrome and the intake of wheat and some other cereal grains through epidemiological analysis. He and his coworkers (van de Kamer *et al.,* 1953) subsequently recognized gluten as the major component of cereals involved in GIE. Finally, Paulley (1954) published an extensive study on the histopathology of this disease.

The major clinical manifestations of GIE result from the malabsorption of nutrients, predominantly involving the proximal small intestine. The disease is defined further by characteristic, but not specific, changes of the small intestinal mucosa, namely deepening of crypts and loss of villi ("flat mucosa"), and by striking improvement of clinical and histological presentation on withdrawal of gluten from the diet (Falchuk, 1983; Cooke and Holmes, 1985; Mike and Asquith, 1987; Trier, 1989b,1991). Diagnostic criteria rely on these characteristics [Working Group of European Society of Pediatric Gastroenterology and Nutrition (WGESPGN), 1991). The additional requirement to demonstrate deterioration of mucosa on gluten challenge (Meuwisse, 1970; Bramble *et al.,* 1985) has been questioned (McNeish *et al.,* 1979; WGESPGN, 1991). A workshop on diagnostic criteria of celiac disease, organized by the European Society of Pediatric Gastroenterology and Nutrition in 1989, stressed the contribution of recently developed serological tests to the diagnosis of GIE (WGESPGN, 1991). Antigluten (Schmitz *et al.,* 1978), anti-reticulin (Mäki *et al.,* 1984), and anti-endomysial (Chorzelski *et al.,* 1984; Kumar *et al.,* 1989) antibodies of the IgA isotype have proved to be reliable indicators of sensitization to gluten at the time of diagnosis (WGESPGN, 1991), with the exception of GIE in individuals with hypogammaglobulinemia or IgA deficiency.

It is important to emphasize that, in addition to full-blown celiac disease, a host of clinical presentations may be associated with gluten hypersensitivity. These include dermatitis herpetiformis (see subsequent text), recurrent aphthae, IgA nephropathy, and arthritides (Ferguson *et al.*, 1993; Marsh, 1993). Some patients may present with more atypical and diffuse symptoms, such as malaise, psychological problems, abdominal pain, and ill-defined growth defects (Collin *et al.*, 1990). Finally, 50–60% of patients with gliadin hypersensitivity are asymptomatic. All these conditions could be subsummarized under the term "gluten sensitivity complex." Ferguson *et al.* (1993) have proposed recently to subdivide "permanent gluten sensitive enteropathy" (i.e., celiac disease) into "active," "silent," "latent," and "potential." This may be helpful in the understanding of the pathogenesis of this group of diseases.

Malabsorption in GIE results from the drastic decrease of absorptive surface and from derangements and loss of the epithelial cell brush border and its enzymes. Clinically, severity of symptoms spans a wide range, reflecting, at least in part, the extent of the intestinal lesions. Thus, GIE may present as isolated iron or folate deficiency anemia without any gastrointestinal symptoms. On the other end of the spectrum are failure to thrive, in pediatric patients, and devastating life-threatening panmalabsorption with secondary involvement of many organ systems. In its long-term evolution, GIE has proven more variable than previously thought (Schmitz *et al.*, 1978; Kamath and Dorney, 1983; Mäki and Visakorpi, 1988; WGESPGN, 1991).

Histology of the small intestinal tissue lesions presents as villous atrophy, crypt epithelial cell hyperplasia, crypt hypertrophy, and changes in the lymphoid-cell population of the mucosa. Mucosa of patients with GIE was shown to produce six times more epithelial cells than healthy mucosa per time unit (Watson and Wright, 1974), with a doubling of the rate of cell division and a 3-fold increase in numbers of proliferating cells. Numbers of undifferentiated crypt cells and frequency of mitoses among crypt cells are increased significantly (Padykula *et al.*, 1961; Yardley *et al.*, 1962). The ultrastructure of crypt epithelial cells usually is normal (Rubin *et al.*, 1966). The populations of goblet and Paneth cells also seem comparable to those of healthy subjects. However, endocrine cells appear to be increased in numbers in the mucosa of GIE patients with severe lesions (Polak *et al.*, 1973). This increase may result from impaired release of cholecystokinin and secretin from such cells. The cuboidal surface epithelial cells display degenerative changes: prominent loss of organelles, accentuation of lysosomes, swelling of mitochondria and endoplasmic reticulum, incomplete development of the terminal web, and staining variability and electron density of the cytoplasm (Rubin *et al.*, 1966). Importantly, microvilli are short, irregular, fused, or absent. In addition, thinning of the glycocalyx occurs. The density of CD8+ and γ/δ TcR+ IELs and mucosal mast cells (Strobel *et al.*, 1983) is increased in untreated patients with GIE; however, the total number of lymphoid cells per area remains in the normal range, reflecting the severely decreased area of intestinal surface (Ferguson and Murray, 1971; Holmes *et al.*, 1974). Plasma cells are much more abundant in the lamina propria mucosae of GIE patients than in that of healthy individuals, whereas lymphocytes tend to appear in lower than normal numbers (Holmes *et al.*, 1974). The mucosal cellular infiltrates usually show high numbers of neutrophilic and eosinophilic granulocytes and mast cells (Marsh and Hinde, 1985). Succinctly, the histopathology of GIE has been described as "extensive villous atrophy with hyperplasia of the crypts and an abnormal surface epithelium" (Marsh, 1988). Remember that the mucosal lesions in GIE are rather variable in character, severity, and extent (Mäki and Visakorpi, 1988), and that the same patients may have, concomitantly, several types of intestinal lesions (Roy-Choudhury *et al.*, 1967). Flat mucosa most often is found only in the proximal portion of the jejunum and, even here, distribution of lesions may be patchy (Thompson, 1974). Recently, the spectrum of the interrelated patterns of mucosal tissue lesions seen in GIE have been classified by Marsh (1992a,1992b) as follows: infiltrative, infiltrative-hyperplastic, flat-destructive, and irreversible hypoplastic atrophic, spanning the gamut of isolated increase of IEL to the end-stage disease with progressive intestinal failure.

The pathophysiological mechanisms leading to malabsorption, in addition to simply decreased absorptive surface, result from a variety of derangements of the intestinal epithelial cell involving the microenvironment defined by the brush border and its enzymes (Padykula *et al.*, 1961; Dissanyake *et al.*, 1974; Bramble *et al.*, 1985) and the glycocalyx (Rubin *et al.*, 1966). The microenvironment (or microclimate) defined by the glycocalyx seems essential to normal absorption of neutral molecules. The pH of the microenvironment has been shown to be changed strikingly in GIE patients compared with healthy subjects (Lucas *et al.*, 1978). In addition, decreased activity or lack of enzymes, most importantly of the brush border, must contribute to impaired uptake of nutrients (Padykula *et al.*, 1961; Dissanyake *et al.*, 1974; Bramble *et al.*, 1985). Indeed, this enzymatic activity may be reduced by 90% in GIE. Further, lysosomal enzymes are increased and may contribute to the production of abnormal, potentially toxic metabolites, as well as to absorption of such moieties. In addition to malabsorption proper, maldigestion also may occur; thus the intraluminal pH in the proximal small intestine is higher than normal in untreated GIE patients, and the bacterial flora of the intestines may be changed.

Intensive research over the last four decades has allowed the formulation of several hypotheses attempting to explain the pathogenesis of GIE. One of the major problems, as is often the case in such endeavors, is the difficulty in differentiating primary pathogenic factors from those arising as secondary phenomena during the disease.

Central in the discussion of pathogenesis is the clearly established association of GIE and gluten. Gluten makes up 90% of wheat flour protein; it is a heterogeneous preparation of proteins that can be separated into an ethanol-soluble fraction termed gliadin and an insoluble fraction, glutenin. Gliadin itself consists of over 40 moieties that can be grouped into four categories (Kasarda *et al.*, 1984). A-gliadin, which is a major component of alpha gliadin, has been shown to activate GIE (Kagnoff, 1989b). Closely related to gliadin are the prolamins of rye, barley, and oats, which also may induce intestinal damage.

Even though demonstration of a direct toxic effect on mature normal enterocytes still is lacking (Davidson and Bridges, 1987), direct toxic action on fetal animal or human intestinal epithelial cells and cultured tumor cells has been documented for enzymatic digests of gluten (gluten fraction III) (Dissanyake *et al.*, 1974) and fraction 9 of gliadin (Townley *et al.*, 1973). Subsequently, lack of a normally present peptidase on jejunal mucosal tissue was suggested to explain the accumulation of these toxic products of gluten. This "missing enzyme hypothesis" still has not received substantial support from available data. Since enzymatic activities that are depressed in untreated GIE return in most cases to normal values, after exclusion of gluten from the diet, with the possible exception of lactase, the enzymatic defects seem likely to be secondary to GIE. A primary lack of peptidases has not been documented yet in patients with GIE. Similarly, carbohydrase deficiency, implicated by others (Phelan *et al.*, 1977) in the toxogenesis of gluten, still remains a possible but rather unlikely candidate. Since lactase levels remain low even after histological normalization of the mucosa, lactase deficiency may be an enhancing or precipitating factor in the pathogenesis of GIE (McNicholl *et al.*, 1976).

Weiser and Douglas (1976) have proposed a lectin-like harmful action of gluten on intestinal epithelial cells; this interaction could involve incomplete glycoproteins on immature epithelial cells. Such moieties do indeed occur in large numbers in GIE mucosa, and immature epithelial cells have been shown to have increased reactivity to several known plant lectins, and lectin interaction can induce cell death. On the other hand, stress to enterocytes during enteric infections, inflammation, or increased gluten intake, could derange glycosyl transferases of intestinal epithelial cells and interfere with the synthesis of oligosaccharide side chains of cell surface glycoproteins. This original hypothesis has gained support by the demonstration that mucosa of patients with celiac disease indeed binds the gluten fraction Glyc-Gli (Douglas, 1976).

Increased permeability of the mucosa has been repeatedly demonstrated in GIE patients (e.g., Parkins, 1960). Green and Wollaenger (1960) showed hypoalbuminemia in 60% of celiac disease patients in the United States; more recently, Bai *et al.* (1991) reported decreased serum albumin in 54% of Argentinian patients. Increased intestinal permeability has been proposed as a factor in the pathogenesis of GIE. It was suggested that facilitated influx of gluten or prolamin-derived peptides may lead to enhanced or deregulated immunological reactivity in the mucosa, or to direct toxicity. However, evaluation of the impact of hyperpermeability on the development of GIE remains difficult. On one hand it seems probable that untreated patients have more permeability disturbances than treated patients (e.g., Bai *et al.*, 1991); this suggests that permeability changes observed in GIE are secondary to the tissue lesions in the mucosa. On the other hand, a recent report (van Elburg *et al.*, 1993) on sugar absorption in patients with celiac disease showed a significantly increased ratio of lactulose vs. mannitol in the urine of patients as well as their relatives; this suggests that asymptomatic relatives of GIE patients may have increased intestinal permeability, and that such hyperpermeability may contribute to the pathogenesis of GIE.

Involvement of immune reactions in the pathogenesis of GIE is evidenced by a large number of observations (Kagnoff 1989a,b; Cole and Kagnoff, 1985; Marsh, 1989; Brandtzaeg *et al.*, 1991). However, it still seems difficult to assign convincingly to any of the collected data a definitive place and value in the pathogenesis of GIE and to formulate a hypothesis compatible with the great majority of observations. Over the past few years, many studies have evaluated exciting aspects of the immune response in GIE. In the following section, we review the major of the findings and hypotheses proposed for an immunopathogenesis of GIE.

Any role for atopic and anaphylactic reactivity in the pathogenesis of GIE remains to be established. Some researchers have reported a significant increase of asthma, eczema, and urticaria in patients with GIE compared with the healthy population (Friedman and Hare, 1965; Hodgson *et al.*, 1976; Williams *et al.*, 1984). Others could not confirm these results (Cooper *et al.*, 1978). However, improvement of eczema has been reported on gluten withdrawal (Cooper *et al.*, 1978). A child on a gluten-free diet was reported to develop systemic anaphylaxis after introduction of small amounts of gluten ("gluten shock"; Krainick *et al.*, 1958). However, no differences in serum IgE concentrations exist between patients with GIE and normal controls (Williams *et al.*, 1984), and antibodies of the IgE isotype that react with wheat proteins were not elevated in the circulation of patients with GIE (Bahna *et al.*, 1980). Immediate hypersensitivity skin tests with gluten were not detectable in these patients (Baker and Read, 1976). On the other hand, IgE-producing cells increase in numbers in the jejunal mucosa of both untreated and treated patients with celiac disease (Scott *et al.*, 1983). Gluten challenge leads to further increase of frequency of IgE-producing plasma cells (O'Donoghue *et al.*, 1979). A Type I hypersensitivity reaction, according to Gell and Coombs, has been described in patients with GIE; mast cell degranulation and increased concentrations of histamine and 5-hydroxytrptamine occur in the intestinal lesional mucosa, followed by influx of eosinophilic granulocytes (McLaughlin *et al.*, 1983; Strobel *et al.*, 1983). Collectively, these data suggest a secondary rather than a primary involvement of atopic reactions in GIE. Atopy in GIE possibly results from increased permeability of the gut to various allergens.

Numbers of IgA, IgG and IgM-producing plasma cells are increased in lesional mucosa of GIE; (Brandtzaeg *et al.*, 1991). Concurrently, the percentage of plasma cells producing antibodies to gliadin is increased in GIE mucosa (Brantzaeg *et al.*, 1991). In some patients with dermatitis herpetiformis, IgA and IgM isotype antibodies to gliadin are demonstrable in the intestinal fluid only (Kett *et al.*, 1990). Since this disease is related closely to, or a variant of, celiac disease, this finding has been interpreted to suggest that IgA and IgM gliadin antibodies in the intestinal lumen are the hallmark of early GIE (O'Mahony *et al.*, 1990;1991; Brandtzaeg *et al.*, 1991; Ferguson *et al.*, 1993; Marsh 1993). As the disease progresses, IgA isotype antibodies to gliadin increase in circulation also, whereas IgM isotype antibodies do not (Baklien *et al.*, 1977). Since IgM has a stronger affinity for secretory component (SC) than IgA, IgM may be excreted efficiently into the intestinal lumen whereas IgA is inhibited from reacting with SC and thus finds its way into circulation (Brandtzaeg, 1985). Importantly, SC shows an enhanced expression on intestinal epithelial cells in GIE (Kvale *et al.*, 1988), and J chains are expressed more densely in IgA-producing cells in GIE patients than in healthy individuals (Kett *et al.*, 1990). Ultimately, however, more IgG- than IgA-producing cells are specific for gliadin (5.7% vs. 1.6%; Brandtzaeg and Baklien, 1976). These antibodies may contribute to the pathogenesis of GIE by interacting with gliadin adsorbed to epithelial cells or by formation of immune complexes. Terminal complement components (TCC) have been demonstrated in subepithelial sites of GIE mucosa (Brandtzaeg *et al.*, 1991). Complement-mediated lysis and sublytic effects of the membrane attack complex (MAC; Morgan *et al.*, 1988) could contribute significantly to the desquamation of surface epithelium observed in GIE (Brandtzaeg *et al.*, 1991). Alternatively, antibodies to gliadin may collaborate with K cells in antibody-dependent cellular cytotoxicity (ADCC). The only skin test reactivity documented to date in patients with GIE is an Arthus-like reaction agaist gliadin (Baker and Read, 1976; Anand *et al.*, 1977), which could suggest a major role for immune complexes in GIE tissue lesions. Finally, polymeric IgA has been shown to activate and degranulate neutrophilic and eosinophilic granulocytes, which could enhance the overall inflammatory response and damage epithelial cells (Abu-Ghazaleh *et al.*, 1989).

In addition to a possible role in the pathogenesis of GIE, several antibodies promise to play increasingly important roles in the diagnosis of celiac disease and related syndromes (WGESPGN, 1991; Ferguson *et al.*, 1993). In addition to antibodies to gliadin (Schmitz *et al.*, 1978), antibodies to reticulin (Mäki *et al.*, 1984), and antibodies to smooth muscle endomysium (Chorzelski *et al.*, 1984; Kumar *et al.*, 1989) have contributed significantly to the confirmation of diagnosis of celiac disease and dermatitis herpetiformis. Antibodies to endomysium (Figure 3) have proven to be of especially high specificity and sensitivity (Kumar *et al.*, 1989); their involvement in the immune reactions of GIE, however, remains to be investigated further.

Great potential for improved understanding of various syndromes of gluten sensitivity as well as for the institution of gluten free diet offer reports on a characteristic pattern of antibodies to food antigens detected in jejunal fluid and whole gut lavage fluids (reviewed in Ferguson *et al.*, 1993 and Marsh, 1993). Gliadin-specific antibodies of the IgA, but most impressively, of the IgM isotype were detected in a small group of patients with *dermatitis herpetiformis* lacking enteropathy (O'Mahony *et al.*, 1990) as well as patients with active, silent, latent, or potential celiac disease (O'Mahony *et al.*, 1991; Ferguson *et al.*, 1993). These pattern of antibodies was termed "celiac-like intestinal antibody" or "celiac-associated intestinal antibody pattern" and given the ominous acronym "CIA." Most recently, an extensive study was conducted on the presence of CIA, with special emphasis on celiac disease patients with normal jejunal biopsy histology

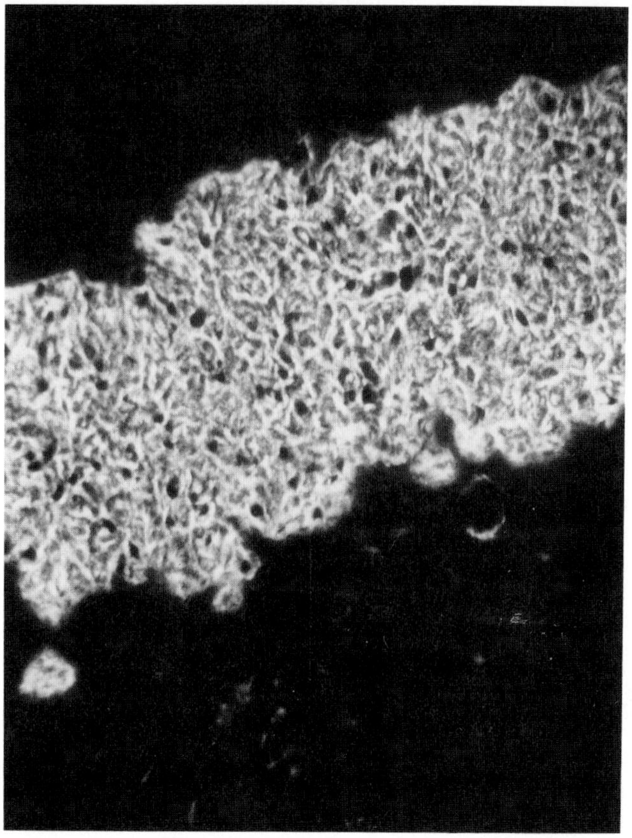

Figure 3 IgA-antibodies to endomysium from a patient with GIE. Indirect immunofluorescence on monkey esophagus. (Microphotograph kindly supplied by Dr. V. Kumar, Buffalo, New York.)

(Arranz and Ferguson, 1993). In addition to antibodies to gliadin, the intestinal fluid contained also increased titers of IgM class antibodies to ovalbumin and β lactoglobulin. Antibodies to food antigens have been described in a number of diseases. Thus, Knoflach *et al.* (1987) showed impressive amounts of circulating IgM-class antibodies to a number of milk antigens, including β lactoglobulin, in adult patients with inflammatory bowel disease (IBD), and a somewhat distinct pattern was seen in sera of pediatric IBD patients by Lerner *et al.* (1989). Occurrence of food antibodies in a variety of intestinal disorders suggests that at least some of them may be secondary to widely shared defects of intestinal function (e.g., increased permeability leading to enhanced penetration of the mucosa by antigens). The preferential increase in IgA and, most impressively, IgM antibodies may represent a characteristic mucosal antibody response pattern present in many diseases. However this may be, studies of CIA and of antigliadin antibodies in circulation (Ferguson *et al.*, 1993; Marsh, 1993) should open up new diagnostic potentials, especially in conjunction with other parameters, and help us define what may be called in future "gluten-sensitive disease complex."

An early influx of lymphocytes into the epithelium of small intestinal crypts has been demonstrated in elegant experiments (Marsh, 1988,1989). This event is followed by crypt cell hyperplasia and crypt hypertrophy, and by villus atrophy.

Especially in flat mucosa, $CD3^+CD45RO^+$ cells are frequent, attesting to T cell activation (Scott *et al.*, 1987). IELs also show morphological signs of activation (Spencer *et al.*, 1989a). The number of T $\gamma\delta$ cells has been shown to be increased among IELs (Halsensten *et al.*, 1989b; Spencer *et al.*, 1989b; Brandtzaeg *et al.*, 1991; Kutlu *et al.*, 1993). A high percentage of these cells employs the variable delta 1 gene ($V\delta - J\delta,2$), suggesting that a large proportion of these cells has a limited specificity (Spencer *et al.*, 1989a). The T $\gamma\delta$ cells could react with heat-shock protein (HSP; Born *et al.*, 1990) on stressed cells (Evans *et al.*, 1990; Brandtzaeg *et al.*, 1991). Indeed, HSP has been detected on jejunal epithelium of patients with GIE.

Enhanced T counter-suppressor cell activity among IELs (Brandtzaeg *et al.*, 1991) could contribute to an abrogation of oral tolerance, including that to gliadin. The abrogation of oral tolerance also could result from the increased expression of HLA-DR antigens on intestinal epithelial cells; several cytokines are known to mediate increased expression of HLA-encoded moieties (Scott *et al.*, 1987). Therefore, that increased HLA-DR antigen expression parallels the increase in numbers of $CD3^+CD45RO^+$ cells in GIE is of special interest (Scott *et al.*, 1987; Schreiber *et al.*, 1991). Obviously, cytokine production by activated T cells may have a wide range of effects, for example, induction of hyperplasia of crypt cells, increase of permeability of the intestinal epithelium, and stimulation of B cells and effector T cells (Brandtzaeg *et al.*, 1991).

Striking is the association of GIE with genetic markers (Falchuk *et al.*, 1972; Keuning *et al.*, 1976; Demarchi *et al.*, 1983). An extended HLA haplotype (Howell *et al.*, 1988) seems characteristic in GIE patients (Tosi *et al.*, 1983; Cole and Kagnoff, 1985; Corazza *et al.*, 1985; Alper *et al.*, 1987). The genetic markers include HLAB8 (Class I region) and SC01 in the adjacent Class III region. The strongest association between disease and major histocompatibility complex (MHC) haplotype is found in Class II moieties; these molecules are also of special interest in relation to immune responses, since Class II molecules participate in cell interactions, especially during antigen presentation. Of Caucasian patients with GIE, 80–90% show HLA-DR3 and HLA-DQw2 markers, whereas these markers are found in only 20% of healthy Caucasians. More recently, restriction fragment length polymorphism (RFLP) analysis using restriction endonuclease *Rsa* I defined a polymorphic 4-kb genomic DNA fragment in over 90% of HLA-DR3-/DQw2$^+$ patients with celiac disease, but only in 30% of healthy patients with this HLA haplotype (Howell *et al.*, 1986). The 4kb fragment is part of a gene encoding a HLA-DP β chain (Howell *et al.*, 1988). In addition, a similar polymorphism was suggested for the HLA-DP α chain-encoding gene (Hitman *et al.*, 1987; Kagnoff, 1989b).

Genes outside the HLA haplotype also seem to be involved in GIE, as was suggested by the much higher concordance rate for GIE among monozygotic twins (~75%) than among HLA-identical siblings (~40%) (Polanco *et al.*, 1981; Schols and Albert, 1983). Similarly, among individuals sharing the susceptibility HLA haplotype, disease manifests more frequently in the patients' family members than in nonrelated subjects (Kagnoff, 1989b). Thus, immunoglobulin heavy chain allotypic markers may show association with celiac disease (Kagnoff *et al.*, 1983; Weiss *et al.*, 1983). Particular MHC Class II gene products may enhance the presentation of selected environmental epitopes to T cells, and distinct immunoglobulin genes may up-regulate the magnitude and increase specificity of host antibody responses. The importance of environmental factors in the pathogenesis of GIE, however, is demonstrated clearly by the discordant pairs of monozygotic twins (Polanco *et al.*, 1981).

Kagnoff and co-workers (1984) have demonstrated a homology between amino acid sequences of A-gliadin and a dodecapeptide of the E1b protein of adenovirus type 12. These authors also showed that untreated patients with celiac disease had significantly more frequently infections with adenovirus type 12 than controls (Kagnoff *et al.*, 1987). Further, the homology region seems to be an antigenic determinant (Kagnoff *et al.*, 1987; Karagiannis *et al.*, 1987). Kagnoff and co-workers (1987) have proposed that such cross-reactive epitopes on microbial, most likely viral, moieties may trigger the reactivity to gliadin.

Several other factors may influence the immune response in GIE. Exorphins, opioid agonists similar to β-casomorphin, have been shown to be generated during digestion of gluten (Zioudrou *et al.*, 1979; Morley *et al.*, 1983). These molecules are known to influence, among others, the proliferation of LPLs. In addition, bacterial and nutrient antigens passing more easily through the intestinal epithelium in GIE patients than in healthy subjects could engage the immune system and contribute to its deregulation.

On the basis of the large but somewhat scattered portfolio of data on the pathogenesis of GIE, a comprehensive hypothesis can be envisioned. The initial event in GIE must be the coming together of genetic predisposition and environmental factors. The genetic predisposition could be some defect of the intestinal enzymes crucial in detoxifying gluten metabolites as well as a predisposition of the immune system, for example, enhanced gliadin presentation to T cells, abnormally active T counter-suppressor cells among IELs, and so on. The triggering event could be a lectin-like or toxic activity of gluten as well as its immunogenic property; alternatively, cross-reactive microbial epitopes, such as adenovirus type 12 E1b protein, could activate an immune response to gluten. The immune reactivity, induced either as a primary pathogenic mechanism or in response to lectin- or toxin-induced tissue damage, could lead to crypt cell hyperplasia and degeneration of surface epithelial cells by the action of cytotoxic T cells, cytokines, and antibodies or immune complexes activating complement or interacting with K cells in ADCC. Stimulating the immune response further, cytokines could enhance expression of MHC Class II antigens and modulate changes in immunologically reactive cells. The deleterious effect of the immune response could be amplified further by the induced expression of HSPs (Born *et al.*, 1990) on stressed cells and the interaction of T $\gamma\delta$ or other cells with these moieties. The destruction of brush border and degenerative changes in intestinal epithelial cells, as well as the ultimate loss of intestinal surface, possibly resulting from a combined onslaught of toxic and lectin-like gluten moieties and immune reactants, then causes malabsorption, which is the major clinical manifestation of GIE.

A two-stage model of GIE pathogenesis has been proposed by O'Mahony *et al.* (1990), comprising latent and fully expressed disease. The first stage is characterized by a genetically determined abnormal interaction of the immune system with gluten, without full-blown lesions in the gut, (e.g., T-cell activation in the mucosa without other changes, or isolated increased density of IEL). The second stage of severe or full intestinal involvement ("celiac disease" proper) could be triggered by a number of environmental factors or changes of endogenous regulatory mechanisms, illustrated by Ferguson *et al.* (1993) as episode of hyperpermeability, nutrient deficiency, increased dietary gluten, impaired intraluminal digestion of ingested gluten, adjuvant effects of intestinal infection and a HLA associated gene. Even though the interphase of these two stages of GIE probably still is very fuzzy, this hypothesis provides a workable framework for further research and is well supported by clinical and animal research. Clinically, the more recent realization of the high frequency of individuals showing abnormal immune response to gluten and other prolamins without manifest enteropathy fits well the two stage concept. In animal experiments, Troncone and Ferguson (1991) have shown that enteropathy in mice sensitized to gliadin does not occur after simple feeding of gliadin, but requires "triggering" factors, such as those associated with intestinal anaphylaxis or graft-versus-host reactions. The exact mechanisms that come to bear in this events are not well understood but could be enhanced antigen presentation, T-cell recruitment, enhanced expression of MHC class II antigens, etc. As such triggering events, obviously, inflammation induced by antibody or cell mediated mechanisms may be of importance.

Avoidance of gluten-containing food is the treatment of choice and results in complete restoration of absorptive function and reparation of the mucosal structure. In severe cases, patients should be supplemented with essential nutrients such as vitamin B_{12}. In some patients with transient adrenal insufficiency resulting from malnutrition, corticosteroids may be beneficial. Importantly, in patients with malnutrition, that is, before the effects of gluten-free diet have set in, parenteral, rather than oral administration of drugs seems preferable since drugs, like nutrients, may be absorbed abnormally in GIE patients (Trier, 1989b).

As bleak as the prognosis may be for unrecognized or inadequately treated GIE, the promptly diagnosed and treated patient with the disease, whether child or adult, has a very good to excellent prognosis. Only seldom may complications of GIE, such as peripheral neuropathy, not resolve completely (Trier, 1989b), and only few patients develop refractory sprue (Rubin *et al.*, 1970; Trier *et al.*, 1978) or ulcerations and strictures of the small intestine (Bayless *et al.*, 1967). A propensity for malignancies, however, is present in an appreciable number of GIE patients (Holmes *et al.*, 1976; Selby and Gallagher, 1979) and their relatives (Stokes *et al.*, 1976; Holmes and Thompson, 1992). Whether gluten-free diet influences these predispositions is not yet fully established (Holmes *et al.*, 1989).

2. Dermatitis Herpetiformis

Dermatitis herpetiformis (Alexander, 1975; Cooke and Holmes, 1985; Jordon and Provost, 1988) is a skin disease closely related in its intestinal manifestations to celiac sprue. This disorder is characterized by chronic papulovesicular lesions located symetrically on elbows, knees, buttocks, sacrum, face, scalp, neck, trunk, and sometimes oral cavity. The vesicles are subepidermal. The lesions are associated with intense pruritus. IgA deposits are found around microfibrillar bundles in the dermal papillary tips and along the anchoring fibrils on the basement membrane (Katz and Strober, 1978). Complement is activated (Provost and Tomasi, 1974; Katz *et al.*, 1980), and circulating immune complexes containing IgA occur in 40% of patients (Hall *et al.*, 1980; Zone *et al.*, 1980). IgA is found in lesional and extralesional skin (Chorzelski *et al.*, 1971), suggesting that the induction of tissue lesions relies on additional pathogenic factors, a situation similar to that seen in GIE (O'Mahony *et al.*, 1990). The etiology and pathogenesis of this disease still remains poorly understood. The hypotheses proposed to explain celiac disease also may apply to dermatitis herpetiformis. Of patients with this skin disorder, 90% have patchy duodenal and jujunal atrophy (Brow *et al.*, 1971) that cannot be distinguished from the lesions of celiac disease. However, gastrointestinal clinical symptoms, that is, diarrhea, fatigue, abdominal distension, and pain, are infrequent. Nevertheless, steatorrhea is seen often, usually combined with iron and folic acid malabsorption (Katz and Strober, 1978). In addition to malabsorption, protein loss into intestines as well as dapsone therapy may contribute to hypoalbuminemia (Cooke and Holmes, 1985; see Section III of this chapter).

Gluten-free diet is successful in restoring the intestinal tissue to normalcy more often than affecting skin lesions. However, all patients that show gluten-dependent improvement of skin lesions also have improvement of mucosal lesions (Cooke and Holmes, 1985). Gluten has not been found in the skin lesions (Cooke and Holmes, 1985).

3. Cow's Milk and Soy Protein Intolerance

Although food allergies may lead sometimes to fatal or near-fatal anaphylactic reactions, most often in children and adolescents (Sampson *et al.*, 1992), most food allergens (e.g., shellfish, fish, eggs, and nuts) do not lead to malabsorption. However, ingestion of cow's milk or soy bean protein may be associated with intestinal symptoms. Both food intolerance (i.e., a process induced by direct toxicity) and food allergy, (i.e., a process involving immune reactivity) could result in deranged mucosal absorption and permeability (F. Shanahan, 1993). Classically a time-limited condition of infancy (Walker-Smith *et al.*, 1978), cow's milk protein intolerance presents with jejunal mucosal lesions comparable to those of GIE (Kuitunen *et al.*, 1973; Walker-Smith *et al.*, 1978). However, the numbers of IELs usually are not as high as those seen in the intestinal epithelium of GIE patients (Walker-Smith *et al.*, 1978). In some patients, milk intolerance is combined with gluten sensitivity. Malabsorption may be induced by mechanisms similar to those operating in GIE (see Section II.C.1.). Patients may respond to soy protein with jejunal mucosal lesions comparable to those of cow's milk protein and gluten intolerance (Donavan and Torres-Pinedo, 1987). The treatment of choice for food intolerance and allergy is avoidance diet.

4. Crohn's Disease

The etiology and pathogenesis of chronic idiopathic IBD still are not well understood (Donaldson, 1989; Kagnoff, 1989a). However, increasing evidence suggests that the immune system plays an important role in the pathogenesis of the diseases. The two main diseases—Crohn's disease and ulcerative colitis—could be caused by two distinct pathogenic mechanisms. This topic is reviewed in detail in Chapter 38 of this volume, so a brief review will suffice here.

The early histopathology of Crohn's disease suggested a link to intestinal tuberculosis (Crohn *et al.*, 1932). This link, however, could not be substantiated. Only recently, a series of reports reawakened the hypothesis that mycobacteria may be an etiological agent in Crohn's disease (Burnham and Lennard-Jones, 1978; Chiodini, 1988). Currently, observations are accumulating which again caution against a pathogenic link between these bacteria and the disease (Ibbotson *et al.*, 1992; Stainsby *et al.*, 1993). Similar was the fate of other bacteria or viruses implicated over the years in the pathogenesis of Crohn's disease, and thus the quest for a microbial pathogenesis of this inflammatory bowel disease still remains in limbo. Both humoral and cell-mediated immune abnormalities have been described in Crohn's disease. Although circulating immune complexes seem not to be increased significantly in frequency or amount in patients with IBD (Soltis *et al.*, 1979; Knoflach *et al.*, 1986b), *in situ* formation of these reactants seems possible (Figure 4; Knoflach *et al.*, 1989), especially since complement activation has been suggested by demonstration of TCC and C3b in lesional tissue of both ulcerative colitis (Halstensen *et al.*, 1990) and Crohn's disease (Halstensen *et al.*, 1989b,c). The histopathological lesion of Crohn's disease consists of deep ulcers in the transmurally inflamed intestinal wall. Sankey *et al.* (1993) have shown that the earliest mucosal changes in Crohn's disease may be an accumulation of eosinophilic macrophages, defective basement membranes and ruptured capillaries with hemorrhages and fibrinol plugs containing platelet antigens. The vascular lesions could be, it seems, immunologically mediated, possibly facilitated by the abnormal reactivity of platelets in Crohn's disease (Webberley *et al.*, 1993). These reports suggest to look more towards the vasculature than the intestinal lumen in the quest for the early pathogenesis of Crohn's disease.

Many features of a response involving $CD4^+$ T cells have been reported. Increased Class II MHC expression is seen on intestinal epithelial cells (Selby *et al.*, 1983; Brandtzaeg *et al.*, 1987,1989; Morise *et al.*, 1991), many of the T cells of the lamina propria express interleukin-2 receptors as markers of activation (Schreiber *et al.*, 1991; Sengu *et al.*, 1991; Choy *et al.*, 1990), and high concentrations of soluble interleukin-2 receptor have been detected in serum of patients with active Crohn's disease (Brynskov and Tvede, 1990; Müller *et al.*, 1990). Macrophages are activated, and tumor necrosis factor (TNF) can be detected in sera from patients with Crohn's disease (Brandtzaeg *et al.*, 1991; Murch *et al.*, 1991), as well as in their lesional mucosa (MacDonald *et al.*, 1990) and feces (Braegger *et al.*, 1992). Lesional endothelin-1 production by activated macrophages and endothelial cells may contribute to vasculitis in chronic IBD by inducing intestinal vasoconstriction and ischemia (Murch *et al.*, 1992). These findings have been interpreted to suggest a primary T-cell hypersensitivity in Crohn's disease. Interestingly, the most exciting studies now are on cytokines (Fiocchi, 1993), adhesion molecules, and immune effectors. Such studies can best be done in animal models, and the re-evaluation of classical, and the search for new, models of IBD should allow dissection of the extremely complex interplay of exogenous and endogenous factors in this disease complex.

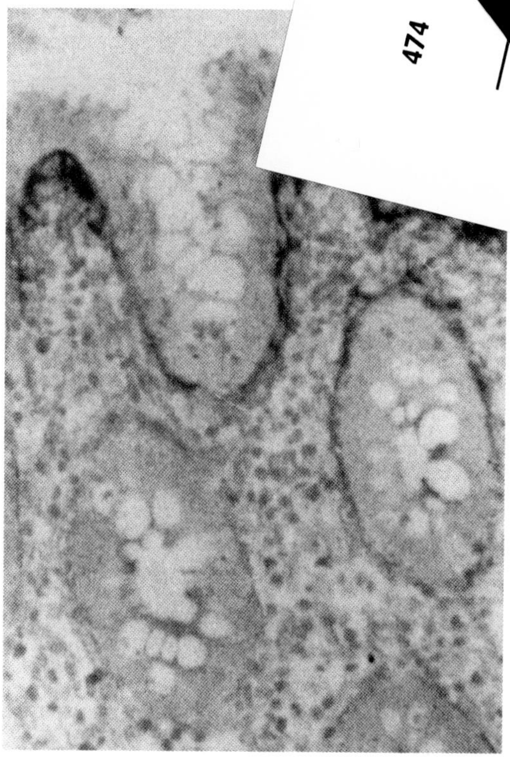

Figure 4 Colon of a patient with Crohn's disease. Granular IgG deposits along the intestinal basement membrane ×80. [Reproduced with kind permission from Knoflach, P., Albini, B. and Weiser, M. M. (1989). Experimental immune complex disease of the intestine. *In* "Immunology and Immunopathology of the Alimentary Canal" (B. Albini, R. J. Genco, P. L. Ogra, and M. M. Weiser, eds), Marcel Dekker, Inc., New York and Basel.]

The severe nutritional problems common in patients with Crohn's disease have a multifactorial pathogenesis (Table IV; Donaldson, 1989). Most important are deficiencies arising from anorexia and dietary restrictions (Sitrin *et al.*, 1980). However, the extensive inflammatory cellular infiltrates and the severe damage to the intestinal tissue impair absorption of several nutrients, especially carbohydrates and lipids, as

Table IV Malabsorption, Mucosal Permeability Change, and Malnutrition in Crohn's Disease

Clinical sign	Primary factor	Mechanisms
Malnutrition	Anorexia	Inadequate intake of nutrients
	Bacterial overgrowth	Altered bile salt metabolism (fat)
		Enhanced intraluminal catabolism (carbohydrates, protein)
Maldigestion	Mucosal inflammation	Disaccharidase deficiency
		Obstruction of lymphatics (fat)
		Derangement of epithelium and lamina propria (panmalabsorption)
		Enhanced catabolism of various moieties
Malabsorption	Therapy	Dietary restrictions
		Surgery: loss of absorptive surface (vitamin B_{12} malabsorption; panmalabsorption; bacterial overgrowth, see above)
		Sulfasalazine: Competition for folate conjugase binding sites (vitamin B_{12} malabsorption)
Mucosal permeability change	Mucosal inflammation	Diarrhea: fluid and electrolyte loss
		Protein loss: disruption of epithelium (ulcers)
		Immunologically mediated change of protein permeability
		Lymphatic obstruction
		Blood loss: iron deficiency, protein deficiency, reduction of lymphocyte numbers.

well as water- and lipid-soluble vitamins. Disaccharidase deficiency is common in these patients. On the other hand, Crohn's disease patients frequently have a normal absorption of vitamin B_{12}.

Stasis of intestinal content caused by stenoses and strictures leads to bacterial overgrowth and panmalabsorption (Donaldson, 1989). Entero-enteric or entero-cutaneous fistulas may dramatically reduce the length of bowel with absorptive capacity. Therapy of Crohn's disease can add to malabsorption; surgical resection or bypass operations reduce further the absorptive surface available (Donaldson, 1989), and administration of sulfasalazine may impair uptake of folate, possibly by competition for sites on intestinal folate conjugase (Franklin and Rosenberg, 1973; Selhub *et al.*, 1978). Lymphatics in these patients are often obstructed, which may impair fat absorption significantly (Donaldson, 1989).

In addition to malabsorption, the changes in intestinal mucosal permeability may lead to protein losing enteropathy (see Section III) and may allow increased stimulation of the immune system to otherwise-excluded antigens, which may explain the significant increase in circulating antibodies to cow's milk reported in adult (Knoflach *et al.*, 1987) and pediatric (Lerner *et al.*, 1989) patients with IBD, It is interesting that the characteristic intestinal fluid pattern of antibody described for celiac disease and its related disorders as well as IBD show impressive increases of IgM class antibodies to food antigens (Arranz and Ferguson, 1993). These similarities may suggest that permeability changes in these intestinal diseases are epiphenomena (i.e., common pathways of pathogenesis). However, some evidence suggests that permeability changes may antedate Crohn's disease (see Section III) and that such changes, as speculated also for celiac disease, may be a predisposing factor for disease manifestation.

5. Immunoproliferative Intestinal Diseases

Especially in countries located around the Mediterranean Sea, premalignant and malignant lymphomes of GALT have been reported, predominantly among underprivileged young adults 10–30 years of age (Rambaud *et al.*, 1968; Seligmann and Rambaud, 1969 Rambaud *et al.*, 1990). These proliferative disorders, primarily of B cells, often are associated with intestinal parasitic infestation (Rambaud and Seligmann, 1976). More than one-third of the patients have *G. lamblia* in their gastrointestinal tract. The disease most often is seen in the small intestines, which can be involved along the whole length; other segments of the gastrointestinal tract are involved only infrequently (Rambaud, 1983). This syndrome has been termed "Mediterranean lymphoma" (ML; Rambaud *et al.*, 1968). A similar presentation has been reported for a nosological entity called "alpha heavy chain disease" (αHCD; Seligmann *et al.*, 1968; Seligmann and Rambaud, 1969). For some time, the exact relationship between ML and αHCD remained open, since 70% of patients with ML were reported to lack α heavy chains in the serum. The lack of demonstrability, however, could be a function of limits on the sensitivity of the assays used to demonstrate α heavy chains (Rachmilewitz and Okon, 1985). In general, αHCD was thought to be either a subclass of immunoproliferative intestinal diseases or the same entity as ML (World Health Organization, 1976). Currently, α HCD, with predominantly B-cell proliferation, is frequently termed immunoproliferative small-intestinal disease (IPSID), whereas the bulk of what was formerly called ML, with diffuse cellular proliferation involving intestinal mucosa and without α heavy chain production, is termed "non-IPSID lymphoma" (Strober and James, 1992). Even though there are histological presentations preferred in IBSID and non-IPSID lymphomas, there is enough overlap to treat them here as one histopathological entity.

The intestines show diffuse thickening and induration of the affected intestinal segments and flat mucosa (Figure 5). Extensive cellular infiltration of the lamina propria is seen and, late in the disease, of the submucosa as well. In the early stages of the disease, infiltrating cells are polymorphic. The infiltrates consist of large and small lymphocytes, immunoblasts, plasma cells, granulocytes, and, sometimes, multinucleated giant cells (Rachmilewitz and Okon, 1985). The plasma cell lineage usually shows a variety of maturation stages, but sometimes rather uniformly mature plasma cells are seen. Later in the disease, the cells infiltrate the muscularis propria and may reach serosal fat (Rachmilewitz and Okon, 1985). Widespread lesions take on the typical appearance of immunoblastic lymphomas (Selzer *et al.*, 1979). Serum electrophoresis detects a protein in the $\alpha 2$ and $\beta 2$ region that reacts with antibodies to the α chain but not with antibodies to κ or λ chains (Selzer *et al.*, 1979). Serum concentrations of IgG and IgM usually are depressed (Rachmilewitz and Okon, 1985). In some patients, other truncated heavy chains (μ and γ) are demonstrable.

The primary clinical manifestation of IPSID and non-IPSID is severe malabsorption and diarrhea. Mild anemia, hypoalbuminemia, electrolyte imbalance, and low serum concentrations of lipids and cholesterol may occur. D-Xylose absorption, Schilling tests, and other assays of absorptive function tend to be abnormal. Serum often contains high concentrations of the intestinal isotype of alkaline phosphatase. Steatorrhea and creatorrhea usually exist (Rachmilewitz and Okon, 1985).

The cellular infiltrates mentioned earlier reduce the number of crypts and villi; in some patients, a flat mucosa as a result of complete villous atrophy is seen. The surface epithelium may be deranged and ulcerated. In this disease, malabsorption seems to be brought about primarily by the direct effect of proliferating cells of the B-cell lineage on the surrounding tissue and cells. In addition, the stagnant loop syndrome seen in this disease may contribute to the derangements of absorption (Doe and Hapel, 1983).

The heavy chains of immunoglobins in IPSID are truncated and often begin at sites of interdomain and exon boundaries (Korsmeyer, 1989). The molecular defects in HCD have been elucidated to some degree for μ- and γHCD (Alexander *et al.*, 1982; Bakhshi *et al.*, 1986; Guglielmi *et al.*, 1988); similar defects can be expected in αHCD, although the defects are multiple and varied. Bakhshi *et al.* (1985) have reported an aberrant RNA splice between the leader sequence and the constant region in μHCD. A small DNA insertion and deletion event removed a J4 donor splice site; thus an aberrant RNA splice between the leader region and the first exon (C_H1) of $C\mu$ arose. A recognition sequence for signal peptidase was created at the fifth amino acid residue of $C\mu$. As a result, a shortened μ chain was produced that lacked the V region and therefore did not bind light chains. In a γHCD, sequences probably of nongenomic origin were placed into a V region by a number of insertion and deletion events. Downstream, the C_H1 splice site was eliminated by an abnormal switch (Guglielmi *et al.*, 1988). A splice resulted between leader and hinge exon; the $\gamma 1$ protein amino-acid sequence indeed began inside the hinge region. In conclusion, the genomic defect in HCD seems to involve elimination of donor or acceptor splice sites through insertion and deletion events, inappropriate rearrangement, or somatic mutation. As a consequence, the leader exon is spliced to the next available Ig exon. Since the synthesized heavy chain proteins always are small, post-synthetic degradation seems not to be prominent as a mechanism of shortening the heavy chain in HCD (Korsmeyer, 1989).

Whereas μHCD plasmacytic elements synthesize light

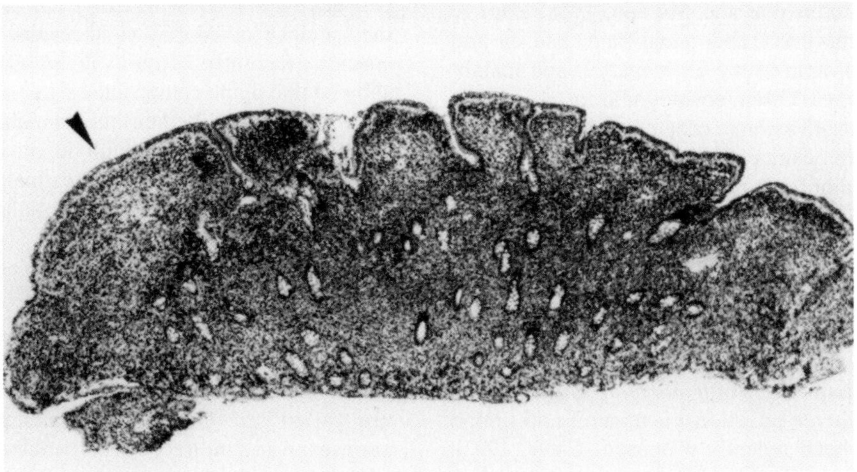

Figure 5 Jejunal biopsy specimen from a patient with alpha heavy chain disease. Extensive infiltration of the lamina propria by a polymorphous infiltrate. Villi are short and wide, number of crypts is reduced, and in one area, there is complete villous atrophy (arrow). [From Rachmilewitz, D. and Okon, E. (1985). Primary small intestinal lymphoma. *In* "Bockus Gastroenterology" (J. E. Berk, ed.), W. B. Saunders, Co., Philadelphia, with kind permission from the authors and the publisher.]

chains and result in Bence–Jones proteins in the urine of the patients (Korsmeyer, 1989), most γ- and αHCD patients do not produce light chains. In the latter, a dual defect involving both heavy and light chains has been postulated. Further, Wilde and Milstein (1980) have shown that free intact γ chains are toxic for cells. Light chain defects are most likely the primary events in γ- and αHCD; the simultaneous defects in heavy and light chains could be the results of hypermutational mechanisms in α- and γ-synthesizing B cells that are absent from μ-producing cells (Korsmeyer, 1989). In α-HCD, a variety of forms of heavy chain molecules appear in intestinal fluid, and a recent case report may shed some light on this aspect of the pathogenesis (Lucidarme *et al.*, 1993).

The diagnosis of IPSID and non-IPSID relies on multiple small intestinal biopsy. In IPSID, Ig heavy chains can be detected in serum and in the jejunal fluid. The serum concentrations of the abnormal protein usually fall as the disease progresses, and the plasmocytic elements become less differentiated. Mild forms of the disease may be treated with antibiotics. This could suggest participation of infectious agents in the pathogenesis of these syndromes. Without significant decrease in the synthesis of the abnormal α heavy chain molecule over 3 months, chemotherapy should be instituted (Rachmilewitz and Okon, 1985). Distinct palpable lymphomas should be removed surgically. The severe malabsorption should be treated by administration of fluids and electrolytes as well as blood units. Hyperalimentation sometimes is necessary (see Chapter 36).

6. Other Malabsorption Syndromes

Several other diseases involve the immune response and may manifest with malabsorption. Eosinophilic gastroenteritis is a disease of unknown etiology, associated with eosinophilic granulocytes infiltrating the mucosa of the esophagus, stomach, and small and large intestines. Peripheral eosinophilia and elevated serum IgE concentrations are common (Klein *et al.*, 1970; Johnstone and Morson, 1978; Zora *et al.*, 1984). The patients have abdominal pain, nausea and vomiting, diarrhea, protein-losing enteropathy, and malabsorption with steatorrhea. Often, eosinophilic gastroenteritis occurs in conjunction with asthma, eczema, or rhinitis (Cello, 1979). Tissue injury in eosinophilic gastroenteritis was suggested to involve a major basic protein released from eosinophilic granulocytes (Zora *et al.*, 1984). Diagnosis is made by biopsy of lesional tissue. Steroid treatment may be beneficial. Attempts to institute elimination diets usually are not successful, but the prognosis is favorable, although the disease may become chronic. (For the discussion of this disease and of food allergies in general we refer the reader to Chapter 40 of this volume.) A possible role of *hypochlorhydria, chronic gastritis,* and *Heliobacter* infection on mineral and amino acid absorption has been recently proposed (Cater, 1992). In chronic alcohol abuse, malabsorption may have several pathogenic roots (Roggin *et al.*, 1961; Rubin *et al.*, 1972). Primarily, pancreatic insufficiency and maldigestion are made responsible for the steatorrhea of alcoholics. Toxic epithelial cell damage may cause D-xylose, thiamine, and methionine malassimilation. In addition, small bowel motility may be increased and contribute to the diarrhea. Since immunological derangements have been described in chronic alcoholic abuse (MacGregor, 1986; Chadha *et al.*, 1991), we cannot exclude a contribution of a deregulated immune system to the malabsorption in such patients. Malabsorption can also be seen in autoimmune diseases of endocrine organs, for example, Grave's disease (Thomas *et al.*, 1973; Shater *et al.*, 1984), thyroiditides (Siurala *et al.*, 1968), Addison's disease (McBrien *et al.*, 1963), hypoparathyroidism (Clarkson *et al.*, 1960; Arulanantham *et al.*, 1979), and diabetes mellitus (Wruble and Kalser, 1964). Connective tissue diseases, such as progressive systemic sclerosis (Akesson *et al.*, 1985), systemic lupus erythematosus (Bazinet and Marin, 1971), rheumatoid arthritis (Dyer *et al.*, 1970), and Reiter's syndrome (Mielants *et al.*, 1985), may show malabsorption. In many of these disorders, increased deposition of collagen fibers in the small intestines may be of importance in the pathogenesis of malabsorption. However, systemic effects of the diseases on the immune system also may contribute significantly to bacterial overgrowth of the intestines and to malabsorption. Finally, many vasculitides may involve the small intestines and lead to malabsorption, for example, polyarteritis nodosa, Wegener's granulomatosis, and Henoch–Schoenlein purpura. In all these syndromes, immune responses likely are involved (Camilleri *et al.*, 1983).

With increasing age, the nutritional status of the individual tends to decrease (Webster *et al.*, 1977; Feibusch and Holt, 1982). This malnutrition of aging can be explained to a large extent by the anorexia that arises in old age. However, bacterial overgrowth also is seen frequently in the intestines of the elderly. Here, immunological changes of old age (DeWeck, 1984) could contribute to the malnutrition by facilitating bacterial infections of the intestines. However, mucosal immunity in aging is only poorly understood and seems not to reflect systemic changes. Using whole gut lavage, Arranz *et al.* (1992) obtained evidence for changes in IgA secretion and numbers of IEL in aged humans. Others have seen little changes of MALT with aging. As in all studies on aging, the species studied may yield results not applicable to other species. Recently, Taylor *et al.* (1992), using monkeys, showed that aging compromises gastrointestinal mucosal immune response. Whether there is malnutrition simply associated with aging in healthy individuals is not clear. Thus, Holt and Balint (1993), reviewing intestinal lipid absorption, could not find conclusive evidence for malabsorption in the aged.

D. Concluding Remarks

Malabsorption thus is observed in a large number of syndromes involving immune reactivity. The mechanisms by which immune reactions may contribute to malabsorption are varied and include humoral and T cell-mediated responses. As an indirect effect, deficiencies and dysregulation of the immune system contribute significantly to bacterial overgrowth and facilitate opportunistic infections and infestations of the small intestines, which then lead to inflammatory changes and malabsorption. On the other hand, infiltration of the small intestinal mucosa with immunoreactive cells, as seen in αHCD, may contribute to malabsorption by the derangement of tissue structure. Further, immune effector mechanisms—be they mediated by cytotoxic antibodies, ADCC, immune complexes, or delayed hypersensitivity mediated by $CD4^+$ or cytotoxic T cells and possibly natural killer (NK) cells—may damage or destroy intestinal epithelial cells and other structures of the mucosa and thus interfere with normal absorption. Proliferation of lymphocytes may obstruct the transport of absorbed nutrients; derangements of lymphatics may have the same effects. Finally, intraluminal antibodies may impede the absorption of nutritional moieties, increase their intraluminal digestion, or react with transport molecules, such as the intrinsic factor for vitamin B_{12}, and thus prevent their uptake. Still understood only in the most superficial way, the interaction of the immune system with gut and other hormones and the nervous system could contribute significantly to disturbances of the homeostasis of the small intestines and, thus, also to malabsorption. Further research is needed to obtain insight into the various pathways of immunologically mediated pathogenesis of malabsorption in the various nosological entities.

III. PROTEIN-LOSING GASTROENTEROPATHY

Many serum proteins are synthesized in the small intestinal mucosa, most importantly lipoproteins, complement components, and immunoglobulins. The gut also seems to play a role in the catabolism of plasma proteins (Waldmann, 1985). Most importantly, protein loss occurs also through the mucosa (i.e., there is an efflux of plasma proteins into the intestinal lumen). Healthy subjects show an enteric loss of plasma proteins of usually less than 1–2% of the body pool per day (Editor, 1959). In addition to being a site of synthesis and catabolism as well as protein loss into the intestines, the mucosa is a primary site of absorption of the products of protein digestion. Therefore, obviously, the gastrointestinal tract plays a significant role in the homestasis of plasma proteins.

Hypoproteinemia without plasma protein loss into the urine and with normal rates of plasma protein synthesis was described in the 1950s. Albright *et al.* (1949) were the first to demonstrate convincingly a major role of catabolism, rather than of deficient synthesis, in this condition. The loss of plasma protein into the intestinal lumen, however, was described first by Citrin *et al.* (1957). Since then, the term "protein-losing gastroenteropathy" denotes a gamut of gastrointestinal syndromes associated with excessive loss of plasma proteins into the intestinal lumen (Editor, 1959).

Protein loss into the intestinal fluid can be demonstrated by several methods (Jeffries, 1989), most of which require the use of radioactive markers. ^{51}Cr-Labeled albumin (Waldmann, 1961); ^{51}CrCl (Rootwelt, 1966; van Tongeren and Majoor, 1966; Walker-Smith *et al.*, 1967), which labels plasma proteins, predominantly albumin and transferrin, *in situ* in the patient; radioiodinated serum proteins (Sterling, 1951); as well as other radiolabeled plasma proteins (MacFarlane, 1957) have been used to measure intestinal loss in humans and animals. Most promising for clinical studies is the use of α_1 antitrypsin, which does not require radioactive markers (Bernier *et al.*, 1978; Thomas *et al.*, 1981). Tc-99m albumin scintigraphy can now be used to localize the site of protein loss in the gut (Oommen *et al.*, 1992).

Many gastrointestinal diseases manifesting malabsorption (see Section II) also show protein-losing enteropathy. Selected syndromes involving responses of immunoreactive cells directly or indirectly and often associated with protein-losing enteropathy are summarized in Table V. The end result of protein-losing enteropathy is hypoproteinemia. This condition manifests as dependent edema following decreased colloidal osmotic pressure of plasma and fluid transudation (Jeffries, 1989). Decreased plasma concentration of albumin in most patients is accompanied by diminished levels of fibrinogen, lipoproteins, α_1 antitrypsin, transferrin, ceruloplasmin, and, importantly, globulin (see Section IV). Blood clotting factors also are lost, but plasma proteins with a long half-life are affected more severely than those with a short life-span. The loss into the intestines, in contrast to many instances of proteinuria, is not selective regarding molecular size of the proteins; small and large proteins seem to be lost without preference (Jeffries, 1989).

With the exception of IgA and IgM bound to SC, intestinal epithelial cells are not known to transport any plasma proteins

Table V Syndromes Associated with Protein-Losing Enteropathy and Probable Involvement of the Immune System

Syndromes with disruption of intestinal epithelium:
Acute infectious enteritis
Chronic ulcerative jejunitis
Crohn's disease
Ulcerative colitis
Kaposi's sarcoma
Enteropathies in immunodeficient patients
Syndromes with impaired transport via lymphatics:
Intestinal lymphangiectasia
Tuberculosis (*tabes mesenterica*)
Infections of mesenteric lymph nodes
Whipple's disease
Lymphomas
Syndromes with unknown mechanism of intestinal protein loss:
Gluten-induced enteropathy
Allergic protein-losing gastroenterpathy
Eosinophilic gastroenteritis
Tropical sprue
Giardiasis
Campylobacter infection
Schistomsoma-associated polyposis coli
Dermatitis herpetiformis
Enteropathies in immunodeficient patients
Connective tissue disease
α Chain disease
Vasculitides
Rheumatoid arthritis
Nephrotic syndrome
Autoimmune diseases
Antibiotica-induced pseudomembranous colitis
Arsenic and heavy metal poisoning

actively into the lumen of the gut. Cells, and the intercellular spaces sealed off by apical junctional complexes, present a formidable barrier to protein efflux. Protein loss seems most likely to occur through rapid shedding of the epithelial cells, especially at the tips of the villi. Granger *et al.* (1976) have shown, in an experiment using Evans blue as an albumin tracer, that the villus tips of canine intestines were the sites of the most active protein transfer into the lumen. Extravasation of protein was detected by this method only with an experimentally increased venous pressure. This mechanism most likely plays a role in mucosal diseases without ulceration and in diseases with lymphatic obstruction (see Table V). With extensive erosions of the intestinal mucosa, protein oozes out of the lesional tissue, often accompanied by bleeding. The mechanisms leading to protein loss into the intestinal lumen can be summarized as follows: (a) lymphatic obstruction; (b) mucosal ulceration or erosion; (c) enterocyte damage or increased turnover; and (d) leakeage between enterocytes. Vascular derangements obviously can contribute to protein loss by increasing tissue fluid pressure, as well as by inflammation.

Immunologically mediated lesions of intestinal epithelial cells and their supportive structure may contribute in a variety of reactions to protein loss. Cellular and humoral immune mechanisms, involving cytokines and inflammatory mediators, are likely to be involved. Protein loss is seen in bacterial overgrowth of the small intestine and in viral and parasitic infections, and often accompanies primary and secondary immunodeficiency syndromes (Waldmann, 1985). Protein loss is frequent in allergic enteropathies, for example, cow's milk intolerance, and often is seen in GIE and dermatitis herpetiformes with intestinal involvement, in vasculitides, and in graft-versus-host disease developing after bone marrow transplantation (Epstein *et al.*, 1980; Jafri *et al.*, 1990). Many patients with IBD show protein loss, even in the absence of ulcerative lesions (Holman *et al.*, 1959; Steinfeld *et al.*, 1961). In Crohn's disease, there is a general hyperpermeability, and molecules can penetrate mucosa from the intestinal lumen easier than in healthy individuals. Interestingly, larger probes penetrate the mucosa better than smaller ones (Hollander, 1993). Of great interest for the understanding of the pathogensis of this disease is the current discussion on altered barrier functions in the mucosa of healthy relatives of patients with Crohn's disease (Mayer *et al.*, 1993). In systemic lupus erythematosus (SLE), the paradigm of a primarily immune complex-mediated connective tissue disease, intestinal protein loss may occur with or without proteinuria and may lead to severe hypoproteinemia (Bazinet and Marin, 1971; Trenthan and Masi, 1976; Brentjens *et al.*, 1977). Weiser *et al.* (1981) have shown the association of intestinal protein loss with intestinal venulitis characterized by immune deposits, that is, most likely, an immune complex-mediated venulitis (Figure 6).

In most of the patients with PLE and SLE—most of them young women— the mechanism leading to PLE is not well understood, since overt signs of intestinal vasculitis are missing (Perednia and Curosh, 1990). Possible candidates for this mechanism are intestinal lymphangiectasia, mucosal defects, chronic lupus enteritis (Nadorra et al., 1987), and cytokine induced capillary leakiness. Protein losing enteropathy may be associated with chronic interstitial cystitis and paralytic ileus in a subgroup of SLE patients usually responsive to steroid therapy (Meulders *et al.*, 1992). Protein losing enteropathy occurs also in Henoch-Schönlein's Purpura (Reif *et al.*, 1991) and other disorders related to the group of connective tissue diseases (e.g., Tsutsumi *et al.*, 1991; Stark *et al.*, 1992).

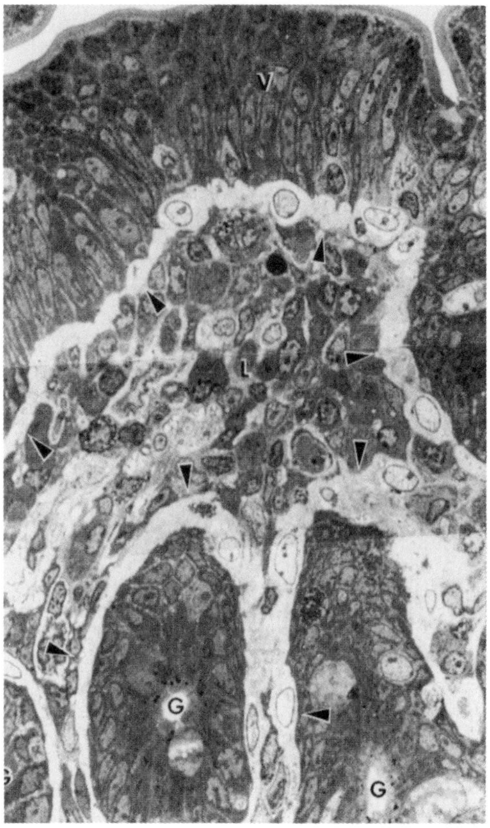

Figure 6 Thickened basement membranes in the intestines of a patient with systemic lupus erythematosus and protein-losing enteropathy. [Reproduced from Weiser, M. M., *et al.* (1981). *Gastroenterology* **81,** 570, with kind permission from authors and the publisher.]

Knoflach *et al.* (1989) studied mercuric chloride-induced enteropathy of rats (Sapin *et al.*, 1977; Knoflach *et al.*, 1986a). In this model, linear immune deposits, predominantly of IgA, had been documented along the intestinal basement membrane by Andres (1984). A shift from these linear and not complement-activating deposits to granular and complement-activating (Figure 7) deposits of IgG along the intestinal basement membrane entails significant increase of protein loss into the intestines (Knoflach *et al.*, 1989) that is accompanied by influx of granulocytes into subepithelial sites of intestinal mucosa and increase of mitotic figures among crypt epithelial cells, suggesting immune complex-mediated tissue injury and accelerated turnover of intestinal epithelial cells. The mechanism responsible for the change in the intestinal immune deposits, especially the switch from complement nonactivating to activating immunoglobulin deposits, is not yet under-

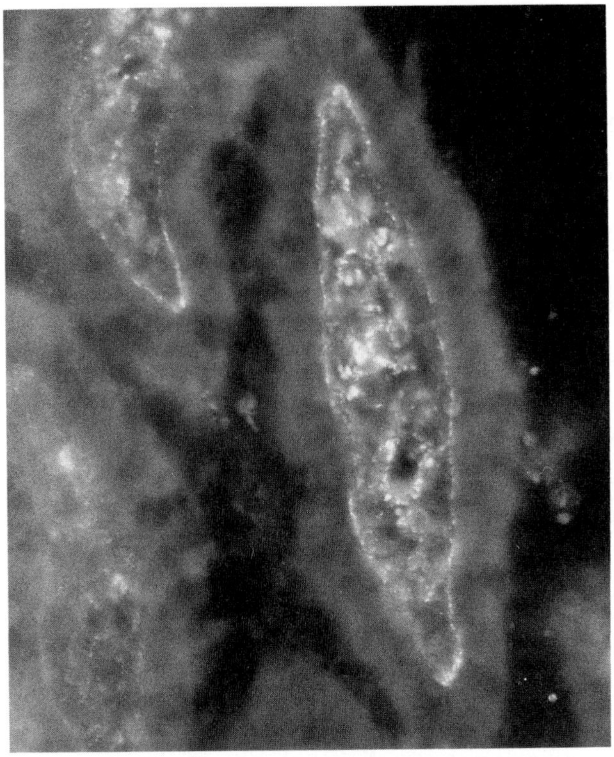

Figure 7 Complement C3 deposits in the small intestines of a rat with HgCl2-induced protein-losing enteropathy.

stood. It may be of importance, however, that rats with mercuric chloride-induced immune complex disease have anti-idiotypic antibodies as well as IgG rheumatoid factors several weeks into the experimental protocol (unpublished observations, Miyata, and Milgrom). This model seems to offer a well-defined approach to the study of immune complex-mediated protein loss into the intestines and may be of interest in increasing our understanding of heavy metal-induced, immunologically mediated injury of the gut. These studies on mercuric chloride-induced mucosal lesions have been confirmed and extended by others (Mathieson *et al.*, 1992; Hultman and Enestrom, 1992; Böhme *et al.*, 1992). Itoi *et al.* (1989) have, indeed, shown deposits of IgG, IgM, and C3 in capillary walls in the intestines of a patient with protein-losing enteropathy. Studies using gut lavage in patients with IBD have shown a close correlation of protein loss into the intestinal fluid and disease activity (O'Mahony *et al.*, 1991b; Choudari *et al.*, 1993). One could speculate that events similar to those leading to protein loss in the experiments of Knoflach *et al.* (1989) could operate also in IBD. Most recently, Halstensen *et al.* (1993) have demonstrated co-localization of IgG_1, terminal complement components and the 40 kDa "putative autoantigen" on the surface of colonic epithelial cells of patients with active ulcerative colitis. This finding supports the notion that an autoimmune reaction contributes to the pathogenesis of ulcerative colitis, and that complement activating antigen-antibody complexes may occur in active disease. Protein loss, especially in the presence of defects of the epithelium and bleeding into the intestines, may be associated with loss of blood cells, including lymphocytes (Douglas *et al.*, 1976).

IV. EFFECTS OF MALABSORPTION AND INTESTINAL PROTEIN LOSS ON THE IMMUNE SYSTEM

Malabsorption and protein-losing gastroenteropathy can lead to severe protein-energy malnutrition. However, even mild protein-energy malnutrition and selected nutrient deficits can have serious effects on the immune system (Doe and Hapel, 1983).

With severe protein loss into the intestinal lumen, hypogammaglobulinemia ensues, usually affecting IgG most severely because of its relatively slow rate of synthesis (Waldman and Strober, 1969). Whereas the hypogammaglobulinemia itself tends to have little impact on the health of the patient, a combination with malabsorption and loss of immunoreactive cells (Douglas *et al.*, 1976)—as observed, for example, in IBD, GIE, and intestinal lymphangiectasia—can induce overt secondary immunodeficiency (Sorensen *et al.*, 1985).

Obviously, malnutrition also influences GALT. Only scant data are available on this aspect of mucosal immunity, but the still preliminary results of human and animal experiments suggest a decreased secretory IgA response (Chandra, 1975); decreased numbers of IELs and LPLs (Barry and Pierce, 1979; Chandra, 1979), especially IgA-producing plasma cells; impeded migration of labeled mesenteric lymphoblasts in the entero-systemic cycle (Chandra, 1983); and decreased mucosal NK-cell activity (Chandra and Wadhwa, 1989). Several reviews are available on the topic of the effect of nutrient deficiency on the immune system (Chandra and Chandra, 1986; Chandra, 1989; Chandra and Wadhwa, 1989). A consequence of malnutrition is atrophy of lymphoid tissue. In the lymph nodes and the spleen, predominantly T cells are diminished in numbers. Helper T cells are affected more than T suppressor cells in protein-losing enteropathy (Muller *et al.*, 1991). Lymphocyte proliferation and other functions seem to be impaired, not only because of lack of nutrients, but also because of possible production of inhibitory factors. Delayed hypersensitivity skin tests are weak or negative in many malnourished individuals. Although humoral antibody-mediated responses tend to remain much longer intact than T cell-mediated reactivity, some evidence is available for inhibition of antibody formation to particular antigens, for example, *Salmonella typhi;* antibodies, even when produced in normal quantities, may have lower affinities. An increased incidence of immune complexes is seen in malnourished patients. Phagocytosis and availability of complement components are decreased by nutrient deficit. Vitamin B_6 deficit also has been shown to decrease lymphocyte stimulation responses (Chandra and Wadhwa, 1989).

Kowdley *et al.* (1992) have shown polyneuropathy and impairment of T-cell function in the wake of intestinal fat malabsorption and subsequent vitamin E deficiency; correction of the vitamin deficiency also led to improvement of the

T cell function. Diseases of the gastrointestinal tract often are associated with defective splenic function (Corazza and Gasbarrini, 1983); malabsorption as well as protein and lymphocyte loss may account for some aspects of these disorders. The combination of immunodeficiency, infection, malnutrition, and malabsorption creates a fatal spiral of mutually enhancing pathological processes, as seen most dramatically in AIDS and in other conditions (e.g., chronic diarrhea of childhood).

V. SUMMARY

Immune reactions may contribute to malabsorption (Section II), intestinal protein and lymphocyte loss (Section III), and increased influx of antigens (Cunningham-Rundles, 1987) in several diseases. Conversely, malabsorption and protein loss may lead to malnutrition and, thus, to derangements and deficiencies of the immune system. A vicious cycle may be established that insures chronicity of disease and continued deterioration. Obviously, infectious agents often participate in this deleterious interaction of the immune system and the gut, leading to derangements of intestinal permeability and absorptive funcions. Improved understanding of mucosal immunity is needed to enhance development of new diagnostic and therapeutic tools in gastroenteropathies associated with malabsorption or protein loss.

Acknowledgments

The authors thank Judy Marino for typing and retyping this manuscript.

References

Abu-Ghazaleh, R. I., Fujisawa, T., Mestecky, J., Kyle, R. A., and Gleich, G. J. (1989). IgA-induced eosinophil degranulation. *J. Immunol.* **142,** 2393–2400.

Ahlstedt, S., Carlsson, B., Fallstrom, S. P., Hanson, L. A., Holmgren, J., Lidin-Janson, G., Lindblad, B. S., Joohal, U., Kaijser, B., Sohl-Åkerlund, A., and Wordsworth, O. (1977). Antibodies in human serum and milk induced by enterobacteria and food proteins. *Ciba Found. Symp.* **46,** 115–129.

Ahnen, D. J., and Brown, W. R. (1982). *Campylobacter* enteritis in immunodeficient patients. *Ann. Intern. Med.* **96,** 187–188.

Akesson, A., Akesson, B., Gustafson, T., and Wollhein, F. (1985). Gastrointestinal function in patients with progressive systemic sclerosis. *Clin. Rheumatol.* **4,** 441–450.

Albright, F., Bartter, F. C., and Forbes, A. P. (1949). The fate of human serum albumin administered intravenously to a patient with idiopathic hypoalbuminemia and hypoglobulinemia. *Trans. Assoc. Amer. Phys.* **62,** 204–213.

Alexander, A., Steinmetz, M., Barritault, D., Frangione, B., Franklin, E. C., Hood, L., and Buxbaum, J. N. (1982). Γ-heavy chain disease in man: cDNA sequence supports partial gene deletion model. *Proc. Natl. Acad. Sci. U.S.A.* **79,** 3260–3264.

Alexander, J. O. D. (1975). "Dermatitis Herpetiformis." Saunders, Philadelphia.

Alper, C. A., Fleischnick, E., Awdeh, Z., Katz, A. J., and Yunis E. J. (1987). Extended major histocompatibility complex haplotypes in patients with gluten-sensitive enteropathy. *J. Clin. Invest.* **79,** 251–256.

Amarenco, P., Roullet, E., Hannoun, L., and Marteau, R. (1991). Progressive supranuclear palsy as the sole manifestation of systemic Whipple's disease treated with perfloxacine (letter) *J. Neurol. Neurosurg. Psychiatry* **54,** 1121–1122.

Ament, E. (1975). Immunodeficiency syndromes and gastrointestinal disease. *Pediatr. Clin. North Am.* **22,** 807–825.

Ament, E., and Ochs, H. D. (1973). Gastrointestinal manifestations of chronic granulomatous disease. *N. Engl. J. Med.* **288,** 382–387.

Ament, M. E., Ochs, H. D., and Davis, S. D. (1973). Structure and function of the gastrointestinal tract in primary immunodeficiency syndromes: A study of 39 patients. *Medicine* **52,** 227–248.

Anand, B. S., Truelove, S. C., and Offord, R. E. (1977). Skin test for coeliac disease using a subfraction of gluten. *Lancet* **I,** 118–120.

Andres, P. (1984). IgA-IgG disease in the intestine of brown Norway rats ingesting mercuric chloride. *Clin. Immunol. Immunopathol.* **30,** 488–494.

Aretaeus the Cappadocian (1856). "The Extant Works of Aretaeus." (I. E. Drabkin, ed. and transl.). Chicago University Press, Chicago.

Arranz, E., and Ferguson, A. (1993). Intestinal antibody pattern of celiac disease: occurance in patients with normal jejunal biopsy histology. *Gastroenterology* **104,** 1263–1272.

Arranz, E., O'Mahony, S., Barton, J. R., and Ferguson, A. (1992). Immunosenescence and mucosal immunity; significant effects of old age on secretory IgA concentrations and intraepithelial lymphocyte counts. *Gut* **33,** 882–886.

Arulanantham, K., Dwyer, J. M., and Genel, M. (1979). Evidence for defective immunoregulation in the syndrome of familial candidiasis endocrinopathy. *N. Engl. J. Med.* **300,** 164–168.

Asquith, P. (1979). "Immunology of the Gastrointestinal Tract." Churchill Livingstone, New York.

Bahna, S. L., Tateno, K., and Heiner, D. C. (1980). Elevated IgD antibodies to wheat in coeliac disease. *Ann. Allergy* **44,** 146–151.

Bai, J. C., Sambuelli, A., Niveloni, S., Sugai, E., Mazure, R., Kogan, Z., Pedreira, S., and Boerr, L. (1991). Alpha-antitrypsin clearance as an aid in the management of patients with celiac disease. *Am. J. Gastroenterol.* **86,** 986–991.

Baker, P. G., and Read, A. E. (1976). Positive skin reactions to gluten in coeliac disease. *Q. J. Med.* **45,** 603–610.

Bakhshi, A., Jensen, J. P., Goldman, P. G., Wright, J. J., McBride, O. W., Epstein, A. L., and Korsmeyer, S. J. (1985). Cloning the chromosomal breakpoint of (14;18) human lymphomas: Clustering around J_H on chromosome 14 and near a transcriptional unit on 18. *Cell* **41,** 899–906.

Bakhshi, A., Guglielmi, P., Siebenlist, U., Ravetch, J. V., Jensen, J. P., and Korsmeyer, S. J. (1986). A DNA insertion/deletion necessitates an aberrant RNA splice accounting for a μ-heavy chain disease protein. *Proc Natl. Acad. Sci. U.S.A.* **83,** 2689–2693.

Baklien, K., Brandtzaeg, P., and Fausa, O. (1977). Immunoglobulins in jejunal mucosa and serum from patients with adult coeliac disease. *Scand. J. Gastroenterol.* **12,** 149–159.

Barry, W. C., and Pierce, N. F. (1979). Protein deprivation causes reversible impairment of mucosal immune response to cholera-toxoid/toxin in rat gut. *Nature (London)* **281,** 64–65.

Baskin, D. H., Lax, J. D., and Barenberg, D. (1987). *Shigella* bacteremia in patients with the acquired immunodeficiency syndrome. *Am. J. Gastroenterol.* **82,** 338–341.

Bayless, T. M., Kapelowitz, R. F., Shelly, W. M., Ballinger, W. F., II., and Hendrix, T. R. (1967). Intestinal ulceration: A complication of celiac disease. *N. Engl. J. Med.* **276,** 996–1002.

Bazinet, P., and Marin, G. (1971). Malabsorption in systemic lupus erythematosus with protein-losing enteropathy. *Dig. Dis. Sci.* **16,** 460–471.

Beiser, W. R. (1987). Metabolic response of host to infections. *In* "Textbook of Pediatric Infectious Diseases." (R. D. Feigin and J. D. Cheny, eds.), pp. 1–16. W. B. Saunders, Philadelphia.

Berheim, A., and Berger, R. (1988). Cytogenetic studies of Burkitt, lymphoma-leukemia in patients with acquired immunodeficiency syndrome. *Cancer Genet. Cytogenet.* **32,** 67–74.

Bernier, J. J., Floerent, C., Desmazures, C., Aymes, C., and L'Hirondel, C. (1978). Diagnosis of protein losing enteropathy by gastrointestinal clearance of alpha antitrypsin. *Lancet* **II,** 763–764.

Bloom, B. R., and Murray, C. J. L. (1992). Tuberculosis: Commentary on a reemergent killer. *Science* **257,** 1055–1064.

Böhme, M., Diener, M., Mestres, P., and Rummel, W. (1992). Direct and indirect actions of $HgCl_2$ and methyl mercury chloride on permeability and chloride secretion across the rat colonic mucosa. *Toxicol. Appl. Pharmacol.* **114,** 285–294.

Born, W., Happ, M. P., Dallas, A., Reardon, C., Kubo, R., Shinnick, T., Brennan, P., and O'Brien, R. (1990). Recognition of heat shock proteins and $T\gamma\delta$ cell function. *Immunol. Today* **11,** 40–43.

Braegger, C. P., Nicholl, S., Murch, S., Stevens, S., and MacDonald, T. T. (1992). Tumour necrosis factor alpha in stool as a marker of intestinal inflammation. *Lancet* **I,** 89–91.

Bramble, M. G., Zucoloto, S., Wright, N. A., and Record, C. O. (1985). Acute gluten challenge in treated adult coeliac disease: A morphometric and enzymatic study. *Gut* **26,** 169–174.

Brandborg, L. L., Tankersley, C. B., Gottlieb, S., Barancik, M., and Sartor, V. E. (1967). Histological demonstration of mucosal invasion by *Giardia lamblia* in man. *Gastroenterology* **52,** 143–150.

Brandt deOliveira, R., Voltarelli, J. C., and Meneghelli, U. G. (1981). Severe strongyloidiasis associated with hypogammaglobulinemia. *Parasite Immunol.* **3,** 165–169.

Brandtzaeg, P. (1985). Role of J chain and secretory component in receptor-mediated glandular and hepatic transport of immunoglobulins in man. *Scand. J. Immunol.* **22,** 111–146.

Brandtzaeg, P., and Baklien, K. (1986). Immunohistochemical studies of the formation and epithelial transport of immunoglobulins in normal and diseased human intestinal mucosa. *Scand. J. Gastroenterol.* **11,** S1–S45.

Brandtzaeg, P., Baklien, K., Bjerke, K., Rognum, T. O., Scott, H., and Valnes, K. (1987). Nature and properties of the human gastrointestinal immune system. *In* "Immunology of the Gastrointestinal Tract" (K. Miller and S. Nicklin, eds.), Vol. 1, pp. 1–85. CRC Press, Boca Raton, Florida.

Brandtzaeg, P., Halstensen, T. S., Kett, K., Krajci, P., Kvale, D., Rognum, T. O., Scott, H., and Sollid, L. M. (1989). Immunobiology and immunopathology of human gut mucosa: Humoral immunity and intraepithelial lymphocytes. *Gastroenterology* **97,** 1562–1584.

Brandtzaeg, P., Farstad, I. N., Halstensen, T. S., Helgeland, L., Kvatum, M., Kett, K., Krajvi, P., Muller, F., Nilssen, D. E., and Scott, H. (1991). Immune functions in the normal and diseased human gut. *In* "Frontiers of Mucosal Immunology" (M. Tsuchiya, H. Nagura, T. Hibi, and I. Moro, eds.), Vol. 1, pp. 29–36. Excerpta Medica, Amsterdam.

Brasitus, T. A., and Sitrin, M. D. (1990). Intestinal malabsorption syndromes. *Annu. Rev. Med.* **41,** 339–347.

Brentjens, J. R., Ossi, E., Albini, B., Sepulveda, M., Kano, K., Sheffer, J., Vasilion, P., Marine, E., Baliah, T., Jockin, H., and Andres, G. (1977). Disseminated immune deposits in lupus erythematosus. *Arthr. Rheum.* **20,** 962–968.

Brow, J. R., Parker, F., Weinstein, W. M., and Rubin, C. E. (1971). The small intestinal mucosa in dermatitis herpetiformis. I. Severity and distribution of small intstinal lesions and associate malabsorption. *Gastroenterology* **60,** 355–361.

Brown, A. P., Lane, J. C., Murayama, S., and Vollmer, D. G. (1990). Whipple's disease presenting with isolated neurological symptoms. Case report. *J. Neurosurg.* **73,** 623–627.

Brown, W. R., and Strober, W. (1988). Immunological diseases of the gastrointestinal tract. *In* "Immunological Diseases" (M. Samter, D. W. Talmage, M. M Frank, K. F. Austen, and H. N. Claman, eds.), 4th Ed. pp. 1995–2033. Little, Brown, Boston.

Brown, W. R., Butterfield, D., Savage, D. C., and Tada, T. (1972a). Clinical, microbiological and immunological studies in patients with immunologlobulin deficiencies and gastrointestinal disorders. *Gut* **13,** 441–449.

Brown, W. R., Savage, D. C., Dubois, R. S., Alp, M. H., Mallory, A., and Kern, F., Jr. (1972b). Intestinal microflora of immunoglobulin deficient and normal subjects. *Gastroenterology* **62,** 1143–1152.

Bruton, O. C. (1952). Agammaglobulinemia. *Pediatrics* **9,** 722–728.

Bryk, D., Farman, J., and Dalleman, S. (1978). Kaposi's sarcoma of the intestinal tract: roentgen manifestations. *Gastroint. Radiol.* **3,** 425.

Brynskov, J., and Tvede, N. (1990). Plasma interleukin-2 and soluble/shed interleukin-2 receptor in serum of patients with Crohn's disease. Effect of cyclosporin. Gut **31,** 795–799.

Budhraja, M., Levndoglu, H., and Sherer, R. (1985). Spectrum of sigmoidoscopic findings in AIDS patients with diarrhea. *Am. J. Gastroenterol.* **80,** 828A.

Burnham, W. R., and Lennard-Jones, J. E. (1978). Mycobacteria as a possible cause of inflammatory bowel disease. *Lancet.* **ii,** 693–696.

Camilleri, M., Pusey, C. D., Chadwick, V. S., and Rees, A. J. (1983). Gastrointestinal manifestations of systemic vasculitis. *Q. J. Med.* **206,** 141–149.

Canturee, A. R. (1982). Histologic observations of variable acid-fast pleomorphic bacteria in systemic sarcoidosis: A report of 3 cases. *Growth* **46,** 113–121.

Castro, G. A., Badial-Aceves, F., Smith, J. W., Dudrick, S. J., and Weisbrodt, N. W. (1976). Altered small bowel propulsion associated with parasitism. *Gastroenterology* **71,** 620–625.

Cater, R. E. III. (1992). The clinical importance of hypochlorhydria (A consequence of chronic Heliobacter infection): Its possible etiological role in mineral and amino acid malabsorption, depression, and other syndromes. *Med. Hypotheses* **39,** 375–383.

Cello, J. P. (1979). Eosinophilic gastroenteritis—A complex disease entity. *Am. J. Med.* **67,** 1097–1104.

Centers for Disease Control (1982). Update on acquired immunodeficiency syndrome (AIDS) in the United States. *Morbid. Mortal. Wkly. Rep.* **24,** 507–509.

Chaisson, R. (1993). Mycobacterial infections and HIV. *Current Opin. Infect. Dis.* **6,** 237–243.

Chadha, K. C., Stadler, I., Albini, B., Nakeeb, S. M., and Thacore, H. R. (1991). Effect of alcohol on spleen cells and their functions in C57B1/6 mice. *Alcohol* **8,** 481–485.

Chandra, R. K. (1975). Reduced secretory antibody response to live attenuated measles and poliovirus vaccines in malnourished children. *Br. Med. J.* **2,** 583–585.

Chandra, R. K. (1979). Nutritional deficiency and susceptibility to infection. *Bull. WHO* **57,** 167–177.

Chandra, R. K. (1983). The nutrition-immunity-infection nexus: The enumeration and functional assessment of lymphocyte subsets in nutritional deficiency. *Nutr. Res.* **3,** 605–615.

Chandra, R. K. (1989). Nutritional regulation of immunity and risk of infection in old age. *Immunology* **67,** 141–147.

Chandra, R. K., and Wadhwa, M. (1989). Nutritional modulation of intestinal mucosal immunity. *Immunol. Invest.* **18,** 119–126.

Chandra, S., and Chandra, R. K. (1986). Nutrition, immune response, and outcome. *Prog. Food Nutr. Sci.* **10,** 1–65.

Char, S. Cevallos, A. M., Yamson, P., Sullivan, P. B., Neale, G., and Farthing, M. J. G. (1993). Impaired IgA response to Giarodia heat shock antigen in children with persistent diarrhoea and giardiasis. *Gut* **34,** 38–40.

Chiodini, R. J. (1988). Identification of mycobacteria from Crohn's disease by restriction polymorphism of the 5s ribosomal DNA genes. *In* Inflammatory Bowel disease. Current status and future approach. (R. P. MacDermott, ed.), pp. 509–514. Elsevier, Amsterdam.

Chorzelski, T. P., Beutner, E. H., Jablonska, S., Blaszczyk, M., and Triftshauser, C. (1971). Immunofluorescent studies in the diagnosis of dermatitis herpetiformis and its differentiation from bullous pemphigoid. *J. Invest. Dermatol.* **56,** 373–380.

Chorzelski, T. P., Beutner, E. H., Sulej, J., Tchorzewska, H., Jablonska, S., Kumar, V., and Kapuscinska, A. (1984). IgA antiendomysium antibody. A new immunologic marker of dermatitis herpetiformis and coeliac disease. *Br. J. Dermatol.* **111,** 395–402.

Choudari, C. P., O'Mahony, S., Brydon, G., Mwantembe, O., and Ferguson, A. (1993). Gut lavage fluid protein concentrations: Objective measures of disease activity in inflammatory bowel disease. *Gastroenterology* **104,** 1064–1071.

Choy, M. Y., Walker-Smith, J. A., Williams, C. B., and MacDonald, T. T. (1990). Differential expression of CD25 (interleukin-2 receptor) on lamina propria T cells and macrophages in the intestinal lesions in Crohn's disease and ulcerative colitis. *Gut* **31,** 1365–1370.

Chuttani, H. K., Kasthuri, D., and Misra, R. C. (1968). Course and prognosis of tropical sprue. *J. Trop. Med. Hyg.* **71,** 96–99.

Citrin, Y., Sterling, K., and Halsted, J. A. (1957). Mechanism of hypoproteinemia associated with giant hypertrophy of gastric mucosa. *N. Engl. J. Med.* **257,** 906–912.

Clarkson, B. O., Kowlessar, O. D., Horwith, M., and Sleisenger, M. H. (1960). Clinical and metabolic study of a patient with malabsorption and hypoparathyroidism. *Metabolism* **9,** 1093–1106.

Clayton, F. (1991). Gross and microscopic pathology of AIDS in the gastrointestinal tract. *In* "Gastrointestinal and Nutritional Manifestions of the Acquired Immunodeficiency Syndrome" (D. P. Kotler, ed.), pp. 141–186. Raven Press, New York.

Cleveland, W. W. (1975). Immunologic reconstitution in the DiGeorge syndrome by fetal thymic transplant. *Birth Defects* **11,** 352–365.

Cole, S. G., and Kagnoff, M. F. (1985). Celiac disease. *Ann. Rev. Nutr.* **5,** 241–266.

Collin, P., Halstrom, O., Maki, M., Viander, M., and Keyrilainen, O. (1990). Atypical coeliac disease found with serologic screening. *Scand. J. Gastronetrol.* **25,** 245–250.

Cooke, W. T., and Holmes, G. K. T. (1985). Gluten-induced enteropathy (celiac disease). *In* "Bockus Gastroenterology" (J. E. Berk, ed.), 4th Ed. pp. 1719–1757. Saunders, Philadelphia.

Cooper, B. T., Holmes, G. K. T., and Cooke, W. T. (1978). Coeliac disease and immunological disorders. *Br. Med. J.* **1,** 537–539.

Corazza, G. R., and Gasbarrini, G. (1983). Defective splenic function and its relation to bowel disease. *Clin. Gastroenterol.* **12,** 651–669.

Corazza, G. R., Tabacchi, P., Frisoni, M., Prati, C., and Gasbarrini, G. (1985). DR and non-DR Ia allotypes are associated with susceptibility to coeliac disease. *Gut* **26,** 1210–1213.

Corcino, J. J., Maldonado, M., and Klipstein, F. A. (1983). Intestinal perfusion studies in tropical sprue. I. Transport of water, electrolytes and D-xylose. *Gastroenterology* **65,** 192–198.

Cortner, J. A. (1959). Giardiasis, a cause of celiac syndrome. *Am. J. Dis. Child* **98,** 311–318, 1959.

Crago, S. S., and Mestecky, J. (1985). Presence of antibodies to food antigens in human milk and milk cells. *Protides Biol. Fluids* **32,** 227–230.

Crohn, B. B., Ginzburg, L., and Oppenheimer, G. D. (1932) Regional ileitis: A pathologic and clinical entity. *JAMA* **99,** 1323–1329.

Cunningham-Rundles, C. (1987). Failure of antigen exclusion. *In* "Food Allergy and Intolerance" (J. Brostoff and S. J. Challacombe, eds.), pp. 223–236. Bailliere Tindall, London.

Cunningham-Rundles, C., Brandeis, W. E., Good, R. A., and Day, N. K. (1979). Bovine antigens and the formation of circulating immune complexes in selective immunoglobulin A deficiency. *J. Clin. Invest.* **64,** 272–279.

Current, W. L., Reese, N. C., Ernst, J. V., Bailey, W. S., Heyman, M. B., and Weinstein, W. M. (1983). Human cryptosporidiosis in immunocompetent and immunodeficient persons. Studies on an outbreak and experimental transmission. *N. Engl. J. Med.* **308,** 1252–1257.

Damsker, B., and Bottone, E. J. (1985). *Mycobacterium avium-intracellulare* from the intestinal tracts of patients with acquired immunodeficiency syndrome: Concepts regarding acquisition and pathogenesis. *J. Infect. Dis.* **151,** 179–181.

Davidson, A. G. F., and Bridges, M. A., (1987). Coeliac disease: A critical review of etiology and pathogenesis. *Clin. Chim. Acta* **163,** 1–40.

DeHovitz, J. A., Pape, J. W., Bohcy, M., and Johnson, W. D., Jr. (1986). Clinical manifestations and therapy of *Isospora belli* infection in patients with the acquired immunodeficiency syndrome. *N. Engl. J. Med* **315,** 87–90.

Demarchi, M., Carbonara, A., Ansaldi, N., Santini, B., Barbera, C., Borelli, I., Rossino, P., and Rendine, S. (1983). HLA-DR3 and DR7 in coeliac disease: Immunogenetic and clinical aspects. *Gut* **24,** 706–712.

Desportes, I., LeCharpentier, Y., Galian, A., Bernard, F., Cochand-Priollet, B., Lavegne, A., Ravisse, P., and Modigliani, R. (1985). Occurrence of a new microsporidium: *Enterocytozoon bieneusi*; n. g., n. sp., in the enterocytes of a human patient with AIDS. *J. Protozool.* **32,** 250–254.

DeWeck, A. (1984). Lymphoid cell function in aging. *In* "Topics in Aging Research in Europe," Vol. 3. Eurage, Rijswijk, Iceland.

Dicke, W. K. (1950). Coeliac disease: Investigation of harmful effects of certain types of cereal on patients with coeliac disease. Ph.D. thesis., University of Utrecht, The Netherlands.

DiGeorge, A. M. (1968). Congenital absence of the thymus and its immunologic consequences: Concurrence with congenital hypoparathyroidism. *Birth Defects* **4,** 116–121.

Dissanyake, A. S., Jerrome, D. W., Offord, R. E., Truelove, S. C., and Whitehead, R. (1974). Identifying toxic fractions of wheat gluten and their effect on the jejunal mucosa in coeliac disease. *Gut* **15,** 931–946.

Dobbins, W. O., III (1985). Whipple's disease. *In* "Bockus Gastroenterology" (J. E. Berk, ed.), 4th Ed., pp. 1803–1813. Saunders, Philadelphia.

Dobbins, W. O. (1986). Human intestinal intraepithelial lymphocytes. *Gut* **27,** 972–985.

Dobbins, W. O., III, and Kawanishi, H. (1981). Bacillary characteristics in Whipple's disease: An electron microscopic study. *Gastroenterology* **80,** 1468–1475.

Dobbins, W. O., III, and Weinstein, W. M. (1985). Electron microscopy of the intestine and rectum in acquired immunodeficiency syndrome. *Gastroenterology* **88,** 738–749.

Doe, W. F. (1983). Immunodeficiency and the gastrointestinal tract. *Clin. Gastroenterol.* **12,** 839–853.

Doe, W. F., and Hapel, A. J. (1983). Intestinal immunity and malabsorption. *Clin. Gastroenterol.* **12,** 415–435.

Donaldson, R. M., Jr. (1989). Crohn's disease. *In* "Gastrointestinal

Disease" (M. H. Sleisenger and J. S. Fordtran, eds.), 4th edition. pp. 1327–1358. Saunders, Philadelphia.

Donovan, G. K., and Torres-Pinedo, R. (1987). Chronic diarrhea and soy formulas. Inhibition of diarrhea by lactose. *Am. J. Dis. Child* **141,** 1069–1071.

Douglas, A. P. (1976). The binding of glycopeptide component of wheat gluten to intestinal mucosa of normal and coeliac human subject. *Clin. Chim. Acta* **73,** 357–361.

Douglas, A. P., Weetman, A. P., and Haggith, J. W. (1976). The distribution and enteric loss of ^{51}Cr-labelled lymphocytes in normal subjects and in patients with coeliac disease and other disorders of the small intestine. *Digestion* **14,** 29–43.

Du Bois, R. M., Kirby, M., Balbi, B., Saltini, C., and Crystal, R. G. (1992). T-lymphocytes that accumulate in the lung in sarcoidosis have evidence of recent stimulation of the T-cell antigen receptor. *Rev. Resp. Dis.* **145,** 1205–1211.

Dubois, R. S., Roy, C. C., Fulginiti, V. A., Merrill, D. A., and Murray, R. L. (1970). Disaccharidase deficiency in children with immunologic deficits. *J. Pediatr.* **76,** 377–385.

Dworkin, B., Warmser, G. P., Abdoo, R. A., Cabello, F., Aquero, M. E., and Sivak, S. L. (1986). Persistence of multiple antibiotic resistant *Campylobacter jejuni* in a patient with the acquired immunodeficiency syndrome. *Am. J. Med.* **80,** 965–969.

Dyer, N. J., Kendall, M. J., and Hawkins, C. J. (1970). Malabsorption in rheumatoid disease. *Ann. Rheum. Dis.* **30,** 626–630.

Editorial (1959). Protein losing gastroenteropathy. *Lancet* **I,** 351–352.

Ehrenpreis, E. D., Patterson, B. K., Brainer, J.A., Yokoo, H., Rademaker, A. W., Glogowski, W., Noskin, G. A., and Craig, R. M. (1992). Histopathologic findings of duodenal biopsy specimens in HIV-infected patients with and without diarrhea and malabsorption. *Am. J. Clin. Pathol.* **97,** 21–28.

Elsagher, A., Lathigre, R., and Ivanyi, J. (1992). Localization of linear epitopes at the carboxy-terminal end of the mycobacterial 71 kDa heat shock protein. *Mol. Immunol.* **29,** 1153–1156.

Epstein, R. J., McDonald, G. B., Sole, G. E., Shulman, H. M., and Thomas, E. D. (1980). The diagnostic accuracy of the rectal biopsy in acute graft-versus-host disease. A prospective study of thirteen patients. *Gastroenterology* **78,** 764–771.

Erickson, R. H., and Kim, Y. S. (1990). Digestion and absorption of dietary protein. *Annu. Rev. Med.* **41,** 133–139.

Erlandsen, S., and Chase, D. G. (1974). Morphological alterations in the microvillous border of villous epithelial cells produced by intestinal microorganisms. *Am. J. Clin. Nutr.* **27,** 1277–1286, 1974.

Falchuk, Z. M. (1983). Gluten-sensitive enteropathy. *Clin. Gastroenterol.* **12,** 475–494.

Falchuk, Z. M., Rogentine, G. N., and Strober, W. (1972). Predominance of histocompatibility antigen HL-A8 in patients with gluten-sensitive enteropathy. *J. Clin. Invest.* **51,** 1602–1605.

Feibusch, J. M., and Holt, P. R. (1982). Impaired absorptive capacity for carbohydrate in the aging human. *Dig. Dis. Sci.* **27,** 1095–1100.

Ferguson, A., and Murray, D. (1971). Quantitation of intraepithelial lymphocytes in human jejunum. *Gut* **12,** 988–994.

Ferguson, A., Arranz, E., and O'Mahony, S. (1993). Clinical and pathological spectrum of coeliac disease—Active, silent, latent, potential. Gut **34,** 150–151.

Feurle, G. E., Volk, B., and Waldherr, R. (1979). Cerebral Whipple's disease with negative jejunal histology. *N. Engl. J. Med.* **300,** 907–908.

Fick, R. B., Jr., and Hunninghake, G. W. (1988). Sarcoidosis. *In* "Immunological Diseases" (M. Samter, D. W. Talmage, M. M. Frank, K. F. Austen, and H. N. Claman, eds.), 4th Ed., pp. 1587–1607. Little, Brown, Boston.

Fiocchi, C., (1993). Cytokines and animal models: A combined path to inflammatory bowel disease pathogenesis. *Gastroenterology* **104,** 1202–1219.

Fišchel, B., Burke, M., Sasson, E., and Felner, S. (1990). Acquired immunodeficiency, malabsorption and lymphoma. *Postgrad. Med. J.* **66,** 122–124.

Fisher, S. E., Smith, W. I., Jr. Robin, B. S., Tomasi, T. B., Jr., Lester, R., and VanThiel, D. H. (1982). Secretory component and serum immunoglobulin A deficiencies with intestinal autoantibody formation and autoimmune disease: A family study. *J. Pediatr. Gastroenterol. Nutr.* **1,** 35–42.

Forte, M., Maartens, G., Rahelu, M., Pasi, J., Ellis, C., Gaston, H., and Kumararatne, D. (1992). Cytolytic T-cell activity against mycobacterial antigens in HIV. *AIDS* **6,** 407–411.

Foucar, E., Mukai, K., Foucar, K., Sutherland, D. E. R., and Van Buren, C. T. (1981). Colon ulceration in lethal cytomegalovirus infection. *Am. J. Clin. Pathol.* **76,** 788–801.

Fox, C. H., Kotler, D., Tierney, A., Wilson, C. S., and Fauci, A. S. (1989). Detection of HIV-1 RNA in lamina propria of patients with AIDS and gastrointestinal disease. *J. Infect. Dis.* **159,** 467–471.

Frank, D., and Raicht, R. F. (1984). Intestinal perforation associated with cytomegalovirus infection in patients with acquired immune deficiency syndrome. *Am. J. Gastroenterol.* **79,**201–205.

Franklin, J. L., and Rosenberg, I. H. (1973). Impaired folic acid absorption in inflammatory bowel disease: Effects of salicylazosulfapyridine. *Gastroenterology* **64,** 517–525.

Frazer, A. C. (1956). Discussion on some problems of steatorrhea and reduced stature. *Proc. R. Soc. Med.* **49,** 1009–1013.

Freier, S., Eran, M., and Alon, I. (1989). A study of stimuli operative in the release of antibodies in the rat intestine. *In* "Immunology and Immunopathology of the Alimentary Canal" (B. Albini, R. T. Genco, P. L. Ogra, and M. M. Weiser, eds.). pp. 431–447. M. Dekker, New York.

Friedman, M., and Hare, P. F. (1965).Gluten sensitive enteropathy and eczema. *Lancet* **I,** 521–524.

Friedman, S. L., and Owen, R. L. (1989). Gastrointestinal manifestations of AIDS and other sexually transmissable diseases. *In* "Gastrointestinal Disease" (M. H. Sleisenger and J. S. Fordtran, eds.), 4th Ed., pp. 1242–1280. Saunders, Philadelphia.

Friedman-Kien, A. E. (1981). Disseminated Kaposi's sarcoma syndrome in young homosexual men. *J. Am. Acad. Dermatol.* **5,** 468–471.

Gardner, R. H. (1958). Tropical sprue. *N. Engl. J. Med* **258,** 791–796.

Gee, S. (1888). On the celiac affection. *St. Bartholomew's Hosp. Rep.* **24,** 17–20.

Glaser, J. B., Morton-Kute, L., Berger, S. R., Weber, J., Siegal, F. P., Lopez, C., Robbins, W., and Landesman, S. H. (1985). Recurrent *Salmonella typhimurium* bacteremia associated with the acquired immunodeficiency syndrome. *Ann. Intern. Med.* **102,** 189–193.

Goodell, S. E., Quinn, T. C., Mkrtichian, E., Schuffler, M. D., Holmes, K. K., and Corey, L. (1983). Herpes simplex proctitis in homosexual men. Clinical, sigmoidoscopic and histopathologic features. *N. Engl. J. Med.* **308,** 868–871.

Gorbach, S. L. (1989). Infectious diarrhea. *In* "Gastrointestinal Disease" (M. H. Sleisenger and J. S. Fordtran, eds.), 4th ed., pp. 1191–1232. Saunders, Philadelphia.

Gorbach, S. L., Mitra, R., Jacobs, B., Banwell, J. G., Chatterjee, B. D., and Guha Mazunder, D. N. (1969). Bacterial contamination of the upper small bowel in tropical sprue. *Lancet* **I,** 74–77.

Gottlieb, M. S., Schroff, R., Schanker, H. M., Weisman, J. D., Fan, P. T., Wolf, R. A. and Saxon, A. (1981). *Pneumocystis carinii* pneumonia and mucosal candidiasis in previously healthy homosexual men: Evidence of a newly acquired cellular immunodeficiency. *N. Engl. J. Med.* **305,** 1425–1431.

Gowen, A. E., and Campbell, C. B. (1973). Giardiasis—A cause of vitamin B12 malabsorption. *Am. J. Digest. Dis.* **18,** 384–390.

Gracey, M. (1981). Chronic diarrhoea in protein-energy malnutrition. *Paediatrica Indonnesiana* **21,** 235–239.

Granger, D. N., Cook, B. H., and Taylor, A. E. (1976). Structural locus of transmucosal albumin efflux in canine ileum. A fluorescent study. *Gastroenterology* **71,** 1023–1027.

Green, P. A., and Wollaeger, E. E. (1960). The clinical behaviour of sprue in the United States. *Gastroenterology* **38,** 399–418.

Greene, J. B. (1988). Clinical approach to weight loss in the patient with HIV infection. *Gastroenterol. Clinics North Am.* **17,** 573–586.

Guglielmi, P., Bakhshi, A., Cogne, M., Seligmann, M., and Korsmeyer, S. J. (1988). Multiple genomic defects result in the alternative RNA splice creating a human Γ H-chain disease protein. *J. Immunol.* **141,** 1762–1768.

Hall, R. P., Lawley, T. J., Heck, J. A., and Kats, S. I. (1980). IgA containing circulating immune complexes in dermatitis herpetiformis, Henoch–Schönlein purpura, systemic lupus erythematosus and other diseases. *Clin. Exp. Immunol.* **40,** 431–437.

Halstensen, T. S., Das, K. M., and Brandtzaeg, P. (1993). Epithelial deposits of immunoglobulin G1 and activated complement colocalise with the M_r40 kDa putative autoantigen in ulcerative colitis. *Gut* **34,** 650–657.

Halstensen, T. S., Scott, H., and Brandtzaeg, P. (1989a). Intraepithelial T cells of the TcR gamma/delta + $CD8^-$ and V delta 1/J delta 1+ phenotypes are increased in coeliac disease. *Scand. J. Immunol.* **30,** 665–672.

Halstensen, T. S., Mollnes, T. E., and Brandtzaeg, P. (1989b). Persistent complement activation in submucosal blood vessels of active inflammatory bowel disease: Immunohistochemical evidence. *Gastroenterology* **97,** 10–19.

Halstensen, T. S., Mollnes, T. E., Fausa, O., and Brandtzaeg, P. (1989). Deposits of terminal complement complex (TCC) in muscularis mucosae and submucosal vessels in ulcerative colitis and Crohn's disease of the colon. *Gut* **30,** 361–366.

Halstensen, T. S., Mollnes, T. E., Garred, P., Gausa, O., and Brandtzaeg, P. (1990). Epithelial deposition of immunoglobulin G1 and activated complement (C3b and terminal complement complex) in ulcerative colitis. *Gastroenterology* **98,** 1264–1271.

Hanauer, S. B., and Kraft, S. C. (1985). Intestinal immunology. *In* "Bockus Gastroenterology" (J. E. Berk, ed.), 4th Ed., pp. 1607–1631. Saunders, Philadelphia.

Hanngren, A., Biberfeldt, G., Carlens, E., Herdfers, E., Nilsson, B. S., Ripe, E., and Wahren, B. (1974). Is sarcoidosis due to an infectious interaction between virus and mycobacterium? *In* "Proceedings of the VI International Conference on Sarcoidosis" (K. Iwai and Y. Hosoda, eds.), pp. 8–11. University Park Press, Baltimore.

Heise, C., Dandekar, S., Kumar, P., Duplantier, R., Donovan, R. M., and Halsted, C. H. (1991). Human immunodeficiency virus infection of enetrocytes and mononuclear cells in human jejunal mucosa. *Gastroenterology* **100,** 1521–1527.

Hermans, P. E., Diaz-Buxo, J. A., and Stobo, J. D. (1976). Idiopathic late onset immunoglobulin deficiency. *Am. J. Med.* **61,** 221–237.

Hitman, G. A., Niven, M. J., Festenstein, H., Cassell, P. G., Awad, F., Walker-Smith, J., Leonard, J. N., Lionel, F., Ciclitira, P., Kumar, P., and Sachs, J. A. (1987). HLA Class II alpha chain gene polymorphisms in patients with insulin dependent diabetes mellitus, dermatitis herpetiformis, and celiac disease. *J. Clin. Invest.* **79,** 609–615.

Hodgson, H. J., and Jewell, D. P. (1977). Selective IgA deficiency and Crohn's disease: Report of two cases. *Gut* **18,** 644–646.

Hodgson, H. J. F., Davies, R. J., Gent, A. E., and Hodson, M. E. (1976). Atopic disorders and adult coeliac disease. *Lancet* **I,** 115–117.

Hollander, D. (1993). Editorial: Permeability in Crohn's disease: Altered barrier functions in healthy relatives? *Gastroenterology* **104,** 1848–1873.

Holman, H., Nickel, W. F., Jr., and Sleisenger, M. H. (1959). Hypoproteinemia antedating intestinal lesions, and possibly due to excessive serum protein loss into the intestine. *Am. J. Med.* **27,** 963–975.

Holmes, G. K. T., and Thompson, H. (1992). Malignancy as a complication of coeliac disease. *In* "Coeliac Disease" (M. N. Marsh, ed.), pp. 105–135. Blackwell Scientific Publ, Oxford.

Holmes, G. K. T., Prior, P., Lane, M. R., Pope, D., and Allan, R. N. (1989). Malignancy in coeliac disease—Effect of gluten free diet. *Gut* **30,** 333–338.

Holmes, G. K. T., Asquith, P., Stokes, P. L., and Cooke, W. T. (1974). Cellular infiltrate of jejunal biopsies in celiac sprue. *Gut* **15,** 278–283.

Holmes, G. K. T., Stokes, P. L., Sorahan, T. M., Prior, P., Waterhouse, J. A. H., and Cooke, W. T. (1976). Coeliac disease, gluten-free diet, and malignancy. *Gut* **17,** 612–619.

Holt, P. R. and Balint, J. A. (1993). Effects of aging on intestinal lipid absorption. *Am. J. Physiol.* **264,** G1-G6.

Hoskins, L. C., Winawer, S. J., Broitman, S. A., Gottlieb, L. S., and Zamcheck, N. (1967). Clinical giardiasis and intestinal malabsorption. *Gastroenterology* **53,** 265–279.

Howell, M. D., Austin, R. K., Kelleher, D., Nepom, G. Y., and Kagnoff, M. F. (1986). An HLA-D region restriction fragment length polymorphism associated with celiac disease. *J. Exp. Med.* **164,** 333–338.

Howell, M. D., Smith, J. R., Austin, R. K., Kelleher, D., Nepom, G. Y., Volk, B., and Kagnoff, M. F. (1988). An extended HLA-D region haplotype associated with celiac disease. *Proc. Natl. Acad. Sci. U.S.A.* **85,** 222–226.

Hultman, P., and Enestrom, S. (1992). Dose-response studies in murine mercury-induced autoimmunity and immune complex disease. *Toxicology Appl. Pharmacol.* **113,** 199–208.

Ibbotson, J. P., Lowes, J. R., Chahal, H., Gaston, J. S., Life. P. Kumararatne, D. S., Sharif, H., Alexander-Williams, J., and Allan, R. N. (1992). Mucosal cell-mediated immunity to mycobacterial and other microbial antigens in inflammatory bowel disease. *Clin. Exp. Immunol.* **87,** 224–230.

Ioachim, H. L., Cooper, M. C., and Hellman, G. C. (1985). Lymphomas in men at high risk for acquired immune deficiency syndrome (AIDS). *Cancer* **56,** 2831–2892.

Itoi, K., Sasaki, T., Sawai, T., Nakamura, M., Hiwatashi, N., Muryoi, T., Yokoyama, N., and Yoshinagi, K. (1989). Protein-losing gastroenteropathy in association with immune deposits in gastrointestinal mucosal capillaries. *Am. J. Gastroenterol.* **84,** 187–191.

Jackson, S., Dawson, L. M., and Kotler, D. P. (1988). IgA_1 is the major immunoglobulin component of immune complexes in the acquired immune deficiency syndrome. *J. Clin. Immunol.* **86,** 64–68.

Jacobs, J. L., Gold, J. W. M., Murray, H. W., Roberts, R. B., and Armstrong, D. (1985). *Salmonella* infections in patients with the acquired immunodeficiency syndrome. *Ann. Intern. Med.* **102,** 186–188.

Jafri, F. M., Mendelow, H., Shadduck, R. K., and Sekas, G. (1990). Jejunal vasculitis with protein-losing enteropathy after bone marrow transplantation. *Gastroenterology* **98,** 1689–1692.

Jeffries, G. H. (1989). Protein-losing gastroenteropathy. *In* "Gastrointestinal Disease" (M. H. Sleisenger and J. S. Fordtran, eds.), 4th ed., pp. 283–290. Saunders, Philadelphia.

Johnstone, J. M., and Morson, B. C. (1978). Eosinophilic gastroenteritis. Histopathology **2,** 335–348.

Jones, T. C., Dean, A. G., and Parker, G. W. (1972). Seasonal gastroenteritis and malabsorption at an American military base in the Philippines. *Am. J. Epidemiol.* **95,** 128–139.

Jordon, R. E., and Provost, T. T. (1988). Bullous skin diseases. *In* "Immunological Diseases" (M. Samter, D. W. Talmage, M. M. Frank, K. F. Austen, and H. N. Claman, eds.), 4th Ed., pp. 1281–1295. Little, Brown, Boston.

Kagnoff, M. F. (1981). Immunology of the digestive system. *In* "Physiology of the Digestive System" (L. R. Johnson, ed.), pp. 1337–1359. Raven Press, New York.

Kagnoff, M. F. (1989a). Immunology and disease of the gastrointestinal tract. *In* "Gastrointestinal Disease" (M. H. Sleisenger and J. S. Fordtran, eds.), 4th Ed., pp. 114–144. Saunders, Philadelphia.

Kagnoff, M. F. (1989b). Immunpathogenesis of celiac disease. *Immunol. Invest.* **18,** 499–508.

Kagnoff, M. F., Weiss, J. B., Brown, R. J., Lee, T., and Schanfield, M. S. (1983). Immunoglobulin allotype makers in gluten-sensitivity enteropathy. *Lancet* **I,** 952–953.

Kagnoff, M. F., Austin, R. K., Hubert, J. J., Bernardin, J. E., and Kasarda, D. D. (1984). Possible role for a human adenovirus in the pathogenesis of celiac disease. *J. Exp. Med.* **160,** 1544–1557.

Kagnoff, M. F., Paterson, Y. J., Kumar, P. J., Kasarda, F. R., Carbone, F. R., Unsworth, D. J., and Austin, R. K. (1987). Evidence for the role of a human intestinal adenovirus in the pathogenesis of coeliac disease. *Gut* **28,** 995–1001.

Kagnoff, M. F., Omary, M. B., Roebuck, K. A., deGrandpre, L., Richman, D. V., and Brenner, D. A. (1991). HIV-1 infection and expression in human colonic epithelial cell lines. *In* "Frontiers of Mucosal Immunology" (M. Tsuchiya, H. Nagura, T. Hibi, and I. Moro, eds.), Vol. 1, pp. 623–625. Excerpta Medica, Amsterdam.

Kalser, M. H. (1985a). Principles of absorption. *In* "Bockus Gastroenterology" (J. E. Berk, ed.), 4th Ed. pp. 1504–1509. Saunders, Philadelphia.

Kalser, M. H. (1985b). Clinical manifestations and evaluation of malabsorption. *In* "Bockus Gastroenterology" (J. E. Berk, ed.) 4th Ed. pp. 1667–1671. Saunders, Philadelphia.

Kalser, M. H. (1985c). Water and mineral transport. *In* "Bockus Gastroenterology" (J. E. Berk, ed.), 4th Ed., pp. 1538–1552. Saunders, Philadelphia.

Kamath, K. R., and Dorney, S. F. A. (1983). Is discordance for coeliac disease in monozygotic twins permanent? *Pediatr. Res.* **17,** 422A.

Kanoh, T. (1991). Gastrointestinal disorders in adult-onset primary immunodeficiency diseases. *In* "Frontiers of Mucosal Immunology" (M. Tsuchiya, H. Nagura, T. Hibi, and I. Moro, eds.), Vol. 1, pp. 611–614. Excerpta Medica, Amsterdam.

Kapembwa, M. S., Bridges, C., Joseph, A. E., Fleming, S. C., Batman, P., and Griffin, G. E. (1990). Ileal and jejunal absorptive function in patients with AIDS and enterococcidial infection. *J. Infect.* **21,** 43–53.

Kaposi, M. (1872). Idiopathisches multiples Pigmentsarkom der Haut. *Arch. Dermatol. Syphil.* **4,** 265–273.

Karagiannis, J. A., Priddle, J. D., and Jewell, D. P. (1987). Cell-mediated immunity to a synthetic gliadin peptide resembling a sequence from adenovirus. 12. *Lancet* **I,** 884–886.

Kasarda, D. D., Okita, T. W., Bernardin, J. E., Baecker, P. A., and Nimmo, C. C. (1984). Nucleic acid (cDNA) and amino acid sequences of alpha gliadin from wheat (Triticum sativum). *Proc. Natl. Acad. Sci. USA* **81,** 4712–4716.

Katz, S. I., and Strober, W. (1978). The pathogenesis of dermatitis herpetiformis. *J. Invest. Dermatol.* **70,** 63–75.

Katz, S. I., Hall, R. P., Lawley, T. J., and Strober, W. (1980). Dermatitis herpetiformis: The skin and the gut. *Ann. Intern. Med.* **93,** 857–874.

Kett, K., Scott, H., Fausa, O., and Brandtzaeg, P. (1990). Secretory immunity in celiac disease. Cellular expression of immunoglobulin A subclass and joining chain. *Gastroenterology* **99,** 386–392.

Keuning, J. J., Pena, A. S., van Hooff, J. P., van Leeuwen, A., and vanRood, J. J. (1976). HLA-DW3 associated with coeliac disease. *Lancet* **I,** 505–507.

Keusch, G. T., Thea, D. M., Kamenga, M., Kakanda, K., Mbala, M., Brown, C., and Davachi, F. (1992). Persistent diarrhea associated with AIDS. *Acta Paediatr. Suppl.* **381,** 45–48.

King, C. E., and Toskes, P. P. (1985). Bacterial overgrowth syndromes. *In* "Bockus Gastroenterology" (J. E. Berk, ed.), 4th Ed., pp. 1781–1791. Saunders, Philadelphia.

Klein, N. C., Hargrove, L., Sleisenger, M. H., and Jeffries, G. H. (1970). Eosinophilic gastroenteritis. *Medicine* **49,** 299–319.

Klein, R. S., Harris, C. A., Small, C. B., Moll, B., Lesser, M., and Friedland, G. H. (1984). Oral candidiasis in high risk patients as the intitial manifestation of the acquired immune deficiency syndrome. *N. Engl. J. Med.* **311,** 354–358.

Klipstein, F. A. (1989). Tropical sprue. *In* "Gastrointestinal Disease" (M. H. Sleisenger and J. S. Fordtran, eds.), 4th Ed., pp. 1281–1289. Saunders, Philadelphia.

Klipstein, F. A., Holdeman, L. V., Corcino, J. J., and Moore, W. E. C. (1973). Enterotoxigenic intestinal bacteria in tropical sprue. *Ann. Intern. Med.* **79,** 632–641.

Klipstein, F. A., Engert, R. F., and Short, H. B. (1978). Enterotoxigenicity of colonising bacteria in tropical sprue and blind-loop syndrome. *Lancet* **I,** 342–344.

Knoflach, P., Albini, B., and Weiser, M. M. (1986a). Autoimmune disease induced by oral administration of mercuric chloride in Brown–Norway rats. *Toxicol. Pathol.* **14,** 188–193.

Knoflach, P., Vladutiu, A. O., Swierczynska, Z., Weiser, M. M., and Albini, B. (1986b). Lack of circulating immune complexes in inflammatory bowel disease. *Int. Arch. Allergy Appl. Immunol.* **80,** 9–16.

Knoflach, P., Park, B. H., Cunningham, R., Weiser, M. M., and Albini, B. (1987). Serum antibodies to cow's milk proteins in ulcerative colitis and Crohn's disease. *Gastroenterology* **92,** 479–485.

Knoflach, P., Albini, B., and Weiser, M. M. (1989). Experimental immune complex disease of the intestine. *Immunol. Invest.* **18,** 473–483.

Knowles, D. M., Inghirami, G., Ubriaco, A., and Dalla-Favera, R. (1989). Molecular genetic analysis of three AIDS-associated neoplasms of uncertain lineage demonstrates their B-cell derivation and the possible pathogenetic role of the Epstein–Barr virus. *Blood* **73,** 792–799.

Koretz, S. H., and the Collaborative DMPG Treatment Group (1986). Treatment of serious cytomegalovirus infections using 9-(1,3-dihydroxy-2propoxymethyl) guanine in patients with AIDs and other immunodeficiencies. *N. Engl. J. Med.* **314,** 801–806.

Korsmeyer, S. J. (1989). Immunoglobulin genes in human lymphoid neoplasms. *In* "Immunoglobulin Genes" (T. Honjo, F. W. Alt, and T. H. Rabbits, eds.), pp. 233–255. Academic Press, London.

Kotler, D. P. (1991a). "Gastrointestinal and Nutritional Manifestations of the Acquired Immunodeficiency Syndrome." Raven Press, New York.

Kotler, D. P. (1991b). Biological and clinical features of HIV infection. *In* "Gastrointestinal and Nutritional Manifestations of the Acquired Immunodeficiency Syndrome" (D. P. Kotler, ed.), pp. 1–16. Raven Press, New York.

Kotler, D., Gaetz, H. P., Lange, M., Klein, E. B., and Holt, P. R. (1984). Enteropathy associated with the acquired immunodeficiency syndrome. *Ann. Intern. Med.* **101,** 421–428.

Kotler, D. P., Francesco, A., and Ramey, W. G. (1986). Intestinal lymphoid composition: Alterations in AIDS. *Clin. Res.* **34,** 442A.

Kotler, D. P., Tierney, A. R., and Scholes, J. V. (1987). Intestinal plasma cell alteration in acquired immunodeficiency syndrome. *Dig. Dis. Sci.* **32,** 129–138.

Kowley, K. U., Mason, J. B., Meydani, S. N., Cornwall, S., and Grand, R. J. (1992). Vitamin E deficiency and impaired cellular immunity related to intestinal fat malabsorption. *Gastroenterology* **102,** 2039–2142.

Krainick, H. G., Debatin, F., and Gauter, E. (1958). Additional research on the injurious effect of wheat flour in coeliac disease. I. Acute gliadin reaction—gliadin shock. *Helv. Paediatr. Acta* **13,** 432–454.

Kuitunen, P., Rapola, J., Savilahti, E., and Visakorpi, J. K. (1973). Response of the jejunal mucosa to cow's milk in the malabsorption syndrome with cow's milk intolerance. *Acta Paediatr. Scand.* **62,** 585–595.

Kumar, V., Lerner, A., Valeski, E., Beutner, E. H., Chorzelski, T. P., and Rossi, T. (1989). Endomysial antibodies in the diagnosis of celiac disease and the effect of gluten on antibody titers. *Immunol. Invest.* **18,** 533–544.

Kutlu, T., Brousse, N., Rambaud, D., Le Deist, F., Schmitz, J., and Cerf-Bensussan, N. (1993). Number of T cell receptor (TCR) α,β + but not TcR γ,δ + intraepithelial lymphocytes correlate with the grade of villous atrophy in coeliac patients on a long term normal diet. *Gut* **34,** 208–214.

Kvale, D., Lovhaug, D., Sollid, L. M., and Brandtzaeg, P. (1988). Tumor necrosis factor-α up-regulates expression of secretory component, the epithelial receptor for polymeric Ig. *J. Immunol.* **140,** 3086–1089.

Laine, L., Politoske, E. J., and Gill, P. (1987). Protein losing enteropathy in acquired immunodeficiency syndrome due to intestinal Kaposi's sarcoma. *Arch. Intern. Med.* **147,** 1174–1175.

Lake, A. M., Bloch, K. J., Sinclair, K. J., and Walker, W. A. (1980). Anaphylactic release of intestinal goblet cell mucus. *Immunology* **39,** 173–178.

Laughon, B. E., Druckman, D. A., Vernon, A., Quian, T. C., Polk, B. F., Modlin, J. F., Yolken, R. H., and Bartlett, O. G. (1988). Prevalence of enteric pathogens in homosexual men with and without acquired immunodeficiency syndrome. *Gastroenterology* **94,** 984–993.

Lerner, A., Rossi, T. M., Park, B., Albini, B., and Lebenthal, E. (1989). Serum antibodies to cow's milk proteins in pediatric inflammatory bowel disease *Acta Paediatr. Scand.* **78,** 384–389.

Levine, N. D. (1980). A newly revised classification of the protozoa. *J. Protozool.* **27,** 37–42.

Longcope, W. T., and Freiman, O. G. (1952). A study of sarcoidosis. *Medicine* **31,** 132–147.

Lucas, M. L., Cooper, B. T., Lei, F. H., Holmes, G. K. T., Blair, J. A., and Cooke, W. T. (1978). Acid microclimate in coeliac disease and Crohn's disease: A model for folate malabsorption. *Gut* **19,** 735–742.

Lucidarme, D., Colombel, J. F., Brandtzaeg, P., Tulliez, M., Chaussade, S., Marteau, P., Dehennin, J. P., Vaerman, J. P., and Rambaud, J. C. (1993). Alpha-chain disease: Analysis of alpha-chain protein and secretory component in jejunal fluid. *Gastroenetrology* **104,** 278–285.

McBrien, D. J., Jones, R. V., and Creamer, B. (1963). Steatorrhoea in Addison's disease. *Lancet* **I,** 25–26.

MacDonald, T. T., Hutchings, P., Choy, M. Y., Murch, S., and Cooke, A. (1990). Tumour necrosis factor alpha and interferon-gamma production measured at the single cell level in normal and inflamed human intestine. *Clin. Exp. Immunol* **81,** 301–305.

MacFarlane, A. S. (1957). The behavior of ^{131}I-labelled plasma proteins in vivo. *Ann. N.Y. Acad. Sci.* **70,** 19–25.

MacGregor, R. R. (1986). Alcohol and immune defense. *J. Am. Med. Assoc.* **256,** 1474–1479.

McLaughlin, P., Hunter, J. O., and Easter, G. B. (1983). Histamine release *in vitro* from jejunal mucosa following challenge with gliadin and also anti-IgE. *In* "Proceedings of the Second Fusions Food Allergy Workshop," pp. 7–9. Oxford Medical Publications, Oxford.

McNeish, A. S., Harms, K., Rey, J., Shmerling, D. H., Visakorpi, J. K., and Walker-Smith, J. A. (1979). The diagnosis of coeliac disease. *Arch. Dis. Child.* **54,** 783–786.

McNicholl, B., Egan-Mitchell, B., Stevens, F., Keane, R., Baker, S., McCarthy, C. F., and Fottrell, P. F. (1976). Mucosal recovery in treated celiac disease (gluten sensitive enteropathy). *J. Pediatr.* **89,** 418–424.

Mäki, M., and Visakorpi, J. K. (1988). Normal small bowel histology does not exclude coeliac disease. *Pediatr. Res.* **24,** 411A.

Mäki, M., Hällström, O., Vesikari, T., and Visakorpi, J. K. (1984). Evaluation of a serum IgA class reticulin antibody test for the detection of childhood coeliac disease. *J. Pediatr.* **105,** 901–905.

Malenbranche, R., Guerin, J. M., Laroche, A. C., Elie, R., Spira, T., Drotman, P., Arnoux, E., Pierre, G. D., Péan-Guichard, C., Morisset, P. H., Mandeville, P. H., Seemeyer, T., and Dupuy, J.-M. (1983). Acquired immunodeficiency syndrome with severe gastrointestinal manifestations in Haiti. *Lancet* **II,** 873–878.

Mansbach, C. M., II, Shelburne, J. D., Stevens, R. D., and Dobbins, W. O., III. (1978). Lymph node bacilliform bodies resembling those of Whipple's disease in a patient without intestinal involvement. *Ann. Intern. Med.* **88,** 64–70.

Marsh, M. N. (1988). Studies on intestinal lymphoid tissue. XI. The immunopathology of cell-mediated reactions in gluten sensitivity and other enteropathies. *Scanning Microsc.* **2,** 1663–1684.

Marsh, M. N. (1989). The immunopathology of the small intestinal reaction in gluten-sensitivity. *Immunol. Invest.* **18,** 509–531.

Marsh, M. N. (1992a) Gluten, major histocompatibility complex, and the small intestine: a molecular and immunobiologic approach to the spectrum of gluten-sensitivity "celiac sprue"). *Gastroenterology* **102,** 330–354.

Marsh, M. N. (1992b). The mucosal pathology of gluten-sensitivity. *In* Coeliac disease. (M. D., Marsh, ed.). pp. 136–191. *Blackwell Sci. Publ.,* Oxford.

Marsh, M. N. (1993). Gluten sensitivity and latency: Can patterns of intestinal antibody secretion define the great "silent majority"? *Gastroenterology* **104,** 1550–1562.

Marsh, M. N., and Hinde, J. (1985). Inflammatory component of celiac sprue mucosa. I. Mast cells, basophils and eosinophils. *Gastroenterology* **89,** 91–101.

Masur, H., and Fauci, A. (1989). Acquired immunodeficiency syndrome (AIDS). *In* "Gastrointestinal Disease" (M. H. Sleisenger and J. S. Fordtran, eds.), 4th Ed., pp. 1233–1242. Saunders, Philadelphia.

Mathieson, P. W., Thiru, S., and Oliviera, D. B. G. (1992). Mercuric chloride-treated brown Norway rats develop widespread tissue injury including necrotizing venulitis. *Lab. Invest.* **67,** 121–129.

Mathijs, J. M., Hing, M., Grierson, J., Dwyer, D. E., Goldschmidt, C., Cooper, D. A., and Cunningham, A. L. (1988). HIV infection of rectal mucosa. *Lancet* **I,** 1111.

May, G. R., Sutherland, L. R., and Meddings, J. B. (1993). Is small intestinal permeability really increased in relatives of patients with Crohn's disease? *Gastroenterology* **104,** 1627–1632.

Meiselman, M. S., Cello, J. P., and Margaretten, W. (1985). Cytomegalovirus colitis: Report of the clinital, endoscopic, and pathologic findings in two patients with acquired immune deficiency syndrome. *Gastroenterology* **88,** 171–175.

Meulders, Q., Michel, C., Marteau, P., Grange, J. D., Mougenot, B., Ronco, P., and Mignon, F. (1992). Association of chronic interstitial cystitis, protein-loosing enteropathy and paralytic ileus with seronegative systemic lupus erythematosus: Case report and review of the literature. *Clin. Nephrology* **37,** 239–244.

Meuwisse, G. W. (1970). Diagnostic criteria in coeliac disease. *Acta Paediatr. Scand.* **59,** 461–463.

Meyer, E. A., and Radulescu, S. (1979). *Giardia* and giardiasis. *Adv. Parasitol.* **17,** 1–47.

Mielants, H., Veys, E. M., Cuvelier, C., De-Vos, M., and Botelberghe, L. (1985). HLA B27 related arthritis and bowel inflammation. II. Ileocolonoscopy and bowel histology in patients with HLA B27 related arthritis. *J. Rheumatol.* **12,** 294–298.

Mike, N. and Asquith, P. (1987). Gluten toxicity in coeliac disease and its role in other gastrointestinal disorders. *In* "Food Allergy and Intolerance" (J. Brostoff and S. J. Challacombe, eds.), pp. 521–548. Bailliere Tindall, London.

Mitchell, I. C., Turk, J. L., and Mitchell, D. N. (1992). Detection of mycobacterial rRNA in sarcoidosis with liquid-phase hybridisation. *Lancet* **339,** 1015–1017.

Mitchell, N., and Feder, I. A. (1949). Kaposi's sarcoma with secondary involvement of the jejunum, perforation and peritonitis. *Ann. Intern. Med.* **31,** 324–329.

Miura, S., Morita, A., Erickson, R. H., and Kim, Y. S. (1983). Content and turnover of rat intestinal microvillus membrane aminopeptidase. *Gastroenterology* **85,** 1340–1349.

Morecki, R., and Parker, J. G. (1967). Ultrastructural studies of the human *Giardia lamblia* and subadjacent mucosa in a subject with steatorrhea. *Gastroenterology* **52,** 151–164.

Morgan, B. P., Daniels, R. H., Watts, M. J., and Williams, D. B. (1988). *In vivo* and *in vitro* evidence of cell recovery from complement attack in rheumatoid synovium. *Clin. Exp. Immunol.* **73,** 467–472.

Morise, K., Kimura, M., Saito, Y., Inagaki, T., Iwase, H., Kanayama, K., Horiuchi, Y., Sakakibara, M., Kusugami, K., and Nagura, H. (1991). Expression of HLA-DR antigens by colonic epithelium and lamina propria dendritic cells in inflammatory bowel disease. *In* "Frontiers of Mucosal Immunology" (M. Tsuchiya, H. Nagura, T. Hibi, and I. Moro, eds.), Vol. 1, pp. 193–194. Excerpta Medica, Amsterdam.

Morley, J. E., Levine, A. S., Yamada, T., Genhard, R. L., Prigge, W. F., Shafer, R. B., Goetz, F. C., and Silvis, S. E. (1983). Effect of exorphins on gastrointestinal function, hormone release, and appetite. *Gastroenterology* **84,** 1517–1523.

Müller, C., Knoflach, P., and Zielinski, C. C. (1990). T-cell activation in Crohn's disease. *Gastroenterology* **98,** 639–646.

Müller, C., Wolf, H., Göttlicher, J., Zielinski, C., and Eibl, M. M. (1991). Cellular immunodeficiency in protein-losing enteropathy. Predominant reduction of $CD3^+$ and $CD4^+$ lymphocytes. *Dig. Dis. Sci.* **36,** 116–122.

Muller, F., Froland, S. S., and Brandtzaeg, P. (1991). Reduced parotid secretory IgA in patients with AIDS. *In* "Frontiers of Mucosal Immunology" (M. Tsuchiya, H. Nagura, T. Hibi, and I. Moro, eds.), Vol. 1, pp. 635–636. Excerpta Medica, Amsterdam.

Murch, S. H., Lamkin, V. A., Savage, M. O., Walker-Smith, J. A., and MacDonald, T. T. (1991). Serum concentrations of tumour necrosis factor alpha in childhood chronic inflammatory bowel disease. *Gut* **32,** 913–917.

Murch, S. H., Braegger, C. P., Sessa, W. C., and MacDonald, T. T. (1992). High endothelin-1 immunoreactivity in Crohn's disease and ulcerative colitis. *Lancet* **I,** 381–385.

Nadorra, R. L., Nakazato, Y., and Landing, B. H. (1987). Pathologic features of gastrointestinal tract lesions in childhood-onset systemic lupus erythematosus: Study of 26 patients with review of the literature. *Pediatr. Pathol.* **7,** 245–259.

Navin, T. R., and Juranek, D. D. (1984). Cryptosporidioidosis: Clinical, epidemiologic and parasitologic review. *Rev. Infect. Dis.* **6,** 313–327.

Nelson, J. A., Wiley, C. A., Reynolds-Kohler, C., Reese, C. E., Margaretten, W., and Levy, J. A. (1988). Human immunodeficiency virus detected in bowel epithelium from patients with gastrointestinal symptoms. *Lancet* **I,** 259–262.

Nemoz, G., Prigent, A. F., Aloui, R., Charpin, G., Gor, and, F., Gallet, H., Debos, A., Biot, N., Perrin-Fayolle, M., Lagarde, M., and Pacheco, Y. (1993). Impaired G-proteins and cyclic nucleotide phosphodiesterase activity in T-lymphocytes from patients with sarcoidosis. *Eur. J. Clin. Invest.* **23,** 18–27.

O'Brien, W., and England, N. W. J. (1971). Tropical sprue amongst British servicemen and their families in South East Asia. *In* "Tropical Sprue and Megaloblastic Anemia," pp. 25–60. Churchill-Livingstone, London.

O'Donoghue, D. R., Swarbrick, E. T., and Kumar, P. J. (1979). Type 1 hypersensitivity reactions in coeliac disease. *Gastroenterology* **76,** 1211A.

Okubo, S., and Yasunaga, K. (1991). Present status of AIDS in Japan with special reference to digestive tract disorders. *In* "Frontiers of Mucosal Immunology" (M. Tsuchiya, H. Nagura, T. Hibi, and I. Moro, eds.), Vol. 1, pp. 627–630. Excerpta Medica, Amsterdam.

O'Mahony, S., Vestey, J. P., and Ferguson, A. (1990). Similarities in intestinal humoral immunity in dermatitis herpetiformis without enteropathy and in coeliac disease *Lancet* **335,** 1487–1490.

O'Mahony, S., Choudari, C. P., Barton, J. R., Walker, S., and Ferguson, A. (1991b). Gut lavage fluid proteins as markers of activity in inflammatory bowel disease. *Scand. J. Gastroenterol.* **26,** 940–944.

O'Mahony, S., Arranz, E., Barton, J. R., and Ferguson, A. (1991a). Dissociation between systemic and mucosal immune responses in coeliac disease *Gut* **32,** 29–35.

Oommen, R., Kurien, G., Balakrishnan, N., and Narasimhan, S. (1992). Tc-99m albumin scintigraphy in the localization of protein loss in the gut. *Clin. Nucl. Med.* **17,** 787–788.

Orenstein, J. M., Chiang, J., Steinberg, W., Smith, P., Rotterdam, H., and Kotler, D. P. (1990). Intestinal microsporidiosis as a cause of diarrhea in HIV-infected patients: A report of 20 cases. *Hum. Pathol.* **21,** 475–481.

Owen, R. L. (1989). Parasitic diseases. *In* "Gastrointestinal Disease" (M. H. Sleisenger and J. S. Fordtran, eds.), 4th Ed., pp. 1153–1191. Saunders, Philadelphia.

Padykula, H. A., Strauss, E. W., Ladman, A. J., and Gardner, F. H. (1961). A morphologic and histochemical analysis of the human jejunal epithelium in non-tropical sprue. *Gastroenterology* **40,** 735–765.

Parkins, R. A. (1960). Protein-losing enteropathy in the sprue syndrome. *Lancet* **2,** 1366–1369.

Paulley, L. W. (1954). Observations on the aetiology of idiopathic steatorrhea. *Br. Med. J.* **2,** 1318–1321.

Perednia, D. A. and Curosh, N. A. (1990). Lupus-associated protein-losing enteropathy. Arch. *Intern. Med.* **150,** 1806–1810.

Perrone, V., Pergola, M., Abate, G., Silvestro, L., Ronga, D., Bruni, G., D'Aprile, M., and Blesi, A. (1981). Protein-losing enteropathy in a patient with generalized Kaposi's sarcoma. *Cancer* **47,** 588–591.

Petersen, J. M., Tubbs, R. R., Savage, R. A., Calabrese, L. C., Proffitt, M. R., Manolova, Y., Manolov, G., Shumaker, A., Tatsumi, E., McClain, K., and Purtilo, D. T. (1985). Small noncleaved B cell Burkitt-like lymphoma with chromosome t(8;14) translocation and Epstein–Barr virus nuclear-associated antigen in a homosexual man with acquired immune deficiency syndrome. *Am. J. Med.* **78,** 141–148.

Peterson, R. D. A., Cooper, M. D., and Good, R. A. (1965). The pathogenesis of the immunologic deficiency diseases. *Am. J. Med.* **38,** 579–604.

Phelan, J. J., Stevens, F. M., McNicholl, B., Fottrell, P. F., and McCarthy, C. F. (1977). Coeliac disease: The abolition of gliadin toxicity by enzymes from *Aspergillus niger*. *Clin. Sci. Mol. Med.* **53,** 35–43.

Polak, J. M., Pearse, A. G. E., van Noorden, S., Bloom, S. R., and Rossiter, M. A. (1973). Secretin cells in coeliac disease. *Gut* **14,** 870–874.

Polanco, I., Biemond, I., van Leeuwen, A., Schreuder, I., Kahn, P. M., Guerrero, J., D'Amaro, J., Vazquez, C., van Rood, J. J., and Peña, A. S. (1981). Gluten sensitive enteropathy in Spain: Genetic and environmental factors. *In* "Genetics of Coeliac Disease" (R. B. McConnell, ed.), pp. 211–230. MTP Press, Lancaster.

Poley, J. R., and Rosenfield, S. (1981). Giardiasis and malabsorption: Presence of an organic mucosal barrier. A scanning (SEM) and transmission (TEM) electron microscopic study of small bowel mucosa. *Gastroenterology* **80,** 1245A.

Potter, D. A., Danforth, D. N., Macher, A. M., Longo, D. L., Steward, L., and Masur, H. (1984). Evaluation of abdominal pain in the AIDS patient. *Ann. Surg.* **199,** 332–339.

Prendville, J., Robinson, A., and Young, M. (1982). Familial sarcoidosis. *Ir. J. Med. Sci.* **151,** 258–260.

Provost, T. T., and Tomasi, T. B., Jr. (1974). Evidence for the activation of complement via the alternate pathway in skin disease. II. Dermatitis herpetiformis. *Clin. Immunol. Immunopathol.* **3,** 178–186.

Pueringer, R. J., Schwartz, D. A., Dayton, C. S., Gilbert, S. R., and Hunninghake, G. W. (1993). The relationship between alveolar macrophage TNF, IL-1, and PGE2 release, alveolitis, and disease severity in sarcoidosis. *Chest* **103,** 832–838.

Rachmilewitz, D., and Okon, E. (1985). Primary small intestinal lymphoma. *In* "Bockus Gastroenterology" (J. E. Berk, ed.), 4th Ed., pp. 1865–1873. Saunders, Philadelphia.

Rambaud, J. C. (1983). Small intestinal lymphomas and alpha chain disease. *Clin. Gastroenterol.* **12,** 743–766.

Rambaud, J. C., and Seligmann, M. (1976). Alpha-chain disease. *Clin. Gastroenterol.* **5,** 341–358.

Rambaud, J. C., Halphen, M., Galian, A., and Tsapis, A. (1990). Immunoproliferative small intestinal disease (IPSID): Relationship with alpha chain disease and "Mediterranean" lymphomas. *Springer Semin. Immunopathol.* **12,** 239–250.

Rambaud, J. C., Bognel, C., Prost, A., Bernier, J. J., LeQuintrec, Y., Lambling, A., Danon, F., Huves, D., and Seligmann, M. (1968). Clinico-pathologic study of a patient with "Mediterranean type of abdominal lymphoma and a new type of IgA abnormality (Alpha-chain disease)." *Digestion* **1,** 321–336.

Reif, S., Jain, A., Santiago, J., and Rossi, T. (1991). Protein losing enteropathy as a manifestation of Henoch-Schönlein purpura. *Acta Paed. Scand.* **80,** 482–485.

Reka, S., Borcich, A., Cronin, W., and Kotler, D. P. (1989). Diarrhea associated with intestinal HIV infection in ARC, *Clin. Res.* **37,** 371A.

Relman, D. A., Schmidt, T, M., McDermott, R. P., and Falkow, S. (1992). Identification of the uncultured *bacillus* of Whipple's disease. *N. Engl. J. Med.* **327,** 346–348.

René, E., Jarry, A., Brousse, N., Vazeux, R., Marche, C., Regnier, B., Saimot, A. G., Rozé, C., Roussel, J. Y., Vallot, T., Mignon, M., Potet, F., and Bonfils, S. (1988). Demonstration of HIV infection in the gut in AIDS patients: Relation with symptoms and other digestive infection. *Gastroenterology* **94,** A373.

René, E., Marche, C., Regnier, B., Saimot, A. G., Vilde, J. G., Perrone, C., Michon, C., Wolf, M., Chevalier, T., Vallot, T., Brun-Vesinet, F., Pangon, B., Deluol, A. M., Camus, F., Roze, C., Pignon, J. P., Mignon, M., and Bonfils, S. (1989). Intestinal infection in patients with acquired immunodeficiency syndrome: A prospective study in 132 patients. *Dig. Dis, Sci.* **34,** 773–780.

René, E., Roze, C., and the AIDS GIT (1991). Diagnosis and treatment of gastrointestinal infections in AIDS, *In* "Gastrointestinal and Nutritional Manifestations of the Acquired Immunodeficiency Syndrome" (D. P. Kotler, ed.), pp. 65–91. Raven Press, New York.

Riecken, E.-O., Zeitz, M., and Ullrich, R. (1991). HIV infection of the gut. *In* "Frontiers of Mucosal Immunology" (M. Tsuchiya, H. Nagura, T. Hibi, and I. Moro, eds.), Vol. 1, pp. 619–622. Excerpta Medica, Amsterdam.

Rinderknecht, H. (1986). Pancreatic secretory enzymes. *In* "The Exocrine Pancreas: Biology, Pathobiology and Diseases" (V. L. W. Go, ed.), pp 375–386. Raven Press, New York.

Rodgers, V. D., and Kagnoff, M. F. (1987). Gastrointestinal manifestations of the acquired immunodeficiency syndrome. *West. J. Med.* **146,** 57–67.

Rodgers, V. D., Fassett, R., and Kagnoff, M. F. (1986). Abnormalities in intestinal mucosal T cells in homosexual populations including those with the lymphoadenopathy syndrome and acquired immunodeficiency syndrome. *Gastroenterology* **90,** 552–558.

Roggin, G. M., Iber, F. L., and Kater, R. M. H. (1961). Malabsorption in the chronic alcoholic. *Johns Hopkins Med. J.* **125,** 321.

Rootwelt, K. (1966). Direct intravenous injection of ^{51}chromic chloride compared with ^{125}I-polyvinylpyrrolidone and ^{131}I-albumin in the detection of gastrointestinal protein loss. *Scand. J. Clin. Lab. Invest.* **18,** 405–416.

Roth, R. I., Owen, R. L., Keren, D. F., and Volberding, P. A. (1985). Intestinal infection with *Mycobacterium avium* in acquired immune deficiency syndrome (AIDS). Histologic and clinical comparison with Whipple's disease. *Dig. Dis. Sci.* **30,** 497–504.

Roy-Choudhury, D. C., Cooke, W. T., Banwell, J. G., and Smits, B. J. (1967). Multiple jejunal biopsies in adult celiac disease. *Am. J. Dig. Dis.* **12,** 657–663.

Rubin, C. E., Eidelman, S., and Weinstein, W. M. (1970). Sprue by any other name. *Gastroenterology* **58,** 409–413.

Rubin, E., Rybac, B. J., Lindenbaum, J., Gerson, C. D., Walker, G., and Lieber, C. S. (1972). Ultra-structural changes in the small intestine induced by ethanol. *Gastroenterology* **63,** 801–814.

Rubin, W., Ross, L. L., Sleisenger, M. H., and Weser, E. (1966). An electron microscopic study of adult celiac disease. *Lab. Invest.* **15,** 1720–1747.

Saboor, S. A., Johnson, N. M., and McFadden, J. (1992). Detection of mycobacterial DNA in sarcoidosis and tuberculosis with polymerase chain reaction. *Lancet* **339,** 1012–1015.

Safrin, S., Crumpacker, C., Chatis, P., Davis, R., Hafner, R., Rush, J., Kessler, H. A., Landry, B., and Mills, J. (1991). A controlled trial comparing Foscarnet with Vidarabine for Acyclovir-resistant mucocutaneous *Herpes simplex* in the acquired immunodeficiency syndrome. (The AIDS Clinical Trial Group). *N. Engl. J. Med.* **325,** 551–555.

Sale, G. E., McDonald, G. B., Shulman, H. M., and Thomas, E. D. (1979). Gastrointestinal graft-versus-host disease in man. *Am. J. Surg. Pathol.* **3,** 291–299.

Sampson, H. A., Mendelson, L. and Rosen, J. P. (1992). Fatal and near-fatal anaphylactic reactions to food in children and adolescents. *N. Engl. J. Med.* **327,** 380–384.

Sankey, E. A., Dhillon, A. P., Anthony, A., Wakefield, A. J., Sim, R., More, L., Hudson, M., Sawyerr, A. M., and Pounder, R. E. (1993). Early mucosal changes in Crohn's disease. *Gut* **34,** 375–381.

Sapin, C., Druet, E., and Druet, P. (1977). Induction of antiglomular basement membrane antibodies in the Brown–Norway rat by mercuric chloride. *Clin. Exp. Immunol.* **28,** 173–179.

Saulsbury, F. T., Winkelstein, J. A., and Yolken, R. H. (1980). Chronic rotavirus infection in immunodeficiency. *J. Pediatr.* **97,** 61–65.

Savilahti, E., Viander, M., Perkkio, M., Vainio, E., Kalimo, K., and Reunala, T. (1983). IgA gliadin antibodies: A marker of mucosal damage in childhood coeliac disease *Lancet* **I,** 320–322.

Scheib, J. S., and Quinet, R. J. (1990). Whipple's disease with axial and peripheral joint destruction. *South Med. J.* **83,** 684–687.

Schmitz, J., Jos, J., and Rey, J. (1978). Transient mucosal atrophy in confirmed coeliac disease. *In* "Perspectives in Coeliac Disease" (B. McNicholl, C. F. MacCarthy, and P. F. Fottrell, eds.), pp. 259–262. MTP, Lancaster, England.

Scholz, S., and Albert, E. (1983). HLA and diseases: Involvement of more than one HLA-linked determinant of disease susceptibility. *Immunol. Rev.* **70,** 77–88.

Schreiber, S., Nash, G. S., Raedler, A., Pinnau, R., Berovich, M., and McDermott, R. P. (1991). Human lamina propria mononuclear cells are activated in inflammatory bowel disease. *In* "Frontiers of Mucosal Immunology" (M. Tsuchiya, H. Nagura, T. Hibi, and I. Moro, eds.), Vol. 1, pp. 749–753. Excerpta Medica, Amsterdam.

Scott, B. B., Goodall, A., Stephenson, P. M., and Jenkins, D. (1983). Is reaginic hypersensitivity involved in coeliac disease? *Gut* **24,** A990.

Scott, H., Brandtzaeg, P., Solheim, B. G., and Thorsby, E. (1981). Relation between HLA-DR-like antigens and secretory component (SC) in jejunal epithelium of patients with coeliac disease or dermatitis herpetiformis. *Clin. Exp. Immunol.* **44,** 233–238.

Scott, H., Sollid, L. M., Fausa, O., Brandtzaeg, P., and Thorsby, E. (1987). Expression of major histocompatibility complex class II subregion products by jejunal epithelium on patients with coeliac disease. *Scand. J. Immunol.* **26,** 563–572.

Selby, W. S., and Gallagher, N. D. (1979). Malignancy in a 19-year experience of adult celiac disease. *Dig. Dis. Sci.* **24,** 684–688.

Selby, W. S., Janossy, G., Mason, D. Y., and Jewell, D. P. (1983). Expression of HLA-DR antigens by colonic epithelium in inflammatory bowel disease. *Clin. Exp. Immunol.* **53,** 614–618.

Selhub, J., Dhar, G. J., and Rosenberg, I. H. (1978). Inhibition of folate enzymes by sulfasalazine. *J. Clin. Invest.* **61,** 221–224.

Seligmann, M., and Rambaud, J. C. (1969). IgA abnormalities in abdominal lymphoma (alpha-chain disease). *Israel J. Med. Sci.* **5,** 151–157.

Seligmann, M., Danon, F., Hurez, D., Mihaesco, E., and Preud'homme, J-L. (1968). Alpha-chain disease: A new immunoglobulin abnormality. *Science* **62,** 1396–1397.

Selzer, G., Sherman, G., Callihan, T. R., and Schwartz, Y. (1979). Primary cell intestinal lymphomas and alpha heavy chain disease: A study of 43 cases from a pathology department in Israel. *Israel J. Med. Sci.* **15,** 111–123.

Senju, M., Umene, Y., Yamasaki, K., Murata, I., Makiyama, K., Hara, K., and Jewell, D. P. (1991). Peripheral blood lymphocyte subsets in inflammatory bowel disease. *In* "Frontiers of Mucosal Immunology" (M. Tsuchiya, H. Nagura, T. Hibi, and I. Moro, eds), Vol. 1, pp. 759–760. Excerpta Medica, Amsterdam.

Seth, V., Kukreja, N., and Saundaram, K. R. (1982). Waning of cell mediated immune response in preschool children given BCG at birth. *Indian J. Med. Res.* **76,** 710–715.

Sewankambo, N., Mugerwa, R. D., and Godgame, R. D. (1987). Enteropathic AIDS in Uganda. An endoscopic, histologic and microbiologic study. *AIDS* **1,** 9–13.

Shafer, R. B., Prentiss, R. A., and Bond, J. H. (1984). Gastrointestinal transit in thyroid disease. *Gastroenterology* **86,** 852–855.

Shakoor, Z., and Hamblin, A. S. (1992). Increased CD11/CD18 expression on peripheral blood leucocytes of patients with sarcoidosis. *Clin. Exp. Immunol.* **90,** 99–105.

Shanahan, F. (1993). Summary: Food allergy: Fact, fiction, and fatality. Gastroenterology **104,** 1229–1231.

Sheehy, T. W. (1985). Tropical sprue. *In* "Bockus Gastroenterology" (J. E. Berk, ed.), 4th ed., pp. 1758–1780. Saunders, Philadelphia.

Sherman, S., Rohwedder, J. J., Ravikrishnan, K. P., and Weg, J. G. (1980). Tuberculous enteritis and peritonitis: Report of 36 general hospital cases. *Arch. Intern. Med.* **140,** 506–508.

Shin, J.-Y., Barnes, P. F., Rea, T. H., and Meyer, P. R. (1988). Immunohistology of tuberculous adenitis in symptomatic HIV infection. *Clin. Exp. Immunol.* **72,** 186–189.

Siegal, F. P., Lopez, C., Hammer, G. S., Brown, A. E., Kornfeld, S. J., Gold J., Hassett, J., Hirschman, S. Z., Cunningham-Rundles, C., Adelsberg, B. R., Parham, D. M., Siegal, M., Cunningham-Rundles, S., and Armstrong, D. (1981). Severe acquired immunodeficiency in male homosexuals manifested by chronic perianal ulcerative herpes simplex lesions. *N. Engl. J. Med.* **305,** 1439–1444.

Sieracki, J. C., and Fine, G. (1959). Whipple's disease: Observation on systemic involvement. I. Gross and histologic observation. *Arch. Pathol.* **67,** 81–93.

Sitrin, M. D., Rosenberg, I. H., Chawla, K., Meredith, S., Sellin, J., Rabb, J. M., Coe, F., Kirsner, J. B., and Kraft, S. C. (1980). Nutritional and metabolic complications in a patient with Crohn's disease and ileal resection. *Gastroenterology* **78,** 1069–1079.

Siurala, M., Varis, K., and Lamberg, B. A. (1968). Intestinal absorption and autoimmunity in endocrine disorders. *Acta. Med. Scand.* **184,** 53–64.

Smith, P. D., Macher, A. M., and Brookman, M. A. (1985). *Salmonella typhimurium* enteritis and bacteremia in the acquired immunodeficiency syndrome. *Ann. Intern. Med.* **102,** 207–208.

Soave, R., Danner, R. L., Honig, C. L., Ma, P., Hart, C. C., Nash, T., and Roberts, R. B. (1984). Cryptosporidiosis in homosexual men. *Ann. Intern, Med.* **100,** 504–511.

Soltis, R. D., Hasz, D., Morris, M. J., and Wilson, J. D. (1979). Evidence against the presence of circulating immune complexes in chronic inflammatory bowel disease. *Gastroenterology* **76,** 1380–1385.

Soothill, J. F., Stikes, C. R., Turner, M. W., Norman, A. P., and Taylor, B. (1976). Predisposing factors and the development of reaginic allergy in infancy. *Clin. Allergy* **6,** 305–319.

Sorensen, R. U., Halpin, T. C., Abramowsky, C. R., Hornick, D. L., Miller, K. M., Naylor, P., and Incefy, G. S. (1985). Intestinal lymphangiectasia and thymic hypoplasia. *Clin. Exp. Immunol.* **59,** 217–226.

Spencer, J., MacDonald, T. T., Diss, T. C., Walker-Smith, J. A., Ciclitira, P. J., and Isaacson, P. G. (1989a). Changes in intraepithelial lymphocyte subpopulations in coeliac disease and enteropathy associated T cell lymphoma (malignant histiocytosis of the intestine). *Gut* **30,** 339–346.

Spencer, J., Isaacson, P. G., Diss, T. C., and MacDonald, T. T. (1989b). Expression of disulfide-linked and non-disulfide-linked forms of the T cell receptor τ/δ heterodimer in human intestinal intraepithelial lymphocytes. *Eur. J. Immunol.* **19,** 1335–1338.

Sperber, S. J., and Schleupner, C. J. (1987). Salmonellosis during infection with human immunodeficiency virus. *Rev. Infect. Dis.* **9,** 925–934.

Sprague, R., Harper, P., McClain, S., Trainer, T., and Beeken, W.

(1984). Disseminated intestinal sarcoidosis. *Gastroenterology* **87,** 421–425.

Stainsby, K. J., Lowes, J. R., Allan, R. N., and Ibbotson, J. P. (1993). Antibodies to *Mycobacterium paratuberculosis* and nine species of environmental mycobacteria in Crohn's disease and control subjects. *Gut* **34,** 371–374.

Stark, M. E., Batts, K. P., and Alexander, G. L. (1992). Protein-losing enteropathy with collagenous colitis. *Am J. Gastroenterol.* **87,** 780–783.

Steinfeld, J. L., Davidson, J. D., Gordon, R. S., Jr., and Greene, F. E. (1961). The mechanism of hypoproteinemia in patients with regional enteritis and ulcerative colitis. *Am. J. Med.* **29,** 405–415.

Sterling, K. (1951). Turnover rate of serum albumin in man as measured by I^{131} tagged albumin. *J. Clin. Invest.* **30,** 1228–1237.

Stiehm, E. R. (1990). Immunodeficiency disorders: General considerations. *In* "Immunologic Disorders in Infants and Children" (E. R. Stiehm, ed.), 3d Ed., pp. 157–195. Saunders, Philadelphia.

Steinhardt, J. J., and Adibi, S. A. (1986). Kinetics and characteristics of absorption from an equimolar mixture of 12 glycyl-dipeptides in the human jejunum. *Gastroenterology* **90,** 577–582.

Stokes, P. L., Prior, P., Sorahan, T. M., McWalter, R. J., Waterhouse, J. A. H., and Cooke, W. T. (1976). Malignancy in relatives of patients with coeliac disease. *Br. J. Prev. Soc. Med.* **30,** 17–21.

Stoll, T., Keusch, G., Jost, R., Burger, H., Oelz, O. (1993). IgA nephropathy and hypercalcemia in Whipple's disease. *Nephron* **63,** 222–225.

Strausz, J., Mannel. D. N., Pfeifer, S., Borkowski, A., Ferlinz, R., and Müller-Quernheim, J. (1991). Spontaneous monokine release by alveolar macrophages in chronic sarcoidosis. *Int. Arch. Allergy Appl. Immunol.* **96,** 68–75.

Strobel, S., Busittil, A., and Ferguson, A. (1983). Human intestinal mucosal mast cells: Expanded population in untreated coeliac disease. *Gut* **24,** 222–227.

Strober, W., and James, S. P. (1992). The immunopathogenesis of gastrointestinal and hepatobiliary diseases. *JAMA* **268,** 2910–2917.

Strober, W., Krakauer, R., Klaeveman, H. L., Reynolds, H. Y., and Nelson, D. L. (1976). Secretory component deficiency. A disorder of the IgA immune system. *N. Engl. J. Med.* **294,** 351–356.

Subar, M., Chadburn, A., and Knowles, D. M. (1991). Gastrointestinal neoplasms in AIDS. *In* "Gastrointestinal and Nutritional Manifestations of the Acquired Immunodeficiency Syndromes" (D. P. Kotler, ed.), pp. 93–117. Raven Press, New York.

Taylor, L. D., Daniels, C. K., and Schmucker, D. L. (1992). Ageing compromises gastrointestinal mucosal immune response in the rhesus monkey. *Immunology* **75,** 614–618.

Tazi, A., Fajac, I., Soler, P., Valeyre, D., Battesti, J. P., and Hance, A. J. (1991). Gamma/delta T lymphocytes are not increased in number in granulomatous lesions of patients with tuberculosis or sarcoidosis. *Am. Rev. Resp. Dis.* **144,** 1373–1375.

Thaysen, T. E. H. (1932). "Non-Tropical Sprue." Oxford University Press, London.

Thomas, D. W., Sinatra, F. R., and Merritt, R. J. (1981). Random fetal $alpha_1$ antitrypsin concentration in children with gastrointestinal disease. *Gastroenterology* **80,** 776–782.

Thomas, F. B., Caldwell, J. H., and Greenberger, N. J. (1973). Steatorrhea in thyrotoxicosis: Relationship to hypermotility and excessive dietary fat. *Ann. Intern. Med.* **78,** 669–675.

Thomas, G., and Clain, D. J. (1976). Endemic tropical sprue in Rhodesia. *Gut* **17,** 877–887.

Thompson, H. (1974). The small intestine at autopsy. *Clin. Gastroenterol.* **3,** 171–181.

Tosi, R., Vismara, D., Tanigaki, N., Ferrara, G. B., Cicimarra, F., Buffolano, W., Follo, D., and Auricchio, S. (1983). Evidence that celiac disease is primarily associated with a DC locus allelic specificity. *Clin. Immunol. Immunopathol.* **28,** 395–404.

Townley, R. R. W., Bhathal, P. S., Cornell, H. J., and Mitchell, J. D. (1973). Toxicity of wheat gliadin fraction in coeliac disease. *Lancet* **I,** 1363–1364.

Trenthan, D. E., and Masi, A. T. (1976). Systemic lupus erythematosus with protein-losing enteropathy. *J. Am. Med. Assoc.* **236,** 287–288.

Trier, J. S. (1989a). Whipple's disease. *In* "Gastrointestinal Disease" (M. H. Sleisenger and J. S. Fordtran, eds.), 4th Ed., pp. 1297–1306. Saunders, Philadelphia.

Trier, J. S. (1989b). Celiac sprue. *In* "Gastrointestinal Disease" (M. H. Sleisenger and J. S. Fordtran, eds.), 4th Ed., pp. 1134–1152. Saunders, Philadelphia.

Trier, J. S. (1991). Celiac sprue. *N. Engl. J. Med.* **325,** 1709–1719.

Trier, J. S., Falchuk, Z. M., Carey, M. C., and Schreiber, D. S. (1978). Celiac sprue and refractory sprue. *Gastroenterology* **75,** 307–316.

Troncone, R., and Ferguson, A. (1991). An animal model of gluten-induced enteropathy in mice. *Gut* **32,** 871–875.

Tsutsumi, A., Sugiyama, T., Matsumura, R., Sueishi, M., Takabayashi, K., Koike, T., Tomioka, H., and Yoshida, S. (1991). Protein losing enteropathy associated with collagen diseases. *Ann. Rheum. Dis.* **50,** 178–181.

Twomey, J. J., Jordan, P. H., Jarrold, T., Trubowitz, S., Ritz, N. R., and Conn, H. O. (1969). The syndrome of immunoglobulin deficiency and pernicious anemia: A study of ten cases. *Am. J. Med.* **47,** 340–350.

Ullrich, R., Heise, W., Bergs, C., L'Age, M., Riecken, E.-O., and Zeitz, M. (1992). Effects of ziduvine treatment on the small intestinal mucosa in patients infected with the human immunodeficiency virus. *Gastroenterology* **102,** 1483–1492.

Ullrich, R., Zeitz, M., Heise, W., L'age, M., Höffken, G., and Riecken, E. O. (1989). Small intestinal structure and function in patients infected with human immunodeficiency virus (HIV): Evidence for HIV-induced enteropathy. *Ann. Intern. Med.* **111,** 15–21.

van de Kamer, J. H., Weijers, H. A., and Dicke, W. K. (1953). Coeliac disease. IV. An investigation into the injurious constituents of wheat in connection with the reaction on patients with coeliac disease. *Acta Paediatr.* **42,** 223–231.

Vanek, J., and Schwarz, J. (1970). Demonstration of acid-fast rods in sarcoidosis. *Am. Rev. Respir. Dis.* **101,** 395–400.

Van Elburg, R. M., Uil, J. J., Mulder, C. J. J., and Heymans, H. S. A. (1993). Intestinal permeability in patients with coeliac disease and relatives of patients with coeliac disease. *Gut* **34,** 354–357.

Van Tongeren, J. H. M., and Majoor, C. L. H. (1966). Demonstration of protein-losing gastroenteropathy. The disappearance rate of ^{51}Cr from plasma and the binding of ^{51}Cr to different serum proteins. *Clin. Chim. Acta* **14,** 31–41.

Veghelyi, P. (1939). Celiac disease imitated by giardiasis. *Am. J. Dis. Child* **57,** 894–902.

Volberding, P. A., Lagakos, S. W., Koch, M. A., Pettinelli, C., Myers, M. W., Booth, D. K., Balfour, H. H., Reichman, R. C., Bartlett, J. A., Hirsch, M. S., Murphy, R. L., Hardy, W. D., Soeiro, R., Fischl, M. A., Bartlett, J. G., Merigan, T. C., Hyslop, N. E., Richman, D. D., Valentine, F. T., Corey, L., and the AIDS clinical trials group of NIAID. (1990). Ziduvine in asymptomatic human immunodeficiency virus infection: A controlled trial in persons with fewer than 500 CD4-positive cells per cubic millimeter. *N. Engl. J. Med.* **322,** 941–949.

Waldman, R. H., and Strober, W. (1969). Metabolism of immunoglobulins. *Progr. Allergy* **13,** 1–110.

Waldmann, T. A. (1961). Gastrointestinal protein loss demonstrated by ^{51}Cr-labelled albumin. *Lancet* **II,** 121–123.

Waldmann, T. A. (1985). Protein-losing gastroenteropathies. *In* "Bockus Gastroenterology" (J. E. Berk, ed.), 4th Ed., pp. 1814–1837. Saunders, Philadelphia.

Walker, W. A., and Bloch, K. J. (1983). Intestinal uptake of macromolecules: *In vitro* and *in vivo* studies. *Ann. N.Y. Acad. Sci.* **409,** 593–601.

Walker, W. A., Wu, M., and Bloch, K. J. (1977). Stimulation by immune complexes of mucus release from goblet cells of the rat small intestine. *Science* **197,** 370–372.

Walker-Smith, J. A., Skyring, A. P., and Mistilis, S. P. (1967). Use of $^{51}CrCl_3$ in the diagnosis of protein-losing enteropathy. *Gut* **8,** 166–168.

Walker-Smith, J., Harrison, M., Kilby, A., Philips, A., and France, N. (1978). Cow's milk-sensitive enteropathy. *Arch. Dis. Child* **53,** 375–380.

Wallis, R. S., Vjecha, M., and Amir-Tahmasseb, M. (1993). Synergy of *Mycobacterium tuberculosis* and HIV-1: Enhanced cytokine expression and elevated beta-2 microglobulin in HIV-positive tuberculosis. *J. Infect. Dis.* **167,** 43–48.

Watson, A. J., and Wright, N. A. (1974). Morphology and cell kinetics of the jejunal mucosa in untreated patients. *Clin. Gastroenterol.* **3,** 11–31.

Webberley, M. J., Hart, M. T., and Melikian, V. (1993). Thromboembolism in inflammatory bowel disease: role of platelets. *Gut* **34,** 247–251.

Weber, J. N., Thom, S., Barrison, I., Unwin, R., Forster, S., Jeffries, D. J., Boylston, A., and Pinching, A. J. (1987). Cytomegalovirus colitis and esophageal ulceration in the context of AIDS: Clinical manifestations and preliminary report on treatment with Foscarnet. *Gut* **28,** 482–487.

Webster, S. G. P., Wilkinson, E. M., and Gowland, E. (1977). A comparison of fat absorption in young and old subjects. *Age Aging* **6,** 113–117.

Weiser, M. M., and Douglas, A. P. (1976). An alternative mechanism for gluten toxicity in coeliac disease. *Lancet* **I,** 567–569.

Weiser, M. M., Andres, G. A., Brentjens, R. T., Evans, R. T., and Reichlin, M. (1981). Systemic lupus erythematosus and intestinal venulitis. *Gastroenterology* **81,** 570–579.

Weiss, J. B., Austin, R. K., Schanfield, M. S., and Kagnoff, M. F. (1983). Gluten-sensitive enteropathy: Immunoglobulin G heavy chain (Gm) allotypes and the immune response to wheat gliadin. *J. Clin. Invest.* **72,** 96–101.

Welch, K., Finkbeiner, W., Alpers, C. E., Blumenfeld, W., Davis, R. L., Smuckler, E. A., and Beckstead, J. H. (1984). Autopsy findings in the acquired immunodeficiency syndrome. *J. Am. Med. Assoc.* **252,** 1152–1159.

Werlin, S. L., Chusid, M. J., Caya, J., and Oechler, H. W. (1982). Colitis in chronic granulomatous disease. *Gastroenterology* **82,** 328–331.

Weser, E. (1976). The management of patients after small bowel resection. *Gastroenterology* **71,** 146–150.

Whimbey, E., Gold, J. W. M., Polsky, B., Dryjanski, J., Hawkins, C., Blevins, A., Brannon, P., Kiehn, T. E., Brown, A. E., and Armstrong, D. (1986). Bacteremia and fungemia in patients with acquired immunodeficiency syndrome. *Ann. Intern. Med.* **104,** 511–514.

Whipple, G. H. (1907). A hitherto undescribed disease characterized anatomically by deposits of fat and fatty acids in the intestinal and mesenteric lymphatic tissues. *Bull. Johns Hopkins Hosp.* **18,** 382–391.

White, J. A. M., and King, M. H. (1964). Kaposi's sarcoma presenting with abdominal symptoms. *Radiology* **46,** 197–201.

Whiteside, M. E., Barkin, J. S., May, R. G., Weiss, S. D., Fischl, M. A., and MacLeod, C. L. (1984). Enteric coccidiosis among patients with the acquired immunodeficiency syndrome. *Am. J. Trop. Med. Hyg.* **33,** 1065–1072.

Wilde, C. D., and Milstein, C. (1980). Analysis of immunoglobulin chain secretion using hybrid myelomas. *Eur. J. Immunol.* **10,** 462–467.

Williams, A., Asquith, P., and Stableforth, D. E. (1984). Asthma, eczema, seasonal rhinitis and skin atopy in adult coeliac disease. *Gut* **25,** A1991.

Wilson, K. H., Blitchington, R., Frothingham, R., and Wilson, J. A. (1991). Phylogeny of the Whipple's-disease-associated bacterium. *Lancet* **II,** 474–475.

Working Group of European Society of Pediatric Gastroenterology and Nutrition (1991). Revised criteria for diagnosis of coeliac disease. *Arch. Dis. Child* **65,** 909–911.

World Health Organization (1976). Report of WHO meeting of investigators. Alpha heavy chain disease. *Arch. Fr. Mal. App. Dig. Malnutr.* **65,** 591–607.

Wright, T. L., and Heyworth, M. F. (1989). Maldigestion and malabsorption. *In* "Gastrointestinal Disease" (M. H. Sleisenger and J. S. Fordtran, eds.), 4th Ed., pp. 263–282. Saunders, Philadelphia.

Wroe, S. J., Pires, M., Harding, B., Youl, B. D., and Shorvon, S. (1991). Whipple's disease confined to the CNS presenting with multiple intracerebral mass lesions. *J. Neurol. Neurosurg. Psychiatry* **54,** 989–992.

Wruble, L. D., and Kalser, M. H. (1964). Diabetic steatorrhea: A distinct entity. *Am. J. Med.* **37,** 118–129.

Yarchoan, R., Klecker, R. W., Weinhold, K. J., Markham, P. D., Lyerly, H. K., Durack, D. T. Gelmann, E., Nusinoff-Lehrmann, S., Blum, R. M., Barry, D. W., Shearer, G. M., Fischl, M. A., Mitsuya, H., and Gallo, R. C. (1986). Administration of 3′-azido-3′-dexythymidine, an inhibitor of HTLVIII/LAV replication, to patients with AIDS or AIDS-related complex. *Lancet* **1,** 575–580.

Yardley, J. B., and Bayless, T. M. (1967). Giardiasis. *Gastroenterology* **52,** 301–304.

Yardley, J. H., Bayless, T. M., Norton, J. H., and Hendrix, T. R. (1962). A study of the jejunal epithelium before and after a gluten-free diet. *N. Engl. J. Med.* **267,** 1173–1179.

Yolken, R. H., Hart, W., Oung, I., Shiff, C., Greenson, J., and Perman, J. A. (1991). Gastrointestinal dysfunction and di-saccharide intolerance in children infected with human immunodeficiency virus. *J. Pediatr.* **118,** 359–363.

Ziegler, J. L., Beckstead, J. A., Volberding, P. A., Abrams, D. I., Levine, A. M. Lukes, R. J., Gill, P. S., Burkes, R. L., Meyer, P. R., Metroka, C. E., Mouradian, J., Moore, A., Riggs, S. A., Butler, J. J., Cabanillas, F. C, Hersh, E., Newell, G. R., Laubenstein, L. J., Knowles, D., Odognyk, C., Raphel, B., Koziner, B., Urmacher, C., and Clarkson, B. D. (1984). Non-Hodgkin's lymphoma in 90 homosexual men: Relation to generalized lymphadenopathy and the acquired immunodeficiency syndrome. *N. Engl. J. Med.* **311,** 565–570.

Zioudrou, C., Streaty, R. A., and Klee, W. A. (1979). Opioid peptides derived from food proteins. *J. Biol. Chem.* **254,** 2446–2449.

Zone, J. J., Lasalle, B. A., and Provost, T. T. (1980). Circulating immune complexes of IgA type in dermatitis herpetiformis. *J. Invest. Dermatol.* **75,** 152–155.

Zora, J. A., O'Connell, E. J., Sachs, M. I., and Hoffman, A. D. (1984). Eosinophilic gastroenteritis: A case report and review of the literature. *Ann. Allergy* **53,** 45–49.

40

Food Allergy

Dean D. Metcalfe

I. INTRODUCTION

Food allergy is a term applied to an immunological reaction to a food or food additive that occurs only in some individuals and is unrelated to a physiological effect of the substance. The term "food allergy" is synonymous with the phrase "food hypersensitivity." "Food intolerance" is a general term describing an abnormal physiological response to an ingested food or food additive that is not immunological in origin (Anderson, 1986). Under the term "food allergy" are several distinct clinicopathological entities, including classic immediate reactions to foods, eczema, eosinophilic gastroenteritis, and the food-induced enterocolitis syndrome.

The prevalence of food allergy in the general population has not been determined. However, two prospective surveys reported that 23–28% of parents believe their children had experienced at least one adverse reaction to food (Kayosaari, 1982; Bock, 1987). After evaluation, only approximately one-third of the complaints could be reproduced and only 2–4% of these children experienced reproducible allergic reactions to foods. Similar studies of food allergy are not available in adult populations, although allergic reactions to foods in adults generally are believed to occur less frequently than in children. The prevalence of reactions to food additives, assessed by questionnaire and compared with the number that could be confirmed by a double-blind challenge in a group of 18,582 respondents, has been estimated at 0.01–0.23% (Young *et al.*, 1987). In summary, 2–4% of children and even fewer adults suffer from food allergies; the prevalence of reactions to food additives is less than 1%.

II. IMMEDIATE REACTIONS TO FOODS

IgE-mediated immediate hypersensitivity reactions are the basis for the majority of allergic reactions to foods. Such reactions occur within minutes of consuming a food to which a given individual is sensitive. These reactions occur in all age groups and may involve multiple target organs. These responses appear to be IgE dependent and involve the release of chemical mediators of inflammation from mast cells and basophils.

Patients who develop immediate reactions to foods are usually atopic to begin with (Atkins *et al.*, 1985). Patients who develop food allergies tend to be individuals with severe respiratory allergies and a greater number of positive skin tests (Fiorini *et al.*, 1990). Thus, patients with food allergies, although representing a subgroup of atopic individuals, appear to have severe allergies in general and more difficulty regulating IgE levels in response to environmental antigens.

A. Pathogenesis

Immediate hypersensitivity reactions to foods are caused by the production of IgE in response to specific food antigens. This food-specific IgE then binds to mast cells in the gastrointestinal mucosa as well as elsewhere. On subsequent exposure to a specific food antigen, the potential exists for IgE-dependent mast cell activation. This process is influenced by age, digestive processes, and gastrointestinal permeability.

Both nonspecific and specific barrier systems limit ingress of intact proteins. After ingestion, food initially is subjected to stomach acid and pepsins, pancreatic enzymes, and intestinal peptidases. Large proteins generally are degraded into peptides and amino acids. Mucosal epithelial cells absorb amino acids and small peptides. Antigenic proteins and peptides that successfully traverse the mucosal epithelial barrier elicit an immune response. This response, in part, leads to the secretion of antigen-specific IgA onto the mucosal surface. This IgA further complexes with specific antigens and helps prevent their absorption. Abnormalities in these systems associated with achlorhydria, cystic fibrosis, selective IgA deficiency, or immaturity of the gut may result in increased antigenic penetration of the gastrointestinal barrier. Substances such as alcohol, aspirin, and tobacco are examples of exogenous substances that may reduce gastric mucus and disrupt the epithelial barrier.

Clinical evidence supports the concept that food antigens do indeed penetrate the normal gastrointestinal tract. When 65 adults were sensitized intradermally with serum from a fish allergic individual and then fed raw fish (Prausnitz–Küstner test), 94% developed a wheal-and-flare response at the sensitized site. Reactions developed within 15–60 min of the ingestion of fish. No reactions were observed at control sites (Brunner and Walzer, 1928). Wilson and Walter (1935) also reported that 74% of children sensitized with serum from an egg-allergic subject exhibited wheal-and-flare responses at sites of sensitization after consuming eggs. Intravenous injection of the protein nitrogen equivalent of 1/44,000 of a peanut kernel reportedly is sufficient to elicit a wheal-and-flare response at a passively sensitized skin site (Walzer, 1942).

Local mucosal reactions reminiscent of those that follow mast cell degranulation in human skin have been reported *in vivo* after passive sensitization of human ileum and colonic mucosa. Local reactions after passive sensitization could be induced by ingestion or by direct application of the antigen. Human jejunal mucosal mast cells also have been reported to degranulate *in vitro* in IgE-dependent reactions (Selbekk *et al.*, 1978).

The increased susceptibility of young infants to food allergic reactions is believed to be the result of both immunological immaturity and immaturity of the gastrointestinal barrier. In genetically predisposed infants, ingested antigens consequently may stimulate production of food-antigen-specific IgE antibodies or other abnormal immune responses. Prospective studies suggest that exclusive breast-feeding promotes the development of oral tolerance and prevents some food allergy and atopic dermatitis in infants and young children (Zeiger *et al.*, 1989). This protective effect may be the result of decreased exposure to foreign proteins, passive protection provided by breast milk SIgA, and soluble factors in breast milk that induce earlier maturation of the gut barrier and the infant immune response.

Several studies have demonstrated increased lymphocyte proliferation after food antigen stimulation *in vitro* in patients with food allergy. However, *in vitro* T-cell responses also commonly are found in normal individuals. Whether these T-cell responses *in vitro* represent an immunopathogenic marker or simply reflect a response to increased antigen penetration of the gastrointestinal tract is not clear.

B. Food Allergens

Only a few foods provoke the majority of immediate hypersensitivity reactions to foods. In children, foods most commonly incriminated include egg, milk, peanut, tree nuts, and, less commonly, fish, soy, shrimp, and pea (Bock, 1986). Other foods also have been incriminated, including wheat, chicken, and turkey, leading to the conclusion that many individuals under the appropriate circumstances can develop IgE-dependent reactions to any one of a number of diverse food groups. The prevalence of reactions to specific foods depends, in part, on the eating habits of a given population; for example, fish allergies appear to be more prevalent in Scandinavian countries (Aas, 1966) and soybean allergy is more common in Japan (Moroz and Yang, 1980).

Infants with food allergies tend to outgrow certain food sensitivities, particularly those to milk and eggs (Bock, 1982). Some adults also may lose food sensitivity if they practice rigorous food avoidance for a period of time. Pastorello *et al.* (1989) demonstrated by a double-blind food challenge that, out of 10 adults with food sensitivity, 1- to 2-yr avoidance of specific foods led to tolerance of the food in 4 patients. Thus, at least a subgroup of adults appears to lose the food allergy after a period of food avoidance. However, the data also show that several adults continued to be sensitive despite food avoidance. Further evidence supporting the latter observation is provided by a study of the natural history of shrimp hypersensitivity (Dual *et al.*, 1990). Baseline levels of shrimp-specific IgE did not appear to be altered in the long term by isolated shrimp challenges.

Several specific food antigens responsible for immediate IgE-mediated food reactions have been isolated and characterized, including allergens from codfish (Aas and Jebsen, 1967; Elsayed and Bennich, 1975), shrimp (Hoffman *et al.*, 1981; Nagpal *et al.*, 1989), peanuts (Sachs *et al.*, 1981), and soybeans (Moroz and Yang, 1980). These water-soluble food allergens tend to be relatively resistant to acid and to proteolytic enzymes (Table I). Protein fractions from cow's milk and egg also have been examined for antigenicity. Cow's milk consists of casein (80%) and whey (20%). β-Lactoglobulin and α-lactalbumin are the principal proteins in whey. β-Lactoglobulin is a glycoprotein with a molecular weight of 18,263; α-lactalbumin has a molecular weight of 14,174; and bovine serum albumin consists of a polypeptide with a molecular weight of 67,000. Positive skin tests have been reported to occur in response to casein, α-lactalbumin, β-lactoglobulin, and bovine serum albumin in milk-allergic children in approximately equal numbers (Goldman *et al.*, 1963b). Positive oral challenges have been reported in response to all fractions tested, but β-lactoglobulin produced the highest rate of positive challenges (Goldman *et al.*, 1963a). Individuals reactive to egg are usually sensitive to the egg white. Oval-

Table I Common Food Allergens

Allergen	Source	Molecular weight	Composition	Characteristics	Reference
Antigen M (Gad c I)	Codfish	12,328	113 Amino acids, 1 glucose	Parvalbumin; chelates calcium; relatively acid and protease resistant	Aas and Jebsen (1967); Elsayed and Bennich (1975)
Antigen I	Shrimp	42,000	Dimer	Heat labile	
Antigen II (Pen i I)	Shrimp	38,000	96% protein; 4% carbohydrate	Heat stable	Hoffman *et al.* (1981); Nagpal *et al.* (1989)
Peanut I	Peanut	20,000; 30,000	Two bands	Relatively acid, protease, and heat resistant	Sachs *et al.* (1981)
Kunitz soybean trypsin inhibitor	Soybean	20,500	Polypeptide chain, two disulfide bridges	Relatively acid and protease resistant	Moroz and Yang (1980)

bumin and ovomucoid are the primary allergens in egg white protein. Both are present in uncooked and cooked egg. Conalbumin (ovotransferrin) is also allergenic. Lysozyme appears to be much less allergenic (Yunginger, 1991).

Related foods sometimes contain allergens that cross-react clinically. Cross-reactive allergens have been reported in certain foods and pollens, for example, in melons, banana, and ragweed pollen; celery and mugwort pollen; and apple, carrot, hazelnut, and birch pollen. Food-allergic patients should be evaluated by history and/or with oral food challenges to determine whether foods within similar food groupings are capable of causing clinical reactions.

C. Clinical Manifestations

Immediate hypersensitivity reactions to food antigens are evidenced by a spectrum of signs and symptoms from abdominal pain to anaphylaxis. Reactions are influenced by factors including the age of the patient and the quality and quantity of food ingested. The presence of other medical problems also must be considered.

The oropharynx is the initial site of exposure to food antigens. Edema and pruritus of the lips, oral mucosa, and pharynx may be reported since the food contacts the mucosal surfaces. Such reactions are transient and may not be followed by other allergic manifestations. The term "oral allergy syndrome" has been suggested for the clinical situation dominated by oropharyngeal symptoms. The oral allergy syndrome consists of the development of oropharyngeal symptoms most commonly associated with the ingestion of fruits or vegetables. Symptoms include tingling, pruritus, and angioedema of the lips, and occasionally throat tightness, facial flushing, and oral mucosal blebs and hoarseness (Enberg, 1991). Symptoms usually occur within 5–30 min of exposure to the inciting food. Foods such as apple, which cross-reacts with birch, or watermelon and cantaloupe, which cross-react with ragweed, have been suggested to be more likely to induce symptoms. This observation suggests a relationship between the oral allergy syndrome and allergic rhinitis. However, oropharyngeal symptoms may be a prelude to other symptoms of food allergy.

Entry of food into the stomach and intestine may result in nausea, cramping, pain, abdominal distension, vomiting, flatulence, and diarrhea. Symptoms of gastrointestinal involvement may be the only expression of food hypersensitivity. However, this condition alone is unusual.

Food allergy usually also is expressed in one or more extraintestinal target tissues. The basis of reactivity of one system over another has not been determined. The skin is a common target organ in food allergy. Skin reactions consist of acute urticaria, acute angioedema, and, much less frequently, chronic urticaria. In one study of adults with recurrent urticaria, food allergy was demonstrated as the cause in only 1.4% (Champion *et al.*, 1969). Clinically significant food hypersensitivity has been estimated to exist in approximately 20% of children and 10% of adults with atopic dermatitis (Hanifin, 1984). Because of the unique features of eczema, this condition is discussed in a separate section. Asthma and rhinitis secondary to food hypersensitivity are more common in children (Bock *et al.*, 1978) than in adults (Van Metre *et al.*, 1968).

Systemic anaphylaxis associated with allergy to ingested foods generally occurs within 1–30 min but rarely has been reported hours after ingestion of the offending food (Golbert *et al.*, 1969). The first anaphylactic episode may be unexpected or may be preceded by minor symptoms such as abdominal discomfort or urticaria on previous exposure to the food. Anaphylaxis may be evidenced clinically by tongue itching and swelling, palatal itching, throat itching and tightness, wheezing and cyanosis, chest pain, urticaria, angioedema, abdominal pain, vomiting, diarrhea, hypotension, and shock. Severe life-threatening reactions most often are associated with the ingestion of peanuts, nuts, fish, and crustacea. Fatal reactions from the onset may progress rapidly or begin with mild symptoms and then progress to cardiorespiratory arrest and shock over 1–3 hr. Systemic anaphylaxis also has been reported only after ingestion of food followed by exercise. In some cases, symptoms occur only after eating certain foods but in other individuals no specific food can be identified, although the association of the meal with exercise did predispose to anaphylaxis (Dohi *et al.*, 1991).

D. Laboratory Procedures

Laboratory procedures supporting the diagnosis of food hypersensitivity rely on the identification of antigen-specific IgE to water-soluble allergens in extracts of foods. In the case of skin testing, the IgE examined is fixed to skin mast cells. *In vitro* tests identify antigen-specific IgE in serum. Laboratory tests such as total IgE determinations and eosinophil counts do not correlate with immediate hypersensitivity reactions to foods.

Skin testing with food extracts consists of the application of extracts to the dermis. Such testing is the most reliable method of demonstrating specific IgE antibodies. The routine method is the puncture or prick skin test, in which a drop of food extract is placed on the skin. The skin is then punctured through the drop with a sterile needle. Extracts for testing usually are supplied as 1:20 w/v extracts in 50% glycerine. Skin testing using 1:1000 or 1:100 w/v extracts may be performed by the intradermal technique. However, intradermal tests are more likely to produce clinically irrelevant positive tests (Bock *et al.*, 1977) and are associated with a higher frequency of systemic reactions that, in rare instances, have been fatal. Allergic reactions to foods are unusual in the face of negative skin tests (false negatives). Food extracts including nuts, egg, milk, soy, and fish induce reactions that correlate reliably with allergic manifestions. Patients should never be advised that they are allergic to certain foods solely on the basis of positive skin tests, because skin tests may be positive in the absence of symptomatic food allergy (false-positive tests). In cases of the oral allergy syndrome, the use of extracts of fresh fruits and vegetables is often necessary to exclude IgE-mediated food hypersensitivity. Skin testing is not feasible or recommended in some clinical situations. Thus, in patients with extensive skin disease or significant and prolonged dermatographism, or in patients in whom exposure to minute quantities of a specific food resulted in a life-threatening reaction, *in vitro* diagnostics are used to demonstrate food-allergen-specific IgE.

The radioallergosorbent test (RAST) is an *in vitro* test that is considered less sensitive than skin testing. Although modifications of the RAST procedure have been made, all involve antigens coupled to a solid phase (e.g., paper disk). Patient sera are reacted with the solid phase and, after washing, the amount of bound IgE antibodies is calculated by adding labeled anti-human IgE antibodies. The enzyme-linked immunosorbent assay (ELISA) is a variation on this theme. The amount of antigen that binds to the plastic surface of a microtiter plate used in the ELISA assay is generally lower than that bound by coupling in the RAST. Thus, the number of available antibody sites may be lower and the test may be more subject to inhibition by antigen-specific IgG.

Basophil degranulation tests sometimes are employed in the evaluation of allergic reactions to foods. In this test, heparinized venous blood (or separated blood leukocytes) is incubated with extracts of suspected foods. Histamine will be released into the supernatant fluid and may be measured as an index of reactivity if antigen-specific IgE is present on the basophils that interacts with allergens in the added food extract. Basophil degranulation tests are comparable in outcome to the RAST. Interestingly, a high spontaneous *in vitro* release of histamine from basophils occurs in subjects allergic to foods who ingest them on a frequent basis (Sampson *et al.*, 1989).

E. Diagnosis

The evaluation of a possible food allergy uses medical history, physical examination, and relevant laboratory studies. Reactions or diseases that sometimes mimic food allergy must be eliminated. The diagnosis in some instances must be confirmed by double-blind food challenge.

A comprehensive history of each reaction is obtained first, including its clinical features, severity, duration, extent, and response to therapeutic intervention. The patient should be questioned to determine whether the reaction was associated with exercise. Details on how the food was prepared, including whether it was consumed raw or cooked, must be determined. A suspected food may fail to lead consistently to an allergic reaction. Reasons for this inconsistency include the amount consumed (larger amounts are more likely to induce reactions), the presence of other simultaneously ingested foods that may delay digestion, and the possibility that concomitant medications such as antihistamines may have masked the reaction. When evaluating an adverse reaction to a food, the patient and physician must consider a number of other diseases, anatomic defects, and reactions to additives, toxins, and contaminants that may in some way mimic an allergic reaction (Table II).

Several enzyme deficiencies mimic or may complicate gastrointestinal inflammatory diseases. For instance, abdominal cramps, bloating, and diarrhea accompany the ingestion of milk and milk products in individuals with lactase deficiency.

Table II Differential Diagnosis of Food Allergy[a]

Enzyme deficiencies	Endogenous chemicals
Lactase deficiency	Caffeine
Sucrase deficiency	Tyramine
Phenylketonuria	Phenylethylamine
Gastrointestinal disease	Theobromine
Hiatal hernia	Tryptamine
Peptic ulcer	Alcohol
Gallbladder disease	Histamine
Postsurgical dumping syndrome	Toxins
Neoplasia	Bacterial toxins
Inflammatory bowel disease	Botulinum
Pancreatic insufficiency	Staphylococcal toxin
Additives and contaminants	Endogenous toxins
Dyes	Certain mushrooms—alpha-amanitine
Tartrazine	"Shellfish"—saxitoxin
Exogenous chemicals	Ichthyotoxin
Monosodium glutamate	Fungi
Sulfiting agents	Aflatoxin
Nitrates and nitrites	Ergot
Antibiotics	Physiological reactions
	Bulemia
	Anorexia nervosa

[a] Adapted with permission from Sampson and Metcalfe (1991).

Deficiencies such as galactose-4-epimerase (galactosemia) may be diagnosed in infancy as a result of vomiting and diarrhea after milk ingestion. Cystic fibrosis initially may be confused with a food-induced malabsorption syndrome because of associated pancreatic enzyme deficiency.

Symptoms accompanying a number of gastrointestinal diseases initially may be attributed to food allergies. Chronic cough and wheezing secondary to aspiration may occur with hiatal hernia, pyloric stenosis, and, rarely, an H-type tracheo-esophageal fistula. Overfeeding and chalasia are estimated to occur in up to 50% of newborns and result in vomiting associated with feeding (Sampson and Metcalfe, 1991). Particularly in adults, abdominal pain following meals may be due to peptic ulcer disease or cholelithiasis.

Drugs, dyes, additives, bacteria, and bacterial products occasionally are present in foods. Milk from cattle has been contaminated with bacitracin, penicillin, and tetracycline used to treat bovine diseases. Tartrazine yellow (FD&C Yellow Dye No. 5) is a rare cause of hives. Sulfiting agents used to reduce spoilage of such foods as lettuce and shrimp; to inhibit undesirable microorganisms during fermentation, as in wine making; to sanitize food containers; and to prevent oxidative discoloration of foods have been demonstrated to induce problems reminiscent of allergic diseases (Taylor *et al.*, 1991). Foods that may have higher amounts of sulfiting agents include salads, dehydrated potatoes, fruits, vegetables, wines, shrimp and other seafood, baked goods, tea mixes, and vegetable and fruit juices. Asthmatic patients in some instances experience wheezing and associated anaphylactoid symptoms and signs after challenge with potassium metabisulfite (Stevenson and Simon, 1981). Monosodium glutamate in sufficient quantity (usually greater than 6 g) can lead to a transient syndrome consisting of a warmth or burning sensation (especially over the head and shoulders), stiffness or tightness, extremity weakness, pressure, tingling, headache, light-headedness, and gastric discomfort, occurring approximately 15 min after ingestion. Monosodium glutamate also is said to induce wheezing in some asthmatics (Allen, 1991).

Toxins ingested in foods may induce signs and symptoms closely resembling allergic reactions. In scombroid poisoning, ingestion of fish containing high levels of histamine is followed shortly by symptoms including diffuse erythema and headaches. Scombroid fish commonly implicated include tuna, skipjack, and mackerel. Nonscombroid fish implicated include mahi mahi, sardines, anchovies, and herring (Saavedra-Delgado and Metcalfe, 1993). Ciguatera poisoning is seen especially in the Caribbean and Pacific islands. Symptoms include tingling of the lips, tongue, and throat, followed by nausea, vomiting, abdominal pain, diarrhea, headache, and chills, fever, and myalgias. The toxin is produced by algae that are eaten by small herbivores off the reef; these in turn are consumed by carnivorous fish. Paralytic shellfish poisoning is caused by ingestion of bivalve mollusks (especially mussels, clams, oysters, and scallops) contaminated with dinoflagellates of the genus *Gonyaulax,* which produce neurotoxins. When these dinoflagellates "bloom," they lead to a red to reddish-brown discoloration of the water known as a "red tide." Amnesic shellfish poisoning is an acute illness characterized by gastrointestinal symptoms and neurological abnormalities including seizures, coma, disorientation, and loss of memory after the ingestion of mussels. This disease is caused by domoic acid, a potent neurotoxin produced by the bloom of the pennate phytoplanktonic diatom *Nitzia pungens.*

If the relationship between ingestion of foods and symptoms is unclear, elimination diets may be warranted. The possibility of establishing a diagnosis by the use of such diets is higher when fewer foods are responsible for the symptoms. Elimination diets followed by the return of suspect foods to the diet should be applied only in situations in which symptoms are not life-threatening, as in chronic hives or rhinitis. Before any elimination diet is initiated, the patient should remain on the usual diet for 1–2 wk. During that time, the patient records the type and amounts of foods ingested and the occurrence and character of adverse reactions. This record is useful in searching for suspect foods and in establishing baseline symptoms against which the success or failure of elimination diets can be measured. If symptoms fail to appear within this baseline period, the occurrence of symptoms is too infrequent to be appreciated during the period of an elimination diet. If no more than a few foods are suspected to cause the symptoms, the initial elimination diet may consist of removing these foods.

If removal of selected foods from the diet is not successful in eliminating symptoms or if symptoms are unlikely to be caused by foods, as in chronic urticaria, a severely limited diet sometimes is warranted. Severe elimination diets, especially in children, are used for only short periods. Extensive elimination diets for infants under 3 months of age consist of milk substitute alone; for 3–6 months of age, milk substitute and rice cereal; for 6 months to 2 yr, milk substitute with vitamin supplement, rice cereal, applesauce, pears, carrots, squash, and lamb (Crawford, 1980); and for older children and adults, lamb and rice. Continuation of symptoms while patients are on restricted diets indicates that the symptoms are not caused by foods. If symptoms resolve on the restricted diet, resumption of a normal diet should be accompanied by a return of symptoms; subsequent resumption of the restricted diet should alleviate these symptoms. Such cycling reproducibly should eliminate or provoke symptoms to allow the conclusion that symptoms are caused by foods. If a relationship to diet is established, foods, representing food groups eaten by the patient during the control period should be returned individually to the diet in normal amounts at intervals of 3–4 days. Foods returned to the diet without induction of symptoms remain in the diet. Foods provoking symptoms are removed until the procedure is completed. If resumption of symptoms is associated with the introduction of specific foods, this cause-and-effect relationship must be verified by the disappearance of symptoms on elimination of that food.

Double-blind placebo-controlled food challenge (DBPCFC) is the diagnostic procedure by which other diagnostic approaches are judged. DBPCFC is employed in difficult cases in children and adults (Bock *et al.,* 1988). Before DBPCFC, suspect foods should be eliminated for 10–14 days. Antihistamines are discontinued long enough to establish a normal histamine skin test. Other medications are minimized to levels sufficient to prevent breakthrough of acute symptoms. The food challenge is administered in a fasting state, starting with a dose unlikely to provoke symptoms. The dose is then doubled every 30–60 min or more, depending on the type of reaction suspected and the length of time required to produce symptoms. Once the patient has tolerated 10 g lyophilized food blinded in capsules or liquid, clinical reactivity generally is ruled out. If the blinded challenge is negative, the food must be given openly in usual quantities under observation to rule out the rare false-negative challenge. To control for a variety of confounding factors, an equal number of placebo and food antigen challenges is necessary; the order of administration should be randomized. DBPCFCs should be conducted in a clinic or hospital setting, especially if an IgE-mediated reaction is suspected, only if trained personnel and equipment for treating systemic anaphylaxis are present and only with informed consent.

The diagnosis of food allergy is dependent on the history, selective skin tests or RASTs, an appropriate exclusion diet, and blinded provocation. No evidence at this time suggest any diagnostic value for food-specific IgG or IgG_4 antibody levels, measurement of food antigen–antibody complexes, evidence of lymphocyte activation or sublingual or intracutaneous provocation. In gastrointestinal disorders in which pre- and post-challenge biopsy studies are performed for diagnosis, blinded challenge may not be essential.

F. Therapy

The only proven therapy for food allergy is strict elimination of the offending allergen. However, severe elimination diets may lead to malnutrition or eating disorders, and should be instituted only with nutritional guidance. Patients must learn to read and understand food labels to detect hidden food allergens. Clinical reactivity to food allergens is generally specific. Patients rarely react to more than one member of a botanical family or animal species. No appropriately designed trial has demonstrated clear efficacy for the use of prophylactic medications, injection immunotherapy, oral desensitization, or subcutaneous provocation and neutralization in the prevention of allergic reactions to foods.

A patient sometimes may consume a food inadvertently to which he or she is sensitive. Treatment for a specific symptom that results from inadvertent exposure is the same as that employed when other factors provoke symptoms. Thus, laryngeal or pulmonary symptoms following an inadvertent food exposure should be treated immediately with epinephrine, bronchodilator therapy, or both. The treatment of food-induced anaphylaxis is essentially the same as that for anaphylaxis caused by a medication or insect sting. A patient with potential anaphylactic reactivity should be taught to self-administer epinephrine, and should have an epinephrine-containing syringe and an antihistamine available at all times. For children, day care centers and schools should have a list of emergency telephone numbers with back-ups to be called in case of incident. Note that a patient may exhibit only mild symptoms in the first few minutes after ingesting a food to which he or she is allergic, but these may be followed 10–60 min later by hypotension and other severe problems. Following self-medication for systemic reactions, the patient should seek medical attention immediately. All patients with IgE-mediated food allergy should be warned about the possiblity of developing a severe anaphylactic reaction and should be educated in the appropriate treatment measures to be taken in case of an accidental ingestion (Sampson and Metcalfe, 1992).

III. ATOPIC DERMATITIS AND FOOD ALLERGENS

A. Pathogenesis

Atopic dermatitis is a form of eczema that usually has its onset in infancy. The rash is a pruritic, erythematous, papulovesicular eruption that progresses to a scaly lichenified state. The dermatitis tends to be relapsing. Atopic dermatitis involves the cheeks and extensor surfaces of the arms and legs of infants. In young children, the condition tends to involve flexor surfaces; in teenagers and young adults, the flexor surfaces, hands, and feet are involved. The association with other atopic disease is remarkable; 50–80% of children with atopic dermatitis develop allergic rhinitis or asthma. In addition, 60–70% of children with atopic dermatitis have a family history of allergic rhinitis or asthma (Marsh *et al.*, 1981). In children with atopic dermatitis, approximately one-third can be found to have food-related hypersensitivity reactions (Sampson, 1989).

The histological findings in atopic dermatitis depend on the chronicity of the lesion. Acute lesions demonstrate intracellular edema (spongiosis) and an inflammatory infiltrate of mononuclear cells in the upper dermis. Chronic lesions show epidermal thickening, increased numbers of mast cells, and decreased numbers of sebaceous glands (Mihn *et al.*, 1976). Dermal deposits of major basic protein have been described (Leiferman *et al.*, 1985). The serum IgE is elevated in most patients with atopic dermatitis. On average, serum IgE levels are higher in patients with atopic dermatitis than in patients with allergic rhinitis or asthma. The serum IgE level typically remains elevated regardless of the clinical state of the atopic dermatitis, although some patients have demonstrated a decrease in serum IgE with healing or remission of their skin lesions.

A relationship between food allergy and atopic dermatitis is supported by the demonstration of rises in plasma histamine after positive oral food challenges in children with atopic dermatitis (Sampson and Jolie, 1984). A relationship of food hypersensitivity to atopic dermatitis also is supported by the results of DBPCFCs in 113 children with severe atopic dermatitis (Sampson and McCaskill, 1985). In this study, 56% of the children exhibited positive food challenges, as manifested by signs and symptoms that included diffuse pruritic erythematous or morbilliform rash, nausea, vomiting, abdominal pain, diarrhea, and bronchospasm. Significantly, egg, peanut, and milk accounted for 42%, 19%, and 11%, respectively, of the positive food challenges. Soy, wheat, fish, chicken, pork, beef, and potato each accounted for 5% or less. When 31 patients were placed on a restrictive diet for 1–2 yr, approximately 40% of the individuals with intitial positive food challenges no longer exhibited a positive challenge; most of them showed improvement in their atopic dermatitis.

B. Clinical Manifestations

Acute lesions of atopic dermatitis are characterized by erythematous papules, edema, and weeping whereas chronic lesions appear scaly with thickening and hyperpigmentation. Typically, the lesions are preceded by an intense pruritis, resulting in the classic description of "the itch that rashes." Approximately 60% of atopic dermatitis is manifested during the first year of life; 95% is seen by 5 years of age. In infants, the lesions predominate in the head and neck region, whereas lesions in the flexural regions of the popliteal and antecubital fossae predominate in older children. Atopic dermatitis can have a fluctuating course with improvement of symptoms in the spring and summer. Children with onset of atopic dermatitis after 2 years of age generally have a worse prognosis. In severe cases of atopic dermatitis, 70% have had persistence of their symptoms for 20 years. Overall, 90% of patients with atopic dermatitis can expect improvement of their symptoms with time.

C. Diagnosis

Demonstration of the relationship between immediate reactions to foods and eczema requires the elicitation of positive skin tests to foods in question as well as clinical reactions in response to these foods on oral food challenge. Associating specific food allergies with atopic dermatitis is difficult. Many foods that provoke skin symptoms during a double-blind challenge do not provoke obvious symptoms when the patients consume them on a regular basis. Urticaria is uncommon in children with atopic dermatitis exacerbated by food allergies.

The avoidance of foods shown to induce a positive response on double-blind controlled challenge leads to substantial improvement in the disease. Once a specific food allergen has been avoided for 6–12 months and the patient's skin largely has returned to a normal state, the re-administration of these foods often will precipitate urticarial skin lesions rather than the morbilliform rash that is seen during challenge procedures during active atopic dermatitis.

The differential diagnosis of atopic dermatitis includes seborrheic dermatitis, contact dermatitis, candidiasis, and histiocytosis X. Similar skin lesions also may be seen in patients with the Wiskott–Aldrich syndrome, ataxia telangiectasia, phenylketonuria, X-linked infantile agammaglobulinemia, the syndrome of elevated serum IgE with recurrent furunculosis, and the hyper-IgE syndrome. Initially, the rash of acrodermatitis enteropathica from zinc deficiency may be confused with atopic dermatitis, although its characteristic distribution, other associated symptoms, and a history of a deficient zinc intake allow for differentiation.

D. Treatment

When exacerbation of atopic dermatitis has been documented to be related to a specific food allergen, that food should be eliminated from the diet. Symptomatic control of pruritis may be attempted with antihistamines. In severe cases, a brief application of a topical steroid to control a flare of the disease may be warranted. When an infection is suspected, an antistaphylococcal antibiotic may be prescribed. Other general measures include avoidance of irritants, such as soaps and wools, as well as of trauma, as from scratching. Maintenance of skin hydration is an important component of therapy.

IV. FOOD PROTEIN-INDUCED GASTROENTEROPATHY

Food protein-mediated gastroenteropathy is a disease of infants and children in which a hypersensitivity reaction to a food protein results in damage to the intestinal mucosa and mucosal dysfunction. The best-known food protein gastroenteropathy is that induced by cow's milk protein (Kuitunen *et al.*, 1975; Lake, 1991). Soy protein gastroenteropathy also has been identified and has a similar clinical and histological pattern (Ament and Rubin, 1972). Intolerances to egg, fish, rice, and chicken have been reported (Iyngkaran *et al.*, 1982; Victoria *et al.*, 1982).

A. Pathogenesis

The pathogenesis of food protein-mediated gastroenteropathy is unknown. The disease typically resolves with age. Thus, the immaturity of the infant gastrointestinal mucosa and immune system appears to be a factor. Immaturity or disruption of the normal gastrointestinal mucosal barrier may allow for sensitization to intact food antigens, as suggested by the observation that a protein gastroenteropathy may follow an acute episode of gastroenteritis (Jackson *et al.*, 1983). Likewise, a transient deficiency of secretory IgA may allow more food antigen access to the gastrointestinal mucosa. Histological examination of intestinal biopsies of untreated children with food protein-induced gastroenteropathy has shown an increased number of plasma cells, lymphocytes, eosinophils, and neutrophils in the mucosa and between epithelial cells, consistent with an evolving immune reaction. A cell-mediated delayed hypersensitivity mechanism has been supported by the demonstration of an *in vitro* lymphoblastic transformation to α-lactalbumin and β-lactoglobulin in 38% of 45 children (1–34 months of age) with cow's milk protein gastroenteropathy. This result compares with a rate of 9.5% in a similar age-matched control group (Scheinmann *et al.*, 1976; Savilahti and Verkasala, 1984).

The role of antibody in the pathogenesis of cow's milk protein gastroenteropathy is unclear. At birth, virtually no infants exhibit serum antibodies against cow's milk proteins but, by age 2 years, 95% of formula-fed children exhibit IgA and IgG antibodies against these antigens. Total serum IgE is often normal, and IgE specific to cow's milk protein is usually absent in affected children (Danneus and Johansson, 1979). Antibodies to cow's milk proteins also have been found in stools of normal children, those recovering from acute gastroenteritis, and those with cow's milk protein gastroenteropathy (Davis *et al.*, 1970).

B. Clinical Manifestations

The predominant symptoms of food protein-mediated gastroenteropathy are vomiting, diarrhea, malabsorption resulting in growth failure, and gross or occult stool blood loss resulting in anemia. Subtle symptoms such as irritability or colic may be the initial manifestations in some infants. Symptoms usually appear within 1 month of introducing cow's milk or a cow's milk-based formula into the diet. Gross intestinal bleeding may occur in infants aged 1–5 wk that may mimic necrotizing enterocolitis. Resolution of the intestinal bleeding occurs 24–48 hr after removal of milk from the diet. Radiologic features of four infants with gross intestinal bleeding secondary to cow's milk consumption suggested segmental colitis with short segment colonic spasm as well as mucosal ulceration in two of the four infants (Swischuk and Hayden, 1985). Occult intestinal bleeding in infants 4–12 months of age can result in a hypochromic microcytic anemia, in which associated occasional protein-losing gastroenteropathy may cause periorbital and gross edema from hypoproteinemia. Gastrointestinal blood loss results in iron deficiency anemia with guaiac-positive stools. Carbohydrate malabsorption may be present secondary to an intestinal mucosal injury, as is manifested by stools containing reducing sugars (lactose or sucrose) as well as by a low stool pH. Eosinophilia may be present in some patients. An unusual manifestation of milk hypersensitivity has been described in which precipitating antibodies to cow's milk protein is associated with chronic pulmonary disease (Heiner's syndrome) in children (Heiner *et al.*, 1962).

C. Diagnosis

The diagnosis of cow's milk protein hypersensitivity requires the demonstration of a relationship between ingestion of cow's milk and symptomatology consistent with intestinal damage. In children exhibiting diarrhea and malabsorption, biopsy of the small intestine usually reveals villous atrophy, primarily in the jejunum. In some children only the colon is involved, manifesting as colitis (Lake, 1991).

Histological evaluation of the intestinal mucosa may be unrevealing in mild cases or may resemble celiac disease. In such instances, oral challenge with cow's milk protein may allow confirmation of the diagnosis. A lactose tolerance test should be performed to rule out lactase deficiency. (If a soy protein gastroenteropathy is being evaluated, a sucrose tolerance test should be performed, since the carbohydrate source in soy formula is sucrose; Ament, 1972). This tolerance test is followed by an oral challenge that is not blinded. The child's stool is carefully followed for weight, presence of blood, pH, and reducing substances. A volume greater than 20 g/kg/day, appearance of blood, or the development of carbohydrate malabsorption as demonstrated by a stool pH below 6.0 or a positive test for reducing sugars is sufficient evidence of cow's milk hypersensitivity. A second approach is to demonstrate a reproducible clinical response in a 48-hr period to three separate cow's milk challenges, with total resolution of symptoms after withdrawal of milk.

D. Treatment

Treatment is dependent on removal of milk or other sensitizing protein from the child's diet. An elemental formula or formulation or total parenteral nutrition may be required to allow repair of and return of normal function to the gastrointestinal mucosa. Reintroduction of offending protein may be attempted, since protein-mediated gastroenteropathy typically resolves by 18–24 months of age (Walker-Smith, 1986).

V. EOSINOPHILIC GASTROENTERITIS

Eosinophilic gastroenteritis is a disease characterized by eosinophilic infiltration of the gastrointestinal wall, peripheral eosinophilia, and gastrointestinal symptoms. The sites of involvement of eosinophilic gastroenteritis include the esophagus, stomach, small intestine, colon, and, rarely, extraintestinal organs. Approximately half the cases have allergic features and may be related to food allergy.

The true incidence of eosinophilic gastroenteritis is not known. Males are affected slightly more often than females. Eosinophilic gastroenteritis may occur at any age, although the peak age of onset is in the third decade. Most individuals with food-dependent disease are under the age of 20 years (Johnstone and Morrison, 1978; Thounce and Tanner, 1985).

A. Pathogenesis

The cause of eosinophilic gastroenteritis is largely unknown, although an IgE-dependent, mast cell-mediated mechanism has been advocated as the immunological basis of this disorder in some patients with an immunological reaction to food antigen (Caldwell *et al.*, 1978). Atopic diseases, such as childhood food allergies, eczema, allergic rhinitis, bronchial asthma, and urticaria, and a positive family background for allergy are common in patients with eosinophilic gastroenteritis. Moreover, many patients have peripheral eosinophilia, an elevated serum IgE level, and positive RASTs for specific IgE antibodies to food antigens. Results of RASTs or skin tests may be accompanied by a symptomatic response to food challenge (Caldwell *et al.*, 1979).

Participation of a similar allergic mechanism has been demonstrated in cow's milk allergy in childhood. Some children with severe milk allergy present with iron-deficiency anemia and hypoprotenemia, demonstrating that ingested bovine milk protein may cause protein and fat malabsorption. Milk challenge results in an increase of IgE-positive plasma cells, mast cell degranulation, and an infiltration of eosinophils in the small intestinal mucosa (Oyaizu *et al.*, 1985). Eosinophils infiltrating the bowel mucosa are both activated and degranulated; in this way, they may induce tissue damage by releasing eosinophil major basic protein (Keshavarzian, 1985). An ultrastructural study of mucosal eosinophils obtained from damaged duodenum also has shown that the electron core density of eosinophil granules is inverted or absent, and tubulovesicular structures appear. Major basic protein is detected diffusely in the matrix of eosinophil granules and outside of granules in tight association with extragranular membrane formations. In contrast, eosinophil cationic protein and eosinophil peroxidase normally are distributed in the granular matrix, supporting a selective release of eosinophil mediators and a role for major basic protein in tissue damage in eosinophilic gastroenteritis (Torpier *et al.*, 1988). Indeed, many pediatric cases of food protein intolerance, such as milk protein or soy protein intolerance, have been classified as allergic gastroenteropathy when convincing evidence of an allergic mechanism was available and when the clinical findings were those of eosinophilic gastroenteritis. In these cases, the elimination of the incriminated food antigen frequently resulted in improvement (Katz *et al.*, 1984).

All patients with eosinophilic gastroenteritis, however, are not atopic, and all cases cannot be explained by food allergy. Only approximately half the patients with eosinophilic gastroenteritis have findings consistent with atopy. Many patients show no personal or family history of allergy, no positive skin tests for food allergens, no elevation in serum IgE, and no adverse reactions to foods. Even in patients who have suspected food allergies, sequential withdrawal of various food substances may fail to provide amelioration of symptoms, and a poor correlation may exist between the results of skin tests to specific food antigens and the results of an elimination diet. In addition, most patients show no abnormality after extensive immunological studies, including serum IgE, IgM, and IgA levels; complement levels; lymphocyte quantification; and lymphocyte responses to nonspecific mitogens (Elkon *et al.*, 1977).

B. Clinical Manifestations

Patients with eosinophilic gastroenteritis experience postprandial nausea with vomiting, abdominal pain, diarrhea, steatorrhea, and weight loss in the adult or growth failure in the child. Both weight loss and growth failure are associated with malabsorption or a restricted caloric intake. Radiologic findings may reveal mucosal edema and coarsening with nodularity of the folds of the small bowel (Goldberg *et al.*, 1973). Muscular disease can precipitate abdominal distress with vomiting from proximal small bowel obstruction. Radiologic features in such cases include evidence of pyloric narrowing and obstruction. Small bowel obstruction is unusual in children. Subserosal disease results in ascites with a marked eosinophilia.

C. Diagnosis

Significant mucosal disease typically presents with evidence of iron-deficiency anemia, hypoalbuminemia, and hypogammaglobulinemia secondary to a protein-losing gastroenteropathy, steatorrhea, and an eosinophilic leukocytosis. Multiple positive skin tests in response to food extracts may be present. The mucosal form of eosinophilic gastroenteritis disease may be confused with celiac disease, regional enteritis, neoplasms (lymphoma), polyarteritis nodosa, parasites, the hypereosinophilic syndrome, or another protein-losing gastroenteropathy (Robert *et al.*, 1977; Greenberger and Gryboski, 1978). The diagnosis of eosinophilic gastroenteritis is established with a gastrointestinal biopsy, demonstrating an eosinophilic infiltration of the gastrointestinal wall (Figure 1). Examination of the stool may reveal Charcot–Leyden crystals. An impaired D-xylose absorption secondary to damage of the intestinal mucosa can be present (Cello, 1979).

Eosinophilic gastroenteritis in children may be difficult to differentiate from a transient cow's milk gastroenteropathy of infancy. In a study of 12 children with symptoms and diagnostic findings of eosinophilic gastroenteritis, two groups were clinically distinguishable (Katz *et al.*, 1984). One group of children, all of whom were less than 1 year of age and had no IgE antibodies to milk protein antigens, responded to withdrawal of milk from their diet with resolution of their symptoms. The other group of children was generally older than 1 year of age, demonstrated other atopic symptoms, exhibited IgE to food antigens, and had a poor response to dietary manipulation; this group required oral steroids to control the symptoms. Clinically, the first group of children who responded to cow's milk exclusion was diagnosed as having a cow's milk gastroenteropathy with eosinophilia. The follow-up of the infants with a cow's milk gastroenteropathy revealed that most of these children were able to have milk reintroduced into their diet by 30 months of age.

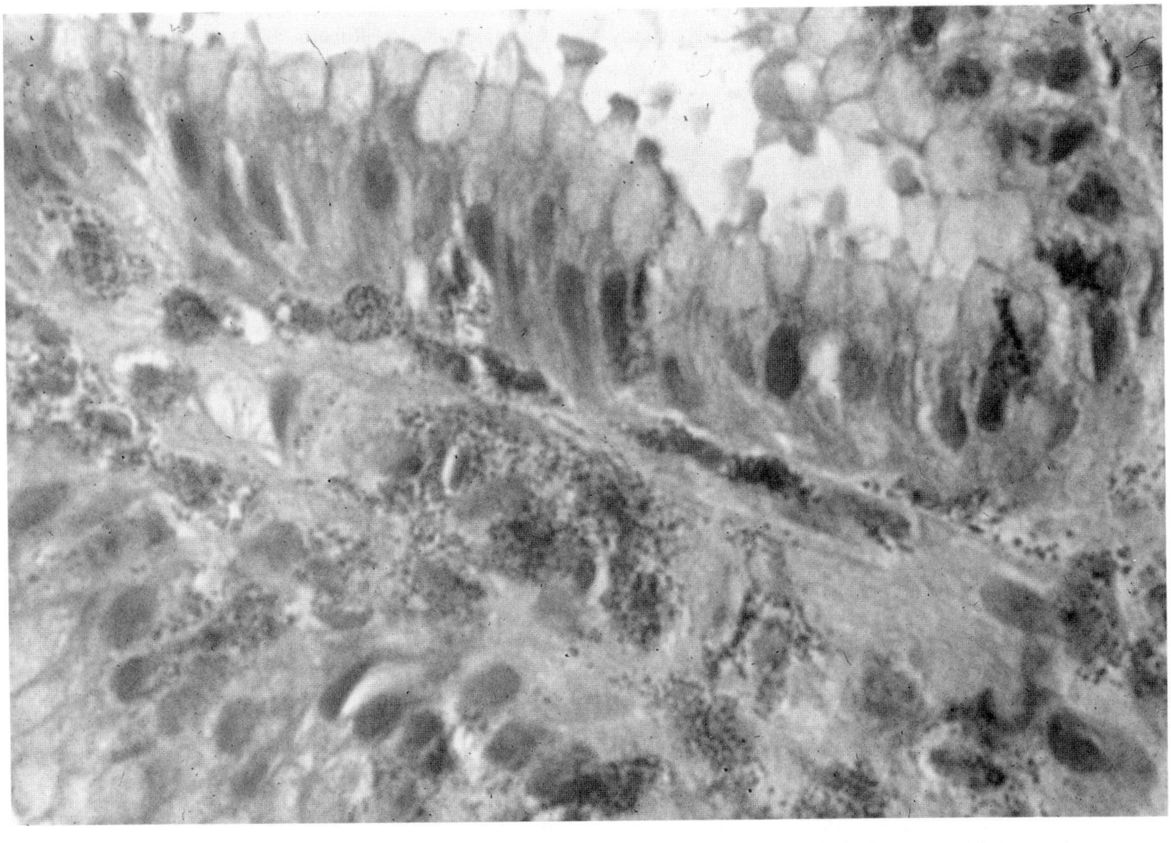

Figure 1 Small bowel biopsy. The lamina propria is infiltrated heavily with eosinophilic leukocytes, which contain many eosinophilic granules. The villous architecture is preserved. Hematoxylin and eosin stain (H & E), ×400. Reprinted with permission from Min and Metcalfe (1991).

D. Treatment

Treatment of eosinophilic gastroenteritis is often unsatisfactory. Food hypersensitivity should be ruled out as the precipitating or exacerbating factor in eosinophilic gastroenteritis. History and skin testing or RAST may identify food allergens for a trial of elimination. A trial diet that eliminates multiple food antigens from the diet in a systematic order may be performed when no clear history or evidence of IgE-mediated hypersensitivity is elicited. In patients with eosinophilic gastroenteritis and food sensitivity, the number of foods involved may preclude the long-term use of an elimination diet for symptom control, although improvement may be demonstrated initially. Patients who respond poorly to dietary restrictions as well as those without evidence of food hypersensitivity may require oral steroid therapy. Although this treatment usually results in clinical improvement, the need for long-term steroid therapy is variable. In some cases, steroids eventually may be withdrawn without recurrence of the symptoms. In other cases, withdrawal of steroids is followed by an exacerbation of disease. Individuals with multiple food sensitivities appear to be less likely to have resolution of their eosinophilic gastroenteritis with treatment, perhaps because of persistence of food antigen-induced immunological responses in the gastrointestinal tract. Initially, in adults, prednisone should be instituted to suppress inflammation. As evidenced by improvement of clinical symptoms and resolution of the histological abnormalities, prednisone may be tapered to an every-other-day regimen. When exacerbations occur, a brief burst of steroids is usually sufficient to bring the symptoms under control (Klein *et al.*, 1970; Min and Metcalfe, 1991).

Acknowledgments

The author would like to thank Belinda Richardson for her assistance in the preparation of this manuscript.

References

Aas, K. A. (1966). Studies on hypersensitivity to fish. A clinical study. *Int. Arch. Allergy Appl. Immunol.* **29,** 346–363.

Aas, K., and Jebsen, J. W. (1967). Studies of hypersensitivity to fish. Partial purification and crystallization of a major allergenic component of cod. *Int. Arch. Allergy Appl. Immunol.* **32,** 1–28.

Allen, D. H. (1991). Monosodium glutamate. *In* "Food Allergy: Adverse Reactions to Foods and Food Additives" (D. D. Metcalfe, H. A. Sampson, and R. A. Simon, eds.), pp. 261–266. Blackwell Scientific Publications, Oxford.

Ament, M. E. (1972). Malabsorption syndromes in infancy and childhood. *J. Pediatr.* **81,** 685–697.

Ament, M. E., and Rubin, C. E. (1972). Soy protein—Another cause of the flat intestinal lesion. *Gastroenterology* **62,** 227–234.

Anderson, J. A. (1986). The establishment of common language concerning adverse reactions to food and food additives. *J. Allergy Clin. Immunol.* **78,** 140–144.

Atkins, F. M., Steinberg, S. S., and Metcalfe, D. D. (1985). Evaluation of immediate adverse reactions to foods in adults. I. Correlation of demographic, laboratory, and prick skin test data with response to controlled oral food challenge. *J. Allergy Clin. Immunol.* **75,** 348–355.

Bock, S. A. (1982). The natural history of food sensitivity. *J. Allergy Clin. Immunol.* **69,** 173–177.

Bock, S. A. (1986). A critical evaluation of clinical trials in adverse reactions to foods in children. *J. Allergy Clin. Immunol.* **78,** 165–174.

Bock, S. A. (1987). Prospective appraisal of complaints of adverse reactions to foods in children during the first 3 years of life. *Pediatrics* **79,** 863–888.

Bock, S. A., Buckley, J., Holst, A., and May, C. D. (1977). Proper use of skin tests with food extracts in diagnosis of hypersensitivity to food in children. *Clin. Allergy* **7,** 375–383.

Bock, S. A., Lee, Y., Remigio, L. K., and May, C. D. (1978). Studies of hypersensitivity reactions to foods in infants and children. *J. Allergy Clin. Immunol.* **62,** 327–334.

Bock, S. A., Sampson, H. A., Atkins, F. M., Zieger, R. S., Lehrer, S., Sachs, M., Bush, R. K., and Metcalfe, D. D. (1988). Double-blind placebo-controlled food challenge as an office procedure: A manual. *J. Allergy Clin. Immunol.* **82,** 986–997.

Brunner, M., and Walzer, M. (1928). Absorption of undigested proteins in human beings: The absorption of unaltered fish protein in adults. *Arch. Int. Med.* **42,** 173–179.

Caldwell, J. H., Mekhjian, H. S., Hurtubise, P. E., and Beman, F. M. (1978). Eosinophilic gastroenteritis with obstruction: Immunological studies of seven patients. *Gastroenterology* **74,** 825–828.

Caldwell, J. H., Sharma, H. M., Hurtubise, P. E., and Colwell, D. L. (1979). Eosinophilic gastroenteritis in extreme allergy: Immunopathological comparison with nonallergic gastrointestinal disease. *Gastroenterology* **77,** 560–564.

Cello, J. P. (1979). Eosinophilic gastroenteritis—A complex disease entity. *Am. J. Med.* **67,** 1097–1104.

Champion, R. H., Roberts, S. O., Carpenter, R. G., and Roger, J. H. (1969). Urticaria and angioedema: A review of 554 patients. *Br. J. Dermatol.* **81,** 588–597.

Crawford, L. V. (1980). Allergy diets. *In* "Allergic Diseases of Infants, Childhood, and Adolescence" (C. W. Bierman and D. S. Pearlman, eds.), pp. 394–406. Saunders, Philadelphia.

Dannaeus, A., and Johansson, S. G. O. (1979). A follow up study of infants with adverse reactions to cow's milk. I. Serum IgE, skin test reactions and RAST in relation to clinical course. Acta. Paediatr. Scand. **68,** 377–382.

Davis, S. D., Bierman, C. W., Pierson, W. E., Maas, C. W., and Iannetta, A. (1970). Clinical nonspecificity of milk coproantibodies in diarrheal stools. *N. Engl. J. Med.* **282,** 612–613.

Dohi, M., Suko, M., Sugiyama, H., Yamshita, N., Tadokoro, K., Juji, F., Okudaira, H,. Sano, Y., Ito, K., and Miyamoto, T. (1991). Food-dependent, exercise-induced anaphylaxis: A study on 11 Japanese cases. *J. Allergy Clin. Immunol.* **87,** 34–40.

Dual, C. B., Morgan, J. E., and Lehrer, S. B. (1990). The natural history of shrimp hypersensitivity. *J. Allergy Clin. Immunol.* **86,** 88–93.

Elkon, K. B., Sher, R., and Seftel, H. C. (1977). Immunological studies of eosinophilic gastroenteritis and treatment with disodium cromoglycate and beclomethasone dipropionate. *S. Afr. Med. J.* **52,** 838–841.

Elsayed, S., and Bennich, H. (1975). The primary structure of allergen M from cod. *Scand. J. Immunol.* **4,** 203–208.

Enberg, R. N. (1991). Food-induced oropharyngeal symptoms: The oral allergy syndrome. *In* "Food Allergy. Immunology and Allergy Clinics of North America" (J. A. Anderson, ed.), Vol. II, pp. 767–772. Saunders, Philadelphia.

Fiorini, G., Rinaldi, G., Bigi, G., Sironi, D., and Cremonini, L. M. (1990). Symptoms of respiratory allergies are worse in subjects with coexisting food sensitization. *Clin. Exp. Allergy* **20,** 689–692.

Golbert, T. M., Patterson, R., and Pruzansky, J. J. (1969). Systemic allergic reactions to ingested antigens. *J. Allergy* **44,** 96–107.

Goldberg, H. I., O'Kieffe, D., Jenis, E. H., and Boyce, H. W. (1973). Diffuse eosinophilic gastroenteritis. *Am. J. Roentgenol. Radium Ther. Nucl. Med.* **119,** 342–351.

Goldman, A. S., Anderson, D. W., Sellars, W. A., Saperstein, S., Kniker, W. T., and Halpern, S. R. (1963a). Milk allergy. I. Oral challenge with milk and isolated milk proteins in allergic children. *Pediatrics* **32,** 425–443.

Goldman, A. S., Sellars, W. A., Halpern, S. R., Anderson, D. W., Furlow, I. E., and Johnson, C. H. (1963b). Milk allergy. II. Skin testing of allergic and normal children with purified milk proteins. *Pediatrics* **32,** 572–579.

Greenberger, N., and Gryboski, J. D. (1978). Allergic disorders of the intestine and eosinophilic gastroenteritis. *In* "Gastrointestinal Disease—Pathophysiology, Diagnosis, and Management" (M. Sleisenger and J. S. Fordtran, eds.), pp. 1228–1239. Saunders, Philadelphia.

Hanifin, J. M. (1984). Atopic dermatitis. *J. Allergy Clin. Immunol.* **73,** 211–222.

Heiner, D. C., Sears, J. W., and Kniker, W. T. (1962). Multiple precipitins to cow's milk in chronic respiratory disease. *Am. J. Dis. Child* **103,** 634–654.

Hoffman, D. R., Day, E. D., and Miller, J. S. (1981). The major heat stable allergen of shrimp. *Ann. Allergy* **47,** 17–22.

Iyngkaran, N., Abidin, Z., Meng, L. L., and Yadav, M. (1982). Egg-protein-induced villous atrophy. *J. Pediatr. Gastroenterol. Nutr.* **1,** 29–31.

Jackson, D., Walker-Smith, J. A., and Phillips, A. D. (1983). Macromolecular absorption by histologically normal and abnormal small intestinal mucosa in childhood: An *in vitro* study using organ culture. *J. Pediatr. Gastroenterol. Nutr.* **2,** 235–242.

Johnstone, J. M., and Morson, B. S. (1978). Eosinophilic gastroenteritis. *Histopathology* **2,** 335–348.

Katz, A. J., Twarog, F. J., Zeiger, R. S., and Falchuk, Z. M. (1984). Milk-sensitive and eosinophilic gastroenteropathy: Similar clinical features with contrasting mechanisms and clinical course. *J. Allergy Clin. Immunol.* **74,** 72–78.

Kayosaari, M. (1982). Food allergy in Finnish children aged 1 to 6 years. *Acta Paediatr. Scand.* **71,** 815–819.

Keshavarzian, A., Saverymuttu, S. H., Tai, P. C., Thompson, M., Barter, S., Spry, C. J. F., and Chadwick, V. S. (1985). Activated eosinophils in familial eosinophilic gastroenteritis. *Gastroenterology* **88,** 1041–1049.

Klein, N. C., Hargrove, R. L., Sleisenger, M. H., and Jeffries, G. H. (1970). Eosinophilic gastroenteritis. *Medicine* (*Baltimore*) **49,** 299–319.

Kuitunen, P., Visakorpi, J. K., Savilahti, E., and Pelkonen, P. (1975). Malabsorption syndrome with cow's milk intolerance. *Arch. Dis. Child* **50,** 351–356.

Lake, A. M. (1991). Food protein-induced gastroenteropathy in infants and children. *In* "Food Allergy: Adverse Reactions to Foods and Food Additives (D. D. Metcalfe, H. A. Sampson, and R. A. Simon, eds.), pp. 173–185. Blackwell Scientific Publications, Oxford.

Leiferman, K. M., Ackerman, S. J., Sampson, H. A., Haugen, H. S., Venencie, P. Y., and Gleich, G. J. (1985). Dermal deposition of eosinophil-granule major basic protein in atopic dermatitis. *N. Engl. J. Med.* **313,** 282–285.

Marsh, D. G., Meyers, D. A., and Bias, W. B. (1981). The epidemiology and genetics of atopic allergy. *N. Engl. J. Med.* **305,** 1551–1559.

Mihm, M. C., Jr., Soter, N. A., Dvorak, H. F., and Austen, K. F. (1976). The structure of normal skin and the morphology of atopic eczema. *J. Invest. Dermatol.* **67,** 305–312.

Min, K-U., and Metcalfe, D. D. (1991). Eosinophilic gastroenteritis. *In* "Food Allergy. Immunology and Allergy Clinics of North America" (J. A. Anderson, ed.), Vol. II, pp. 799–813. Saunders, Philadelphia.

Moroz, L. A., and Yang, W. H. (1980). Kunitz soybean trypsin inhibitor. A specific allergen in food anaphylaxis. *N. Engl. J. Med.* **302,** 1126–1128.

Nagpal, S., Rajappa, L., Metcalfe, D. D., and Subba Rao, P. V. (1989). Isolation and characterization of heat stable allergens from shrimp (*Penaeus indicus*). *J. Allergy Clin. Immunol.* **83,** 26–36.

Oyaizu, N., Uemura, Y., Izumi, H., Morii, S., Nishi, M., and Hioki, K. (1985). Eosinophilic gastroenteritis: Immunochemical evidence for IgE mast cell-mediated allergy. *Acta. Pathol. Jpn.* **35,** 759–766.

Pastorello, E. A., Stocchi, L., Pravettoni, V., Bigi, A., Schilke, M. L., Incorvala, C., and Zanussi, C. (1989). Role of the elimination diet in adults with food allergy. *J. Allergy Clin. Immunol.* **84,** 475–483.

Robert, F., Omura, E., and Durant, J. (1977). Mucosal eosinophilic gastroenteritis with systemic involvement. *Am. J. Med.* **62,** 139–143.

Saavedra-Delgado, A-M., and Metcalfe, D. D. (1993). Seafood toxins. *Clin. Rev. Allergy,* in press.

Sachs, M. I., Jones, R. T., and Yunginger, J. W. (1981). Isolation and partial characterization of a major peanut allergen. *J. Allergy Clin. Immunol.* **67,** 27–34.

Sampson, H. A. (1989). Role of food allergy and mediator release in atopic dermatitis. *J. Allergy Clin. Immunol.* **81,** 635–645.

Sampson, H. A., and Jolie, P. L. (1984). Increased plasma histamine concentrations after food challenges in children with atopic dermatitis. *N. Engl. J. Med.* **31,** 372–376.

Sampson, H. A., and McCaskill, C. C. (1985). Food hypersensitivity and atopic dermatitis: Evaluation of 113 patients. *J. Pediatr.* **107,** 669–675.

Sampson, H. A., and Metcalfe, D. D. (1991). Immediate reactions to foods. *In* "Food Allergy: Adverse Reactions to Foods and Food Additives" (D. D. Metcalfe, H. A. Sampson, and R. A. Simon, eds.), pp. 99–112. Blackwell Scientific Publications, Oxford.

Sampson, H. A., and Metcalfe, D. D. (1992). Food allergies. *J. Am. Med. Assoc.* **25,** 2840–2844.

Sampson, H. A., Broadbent, K. R., and Bernhisel-Broadbent, J. (1989). Spontaneous release of histamine from basophils and histamine-releasing factor in patients with atopic dermatitis and food hypersensitivity. *N. Engl. J. Med.* **321,** 228–232.

Savilahti, E., and Verkasalo, M. (1984). Intestinal cow's milk allergy: Pathogenesis and clinical presentation. *Clin. Rev. Allergy* **2,** 7–23.

Scheinmann, P., Gendrel, D., Charlas, J., and Paupe, J. (1976). Value of lymphoblast transformation test in cow's milk protein intestinal intolerance. *Clin. Allergy* **6,** 515–521.

Selbekk, B. H., Aas, K., and Myren, J. (1978). *In vitro* sensitization and mast cell degranulation in human jejunal mucosa. *Scand. J. Gastroenterol.* **13,** 87–92.

Shibaski, M., Suzuki, S., Tajima, S., Nemoto, H., and Kuroume, T. (1980). Allergenicity of major components of soybeans. *Int. Arch. Allergy Appl. Immunol.* **61,** 441–448.

Stevenson, D. D., and Simon, R. A. (1981). Sensitivity to ingested metabisulfites in asthmatic subjects. *J. Allergy Clin. Immunol.* **68,** 26–32.

Swischuk, L. E., and Hayden, C. K., Jr. (1985). Barium enema findings (? segmental colitis) in four neonates with bloody diarrhea—Possible cow's milk allergy. *Pediatr. Radiol.* **15,** 34–37.

Taylor, S. L., Bush, R. K., and Nordlee, J. A. (1991). Sulfites. *In* "Food Allergy: Adverse Reactions to Foods and Food Additives" (D. D. Metcalfe, H. A. Sampson, and R. A. Simon, eds.), pp. 239–260. Blackwell Scientific Publications, Oxford.

Thounce, J. Q., and Tanner, M. S. (1985). Eosinophilic gastroenteritis. *Arch. Dis. Child* **60,** 1186–1188.

Torpier, G., Colombel, J. F., Mathieu-Chandelier, C., Capron, M., Dessaint, J. P., Cortot, A., Paris, J. C., and Capron, A. (1988). Eosinophilic gastroenteritis: Ultrastructural evidence for a selective release of eosinophil major basic protein. *Clin. Exp. Immunol.* **74,** 404–408.

Van Metre, T. E., Anderson, S. A., Barnard, J. H., Bernstein, I. L., Chafee, F. H., Crawford, L. V., and Wittig, H. J. (1968). A controlled study of the effects on manifestations of chronic asthma of a rigid elimination diet based on Rowe's cereal-free diet 1, 2, 3. *J. Allergy* **41,** 195–208.

Victoria, J. C., Camarero, C., Sojo, A., Ruiz, A., and Rodriquez-Soriano, T. (1982). Enteropathy related to fish, rice and chicken. *Arch. Dis. Child* **57,** 44–48.

Walker-Smith, J. A. (1986). Food sensitive enteropathies. *Clin. Gastroenterol.* **15,** 55–69.

Walzer, M. (1942). Absorption of allergens. *J. Allergy* **13,** 554–562.

Wilson, S. J., and Walzer, M. (1935). Absorption of undigested proteins in human beings. IV. Absorption of unaltered egg protein in infants. *Am. J. Dis. Child* **50,** 49–54.

Young, E., Patel, S., Stoneham, M., Rona, R., and Wilkinson, J. D. (1987). The prevalence of reaction to food additives in a survey population. *J. R. Coll. Phys. London* **21,** 241–247.

Yunginger, J. W. (1991). Food antigens. *In* "Food Allergy: Adverse Reactions to Foods and Food Additives" (D. D. Metcalfe, H. A. Sampson, and R. A. Simon, eds.), pp. 36–51. Blackwell Scientific Publications, Oxford.

Zeiger, R. S., Heller, S., Mellon, M. H., Forsyth, A. B., O'Connor, R. D., Hamburger, R. N., and Schatz, M. (1989). Effect of combined maternal and infant food-allergen avoidance on development or atopy in early infancy: A randomized study. *J. Allergy Clin. Immunol.* **84,** 72–89.

41

Intestinal Infections

Myron M. Levine • James P. Nataro

I. INTRODUCTION

Various bacteria, viruses, protozoa, and helminths are capable of causing intestinal infections accompanied by clinical illness in immunologically competent individuals (Table I); this list would lengthen considerably with the inclusion of agents known to cause illness in immunocompromised hosts. These various pathogens cause an array of diarrheal illnesses, dysenteries, enteric fevers, and malabsorptive states. Clearly, discussing every known enteric pathogen or even mentioning them is beyond the scope of this chapter. Instead, we emphasize the common themes encountered among diverse intestinal infections with respect to virulence properties of the etiologic agents, steps in pathogenesis, modes of interaction with the host intestinal mucosa, resultant clinical syndromes, and components of the host immune system that mount putatively protective responses.

Table I Some Bacteria, Viruses, Protozoa, and Helminths That Are Incriminated as Causes of Intestinal Illness

Bacteria	
Shigella	*Vibrio cholerae*
Escherichia coli	O1
enterotoxigenic	non-O1
enteroinvasive	*Campylobacter jejuni*
enteropathogenic	*Yersinia enterocolitica*
enterohemorrhagic	*Salmonella,* nontyphoidal
enteroaggregative	*Vibrio parahemolyticus*
diffuse-adherent	*Vibrio mimicus*
Aeromonas hydrophila	*Plesiomonas shigelloides*
Clostridium dificile	*Bacterioides fragillis,* enterotoxigenic
Viruses	
Group A rotaviruses	Norwalk-like 27-nm gastroenteritis viruses
Group B rotaviruses	Enteric adenoviruses
Astroviruses	Caliciviruses
Pestiviruses	Picobirnaviruses
Protozoa	
Giardia lamblia	*Cryptosporidium parvum*
Entameba histolytica	*Isospora belli*
Balantidium coli	
Helminths	
Capillaria philippinensis	*Strongyloides stercoralis*

II. EPIDEMIOLOGY

On the global level, diarrheal diseases, dysenteries, and enteric fever are predominantly problems of populations living in less-developed areas of the world, where infants and young children suffer the highest incidence rates. Travelers of all ages from industrialized countries experience high attack rates of diarrheal illness and other enteric infections when they visit such less-developed areas of the world. Intestinal infections constitute a much smaller health problem in industrialized countries. Nevertheless, problems that remain include viral gastroenteritis (e.g., rotavirus in infants), certain foodborne infections (e.g., salmonellosis and campylobacteriosis), and shigellosis in subpopulations in which hygiene is compromised (e.g., children in day care, patients in custodial institutions).

Although the list of etiologic agents capable of causing intestinal infection and disease is long, a relatively small number of pathogens worldwide accounts for the majority of intestinal diseases of public health importance. Those that have been cited as being of paramount public health importance include enterotoxigenic *Escherichia coli,* enteropathogenic *E. coli, Shigella,* and rotavirus as causes of endemic diarrheal disease; *Vibrio cholerae* O1 and *Shigella dysenteriae* 1 as causes of epidemic disease; and *Salmonella typhi* as the predominant cause of enteric fever. Agents of lesser importance include *Campylobacter jejuni,* enteric adenoviruses, and *Entamoeba histolytica.* In many industrialized countries, enterohemorrhagic *E. coli,* which causes hemorrhagic colitis and (more rarely) the hemolytic–uremic syndrome, increasingly is being recognized as an important enteric pathogen.

III. PATHOGENESIS

A. Virulence Properties

Bacterial enteric pathogens are, arguably, better understood than viral or parasitic infections with respect to their virulence properties and the manner in which they interact with the host intestinal mucosa. Therefore, bacterial enteropathogens are used as examples to illustrate certain fundamental concepts (e.g., the interaction of pathogens with mucosal epithelial cells).

Among the recognized virulence properties elaborated by bacterial enteropathogens are cytotonic enterotoxins that lead to intestinal secretion (Levine *et al.*, 1983), fimbrial attachment factors that permit adherence to epithelial cells (Knutton *et al.*, 1985), expression of proteins that lead to effacement of the microvilli of enterocytes (Jerse *et al.*, 1991), expression of certain outer membrane proteins that allow the bacteria to be internalized by epithelial cells (Isberg and Leong, 1990; Miller *et al.*, 1990), cytotoxins that suppress protein synthesis and lead to cell death (Brown *et al.*, 1980), and expression of proteins that allow survival within the phagolysosomes of macrophages (Fields *et al.*, 1989; Miller, 1991). Bacterial enteropathogens often possess several distinct virulence properties, the particular array of which markedly affects the mode of interaction of the pathogen with the intestinal mucosa of the host as well as the clinical syndromes caused, Table II lists some of the most important bacterial enteric pathogens and the virulence properties they are known to possess.

Two pathogenic motifs encountered recurrently among diverse bacteria are (1) mechanisms to adhere to mucosa and (2) elaboration of toxins. Adherence to mucosal epithelium allows the bacteria to counteract peristalsis, an important and effective nonspecific defense mechanism of the proximal small intestine. Bacteria have developed a variety of distinct means to achieve adherence; sometimes initial adherence represents a preliminary step to more intimate attachment or to actual invasion of epithelial cells. Many bacterial enteropathogens express fimbrial attachment factors. Fimbriae (also called pili) are hairlike appendages that radiate from the surface of bacteria and are composed of thousands of protein subunits stacked end-on-end to result in long filaments that can bind to specific receptors on enterocytes. Fimbriae that serve as attachment factors are found, for example, in enterotoxigenic *E. coli* (Evans *et al.*, 1975; Levine *et al.*, 1983,1984), enteropathogenic *E. coli* (Giron *et al.*, 1991), enterohemorrhagic *E. coli* (Karch *et al.*, 1987), enteroaggregative *E. coli* (Vial *et al.*, 1988; Nataro *et al.*, 1992), diffuse adherence *E. coli* (Bilge *et al.*, 1989), and *V. cholerae* O1 (Taylor *et al.*, 1987). After contact with epithelial cells, some bacteria, such as *Shigella, Salmonella,* and *Yersinia enterocolitica,* are internalized by the epithelial cells (Levine *et al.*, 1983). In each instance, the bacteria must express specific outer membrane proteins that are involved in the internalization process (Hale *et al.*, 1983; Elsinghorst *et al.*, 1989; Isberg and Leong, 1990; Miller *et al.*, 1990) the epithelial cell plays an active role in the process. Certain other bacterial enteropathogens demonstrate an intimate form of attachment to epithelial cells in which the outer membrane of the enterocyte appears to wrap partially around the bacterium, giving the impression that the bacterium is perched on a pedestal of enterocyte membrane (Rothbaum *et al.*, 1983).

The second recurring pathogenic motif is the elaboration of toxins. Enterotoxins that resemble cholera toxin and LT (the heat-labile enterotoxin of enterotoxigenic *E. coli*) in structure, pharmacological properties, and immunological properties are produced by *C. jejuni* (Ruiz-Palacios *et al.*, 1983), *S. typhimurium* (Finkelstein *et al.*, 1983), and *Vibrio mimicus* (Chowdhury *et al.*, 1987), for example. Small peptide heat-stable enterotoxins (ST) are elaborated by enterotoxigenic *E. coli, Y. enterocolitica* (Delor *et al.*, 1990), *Citrobacter freundii* (Guarino *et al.*, 1987), non-O1 *V. cholerae* (Arita *et al.*, 1986), and enteroaggregative *E. coli* (Savarino *et al.*, 1991). Enteroinvasive *E. coli* and *Shigella* now are recognized to elaborate enterotoxins as well (Fasano *et al.*, 1990).

The genes encoding virulence properties of bacterial enteropathogens often are located on plasmids. Genes encoding other virulence factors, as well as regulatory genes that control the plasmid genes, often are found on the bacterial chromosome. Some bacterial pathogens exhibit "coordinate regulation of virulence properties," in which regulatory genes sense a change in the environment and generate a cascade effect in which the transcriptional promoters of certain genes are activated while those of others are suppressed (Miller *et al.*, 1989).

Table II Virulence Properties of Some Major Bacterial Enteropathogens

Pathogen	Fimbrial colonization factor	Intimate attachment	Effacement of microvilli	Enterocyte invasion	Toxins: LT	Toxins: ST or ST-like	Toxins: Other	Toxins: Potent cytotoxins
Escherichia coli								
enterotoxigenic	+	−	−	−	+	+	−	−
enteroinvasive	−	−	−	+	−	−	+	−
enteropathogenic	+	+	+	+/−	−	−	?	−
enterohemorrhagic	+	+	+	−	−	−	−	+
enteroaggregative	+	−	−	−	−	+	−	?
diffuse adherence	+	−	−	−	−	−	?	?
Shigella dysenteriae 1	−	−	−	+	−	−	+	+
Shigella, other	−	−	−	+	−	−	+	−
Salmonella, nontyphoidal	?	−	−	+	Some	−	−	−
Yersinia enterocolitica	−	−	−	+	−	Some	−	−
Campylobacter jejuni	−	−	−	+	+	−	−	+/−

B. Modes of Interaction with the Host Mucosa

The various bacterial enteric pathogens can be categorized on the basis of the manner in which their virulence properties interact with the intestinal mucosa of the host and on their degree of invasiveness.

1. Mucosal Adherence and Enterotoxin Production

Pathogens in this class, exemplified by *V. cholerae* O1 and enterotoxigenic *E. coli* (ETEC), adhere to the mucosa of the proximal small intestine before elaborating enterotoxins that lead to intestinal secretion (Levine *et al.*, 1983). In each instance, the attachment or colonization factor consists of one or another type of fimbria that adheres to specific receptors on the enterocytes. The fimbrial colonization factor of *V. cholerae* O1 is the toxin co-regulated pilus (TCP), so-called because its expression is controlled by the same regulatory gene (*tox*R) that controls expression of cholera toxin (Taylor *et al.*, 1987). A series of antigenically distinct fimbrial colonization factors is found in ETEC. Some fimbriae are rigid structures 6–7 nm in diameter, whereas others consist of thin flexible fibrillae that are ~3 nm in diameter (Levine *et al.*, 1984). The plasmids that encode the fimbrial subunits often also carry genes encoding enterotoxins (Levine *et al.*, 1983). Certain colonization factor antigen fimbriae are associated with particular O:H serotypes of ETEC.

Although cholera or ETEC infection can result in copious diarrhea, virtually no morphological damage to the intestinal mucosa is evident in such infections; functionally, such infections can be considered intracellular intoxications leading to disruption of biochemical pathways within enterocytes. Cholera toxin and LT activate adenylate cyclase within enterocytes, leading to an intracellular accumulation of AMP. The consequence is that enterocytes in the crypts secrete and those of the villus tips manifest diminished absorption. The ST of ETEC is a small peptide consisting of 18 or 19 amino acids, rich in cysteines. ST activates guanylate cyclase, leading to an intracellular accumulation of GMP; this effect also culminates in net secretion to the gut.

2. Intimate Mucosal Adherence and Effacement of Microvilli

Enteropathogenic *E. coli* (EPEC) of classical O:H serotypes that originally were incriminated as causes of infant diarrhea in the 1940s and 1950s exhibit a multistep pathogenesis. Plasmid-encoded bundle-forming fimbriae (BFP, bearing some genetic relatedness to TCP) result in a preliminary adherence to epithelial cells (Giron *et al.*, 1991). This is followed by an intimate attachment mediated by a 94-kDa outer membrane protein called intimin (Jerse *et al.*, 1990; Donnenbert and Kaper, 1992). The gene encoding this protein is located on the EPEC chromosome (Jerse *et al.*, 1990). Nevertheless, the same EPEC Adherence Factor (EAF) plasmid (Nataro *et al.*, 1987) that carries genes encoding the fimbrial attachment factor (Giron *et al.*, 1991) also regulates expression of the 94-kDa protein. Yet other genes encode proteins that result in the effacement of the microvilli of the enterocyte. This process may be mediated by protein kinases that cause an intracellular accumulation of Ca^{2+} (Baldwin *et al.*, 1991). Transmission electron microscopy reveals occasional EPEC bacteria within vacuoles internalized by the enterocytes (Donnenberg *et al.*, 1990). Note that the 94-kDa protein intimin bears considerable DNA homology to invasins, outer membrane proteins expressed by *Yersinia pseudotuberculosis* and *Y. enterocolitica* (Jerse *et al.*, 1990) that are involved in invasion of epithelial cells.

3. Intimate Mucosal Adherence, Effacement of Microvilli, and Production of Potent Cytotoxins

Enterohemorrhagic *E. coli* (EHEC), a new category of pathogen recognized only since the early 1980s, manifests an unusual interaction with the intestinal mucosa consequent to the interplay of several virulence properties. Novel fimbriae (the expression of which requires the presence of a 60-MDa plasmid) are believed to foster initial attachment to epithelial cells (Karch *et al.*, 1987). Ultimately, the expression of phage-encoded potent Shiga-like cytotoxins (O'Brien *et al.*, 1984) is thought to cause death of enterocytes in the colon, leading to sloughing of these epithelial cells and denudation of the mucosa (Pai *et al.*, 1986). In animal models of EHEC infection (Tzipori *et al.*, 1986,1987), intimate attachment and effacement of microvilli is observed. Indeed, the EHEC chromosome harbors a gene bearing close homology to *eae* of EPEC and is believed to encode a protein similar to intimin. Note, however, that although intimate attachment and effacement of microvilli are prominent in animal models of EHEC, they not been observed in biopsy or autopsy specimens of patients with hemorrhagic colitis or hemolytic–uremic syndrome caused by EHEC (Griffin and Tauxe, 1991).

4. Expression of Enterotoxin and Potent Cytotoxin

Some enteric pathogens, typified by *Clostridium difficle*, elaborate enterotoxins and potent cytotoxins that lead to enterocyte death and denudation of mucosa, particularly in the colon. *Clostridium difficile* is the predominant pathogen in cases of antibiotic-associated diarrhea and pseudomembranous colitis. The ability of *C. difficile* to grow vigorously in the intestine and to cause disease is promoted strongly by derangement of the normal microflora (Rolfe *et al.*, 1981). *Clostridium difficile* produces at least two exotoxins: the cell-associated cytotoxin/enterotoxin toxin A and the cytotoxin toxin B (Mitchell *et al.*, 1986). When fed intragastrically in animal models, these toxins appear to work synergistically to induce mucosal damage and to induce fluid secretion (Lyerly *et al.*, 1985). In contrast to the bacterial pathogens described earlier, adherence of *C. difficile* to the intestinal mucosa has not been recognized as a prominent component of the organism's pathogenic nature. Few bacteria are noted on pathologic examination of *C. difficile* lesions.

5. Enterotoxin Production, Epithelial Cell Invasion, and Intraenterocytic Proliferation

The cardinal feature of *Shigella* and of enteroinvasive *E. coli* (EIEC) is their ability to invade epithelial cells, multiply therein, invoke an inflammatory response characterized by immigration of polymorphonuclear neutrophilic leukocytes, and cause mucosal ulcerations (Dupont *et al.*, 1971; Hale and Formal, 1986; Yoshikawa *et al.*, 1988). The major sites of intestinal pathology caused by *Shigella* are the colon and terminal ileum. The invasion process is complex and requires the involvement of genes located on the 120- to 140-MDa *Shigella* invasiveness plasmid, as well as chromosomal regulatory genes, and the active participation of the host epithelial cell (Hale and Formal, 1986; Yoshikawa *et al.*, 1988).

Shigella flexneri 2a and EIEC have been shown to elaborate enterotoxins that cause intestinal secretion (Fasano *et al.*, 1990). Such enterotoxins can explain the early phase of clinical shigellosis, when watery diarrhea is prominent, prior to the onset of dysentery.

6. Mucosal Translocation Followed by Proliferation in the Lamina Propria and Mesenteric Lymph Nodes

Nontyphoidal *Salmonella, Y. enterocolitica,* and *C. jejuni* invade enterocytes in membrane-bound vesicles. These organisms migrate intracellularly through the enterocytes in these pinocytotic vesicles from the apical end to the basal extremity to exit finally into the lamina propria, where they elicit a chemotactic response resulting in an influx of polymorphonuclear leukocytes (Levine *et al.*, 1983). These enteric pathogens readily reach the mesenteric lymph nodes, but further invasion accompanied by bacteremia is believed to be relatively uncommon, except in immunocompromised hosts (or in very young infants). *Salmonella* also gains entry to the gut lymphoid tissue after active uptake by M cells that cover the Peyer's patches and other lymphoid tissue.

7. Mucosal Translocation Followed by Generalized Infection of the Reticuloendothelial System

Salmonella typhi and *Salmonella paratyphi* A and B pass through the mucosa like other *Salmonella,* both by M-cell uptake (Yokoyama *et al.*, 1989) and by pinocytotic vesicles that transmigrate through enterocytes (Levine *et al.*, 1983). However, on reaching the lamina propria, these organisms elicit a chemotactic response that leads to an influx of macrophages (Harris *et al.*, 1972) rather than polymorphonuclear leukocytes. These macrophages ingest the *Salmonella* but, in the nonimmune host, not only do *S. typhi* and *S. paratyphi* readily drain to the mesenteric lymph nodes but some reach the bloodstream via lymphatic drainage through the thoracic duct (Levine *et al.*, 1983). During this silent primary bacteremia, these *Salmonella* spp. are removed by fixed phagocytic cells of the reticuloendothelial system in the spleen, liver, bone marrow, and so on. In the susceptible host, virulence properties possessed by these *Salmonella* allow them to survive within the phagolysosomes of the macrophages (Fields *et al.*, 1989; Miller, 1991). Following an incubation period that usually lasts 8–14 days, the clinical features of enteric feaver (typhoid or paratyphoid fever) commence, accompanied by secondary bacteremia.

8. Viruses

Among the viruses that cause gastrointestinal disease (Table I), the pathogenesis of rotavirus infection is the best studied (Table I) (Davidson *et al.*, 1977; Mebus *et al.*, 1977; Estes and Cohen, 1989). Specific rotaviruses of one type or another cause diarrheal disease in many mammals. Rotaviruses consist of nonenveloped double-shelled capsids, ~70 nm in diameter, that enclose an RNA core that is divided into 11 separate segments. Each of the 11 genes encodes a protein, of which 6 form part of the structure of the virus particle. Viral proteins VP1, VP2, VP3, and VP6 form the inner shell of the virus, whereas glycosylated viral proteins VP7 and VP4 on the surface of the virus play critical roles in the attachment and internalization of rotaviruses into enterocytes. The surface-exposed proteins VP4 and VP7, which make up the outer shell of the virion, constitute the major neutralization antigens against which protective antibodies are directed. VP7 contains 326 amino acids, whereas VP4 consists of 775 or 776 amino acids. For rotavirus to be able to infect enterocytes, VP4 must be split by intestinal trypsin into two components (Espejo *et al.*, 1981).

Rotavirus invades enterocytes of the villus tips leading to cell death, sloughing of the dead enterocytes, and denudation of the villus tips (Mebus *et al.*, 1977; Estes and Cohen, 1989). This behavior is accompanied by striking diminutions in the activities of disaccharidases and other enzymes in the affected areas of the intestine. Since villus tip cells represent mature enterocytes that are important for absorption, the loss of absorptive capacity that follows destruction of these cells creates an imbalance with the secreting cells of the villus crypts; the result is net secretion. Visualization of the human infant intestine infected by rotavirus reveals foci of severe pathology intermingled with virtually unaffected areas.

9. Protozoa

The best-studied protozoa that cause intestinal disease are *Giardia lamblia, E. histolytica,* and *Cryptosporidium parvum.* These protozoa possess adhesion factors that allow them to attach to enterocytes. *Entamoeba histolytica* has been shown to effect mucosal colonization using specific adherence factors and also has been shown to elaborate soluble toxins (Ravdin, 1989). *Giardia lamblia* also adheres strongly to the intestinal mucosa, in this case in the small bowel (Farthing *et al.*, 1986). However, neither invasion nor enterotoxin production has been demonstrated conclusively. Instead, data suggest that the immune response of the host may be important in pathogenesis, as may the ability of the parasite to promote deconjugation of bile salts (Farthing *et al.*, 1985). *Cryptosporidium* effaces microvilli, leading to host–parasite interaction that resembles that of EPEC (Tzipori *et al.*, 1983).

IV. CLINICAL SYNDROMES

With few exceptions, when the various enteric pathogens listed in Table I cause clinical disease, the result is one or another of the seven distinct syndromes shown in Table III. By far the most common clinical syndrome is "simple diarrhea," characterized by the passage of multiple loose stools (without blood), low-grade fever, malaise, nausea, and some vomiting. Simple diarrheal illnesses usually are self-limited and require only oral rehydration therapy. Most of the patho-

Table III Most Common Clinical Syndromes Caused by Enteric Pathogens

Syndrome	Features	Pathogens[a]
Simple diarrhea	Watery diarrhea; nausea; low grade fever	Rotavirus, ETEC, EPEC, *Campylobacter jejuni,* enteric adenovirus, astroviruses, *Shigella, Salmonella, Yersinia enterocolitica, Cryptosporidia,* EIEC
Dysentery	Scanty stools with gross blood and mucus; high fever; toxemia; sheets of fecal leukocytes	*Shigella, C. jejuni,* EIEC, *Y. enterocolitica*
Persistent diarrhea	Diarrhea > 14 days	EAggEC, EPEC, *Giardia lamblia*
Hemorrhagic colitis	Copious bloody diarrhea; no fever; no fecal leukocytes	EHEC
Rice water purging	Voluminous Na^+-rich "rice water" stools	*Vibrio cholerae* O1, ETEC
Vomiting without diarrhea	Acute, short-lived	27-nm Norwalk-like gastroenteritis viruses
	Persistent	*G. lamblia, Strongyloides stercoralis*
Enteric fever	Persisting fever; malaise; headache; abdominal discomfort	*Salmonella typhi; Salmonella paratyphi* A, B

[a] Abbreviations: ETEC, enterotoxigenic *E. coli;* EPEC, enteropathogenic *E. coli;* EIEC, enteroinvasive *E. coli;* EAggEC, enteroaggregative *E. coli;* EHEC, enterohemorrhagic *E. coli.*

gens listed in Table I can cause this syndrome; perhaps 85% of health care visits for diarrheal illness are the result of clinical infections of this nature and severity.

Some agents, particularly invasive bacterial pathogens, are capable of causing the syndrome of dysentery, that is, the passage of scanty stools containing gross blood and mucus. Dysenteric illnesses tend to be severe and commonly are accompanied by high fever, toxemia, and notable malaise. Approximately 5–10% of patients with diarrheal illness visiting health care facilities in less-developed countries suffer from dysentery. Although *Shigella* is the most common cause of dysentery, *C. jejuni, Y. enterocolitica,* and occasionally nonthphoidal *Salmonella* can cause an identical clinical picture. *Entamoeba histolytica* infection also leads to dysentery, but such infections usually are not associated with the high fever, malaise, and toxemia seen with the bacterial dysenteries.

Approximately 5% of episodes of acute diarrhea in less-developed countries persist for more than 14 days, at which point they become defined as "persistent diarrhea." The clinical–epidemiological syndrome of persistent diarrhea carries a poor prognosis for afflicted infants and young children in the developing world (Bhan *et al.,* 1989a); the consequences include malnutrition and death. Until recently, no specific pathogen was associated with this syndrome. However, several reports now have shown a statistically significant association between enteroaggregative *E. coli* (EAggEC) and persistent diarrhea; up to 51% of cases have been attributed to this etiology (Cravioto *et al.,* 1991).

Hemorrhagic colitis is a syndrome caused by EHEC. The salient clinical features include copious bloody diarrhea in the absence of fever (Riley *et al.,* 1983; Griffin and Tauxe, 1991). The copious nature of the bloody diarrheal stools, the lack of fever, and the absence of fecal leukocytes differentiate this syndrome from dysentery caused by *Shigella* or other organisms, which consists of scanty stools, accompanying high fever, and sheets of fecal leukocytes that can be visualized in simple stains of stool mucus. Occasionally, patients with hemorrhagic colitis (or milder diarrheal illness) caused by EHEC proceed to develop the hemolytic–uremic syndrome that includes hemolytic anemia, fragmented erythrocytes (schistocytes), severe thrombocytopenia, and acute renal failure (Karmali *et al.,* 1985)

Some intestinal infections, particularly in cholera-endemic areas, are characterized by the passage of voluminous stools resembling "rice water." An older child or adult with cholera can pass stools of 1.0–1.25 liters hourly. Such diarrheal infections, which rapidly lead to severe dehydration, acidosis, and circulatory collapse, must be treated aggressively with rehydration.

Another uncommon syndrome caused by intestinal infection is vomiting in the absence of diarrhea or accompanied by scanty diarrhea. Acute short-lived bouts of "winter vomiting disease" are mainly caused by 27-nm gastroenteritis viruses typified by the Norwalk agent. Persistent vomiting in the absence of diarrheal illness, a particularly uncommon syndrome, usually is associated with duodenitis or jejunitis caused by *G. lamblia* or *Strongyloides stercoralis* infection.

Salmonella typhi and *S. paratyphi* A and B cause typhoid and paratyphoid fever, respectively. These conditions represent generalized infections that involve the intestinal lymphoid tissue, the reticuloendothelial system, and the gall bladder. Following a relatively long incubation (usually 8–14 days), the clinical illness commences with fever (that increases in stepwise fashion), abdominal discomfort, and headache. Because these infections are generalized, inappropriate or delayed treatment can result in a wide array of complications. In the pre-antibiotic era, the case fatality rate of typhoid fever was 10–20%.

V. IMMUNE RESPONSES

The immune responses elicited by various enteric pathogens and their role in protection against subsequent infection vary and depend, to a large extent, on the virulence properties of the agent, the type of host–parasite interaction as described earlier, and the degree of invasiveness. Virtually all intestinal infections prime the intestinal immune system (as measured by gut-derived IgA-antibody-secreting cells detected in peripheral blood) (Van de Verg *et al.*, 1990; Kantele and Makela, 1991; Quiding *et al.*, 1991) to respond to subsequent contact with antigen by producing specific SIgA antibodies. The impressive capacity of mucosal antibodies to protect is evidenced by the fact that, in experimental challenge studies, passively administered milk immunoglobulin concentrates conferred a very high level of protection to adult volunteers against challenge with ETEC or *Shigella* (Tacket *et al.*, 1988,1992). Similarly, in veterinary studies, piglets or calves nursed by sows or cows that received intramammary immunization with vaccines consisting of purified colonization factor fimbriae were protected highly against otherwise lethal challenge with ETEC bearing the homologous antigenic type of fimbriae (Rutter and Jones, 1973; Acres *et al.*, 1979; Levine, 1981).

Serum antibodies commonly are detected, even after noninvasive intestinal infections. Although serum antibodies are not believed to play an important role in protection against noninvasive infections of the gut, such antibodies often show strong correlations with protection. An example is the correlation between serum vibriocidal antibody and protection against cholera (Mosley *et al.*, 1968a,b; Glass *et al.*, 1985).

An unusual form of antibody-dependent cellular cytotoxicity (ADCC) is seen in *Salmonella* and *Shigella* infections in which antibodies provide the specificity and mononuclear cells mediate the killing of these bacteria (Lowell *et al.*, 1980; Tagliabue *et al.*, 1986; Levine *et al.*, 1987). In general, cytokine-mediated cellular immune responses are important in immunity to *Salmonella,* particularly *S. typhi.*

Increasingly scientists are recognizing that infection with intracellular bacteria can elicit major histocompatibility complex (MHC) Class I-restricted cytotoxic lymphocyte responses of a type that once were thought to occur only in infections by viruses (Kaufmann, 1988). Attenuated *Salmonella* are attractive candidates for "live vectors" or "carrier vaccines" for the expression of foreign antigens (Dougan *et al.*, 1987; Levine *et al.*, 1990). In this regard, note that animals immunized with attenuated *S. typhimurium* expressing the circumsporozoite protein of *Plasmodium falciparum* were shown to develop MHC I-restricted $CD8^+$ cytotoxic lymphocytes that recognized epitopes of the *P. falciparum* circumsporozoite protein (Aggarwal *et al.*, 1990).

References

Acres, S. D., Isaacson, R. E., Babuik, L. A., and Kapitany, R. A. (1979). Immunization of calves against enterotoxigenic colibacillosis by vaccinating dams with purified K99 antigen and whole cell bacterins. *Infect. Immun.* **25,** 121–126.

Aggarwal, A., Kumar, S., Jaffe, R., Hone, D., Gross, M., and Sadoff, J. (1990). Oral *Salmonella:*malaria circumsprozoite recombinants induce specific $CD8^+$ cytotoxic T cells. *J. Exp. Med.* **172,** 1083–1090.

Arita, M., Takeda, T., Honda, T., and Miwatani, T. (1986). Purification and characterization of *Vibrio cholerae* non-O1 and heat-stable enterotoxin. *Infect. Immun.* **52,** 45–49.

Baldwin, T. J., Ward, W., Aitken, A., Knutton, S., and Williams, P. H. (1991). Elevation of intracellular free calcium levels in HEp-2 cells infected with enteropathogenic *Escherichia coli. Infect. Immun.* **59,** 1599–1604.

Bhan, M. K., Bhandari, N., Sazawal, S., Clemens, J., Raj, P., Levine, M. M., and Kaper, J. B. (1989a). Descriptive epidemiology of persistent diarrhoea among young children in rural northern India. *Bull. WHO* **67,** 281–288.

Bhan, M. K., Raj, P., Levine, M. M., Kaper, J. B., Bhandari, N., Srivastava, R., Kumar, R., and Sazawal, S. (1989b). Enteroaggregative *Escherichia coli* associated with persistent diarrhea in a cohort of rural children in India. *J. Infect. Dis.* **159,** 1061–1064.

Bilge, S. S., Clausen, C. R., Lau, W., and Moseley, S. L. (1989). Molecular characterization of a fimbrial adhesin, F1845, mediating diffuse adherence of diarrhea-associated *Escherichia coli* to HEp-2 cells. *J. Bacteriol.* **171,** 4281–4289.

Brown, J. E., Rothman, S. W., and Doctor, B. P. (1980). Inhibition of protein synthesis in intact HeLa cells by *Shigella dysenteriae* 1 toxin. *Infect. Immun.* **29,** 98–107.

Chowdhury, M. A. R., Aziz, K. M. S., Kay, B. A., and Rahim, Z. (1987). Toxin production by *Vibrio mimicus* strains isolated from human and environmental sources in Bangladesh. *J. Clin Microbiol.* **25,** 2200–2203.

Cravioto, A., Tello, A., Navarro, A., Ruiz, J., Villafan, H., Uribe, F., and Eslava, C. (1991). Association of *Escherichia coli* HEp-2 adherence patterns with type and duration of diarrhoea. *Lancet* **337,** 262–264.

Davidson, G. P., Gall, D. G., Petric, M., Butler, D. G., and Hamilton, J. R. (1977). Human rotavirus enteritis induced in conventional piglets. *J. Clin. Invest.* **60,** 1402–1409.

Delor, I., Kaeckenbeeck, A., Wauters, G., and Cornelius, G. R. (1990). Nucleotide sequence of *yst,* the *Yersinia enterocolitica* gene encoding the heat-stable enterotoxin, and prevalence of the gene among pathogenic and non-pathogenic yersiniae. *Infect. Immun.* **58,** 2983–2988.

Donnenberg, M. S., and Kaper, J. B. (1992). Enteropathogenic *Escherichia coli. Infect. Immun.* **60,** 3953–3961.

Donnenberg, M. S., Calderwood, S. B., Donohue-Rolfe, A., Keusch, G. T., and Kaper, J. B. (1990). Construction and analysis of Tn*pho*A mutants of enteropathogenic *Escherichia coli* unable to invade HEp-2 cells. *Infect. Immun.* **58,** 1565–1571.

Dougan, G., Hormaeche, C. E., and Maskell, D. J. (1987). Live oral *Salmonella* vaccines: Potential use of attenuated strains as carriers of heterologous antigens to the immune system. *Parasite Immunol.* **9,** 151–160.

DuPont, H. L., Formal, S. B., Hornick, R. B., Snyder, M. J., Libonati, J. P., Sheahan, D. G., LaBrec, E. H., and Kalas, J. P. (1971). Pathogenesis of *Escherichia coli* diarrhea. *N. Engl. J. Med.* **285,** 1–9.

Elsinghorst, E. A., Baron, L. S. and Kopecko, D. J. (1989). Penetration of human intestinal epithelial cells by *Salmonella:* Molecular cloning and expression of *Salmonella typhi* invasion determinants in *Escherichia coli. Proc. Natl. Acad. Sci. U.S.A.* **86,** 5173–5177.

Espejo, R. T., Lopez, S., and Arias, C. (1981). Structural peptides of simian rotavirus SA11 and the effect of trypsin. *J. Virol.* **37,** 156–160.

Estes, M. K., and Cohen, J. (1989). Rotavirus gene structure and function. *Microbiol. Rev.* **53,** 410–449.

Evans, D. G., Silver, R. P., Evans, D. J., Jr., Chase, D. G., and Gorbach, S. L. (1975). Plasmid-controlled colonization factor associated with virulence in *Escherichia coli* enterotoxigenic for humans. *Infect. Immun.* **12,** 656–667.

Farthing, M. J. G., Keusch, G. T., and Carey, M. C. (1985). Effect of bile and bile salts on growth and membrane lipid uptake by *Giardia lamblia;* Possible implications for pathogenesis of intestinal disease. *J. Clin. Invest.* **76,** 1727–1732.

Farthing, M. J. G., Periera, M. E. A., and Keusch, G. T. (1986).

Description and characterisation of surface lectin from *Giardia lamblia*. *Infect. Immun.* **51,** 661–667.

Fasano, A., Kay, B. A., Russell, R. G., Maneval, D. R., and Levine, M. M. (1990). Enterotoxin and cytotoxin production by enteroinvasive *Escherichia coli*. *Infect. Immun.* **58,** 3717–3723.

Fields, P. I., Groisman, E. A., and Heffron, F. (1989). A *Salmonella* locus that controls resistance to microbicidal proteins from phagocytic cells. *Science* **243,** 1059–1062.

Finkelstein, R. A., Marchilewicz, B. A., McDonald, R. J., and Boesman-Finkelstein, M. (1983). Isolation and characterization of a cholera-related enterotoxin from *Salmonella typhimurium*. *FEMS Microbiol. Lett.* **17,** 239–241.

Glass, R. I., Svennerholm, A.-M., Khan, M. B., Huda, S., Huq, I., and Holmgren, J. (1985). Seroepidemiological studies of El Tor cholera in Bangladesh: Association of serum antibody levels with protection. *J. Infect. Dis.* **151,** 236–242.

Giron, J., Ho, A. S. Y., and Schoolnik, G. (1991). An inducible bundle-forming pilus of enteropathogenic *Escherichia coli*. *Science* **254,** 710–713.

Griffin, P., and Tauxe, R. (1991). The epidemiology of infections cause by *Escherichia coli* O157:H7 or other enterochemorrhagic *E. coli* and the associated hemolytic-uremic syndrome. *Epidemiol. Rev.* **13,** 60–98.

Guarino, A., Capano, G., Malamisura, B., Alessio, M., Gundalini, S., and Rubino, A. (1987). Production of *Escherichia coli* STa-like heat-stable enterotoxin by *Citrobacter freundii* isolated from humans. *Infect. Immun.* **25,** 110–114.

Hale, T. L., and Formal, S. B. (1986). Genetics of virulence in *Shigella*. *Microb. Pathogen.* **1,** 511–518.

Hale, T. L., Sanosonetti, P. J., Schad, P., Austin, S., and Formal, S. B. (1983). Characterization of virulence plasmids and plasmid-associated outer membrane proteins in *Shigella flexneri, Shigella sonnei,* and *Escherichia coli Infect. Immun.* **40,** 340–350.

Harris, J. C., DuPont, H. L., and Hornick, R. B. (1972). Fecal leukocytes in diarrheal illness. *Ann. Intern. Med.* **76,** 697–703.

Isberg, R. R., and Leong, J. M. (1990). Multiple B_1 chain integrins are receptors for invasin, a protein that promotes bacterial penetration into mammalian cells. *Cell* **60,** 861–871.

Jerse, A. E., Yu, J., Tall, B. D., and Kaper, J. B. (1990). A genetic locus of anteropathogenic *Escherichia coli* necessary for the production of attaching and effacing lesions on tissue culture cells. *Proc. Natl. Acad. Sci. U.S.A.* **87,** 7839–7843.

Jerse, A. E., Gicquelais, K. G., and Kaper, J. B. (1991). Plasmid and chromosomal elements involved in the pathogenesis of attaching and effacing *Escherichia coli*. *Infect. Immun.* **59,** 3869–3875.

Kantele, A., and Makela, P. H. (1991). Different profiles of the human immune response to primary and secondary immunization with an oral *Salmonella typhi* Ty21 a vaccine. *Vaccine* **9,** 423–427.

Karch, H., Heeseman, J., Laufs, R., O'Brien, A. D., Tacket, C. O., and Levine, M. M. (1987). A plasmid of enterochemorrhagic *Escherichia coli* 0157:H7 is required for expression of a new fimbrial antigen and for adhesion to epithelial cells. *Infect. Immun.* **55,** 455–461.

Karmali, M. A., Petric, M., Lim, C., Fleming, P. C., Arbus, G. S., and Lior H. (1985). The association between idiopathic hemolytic uremic syndrome and infection by verotoxin-producing *Escherichia coli*. *J. Infect. Dis.* **151,** 775–782.

Kaufmann, S. H. E. (1988). $CD8^+$ T lymphocytes in intracellular microbial infections. *Immunol. Today* **9,** 168–174.

Knutton, S., Lloyd, D. R., Candy, C. D. A., and McNeish, A. S. (1985). Adhesion of enterotoxigenic *Escherichia coli* to human small intestinal enterocytes. *Infect. Immun.* **48,** 824–831.

Levine, M. M. (1981). Adhesion of enterotoxigenic *Escherichia coli* in man and animals. *In* "Adhesion and Pathogenicity" (D. Taylor-Robinson, ed.), pp. 142–154. Pitman Medical, London.

Levine, M. M., Kaper, J. B., Black, R. E., and Clements, M. L. (1983). New knowledge on pathogenesis of bacterial enteric infections as applied to vaccine development. *Microbiol. Rev.* **47,** 510–550.

Levine, M. M., Ristaino, P., Marley, G., Smyth, C., Knutton, S., Boedeker, E., Black, R., Young, C., Clements, M, L., Cheney, C., and Patnaik, R. (1984). Coli surface antigens 1 and 3 of colonization factor antigen II-positive enterotoxigenic *Escherichia coli:* Morphology, purification, and immune responses in humans. *Infect. Immun.* **44,** 409–420.

Levine, M. M., Herrington, D., Murphy, J. R., Morris, J. G., Losonsky, G., Tall, B., Lindberg, A., Svenson, S., Baqar, S., Edwards, M. F., and Stocker, B. (1987). Safety, infectivity, immunogenicity and *in vivo* stability of two attenuated auxotrophic mutant strains of *Salmonella typhi,* 541Ty and 543Ty, as live oral vaccines in man. *J. Clin. Invest.* **79,** 888–902.

Levine, M. M., Hone, D., Heppner, D. G., Noriega, F., and Sriwathana, B. (1990). Attenuated *Salmonella* as carriers for the expression of foreign antigens. *Microecol. Ther.* **19,** 23–32.

Lowell, G. H., MacDermott, R. P., Summers, P. L., Reeder, A. A., Bertovich, M. J., and Formal, S. B. (1980). Antibody-dependent cell-mediated antibacterial activity: K lymphocytes, monocytes and granulocytes are effective against *Shigella*. *J. Immunol.* **125,** 2778–2784.

Lyerly, D. M., Saum, K. E., MacDonald, D. K., and Wilkins, T. D. (1985). Effects of *Clostridium difficile* toxins given intragastrically to animals. *Infect. Immun.* **47,** 349–352.

Mebus, C. A., Wyatt, R. G., and Kapikian, A. Z. (1977). Intestinal lesions induced by gnotobiotic calves by the virus of human infantile gastroenteritis. *Vet. Pathol.* **14,** 273–282.

Miller, J., Mekalanos, J. J., and Falkow, S. (1989). Coordinate regulation and sensory transduction in the control of bacterial virulence. *Science* **243,** 916–922.

Miller, S. (1991). PhoP/PhoQ: Macrophage-specific modulators of *Salmonella* virulence. *Mol. Microbiol.* **5,** 2073–2078.

Miller, V. L., Bliska, J. B., and Falkow, S. (1990). Nucleotide sequence of the *Yersinia enterocolitica ail* gene and characterization of the Ail protein product. *J. Bacteriol.* **172,** 1062–1069.

Mitchell, T. J., Ketley, J. M., Haslam, S. C., Stephen, J., Burdon, D. W., Candy, D. C. A., and Daniel, R. (1986). Effect of toxin A and B of *Clostridium difficile* on rabbit ileum and colon. *Gut* **27,** 78–85.

Mosley, W. H., Benenson, A. S., and Barui, R. (1968b). A serological survey for cholera antibodies in rural East Pakistan. 1. The distribution of antibody in the control population of a cholera-endemic field trial area and the realtion of antibody titre to the pattern of endemic cholera. *Bull. WHO* **38,** 327–334.

Nataro, J. P., Maher, K. O., Mackie, P., and Kaper, J. B. (1987). Characterization of plasmids encoding the adherence factor of enteropathogenic *Escherichia coli*. *Infect. Immun.* **55,** 2370–2377.

Nataro, J. P., Deng, Y., Maneval, D. R., German, A. L., Martin, W. C., and Levine, M. M. (1992). Aggregative adherence fimbriae I of enteroaggregative *E. coli* mediate adherence to HEp-2 cells and hemagglutination of human erythrocytes. *Infection and Immunity* **60,** 2297–2304.

O'Brien, A. D., Newland, J. W., Miller, S. F., Holmes, R. K., Smith, H. W., and Formal, S. B. (1984). Shiga-like toxin converting phages that cause hemorrhagic colitis or infantile diarrhea. *Science* **226,** 694–696.

Pai, C. H., Kelly, J. K., and Meyers, G. L. (1986). Experimental infection of infant rabbits with verotoxin-producing *Escherichia coli*. *Infect. Immun.* **51,** 16–23.

Quiding, M., Nordstrom, I., Kilander, A., Andersson, G., Hanson, L. A., Holmgren, J., and Czerkinsky, C. (1991). Oral cholera vaccination induces strong intestinal antibody responses and intereferon-gamma production and evokes local immunological memory. *J. Clin. Invest.* **88,** 143–148.

Ravdin, J. I. (1989). *Entameba histolytica:* From adherence to enteropathy. *J. Infect. Dis.* **159,** 420–429.

Riley, L. W., Remis, R. S., Helgerson, S. D., McGee, H. B., Wells, J. G., Davis, B. R., Hebert, R. J., Olcott, E. S., Johnson, L. M., Hargrett, N. T., Blake, P. A., and Cohen, M. L. (1983). Hemorrhagic colitis associated with a rare *Escherichia coli* serotype. *N. Engl. J. Med.* **308,** 681–685.

Rolfe, R. D., Helebian S., and Finegold, S. M. (1981). Bacterial interference between *Clostridium difficile* and normal fecal flora. *J. Infect. Dis.* **143,** 470–475.

Rothbaum, R. J., Partin, J. C., Saalfield, K., and McAdams, A. J. (1983). An ultrastructural study of enteropathogenic *Escherichia coli* infection in human infants. *Ultrastruct. Pathol.* **4,** 291–304.

Ruiz-Palacios, G. M., Torres, J., Torres, N. I., Escamilla, E., Ruiz-Palacios, B. R., and Tamayo, J. (1983). Cholera-like enterotoxin produced by *Campylobacter jejuni. Lancet* **II,** 250–252.

Rutter, J. M., and Jones, G. W. (1973). Protection against enteric disease caused by *Escherichia coli*—A model for vaccination with a virulence determinant? *Nature (London)* **242,** 531–532.

Savarino, S. J., Fasano, A., Robertson, D. C., and Levine, M. M. (1991). Enteroaggregative *Escherichia coli* elaborate a heat-stable enterotoxin demonstrable in an *in vitro* rabbit intestinal model. *J. Clin. Invest.* **87,** 1450–1455.

Tacket, C. O., Losonsky, G., Link, H., Hoang, Y., Guesry, P., Hilpert, H., and Levine, M. M. (1988). Protection by milk immunoglobulin concentrate against oral challenge with enterotoxigenic *Escherichia coli. N. Eng. J. Med.* **318,** 1240–1243.

Tacket, C. O., Binion, S. B., Bostwick, E., Losonsky, G., Roy, M. J., and Edelman, R. (1992). Efficacy of bovine milk immunoglobulin concentrate in preventing illness after *Shigella flexneri* challenge. *Am. J. Trop. Med. Hyg.* **47,** 276–283.

Tagliabue, A., Villa, L., De Magistris, M. T., Romano, M., Silvestri, S., Boraschi, D., and Nencioni, L. (1986). IgA-driven T cell-mediated anti-bacterial immunity in man after live oral Ty21a vaccine. *J. Immunol.* **137,** 1504–1510.

Taylor, R. K., Miller, V. L., Furlong, D. B., and Mekalanos, J. J. (1987). Use of *pho*A gene fusions to identify a pilus colonization factor coordinately regulated with cholera toxin. *Proc. Nat. Acad. Sci. U.S.A.* **84,** 2833–2837.

Tzipori, S. (1983). Cryptosporidiosis in animals and humans. *Microbiol. Rev.* **47,** 84–96.

Tzipori, S., Wachsmuth, I. K., Chapman, C., Birner, R., Brittingham, J., Jackson, C., and Hogg, J. (1986). The pathogenesis of hemorrhagic colitis caused by *Escherichia coli* O157:H7 in gnotobiotic piglets. *J. Infect. Dis.* **154,** 712–716.

Tzipori, S., Karch, H., Wachsmuth, K. I., Robins-Browne, R. M., O'Brien, A. D., Lior, H., Cohen, M. L., Smithers, J., and Levine, M. M. (1987). Role of a 60-megadalton plasmid and shiga-like toxins in the pathogenesis of infection caused by enterohemorrhagic *Escherichia coli* 0157:H7 in gnotobiotic piglets *Infect. Immun.* **55,** 3117–3125.

Van de Verg, L., Herrington, D. A., Murphy, J. R., Wasserman, S. S., Formal, S. B., and Levine, M. M. (1990). Specific IgA secreting cells in peripheral blood following oral immunization with bivalent *Salmonella typhi/Shigella sonnei* vaccine or infection with pathogenic *S. sonnei* in humans. *Infect. Immun.* **58,** 2002–2004.

Vial, P., Robins-Browne, R., Lior, H., Prado, V., Nataro, J., Kaper, J., Elsayed, A., Maneval, D., and Levine, MM. (1988). Characterization of enteroadherent-aggregative *Escherichia coli:* A newly-defined agent of diarrheal disease. *J. Infect. Dis.* **158,** 70–79.

Yokoyama, H., Ikedo, M., Kohbata, S., Ezaki, T., and Yabuuchi, E. (1989). An ultrastructural study of HeLa cell invasion with *Salmonella typhi* GIFU 10007. *Microbiol. Immunol.* **31,** 1–11.

Yoshikawa, M., Sasakawa, C., Makino, S., Okada, N., Lett, M.-C., Sakai, T., Yamada, M., Komatsu, K., Kamata, K., Kurata, T., and Sata, T. (1988). Molecular genetic approaches to the pathogenesis of bacillary dysentery. *Microbiol. Sci.* **5,** 333–339.

42

Liver and Biliary Tract

William R. Brown • Charles D. Howell

I. IgA IN HEPATOBILIARY DISEASES

A. Alcoholic Liver Disease

Many attempts have been made to implicate abnormalities in the IgA immune system in diseases of the liver and biliary tract. The most provocative of the putative associations is that of alcoholic liver disease (ALD), which some writers refer to as an IgA-associated disease (Van de Wiel *et al.*, 1987a). Several alterations in serum IgA have been described in ALD. Total serum IgA levels may be elevated (Kutteh *et al.*, 1982; Chandy *et al.*, 1983; Kalsi *et al.*, 1983; Newkirk *et al.*, 1983); the proportions of serum IgA present as polymeric IgA (pIgA) and secretory IgA (SIgA) may be increased, and the ratio of IgA1 to IgA2 may be decreased (Delacroix *et al.*, 1983; Van de Wiel *et al.*, 1987b). Most of these changes, however, are mild and not specific. One piece of evidence favoring a unique link between IgA abnormalities and ALD is that serum IgA concentrations may be increased even in mild ALD (steatosis). In contrast, increased concentrations do not occur in other disease until later, when histopathological abnormalities are more severe. The causes of elevated levels of serum IgA in ALD seem to include a selective and significant reduction in the catabolic rate in conjunction with increased synthesis of pIgA (Delacroix and Vaerman, 1983; Delacroix *et al.*, 1983), impaired removal of plasma pIgA by hepatocytes (Delacroix *et al.*, 1983), and increased spontaneous production of IgA by peripheral blood mononuclear cells (Kalsi *et al.*, 1983; Van de Wiel *et al.*, 1987c). Increased amounts of IgA antibodies against dietary and microbial antigens have been reported in ALD (Bjorneboe *et al.*, 1972; Nolan *et al.*, 1986), leading to the suggestion that the liver fails to extract circulating antigens and gut-derived endotoxins properly, perhaps because of impaired function of hepatic macrophages (Staun-Olsen *et al.*, 1983).

Far more interesting and potentially important than alterations in serum IgA in ALD are the deposits of IgA in the liver, skin, and kidneys of many such patients. IgA deposited in a continuous pattern along the margins of liver sinusoids has been described in about 75% of patients with ALD compared with less than 10% in non-ALD patients (Swerdlow and Chowdhury, 1984,1983; Van de Wiel *et al.*, 1987b). In addition, the presence of the IgA deposits has been associated with a higher likelihood of progressive hepatic injury (Swerdlow and Chowdhury, 1984); some authors, however, have reported the common occurrence of IgA deposits in non-ALD individuals, especially those with chronic hepatitis (Amano *et al.*, 1988). The hepatic deposition of IgA in ALD occurs about equally often in all histological expressions (steatosis, fibrosis, hepatitis, and cirrhosis), so this condition may be a consequence of alcohol-induced changes in the liver per se.

Most evidence now indicates that the hepatic IgA deposits in ALD are of the IgA1 subclass (Van de Wiel *et al.*, 1986,1987b; Amano *et al.*, 1988). The IgA also lacks J chain, does not bind to the polymeric immunoglobulin receptor (secretory component), and therefore appears to be mostly in a monomeric form. That the IgA deposits are predominantly IgA1 raises the intriguing possibility that the deposition is linked to an abnormality in the handling of IgA1 by the asialoglycoprotein receptor. The receptor, expressed on the sinusoidal surface of hepatocytes, functions to remove desialylated glycoproteins from plasma and degrades them in the liver (Ashwell and Harford, 1982). Because of its high content of galactose residues, IgA1 can bind to the receptor (Stockert *et al.*, 1982; Tomana *et al.*, 1988) and stimulate receptor-mediated clearance of the IgA (Tomana *et al.*, 1988). Conceivably, alcohol-induced damage to the hepatocyte membrane could impair such a clearance mechanism and lead to accumulation of IgA1 on the sinusoidal margin. The reported frequency of renal deposits of IgA in ALD varies from more than 50% (Berger *et al.*, 1977; Woodroffe *et al.*, 1981) to less than 20% (Montoliu *et al.*, 1986). Likewise, the severity of the disease also varies from a latent asymptomatic state to a very active proliferative condition. The prevailing opinion is that the deposits are complexes of IgA with various antigens, but no specific antigen has been identified consistently. The characteristics of the IgA renal deposits are now defined fairly conclusively. The IgA most likely is not associated with the polymeric immunoglobulin receptor and is IgA1 (Russell *et al.*, 1986). We have suggested that an abnormality in the handling of IgA1 by the liver in ALD is responsible for the renal accumulation of IgA (Brown and Kloppel, 1989). We speculate that complexes of IgA and the receptor, released from the liver or formed in the circulation, are "trapped" in the renal mesangium.

B. Primary Biliary Cirrhosis

Marked elevations of SIgA are common in primary biliary cirrhosis (PBC); values greater than 118 mg/ml have been called specific for the disease (Homburger *et al.*, 1984). However, on the basis of several reports, measurement of serum SIgA does not appear to distinguish PBC reliably from other cholestatic diseases. Also, IgA seems unlikely to be linked in any way pathogenically to the biliary ductule injury in PBC, since the disease has been reported in patients with selective and severe IgA deficiency (James *et al.*, 1986; Logan, 1987). However, an interesting relationship between IgA and biliary epithelium has been described. IgA allegedly stimulated the proliferation of extrahepatic bile duct epithelium in mice (Fallon-Friedlander *et al.*, 1987), but that observation subsequently has been refuted convincingly (Solbreux *et al.*, 1991).

C. Other Obstructive Biliary Tract Disease

Early reports suggested that measurement of IgA, especially SIgA, in serum would be useful in diagnosing extrahepatic biliary obstruction (Thompson *et al.*, 1973; Goldblum *et al.*, 1980) but, regrettably, that is not the case (Kutteh *et al.*, 1982; Delacroix *et al.*, 1983). The failure of SIgA and secretory component to reach high levels in biliary obstructive disease in humans, as they do after bile duct ligation in the rat (Lemaitre-Coelho *et al.*, 1978), no doubt reflects the fact that the human liver normally does not clear much IgA from the circulation (Delacroix *et al.*, 1982).

II. IMMUNODEFICIENCY AND HEPATOBILIARY DISEASES

Although congenital immunodeficiency states commonly have associated gastrointestinal abnormalities, diseases of the biliary tract and liver ordinarily are not prominently associated. Infrequently, however, selective IgA deficiency may be accompanied by an autoimmune-type liver disease (Brown *et al.*, 1972). Biliary tract sepsis evidently is not a feature of congenital immunodeficiencies or acquired hypogammaglobulinemia.

In contrast to the apparent sparing of hepatobiliary tissues in the immunodeficiencies just mentioned, these tissues are not spared in the acquired immunodeficiency syndrome (AIDS), in which numerous infectious and neoplastic manifestations have been described (Lebovics *et al.*, 1985; Gordon *et al.*, 1986; Cappell *et al.*, 1990; Schaffner, 1990). Since all persons at risk for infection with the human immunodeficiency virus (HIV) also are at risk for hepatitis B virus, this type of hepatitis is, not surprisingly, very commonly associated with the HIV positive condition. However, histological sequelae of the infection (chronic hepatitis) are not common in AIDS patients, perhaps because of the underlying immunoincompetent state. A common finding in the liver of AIDS patients are hepatic granulomas. Often the granulomas are ill defined or composed of foamy histiocytes, perhaps reflecting the decreased ratio of helper to suppressor type T cells. Infection of the gall bladder or biliary ducts with cytomegalovirus, *Cryptosporidium*, or both agents may occur in AIDS, and obstruction of the ducts with a sclerosing cholangitis-like lesion is a feature of these infections (Margulis *et al.*, 1986; Viteri and Green, 1987). Biopsy of the liver in AIDS patients who have hepatomegaly and unexplained fever often is recommended and may yield a diagnosis but, regrettably, this information usually does not lead to an effective treatment (Cappell *et al.*, 1990; Schaffner, 1990). Kaposi's sarcoma and lymphoma are the most common neoplasms of the liver in AIDS (Friedman, 1988). A list of many of the recognized infections of the liver and bile ducts in AIDS is given in Table I.

III. AUTOIMMUNE LIVER DISEASES

Primary biliary cirrhosis and idiopathic "autoimmune" chronic active hepatitis are hypothesized to be autoimmune in origin. Both disorders fulfill several of the proposed criteria for an autoimmune disease (Shoenfeld and Isenberg, 1989), including the presence of circulating autoantibodies, cell-mediated immunity to autoantigens, induction of disease in experimental animals by adoptive transfer of T cells or by immunization with self antigens, and the production of autoantibodies and autoreactive cells after immunization of mice. However, the role of the identified autoantigen(s) in disease induction and the immune effector mechanisms responsible for liver injury in both disorders remain undefined. Primary sclerosing cholangitis also is hypothesized to be autoimmune in origin, but will not be reviewed here.

Table I Infections of the Liver and Bile Ducts Associated with AIDS

Viral infections
Hepatitis B, nonA, nonB (C), D
Herpes (I, II, and Varicella zoster)
Cytomegalovirus
Epstein–Barr virus
Bacterial infections
Mycobacteria (*M. avium-intracellulare, M. kansasii, M. tuberculosis*)
Salmonella species
Vibrio species
Fungal infections
Cryptococcosis
Candidiasis
Histoplasmosis
Coccidioidomycosis
Parasitic infections
Toxoplasma gondii
Cryptosporidium

A. Primary Biliary Cirrhosis

PBC is a chronic cholestatic disease (characterized by impaired excretion of bile acids) of unknown etiology that primarily affects middle-aged females (Sherlock and Scheuer, 1973; Christensen *et al.*, 1980). The fundamental pathological process is T cell-mediated inflammation and destruction of interlobular and septal bile ducts, a process referred to as nonsuppurative destructive cholangitis (Rubin *et al.*, 1965). Similar lesions are observed during chronic graft-versus-host disease (Shulman *et al.*, 1988) and liver allograft rejection (Vierling and Fennell, 1985).

1. Clinical Features of PBC

The natural history of PBC includes a preclinical period in which no symptoms of liver disease are apparent (Long *et al.*, 1977; Fleming *et al.*, 1978; Beswick *et al.*, 1985). Up to 50% of patients are diagnosed during this phase of the disorder and may remain free of liver symptoms for at least 10 years. These "asymptomatic" patients are discovered because of elevated liver tests or symptoms of the extrahepatic autoimmune diseases associated with PBC (keratoconjunctivitis sicca or Sjögren's syndrome, scleroderma, autoimmune thyroidits, seronegative nondestructive arthritis, and Raynaud's phenomenon). As bile duct destruction progresses, symptoms (pruritus and jaundice) and signs of cirrhosis ultimately develop and result in either death or the need for liver transplantation (Christensen *et al.*, 1980; Balasubramaniam *et al.*, 1990).

2. Hypergammaglobulinemia and Autoantibodies

In addition to biochemical markers of liver disease (elevated fasting serum bile acids, copper, ceruloplasmin, liver alkaline phosphatase, bilirubin), PBC is characterized by polyclonal hypergammaglobulinemia. Serum IgM, IgG, and IgA all are elevated, but the most striking elevation is in IgM levels, which may be higher than 5 times the normal level (Christensen *et al.*, 1980). Several autoantibodies, including antinuclear, antithyroid, and anti-smooth muscle antibodies, have been reported in PBC; the most notable and relatively disease-specific are the M2 antimitochondrial antibodies (AMA) found in 83–99% of patients (discussed subsequently). The natural history of PBC is the same in patients with and without serum AMA.

3. Pathogenesis of PBC

a. Genetic susceptibility and environmental factors. The pathogenesis of PBC is undefined. The increased frequency of extrahepatic autoimmune disorders, autoantibody production, abnormalities of T-cell immunity, and absence of a defined infectious, toxic, or metabolic etiology led to the hypothesis that PBC is mediated by autoimmune mechanisms (James *et al.*, 1983). The induction of liver injury is hypothesized to involve an interplay between host susceptibility and an environment factor(s) that triggers the onset of disease. Indeed, an increased frequency of HLA-DRw8 (Gores *et al.*, 1987), -DRw3 (Ercilla *et al.*, 1979), and -DR2 (Miyamori *et al.*, 1983) in patients compared with controls has been reported. Further, patients and their first-degree relatives have an increased frequency of autoantibodies as well as defective T-cell suppressor activity (Galbraith *et al.*, 1974; Miller *et al.*, 1983). These observations suggest that susceptibility to PBC may be determined by (or linked to) genetic factors.

Clusters of cases in urban areas and near a common water source in one report is consistent with the existence of a yet-to-be defined environmental agent (Hamlyn and Sherlock, 1974), yet such clustering usually is not observed (Lofgren *et al.*, 1985). In addition, reports of an increased frequency of gram-negative bacterial urinary infections (a potential source of sensitization to mitochondrial antigens) in PBC have been refuted (Floreani *et al.*, 1989; Morreale *et al.*, 1989). Nonetheless, AMA-positive sera react with mitochondrial antigens from rough-mutant gram-negative bacteria. Hopf (1989) reported that the feces of PBC patients have increased numbers of rough mutants and that PBC patients have lipid A (endotoxin) deposits in the liver. These results have not been confirmed by others. However, since immunization of rabbits with rough mutants but not wild-type gram-negative organisms results in production of AMAs, sensitization to mitochondria of mutant gram-negative bacteria may be involved in induction of AMA and, possibly, in the pathogenesis of bile duct destruction.

b. Histological features of PBC. Liver histology in PBC is characterized by accumulation of mononuclear inflammatory cells in portal triads and inflammation of septal and interlobular bile ducts (Rubin *et al.*, 1965; Ludwig, 1978). Inflammation of bile ducts is associated with necrosis of biliary epithelial cells and ultimately results in destruction of the ducts. Bile duct inflammation occurs in a segmental distribution and varies in intensity along the length of the ducts. Piecemeal necrosis of periportal hepatocytes, portal lymphoid aggregates, and granulomas also are observed. Progressive destruction of bile ducts is accompanied by proliferation of bile ductules and liver fibrosis, and ultimately results in cirrhosis.

T cells with receptors for antigen–major histocompatibility complex (MHC) composed of α and β heterodimers constitute 81–99% of mononuclear cells in the liver in PBC (Shimizu *et al.*, 1986; Yamada *et al.*, 1986; Krams *et al.*, 1990). The percentage of $CD4^+$ (MHC Class II-restricted) T cells is generally equal to or greater than that of $CD8^+$ (MHC Class I-restricted) T cells. $CD4^+$ and $CD8^+$ T cells infiltrate the bile duct epithelium, but $CD8^+Leu15^-$ (cytotoxic) T cells appear to predominate. Lymphocytes frequently are observed in intercellular spaces between injured and necrotic biliary epithelial cells. Biliary epithelial cells show increased expression of MHC Class I (Shimizu *et al.*, 1986; Calmus *et al.*, 1990) as well as new expression of Class II antigens (Spengler, 1988) and intracellular adhesion molecule 1 (ICAM-1) (Calmus *et al.*, 1990). Periportal hepatocytes also show increased expression of MHC Class I antigens. Increased HLA antigen and ICAM-1 expression, presumably induced by cytokines released locally (Paradis and Sharp, 1989), may allow biliary epithelial cells and hepatocytes to present antigen(s) more efficiently and to stimulate the T-cell response to bile duct cells and periportal hepatocytes. However, the functions of liver T cells and the significance of increased MHC antigen and ICAM-1 expression in the liver during PBC remain to be clarified.

The hepatic non-T-cell population is composed primarily of plasma cells, with a smaller percentage of natural killer and interstitial dendritic cells (Krams *et al.*, 1990). Deposits of IgG, IgA, and IgM have been observed on biliary epithelial cells (Ghadiminejad and Baum, 1987; Krams *et al.*, 1990). These results suggest that antibody-mediated cellular cytotoxicity, either through complement activation (IgG and IgM) or through the activation of antigen-nonspecific FcR γ positive (NK, macrophage, or K) cells, may be involved in bile duct injury.

c. Autoantigens in PBC. The bile duct antigen(s) recognized in PBC is (are) unknown. The large number of autoantibodies in PBC is indicative of a lack of immunological tolerance to the respective antigens. Elucidation of the mechanisms responsible for lack (or loss) of immune tolerance may provide insight into the pathogenesis of bile duct destruction in this disorder. However, only one of the autoantigens identified in PBC (the asialoglycoprotein receptor) is liver specific; only the M2 mitochondrial autoantigens are nearly disease specific. Serum autoantibodies and T-cell sensitization to the asialoglycoprotein receptor (ASGR), a hepatocyte-specific glycoprotein expressed in hepatocyte plasma membranes, have been reported (McFarland *et al.*, 1985; Vento *et al.*, 1986). Recognition of the peptide fragments of ASGR by autoreactive T cells could contribute to destruction of periportal hepatocytes by T cells. However, the ASGR is not expressed by bile duct epithelial cells. ASGR may be shed by periportal hepatocytes, processed by bile duct cells, and presented to ASGR-specific T cells. However, evidence of such a phenomenon is lacking. Further, since sensitization to the ASGR is not specific to PBC, this receptor is not likely to play a primary (initiating) role in the pathogenesis of bile duct destruction.

d. M2 mitochondrial autoantigens. Serum complement-fixing antibodies to mitochondria in PBC first were reported by Walker *et al.* (1965). Subsequent studies indicated that AMAs recognize antigens located in the inner membrane of the mitochondria. Based on the pattern of immunofluorescence and reactivity with submitochondrial particles, AMAs can be subdivided into 9 subtypes (M1–9; Berg and Klein, 1989). Subtypes 2, 4, 8, and 9 are observed in PBC. The M2 pattern is most specific for PBC. Immunoblots of submitochondrial fractions with PBC sera show reactivity with five major bands at 70–75, 55–56, 51–52, 48, and 36 kDa (referred to as M2a–e; Bassendine *et al.*, 1989). The genes for the 74-kDa and 52-kDa antigens have been cloned, and recombinant M2 proteins have been produced (Gershwin *et al.*, 1987; Coppel *et al.*, 1988; Yeaman *et al.*, 1988; Van de Water *et al.*, 1989). The M2 antigens are subunits or components of inner membrane enzymes of the 2-oxo acid dehydrogenase complex. This complex includes three enzymes of similar structure and function—pyruvate dehydrogenase (PDH), alpha-keto acid dehydrogenase, and the oxoglutarate dehydrogenase complex. Each enzyme plays a critical role in intermediary metabolism. Each complex consists of several copies of three subunits termed E1, E2, and E3. The 74-kDa and 56-kDa antigens are the E2 of PDH and a protein X that co-purifies with it. The 52-kDa antigen has been found to be the E2 of alpha-keto acid dehydrogenase; the 48- and 36-kDa antigens are the E1 α and β subunits of PDH (Fussey *et al.*, 1989). Approximately 100% of AMA-positive sera react with at least one of these antigens (90–95% react with the 74- and 52-kDa antigens). Alderrucio *et al.* (1986) have reported that sera from patients with scleroderma also react with the 70–74-kDa submitochondrial antigen recognized by PBC sera. AMA reactivity also is found in other disorders (chronic active hepatitis, systemic lupus erythematosus, rheumatoid arthritis, and Sjögren's syndrome), indicating that M2 AMAs are not specific to PBC. The ability of M2 AMAs to inhibit the activity of inner mitochondrial enzymes indicates that the active sites of the enzymes may be recognized (Van de Water, 1988; Fregeau *et al.*, 1989,1990a,b). Alternatively, binding of the AMA to its epitope may induce a conformational change that prevents the enzyme from binding to its substrates. The immunoglobulin or B-cell epitope of the 74-kDa E2 of PDH consists of a 75–93 amino acid segment of the lipoic acid domain (Surh *et al.*, 1990). The T-cell epitope(s) has (have) not been identified. Like many autoantigens, the mitochondrial autoantigens in PBC are highly conserved in nature and are present in prokaryotic as well as eukaryotic cells. Additional similarities to other autoantigens include (1) that they are intracellular enzymes composed of multiple subunits and (2) that autoantibodies directed toward these enzymes are directed toward functional sites or domains. However, the role of sensitization to mitochondrial autoantigens in the pathogenesis of PBC is unclear. The occurrence of PBC in the absence of M2 AMA reactivity suggests that an AMA response is not required for induction of PBC. Indeed, immunization of mice with the recombinant 70-kDa human mitochondrial autoantigen results in a high titer AMA response but no liver inflammation. Transfer of peripheral blood mononuclear cells (PBMC) from patients with PBC into severe combined immunodeficient (SCID) mice results in liver lesions that are histologically similar to those in PBC (Krams *et al.*, 1989a). Similar lesions were induced also (albeit much less frequently) by PBMCs from normal subjects, suggesting that graft-versus-host disease may be in part responsible. Van de Water *et al.* (1991) reported that $CD4^+$ T-cell clones derived from the liver during PBC are sensitized to mitochondrial autoantigens. Whether T-cell sensitization to these antigens is a primary or secondary event in the pathogenesis of bile duct destruction remains to be defined.

e. Plasma membrane expression of mitochondrial antigens by bile duct. Studies in yeast indicate that the M2 mitochondrial antigens are encoded by nuclear (and not mitochondrial) DNA, synthesized in the cytoplasm, and transported to the mitochondria. For mitochondrial antigens to be recognized by T cells, they must be presented in association with self-MHC Class I or II antigens on the plasma membrane of antigen-presenting cells (macrophages, dendritic cells, B cells) or biliary epithelial cells. Two studies suggest that AMAs recognize antigens expressed on the plasma membranes of mammalian hepatocytes (Ghadiminejad and Baum, 1987) and intrahepatic bile duct cells (Krams *et al.*, 1990). These observations suggest that mitochondrial autoantigens are transported aberrantly to the plasma membrane, where they can be recognized by effector T cells or AMAs. Alternatively, a cross-reactive plasma membrane antigen may be recognized. The plasma membrane antigen(s) recognized by AMA-positive sera and the mouse antibody to recombinant autoantigens used in these studies have not been identified. In addition, hepatocytes and biliary epithelial cells from normal subjects and patients with other liver diseases show less intense but similar patterns of staining when reacted with antibodies to mammalian E2 of PDH. Therefore, plasma membrane expression of E2 by bile duct cells and hepatocytes is not sufficient to initiate PBC. Consistent with this notion, Joplin (1991) reported that macrophages in lymph nodes draining the livers of PBC patients stain more intensely with antibodies to E2 than do macrophages from normal subjects and patients with other liver disease. These observations suggest that the release of mitochondrial antigen (and presumably other self components) from senescent and injured liver cells into hepatic lymph is a normal physiological phenomenon. A comparison of the handling of mitochondrial antigens (processing, presentation, accessory signal production) by macrophages of PBC patients compared with that of control subjects may provide insight into the process by which loss of immunological tolerance to self antigens occurs in PBC.

f. Peripheral blood B- and T-cell activity. An increase in the mean number of peripheral blood B cells that spontaneously secrete immunoglobulins has been reported in PBC (James *et al.*, 1985; Bird *et al.*, 1988). Immunoglobulin secretion after mitogen stimulation has been either normal or slightly diminished. The percentage of activated peripheral blood B cells in PBC is not increased. These results suggest that immunoglobulin secretion is not the result of an intrinsic defect in B-cell functions. James, 1980a and Suou *et al.*, 1989 have reported that increased Ig secretion is the result of defective $CD4^+$ (suppressor–inducer) T-cell function. Others (Zetterman and Woltjen, 1980) also have reported defects in inducible T-cell suppressor activity in PBC. However, defective suppressor–inducer T-cell function is not present in all patients. Therefore, other mechanisms must be involved in the induction of hypergammaglobulinemia. Since a similar defect in T-cell suppressor function occurs in disease-free relatives of PBC patients (Galbraith *et al.*, 1974; Miller *et al.*, 1983), other yet-to-be defined factors maybe required for the expression of the disease.

Other manifestations of altered immunity in PBC include impaired cutaneous delayed hypersensitivity (skin test anergy) (Fox *et al.*, 1969), decreased mean antibody response after immunization (Fox *et al.*, 1969), defective mitogen-induced lymphocyte blastogenesis (Fox *et al.*, 1973; MacSween and Thomas, 1973), defective recognition of self in autologous mixed-lymphocyte culture (Lindor *et al.*, 1988), circulating immune complexes, and impaired clearance of C3b-containing immune complexes by Kupffer cells. The role of these factors in the pathogenesis of PBC is also unknown.

g. Activity of liver-derived T cells. Studies of T-cell lines propagated from liver biopsies of patients suggest that PBC may be mediated by a limited number of T-cell clones (Moebius, 1990). However, cloned liver T cells consistently show only lectin-dependent cellular cytotoxicity (LDCC) and minimal natural killer and antibody-dependent cellular cytotoxicity (ADCC) activities (Meuer *et al.*, 1988; Hoffman *et al.*, 1989). No spontaneous T cell-mediated cytotoxicity toward a number of mammalian cell lines, including a well-differentiated bile duct carcinoma, has been reported. The lack of classic cytotoxic T lymphocyte (CTL) activity by T-cell lines that presumably are sensitized to bile duct cells is puzzling, but may reflect the use of allogeneic target cells that either do not express the antigen(s) recognized in PBC or do not present the antigen(s) in association with syngeneic HLA antigens. Alternatively, these liver T lymphocytes (LTLs) are propagated in the absence of specific antigen and may not play a role in bile duct destruction. Whether LDCC in these studies is mediated by bile duct-specific T cells is not clear since mitogens may stimulate nonspecific cytotoxic activity *in vitro*. T-cell reactivity toward intrahepatic bile duct epithelial cells has not been reported in PBC, primarily because of the difficulty in obtaining autologous or syngeneic biliary epithelial cells. Saidman *et al.* (1990) have reported that a liver T-cell line proliferates when stimulated with autologous extrahepatic biliary epithelial cells. Since extrahepatic bile ducts are not affected in PBC, the meaning of this observation is unclear.

4. Conclusion

The features of PBC mentioned earlier do not generate a unified hypothesis of its etiology. However, susceptibility to PBC appears to be determined genetically. The factor(s) that acts in association with genetic susceptibility to induce disease is (are) unknown. Bile duct destruction appears to be mediated by $CD4^+$ and $CD8^+$ T-cells. Although T-cell destruction of bile ducts appears to be the primary pathogenic process, a bile duct-specific antigen has not been identified and the mechanisms by which T cells mediate bile duct injury are not defined. Circumstantial evidence also suggests that ADCC also may be involved. A better understanding of the function of liver-derived T and non-T cells is necessary to elucidate the immunological effector mechanisms responsible for bile duct destruction. Such studies are not feasible in humans because intrahepatic bile duct cells are not readily available. The surface membrane expression of M2 mitochondrial autoantigens by hepatocytes, bile duct cells, and macrophages of normal individuals as well as patients, and the presence of AMAs in disease-free relatives of patients, casts doubt on (but does not exclude) a primary role for sensitization to mitochondrial antigens in the pathogenesis of PBC. On the other hand, recognition of mitochondrial or other self-peptide fragments may be a secondary mechanism that helps perpetuate or amplify the immune response to bile ducts. Pursuit of these issues using animal models (graft-versus-host diseases, SCID mouse) of nonsuppurative destructive cholangitis may overcome the limitations of human studies.

B. Autoimmune Chronic Active Hepatitis

Autoimmune chronic active hepatitis (ACAH) is a clinical syndrome defined by idiopathic, hepatitis B and C virus-negative, chronic active hepatitis that is associated with marked hypergammaglobulinemia, circulating autoantibodies, immune-mediated extraintestinal organ injury, and responsiveness to treatment with immunosuppressive medications (Joske and King, 1955; Bearn *et al.*, 1956; Mackay *et al.*, 1956). In untreated patients with severe ACAH, the natural history is characterized by progressive hepatocyte destruction that results in cirrhosis and high mortality. The clinical and serological features of this syndrome have led to the hypothesis that hepatocyte injury in ACAH is mediated by autoimmune mechanisms. The targeted hepatocyte antigen(s) have not been identified conclusively and the autoimmune effector mechanism(s) responsible for liver injury are undefined.

1. Pathogenesis of ACAH

a. Genetic susceptibility and environmental factors. The pathogenesis of ACAH also is not defined completely. An increased frequency of HLA-A1, -B8, -DR3, -DR4, and IgG heavy chain Gm a^+x^+ alleles suggests that susceptibility to ACAH may be determined genetically (Whittingham *et al.*, 1981; O'Brien *et al.*, 1986; Krawitt *et al.*, 1988; Johnson *et al.*, 1991). The occurrence of decreased serum complement components (Vergani *et al.*, 1985) and decreased peripheral blood T suppressor-cell activity (Nouri-Aria *et al.*, 1985; O'Brien *et al.*, 1986; Vento *et al.*, 1986; Krawitt *et al.*, 1988) in patients and first-degree relatives provides additional support for inherited susceptibility to ACAH.

Much attention has focused on the role of environmental agents (especially medications and viral infections) in ACAH. Chronic active hepatitis (CAH) that is both clinically and histologically similar to that in idiopathic autoimmune CAH occurs as idiosyncratic reactions to several prescription medications (i.e., alpha-methyl DOPA, oxyphenistatin, nitrofurantoin; Johnson *et al.*, 1991). In addition, liver lesions during chronic hepatitis B, C, and non-A, non-B infections are frequently indistinguishable from those in ACAH. Therefore, much attention has been focused on a search for a viral etiology of ACAH. An increased frequency of antibodies to measles and persistence of the measles virus genome in lymphocytes (but not hepatocytes) of ACAH patients has been reported (Robertson *et al.*, 1987). Vento and colleagues (1991) have reported that acute hepatitis A may trigger ACAH in disease-free relatives who have defective T-cell suppressor activity. The role of the hepatitis C virus (HCV), the etiologic agent for 70–90% of chronic non-A, non-B hepatitis (both transfusion-related and sporadic cases) has become the focus of many studies. Depending on the population, up to 80% of patients with ACAH have antibodies to recombinant HCV c100 antigen. In most patients, anti-c100 reactivity appears to be falsely positive (McFarlane *et al.*, 1990; Schvarcz *et al.*, 1990; Czaja *et al.*, 1991; Pohjanpelto *et al.*, 1991), since the antibody HCV titer correlates with the degree of hypergammaglobulinemia and antibody reactivity disappears when disease activity and serum γ globulin levels decrease in response to immunosuppressive therapy. More importantly, in ACAH patients, most anti-c100-positive sera are nonreactive in supplemental HCV antibody tests (i.e., immunoblot and neutralization assays) and do not contain HCV RNA. This result does not apply to Italians with ACAH, in whom antibody to HCV is confirmed using supplemental anti-HCV assays in up to 73% of cases (Lenzi *et al.*, 1990; Magrin *et al.*, 1991; Todros *et al.*, 1991). In addition, Garson *et al.* (1991) have reported HCV RNA in sera of 9 of 13 (69%) selected Italian patients with ACAH. Further, some of these patients have responded to antiviral (but not immunosuppressive) therapy, suggesting that active HCV is responsible for liver disease. Although chronic HCV in Italians can mimic some of the clinical features of ACAH, the lack of response to immunosuppressive medications by definition excludes a diagnosis of ACAH.

In Japanese patients, chronic HCV is associated with production of antibodies to a host (GOR 47-1) autoantigen (Mishiro *et al.*, 1990), suggesting that the hepatitis C infection can induce autoantibody formation. Indeed, GOR and the polyprotein of HCV share considerable homology with the kidney microsomal autoantigen-1 (cytochrome P450 II D6; Manns *et al.*, 1991a,b) that is associated with ACAH. These results provide circumstantial evidence that molecular mimicry of self by viral antigens may result in autoantibody formation in some instances. However, anti-GOR antibodies were not found in patients with ACAH (or PBC). Therefore, no direct evidence is available that HCV infection is an etiological agent in rigorously defined cases of ACAH.

b. Histological features. Liver histology shows infiltration and expansion of portal triads by mononuclear inflammatory cells. These cells infiltrate the limiting plate of hepatocytes and induce necrosis of periportal hepatocytes. In severe cases, bridging and multilobular hepatocyte necrosis are observed and indicate a high risk for rapid progression from CAH to cirrhosis. Most lymphocytes in portal tracts and areas of periportal hepatocyte piecemeal necrosis are mature T cells. The representation of T-cell subsets is somewhat controversial. Eggink *et al.* (1982) have reported that $CD8^+$ cells predominate. Others have shown a more equal percentage of $CD4^+$ and $CD8^+$ cells. Natural killer (NK) cells and plasma cells also are present, but at frequencies less than 10%. ACAH is associated with increased expression of Class I and new expression of Class II MHC antigens by hepatocytes, which may allow hepatocytes to present the relevant antigen to liver T cells. T-cell recognition of autologous antigens in association with induced MHC antigens on hepatocytes is hypothesized to be a mechanism of liver cell injury during ACAH. However, the significance of aberrant expression of MHC antigens by hepatocytes is unknown. The presence of NK and plasma cells and immunoglobulin deposits on hepatocytes (Hopf *et al.*, 1976; Kawanishi and McDermott, 1979; Frazer *et al.*, 1983) also suggest that non-MHC-restricted cytotoxic activity and ADCC may be involved.

c. Autoantigens in ACAH. The specific hepatocyte antigen(s) and autoimmune effector mechanism(s) that mediate liver cell injury in ACAH also are undefined. Several autoantibodies and corresponding autoantigens have been identified in ACAH. The list includes antibodies to nuclear (Joske and King, 1955; Penner *et al.*, 1986), mitochondrial (Walker, 1965), smooth muscle (actin) (Whittingham *et al.*, 1966), liver kidney microsomal-1 (i.e., cytochrome P450 II D6; Kyriatsoulis *et al.*, 1987; Peakman *et al.*,1987; Franch-Codoner *et al.*, 1989), ASGR (McFarlane *et al.*, 1985), and soluble liver (Manns *et al.*, 1987) antigens. In general, these autoantigens and autoantibodies are neither liver, species, nor disease specific. With few exceptions, antibody titers do not correlate with disease activity. Further, all autoantigens identified to date, except the ASGR, are localized to intracellular organelles and not the plasma membrane where they can be recognized by autoantibodies or antigen-specific T cells. Nonetheless, two autoantigens (ASGR and cytochrome P450 II D6) are particularly worthy of further discussion.

The ASGR is a hepatocyte-specific glycoprotein located in the basolateral plasma membrane. Antibodies to the ASGR have been reported during ACAH, chronic active hepatitis B, and PBC and, therefore, are not disease specific (McFarlane *et al.*, 1985). Nonetheless, a feature common to these disorders is inflammatory necrosis of periportal hepatocytes that appear to express more ASGR than do hepatocytes in the centrilobular zone. In addition, peripheral blood and liver T cells of ACAH patients are sensitized to the ASGR (Vento *et al.*, 1986; Wen *et al.*, 1990), and peripheral blood mononuclear cells lyse autologous hepatocytes *in vitro*. Although whether the ASGR is the targeted antigen is not clear in these studies, these observations keep alive the possibility that recognition of the ASGR may result in immune-mediated liver injury in ACAH.

A subgroup of patients with ACAH has been described in whom antinuclear and anti-actin antibodies are absent but in whom antibodies that, by immunofluorescence, react with liver and kidney microsomes (anti-LKM-1; Manns, 1991; Manns *et al.*, 1991a) are present. The antigen recognized by anti-LKM-1 is a 33-amino-acid segment of cytochrome P450 II D6. The smallest epitope is an 8-amino-acid peptide in which a 6-amino-acid sequence is identical to that found in the herpes simplex 1 immediate early antigen 175. In addition, the 33-amino-acid segment includes segments highly homologous to the polyprotein of HCV and the GOR 47-1 autoantigen associated with HCV infection. This finding raises the possibility that sensitization to herpes simplex or HCV antigens triggers induction of antibodies to LKM. Autoantibodies to cytochrome P450 inhibit enzyme activity *in vitro*. However, the enzymatic activity of cytochrome P450 isolated from the livers of patients with antibodies to LKM-1 is normal. Therefore, inhibition of cytochrome P450 by anti-LKM-1 is not significant *in vito*. Further, a report that LKM-1 antigen is expressed in liver plasma membrane has been disputed (Peakman *et al.*, 1987). In light of these results, hypothesizing a role for anti-LKM-1 in the pathogenesis of liver injury in ACAH is difficult.

d. Peripheral blood B- and T-cell activity. Increased spontaneous and pokeweed mitogen-induced polyclonal IgG production by PBMCs isolated during ACAH has been reported (Kayhan, 1985). Increased Ig secretion has been attributed to an abnormality in regulatory T-cell function. Indeed, decreased concanavalin A (Con A)-induced and antigen-specific T-cell suppressor activity in patients and first- and second-degree relatives has been reported (Hodgson *et al.*, 1978; O'Brien *et al.*, 1986; Krawitt *et al.*, 1988). However, the relationship between increased Ig secretion and decreased T-cell suppressor activity is undefined.

PBMCs from patients with ACAH are capable of mediating cytotoxic activity toward xenogeneic, allogeneic, and autologous hepatocytes *in vitro* (Thompson *et al.*, 1974; Wands and Isselbacher, 1975; Cochrane *et al.*, 1976; Geubel *et al.*, 1976; Kawanishi, 1977; Kawanishi, and McDermott, 1979). The mononuclear cell subpopulation responsible for peripheral blood cytotoxic activity is a non-T cell that expresses Fc receptor for IgG and mediates ADCC *in vitro* (Vergani *et al.*, 1979; Stefanini *et al.*, 1983; Mondelli *et al.*, 1985. T-cell cytotoxic activity appears to be less important. PBMCs from patients with ALD and chronic non-A, non-B hepatitis also show cytotoxic activity toward autologous hepatocytes (Izumi *et al.*, 1983; Poralla *et al.*, 1984). Further, most of these experiments have assayed adherence of cocultured hepatocytes to measure cytotoxicity. The high rate of spontaneous hepatocyte death in control cultures (Stefanini *et al.*, 1983) suggests that cytotoxicity as defined in these experiments in part reflects cell death of a nonimmune nature. Given the predominance of T cells in the liver during ACAH, the lack of CTL activity toward autologous hepatocytes is perplexing. However, the functions of peripheral T cells may not reflect the functions of liver T cells accurately.

e. Activity of liver-derived T-cell clones. T-cell clones derived from the liver during ACAH are also predominantly (75%) $CD4^+$. Like peripheral blood T cells, liver T-cell clones also are sensitized to the ASGR and LKM-1 antigen (Lohr et al., 1991; Poralla *et al.*, 1991). However, of 89 liver LKM-specific T-cell clones tested, 24 of 26 $CD8^+$ and 20 of 63 $CD4^+$ clones showed only LDCC (Lohr *et al.*, 1991) toward autologous but not allogeneic B cells. Of the remaining clones, 14 showed non-MHC-restricted cytotoxic activity toward NK-sensitive K562 cells. The cytotoxic activity of 5 $CD8^+$ clones was restricted to autologous Epstein–Barr virus-transformed B cells. Since cytotoxic activity against autologous human hepatocytes was not assessed, the meaning of these results is unclear. The requirement for lectins to induce cytotoxicity and the high rate of non-MHC-restricted killing are perplexing but may be explained by propagation of clones in high dose interleukin-2 in the absence of antigen (autologous hepatocytes). Further, in the absence of challenge with hepatocyte antigens, B cells (normal or immortalized) are unlikely to express the antigens recognized by "hepatocyte-specific" T cells.

2. Conclusion

The pathogenesis of ACAH is undetermined. Susceptibility appears to be determined by genetic factors. In some susceptible individuals, a number of environmental agents (medications, viral infections) appear to trigger the onset of disease. However, in the majority of cases, no specific environmental trigger can be identified. In addition, the hepatocyte antigen(s) targeted by the immune system in ACAH has not been identified conclusively. Contrary to histochemical studies, which show a predominance of T cells in the liver, studies of PBMCs suggest that non-T cells are primarily responsible for liver injury in ACAH. However, a complete understanding of the mechanisms involved must include investigations of the functions of T cells isolated from the liver. The ability to clone liver T cells should allow better definition of the roles of T cells in the pathogenesis of ACAH.

References

Alderuccio, F., Toh, B.-H., Barnett, A., and Pedersen, J. (1986). Identification and characterization of mitochondria autoantigens in progressive systemic sclerosis: Identity with the 72,000 Dalton autoantigen in primary biliary cirrhosis. *J. Immunol.* **137,** 1855–1859.

Amano, K., Tsukada, K., Takeuchi, T., Fukuda, Y., and Nagura, H. (1988). IgA deposition in alcoholic liver disease. An immunoelectron microscopic study. *Am. J. Clin. Pathol.* **89,** 22–28.

Ashwell, G., and Harford, J. (1982). Carbohydrate-specific receptors of the liver. *Ann. Rev. Biochem.* **51,** 531–554.

Balasubramaniam, K., Grambsch, P., Wiesner, R., Lindor, K., and Dickson, E. (1990). Diminished survival in asymptomatic primary biliary cirrhosis. *Gastroenterology* **98,** 1567–1571.

Bassendine, M., Dewar, P., and James, O. (1985). HLA-DR antigens in primary biliary cirrhosis: Lack of association. *Gut* **26,** 625–628.

Bassendine, M., Fussey, S., Mutimer, D., James, O., and Yeaman, S. (1989). Identification and characterization of four M2 mitochondrial autoantigens in primary biliary cirrhosis. *In* "Seminars in Liver Disease" (M. A. Rothschild, ed.), Vol. 9, pp. 124–131. Thieme Medical Publishers, New York.

Baum, H. (1989). Nature of the mitochondrial antigens of primary biliary cirrhosis and their possible relationships to the etiology of the disease. *In* "Seminars in Liver Disease" (M. A. Rothschild, ed.), Vol. 9, pp. 117–123. Thieme Medical Publishers, New York.

Bearn, A., Kunkel, H., and Slater, R. (1956). The problem of chronic liver disease in young women. *Am. J. Med.* **7,** 3–15.

Berg, P., and Klein, R. (1989). Heterogeneity of antimitochondrial antibodies. *In* "Seminars in Liver Disease" (M. A. Rothschild, ed.), Vol. 9, pp. 124–131. Thieme Medical Publishers, New York.

Berger, J., Yaneva, H., and Nabarra, B. (1977). Glomerular changes in patients with cirrhosis of the liver. *Adv. Nephrol.* **7,** 3–14.

Bernuau, D., Feldmann, G., Degott, C., and Gisselbrecht, C. (1981). Ultrastructural lesions of bile ducts in primary biliary cirrhosis. *Hum. Pathol.* **12,** 782–793.

Beswick, D., Klatskin, G., and Boyer, J. (1985). Asymptomatic primary biliary cirrhosis. *Gastroenterology* **89,** 267–271.

Bird, P., Calvert, J., Mithison, H., Ling, N., Basendine, M., and James, O. (1988). Lymphocytes from patients with primary biliary cirrhosis spontaneously secrete high levels of IgG3 in culture. *Clin. Exp. Immunol* **71,** 475–480.

Bjorneboe, M., Prytz, H., and Orskov, F. (1972). Antibodies to intestinal microbes in serum of patients with cirrhosis of the liver. *Lancet* **8,** 58–60.

Bradford, A., Howell, S., Aitken, A., James, L., and Yeaman, S. (1987). Primary structure around the lipoate-attachment site on the E2 component of bovine heart pyruvate dehydrogenase complex. *Biochem. J.* **245,** 919–922.

Brown, W. R., and Kloppel, T. M. (1989). The liver and IgA: Immunological, cell biological and clinical implications. *Hepatology* **9,** 763–784.

Brown, W. R., Butterfield, D., Savage, D., and Tada, T. (1972). Clinical, microbiological, and immunological studies in patients with immunoglobulin deficiencies and gastrointestinal disorders. *Gut* **13,** 441–449.

Calmus, Y., Gane, P., Rouger, P., and Poupon, R. (1990). Hepatic expression of class I and class II major histocompatibility complex molecules in primary biliary cirrhosis, effect of ursodeoxycholic acid. *Hepatology* **11,** 12–15.

Cappell, M. S., Schwartz, M. S., and Biempica, L. (1990). Clinical utility of liver biopsy in patients with serum antibodies to the human immunodeficiency virus. *Am. J. Med.* **88,** 123–130.

Chandy, K. G., Hubscher, S. G., Elias, E., Berg, J., Khan, M., and Burnett, D. (1983). Dual role of the liver in regulating circulating polymeric IgA in man: Studies on patients with liver disease. *Clin. Exp. Immunol* **52,** 207–218.

Christensen, E., Crowe, J., Doniach, D., Popper, H., Ranek, L., Rodes, J., Tygstrup, N., and Williams, R. (1980). Clinical pattern and course of disease in primary biliary cirrhosis based on an analysis of 236 patients. *Gastroenterology* **78,** 236–246.

Cochrane, A., Moussouros, A., Thomson, A., Eddleston, A., and Williams, R. (1976). Antibody-dependent cell-mediated (K cell) cytotoxicity against isolated hepatocytes in chronic active hepatitis. *Lancet* **1,** 441–444.

Coppel, R., McNeilage, L., Surh, C., Van de Water, J., Spithill, T., Whittingham, S., and Gershwin, M. (1988). Primary structure of the human M2 mitochondrial autoantigen of primary biliary cirrhosis: Dihydrolipoamide acetyltransferase. *Proc. Natl. Acad. Sci. U.S.A.* **85,** 7317–7321.

Crowe, J., Christensen, E., Butler, J., Wheeler, P., Doniach, D., Keenan, J., and Williams, R. (1980). Primary biliary cirrhosis: The prevalence of hypothyroidism and its relationship to thyroid autoantibodies and sicca syndrome. *Gastroenterology* **78,** 1437–1441.

Czaja, A., Rakela, J., Hay, J., and Moore, S. (1990). Clinical and prognostic implications of HLA B8 in corticosteroid-treated severe autoimmune chronic active hepatitis. *Gastroenterology* **98,** 1587–1593.

Czaja, A. J., Taswell, H. F., Rakela, J., and Schimek, C. M. (1991). Frequency and significance of antibody to hepatitis C virus in severe corticosteroid-treated autoimmune chronic active hepatitis. *Mayo Clin. Proc.* **66,** 572–582.

Danielssen, A. (1990). Epidemiology of primary biliary cirrhosis in a defined rural population in the northern part of Sweden. *Hepatology* **11,** 458–464.

Delacroix, D. L., and Vaerman, J. P. (1983). Function of the human liver in IgA homeostasis in plasma. *Ann. N.Y. Acad. Sci.* **409,** 383–401.

Delacroix, D. L., Hodgson, H. J. F., McPherson, A., Dive, C., and Vaerman, J. P. (1982). Selective transport of polymeric immunoglobulin A in bile. *J. Clin. Invest.* **70,** 230–241.

Delacroix, D. L., Elkon, K. B., Geubel, A. P., Hodgson, H. F., Dive, C., and Vaermon, J. P. (1983). Changes in size, subclass, and metabolic properties of serum immunoglobulin A in liver diseases and in other diseases with high serum immunoglobulin A. *J. Clin. Invest.* **71,** 358–367.

Douglas, J., and Finlayson, N. D. C. (1979). Are increased individual susceptibility and environmental factors both necessary for the development of primary biliary cirrhosis? *Br. Med. J.* **2,** 419–420.

Eggink, H., Houthoff, H., Huitema, S., Gips, C., and Poppema, S. (1982). Cellular and humoral immune reactions in chronic active liver disease. I. Lymphocyte subsets in liver biopsies of patients with untreated idiopathic autoimmune hepatitis, chronic active hepatitis B, and primary biliary cirrhosis. *Clin. Exp. Immunol.* **50,** 17–24.

Ercilla, G., Pares, A., Arriaga, F., Bruguera, M., Castillo, R., Rodes, J., and Vives, J. (1979). Primary biliary cirrhosis associated with HLA-DRw3. *Tissue Antigens* **14,** 449–452.

Esquivel, C., Van Thiel, D., Demetris, A., Bernardos, A., Iwatsuki, S., Markus, B., Gordon, R., Marsh, J., Makowka, L., Tzakis, A., Todo, S., Gavaler, J., and Starzl, T. (1988). Transplantation for primary biliary cirrhosis. *Gastroenterology* **94,** 1207–1216.

Fallon-Friedlander, S., Boscamp, J. R., Morecki, R., Lilly, F., Horwitz, M. S., and Glaser, J. H. (1987). Immunoglobulin A stimulates growth of the extrahepatic bile duct in BALB/c mice. *Proc. Natl. Acad. Sci. U.S.A.* **84,** 3244–3248.

Feizi, T., Naccarato, R., Sherlock, S., and Doniach, D. (1972). Mitochondrial and other tissue antibodies in relatives of patients with primary biliary cirrhosis. *Clin. Exp. Immunol.* **10,** 609–622.

Flannery, G. (1989). Antimitochondrial antibodies in primary biliary cirrhosis recognize both specific peptides and shared epitopes of the M2 family of antigens. *Hepatology* **9,** 370–374.

Fleming, C., Ludwig, J., and Dickson, E. (1978). Asymptomatic primary biliary cirrhosis: Presentation, histology and results with *d*-penicillamine. *Mayo Clin. Proc.* **53,** 587–593.

Floreani, A., Bassendine, M., Mitchison, H., Freeman, R., and James, O. (1989). No specific association between primary biliary cirrhosis and bacteriuria? *J. Hepatol.* **8,** 201–207.

Fox, R., James, D., Scheuer, P., and Sharma, O. (1969). Impaired delayed hypersensitivity in primary biliary cirrhosis. *Lancet* **1,** 959–962.

Fox, R., Dudley, F., Samuels, M., Milligan, J., and Sherlock, S. (1973). Lymphocyte transformation in response to phytohaemagglutinin in primary biliary cirrhosis: The search for a plasma inhibitory factor. *Gut* **24,** 89–93.

Franch-Codoner, P., Paradis, K., Gueguen, M., Bernard, O., Costesec, A., and Alvarez, F. (1989). A new antigen recognized by anti-liver-kidney-microsome antibody (LKMA). *Clin. Exp. Immunol.* **75,** 354–358.

Frazer, I., Kronborg, I., and Mackay, I. (1983). Antibodies to liver membrane antigens in chronic active hepatitis (CAH). II. Specificity for autoimmune CAH. *Clin. Exp. Immunol.* **54,** 213–218.

Fregeau, D., Davis, P., Danner, D., Ansari, A., Coppel, R., Dickson, E., and Gershwin, M. (1989). Antimitochondrial antibodies of primary biliary cirrhosis recognize dihydrolipoamide acyltransferase and inhibit enzyme function of the branched chain alphaketoacid dehydrogenase complex. *J. Immunol.* **142,** 3815–3820.

Fregeau, D., Prindiville, T., Coppel, R., Kaplan, M., Dickson, E., and Gershwin, M. (1990a). Primary biliary cirrhosis. Inhibition of pyruvate dehydrogenase complex activity by autoantibodies specific for E1 alpha, a non-lipoic acid containing mitochondrial enzyme. *J. Immunol.* **144,** 1671–1676.

Fregeau, D., Roche, T., Davis, P., Coppel, R., and Gershwin, M. (1990b). Inhibition of alpha-ketoglutarate dehydrogenase activity by a distinct population of autoantibodies recognizing dihydrolipoamide succinyltransferase in primary biliary cirrhosis. *Hepatology* **11,** 975–981.

Friedman, S. L. (1988). Gastrointestinal and hepatobiliary neoplasms in AIDS. *Gastroenterol. Clin. North Am.* **17,** 465–487.

Frostell, A., Mendel-Harttvig, Il, Nelson, B., Totterman, T., Bjorkland, A., and Ragan, I. (1988a). Evidence that the major primary biliary cirrhosis-specific mitochondrial autoantigen is a subunit of complex I of the respiratory chain. *Scand. J. Immunol.* **28,** 157–165.

Frostell, A., Mendel-Hartvig, I., Nelson, B., Totterman, T., Bjorkland, A., Ragan, I., Cleeter, M., and Patel, S. (1988b). Mitochondrial autoantigens in primary biliary cirrhosis. *Scand. J. Immunol.* **28,** 645–652.

Fusconi, M., Ghadiminejad, I., Bianchi, F., Baum, H., Bottazzo, G., and Pisi, E. (1988). Heterogeneity of antimitochondrial antibodies with the M2-M4 pattern by immunofluorescence as assessed by Western immunoblotting and enzyme linked immunosorbent assay. *Gut* **29,** 440–447.

Fussey, S., Guest, J., James, O., Bassendine, M., and Yeaman, S. (1988). Identification and analysis of the major M2 autoantigens in primary biliary cirrhosis. *Proc. Natl. Acad. Sci. U.S.A.* **11,** 8654–8658.

Fussey, S., Guest, J., James, O., Bassendine, M., and Yeaman, S. (1989). The E1 alpha and beta subunits of the pyruvate dehydrogenase complex are M2′d′ and M2′e′ autoantigens in primary biliary cirrhosis. *Clin. Sci.* **10,** 365–368.

Fussey, S., Ali, S., Guest, J., James, O., Bassendine, M., and Yeaman, S. (1990). Reactivity of primary biliary cirrhosis sera with *Escherichia coli* dihydrolipoamide acetyltransferase (E2p): Characterization of the main immunogenic region. *Proc. Natl. Acad. Sci. U.S.A.* **5,** 3987–3991.

Galbraith, R., Smith, M., Mackenzie, R., Tee, D., Doniach, D., and Williams, R. (1974). High prevalence of seroimmunologic abnormalities in relatives of patients with active chronic hepatitis or primary biliary cirrhosis. *N. Engl. J. Med.* **290,** 63–69.

Garson, J., Lenzi, M., Ring, C., Cassani, F., Ballardini, G., Briggs, M., Tedder, R., and Bianchi, F. (1991). Hepatitis C viraemia in adults with type 2 autoimmune hepatitis. *J. Med. Virol.* **34,** 223–226.

Gershwin, M., Mackay, I., Sturgess, A., and Coppel, R. (1987). Identification and specificity of a cDNA encoding the 70 KD mitochondrial antigen recognized in primary biliary cirrhosis. *J. Immunol.* **138,** 3525–3531.

Geubel, A., Keller, R., Summerskill, W., Dickson, E., Thomasi, T., and Shorter, R. (1976). Lymphocyte cytotoxicity and inhibition studies with autologous liver cells: Observations in chronic active liver disease and the primary biliary cirrhosis syndrome. *Gastroenterology* **71,** 450–456.

Ghadiminejad, I. (1988). Expression of the primary biliary cirrhosis antigens in yeast: Aspects of mitochondrial control. *J. Bioenerg. Biomembr.* **20,** 243–259.

Ghadiminejad, I., and Baum, H. (1987). Evidence for the cell-surface localization of antigens cross-reaching with the "mitochondrial antibodies" of primary biliary cirrhosis. *Hepatology* **7,** 743–749.

Goldblum, R. M., Powell, G. K., and Van Sickle, G. (1980). Secretory IgA in the serum of infants with obstructive jaundice. *J. Pediatr.* **97,** 33–36.

Gordon, S. C., Reddy, K. R., Gould, E. E., McFadden, R., O'Brien, C., De Medina, M., Jeffers, L. J., and Schiff, E. R. (1986). The spectrum of liver disease in the acquired immunodeficiency syndrome. *J. Hepatol.* **2,** 475–484.

Gores, G. (1989). Prospective evaluation of esophageal varices in primary biliary cirrhosis: Development, natural history, and influence on survival. *Gastroenterology* **96,** 1552–1559.

Gores, G., Moore, S., Fisher, L., Powell, F., and Dickson, E. (1987). Primary biliary cirrhosis: Associations with class II major histocompatibility complex antigens. *Hepatology* **7,** 889–892.

Hamlyn, A., and Sherlock, S. (1974). The epidemiology of primary biliary cirrhosis: A survey of mortality in England and Wales. *Gut* **15,** 473–479.

Hanik, L., and Eriksson, S. (1977). Presymptomatic Primary Biliary Cirrhosis. *Acta Med. Scand.* **202,** 277–281.

Hartvig-Mendel, I. (1988). Primary biliary cirrhosis: Indication for a single mitochondrial antigenic epitope detected by patient autoantibodies and a novel monoclonal antibody. *Scand. J. Immunol.* **28,** 403–410.

Hodgson, H., Wands, J., and Isselbacher, K. (1978). Alteration in suppressor cell activity in chronic active hepatitis. *Proc. Natl. Acad. Sci.* **75,** 1549–1553.

Hoff, U., Meyer von Buschenfelde, K., and Wolfgang, A. (1976). Detection of a liver-membrane autoantibody in HB_s ag-negative chronic active hepatitis. *N. Engl. J. Med.* **294,** 578–582.

Hoffman, R., Pape, G., Spengler, U., Rieber, E., Eisenburg, J., Dohrmann, J., Paumgartner, G., and Riethmuller, G. (1989). Clonal analysis of liver-derived T cells of patients with primary biliary cirrhosis. *Clin. Exp. Immunol.* **76,** 210–215.

Homburger, H. A., Casey, M., Jacob, G. L., *et al.* (1984). Measurement of secretory IgA in serum by radioimmunoassay in patients with chronic nonalcoholic liver disease or carcinoma. *Am. J. Clin. Pathol.* **81,** 569–574.

Hopf, U., Meyer zum Büschenfelde, K.-H., and Arnold, W. (1976). Detection of a liver-membrane autoantibody in HB_s Ag-negative chronic active hepatitis. *N. Engl. J. Med.* **294,** 578–582.

Hopf, U. (1989). Relation between *Escherichia coli* R (rough)-forms in gut, lipid A in liver, and primary biliary cirrhosis. *Lancet* **2,** 1419–1422.

Ikeda, T. (1989). *In vitro* effect of corticosteroid on immunoregulatory functions in primary biliary cirrhosis. *J. Clin. Immunol.* **53,** 192–201.

Izumi, N., Hasumura, Y., and Takeuchi, J. (1983). Lymphocyte cytotoxicity for autologous human hepatocytes in alcoholic liver disease. *Clin. Exp. Immunol.* **53,** 219–224.

James, S., Elson, C., Jones, E., and Strober. (1980a). Abnormal regulation of immunoglobulin synthesis *in vitro* in primary biliary cirrhosis. *Gastroenterology* **79,** 242–254.

James, S., Elson, C., Waggoner, J., Jones, E., and Strober, W. (1980b). Deficiency of the autologous mixed lymphocyte reaction in patients with primary biliary cirrhosis. *J. Clin. Invest.* **66,** 1305–1310..

James, S., Hoofnagle, J., Strober, W., and Anthony, E., (1983). Primary biliary cirrhosis: A model autoimmune disease. *Ann. Int. Med.* **99,** 500–512.

James, S., Jones, E., Hoofnagle, J., and Strober, W. (1985). Circulating activated B cells in primary biliary cirrhosis. *J. Clin. Inv.* **5,** 254–260.

James, S. P., Jones, E. A., Schafer, D. F., Hoofnagle, J. H., Varma, R. R., and Strober, W. (1986). Selective immunoglobulin A deficiency associated with primary biliary cirrhosis in a family with liver disease. *Gastroenterology* **90,** 283–288.

Janossy, G., Montano, L., Selby, W., Duke, O., Panayi, G., Lampert, I., Thomas, J., Granger, S., Bonfill, M., Tidman, N., Thomas, H., and Goldstein, G. (1982). T-cell subset abnormalities in tissue lesions developing during autoimmune disorders, viral infection, and graft-vs-host disease. *J. Clin. Immunol.* **2,** 42S–56S.

Johnson, P., McFarlane, I., and Eddleston, A. (1991). The natural course and heterogeneity of autoimmune-type chronic active hepatitis. *In* "Seminars in Liver Disease" (M. A. Rothschild, ed.), Vol. 11, pp. 187–196. Thieme Medical Publishers, New York.

Joplin, R., Lindsay, J., Hubscher, S., Johnson, G., Shar, J., Strain, A., and Neuberger, J. (1991). Distribution of dihydrolipoamide acetyltransferase (E2) in the liver and portal lymph nodes of patients with primary biliary cirrhosis: An immunohistochemical study. *Hepatology* **14,** 442–453.

Joske, R., and King, W. (1955). The "L.E.-Cell" phenomenon in active chronic viral hepatitis. *Lancet* **2,** 477–479.

Kalsi, J., Delacroix, D. L., and Hodgson, H. J. (1983). IgA in alcoholic cirrhosis. *Clin. Exp. Immunol.* **52,** 499–504.

Katkov, W., Dienstag, J., Cody, H., Evans, A., Choo, Q., Houghton, M., and Kuo, G. (1991). Role of hepatitis C virus in non-B chronic liver disease. *Arch. Intern. Med.* **151,** 1548–1552.

Kawanishi, H. (1977). In vitro studies in IgG-mediated lymphocyte cytotoxicity in chronic active liver disease. *Gastroenterology* **73,** 549–555.

Kawanishi, H., and MacDermott, R. (1979). K-Cell-mediated antibody-dependent cellular cytotoxicity in chronic active liver disease. *Gastroenterology* **76,** 151–158.

Klein, R., and Berg, P. (1988). Characterization of a new mitochondrial antigen-antibody system(M9/anti-M9) in patients with anti-M2 positive and anti-M2 negative primary biliary cirrhosis. *Clin. Exp. Immunol.* **74,** 68–74.

Klein, R., Kloopel, G., Fischer, R., Fintelmann, V., Miting, D., and Berg, R. (1988). The antimitochondrial antibody anti-M9. A marker for the diagnosis of early primary biliary cirrhosis. *J. Hepatol.* **6,** 299–306.

Krams, S., Surh, C., Coppel, R., Ansari, A., Ruebner, B., and Gershwin, M. (1989a). Immunization of experimental animals with dihydrolipoamide acetyltransferase, as a purified recombinant polypeptide, generates mitochondrial antibodies but not primary biliary cirrhosis. *Hepatology* **9,** 411–416.

Krams, S., Dorshkind, K., and Gershwin, M. (1989b). Generation of biliary lesions after transfer of human lymphocytes into severe combined immunodeficient (SCID) mice. *J. Exp. Med.* **170,** 1919–1930.

Krams, S., Van de Water, J., Coppel, R., Esquivel, C., Roberts, J., Ansari, A., and Gershwin, M. (1990). Analysis of hepatic T lymphocyte and immunoglobulin deposits in patients with primary biliary cirrhosis. *Hepatology* **12,** 306–313.

Krawitt, E., Kilby, A., Albertini, R., Schanfield, M., Chastenay, B., Harper, P., Mickey, R., and McAuliffe, T. (1988). An immunogenetic study of suppressor cell activity in autoimmune chronic active hepatitis. *J. Clin. Immunol.* **46,** 249–257.

Kutteh, W. H., Prince, B. J., Phillips, J. O., Spenney, J. G., and Mestecky, J. (1982). Properties of immunoglobulin A in serum of individuals with liver diseases and in hepatic bile. *Gastroenterology* **82,** 184–193.

Kyriatsoulis, A., Manns, M., Gerken, G., Lohse, A., Ballhausen, W., Reske, K., and Buschenfelde, K. (1987). Distinction between natural and pathological autoantibodies by immunoblotting and densitometric subtraction: Liver-kidney microsomal antibody (LKM) positive sera identify multiple antigens in human liver tissue. *Clin. Exp. Immunol.* **70,** 53–60.

Lebovics, E., Thung, S. N., Schaffner, F., and Radensky, P. W. (1985). The liver in the acquired immunodeficiency syndrome: A clinical and histological study. *Hepatology* **2,** 293–298.

Lemaitre-Coelho, I., Jackson, G. D. F., and Vaerman, J-P. (1978). High levels of secretory IgA and free secretory component in the serum of rats with bile duct obstruction. *J. Exp. Med.* **147,** 934–939.

Lenzi, M., Ballardini, G., Fusconi, M., Cassani, F., Selleri, L., Volta, U., Zauli, D., and Bianchi, F. (1990). Type 2 autoimmune hepatitis and hepatitis C virus infection. *Lancet* **335,** 258–259.

Lindor, K., Wiesner, R., Dickson, E., and Homburger, H. (1988). The autologous mixed lymphocyte reaction in primary biliary cirrhosis: Analysis of activation and blastogenesis of autoreactive T lymphocytes. *Hepatology* **8,** 1555–1559.

Lofgren, J., Jarnerot, G., Danielssen, D., and Hemdal, I. (1985). Incidence and prevalence of primary biliary cirrhosis in a defined population in Sweden. *Scand. J. Gastroenterol.* **20,** 647–650.

Logan, R. F. (1987). Selective IgA deficiency and primary biliary cirrhosis (letter). *Gastroenterology* **92,** 270–271.

Lohr, H., Manns, M., Kyriatsoulis, A., Lohse, A., Trautwein, C., Meyer Von, Buschenfelde, K., and Fleischer, B. (1991). Clonal analysis of liver-infiltrating T cells in patients with LKM-1 antibody-positive autoimmune chronic active hepatitis. *Clin. Exp. Immunol.* **84,** 297–302.

Long, R., Scheuer, P., Path, F., and Sherlock, S. (1977). Presentation and course of asymptomatic primary biliary cirrhosis. *Gastroenterology* **72,** 1204–1207.

Lucey, M., Neuberger, J., and Williams, R. (1986). Primary biliary cirrhosis in men. *Gut* **27,** 1373–1376.

Ludwig, J. (1978). Staging of chronic nonsuppurative destructive cholangitis (syndrome of primary biliary cirrhosis). *Virchow's Arch. Pathol. Anat. Histol.* **379,** 103–112.

McFarlane, B., McSorley, C., McFarlane, I., and Williams, R. (1985). A radioimmunoassay for detection of circulating antibodies reacting with the hepatic asialoglycoprotein receptor protein. *J. Immunol. Meth.* **77,** 219–228.

McFarlane, I., Smith, H., Johnson, P., Bray, G., Vergani, D., and Williams, R. (1990). Hepatitis C virus antibodies in chronic active hepatitis: Pathogenic factor or false-positive result? *Lancet* **335,** 754–757.

Mackay, I. (1989). The first international symposium on primary biliary cirrhosis. *In* "Seminars in Liver Disease" (M. A. Rothschild, ed.), Vol. 9, pp. 124–131. Thieme Medical Publishers, New York.

Mackay, I., Taft, L., and Cowling, D. (1956). Lupoid hepatitis. *Lancet* **2,** 1323–1326.

MacSween, R., and Thomas, M. (1973). Lymphocyte transformation by phytohaemagglutinin (PHA) and purified protein derivative (PPD) in primary biliary cirrhosis. *Clin. Exp. Immunol.* **15,** 523–533.

Magrin, S., Craxi, A., Fiorentino, G., Fabiano, C., Provenzano, G., Pinzello, G., Palazzo, U., Almasio, P., and Pagliaro, L. (1991). Is autoimmune chronic active hepatitis a HCV-related disease? *J. Hepatol.* **13,** 56–60.

Manns, M. (1991). Cytoplasmic autoantigens in autoimmune hepatitis: Molecular analysis and clinical relevance. *In* "Seminars in Liver Disease" (M. A. Rothschild, ed.), Vol. 11, pp. 205–214. Thieme Medical Publishers, New York.

Manns, M., Gerken, G., Kyriatsoulis, A., Staritz, M., and Meyer von Buschenfelde, K. (1987). Characterization of a new subgroup of autoimmune chronic active hepatitis by autoantibodies against a soluble liver antigen . *Lancet* **i,** 292–294.

Manns, M., Bremm, A., Schneider, P., Notghi, A., Gerken, G., Eberle, M., Bellinghausen, B., Meyer von Buschenfelde, K., and Rittner, C. (1991a). HLA DRw8 and complement C4 deficiency as risk factors in primary biliary cirrhosis. *Gastroenterology* **101,** 1367–1373.

Manns, M., Griffin, K., Sullivan, K., and Johnson, E. (1991b). LKM-1 autoantibodies recognize a short linear sequence in P45011D6, a cytochrome P-450 monooxygenase. *J. Clin. Invest.* **88,** 1370–1378.

Margulis, S. J., Honig, C. L., Soave, R., Govoni, A. F., Mouradian, J. A., and Jacobson, I. M. (1986). Biliary tract obstruction in the acquired immunodeficiency syndrome. *Ann. Intern. Med.* **105,** 207–210.

Meuer, S., Moebius, U., Manns, M., Dienes, H., Ramadori, G., Hess, G., Hercend, T., and Meyer zum Buschenfelde, K. (1988). Clonal analysis of human T lymphocytes infiltrating the liver in chronic active hepatitis B and primary biliary cirrhosis. *Eur. J. Immunol.* **18,** 1447–1452.

Miller, J., Smith, M., Mitchell, C., Reed, W., Eddleston, A., and Williams, R. (1972). Cell-mediated immunity to a human liver-specific antigen in patients with active chronic hepatitis and primary biliary cirrhosis. *Lancet* **8,** 296–297.

Miller, K., Sepersky, R., Brown, K., Goldberg, M., and Kaplan, M. (1983). Genetic abnormalities of immunoregulation in primary biliary cirrhosis. *Am. J. Med.* **75,** 75–80.

Mishiro, S., Hoshi, Y., Takeda, K., Yoshikawa, A., Gotanda, T., Takahashi, K., Akahane, Y., Yoshizawa, H., Okamoto, H., Tsuda, F., Peterson, D., and Muchmore, E. (1990). Non-A, non-B hepatitis specific antibodies directed at host-derived epitope: Implication for an autoimmune process. *Lancet* **336,** 1400–1403.

Miyamori, H., Kato, Y., Kobayashi, K., and Hattori, N. (1983). HLA antigens in Japanese patients with primary biliary cirrhosis and autoimmune hepatitis. *Digestion* **26,** 213–217.

Moebius, U. (1990). T cell receptor gene rearrangements of T lymphocytes infiltrating the liver in chronic active hepatitis B and primary biliary cirrhosis (PBC): Oligoclonality of PBC-derived T cell clones. *Eur. J. Immunol.* **20,** 889–896.

Mondelli, M., Vergani, G., Bortolotti, F., Cadrobbi, P., Portmann, B., Alberti, A., Realdi, G., Eddleston, A., and Mowat, A. (1985). Different mechanisms responsible for in vitro cell-mediated cytotoxicity to autologous hepatocytes in children with autoimmune and Hbs Ag-positive chronic liver disease. *Pediatrics* **106,** 899–906.

Montoliu, J., Darnell, A., Torras, A., and Revert, L. (1986). Glomerular disease in cirrhosis of the liver: low frequency of IgA deposits. *Am. J. Nephrol.* **6,** 199–205.

Morreale, M., Tsirigotis, M., Hughes, M., Brumfitt, W., McIntyre, N., and Burroughs, A. (1989). Significant bacteriuria has prognostic significance in primary biliary cirrhosis. *J. Hepatol.* **9,** 149–158.

Mu, F., Alderuccio, F., Toh, B., Gershwin, M., Coppol, R., and Mackay, I. (1989). Murine monoclonal antibody to mitochondria reacts with the 72kD antigen of primary biliary cirrhosis. *Clin. Exp. Immunol.* **71,** 100–106.

Mutimer, D. (1989). Frequency of IgG and IgM autoantibodies to four specific M2 mitochondrial autoantigens in primary biliary cirrhosis. *Hepatology* **10,** 403–407.

Nakanuma, Y. (1988). Expression of beta 2-macroglobulin on interlobular bile ducts in primary biliary cirrhosis and other hepatobiliary diseases. *Acta Pathol. Jpn.* **38,** 853–860.

Newkirk, M. M., Klein, M. H., Katz, A. (1983). Estimation of polymeric IgA in human serum: An assay based on binding of radiolabeled human secretory component with applications in the study of IgA nephropathy, IgA monoclonal gammopathy, and liver disease. *J. Immunol.* **130,** 1176–1181.

Nolan, J. P., DeLissio, M. G., Camara, D. S., Feind, D. M., and Gagliardi, N. C. (1986). IgA antibody to lipid A in alcoholic liver disease. *Lancet* **i,** 176–179.

Nouri-Aria, K., Lobo-Yeo, A., Vergani, D., Mieli-Vergani, G., Kayhan, T., Eddleston, A., and Mowat, A. (1985). T. suppressor cell function and number in children with disease. *Clin. Exp. Immunol.* **61,** 283–289.

Nouri-Aria, K. T., Hegarty, J. E., Alexander, G. J., Eddleston, A. L., William, R. (1985). IgG production in autoimmune chronic active hepatitis. Effect of prednisolone on T and B cell function. *Clin. Exp. Immunol.* **61(2),** 290–296.

O'Brien, C., Vento, S., Donaldson, P., McSorley, C., McFarlane, I., Williams, R., and Eddleston, A. (1986). Cell-mediated immunity and suppressor T-cell defects to liver-derived antigens in families of patients with autoimmune chronic active hepatitis. *Lancet* **1,** 350–353.

Paradis, K., and Sharp, H. (1989). In vitro duct-like structure formation after isolation of bile ductular cells from a murine model. *J. Lab. Clin. Med.* **113,** 689–694.

Peakman, M., Lobo-Yeo, A., Mieli-Vergani, G., Davis, E., Mowat, A., and Vrgani, D. (1987). Characterization of anti-liver kidney microsomal antibody in childhood autoimmune chronic active hepatitis: Evidence for IgG1 subclass restriction, polyclonality and non cross-reactivity with hepatocyte surface antigens. *Clin. Exp. Immunol.* **69,** 543–549.

Penner, E., Kindas-Mugge, I., Hitchman, E., and Sauermann, G. (1986). Nuclear antigens recognized by antibodies present in liver disease sera. *Clin. Exp. Immunol.* **63,** 428–433.

Pohjanpelto, P., Tallgren, M., Farkkila, M., Miettinen, K., Nuutinen, H., Vuoristo, M., Heinala, P., and Makela, T. (1991). Low prevalence of hepatitis C antibodies in chronic liver disease in Finland. *Scand. J. Infect. Dis.* **23,** 139–142.

Poralla, T., Hutteroth, T., and Buschenfelde, K. (1984). Cellular cytotoxicity against autologous hepatocytes in acute and chronic non-A, non-B hepatitis. *Gut* **25,** 114–120.

Poralla, T., Treichel, U., Lohr, H., and Fleischer, B. (1991). The asialoglycoprotein receptor as target structure in autoimmune liver diseases. *In* "Seminars in Liver Disease" (M. A. Rothschild, ed.), Vol. 11, pp 215–222. Thieme Medical Publishers, New York.

Robertson, C. (1990). The relative affinity of recombinant dihydrolipoamide transacetylase for autoantibodies in primary biliary cirrhosis. *Hepatology* **11,** 717–722.

Robertson, D., Zhang, S., Guy, E., and Wright, R. (1987). Persistent measles virus genome in autoimmune chronic active hepatitis. *Lancet* **2,** 9–11.

Roll, J. (1983). The prognostic importance of clinical and histologic features in asymptomatic and symptomatic primary biliary cirrhosis. *N. Engl. J. Med.* **308,** 3–6.

Rubin, E., Schaffner, F., and Popper, H. (1965). Primary biliary cirrhosis. Chronic non-suppurative destructive cholangitis. *Am. J. Pathol.* **46,** 387–407.

Russell, M. W., Mestecky, J., Julian, B. A., and Golla, J. H. (1986). IgA-associated renal diseases: Antibodies to environmental antigens in sera and deposition of immunoglobulins and antigens in glomeruli. *J. Clin. Immunol.* **6,** 74–86.

Saidman, S., Demetris, A., Zeevi, A., and Duquesnoy, R. (1990). Propagation and characterization of lymphocytes infiltrating livers of patients with primary biliary cirrhosis and autoimmune hepatitis. *Hum. Immunol.* **28,** 237–244.

Schaffner, F. (1990). The Liver in HIV infection. *Prog. Liver Dis.* **9,** 505–522.

Schvarcz, R., von Sydow, M., and Weiland, O. (1990). Autoimmune chronic active hepatitis: Changing reactivity for antibodies to hepatitis C virus after immunosuppressive treatment. *Scand. J. Gastroenterol.* **25,** 1175–1180.

Schvarcz, R., von Sydow, M., and Weiland, O. (1991). Positive reactivity with anti-HCV ELISA in patient with autoimmune hepatitis-not confirmed with a neutralization test. *Scand. J. Infect. Dis.* **23,** 127–128.

Shapiro, J., Scheir, M., Smith, H., and Schaffner, F. (1979). Serum bilirubin: A prognostic factor in primary biliary cirrhosis. *Gut* **20,** 137–140.

Shelley, P., Fussey, M., Sohail, T., Ali, S., Guest, J., James, O., Bassendine, M., and Yeaman, S. (1990). Reactivity of primary biliary cirrhosis sera with *Escherichia coli* dihydrolipoamide acetyltransferase (E2p): Characterization of the main immunogenic region. *Proc. Natl. Acad. Sci. U.S.A* **87,** 3987–3991.

Sherlock, S., and Scheuer, P. (1973). The presentation and diagnosis of 100 patients with primary biliary cirrhosis. *N. Engl. J. Med.* **289,** 674–678.

Shimizu, M., Yuh, K., Aoyama, S., Ichihara, I., Watanabe, H., Shijo, H., and Okumura, M. (1986). Immunohistochemical characterization of inflammatory infiltrates at the site of bile duct injury in primary biliary cirrhosis. *Liver* **6,** 1–6.

Shoenfeld, Y., and Isenberg, D. (1989). "The Mosaic of Autoimmunity." Elsevier Science Publishers, New York.

Shulman, H., Sharma, P., Amos, D., Fenster, L., and McDonald, G. (1988). A coded histologic study of hepatic graft-versus-host disease after human bone marrow transplantation. *Hepatology* **8,** 463–470.

Sieber, G. (1988). Abnormalities of B cell activation and immunoregulation in patients with chronic inflammatory liver disease. *Immunobiology* **178,** 215–223.

Solbreaux, P., Maldogine, P., and Vaerman, J. (1991). Immunoglobin a (IgA) as growth factor for the extra-hepatic bile duce in susceptible mice. Fact or fiction? *In* "Frontiers in Mucosal Immunology" (M. Tsuchiya, H. Naguara, T. Hibi, and I. Moro, eds.), Vol. 1, pp. 45–52. Excerpta Medica, Amsterdam.

Spengler, U. (1988). Differential expression of MHC class II subregion products on bile duct epithelial cells and hepatocytes in patients with primary biliary cirrhosis. *Hepatology* **8,** 459–462.

Staun-Olsen, P., Bjorneboe, M., Prytz, H., Thomsen, A. C., and Orskov, F. (1983). *Escherichia coli* antibodies in alcoholic liver disease. *Scand. J. Gastroenterol.* **18,** 889–896.

Stefanini, G., Meliconi, R., Miglio, F., Mazzetti, M., Baraldini, M., Facchini, A., and Gasbarrini, G. (1983). Lymphocytoxicity against autologous hepatocytes and membrane-bound IgG in viral and autoimmune chronic active hepatitis. *Liver* **3,** 36–45.

Stemerowicz, R., Bernd, M., Rodloff, A., Freudenberg, M., Hopf, U., Wittenbrink, C., Reinhardt, R., and Galanos, C. (1988). Are antimitochondrial antibodies in primary biliary cirrhosis induced by R(rough)-mutants of enterobacteriaceae? *Lancet* **2,** 1166–1170.

Stockert, R. J., Kressner, M. B., Collins, J. C., Sternlieb, I., and Morrell, A. G. (1982). IgA interaction with the asialoglycoprotein receptor. *Proc. Natl. Acad. Sci. U.S.A,* **79,** 6229–6231.

Suou, T., Civeira, M., Kanof, M., Moreno-Otero, R., Jones, E., and James, S. (1989). Defective immunoregulation in primary biliary cirrhosis: CD4+, Leu−8+ T cells have abnormal activation and suppressor function *in vitro*. *Hepatology* **10,** 408–413.

Surh, C. (1988). The predominance of IgG3 and IgM isotype antimitochondrial autoantibodies against recombinant fused mitochondrial polypeptide in patient with primary biliary cirrhosis. *Hepatology* **8,** 290–295.

Surh, C. (1989a). Reactivity of primary biliary cirrhosis sera with a human fetal liver cDNA clone of branched-chain alpha-keto acid dehydrogenase dihydrolipoamide acyltransferase, the 52-kD mitochondrial autoantigen. *Hepatology* **9,** 63–68.

Surh, C. (1989b). Antimitochondrial autoantibodies in primary biliary cirrhosis recognize cross-reactive epitope(s) on protein X and dihydrolipoamide acetyltransferase of pyruvate dehydrogenase complex. *Hepatology* **10,** 127–133.

Surh, C. (1990). Comparative epitope mapping of murine monoclonal and human autoantibodies to human PDH-E2, the major mitochondrial autoantigen of primary biliary cirrhosis. *J. Immunol.* **144,** 2647–2652.

Surh, C., Coppel, R., and Gershwin, M. (1990). Structural requirement for autoreactivity on human pyruvate dehydrogenase-E2, the major autoantigen of primary biliary cirrhosis. Implication for a conformational autoepitope. *J. Immunol.* **144,** 3367–3374.

Swerdlow, M. A., and Chowdhury, L. N. (1983). IgA subclasses in liver tissue in alcoholic liver disease. *Am. J. Clin. Pathol.* **80,** 283–289.

Swerdlow, M. A., and Chowdhury, L. N. (1984). IgA deposition in liver in alcoholic liver disease. An index of progressive injury. *Arch. Pathol. Lab. Med.* **108,** 416–419.

Thomas, H., Brown, D., Labrooy, J., and Epstein, O. (1982). T cell subsets in autoimmune and HBV-induced chronic liver disease, HBs antigen carriers with normal histology and primary biliary cirrhosis: A review of the abnormalities and the effects of treatment. *J. Clin. Immunol.* **2,** 57S–60S.

Thompson, R. A., Carter, R., Stokes, R. P., Geddes, A. M., and

Goodall, J. A. D. (1973). Serum immunoglobuline complement component levels and autoantibodies in liver disease. *Clin. Exp. Immunol.* **14,** 335–346.

Thompson, A., Cochrane, M., McFarland, I., Eddleston, A., and Williams. R. (1974). Lymphocyte cytotoxicity to isolated hepatocytes in chronic active hepatitis. *Nature (London)* **252,** 721–722.

Todros, L., Touscoz, G., Urso, N., Durazzo, M., Albano, E., Poli, G., Baldi, M., and Rizzetto, M. (1991). Hepatitis C virus-related chronic liver disease with autoantibodies to liver-kidney microsomes (LKM). *J. Hepatol.* **13,** 128–131.

Tomana, M., Kulhavy, R., and Mestecky, J. (1988). Receptor-mediated binding and uptake of immunoglobulin A by human liver. *Gastroenterology* **94,** 762–770.

Triger, D. (1980). Primary biliary cirrhosis: An epidemiological study. *Br. Med. J.* **281,** 772–775.

Uibo, R. (1990). Inhibition of enzyme function by human autoantibodies to an autoantigen pyruvate dehydrogenase E2: Different epitope for spontaneous human and induced rabbit autoantibodies. *Clin. Exp. Immunol.* **80,** 19–24.

Uwe, H., Stemerowicz, R., Rodloff, A., Galanos, C., Moller, B., Lobeck, H., Freudenberg, M., and Huhn, D. (1989). Relation between *Escherichia coli* r (rough)-forms in gut, lipid a in liver, and primary biliary cirrhosis. *Lancet* **2,** 1419–1421.

Van de Water, J. (1988). Autoantibodies of primary biliary cirrhosis recognize dihydrolipoamide acetyltransferase and inhibit enzyme function. *J. Immunol.* **141,** 2321–2324.

Van de Water, J. (1989). Detection of autoantibodies to recombinant mitochondrial proteins in patients with primary biliary cirrhosis. *N. Engl. J. Med.* **320,** 1377–1380.

Van de Water, J., Surh, C., Leung, P., Krams, S., Fregeau, D., Davis, P., Coppel, R., Mackay, I., and Gershwin, M. (1989). Molecular definitions, autoepitopes, and enzymatic activities of the mitochondrial autoantigens of primary biliary cirrhosis. *In* "Seminars in Liver Disease" (M. A. Rothschild, ed.), Vol. 9, pp 132–137. Thieme Medical Publishers, New York.

Van de Water, J., Ansari, A., Surh, C., Coppel, R., Roche, T., Bankovsky, H., Kaplan, M., and Gershwin, M. (1991). Evidence for the targeting by 2-oxo-dehydrogenase enzymes in the T cell reponse of primary biliary cirrhosis. *J. Immunol.* **146,** 89–94.

Van de Wiel, A., Schuurman, H.-J., van Riessen, D., Haaijman, J. J., Radl, J., Delacroix, D. L. van Hattum, J., Roeland Blok, A. P., and Kater, L. (1986). Characteristics of IgA deposits in liver and skin of patients with liver disease. *Am. J. Clin. Pathol.* **86,** 724–730.

Van de Wiel, A., Schuurman, H. J., and Kater, L. (1987a). Alcoholic liver disease: An IgA-associated disorder. *Scand. J. Gastroenterol.* **22,** 1025–1030.

Van de Wiel, A., Delacroix, D. L., van Hattum, J., Schuurman, H.-J., and Kater, L. (1987b). Characteristics of serum IgA and liver IgA deposits in alcoholic liver disease. *Hepatology* **7,** 95–99.

Van de Wiel, A., Seifert, W. F., Van der Linden, J. A., Gmelig-Meyling, F. H. J., Kater, L., and Schuurman, H.-J. (1987c). Spontaneous IgA synthesis by blood mononuclear cells in alcoholic liver disease. *Scand. J. Immunol.* **25,** 181–187.

Vento, S., O'Brien, C., McFarlane, B., McFarlane, I., Eddleston, A., and Williams, R. (1986). T-Lymphocyte sensitization to hepatocyte antigens in autoimmune chronic active hepatitis and primary biliary cirrhosis. *Gastroenterology* **91,** 810–817.

Vento, S., Garofano, T., Di Perri, G., Dolci, L., Concia, E., and Bassetti, D. (1991). Identification of hepatitis A virus as a trigger for autoimmune chronic hepatitis type 1 in susceptible individuals. *Lancet* **337,** 1183–1187.

Vergani, G., Vrgani, D., Jenkins, P., Portmann, B., Mowat, A., Eddleston, A., and Williams, R. (1979). Lymphocyte cytotoxicity to autologous hepatocytes in HBsAg-negative chronic active hepatitis. *Clin. Exp. Immunol.* **38,** 16–21.

Vergani, D., Wells, L., Larcher, V., Nasaruddin, B., Davies, E., Mieli-Vergani, G., and Mowat, A. (1985). Genetically determined low C: A predisposing factor to autoimmune chronic active hepatitis. *Lancet* **2,** 294–297.

Viteri, A. L., and Greene, J. F., Jr. (1987). Bile duct abnormalities in the acquired immune deficiency syndrome. *Gastroenterology* **92,** 2014–2018.

Walker, J., Lond, M., Doniach, D., Roitt, I., Phil, M., and Sherlock, S. (1965). Serological tests in diagnosis of primary biliary cirrhosis. *Lancet* **1,** 827–831.

Wands, J., and Isselbacher, K. (1975). Lymphocyte cytotoxicity to autologous liver cells in chronic active hepatitis. *Proc. Natl. Acad. Sci. U.S.A.* **72,** 1301–1303.

Wen, L., Peakman, M., Lobo-Yeo, A., McFarlane, B., Mowat, A., Vergani, G., and Vergani, D. (1990). T-cell-directed hepatocyte damage in autoimmune chronic active hepatitis. *Lancet* **336,** 1527–1530.

Whittingham, S., Irin, J., Mackay, I., and Smalley, M. (1966). Smooth muscle autoantibody in "autoimmune" hepatitis. *Gastroenterology* **51,** 499–505.

Whittingham, S., Mathews, J., Schanfield, M., Tait, B., and MacKay, R. (1981). Interaction of HLA and Gm in autoimmune chronic active hepatitis. *Clin. Exp. Immunol.* **43,** 80–86.

Woodroffe, A. J. (1981). IgA, glomerulonephritis and liver disease. *Aust. N.Z. J. Med.* **11,** 109–111.

Yamada, G., Hyodo, I., Tobe, K., Mizuno, M., Nishihara, T., Kobayashi, T., and Nagashima, H. (1986). Ultrastructural immunocytochemical analysis of lymphocytes infiltrating bile duct epithelia in primary biliary cirrhosis. *Hepatology* **6,** 385–391.

Yeaman, S., Danner, D., Mutimer, D., Fussey, S., James, O., and Bassendine, M. (1988). Primary biliary cirrhosis: Identification of two major M2 mitochondrial autoantigens. *Lancet* **1,** 1067–1069.

Yoshida, T. (1990). Antibodies against mitochondrial dehydrogenase complexes in primary biliary cirrhosis. *Gastroenterology* **99,** 187–194.

Zetterman, R., and Woltjen, J. (1980). Suppressor cell activity in primary biliary cirrhosis. *Dig. Dis. Sci.* **25,** 104–107.

Section F

Lungs and Airways

Section Editor: John Bienenstock

(Chapters 43 through 46)

43

Bronchial Mucosal Lymphoid Tissue

John Bienenstock • Robert Clancy

I. INTRODUCTION

The lymphoid tissue of the bronchus is linked primarily to mucosal defense against inhaled microbes. Therefore, this tissue is one of a series of integrated units that operate to insure that sterile air is delivered into the gas exchange apparatus of the lungs in such a way that sensitization to inhaled antigen is avoided. The cooperative activity between these different lymphoid units, and their involvement in generating down-regulation of the inflammatory response within various compartments of the bronchopulmonary system, suggests the value of reviewing the bronchial mucosal lymphoid tissue in terms of its relationship with these additional pools of lymphocytes. A second general issue requiring discussion is the relationship within the bronchial mucosa itself between the aggregated collections of bronchial lymphoid tissue that originally were termed the bronchus-associated lymphoid tissue (BALT; Bienenstock, 1984), which constitutes the majority of bronchial mucosal lymphocytes in some species, and the less-organized lymphoid tissue that predominates in others, such as humans (Kyriazis and Esterly, 1970; Emery and Dinsdale, 1973,1974).

T and B lymphocyte effector mechanisms are generated from bronchial mucosal lymphoid tissue and delivered into the bronchial lumen. The secretory IgA system initially focused attention on a discrete mucosal defense mechanism. An IgA response to luminal antigen plays a key role in local defense in the initial control of microbial colonization (Waldmann and Henney, 1971). The susceptibility of secreted IgA antibody to high zone tolerance (Clancy *et al.*, 1987), the relatively poor immunological memory associated with this isotype (Clancy and Bienenstock, 1976), and the reasonable health of most subjects with IgA deficiency suggest that additional immune mechanisms are crucial to mucosal defense. The vigorous T-cell response to inhaled antigen (Clancy and Bienenstock, 1974) and the capacity of $CD4^+$ T cells to transfer immunity in animal models of colonization (Wallace *et al.*, 1989,1991) suggest T cells as candidates for the controllers of infection involving persistent microbes or under circumstances under which a large inoculum of antigen is inhaled.

Communication between the bronchial mucosal lymphoid tissue and distant mucosal sites through an intermucosal cell circuit known as the common mucosal immune system (McDermott and Bienenstock, 1979) involves predominantly a "gut to bronchus" flow of cells originating in Peyer's patches (Scicchitano *et al.*, 1984). Depending on antigen dose and previous immunological experience, antigen-reactive T cells (Husband *et al.*, 1984) and antibody-secreting B cells (Rudzik *et al.*, 1975a; Scicchitano *et al.*, 1984) can populate bronchial mucosa to modulate immunity, a principle used successfully to develop an oral vaccine that protects against acute bronchitis (Clancy *et al.*, 1985,1989; Lehmann *et al.*, 1991). Study of animal models in which activated T lymphocytes contribute to mucosal defense suggests that T-dependent neutrophil recruitment is important (Wallace *et al.*, 1991), although additional mechanisms such as secretion of lysozyme from T-cell activated macrophages have been implicated (Taylor *et al.*, 1990).

Communication with other effector mechanisms within the bronchial lumen is indicated by these latter observations. An ascending carpet of mucus contains cells derived mainly from the bronchoalveolar compartment. About 90% of these cells are bone marrow-derived macrophages, whereas the remaining cells are predominantly lymphocytes (Young and Reynolds, 1984). The relationship between the bronchoalveolar lymphocytes and macrophages the two large pools of lymphocytes within the lung interstitum, and the pulmonary circulation are not known (Pabst, 1990), but these larger collections almost certainly play a role in determining the constitutional make-up and function of the bronchoalveolar cell population. The vascular and interstitial pools of cells represent both selective contributions from the systemic pool and an inductive effect of the pulmonary macrophages whereas about half the resident macrophage population is derived from local cell proliferation (Mezzette *et al.*, 1990). About 10–20% of the mucosal interstitium lymphocyte pool is composed of T cells—the expansion of cells bearing V chain determinants in a nonrandom way is consistent with further tissue restrictive elements operating in the lung interstitium (Augustin *et al.*, 1989.

That these effector mechanisms normally operate with minimal inflammation within the bronchial lumen or the bronchial mucosa depends on two factors. First, a series of down-regulating mechanisms restricts cell division and recruitment of nonspecific inflammatory cells. Second, regional lymph nodes rather than the mucosa are primary sites for both antigen handling (Yoshizawa *et al.*, 1989) and induction of immune responses (van der Brugge-Gamelkoorn *et al.*, 1986). The down-regulating mechanisms are linked to the site of deposition of antigen. Thus, allergens deposited in the nasopharynx initiate a series of suppressor-cell loops within regional lymph nodes that regulate immediate and delayed hypersensitivity reactions (Sedgwick and Holt, 1985), whereas colonization of the bronchial mucosa is associated with an expanded suppressor T-cell population that inhibits antigen-induced T-lymphocyte proliferation (Pucci *et al.*, 1982; Figure 1). Whether mucosal suppressor cells within the bronchus are activated by presentation of antigen by Class II-bearing epithelial cells, as has been suggested for the gut (Pang *et al.*, 1990), or through the aggregated BALT is not clear. The lumen is protected from inflammation by the antiproliferative effect of T cell-activated alveolar macrophages, which also carry antigen away from the mucosa, to regional lymph nodes (Warner *et al.*, 1981), and upward over the epiglottis into the gut, where aspirated antigen can activate Peyer's patches.

The bronchial mucosal lymphocyte compartment has, therefore, a complex relationship with various lymphocyte populations important in the activation and regulation of bronchial immunity. This collection of cells is a mixture of antigen-reactive, effector, and regulatory lymphocytes, as well as ancillary cells, derived from various mucosal and systemic sources. Early studies on bronchial mucosal lymphoid tissue used animal species with organized BALT, which facilitated on understanding of function, in part by analogy with Peyer's patches in the gut (Bienenstock *et al.*, 1973a,b). Differences between species in the degree of organization of bronchial mucosal lymphoid tissue have led to the idea that early studies on aggregated structures may not be relevant to bronchial immune function, at least in species such as humans, who are not characterized by major BALT development (Pabst and Gehrke, 1990). However, failure to detect BALT in some studies (Pabst and Gehrke, 1990), may reflect sampling error, since BALT has been well described in normal human bronchus (Jeffery and Corrin, 1984), and epithelium covering less-organized aggregates, and even some areas without lymphoid accumulations, including cells that are flattened and possess irregular microvilli and no cilia (Jeffery and Corrin, 1984). Since these cells may transport antigen by pinocytosis (Owen, 1977) and since a network of Ia antigen-bearing dendritic cells and processes penetrating into the lumen exists (Holt *et al.*, 1985,1988), a classical lymphoepithelium with M cells may not be essential for antigen processing. This chapter continues by describing knowledge gained from the study of classical BALT, and subsequently addresses the issue of interspecies variation in mucosal lymphoid tissue morphology and bronchial mucosal immune function.

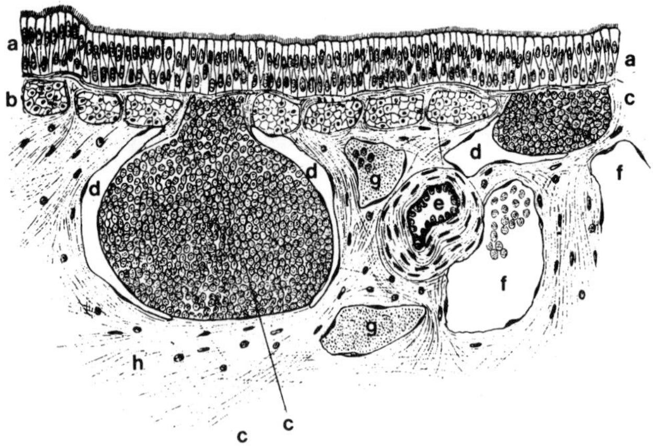

Figure 1 The nature of the mucosal lymphoid follicle and the epithelial relationship are seen clearly. Reprinted with permission from Klein (1875).

II. CLASSICAL BRONCHUS-ASSOCIATED LYMPHOID TISSUE

The existence of lymphoid aggregates in the bronchial wall was noted in 1867 by Burdon-Sanderson; the observation that they were analogous to the lymphoid follicles found in other mucous membranes such as the tonsil and intestine was made by Klein in 1875 (see Bienenstock, 1984). Recent interest in the lymphoid tissue of the bronchial mucosa began with a systematic study of lymphoid aggregates in experimental animals in 1973 (Bienenstock *et al.*, 1973a,b), when their similarity to Peyer's patches in the gut was noted. Subsequently, BALT was described in a number of species including rats (Bienenstock *et al.*, 1973a; Chamberlain *et al.*, 1973; Fournier *et al.*, 1977), rabbits (Bienenstock *et al.*, 1973a,b; Racz *et al.*, 1977; Tenner-Racz *et al.*, 1979), and mice (Milne *et al.*, 1975), as well as sheep, chickens, and guinea pigs, but has been characterized best in rats and rabbits. Other species, such as pigs, cats, and humans, have few classical BALT aggregates (Jeffery and Corrin, 1984; Daniele, 1988a), although in humans BALT aggregates are well described and, in the pig, infection with mycoplasma was linked to the regular development of BALT (Chu *et al.*, 1989). These and other studies (Bienenstock *et al.*, 1973a,b; Weisz-Carrington *et al.*, 1987) emphasize the importance of antigenic stimulation in the full expression of organized BALT, with, however, considerable species variation. Since much of the current understanding of bronchial mucosal lymphoid tissue comes from study either directly of BALT aggregates or indirectly of lymphocytes derived from bronchial tissues containing numerous BALT aggregates, review of these studies on structure and function provides an excellent model for understanding bronchial mucosal lymphoid tissue.

BALT develops in early postnatal life in most species (Bienenstock *et al.*, 1973a; Milne *et al.*, 1975). Antigen is not necessary for this development since BALT is present in germ-free rats (Bienenstock *et al.*, 1973a) and mice (Milne *et al.*, 1975) as well as in fetal lungs transplanted into syngeneic adults (Milne *et al.*, 1975). BALT development under these circumstances is primitive compared with conventionally raised animals (Bienenstock *et al.*, 1973a), and antigenic challenge (Rudzik *et al.*, 1975a) induces early and hyperplastic BALT. Lymphoreticular aggregates appear at 1 week in humans (Weisz-Carrington *et al.*, 1987), although larger and more confluent aggregates are described with a lymphoepithelium in sudden infant death syndrome (Emery and Dinsdale, 1973), in which intercurrent infection is common. BALT can be identified macroscopically in experimental animals including rabbits, rats, guinea pigs, and chickens (Bienenstock *et al.*, 1973a) as white patches after acetic acid fixation (Cornes, 1965) for example, 30–50 BALT aggregates appear in adult rats (Plesch, 1982), concentrated around bifurcations in the major bronchus divisions that are, additionally, the sites of impaction of inhaled particles.

Although classical BALT has a structure similar to that of Peyer's patches, division into distinct structural and functional areas is less apparent. The epithelium overlying BALT aggregates is not as specialized and is infiltrated heavily with lymphocytes; scanning electron microscopy shows the presence of M (microfold) cells similar to those described in the Peyer's patch and the bursa of Fabricius (Figure 2) (Bienenstock *et al.*, 1973a,b; Bockman and Cooper, 1973; Bockman and Stevens, 1977). Cells of BALT cluster within a reticulin framework into a "dome" beneath the epithelium and a follicle that is usually single (Bienenstock *et al.*, 1973; Owen and Bhalla, 1983). In the mammalian BALT, germinal centers usually are found only after antigenic stimulation (Bienenstock *et al.*, 1973a). Tenner-Racz and colleagues (1979) described a parafollicular area after immunization, considered to be populated by T cells. Plasma cells are found around the periphery (Bienenstock *et al.*, 1973a; Milne *et al.*, 1975), whereas cells capable of presenting antigen, including macrophages (Owen, 1977) and follicular dendritic cells (Milne *et al.*, 1975; Holt *et al.*, 1988), appear within BALT. Efferent but not afferent lymphatic vessels are described (van der Brugge-Gamelkoorn and Kraal, 1985).

In rabbit BALT, about 20% of lymphocytes have the T-cell marker rabbit thymic lymphocyte antigen (RTLA), a percentage similar to that in the Peyer's patch, but location in a distinct parafollicular area can be recognized only under conditions of antigenic stimulation (Bienenstock *et al.*, 1973b). The presence of high endothelial venules (HEV) and interdigitating dendritic cells are characteristic of T-dependent areas in other lymphoid structures, although the HEV in BALT tends to be more like the structures in mesenteric lymph nodes than those in Peyer's patches (Nash and Holle, 1973), with respect to the immunohistochemical definition of T and B cells clustered about them (Bienenstock *et al.*, 1973a,b). About 50% of the lymphocytes in the BALT of rabbit (Rudzik *et al.*, 1975b) and rat (Plesch, 1982) bear surface immunoglobulin. In the rabbit, equal proportions stain with anti-IgM and anti-IgA, whereas in the rat a minority (15%) reacts with anti-IgA and few (5%) stain with anti-IgE.

Study of the function of BALT has focused on analogy

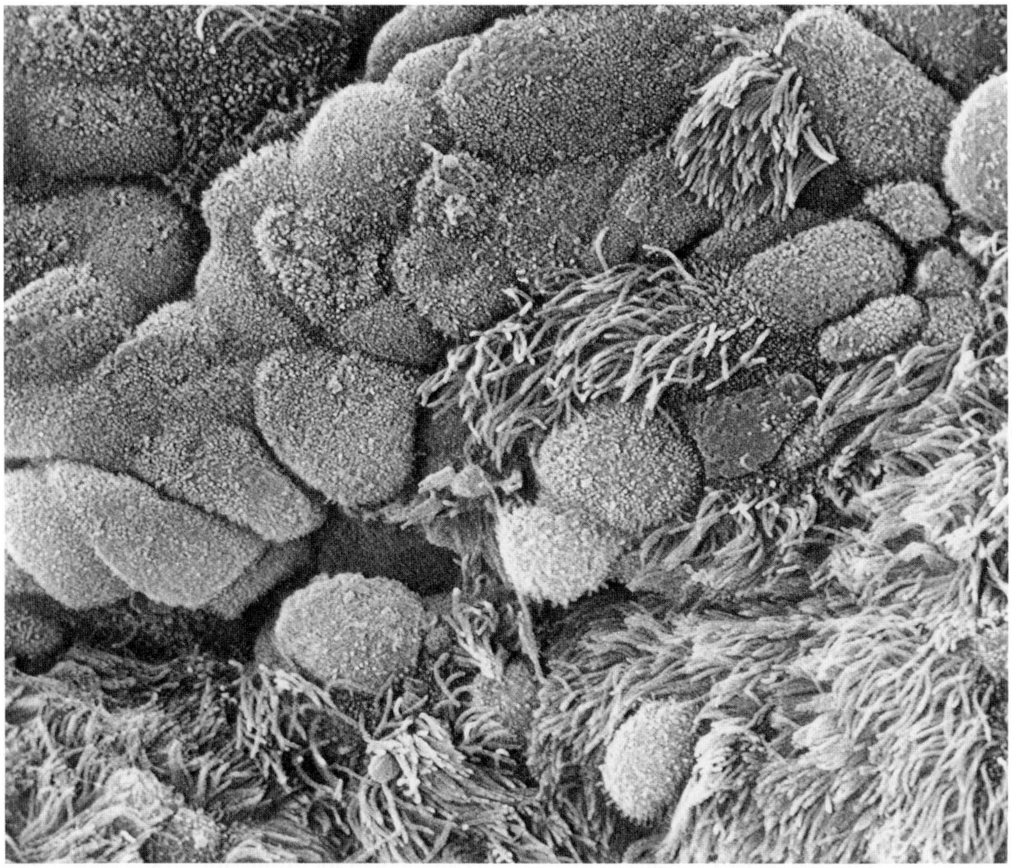

Figure 2 A scanning electron micrograph showing the junction between the ciliated and nonciliated lymphoepithelium overlying the BALT follicle immediately below. Note the microprojections on the M cells and the crevices between cells. ×378. Reprinted with permission from Bienenstock and Johnston (1976). A morphologic study of rabbit bronchial lymphoid aggregates and lymphoepithelium. *Lab. Invest.* **35,** 343–348. © the US and Canadian Academy of Pathology.

with Peyer's patches. Thus, induction of a mucosal immune response and use of the common mucosal system to deliver this response have been prominent. Horseradish peroxidase (HRP) is taken up preferentially by the epithelium over BALT (Fournier *et al.*, 1977), a process that can be enhanced after antigen stimulation with *Bacillus* Calmette–Guerin (BCG), which causes hypertrophy of the specialized epithelium (Tenner-Racz *et al.*, 1979). In this latter study, bacteria were found within BALT macrophages, supporting earlier work (Bienenstock, 1984) that identified BALT as an early site for the uptake of particulate material. Other studies that have demonstrated that epithelial cells can present soluble antigen (Pang *et al.*, 1990) and that a carpet of dendritic cells bearing Class II antigen lies within and beneath the epithelium of species bearing numerous BALT aggregates (Holt *et al.*, 1988), as well as of species such as humans (Holt *et al.*, 1986), raises important questions about the qualitative and quantitative contributions of BALT aggregates to the development of local immunity. The description of numerous nonspecialized epithelial cells in the normal human respiratory tract (Daniele, 1988b), and the clear link between the amount of BALT and antigenic stimulus (Meuwissen and Hussain, 1982; Delventhal *et al.*, 1992a,b; Pabst, 1991) support the concept that "classical" BALT is, in part, an adaptation to antigen load, with variable degrees of expression of aggregate structure appearing constitutively. The transformation of young mature epithelial cells into M cells induced by lymphocyte–epithelial contact (Craig and Cebra, 1971) is consistent with this view. Of particular interest with respect to human BALT was a study on chronically inflamed human lungs, in which classical BALT was noted in 8% of 100 patients; in those with an occlusive tumor, BALT was confined to the poststenotic segments (Delventhal *et al.*, 1992b).

A study by Craig and Cebra (1971) gave the first clear indication of the major role mucosal aggregates of lymphoid tissue play in generating mucosal immunity. These investigators used allotypic markers and adoptive transfer of Peyer's patch cells in rabbits to demonstrate that this tissue was an enriched source of IgA plasma cell precursors. Cebra suggested that environmental factors, including antigen and bacterial lipopolysaccharide (LPS), drove B-cell differentiation during an antigen-stimulated clonal expansion, a concept that was consistent with the observation that oral immunization induced an increase in numbers of B cells expressing surface IgA in the Peyer's patch (Fuhrman and Cebra, 1981). Subsequently, Elson *et al.* (1979) demonstrated that IgA "switch" T helper cells within the Peyer's patch directed clonal expansion of IgA-secreting B cells. The isolation of T-cell clones from the Peyer's patch (Kiyono *et al.*, 1982; Kawanishi *et al.*, 1983) that bore receptors for IgA suggested that a number of T-lymphocyte populations may be involved in immunoregulation, possibly by secreting type-specific immunoglobulin-binding factors (Kiyono *et al.*, 1985). The repopulation studies of Rudzik *et al.* (1975a,c), in which bronchial lamina propria cells were transferred to lethally irradiated rabbits, demonstrated IgA-containing plasma cells repopulating the gut and bronchial mucosa. These studies identified the BALT analogous to the Peyer's patch, and provided the information on which the concept of a "common mucosal immune system" was developed (McDermott and Bienenstock, 1979). Inhaled antigen stimulated T-cell proliferation within the bronchial mucosal lymphocyte population that correlated in time with the appearance of proliferating T cells in the bronchial lumen (Waldman and Henry, 1971; Clancy and Bienenstock, 1974), as well as of T cells secreting cytokines (Clancy *et al.*, 1977) and of cytotoxic T cells (Husband *et al.*, 1983). The contribution of specific T lymphocytes to the common mucosal immune system (Clancy *et al.*, 1977), as well as the specific relocation of influenza-specific T-cell clones to the lung (Bienenstock *et al.*, 1983), is consistent with the observed circulation pathway of T lymphoblasts from mediastinal lymph nodes and thoracic duct lymph that included mucosal surfaces (Guy-Grand *et al.*, 1974; Sprent, 1986), and their origin in part from Peyer's patches (Guy-Grand *et al.*, 1978). The specific role played by aggregates of BALT in the localization of T and B cells in bronchial mucosa is uncertain. The immune functions localized to aggregated lymphoid tissue in the bronchus may be restricted to the generation and distribution of specific T- and B-cell responses to inhaled antigen. The potential for aggregated lymphoid structures to generate suppression within mucosal (Pucci *et al.*, 1982) or systemic tissues (Ngan and Kind, 1978; Richman *et al.*, 1981) is raised by the appearance of antigen-specific suppressor T cells within Peyer's patches. Down-regulation within bronchopulmonary tissues suggests that, indeed, a similar function exists in BALT, as does the rapid development of a state of nonresponsiveness in mucosal T-cell populations following inhalation of antigen (Clancy and Bienenstock, 1974).

Important cells linked to BALT and the bronchial epithelium are the "granulated lymphocytes" and mast cells in the adjoining mucosa (Sprent, 1986). The heterogeneity of mast cells based on differential sensitivity of rat mast cells in different tissues to various fixation procedures (Enerback, 1966) was extended to demonstrate functional heterogeneity (Befus *et al.*, 1986). Similar heterogeneity based on distinct neutral protease contents (Irani *et al.*, 1986) has been described in humans, particularly for cells within the bronchial mucosa (Shanahan *et al.*, 1987). We described granulated basophil-like cells in and adjacent to BALT follicles and in the epithelium lateral to these follicles (Bienenstock, 1984). Similar cells can be washed from the bronchial lumen; such cells contain histamine and may be sensitized by IgE to release ρ histamine in response to antigen (Patterson *et al.*, 1974,1977). Ahlstedt *et al.* (1983) showed an increase in these cells after inhalation of antigen that is likely to be influenced by T cells (Ruitenberg and Elgersma, 1976). Of particular interest is the association between the mast cells in and below the epithelium of the respiratory tract and the nerves, forming a homeostatic regulatory unit (Bienenstock *et al.*, 1988). Many of these epithelial leukocytes have an unusual phenotype related to, but not conclusively demonstrated to be, a part of the T-lymphocyte population (Petit *et al.*, 1985). Indeed the whole question of origin and function of the intraepithelial lymphocyte pool in the respiratory tract is even less clear than it is in the intestine, on which most work has been focused. The demonstration of an expanded population of T-cell receptor-expressing cells in this population (Goodman and Lefrancois,

1988) added an additional facet to the puzzle presented by these cells. Are these cells a population uniquely geared to cope with intraluminal pathogens? Do they represent a thymic-independent T-cell population, developed in a mucosal epithelial environment? Do the variously demonstrated cytotoxic activities have a physiological role (Ernst *et al.*, 1985)?

III. BRONCHUS ASSOCIATED LYMPHOID TISSUE REVISITED

BALT has been defined classically as an aggregated lymphoid structure separated from the bronchial lumen by a specialized lymphoepithelium. The availability of this relatively organized structure has allowed structural and functional analysis, which has focused in particular on its role in the development of a local immune response to inhaled antigen (Rudzik *et al.*, 1975a). The similarity in structural relationships between BALT and Peyer's patches that have been identified by these studies have given us, by extension, a better understanding of respiratory tract immunity, as was discussed already. Certain differences observed between the two lymphoid structures, often quantitative in nature, have been explained in terms of environmental stimuli associated with gut content. The similarity of structure, however, led to the concept of a common mucosal immune system when the morphological similarities between Peyer's patches and BALT were extended to include the observation that both contained an enriched precursor population of IgA-committed lymphocytes (Rudzik *et al.*, 1975a), that were capable of repopulating mucosal sites of irradiated recipient rabbits. Subsequent studies in sheep (Scicchitano *et al.*, 1984) and rats (van der Brugge-Gamelkoorn *et al.*, 1986) modified the general concept to emphasize a "gut to bronchus" directional flow of activated lymphocytes. Based on these observations, an orally administered, killed, nontypable *Haemophilus influenzae* vaccine was shown to be protective against recurrent episodes of acute bronchitis in carriers of this bacteria with chronic lung disease; the vaccine functioned by reducing the level of bronchial colonization (Clancy *et al.*, 1985,1989; Lehmann *et al.*, 1991). In an animal model, protection was transferred with primed thoracic duct T cells (Wallace *et al.*, 1989; Lehmann *et al.*, 1991). These observations raise the question of the role played by BALT in localizing gut-derived T and B lymphocytes. Since no afferent lymphatics have been described in BALT, the majority of lymphocytes are likely to reach the bronchial mucosa via binding of specific adhesions to receptors on postcapillary venules with high cuboidal endothelium (Sminia and van der Brugge-Gamelkoorn, 1989), which is the mechanism used by lymphocytes for entry into other lymphoid organs. Adherence *in vitro* by lymphocytes to the HEVs in BALT differs from that in the Peyer's patches, where the majority of adhering cells are B cells (Kieran *et al.*, 1989). The BALT HEVs function more like those of mesenteric lymph nodes (van der Brugge-Gamelkoorn and Kraal, 1985), with equal numbers of T and B lymphocytes adhering. Using peroxidase staining, a selective attachment of B cells bearing μ and L chains was described (Otuski *et al.*, 1989) that is consistent with the pattern of localization of gut-derived IgA-secreting B cells in the sheep respiratory tract, which in form corresponds to the geographic distribution of BALT (Scicchitano *et al.*, 1984).

BALT is likely to play a key role in the localization of both T and B lymphocytes within the bronchial mucosa where, additionally, regulatory T cells (Iwata and Sato, 1991) and a transport epithelium, allowing migration into the bronchial lumen (Bienenstock *et al.*, 1973a,b), are sited conveniently.

Early studies suggesting a regulatory role for BALT (Clancy and Bienenstock, 1974) have been extended by infection and immunization models that have confirmed the narrow antigen dose range that stimulates a local antibody response and a time-frame of T-cell help followed by immune suppression (Iwata and Sato, 1991). Thus, in a rat model of pulmonary infection with *Pseudomonas aeruginosa,* an early dominance of $SIgA^+$ cells correlated with a predominance of $W3/25^+$ T cells, which gave way to a dominance of $OX8^+$ suppressor T cells after 2 weeks, correlating with a decrease in both $SIgA^+$ cells and inflammatory changes in the lung (Iwata and Sato, 1991). A pro-inflammatory cytokine profile, detected as both RNA expression and cytokine secretion, by T cells cloned from sputum in subjects with chronic bronchial inflammation (G. Pang and R. Clancy, unpublished observations) would indicate that T cells derived from bronchial mucosa that migrate into the bronchial lumen, may play a more prominent role in mucosal defense under circumstances of high dose or chronic antigenic stimulation. A regional distribution of peptidergic nerve fibers within classical BALT, and localization of immunoreactive neuropeptides known to influence lymphocyte physiology in different zones of the BALT (Inoue *et al.*, 1990), suggest important neuroimmunological control mechanisms in the bronchial mucosa. The close connection between BALT and regional lymph nodes, involving efferent lymphatics (van der Brugge-Gamelkoorn *et al.*, 1986), is reflected in the compartmentalized response to bronchial infection that includes both lymphoid structures (Weisz-Carrington *et al.*, 1987). The regional lymph nodes relating to BALT appear to have several important roles. The migratory patterns of lymphocytes in efferent lymphatics are more eclectic than those from mesenteric nodes (Rudzik *et al.*, 1975a; Butler *et al.*, 1982; Spencer and Hall, 1984; Joel and Chanana, 1987; Scicchitano *et al.*, 1988). Clearly, despite the potential of BALT B cells to populate intestinal mucosa (Scicchitano *et al.*, 1988), respiratory tract immunization has little influence on the intestinal immune response (Scicchitano *et al.*, 1984; Bice and Shopp, 1988). The regional node, however, has an important role in establishing a generalized immune response within the lung (Scicchitano *et al.*, 1984) as well as systemic sensitization (Butler *et al.*, 1982; Kattreider *et al.*, 1987; Muggenburg *et al.*, 1987). A second role relates to the generation of an immune response to inhaled antigen. Macrophage-associated antigen transported from the lumen requires cytokine activation for T-cell presentation (Thomas *et al.*, 1974), which occurs within regional nodes. Down-regulation of IgE- and T cell-dependent hyposensitization after inhalation of allergens involves the generation of a suppressor T-cell population in regional nodes of the upper respiratory tract (Holt *et al.*,

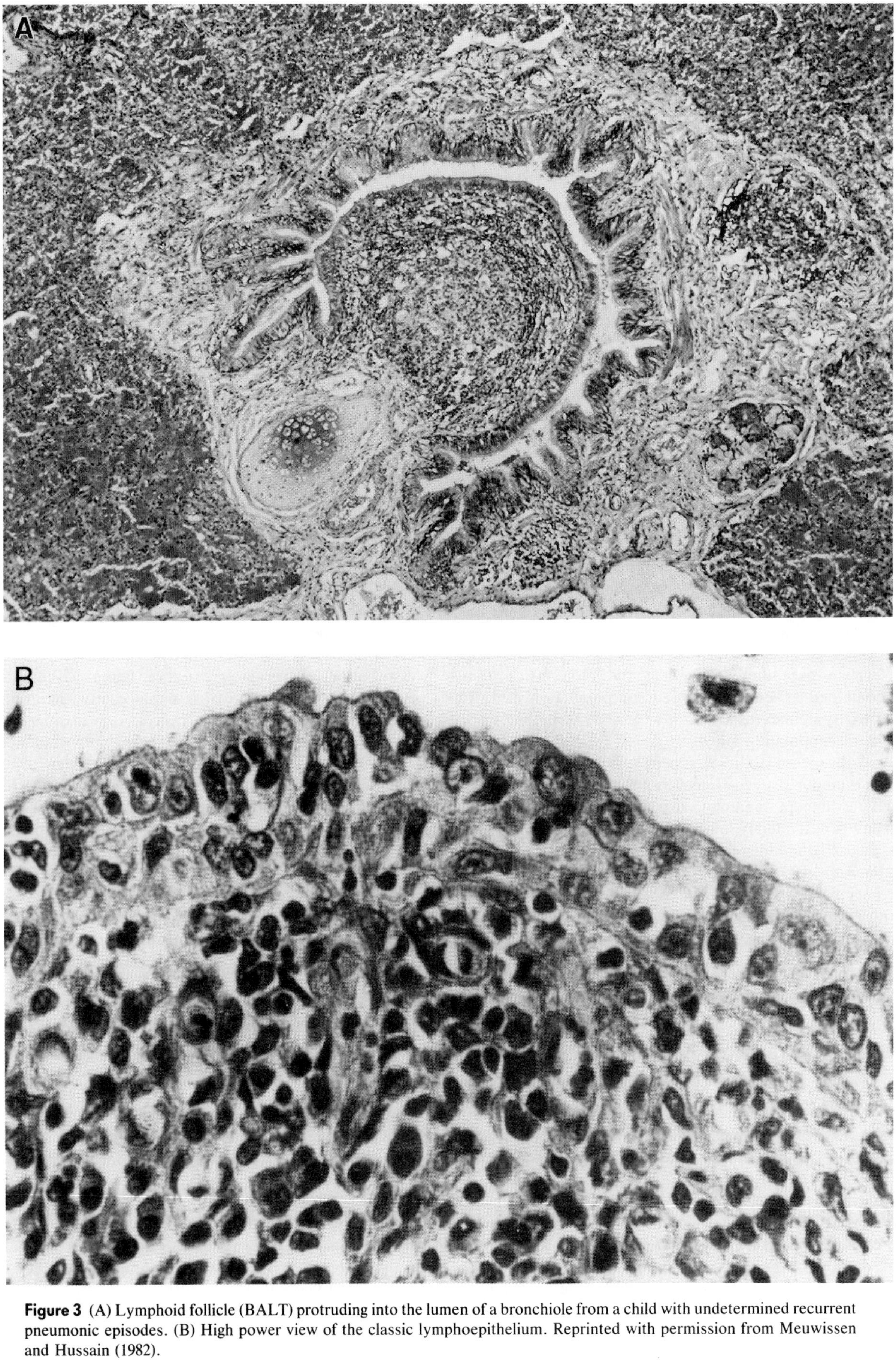

Figure 3 (A) Lymphoid follicle (BALT) protruding into the lumen of a bronchiole from a child with undetermined recurrent pneumonic episodes. (B) High power view of the classic lymphoepithelium. Reprinted with permission from Meuwissen and Hussain (1982).

1981). The detection of T-cell populations in Peyer's patches that are capable of mediating down-regulation (Clancy and Pucci, 1978; Kiyono *et al.*, 1980), and the switch toward a T-suppressor phenotype (Iwata and Sato, 1991) in chronic infection in the lung, indicates a regulatory role for BALT, but the relative contribution of BALT compared with the regional lymph node is not clear.

Much of the discussion in this chapter is based on studies involving a variety of species, including humans, that vary considerably in their expression of organized BALT in a physiological state. Several general observations can be made. First, no major differences in mucosal handling of antigen, nor in the development of a local immune response nor participation in a gut-driven common mucosal immune system, are noted among those species in which bronchial lymphoid tissue predominantly occurs in organized BALT and those in which the bronchial lymphoid tissue has less structure. Second, most, if not all, species (including humans) can develop classical BALT structures including a lympho-epithelium under conditions of increased antigen load. In those species with small amounts of BALT, under normal conditions, an adaptive immune function would focus the elements of an immune response into an efficient mechanism for the induction, capture, and delivery of a local mucosal immune response, as well as its control and integration within a broader defense network of lymphoid structures. Third, study of aggregated BALT and cells obtained essentially from these aggregates have given much insight into mechanisms of mucosal defense, both within the bronchopulmonary system and within mucosal tissues in general.

The presence of additional antigen-handling mechanisms within the bronchial mucosa that involve dendritic cells and epithelial cells, and the presence of T- and B-cell effector and regulatory lymphocytes within the bronchial mucosa, however, requires a dissection of the various components of mucosal immunity to determine the degree to which BALT in its classical form encompasses all these functions in one efficient unit. Further, the interdependence of various "pools" of lymphocytes within the lungs (Figure 4), and their functional interaction in health and disease, must be studied carefully. Perhaps particular insight into these interactions could come from careful analysis of cell traffic through the often forgotten regional lymph node, which not only represents a crossroad for lymphocyte traffic but appears to be central to the generation of mucosa-related immune responses, the up- and down-regulation of immune pathways, and the expansion of lung-specific immunity.

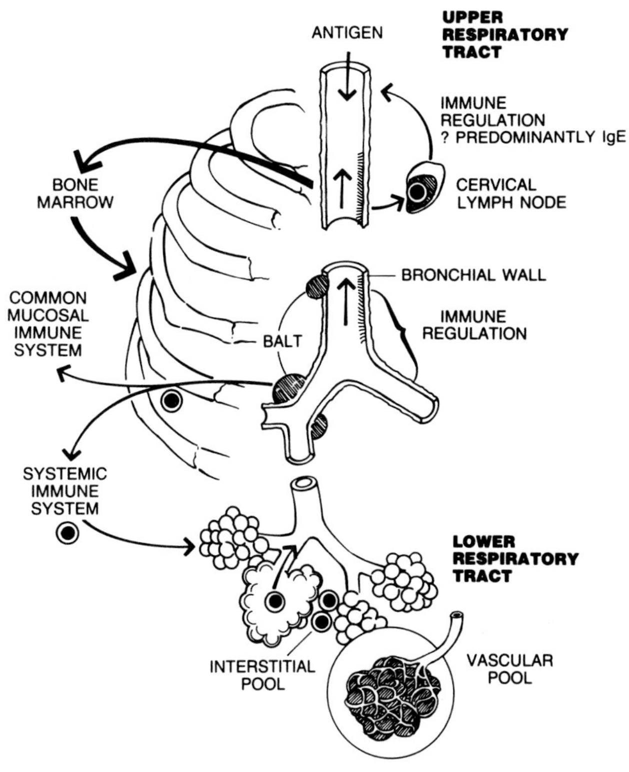

Figure 4 Schematic drawing of the elements of the lung lymphoid tissue. An immune regulation loop involves cervical lymph nodes, particularly relevant to the down regulation of IgE (Holt *et al.*, 1981). The immune regulation loop involving mucosal T lymphocytes is particularly relevant to the inhibition of T cell proliferation (Pucci *et al.*, 1982). The bronchus associated lymphoid tissue (BALT) is a mechanism for effectively generating both T and B lymphocyte immunity in response to luminal antigen, both locally and at distinct mucosal sites. The role of the mesenteric regional lymph node appears crucial to the expansion of mucosa-associated immunity. The exact role of the bronchial and mediastinal nodes is less clear. The interstitial lymphocyte pool is modified in function from that of the circulating blood pool and is at least as large as the latter. Its role within the lung, and its relationship to other "pulmonary lymphocyte" pools, is undefined (Pabst, 1990). The vascular lymphocyte pool has been identified on the basis of cell sequestration studies. Whether this pool represents more than differential cell sequestration or has an important modulatory effect on cell traffic within other lymphocyte pools is not known (Pabst, 1990). The broncho-alveolar cell pool contains 5–10% lymphocytes, whose functions probably involve immunoregulating activities that range from afferent to efferent limbs of the inflammatory response.

References

Ahlstedt, S., Smedegard, G., Nygen, H., and Bjorksten, B. (1983). Immune response in rats immunized with aerosolized antigen. Antibody formation, lymphoblastic response and mast cell and goblet cell development related to bronchial reactivity. *Int. Arch. Appl. Immunol.* **72,** 71–78.

Augustin, A., Kubo, R., and Sim. G. (1989). Resident pulmonary lymphocytes expressing the gamma/delta T cell receptor. *Nature (London)* **340,** 239–241.

Befus, A. D., Lee, T., Goto, T., Goodacre, R., Shanahan, F., and Bienenstock, J. (1986). Histologic and Functional properties of mast cells in rats and humans. *In* Mast Cell Differentiation and Heterogeneity. (A. D. Befus, J. Bienenstock, and J. A. Denburg, eds.) pp. 205–213. Raven Press, New York.

Bice, D. E., and Shopp, G. M. (1988). Antibody responses after lung immunization. *Exp. Lung Res.* **14,** 133–155.

Bienenstock, J. (1984). Bronchus-associated lymphoid tissue. *In* "Immunology of the Lung and Upper Respiratory Tract" (J. Bienenstock, ed.), pp. 96–118. McGraw-Hill, New York.

Bienenstock, J., and Johnson, N. (1976). A morphologic study of rabbit bronchial lymphoid aggregates and lymphoeipthelium. *Lab. Invest.* **35,** 343–348.

Bienenstock, J., Johnston, N., and Perey, D. Y. E. (1973a). Bron-

chial lymphoid tissue. I. Morphologic characteristics. *Lab. Invest.* **28,** 686–692.
Bienenstock, J., Johnston, N., and Perey, D. Y. E. (1973b). Bronchial lymphoid tissue. II. Functional characteristics. *Lab. Invest.* **28,** 693–698.
Bienenstock, J., Befus, A. D., McDermott, M. R., Mirski, S., Rosenthal, K., and Tagliabue, A. (1983). The mucosal immunologic network: Compartmentalization of lymphocytes, natural killer cells, and mast cells. *Ann. N. Y. Acad. Sci.* **409,** 164–170.
Bienenstock, J., Perdue, M., Blennerhassett, M., Stead, R., Kakuta, Y., Sestini, P., Vancheri, C., and Marshall, J. (1988). Inflammatory cells and the epithelium: Mast cell/nerve interactions in the lung in vitro and in vivo. *Am. Rev. Resp. Dis.* **138,** s31–s34.
Bockman, D. E., and Cooper, M. D. (1973). Pinocytosis by epithelium associated with lymphoid follicles in the bursa of Fabricius, appendix and Peyer's patches. An electron microscopic study. *Am. J. Anat.* **136,** 455–477.
Bockman, D. E., and Stevens, W. (1977). Gut-associated lymphoepithelial tissue: Bidirectional transport of tracer by specialized epithelial cells associated with lymphoid follicle. *J. Reticuloendothel. Soc.* **21,** 245–254.
Burdon-Sanderson, J. (1870). Recent researches on tuberculosis. *Edinburgh Med.* **15,** 385.
Butler, J. E., Swanson, P. A., Richerson, H. B., Ratajczak, H. V., Richards, D. W., and Suelzer, M. T. (1982). The local and systemic IgA and IgG antibody responses of rabbits to a soluable inhaled antigen. Measurement of responses in a model of acute hypersensitivity pneumonitis. *Am. Rev. Respir. Dis.* **126,** 80–85.
Chamberlain, D. W., Nopajaroonsri, C., and Simon, G. T. (1973). Ultrastructure of the pulmonary lymphoid tissue. *Am. Rev. Respir. Dis.* **108,** 621–631.
Chu, R. M., Huange, Y. T., and Weng, C. N. (1989). Changes of epithelial cells covering the intrapulmonary airway-associated lymphoid tissues after mycoplasma hyponeumoniae innoculation. *Immunobiol.* **4,** 75.
Clancy, R. L., and Bienenstock. (1974). The proliferative response of bronchus associated lymphoid tissue following local and systemic immunization. *J. Immunol.* **112,** 1997–2001.
Clancy, R., and Bienenstock, J. (1976). Secretion immunoglobulins. *Clin. Gastroenterol.* **5,** 229–249.
Clancy, R. L., and Pucci, A. (1978). Human mucosal lymphocytes—memory for "recall" antigens and non-specific suppression by T-lymphocytes. *Adv. Exp. Med. Biol.* **107,** 575–582.
Clancy, R., Rawls, W. E., and Jagannaths, S. (1977). Appearance of cytotoxic cells within the bronchus after local infection with herpex simplex virus. *J. Immunol.* **119,** 1102–1105.
Clancy, R., Cripps, A., Murree-Allen, K., Yeung, S., and Engel, M. (1985). Oral immunization with killed *Haemophilus influenzae* for protection against acute bronchitis in chronic obstructive lung disease. *Lancet* **2,** 1395–1397.
Clancy, R., Cripps, A., Yeung, S., Standish-White, S., Pang, G., Gratten, H., Koki, G., Gratten, M., Smith, D., and Alpers, M. (1987). Salivary and serum antibody responses to Haemophilus influenzae infection in Papua New Guinea. *Papua New Guinea Med. J.* **30,** 271–276.
Clancy, R., Cripps, A. W., and Gebski, V. (1989). Protection against recurrent acute bronchitis following oral immunization with killed Haemophilus influenzae. *Med. J. Aust.* **152,** 413–416.
Cornes, J. S. (1965). Number, size and distribution of Peyer's patches in the human small intestine. I. The development of Peyer's patches. *Gut* **6,** 225–229.
Craig, S. W., and Cebra, J. J. (1971). Peyer's patches: an enriched source of precursors for IgA-producing immunocytes in the rabbit. *J. Exp. Med.* **134,** 188–200.
Daniele, R. P. (1988a). The secretory immune system of the lung. *In* "Immunology and Immunologic Diseases of the Lung," 2nd ed. McGraw-Hill, New York.
Daniele, R. P. (1988b). Immune defenses of the lung. *In* "Pulmonary Diseases and Disorders," 2d Ed, pp. 589–598. McGraw-Hill, New York.
Delventhal, S., Hensel, A., Petzoldt, K., and Pabst, R. (1992a). Effects of microbial stimulation on the number size and activity of bronchus associated lymphoid tissue (BALT) structures in the pig. *Int. J. Exp. Pathol.* **73,** 351–357.
Delventhal, S., Brondis, A., Osterlay, H., and Pabst, R. (1992b). Low incidence of bronchus-associated lymphoid tissue (BALT) in chronically inflamed human lungs. *Virchow Arch B Cell. Pathol.* **64,** 271–274.
Elson, C. O., Heck, J. A., and Strober, W. (1979). T-cell regulation of murine IgA synthesis. *J. Exp. Med.* **149,** 632–643.
Emery, J. L., and Dinsdale, F. (1973). The postnatal development of lymphorecticular aggregates and lymph nodes in infants' lungs. *J. Clin. Pathol.* **26,** 539–545.
Emery, J. L., and Dinsdale, F. (1974). Increased incidence of lymphoreticular aggregates in lungs of children found unexpectedly dead. *Arch. Dis. Child.* **49,** 107–111.
Enerback, L. (1966). Mast cells in rat gastrointestinal mucosa. Effects of fixation. *Acta Pathol. Microbiol. Scand.* **66,** 289–302.
Ernst, P., Befus, A., and Bienenstock, J. (1985). Leucocytes in the intestinal epithelium. *Immunol. Today* **6,** 50–55.
Fournier, M., Vai, F., Dereene, J. P., and Pariente, R. (1977). Lymphoepithelial nodules in the rat: Morphologic featues and uptake and transport of exogenous protein. *Am. Rev. Respir. Dis.* **116,** 685–694.
Fuhrman, J. A., and Cebra, J. J. (1981). Special features of the priming process for a secretory IgA response. B cell priming with cholera toxin. *J. Exp. Med.* **153,** 534–544.
Goodman, T., and Lefrancois, L. (1988). Expression of the T cell receptor on intestinal CD+ intraepithelial lymphocytes. *Nature (London)* **333,** 855–858.
Guy-Grand, D., Griscelli, C., and Vassalli, P. (1974). The gut-associated lymphoid system: nature and properties of large dividing cells. *Eur. J. Immunol.* **4,** 435–443.
Guy-Grand, D., Griscelli, C., and Vassalli, P. (1978). The mouse gut T lymphocyte, a novel type of T cell. Nature, origin and traffic in mice in normal and graft-versus-host conditions. *J. Exp. Med.* **148,** 1661–1667.
Holt, P. G., Warner, L. A., and Mayrhofer, G. (1981a). Macrophages as effectors of T suppression: T-lymphocyte-dependent macrophage-mediated suppression of mitogen-induced blastogenesis in the rat. *Cell. Immunol.* **63,** 57–70.
Holt, P. G., Batty, S. E., and Turner, K. (1981b). Inhibition of specific IgE responses in mice by pre-exposure to inhaled antigen. *Immunology* **42,** 409–417.
Holt, P. G., Degebrodt, A., Venaille, T., O'Leary, C., Krsaka, K., Flexman, J., Farrell, H., Shellam, G., Young, P., Penhale, J., Robertson, T., and Papdimitriou, J. M. (1985). Preparation of interstitial lung cells by enzymatic digestion of tissue slices: Preliminary characteristics by morphology and performances in functional assays. *Immunology* **54,** 139–147.
Holt, P., Schon-Hegrad, M., and Oliver, J. (1988). MHC Class II antigen-bearing dendritic cells in pulmonary tissues of the rat. Regulation of antigen presentation activity by endogenous macrophage populations. *J. Exp. Med.* **167,** 262–274.
Husband, A., Cripps, A., Clancy, R., and Gleeson, M. (1983). Restrictions on mucosal B-lymphocytes function in man. *Ann. N.Y. Acad. Sci.* **409,** 745–750.
Husband, A. J., Dunkley, M. L., Cripps, A. W., and Clancy, R. L.

(1984). Antigen-specific response among T lymphocytes following intestinal administration of alloantigens. *Aust. J. Exp. Biol. Med. Sci.* **62,** 687–699.

Inoue, N., Magari, S., and Sakanaka, M. (1990). Distribution of peptidergic nerve fibres in rat bronchus-associated lymphoid tissue: Light microscopic observations. *Lymphology* **23,** 155–160.

Irani, A. A., Schechter, N. M., Craig, S. S., DeBlois, E., and Schwartz, L. B. (1986). Two types of human mast cells that have distinct neutral protease compositions. *Proc. Natl. Acad. Sci. U.S.A.* **83,** 4464–4468.

Iwata, M., and Sato, A. (1991). Morphological and immunohistochemical studies of the lungs and bronchus-associated lymphoid tissue in a rat model of chronic pulmonary infection with Pseudomonas aeruginosa. *Infect. Immunol.* **59,** 1514–1520.

Jeffery, P. K., and Corrin, B. (1984). Structural analysis of the respiratory tract. *In* "Immunology of the Lung and Upper Respiratory Tract" (J. Bienenstock, ed.), pp. 1–27. McGraw-Hill, New York.

Joel, D. D., and Chanana, A. D. (1987). Distribution of lung-associated lymphocytes from the caudal mediastinal lymph node: Effect of antigen. *Immunology* **62,** 641–646.

Kaltreider, H. B., Curtis, J. L., and Arraj, S. M. (1987). The mechanism of appearance of specific antibody-forming cells in lungs of inbred mice after immunization with sheep erythrocytes intratracheally. II. Dose-dependence and kinetics of appearance of antibody-forming cells in hilar lymph nodes and lungs of unprimed mice. *Am. Rev. Respir. Dis.* **135,** 87–92.

Kawanishi, H., Saltzman, L. E., and Strober, W. (1983). Mechanisms regulating IgA-class specific immunoglobulin production in murine gut-associated lymphoid tissues. I. T cells derived from Peyer's patches that switch sIgM cells in vitro. *J. Exp. Med.* **157,** 433–450.

Kieran, M. W., Blank, V., le Bail, O., and Israel, A. (1989). Lymphocyte homing. *Res. Immunol.* **140,** 399–450.

Kiyono, H., Babb, J. L., Michalek, S. M., and McGhee, J. R. (1980). Cellular basis for elevated IgA response in C3H-HeJ mice. *J. Immunol.* **125,** 732–737.

Kiyono, H., McGhee, J. R., Mosteller, L. M., Eldridge, J. H., Koopman, W. J., Kearney, J. F., and Michalek, S. M. (1982). Murine Peyer's patch T cell clones. Characterization of antigen-specific helper T cells for immunoglobulin A responses. *J. Exp. Med.* **156,** 1115–1130.

Kiyono, H., Mosteller-Barnum, L. M., Pitts, A. M., Williamson, S. L., and McGhee, J. R. (1985). Isotype specific immunoregulation. IgA-binding factors produces by Fca receptor-positive T cell hybridomas regulate IgA responses. *J. Exp. Med.* **161,** 731–747.

Klein, E. (1875). The anatomy of the lymphatic system. *In* "The Lung." Smith Elder, & Co., London.

Kyriazis, A. A., and Esterly, J. R. (1970). Development of lymphoid tissues in the human embryo and early fetus. *Arch. Pathol.* **90,** 348–353.

Lehmann, D., Coakley, K. J., Coakley, C. A., Spooner, V., Montgomery, J. M., Michael, A., Riley, I. D., Smith, T., Clancy, R. L., Cripps, A. W., and Alpers, M. P. (1991). Reduction in the incidence of acute bronchitis by an oral Haemophilus influenzae vaccine in patients with chronic bronchitis in the Highlands of Papua New Guinea. *Am. Rev. Respir. Dis.* **144,** 324–330.

McDermott, M. R., and Bienenstock, J. (1979). Evidence for a common mucosal immunologic system. I. Migration of B immunoblasts into intestinal, respiratory and genital tissues. *J. Immunol.* **122,** 1892–1898.

Meuwissen, H. J., and Hussain, M. (1982). Bronchus associated lymphoid tissue in the human lung: correlation of the hyperplasia with chronic pulmonary disease. *Clin. Immunol. Immunopathol.* **23,** 548–561.

Mezzette, M., Soloperto, M., Fasoli, A., and Mattoli, S. (1990). Human bronchial epithelial cells modulate CDE and mitogen-induced DNA synthesis in T cells but function poorly as antigen-presenting cell compared to pulmonary macrophages. *J. Allergy Clin. Immunol.* **87,** 930–938.

Milne, R. W., Bienenstock, J., and Perey, D. Y. E. (1975). The influence of antigenic stimulation on the ontogeny of lymphoid aggregates and immunoglobulin-containing cells in mouse bronchial and intestinal mucosa. *J. Reticuloendothel. Soc.* **17,** 361–369.

Muggenburg, B. A., Bice, D. E., Haley, P. J., Mauderley, J. L., Dauber, J. J., Herlan, K., and Griffith, B. P. (1987). Immune response in the transplanted canine lung. *Am. Rev. Respir. Dis.* **135,** A103.

Nash, D. R., and Holle, B. (1973). Local and systemic cellular immune responses in guinea-pigs given antigen parenterally or directly into the lower respiratory tract. *Clin. Exp. Immunol.* **13,** 573–583.

Ngan, J., and Kind, L. S. (1978). Suppressor T cells for IgE and IgG in Peyer's patches of mice made tolerant by the oral administration of ovalbumin. *J. Immunol.* **120,** 861–865.

Otuski, Y., Ito, Y., and Magari, S. (1989). Lymphocyte subpopulations in high endothelial venules and lymphatic capillaries of bronchus-associated lymphoid tissue (BALT) in the rat. *Am. J. Anat.* **184,** 139–146.

Owen, R. L. (1977). Sequential uptake of horseradish peroxidase by lymphoid follicle epithelium of Peyer's patches in the normal unobstructed mouse intestine: An ultrastructural study. *Gastroenterology* **72,** 440–451.

Owen, R. C., and Bhalla, D. H. (1983). Lympho-epithelial organs and lymph nodes. *Biomed. Res. Appl. Sem.* **3,** 79–169.

Owen, R. L., and Jones, A. L. (1974). Epithelial cell specialization within human Peyer's patches: an ultrastructural study of intestinal lymphoid follicles. *Gastroenterol.* **66,** 189–203.

Pabst, R. (1990). Compartmentalization and kinetics of lymphoid cells in the lung. *Reg. Immunol.* **3,** 62–71.

Pabst, R. (1992). Is BALT a major component of the human lung immune system. *Immunol. Today* **13,** 119–122.

Pabst, R., and Gehrke, I. (1990). Is the bronchus-associated lymphoid tissue (BALT) an integral structure of the lung in normal mammals, including humans? *Am. J. Resp. Cell. Mol. Biol.* **3,** 131–135.

Pang, G. T., Clancy, R., and Saunders, H. (1990). Dual inhibition of the immune response by enterocytes isolated from the rat small intestine. *Immunol. Cell. Biol.* **68,** 387–396.

Patterson, R., Tomita, Y., Oh, S. H., Suszko, I. M., and Pruzansky, J. J. (1974). Respiratory mast cells and basophiloid cells. I. Evidence that they are secreted into the bronchial lumen, morphology, degranulation and histamine release. *Clin. Exp. Immunol.* **16,** 223–224.

Patterson, R., McKenna, J. M., Suszko, I. M., *et al.* (1977). Living histamine-containing cells from the bronchial lumens of humans. *J. Clin. Invest.* **59,** 217–225.

Petit, A., Ernst, P., Befus, A., and Bienenstock, J. (1985). Murine intestinal intraepithel lymphocytes. I Relationship of a novel Thy-1, Lyt-1, Lyt-2+. granulated sub-population to natural killer cells and mast cell precursors. *J. Immunol.* **15,** 122–125.

Plesch, B. E. (1982). Histology and immunochemistry of bronchus associated lymphoid tissue (BALT) in the rat. *Adv. Exp. Med. Biol.* **149,** 491–497.

Pucci, A., Clancy, R., and Jackson, G. (1982). Quantitation of T lymphocyte subsets in human bronchus mucosa. *Am. Rev. Respir. Dis.* **126,** 364–366.

Racz, P., Tenner-Racz, K., Myrvik, Q. N., and Fainter, L. K. (1977). Functional architecture of BALT and lymphoepithelium in pulmonary cell-mediated reactions in the rabbit. *J. Reticuloendothel. Soc.* **22,** 59–83.

Richman, L. K., Graeff, A. S., Yarchoan, R., and Strober, W. S. (1981). Simultaneous induction of antigen-specific IgA helper T cells and IgG suppressor T cells in the murine Peyer's patches after protein feeding. *J. Immunol.* **126,** 2079–2083.

Rudzik, O., Clancy, R., Perey, D. Y. E., Day, R. P., and Bienenstock, J. (1975a). Repopulation with IgA-containing cells of bronchial and intestinal lamina propria after the transfer of homologous Peyer's patches and bronchial lymphocytes. *J. Immunol.* **114,** 1599–1604.

Rudzik, O., Clancy, R. L., Perey, D. Y. E., Bienenstock. J., and Singal, D. P. (1975b). The Distribution of a rabbit thymic antigen and membrane immunoglobulins in lymphoid tissue with special reference to mucosal lymphocytes. *J. Immunol.* **114,** 1–4.

Rudzik, O., Perey, D. Y. E., and Bienenstock, J. (1975c). Differential IgA repopulation after transfer of autologons and allogeneic rabbit Peyer's patch cells. *J. Immunol.* **114,** 40–44.

Ruitenberg, E. J., and Elgersma, A. (1976). Absence of intestinal mast cell response in congenitally athymic mice during *Trichinella spiralis* infection. *Nature (London)* **264,** 258–260.

Scicchitano, R., Husband, A. J., and Clancy, R. (1984). Contribution of gut immunization to the local response in the respiratory tract. *Immunology* **53,** 375–384.

Scicchitano, R., Stanisz, A., Ernst, P., and Bienenstock, J. (1988). A common mucosal immune system revisited. *In* "Migration and Homing of Lymphoid Cells" (A. J. Husband, ed.), pp. 1–34. CRC Press, Boca Raton, Florida.

Sedgwick, J. D., and Holt, P. G. (1985). Down-regulation of immune response to inhaled antigen: Studies on the mechanism of induced suppression. *Immunology* **56,** 635–642.

Shanaban, F., MacNiven, I., Dyck, N., Denburg, J., Bienenstock, J., and Befus, A. (1987). Human lung mast cells: Distribution and abundance of histochemically distinct subpopulations. *Int. Arch. Allergy Appl. Immunol.* **83,** 3290–3331.

Sminia, T., and van der Brugge-Gamelkoorn, G. J. (1989). Structure and function of bronchus-associated lymphoid tissue (BALT). *Crit. Rev. Immunol.* **9,** 119–150.

Spencer, J., and Hall, J. G. (1984). Studies on the lymphocytes of sheep. IV. Migration patterns of lung-associated lymphocytes efferent from the caudal mediastinal lymph node. *Immunology* **52,** 1–5.

Sprent, J. (1986). Fate of H2-activated T lymphocytes in syngeneic hosts. I. Fate in lymphoid tissues and intestines traced with H-thymine, 1-deoxyuridine and chromium. *Cell. Immunol.* **21,** 278–302.

Taylor, D. C., Cripps, A. W., and Clancy, R. (1990). Interaction of bacteria and the epithelial surface in chronic bronchitis. *In* "Advances in Mucosal Immunology" (T. T. MacDonald and S. J. Challacombe, eds.), pp. 806–807. Kluwer Academic Publishers, London.

Tenner-Racz, K., Racz, P., Myrvik, Q. N., Ockers, J. R., and Geister, R. (1979). Uptake and transport of horseradish peroxidase by lymphoepithelium of the bronchus associated lymphoid tissue in normal and *Bacillus* Calmette-Guerin immunized and challenged rabbits. *Lab. Invest.* **41,** 106–115.

Thomas, W. R., Holt, P. G., Papadimitriou, J. M., and Keast, D. (1974). The growth of transplanted tumours in mice after chronic inhalation of fresh cigarette smoke. *Br. J. Cancer* **30,** 459–462.

van der Brugge-Gamelkoorn, G. J., and Kraal, G. (1985). The specifity of the high endothelial venule in bronchus-associated lymphoid tissue (BALT). *J. Immunol.* **134,** 3746–3750.

van der Brugge-Gamelkoorn, G. J., Claassen, E., and Sminia, T. (1986). Anti-TNP-forming cells in bronchus-associated lymphoid tissue (BALT) and paratracheal lymph node (PTLN) of the rat after intratracheal priming and boosting with TPN-KLH. *Immunology* **57,** 405–409.

Waldman, R. H., and Henney, C. S. (1971). Cell-mediated immunity and antibody responses in the respiratory tract after local and systemic immunization. *J. Exp. Med.* **134,** 482–489.

Wallace, F. J., Clancy, R., and Cripps, A. W. (1989). An animal model demonstration of enhanced clearance of non-typable *Haemophilus influenzae* from the respiratory tract after antigen stimulation of gut associated lymphoid tissue. *Am. Rev. Respir. Dis.* **140,** 311–316.

Wallace, F. J., Cripps, A. W., Clancy, R. L., Husgand, A. J., and Witt, C. S. (1991). A role for intestinal T lymphocytes in bronchial mucosal immunity. *Immunology* **74,** 68–73.

Warner, L. A., Holt, P. G., and Mayrhofer, G. (1981). Alveolar macrophage. VI. Regulation of alveolar macrophage-mediated suppression of lymphocyte proliferation by a putative T cell. *Immunology* **42,** 137–147.

Weisz-Carrington, P., Grimes, S. R., and Lamm, M. E. (1987). Gut-associated lymphoid tissue as source of an IgA immune response in respiratory tissues after oral immunization and intrabronchial challenge. *Cell. Immunol.* **106,** 132–138.

Yoshizawa, I., Norma, T., and Kawano, Y. (1989). Allergen-specific induction of interleukin-2 (IL-2) responsiveness in lymphocytes from children with asthma. *J. Allergy Clin. Immunol.* **84,** 246–255.

Young, K. R., and Reynolds, H. Y. (1984). Bronchoalveolar washings: Proteins and cells from normal lungs. *In* "Immunology of the Lung and Upper Respiratory Tract" (J. Bienenstock, ed.), pp. 157–173. McGraw-Hill, New York.

44

Mucosal Immune Function in Asthma

A. E. Redington • D. B. Jones • S. T. Holgate

The pathogenesis of the asthmatic state represents a complex disease process that involves mast cells, eosinophils, neutrophils, basophils, macrophages, platelets, and T cells in a complex series of cross-interactions, with the participation of a cascade of cytokines, complement factors, and other inflammatory mediators.

The understanding of the cellular interactions in the mucosal compartment of human lung is central to our understanding of the development of the asthmatic process. Studies of immune interactions in the pathological lung must be seen against the background of immune function in normal tissue. Largely for technical reasons, our understanding of the mucosal immune process has lagged behind that of the peripheral immune system. Clearly, however, with respect specifically to the mucosal compartment, the T cell is the major orchestrator of immune function and also represents the cellular component that exhibits antigenic specificity. In this chapter, we initially describe features of the T-cell populations that are characteristic of mucosal sites and subsequently describe changes in these populations and the various cellular interactions that are known to occur after the development of the asthmatic condition.

I. MUCOSAL T LYMPHOCYTE POPULATIONS

In the literature, investigations of the T-cell component of the mucosal compartment of the gut appear to have proceeded at a faster rate than those relating to lung mucosa. However, based on the rapidly expanding lung literature, clearly general statements can be made that are relevant to both sites. We have adopted this approach to our discussion of mucosal T cells.

A. T-Cell Development

T lymphocytes undergo maturation within the cortical area of the human thymus, which they enter as committed T-lymphocyte precursors (Janossy *et al.*, 1981). During their passage through the thymus, two important events occur. First, shuffling of genes encoding various components of the T-cell receptors allows the random development of the T-cell repertoire. Second, individual T cells that express self (host)-directed specificity are deleted or inactivated.

The majority of T cells present in the peripheral compartment of the lymphoid system express a surface receptor composed of α and β polypeptides that are bonded covalently. A minority population expresses a receptor composed of γ/δ polypeptide chains that may or may not show disulfide linkage. The significance of this population in relation to mucosal sites will be discussed subsequently. In addition to the expression of antigen-specific receptor molecules, the maturation of T cells involves the production of the CD3 molecular complex and its association with the T-cell receptor, as well as the expression of membrane CD4 or CD8 glycoproteins. These molecules, which are members of the immunoglobulin gene superfamily, dictate aspects of antigen recognition by T cells and, in conjunction with CD3, form the basis of early studies of T-lymphocyte subset function.

B. T-Lymphocyte Subset Markers in Relation to Antigen Experience

Exposure of T cells to antigen is accompanied by changes in the molecular species of CD45 expressed on their surface. CD45, formerly known as leukosialin or leukocyte common antigen, has a short intracellular tail and an extended, heavily glycosylated, extracellular portion that varies in length (Akbar *et al.*, 1988). Changes in CD45 isoforms, which can be expressed variably on different leukocyte subtypes, are achieved largely by alternative splicing but also, as more recent comparisons of human and neonatal T cells have shown, by changes in the rate of turnover of the different subspecies of the molecule (Yamada *et al.*, 1992). Within T cells, the most significant isoform change is from CD45RA to CD45RO, demonstrating the switch from immunological immaturity to immunological experience. The CD45RO population contains the bulk of T cells reactive to recall antigens (Akbar *et al.*, 1988). The CD45RA–CD45RO switch is accompanied by a change in the cytokine profile secreted by the cells on activation (Ferrer *et al.*, 1992).

In mice, $CD4^+$ T cells are known to be subdivided into two categories, Th1 and Th2, which differ in their capacity to secrete cytokines and also in the efficiency with which they can support delayed type hypersensitivity (Th1) or IgE synthesis (Th2). Experimental studies of these two $CD4^+$ subsets suggest that the functional differences shown may be significant in the pathogenesis of the asthmatic state (Frew and Kay, 1991; Robinson *et al.*, 1992). Currently, CD45RA and CD45R0 human T-cell subsets have not been definitively characterized as direct human correlates to murine Th1 and Th2 T cells. Nevertheless, studies of cytokine mRNA production suggest that human T-cell populations containing a high proportion of CD45R0$^+$ lymphocytes show cytokine secretion patterns that closely resemble those of the murine Th2 subpopulation (Ferrer *et al.*, 1992).

C. Phenotype of the Intraepithelial T-Lymphocyte Population

The intraepithelial lymphocyte (IEL) population of the human intestine has been investigated extensively; numerous reviews on this topic exist. Both phenotypic and functional investigations of IELs demonstrate selective recruitment of functionally distinct T-lymphocyte subsets (Selby *et al.*, 1981; Harvey and Jones, 1991). In the human intestine, the majority of CD3$^+$ IELs strongly express CD7, a 40-kDa antigen that has been considered to represent an activation marker (Spencer *et al.*, 1989a). Between 70 and 90% of small intestinal IELs are CD8$^+$, although CD8 dominance is less marked in the colon (Trejdosiewicz *et al.*, 1987). A large proportion of intestinal IELs is positive for CD45R0, demonstrating selective recruitment of an antigen-experienced population, and also expresses the antigen recognized by the monoclonal antibody HML1. The molecule identified by HML1 is claimed to be associated intimately with recruitment of lymphocytes into mucosal surfaces (Cerf-Bensussan *et al.*, 1987; Schieferdecker *et al.*, 1990). IELs also show positivity for the β_1 integrin VLA-4 (Choy *et al.*, 1990). IELs would, therefore, appear to be well adapted to cell–stroma and cell–cell interactions. Functional studies of intestinal IELs show widely varying results among and within species (Bland and Warren, 1986; Mayer and Shlien, 1987). These differences presumably relate to some genuine interspecies variation but also reflect difficulties inherent in the extraction of IELs from tissue biopsies, as well as wide variation in the experimental design of the functional studies performed. To date, the immunological consensus would appear to be that CD3$^+$ IELs are, at least in part, responsible for the regulation of oral tolerance in humans. Beneath the intestinal mucosal compartment lies the lamina propria, which contains a much more complex cell mixture in which CD4$^+$ T cells are more common, as are B lymphocytes, plasma cells, basophils, mast cells, and eosinophils (reviewed by Harvey and Jones, 1991).

In comparison with studies of the human intestine or investigations conducted on bronchoalveolar lavage fluid, immunophenotypic analysis of lymphocyte populations present within human lung tissue of normal histology are infrequent (Azzawi *et al.*, 1990). From the studies that do exist, based either on tissue removed from resection specimens or on biopsies obtained during bronchoscopy, the following general statements can be made. T cells are relatively abundant both in the lung parenchyma and within the epithelial lining of the bronchial wall (Azzawi *et al.*, 1990). Unlike the human intestine, CD8$^+$ cells are not present in great excess. At least with respect to parenchymal tissue, this absence may reflect dilution by circulating peripheral blood. HML1 is expressed widely on lung T cells (Cerf-Bensussan *et al.*, 1987); up to 80% of bronchial wall T lymphocytes are CD45R0$^+$. As in the human intestine, CD7 is expressed strongly and, at least in histologically normal tissue, CD25 [the interleukin 2 (IL-2) receptor] is shown very infrequently on CD3$^+$ T cells. From these data, the mucosal compartments of histologically normal human lung and intestine could be considered to contain phenotypically equivalent IEL populatons.

D. T-Cell Receptor Gene Expression in Intraepithelial Lymphocytes

In mice and birds, γ/δ T-cell receptor-carrying lymphocytes appear to predominate at all mucosal surfaces. These cells have been considered to have a specialized function in the immune surveillance of epithelia (Janeway, 1988). In humans, however, α/β- expressing T lymphocytes represent the predominant mucosal T-cell population in gut (Brandtzaeg *et al.*, 1989; Trejdosiewicz *et al.*, 1989) and in lung (Augustin *et al.*, 1989). γ/δ Receptors exist in biochemically distinct forms. In the intestine, γ/δ-positive cells appear to carry the nondisulfide linked heterodimer (Spencer *et al.*, 1989b), in contrast to peripheral blood, suggesting that the small population of γ/δ positive cells present in humans may have some specialized function. γ/δ-Positive T cells have been claimed to represent an early form of immune surveillance of epithelial surfaces (Janeway, 1988), based on their appearance early in ontogeny, the demonstration in nude mice that their development may occur independently of thymic influences, and their claimed restricted gene repertoire. Note, however, that a high level of junctional diversity could produce a much higher level of receptor variability than is apparent from the numbers of coding genes.

In contrast to the γ/δ T-cell receptor, the genomic information encoding the α/β receptor encompasses a large number of Vβ genes. These genes have been placed into 24 subfamilies based on the presence of 75% homology between individual genes at the sequence level (Robinson, 1991). Monoclonal antibodies have been produced that identify a proportion of these Vβ gene families. Although our data are preliminary, by comparison with the peripheral lymphoid system, the Vβ_6 and Vβ_8 subfamilies appear to be overrepresented in the lung (S. Berry, S. T. Holgate, and D. B. Jones, unpublished observations). Should this prove to be true, preferential usage of individual V gene segments may occur at mucosal sites in addition to preferential selection of T cells with specialized function and phenotype.

E. Macrophages and Accessory Cells

Macrophages and dendritic cells show much greater phenotypic heterogeneity than lymphocytes. Surface markers vary during maturation, and this plasticity is compounded by the effects of macrophage–mediator and macrophage–cell interactions in tissue sites. The intestinal mucosa contains a population of cells resembling interdigitating reticulum cells that may have a role in the sampling of incoming antigen (Tseng, 1984; Mahida *et al.*, 1989; Harvey *et al.*, 1990). Scavenging macrophages are described also that differ in phenotype. Many of these show up-regulation of a range of surface receptors, suggesting an activated state (Selby *et al.*, 1983; Trejdosiewicz *et al.*, 1987). Within the lung, populations can be identified that have the characteristics of antigen-presenting (dendritic) cells as well as phagocytes with varying phenotypes (Spiteri and Poulter, 1991). The precise interaction of these cell populations, in terms of allergen presentation, antigen and cell clearance, and production of inflammatory mediators, and their overall contribution toward the asthmatic process have yet to be determined.

F. Synthesis

The preceding data clearly demonstrate that unique populations of lymphocytes are recruited selectively to mucosa-associated lymphoid tissue. Also clearly, from the pathological picture seen in asthma, these cells operate in conjunction with a range of inflammatory cells types. In addition, complex mediator interactions occur during the development of lung pathology. In the following sections, we discuss a variety of different cell types and their actions in terms of mediator production and response in the context of asthmatic disease.

II. IMMUNOLOGICAL MECHANISMS IN ASTHMA

Until recently, asthma was viewed primarily in terms of contraction of bronchial smooth muscle; relatively little attention was paid to the underlying processes responsible. Attempts to define asthma focused on disordered airway function rather than on pathological abnormalities. However, although bronchoconstriction is undeniably important, the causes of airway narrowing are multiple and include, in addition, airway wall edema and hypersecretion of mucus. Another feature characteristic of asthma is nonspecific bronchial hyperresponsiveness, the ability of the airways to respond to a wide variety of stimuli in an exaggerated manner. Using modern techniques, real progress is now being made in unraveling the complex and interrelated events that can explain these disparate features.

Increasing clinical and pathological evidence points to airway inflammation as a basic underlying abnormality. For over a century, scientists have known that the airways of patients with asthma are inflamed. Early postmortem studies on the lungs of patients who died of asthma (Dunnill, 1960; Dunnill *et al.*, 1969) demonstrated extensive inflammation of the airway wall, characterized by infiltration of the tissue with eosinophils and mononuclear cells, extensive loss of the bronchial epithelium, hyperplasia of mucus-secreting cells, hypertrophy of bronchial smooth muscle, and the presence of an exudate within the lumen containing mucus and cellular debris. Asthma also frequently is associated with atopy—the genetic predisposition to produce IgE in response to common enviornmental allergens—suggesting an association between asthma and immediate hypersensitivity. Finally, drugs with the predominant action of suppressing inflammatory responses, for example, corticosteroids, sodium cromoglycate, and cyclosporin, are all effective in the treatment of asthma.

Considering these lines of evidence together builds a strong case for implicating inflammatory responses in the disordered airway function of asthma. Until recently, testing this hypothesis directly has not been possible; however, the advent of fiber-optic bronchoscopy has provided an opportunity to obtain bronchoalveolar lavage fluid and mucosal biopsy specimens from patients with asthma, thereby enabling a detailed characterization of the inflammatory response. This approach has been applied both in day-to-day asthma and following bronchial provocation with specific allergen, which results in both early and late phases of airway constriction as well as in an acquired increase in bronchial responsiveness.

Using these techniques, a number of specific cells and mediators stand out as particularly important. These cells and mediators are considered in more detail.

A. Mast Cells

Mast cells play a central role in allergic reactions involving immediate or type I hypersensitivity responses; asthma is no exception. Good evidence exists that mediators released on activation of mast cells are responsible for the early bronchoconstrictor response provoked by inhaled allergen. These mediators include histamine, prostaglandin (PG) D_2 and its metabolite $9\alpha,11\beta$-PGF_2, and the sulfidopeptide leukotrienes (LTs) C_4, D_4, and E_4. All these molecules are powerful contractile agonists of bronchial smooth muscle and, in addition, are vasodilators and increase microvascular permeability.

Mast cells are found throughout the airway wall, particularly beneath the bronchial epithelium and surrounding the airway smooth muscle. Most of these cells contain tryptase as their only neutral protease, in contrast to mast cells from skin and other connective tissue sites which contain both tryptase and chymase. Although the total number of mast cells does not differ greatly between patients with mild-to-moderate asthma and normal subjects, increased activation of these cells is believed to occur in asthma.

Several lines of evidence support the view that mast cell activation occurs in asthma. First, transmission electron microscopy (Figure 1) demonstrates ultrastructural evidence of mast cell degranulation, with loss of electron density of the characteristic scroll-containing granules and the formation of secretory channels (Beasley *et al.*, 1989a). Second, mast cell-derived mediators such as histamine (Casale *et al.*, 1987), tryptase (Wenzel *et al.*, 1988), and LTC_4 (Lam *et al.*, 1988) are found in increased quantities in lavage from asthmatics compared with normal controls. Finally, bronchial provocation of the airway, either by inhalation challenge or by introduction of the allergen directly onto the airway surface via a bronchoscope, results in an early bronchoconstrictor response accompanied by the release of mast cell-derived mediators including histamine, tryptase, PGD_2, and leukotrienes (Murray *et al.*, 1986; Wenzel *et al.*, 1988; Miadonna *et al.*, 1990).

Pharmacological manipulation also supports a role for mast cells in mediating the early bronchoconstrictor response. This

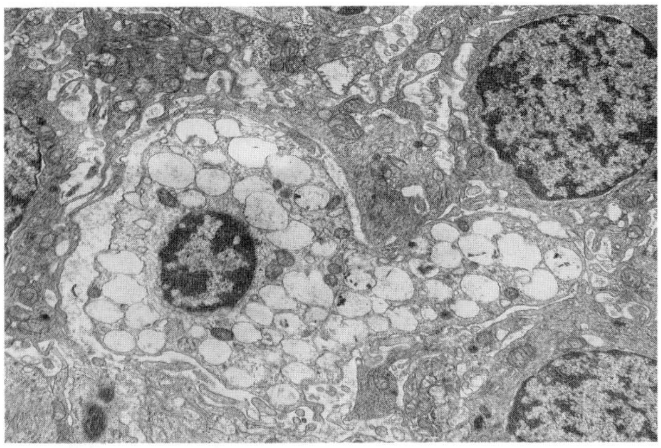

Figure 1 Electron micrograph of a mast cell showing evidence of extensive degranulation.

response can be inhibited effectively by drugs known to inhibit mast cell function, for example, sodium cromoglycate (Atkins *et al.*, 1978), and can be attenuated markedly by mediator antagonists, specifically those directed against histamine H1 (Rafferty *et al.*, 1987), prostanoid TP (Beasley *et al.*, 1989), and leukotriene (Taylor *et al.*, 1991) receptors. β2 Adrenoceptor agonists such as salbutamol are also powerful inhibitors of the immediate reaction (Cockcroft and Murdock, 1987), probably by a combination of a direct action on bronchial smooth muscle and inhibition of mast cell mediator release. The ability of histamine H1 antagonists (Rafferty *et al.*, 1990) and leukotriene antagonists (Hui and Barnes, 1991) to produce a degree of bronchodilation in symptomatic asthma suggests that mast cell products contribute to airflow obstruction even in the absence of specific antigen challenge.

In addition to the traditional mediators just discussed, evidence indicates that mast cells are also a source of a number of cytokines. Initial work showed that activated murine mast cells generate a wide range of cytokines including IL-1, IL-3, IL-4, IL-5, IL-6, and GM-CSF (Burd *et al.*, 1989; Plaut *et al.*, 1989; Wodnar-Filipowicz *et al.*, 1989). These findings have now been in part extended to human lung mast cells which have been shown to produce TNFα (Ohkawara *et al.*, 1992) and IL-4 (Bradding *et al.*, 1992). The potential implications of these molecules in the inflammatory processes of asthma is currently under investigation but the likelihood is that the role of the mast cell is more far-reaching than has recently been supposed.

Finally, mast cells probably play an important role in exercise-induced asthma (McFadden, 1987). In this case, the immediate stimulus for mast cell activation is believed to be provided by local hypertonicity resulting from water loss from the airway surface. Therefore, not surprisingly drugs such as histamine H1 antagonists (Finnerty and Holgate, 1990) and leukotriene antagonists (Manning *et al.*, 1990) are able to attenuate the bronchoconstrictor response when administered prior to exercise. Sodium cromoglycate, nedocromil sodium, and β agonists are also effective inhibitors of exercise-induced asthma, consistent with their known inhibitory effects on mast cells. Reflex bronchoconstriction produced by cooling of the airway by inspired air also may contribute to exercise-induced asthma.

B. Eosinophils

At one time, the eosinophil was believed to be a protective cell in allergic responses but now the opposite is known to be true. The frequent association of asthma with peripheral blood and sputum eosinophilia, the extensive infiltration of eosinopils into the airways of patients dying of acute severe asthma, and the demonstration of the release of eosinophil-derived pro-inflammatory mediators all point to a central role for this cell in contributing to the inflammatory response characteristic of asthma.

Recruitment of eosinophils from the circulation entails a series of separate processes. Initial adherence to endothelium is followed by transendothelial migration and chemotaxis toward the site of inflammation. The process by which eosinophils are slowed down and eventually arrested against the endothelium as they traverse postcapillary venules is dependent on the induction or up-regulation of specific adhesion molecules by activated endothelial cells. These molecules are E-selectin (formerly known as endothelial leukocyte adhesion molecule 1 or ELAM-1; Bevilacqua *et al.*, 1989), which interacts with a carbohydrate ligand known as sialyl Lewis X that is expressed on eosinopils and neutrophils; intercellular adhesion molecule 1 (ICAM-1; Pober *et al.*, 1986), which interacts with molecules of the integrin family, LFA-1 and Mac-1, again expressed on both types of leukocyte; and, finally, vascular cell adhesion molecule (VCAM-1; Bochner *et al.*, 1991), a member of the immunoglobulin superfamily, the ligand of which on the eosinophil is the β1 intergrin VLA-4, which has been shown to be more specific to eosinophil recruitment. endobronchial provocation of the airways of atopic asthmatics with allergen results in the increased expression of E-selectin and ICAM-1 (evident at 5–6 hr; S. Montefort, unpublished observations) and VCAM-1 (apparent at 24 hr postchallenge; Bentley *et al.*, 1992). Transendothelial migration of leukocytes also is believed to be dependent on interactions with adhesion molecules including ICAM-1 (Smith, 1988).

Within the perivascular space, eosinophils are capable of responding to a variety of chemoattractant factors including C5a, LTB_4, platelet activating factor (PAF), and IL-5. Two factors that have generated interest as potent chemoattractant stimuli for eosinophils are IL-2 (Rand *et al.*, 1991a) and lymphocyte chemoattractant factor (LCF; Rand *et al.*, 1991b). LCF is a 14-kDa highly cationic protein that is thought to be released by activated $CD8^+$ lymphocytes. This glycoprotein interacts with eosinophils at extremely low concentrations (10^{-11}–$10^{-12}M$) in a process involving CD4, which is expressed on eosinophils as well as on T lymphocytes. An additional finding is that allergen itself can provide a chemotactic stimulus for eosinophils via an interaction with IgE bound to low-affinity cell-surface IgE receptors.

To survive in the airways, eosinophils require the presence of certain cytokines and growth factors. IL-3, granulocyte–macrophage colony stimulating factor (GM-CSF), and

IL-5 all can maintain eosinophils in a viable state in culture (Tai *et al.*, 1991) and are known to be generated within the airway wall in asthma. T lymphocytes probably provide the majority of the IL-5, whereas GM-CSF is likely to be derived additionally from both the monocyte–macrophage population and the bronchial epithelium. Stimulated fibroblasts also can produce GM-CSF (Kaushansky *et al.*, 1988). Eosinophil survival *in vitro* is prolonged by coculture with fibroblasts, an effect mediated by GM-CSF (Owen *et al.*, 1987). This result may be important in light of the population of myofibroblasts beneath the bronchial epithelium.

The mechanisms by which eosinophils become activated are not understood completely. However, these cells appear to possess at least two types of IgE binding site on their surface—low-affinity FcεR2 receptors and the carbohydrate binding protein MAC-2 described previously on macrophages (Cherayil *et al.*, 1989)—as well as FcγR2 receptors for IgG, receptors for IgA, and receptors for certain components of the complement cascade. Different receptors have been shown to be able to mediate the release of different mediators (Tomassini *et al.*, 1991). Further, IL-3 (Rothenberg *et al.*, 1988), IL-5 (Lopez *et al.*, 1988), and GM-CSF (Owen *et al.*, 1987) all can increase the functional activation status of eosinophils.

Once activated, eosinophils represent a potent source of pro-inflammatory mediators (Figure 2), including oxygen radicals, lipids such as LTC_4 15-HETE and PAF, and the arginine-rich proteins of the eosinophil granule: major basic protein (MBP), eosinophil cationic protein (ECP), eosinophil-derived neurotoxin (EDN), and eosinophil peroxidase (EPO). These proteins are directly toxic to airway epithelial cells, but an additional source of damage to the epithelium may result from a cognate interaction between eosinophils and epithelial cells, resulting in the induction of epithelial cell-derived proteases (Herbert *et al.*, 1991).

Finally, evidence suggests that eosinophils are an important source of cytokines, in particular IL-3 (Kita *et al.*, 1991), GM-CSF (Kita *et al.*, 1991; Moqbel *et al.*, 1991), IL-5 (Desreumaux *et al.*, 1992), IL-6 (Hamid *et al.*, 1992), transforming growth factor (TGF)α (Wong *et al.*, 1990), and TGFβ (Ohno *et al.*, 1992; Wong *et al.*, 1991). These cytokines may, in some cases, have important autocrine effects, but also would amplify and prolong the inflammatory response and perhaps contribute to airway fibrosis.

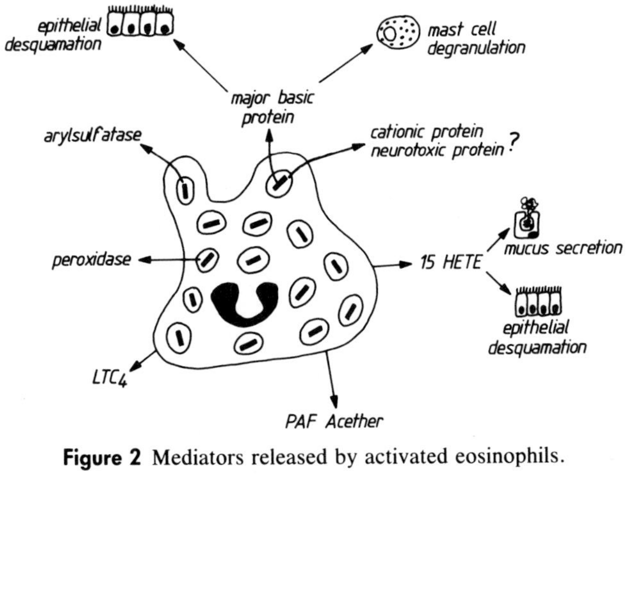

Figure 2 Mediators released by activated eosinophils.

C. Neutrophils

Traditionally, neutrophils have not been associated with the inflammatory response of asthma, although some evidence implicates them in both occupational asthma (Fabbri *et al.*, 1987) and the late-phase response of allergic asthma (Metzger *et al.*, 1987).

As with eosinophils, their initial recruitment involves the increased expression of endothelial adhesion molecules, including E-selectin and ICAM-1 (Kyan-Aung *et al.*, 1991), and they are influenced by a number of chemotactic factors such as C5a, LTB_4, PAF, and IL-8. Some of these factors—including C5a, LTB_4, and PAF—also have the capacity to prime neutrophils for enhanced mediator release. A number of other neutrophil chemotactic activities have been recognized in the serum and lavage fluid of patients with asthma. The molecular identity of these activities will, no doubt, be discovered, as was the newly described monocyte-derived neutrophil-activating peptide 2 (NAP-2) (Walz *et al.*, 1989). Activated neutrophils are capable of generating a number of mediators that might be relevant to the pathogenesis of asthma, including oxygen radicals, LTB_4, and various granule-derived enzymes such as myeloperoxidase.

Currently, however, the possible importance of neutrophils and of novel mediators such as IL-8 and NAP-2 in asthma remains unclear.

D. Basophils

Basophils once were considered to be circulating precursors of mast cells, but recently more emphasis has been placed on the differences between these two cells (Henderson, 1990). Like mast cells, however, basophils possess high-affinity IgE receptors and can be activated directly by allergen. Several "histamine releasing factors" also have been described, including NAP-2 (Kaplan *et al.*, 1991) and monocyte chemotactic activating factor (MCAF) (Kuna *et al.*, 1992). Once activated, basophils are capable of releasing a range of inflammatory mediators including histamine, LTB_4, LTC_4 (but not PGD_2), as well as various proteases.

A late increase in basophils has been demonstrated in bronchoalveolar lavage fluid after direct allergen challenge via the bronchoscope (Liu *et al.*, 1991). Evidence also exists from the upper airway to implicate basophils in the late-phase response (Bascom *et al.*, 1988). However, the true importance of this potential pro-inflammatory cell in asthma is unknown.

E. T Lymphocytes

An important advance has been our increasing knowledge about the role of T lymphocytes in initiating and prolonging the inflammatory response in asthmatic airways.

Evidence for the involvement of T lymphocytes in asthma derives from a number of sources. Increased numbers of T lymphocytes expressing activation markers (IL-2R VLA-1 and HLA-DR) (Corrigan *et al.*, 1988) and elevated levels of T-lymphocyte-derived cytokines (Corrigan and Kay, 1990) have been described in the blood of patients with acute severe asthma. Markers of T-lymphocyte activation also have been shown to be increased in bronchoalveolar lavage fluid (Mattoli *et al.*, 1991) and in bronchial biopsies (Azzawi *et al.*, 1990) from asthmatics.

Dendritic cells of macrophage lineage are present in large numbers within the bronchial epithelium (Holt *et al.*, 1990) and are responsible for processing antigen and presenting it to T lymphocytes in association with Class II major histocompatibility complex (MHC) determinants. This process may take place locally in the bronchial epithelium, but a more important site is probably local lymphoid tissue after migration of the dendritic cells to that location. Once activated, antigen-specific T lymphocytes undergo selective clonal expansion and proliferation.

In response to allergen challenge, $CD4^+$ T lymphocytes are recruited from the circulation over a period of 1–12 hr, a process again involving the up-regulation of endothelial adhesion molecules such as VCAM-1 and their interaction with cell-surface ligands. As discussed in the previous section, two types of $CD4^+$ T lymphocytes have been described in the mouse that differ in their pattern of cytokine secretion (Mosmann and Coffman, 1989). Comparable subsets are believed to exist in humans, and the Th2 subset is believed to be important in asthma. These cells express (in addition to IL-3 and GM-CSF) IL-4, IL-5, IL-6, and IL-10, cytokines that are important for regulation of IgE synthesis by B lymphocytes; for mast cell growth and differentiation; for eosinophil recruitment, survival, and activation; and, in the case of IL-10 (Fiorentino *et al.*, 1989), for inhibition of production of the Th1 subset cytokines, namely IL-2, interferon (IFN)γ, and lymphotoxin (LT). Th1 lymphocytes are believed to be involved in delayed type hypersensitivity, so a reciprocal relationship would appear to exist between this type of immune response and allergic inflammation.

F. Monocytes and Macrophages

Human airway macrophages are derived from circulating monocytes and normally are resident throughout the respiratory tract, both in the lumen and in the airway wall.

The ability of these cells to act as antigen-presenting cells is limited in comparison to that of dendritic cells and their main role in asthma seems to be as primary mediator-secreting cells after activation via their low-affinity IgE receptors. Increased release of macrophage products has indeed been demonstrated in bronchoalveolar lavage fluid from asthmatics after allergen challenge (Tonnel *et al.*, 1983). Increased numbers of macrophages also have been reported in bronchial biopsies from asthmatics (Poston *et al.*, 1992).

Activated macrophages are capable of generating numerous inflammatory mediators including oxygen radicals, leukotrienes, and PAF, as well as many enzymes such as β-glucuronidase. However, the relative importance of these molecules in comparision with mediators derived from other inflammatory cells is unclear. In addition, macrophages are a potential source of cytokines—both pro-inflammatory, such as IL-1 and TNFα, and fibrogenic, including platelet-derived growth factor (PDGF) and TGFβ.

Macrophages also may play a part in terminating the inflammatory response in a process known as apoptosis (Cohen, 1991). Aging neutrophils and eosinophils express specific cell-surface markers that are recognized by macrophages. This process is not well understood but appears to involve the macrophage vitronectin receptor and, perhaps, recognition of membrane phosphatidylserine. These granulocytes are phagocytosed and degraded. It is possible to speculate that in asthma, a defect in leuykocyte removal may contribute to the disease state.

G. Platelets and Platelet Activating Factor

During the 1980s, researchers suggested that platelets might have an important pro-inflammatory action in asthma via the production of PAF (Morley *et al.*, 1984). Inhalation of PAF by normal volunteers was reported to be capable of inducing not only acute bronchoconstriction but also a prolonged increase in bronchial responsiveness (Cuss *et al.*, 1986). Other studies, however, have been unable to confirm this result (Lai *et al.*, 1990). More recently, the PAF antagonist WEB 2086 failed to attenuate late-phase bronchoconstriction (Wilkens *et al.*, 1991) and also failed to demonstrate any evidence of therapeutic benefit (Johnston *et al.*, 1992). Despite its undoubted relevant biological actions, PAF now seems unlikely to play a central role in the inflammatory response of asthma.

H. Bronchial Epithelium

The bronchial epithelium is a major target for the inflammatory response of asthma. Many studies indicate that the bronchial epithelium in asthma is either disrupted or completely absent (Dunnill, 1960; Beasley *et al.*, 1989a; Jeffery *et al.*, 1989).

Under normal circumstances, the integrity of the epithelium is maintained by a variety of adhesive mechanisms (S. Montefort, J. Baker, W. R. Roche, and S. T. Holgate, in press). Tight junctions connect the suprabasal cells distally to form a selectively permeable barrier. Below these connections are intermediate junctions which contain adhesion molecules of the cadherin family, the most important of which is L-CAM or uvomorulin, connected intracellularly to actin filaments. Desmosomes connected the suprabasal cells to each other and to the basal cells. These junctions contain cadherin-like desmosomal glycoproteins or desmogleins linked to an intracellular plaque, made up of at least three desmosomal proteins or desmoplakins, which is itself attached to intracellular intermediate filaments composed of keratin. Finally, hemidesmosomes connect the basal epithelial cells to the basement membrane and contain the integrin $\alpha_6\beta_4$.

As discussed previously, the highly cationic proteins of the eosinophil granule are directly toxic to airway epithelial cells. However, a more subtle damaging effect might arise from an interaction between eosinophil and epithelial cells resulting in the induction of epithelial cell-derived proteases (Herbert *et al.,* 1991) such as collagenase, gelatinase, and stromolysin. These enzymes would have the capacity to break the desmosomal links, thereby releasing suprabasal cells from their attachment; indeed, such isolated clumps of suprabasal cells have been observed in bronchoalveolar lavage fluid from asthmatics (Montefort *et al.,* 1992).

The net result of this disruption is impairment of the ability of the epithelium to maintain homeostasis with respect to permeability. Using ^{99m}Tc-labeled DTPA clearance, increased epithelial permeability has been demonstrated both in stable asthmatics (Ilowite *et al.,* 1989) and during acute attacks (Urzua *et al.,* 1992). Clearly, this event will expose the airway to a range of environmental insults including viral infections and hyperosmolar stimuli provided by exercise.

Myofibroblast proliferation has been demonstrated beneath the epithelium in asthmatic airways (Brewster *et al.,* 1990). These cells may be important in prolonging the survival of both mast cells and eosinophils, thereby maintaining the chronicity of the response, and are also believed responsible for the deposition of collagen types III and V and fibronectin immediately below the basement membrane (Roche *et al.,* 1989; Figure 3). In longstanding poorly controlled asthma, this subepithelial fibrosis could contribute to the development of fixed airways obstruction.

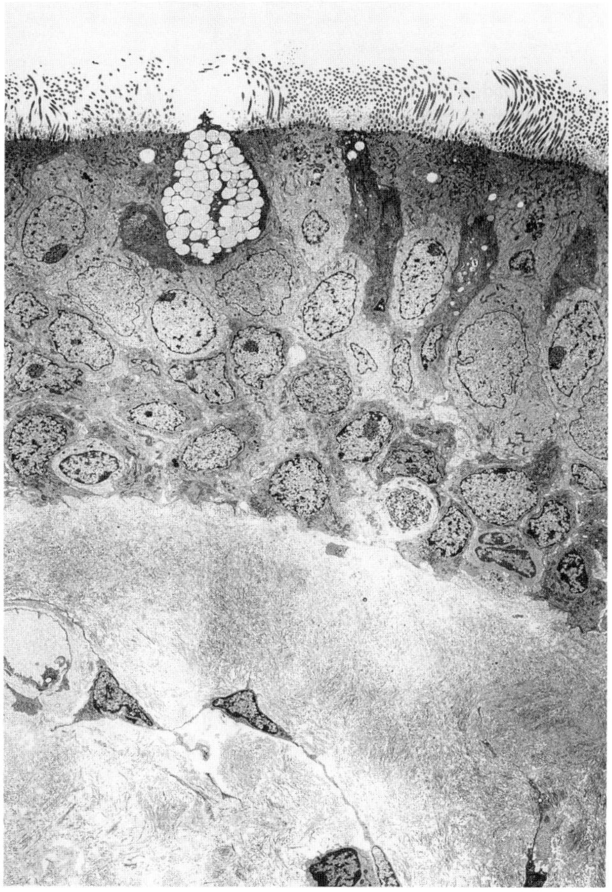

Figure 3 Electron micrograph showing subepithelial collagen deposition.

I. Smooth Muscle

Although recent attention has focused on underlying pathogenic mechanisms, contraction of airway smooth muscle still is of critical importance in producing airway obstruction, both during the early phase and, to a lesser extent, during the late-phase response.

Bronchial smooth muscle is clearly under autonomic control, allowing manipulation by bronchodilator drugs such as β-agonists and anticholinergics. However, this muscle is also under the influence of certain cytokines and growth factors. The actions of PDGF and TGFβ might account for the smooth muscle hypertrophy and hyperplasia that characterize persistent asthma. TNFα and IL-8 have been shown to be able to up-regulate the expression of substance P and muscarinic M3 receptors on airway smooth muscle, possibly contributing to the pathogenesis of bronchial hyperresponsiveness. A number of other mediators, including tryptase (Sekizawa *et al.,* 1989), also can increase airway smooth muscle responsiveness by a mechanism not currently understood.

J. Airway Nerves

Sensory nerve endings in the airway have been determined to contain many neuropeptides with important biological effects. These peptides can be released by the spread of nerve impulses antidromically along the nerve plexus in the airway wall, so these nonmyelinated C-fibers can cause neurogenic inflammation (Barnes, 1991). For example, calcitonin gene-related peptide (CGRP) and the related tachykinins substance P and neurokinin A (NKA) are all bronchoconstrictors. In addition, these molecules have actions on the microvasculature; CGRP is a particularly potent and long-lasting vasodilator whereas substance P and NKA increase microvascular permeability. Substance P is also a potent stimulus to mucus secretion and can activate inflammatory cells.

Direct evidence for the involvement of neurogenic inflammation in asthma has been obtained only recently. After allergen challenge, for example, the airway response to inhaled bradykinin, which mediates its effects through stimulation of C-fibers, is increased by several orders of magnitude in comparison with the 2- to 3-fold enhancement observed for methacholine (DjuKanovic *et al.,* 1992), suggesting that, in response to allergen challenge, a change occurs in the sensitivity of the afferent nerves so they respond to lower concentrations of bradykinin.

Nerve growth factors released by T lymphocytes or other inflammatory cells could lead to proliferation of neuropeptide-containing nerves, which might explain why a component of bronchial hyperresponsiveness in chronic asthma appears to be relatively resistant to resolution by

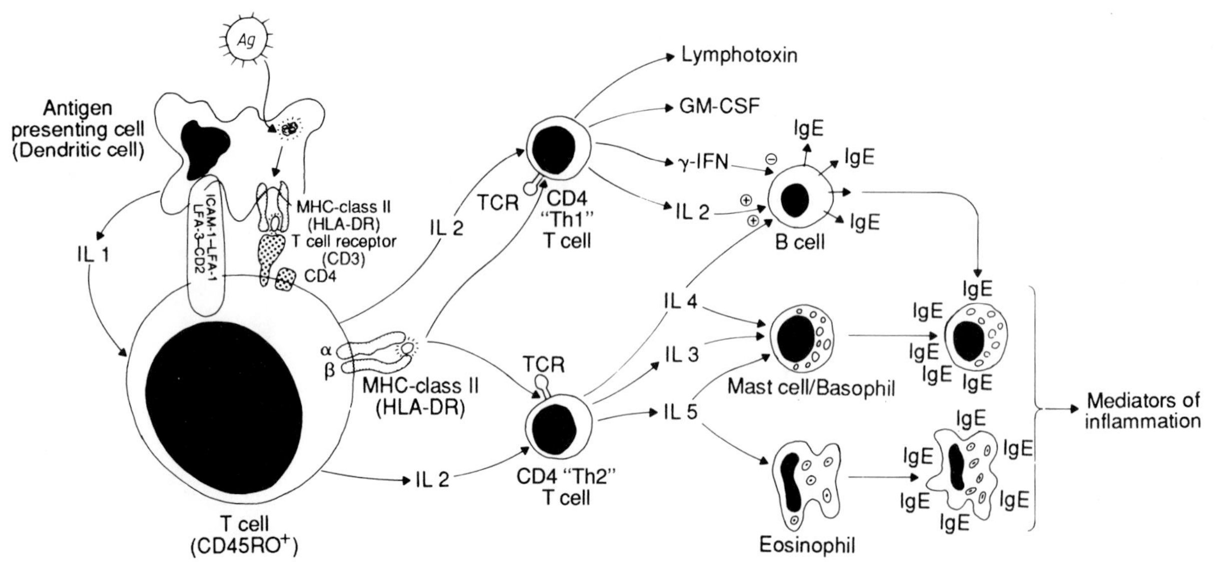

Figure 4 Network of cellular interactions occuring in allergic inflammation.

corticosteroids (Lundgren *et al.*, 1988). However, currently our understanding of the importance of neuropeptides and neurogenic inflammation in asthma is still at an early stage.

K. Clinical Implications

Figure 4 shows how the various inflammatory cells in asthma are thought to interact via the generation of cytokines. T lymphocytes are involved centrally through the secretion of cytokines that are responsible for isotype switching of B lymphocytes to make IgE and that have specific activities for mast cells and eosinophils. However, asthma is more than simple inflammation involving mast cells and eosinophils since nerves, smooth muscle, and myofibroblasts are all also important in the response.

Using this diagram as a framework, we can consider the actions of the various anti-asthma drugs. β-Agonists, as powerful bronchodilators and inhibitors of mast cell function, attenuate the early bronchconstrictor response to allergen challenge but have relatively little effect on the late-phase response (Cockcroft and Murdock, 1987). In contrast, corticosteroids and cyclosporin down-regulate cytokine expression by T lymphocytes, which in turn leads to a decrease in mast cell and eosinophil numbers. Finally, sodium cromoglycate (Holgate, 1989) and nedocromil sodium, long recognized as mass cell stabilizers, now are known to have additional effects on various other cell types.

Clearly, with our improved knowledge about the mucosal immune system and how it becomes disturbed in asthma, real advances are now being made, not only in understanding the nature of this disease but also in providing opportunities for novel therapeutic strategies designed to intervene in the inflammatory cascade in a more specific manner than currently possible.

Acknowledgments

The authors wish to thank William Roche and David A. Goulding for kindly supplying the electron micrographs used in this manuscript.

References

Akbar, A. N., Terry, L., Timms, A., Beverley, P., and Janossy, G. (1988). Loss of CD45R and gain of UCHL1 reactivity is a feature of primed T-cells. *J. Immunol.* **140,** 2171–2178.

Atkins, P. C., Norman, M. E., and Zweiman, B. (1978). Antigen-induced neutrophil chemotactic activity in man: Correlation with bronchospasm and inhibition by disodium chromoglycate. *J. Allergy Clin. Immunol.* **52,** 149–155.

Augustin, A., Kibo, R. T., and Sim, G. K. (1989). Resident pulmonary lymphocytes expressing the gamma/delta T-cell receptor. *Nature (London)* **340,** 238–241.

Azzawi, M., Bradley, B., Jeffery, P. K., Frew, A. J., Wardlaw, A. J., Knowles, G., Assoufi, B., Collins, J. V., Durhams, S., and Kay, A. B. (1990). Identification of activated T-lymphocytes in bronchial biopsies in stable asthma. *Am. Rev. Respir. Dis.* **142,** 1407–1413.

Barnes, P. J. (1991). Neurogenic inflammation in airways. *Int. Arch. Allergy Appl. Immunol.* **94,** 303–309.

Bascom, R., Wachs, M., Naclerio, R. M., Pipkorn, U., Galli, S., and Lichtenstein, L. M. (1988). Basophil influx occurs after nasal antigen challenge: Effects of topical corticosteroid pretreatment. *J. Allergy Clin. Immunol.* **81,** 580–589.

Beasley, R., Roche, W. R., Roberts, J. A.,. and Holgate, S. T. (1989a). Cellular events in the bronchi in mild asthma and after bronchial provocation. *Am. Rev. Respir. Dis.* **139,** 806–817.

Beasley, R. C. W., Featherstone, R. L., Church, M. K., Rafferty, P., Varley, J. G., Harris, A., Robinson, C., and Holgate, S. T. (1989b). Effect of a thromboxane antagonist on PGD_2- and allergen-induced broncho constriction. *J. Appl. Physiol.* **66,** 1685–1693.

Bentley, A. M., Durham, S. R., Robinson, D. S., Cromwell, O., Kay, A. B., and Wardlaw, A. J. (1992). Expression of the endothelial and leucocyte adhesion molecules ICAM-1, E-selectin and VCAM-1 in the bronchial mucosa in steady state asthma and allergen induced asthma. *Thorax* **47,** 852.

Bevilacqua, M. P., Stengelin, S., Gimbrone, M. A., and Seed, B. (1989). Endothelial leukocyte adhesion molecule 1: An inducible receptor for neutrophils related to complement regulatory proteins and lectins. *Science* **243,** 1160–1165.

Bland, P. W., and Warren, L. G. (1986). Antigen presentation by epithelial cells of the rat small intestine. II. Selective induction of suppressor T-cells. *Immunology* **58,** 9–14.

Bochner, B. S., Luscinskas, F. W., Gimbrone, Jr., M. A., Newman, W., Sterbinsky, S. A., Derse-Anthony, C. P., Klunk, D., and Schleimer, R. P. (1991). Adhesion of human basophils, eosinophils, and neutrophils to interleukin 1-activated human vascular endothelial cells: Contribution of endothelial cell adhesion molecules. *J. Exp. Med.* **173,** 1553–1556.

Bradding, P., Feather, I. H., Howarth, P. H., Mueller, R., Roberts, J. A., Britten, K., Bews, J. P. A., Hunt, T. C., Okayama, Y., Heusser, C. H., Bullock, G. R., Church, M. K., and Holgate, S. T. (1992). Interleukin 4 is localised to and released by human mast cells. *J. Exp. Med.* **176,** 1381–1386.

Brandtzaeg, P., Halstensen, T., Keh, K., Urajci, P., Kuale, D., Rognum, T. O., Scott, H., and Sollid, L. M. (1989). Immunobiology and immunopathology of human gut mucosa: Humoral immunity and intraepithelial lymphocytes. *Gastroenterology* **97,** 1562–1584.

Brewster, C. E. P., Howarth, P. H., Djukanovic, R., Wilson, J., Holgate, S. T., and Roche, W. R. (1990). Myofibroblasts and supepithelial fibrosis in bronchial asthma. *Am. J. Resp. Cell Mol. Biol.* **3,** 507–511.

Burd, P. R., Rogers, H. W., Gordon, J. R., Martin, C. A., Jayaraman, S., Wilson, S. D., Dvorak, A. M., Galli, S. J., and Dorf, M. E. (1989). Interleukin 3-dependent and -independent mast cells stimulated with IgE and antigen express multiple cytokines. *J. Exp. Med.* **170,** 245–247.

Casale, T. B., Wood, D., Richerson, H. B., Trapp, S., Metzger, W. J., Zavala, D., and Hunninghake, G. W. (1987). Elevated bronchoalveolar lavage fluid histamine levels in allergic asthmatics are associated with methacholine bronchial hyper responsiveness. *J. Clin. Invest.* **79,** 1197–1203.

Cerf-Bensussan, N., Jarry, A., Brousse, N., Lisowska-Grospierre, B., Guy-Grand, D., and Griscelli, C. (1987). A monoclonal antibody HML-1 defining a novel membrane molecule present on human intestinal lymphocytes. *Eur. J. Immunol.* **17,** 1279–1285.

Cherayil, B. J., Weiner, S. J., and Pillai, S. (1989). The Mac-2 antigen is a galactose-specific lectin that binds IgE. *J. Exp. Med.* **170,** 1959–1972.

Choy, M. Y., Richman, P. I., Horton, M. A., and MacDonald, T. T. (1990). Expression of the VLA family of integrins in human intestine. *J. Pathol* **160,** 35–40.

Cockroft, D. W., and Murdock, K. Y. (1987). Comparative effects of inhaled salbutamol, sodium cromoglycate, and beclomethasone dipropionate on allergen-induced early asthmatic responses, late asthmatic responses and increased bronchial responsiveness to histamine. *J. Allergy Clin. Immunol.* **79,** 734–740.

Cohen, J. J. (1991). Programmed cell death in the immune system. *Adv. Immunol.* **50,** 55–85.

Corrigan, C. J., and Kay, A. B. (1990). CD4 T-lymphocyte activation in acute severe asthma. Relationship to disease activity and atopic status. *Am. Rev. Respir. Dis.* **141,** 970–977.

Corrigan, C. J., Hartnell, A., and Kay, A. B. (1988). T-lymphocyte activation in acute severe asthma. *Lancet* **1,** 1129–1132.

Cuss, F. M., Dixon, C. M. J., and Barnes, P. J. (1986). Effect of inhaled platelet activating factor on pulmonary function and bronchial responsiveness in man. *Lancet* **2,** 189–192.

Desreumaux, P., Janin, A., Colombel, J. F., Prin, L., Plumas, J., Emilie, D., Torpier, G., Capron, A., and Capron, M. (1992). Interleukin 5 messenger RNA expression by eosinophils in the intestinal mucosa of patients with coeliac disease. *J. Exp. Med.* **175,** 293–296.

Djukanovic, R., Polosa, R., and Holgate, S. T. (1991). The effect of bronchial allergen challenge on methacholine (MCh) and bradykinin (BK) airway responsiveness. *Eur. Respir. J.* **4 Suppl. 14,** 340s.

Dunnill, M. S. (1960). The pathology of asthma with special reference changes in the bronchial mucosa. *J. Clin. Pathol.* **13,** 27–33.

Dunnill, M. S., Massarella, G. R., and Anderson, J. A. (1969). A comparison of the quantitative anatomy of the bronchi in normal subjects, in status asthmaticus, in chronic bronchitis and in emphysema. *Thorax* **24,** 176–179.

Fabbri, L. M., Boschetto, P., Zocca, E., Milani, G., Pivirotto, F., Plebani, M., Burlina, A., Licata, B., and Mapp, C. E. (1987). Bronchoalveolar neutrophilia during late asthmatic reactions induced by toluene diisocyanate. *Am. Rev. Respir. Dis.* **136,** 36–42.

Ferrer, J. M., Plaza, A., Kreisler, M., and Diaz-Espada, F. (1992). Differential interleukin secretion by *in vitro* activated human CD45TA and CD45RO CD4+ T-cell subsets. *Cell. Immunol.* **141,** 10–20.

Finnerty, J. P., and Holgate, S. T. (1990). Evidence for the roles of histamine and prostaglandins as mediators in exercise-induced asthma: The inhibitory effects of terfenadine and flurbiprofen alone and in combination. *Eur. Resp. J.* **3,** 540–547.

Fiorentino, D. F., Bond, M. W., and Mosmann, T. R. (1989). Two types of mouse T helper cells. IV. Th_2 clones secrete a factor that inhibits cytokine production by Th_1 clones. *J. Exp. Med.* **170,** 65–80.

Frew, A. S., and Kay, A. B. (1991). UCHL1+ (CD45RO+) 'memory' T-cells predominate in the CD4+ cellular infiltrate associated with allergen-induced late-phase skin reactions in the atopic subjects. *Clin. Exp. Immunol.* **84,** 270–274.

Hamid, Q., Barkans, J., Meng, Q., Ying, S., Abrams, J. S., Kay, A. B., and Moqbel, R. (1992). Human eosinophils synthesize and secrete interluekin-6, in vitro. *Blood* **80,** 1496–1501.

Harvey, J., and Jones, D. B. (1991). Human mucosal T-lymphocyte and macrophage sub-populations in normal and inflamed intestine. *Clin. Exp. Allergy* **21,** 549–560.

Harvey, J., Jones, D. B., and Wright, D. H. (1990). Differential expression of MHC- and macrophage-associated antigens in human fetal and post-natal small intestine. *Immunology* **69,** 409–415.

Henderson, W. R. (1990). Basophils. *Immunol. Allergy Clin. North Am.* **10,** 273–282.

Herbert, C. A., Edwards, D., Boot, J. R., and Robinson, C. (1991). *In vitro* modulation of the eosinophil-dependent enhancement of the permeability of the bronchial epithelium. *Br. J. Pharmacol.* **104,** 391–398.

Holgate, S. T. (1989). Reflections on the mechanism(s) of action of sodium cromoglycate (Intal) and the role of mast cells in asthma. *Respir. Med. (Suppl.)* **83,** 231–254.

Holt, P. G., Schon-Hegrad, M. A., Oliver, J., Holt, B. J., and McMenamin, P. G. (1990). A contiguous network of dendritic antigen-presenting cells within the respiratory epithelium. *Int. Arch. Allergy Appl. Immunol.* **91,** 155–159.

Hui, K. P., and Barnes, N. C. (1991). Lung function improvement in asthma with a cysteinyl-leukotriene receptor antagonist. *Lancet* **337,** 1062–1063.

Ilowite, J. J., Bennett, W. D., Sheetz, M. J., Groth, M. L., and Nierman, D. M. (1989). Permeability of the bronchial mucosa to 99m-Tc DTPA in asthma. *Am. Rev. Respir. Dis.* **139,** 1139–1143.

Janeway, C. A. (1988). Frontiers of the immune system. *Nature (London)* **333,** 804–806.

Janossy, G., Tidman, N., Papageorgion, E. S., Kung, P. C., and Goldstein, G. (1981). Distribution of human T-cell lymphocyte subsets in the human bone marrow and thymus, an analysis with monoclonal antibodies. *J. Immunol.* **126,** 1608.

Jeffery, P. K., Wardlaw, A. J., Nelson, F. C., Colins, J. V., and Kay, A. B. (1989). Bronchial biopsies in asthma—An ultrastructural, quantitative study and correlation with hyperreactivity. *Am. Rev. Respir. Dis.* **140,** 1745–1753.

Johnston, S., Spence, D., Calverley, P., Winter, J., Dhillon, P., Winning, A., Ramhamadany, E., Higgins, C., Turner, S., and Holgate, S. (1992). WEB 2086, a PAF antagonist, has no steroid-sparing effect in asthmatics requiring inhaled corticosteroids. *Thorax* **47,** 871p.

Kaplan, A. P., Baeza, M., Reddigari, S., and Kuna, P. (1991). Histamine-releasing factors. *Int. Arch. Allergy Appl. Immunol.* **94,** 148–153.

Kaushansky, K., Lin, N., and Adamson, J. W. (1988). Interleukin-1 stimulates fibroblasts to synthesise granulocyte/macrophage and granulocyte colony-stimulating factors. *J. Clin. Invest* **81,** 92–97.

Kita, H., Ohnishi, T., Okubo, Y., Weiler, D., Abrams, J. S., and Gleich, G. J. (1991). Granulocyte/macrophage colony-stimulating factor and interleukin 3 release from human peripheral blood eosinophils and neutrophils. *J. Exp. Med.* **174,** 745–748.

Kuna, P., Reddigari, S. R., Rucinski, D., Oppenheim, J. J., and Kaplan, A. P. (1992). Monocyte chemotactic and activating factor is a potent histamine-releasing factor for human basophils. *J. Exp. Med.* **175,** 489–493.

Kyan-Aung, U., Haskard, D. O., Poston, R. N., Thornhill, M. H., and Lee, T. H. (1991). Endothelial leukocyte adhesion molecule-1 and intercellular adhesion molecule-1 mediate the adhesion of eosinophils to endothelial cells in vitro and are expressed by endothelium in allergic cutaneous inflammation in vivo. *J. Immunol.* **146,** 521–528.

Lai, C. K. W., Jenkins, J. R., Polosa, R. J., and Holgate, S. T. (1990). Inhaled PAF fails to induce airway hyper-responsiveness in normal human subjects. *J. Appl. Physiol.* **68,** 919–926.

Lam, S., Chan, H., Le Riche, J. C., Chan-Yeung, M., and Salari, H. (1988). Release of leukotrienes in patients with bronchial asthma. *J. Allergy Clin. Immunol.* **81,** 711–717.

Liu, M. C., Hubbard, W. C., Proud, D., Stealey, B. A., Galli, S. J., Kagey-Sobotka, A., Bleecker, E. R., and Lichtenstein, L. M. (1991). Immediate and late inflammatory responses to ragweed antigen challenge of the peripheral airways in allergic asthmatics. *Am. Rev. Respir. Dis.* **144,** 51–58.

Lopez, A. F., Sanderson, C. J., Gamble, J. R., Campbell, H. D., Young, I. G., and Vadas, M. A. (1988). Recombinant human interleukin 5 is a selective activator of human eosinophil function. *J. Exp. Med.* **167,** 219–224.

Lundgren, R., Soderberg, M., Horstedt, P., and Stenling, R. (1988). Morphological studies of bronchial mucosal biopsies from asthmatics before and after ten years of treatment with inhaled steroids. *Eur. Respir. J.* **1,** 883–889.

McFadden, E. R. (1987). Exercise-induced asthma. Assessment of current etiologic concepts. *Chest* **915,** 1515–1575.

Mahida, Y. R., Patel, S., Gionchetti, P., Vaux, D., and Jewell, D. P. (1989). Macrophage sub-populations in the lamina propria of normal and inflamed colon and terminal ileum. *Gut* **30,** 826–834.

Manning, P. J., Watson, R. M., Margolskee, D. J., Williams, V. C., Schwartz, J. I., and O'Byrne, P. M. (1990). Inhibition of exercise-induced broncho-constriction by MK-571, a potent leukotriene D_4 receptor antagonist. *N. Engl. J. Med.* **32,** 1736–1739.

Mattoli, S., Mattoso, V. L., Soloperto, M., Allegra, L., and Fasoli, A. (1991). Cellular and biochemical characteristics of bronchoalveolar lavage fluid in symptomatic nonallergic asthma. *J. Allergy Clin. Immunol.* **87,** 794–802.

Mayer, L., and Schlein, R. (1987). Evidence for function of Ia molecules on gut epithelial cells in man. *J. Exp. Med.* **166,** 1471–1483.

Metzger, W. J., Zavala, D., Richerson, H. B., Moseley, P., Iwamota, P., Monick, M., Sjoerdsma, K., and Hunninghake, G. W. (1987). Local allergen challenge and bronchoaveolar lavage of allergic asthmatic lungs. Description of the model and local airway inflammation. *Am. Rev. Respir. Dis.* **135,** 433–440.

Miadonna, A., Tedeschi, A., Brasca, C., Folco, G., and Sala, A. (1990). Mediator release after endobronchial challenge in patients with respiratory allergy. *J. Allergy Clin. Immunol.* **85,** 906–913.

Montefort, S., Roberts, J. A., Beasley, R., Holgate, S. T., and Roche, W. R. (1992). The site of disruption of the bronchial epithelium in asthmatic and non-asthmatic subjects. *Thorax* **47,** 499–503.

Moqbel, R., Hamid, Q., Ying, S., Barkans, J., Hartnell, A., Tsicopoulos, A., Wardlaw, A. J., and Kay, A. B. (1991). Expression of mRNA and immunoreactivity for the granulocyte/macrophage colony-stimulating factor in activated human eosinophils. *J. Exp. Med.* **174,** 749–752.

Morley, J., Sanjar, S., and Page, C. P. (1984). The platelet in asthma. *Lancet* **2,** 1142–1144.

Mosmann, T. R., and Coffman, R. L. (1989). Th_1 and TH_2 cells: Different patterns of lymphocyte secretion lead to different functional properties. *Annu. Rev. Immunol.* **7,** 145–173.

Murray, J. J., Tonnel, A. B., Brash, A. R., Roberts, L. J., Gosset, P., Workman, R., Capron, A., and Oates, J. A. (1986). Release of prostaglandins D2 into human airways during acute antigen challenge. *N. Engl. J. Med.* **315,** 800–804.

Ohkawara, Y., Yamauchi, K., Tanno, Y., Tamura, G., Ohtani, H., Nagura, H., Ohkuda, K., and Takishima, T. (1992). Human lung mast cells and pulmonary macrophages produce tumor necrosis factor-α in sensitized lung tissue after IgE receptor triggering. *Am. J. Respir. Cell Mol. Biol.* **7,** 385–392.

Ohno, I., Lea, R. G., Flanders, K. C., Clark, D. A., Banwatt, D., Dolovich, J., Denburg, J., Harley, C. B., Gauldie, J., and Jordana, M. (1992). Eosinophils in chronically inflamed human upper airway tissues express transforming growth factor β1 gene (TGFβ1). *J. Clin. Invest* **89,** 1662–1668.

Owen, Jr., W. F., Rothenberg, M. E., Silberstein, D. S., Gasson, J. C., Stevens, R. L., Austen, K. F., and Soberman, R. J. (1987). Regulation of human eosinophil viability, density and function by granulocyte/macrophage colony-stimulating factor in the presence of 3T3 fibroblasts. *J. Exp. Med.* **166,** 129–141.

Plaut, M., Pierce, J. H., Watson, C. J., Hanley-Hide, J., Nordan, R. P., and Paul, W. E. (1989). Mast cells produce lymphokines in response to cross-linkage of FcεR1 or to calcium ionophores. *Nature (London)* **339,** 64–67.

Pober, J. S., Gimbrone, Jr., M. A., Lapieree, L. A., Mendrick, D. L., Fiers, W., Rothlein, R., and Springer, T. A. (1986). Overlapping patterns of activation of human endothelial cells by interleukin 1, tumour necrosis factor, and immune interferon. *J. Immunol.* **137,** 1893–1896.

Poston, R. N., Chanez, P., Lacoste, J. Y., Lichfield, T., Lee, T. H., and Bousquet, J. (1992). Immunohistochemical characterization of the cellular infiltration in asthmatic bronchi. *Am. Rev. Respir. Dis.* **145,** 918–921.

Rafferty, P., Beasley, C. R., and Holgate, S. T. (1987). The contribution of histamine to bronchoconstriction produced by inhaled allergen and adenosine 5 monophosphate in asthma. *Am. Rev. Respir. Dis.* **136,** 369–373.

Rafferty, P., Jackson, L., Smith, R., and Holgate, S. T. (1990). Terfenadine, a potent histamine H1 antagonist in the treatment of grass pollen sensitive asthma. *Br. J. Clin. Pharmacol.* **50,** 220–235.

Rand, T. H., Silberstein, D. S., Kornfeld, H., and Weller, P. F. (1991a). Human eosinophils express functional interleukin 2 receptors. *J. Clin. Invest.* **88,** 825–832.

Rand, T. H., Cruikshank, W. W., Center, D. M., and Weller, P. F. (1991b). CD4-mediated stimulation of human eosinophils: Lymphocyte chemoattractant factor and other CD4-binding ligands elicit eosinophil migration. *J. Exp. Med.* **173,** 1521–1528.

Robinson, D. S., Hamid, Q., Ying, S., Tsicopoulos, A., Barkans, J., Bentley, A. M., Corrigan, C., Durham, S. R., and Kay, A. B. (1992). Predominant TH2-like bronchoalveolar T-lymphocyte population in atopic asthma. *N. Engl. J. Med.* **326,** 298–304.

Robinson, M. A. (1991). The human T-cell receptor beta-chain gene complex contains at least 57 variable gene segments. *J. Immunol.* **146,** 4392–4397.

Roche, W. R., Beasley, R., Williams, J. H., and Holgate, S. T. (1989). Subepithelial fibrosis in the bronchi of asthmatics. *Lancet* **1,** 520–524.

Rothenberg, M. E., Owen, Jr, W. F., Silberstein, D. S., Woods, J., Soberman, R. J., Austen, K. R., and Stavens, R. L. (1988). Human eosinophils have prolonged survival, enhanced functional properties, and become hypodense when exposed to human interleukin 3. *J. Clin Invest* **81,** 1986–1992.

Schieferdecker, H. L., Ulrich, B., Weiss-Breckwoldt, A. N., Schwarting, R., Stein, H., Reicken, E. D., and Zeitz, M. (1990). The HML-1 antigen of intestinal lymphocytes is an activation antigen. *J. Immunol.* **144,** 2541–2549.

Sekizawa, K., Caughey, G. H., Lazarus, S. C., Gold, W. M., and Nadel, J. A. (1989). Mast cell tryptase causes airway smooth muscle hyper-responsiveness in dogs. *J. Clin. Invest.* **83,** 175–179.

Selby, W. S., Janossy, G., and Jewell, D. P. (1981). Immunohistological characterization of the intraepithelial lymphocytes of the human gastrointestinal tract. *Gut* **22,** 169–176.

Selby, W. S., Janossy, G., Bofill, M., and Jewell, D. P. (1983). Lymphocyte populations in the human small intestine. The findings in normal mucosa and in the mucosa of patients with adult coeliac disease. *Clin. Exp. Immunol.* **52,** 219–228.

Smith, C. W., Rothlein, R., Hughes, B. J., Mariscalco, M. M., Rudloff, H. E., Schmalstieg, F. C., and Anderson, D. C. (1988). Recognition of an endothelial determinant for CD18-dependent human neutrophil adherence and transendothelial migration. *J. Clin. Invest* **82,** 1746–1756.

Spencer, J., MacDonald, T. T., Diss, T. C., Walker-Smith, J. A., Ciclitira, P. J., and Isaacson, P. G. (1989a). Changes in intraepithelial lymphocyte sub-populations in coeliac disease and enteropathy-associated T-cell lymphoma (malignant histiocytosis of the intestine). *Gut* **30,** 339–346.

Spencer, J., Isaacson, P. G., Diss, T. C., and MacDonald, T. (1989b). Expression of disulfide-linked and non-disulfide-linked forms of the T cell receptor γ/δ heterodimer in human intestinal intraepithelial lymphocytes.

Spiteri, M. A., and Poulter, L. W. (1991). Characterization of immune inducer and suppressor macrophages from the normal human lung. *Clin. Exp. Immunol.* **83,** 157–162.

Tai, P.-C., Sun, L., and Spry, C. J. F. (1991). Effects of IL-5, granulocyte/macrophage colony-stimulating factor (GM-CSF) and IL-3 on the survival of human blood eosinophilis in vitro. *Clin. Exp. Immunol.* **85,** 312–316.

Taylor, I. K., O'Shaughnessy, K. M., Fuller, R. W., and Dollery, C. T. (1991). Effect of a cysteinyl-leukotriene antagonist ICI204.219 on allergen-induced broncho-constriction and airway hyperresponsiveness in atopic subjects. *Lancet* **337,** 690–694.

Tomassini, M., Tsicopoulos, A., Tai, P. C., Gruart, V., Tonnel, A. B., Prin, L., Capron, A., and Capron, M. (1991). Release of granule proteins by eosinophils from allergic and non-allergic patients with eosinophilia on immunoglobulin-dependent activation. *J. Allergy Clin. Immunol.* **88,** 365–375.

Tonnel, A. B., Gosset, Ph., Joseph, M., Fournier, E., and Capron, A. (1983). Stimulation of alveolar macrophages in asthmatic patients after local provocation test. *Lancet* **1,** 1406–1408.

Trejdosiwicz, L. K., Maliza, G., Badr-el-Dan, S., Smart, C. J., Oaks, D. J., and Southgate, J. (1987). T-cell and mononuclear phagocyte populations of the human small and large intestine. *Adv. Exp. Med. Biol.* **216A,** 465–473.

Trejdosiewicz, L. K., Smart, C. J., Oakes, D. J., Howdle, P. G., Malizioi, G., and Campana, D. (1989). Expression of T-cell receptors TCR1 (gamma-delta) and TCR2 (alpha-beta) in human intestinal mucosa. *Immunology* **68,** 7–12.

Tseng, J. (1984). Re-population of the gut lamina propria with IgA-containing cells by lymphoid cells isolated from the gut lamina propria. *Eur. J. Immunol* **14,** 420–425.

Urzua, G., Barritault, L., Huchon, G. J., Lemarchand, P., Chinet, T., and Collignon, M. (1992). Bronchial clearance of DTPA is increased in acute asthma but not in chronic asthma. *Am. Rev. Respir. Dis.* **145,** 147–152.

Walz, A., Deward, B., von Tscharner, V., and Baggiolini, M. (1989). Effects of the neutrophil-activating peptide NAP-2, platelet basic protein, connective tissue-activating peptide III, and platelet factor 4 on human neutrophils. *J. Exp. Med.* **170,** 1745–1750.

Wenzel, S. E., Fowler III, A. A., and Shwartz, L. B. (1988). Activation of pulmonary mast cells by bronchoalveolar challenge. In vivo release of histamine and tryptase in atopic subjects with and without asthma. *Am. Rev. Rspir. Dis.* **137,** 1002–1006.

Wilkens, H., Wilkens, J. H., Bosse, S., Kempe, F., Fritz, S., Frolich, J. C., and Fabel, H. (1991). Effects of an inhaled PAF-antagonist (WEB 2086 BS) on allergen-induced early and late asthmatic responses and increased bronchial responsiveness to methacholine. *Am. Rev. Respir. Dis.* **143,** A812.

Woodnar-Filipowicz, A., Heusser, C., and Moroni, C. (1989). Production of the haematopoietic growth factors GM-CSF and interleukin-3 by mast cells in response to IgE receptor-mediated activation. *Nature* (*London*) **339,** 150–152.

Wong, D. T. W., Elovic, A., Matossian, K., Nagura, N., McBride, J., Chou, M. Y., Gordon, J. R., Rand, T. H., Galli, S. J., and Weller, P. F. (1991). Eosinophils from patients with blood eosinophilia express transforming growth factor $\beta 1$. *Blood* **78,** 2702–2707.

Wong, D. T. W., Weller, P. F., Galli, S. J., Elovic, A., Rand, T. H., Gallagher, G. T., Chiang, T., Chou, M. Y., Matossian, K., McBride, J., and Todd, R. (1990). Human eosinophils express transforming growth factor α. *J. Exp. Med.* **172,** 673–681.

Yamada, A., Kaneyuki, T., Hara, A., Rothstein, D. M., and Yokoyama, M. M. (1992). CD45 isoform expression on human neonatal T-cells: Expression and turnover of CD45 isoforms on neonatal versus adult T-cells after activation. *Cell. Immunol.* **142,** 114–124.

45

Respiratory Infections

Robert C. Welliver

I. INTRODUCTION

The respiratory tract is the primary site of entry for numerous microbial pathogens. Many agents initiate replication events on the respiratory mucosa, leading to eventual systemic spread, without producing any clinical disease locally. In other cases, the respiratory tract is the principal target organ of the disease-producing microbe (Table I). Colonization of the respiratory tract with a potentially infectious organism represents a situation in which the invasiveness or virulence of the organism is opposed by local or systemic immunity. In most cases, little or no clinical illness occurs and some persistent immunity may develop, even in the absence of clinically evident infection. Clinical illness apparently results from infection of the uniquely susceptible host, or inoculation with an organism in sufficent quantity or with sufficient virulence to overcome the natural or acquired immunity of the host.

In the United States, upper respiratory tract infections are a common nuisance, representing the most frequent reason for seeking medical attention and disrupting lifestyles by requiring absence from school or employment. Lower respiratory tract infections are relatively uncommon and are usually only life-threatening at the extremes of age. In contrast, in developing countries, respiratory tract infections are second only to gastrointestinal infections as the leading cause of death in infants and children in the first few years of life.

This chapter summarizes the clinical features of viral, bacterial, and mycobacterial infections of the respiratory tract. In addition, the contribution of the immune system to recovery from the infection as well as its role in the pathogenesis of the disease is described.

II. EPIDEMIOLOGY OF COMMON RESPIRATORY INFECTIONS

Although numerous viruses can result in minor upper respiratory infections, respiratory syncytial virus (RSV) and influenza virus account for the most severe infections in infants and adults, respectively. An estimated 50% of infants in the first year of life acquire RSV infection during their first epidemic exposure; 1–2% of all infants will be admitted to a hospital in the first year of life for lower respiratory disease caused by RSV infection (Beem *et al.*, 1934; Clarke *et al.*, 1978). Influenza viruses cause yearly outbreaks of respiratory illness of varying severity. During 10-wk epidemic periods in 1982 and 1983, approximately 2500 hospitalizations for acute respiratory disease occurred in the Houston area (Glezen *et al.*, 1987). Weekly tabulations of deaths from pneumonia and influenza from large United States cities permit an accurate estimation of influenza virus activity in the community. Reported deaths in excess of expected thresholds correlate well with the occurrence of widespread influenza activity (Langmuir and Housworth, 1969; Glezen *et al.*, 1982). Mortality from infection with each of these agents is most common in individuals with pre-existing heart or lung disease or other underlying illnesses, or in the elderly (Eickhoff *et al.*, 1961; McDonald *et al.*, 1982; Groothuis *et al.*, 1988). *Streptococcus pneumoniae* is the leading cause of otitis media in children, is a major cause of mortality due to pneumonia in infants and the elderly, and is still a common cause of overwhelming bacterial sepsis and meningitis (Austrian and Golb, 1964; Klein, 1981). Tuberculosis, however, probably has accounted for more chronic respiratory illness than any infectious agent, particularly since the era of urbanization and industrialization in the 18th and 19th centuries (Dubos and Dubos, 1952).

III. VIRAL INFECTIONS

An impressive amount of information has been gathered concerning the role of the immune system in influenza and RSV infections with respect to mechanisms of eradication of primary infection, pathogenesis of severe disease, and prevention of reinfection (Table II). A review of the immune response to infection with these specific agents provides an overall perspective that probably can be applied to infection with other viral agents.

A. Respiratory Syncytial Virus

1. Clinical Presentation

RSV is the major cause of serious lower respiratory disease in infancy and early childhood. An estimated 28 episodes of lower respiratory disease caused by RSV occur for every 100 children followed through the first 12 months of life. Reinfections in the second year of life are extremely common

Table I Pathogens Associated with Different Forms of Respiratory Illness[a]

Form of illness	Pathogen							
	Rhinovirus	Influenza virus	Respiratory syncytial virus	Parainfluenza virus	Adenovirus	*Streptococcus pyogenes*	*Streptococcus pneumoniae*	*Staphylococcus aureus*
Upper respiratory illness	+ + +	+ +	+ +	+ +	+	0	0	0
Pharyngitis	+	+ +	+	+	+ +	+ + +	0	0
Croup	0	+	+	+ + +	+	0	0	0
Bronchiolitis or "infectious asthma"	+ +	+	+ + +	+ +	+	0	0	0
Pneumonia	+	+	+ +	+	+ +	+	+ + +	+

[a] 0, Little or no causal relationship to disease at this site; +, occasional relationship; + +, frequent relationship; + + +, very common relationship.

and occur with some frequency at all ages (Glezen *et al.*, 1986). Therefore, although most individuals develop relatively mild symptoms at the time of RSV infection, certain individuals seem more prone to develop lower respiratory illness (in particular, bronchiolitis) at the time of RSV infection. The fact that bronchiolitis (as well as croup) can be seen with a wide variety of viral agents suggests that the development of these illnesses is not entirely specific to any feature of RSV, but to a similar feature of a variety of viruses as well as to some unique host component.

Inoculation of RSV occurs through the nasal mucosal surface or through the eye (Hall *et al.*, 1981). The incubation period is assumed to be 4–5 days, at which time the infected child develops symptoms of rhinorrhea, nasal obstruction, and low-grade fever. In most patients, the illness resolves over 7–10 days, but in others the cough becomes progressive and eventually signs of lower respiratory tract involvement appear. At this point, secretions and profuse and contain 10^5–10^6 infectious units of virus per milliliter of secretion (Hall *et al.*, 1976). In cases of pneumonia, descent of virus to the lower respiratory tract probably occurs as a result of aspiration. In the syndrome of bronchiolitis, whether disease is entirely the result of spread of virus to the bronchioles or the result of the involvement of the immune response simultaneously is not yet clear. In any case, the child at this point manifests respiratory distress that may be severe. Nasal flaring, dyspnea, and retractions are noted, and auscultation of the chest reveals rhonchi and harsh wheezing. Otherwise the child remains remarkably free of other symptoms. Fevers are usually not marked and the child may be quite active despite the presence of moderate to severe hypoxia, again suggesting that severe illness may be mediated, at least in part, by mechanisms other than progressive viral infection.

2. Histopathology

The histological picture of interstitial pneumonia reveals lymphocytes within the alveolar walls and small airways. Engorgement of the capillary bed with edema is also noted. Lymphocytes and plasma cells are recruited into alveolar walls. The alveolar walls may become increasingly thick and filled with proteinaceous material, and intranuclear or cytoplasmic inclusions and giant cells may be observed (Aherne *et al.*, 1970). Bronchiolitis, in contrast, is characterized by necrosis and sloughing of the respiratory epithelium and plugging of the small bronchioles with fibrin and mucus. An intense peribronchiolar infiltration of lymphocytes and plasma cells occurs, with considerable edema. Localized hyperinflation due to airflow obstruction is characteristic, and atelectasis is common.

3. Protective Immune Response

The precise role of RSV-specific antibody in recovery from primary infection is controversial. Local antibody responses, predominantly in the secretory IgA class, appear in the respiratory tract shortly after the onset of primary infection (McIntosh *et al.*, 1979; Kaul *et al.*, 1981). In some studies (McIntosh *et al.*, 1979), viral shedding is terminated at about the time of appearance of antibody-free secretions. However, in other studies (Kaul *et al.*, 1981), antibody is present at a time when substantial quantities of virus are still recoverable from the respiratory tract. Administration of very high concentrations of neutralizing antibody of the IgG isotype to infants with RSV infection did not have a dramatic effect on viral shedding (Hemming *et al.*, 1987). In contrast, the presence of neutralizing antibody in serum correlates with resistance to reinfection (Hall *et al.*, 1991). Although repeated infection tends to result in accelerated local antibody responses (Kaul *et al.*, 1981) and reduced severity of illness, whether local antibody is responsible for protection is not clear. In one study of adults undergoing experimental RSV challenge, specific nasal IgA antibody titers did not correlate with protection against infection (Hall *et al.*, 1991). In other investigations (Mills *et al.*, 1971), neutralizing activity in nasal secretions apparently was related to partial resistance to infection. However, subsequent studies (McIntosh *et al.*, 1979) demonstrated that such neutralizing activity is not necessarily antibody related. Therefore, serum antibody, presumably appearing in the respiratory tract by transudation following infection with RSV, appears to be better associated with protection against detectable infection than locally synthesized IgA antibody. Nevertheless, even the highest titers of antibody in serum or respiratory secretions do not seem to provide absolute protection against RSV, since as many as 25% of adults can be infected despite very high antibody titers (Mills *et al.*, 1971; Hall *et al.*, 1991).

RSV-specific IgE antibody responses have been documented in respiratory secretions of infants and young children undergoing natural RSV infection (Welliver *et al.*, 1980,1981; Bui *et al.*, 1987). As with secretory IgA, IgE appears first bound to the surface of RSV-infected cells and later free in secretions (Welliver *et al.*, 1980,1981). Higher concentrations of RSV–IgE were observed in infants with bronchiolitis in comparison with infants with upper respiratory illness alone (Welliver *et al.*, 1981; Bui *et al.*, 1987). In addition, histamine and various leukotrienes also have identified in secretions of infants with bronchiolitis Welliver *et al.*, 1981; Garofalo *et al.*, 1991). Therefore, in certain individuals, RSV infection may elicit the release of chemical mediators of airway obstruction, either directly or by IgE-dependent mechanisms.

Cell-mediated immune mechanisms also may be important in recovery from RSV infection. Individuals with congenital or acquired defects in cell-mediated immune function shed virus for prolonged periods of time and seem to have a greater frequency of development of pneumonia than immunologically intact individuals (Fishaut *et al.*, 1980; Hall *et al.*, 1986). T lymphocytes expressing cytotoxic activity against RSV-infected cells have been demonstrated in human infants, and appear at about the time that viral shedding begins to decrease (Issacs *et al.*, 1987; Chiba *et al.*, 1989). No studies of lymphocytes obtained from the respiratory tract have been completed

Evidence also suggests exaggerated T-cell responses may result in enhanced lung disease after RSV infection. Reconstitution of RSV-infected mice with cytotoxic T cells that have been stimulated repeatedly with RSV antigen clears virus rapidly from lungs, but results in enhanced mortality and increases histopathological changes in the lungs (Cannon *et al.*, 1988). Whether similar events occur in humans is not known, but infants with RSV bronchiolitis have been reported to have peripheral blood lymphocytes that are more responsive to RSV antigen than similar cells from infants with upper respiratory infection alone due to RSV (Welliver *et al.*, 1979). In addition, recipients of an inactivated RSV vaccine developed evidence of cell-mediated hypersensitivity to RSV after vaccination, and subsequently developed enhanced lung disease when naturally infected with RSV (Kim *et al.*, 1976).

B. Influenza Virus Infections

1. Clinical Presentation

Influenza viruses are responsible for yearly outbreaks of respiratory illness among all age groups. The highest mortality rates are observed in infants and in the elderly. Characteristic "flu-like" symptoms include fever, headache, intense myalgia, and prolonged malaise. Cough may or may not be a prominent finding, especially early in the illness. The principal sites of involvement in most influenza virus infections are the trachea and the bronchi. As with RSV infections, lower respiratory tract illnesses such as pneumonia or wheezing are not as common in otherwise healthy persons. Nevertheless, croup and bronchiolitis may occur in infancy and pneumonia may occur at any age.

2. Histopathology

Influenza infection of the respiratory tract results in swelling and desquamation of infected ciliated cells. Airway edema and infiltration by mononuclear and polymorphonuclear cells follows, with extensive sloughing to the layer of the basal cells. Influenza pneumonia is characterized by hemorrhagic alveolar infiltrates, formation of hyaline membranes, and marked lymphocytic infiltration of the interstitium and alveolar walls (Kilbourne, 1987). Increased bronchial reactivity is a frequent complication of influenza infection (Little *et al.*, 1978; Laitenen and Kava, 1980). The increase in bronchial reactivity is associated with loss of the epithelium and may be caused by either exposure of airway irritant receptors (Empey *et al.*, 1976) or a loss of natural inhibitors of airway reactivity (Jacoby *et al.*, 1988). The role of influenza-specific

Table II Role of Aspects of the Immune System in Infection Caused by Various Pathogens

Immune system component	Pathogen: Respiratory syncytial virus	Influenza virus	*Streptococcus pneumoniae*	*Mycobacterium tuberculosis*
Serum IgG antibody	Partially protective	Strongly protective	Strongly protective	Probably not protective
Secretory IgA antibody	Partially protective	Possibly protective	Probably not protective	Probably not protective
Mucosal IgE antibody	Potentially pathogenic	Unknown	Unknown	Unknown
Cell-mediated immunity	Clears primary infection, potentially pathogenic	Clears primary infection, potentially pathogenic	Unknown	Related to immunity

IgE responses and mediator release has not been evaluated extensively for a possible role in inducing bronchial hyperreactivity.

In contrast to infection with RSV and most other viruses, influenza infection is accompanied by an increased frequency of bacterial superinfection that may be the result of reduced mucociliary clearance after influenza virus infection (Camner *et al.*, 1973), greater damage to the mucosa with resultant diminished resistance to bacterial invasion (Kilbourne, 1987), or suppression of activity of phagocytic cells (Casali *et al.*, 1984; Hartshorn and Tauber, 1988).

3. Protective Immune Response

Initial infection with one strain of influenza virus provides partial immunity to reinfection with the same strain. Reinfections are generally asymptomatic (Frank *et al.*,1979; Sonoguchi *et al.*, 1986). Resistance to reinfection has been attributed to the presence of antibody in serum or respiratory secretions; high titers of antibody at either site appear to be capable of conferring resistance (Clements *et al.*, 1986). Whether local or serum antibody is most efficient in providing protection against reinfection in humans is uncertain.

Antibody to the hemagglutinin of influenza appears to contribute to immunity by preventing attachment of the virus to the respiratory epithelium, whereas antibody to the neuraminidase antigen inhibits cleavage of preformed virus from the cell membrane (Ogra *et al.*, 1977). Virtually no data are available on the role of serum or secretory antibody in recovery from primary influenza virus infection. Minor changes in hemagglutinin structure by variation in amino acid sequences ("antigenic drift") or major changes via genetic reassortment ("antigenic shift") enable the virus to infect previously exposed individuals.

The role of cell-mediated immunity in influenza virus infection has been investigated extensively in mice and, to a lesser extent, in humans, Transfer of primary or secondary influenza-immune splenic cells to mice infected intranasally with influenza virus results in significant clearance of virus from the lung and protection against death in the recipients. T lymphocytes represent the cell population primarily responsible for this immunity (Yap and Ada, 1978). Evidence suggests that the pathogenesis of influenza virus infection may be a reflection of the cell-mediated immune response in the lung. First, influenza virus replicates in and is released from the cells without causing cell death. Second, mice without functioning T cells develop extensive replication of virus in the lung with dissemination to other organs, but develop minimal pulmonary infiltration after influenza virus challenge (Wyde *et al.*, 1977). In contrast, cytotoxic T cells appear in the lungs of immunocompetent mice at the peak of respiratory symptoms and when histopathology in the lung is most prominent (Ennis *et al.*, 1977).

Although such definitive studies have not been repeated in humans, cytotoxic T-cell responses are known to develop in humans after influenza virus infection. Maximal responses occur in the second week after infection (Greenberg *et al.*, 1978). These cytotoxic cells apparently recognize all influenza type A strains but not influenza viruses of other types or non-influenza viruses. These cytotoxic cells appear to be HLA-restricted and apparently are capable of providing protection against subsequent influenza virus infection, even when influenza-specific serum antibody is undetectable in serum or secretions. These cytotoxic responses are apparently short lived, since only 30% of individuals exposed to a given strain of influenza virus had inducible cytotoxic T-cell activity when tested 5 years later (McMichael *et al.*, 1983). The majority of the cytotoxic T-cell responses appear to be mediated by $CD8^+$ cells with major histocompatibility complex (MHC) restriction Class I (Fleischer *et al.*, 1985; Yamada *et al.*, 1986).

In addition to specific cytotoxic T cells, nonspecific natural killer cell activity also increases after influenza virus infection in humans. However, the same increase in natural killer activity is observed in humans who continue to shed virus as in those individuals who do not continue to shed virus (Ennis *et al.*, 1981). A sufficiently large viral inoculum may be able to overcome natural killer cell resistance.

Therefore, although data on mucosal cell-mediated immune responses are lacking, cytotoxic T cells circulating in the blood appear to be important in restricting primary viral infection by RSV and influenza, and probably by other viruses. These cytotoxic cells may play some role in protection against reinfection, and are almost undoubtedly responsible for much of the histopathology seen with viral infections of the lung. Some evidence suggests that exaggerated T-cell responses may be responsible for unusually severe forms of infection, both by RSV and by influenza virus.

C. Bacterial Infections

1. Clinical Presentations

Pharyngitis is the most frequent infection caused by direct bacterial effects on the respiratory tract. However, these infections are generally sources of only temporary discomfort and not serious morbidity, in comparison with bacterial infections of the lower respiratory tract. Bacterial infections in the lung and, to a lesser extent, of the trachea are less common but are of greater severity. Most of these infections represent secondary bacterial infection following a precipitating viral infection. Bacterial infections of the lung usually are associated with more prominent fever than are viral infections, with more dyspnea, greater degrees of hypoxia, more prominent radiologic infiltrates, and higher mortality. Typical patients are infants or the elderly, who may or may not provide a history of antecedent viral upper respiratory tract illness. Cough and dyspnea become progressively more prominent, and patients appear more acutely ill.

The mechanism by which viral infections predispose to bacterial superinfection is not yet clear (Table III). Viral infections promote Desquamation of Ciliated Epithelial Cells (Reynolds, 1987) and Diminish Ciliary Function (Carson, 1983) Theraby Promoting Bacterial Adherence. However, bacterial superinfection occurs at a later time in the lung. Influenza virus infection down-regulates the antibacterial function of neutrophils (Hartshorn and Tauber, 1988). In addition, virus infections of the lung result in a progressive

Table III Secondary Bacterial Invasion of the Lung: Relationship to Viral and Immunologic Events[a]

	Stage of viral infection			
	Infection	Incubation	Replication in lung	Recovery phase
Viral growth	Undetectable	Slight	Maximal	Reduced
Histopathology	Unchanged	Unchanged	Sloughing of epithelium	Inflammation maximal
Cytotoxic lymphocyte response	Undetectable	Undetectable	Detectable	Maximal
Macrophage function	Unchanged	Unchanged	Increased	Reduced
Bacterial growth	Not present	Not present	Adherent to damaged	Maximum potential

[a] See Jakab *et al.* (1980); Jakab (1982).

decrease in virtually all antibacterial functions of pulmonary macrophages. This dysfunction of phagocytic cells coincides with the time at which the lung is most susceptible to secondary bacterial pneumonias, that is, about 7 days after viral infection (Jakab *et al.,* 1980) and a few days after the peak lung titers of virus are achieved. This result implies that susceptibility to bacterial infections is not simply a function of viral replication and tissue destruction in the lung. Cytotoxic immune activity peaks in the lung at about the time that the titer of virus replicating in the lung disappears. Pulmonary macrophage function becomes abnormal at this time, suggesting that cytotoxic activity may suppress macrophage function. Treatment with antilymphocyte serum ameliorates the virus-induced suppression of pulmonary bacterial defenses. However, this phagocytic defect can be re-established after antilymphocyte treatment by addition of specific antiviral immunoglobulin (Jakab, 1982). Although a clear explanation for these findings is not evident, the normal immune response to viral infection does appear in some ways to suppress antibacterial defenses, probably by direct immunological attack on the alveolar macrophages.

2. Histopathology

Streptococcus pneumoniae is the most frequent cause of bacterial pneumonia. In the earliest stages of pneumococcal pneumonia, bacteria are present in the alveolar spaces. Alveolar capillaries become intensely congested, with extravasation of erythrocytes and neutrophils through the interstitium into the alveolar spaces. The alveoli eventually fill with red cells, white cells, and fibrin. The lesion generally heals without scarring or disruption of the normal architecture (Loosli and Baker, 1962). In pneumonia caused by *Staphylococcus aureus,* persistent scarring of the lung is more likely to occur.

The strikingly toxic appearance of individuals with pneumococcal pneumonia suggests to some investigators that the release of some biologically active compound by pneumococci contributes heavily to the clinical appearance. This possibility is supported by the fact that death can occur days after antibiotic therapy for pneumococcal pneumonia has been started, when tissues are sterile and when the pneumonia is clearing (Austrian and Golb, 1964), The polysaccharide capsule is nontoxic and, to date, no evidence exists that pneumococci produce a toxin that is related to clinical illness (MacLoud, 1970) nor is evidence available that pneumococci are more readily able to provoke release of tumor necrosis factor (cachectin) or other inflammatory substances than any other bacterial species.

3. Protective Immune Response

In adults and children, most pneumococcal infections occur after the recent acquisition of a particular serotype rather than after prolonged carriage of a given serotype (Gray *et al.,* 1980). In addition, overwhelming infection is more common in infants who lack antibody to pneumococcal antigens (Mufson *et al.,* 1974) and in adults with hypogammaglobulinemia or complement deficiencies (Winkelstein, 1984; Gray and Dillon, 1988). These findings suggest that antibody and complement play a major role in resistance to pneumococcal infection. The virulence of pneumococci appears to be related to the polysaccharide capsule. Certain capsular serotypes are highly associated with potential for invasive disease (Austrian and Golb, 1964; Grey *et al.,* 1980). Virulence of encapsulated strains appears to be related to their resistance to phagocytosis. Indeed, the presence of opsonic antibody to a given capsular serotype in serum is required for protection against illness after challenge. Antibodies to cell wall polysaccharides, surface proteins, and phosphocholine also provide lesser degrees of resistance (Briles *et al.,* 1989; Musher *et al.,* 1990). In addition to its antiphagocytic effect, incubation of the pneumococcal capsule with serum destroys some natual antipneumococcal activity (Schweinle, 1986).

Pneumococcal infections, particularly otitis media, also can result in mucosal immune responses. Antipneumococcal antibody of the IgA isotype has been demonstrated in middle ear fluids (Giebink, 1981; Karjalainen *et al.,* 1990), in colostrum, in saliva, and in nasal secretions (Mouton *et al.,* 1970). However, protection against otitis media is correlated with IgG antibody present via transudation rather than with locally formed IgA antibody (Giebink, 1981; Karjalainen *et al.,* 1990).

Immunization with polyvalent pneumococcal vaccines apparently has reduced the mortality from pneumonia in developing countries (Reilly *et al.,* 1981). Whether local or systemic antibody is more important in providing resistance to pneumococcal infection in the lung remains unclear (Bull and McKee, 1929).

D. Tuberculosis

1. Clinical Presentation

Although *Mycobacterium tuberculosis* can spread to virtually all body organs under appropriate circumstances, the primary target organ for disease is the lung. Asymptomatic primary infection occurs after inhalation of bacteria suspended in aerosols. Infection of the lung occurs initially in the subpleural area. A primary complex consisting of the primary subpleural focus, lymphangitis, and regional lymphadenitis is a regular feature of primary lung involvement (Ghon, 1916). Pulmonary tuberculosis also can be arrested at this stage, or it can become progressive with the development of larger alveolar ilfiltrates or extension of the inflammatory focus into the bronchus, causing bronchial obstruction or atelectasis. The location of the primary focus close to the pleural area frequently results in irritation of the pleural surface and development of pleural effusions. The initial primary focus can undergo liquefaction and the development of cavitary lesions. These lesions contain high numbers of tubercle bacilli with a propensity to spread to other areas of the lung. Enlarging primary foci also can rupture into the pleural cavity, causing pneumothorax or even a fistula through the chest wall. Children and adults with primary foci alone may remain asymptomatic or develop only progressive weight loss. In contrast, individuals with primary progressive pulmonary tuberculosis or cavitary lesions usually have much higher fevers, much more prominent cough, and profound malaise and weight loss. Tuberculosis was often fatal in the pre-antibiotic era, and profound scarring of the lung was prominent among survivors. In addition, dissemination to bones, joints, and other organs including the brain was not unusual, with severe long-term consequences.

2. Histopathology

An inflammatory focus consisting primarily of macrophages occurs in the area where tubercle bacilli are inhaled into the alveoli. These macrophages then change into epithelioid cells, forming tubercules. These nodules may disappear or develop central caseation. The caseous lesions, characteristic of tuberculosis, contain enormous numbers of tubercle bacilli. These bacilli may enter the regional lymphatic vessels and spread to regional lymph nodes. Caseating granulomas, appearing at the primary site or along the routes of drainage to the lymph nodes, also may calcify. Evidence of dermal hypersensitivity develops within 3–10 weeks of initial infection. The radiographic appearance of prominent lymphadenitis, in contrast to the relatively insignificant size of the initial focus, suggests that hypersensitivity responses also occur in the lungs. As noted earlier, bronchial obstruction can result from compression of the airway by the enlarged lymph nodes. Alternatively, the adjacent infection can destroy the cartilaginous component of the airway or caseous material may perforate into the bronchus, forming semiliquid plugs. Collapse of the lung distal to the site of the obstruction is common.

In adults, reactivation of pulmonary tuberculosis acquired in earlier life is the most common form of tuberculosis. The lesions in the lung in active ''adult'' tuberculosis are probably caused by reactivation of primary foci with spread to new areas of lung (Stead, 1967). The lesions in adults are smaller than those in children and are less likely to spread to lymph nodes or to other organs. Protracted cough, persistent high fevers, chest pain, and hemoptysis are the most common clinical manifestations of tuberculosis in adults.

Certain races appear to be more disposed to infection with *M. tuberculosis* than others on similar exposures (Stead *et al.,* 1990). Malnutrition appears to be associated with an increased risk of infection and, in particular, vitamin D deficiency may be associated with increased susceptibility to tuberculosis (Rook, 1988). In addition, patients on immunosuppressive medications or with underlying diseases associated with immunosuppression are at a greater risk for developing severe forms of tuberculosis.

3. Protective Immune Response

The findings just described suggest that cell-mediated immunity is important in resistance to tuberculosis and in recovery from infection. Tuberculin-specific cell-mediated and humoral immune responses have been evaluated in individuals with various forms of tuberculosis (Table IV). Anergy, both to tuberculin and to unrelated antigens, seems to be related to the severity of illness. In one study, only 2 of 10 individuals with miliary tuberculosis had positive cutaneous reactions to tuberculin, whereas 14 of 15 individuals with active pulmonary tuberculosis and 20 of 22 healthy controls who probably had been infected with tuberculosis early in life had positive cutaneous reactions (Bhatnagar *et al.,* 1977). Tuberculin anergy apparently is more likely to be noted during the first few weeks of acute pulmonary tuberculosis than during convalescence (Daniel *et al.,* 1981). *In vitro* lymphocyte transformation assays also have been used to assess cell-mediated immune function in tuberculosis (Cox *et al.,* 1981). These *in vitro* responses correlate quite well with skin test reactivity, and are occasionally positive when skin tests are negative.

Serologic tests also have been developed for diagnosis of tuberculosis. These tests include passive hemagglutination techniques using PPD-coated red blood cells (Bhatnagar *et al.,* 1977) and enzyme-linked immunosorbent assays (ELISA) (Daniel *et al.,* 1981; Benjamin and Daniel, 1982). These serologic tests have not been useful in the diagnosis of tuberculosis because of a high degree of cross-reactivity of antibodies directed against *M. tuberculosis* with other environmental or ''atypical'' mycobacteria. Antigen 5 appears to be somewhat more specific for *M. tuberculosis* than for other mycobacterial antigens (Benjamin and Daniel, 1982). Analaysis of antibody responses in individuals with tuberculosis reveals the opposite of the findings for cell-mediated immunity, that is, individuals with remote asymptomatic infection have very low levels of antibody despite their strong cutaneous reactivity. Antibody titers are somewhat higher in individuals with acute or resolving primary pulmonary tuberculosis, and are the highest in individuals with miliary tuberculosis (Bhatnagar *et al.,* 1977; Lenzini *et al.,* 1977; Daniel *et al.,* 1981).

The observed immunological aberrations in tuberculosis return to normal with recovery from disease, that is, evidence of cell-mediated immunity is present in essentially all individ-

Table IV Humoral and Cell-Mediated Immunity to *Mycobacterium tuberculosis* in Different Stages of Illness[a]

	Asymptomatic infection	Primary pulmonary tuberculosis	Miliary or disseminated disease	Convalescence
Antibody titers to *M. tuberculosis*	Low	Mildly increased	Markedly increased	Mildly increased
Cell-mediated responsiveness	Present	Generally present	Diminished	Generally present

[a] See Bhatnager *et al.* (1977); Lenzini *et al.* (1977); Daniel *et al.* (1981).

uals who have recovered from acute tuberculosis whereas antibody titers fall with recovery (Bhatnagar *et al.,* 1977; Daniel *et al.,* 1981). These observations suggest that the immunological abnormalities are a result of tuberculosis rather than a cause of invasive infection.

Although cell-mediated immunity appears to be the principal means of protection against invasive tuberculosis, whether macrophages (Patterson and Youmans, 1970) or lymphocytes (Lefford *et al.,* 1973) are primarily responsible for tuberculocidal activity is not clear. Each of these cell types has been shown to have some activity in eradication of infection, but has not been shown clearly to have tuberculocidal activity. In addition, humans appear to have significant natural immunity to tuberculosis (Kallmann and Reisner, 1943; Skamene, 1989). When one monozygotic twin became infected with tuberculosis, the other twin was more likely to be infected than when one of a pair of dizygotic twins became infected (Kallmann and Reisner, 1943).

Despite the correlation of cell-mediated hypersensitivity with clinical phases of illness, cell-mediated hyperresponsiveness has never been demonstrated conclusively to be responsible for immunity. In fact, numerous experiments have demonstrated a clear dissociation of hypersensitivity and immunity in tuberculosis (Rich and McCordock, 1929). Some experiments have indicated that macrophages have minor intrinsic ability to inactivate *M. tuberculosis,* and that this capability can be enhanced by interaction of macrophages with tuberculin-sensitized T cells (Wilson *et al.,* 1940). However, this degree of tuberculocidal activity is rather limited and probably does not account for the fairly solid immunity resulting from tuberculous infection. Production of lymphokines from sensitized T lymphocytes seems more likely to play an important role in restriction of immunity to tuberculosis (Youmans, 1975, Rook *et al.,* 1986), perhaps recruiting a variety of inflammatory cell types.

References

Aherne, W., Bird, T., Court, S. D. M., Gardner, P. S., and McQuillin, J. (1970). Pathologic changes in virus infections of the lower respiratory tract in children. *J. Clin. Pathol.* **23,** 7–18.

Austrian, R., and Golb, J. (1964). Pneumococcal bacteremia with a special reference to bacteremic pneumococcal pneumonia. *Ann. Intern. Med.* **60,** 759–776.

Beem, M., Egerer, R., and Anderson, J. (1934). Respiratory syncytial virus neutralizing antibodies in persons residing in Chicago, IL. *Pediatrics* **34,** 761–770.

Benjamin, R. G., and Daniel, T. M. (1982). Serodiagnosis of tuberculosis using the enzyme-linked immunoabsorbent assay of antibody to *Mycobacterium tuberculosis* antigen 5. *Am. Rev. Resp. Dis.* **126,** 1013–1016.

Bhatnagar, R., Malaviya, A. N., Narayanan, S., Rajgopalan, P., Kumar, R., and Bharadwaj, O. P. (1977). Spectrum of immune response abnormalities in different clinical forms of tuberculosis. *Am. Rev. Resp. Dis.* **115,** 207–212.

Briles, D. E., Forman, C., Horowitz, J. C., Volanakis, J. E., Benjamin, W. H., Jr., McDaniel, L. S., Eldridge, J., and Brooks, J. (1989). Antipneumococcal effects of C-reactive protein and monoclonal antibodies to pneumococcal cell wall and capsular antigens. *Infect. Immun.* **57,** 1457–1464.

Bui, R. H. D., Molinaro, G. A., Kittering, J. D., Heiner, D. C., Imagawa, D. T., and St. Geme, J. W., Jr. (1987). Virus-specific IgE and IgG_4 antibodies in serum of children infected with respiratory syncytial virus. *J. Pediatr.* **110,** 87–90.

Bull, C. G., and McKee, C. M. (1929). Respiratory immunity in rabbits. VII. Resistance to intranasal infection in the absence of demonstrable antibodies. *Am. J. Hyg.* **9,** 490–499.

Camner, P., Jarstrand, C., and Philipson, K. (1973). Tracheobronchial clearance in patients with influenza. *Am. Rev. Resp. Dis.* **108,** 131–135.

Cannon, M. J., Openshaw, P. J. M., and Askonas, B. A. (1988). Cytotoxic T cells clear virus but augment lung pathology in mice infected with respiratory syncytial virus. *J. Exp. Med.* **168,** 1163–1168.

Carson, J. L., Collier, A. M., and Hu, S. S. (1985). Acquired ciliary defects in nasal epithelium of children with acute viral upper respiratory infections. *N. Engl. J. Med.* **312,** 463–468.

Casali, P., Rice, G. P. A., and Oldstone, M. B. A. (1984). Viruses disrupt functions of human lymphocytes: Effects of measles virus and influenza virus on lymphocyte-mediated killing and antibody production. *J. Exp. Med.* **159,** 1322–1327.

Chiba, Y., Higashidate, Y., Suga, K., Honjo, K., Tsutsumi, H., and Ogra, P. L. (1989). Development of cell-mediated cytotoxic immunity to respiratory syncytial virus in human infants following naturally acquired infection. *J. Med. Virol.* **28,** 133–139.

Clarke, S. K. R., Gardner, P. S., Poole, P. M., Simpson, H., and Tobin, J. (1978). Respiratory syncytial virus infection: Admissions to hospital, industrial, urban and rural areas. Report to the Medical Research Council Subcommittee on Respiratory Syncytial Virus Vaccines. *Brit. Med. J.* **2,** 796–798.

Clements, M. L., Betts, R. S., Tierney, E. L., and Murphy, B. R. (1986). Serum and nasal wash antibodies associated with resistance to experimental challenge with influenza A wild-type virus. *J. Clin. Microbiol.* **24,** 157–160.

Cox, R., Lundberg, D. I., and Arnold, D. L. (1981). Lymphocyte transformation assays as a diagnostic tool in tuberculosis of children. *Am. Rev. Resp. Dis.* **123,** 627–630.

Daniel, T. M., Oxtoby, M. J., Pinto, E. M., and Moreno, E. S. (1981). The immune spectrum in patients with pulmonary tuberculosis. *Am. Rev. Resp. Dis.* **123,** 556–559.

Dubos, R., and Dubos, J. (1952). "The White Plague: Tuberculosis, Man and Society." Little, Brown, Boston.

Eickhoff, T. C., Sherman, I. L., and Serfling, R. E. (1961). Observations on excess mortality associated with epidemic influenza. *J. Am. Med. Assoc.* **176,** 776–782.

Empey, D. W., Laitenen, L. A., Jacobs, L., Gold, W. M., and Nadel, J. A. (1976). Mechanisms of bronchial hyperreactivity in normal subjects after upper respiratory tract infection. *Am. Rev. Resp. Dis.* **113,** 131–138.

Ennis, F. A., Martin, W. J., and Verbonitz, M. W. (1977). Specificity studies on cytotoxic thymus-derived lymphocytes reactive with influenza virus infected cells: Evidence for dual recognition of H2 and the viral hemagglutinin antigens. *Proc. Natl. Acad. Sci. U.S.A.* **74,** 3006–3010.

Ennis, F. A., Meager, A., Beare, S. Yi-Hua, Q., Reilly, B., Schwarz, G., Schild, G. C., and Rook, A. H. (1981). Interferon induction in increased natural killer cell activity in influenza infections in man. *Lancet* **II,** 891–895.

Fishaut, M., Tubergen, D., and McIntosh, K. (1980). Cellular response to respiratory viruses with particular reference to children with disorders of cell-mediated immunity. *J. Pediatr.* **96,** 179–186.

Fleischer, B., Becht, H., and Rott, R. (1985). Recognition of viral antigens by human influenza A virus-specific T lymphocyte clones. *J. Immunol.* **135,** 2800–2804.

Frank, A. L., Taber, L. H., Glezen, W. P., Parades, A., and Couch, R. B. (1979). Reinfection with influenza A (H3N2) virus in young children and their families. *J. Infect. Dis.* **140,** 829–836.

Garofalo, R., Welliver, R. C., and Ogra, P. L. (1991). Concentrations of LTB_4, LTC_4, LTB_4 and LTE_4 in bronchiolitis due to respiratory syncytial virus. *Pediatr. Allerg. Immunol.* **2,** 30–37.

Ghon, A. (1916). "The Primary Lung Focus of Tuberculosis in Children." Churchill, London.

Giebink, G. S. (1981). The pathogenesis of pneumococcal otitis media in chinchillas and the efficacy of vaccination in prophylaxis. *Rev. Infect. Dis.* **3,** 342–351.

Glezen, W. P., Payne, A. A., Snyder, D. N. (1982). Mortality and influenza. *J. Infect. Dis.* **146,** 313–321.

Glezen, W. P., Taber, L. H., Frank, A. L., and Kasel, J. A. (1986). Risk of primary infection and reinfection with respiratory syncytial virus. *Am. J. Dis. Child,* **140,** 543–546.

Glezen, W. P., Decker, M., Joseph, S., and MacCready, R. G., Jr. (1987). Acute respiratory disease associated with influenza epidemics in Houston 1981–83. *J. Infect. Dis.* **155,** 1119–1126.

Greenberg, S. B., Criswell, B. S., Six, H. R., and Couch, R. B. (1978). Lymphocyte cytotoxicity to influenza virus-infected cells: Response to vaccination in virus infection. *Infect. Immun.* **20,** 640–645.

Gray, B. M., and Dillion, H. C., Jr. (1988). Epidemiological studies of *Streptococcus pneumoniae* in infants: Antibody to types 3, 6, 14 and 23 in the first two years of life. *J. Infect. Dis.* **158,** 948–955.

Gray, B. M., Converse, G. M., III, and Dillon, H. C., Jr. (1980). Epidemiologic studies of *Streptococcus pneumoniae* in infants: Acquisition, carriage and infection during the first 24 months of life. *J. Infect. Dis.* **142,** 923–933.

Groothuis, J. R., Gutierrez, K. M., and Lauer, B. A. (1988). Respiratory syncytial virus infection in children with bronchopulmonary dysplasia. *Pediatrics* **82,** 199–203.

Hall, C. B., Douglas, R. G., Jr., and Geiman, J. M. (1976). Respiratory syncytial virus infection in infants: quantitation and degration of shedding. *J. Pediatr.* **89,** 11–15.

Hall, C. B., Douglas, R. G., Jr., Schnabel, K. C., and Geiman, J. M. (1981). Infectivity of respiratory syncytial virus by various routes of inoculation. *Infect. Immun.* **33,** 779–783.

Hall, C. B., Powell, K. R., McDonald, N. E., Gala, C. L., Menegus, M. E., Suffin, S. C., and Cohen, H. J. (1986). Respiratory syncytial viral infection in children with compromised immune function. *N. Engl. J. Med.* **315,** 77–81.

Hall, C. B., Walsh, E. E., Long, C. E., and Schnabel, K. C. (1991). Immunity to and frequency of reinfection with respiratory syncytial virus. *J. Infect. Dis.* **163,** 693–698.

Hartshorn, K. L., and Tuber, A. I. (1988). The influenza virus-infected phagocyte: A model of deactivation. *Hematol. Oncol. Clin. North Am.* **2,** 301–315.

Hemming, V. G., Rodriguez, W., and Kim, H. W. (1987). Intravenous immunoglobulin treatment of respiratory syncytial virus infections in infants and young children. *Antimicrob. Agents Chemother.* **31,** 1882–1886.

Issacs, D., Bangham, C. R. M., and McMichael, A. J. (1987). Cell-mediated cytotoxic response to respiratory syncytial virus in infants with bronchiolitis. *Lancet* **2,** 769–771.

Jacoby, D. B., Tamaoki, J., Borson, B. B., and Nadel, J. A. (1988). Influenza infection causes airway hyperresponsiveness by decreasing enkephalinase. *J. Appl. Physiol.* **64,** 2653–2658.

Jakab, G. J. (1982). Immune impairment of alveolar macrophage phagocytosis during pneumonia. *Am. Rev. Resp. Dis.* **126,** 778–782.

Jakab, G. J., Warr, G. A., and Sannes, P. L. (1980). Alveolar macrophage ingestion and phagosome-lysosome fusion defect associated with virus pneumonia. *Infect. Immun.* **27,** 960–968.

Kallmann, F. J., and Reisner, D. (1943). Twin studies on the significance of genetic factors in tuberculosis. *Am. Rev. Tuberculosis* **47,** 549–574.

Karjalainen, H., Koskela, M., Luotonen, J., Herba, E., and Sipila, P. (1990). Antibodies against *Streptococcus pneumoniae, Hemophilus influenzae, Branhamella catarrhalis* in middle ear effusion during early phase of acute otitis media. *Acta Otolaryngol.* **109,** 111–118.

Kaul, T. N., Welliver, R. C., Wong, D., Udwadia, R. A., Riddlesberger, K., and Ogra, P. L. (1981). Secretory antibody response to respiratory syncytial virus infection. *Am. J. Dis. Child.* **135,** 1013–1016.

Kilbourne, E. D. (1987). Influenza in man. *In* "Influenza" (E. D. Kilbourne, ed.), pp. 157–218. Plenum, New York.

Kim, H. W., Leikin, S. L., Arrobio, J., Brandt, C. D., Chanock, R. M., and Parrott, R. H. (1976). Cell-mediated immunity to respiratory syncytial virus induced by inactivated vaccine or by infection. *Pediatr. Res.* **10,** 75–78.

Klein, J. O. (1981). The epidemiology of pneumococcal disease in infants and children. *Rev. Infect. Dis.* **3,** 246–253.

Laitenen, L. A., and Kava, T. (1980). Bronchial reactivity following uncomplicated influenza A infection in healthy subjects and in asthmatic patients. *Eur. J. Resp. Dis.* **61,** 51–58.

Langmuir, A. D., and Housworth J. (1969). A critical evaluation of influenza surveillance. *Bull. W.H.O.* **41,** 393–398.

Lefford, M. J., McGregor, D. D., and Mackaness, G. B. (1973). Immune response to *Mycobacterium tuberculosis* in rats. *Infect. Immun.* **8,** 182–190.

Lenzini, L., Rottoli, P., and Rottoli, L. (1977). The spectrum of human tuberculosis. *Clin. Exp. Immunol.* **27,** 230–237.

Little, J. W., Hall, W. J., Douglas, R. G., Jr., Mudholkar, G. S., Spears, D. M., and Patel, K. (1978). Airway hyperreactivity and peripheral airway dysfunction in influenza A infection. *Am. Rev. Resp. Dis.* **118,** 295–303.

Loosli, C. G., and Baker, R. F. (1962). Acute experimental pneumococcal pneumonia in the mouse: The migration of leukocytes from the pulmonary capillaries into the alveolar spaces as revealed by the electron microscope. *Trans. Am. Clin. Climatol. Assoc.* **74,** 15–28.

McDonald, N. E., Hall, C. B., Suffin, S. C., Alexson, C., Harris, P. J., and Manning, J. A. (1982). Respiratory syncytial virus infection in infants with congenital heart disease. *N. Engl. J. Med.* **307,** 397–400.

McIntosh, K., McQuillin, J., and Gardner, P. S. (1979). Cell-free and cell-bound antibody in nasal secretions from infants with respiratory syncytial virus infection. *Infect. Immun.* **23,** 276–281.

MacLoud, C. M. (1970). Prevention of pneumococcal pneumonia by immunization with specific capsular polysaccharides. *In* "Infectious Agents and Host Reactions" (S. Mudd, ed.), pp. 165–173. Saunders, Philadelphia.

McMichael, A. J., Gotch, F. M., Noble, G. R., and Beare, P. A. (1983). Cytotoxic T cell immunity to influenza. *N. Engl. J. Med.* **309,** 13–17.

Mills, B. J., VanKirk, J. E., Wright, P. F., and Chanock, R. M. (1971). Experimental respiratory syncytial virus infection of adults. *J. Immunol.* **107,** 123–130.

Mouton, R. P., Stoop, J. W., Ballieux, R. E., and Mul, N. A. J. (1970). Pneumococcal antibodies in IgA of serum and external secretions. *Clin. Exp. Immunol.* **7,** 201–210.

Mufson, M. A., Kruss, D. M., Wasil, R. E., and Metzger, W. I. (1974). Capsular types and outcome of bacteremic pneumococcal disease in the antibiotic era. *Arch. Intern. Med.* **134,** 505–510.

Musher, D. M., Watson, D. A., and Vaughn, R. E. (1990). Does naturally acquired IgG antibody to cell wall polysaccharide protect human subjects against pneumococcal infection? *J. Infect. Dis.* **161,** 736–740.

Ogra, P. L., Chow, T., and Beutner, K. R. (1977). Clinical evaluation of neuraminidase specific influenza A virus vaccine in humans. *J. Infect. Dis.* **135,** 499–506.

Patterson, R. J., and Youmans, G. R. (1970). Demonstration in tissue culture of lymphocyte-mediated immunity in tuberculosis. *Infect. Immun.* **1,** 600–608.

Reilly, I. D., Everingham, F. A., Smith, D. E., and Douglas, R. M. (1981). Immunization with a polyvalent pneumococcal vaccine: Effect on respiratory mortality in children living in the New Guinea highlands. *Arch. Dis. Child.* **56,** 354–357.

Reynolds, H. Y. (1987). Host defense impairments that may lead to respiratory reinfections. *Clin. Chest Med.* **8,** 339–358.

Rich, A. J., and McCordock, H. A. (1929). An inquiry concerning the role of allergy, immunity and other factors of importance in the pathogenesis of human tuberculosis. *Bull. Johns Hopkins Hosp.* **44,** 273–280.

Rook, G. A. W. (1988). The role of vitamin D in tuberculosis. *Am. Rev. Resp. Dis.* **138,** 768–770.

Rook, G. A. W., Steele, J., Ainsworth, M., and Champion, B. R. (1986). Activation of macrophages to inhibit proliferation of mycobacterium tuberculosis: Comparison of the effects of recombinant gamma-interferon on human monocytes and murine peritoneal macrophages. *Immunology* **59,** 333–338.

Schweinle, J. E. (1986). Pneumococcal intracellular killing is abolished by polysaccharides despite serum complement activity. *Infect. Immun.* **54,** 876–881.

Skamene, E. (1989). Genetic control of susceptibility to mycobacterial infections. *Rev. Infect. Dis.* (*Suppl. 2*) **11,** 394–399.

Sonoguchi, T., Sakoh, M., Kunita, N., Satsuta, K., and Noriki, H. (1986). Reinfection with influenza A (H2N2, H3N2 and H1N1) viruses in soldiers and students in Japan. *J. Infect. Dis.* **153,** 33–40.

Stead, W. W. (1967). Pathogenesis of a first episode of chronic pulmonary tuberculosis in man: Recrudescence of residuals of the primary infection or exogenous reinfection? *Am. Rev. Resp. Dis.* **95,** 729–745.

Stead, W. W., Cenner, J. W., Reddick, W. T., and Lofgren, J. P. (1990). Racial differences in susceptibility to infection by mycobacterium tuberculosis. *N. Engl. J. Med.* **322,** 422–427.

Welliver, R. C., Kaul, A., and Ogra, P. L. (1979). Cell mediated immune response to respiratory syncytial virus infection: Relationship to the development of reactive airway disease. *J. Pediatr.* **94,** 370–519.

Welliver, R. C., Kaul, T. N., and Ogra, P. L. (1980). The appearance of cell-bound IgE in respiratory tract epithelium after respiratory syncytial virus infection. *N. Engl. J. Med.* **303,** 1198–1202.

Welliver, R. C., Wong, D. T., Sun, M., Middleton, E., Jr., Vaughan, R. S., and Ogra, P. L. (1981). The development of respiratory syncytial virus-specific IgE on the release of histamine in nasopharyngeal secretions after infection. *N. Engl. J. Med.* **305,** 841–846.

Wilson, G. S., Schwabacher, H., and Maier, I. (1940). The effect of desensitization of tuberculous guinea pigs. *J. Pathol. Bacteriol.* **50,** 89–97.

Winkelstein, J. A. (1984). Complement and the host defense against the pneumococcus. *Crit. Rev. Microbiol.* **11,** 187–208.

Wyde, P. R., Couch, R. B., and Mackler, B. F. (1977). Effects of low and high passage influenza virus infection in normal and nude mice. *Infect. Immun.* **15,** 221–229.

Yamada, Y. K., Mager, A., Yamada, A., and Ennis, F. A. (1986). Human interferon alpha and gamma production by lymphocytes during the generation of influenza virus-specific cytotoxic T lymphocytes. *J. Gen. Virol.* **67,** 2325–2334.

Yap, K. L., and Ada, G. L. (1978). The recovery of mice from influenza virus infection: Adoptive transfer of immunity with immune T lymphocytes. *Scand. J. Immunol.* **7,** 389–397.

Youmans, G. P. (1975). Relation between delayed hypersensitivity and immunity in tuberculosis. *Am. Rev. Resp. Dis.* **111,** 109–118.

46

Inhalant Allergy and Hypersensitivity Disorders

Bengt Björkstén

I. INTRODUCTION

Asthma is the most common chronic debiliating disease in children and one of the major causes of repeated absence from work in adults. IgE antibodies play an important role in childhood asthma and are considered to be at least a contributing factor in over 80% of the cases. In adults, atopy and other confirmed allergy are much less common causes of asthma.

Immunologically triggered immediate type hypersensitivity reactions seem to be mediated exclusively by IgE antibodies. Although other homocytotropic antibodies have been described in humans, their role in disease is still obscure. Other hypersensitivity diseases of the lung are much less common in children. In adults, however, allergic alveolitis and other hypersensitivity disorders constitute a large proportion of occupational diseases of the respiratory tract. The pathogenesis of these conditions includes a strong immunological component, although the precise underlying mechanisms are not fully understood.

The presentation in this chapter is limited to disorders of the respiratory tract in which immunological mechanisms and allergic reactions play a dominating role. Although inhaled allergens are well established to cause symptoms not only in the respiratory tract, for example, dermatitis and severe systemic reactions such as anaphylaxis, these conditions are beyond the scope of this chapter.

II. DEFINITIONS

In this chapter, asthma is defined as reversible episodes of severe wheezy breathlessness. Such patients may be atopic or nonatopic, depending on whether antibodies of the IgE isotype are involved. However, even in atopic patients, the allergens precipitating an attack are not always known. No clinically discernible difference exists between the two. Further, in both types of patients, attacks of varying severity usually are triggered by inhaled irritants, and airway hyperresponsiveness (BHR) is characteristic of all patients. This hyperreactivity expresses itself clinically by bronchial and nasal obstruction after exposure to various nonspecific stimuli such as cold, humid, or polluted air, physical exercise, and emotional stress. BHR can be verified objectively in the laboratory by provocation tests with cold air, various compounds including histamine, and exercise.

Sensitization, as proven by the demonstration of low levels of IgE antibodies directed against environmental allergens, appears to be part of the normal immune response. In most instances, at least in children, these antibodies are only temporary since continued IgE antibody formation is suppressed rapidly. However, when genetically predisposed individuals are exposed to an allergen at a time when the regulation of the immune system is impaired, higher levels of IgE antibodies that persist for a long time may appear. The more susceptible to sensitization the individual is, the lower the allergen dose needed for this response to occur. The fact that an individual is sensitized does not, however, mean that clinical symptoms such as allergic disease will develop.

III. GENETIC BACKGROUND OF ALLERGIC DISEASE

Phenotype and genotype are two terms used when describing the genetics of an illness. The first term represents the observed manifestations of the disease, whereas genotype describes the underlying structural lesion in the DNA. Allergy (atopy) can be defined in several ways, and the phenotype is highly variable. Nevertheless, however defined, allergy is well known to be much more common in individuals with a family history of allergy. Thus, the likelihood of allergy appearing in a child is elevated if one of the parents is allergic, and reaches over 50% if both parents are allergic (Björkstén and Kjellman, 1992). If both parents are allergic with the same disease, then the chance of allergy in their child is increased further and reaches over 70%. A strong genetic influence also is seen in asthma, independent of other atopic manifestations.

Several studies have addressed the mode of inheritance for elevated serum IgE and for IgE antibody formation against individual allergens. Studies of serum IgE levels in families with allergic individuals have not revealed any simple pattern of Mendelian inheritance, although in most of the studies data best fit a condition of one or two loci that determine high IgE levels and are, in turn, influenced by other genes.

Immune responses, including IgE antibody formation, against at least some major allergens are partially HLA determined (Marsh, 1990). Thus, significant relationships have been demonstrated between haplotypes DR2/Dw2 and DR5 and responsiveness to some major ragweed allergens and between DR3/Dw3 and antibody responses to grass. A genetic linkage was suggested in some atopic families between allergy and a gene on the long arm of chromosome 11. However, this result could not be confirmed in any of three other studies performed by other investigators. Thus, the genetics of allergy remain poorly understood.

IV. NATURAL HISTORY OF ALLERGIC DISEASE AND EPIDEMIOLOGICAL ASPECTS

The highest incidence (new cases appearing during a given year) of allergy appears in infants and adolescents. The prevalence of a disease, that is, the presence of symptoms at any time during the past 12 months, depends on the incidence, the age of the subjects, and the natural history of the disease, including healing and change to a latent phase. The accumulated incidence (sick presently or previously) of a disease in a particular region therefore should increase with age, unless a dramatic reduction has occurred in the prevalence as a consequence of efficient prevention, reduced exposure to allergens, or adjuvant factors, or improved treatment.

The clinical symptoms of allergic disease vary with age. Symptoms from the skin, such as dermatitis and urticaria, and gastrointestinal tract dominate in infants and the offending allergens mainly are introduced with food. After infancy, inhaled allergens become increasingly more common as triggers of symptoms, and after the age of 3 the appearance of new food allergies is not common.

From the second year of life, wheezing becomes increasingly common. Wheezy bronchitis occurs before 18 months of age in up to 20% of all young children. In most cases, the episodes of wheezing are not associated with development of asthma. The wheezing is, however, diagnosed as asthma when the episodes of wheezing recur three times, and as soon as a relationship is determined to exposure to a particular allergen. Wheezing in older children often is associated with asthma. The prevalence of asthma then increases to a peak level in school children and declines after puberty. Through adolescence, asthma is associated with allergy in up to 80% of the patients and IgE antibodies can be demonstrated in most patients. In young adults with asthma, an IgE-mediated component is also present in the majority of the patients. After the age of 50, however, allergy is less common.

Allergic rhinoconjunctivitis is not commonly seen before 5–6 years of age, and then increases to a peak prevalence in adolescence. In adults, particularly in middle-aged and old patients, the etiology of rhinitis is usually nonallergic.

Scandinavian studies show a total accumulated incidence of one or more of the allergic diseases in over 30% of adolescents and young adults (Björkstén and Kjellman, 1989). In prospective studies, the prevalence of asthma in childhood is 3–5% whereas the accumulated incidence is around 8%. Similar and higher figures have been reported from other industrialized countries. In a few studies, the incidence of allergic disease has been studied repeatedly over 10–20 years with a similar methodology. These studies all indicate a true increased incidence over time, although none of the investigations conclusively proves this statement. The incidence of allergic disease is higher in boys than in girls, at least in infants and young children. In adolescents, however, no sex differences seem apparent. Children with biparental family history of allergic disease begin to have symptoms at an earlier age than children with less pronounced or no family history of allergy.

V. ENVIRONMENTAL FACTORS IN THE DEVELOPMENT OF ALLERGIC DISEASE

Several studies strongly indicate that the prevalence of allergic diseases is increasing in many parts of the world. Since the human genotype has not changed appreciably over the past few generations, we can assume that the increase is caused by environmental influence. Available epidemiological data strongly suggest that the development of allergic disease is enhanced when a genetically predisposed individual is exposed to allergens in the presence of various environmental adjuvant factors that may enhance sensitization (Munir and Björkstén, 1992). According to this hypothesis, the impact of the environment is best studied in individuals with a family history of allergy or in individuals who previously have shown allergic symptoms. The impact of the environment may begin before birth. Thus, maternal immunity, tobacco, smoking, and medication appear to affect the likelihood of allergic disease in the offspring (Hattevig and Björkstén, 1993).

A. Early Exposure to Antigens

Early weaning to cow's milk formulas has been associated with an increased rate of allergic disease. However, many studies also have been done in which prolonged breast-feeding was not associated with less allergy than early administration of cow's milk formulas. The explanation for the apparently conflicting results seems to lie in selection of patients for the studies, the necessity for other dietary precautions, and self-selection bias. Studies showing a protective effect of prolonged exclusive breast-feeding have included infants with a genetic propensity to allergy rather than an unselected group of infants. Also, the breast-feeding in these cases was associated with an avoidance of other foods, for example, juices and solid foods. Critical reviews indicate, however, that even under the best circumstances the effect of breast-feeding on the development of atopy or allergy is limited to risk individuals and that it appears merely to delay rather than prevent the onset of allergy.

Several possible explanations are available for the protective role of breast milk against allergy, including low content of allergens, protection against intestinal and respiratory infections, passive transfer of immunity from the mother by secretory IgA antibodies, and transfer of components that stimulate the maturation of the infantile immune system. Human milk is well established to contain food antigens similar to cow's milk proteins and egg if these items are ingested by the mother, which may sensitize the breast-fed baby. The small amounts of allergens that may be present in breast milk can, thus, be sufficient to cause a high grade of sensitization in a genetically predisposed infant, and even to evoke allergic symptoms during lactation.

The effect of maternal hypoallergenic diet during the lactation period has been addressed recently. Both studies show that maternal avoidance of certain allergenic foods such as eggs, cow's milk, fish, soy, and peanuts was associated with less allergic disease for the first years of life in their babies. Also, the disease tended to be less severe in babies of mothers who had adhered to the diet (Hattevig *et al.*, 1989; Zeiger *et al.*, 1992).

Similar to early exposure to foreign antigenic foods, exposure of infants to inhaled allergens may result in sensitization that becomes manifested clinically only several years later. Thus, several clinical studies indicate a period in early infancy during which exposure to inhalant allergens readily may sensitize the baby. The relationship between early exposure to inhalant allergens and allergic disease seems, however, to be limited to children with a congenital propensity for allergy, rather than being present in all children. Reasons for the association between early exposure and disease are poorly understood, since clinical symptoms in response to inhalant allergens usually only appear several years after infancy. Animal experiments may, however, offer an explanation. Holt and associates (1990) have shown that, when young rats of a strain with a low propensity for IgE antibody formation inhale an allergen, they initially respond with a low-grade IgE antibody formation. On repeated exposure, the IgE antibody response is suppressed. In contrast, rats of a strain with a higher tendency to IgE antibody formation respond to repeated exposure with increasing levels of IgE antibodies. Cloning experiments have shown that repeated allergen exposure of normal low-responder rats induces T cells with the capacity to suppress IgE antibody formation, whereas T helper cells are induced in young high-responder rats.

The normal induction of tolerance can be disturbed by exposure to various environmental agents. Thus, if young rats of the low-responder genotype are exposed to tobacco smoke, ozone, or SO_2 (for example) at the time of initial antigen exposure, then repeated exposure to antigen results in prolonged IgE antibody formation. As indicated by clinical observations, these findings in rats also may be relevant for humans.

B. Nonspecific Factors

In addition to allergens, several environmental factors facilitate sensitization to almost any allergen to which the individual is exposed (Table I). Among these "adjuvant" factors, exposure to tobacco smoke and certain infections appear to play a particular role in early infancy (Munir and Björkstén, 1992). The role of tobacco smoke has been substantiated in several studies in infants, young children, and adults. Therefore, strongly discouraging parents from smoking near a young infant, particularly in families with allergic disease, and regarding smoking and passive smoking as occupational health hazards in adults is reasonable. Other nonspecific factors that appear to play a role in allergy include industrial air pollution and living in modern, tight, poorly ventilated houses.

Table I Environmental Factors Encountered during Fetal Life and Early Infancy That May Influence the Development of Allergy

Prenatally	In infancy	In children and adults
Placental barrier function?	Early introduction of formula	Exposure to tobacco smoke
Maternal immunity	Amount and quality of breast milk	Exposure to air pollution
Maternal smoking?	Exposure to tobacco smoke	Psychological stress?
Maternal medication	Exposure to outdoor air pollutants	
Maternal health?	Living in tight, poorly ventilated buildings	
	Early exposure to inhalant allergens	
	Infections	
	Neonatal complications	

Several studies suggest an association between respiratory infections and appearance of allergic disease. Possible explanations for these observations include that infectious agents may induce an inflammatory reaction in the airways, may alter immune defense, and may act as adjuvants or as allergens. From animal studies, pertussis bacteria are well known to be adjuvants for the induction of IgE antibody formation against various antigens. In humans, whooping cough is associated with a prolonged period of bronchial hyperreactivity, and IgE antibodies against pertussis toxin commonly are encountered in children with whooping cough and after immunization.

All these specific nonallergen environmental influences seem to play a major role only in individuals with a genetically predetermined tendency toward allergic disease. Based on extensive experimental work in rodents and analysis of epidemiological data on the appearance of IgE antibodies in infants and children, researchers have proposed that the capacity to produce IgE antibodies in response to environmental allergens is controlled genetically through the T-cell system (Holt, 1990). The ultimate expression of a genetic potential for high IgE production requires the intervention of additional environmental risk factors (e.g., air pollution). Many of those factors described so far appear to function at a level that enhances contact between the allergen and the immune system, particularly by increasing net flux of inhalant allergen across respiratory mucous membranes. At the time of initial contact with an allergen not previously encountered, the immune system responds to it. A transient IgE production is part of this normal response. In nonatopic individuals, the initial IgE response is self-limiting and is replaced by a lifelong tolerance to the allergen. However, if the individual at the time of initial exposure, for example, in early infancy, is exposed simultaneously to appropriate risk factors, the immune response may, instead, increase steadily and give rise to an expanding pool of memory T cells that effectively prime the immune system, laying the foundation for a state of hyersensitivity to the allergen. Once in allergic inflammatory response to an allergen occurs, this process enhances sensitization to new allergens encountered during the reaction.

VI. PREVENTION AND TREATMENT OF RESPIRATORY ALLERGY

Obviously the best treatment for all diseases would be prevention. Through primary prevention, sensitization to allergens is avoided. In principle, prevention is only possible in early childhood. As discussed earlier, a period seems to exist early in life during which an individual is particularly susceptible to sensitization. The conditions under which the first exposure to allergens occurs may influence the immune system for a long time, possibly even for life.

Secondary prevention aims at the prevention of symptoms of disease in the already sensitized individual, which can be achieved by avoiding exposure to triggering factors and to allergens against which the individual is sensitized, by drugs, and by other means to reduce hyperreactivity. Clean air, air filters, and elimination of allergen sources at home, in schools, and in working places are all important in this respect. Also, several prophylactic drugs are available on the market, including sodium cromoglycate.

Asthma induced by exercise and cold air often may be prevented by a prolonged warming-up period before exercising and by prophylactic medication through inhalation of a β-2-stimulating agent.

Tertiary prevention aims at reducing permanent damage as a consequence of the allergic disease. The most important measure in this respect is reducing inflammation in the lungs by adequate treatment with corticosteroids. Usually, this treatment can be achieved by inhalation therapy. If such medication is insufficient, oral prednisone should be considered, bearing in mind the potential harmful effects of prolonged systemic treatment with corticosteroids. Other treatment possibilities in severe asthma, if steroid treatment fails or is associated with unacceptable side effects, include methotrexate, chloroquine, cyclosporin A, and intravenous infusion of immunoglobulin. None of these procedures, however, is established in clinical practice and each should be considered only in highly selected cases, preferably as part of clinical research.

VII. NONALLERGIC RHINITIS

The nose is exposed constantly to allergenic particles as it filters them from inhaled air. Accordingly, it is the site of more allergic symptoms and illnesses than any other organ. In some patients with chronic noninfectious rhinitis, neither an allergic etiology nor evidence of inflammation can be found. Such patients often act as though they have hyperreactive nasal ucosa with exaggerated responses to a large number of stimuli that are ordinarily tolerated. (Anderson and Pipkorn, 1990).

In the lower airways, bronchial challenge tests with histamine and metacholine can be used to differentiate normal subjects from patients with hyperreactive airways. A similar approach has been taken to test for hyperreactivity of the upper airways with the same agents given in nasal challenge procedures.

Treatment includes environmental control, for example, avoidance of known irritating agents, short-term treatment with nasal decongestants, local steroids, and cromolyn sodium.

VIII. ALLERGIC ALVEOLITIS OR HYPERSENSITIVITY PNEUMONITIS

Several eponyms for this condition are used in the literature, including farmer's lung, bird fancier's lung, pigeon breeder's disease, saw dust disease, and byssinosis. (Fink, 1983,1984). All the names give an indication of the conditions under which this disease appears. Some overlap exists between occupational asthma and allergic alveolitis, and episodes of bronchiolitis obliterans can cause diagnostic difficulty. The condition is characterized clinically by acute episodes of tachypnea and dyspnea, often with inspiratory rales and fever, appearing several hours after inhalation of organic dust that contains a wide variety of antigenic material from thermophilic organisms, birds, animal proteins, chemicals, or drugs.

Some of these antigens are encountered only in the working environment. Hypersensitivity pneumonitis also may be caused by inhalation of high doses of fungi, including *Trichosporum, Alternaria, Aspergillus,* and *Penicillium.* Allergic alveolitis is an important occupational disease and is seen only rarely in children and adolescents. Exposure to birds (pigeon breeder's disease) is the most common and best studied pediatric hypersensitivity pneumonitis. Severe alveolitis has been recorded in mushroom workers. Of more general importance is the occurrence of sensitivity reactions to thermophilic actinomycetes and *Aspergillus* in office cooling systems that use water contaminated with these organisms. Certain drugs, including belomycin, furazolidine, hydrochlorthiazide, and tetracyclines, also have been reported to cause allergic alveolitis after oral ingestion. Because of a delay in onset of symptoms following exposure to the causative agent, the patient may fail to notice a relationship. The symptoms usually resolve within 18 hr of onset but occasionally may persist for several days, unless treated with corticosteroids.

From the clinical perspective, the diagnosis should be suspected from a careful history. Typically, a person working in an exposed environment experiences increasing respiratory symptoms during the week and then improves remarkably over the weekend. Radiologic changes usually consist of patchy diffuse interstitial infiltrates, often more evident in the lower zones of the lungs. Lung function tests reveal restrictive impairment of pulmonary function with reduced forced vital capacity. Morphological findings always include an interstitial infiltrate. In most cases, pneumonitis, interstitial fibrosis, and bronchiolitis are seen. Edema and pleural fibrosis are other common microscopic findings. Since the clinical radiologic and functional characteristics are sufficiently well defined, a lung biopsy is not usually required to confirm the diagnosis in the presence of a clear history of exposure to a known precipitating agent.

The condition is, at least in part, immunologically mediated. Antigens inducing reactions are small enough to reach the bronchial tree, where they are processed by pulmonary macrophages. High titers of precipitating IgG antibodies against the causative antigens usually are found in the serum. Therefore, a type III reaction long was thought to be the major underlying pathogenic mechanism. These antibodies, however, may also be detected in up to 50% of asymptomatic similarly exposed individuals; therefore their presence is not conclusively indicative of the disease. Patients with farmer's lung disease have broad immune responses with elevated specific antibody levels against many common respiratory viruses and miocroorganisms compared with healthy persons, possibly indicating abnormal host responsiveness. More likely, the presence of precipitating IgG antibodies simply reflects antigen exposure. Although type III reactions appear to occur in these diseases, experimental and clinical studies indicate that type IV reactions involving monocytes and lymphocytes are more important in the pathogenesis of the pulmonary reaction. Possibly, the precipitating antibodies may play a protective role in antigen-clearing mechanisms. The antibody titers are, however, generally higher in symptomatic individuals.

Like asthma and atopic disease, genetic control of the pulmonary immune response is suggested by studies in humans and animals. However, no link to a particular haplotype has been confirmed to date. Pulmonary damage appears to develop after an immune response that combines both antigen-specific humoral antibodies and cellular hypersensitivity with mononuclear cells releasing lymphokines. Complement activation in the lung and irritant effects of thermophilic agents also may be important. Cellular hyerpsensitivity to organic dusts may lead to hypersensitivity pneumonitis, after being triggered by a nonspecific inflammatory process such as respiratory infection.

Allergic alveolitis often is associated strongly with the conditions of the workplace. As indicated by the many names given to the condition, a continued exposure to inhalation of organic material, for example, on farms and in saw mills, once was very common. Today, home and office air conditioning systems may present specific hazards of hypersensitivity pneumonitis. This disorder may be a contributing factor to the "sick building" syndrome and, thus, be one of several diseases and symptoms associated with poorly ventilated, faultily constructed buildings.

Although complete recovery from allergic alveolitis does occur, residual abnormality with dyspnea is common. Suspected causative agents may be confirmed by challenge testing after the acute episode is over. The disease can cause long-term effects if repeated exposures occur. Farmer's lung can be prevented entirely by an intensive educational program and by wearing a mask when exposure is likely. Families in which severe cases of allergic alveolitis occur as a result of exposure to pet birds should be advised on the importance of avoiding exposure. In homes and offices, care should be taken to avoid microbial contamination of humidifiers, if the machines are used at all.

IX. OTHER HYPERSENSITIVITY DISORDERS OF THE RESPIRATORY TRACT

Allergic bronchopulmonary aspergillosis (ABA) is an immune bronchial disease that occurs in asthmatics and is characterized by pulmonary infiltrates and eosinophilia in blood and sputum (Slavin, 1985; Massie, 1988). Skin testing with *Aspergillus fumigatus* antigen usually reveals a dual reaction with an immediate (within 20 min) and a late (after 4–8 hr) response. The immediate, and possibly also the late, response is IgE mediated. Also IgG, IgM, and IgA antibodies against the fungus are often detectable, but histological examination does not support their role in the pathogenesis. Roentgenographic findings in ABA vary according to disease activity, and include bronchial wall edema, inflammation, obstruction, and infiltrates, predominantly in the upper lobes. In advanced cases, central bronchiectasia appears as hilar shadows, cavitation, fibrosis, and contracted upper lobes. Determined corticosteroid therapy is the preferred treatment.

The typical patient with chronic obstructive pulmonary disease (COPD) in adults presents with a mixed form of chronic bronchitis and emphysema, with wheezing similar to that in asthma. This condition may be complicated by manifestations of right-sided heart failure. Cigarette smoking is the major cause of COPD. The condition often is lumped together with other obstructive lung disease, including chronic bronchitis and emphysema of various etiologies. Although this assessment may be reasonable with respect to clinical symptoms, this tendency may result in overmediation for the severely emphysematic patient and in inadequate therapy for those with predominant chronic bronchitis. Clinically, physicians often recognize the reversible component of airway obstruction in elderly patients with COPD. Elevated IgE levels in serum also are a common finding, although a search for IgE antibodies against defined allergens in sera is usually negative (Itabaskis *et al.*, 1991). Possibly, the elevated IgE levels are secondary to increased airway mucosal permeability caused by mucosal epithelial damage from chronic inflammation. The goals of treatment of COPD include prevention of progression of the disease, treatment of potentially reversible components of the disease, and teaching patients to participate in their own management.

References

Andersson, M., and Pipkorn, U. (1990). Nasal hyperreactivity. *In* "Rhinitis and Asthma" (N. Mygind, U. Pipkorn, and R. Dahl, eds.), pp. 156–171. Munksgaard, Copenhagen.

Björkstén, B., and Kjellman, N.-I. M. (1992). Epidemiology of allergic diseases in children. Proceedings of the XIVth IAACI Congress, pp. 16–20. Hogrefe & Huber Publishers, Toronto.

Fink, J. N. (1983). Pigeon breeder's disease. *Clin. Rev. Allergy* **1,** 497–508.

Fink, J. N. (1984). Hypersensitivity pneumonitis. *J. Allergy Clin. Immunol.* **74,** 1–9.

Hattevig, G., and Björkstén, B. (1993). Environmental factors in the development of allergy. *In* "Asthma and Allergy in Pregnancy and Early Infancy," (M. Schatz, R. N. Zeiger, eds.), pp. 395–412. Marcel Dekker, Inc., New York.

Hattevig, G., Kjellman, B., Sigurs, N., and Björkstén, B. (1989). Effect of maternal avoidance of eggs, cow's milk and fish during lactation upon allergic manifestations in infants. *Clin. Exper. Allergy,* **19,** 27–32.

Holt, P. (1990). Primary sensitisation to inhalant ellergens during infancy. *Pediatr. Allergy Immunol.* **1,** 3–13.

Itabaskis, I. K. *et al.* (1991). Allergic sensitization in elderly patients with chronic obstructive pulmonary disease. *Respiration* **57,** 384–388.

Marsh, D. G. (1990). Immunogenetic and immunogenetic factors determining immune responsiveness to allergens: Studies in unrelated subjects. *In* "Genetic and Environmental Factors in Clinical Allergy (D. G. Marsh and M. Blumenthal, eds.), pp. 97–123. Univ. of Minnesota Press, Minneapolis.

Massie, F. S. (1988). Hypersensitivity pneumonitis and allergic bronchopulmonary aspergillosis. *In* "Allergic Diseases from Infancy to Adulthood" (C. W. Bierman and D. S. Pearlman, ed.), pp. 617–625. Saunders, Philadelphia.

Munir, A. K. M., and Björkstén, B. (1992). Indoor pollution and allergic sensitization. *In* "Chemical, Microbiol, Health and Comfort. Aspects of Indoor Air Quality. State of the Art in SBS" (H. Knöppel, and P. Wolkoff, eds.), pp. 181–199. Kluwer Academic Publishers, London.

Slavin, R. G. (1985). Allergic bronchopulmonary aspergillosis. *Clin. Rev. Allergy* **3,** 167–182.

Zeiger, R. S., Heller, S., Mellon, M. H., Halsey, J. F., Hamburger, R. N., and Sampson, H. A. (1992). Genetic and environmental factors affecting the development of atopy through the age 4 in children of atopic parents: A prospective randomized study of food allergen avoidance. *Pediatr. Allergy Immunol.* **3,** 110–127.

Section G

Oral Cavity, Upper Airway, and Head and Neck

Section Editor: John Bienenstock

(Chapters 47 through 50)

47

Ocular Mucosal Immunity

David A. Sullivan

I. INTRODUCTION

The secretory immune system of the eye defends the ocular surface against antigenic challenge (Franklin, 1989; Friedman, 1990; Sullivan, 1990). This immunological role is mediated primarily through secretory IgA (SIgA) antibodies, which are known to inhibit viral adhesion and internalization; prevent bacterial attachment, colonization, and activity; interfere with parasitic infestation; and reduce antigen-related damage in mucosal sites (Underdown and Schiff, 1986; Brandtzaeg, 1985; Mestecky, 1987; Mestecky and McGhee, 1987; Brown and Kloppel, 1989; Childers *et al.*, 1989; McGhee *et al.*, 1989; MacDonald *et al.*, 1990). Thus, the ocular secretory immune system appears to protect the eye against allergic, inflammatory, and infectious disease, thereby promoting conjunctival and corneal integrity and preserving visual acuity.

This chapter reviews the immunological architecture and regulation of the secretory immune system of the eye, and explores the impact of ocular infection and autoimmune disease on the structure and function of this system. For information on nonmucosal aspects of ocular immunity, for example, anterior chamber-associated immune deviation and retinal immunology, the reader is referred to several excellent reports (Gery *et al.*, 1986; Streilein, 1987; Usui *et al.*, 1990).

II. ARCHITECTURE OF THE SECRETORY IMMUNE SYSTEM OF THE EYE

A. *Tissues Involved in Ocular Mucosal Immunity*

The principal tissues involved in immunological protection of the ocular surface are the lacrimal gland and the conjunctiva. The lacrimal gland, which serves as the predominant source of tear SIgA antibodies (Sullivan and Allansmith, 1984; Peppard and Montgomery, 1987), is the primary effector tissue in the secretory immune defense of the eye (Franklin, 1989; Friedman, 1990; Sullivan, 1990). This gland contains a diverse array of lymphocytes, including plasma cells, T cells, B cells, dendritic cells, and macrophages (Table I; Figure 1). In humans, plasma cells represent the most numerous lymphocytic population, accounting for more than 50% of all mononuclear cells in lacrimal tissue (Weiczorek *et al.*, 1988). The vast majority of these plasma cells are IgA positive (Franklin *et al.*, 1973; Allansmith *et al.*, 1976a,1985; Brandtzaeg *et al.*, 1979,1987; Gillette *et al.*, 1980; Crago *et al.*, 1984; Damato *et al.*, 1984; Brandtzaeg, 1985; Kett *et al.*, 1986; Weiczorek *et al.*, 1988) and express an IgA1/IgA2 subclass distribution that is either different from (Kett *et al.*, 1986) or similar to (Crago *et al.*, 1984; Allansmith *et al.*, 1985) that of other mucosal tissues. In addition, a high percentage of lacrimal IgA plasma cells, which are located in the gland's interstitium, synthesizes both J chain and polymeric IgA (pIgA; Brandtzaeg, 1985) that may bind secretory component (SC; Brandtzaeg, 1983). These cells are complemented by limited numbers of IgG, IgM, IgE, and IgD plasma cells (Franklin *et al.*, 1973; Allansmith *et al.*, 1976; Brandtzaeg *et al.*, 1979,1987; Gillete *et al.*, 1980; Damato *et al.*, 1984; Wieczorek *et al.*, 1988), although the IgD-containing subset may increase during IgA deficiency (Brandtzaeg *et al.*, 1979). The second most frequent lymphocyte population in human lacrimal tissue consists of T cells, which are situated between acinar and ductal epithelial cells, throughout glandular interstitial regions, and within small periductular lymphoid aggregates (Weiczorek *et al.*, 1988; Pepose *et al.*, 1990). The distribution of T cells appears to vary topographically according to specific subclasses, including suppressor/cytotoxic and helper T cells (Weiczorek *et al.*, 1988; Pepose *et al.*, 1990), and presents with an overall helper : suppressor ratio of approximately 0.56 (Weiczorek *et al.*, 1988). Minor or rare populations of lacrimal lymphocytes include surface Ig-bearing B cells, Langerhans-type dendritic cells, monocyte–macrophages, and activated IL-2^+ T cells, which occur almost exclusively in periductular lymphocyte foci (Weiczorek *et al.*, 1988; Pepose *et al.*, 1990). These latter lymphoid aggregates, when present, typically appear as primary follicles without germinal center formation and, theoreticaly, may be involved in antigen processing (Weiczorek *et al.*, 1988).

The human lacrimal gland also

1. produces lysozyme (Gillette *et al.*, 1980,1981), and SC (Franklin *et al.*, 1973; Allansmith and Gillette, 1980; Gillette *et al.*, 1980), the pIgA antibody receptor (Underdown and Schiff, 1986; Brandtzaeg *et al.*, 1987; Brown and Kloppel, 1989) in acinar and ductal epithelium
2. synthesizes lactoferrin (Gillette and Allansmith, 1980; Gillette *et al.*, 1980) and convertase decay-accelerating factor, which protects against autologous complement activation (Lass *et al.*, 1990), in acinar cells
3. expresses HLA-DR antigens on B cells, dendritic cells,

Table I Lymphocyte Populations Identified in Lacrimal Glands of Various Species

Species	References
Human	
IgA (predominant; both IgA1 and IgA2), IgG, IgM, IgD, and IgE plasma cells Suppressor/cytotoxic (predominant), helper, and activated (IL2$^+$) T cells Surface IgM- (predominant), IgD-, IgG-, or IgA-bearing B cells Macrophages and dendritic cells	Franklin *et al.* (1973); Allansmith *et al.* (1976a,1985); Brandtzaeg *et al.* (1979,1987); Gillette *et al.* (1980); Crago *et al.* (1984); Damato *et al.* (1984); Brandtzaeg (1985); Kett *et al.* (1986); Wieczorek *et al.* (1988)
Rabbit	
IgA (predominant) and IgG plasma cells	Shimada and Silverstein (1974); Franklin *et al.* (1979); Jackson and Mestecky (1981)
Rat	
IgA (predominant), IgG, IgG1, IgG2a, IgG2b, IgG2c, and IgM plasma cells Immature, suppressor/cytotoxic, and helper T cells Surface IgM-, IgA-, and IgG-bearing B cells Macrophages and mast cells (rare)	Gudmundsson *et al.* (1984,1985a,1988); Sullivan *et al.* (1986,1990a, 1990/91); Allansmith *et al.* (1987); Hann *et al.* (1988); Pappo *et al.* (1988); Montgomery *et al.* (1989,1990); Sullivan and Hann (1989a)
Mouse	
IgA (predominant), IgG, and IgM plasma cells Surface IgA-, IgG-, or IgM-bearing B cells	McGee and Franklin (1984); Montgomery *et al.* (1985)

ductule epithelium (Weiczorek *et al.*, 1988) and certain acini (Mircheff *et al.*, 1991)

4. contains lymphatic channels that drain into local cervical and preauricular lymph nodes (Iwamoto and Jakobiec, 1989)

With respect to human accessory lacrimal tissue, its immunological characteristics appear to be identical to those of the major lacrimal gland (Gillette *et al.*, 1980,1981; Sacks *et al.*, 1986).

Lacrimal tissues of rats, rabbits, cows, and mice also seem to share the immune features of the human gland (Table I). Thus, rat lacrimal glands contain a pronounced population of IgA plasma cells (Gudmundsson *et al.*, 1985a; Sullivan *et al.*, 1986,1990a,1990/91; Allansmith *et al.*, 1987; Hann *et al.*, 1988; Sullivan and Hann, 1989), which undergo a striking age-related increase in density from infancy to adulthood (Hann *et al.*, 1988; Sullivan *et al.*, 1990a). These cells are accompanied by IgG and IgM plasma cells (Gudmundsson *et al.*, 1985a; Allansmith *et al.*, 1987; Hann *et al.*, 1988; Sullivan *et al.*, 1990a), immature suppressor/cytotoxic and helper T cells (Gudmundsson *et al.*, 1988; Pappo *et al.*, 1988; Montgomery *et al.*, 1989,1990), surface Ig-bearing B cells (Pappo *et al.*, 1988; Montgomery *et al.*, 1989,1990) that proliferate in response to mitogen exposure (Pappo *et al.*, 1988), phagocytic macrophages that express Fc receptors and Ia antigens (Pappo *et al.*, 1988), and rare mast cells (Gudmundsson *et al.*, 1984). Moreover, acinar cells from rat lacrimal tissue synthesize and secrete SC (Sullivan *et al.*, 1984b,1990b; Gudmundsson *et al.*, 1985a; Hann *et al.*, 1989, 1991; Kelleher *et al.*, 1991; Lambert *et al.*, 1993) which appears to transport pIgA into tears against an apparent concentration gradient (Allansmith *et al.*, 1987; Sullivan and Allansmith, 1988; Sullivan and Hann, 1989b). Similarly, lacrimal glands of cows (Butler *et al.*, 1972), rabbits (Shimada and Silverstein, 1975; Franklin *et al.*, 1979), and mice (McGee and Franklin, 1984) either produce IgA or harbor plasma cell populations that are predominantly IgA positive and, at least in rabbits, contain acinar and ductal cells that produce SC (Franklin *et al.*, 1979). However, periductular lymphoid aggregates appear to be very uncommon in lacrimal tissues of these species, except under pathological conditions (e.g., autoimmune disorders; Kessler, 1968; Mizejewski, 1978; Hoffman *et al.*, 1984; Jabs *et al.*, 1985; Liu *et al.*, 1987; Jabs and Prendergast, 1988; Ariga *et al.*, 1989; Liu, 1989; Vendramini *et al.*, 1991; Sato *et al.*, 1991).

The primary origin of IgA-containing lymphocytes and T cells in the lacrimal gland remains to be determined, but may, in part, be local cervical (Brandtzaeg *et al.*, 1979; Ebersole *et al.*, 1983), distant peripheral (Montgomery *et al.*, 1985; O'Sullivan and Montgomery, 1990), and gut-associated lymphoid tissue (Montgomery *et al.*, 1983; O'Sullivan and Montgomery, 1990), as well as the thoracic duct (O'Sullivan and Montgomery, 1990), spleen (McGee and Franklin, 1984), and mammary gland (Montgomery *et al.*, 1985). The migration of lymphocytes into the lacrimal gland appears to be random (McGee and Franklin, 1984), yet the selective retention and heterogeneous distribution of IgA-containing cells within lacrimal tissue is not random (Sullivan *et al.*, 1990/91) and may be stimulated by antigenic challenge (Jackson and Mestecky, 1981; Allansmith *et al.*, 1987) and regulated by microenvironmental (Franklin, 1981; Pockley and Montgomery, 1990/91a), endocrine (Sullivan *et al.*, 1986; Hann *et al.*, 1988; Sullivan and Hann, 1989a), neural (Walcott *et al.*, 1986; Franklin *et al.*, 1988,1989; Oeschger *et al.*, 1989; Sullivan *et al.*, 1990/91), T-cell (Franklin *et al.*, 1985; Franklin, 1989; Franklin and Shepard, 1990/91), or acinar epithelial-cell (Franklin *et al.*, 1985) signals. The lymphocytic accumulation

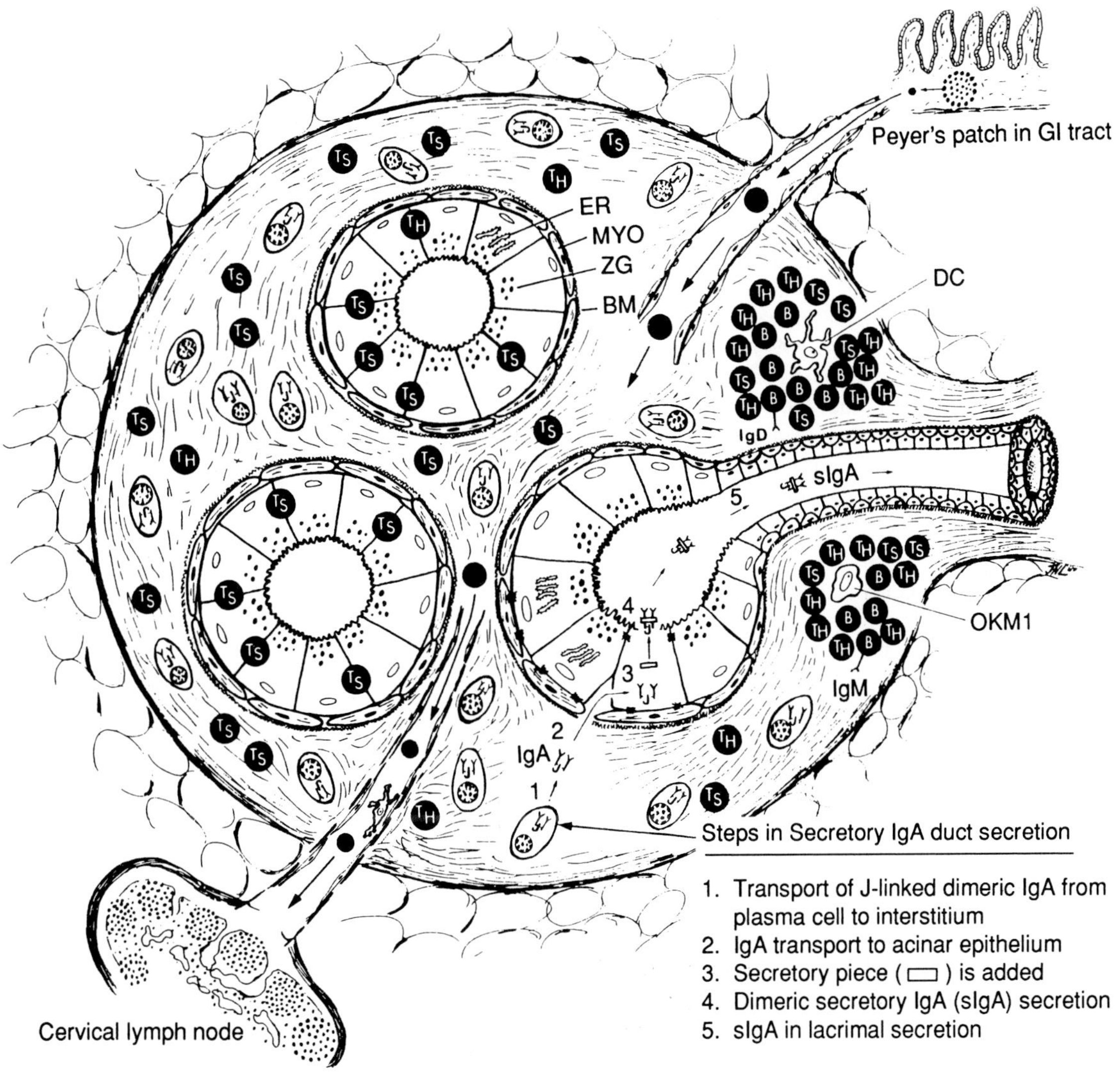
Peyer's patch in GI tract
ER
MYO
ZG
BM
DC
IgD
sIgA
OKM1
IgM
IgA
Cervical lymph node
Steps in Secretory IgA duct secretion
1. Transport of J-linked dimeric IgA from plasma cell to interstitium
2. IgA transport to acinar epithelium
3. Secretory piece (▭) is added
4. Dimeric secretory IgA (sIgA) secretion
5. sIgA in lacrimal secretion

Figure 1 Schematic representation of the secretory immune system of the human lacrimal gland. Topographical features include acinar cells, which contain endoplasmic reticulum (ER) and lysozyme- and lactoferrin-positive zymogen granules (ZG), and synthesize and secrete SC (termed secretory piece); myoepithelial cells, which are adjacent to acinar cells and surrounded by a basement membrane (BM); interstitial plasma cells, which are the primary lymphoid cell and produce principally IgA, but also some IgG, IgM, or IgD; T helper (Th) and suppressor (T_S) cells, which are distributed throughout the interstitium, the intercellular spaces between acinar or ductal cells, and the periductular lymphoid aggregates; B cells (B), OKT6$^+$ Langerhans-type dendritic cells (DC), and OKM1$^+$ monocyte-macrophages, predominantly located in periductular lymphoid aggregates, which most often appear as primary follicles without germinal center formation and may be active in antigen processing; and unlabeled darkened cells, which refer to circulating T or B lymphocytes, which may originate in other mucosal tissues (e.g., intestinal Peyer's patch) and, if not retained locally, possibly exit the lacrimal gland through lymphatic channels to regional cervical ro preauricular lymph nodes. Immunoglobulin A is secreted by plasma cells (1), bound by SC on the acinar cell basolateral membrane (2,3), transported in distinct vesicles (4), and released at the apical surface as SIgA into tear-containing lumina (5). [This figure has been reproduced and published, courtesy of *Ophthalmology* (1988). 95:100–109.]

in, or adherence to, lacrimal tissue appears to require calcium as well as functional oxidative phosphorylation and contractile microfilament systems, and to depend on cell-surface protein and carbohydrate determinants (O'Sullivan and Montgomery, 1990).

In addition to the lacrimal gland, the conjunctiva has been postulated to play an active role in both inductive and effector actions of the ocular secretory immune system (Chandler and Gillette, 1983; Franklin and Remus, 1984; Franklin, 1989; Tagawa *et al.*, 1989; Allansmith and Ross, 1991). In support of this hypothesis, the rabbit conjunctiva contains a substantial number of IgA, and occasional IgG and IgM, plasma cells in the substantia propria and numerous T and B cells in specialized lymphoid follicles (Shimada and Silverstein, 1975;

Franklin *et al.*, 1979; Franklin and Remus, 1984). Moreover, rabbit conjunctival B cells may be induced to differentiate into IgA-positive cells by mitogen stimulation (Franklin and Remus, 1984) and the rabbit conjunctival epithelium produces SC (Franklin *et al.*, 1979; Liu *et al.*, 1981). Since investigators also have reported the presence of plasma cells (Allansmith *et al.*, 1976a; Bhan *et al.*, 1982; Tagawa *et al.*, 1989); T cells (Bhan *et al.*, 1982; Sacks *et al.*, 1986; Tagawa *et al.*, 1989); HLA-DR-positive epithelial, stromal (Lee *et al.*, 1990/91), and Langerhans cells; interdigitating dendritic cells; macrophages; neutrophils (Sacks *et al.*, 1986); mast cells (Allensmith *et al.*, 1978a; Allansmith and Ross, 1991); and lymphatic channels (Srinivasan *et al.*, 1990) in human conjunctival tissue, these findings might indicate that the conjunctiva is involved in antigen processing, lymphocyte migration, and ocular secretory immune defense (Chandler and Gillette, 1983). However, this conclusion is somewhat controversial and perhaps not entirely correct.

1. The evidence for plasma cell existence in normal human conjunctiva appears tenuous: plasma cell identification by light microscopy could not be verified by immunofluorescent staining for cell-associated IgA, IgG, IgM, IgD, or IgE (Allensmith *et al.*, 1976b) and plasma cell enumeration in another study was performed with an antibody that cross-reacted with T cells (Bhan *et al.*, 1982). In contrast, more recent investigations have demonstrated a complete absence of plasma cells in conjunctival tissue of humans (Sacks *et al.*, 1986) and rats (Gudmundsson *et al.*, 1985a). Instead, the majority of lymphocytes in human conjunctiva appears to be primarily suppressor/cytotoxic T cells, with a smaller population of helper T cells that are distributed in a subclass-dependent manner throughout the epithelium and substantia propria of the forniceal, tarsal, and epibulbar conjunctiva (Sacks *et al.*, 1986.
2. B cells (Bhan *et al.*, 1982; Sacks *et al.*, 1986) and activated T cells (Sacks *et al.*, 1986) rarely are observed in human conjunctiva.
3. SC is not synthesized or expressed in either human (Allansmith and Gillette, 1980) or rat (Sullivan *et al.*, 1984b; Gudmundsson *et al.*, 1985a) conjunctival epithelium. Although one study has reported SC, as well as IgA and IgG, synthesis in human conjunctival biopsies (Lai *et al.*, 1973), tissue samples may have contained accessory lacrimal tissue.
4. The conjunctival epithelium in humans (Sacks *et al.*, 1986) and rats (Setzer *et al.*, 1987) does not possess specialized cells for antigen sampling, as found in the intestine (Owen, 1977), or lung (Bienenstock, 1985), and appears to limit severely the passage of most antigens because of structural size and molecular weight restrictions (Huang *et al.*, 1989; Kahn *et al.*, 1990). Therefore, the normal human or rat conjunctiva seems unlikely to synthesize IgA, transport IgA antibodies to the ocular surface, or play a direct and significant role in B-cell maturation or migration.

Nevertheless, the conjunctiva does contain the immunological capacity for antigen processing, cell-mediated immunity, and hypersensitivity responses (e.g., Allansmith *et al.*, 1981,1983; Chandler and Gillette, 1983; Hann *et al.*, 1985; Cornell-Bell *et al.*, 1986; Sacks *et al.*, 1986; Abelson and Smith, 1991).

As concerns the cornea, this tissue does not actively provide immune protection for the anterior surface of the eye. The cornea possesses interstitial IgA, IgG, IgM, IgD, and IgE (Allansmith *et al.*, 1978b), which appear to originate from serum, diffuse from the limbal to central regions, and require extended time periods (months) for complete turnover (Verhagen *et al.*, 1990). However, lymphocytes (Allansmith *et al.*, 1978b) and differentiated Langerhans cells (Seto *et al.*, 1987) are essentially absent from, and SC is not produced by (Allansmith and Gillette, 1980), the avascular corneal epithelium and stroma. The cornea, though, is certainly susceptible to viral (e.g., Sabbaga *et al.*, 1988; Bale *et al.*, 1990; Pavan-Langston, 1990), bacterial (e.g., Hazlett *et al.*, 1981a; Snyder and Hyndiuk, 1988) or other antigenic (e.g., graft; Smolin and O'Connor, 1981) challenge, and the possible ensuing vascularization or inflammation may impair corneal function and vision significantly (Smolin and O'Connor, 1981; Theodore *et al.*, 1983).

Other tissues, organisms, and factors involved in mucosal defense of the eye (Smolin, 1985) include:

1. the orbital skeletal structure, which minimizes potential trauma
2. the eyelid architecture, which is relatively impermeable to macromolecules
3. the eyelid blink reflex and ciliary movement, which rapidly clear foreign objects from the ocular surface
4. the resident conjunctival populations of nonpathogenic bacteria, consisting of aerobes and facultative and obligate anaerobes, which may curtail the ability of invasive bacteria to attach and colonize (McNatt *et al.*, 1978
5. the continuous tear flow and reflex tearing, which act to remove microorganisms and cellular debris through hydrokinetics and eventual drainage into the nasolacrimal duct

B. Role of the Tear Film in Ocular Surface Defense

The preocular tear film plays a critical role in the defense of the eye against microbial and antigenic exposure, as well as in the maintenance of corneal clarity and visual ability (Holly, 1987). These functions are extremely dependent on the stability, tonicity, and composition of the tear film structure, which includes an underlying mucin foundation, a considerable middle aqueous component, and an overlying lipid layer (Holly, 1987; Whitcher, 1987). Alteration, deficiency, or loss of the tear film may increase significantly the susceptibility to ocular surface desiccation and infection, corneal ulceration and perforation, and marked visual impairment and blindness (Lamberts, 1983; Whitcher, 1987; Lubniewski and Nelson, 1990).

With respect to immune protection, the tear film contains numerous components (Gachon *et al.*, 1979; van Haeringen, 1981; Bron and Seal, 1986; Smolin, 1987) that combine to provide both specific and nonspecific immunological activity (Tables II and III). Specific immunity is mediated primarily through the action of IgA antibodies, which are the predominant immunoglobulin in tears of humans (Josephson and Weiner, 1968; Table III) and experimental animals (Butler *et al.*, 1972; Hazlett *et al.*, 1981b; Sullivan and Allansmith, 1985,1987; Gudmundsson *et al.*, 1985; Wells and Hazlett, 1985; Sullivan and Hann, 1989a; Sullivan *et al.*, 1992a), occur almost entirely in polymeric form (Delacroix *et al.*, 1982; Delacroix and Vaerman, 1983; Gudmundsson *et al.*, 1985a; Allansmith *et al.*, 1985; Coyle *et al.*, 1987,1989), and originate from local production in lacrimal gland plasma cells (Butler *et al.*, 1972; Chao *et al.*, 1980; Janssen and van Bijisterveld, 1983; Sullivan and Allansmith, 1984; Peppard and Montgomery, 1987). In humans, tear IgA is distributed almost equally among IgA1 and IgA2 subclasses (Delacroix *et al.*, 1982; Fullard and Snyder, 1990; Fullard and Tucker, 1991). Most tear IgA appears to be transported by and bound to SC, which is synthesized and secreted by lacrimal epithelial cells (Franklin *et al.*, 1973; Allansmith and Gillette, 1980; Gillette *et al.*, 1980; Sullivan *et al.*, 1984b; Gudmundsson *et al.*, 1985a; Hann *et al.*, 1989,1991; Sullivan *et al.*, 1990b; Kelleher *et al.*, 1991; Lambert *et al.*, 1993) and is present in the tear film as an SIgA conjugate or as free SC (Gachon *et al.*, 1979; Delacroix and Vaerman, 1983; Sullivan *et al.*, 1984a; Sullivan and Allansmith, 1984,1987,1988; Gudmundsson *et al.*, 1985a; Watson *et al.*, 1985; Sullivan *et al.*, 1988; Coyle *et al.*, 1989; Sullivan and Hann, 1989a). The high concentrations of SIgA coexist with low levels of IgG and very limited quantities of IgM and IgE (Table III; Sullivan and Hann, 1989a; Sullivan *et al.*, 1990c). Tear IgG may be derived, in part, from lacrimal tissue synthesis (Butler *et al.*, 1972; Chao *et al.*, 1980; Janssen and van Bijsterveld, 1983), after which it moves down a steep concentration gradient into tears (Sullivan and Allansmith, 1988; Sullivan and Hann, 1989a; Sullivan *et al.*, 1990c), as well as from serum, after deposition in and passage through the conjunctival or lacrimal gland interstitium (McGill *et al.*, 1984; Fullard and Snyder, 1990; Fullard and Tucker, 1991; D. A. Sullivan, unpublished data). The source of tear IgM may be lacrimal tissue (Fullard and Snyder, 1990; Fullard and Tucker, 1991), whereas the origin of IgE in normal tears has yet to be determined. No IgD has been detected in the tear film (McClellan *et al.*, 1973; Bluestone *et al.*, 1975; Sen *et al.*, 1976,1978). It is important to note that the concentration of tear immunoglobulins, as shown in Table III, may be influenced significantly by the method of tear collection, the extent of tear stimulation, and the procedures that involve processing of tear samples (van Haeringen, 1981; Stuchell *et al.*, 1984; Fullard, 1988; Tuft and Dart, 1989; Fullard and Snyder, 1990; Fullard and Tucker, 1991; Kuizenga *et al.*, 1991). In addition, although tear Ig levels do not appear to display diurnal rhythms (Horwitz *et al.*, 1978), IgA concentrations may be exceedingly high after prolonged closure of the eyelids (Sack *et al.*, 1991).

Table II Specific and Nonspecific Immunological Factors in Tears of Individuals without Ocular Pathology

Secretory immunoglobulin A	Ceruloplasmin
Monomeric immunoglobulin A	Prostaglandin E_2
Immunoglobulin G	Tear-specific prealbumin
Immunoglobulin M	Histamine
Immunlglobulin E	Properdin factor B
Secretory component	Leukotrienes
Lysozyme	Complement (C3, C3 activator)
Lactoferrin	Anti-complement factor
β-Lysin	Complement decay-accelerating factor
Peroxidase	Superoxide radical producing system
Transferrin	Anti-chlamydial factor
Plasminogen activator	Lysosomal enzymes
α1-Antitrypsin	Antibiotic-producing bacteria
β2-Macroglobulin	T cells
α1-Antichymotrypsin	B cells
Inter-α-trypsin inhibitor	Macrophages
α2-Macroglobulin	Polymorphonuclear leukocytes

Additional specific and nonspecific agents in human tears that support ocular mucosal immunity follow.

1. Lysozyme and lactoferrin, which are secreted by the lacrimal gland (Gillette and Allansmith, 1980; Gillette *et al.*, 1980,1981), represent major tear components (van Haeringen, 1981; Gachon, 1982/83) and possess antibacterial activity (Smolin, 1987). Lactoferrin also may prevent activation of the classical complement pathway through inhibition of C3 convertase and may modulate ocular inflammatory reactions (Kijlstra, 1990/91).
2. β-Lysin may rupture bacterial cell membranes (Ford *et al.*, 1976). The presence of this substance in human tears is controversial (Selsted and Rafael, 1982; Janssen *et al.*, 1984).
3. Complement factors C3 and C3 activator, properdin and properdin factor B (Chandler *et al.*, 1974; Bluestone *et al.*, 1975; Yamamoto and Allansmith, 1979; Liotet *et al.*, 1982; Ballow *et al.*, 1985; Smolin, 1987), as well as anti-complement (Kijlstra and Veerhuis, 1981) and convertase decay-accelerating (Medof *et al.*, 1987; Lass *et al.*, 1990) factors are present. In certain eye diseases, tear IgA appears to fix complement (Barnett, 1968).
4. Nonlysozyme antibacterial factor (NLAF), which inhibits growth of staphylococci (Thompson and Gallardo, 1941) actually may be β-lysin (Ford *et al.*, 1976); its presence is controversial (van Haeringen, 1981; Selsted and Rafael, 1982; Janssen *et al.*, 1984).
5. Anti-chlamydial factor is a heat-stable substance that reduces *Chlamydia* attachment (Elbagir *et al.*, 1989).
6. Peroxidase (van Haeringen *et al.*, 1979; Fullard and Snyder, 1990; Fullard and Tucker, 1991) may exert bactericidal, viricidal, and fungicidal activity, as observed in other secretions, given appropriate levels of H_2O_2 and oxidizable cofactors (De *et al.*, 1987). Such peroxidase functions, however, may not operate

Table III Immunlglobulin Concentrations in Tears of Individuals without Ocular Pathology

Reference		Number of samples	Tear concentration (μg/ml)						
			IgA	SIgA	mIgA	IgG	IgM	IgE	IgD
Chordiker and Tomasi	(1963)	7	70			trace			
Douglas *et al.*	(1967)	4	118						
Bracciolini	(1968)	40	850			trace	0		
Little *et al.*	(1969)	10	212			trace	0		
Bazzi *et al.*	(1970)	9	230			790	0		
Knopf *et al.*	(1970)	7	125			36			
Brauninger and Centifanto	(1971)	24	88–500					detectable	
McClellan *et al.*	(1973)	74	170			140	0/trace	0.25	0
Chandler *et al.*	(1974)	3	230–300				0–12		
Bluestone *et al.*	(1975)	5		70.6		trace	0		0
Allansmith *et al.*	(1976b)	10						0.061	
Sen *et al.*	(1976)	50	246			trace	~0		0
Sen *et al.*	(1978)	220	307			<10	~0		0
Zavaro *et al.*	(1980)	26	199			31	<6.0		
Delacroix *et al.*	(1982)	6	124						
Donshik and Ballow	(1983)	10	123			10	0/trace	2.1[a]	
Gachon *et al.*	(1982/83)	38–101	411			32			
Gupta and Sarin	(1983)	5–35	233			trace	18		
Mackie and Seal	(1984)	54	<100			400–600			
Mannucci *et al.*	(1984)	17	113			32	0	<5.0[a]	
McGill *et al.*	(1984)	55	410–630			7–65			
Samra *et al.*	(1984)	54						0.82[a]	
Aalders-Deenstra *et al.*	(1985)	16						0.058[a]	
Coyle and Sibony	(1986)	20	186			6.7	5.6		
Sand *et al.*	(1986)	25		795					
Coyle *et al.*	(1987a)	23	198						
Coyle and Sibony	(1987)	12	200			2.0	4.9		
Vinding *et al.*	(1987)	42		2420					
Fullard	(1988)	6	398	542		0.54	0.31		
Lue *et al.*	(1988)	3	83			2.1	1.2		
Coyle	(1989)	19		374					
Hoebeke *et al.*	(1989)	8							0
Yuasa *et al.*	(1989)	8							0
Fullard and Snyder	(1990)	30		793	12.15	1.50	2.94		
Lal *et al.*	(1990)	15	350			110	120		
Mavra	(1990)	5				18.5			
Fullard and Tucker	(1991)	6		1930	13.21	3.66	18.3		
Temel *et al.*	(1991)	22	80			70	9		

[a] International Units/ml.

through the thiocyanate–H_2O_2 system, because tear thiocyanate concentrations are suboptimal (van Haeringen *et al.*, 1979).

7. Plasminogen activator (van Haeringen, 1981) is chemotactic for leukocytes (Bron, 1988).
8. Histamine, prostaglandins, and leukotrienes most likely derive from conjunctival mast cell production (van Haeringen, 1981; Gluud *et al.*, 1985; Abelson and Smith, 1991; Allansmith and Ross, 1991).
9. Antiproteases (e.g., α1-antitrypsin) are found (Zirm *et al.*, 1976; van Haeringen, 1981; Liotet *et al.*, 1982).
10. Lysosomal enzymes are present (Yamaguchi *et al.*, 1989).
11. Specific tear prealbumin and transferrin may have antibacterial actions (van Haeringen, 1981; Selsted and Rafael, 1982).
12. Ceruloplasmin may reduce viral infectivity and also may act as a superoxide dismutase (Bron and Seal, 1986).
13. Antibiotic-producing bacteria, primarily staphylococci, apparently occur frequently among ocular flora (Halbert and Swick, 1952).
14. A superoxide radical-producing system, which exhibits bactericidal activity, is situated within conjunctival mucus threads (Proctor *et al.*, 1977)
15. A low density of T and B lymphocytes, plasma cells, macrophages, and polymorphonuclear leukocytes has been identified in the normal tear film (Coyle and Bulbank, 1989).

III. IMMUNE RESPONSE OF THE OCULAR SECRETORY IMMUNE SYSTEM TO ANTIGENIC CHALLENGE

A. Organisms and Naturally Occurring or Induced Antibodies in Human Tears

In human tears, a diverse array of bacterial and viral organisms has been identified, including *Staphylococcus epidermidis, Corynebacterium* (Gregory and Allansmith, 1986,1987), *Staphylococcus aureus, Pneumococcus, Pseudomonas pyocyanea, Streptococcus viridans, Streptococcus pyogenes, Proteus vulgaris, Klebsiella pneumoniae, Escherichia coli,* α-hemolytic streptococci (Sen and Sarin, 1982), HTLV-III (Ablashi *et al.*, 1987), hepatitis B virus (Gastaud *et al.*, 1989), coxsackievirus (Langford *et al.*, 1980), herpesvirus 1 (Shani *et al.*, 1985; Fox *et al.*, 1986; Wilhelmus *et al.*, 1986), and cytomegalovirus (Cox *et al.*, 1975). Moreover, lacrimal tissue of healthy adults may contain both cytomegalovirus and Epstein–Barr virus (Pepose *et al.*, 1990; Pflugfelder *et al.*, 1990a,b). Perhaps in response to these and other microbial exposures, tears may harbor a variety of naturally occurring or induced IgG or SIgA antibodies against numerous antigens, including herpes simplex virus 1 (Little *et al.*, 1969; Norrild *et al.*, 1982; Pedersen *et al.*, 1982; Fox *et al.*, 1986; Coyle and Sibony, 1988), Epstein–Barr virus, varicella zoster virus, rubella, mumps, cytomegalovirus (Coyle and Sibony, 1988), measles (Coyle and Sibony, 1988; Friedman *et al.*, 1989), adenovirus (Nordbo *et al.*, 1986), influenza virus (Waldman and Bergman, 1987), rhinovirus (Douglas *et al.*, 1967), human immunodeficiency virus (HIV; Liotet *et al.*, 1987), *S. epidermidis, Streptococcus mutans* serotypes c and d, a *Corynebacterium* species (Burns *et al.*, 1982; Gregory *et al.*, 1984; Gregory and Allansmith, 1986,1987), *Chlamydia trachomatis* (Treharne *et al.*, 1978; Herrmann *et al.*, 1991), and other allergens (Ballow *et al.*, 1983; Kari *et al.*, 1985). These antibodies, although sometimes expressed in quiescent eyes (Waldman and Bergman, 1987; Coyle and Sibony, 1988), may increase in concentration significantly during active infection (refer to Table VI). The levels of natural tear IgA antibodies against bacterial organisms have been suggested to be either dependent on (Gregory and Allansmith, 1987) or independent of (Burns *et al.*, 1982) local antigenic stimulation.

B. Ocular Immune Response to Defined Antigens

Antigenic challenge to the surface of the eye may result in a marked accumulation of specific SIgA, IgG, and IgM antibodies in tears (Table IV); an accelerated and enhanced anamnestic response after secondary exposure (Mestecky *et al.*, 1978; Gregory *et al.*, 1984; MacDonald *et al.*, 1984; Gregory and Filler, 1987; Levenson *et al.*, 1988); and the generation of immune resistance to, and protection against, antigen reapplication (Table V; also Malaty *et al.*, 1988). In addition, definitive ocular immune responses, as well as the possible accumulation of Ig-containing cells in lacrimal tissue (Jackson and Mestecky, 1981; Allansmith *et al.*, 1987), may be stimulated by antigenic challenge to other sites, including subconjunctival, intracorneal, intravitreal, oral, intrabronchial, gastric, intraduodenal, intravenous, subcutaneous, intradermal, or intramuscular sites (Table IV). The nature (e.g., antibody isotype), extent, and kinetics of these immune reactions appear to be very dependent on the form (e.g., live versus inactivated microorganisms; strain), concentration, route, duration, and frequency of antigen administration: potential immune responses may be augmented, intermittent, suppressed, or absent (Banyard and Morris, 1980; Montgomery *et al.*, 1983,1984a,b; Mondino *et al.*, 1987a, 1991; Peppard *et al.*, 1988; Centifanto *et al.*, 1989; Hall and Pribnow, 1989). Moreover, the magnitude of induced ocular immunity may be altered by the use of adjuvants (e.g., Peppard *et al.*, 1988; Peppard and Montgomery, 1990) and may be influenced by the concurrent state of systemic immunity (Waldman and Bergmann, 1987; Bergmann *et al.*, 1987).

The mechanism by which antigenic exposure to the surface of the eye stimulates a local (e.g., IgA) immune response remains to be elucidated. Direct antigen transfer across the conjunctival epithelium (Huang *et al.*, 1989; Kahn *et al.*, 1990) or countercurrent passage through the lacrimal duct (Sullivan *et al.*, 1990c) appears to be restricted severely. Further, the immunological architecture of healthy lacrimal tissue appears to be limited in its capacity to process and present antigen effectively (Weiczorek *et al.*, 1988). Conse-

Table IV Ocular Secretory Immune Response to Defined Antigenic Challenge

Species	Antigen	Route[a,b]	Ocular response	Reference
Rat	Dinitrophenylated type III pneumococcal vaccine	Intravenous	Infrequent tear IgA antibodies	Montgomery *et al.* (1983,1984a)
		Subcutaneous	↑ Tear IgA, IgG, and IgM antibodies	
		Gastric	↑ Tear IgA antibodies	
		Ocular	↑ Tear IgA antibodies	
Rat	Cholera toxin	Ocular/Ocular	↑ Conjunctival antitoxin-containing cells	Pu *et al.* (1983)
		—/Ocular	No cellular response	
		Intraduodenal/—	No cellular response	
		Intraduodenal/intraduodenal	No cellular response	
		Intraduodenal/ocular	↑ Conjunctival antitoxin-containing cells	
		Intragastric/ocular	↑ Conjunctival antitoxin-containing cells	
Rat	Dinitrophenylated type III pneumococcal vaccine	Ocular	↑ Tear IgA antibodies	Montgomery *et al.* (1984b)
		Ocular/gastric	↑ Tear IgA antibodies	
		Gastric	↑ Tear IgA antibodies	
		Gastric/ocular	↑ Tear IgA antibodies	
Rat	Dinitrophenylated *Pneumococcus* (inactivated)	Ocular	↑ Tear IgA antibodies	Peppard *et al.* (1988)
		Gastric	↑ Tear IgA antibodies	
Rat	Dinitrophenylated *Streptococcus pneumoniae* (inactivated)	Gastric/ocular	↑ Tear IgA antibodies	Peppard and Montgomery (1990)
Guinea pig	Live guinea pig inclusion conjunctivitis organisms	Ocular	↑ Tear SIgA antibodies	Murray *et al.* (1973)
	Inactivated guinea pig inclusion conjunctivitis organisms	Intraperitoneal	No tear SIgA antibodies	
Guinea pig	Live guinea pig inclusion conjunctivitis organisms	Ocular	↑ Tear SIgA antibodies	Watson *et al.* (1977)
Guinea pig	Live guinea pig inclusion conjunctivitis organisms	Ocular	↑ Tear IgA and IgG antibodies	Malaty *et al.* (1981)
	Inactivated guinea pig inclusion conjunctivitis organisms	Ocular	No tear IgA or IgG antibodies	
Guinea pig	Live guinea pig inclusion conjunctivitis organisms	Ocular	↑ Tear SIgA antibodies	Finney and Bushell (1986)
Guinea pig	*Shigella* ribosomal vaccine	Subcutaneous	↑ Tear IgA 'O' antibodies	Levenson *et al.* (1988)
	Lipopolysaccharide	Subcutaneous	↑ Tear IgA 'O' antibodies	
Rabbit	Human serum albumin	Oral and intravenous	↑ Lacrimal gland IgA antibody-producing cells	Jackson and Mestecky (1981)
Rabbit	Herpes simplex virus 1	Ocular	↑ Tear IgG, no IgA or IgM antibodies	Willey *et al.* (1985)
Rabbit	Peptidoglycan–ribitol teichoic acid (from *Staphylococcus aureus*)	Intradermal with CFA	↑ Tear IgG and SIgA antibodies	Mondino *et al.* (1987a,b)
		Subconjunctival with CFA	↑ Tear IgG and SIgA antibodies	
	Live *S. aureus*	Ocular	↑ Tear IgG and SIgA antibodies	
		Ocular	↑ Tear IgG and SIgA antibodies	
Rabbit	Herpes simplex virus 1	Scarified cornea	↑ Tear IgA, IgM, and IgG antibodies	Centifanto *et al.* (1989)

(continues)

Table IV *(continued)*

Species	Antigen	Route[a,b]	Ocular response	Reference
Rabbit	Ovalbumin	Ocular	↑ Tear IgG, infrequent IgA antibodies; ↑ IgG and IgM antibody-producing cells in conjunctiva but not in lacrimal gland	Hall and Pribnow (1989)
		Intravitreous	↑ Tear IgG antibodies	
		Intravenous	No IgG or IgA antibodies	
Rabbit	Peptidoglycan-ribitol teichoic acid (from *S. aureus*)	Intradermal with CFA	↑ Tear IgG and SIgA antibodies	Mondino *et al.* (1991)
		Subconjunctival with CFA	↑ Tear IgG and SIgA antibodies	
		Intradermal with CFA/ocular	↑ Tear IgG and SIgA antibodies	
		Subconjunctival with CFA/ ocular	↑ Tear IgG and SIgA antibodies	
	Live *S. aureus*	Ocular	↑ Tear IgG and SIgA antibodies	
Cattle	Keyhole limpet hemocyanin	Subconjunctival with IFA	↑ Tear antibodies	Banyard and Morris (1980)
		Intramuscular with IFA	↑ Tear antibodies	
		Ocular (3 months)	↑ Tear antibodies	
		Ocular (3 days)	No tear antibody response	
Calves	Live rotavirus	Oral	↑ Tear IgA and IgM antibodies	van Zaane *et al.* (1987)
		Oral/oral	No tear antibodies	
		Oral/oral/ocular	↑ Tear IgA antibodies	
		Oral(2)/ocular/intrabronchial	↑ Tear IgA and IgM antibodies	
		Intrabronchial	↑ Tear IgA and IgM antibodies	
		Intrabronchial/oral	↑ Tear IgA and IgM antibodies	
Horse	*Leptospira interrogans*	Intramuscular	↑ Tear antibodies	Parma *et al.* (1987)
Monkey	Inactivated *Chlamydia trachomatis*	Ocular	↑ Tear antibodies	MacDonald *et al.* (1984)
	Inactivated *C. trachomatis*/ Live *C. trachomatis*	Ocular	↑ Tear antibodies	
Monkey	*C. trachomatis*	Ocular	↑ Conjunctival suppressor/ cytotoxic and helper T cells; ↑ lymphoid follicles containing IgM-positive B cells, some IgG- and IgA-positive B cells	Whittum-Hudson *et al.* (1986)
Monkey	Inactivated *C. trachomatis*	Oral	No IgA, IgG, IgM antibodies	Taylor *et al.* (1987)
	Live C. trachomatis	Ocular	↑ Tear IgA, IgG and IgM antibodies	
		Oral	No IgA antibodies	
		Rectal	No IgA antibodies	
		Rectal/oral/intramuscular	↑ Tear IgA and IgG antibodies	
		Rectal/oral/intramuscular/ ocular	↑ Tear IgA, IgG and IgM antibodies	
Monkey	*C. trachomatis* lipopolysaccaride expressed in recombinant *Escherichia coli*	Oral	No IgA, IgG, IgM antibodies	Taylor and Prendergast (1987)

(continues)

Table IV *(continued)*

Species	Antigen	Route[a,b]	Ocular response	Reference
Monkey	*C. trachomatis* major outer membrane protein/[live *C. trachomatis*][c,d]	Ocular/[ocular] Intraperitoneal/oral/[ocular] Intraperitoneal/oral/ocular/[ocular] [ocular]/[ocular] —/[ocular]	↑ Tear IgA antibodies Rare antibodies ↑ Tear IgA antibodies ↑ Tear IgA antibodies ↑ Tear IgA antibodies	Taylor *et al.* (1988)
Monkey	*C. trachomatis*/chlamydial antigen extract	Ocular	↑ *Chlamydia*-specific lymphocytes in conjunctiva	Pal *et al.* (1990/91)
Human	Live rhinovirus	Intranasal	↑ Tear IgA neutralizing antibodies	Douglas *et al.* (1967)
Human	Live rhinovirus Inactivated rhinovirus	Intranasal Intranasal	↑ Tear IgA and IgG antibodies ↑ Tear IgA antibodies	Knopf *et al.* (1970)
Human	Inactivated *streptococcus mutans*	Oral	↑ Tear IgA antibodies	Mestecky *et al.* (1978)
Human	Inactivated *S. mutans* type c whole cells	Oral	↑ Tear IgA antibodies	Gregory *et al.* (1984)
Human	Influenza virus vaccine	Oral	↑ IgA antibodies	Bergmann *et al.* (1986)
Human	Influenza virus vaccine	Oral	↑ Tear IgA antibodies	Bergmann *et al.* (1987)
Human	Inactivated *S. mutans* whole cells	Oral	↑ Tear IgA antibodies	Gregory and Filler (1987)
Human	Inactivated *S. mutans* type c	Oral	↑ Tear IgA, IgG and IgM antibodies	Czerkinsky *et al.* (1987)
Human	Influenza virus vaccine	Oral Intramuscular	↑ Tear IgA antibodies ↑ Tear IgA antibodies	Waldman and Bergmann (1987)
Human	Pneumococcal vaccine	Subcutaneous	↑ Tear IgA, IgG, and IgM antibodies	Lue *et al.* (1988)

[a] The route of antigen exposure does not convey information about the frequency of antigen application, that is, antigens may have been administered once or multiple times via the specific route. If different routes were used, the sequence of use is given and the routes are separated by a slash. In addition, if primary and secondary immunizations by one route yielded different responses, a distinction is made between these challenges.
[b] Abbreviations: CFA, complete Freund's adjuvant; IFA, incomplete Freund's adjuvant.
[c] The use of sequential antigen administration at different times is designated by a slash.
[d] Note, oral doses given with cholera toxin.

quently, the ocular secretory immune response to infectious or toxic substances may require antigenic clearance through the nasolacrimal duct and stimulation of gut-associated lymphoid tissue. Consistent with this hypothesis are the following observations:

1. Topical application of noninvasive antigens to the rat ocular surface appears to result in passage through the nasolacrimal canal into the gastrointestinal tract, and not retrograde transfer to the lacrimal gland or lymphatic drainage into local lymph nodes (Sullivan *et al.*, 1990a).
2. Intranasal, oral, or gastric administration of bacteria, viruses, or other antigens may induce the accumulation of specific tear IgA antibodies and the generation of ocular surface protection (Mestecky *et al.*, 1978; Nichols *et al.*, 1978; Montgomery *et al.*, 1983,1984a,b; Gregory *et al.*, 1984; Bergmann *et al.*, 1986,1987; Czerkinsky *et al.*, 1987; van Zaane *et al.*, 1987; Waldman and Bergman, 1987; Peppard *et al.*, 1988; Peppard and Montgomery, 1990).

This remote-site stimulation most likely would involve IgA lymphoblast migration from mesenteric and peripheral lymph nodes, spleen, and thoracic duct lymph to the lacrimal gland (Montgomery *et al.*, 1983,1985; McGee and Franklin, 1984; O'Sullivan and Montgomery, 1990), followed by local antibody production and transport to the ocular surface. In contrast, the contribution of serum IgA antibodies to ocular surface defense appears to be minimal or nonexistent (Sullivan and Allansmith, 1984; Montgomery *et al.*, 1984a,b; Bergmann *et al.*, 1987; Czerkinsky *et al.*, 1987; Peppard and Mont-

Table V Influence of Prior Immunization on Subsequent Ocular Response to Infectious Organisms

Species	Immunogen[a]	Immunization route[b]	Clinical response to ocular challenge	Reference
Guinea pig	Live GPIC	Ocular	↑ Resistance to GPIC infection	Murray *et al.* (1973)
	Inactivated GPIC	Intraperitoneal	No resistance to GPIC infection	
Guinea pig	Live GPIC	Oral	↑ Resistance to GPIC infection	Nichols *et al.* (1978)
Guinea pig	Live GPIC	Ocular	↑ Resistance to GPIC infection	Malaty *et al.* (1981)
	Inactivated GPIC	Ocular	No resistance to GPIC infection	
Guinea pig	Live GPIC	Ocular	↑ Resistance to GPIC infection	Finney and Bushell (1986)
Guinea pig	*Shigella* ribosomal vaccine	Subcutaneous	↑ Resistance to *Shigella sonnei* infection	Levenson *et al.* (1988)
Guinea pig	SOMP	Subcutaneous with CFA[c]	↑ Resistance to *Shigella* infection	Adamus *et al.* (1980)
Rabbit	SOMP	Subcutaneous with CFA	↑ Resistance to *Shigella* infection	Adamus *et al.* (1980)
	Rabbit antiserum to SOMP	Intravenous	↑ Resistance to *Shigella* infection	
Calves	Modified live bovine rhinotracheitis virus vaccine	Ocular	↓ Resistance to *Moraxella bovis* infection	George *et al.* (1988)
		Intranasal	↓ Resistance to *M. bovis* infection	
Monkey	Inactivated *Chlamydia trachomatis*	Ocular	↓ Resistance to *C. trachomatis* infection	MacDonald *et al.* (1984)
Monkey	Inactivated *C. trachomatis*	Oral	No resistance to *C. trachomatis* infection	Taylor *et al.* (1987)
	Live *C. trachomatis*	Ocular	↑ Resistance to *C. trachomatis* infection	
		Oral	Mild or no resistance to *C. trachomatis* infection	
		Rectal/oral/intramuscular	↑ Resistance to *C. trachomatis* infection	
Monkey	Lipopolysaccaride from *C. trachomatis* expressed in recombinant *Escherichia coli*	Oral	No resistance to *C. trachomatis* infection	Taylor and Prendergast (1987)
Monkey	*C. trachomatis* major, outer membrane protein[d]	Ocular	Partial resistance to *C. trachomatis* infection	Taylor *et al.* (1988)
		Intraperitoneal/oral	Partial resistance to *C. trachomatis* infection	
		Intraperitoneal/oral/ocular	Partial resistance to *C. trachomatis* infection	

[a] GPIC, Guinea pig inclusion conjunctivitis organisms; SOMP, *Shigella* outer membrane protein.
[b] The route of antigen exposure does not convey information about the frequency of antigen application, that is, antigens may have been administered once or multiple times via the specific route. If different routes were used, the sequence of use is given and the routes are separated by a slash.
[c] CFA, Complete Freund's adjuvant.
[d] Note, oral doses are given with cholera toxin.

gomery, 1987; Lue *et al.*, 1988). IgG antibodies from serum, however, may play a significant role in certain inflammatory disorders of the eye (Chandler *et al.*, 1974; Mackie and Seal, 1984; Seal, 1985; Wilhelmus *et al.*, 1986; Gupta and Sarin, 1983). Overall, ocular immune protection may be conferred by both local and distant antigenic exposure; lacrimal tissue acts at least as a recipient of committed IgA-containing cells that elaborate antigen-specific antibodies. However, the development of an optimal strategy to promote secretory immunity in the eye has yet to be established.

C. Influence of Ocular or Systemic Disease or Contact Lens Wear on the Secretory Immune System of the Eye

As demonstrated in Table VI, various ocular and systemic diseases, as well as contact lens wear, may influence secretory immune expression in the human eye significantly. Thus, bacterial, viral, and fungal infections of the ocular surface; exposure to allergens; endocrine abnormalities; or graft-versus-host disorders may increase levels of specific antibodies, total immunoglobulins, complement proteins, and nonspecific immune factors significantly or may induce changes in the lymphocytic profile of the conjunctiva. Interestingly, if pathological alterations are evident in only one eye, immune responses may (Krichevskaya *et al.*, 1980; Shani *et al.*, 1985) or may not (Centifanto *et al.*, 1970; Hall and O'Connor, 1970) occur in the contralateral unaffected eye. With respect to contact lenses, these may bind (Gudmundsson *et al.*, 1985b) and also cause modifications in the concentrations of (Table VI) immune components in the tear film; the precise immunological effects may depend on the composition of lens material, the efficacy of cleaning regimens, and the length of wear (Manucci *et al.*, 1984; Vinding *et al.*, 1987; Temel *et al.*, 1991).

In contrast, such conditions as IgA deficiency, intrauterine infection, ocular surgery, keratoconjunctivitis sicca, malnutrition, and autoimmune disease often may suppress ocular mucosal immunity (Table VI). For example, severe malnutrition may lead to a significant decrease in tear IgA and SC concentrations, a diminished number of IgA-containing cells in lacrimal tissue, and a blunted SIgA antibody response to infectious challenge (McMurray *et al.*, 1977; Watson *et al.*, 1977,1985; Sullivan *et al.*, 1990d; Sullivan *et al.*, 1993). Similarly, autoimmune disorders such as multiple sclerosis or Sjögren's syndrome may alter or disrupt immune function in the eye significantly. Multiple sclerosis, an autoimmune disease of possible viral origin, is associated with heightened levels of monomeric IgA and lymphocytes, and reduced amounts of SC, in tears of afflicted individuals (Coyle and Sibony, 1987; Coyle, 1989; Coyle and Bulbank, 1989). Sjögren's syndrome, an autoimmune disease that occurs almost exclusively in females, is characterized by a progressive lymphocytic infiltration into the lacrimal gland, an immune-mediated destruction of lacrimal acinar and ductal epithelial cells, decreased tear IgA content, and keratoconjunctivitis, sicca (Tabbara, 1983; Boukes *et al.*, 1987; Moutsopoulos and Talal, 1987; Talal and Moutsopoulos, 1987; Kincaid, 1987). Further, in experimental models of this complex disorder, generation of autoantibodies to (Ohashi *et al.*, 1985) and deposition of IgG, IgA, and complement in ductal epithelial cells of (DeLuise *et al.*, 1982) lacrimal tissue may accompany the striking glandular inflammation (Kessler, 1968; Hoffman *et al.*, 1984; Jabs *et al.*, 1985; Jabs and Prendergast, 1988; Ariga *et al.*, 1989; Vendramini *et al.*, 1991; Sato *et al.*, 1992). The etiology of Sjögren's syndrome may involve the endocrine system (Ahmed *et al.*, 1985,1989; Raveche and Steinberg, 1986; Nelson and Steinberg, 1987; Talal and Ahmed, 1987; Ahmed and Talal, 1990; Carlsten *et al.*, 1990), but also may be the result of primary infection with and reactivation of Epstein–Barr virus, cytomegalovirus, herpes virus-6, or retroviruses. These viruses have been identified in lacrimal or salivary tissues of Sjögren's syndrome patients (Burns, 1983; Fox *et al.*, 1986; Fox, 1988; Garry *et al.*, 1990; Krueger *et al.*, 1990; Prepose *et al.*, 1990; Pflugfelder *et al.*, 1990a,b; Mariette *et al.*, 1991) and may stimulate the inappropriate epithelial-cell HLA-DR expression, T helper/inducer-cell activation, B-cell hyperactivity, and autoantibody production evident in these affected tissues (Maini, 1987; Moutsopoulos and Talal, 1987; Fox, 1988; Venables, 1989). In support of this possibility, certain viral infections in experimental animals exert a striking impact on the lacrimal gland and induce a periductular infiltration of plasma cells, lymphocytes, and macrophages; distinct nonsuppurative periductular inflammation; significant interstitial edema; widespread necrosis of the acinar and ductal epithelium; degenerative and atrophic alterations in epithelial cells; diminished tear flow; and keratoconjunctivitis sicca (Jacoby *et al.*, 1975; Lai *et al.*, 1976; Percy *et al.*, 1984,1990; Green *et al.*, 1989). Moreover, research has demonstrated that herpes viruses (e.g., cytomegalovirus) and coronaviruses (e.g., sialodacryoadenitis virus) may invade and replicate in rat lacrimal gland acinar cells (Huang *et al.*, 1993, Wickham *et al.*, 1992); Epstein–Barr virus may bind to specific receptors in ductal epithelium of the human lacrimal gland (Levine *et al.*, 1990/91); and HIV infection may predispose patients to keratoconjunctivitis sicca (Couderc *et al.*, 1987; Ulirsch and Jaffe, 1987; deClerck *et al.*, 1988; Lucca *et al.*, 1990). However, the precise role of viruses in the induction of autoimmune disease, as well as the mechanism by which viral infection may interfere with lacrimal gland function and immune expression, remains to be determined.

IV. ENDOCRINE, NEURAL, AND IMMUNE MODULATION OF THE OCULAR SECRETORY IMMUNE SYSTEM

During the past three decades, scientists have recognized increasingly that the endocrine and nervous systems regulate multiple aspects of cellular and humoral immunity. The exact nature of this hormonal and neural control—which influences significantly such parameters as lymphocyte maturation, antigen presentation, lymphokine production, and antibody synthesis—critically depends on the specific signal, target cell, and local microenvironment (Besedovsky and Sorkin, 1977; Comsa *et al.*, 1982; Grossman, 1984; Munck *et al.*, 1984; Payan *et al.*, 1984; Ahmed *et al.*, 1985; Besedovsky *et al.*, 1985; Berczi, 1986; Berczi and Kovacs, 1987; Felten *et al.*, 1987; Jancovik *et al.*, 1987; Weigent and Blalock, 1987; Freier, 1989; Hadden *et al.*, 1989; Talal and Ahmed, 1987; Ahmed and Talal, 1990; Ader *et al.*, 1991). Moreover, this neuroendocrine–immune interrelationship is bidirectional, that is, antigenic exposure also may induce the lymphocytic secretion of lymphokines, hormones, and neuropeptides that directly modulate endocrine and neural function (Besedovsky and Sorkin, 1977; Besdovsky *et al.*, 1985; Cotman *et al.*,

Table VI Impact of Ocular or Systemic Disease or Contact Lens Wear on the Secretory System of the Human Eye

Disease	Ocular immune response in the tear film[a]	Reference
Acute adenovirus conjunctivitis	~IgA, ↑ IgG, ~IgM	Gupta and Sarin (1983)
Acute bacterial conjunctivitis	~Lysozyme, ↑ IgA	Sen and Sarin (1979,1982)
Acute bacterial corneal ulcer	~IgA	Sen and Sarin (1979)
Acute endogenous uveitis	~IgA	Sen and Sarin (1979)
Acute follicular conjunctivitis	↑ IgA, ↑ IgG, ↑ IgM	McClellan *et al.* (1973)
	↑ SIgA and ↑ IgG antibodies to herpes simplex virus	Fox *et al.* (1986)
Acute hemorrhagic conjunctivitis	↑ Neutralizing activity to enterovirus and coxsackie virus; ↑ fibroblast interferon	Langford *et al.* (1985)
Acute keratoconjunctivitis	↑ IgA	Sen and Sarin (1979)
Allergic conjunctivitis	~IgG, ~IgE	Donshik and Ballow (1983)
	↑ IgE	Hoebeke *et al.* (1989)
	↑ IgE	Yuasa *et al.* (1989)
	↑ IgE	Kari *et al.* (1985)
	~Complement C3, factor B, and C3 des Arg	Ballow *et al.* (1985)
contact lens	No IgE	Hoebeke *et al.* (1989)
Atopic asthma without conjunctivitis	↑ IgE	Aalders-Deenstra *et al.* (1985)
Atopic conjunctivitis		
chronic	↑ IgE	Aalders-Deenstra *et al.* (1985)
seasonal	↑ IgE	Aalders-Deenstra *et al.* (1985)
Bacterial corneal ulcer	↑ IgA, ~IgG, ~IgM	Lal *et al.* (1990)
Blepharoconjunctivitis	~IgA, ~IgG	McClellan *et al.* (1973)
	↑ IgA	Sen and Sarin (1979)
	~IgA, ↑ IgG, ↑ IgM	Zavaro *et al.* (1980)
Bronchopneumonia	~IgA, ~lysozyme	Bhaskaram *et al.* (1986)
Chronic conjunctivitis	~IgA, ~Iactoferrin, ~lysozyme	Boukes *et al.* (1987)
Chronic graft versus host disease	↑ IgG	Heitman *et al.* (1988)
	↑ T cells in conjunctiva	Bhan *et al.* (1982)
Chronic irritative conjunctivitis	↓ Lysozyme	Sen and Sarin (1982)
Chronic nonulcerative blepharitis and meibomianitis	~IgA, ~IgG, ~lysozyme, ~lactoferrin	Seal (1985)
Contact lens wear	↓ IgA	Suttorp-Shelton *et al.* (1989)
	~Complement C3, factor B, and C3 des Arg	Ballow *et al.* (1985)
extended wear	↓ IgA, ~lysozyme	Vinding *et al.* (1987)
	↑ IgA, ~IgG, ~IgM, ~IgE	Mannucci *et al.* (1984)
rigid	↑ IgA, ~IgG, ~IgM	Temel *et al.* (1991)
soft	~IgA, ~IgG, ~IgM	Temel *et al.* (1991)
	~lactoferrin	Ballow *et al.* (1987)
Corneal dendritic ulcers	↑ SIgA and ↑ IgG antibodies to herpes simplex virus	Fox *et al.* (1986)
Corneal graft reaction	↑ IgA	Sen and Sarin (1979)
Follicular conjunctivitis (+/-trachoma)	IgA and IgG plasma cells in conjunctiva	Tagawa *et al.* (1989)
	↑ IgA, ↑ IgG, ↑ IgM	Zavaro *et al.* (1980)
Fungal corneal ulcer	↑ IgA, ~IgG, ~IgM	Lal *et al.* (1990)
Fungal ulcer—active	↑ IgG	Chandler *et al.* (1974)
Giant papillary conjunctivitis	~IgA, ↑ IgG, ↑ IgM, ↑ IgE	Donshik and Ballow (1983)
	↓ Lactoferrin	Ballow *et al.* (1987)
	↓ IgA	Suttorp-Shelton *et al.* (1989)
	↑ Complement C3, factor B, and C3 des Arg	Ballow *et al.* (1985)
Grave's ophthalmopathy	↑ SIgA	Khalil *et al.* (1989)
Herpes simplex virus keratitis	~IgA, ↑ IgG	McClellan *et al.* (1973)
	↑ Antibodies to HSV	Krichevskaya *et al.* (1980)
	↑ IgA antibodies	Shani *et al.* (1985)

(continues)

Table VI *(continued)*

Disease	Ocular immune response in the tear film[a]	Reference
active	↑ SIgA and ↑ IgG antibodies to HSV, ↑ serum albumin	Pedersen *et al.* (1982)
	↑ SIgA antibodies to HSV	Fox *et al.* (1986)
dendritic	↑ IgG antibodies to HSV, ~IgA antibodies	Wilhelmus *et al.* (1986)
Herpetic keratoconjunctivitis	~IgA, IgA HSV neutralizing antibodies present	Little *et al.* (1969)
HIV-1 infection	↑ Incidence of keratoconjunctivitis sicca	Lucca *et al.* (1990)
Idiopathic dry eye	↓ IgA, ↓ lactoferrin, ↓ lysozyme	Boukes *et al.* (1987)
IgA deficiency	Recurrent or chronic conjunctivitis	South *et al.* (1968)
IgG multiple myeloma	↑ Oligoclonal IgG	Mavra *et al.* (1990)
Keratoconjunctivitis sicca	↓ Lysozyme	Scharf *et al.* (1982)
	↓ IgA, ↑ IgG, ↓ lysozyme, ↓ lactoferrin	Seal (1985)
	↑ Superoxide	Bron (1988)
	↑ IgA, ↑ IgG, ↑ IgM	Zavaro *et al.* (1980)
Keratomalacia	↑ IgA	Sen and Sarin (1979)
Malnutrition—severe	↓ IgA, ↓ free secretory component (FSC), ↓ lysozyme	Watson *et al.* (1985)
	↓ IgA, ↑ IgG	McMurray *et al.* (1977)
Malnutrition with epithelial xerosis	↓ Lysozyme	Sen and Sarin (1982)
Measles	↓ SIgA, ↓ lysozyme, ↑ bacterial pathogens	Bhaskaram *et al.* (1986)
	↑ SIgA and ↑ IgA antibodies to measles	Friedman *et al.* (1989)
Mooren's ulcer	↑ IgG	Chandler *et al.* (1974)
Multiple sclerosis	No oligoclonal IgG	Mavra *et al.* (1990)
	↑ Monomeric IgA	Coyle *et al.* (1987a)
	↑ Monomeric IgA, ↓ secretory component	Coyle (1989)
	↑ Oligoclonal IgG	Coyle *et al.* (1987b)
	↑ Total lymphocytes, ↑ T cells, null cells	Coyle and Bulbank (1989)
	↑ SIgA and ↑ IgG antibodies to measles, herpes simplex virus, and rubella virus	Coyle and Sibony (1987)
Myotonic muscular dystrophy	↓ Lactoferrin	Tsung *et al.* (1983)
Neurosarcoidosis	↑ Oligoclonal IgG	Mavra *et al.* (1990)
Nonatopic conjunctivitis	~IgE	Aalders-Deenstra *et al.* (1985)
Ocular pemphigoid	↑ T cells in conjunctiva	Bhan *et al.* (1982)
mild	↑ IgA, ~lysozyme, ~lactoferrin	Seal (1985)
severe	↑ IgG, ~lysozyme, ~lactoferrin	Seal (1985)
dry eye	↓ IgA, ↑ IgG, ↓ lysozyme, ↓ lactoferrin	Seal (1985)
Ocular cicatricial pemphigoid	↑ IgG or ↑ IgA in conjunctival basement membrane	Furey *et al.* (1975)
Orofacial herpetic vesicles	↑ SIgA and ↑ IgG antibodies to herpes simplex virus	Fox *et al.* (1986)
Pemphigus	↓ IgA, ↑ IgG, ↓ lysozyme, ↓ lactoferrin	Seal (1985)
Perrenial conjunctivitis (dry eye)	~IgG, ~IgE	Donshik and Ballow (1983)
Phlyctenular conjunctivitis	~IgA, ~lysozyme	Sen and Sarin (1979,1982)
Picornavirus epidemic conjunctivitis	Human fibroblast interferon	Langford *et al.* (1980)
Postintrauterine infection (infant)	↓ IgA, ↓ IgG	McMurray and Rey (1981)
Postoperative cataract surgery	↓ IgA	Sand *et al.* (1986)
	↓ Lactoferrin, ↑ neutrophils	Jensen *et al.* (1985)
	↑ PGE_2	Gluud *et al.* (1985)
	↑ Superoxide	Bron (1988)
Rheumatoid arthritis and keratoconjunctivitis sicca	↓ Lysozyme	Sharf *et al.* (1982)
Sicca syndrome	↓ Lactoferrin	Mackie and Seal (1984)
	↓ Antimicrobial properties	Liotet *et al.* (1980)
Sjögren's syndrome	↓ IgA, ↓ lactoferrin, ↓ lysozyme	Boukes *et al.* (1987)
	↓ Globulins	Suarez (1987)
	↑ B and ↑ T cell infiltration into lacrimal tissue	Pepose *et al.* (1990)

(continues)

Table VI *(continued)*

Disease	Ocular immune response in the tear film[a]	Reference
Specific granule deficiency	~Lactoferrin	Raphael *et al.* (1989)
Steven's Johnson syndrome	~IgA, ↑ IgG, ~IgM	Zavaro *et al.* (1980)
Subacute sclerosing panencephalitis	↑ Oligoclonal IgG	Mavra *et al.* (1990)
Systemic lupus erythematosus	↑ Oligoclonal IgG	Mavra *et al.* (1990)
Thygeson's conjunctivitis	No IgE	Hoebeke *et al.* (1989)
Trachoma	↓ Lysozyme	Sen and Sarin (1982)
	↑ Histamine, ↑ PGF_2	Bron (1988)
	↑ Serotype-specific antibodies	Treharne *et al.* (1978)
Trachoma-induced conjunctivitis	↑ IgA antibodies to *Chlamydia trachomatis*	Herrmann *et al.* (1991)
Vernal conjunctivitis	~IgA, ~lysozyme	Sen and Sarin (1979,1982)
	~IgA, ↑ IgG	McClellan *et al.* (1973)
	~IgE	Allansmith *et al.* (1976b)
	↓ Lactoferrin	Ballow *et al.* (1987)
	↑ Antibodies to pollen, ↑ IgG, ↑ IgM, ~IgA	Ballow *et al.* (1983)
	↑ Histamine, ↑ PGF_2	Bron (1988)
	↑ IgA, ↑ IgD, ↑ IgE conjunctival plasma cells	Allansmith *et al.* (1976)
	↑ IgE, ~IgA	Brauninger and Centifanto (1971)
	↑ IgG, ↑ IgE	Donshik and Ballow (1983)
	↑ Major basic protein	Udell *et al.* (1981)
	↑ T cells in conjunctiva	Bhan *et al.* (1982)
	↑ Complement C3, factor B, and C3 des Arg	Ballow *et al.* (1985)
	↑ IgA, ↑ IgG, ↑ IgM	Zavaro *et al.* (1980)
Vernal keratoconjunctivitis	↑ IgE	Yuasa *et al.* (1989)
	↑ IgE	Samra *et al.* (1984)
	↑ IgE	Aalders-Deenstra *et al.* (1985)
Viral corneal ulcer	↑ IgA, ↑ IgG, ↑ IgM	Lal *et al.* (1990)
Viral meningitis	↑ Oligoclonal IgG	Mavra *et al.* (1990)

[a] Symbols: ↑: increase; ↓: decrease; ~: no detectable change.

1987; Weigent and Blalock, 1987; Raine, 1988; Freier, 1989; Hadden *et al.*, 1989; Ader *et al.*, 1990,1991; D'Orisio and Panerai, 1990). In fact, researchers have proposed that the immune system serves as a sensory organ, providing input to the endocrine and nervous compartments in response to noncognitive stimuli such as infection (Blalock, 1984). Consequently, an extensive triangular association appears to exist between the endocrine, nervous, and immune systems that acts to promote and maintain homeostasis.

In the secretory immune system, diverse hormones and neural agonists are known to exert a tissue-selective influence that may augment, antagonize, or curtail immunological processes (Stead *et al.*, 1987,1991; Sullivan, 1990; Kelleher *et al.*, 1991; Lambert *et al.*, 1993). Thus, depending on the precise agent and the specific mucosal site, neuroendocrine interactions may significantly modify

1. the accumulation, proliferation, retention, or function of IgA- and IgG-positive cells, T cells, mast cells, eosinophils, basophils, natural killer cells, polymorphonuclear leukocytes, and/or macrophages
2. the synthesis or secretion of IgA and IgG antibodies and cytokines, the expression of major histocompatibility complex (MHC) Class II antigens, the elaboration and release of SC, and the uptake and transport of pIgA into luminal secretions
3. the adherence and presentation of microorganisms to mucosal cells, the magnitude of neurogenic inflammation, and the extent of local immune protection against infectious agents

In addition, antigen-induced immune responses may alter mucosal neuroendocrine structure, sensitivity, or function significantly (Rowson *et al.*, 1953; Baker and Plotkin, 1978; Botta, 1979; Forslin *et al.*, 1979; Stead *et al.*, 1987,1991; Weisz-Carrington, 1987; Sullivan, 1990; Ader *et al.*, 1991; Kelleher *et al.*, 1991; Bienenstock, 1992; Lambert *et al.*, 1993; McKay *et al.*, 1992; Wira and Prabhala, 1992; Wood, 1992).

With respect to the ocular secretory immune system, endocrine and neural factors appear to exert a dramatic effect on immunological expression and activity (Table VII). However, although this neuroendocrine–immune interrelationship has been shown definitively in eyes of experimental animals, it has yet to be evaluated in humans. In rats, androgens elicit a marked increase in the production and secretion

Table VII Neural, Endocrine, and Immune Regulation of IgA and Secretory Component Levels in the Rat Ocular Secretory Immune System[a]

	Lacrimal gland		Tears		
Treatment	IgA	SC	IgA	SC	Reference
Neural					
Vasoactive intestinal peptide		↑			Kelleher *et al.* (1991)
Calcitonin gene-related peptide		—			Kelleher *et al.* (1991)
Cholinergic agonist (carbachol)		↓			Kelleher *et al.* (1991); Lanbert *et al.* (1993)
β-Adrenergic agonist (isoproterenol)		↑			Kelleher *et al.* (1991)
α-Adrenergic agonist (phenylephrine)		—			Kelleher *et al.* (1991)
α-Endorphin		—			Kelleher *et al.* (1991)
β-Endorphin		—			Kelleher *et al.* (1991)
Leucine-enkephalin		—			Kelleher *et al.* (1991)
Methionine-enkephalin		—			Kelleher *et al.* (1991)
Neuropeptide Y		—			Kelleher *et al.* (1991)
Somatostatin		—			Kelleher *et al.* (1991)
Substance P		—			Kelleher *et al.* (1991)
Endocrine					
Testosterone	↑	↑	↑	↑	Sullivan *et al.* (1984a,b;1988,1990b); Sullivan and Allansmith (1985,1987); Sullivan (1988); Sullivan and Hann (1989a)
Dihydrotestosterone		↑		↑	Sullivan *et al.* (1984a,1990b); Hann *et al.* (1991); Kelleher *et al.* (1991); Lambert *et al.* (1993)
Dihydrotestosterone/carbachol		↑[b]			Kelleher *et al.* (1991); Lambert *et al.* (1993)
Cyproterone acetate		—			Lambert *et al.* (1992)
Dihydrotestosterone/cyproterone acetate		—			Lambert *et al.* (1993)
Dihydrotestosterone/actinomycin D		—			Lambert *et al.* (1993)
4-Estren-7α-methyl-17β-ol-3-one	↑		↑	↑	Sullivan *et al.* (1988); Sullivan and Hann (1989a)
5α-Androstan-17β-ol			—	↑	Sullivan *et al.* (1988)
Danazol			—	—	Sillivan *et al.* (1988)
Estradiol		—	—	—	Sullivan *et al.* (1984a,1990b); Sullivan and Allansmith (1985)
Testosterone/estradiol			↑	↑	Sullivan and Allansmith (1987)
Progesterone		—	—	—	Sullivan *et al.* (1984a,1990b); Sullivan and Allansmith (1987)
Testosterone/progesterone			↑	↑	Sullivan and Allansmith (1987)
Cortisol			—	—	Sullivan *et al.* (1984a); Sullivan and Allansmith (1985)
Dexamethasone[c]		—	—	—	Sullivan and Hann (1989b); Sullivan *et al.* (1990b)
Aldosterone		—			Sullivan *et al.* (1990b)
Prolactin		—	—	—	Sullivan *et al.* (1988); Kelleher *et al.* (1991)
Growth hormone		—	—	—	Sullivan *et al.* (1988); Kelleher *et al.* (1991)
α-Melanocyte stimulating hormone		—	—		Sullivan *et al.* (1988); Kelleher *et al.* (1991)
Adrenocorticotrophic hormone		—			Kelleher *et al.* (1991)
Arginine vasopressin		—			Kelleher *et al.* (1991)
Oxytocin		—			Kelleher *et al.* (1991)
Insulin[d]	↑	↑	↑	↑	Sullivan and Hann (1989a); Hann *et al.* (1991)
Melatonin		—			Kelleher *et al.* (1991)
Human chorionic gonadotropin		—			Kelleher *et al.* (1991)
Bovine pituitary extract		—			Kelleher *et al.* (1991)
Rat hypothalamic extract		—			Kelleher *et al.* (1991)
Cyclic adenosine monophosphate		↑			Kelleher *et al.* (1991); R. W. Lambert *et al.* (1993)
cAMP Inducer (cholera toxin)		↑			Hann *et al.* (1991); Kelleher *et al.* (1991); Lambert *et al.* 1993
Cholera toxin/carbachol		↑			Lambert *et al.* (1993)
Cyclic guanosine monophosphate		—			Kelleher *et al.* (1991)
Phosphodiesterase inhibitor (IBMX)		↑			Kelleher *et al.* (1991)
Prostaglandin E_2		↑			Kelleher *et al.* (1991)

(*continues*)

Table VII *(continued)*

Treatment	Lacrimal gland IgA	Lacrimal gland SC	Tears IgA	Tears SC	Reference
Immune					
γ-Interferon		—			Kelleher *et al.* (1991)
Interleukin 1α		↑			Kelleher *et al.* (1991)
Interleukin 1β		↑			Kelleher *et al.* (1991)
Interleukin 5	↑				Pockley and Montgomery (1990/91b)
Interleukin 6	↑	—			Pockley and Montgomery (1990/91b); Kelleher *et al.* (1991)
Tumor necrosis factor α		↑			Kelleher *et al.* (1991)

[a] Symbols: ↑: increase; ↓: decrease; —: no change; blank: not determined.
[b] The stimulatory effects of dihydrotestosterone and cholera toxin were reduced significantly by the presence of carbachol.
[c] Low concentrations of glucocorticoid are required for optimal acinar cell production of SC *in vitro* (Hann *et al.*, 1991).
[d] Insulin's influence has been observed *in vitro* or inferred from studies with diabetic rats (Sullivan and Hann, 1989a; Hann *et al.*, 1991).

of SC by lacrimal gland acinar cells (Sullivan *et al.*, 1984b,1990b; Kelleher *et al.*, 1991; Hann *et al.*, 1991), enhance the concentration of IgA in lacrimal tissue (Sullivan and Hann, 1989a), and stimulate the transfer and accumulation of SC and IgA, but not IgG, in tears (Sullivan *et al.*, 1984a; Sullivan and Allansmith, 1985; Sullivan and Hann, 1989a). These hormone actions, which may be induced by various andogenic compounds (Sullivan *et al.*, 1988), are not duplicated by estrogen, progestin, glucocorticoid, or mineralocorticoid treatment (Sullivan *et al.*, 1984a,1990b; Sullivan and Allansmith, 1985). Morevoer, the immunological effects of androgens appear to be unique to the eye, because androgen administration does not seem to influence IgA or SC levels in salivary, respiratory, intestinal, uterine, or bladder tissues (Sullivan *et al.*, 1988) and actually suppresses mucosal immunity in the mammary gland (Weisz-Carrington *et al.*, 1978). The mechanism by which androgens regulate ocular SC dynamics may involve hormone association with specific nuclear receptors in lacrimal gland acinar cells, binding of these androgen–receptor complexes to genomic acceptor sites, and promotion of SC mRNA transcription and translation. In support of this hypothesis:

1. saturable, high-affinity, and androgen-specific receptors, which adhere to DNA, have been identified in lacrimal tissue (Ota *et al.*, 1985; Edwards *et al.*, 1990; Rocha *et al.*, 1993)
2. androgens increase mRNA levels in lacrimal glands and stimulate lacrimal glycoprotein synthesis (Quintarelli and Dellovo, 1965; Shaw *et al.*, 1983; Gubits *et al.*, 1984)
3. androgen-induced SC production by acinar cells may be inhibited by androgen receptor (cyproterone acetate), transcription (actinomycin D), or translation (cycloheximide) antagonists (Sullivan *et al.*, 1984b; Lambert *et al.*, 1993). In contrast, the processes underlying androgen action on IgA in the rat eye, as well as hormone enhancement of tear IgA levels in the mouse (Sullivan *et al.*, 1992a) remain to be determined.

Androgen activity also may explain the pronounced gender-related differences in the rat ocular secretory immune system. The number of IgA-containing cells (Sullivan *et al.*, 1986; Hann *et al.*, 1988) and the IgA and SC output (Sullivan *et al.*, 1984b; Sullivan and Allansmith, 1985,1988) are significantly greater in adult male lacrimal tissue than in that of adult females. This sexual dimorphism also extends to tears in which, from puberty to senescence, free SC and IgA but not IgG occur at considerably higher levels in male rats (Sullivan *et al.*, 1984a,1990c; Sullivan and Allansmith, 1985,1988). Indeed, androgen influence may be involved in the distinct gender-associated differences in the structural appearance, histochemistry, biochemistry, immunology, and molecular biological expression of the lacrimal gland in a variety of species, including mice, hamsters, guinea pigs, rats, rabbits, and humans (e.g., Tier, 1944; Martinazzi and Baroni, 1963; Cavallero, 1967; Shaw *et al.*, 1983; Cornell-Bell *et al.*, 1985; Mhatre *et al.*, 1988; Pangerl *et al.*, 1989; Warren *et al.*, 1990; Sullivan and Sato, 1992a). With respect to humans, gender appears to influence (1) the degree of lymphocyte accumulation in the lacrimal gland (Waterhouse, 1963); (2) the IgA concentrations in tear of adults (Sen *et al.*, 1978), but not elderly (Sand *et al.*, 1986); and (3) the frequency of Sjögren's syndrome-related lacrimal gland imjunopathology (Tabbara, 1983; Moutsopoulos and Talal, 1987; Kincaid, 1987). Interestingly, androgen administration to animal models of Sjögren's syndrome (i.e., MRL/Mp-lpr/lpr and NZB/NZW F1 female mice) results in an almost complete suppression of autoimmune sequelae in lacrimal tissue (Ariga *et al.*, 1989; Vendramini *et al.*, 1991; Sato *et al.*, 1991,1992; Sullivan and Sato, 1992a); and an increased output of IgA (Sullivan *et al.*, 1992b).

In addition to androgens, the hypothalamic–pituitary axis appears to play an important role in the expression of the rat ocular secretory immune system. Disruption of this axis by hypophysectomy or extirpation of the anterior pituitary significantly reduces the number of IgA plasma cells in lacrimal tissue, diminishes the acinar cell production of SC, causes a striking decrease in the levels of tear IgA and SC, and almost completely curtails androgen action on ocular mucosal immunity (Sullivan and Allansmith, 1987; Sullivan, 1988; Sullivan and Hann, 1989a). Moreover, this endocrine disturbance has a marked effect on lacrimal gland structure and function, leading to both acinar cell atrophy (Martinazzi, 1962) and diminished tear output (Sullivan and Allansmith, 1986). The physiological mechanisms responsible for hypothalamic–pituitary involvement in the ocular secretory immune system remain to be elucidated, but may include numerous neuroendocrine and immunological pathways: the hypothalamus and pituitary regulate multiple endocrine circuits, directly influence neural innervation in the lacrimal gland, and clearly modulate immune activity (Hosoya *et al.*, 1983; Wilson and Foster, 1985; Berczi, 1990; Berczi and Nagy, 1990). Further, the hypothalamic–pituitary axis is known to control many hormones, neurotransmitters, and lymphokines that modify androgen and acinar cell function and control mucosal immunity (Mooradian *et al.*, 1987; Sullivan, 1990).

Other studies in experimental animals also have demonstrated that (1) sex steroids may alter the development of allergic conjunctivitis in rabbits significantly (Saruya, 1968) and (2) diabetes may diminish significantly the expression of the secretory immune system of the eye. Thus, in diabetic rats, the density of IgA-containing cells in lacrimal tissue and the concentrations of IgA and SC in tears are reduced significantly (Sullivan and Hann, 1989a). These diabetic effects most likely relate to the absence of insulin, which is essential for optimal SC synthesis by acinar (Hann *et al.*, 1991) as well as intestinal (Buts *et al.*, 1988) cells, and apparently is required for maximal androgen action on target tissues (Jackson and Hutson, 1984). Similarly, both the thyroid and the adrenal glands are necessary to achieve the full magnitude of androgen-induced effects on the secretory immune system of the eye (Sullivan and Allansmith, 1987).

From the perspective of neural regulation, the stromal, periductal, perivascular, and acinar areas of lacrimal tissue are innervated by many parasympathetic, sympathetic, and peptidergic fibers that harbor numerous immunoactive transmitters, including vasoactive intestinal peptide (VIP), substance P, methionine enkephalin, leucine enkephalin, calcitonin gene-related peptide, and adrenergic and cholinergic agents (Ruskell, 1971,1975; Uddman *et al.*, 1980; Nikkinen *et al.*, 1984,1985; Lehtosalo *et al.*, 1987; Uusitalo *et al.*, 1990; Walcott, 1990). These neural agonists are known to control lymphocyte retention or function at other mucosal sites (Ottoway, 1984; Stanisz *et al.*, 1986; Walcott *et al.*, 1986; Freier *et al.*, 1987; Scicchitano *et al.*, 1988; Hart *et al.*, 1990) and their release may influence the adherence, distribution, or activity of IgA plasma cells or T cells in the lacrimal gland (Franklin *et al.*, 1988,1989; Oeschger *et al.*, 1989; Sullivan *et al.*, 1990/91). Consistent with this possibility, VIP appears to augment T-cell attachment to murine lacrimal tissue (Oeschger *et al.*, 1989) and systemic administration of the β-adrenergic blocker practolol suppresses human tear IgA levels (Wright, 1975; Garner and Rahi, 1976). However, the nature of the sympathetic–immune interaction requires further clarification, because ocular application of the β-blocker timolol to humans (Coakes *et al.*, 1981) and sympathetic denervation in rats (Sullivan *et al.*, 1990/91) have no apparent effect on tear IgA content.

VIP and the β-adrenergic agent isoproterenol have been demonstrated to increase, whereas the cholinergic agonist carbamyl choline has been shown to decrease, basal and androgen-stimulated SC production by rat acinar cells (Kelleher *et al.*, 1991). This neural regulation of SC synthesis may be mediated through the modulation of intracellular adenylate cyclase and cAMP activity. In support of this hypothesis, VIP and adrenergic agents are known to enhance (Mauduit *et al.*, 1984; Dartt, 1989), and cholinergic agents possibly suppress (Jumblatt *et al.*, 1990), the generation of cellular cAMP. Further, exposure of lacrimal gland acinar cells to cAMP analogs, cAMP inducers (i.e., PGE_2 and cholera toxin), or phosphodiesterase inhibitors may elevate SC production (Kelleher *et al.*, 1991). This cAMP influence on SC elaboration, although pronounced in the lacrimal gland, is not necessarily reproduced in other mucosal epithelial cells (Lambert *et al.*, 1993).

Additionally, neural pathways are extremely important in the spread of herpes virus infection in the eye (Shimeld *et al.*, 1987) and ocular viral transmission and activity may be modulated by neuropeptides (Herbort *et al.*, 1989). Moreover, although the optic nerve does not appear to regulate the ocular secretory immune system (Sullivan *et al.*, 1990/91), light does seem to control anterior chamber-associated immune deviation (Ferguson *et al.*, 1988), herpes virus-related retinitis (Hayashi *et al.*, 1988), and various parameters of systemic immunity (Maestroni *et al.*, 1987).

The secretory immune system of the eye in experimental animals also may be regulated by lymphokines. For example, interleukins (IL) 1α and 1β and tumor necrosis factor α (TNFα), but not IL-6 or interferon γ (IFNγ), stimulate the acinar cell synthesis and secretion of SC (Kelleher *et al.*, 1991). The regulatory effect of TNFα on acinar cell SC production is similar to that found in colonic cell lines, in which TNFα increases the production, surface expression, and release of SC (Kvale *et al.*, 1988a,b). However, the absence of IFNγ effect on SC output by acinar cells is notable because this lymphokine regulates SC dynamics in both intestinal (Sollid *et al.*, 1987; Kvale *et al.*, 1988a) and uterine (Wira and Prabhala, 1992) epithelial cells. Although IL-6 appears to have no influence on lacrimal SC production (Kelleher *et al.*, 1991), both IL-6 and IL-5 stimulate the synthesis of IgA in lacrimal tissue explants (Pockley and Montgomery, 1990/91b) and, in combination, augment the secondary tear IgA antibody response to pneumococcal antigen (Pockley and Montgomery, 1991) and suppress IgG and IgM synthesis in lacrimal tissue (Pockley and Montgomery, 1990/91a). As a further consideration, androgens, VIP, and IL-1 all share the capacity to increase IgA production in specific tissues (Drew and Shearman, 1985; Stanisz *et al.*, 1986; Crowdery *et al.*, 1988; Sullivan and Hann, 1989a); pIgA, in turn, may heighten the monocytic output of TNFα (Deviere *et al.*, 1991). If analogous activity occurs in the lacrimal gland, then various neuroimmunoendocrine factors may control the synthesis of both IgA antibodies and the IgA receptor, leading to enhanced antibody transfer to tears and improved ocular surface defense.

Acknowledgments

This research review was supported by NIH Grants EY05612 and EY02882.

References

Aalders-Deenstra, V., Kok, P. T. M., and Bruynzeel, P. L. B. (1985). Measurement of total IgE antibody levels in lacrimal fluid of patients suffering from atopic and nonatopic eye disorders. Evidence for local IgE production in atopic eye disorders? *Brit. J. Ophthalmol.* **69,** 380–384.

Abelson, M. B., and Smith, L. M. (1991). Mediators of ocular inflammation. *In* "Duanes's Biomedical Foundations of Ophthalmology" (W. Tasman and E. A. Jaeger, eds.), pp. 1–10. Lippincott, New York.

Ablashi, D. V., Sturzenegger, S., Hunter, E. A., Palestine, A. G., Fujikawa, L. S., Kim, M. K., Nussenblatt, R. B., Markham, P. D., and Salahuddin, S. Z. (1987). Presence of HTLV-III in tears and cells from the eyes of AIDS patients. *J. Exp. Pathol.* **3,** 693–703.

Adamus, G., Mulczyk, M., Witkowska, D., and Romanowska, E. (1980). Protection against keratoconjunctivitis shigellosa induced by immunization with outer membrane proteins of *Shigella* spp. *Infec. Immun.* **30,** 321–324.

Ader, R., Felten, D., and Cohen, N. (1990). Interactions between the brain and immune system. *Annu. Rev. Pharmacol. Toxicol.* **30,** 561–602.

Ader, R., Felten, D. L., and Cohen, N., eds. (1991). "Psychoneuroimmunology," 2d Ed. Academic Press, San Diego.

Ahmed, S. A., and Talal, N. (1990). Sex hormones and the immune system—Part 2. Animal data. *Bailliere's Clin. Rheum.* **4,** 13–31.

Ahmed, S. A., Penhale, W. J., and Talal, N. (1985). Sex hormones, immune responses, and autoimmune diseases. *Am. J. Pathol.* **121,** 531–551.

Ahmed, S. A., Aufdemorte, T. B., Chen, J. R., Montoya, A. I., Olive, D., and Talal, N. (1989). Estrogen induces the development of autoantibodies and promotes salivary gland lymphoid infiltrates in normal mice. *J. Autoimmun.* **2,** 543–552.

Allansmith, M. R., and Gillette, T. E. (1980). Secretory component in human ocular tissues. *Am. J. Ophthalmol.* **89,** 353—361.

Allansmith, M. R., and Ross, R. N. (1991). Immunology of the anterior segment. *In* "Clinical Contact Lens Practice" (E. S. Bennett and B. A. Weissman, eds.), pp. 1–6. Lippincott, Philadelphia.

Allansmith, M. R., Kajiyama, G., Abelson, M. B., and Simon, M. A. (1976a). Plasma cell content of main and accessory lacrimal glands and conjunctiva. *Am. J. Ophthalmol.* **82,** 819–826.

Allansmith, M. R., Hahn, G. S., and Simon, M. A. (1976b). Tissue, tear, and serum IgE concentrations in vernal conjunctivitis. *Am. J. Ophthalmol.* **81,** 506–511.

Allansmith, M. R., Kashima, K., and Yamamoto, G. K. (1978a). Immunoglobulins in the cornea. *Doc. Ophthal. Proc. Series* **20,** 23–28.

Allansmith, M. R., Greiner, J. V., and Baird, R. S. (1978b). Number of inflammatory cells in the normal conjunctiva. *Am. J. Ophthalmol.* **86,** 250–259.

Allansmith, M. R., Bloch, K. J., Baird, R. S., and Sinclair, K. (1981). Ocular anaphylaxis induction by local injection of antigen. *Immunology* **44,** 623–627.

Allansmith, M. R., Baird, R. S., Henriquez, A. S., and Bloch, K. J. (1983). Sequence of mast-cell changes in ocular anaphylaxis. *Immunology* **49,** 281–287.

Allansmith, M. R., Radl, J., Haaijman, J. J., and Mestecky, J. (1985). Molecular forms of tear IgA and distribution of IgA subclasses in human lacrimal glands. *J. Allergy Clin. Immunol.* **76,** 569–576.

Allansmith, M. R., Gudmundsson, O. G., Hann, L. E., Keys, C., Bloch, K. J., and Sullivan, D. A. (1987). The immune response of the lacrimal gland to antigenic exposure. *Curr. Eye Res.* **6,** 921–927.

Ariga, H., Edwards, J., and Sullivan, D. A. (1989). Androgen control of autoimmune expression in lacrimal glands of MRL/Mp-lpr/lpr mice. *Clin. Immunol. Immunopathol.* **53,** 499–508.

Baker, D. A., and Plotkin, S. A. (1978). Enhancement of vaginal infection in mice by Herpes simplex virus type II with progesterone. *Proc. Soc. Exp. Biol. Med.* **158,** 131–134.

Bale, J. F., Jr., O'Neill, M. E., Lyon, B., and Perlman, S. (1990). The pathogenesis of murine cytomegalovirus ocular infection. Anterior chamber inoculation. *Invest. Ophthalmol. Vis. Sci.* **31,** 1575–1581.

Ballow, M., Donshik, P. C., Mendelson, L., Rapacz, P., and Sparks, K. (1983). IgG specific antibodies to rye grass and ragweed pollen antigens in the tear secretions of patients with vernal conjunctivitis. *Am. J. Ophthalmol.* **95,** 161–168.

Ballow, M., Donshik, P. C., and Mendelson, L. (1985). Complement proteins and C3 anaphylatoxin in the tears of patients with conjunctivitis. *J. Allergy Clin. Immunol.* **76,** 473–476.

Ballow, M., Donshik, P. C., Rapacz, P., and Samartino, L. (1987). Tear lactoferrin levels in patients with external inflammatory ocular disease. *Invest. Ophthalmol. Vis. Sci.* **28,** 543–545.

Banyard, M. R. C., and Morris, B. (1980). A genetic influence on the appearance of specific antibodies in serum and secretions following challenge with antigen. *Austr. J. Exp. Biol. Med. Sci.* **58,** 357–371.

Barnett, E. I. (1968). Quantitation of immunoglobulins and L-chains by complement fixation tests. *J. Immunol.* **100,** 1093–1100.

Bazzi, C., Cattaneo, G., Migone, V., and Farina, M. (1970). Further observations on immunoglobulins of external secretions. *Progr. Immunobiol. Standardization* **4,** 333–335.

Berczi, I., ed. (1986). "Pituitary Function and Immunity." CRC Press, Boca Raton, Florida.

Berczi, I. (1990). Neurohormonal-immune interaction. *In* "Functional Endocrine Pathology" (K. Kovacs and S. Asa, eds.), pp. 990–1004. Blackwell Scientific, Edinburgh.

Berczi, I., and Kovacs, K., eds. (1987). "Hormones and Immunity." MTP Press, Lancaster, England.

Berczi, I., and Nagy, E. (1990). Effects of hypophysectomy on immune function. *In* "Psychoneuroimmunology II" (R. Ader, D. L. Felten, and N. Cohen, eds.), pp. 339–375. Academic Press, San Diego.

Bergmann, K. C., Waldman, R. H., Tischner, H., and Pohl, W. D. (1986). Antibody in tears, saliva and nasal secretions following oral immunization of humans with inactivated influenza vaccine. *Int. Archs. Allergy Appl. Immunol.* **80.** 107–109.

Bergmann, K. C., Waldman, R. H., Reinhöfer, W. D., Pohl, W. D., Tischner, H., and Werchan, D. (1987). Oral immunization against influenza in children with asthma and chronic bronchitis. *Adv. Exp. Med. Biol.* **216,** 1685–1690.

Besedovsky, H., and Sorkin, E. (1977). Network of immune-neuroendocrine interactions. *Clin. Exp. Immunol.* **27,** 1–12.

Besedovsky, H. O., del Rey, A. E., and Sorkin, E. (1985). Immune-neuroendocrine interactions. *J. Immunol.* **135,** 750–754.

Bhan, A. K., Fujikawa, L. S., and Foster, C. S. (1982). T-Cell subsets and Langerhans cells in normal and diseased conjunctiva. *Am. J. Ophthalmol.* **94,** 205–212.

Bhaskaram, P., Mathur, R., Rao, V., Madhusudan, J., Radhakrishna, K. V., Rhaguramulu, N., and Reddy, V. (1986). Pathogenesis of corneal lesions in measles. *Human Nutr. Clin. Nutr.* **40C,** 197–204.

Bienenstock, J. (1985). Bronchus-associated lymphoid tissue. *Int. Archs Allergy Appl. Immunol.* **76,** (Suppl. 1) 62–69.

Bienenstock, J. (1992). Neuroimmune interactions in the regulation of mucosal immunity. *In* "Immunophysiology of the Gut" (W. A. Walker, ed.). pp. 171–181. Academic Press, San Diego.

Blalock, J. E. (1984). The immune system as a sensory organ. *J. Immunol.* **132,** 1067–1070.

Bluestone, R., Easty, D. L., Goldberg, L. S., Jones, B. R., and Pettit, T. H. (1975). Lacrimal immunoglobulins and complement quantified by counter-immunoelectrophoresis. *Brit. J. Ophthalmol.* **59,** 279–281.

Botta, G. A. (1979). Hormonal and type-dependent adhesion of group B streptococci to human vaginal cells. *Infect. Immun.* **25,** 1084–1086.

Boukes, R. J., Boonstra, A., Breebart, A. C., Reits, D., Glasius, E., Luyendyk, L., and Kijlstra, A. (1987). Analysis of human tear protein profiles using high performance liquid chromatography. *Doc. Ophthalmol.* **67,** 105–113.

Bracciolini, M. (1968). Le immunoglobuline nelle lacrime. *Ann. Ottalmol. Clin. Ocul.* **94,** 490–496.

Brandtzaeg, P. (1983). Immunohistochemical characterization of intracellular J-chain and binding sites for secretory component (SC) in human immunoglobulin (Ig)-producing cells *Mol. Immunol.* **20,** 941–966.

Brandtzaeg, P. (1985). Role of J chain and secretory component in receptor-mediated glandular and hepatic transport of immunoglobulins in man. *Scand. J. Immunol.* **22,** 111–145.

Brandtzaeg, P. (1993). Immunohistochemical characterization of intracellular J-chain and binding sites for secretory component (SC) in human immunoglobulin (Ig)-producing cells. *Mol. Immunol.* **20,** 941–966.

Brandtzaeg, P., Gjeruldsen, S. T., Korsrud, F., Baklian, K., Berdal, P., and Ek, J. (1979). The human secretory immune system shows striking heterogeneity with regard to involvement of J chain-positive IgD immunocytes. *J. Immunol.* **122,** 503–510.

Brandtzaeg, P., Kett, K., and Rognum, T. O. (1987). Subclass distribution of IgG- and IgA-producing cells in secretory tissues and alterations related to gut diseases. *Adv. Exp. Med. Biol.* **216,** 321–333.

Brauninger, G. E., and Centifanto, Y. M. (1971). Immunoglobulin E in human tears. *Am. J. Ophthalmol.* **72,** 588–561.

Bron, A. J. (1988). Eyelid secretions and the prevention and production of disease. *Eye* **2,** 164–171.

Bron, A. J., and Seal, D. V. (1986). The defences of the ocular surface. *Trans. Ophthalmol. Soc. U. K.* **105,** 18–25.

Brown, W. R., and Kloppel, T. M. (1989). The liver and IgA: Immunological, cell biological, and clinical implications. *Hepatology* **9,** 763–784.

Burns, C. A., Ebersole, J. L., and Allansmith, M. R. (1982). Immunoglobulin A antibody levels in human tears, saliva, and serum. *Infect. Immun.* **36,** 1019–1022.

Burns, J. C. (1983). Persistent cytomegalovirus infection—The etiology of Sjögren's syndrome. *Med. Hypotheses* **10,** 451–460.

Butler, J. E., Maxwell, C. F., Pierce, C. S., Hylton, M. B., Asofsky, R., and Kiddy, C. A. (1972). Studies on the relative synthesis and distribution of IgA and IgG1 in various tissues and body fluids of the cow. *J. Immunol.* **109,** 38–45.

Buts, J. P., de Keyser, N., and Dive, C. (1988). Intestinal development in the suckling rat: Effect of insulin on the maturation of villus and crypt cell functions. *Eur. J. Clin. Invest.* **18,** 391–398.

Carlsten, H., Tarkowski, A., Holmdahl, R., and Nilsson, L. A. (1990). Oestrogen is a potent disease accelerator in SLE-prone MRL lpr/lpr mice. *Clin. Exp. Immunol.* **80,** 467–473.

Cavallero, C. (1967). Relative effectiveness of various steroids in an androgen assay using the exorbital lacrimal gland of the castrated rat. *Acta Endocrinol. (Copenh.)* **55,** 119–131.

Centifanto, Y. M., Little, J. M., and Kaufman, H. E. (1970). The relationship between virus chemotherapy, secretory antibody formation and recurrent herpetic disease. *Ann. N.Y. Acad. Sci.* **173,** 649–656.

Centifanto, Y., Norrild, B., Andersen, S. M., Karcioglu, Z. A., Porretta, E., and Caldwell, D. R. (1989). Herpes simplex virus-specific antibodies present in tears during herpes keratitis. *Proc. Soc. Exp. Biol. Med.* **192,** 87–94.

Chandler, J. W., and Gillette, T. E. (1983). Immunologic defense mechanisms of the ocular surface. *Ophthalmology* **90,** 585–591.

Chandler, J. W., Leder, R., Kaufman, H. E., and Caldwell, J. R. (1974). Quantitative determinations of complement components and immunoglobulins in tears and aqueous humor. *Invest. Ophthalmol.* **13,** 151–153.

Chao, C.-C. W., Vergnes, J.-P., Freeman, I. L., and Brown, S. I. (1980). Biosynthesis and partial characterization of tear film glycoproteins, incorporation of radioactive precursors by human lacrimal gland explants. *Exp. Eye Res.* **30,** 411–425.

Childers, N. K., Bruce, M. G., and McGhee, J. R. (1989). Molecular mechanisms of immunoglobulin A defense. *Annu. Rev. Microbiol.* **43,** 503–536.

Chordiker, W. B., and Tomasi, T. B., Jr. (1963). Gamma globulins: Quantitative relationships in human serum and nonvascular fluids. *Science* **142,** 1080–1081.

Coakes, R. L., Mackie, I. A., and Seal, D. V. (1981). Effects of long-term treatment with timolol on lacrimal gland function. *Brit. J. Ophthalmol.* **65,** 603–605.

Comsa, J., Leonhardt, H., and Wekerle, H. (1982). Hormonal coordination of the immune response. *Rev. Physiol. Biochem. Parmacol.* **92,** 115–191.

Cornell-Bell, A. H., Sullivan, D. A., and Allansmith, M. R. (1985). Gender-related differences in the morphology of the lacrimal gland. *Invest. Ophthalmol. Vis. Sci.* **26,** 1170–1175.

Cornell-Bell, A. H., Hann, L. E., Bloch, K. J., and Allansmith, M. R. (1986). Characterization of a localized basophil hypersensitivity lesion in guinea pig conjunctiva. *Cell. Immunol.* **97,** 1–12.

Cotman, C. W., Brinton, R. E., Galaburda, A., McEwen, B., and Schneider, D. M., eds. (1987). "The Neuro-Immune-Endocrine Connection." Raven Press, New York.

Couderc, L.-J., D'Agay, M.-F., Danon, F., Harzic, M., Brocheriou, C., and Claubel., J. P. (1987). Sicca complex and infection with human immunodeficiency virus. *Arch. Intern. Med.* **147,** 898–901.

Cowdery, J. S., Kemp, J. D., Ballas, Z. K., and Weber, S. P. (1988). Interleukin 1 induces T cell-mediated differentiation of murine Peyer's patch B cells to IgA secretion. *Reg. Immunol.* **1,** 9.

Cox, F., Meyer, D., and Hughes, W. T. (1975). Cytomegalovirus in tears from patients with normal eyes and with acute cytomegalovirus chorioretinitis. *Am. J. Ophthalmol.* **80,** 817–824.

Coyle, P. K. (1989). Molecular analysis of IgA in multiple sclerosis. *J. Neuroimmunol.* **22,** 83–92.

Coyle, P. K., and Bulbank, M. (1989). Immune-reactive cells in multiple sclerosis mucosal secretions. *Neurology,* **39,** 378–380.

Coyle, P. K., and Sibony, P. A. (1986). Tear immunoglobulins measured by ELISA. *Invest. Ophthalmol. Vis. Sci.* **27,** 622–625.

Coyle, P. K., and Sibony, P. A. (1987). Viral specificity of multiple sclerosis tear immunoglobulins. *J. Neuroimmunol.* **14,** 197–203.

Coyle, P. K., and Sibony, P. A. (1988). Viral antibodies in normal tears. *Invest. Ophthalmol. Vis. Sci.* **29,** 1552–1558.

Coyle, P. K., Sibony, P. A., and Johnson, C. (1987a). Increased monomeric immunoglobulin A levels in tears from multiple sclerosis patients. *Ann. Neurol.* **21,** 211–214.

Coyle, P. K., Sibony, P. A., and Johnson, C. (1987b). Oligoclonal IgG in tears. *Neurology* **37,** 853–856.

Coyle, P. K., Sibony, P. A., and Johnson, C. (1989). Electrophoresis combined with immunologic identification of human tear proteins. *Invest. Ophthalmol. Vis. Sci.* **30,** 1872–1878.

Crago, S. S., Kutteh, W. H., Moro, I., Allansmith, M. R., Radl, J., Haaijman, J. J., and Mestecky, J. (1984). Distribution of IgA1-, IgA2-, and J chain-containing cells in human tissues. *J. Immunol.* **132,** 16–18.

Czerkinsky, C., Prince, S. J., Michalek, S. M., Jackson, S., Moldoveanu, Z., Russell, M. W., McGhee, J. R., and Mestecky, J. (1987). Oral immunization with bacterial antigen induces IgA-secreting cells in peripheral blood in humans. *Adv. Exp. Med. Biol.* **216,** 1709–1719.

Damato,, B. E., Allan, D., Murray, S. B., and Lee, W. R. (1984). Senile atrophy of the human lacrimal gland: The contribution of chronic inflammatory disease. *Brit. J. Ophthalmol.* **68,** 674–680.

Dartt, D. (1989). Signal transduction and control of lacrimal gland protein secretion: a review. *Curr. Eye Res.* **8,** 619–636.

De, P. K., Roy, A., and Banerjee, R. K. (1987). Immunological characterization of soluble peroxidases from rat tissues including preputial gland. *Mol. Cell. Biochem.* **77,** 127–134.

de Clerck, L. S., Couttenye, M. M., deBroe, M. E., and Stevens, W. J. (1988). Acquired immunodeficiency syndrome mimicking Sjögren's syndrome and systemic lupus erythematosus. *Arthritis Rheum.* **31,** 272–275.

Delacroix, D. L., and Vaerman, J. P. (1983). Function of the human liver in IgA homeostasis in plasma. *Ann. N.Y. Acad. Sci.* **409,** 383–401.

Delacroix, D. L., Dive, C., Rambaud, J. C., and Vaerman, J. P. (1982). IgA subclasses in various secretions and in serum. *Immunology* **47,** 383–385.

deLuise, V. P., Ghoshe, R., and Tabbara, K. F. (1982). The effects of age, sex, and pregnancy on the histopathology and immunopathology of lacrimal glands of NZB/NZW F1 hybrid mice. *Invest. Ophthalmol. Vis. Sci. Suppl.* **22,** 211.

Deviere, J., Vaerman, J. P., Content, J., Denys, C., Schandene, L., Vandenbussche, P., Sibille, Y., and Dupont, E. (1991). IgA triggers tumor necrosis factor α secretion by monocytes: A study in normal subjects and patients with alcoholic cirrhosis. *Hepatology* **13,** 670–675.

Donshik, P. C., and Ballow, M. (1983). Tear immunoglobulins in giant papillary conjunctivitis induced by contact lenses. *Am. J. Ophthalmol.* **96,** 460–466.

D'Orisio, S., and Panerai, A., eds. (1990). Neuropeptides and Immunopeptides: Messengers in a Neuroimmune Axis. *Ann. N.Y. Acad. Sci.* 594.

Douglas, R. G., Rossen, R. D., Butler, W. T., and Couch, R. B. (1967). Rhinovirus neutralizing antibody in tears, parotid saliva, nasal secretions and serum. *J. Immunol.* **99,** 297–303.

Drew, P. A., and D. J. Shearman. (1985). Vasoactive intestinal peptide: a neurotransmitter which reduces human NK cell activity and increases Ig synthesis. *Austr. J. Exp. Biol. Med. Sci.* **63,** 313–318.

Ebersole, J. L., Taubman, M. A., and Smith, D. J. (1983). Cellular and humoral IgA responses after single and multiple local injections of antigen. *Cell. Immunol.* **77,** 372–384.

Edwards, J. A., Kelleher, R. S., and Sullivan, D. A. (1990). Identification of dihydrotestosterone binding sites in the rat lacrimal gland. *Invest. Ophthalmol. Vis. Sci. Suppl.* **31,** 541.

Elbagir. A. N., Stenberg, K., Fröman, G., and Mardh. P.-A. (1989). Antichlamydial activity of tear fluid. *Eye* **3,** 854–859.

Felten, D. L., Felten, S. Y., Bellinger, D. L., Carlson, S. L., Ackerman, K. D., Madden, K. S., Olschowski, J. A., and Livnat, S. (1987). Noradrenergic sympathetic neural interactions with the immune system: structure and function. *Immunol. Rev.* **100,** 225–260.

Ferguson, T. A., Hayashi, J. D., and Kaplan, H. J. (1988). Regulation of the systemic immune response by visible light and the eye. *FASEB J.* **2,** 3017–3021.

Finney, P. M., and Bushell, A. C. (1986). An enzyme-linked immunoassay (ELISA) for anti-chlamydial secretory immunoglobulin A in guinea pig tears. *J. Immunol. Meth.* **86,** 71–74.

Ford, L. C., Delange, R. J., and Petty, R. W. (1976). Identification of a nonlysozomal bacterial factor (β-lysin) in human tears and aqueous humour. *Am. J. Ophthalmol.* **81,** 30–33.

Forslin, L., Danielsson, D., and Falk, V. (1979). Variations in attachment of Neisseria gonorrhoeae to vaginal epithelial cells during the menstrual cycle and early pregnancy. *Med. Microbiol. Immunol.* **167,** 23–38.

Fox, P. D., Khaw, P. T., McBride, B. W., McGill, J. I., and Ward, K. A. (1986). Tear and serum antibody levels in ocular herpetic infection: Diagnostic precision of secretory IgA. *Brit. J. Ophthalmol.* **70,** 584–588.

Fox, R. (1988). Epstein-Barr virus and human autoimmune disease: Possibilities and pitalls. *J. Viral. Meth.* **21,** 19–27.

Fox, R. I., Pearson, G., and Vaughan, J. H. (1986). Detection of Epstein–Barr virus-associated antigens and DNA in salivary gland biopsies from patients with Sjögren's syndrome. *J. Immunol.* **137,** 3162–3168.

Franklin, R. M. (1981). A mechanism for localization of IgA-producing cells in the lacrimal gland. *In* "Immunology of the Eye: Workshop III" (A. Suran, I. Gery, and R. B. Nussenblatt, eds.), pp. 143–149. IRL Press, London.

Franklin, R. M. (1989). The ocular secretory immune system: A review. *Curr. Eye Res.* **8,** 599–606.

Franklin, R. M., and Remus, L. E. (1984). Conjunctival-associated lymphoid tissue: Evidence for a role in the secretory immune system. *Invest. Ophthalmol. Vis. Sci.* **25,** 181–187.

Franklin, R. M., and Shepard, K. F. (1990/91). T-cell adherence to lacrimal gland: The event responsible for IgA plasma cell predominance in lacrimal gland. *Reg. Immunol.* **3,** 213–216.

Franklin, R. M., Kenyon, K. R., and Tomasi, T. B., Jr. (1973). Immunohistologic studies of human lacrimal gland: Localization of immunoglobulins, secretory component and lactoferrin. *J. Immunol.* **110,** 984–992.

Franklin, R. M., Prendergast, R. A., and Silverstein, A. M. (1979). Secretory immune system of rabbit ocular adnexa. *Invest. Ophthalmol. Vis. Sci.* **18,** 1093–1096.

Franklin, R. M., McGee, D. W., and Shepard, K. F. (1985). Lacrimal gland directed B cell responses. *J. Immunol.* **135,** 95–99.

Franklin, R. M., Malaty R., Amirpanahi, F., and Beuerman, R. (1988). Neuroregulation of lacrimal gland function. *Invest. Ophthalmol. Vis. Sci. Suppl.* **29,** 66.

Franklin, R., Malaty, R., Amirphanahi, F., and Beuerman, R. (1989). The role of substance P on neuro-immune mechanisms in the lacrimal gland. *Invest. Ophthalmol. Vis. Sci. Suppl.* **30,** 467.

Freier, S. (1989). "The Neuroendocrine-Immune Network." CRC Press, Boca Raton, Florida.

Freier, S., Eran, M., and Faber, J. (1987). Effect of cholecystokinin and of its antagonist, of atropine, and of food on the release of immunoglobulin A and immunoglobulin G specific antibodies in the rat intestine. *Gastroenterology* **93,** 1242–1246.

Friedman, M. G. (1990). Antibodies in human tears during and after infection. *Surv. Ophthalmol.* **35,** 151–157.

Friedman, M. G., Phillip, M., and Dagan, R. (1989). Virus-specific IgA in serum, saliva, and tears of children with measles. *Clin. Exp. Immunol.* **75,** 58–63.

Fullard, R. J. (1988). Identification of proteins in small tear volumes with and without size exclusion HPLC fractionation. *Curr. Eye Res.* **7,** 163–179.

Fullard, R. J., and Snyder, C. (1990). Protein levels in nonstimulated and stimulated tears of normal human subjects. *Invest. Ophthalmol. Vis. Sci.* **31,** 1119–1126.

Fullard, R. J., and Tucker, D. L. (1991). Changes in human tear protein levels with progressively increasing stimulus. *Invest. Ophthalmol. Vis. Sci.* **32,** 2290–2301.

Furey, N., West, C., Andrew, T., Paul, P. D., and Bean, S. F. (1975). Immunofluorescent studies of ocular cicatricial pemphigoid. *Am. J. Ophthalmol.* **80,** 825–831.

Gachon, A. M. (1982/1983). Human tears: Normal protein pattern and individual protein determinations in adults. *Curr. Eye Res.* **2,** 301–308.

Gachon, A. M., Verrelle, P., Betail, G., and Dastugue, B. (1979). Immunological and electrophoretic studies of human tear proteins. *Exp. Eye Res.* **29,** 539–553.

Garner, A., and Rahi, A. H. S. (1976). Practolol and ocular toxicity. Antibodies in serum and tears. *Brit. J. Ophthalmol.* **60,** 684–686.

Garry, R. F., Fermin, C. D., Hart, D. J., Alexander S. S., Donehower, L. A., and Luo-Zhang, H. (1990). Detection of a human intracisternal A-type retroviral particle antigenically related to HIV. *Science* **250,** 1127–1129.

Gastaud, P., Baudouin, C. H., and Ouzan, D. (1989). Detection of HBs antigen, DNA polymerase activity, and hepatitis B virus DNA in tears; Relevance to hepatitis B transmission by tears. *Brit. J. Ophthalmol.* **73,** 333–336.

George, L. W., Ardans, A., Mihalyi, J., and Guerra, M. R. (1988). Enhancement of infectious bovine keratoconjunctivitis by modified-live infectious bovine rhinotracheitis virus vaccine. *Am. J. Vet. Res.* **11,** 1800–1806.

Gery, I., Mochizuki, M., and Nussenblatt, R. B. (1986). Retinal specific antigens and immunopathogenic processes they provoke. *In* "Progress in Retinal Research" (N. Osborne and J. Chader, eds.), pp. 75–109. Pergamon Press, New York.

Gillette, T. E., and Allansmith, M. R. (1980). Lactoferrin in human ocular tissues. *Am. J. Ophthalmol.* **90,** 30–37.

Gillette, T. E., Allansmith, M. R., Greiner, J. V., and Janusz, M. (1980). Histologic and immunohistologic comparison of main and accessory lacrimal tissue. *Am. J. Ophthalmol.* **89,** 724–730.

Gillette, T. E., Greiner, J. V., and Allansmith, M. R. (1981). Immunohistochemical localization of human tear lysozyme. *Arch. Ophthalmol.* **99,** 298–300.

Gluud, B. S., Jensen, O. L., Krogh, E., and Birgens, H. S. (1985). Prostaglandin E_2 levels in tears during postoperative inflammation of the eye. *Acta Ophthalmol.* **63,** 375–379.

Green, J. E., Hinrichs, S. H., Vogel, J., and Jay, G. (1989). Exocrinopathy resembling Sjögren's syndrome in HTLV-1 *tax* transgenic mice. *Nature* (*London*) **341,** 72–74.

Gregory, R. L., and Allansmith, M. R. (1986). Naturally occuring IgA antibodies to ocular and oral microorganisms in tears, saliva, and colostrum: Evidence for a common mucosal immune system and local immune response. *Exp. Eye. Res.* **43,** 739–749.

Gregory, R. L., and Allansmith, M. R. (1987). Local immune responses in the ocular secretory immune system of humans. *Adv. Exp. Med. Biol.* **216,** 1749–1757.

Gregory, R. L., and Filler, S. J. (1987). Protective secretory immunoglobulin A antibodies in humans following oral immunization with *Streptococcus mutans. Infect. Immun.* **55,** 2409–2415.

Gregory, R. L., Scholler, M., Filler, S. J., Crago, S. S., Prince, S. J., Allansmith, M. R., Michalek, S. M., Mestecky, J., and McGhee, J. R. (1984). IgA antibodies to oral and ocular bacteria in human external secretions. *Protides Biol. Fluids* **32,** 53–56.

Grossman, C. J. (1984). The regulation of the immune system of sex steroids. *Endocr. Rev.* **5,** 435–455.

Gubits, R. M., Lynch, K. R., Kulkarni, A. B., Dolan, K. P., Gresik, E. W., Hollander, P., and Feigelson, P. (1984). Differential regulation of α2u globulin gene expression in liver, lachrymal gland, and salivary gland. *J. Biol. Chem.* **259,** 12803–12809.

Gudmundsson, O. G., Cohen, E. J., Greiner, J. V., Taubman, M. A., and Allansmith, M. R. (1984). Mononuclear and IgA-containing cells in the lacrimal gland of germ-free and conventional rats. *Exp. Eye Res.* **39,** 575–581.

Gudmundsson, O. G., Sullivan, D. A., Bloch, K. J., and Allansmith, M. R. (1985a). The ocular secretory immune system of the rat. *Exp. Eye Res.* **40,** 231–238.

Gudmundsson, O. G., Woodward, D. F., Fowler, S. A., and Allansmith, M. R. (1985b). Identification of protein in contact lens surface deposit by immunofluorescence microscopy. *Arch. Ophthalmol.* **103,** 193–197.

Gudmundsson, O. G., Bjornsson, J., Olafsdottir, K., Bloch, K. J., Allansmith, M. R., and Sullivan, D. A. (1988). T cell populations in the lacrimal gland during aging. *Acta Ophthalmol.* **66,** 490–497.

Gupta, A. K., and Sarin, G. S. (1983). Serum and tear immunoglobulin levels in acute adenovirus conjunctivitis. *Brit. J. Ophthalmol.* **67,** 195–198.

Hadden, J. W., Masek, K., and Nistico, G. (1989). "Interactions among Central Nervous System, Neuroendocrine and Immune Systems." Pythagora Press, Rome.

Halbert, S. P., and Swick, L. S. (1952). Antibiotic-producing bacteria of the ocular flora. *Am. J. Ophthalmol.* **35(2),** 73–81.

Hall, J. M., and O'Connor, G. R. (1970). Correlation between ocular inflammation and antibody production. *J. Immunol.* **104,** 440–447.

Hall, J. M., and Pribnow, J. F. (1989). IgG and IgA antibody in tears of rabbits immunized by topical application of ovalbumin. *Invest. Ophthalmol. Vis. Sci.* **30,** 138–144.

Hann, L. E., Cornell-Bell, A. H., Marten-Ellis, C., and Allansmith, M. R. (1985). Conjunctival basophil hypersensitivity lesions in guinea pigs. Analysis of upper tarsal epithelium. *Invest. Ophthalmol. Vis. Sci.* **27,** 1255–1260.

Hann, L. E., Allansmith, M. R., and Sullivan, D. A. (1988). Impact of aging and gender on the Ig-containing cell profile of the lacrimal gland. *Acta Ophthalmol.* **66,** 87–92.

Hann, L. E., Tatro, J., and Sullivan, D. A. (1989). Morphology and function of lacrimal gland acinar cells in primary culture. *Invest. Ophthalmol. Vis. Sci.* **30.** 145–158.

Hann, L. E., Kelleher, R. S., and Sullivan, D. A. (1991). Influence of culture conditions on the androgen control of secretory component production by acinar cells from the lacrimal gland. *Invest. Ophthalmol. Vis. Sci.* **32,** 2610–2621.

Hart, R., Dancygier, H., Wagner, F., Lersch, C., and Classen, M. (1990). Effect of substance P on immunoglobulin and interferon-gamma secretion by cultured human duodenal mucosa. *Immunol. Lett.* **23,** 199–204.

Hayashi, J. D., Kaplan, H. J., and Ferguson, T. A. (1988). Contralateral HSV-1 retinitis is dependent upon visible light. *Invest. Ophthalmol. Vis. Sci.* **29,** 152.

Hazlett, L. D., Berk, R. S., and Iglewski, B. H. (1981a). Microscopic characterization of ocular damage produced by *Pseudomonas aeruginosa* toxin A. *Infect. Immun.* **34,** 1025–1035.

Hazlett, L. D., Wells, P., and Berk, R. S. (1981b). Immunocytochemical localization of IgA in the mouse cornea. *Exp. Eye Res.* **32,** 97–104.

Heitman, K. F., Lam, K.-W., Maskin, S. L., Yee, R. W., and Lawton, A. W. (1988). Elevated tear IgG and conjunctival plasma cell infiltrate in a graft versus host disease patient. *Cornea* **7,** 51–62.

Herbort, C. P., Weissman, S. S., and Payan, D. G. (1989).Role of peptidergic neurons in ocular herpes simplex infection in mice. *FASEB J.* **3,** 2537–2541.

Herrmann, B., Stenberg, K., and Mardh, P.-A. (1991). Immune response in chlamydial conjunctivitis among neonates and adults with special reference to tear IgA. *Acta Pathologica, Microbiologica, et Immunologica Scandinavica* **99,** 69–74.

Hoebeke, M., Magnusson, C. G. M., and Dernouchamps, J. P. (1989). Clinical interest in the detection of IgE in tears. *In* "Modern Trends in Immunology and Immunopathology of the Eye" (A. G. Secchi and I. A. Fregona, eds.), pp. 371–373. Masson S.p.A.-Milano, Italy.

Hoffman, R. W., Alspaugh, M. A., Waggie, K. S., Durham, J. B., and Walker, S. E. (1984). Sjögren's syndrome in MRL/l and MRL/n mice. *Arthritis Rheum.* **27,** 157–165.

Holly, F. J. (1987). Tear film physiology. *Int. Ophthalmol. Clin.* **27,** 2–6.

Horwitz, B. L., Christensen, G. R., and Ritzmann, S. R. (1978). Diurnal profiles of tear lysozyme and gamma A globulin. *Ann. Ophthalmol.* **10,** 75–80.

Hosoya, Y., Matsushita, M., and Sugiura, Y. (1983). A direct hypothalamic projection to the superior salivatory nucleus neurons in the rat. A study using anterograde autoradiographic and retrograde HRP methods. *Brain Res.* **266,** 329–333.

Huang, A. J. W., Tseng, S. C. G., and Kenyon, K. R. (1989). Paracellular permeability of corneal and conjunctival epithelia. *Invest. Ophthalmol. Vis. Sci.* **30,** 684–689.

Huang, Z., Lambert, R. W., Wickham, L. A., and Sullivan, D. A. (1993). Influence of the endocrine environment on herpes virus infection in rat lacrimal gland acinar cells. *In* "Lacrimal Gland, Tear Film and Dry Eye Syndromes: Basic Science and Clininal Relevance" (D. A. Sullivan, B. B. Bromberg, M. M. Cripps, D. A. Dartt, D. L. MacKeen, A. K. Mircheff, P. C. Montgomery, K. Tsubota, and B. Walcott, eds.), Plenum Press, New York, in press.

Iwamoto, T., and Jakobiec, F. A. (1989). Lacrimal glands. *In* Duanes's Biomedical Foundations of Ophthalmology" (W. Tasman and E. A. Jaeger, eds.), pp. 1–21. Lippincott, New York.

Jabs, D. A., and Prendergast, R. A. (1988). Murine models of Sjögren's syndrome. *Invest. Ophthalmol. Vis. Sci.* **29,** 1437–1443.

Jabs, D. A., Alexander, E. L., and Green, W. R. (1985). Ocular inflammation in autoimmune MRL/Mp mice. *Invest. Ophthalmol. Vis. Sci.* **26,** 1223–1229.

Jackson, F. L., and Hutson, J. C. (1984). Altered responses to androgen in diabetic male rats. *Diabetes* **33,** 819–824.

Jackson, S., and Mestecky, J. (1981). Oral-parenteral immunization leads to the appearance of IgG auto-anti-idiotypic cells in mucosal tissues. *Cell, Immunol.* **60,** 498–502.

Jacoby, R. O., Bhatt, P. N., and Jonas, A. M. (1975). Pathogenesis of sialodacryoadenitis in gnotobiotic rats. *Vet. Pathol.* **12,** 196–209.

Jancovik, B. D., Markovic, B. M., and Spector, N. H., eds. (1987). Neuroimmune Interactions. *Ann. N.Y. Acad. Sci.* **496.**

Janssen, P. T., and van Bijsterveld, O. P. (1983). Origin and biosynthesis of human tear fluid proteins. *Invest. Ophthalmol. Vis. Sci.* **24,** 623–630.

Janssen, P. T., Muytjens, H. L., and van Bijsterveld, O. P. (1984). Nonlysozyme antibacterial factor in human tears. Fact or fiction? *Invest. Opthalmol. Vis. Sci.* **25,** 1156–1160.

Jensen, O. L., Gluud, B. S., and Birgens, H. S. (1985). The concentration of lactoferrin in tears during post-operative ocular inflammation. *Acta Ophthalmol.* **63,** 341–345.

Josephson, A. S., and Weiner, R. S. (1968). Studies of the proteins of lacrimal secretions. *J. Immunol.* **100,** 1080–1092.

Jumblatt, J. E., North, G. T., and Hackmiller, R. C. (1990). Muscarinic cholinergic inhibition of adenylate cyclase in the rabbit irisciliary body and ciliary epithelium. *Invest. Ophthalmol. Vis. Sci.* **31,** 1103–1108.

Kahn, M., Barney, N. P., Briggs, R. M., Bloch, K. J., and Allansmith, M. R. (1990). Penetrating the conjunctival barrier: the role of molecular weight. *Invest. Ophthalmol. Vis. Sci.* **31,** 258–261.

Kari, O., Salo, O. P., Björkstéin, F., and Backman, A. (1985). Allergic conjunctivitis, total and specific IgE in the tear fluid. *Acta Ophthalmol.* **63,** 97–99.

Kelleher, R. S., Hann, L. E., Edwards, J. A., and Sullivan, D. A. (1991). Endocrine, neural and immune control of secretory component output by lacrimal gland acinar cells. *J. Immunol.* **146,** 3405–3412.

Kessler, H. S. (1968). A laboratory model for Sjögren's syndrome. *Am. J. Pathol.* **52,** 671–678.

Kett, K., Brandtzaeg, P., Radl, J., and Haiijman, J. J. (1986). Different subclass distribution of IgA-producing cells in human lymphoid organs and various secretory tissues. *J. Immunol.* **136,** 3631–3635.

Khalil, H. A., de Keizer, R. J. W., Bodelier, V. M. W., and Kijlstra A. (1989). Secretory IgA and lysozyme in tears of patients with Graves' ophthalmopathy. *Doc. Ophthalmol.* **72,** 329–224.

Kijlstra, A. (1990/91). The role of lactoferrin in the nonspecific immune response on the ocular surface. *Reg. Immunol.* **3,** 193–197.

Kijlstra, A., and Veerhuis, R. (1981). The effect of an anticomplementary factor on normal human tears. *Am. J. Ophthalmol.* **92,** 24–27.

Kincaid, M. C. (1987). The eye in Sjögren's syndrome. *In* "Sjögren's Syndrome. Clinical and Immunological Aspects" (N. Talal, H. M. Moutsopoulos, and S. S. Kassan, eds.), pp. 25–33. Springer Verlag, Berlin.

Knopf, H. L. S., Bertran, D. M., and Kapikian, A. Z. (1970). Demonstration and characterization of antibody in tears following intranasal vaccination with inactivated type 13 rhinovirus: A preliminary report. *Invest. Ophthalmol.* **9,** 727–734.

Krichevskaya, G. I., Zaitseva, N. S., Kainarbaeva, K. A., Basova, N. N., and Vinogradova, V. L. (1980). The use of passive hemagglutination test (PHA) in the diagnosis of viral eye diseases. Investigation of lacrimal fluid for the presence of antibody to herpes simplex virus (HSV). *Albrecht von Graefes Arch. Klin. Ophthalmol.* **214,** 239–244.

Krueger, G. R. F., Wasserman, K., de Clerck, L. S., Stevens, W. J., Bourgeois, N., Ablashi, D. V., Josephs, S. F., and Balachandran, N. (1990). Latent herpesvirus-6 in salivary and bronchial glands. *Lancet* **336,** 1255–1256.

Kuizenga, A., van Haeringen, N. J., and Kijlstra, A. (1991). SDS-minigel electrophoresis of human tears. Effect of sample treatment on protein patterns. *Invest. Ophthalmol. Vis. Sci.* **32,** 381–386.

Kvale, D., Brandtzaeg, P., and Lovhaug, D. (1988a). Up-regulation of the expression of secretory component and HLA molecules in a human colonic cell line by tumour necrosis factor-α and gamma interferon. *Scand. J. Immunol.* **28,** 351–357.

Kvale, D., Lovhaug, D., Sollid, L. M., and Brandtzaeg, P. (1988b). Tumor necrosis factor-α up-regulates expression of secretory component, the epithelial receptor for polymeric Ig. *J. Immunol.* **40,** 3086–3089.

Lai, A., Fat, R. F. M., Suurmond, D., and van Furth, R. (1973). *In vitro* synthesis of immunoglobulins, secretory component and complement in normal and pathological skin and the adjacent mucous membranes. *Clin. Exp. Immunol.* **14,** 377–395.

Lai, Y. L., Jacoby, R. O., Bhatt, P. N., and Jonas, A. M. (1976). Keratoconjunctivitis associated with sialodacryoadenitis in rats. *Invest. Ophthalmol.* **15,** 538–541.

Lal, H., Ahluwalia, B. K., Khurana, A. K., Aggarwal, D. C., and Sharma A. (1990). Serum and tear immunoglobulins in bacterial, fungal and viral corneal ulcers. *Acta Ophthalmol.* **68,** 71–74.

Lambert, R. W., Kelleher, R. S., Wickham, L. A., Gao, J., and Sullivan, D. A. (1993). Neural-endocrine control of secretory component synthesis by lacrimal gland acinar cells: specificity, temporal characteristics and molecular basis. *In* "Lacrimal Gland, Tear Film and Dry Eye Syndromes: Basic Science and Clininal Relevance" (D. A. Sullivan, B. B. Bromberg, M. M. Cripps, D. A. Dartt, D. L. MacKeen, A. K. Mircheff, P. C. Montgomery, K. Tsubota, and B. Walcott, eds.), Plenum Press, New York, in press.

Lamberts, D. W. (1983). Keratoconjunctivitis sicca. *In* "The Cornea. Scientific Foundations and Clinical Practice" (G. Smolin, and R. A. Thoft, eds.), pp. 293–308.

Langford, M. P., Yin-Murphy, M., Ho, Y. M., Barber, J. C., Baron, S., and Stanton, G. J. (1980). Human fibroblast interferon in tears of patients with picornavirus epidemic conjunctivitis. *Infect. Immun.* **29,** 995–998.

Langford, M. P., Barber, J. C., Sklar, V. E. F., Clark, S. W., III, Patriarca, P. A., Onarato, I. M., Yan-Murphy, M., and Stanton, G. J. (1985). Virus-specific, early appearing neutralizing activity and interferon in tears of patients with acute hemorrhagic conjunctivitis. *Curr. Eye Res.* **4,** 233–239.

Lass, J. H., Walter, E. I., Burris, T. E., Grossniklaus, H. E., Roat, M. I., Skelnik, D. L., Needham, L., Singer, M., and Medof, M. E. (1990). Expression of two molecular forms of the complement decay-accelerating factor in the eye and lacrimal gland. *Invest. Ophthalmol. Vis. Sci.* **31,** 1136–1148.

Lee, S. J., Rice, B. A., and Foster, C. S. (1990/91). HLA class II expression in normal and inflamed conjunctiva. *Reg. Immunol.* **3,** 177–185.

Lehtosalo, J., Uusitalo, H., Mahrberg, T., Panula, P., and Palkama, A. (1987). Enkephalin-like immunoreactive nerve fibers in the lacrimal glands of the guinea pig. *Invest. Ophthalmol. Vis. Sci. Suppl.* **28,** 23.

Levenson, V. I., Chernokhvostova, E. V., Lyubinskaya, M. M., Salamatova, S. A., Dzhikidze, E. K., and Stasilevitch, Z. K. (1988). Parenteral immunization with *Shigella* ribosomal vaccine elicits local IgA response and primes for mucosal memory. *Int. Arch. Allergy Appl. Immunol.* **87,** 25–31.

Levine, J., Pflugfelder, S. C., Yen, M., Crouse, C. A., and Atherton, S. S. (1990/91). Detection of the complement (CD21)/Epstein–Barr virus receptor in human lacrimal gland and ocular surface epithelia. *Reg. Immunol.* **3,** 164–170.

Liotet, S., Hamard, H., Beranger, A., and Arrata, M. (1980). Etude des protéines lacrymales au cours des syndromes secs. *J. Fr. Ophtalmol.* **3,** 263–266.

Liotet, S., Warnet, V. N., and Schroeder, A. (1982). Etude de la barrière hémato-lacrymale humaine normale. *J. Fr. Ophtalmol.* **11,** 707–710.

Liotet, S., Hartmann, C., Batellier, L., Chaumeil, C., and Frottier, J. (1987). Anti-HIV antibodies in tears of patients with AIDS. *Fortschr. Ophthalmol.* **84,** 340–341.

Little, J. M., Centifanto, Y. M., and Kaufman, H. E. (1969). Immunoglobulins in human tears. *Am. J. Ophthalmol.* **68,** 898–905.

Liu, S. H. (1989). Experimental autoimmune dacryoadenitis: III. Induction by immunization with extracts of intraorbital lacrimal gland. *In* "Modern Trends in Immunology and Immunopathology of the Eye" (A. G. Secchi and I. A. Fregona, eds.), pp. 92–96. Masson S.p.A.-Milano, Italy.

Liu, S. H., Tagawa, Y., Prendergast, R. A., Franklin, R. M., and Silverstein, A. M. (1981). Secretory component of IgA: A marker for differentiation of ocular epithelium. *Invest. Ophthalmol. Vis. Sci.* **20,** 100–119.

Liu, S. H., Prendergast, R. A., and Silverstein, A. M. (1987). Experimental autoimmune dacryoadenitis. I. Lacrimal gland disease in the rat. *Invest. Ophthalmol. Vis. Sci.* **28,** 270–275.

Lubniewski, A. J., and Nelson, J. D. (1990). Diagnosis and management of dry eye and ocular surface disorders. *Ophthalmol. Clin. North Am.* **3,** 575–594.

Lucca, J. A., Farris, R. Linsy, Bielory, L., and Caupto, A. R. (1990). Keratoconjunctivitis sicca in male patients infected with human immunodeficiency virus type 1. *Ophthalmol.* **97,** 1008–1010.

Lue, C., Tarkowski, A., and Mestecky, J. (1988). Systemic immunization with pneumococcal polysaccharide vaccine induces a predominant IgA2 response of peripheral blood lymphocytes and increases of both serum and secretory antipneumococcal antibodies. *J. Immunol.* **140,** 3793–3800.

McClellan, B. H., Whitney, C. R., Newman, L. P., and Allansmith, M. R. (1973). Immunoglobulins in tears. *Am. J. Ophthalmol.* **76,** 89–101.

MacDonald, A. B., McComb, D., and Howard, L. (1984). Immune response of owl monkeys to topical vaccination with irradiated *Chlamydia trachomatis. J. Infect. Dis.* **149,** 439–442.

MacDonald, T. T., Challacombe, S. J., Bland, P. W., Stokes, C. R., Heatley, R. V., and McI Mowat, A. (1990). "Advances in Mucosal Immunology." Kluwer, London.

McGee, D. W., and Franklin, R. M. (1984). Lymphocyte migration into the lacrimal gland is random. *Cell. Immunol.* **86,** 75–82.

McGhee, J. R., Mestecky, J., Elson, C. O., and Kiyono, H. (1989). Regulation of IgA synthesis and immune response by T cells and interleukins. *J. Clin. Immunol.* **9,** 175–199.

McGill, J. I., Liakos, G. M., Goulding, N., and Seal, D. V. (1984). Normal tear protein profiles and age-related changes. *Brit. J. Ophthalmol.* **68,** 316–320.

McKay, D. M., Crowe, S. E., Benjamin, M., Masson, S., Kosecka-Janiszewska, U., Williams, K., and Perdue, M. H. (1992). Neuroimmune amplification and inhibition of mucosal immune function. *In* "Immunophysiology of the Gut" (W. A. Walker, ed.). pp. 229–240. Academic Press, San Diego.

Mackie, I. A., and Seal, D. V. (1984). Diagnostic implications of tear protein profiles. *Br. J. Ophthalmol.* **68,** 321–324.

McMurray, D. N., and Rey, H. (1981). Immunological sequelae of intrauterine infection. *Clin. Exp. Immunol.* **44,** 389–395.

McMurray, D. N., Rey, H., Casazza, L. J., and Watson, R. R. (1977). Effects of moderate malnutrition on concentrations of immunoglobulins and enzymes in tears and saliva of young Colombian children. *Am. J. Clin. Nutr.* **30,** 1944–1948.

McNatt, J., Allen, S. D., Wilson, L. A., and Dowell, V. R., Jr. (1978). Anaerobic flora of the normal human conjunctival sac. *Arch. Ophthalmol.* **96,** 1448–1450.

Maestroni, G. J., Conti, A., and Pierpaoli, W. (1987). The pineal gland and the circadian, opiatergic, immunoregulatory role of melatonin. *Ann. N.Y. Acad. Sci.* **496,** 67–77.

Maini, R. N. (1987). The relationship of Sjögren's syndrome to rheumatoid arthritis. *In* "Sjögren's Syndrome. Clinical and Immunological Aspects" (N. Talal, H. M. Moutsopoulos, and S. S. Kassan, eds.), pp. 165–176. Springer Verlag, Berlin.

Malaty, R., Dawson, C. R., Wong, I., Lyon, C., and Schechter, J. (1981). Serum and tear antibodies to *Chlamydia* after reinfection with guinea pig inclusion conjunctivitis agent. *Invest. Ophthalmol. Vis. Sci.* **21,** 833–841.

Malaty, R., Gebhardt, B. M., and Franklin, R. M. (1988). HSV-specific IgA from tears blocks virus attachment to the cell membrane. *Curr. Eye Res.* **7,** 313–320.

Mannucci, L. L., Pozzan, M., Fregona, I., and Secchi, A. G. (1984). The effect of extended wear contact lenses on tear immunoglobulins. *Contact Lens Association Opthalmologists J.* **10,** 163–165.

Mariette, X., Gozlan, J., Clerc, D., Bisson, M., and Morinet, F. (1991). Detection of Epstein–Barr virus DNA by *in situ* hybridization and polymerase chain reaction in salivary gland biopsy specimens from patients with Sjögren's syndrome. *Am. J. Med.* **90,** 286–294.

Martinazzi, M. (1962). Effetti dell'ipofisectomia sulla ghiandola lacrimale extraorbitale del ratto. *Folia Endocrinol.* **150,** 120–129.

Martinazzi, M., and Baroni, C. (1963). Controllo ormonale delle ghiandola lacrimale extraorbitale nel topo con nanismo ipofisario. *Folia Endocrinol.* **16,** 123–132.

Mauduit, P., Herman, G., and Rossignol, B. (1984). Protein secretion induced by isoproterenol or pentoxifylline in lacrimal gland: Ca^{2+} effects. *Am. J. Physiol.* **246,** C37–C44.

Mavra, M., Thompson, E. J., Nikolic, J., Krunic, A., Ranin, J., Levic, Z., Keir, G., Luxton, R., and Youl, B. D. (1990). The occurrence of oligoclonal IgG in tears from patients with MS and systemic immune disorders. *Neurology* **40,** 1259–1262.

Medof, M. E., Walter, E. I., Rutgers, J. L., Knowles, D. M., and Nussenzweig, V. (1987). Identification of the complement decay-accelerating factor (DAF) on epithelium and glandular cells and in body fluids. *J. Exp. Med.* **165,** 848–864.

Mestecky, J. (1987). The common mucosal immune system and current strategies for induction of immune response in external secretions. *J. Clin. Immunol.* **7,** 265–276.

Mestecky, J., and McGhee, J. R. (1987). Immunoglobulin A (IgA): Molecular and cellular interactions involved in IgA biosynthesis and immune response. *Adv. Immunol.* **40,** 153–245.

Mestecky, J., McGhee, J. R., Arnold, R. R., Michalek, S. M., Prince, S. J., and Babb, J. C. (1978). Selective induction of an immune response in human external secretions by ingestion of bacterial antigen. *J. Clin. Invest.* **61,** 731–737.

Mhatre, M. C., van Jaarsveld, A. S., and Reiter, R. J. (1988). Melatonin in the lacrimal gland: First demonstration and experimental manipulation. *Biochem. Biophys. Res. Comm.* **153,** 1186–1192.

Mircheff, A. K., Gierow, J. P., Lee, L. M., Lambert, R. W., Akashi, R. H., and Hofman, F. M. (1991). Class II antigen expression by lacrimal epithelial cells. *Invest. Ophthalmol. Vis. Sci.* **32,** 2302–2310.

Mizejewski, G. J. (1978). Studies of autoimmune induction in the rat lacrimal gland. *Experientia* **34,** 1093–1095.

Mondino, B. J., Brawman-Mintzer, O., and Adamu, S. A. (1987a). Corneal antibody levels to ribitol teichoic acid in rabbits immunized with staphylococcal antigens using various routes. *Invest. Ophthalmol. Vis. Sci.* **28,** 1553–1558.

Mondino, B. J., Laheji, A. J., and Adamu, S. A. (1987b). Ocular immunity to *Staphylococcus aureus*. *Invest. Ophthalmol. Vis. Sci.* **28,** 560–564.

Mondino, B. J., Adamu, S. A., and Pitchekian-Halabi, H. (1991). Antibody studies in a rabbit model of corneal phlyctenulosis and catarrhal infiltrates related to *Staphylococcus aureus*. *Invest. Ophthalmol. Vis. Sci.* **32,** 1854–1863.

Montgomery, P. C., Ayyildiz, A., Lemaitre-Coelho, I. M., Vaerman, J. P., and Rockey, J. H. (1983). Induction and expression of antibodies in secretions. *Ann. N.Y. Acad. Sci.* **409,** 428–440.

Montgomery, P. C., Rockey, J. H., Majumdar, A. S., Lemaitre-Coelho, I. M., Vaerman, J. P., and Ayyildiz, A. (1984a). Parameters influencing the expression of IgA antibodies in tears. *Invest. Ophthalmol. Vis. Sci.* **25,** 369–373.

Montgomery, P. C., Majumdar, A. S., Skandera, C. A., and Rockey, J. H. (1948b). The effect of immunization route and sequence of stimulation on the induction of IgA antibodies in tears. *Curr. Eye Res.* **3,** 861–865.

Montgomery, P. C., Skandera, C. A., and Majumdar, A. S. (1985). Evidence for migration of IgA bearing lymphocytes between peripheral mucosal sites. *Protides Biol. Fluids* **32,** 43–46.

Montgomery, P. C., Peppard, J. V., and Skandera, C. A. (1989). Isolation and characterization of mononuclear cell populations from lacrimal glands. *In* "Modern Trends in Immunology and Immunopathology of the Eye" (A. G. Secchi and I. A. Fregona, eds.), pp. 339–343. Masson S.p.A.-Milano, Italy.

Montgomery, P. C., Peppard, J. V., and Skandera, C. A. (1990). A comparison of lymphocyte subset distribution in rat lacrimal glands with cells from tissues of mucosal and non-mucosal origin. *Curr. Eye Res.* **9,** 85–93.

Mooradian, A. D., Morley, J. E., and Korenman, S. G. (1987). Biological actions of androgens. *Endocr. Rev.* **8,** 1–28.

Moutsopoulos, H. M., and Talal, N. (1987). Immunologic abnormalities in Sjögren's syndrome. *In* "Sjögren's Syndrome. Clinical and Immunological Aspects" (N. Talal, H. M. Moutsopoulos, and S. S. Kassan, eds.), pp. 258–265. Springer Verlag, Berlin.

Munck, A., Guyre, P. M., and Holbrook, N. J. (1984). Physiological functions of glucocorticoids in stress and their relation to pharmacological actions. *Endocr. Rev.* **5,** 25–44.

Murray, E. S., Charbonnet, L. T., and MacDonald, A. B. (1973). Immunity to chlamydial infections of the eye. I. The role of circulatory and secretory antibodies in resistance to reinfection with guinea pig inclusion conjunctivitis. *J. Immunol.* **110,** 1518–1525.

Nelson, J. L., and Steinberg, A. D. (1987). Sex steroids, autoimmunity, and autoimmune diseases. *In* "Hormones and Immunity" (I. Berczi, and K. Kovacs, eds.), pp. 93–119. MTP Press, Lancaster, England.

Nichols, R. L., Murray, E. S., and Nisson, P. E. (1978). Use of enteric vaccines in protection against chlamydial infection of the genital tract and the eye of guinea pigs. *J. Infect. Dis.* **138,** 742–746.

Nikkinen, A., Lehtosalo, J. I., Uusitalo, H., Palkama, A., and Panula, P. (1984). The lacrimal glands of the rat and the guinea pig are innervated by nerve fibers containing immunoreactivities for substance P and vasoactive intestinal polypeptide. *Histochem.* **81,** 23–27.

Nikkinen, A., Uusitalo, H., Lehtosalo, J. I., and Palkama, A. (1985). Distribution of adrenergic nerves in the lacrimal glands of guinea-pig and rat. *Exp. Eye Res.* **40,** 751–756.

Nordbo, S. A., Nesbakken, T., Skaug, K., and Rosenblund, E. F. (1986). Detection of adenovirus-specific immunoglobulin A in tears from patients with keratoconjunctivitis. *Eur. J. Clin. Microbiol.* **5,** 678–680.

Norrild, B., Pedersen, B., and Moller-Andersen, S. (1982). Herpes simplex virus specific secretory IgA in lacrimal fluid during herpes keratitis. *Scand. J. Clin. Lab. Invest.* **42** (Suppl. 161), 29–33.

Oeschger, N. S., Amipanahi, F., Malaty, R., and Franklin, R. (1989). Regulation of T-cell migration: Effect of neuropeptides and cell factors on the binding of T-cells to lacrimal gland epithelial cells. *Invest. Ophthalmol. Vis. Sci. Suppl.* **30,** 82.

Ohashi, Y., Simpson, K. S., Minasi, P. N., and Tabbara, K. F. (1985). The presence of cytotoxic autoantibody to lacrimal gland cells in NZB/W mice. *Invest. Ophthalmol. Vis. Sci.* **26,** 214–219.

O'Sullivan, N. L., and Montgomery, P. C. (1990). Selective interactions of lymphocytes with neonatal and adult lacrimal tissues. *Invest. Ophthalmol. Vis. Sci.* **31,** 1615–1622.

Ota, M., Kyakumoto, S., and Nemoto, T. (1985). Demonstration and characterization of cytosol androgen receptor in rat exorbital lacrimal gland. *Biochem. Internat.* **10,** 129–135.

Ottaway, C. A. (1984). In vitro alteration of receptors for vasoactive intestinal peptide changes the in vivo localization of mouse T cells. *J. Exp. Med.* **160,** 1054–1069.

Owen, R. L. (1977). Sequential uptake of horseradish peroxidase by lymphoid follicle epithelium of Peyer's patches in the normal unobstructed mouse intestine: An ultrastructural study. *Gastroenterology* **72,** 440–451.

Pal, S., Pu, Z., Huneke, R. B., Taylor, H. R., and Whittum-Hudson, J. A. (1990/91). *Chlamydia*-specific lymphocytes in conjunctiva during ocular infection: limiting dilution analysis. *Reg. Immunol.* **3,** 171–176.

Pangerl, A., Pangerl, B., Jones, D. J., and Reiter, R. J. (1989). β-Adrenoreceptors in the extraorbital lacrimal gland of the Syrian hamster. Characterization with [125I]iodopindolol and evidence of sexual dimorphism. *J. Neural Transm.* **77,** 153–162.

Pappo, J., Ebersole, J. L., and Taubman, M. A. (1988). Phenotype and mononuclear leucocytes resident in rat major salivary and lacrimal glands. *Immunology* **64,** 295–300.

Parma, A. E., Fernandez, A. S., Santisteban, C. G., Bowden, R. A., and Cerone, S. I. (1987). Tears and aqueous humor from horses inoculated with *Leptospira* contain antibodies which bind to cornea. *Vet. Immunol. Immunopathol.* **14,** 181–185.

Pavan-Langston, D. (1990). Major ocular viral infections. *In* "Antiviral Agents and Viral Diseases" (G. J. Galasso, R. J. Whitley, and T. C. Merigan, eds.), pp. 183–233. Raven Press, New York.

Payan, D. G., Levine, J. D., and Goetzl, E. J. (1984). Modulation of immunity and hypersensitivity by sensory neuropeptides. *J. Immunol.* **132,** 1601–1604.

Pedersen, B., Moller-Andersen, S., Klauber, A., Ottovay, E., Prause, J. U., Zhong, C., and Norrild, B. (1982). Secretory IgA specific for herpes simplex virus in lacrimal fluid from patients with herpes keratitis—A possible diagnostic parameter. *Brit. J. Ophthalmol.* **66,** 648–653.

Pepose, J. S., Akata, R. F., Pflugfelder, S. C., and Voigt, W. (1990). Mononuclear cell phenotypes and immunoglobulin gene rearrangements in lacrimal gland biopsies from patients with Sjögren's syndrome. *Ophthalmology* **97,** 1599–1605.

Peppard, J. V., and Montgomery, P. C. (1987). Studies on the origin and composition of IgA in rat tears. *Immunology* **62,** 194–198.

Peppard, J. V., and Montgomery, P. C. (1990). Optimising the expression of antibody in tears: Manipulation of the common mucosal immune respone? *In* "Advances in Mucosal Immunology" (T. T. MacDonald, S. J. Challacombe, P. W. Bland, C. R. Stokes, R. V. Heatley, and A. McI Mowat, eds.), pp. 513–517. Kluwer, London.

Peppard, J. V., Mann, R. V., and Montgomery, P. C. (1988). Antibody production in rats following ocular-topical or gastrointestinal immunization: Kinetics of local and systemic antibody production. *Curr. Eye Res.* **7,** 471–481.

Percy, D. H., Hanna, P. E., Paturzo, F., and Bhatt, P. N. (1984). Comparison of strain susceptibility to experimental sialodacryoadenitis in rats. *Lab. Animal Sci.* **34,** 255–260.

Percy, D. H., Bond, S. J., Paturzo, F. X., and Bhatt, P. N. (1990). Duration of protection from reinfection following exposure to sialodacryoadenitis virus in Wistar rats. *Lab. Animal Sci.* **40,** 144–149.

Pflugfelder, S. C., Crouse, C., Pereira, I., and Atherton, S. (1990a). Amplification of Epstein–Barr virus genomic sequences in blood cells, lacrimal glands, and tears from primary Sjögren's syndrome patients. *Ophthalmology* **97,** 976–984.

Pflugfelder, S. C., Tseng, S. C. G., Pepose, J. S., Fletcher, M. A., Klimas, N., and Feuer, W. (1990b). Epstein–Barr virus infection and immunological dysfunction in patients with aqueous tear deficiency. *Ophthalmology* **97,** 313–323.

Pockley, A. G., and Montgomery, P. C. (1990/91a). Identification of lacrimal gland associated immunomodulatory activities having differential effects on T and B cell proliferative responses. *Reg. Immunol.* **3,** 198–203.

Pockley, A. G., and Montgomery, P. C. (1990/91b). The effects of interleukins 5 and 6 on immunoglobulin production in rat lacrimal glands. *Reg. Immunol.* **3,** 242–246.

Pockley, A. G., and Montgomery, P. C. (1991). In vivo adjuvant effect of interleukins 5 and 6 on rat tear IgA antibody responses. *Immunology* **73,** 19–23.

Proctor, P., Kirkpatrick, D., and McGinness, J. (1977). A superoxide-producing system in the conjunctival mucus thread. *Invest. Ophthalmol. Vis. Sci.* **16,** 763–765.

Pu, Z., Pierce, N. F., Silverstein, A. M., and Prendergast, R. A. (1983). Conjunctival immunity: Compared effects of ocular or intestinal immunization in rats. *Invest. Ophthalmol. Vis. Sci.* **24,** 1411–1412.

Quintarelli, G., and Dellovo, M. C. (1965). Activation of glycoprotein biosynthesis by testosterone propionate on mouse exorbital glands. *J. Histochem. Cytochem.* **13,** 361–364.

Raine, C. S., ed. (1988). Advances in Neuroimmunology. *Ann. N.Y. Acad. Sci.* **540.**

Raphael, G. D., Davis, J. L., Fox, P. C., Malech, H. L., Gallin, J. I., Baraniuk, J. N., and Kaliner, M. A. (1989). Glandular secretion of lactoferrin in a patient with neutrophil lactoferrin deficiency. *J. Allergy Clin. Immunol.* **84,** 914–919.

Raveche, E. S., and Steinberg, A. D. (1986). Sex hormones in autoimmunity. *In* "Pituitary Function and Immunity" (I. Berczi, ed.), pp. 283–301. CRC Press, Boca Raton, Florida.

Rocha, F. J., Kelleher, R. S., Edwards, J. A., Pena, J. D. O., Ono, M., and Sullivan, D. A. (1993). Binding characteristics, immunocytochemical location and hormonal regulation of androgen receptors in lacrimal tissue. *In* "Lacrimal Gland, Tear Film and Dry Eye Syndromes: Basic Science and Clinical Relevance" (D. A. Sullivan, B. B. Bromberg, M. M. Cripps, D. A. Dartt, D. I. MacKeen, A. K. Mircheff, P. C. Montgomery, K. Tsubota, and B. Walcott, eds.), Plenum Press, New York, in press.

Rowson, L. E., Lamming, G. E., and Fry, R. M. (1953). Influence of ovarian hormones on uterine infection. *Nature (London)* **171,** 749–750.

Ruskell, G. L. (1971). The distribution of autonomic post-ganglionic nerve fibers to the lacrimal gland in monkeys. *J. Anat.* **109,** 229–242.

Ruskell, G. L. (1975). Nerve terminals and epithelial cell variety in the human lacrimal gland. *Cell Tissue Res.* **158,** 121–136.

Sabbaga, E. M. H., Pavan-Langston, D., Bean, K. M., and Dunkel, E. C. (1988). Detection of HSV nucleic acid sequences in the cornea during acute and latent ocular disease. *Exp. Eye Res.* **47,** 545–553.

Sack, R. A., Tan, K., and Tan, A. (1991). The closed eye tear film. Evidence for a compliment activated inflammatory tear layer. *Invest. Ophthalmol. Vis. Sci. Suppl.* **32,** 773.

Sacks, E. H., Wieczorek, R., Jakobiec, F. A., and Knowles, D. M. (1986). Lymphocytic subpopulations in the normal human conjunctiva. A monoclonal antibody study. *Ophthalmology* **93,** 1276–1283.

Samra, Z., Zavaro, A., Barishak, Y., and Sompolinsky, D. (1984). Vernal keratoconjunctivitis: The significance of immunoglobulin E levels in tears and serum. *Int. Archs. Allergy Appl. Immun.* **74,** 158–164.

Sand, B., Jensen, O. L., Eriksen, J. S., and Vinding, T. (1986). Changes in the concentration of secretory immunoglobulin A in tears during post-operative inflammation of the eye. *Acta Ophthalmol.* **64,** 212–215.

Saruya, S. (1968). Studies on allergic conjunctivitis. Effects of castration and sex hormone administration on experimental allergic conjunctivitis. *Acta Soc. Ophthalmol. Jap.* **72,** 833–845.

Sato, E. H., and Sullivan, D. A. (1991). Effect of steroids and immunosuppressive agents on lacrimal autoimmune disease in a mouse model of Sjögren's syndrome. Abstracts of the Seventeenth Cornea Research Conference, Eye Research Institute and Massachusetts Eye and Ear Infirmary, p. 33. Boston, Massachusetts.

Sato, E. H., Ariga, H., and Sullivan, D. A. (1992). Impact of androgen therapy in Sjögren's syndrome: hormonal influence on lymphocyte populations and Ia expression in lacrimal glands of MRL/Mp-lpr/lpr mice. *Invest. Ophthalmol. Vis. Sci.* **33,** 2537–2545.

Scharf, J., Meshulam, T., Obedeanu, N., Nahir, M., Zonis, S., and

Merzbach, D. (1982). Lysozyme concentration in tears of patients with sicca syndrome. *Ann. Ophthalmol.* **14,** 1063–1064.

Scicchitano, R., Bienenstock, J., and Stanisz, A. M. (1988). In vivo immunomodulation by the neuropeptide substance P. *Immunology* **63,** 733–735.

Seal, D. V. (1985). The effect of ageing and disease on tear constituents. *Trans. Ophthalmol. Soc. U. K.* **104,** 355–362.

Selsted, M. E., and Rafael, J. (1982). Isolation and purification of bactericides from human tears. *Exp. Eye Res.* **34,** 305–318.

Sen, D. K., and Sarin, G. S. (1979). Immunoglobulin concentrations in human tears in ocular diseases. *Brit. J. Ophthalmol.* **63,** 297–300.

Sen, D. K., and Sarin, G. S. (1982). Immunoassay of tear lysozyme in conjunctival diseases. *Brit. J. Ophthalmol.* **66,** 732–735.

Sen, D. K., Sarin, G. S., Mani, K., and Saha, K. (1976). Immunoglobulins in tears of normal Indian people. *Brit. J. Ophthalmol.* **60,** 302–304.

Sen, D. K., Sarin, G. S., Mathur, G. P., and Saha, K. (1978). Biological variation of immunoglobulin concentrations in normal human tears related to age and sex. *Acta Ophthalmol. (Copehh.)* **56,** 439–444.

Seto, S. K., Gillette, T. E., and Chandler, J. W. (1987). HLA-DR^+/ $T6^-$ Langerhans cells of the human cornea. *Invest. Ophthalmol. Vis. Sci.* **28,** 1719–1722.

Setzer, P. Y., Nichols, B. A., and Dawson, C. R. (1987). Unusual structure of rat conjunctival epithelium. *Invest. Ophthalmol. Vis. Sci.* **27,** 531–537.

Shani, L., Szanton, E., David, R., Yassur, Y., and Sarov, I. (1985). Studies on HSV specific IgA antibodies in lacrimal fluid from patients with herpes keratitis by solid phase radioimmunoassay. *Curr. Eye Res.* **4,** 103–111.

Shaw, P. H., Held, W. A., and Hastie, N. D. (1983). The gene family for major urinary proteins: Expression in several secretory tissues of the mouse. *Cell* **32,** 755–761.

Shimada, K., and Silverstein, A. M. (1975). Local antibody formation within the eye: A study of immunoglobulin class and antibody specificity. *Invest. Ophthalmol.* **14,** 573–583.

Shimeld, C., Dyson, H., Lewkowicz-Moss, S., Hill, T. J., Blyth, W. A., and Easty, D. L. (1987). Spread of HSV-1 to the mouse eye after inoculation in the skin of the snout requires an intact nerve supply to the inoculation site. *Curr. Eye Res.* **6,** 9–12.

Smolin, G. (1985). The defence mechanism of the outer eye. *Trans. Ophthalmol. Soc. U. K.* **104,** 363–366.

Smolin, G. (1987). The role of tears in the prevention of infections. *Int. Ophthalmol. Clin.* **27,** 25–26.

Smolin, G., and O'Connor, R. G. (1981). "Ocular Immunology," Lei & Febiger, Philadelphia.

Snyder, R. W., and Hyndiuk, R. A. (1988). Mechanisms of bacterial invasion of the cornea. *In* "Duanes's Biomedical Foundations of Ophthalmology" (W. Tasman and E. A. Jaeger, eds.), Chapter 49, pp. 1–7. Lippincott, New York.

Sollid, L. M., Kvale, D., Brandtzaeg, P., Markussen, G., and Thorsby, E. (1987). Interferon-γ enhances expression of secretory component, the epithelial receptor for polymeric immunoglobulins. *J. Immunol.* **138,** 4303–4306.

South, M. A., Cooper, M. D., Wolheim, F. A., and Good, R. A. (1968). The IgA system. II. The clinical significance of IgA deficiency: Studies in patients with agammaglobulinemia and ataxia telangiectasia. *Am. J. Med.* **44,** 168–178.

Srinivasan, B. D., Jakobiec, F. A., and Iwamoto, T. (1990). Conjunctiva. *In* "Duanes's Biomedical Foundations of Ophthalmology" (W. Tasman and E. A. Jaeger, eds.), Chapter 29, pp. 1–28. Lippincott, New York.

Stanisz, A. M., Befus, D., and Bienenstock, J. (1986). Differential effects of vasoactive intestinal peptide, substance P, and somatostatin on immunoglobulin synthesis and proliferation by lymphocytes from Peyer's patches, mesenteric lymph nodes, and spleen. *J. Immunol.* **136,** 152–156.

Stead, R. H., Bienenstock, J., and Stanisz, A. M. (1987). Neuropeptide regulation of mucosal immunity. *Immunol. Rev.* **100,** 333–359.

Stead, R. H., Tomioka, M., Pezzati, P., Marshall, J., Croitoru, K., Perdue, M., Stanisz, A., and Bienenstock, J. (1991). Interaction of the mucosal immune and peripheral nervous systems. *In* "Psychoneuroimmunology" (R. Ader, D. L. Felten, and N. Cohen, eds.), 2d Ed., pp. 177–207. Academic Press, San Diego.

Streilein, J. W. (1987). Immune regulation and the eye: A dangerous compromise. *FASEB J.* **1,** 199–208.

Stuchell, R. N., Feldman, J. J., Farris, R. L., and Mandel, I. D. (1984). The effect of collection technique on tear composition. *Invest. Ophthalmol. Vis. Sci.* **25,** 374–377.

Suarez, J. C. (1987). Lacrimal proteins in Sjögren's syndrome. *Ophthalmol. Basel* **194,** 188–190.

Sullivan, D. A. (1988). Influence of the hypothalamic–pituitary axis on the androgen regulation of the ocular secretory immune system. *J. Steroid Biochem.* **30,** 429–433.

Sullivan, D. A. (1990). Hormonal influence on the secretory immune system of the eye. *In* "The Neuroendocrine–Immune Network" (S. Freier, ed.), pp. 199–237. CRC Press, Boca Raton, Florida.

Sullivan, D. A., and Allansmith, M. R. (1984). Source of IgA in tears of rats. *Immunology* **53,** 791–799.

Sullivan, D. A., and Allansmith, M. R. (1985). Hormonal influence on the secretory immune system of the eye: Androgen modulation of IgA levels in tears of rats. *J. Immunol.* **134,** 2978–2982.

Sullivan, D. A., and Allansmith, M. R. (1986). Hormonal modulation of tear volume in the rat. *Exp. Eye Res.* **42,** 131–139.

Sullivan, D. A., and Allansmith, M. R. (1987). Hormonal influence on the secretory immune system of the eye: Endocrine interactions in the control of IgA and secretory component levels in tears of rats. *Immunology* **60,** 337–343.

Sullivan, D. A., and Allansmith, M. R. (1988). The effect of aging on the secretory immune system of teh eye. *Immunology* **63,** 403–410.

Sullivan, D. A., and Hann, L. E. (1989a). Mechanisms involved in the endocrine regulation of the ocular secretory immune system. *In* "Interactions among CNS, Neuroendocrine and Immune Systems" (J. W. Hadden and G. Nistico, eds.), pp. 395–428. Pythagora Press, Rome-Milan.

Sullivan, D. A., and Hann, L. E. (1989b). Hormonal influence on the secretory immune system of the eye: Endocrine impact on the lacrimal gland accumulation and secretion of IgA and IgG. *J. Steroid Biochem.* **34,** 253–262.

Sullivan, D. A., and Sato, E. H. (1993). Immunology of the lacrimal gland. *In* "Principles and Practice of Ophthalmology" (D. M. Albert, and F. A. Jakobiec, eds.). Saunders, Philadelphia, in press.

Sullivan, D. A., and Sato, E. H. (1992a). Potential therapeutic approach for the hormonal treatment of lacrimal gland dysfunction in Sjögren's syndrome. *Clin. Immunol. Immunopathol.* **64,** 9–16.

Sullivan, D. A., Vaerman, J. P., and Soo, C. (1993). Influence of severe protein malnutrition on rat lacrimal, salivary and gastrointestinal immune expression during development, adulthood and aging. *Immunology* **78,** 308–317.

Sullivan, D. A., Bloch, K. J., and Allansmith, M. R. (1984a). Hormonal influence on the secretory immune system of the eye: Androgen regulation of secretory component levels in rat tears. *J. Immunol.* **132,** 1130–1135.

Sullivan, D. A., Bloch, K. J., and Allansmith, M. R. (1984b). Hormonal influence on the secretory immune system of the eye: Androgen control of secretory component production by the rat exorbital gland. *Immunology* **52,** 239–246.

Sullivan, D. A., Colby, E. B., Hann, L. E., Allansmith, M. R., and Wira, C. R. (1986). Production and utilization of a mouse monoclonal antibody to rat IgA: Identification of gender-related differences in the secretory immune system. *Immunol. Invest.* **15,** 311–325.

Sullivan, D. A., Hann, L. E., and Vaerman, J. P. (1988). Selectivity, specificity and kinetics of the androgen regulation of the ocular secretory immune system. *Immunol. Invest.* **17,** 183–194.

Sullivan, D. A., Yee, L., Conner, A. S., Hann, L. E., Olivier, M., and Allansmith, M. R. (1990a). Influence of ocular surface antigen on the postnatal accumulation of immunoglobulin-containing cells in the rat lacrimal gland. *Immunology* **71,** 573–580.

Sullivan, D. A., Kelleher, R. S., Vaerman, J. P., and Hann, L. E. (1990b). Androgen regulation of secretory component synthesis by lacrimal gland acinar cells in vitro. *J. Immunol.* **145,** 4238–4244.

Sullivan, D. A., Hann, L. E., Yee, L., and Allansmith, M. R. (1990c). Age- and gender-related influence on the lacrimal gland and tears. *Acta Ophthalmol.* **68,** 189–194.

Sullivan, D. A., Soo, C., and Allansmith, M. R. (1990d). Severe protein malnutrition: impact on tear IgA levels during development and aging. *In* "Ocular Immunology Today" (M. Usui, S., Ohno and K. Aoki, eds.), pp. 325–328. Elsevier Science, New York.

Sullivan, D. A., Hann, L. E., Soo, C. H., Yee, L., Edwards, J. A., and Allansmith, M. R. (1990/91). Neural-immune interrelationship: Effect of optic, sympathetic, temporofacial or sensory denervation on the secretory immune system of the lacrimal gland. *Reg. Immunology* **3,** 204–212.

Sullivan, D. A., Edwards, J., Soo, C., Sullivan, B. D., Rocha, F. J., and Sato, E. H. (1992b). Influence of steroids and immunosuppressive compounds on tear IgA levels in a mouse model of Sjögren's syndrome. *Invest. Ophthalmol. Vis. Sci. Suppl.* **33,** 845.

Sutthorp-Shelton, M. S., Luyendijk, L., Koh, J. H., and Kijlstra, A. (1989). HPLC analysis of tear proteins in giant papillary conjunctivitis. *Doc. Ophthalmol.* **72,** 235–240.

Tabbara, K. F. (1983). Sjögrens syndrome. *In* "The Corneas: Scientific Foundations and Clinical Practice" (G. Smolin and R. A. Thoft, eds.), pp. 309–314. Little, Brown, Boston.

Tagawa, Y., Saito, M., Kosaka, T., and Matsuda, H. (1989). Lymphocyte subsets of human conjunctival follicles. *In* "Modern Trends in Immunology and Immunopathology of the Eye" (A. G. Secchi and I. A. Fregona, eds.), pp. 344–345. Masson S.p.A.-Milano, Italy.

Talal, N., and Ahmed, S. A. (1987). Sex hormones and autoimmune disease: A short review. *Int. J. Immunotherapy* **3,** 65–70.

Talal, N., and Moutsopoulos, H. M. (1987). Treatment of Sjögren's syndrome. *In* "Sjögren's Syndrome. Clinical and Immunological Aspects" (N. Talal, H. M. Moutsopoulos, and S. S. Kassan, eds.), pp. 291–295. Springer Verlag, Berlin.

Taylor, H. R., and Prendergast, R. A. (1987). Attempted oral immunization with chlamydial lipopolysaccharide subunit vaccine. *Invest. Ophthalmol. Vis. Sci.* **28,** 1722–1726.

Taylor, H. R., Young, E., MacDonald, A. B., Schachter, J., and Prendergast, R. A. (1987). Oral immunization against chlamydial eye infection. *Invest. Ophthalmol. Vis. Sci.* **28,** 249–258.

Taylor, H. R., Whittum-Hudson, J., Schachter, J., Caldwell, H. D., and Prendergast, R. A. (1988). Oral immunization with chlamydial major outer membrane protein (MOMP). *Invest. Ophthalmol. Vis. Sci.* **29,** 1847–1853.

Temel, A., Kazokoglu, H., Taga, Y., and Orkan, A. L. (1991). The effect of contact lens wear on tear immunoglobulins. *Contact Lens Association Ophthalmologists* **17,** 69–71.

Theodore, F. H., Bloomfield, S. E., and Mondino, B. J. (1983). "Clinical Allergy and Immunology of the Eye," Williams & Wilkins, Baltimore.

Thompson, R., and Gallardo, E. (1941). The antibacterial action of tears on staphylococci. *Am. J. Ophthalmol.* **24,** 635–640.

Tier, H. (1944). Über Zeilteilung and Kernklassenbildung in der Glandula orbitalis externa der Ratte. *Acta Pathol. Microbiol. Scan. Suppl.* **50,** 1–185.

Treharne, J. D., Dwyer, R., St. C., Darougar, S., Jones, B. R., and Daghfous, T. (1978). Antichlamydial antibody in tears and sera, and serotypes of *Chlamydia trachomatis* isolated from schoolchildren in Southern Tunisia. *Brit. J. Ophthalmol.* **62,** 509–515.

Tsung, P. K., Hong, B. S., Holly, F. J., and Gordon, W., Jr. (1983). Decrease of lactoferrin concentration in the tears of myotonic muscular dystrophy patients. *Clin. Chim. Acta* **134,** 213–219.

Tuft, S. J., and Dart, J. G. K. (1989). The measurement of IgE in tear fluid: A comparison of collection by sponge or capillary. *Acta Ophthalmol.* **67,** 301–305.

Uddman, R., Alumets, J., Ehinger, B., Hakanson, R., Loren, I., and Sundler, F. (1980). Vasoactive intestinal peptide nerves in ocular and orbital structures of the cat. *Invest. Ophthalmol. Vis. Sci.* **19,** 878–885.

Udell, I. J., Gleich, G. J., Allansmith, M. R., Ackerman, S. J., and Abelson, M. B. (1981). Eosinophil granule major basic protein and Charcot–Leyden crystal protein in human tears. *Am. J. Ophthalmol.* **92,** 824–828.

Ulirsch, R. C., and Jaffe, E. S. (1987). Sjögren's syndrome-like illness associated with acquired immunodeficiency syndrome-related complex. *Hum. Pathol.* **18,** 1063–1068.

Underdown, B. J., and Schiff, J. M. (1986). Immunoglobulin A: Strategic defense initiative at the mucosal surface. *Ann. Rev. Imm.* **4,** 389–417.

Usui, M., Ohno, S., and Aoki, K. (1990). "Ocular Immunology Today," Elsevier Science, Amsterdam.

Uusitalo, H., Mahrberg, T., and Palkama, A. (1990). Neuropeptides in the autonomic and sensory nerves of the lacrimal gland. An immunohistochemical study. *Invest. Ophthalmol. Vis. Sci. Suppl.* **31,** 44.

van Haeringen, N. J. (1981). Clinical biochemistry of tears. *Sur. Ophthalmol.* **26,** 84–96.

van Haeringen, N. J., Ensink, F. T. E., and Glasius, E. (1979). The peroxidase–thiocyanate–hydrogen peroxide system in tear fluid and saliva of different species. *Exp. Eye Res.* **28,** 343–347.

van Zaane, D., Ijzerman, J., and de Leeuw, P. W. (1987). Mucosal antibody responses of calves after oral and intrabronchial administration of rotavirus. *Adv. Exp. Med. Biol.* **216,** 1855–1862.

Venables, P. J. W., Teo, C. G., Baboonian, C., Griffin, B. E., Hughes, R. A., and Maini, R. N. (1989). Persistence of Epstein–Barr virus in salivary gland biopsies from healthy individuals and patients with Sjögren's syndrome. *Clin. Exp. Immunol.* **75,** 359–364.

Vendramini, A. C., Soo, C. H., and Sullivan, D. A. (1991). Testosterone-induced suppression of autoimmune disease in lacrimal tissue of a mouse model (NZB/NZW F1) of Sjögren's Syndrome. *Invest. Ophthalmol. Vis. Sci.* **32,** 3002–3006.

Verhagen, C., Breeboart, A. C., and Kijlstra, A. (1990). Diffusion of immunoglobulin G from the vascular compartment into the normal rabbit cornea. *Invest. Ophthalmol. Vis. Sci.* **31,** 1519–1525.

Vinding, T., Sindberg, J., and Nielsen, N. V. (1987). The concentration of lysozyme and secretory IgA in tears from healthy persons with and without contact lens use. *Acta Ophthalmol.* **65,** 23–26.

Walcott, B. (1990). Leu Enkephalin-like immunoreactivity and the innervation of the rat exorbital gland. *Invest. Ophthalmol. Vis. Sci. Suppl.* **31,** 44.

Walcott, B., Sibony, P. A., Coyle, P. K., McKeon, C., and Keyser, K. T. (1986). Protein and immunoglobulin release from lacrimal gland fragments. *Invest. Ophthalmol. Vis. Sci. Suppl.* **27,** 25.

Waldman, R. H., and Bergmann, K. C. (1987). Stimulation of secretory antibody following oral antigen administration. *Adv. Exp. Med. Biol.* **216,** 1677–1684.

Warren, D. W., Kaswan, R. L., Wood, R. L., Tortoriello, J., and Mircheff, A. K. (1990). Prolactin binding and effects on peroxidase release in rat exorbital lacrimal gland. *Invest. Ophthalmol. Vis. Sci. Suppl.* **31,** 540.

Waterhouse, J. P. (1963). Focal adenitis in salivary and lacrimal glands. *Proc. R. Soc. Med.* **56,** 911–918.

Watson, R. R., Horton, R. G., and Clinton, J. M. (1977). Suppression of secretory IgA antibodies in protein malnourished guinea pigs following a chlamydial eye and vaginal infection. *Fed. Proc.* **36,** 1251.

Watson, R. R., McMurray, D. N., Martin, P., and Reyes, M. A. (1985). Effect of age, malnutrition and renutrition on free secretory component and IgA in secretions. *Am. J. Clin. Nutr.* **42,** 281–288.

Weigent, D. A., and Blalock, J. (1987). Interactions between the neuroendocrine and immune systems: Common hormones and receptors. *Immunol. Rev.* **100,** 79–108.

Weisz-Carrington, P. (1987). Secretory immunology in the mammary gland. *In* "Hormones and Immunity" (I. Berczi and K. Kovacs, eds.), pp. 172–202. MTP Press, Lancaster, England.

Weisz-Carrington, P., Roux, M. E., McWilliams, M., Phillips Quagliata, J. M., and Lamm, M. E. (1978). Hormonal induction of the secretory immune system in the mammary gland. *Proc. Natl. Acad. Sci. U.S.A.* **75,** 2928–2932.

Wells, P. A., and Hazlett, L. D. (1985). Quantitation of immunoglobulins in mouse tears using enzyme-linked immunosorbent assay (ELISA). *Curr. Eye Res.* **4,** 1097–1105.

Whitcher, J. P. (1987). Clinical diagnosis of the dry eye. *Int. Ophthalmol. Clin.* **27,** 7–24.

Whittum-Hudson, J. A., Taylor, H. R., Farazdaghi, M., and Prendergast, R. A. (1986). Immunohistochemical study of the local inflammatory response to chlamydial ocular infection. *Invest. Ophthalmol. Vis. Sci.* **27,** 64–69.

Wickham, L. A., Huang, Z., Lambert, R. W., and Sullivan, D. A. (1993). Sialodacryoadenitis virus infection of rat lacrimal gland acinar cells. *In* "Lacrimal Gland, Tear Film and Dry Eye Syndromes: Basic Science and Clininal Relevance" (D. A. Sullivan, B. B. Bromberg, M. M. Cripps, D. A. Dartt, D. L. MacKeen, A. K. Mircheff, P. C. Montgomery, K. Tsubota, and B. Walcotts, eds.), Plenum Press, New York, in press.

Wieczorek, R., Jakobiec, F. A., Sacks, E. H., and Knowles, D. M. (1988). The immunoarchitecture of the normal human lacrimal gland. Relevancy for understanding pathologic conditions. *Ophthalmology* **95,** 100–109.

Wilhelmus, K. R., Darougar, S., Forsey, T., and Treharne, J. D. (1986). Sequential antibody changes following ulcerative herpetic keratitis. *Brit. J. Ophthalmol.* **70,** 354–356.

Willey, D. E., Smith, M. D., Nesburn, A. B., and Trousdale, M. D. (1985). Sequential analysis of antibody responses in serum, aqueous humor and tear film during latent and induced recurrent HSV infections. *Curr. Eye Res.* **4,** 1235–1240.

Wilson, J. D., and Foster, D. W., eds. (1985). "Williams Textbook of Endocrinology," Saunders, Philadelphia.

Wira, C. R., and Prabhala, R. H. (1992). Sex hormone, glucocorticoid, and cytokine regulation of mucosal immunity: Hormonal influences on antibody levels and antigen presentation in the female genital tract. *In* "Immunophysiology of the Gut" (W. A. Walker, ed.). pp. 183–205. Academic Press, San Diego.

Wood, J. D. (1992). Enteric neuroimmune interactions. *In* "Immunophysiology of the Gut" (W. A. Walker, ed.), pp. 207–227. Academic Press, San Diego.

Wright, P. (1975). Untoward effects associated with practolol administration: Oculomucocutaneous syndrome. *Brit. Med. J.* **i,** 595–598.

Yamaguchi, K., Hayasaka, S., Hara, S., Kurobane, I., and Tada, K. (1989). Improvement of tear lysosomal enzyme levels after treatment with bone marrow transplantation in a patient with I-cell disease. *Ophthalmic Res.* **21,** 226–229.

Yamamoto, G. K., and Allansmith, M. R. (1979). Complement in tears from normal humans. *Am. J. Ophthalmol.* **88,** 758–763.

Yuasa, T., Nakagawa, Y., Tada, R., and Mimura, Y. (1989). Tear IgE in allergic conjunctival disorders. *In* "Modern Trends in Immunology and Immunopathology of the Eye" (A. G. Secchi and I. A. Fregona, eds.), pp. 346–349. Masson S.p.A.-Milano, Italy.

Zavaro, A., Samra, Z., Baryishak, R., and Sompolinsky, D. (1980). Proteins in tears from healthy and diseased eyes. *Doc. Ophthalmol.* **50,** 185–199.

Zirm, M., Schmut, O., and Hofmann, H. (1976). Quantitative Bestimmung der Antiproteinasen in der menschlichen Tränenflüssigkeit. *Albrect von Graefes Arch. Ophthalmol.* **198,** 89–94.

48

Mucosal Immunology of the Middle Ear and Eustachian Tube

David J. Lim • Goro Mogi

I. INTRODUCTION

Our understanding of middle ear immunology is based largely on studies conducted using middle ear effusions and mucosal biopsies collected from patients with otitis media. With the availability of a number of animal models for otitis media, for example, mice, rats, gerbils, and chinchillas, systematic data have been added to our current understanding of the immune mechanisms of the middle ear and eustachian tube (tubotympanum) and of tubotympanum development.

Studies conducted in the early 1970s showed that elevated levels of immunoglobulins, particularly IgG and IgA, in middle ear effusion (MEE) suggested the local synthesis of these immunoglobulins in the mucosa of middle ear (Ishikawa *et al.*, 1972; Mogi *et al.*, 1973; Veltri and Sprinkle, 1973). Liu *et al.* (1975) further demonstrated that the effusion levels of immunoglobulin and lysozyme are much higher than those of the sera and that they increase steadily with advancing age in children, reflecting the development of the local middle ear immune system.

Findings of secretory IgA in MEE (Mogi *et al.*, 1973;1974; Ogra *et al.*, 1974) further confirmed the presence of a local middle ear mucosal immune system similar to that of other mucosal epithelia. Mogi *et al.* (1974a) isolated secretory IgA from pooled MEEs and demonstrated that its antigenicity and subunit structure are identical or very similar to those of secretory IgA obtained from other external secretions such as saliva, nasal secretion, colostrum, and bronchial fluid. Ogra *et al.* (1974) also detected secretory IgA and secretory component in MEEs and demonstrated that specific antibody activity in MEEs against mumps, measles, rubella, and poliovirus, essentially is limited to IgA. Fluorescent antibody staining of mucosal tissues of the tympanic cavity showed characteristic staining for a secretory component in the surface epithelium (Mogi *et al.*, 1974; Ogra *et al.*, 1974). These data suggest the existence of a distinct secretory immune system in the human middle ear.

The purpose of this chapter is to review available data on immune mechanisms, particularly mucosal immunology of the tubotympanum, and the clinical implications of understanding the immunologic aspects of otitis media.

II. MUCOUS MEMBRANE OF THE TUBOTYMPANUM

The middle ear consists of the eustachian tube, tympanic cavity, antrum, and mastoid air cells. The eustachian tube can be divided into two parts, cartilaginous and bony. Secretory glands of mixed type exist only in the cartilaginous portion of the eustachian tube (Figure 1). Although these tubotympanal structures are very similar among different species, rodents lack air cells.

Although the nasopharynx is not a part of the middle ear, this site also affects middle ear pathophysiology. Mucous membranes of the tympanic cavity, antrum, and air cells communicate via the eustachian tube with nasopharyngeal mucosa.

The tubotympanal mucosa are basically a respiratory type, although the tympanic cavity, antrum, and air cells are covered mostly by cuboidal or squamous cells with few secretory and ciliated cells (Lim, 1974; Figure 2).

III. IMMUNOCOMPETENT CELLS IN THE TUBOTYMPANAL MUCOSA

Although many lymphocytes, plasma cells, macrophages, leukocytes, and other inflammatory cells accumulate in inflamed mucosa (Hussi and Lim, 1974; Lim 1974; Mogi *et al.*, 1980), only a few immunocompetent cells (without organized lymphoid follicles) are found in the normal middle ear mucosa. Takahashi *et al.* (1989) investigated immunocompetent cells and inflammatory cells in the middle ear mucosa of normal and nonsensitized BALB/c mice, demonstrating the presence of (in the order of frequency) Mac-1$^+$, Lyt-1$^+$, IgA$^+$, Lyt-2$^+$, IgG$^+$, and IgM$^+$ cells. Ichimiya *et al.* (1990) also analyzed quantitatively the immunocompetent cells in the middle ear mucosa of mice bred under germ-free, specific pathogen-free, and conventional conditions. According to their results, mast cells and Mac-1$^+$ cells exist in the middle ear mucosa of mice bred under all three conditions. The number of mast cells was highest, followed by Mac$^+$ cells and lymphocytes. As seen in Figure 3, the numbers of lymphocyte subsets are fewer in the middle ear mucosa than in the nasal

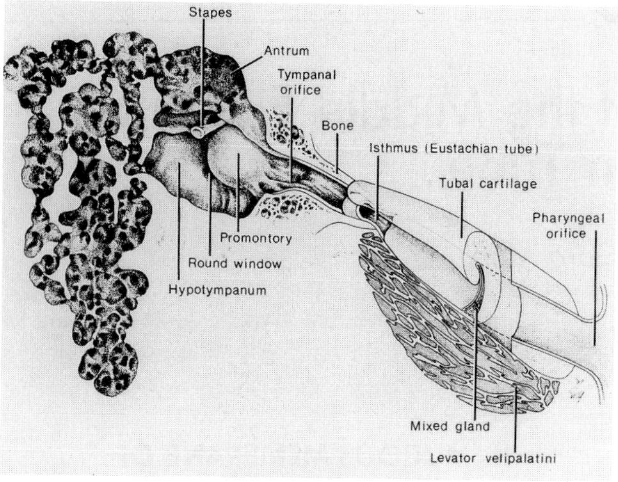

Figure 1 Middle ear, mastoid, and Eustachian tube, demonstrating anatomical landmarks. Reprinted with permission from Lim (1974).

mucosa. Although IgA^+, IgM^+, and Lyt-1^+ cells are seen in the middle ear mucosa of conventional mice, IgM^+ cells exist only in mucosae of specific pathogen-free and germ-free mice. This finding can be interpreted to indicate that, anatomically, the middle ear has less frequent opportunity to be exposed to antigenic stimulation than other areas of the upper respiratory and alimentary tracts. In otitis media-induced mice that have been inoculated with nontypable *Haemophilus influenzae* or lipopolysaccharide (LPS), Mac-1^+ cells were dominant. Although the numbers of IgM^+ and Lyt-1^+ cells increased markedly, the numbers of other lymphocyte subsets did not increase until 14 days after inoculation (Ichimiya *et al.*, 1990). Takahashi *et al.* (1992) induced immune-mediated otitis media in mice using keyhole limpet hemocyanin (KLH) as an antigen and observed immunocytes appearing in the middle ear and eustachian tube. Their results showed that Mac-1^+ cells are the predominant cell type, followed by helper T cells, IgG^+ cells, IgA^+ cells, and IgM^+ cells. Although the difference of infiltrating cell types between these two studies may be related to differences in the procedures to induce otitis media, these findings suggest that the tubotympanum is a potentially immuno-competent organ that can be activated with appropriate antigenic stimulation.

IV. MAST CELLS IN THE MIDDLE EAR

Although few immunocompetent cells exist in the normal middle ear mucosa, mast cells have been demonstrated to be found often in the lamina propria of the pars flaccida of the tympanic membrane (Alm *et al.*, 1982) and middle ear mucosa (Widemar *et al.*, 1986). Almost all mast cells that are distributed in the middle ear and eustachian tube mucosa are of the connective tissue type (Watanabe *et al.*, 1991). The exact role of mast cells in normal middle ear mucosa is not yet known. Since mast cells are involved in type I and III allergic inflammatory reactions, these mast cells may be involved in the pathogenesis of otitis media with effusion (OME). Watanabe *et al.* (1991) investigated the distribution of mast cells in the tubotympanum of both adult and developing guinea pigs, and found a large number of mast cells in the tubotympanic mucosal membrane of the adult but only a few in that of the fetal guinea pig. The middle ear mucosal mast cells accumulate in areas covered with ciliated cells or in areas richly vascularized (Albiin *et al.*, 1986; Watanabe *et al.*, 1991). Jeffrey (1983) suggested that the appearance of mast cells in the airway epithelium is indicative of disease and not a normal feature. One of the major mediators responsible for mast cell accumulation is interleukin 3 (IL-3; Ernst *et al.*, 1987). This lymphokine is derived from many different cells such as T lymphocytes, myeloid cells, and epidermal cells. Judging from the distribution pattern of mast cells in the tubotympanum of developing and adult guinea pigs, one

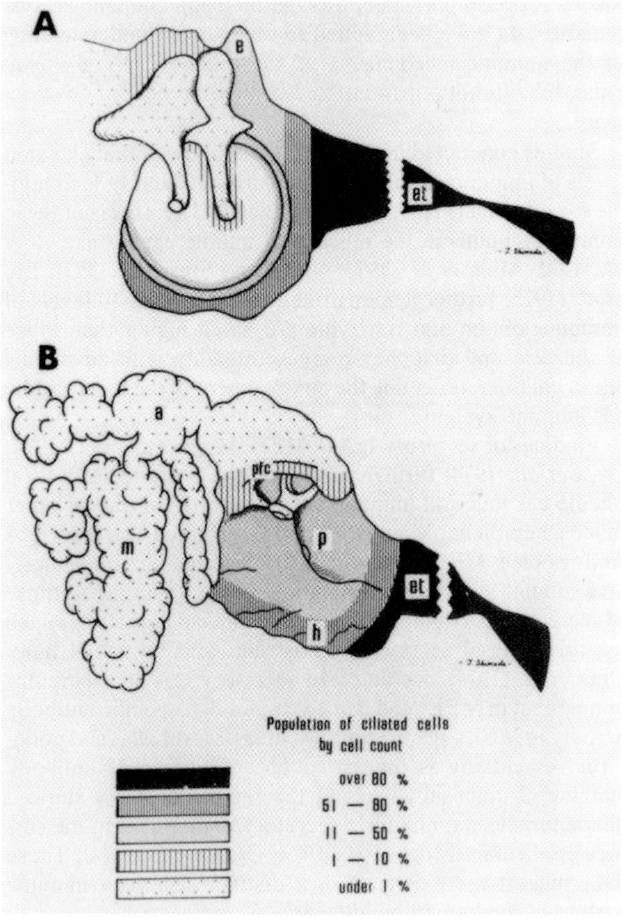

Figure 2 Distribution of ciliated cells in the normal human ear, shown graphically between lateral and medial side. Eustachian tube, et; hypotympanum, h; promontory, p; epitympanic recess, e; prominence of facial canal, pfc; antrum, a; mastoid air cells, m. Reprinted with permission from Shimada and Lim (1972).

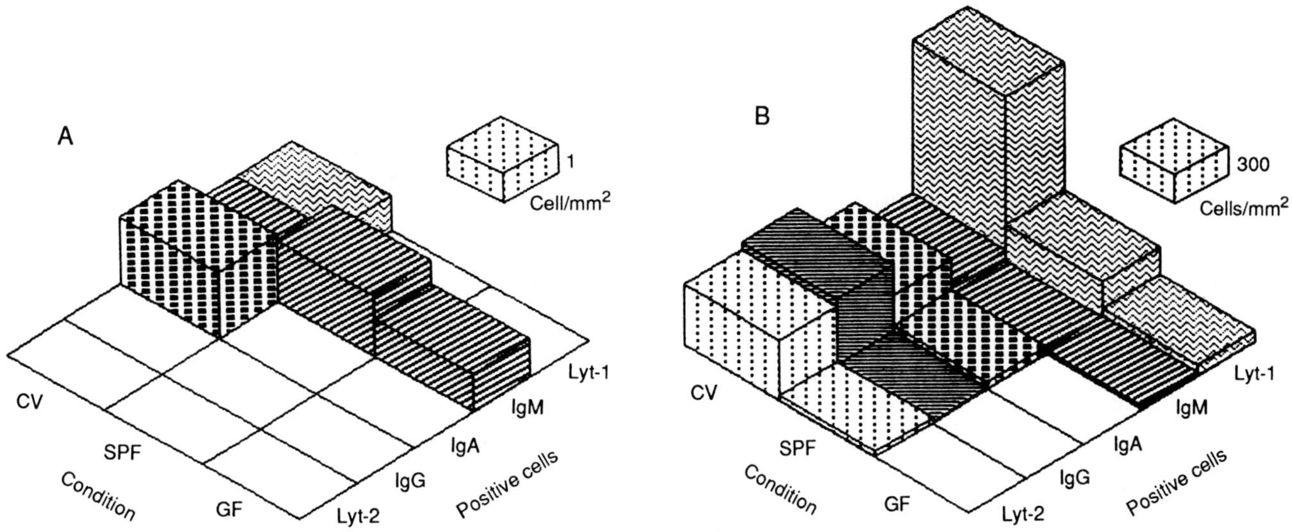

Figure 3 Distribution of lymphocyte subsets in the mucosa of murine middle ear and nose. (A) Middle ear. (B) Nose. Conventional mice, CV; specific pathogen-free mice, SPF; germ-free mice, GF. Note that in the nasal mucosa, all lymphocyte subsets are seen in higher numbers than in the middle ear.

can suggest that mast cell precursors are recruited to the tubotympanal mucosa as a result of antigenic stimulation during development, and differentiate into mast cells locally. These cells also may play a role in the local defense system of the tubotympanum. Mast cells may be recruited to the tubotympanum as part of biological defense mechanism in response to the continuous presence of antigenic stimuli. Biologically active compounds of mast cells induce changes in blood flow and permeability, causing the flooding of plasma and leukocytes that facilitates the removal of antigenic substances (Lembeck, 1983).

V. ROLE OF CIRCULATING ANTIBODIES IN OTITIS MEDIA

Immunity is an important defense system against bacterial otitis media. Immunodeficiency and immaturity of the immune system lead to otitis proneness. Congenital immunodeficiency is causally related to recurrent otitis media (Mogi and Maeda, 1982). Prellner *et al.* (1984) reported that infants with recurrent otitis media have significantly lower IgG antibody levels against pneumococcal capsular polysaccharide 6A or 19F at 1 year of age than those of the control group, but attain normal levels at 8 years of age. Freijd *et al.* (1985) also found that otitis-prone children have lower levels of serum IgG2 subclass, both at 12 months and at 32 months of age, than do age-matched non-otitis-prone children. These findings support the idea that systemic humoral immunity protects the middle ear from bacterial infection, and that certain populations of children may have a delayed immune development of the IgG subclass.

Although overwhelming evidence indicates that specific antibodies are protective against bacterial otitis media, some evidence also suggests that an immune mechanism may be involved in inducing or sustaining MEE. Experimentally, OME can be produced by inoculating the tympanic cavity with a protein antigen after systemic immunization with the same antigen. Smirnov (1938) induced OME in guinea pigs by inoculating horse serum into the middle ear after systemic immunization. Subseqently, Koch (1947) and Hopp *et al.* (1964) were successful in reproducing these results. Ryan *et al.* (1982,1986) and Suzuki *et al.* (1988) further investigated immunologically induced otitis media and demonstrated that immune-mediated otitis media cannot be produced without prior systemic challenge. Inoculation of protein antigen into the tympanic cavity after systemic sensitization of the host with the same antigen induced immune-mediated otitis media (Ryan *et al.*, 1986). These data are interpreted to mean that the afferent limb of systemic immunity from the middle ear appears to operate less effectively and rapidly than that from the dermis. Middle ear mucosa responds in a manner that is more similar to that of oral and nasal mucosa than to that of tracheal mucosa (Kasturi and Hannoun, 1977). Immune-mediated otitis media also is produced by injecting a protein antigen into the tympanic cavity of animals that are sensitized passively with antigen-specific IgG antibodies. However, no OME is produced by inoculating the antigen into the tympanic cavity of hosts that are transfused passively with sensitized lymphocytes (Ryan and Catanzaro, 1983; Mogi, 1989). Formation of immune complex, followed by complement activation and the release of granulocyte proteases from neutrophils, is the key factor in the production of immune-mediated OME (Suzuki *et al.*, 1988; Mogi, 1989). Mravic *et al.* (1978) produced inflammatory response in the middle ear by inoculation of the chinchilla bulla with immune complex. Inoculation of immune complexes of pneumococcal antigens (but not IgG antibodies) into the normal tympanic cavity of nonsensitized chinchillas also produced MEE (G. Mogi *et al.*, in press). Palva *et al.* (1985) found pneumococcal immune complexes in at least 25% of MEEs in patients with chronic OME (secretory otitis media).

Epidemiological and clinical evidence indicates that chronic OME is associated closely with prior episodes of acute otitis media (Groothuis *et al.*, 1979; J. Schwin *et al.*, 1979). In a chinchilla animal model, acute otitis media becomes chronic OME in certain cases (G. Mogi, unpublished data). In this study, chinchillas were immunized systemically with killed *Streptococcus pneumoniae* 19F and then inoculated with live bacteria of the same strain into the middle ear. Of 20 chinchillas, 7 cases became chronic OME, 5 cases showed a drumhead perforation following acute otitis media, 5 animals died, and 2 cases healed within 14 days, and one showed no otitis media. However, of 12 control chinchillas (normal and nonimmunized) receiving live *S. pneumoniae* 19F, 4 chinchillas died, 6 chinchillas healed within 11 days, 1 chinchilla had a drumhead perforation, and one showed no otitis media. None of the control animals developed chronic OME. The formation of the immune complex itself can be viewed as a host defense mechanism to eliminate the antigens. However, during the activation process of this defense mechanism, the activation of the complement system also may have contributed to the initiation and sustenance of inflammatory reactions. Therefore, although humoral systemic immunity is an important defense against infection, its immune reactions can, at the same time, contribute to the pathogenic mechanisms of chronic OME.

VI. SUPPRESSION OF IMMUNE-MEDIATED OTITIS MEDIA

Oral administration of antigens has been known to lead to immune tolerance. Ueyama *et al.* (1988) investigated the effects of mucosa-derived T suppressor cells on the induction of immune-mediated OME in C3H/Hen mice bred under specific pathogen-free conditions. Splenic T suppressor cells, which were obtained after oral administration of ovalbumin (OVA), were transferred intravenously into syngeneic mice. The mice receiving the T suppressor cells were immunized with OVA intraperitoneally, followed by instillation of OVA into the tympanic cavity. OME was seen in only 1 of 10 mice receiving splenic T cells from OVA-fed mice, whereas 9 of 10 control mice to which splenic T cells from saline-fed mice were administered developed OME. IgG-mediated OME can be suppressed to a certain extent by the induction of antigen-specific, mucosa-derived T suppressor cells.

VII. SECRETORY IgA IN MIDDLE EAR EFFUSIONS AND NASOPHARYNGEAL SECRETIONS

A previous study, using a radioactive single radial diffusion technique, reported that the mean value of secretory IgA concentration in the serous effusions is 212.7 ± 13.5 μg/ml and 357.7 ± 13.2 μg/ml in the mucoid effusions (Mogi *et al.*, 1974). Mogi *et al.* (1984) measured secretory IgA and serum type IgA in MEEs using an electro-immunodiffusion method. As shown in Table I, the mean concentration in mucoid MEEs is significantly greater than that in the serous MEEs. Although not statistically significant, the mean concentration of serum type IgA exceeded the value of secretory IgA in both types of MEEs. This finding is in accordance with that reported by Sorensen (1982), who also summarized reported data of concentrations of secretory IgA and IgA in MEEs, nasopharyngeal secretions, and nasal secretions (Sorensen, 1990).

VIII. LOCAL PRODUCTION OF ANTIBODIES IN THE MIDDLE EAR

Streptococcus pneumoniae, nontypable *H. influenzae*, and *Moraxella catarrhalis* are the major pathogens for acute otitis media. On the basis of the presence of specific antibodies in MEEs, these bacteria are also considered causative factors for OME, although bacterial cultures only occasionally demonstrate these bacteria in the MEE (Lim and DeMaria, 1982; Kurono *et al.*, 1988). Investigations of specific antibody activities against these bacteria in the effusions have contributed to our current understanding of the immune mechanism of the middle ear. Whereas specific antibodies in MEE against certain viruses are restricted mainly to IgA class antibodies (Ogra *et al.*, 1974; Meurman *et al.*, 1980; Yamaguchi *et al.*, 1984), those against bacterial antigens belong to IgG, IgA, and IgM classes (Sloyer *et al.*, 1974;1975; Faden *et al.*, 1989a). Liu *et al.* (1975) investigated, immunochemically and bacteriologically, MEEs from children with chronic OME and found that IgA levels are significantly higher in the culture-negative fluids than in the positive effusions, and that bacterial recovery rate is related inversely to the dramatic increase with age of IgA and IgG levels in effusions. Sloyer *et al.* (1974,1975) found specific antibodies against causative pneumococcal serotype in 27% of effusions of patients with acute otitis media taken at the time of diagnosis. These antibodies were IgG, IgM, and IgA classes, but IgA class antibodies were detected more often in MEEs without the simultaneous presence of IgA antibodies in serum. These investigators also found the same results in acute otitis media caused by *H. influenzae*. Faden *et al.* (1989a,b) investigated systemic and local immune responses of young children with recurrent otitis media caused by nontypable *H. influenzae* during and after the infection. However, their results showed that the titer of strain-specific antibody against *H. influenzae* was much higher for the IgG class than for the IgM and IgA classes. Although antibody titers in MEEs declined over time, serum antibody titers remained stable. These researchers suggested that immunity to nontypable *H. influenzae* in the middle ear, in part, reflects systemic immunity. These clinical findings indicate that the local immunity in the middle ear, in conjunction with systemic

Table I Mean Levels of Secretory IgA and Serum Type IgA in Middle Ear Effusion[a,b,c]

	Mucoid group (N = 77)		Serous group (N = 41)	
	MEE	Serum	MEE	Serum
Secretory IgA	(1) 2045.5 ± 1560.0	—	(4) 1326.6 ± 1240.0	—
Serum-type IgA	(2) 2367.3 ± 1461.0	(3) 2867.4 ± 1347.0	(5) 2832.7 ± 2011.0	(6) 3179.0 ± 1382.8

[a] Mean ± SD, μg/ml.
[b] Significant difference: (1) > (2), $p < 0.05$; (3) > (2), $p < 0.01$; (5) > (4), $p < 0.05$.
[c] Significant correlation between: (1) and (2), $p < 0.05$, $r = 0.236$; (2) and (3), $p < 0.01$, $r = 0.330$; (4) and (5), $p < 0.05$, $r = 0.527$.

immunity, plays an important role in middle ear infection.

IX. ROLE OF SECRETORY IgA IN BACTERIAL ADHERENCE

Colonization of pathogenic bacteria in the nasopharynx is an important etiological factor of middle ear infection (Kurono *et al.*, 1988; Stenfors and Raisanen 1990). Nasopharyngeal bacterial adherence is known to be of crucial importance in the pathogenesis of otitis media. The adherence of both nontypable *H. influenzae* and *S. pneumoniae* to nasopharyngeal epithelial cells *in vitro* was reported to be significantly greater in children with OME than in normal control children (Mogi, 1988). Shimamura *et al.* (1990) detected secretory IgA antibody activities in nasopharyngeal secretions against nontypable *H. influenzae* and *S. pneumoniae,* and reported that adherence of both bacteria is significantly less in the group of patients with secretory IgA antibody activity than in the group of patients with no activity. Kurono *et al.* (1991) further investigated bacterial adherence to nasopharyngeal epithelial cells *in vitro* and found that adherence is reduced remarkably by treating bacteria (*H. influenzae* or *S. pneumoniae*) with nasopharyngeal secretions and that the adhesion-blocking activity is significantly greater in nasopharyngeal secretions with secretory IgA antibody activity against bacteria than in those with no activity. These findings suggest that secretory IgA in nasopharyngeal secretions may inhibit bacterial adherence, thus significantly reducing nasopharyngeal bacterial colonization, a first important step in the process of otitis media. Results of an animal study support this concept (Y. Kurono, K. Shimamura, and G. Mogi, unpublished results). When nontypable *H. influenzae* was inoculated into the nasopharynx of BALB/c mice immunized by oral administration of formalin-killed bacteria, salivary IgA antibody titers against *H. influenzae* were increased significantly by oral immunization but salivary IgG antibody titers were not. The bacteria inoculated to the nasopharynx were eliminated more rapidly in immunized mice than in control mice (Figure 4). Further, systemic immunization of mice with *H. influenzae* was found to raise serum IgG antibody titer, but nasopharyngeal colonization of the bacteria was not inhibited (G. Mogi *et al.* unpublished data). Oral immunization that enhances mucosal immunity may be useful in preventing otitis media by inhibiting the colonization of pathogenic bacteria in the nasopharynx.

X. SOURCE OF IgA PRECURSORS IN MIDDLE EAR

The presence of secretory IgA in MEE and the existence of IgA immunocytes in the inflamed middle ear mucosa (rarely in normal mucosa) indicate that mucosal immunity is activated in the tubotympanic cavity under inflammatory conditions. In humans, the tonsils and adenoids were proposed to be possible sources of antibody-producing cells in the tubotympanum (Sorensen, 1983; Brandtzarg, 1984). Watanabe *et al.* (1988) induced antigen-specific IgA-forming cells in the middle ear mucosa of guinea pigs by immunizing the animals intraduodenally or intratracheally with protein antigen after systemic priming. Antigen-specific IgA-forming cells were detected in the inflamed middle ear mucosa, whereas these cells could not be found in animals that received only intratympanic inoculation after systemic priming (Figure 5). However, the number of IgA-forming cells in the inflamed middle ear mucosa was apparently smaller than that of cells induced in the mucosa of the alimentary tract and other sites of the respiratory tracts. These findings show that gut-associated lymphoid tissues (GALT) and bronchus-associated lymphoid tissues (BALT) are two of the sources of IgA precursors for inflamed tubotympanic mucosa and that the tubotympanum shares common mucosal immunity. The selective recruitment of precursors of IgA-forming cells to mucosal sites is thought to be influenced by factors such as hormones and organ-specific endothelial-cell determinants of high endothelial venules (Butcher and Scollary, 1980). Although the number of determinants is extremely small compared with that in the small intestine and spleen (Mogi *et al.*, 1990), a further study suggested that the inflamed mucous membrane of the middle ear possesses determinants to which lymphocytes bind. Normal middle ear mucosa does not express such determinants. Ryan *et al.* (1990) investigated the homing mechanism of middle ear lymphocytes and found that they do not appear to have specialized ligands or receptors that can recruit mucosal lymphocytes selectively to the middle ear sites, since lymphocytes of difference origin show no preferential homing during active recuitment of lymphocytes to the middle ear cavity.

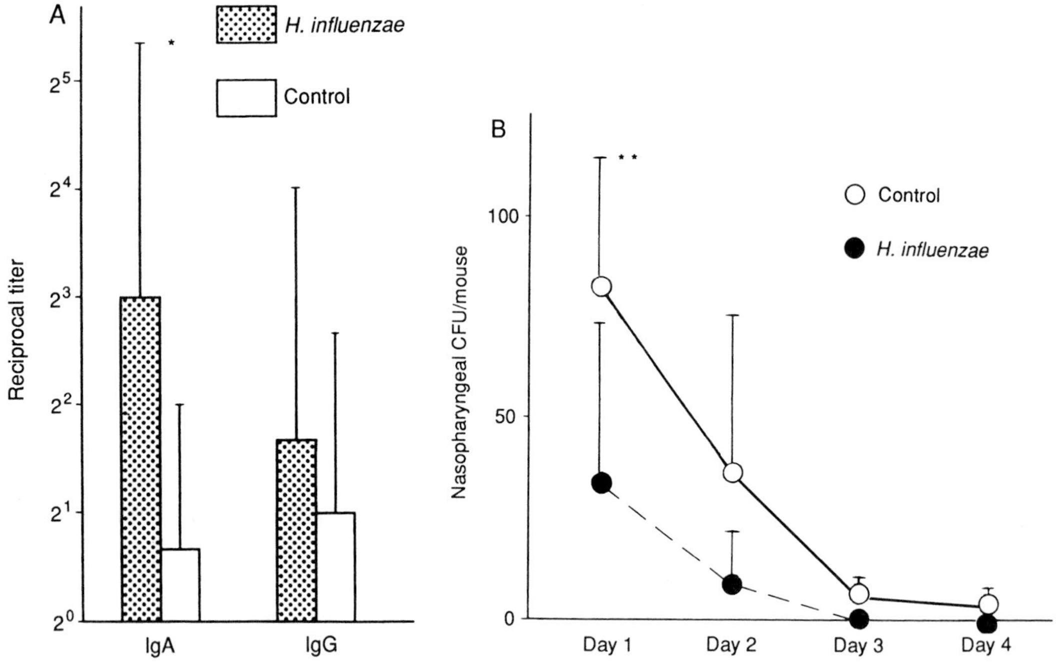

Figure 4 Secretory antibody production by oral immunization and effects of oral immunization on nasopharyngeal colonization of *Haemophilus influenzae*. (A) Salivary antibody activities against *H. influenzae* after oral immunization. Mice immunized orally with GM 53 (adjuvant) only, ○; mice immunized orally with liposomes containing *H. influenzae* and GM 53 (●). (B) Numbers of *H. influenzae* detected from the nasopharynx after nasopharyngeal inoculation of bacteria. Mice immunized with *H. influenzae*, shaded bars; mice immunized with adjuvant only, open bars.

XI. PREVENTION OF IMMUNE-MEDIATED OTITIS MEDIA BY ORAL IMMUNIZATION

Antigen loading onto the duodenal mucosa enhances the mucosal immunity of various mucosal sites, including the nasopharynx and tubotympanum (Watanabe *et al.*, 1988,1989). Moreover, the mucosal immunization that stimulates GALT prevents the occurrence of immune-mediated otitism media (Watanabe *et al.*, 1988), Yoshimura *et al.* (1991) investigated the efficacy of oral immunization of killed bacte-

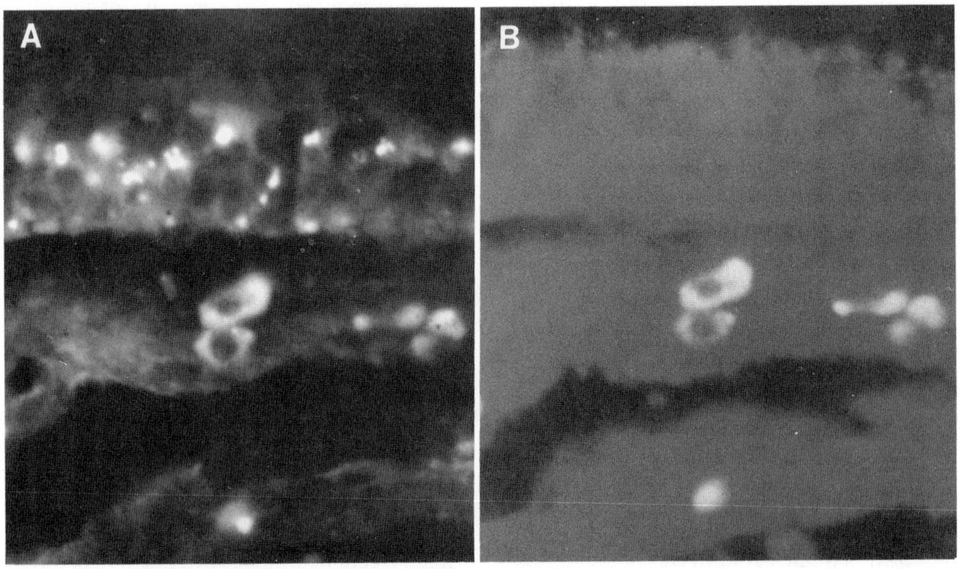

Figure 5 Localization of antigen-specific IgA-forming cells in middle ear mucosa of guinea pigs immunized intraduodenally with protein antigen after systemic priming. Same section was treated with fluoresceinated isothiocyanate conjugates for antigen-specific antibody-forming cells (A) and consequently stained with rhodamine conjugates for IgA-forming cells (B).

ria on the prevention of bacterial otitis media in guinea pigs. With intratympanic inoculation of 10^5 and 10^6 live *S. pneumoniae,* the occurrence of pneumococcal otitis media significantly decreased in guinea pigs that received intraduodenal or intragastric immunization by enteric capsules containing killed bacteria of the same strain. In these guinea pigs, the values of salivary IgA antibody titers against *S. pneumoniae* were increased significantly. These findings indicate that oral vaccination by enteric capsules elicits mucosal IgA responses, presenting an opportunity for clinical application of oral vaccination by enteric capsules for the prevention of middle ear infection.

XII. SUMMARY

The middle ear is anatomically and immunologically unique. Because the normally functioning eustachian tube protects the tympanic cavity, antrum, and mastoid cavities from bacterial invasion, these compartments are aseptic and only a few immunocompetent cells are present in the normal healthy middle ear. Tubotympanal encounters of antigens (bacteria/viruses) stimulate the development of local and systemic immune systems in an age-dependent manner, thus contributing to the protection of the tubotympanum from pathogenic bacteria. Whereas IgG (to a lesser extent IgM) is the main immunoglobulin affording protection, some evidence suggests that IgG-mediated immune reactions in the tympanic cavity also may contribute to the chronicity of MEEs. The role of IgA in protection against otitis media is not well defined. Evidence suggests that the secretory IgA response is beneficial in reducing bacterial adherence in the nasopharynx and in recovery from otitis media.

References

Albiin, N., Hellstrom, S., Stenfors, L.-E., and Cerne, A. (1986). Middle ear mucosa in rats and humans. *Ann. Otol. Rhinol. Laryngol.* **95, (Suppl. 126),** 1–15.

Alm, P. E., Bloom, G. D., Hellstrom, S., Salen, B., and Stenfors, L.-E. (1982). The release of histamine from the pars flaccida mast cells. One cause of otitis media with effusion? *Acta Otolaryngol. (Stockh.)* **94,** 517–522.

Brandtzaeg, P. (1984). Immune functions of human nasal mucosa and tonsils in health and disease. *In* "Immunology of the Lung and Upper Respiratory Tract" (J. Bienenstock, ed.), pp. 28–95. McGraw-Hill, New York.

Butcher, E. C., Scollary, R. G., and Weissman, I. L. (1980). Organ specificity of lymphocyte migration: Meditation by highly selective lymphocyte interaction with organ-specific determinants on the high endothelial venules. *Eur. J. Immunol.* **10,** 559–561.

Ernst, P. B., Otsuka, H., Dolovich, J., Denburg, J. A., and Bienenstock, J. (1987). Update on mast cell. *In* "Immunobiology, Histophysiology and Tumor Immunology in Otolaryngology" (J. E. Veldman, ed.), pp. 281–291. Kugler, Amsterdam.

Faden, H., Brodsky, L., Bernstein, J., Stanievich, J., Krystofik, D., Shuff, C., Hong, J. J., and Ogra, P. L. (1989a). Otitis media in children: Local immune response to nontypable haemophilus influenzae. *Infect. Immun.* **57,** 3555–3559.

Faden, H., Bernstein, J., Brodsky, L., Stanievich, J., Krystofik, D., Shuff, C., Hong, J. J., and Ogra, P. L. (1989b). Otitis media in children. I. The systemic immune response to nontypable hemophilus influenzae. *J. Infect. Dis.* **160,** 999–1004.

Freijd, A., Oxelius, V. A., and Rynnel-Dagoo, B. (1985). A presepective study demonstrating and association between plasma IgG2 concentrations and susceptibility to otitis media in children. *Scand. J. Infect. Dis.* **17,** 115–120.

Groothuis, J. R., Sell, S. H., Wright, P. F., Thompson, J. M., and Altemeier, W. A. (1979). Otitis media in infancy: Tympanometric findings. *Pediatr.* **63(3),** 435–442.

Hopp, E. S., Elevitch, F. R., Pumphrey, R. E., Irving, T. E., and Hoffman, P. W. (1964). Serous otitis media—An "immune" theory. *Laryngoscope* **74,** 1149–1159.

Hussl, B., and Lim, D. J., (1974). Experimental middle ear effusions: An immunofluorescent study. *Ann. Otol. Rhinol. Laryngol.* **83,** 322–342.

Ichimiya, I., Kawauchi, H., and Mogi, G. (1990). Analysis of immunocompetent cells in the middle ear mucosa. *Arch. Otolaryngol. Head Neck Surg.* **116,** 324–330.

Ishikawa, T., Bernstein, J., Reisman, R. E., and Arbesman, C. E. (1972). Secretory otitis media: Immunologic studies of middle ear secretions. *J. Allergy Immunol.* **50,** 319–325.

Jeffery, P. K. (1983). Morphologic features of airway surface epithelial cells and glands. *Am. Rev. Resp. Dis.* **128,** 14–20.

Kasturi, K., and Hannoun, C. (1977). Immune responses to influenza virus in rabbits after local immunization. *Ann. Microbiol.* **128,** 97–117.

Koch, H. (1947). Allergical investigations of chronic otitis media. *Acta Otolaryngol. (Suppl.)* **62,** 1–207.

Kurono, Y., Tomonaga, K., and Mogi, G. (1988). Staphylococcus epidermidis and Staphlococcus aureus in otitis media with effusion. *Arch. Otolaryngol. Head Neck Surg.* **114,** 1262–1265.

Kurono, Y., Shimada., K., and Mogi, G. (1992). Inhibition of nasopharyngeal colonization of *Hemophilus influenzae. Laryngol.* **101(Suppl. 157),** 11–15.

Kurono, Y., Shimamura, K., Shigemi, H., and Mogi, G. (1991). Inhibition of bacterial adherence by nasopharyngeal secretions. *Ann. Otol. Rhinol. Laryngol.* **100,** 455–458.

Lembeck, F. (1983). Thomas Lewis's Nocifensor system, histamine and substance P-containing primary afferent nerves. *Trends neurosci.* **6,** 106–108.

Lim, D. J. (1974). Functional morphology of the lining membranes of the middle ear and Esutachian tube. An overview. *Ann. Otol. Rhinol. Laryngol.* **83,** (Suppl. 11), 5–22.

Lim, D. J., and DeMaria, T. F. (1982). Pathogenesis of otitis media: Bacteriology and immunology. *Laryngoscope* **92,** 278–286.

Liu, Y. S., Lim, D. J., Lang, R. W., and Birck, H. G. (1975). Chronic middle ear effusions. Immunochemical and bacteriological investigations. *Arch. Otolaryngol.* **101,** 278–286.

Meurman, O. H., Sarkkinen, H. K., Puhakka, H. J., Virolainen, E. S., and Meuman, O. H. (1980). Local IgA-class antibodies against respiratory viruses in middle ear and nasopharyngeal secretions of children with secretory otitis media. *Laryngoscope* **90,** 304–311.

Mogi, G. (1989). Immunology of the middle ear—Etiology and prophylaxis of otitis media with effusion. *In* "The 90th Japanese Otorhinolaryngological Society Annual Meeting Research Report." Department of Otolaryngology, Medical College of Oita.

Mogi, G., and Maeda, S. (1982). Recurrent otitis media in association with immuno-deficiency. *Arch. Otolaryngol.* **108,** 204–207.

Mogi, G., Honjo, S., Yoshida, T., and Maeda, S. (1973a). Middle ear effusion. Quantitative analysis of immunoglobulins. *Ann. Otol. Rhinol. Laryngol.* **82,** 196–202.

Mogi, G., Honjo, S., Maeda, S., and Yoshida, T. (1973b). Secretory immunoglobulin A (SIgA) in middle ear effusions. Observation of 160 specimens. *Ann. Otol. Rhinol. Laryngol.* **82,** 302–310.

Mogi, G., Honjo, S., Maeda, S., Yoshida, T., and Watanabe, N.

(1974a). Secretory immunoglobulin A (Siga) in middle ear effusions. A further report. *Ann. Otol. Rhinol. Laryngol.* **83,** 92–101.

Mogi, G., Kawauchi, H., and Kurono, Y. (1993). Role of bacterial infection and immune response. *In* "Otitis Media—Acute Otitis Media and Otitis Media with Effusion," Proc. of 2nd Extraordinary International Symposium on Recent Advances in Otitis Media. (G. Mogi, ed.). Kugler Pub. Amsterdam/New York, in press.

Mogi, G., Maeda, S., and Watanabe, N. (1980). The development of mucosal immunity in guinea pig middle ears. *Int. J. Pediatr. Otorhinolaryngol.* **1,** 331–349.

Mogi, G., Honjo, S., Maeda, S., Yoshida, T., and Watanabe, N. (1974b). Quantitative determination of secretory immunoglobulin A (Siga) in middle ear effusions. *Ann. Otol. Rhinol. Laryngol.* **83,** 239–247.

Mogi, G., Maeda, S., Umehara, T., Fujiyoshi, T., and Kurono, Y. (1984). Secretory IgA, serum IgA, and free secretory component in middle ear effusion. *In* "Recent Advances in Otitis Media with Effusion" (D. J. Lim, C. D. Bluestone, J. O. Klein, and J. D. Nelson, eds.), pp. 147–149. Decker, Philadelphia.

Mogi, G., Watanabe, N., Kawauchi, H., Suzuki, M., Ichimiya, I., and Ueyama, S. (1990). Mucosal immunity of the middle ear and upper respiratory tract. Third International Academic Conference of Immunobiology in Otology, Rhinology, Laryngology; San Diego, November.

Mravec, J., Lewis, D. M., and Lim, D. J. (1978). Experimental otitis media: An immune-complex-mediated response. *Otolaryngol.* ORL258–ORL268.

Ogra, P. L., Bernstein, J. M., Yurchak, A. M., Coppola, P. R., and Tomasi, T. B., Jr. (1974). Characteristics of secretory immune system in human middle ear: Implications in otitis media. *J. Immunol.* **112,** 488–495.

Palva, T., Tuohimaa, P., and Lehtinen, T. (1985). Pneumococcal immune complexes and clinical course of secretory otitis media. *Int. J. Pediatr. Otorhinolaryngol.* **10,** 21–26.

Prellner, K., Kalm, O., and Pedersen, F. K. (1984). Pneumococcal antibodies and complement during and after periods of recurrent otitis. *J. Pediatr. Otorhinolaryngol.* **7,** 39–49.

Ryan, A. F., and Catanzaro, A. (1983). Passive transfer of Immune-mediated middle ear inflammation and effusion. *Acta Otolaryngol. (Stockh.)* **95,** 123–130.

Ryan, F. R., Cleveland, P. H., Hartman, M. T., and Catanzaro, A. (1982). Humoral and cell-mediated immunity in peripheral blood following introduction of antigen into the middle ear. *Ann. Otol. Rhinol. Laryngol.* **91,** 70–75.

Ryan, A. F., Cantanzaro, A., Wasserman, S. I., and Harris, J. P. (1986). Secondary immune response in the middle ear: Immunological morphological, and physiological observations. *Ann. Otol. Rhinol. Laryngol.* **95,** 242–249.

Ryan, A. F., Sharp, P. A., and Harris, J. P. (1990). Lymphocyte circulation to the middle ear. *Acta Otolaryngol. (Stockh.)* **109,** 278–287.

Shimada, T., and Lim, D. J. (1972). Distribution of ciliated cells in the human middle ear: Electron and light microscopic observations. *Ann. Otol. Rhinol. Laryngol.* **81,** 203–211.

Shimaura, K., Shigemi, H., Surono, Y., and Mogi, G. (1990). The role of bacterial adherence in otitis media with effusion. *Arch. Otolaryngol. Head Neck Surg.* **116,** 1143–1146.

Schurin, P. A., Pelton, S. I., Donner, A., and Klein, Jo (1979). Persistence of middle ear effusion after acute otitis media in children. *N. Engl. J. Med.* **17, 300(20),** 1121–1123.

Sloyer, J. L., Jr., Howie, V. M., Ploussard, J. H., Amman, A. J., Austrian, R., and Johnston, R. B. (1974). Immune response to acute otitis media in children. I. Serotypes isolated and serum and middle ear fluid antibody in pneumococcal otitis media. *Infect. Immun.* **9,** 1028–1032.

Sloyer, J. L., Jr., Howie, V. M., Ploussard, J. H., and Johnston, R. B., Jr. (1975). The immune response to acute otitis media in children. II. Serum and middle ear fluid antibody in otitis media due to haemophilus influenzae. *J. Infect. Dis.* **132,** 685–688.

Smirnov, P. P. (1938). Experiences visant a obtenir L'anaphylaxie des animaux au moyen des microbes et des histolysats de l'oreille humanie. *Acta Otololaryngol. (Stockh.)* **26,** 12–17.

Sorensen, C. H. (1982). The ratio of secretory IgA to IgA in middle ear effusions and nasopharyngeal secretions. *Acta Otolaryngol. (Stockh.)* **386**(Suppl.), 91–93.

Sorensen, C. H. (1983). Quantitative aspects of IgE and secretory immunoglobulins in middle ear effusions. *Int. Pediatr. Otorhinolayngol.* **6,** 247–253.

Sorensen, C. H. (1990). Quantitative aspects of the mucosal immunity and bacteriology of the nasopharynx and middle ear cavity. Studies on children with clinically different forms of otitis media. *Acta Pathol. Microbiol. Immunol. Scand.* **98,**(Suppl. 16), 1–41.

Stenfors, L.-E., and Raisanen, S. (1990). Occurrence of middle ear pathogens in the nasopharynx of young individuals—A quantitative study in four groups. *Acta Otolaryngol. (Stockh.)* **109,** 142–148.

Suzuki, M., Kawauchi, H., and Mogi, G. (1988). Immune-mediated otitis media with effusion. *Am. J. Otolaryngol.* **9,** 199–209.

Takahashi, M., Peppard, J., and Harris, J. P. (1989). Immunohistochemical study of murine middle ear and Eustachian tube. *Acta Otolaryngol. (Stockh.)* **107,** 97–103.

Takahashi, M., Kanai, N., Watanabe, A., Oshima, O., and Ryan, A. F. (1992). Lymphocyte subsets in immune-mediated otitis media with effusion. *Eur. Arch. Oto-Rhino-Laryngol.* **249,** 24–27.

Ueyama, S., Kawauchi, H., and Mogi, G. (1988). Suppression of immune-mediated otitis media by T-suppressor cells. *Arch. Otolaryngol. Head Neck Surg.* **114,** 878–882.

Veltri, R. W., and Sprinkle, P. M. (1973). Serous otitis media. Immunoglobulin and lysozyme levels in middle ear fluids and serum. *Ann. Otol. Rhinol. Laryngol.* **82,** 297–301.

Watanabe, N., Yoshimura, H., and Mogi, G. (1988). Induction of antigen-specific IgA forming cells in the middle ear mucosa. *Arch. Otolaryngol. Head Neck Surg.* **114,** 758–762.

Watanabe, N., Kato, H., and Mogi, G. (1989). Induction of antigen-specific IgA-forming cells in the upper respiratory mucosa. *Ann. Otol. Rhinol. Laryngol.* **98,** 523–529.

Watanabe, T., Kawauchi, H., Fujiyoshi, T., and Mogi, G. (1991). Distribution of mast cells in the tubotympanum of guinea pigs. *Ann. Otol. Rhinol. Laryngol.* **100,** 407–412.

Widemar, L., Hellstrom, S., Stenfors, L.-E., and Bloom, G. D. (1986). An overlooked site of tissue mast cells—The human tympanic membrane. Implications for middle ear affections. *Acta Otolaryngol. (Stockh.)* **102,** 391–395.

Yamaguchi, T., Urasawa, T., and Kataura, A. (1984). Secretory immunoglobulin A antibodies to respiratory viruses in middle ear effusion of chronic otitis media with effusion. *Ann. Otol. Rhinol. Laryngol.* **93,** 73–75.

Yoshimura, H., Watanabe, N., Bundo, J., Shinoda, M., and Mogi, G. (1991). Oral vaccine therapy for pneumococcal otitis media in an animal model. *Arch. Otolaryngol. Head Neck Surg.* **117,** 884–894.

49

Immunology of Diseases of the Oral Cavity

S. J. Challacombe • P. J. Shirlaw

I. INTRODUCTION

Oral health is dependent on the integrity of the oral mucosa which normally prevents the penetration of microorganisms and macromolecules that might be antigenic. The mucosa is protected by both nonspecific and specific defense mechanisms. The former include mucins, lysozyme, lactoferrin, and lactoperoxidase; specific immunity includes the systemic immune system and the secretory immune system, both of which play a role in local immune defense in the oral cavity.

The mouth is part of the mucosal lining of the body, and structurally shows similarities with those tissues of the gut and lungs, among others. The most striking difference between the mouth and the tissue lining the remainder of the gastrointestinal tract is the presence of teeth. The junction between the teeth and mucosa not only allows a greater access of serum proteins to the mucosal surface than is found in other mucosae, but also results in exposure of a unique epithelium, the junctional epithelium, to microbial challenge. This epithelium is affected in periodontal diseases. As are other parts of the mucosal system, oral mucosa is exposed to both the systemic and the secretory immune systems but some immune mechanisms are found there that differ from those found elsewhere. Local immune responses include those that are part of the secretory immune system, emanating from major and minor salivary glands, and those of the systemic immunue system, emanating from crevicular fluid or within the gingival and mucosal tissues.

The oral mucosa is bathed constantly in antigens; any deficiency in the surface mucosal systems may result in increased antigen access, as does trauma or inflammation. Such antigens and microorganisms may contain B-cell mitogens, for example, the polysaccharide capsules or antigens of some fungi and bacteria in plaque. If antigen is not cleared from the mucosal site or if additional antigen gains access, locally activated T and B cells may release various cytokines and interact with associated macrophages and neutrophils, resulting in localized inflammatory reactions that cause damage to the host as a by-product of an attempt to clear antigen from the area. The pathogenesis of some mucosal diseases may be related to cross reaction of some microbial components with host antigens, resulting in host damage subsequent to a normal immune response.

The main salivary immunoglobulin is secretory IgA (SIgA). Whole saliva is made of the secretions of the parotid gland (40%), the submandibular glands (40%), the sublingual glands (10%), and the minor salivary glands (10%) of which many dozens occur around the oral mucosa, especially in the labial and buccal mucosae. A small but significant contribution to whole saliva is made by crevicular fluid (see subsequent text). The total volume of saliva produced per day is probably between 750 and 1000 ml. The majority of the IgA in saliva is dimeric, but 5–10% is monomeric. The IgA1:IgA2 ratio is about 55:45. The concentration of SIgA differs in various secretions but is always greater than that of IgG. In whole saliva, the contributions of SIgA, IgG, and IgM are approximately 200, 1, and 1 mg per 1000 ml, respectively.

A. Induction of Salivary IgA Antibodies

Antibodies in saliva can be stimulated at remote sites (centrally) or locally. Locally, direct application of antigen to the mucosa may lead to the induction of antibodies in minor salivary glands (Krasse *et al.*, 1988) whereas injection of antigen submucosally or instillation into the ducts of the glands (Emmings *et al.*, 1975) may lead to antibodies in the saliva from major salivary glands. Centrally, the most effective method of inducing antibodies in saliva seems to be by intragastric or intraduodenal immunization (reviewed by Challacombe, 1987). Salivary antibody induction has been used widely as a model to study secretory responses, primarily because saliva is an easy secretion to collect and analyze. The induction of salivary antibodies after intragastric immunization has been demonstrated in a variety of species including humans (Mestecky *et al.*, 1978), rhesus monkeys (Challacombe and Lehner, 1980), rabbits (Montgomery *et al.*, 1978), rats (Michalek *et al.*, 1977), and mice (Challacombe and Tomasi, 1980). Most of these studies have used particulate antigens. Scientists now generally accept that, in the absence of adjuvants, antigen in particulate form is more effective than antigen in soluble form in the induction of salivary antibodies by remote site stimulation. However, salivary antibodies after intragastric immunization with soluble antigens have been reported in rabbits with bovine gamma globulin (Montgomery *et al.*, 1978) and in mice with ovalbumin (Challacombe and Tomasi, 1980) and streptococcal antigen I/II (Challacombe, 1983).

A feature of salivary antibodies shared with secretory antibodies elsewhere in the mucosal immune system is that antibodies are generally short lived and of low titer (Mestecky *et al.*, 1978). In humans (Mestecky *et al.*, 1978) and in monkeys

(Challacombe and Lehner, 1980), even secondary immunizations only lead to a salivary response slightly greater than that after the primary immunization. These studies suggest that either large doses of antigen or more persistent antigen presentation are needed to mount longer lasting salivary responses to central immunization. Several groups have examined the potential of biodegradable microparticles containing antigen to induce longer lasting secretory antibody responses using saliva as the mucosal model (Eldridge *et al.*, 1991; O'Hagan *et al.*, 1991; Challacombe *et al.*, 1992). These studies suggest that intragastric immunization with antigen incorporated in biodegradable particles not only gives rise to enhanced salivary antibodies, but also induces serum IgG, IgA, and IgM responses. Thus, oral immunization of this type would seem to lead to antibodies in serum and saliva as well as in other secretions and to have great potential in the development of vaccines against mucosal pathogens.

B. Major and Minor Salivary Glands

Salivary gland lymphoid tissue, particularly that surrounding minor salivary glands (DALT), is thought to play a role in local production to secretory antibody (Nair and Schroeder, 1986). Minor salivary glands contribute only about 10% to the total volume of saliva (Dawes and Wood, 1973) but, since the secretory IgA content is much greater than in the main salivary glands (Crawford *et al.*, 1975), the contribution to the total salivary IgA could be as great as 25%. Bacteria have been observed in DALT (Nair and Schroeder, 1986) and direct access of antigens in the oral cavity to lymphoid aggregates may occur via the short ducts of the minor salivary glands.

C. Mechanisms of Action of Salivary IgA

SIgA does not rely on opsonization or complement fixation for its biological activity since neither complement components nor phagocytes normally are found in abundance in secretions such as saliva. The main actions of SIgA in saliva are thought to be:

1. virus neutralization (e.g., polio virus)
2. neutralization of toxins or enzymes (e.g., streptococcal glucosyltransferase); note that the interaction of SIgA antibody and enzymes may, on occasion, lead to enhanced rather than inhibited enzyme activity (Russell and Challacombe, 1976)
3. inhibition of adherence (or growth) of microorganisms on epithelial cells or on teeth
4. antigen trapping and antigen exclusion by preventing the access of antigen to the systemic immune system; antigens are removed from the oral cavity by swallowing of saliva and mucins
5. interaction of IgA with nonspecific defense mechanisms

1. Salivary IgA and Mucin

Secretory IgA will bind to mucins through cysteine residues. Salivary IgA can be found in a complex of very high molecular weight that has agglutinin activity and presumably reflects an IgA–mucin complex. In the intestinal mucosa, *in vivo* challenge of orally immunized rats has been shown to lead to intestinal goblet cell release of mucins. In addition, antigen–antibody complexes or IgE–mast cell reactions can lead to the release of mucins, which may contribute to inhibition of adherence of bacteria or viruses and to immune exclusions of antigens and of toxic substances. Although no such release of mucins by antigen complexes has been demonstrated within the oral cavity, the association of salivary IgA and mucins and the observation that salivary glycoproteins may inhibit the adherence of bacteria strongly suggest that a similar mechanism is operative (Biesbrock *et al.*, 1991).

2. Salivary IgA and Lactoferrin

Lactoferrin is an iron binding protein that has bacteriostatic activity. This activity can be enhanced or, under some circumstances, reduced by SIgA antibodies. Experiments have used purified colostral IgA; investigators assume that IgA from saliva acts in a similar manner. Presumably, when enhancement of lactoferrin activity is found, the synthesis of iron binding proteins (or their release) is prevented by the antibodies and, as a result, the lactoferrin binds the iron that is required as a growth factor for the bacteria.

3. Salivary IgA and Lysozyme

Purified SIgA from colostrum has been shown to inhibit *Escherichia coli* in the presence of complement and lysozyme, whereas either component on its own was ineffective (Hill and Porter, 1974). These observations suggest that a similar mechanism might be operative within the oral cavity, although the concentrations of complement in whole saliva would seem too small for this to be a major defense mechanism unless inflammation is present. Also, salivary mucins may inhibit lysozyme activity; thus, the effectiveness of lysozyme as an antibacterial mechanism in the oral cavity is in some doubt.

4. Salivary IgA and Lactoperoxidase

Salivary IgA can enhance the antimicrobial effect of lactoperoxidase (LPO; Crawford *et al.*, 1975). Interestingly, either IgA1 or IgA2 is effective but serum IgG of IgM has no effect, suggesting a specific relationship between IgA and LPO that might be of great importance at mucosal surfaces.

D. Gingival Crevicular Fluid

Components of blood can reach the tooth surface through the junctional epithelium of the gingiva and is referred to subsequently as the crevicular fluid. This fluid contains both the humoral and cellular elements of blood, although in lower amounts and in different proportions (Shillitoe and Lehner,

1972). Much of the flow is likely to be secondary to the local inflammation in response to bacterial plaque that accumulates continuously, even within minutes of its removal, and causes a physiological inflammatory response in the gingiva. Even in subjects with no clinically detectable inflammation, a crevicular fluid flow rate of about 1–2 μl per tooth per hour has been calculated (Challacombe, 1980b). Crevicular flow increases greatly with the inflammatory changes caused by gingivitis and periodontitis. The total surface area of crevicular epithelium around 28 teeth is approximately 760 mm^2 and can increase 10-fold with periodontal disease.

Many experiments have shown that both humoral (e.g., immunoglobulins) and cellular (e.g., lymphocytes and macrophages) components from blood can reach the tooth surface (Challacombe *et al.,* 1978). The immunological reactions of blood are, therefore, directly relevant to those found in crevicular fluid and may affect the health of the tooth and gingiva, and perhaps other mucosa. Crevicular fluid passes from the gingival crevice into the mouth, where it is mixed with saliva from the major and minor glands at a dilution of 1:500 to 1:1000. Thus, in addition to salivary IgA derived from the major and minor salivary glands, IgG derived from serum via crevicular fluid also could play a role in defense at mucosal surfaces.

II. ORAL MUCOSAL DISEASES

A. Recurrent Aphthous Stomatitis

1. Characterization

Recurrent aphthous stomatitis (RAS; or recurrent oral ulceration, ROU) is one of the most common oral mucosal diseases and is characterized by oral ulcers, occurring singly or in crops, that usually persist for 7–21 days before healing spontaneously. These ulcers recur after a variable period of time, which may be a few days or several weeks. RAS can be separated clinically into three types: minor aphthous ulcers (MiAU), major aphthous ulcers (MjAU; Figure 1), and herpetiform ulcers (HU; Table I). Clinicians have shown a tendency to describe any ulcer occurring in the mouth as aphthous. However, aphthous ulcers have been defined carefully to allow differentiation from the many other types of ulcers occurring in the oral cavity (Table II) (Challacombe and Shirlaw, 1991).

The prevalence of RAS is on the order of 10% of the population, with a wide range reported in the literature. The peak age of onset of MiAU is in the second decade of life, MjAU in the first decade of life, and HU in the third decade

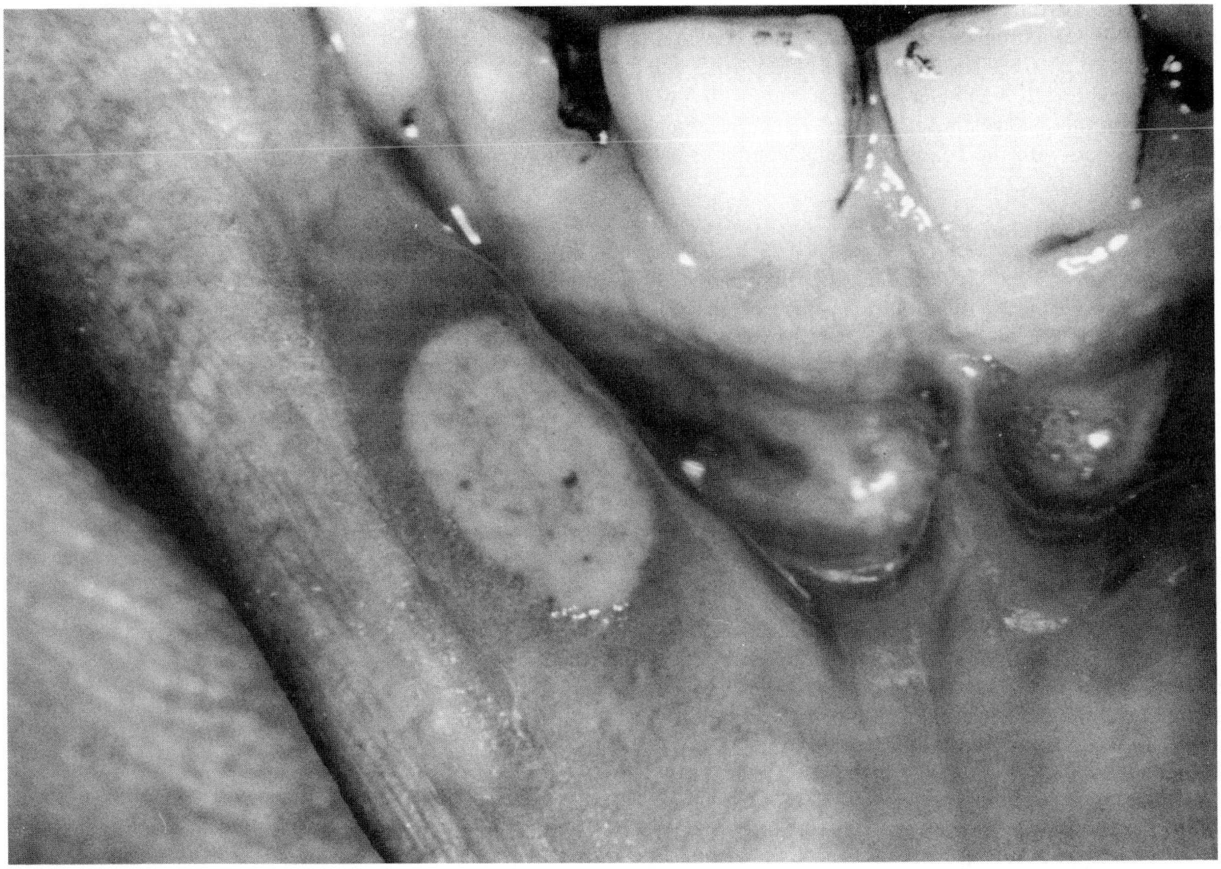

Figure 1 Major aphthous ulcer showing periulcer erythema.

Table I Characteristics of Recurrent Aphthae

	Size	Shape	Color	Duration	Site	Ulcers/crop	Age of onset
Major	>0.5 cm	irregular/oval	gray base with indurated edges that may resemble a carcinoma	2/52–3/12; heal with scarring	most oral mucosa, but particularly fauces and soft palate	1–0	5–20 years
Herpetiform	0.5–3 mm	round/may coalesce to form irregular shape	yellow with marked periulcer erythema	1/52–2/52; heal without scarring	nonkeratinized oral mucosa, but particularly ventral surface of tongue, anterior labial sulci, and soft palate	5–20	20–35 years
Minor	2–7.5 mm	oval	yellow/gray base with thin erythematous border	1/52–2/52; heal without scarring	most nonkeratinizing oral mucosa, but particularly labial and buccal mucosa	1–5	5–45 years

of life. Thus some 85% of patients have developed RAS in the first three decades of life.

2. Genetic Aspects

A family history of ulcers is found in approximately 40% of patients. The highest incidence is found in sibling offspring of parents both of whom have RAS (Ship, 1965). Identical twins show a 90% concordance, implicating a genetic component (Miller *et al.*, 1977). The prevalence of HLA-A2 and B12 (B44) was shown to be higher in 100 patients with RAS than in 100 controls, suggesting that Class I gene products may be associated with the condition (Challacombe *et al.*, 1977b).

3. Etiology of Aphthous Ulceration

An impressive array of factors has been implicated as potentially causative in RAS, although many factors are likely to influence the nature of the disease rather than cause it (Table III). These factors include hereditary factors, hypersensitivity predisposition, socioeconomic status, psychological factors, endocrine factors, microbial agents, and chemical factors in foods (Wilson, 1980). No evidence exists that food allergy is causative in the majority of cases of aphthous ulceration although food allergy or intolerance is likely to initiate some cases of oral ulceration. Whether these cases can be distinguished clinically from the majority of cases of RAS is not clear.

Hematological deficiencies (Wray *et al.*, 1975; Challacombe 1977a); may not only cause some types of oral ulceration but also may influence susceptibility to other types of ulceration. In addition, lesions clinically consistent with RAS are found in association with some systemic or multisystem illnesses such as Behcet's syndrome, clinical neutropenia, vitamin B_{12} deficiency, and celiac disease.

Little evidence exists to support a viral etiology for RAS. Typical RAS lesions fail to show any significant relationship to herpes virus on the basis of histopathology, culture, or serological investigations (Lehner, 1978). However, deoxyribonucleic acid (DNA) hybridization experiments have indicated some homology between DNA of herpes type 1 virus and the DNA in mitogen-transformed lymphocytes from some cases of Behcet's syndrome and MiAU (Eglin *et al.*, 1982). Adenovirus has been identified in some aphthous lesions by immunofluorescence techniques, but no causative role has been determined (Sallay *et al.*, 1973).

4. Theory of Pathogenesis of RAS

Although no definitive infective microorganism has been identified, a currently accepted hypothesis for the etiology of RAS is that patients are exposed to an unidentified infective agent that, in susceptible patients, triggers an autoimmune response against oral mucosa (Donatsky, 1976). Therefore, the agent either is in or cross-reacts with oral mucosa in these patients. Autoantibodies, cytotoxic lymphocytes, and circulating sensitized lymphocytes to oral mucosa can be demonstrated in RAS patients (Lehner, 1978). In the majority of RAS patients, anti-epithelial antibodies that are cytotoxic to oral epithelial cells can be found (Thomas *et al.*, 1990).

5. Behcet's Syndrome

ROU, genital ulcers, and uveitis are the major features of Behcet's syndrome (BS; Behcet, 1937). Cutaneous, vascular, arthritic, neurological, and gastrointestinal manifestations may occur also (Lehner and Barnes, 1979). BS is an uncommon condition in the United Kingdom and the United States but is probably underdiagnosed. A high prevalence has been reported in Japan and in Eastern Mediterranean countries. Patients may suffer a variety of manifestations and, since only some may have the classical triad of ROU, genital ulcers, and iridocyclitis, involvement of a minimum of two of the major sites is sufficient for diagnosis. BS can be separated on clinical and prognostic bases into four types (Lehner and Barnes, 1979):

1. mucocutaneous type, in which the mouth, genitals, skin, and conjunctiva may be involved

Table II Classification of Oral Ulcers Related to Cause

Recurrent ulceration
Recurrent aphthous ulcers
Minor
Major
Herpetiform
Recurrent aphthous ulcers associated with Behcet's disease
Smoking-related aphthous ulcers
Atypical recurrent oral ulceration
Recurrent erythema multiforme
Recurrent/persistent oral ulceration
Secondary to haematological deficiency state/anemia
B_{12}/Folate/Iron
Secondary to a gastrointestinal enteropathy
Ulcerative colitis
Crohn's disease
Celiac disease
Secondary to a dermatological condition
Benign mucous membrane/bullous pemphigoid
Pemphigus
Erosive lichen planus
Dermatitis herpetiformis and linear IgA disease
Secondary to connective tissue disease
Systemic/discoid lupus erythematosus
Oral ulcers as part of Reiter's syndrome
Single episode of ulceration
Infective
Viral (may also be recurrent)
Syphilitic
Tuberculous
Traumatic
Physical/mechanical
Chemical
Drug reaction
Single persistent ulcer
Neoplastic

2. arthritic type, in which one or more of the large joints is involved in addition to one or more of the mucocutaneous manifestations
3. neurological type, in which neurological involvement exists without ocular lesions
4. ocular type, which shows ocular involvement in addition to any of the mucocutaneous or arthritic features; of those with neurological manifestations, 92% show ocular involvement

Behcet (1937) proposed a viral etiology, but attempts to isolate viruses have been largely unsuccessful. However, several studies using DNA hybridization again have suggested a viral involvement (Denman *et al.*, 1986). Histopathological examination shows an early intense mononuclear cell infiltration, prominent vascular lesions, endarteritis obliterans, fibrinoid necrosis, and thromboses. The basic underlying histopathological lesion, therefore, is consistent with a vasculitis (Chajek and Fainaru, 1975).

6. Immunological Findings

No obvious association with classical autoimmune diseases has been demonstrated. Cellular immunity and hemagglutinating antibodies to fetal oral mucosa homogenates can be found in the majority of patients (Lehner, 1978). Antibodies against polymorphonuclear leukocytes and increased leukocyte chemotaxis (Matsumura and Mizushima, 1975) have been reported as well. Serum C9 levels may be increased (Adinolfi and Lehner, 1976) and C3 and C4 levels may be depressed before an attack of uveitis (Shimada *et al.*, 1974). Since C2 is reduced also, the classical pathway of complement may be activated. Immune complexes have been detected in the serum of 60% of patients, especially in those with the active form of neuroocular and arthritic types of BS (Williams and Lehner, 1977).

The abnormalities in the complement components and the clinical manifestations of uveitis, arthritis, and erythema nodosum suggest that such immune complexes may play a role in the pathogenesis of BS. The size and nature of the immune complexes may differ in the different types of BS. Recently an association between antibodies to a bacterial 65 kDa heat shock protein and Behcet's syndrome has been described (Lehner *et al.*, 1991).

BS has a well-established association with the major histocompatibility complex (MHC). The Class I gene product HLA-B51 (B5) is raised in all ethnic groups with BS studied to date (Spitler *et al.*, 1974; Lehner *et al.*, 1982). The Class II products DRw52 and DR7 also have raised prevalences, although this might be because of linkage disequilibrium with the Class I genes (Sun *et al.*, 1991).

B. Lichen Planus

Lichen planus is a common and distinctive mucocutaneous disease that usually presents in the mouth as bilateral symmetrical white patches or striae on the mucosa, but may present as a bullous, ulcerative, or erosive condition, or even as desquamation of the gingivae. The most common form is a reticular pattern with a network of white striae, principally on the buccal mucosa (Wickham's striae: Figure 2). The lesions sometimes appear as white plaques on mucosa or

Table III Etiological Factors in Recurrent Aphthous Stomatitis

Immunological
Hematological
L forms of bacteria
Mycoplasma
Viruses
Trauma
Food allergy
Hormones

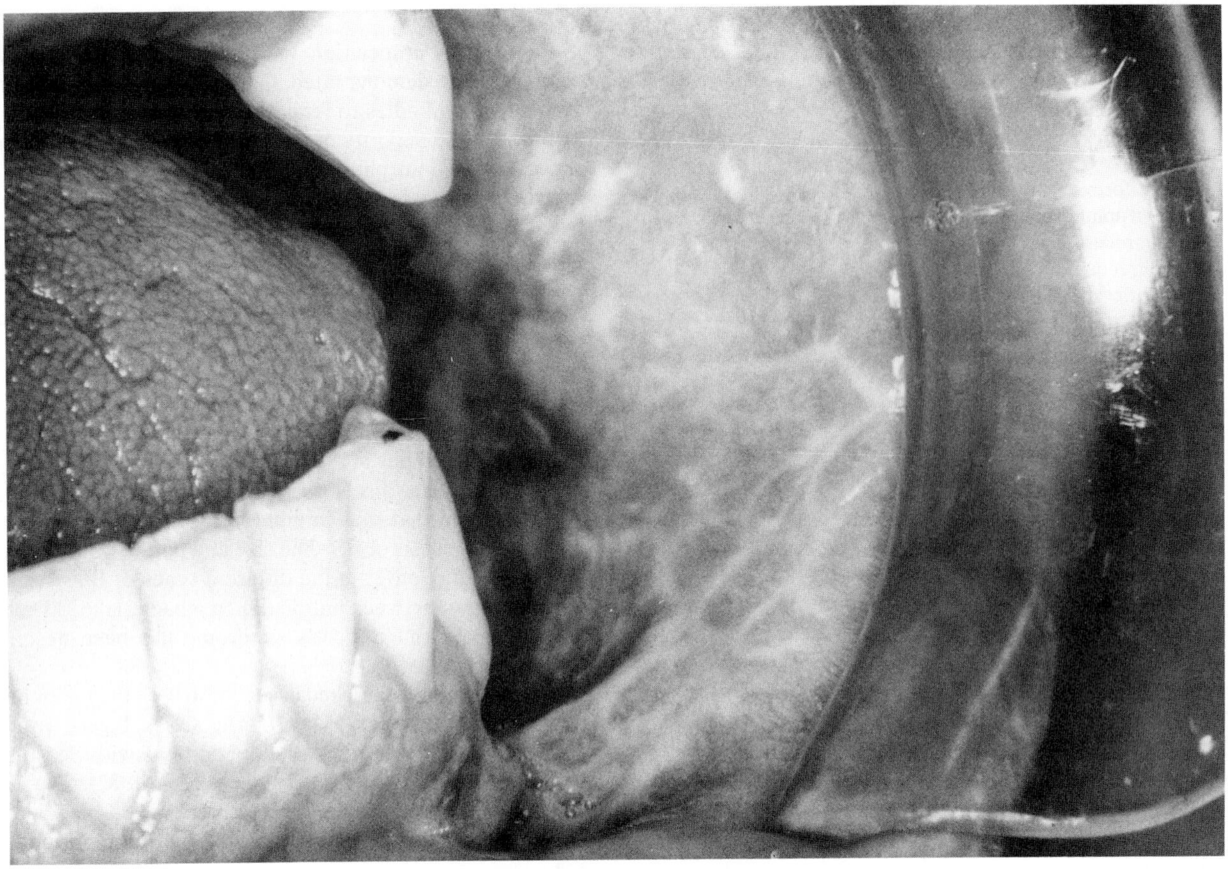

Figure 2 Classical reticular white striae in the buccal mucosa in lichen planus. Note also the erosive lesions medially in the buccal mucosa.

tongue, but often are associated with radiating peripheral white striae. Desquamative gingivitis is essentially an atrophic form of lichen planus. About 10% of patients presenting with oral lesions have cutaneous manifestations that appear as a papular rash, predominantly affecting the flexor surfaces of the arms. This condition is common and has a peak incidence in middle age. The lesions of the mucosa may persist for several years.

Lichenoid drug eruptions, which closely resemble lichen planus, can be precipitated by a number of drugs including methyl-DOPA, β blockers, and nonsteroidal anti-inflammatories and some antimalarials. Clinically, the lesions are often asymmetrical and histologically they may have a greater plasma cell or eosinophilic component, but distinguishing between true lichen planus and such lichenoid reactions often has been difficult.

1. Histopathological Features

Histologically, lichen planus is characterized by a dense, often band-like connective tissue infiltrate of lymphocytes that hugs the epithelium. This tissue formation is associated with widening of the basement membrane zone and loss of the basal cell layer, a phenomenon referred to as liquefaction degeneration. Also hyperparakeratosis, acanthosis, and, classically, a saw-tooth configuration of the rete pegs occur. In the lower epithelial layers, circular eosinophilic Civatte bodies, which are probably degenerating epithelial cells, may be found. Alternating with acanthosis, epithelial atrophy may be found and, in some cases, is the predominant feature (Barnett, 1976).

2. Immunological Findings

Little evidence suggests that lichen planus is a classical autoimmune disease, but the finding of an intense lymphocytic infiltrate in addition to degeneration of the basal cell layer clearly suggests that immunological mechanisms may be of major importance in the pathogenesis. An early increase in the number of Langerhans cells in the epithelium (Ragaz and Ackerman, 1981) suggests that these cells may be functioning as antigen-presenting cells interacting with the lymphocytes. Contact between the Langerhans cells and mononuclear cells in lichen planus has been reported (Medenica and Lorincz, 1977). The antigen that might be responsible is unknown, but some studies have reported a lichen planus-specific epidermal antigen in the granular and deep-prickle epithelial cells in cutaneous lichen planus (Olson *et al.*, 1983).

Another early change in lichen planus is the expression of HLA-DR by keratinocytes. This expression by keratinocytes also provides a possible mechanism by which epithelium-associated antigen could be presented to the lymphocytic infiltrate. However, this expression of HLA-DR by keratinocytes might be secondary to inflammation and switched on by interferon γ (IFNγ) produced by infiltrating lymphocytes rather than being a primary event.

The lymphocytic infiltrate is almost entirely composed of T cells (Dockrell and Greenspan, 1979). These T cells in the infiltrate are Ia antigen positive, suggesting they are activated T lymphocytes (DePanfilis *et al.*, 1983). The phenotype of the lymphocytes in established oral lichen planus appears to be predominantly $CD8^+$ or suppressor cytotoxic (Matthews *et al.*, 1984), although early lichen planus lymphocytes may be mainly $CD4^+$. Predominantly helper–inducer $CD4^+$ T cells have been reported in cutaneous lesions (Bhan *et al.*, 1981). An antigen in the epithelium, possibly associated with local virus infection or induced by drugs, may be presented to lymphocytes in the connective tissue by Langerhans cells migrating from the epithelium. Reacting helper–inducer T cells then lead to the accumulation and retention of cytotoxic T cells that effect the keratinocyte damage. HLA-DR expression by keratinocytes is induced by IFNγ and allows the keratinocytes to become involved in the persistence of the lesion by further presentation of antigen.

C. Oral Candida Infections

Species of *Candida* can be found in the mouths of some 40% of normal subjects in amounts up to approximately 800 per ml. However, in patients with the various forms of candidiasis, these amounts are increased greatly; counts of more than 10^4 may be found. A classification of *Candida* infections is shown in Table IV.

1. Acute pseudomembranous candidiasis (thrush) is a common infection in the young, elderly, or debilitated. The white plaques are easily removable and contain candidal hyphae, spores, epithelial cells, and polymorphs.
2. Acute atrophic candidiasis also is known as antibiotic sore mouth because it frequently occurs during antibiotic therapy. This condition is a response to the suppression of the normal bacterial flora and is characterized by widespread erythematous stomatitis with accompanying depapillation of the tongue.
3. Chronic atrophic candidiasis (Figure 3A) also is known as denture sore mouth and presents as a relatively asymptomatic confluent erythema and inflammation of the entire denture-bearing mucosa of the palate. This condition results from candidal colonization of the surface of the denture, usually in patients who wear their prosthesis continuously day and night.
4. Chronic hyperplastic candidiasis (candidal leukoplakia; Figure 3B) is a speckled or nodular chronic leukoplakia usually found in middle-aged or elderly patients. This invasive form of candidiasis shows hyphae present often throughout the depth of the epithelium, and carries a significant risk of malignant transformation.

Infection with *Candida albicans* is an almost universal finding in patients with severe immunodeficiency of the T-cell type. However, this condition is not seen in patients with B-cell defects in the absence of concomitant T-cell defects. *Candida* infections are found in about 40% of human immunodeficiency virus (HIV)-infected individuals and in over 75% of patients who suffer from acquired immunodeficiency syndrome (AIDS). Acute pseudomembranous candidiasis is found particularly in association with low CD4 counts, but a newly recognized entity, erythematous candidiasis, is found often. This condition presents as areas of erythema, usually of the palate or tongue, in the absence of white plaques (Challacombe, 1991).

Theoretically, IgA and cellular immunity might be expected to play a role in the protection of mucosal surfaces against candidal infections. Certainly in IgA-deficient individuals, a markedly increased prevalence of *Candida* infection is apparent. Animal studies using the rhesus monkey have emphasized the role of cellular immunity in chronic *Candida* infections (Budtz-Jorgensen, 1973). In this model, azathioprine-treated monkeys showed a depression of cellular immunity to *Candida* but a normal humoral antibody response. These animals had a prolonged and severe *Candida* infection, suggesting that cellular immunity to *Candida,* not serum antibody titer, is of primary importance in host resistance. *Candida* infection is not a noted feature of selected IgA deficiency although, in patients with chronic mucocutaneous candidiasis, over 50% appear to have reduced salivary IgA antibodies (Lehner *et al.*, 1972). Although serum IgG antibodies against *Candida* can be detected readily in humans, serodiagnosis of candidal infections is inconsistent.

In chronic mucocutaneous candidiasis (CMCC), a wide spectrum of immune abnormalities has been reported that ranges from lowered serum IgM and IgG antibodies to defects

Table IV Classification of Oral Candidiasis

Acute	Acute/chronic	Chronic
Pseudomembranous candidiasis Thrush	Erythematous candidiasis (HIV associated)	Hyperplastic candidiasis Candidal leukoplakia Median rhomboid glossitis
Atrophic candidiasis Antibiotic sore mouth	Angular cheilitis Mucocutaneous candidiasis	Atrophic candidiasis Denture induced stomatitis (Denture sore mouth)

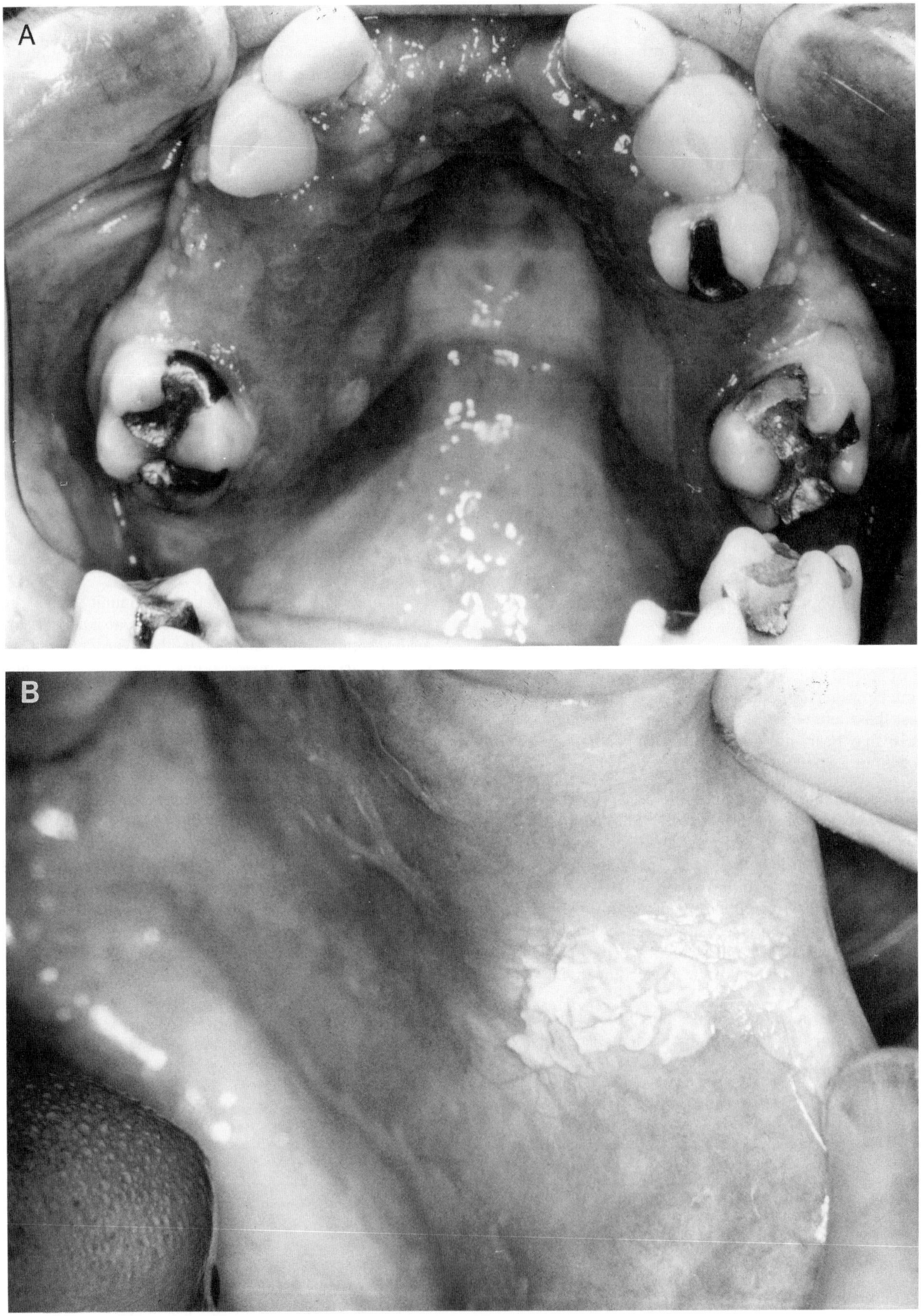

Figure 3 (A) Chronic atrophic candidiasis (denture-induced stomatitis) with marked erythema of palate corresponding to the denture outline. (B) Adherent nodular white patch at angle of mouth—histologically hyperplastic candidiasis.

in lymphocyte transformation and mitogen stimulation in the most severe types of CMCC (Lehner *et al.*, 1972). However, whether these immune defects are primary to the disease or a consequence of it is not clear. Several studies have shown restoration of immune functions once *Candida* has been cleared by antifungal therapy (Valdimarrson *et al.*, 1973).

D. Immunology of Dental Caries

Dental caries is one of the most prevalent diseases of humans. Despite reductions in the rate of decay in Western societies, the prevalence of caries in developed countries remains at greater than 95% of the population. Caries is still increasing in the developing countries. Thus, for practical purposes, the condition can be considered ubiquitous in developed countries. The cost of treatment of dental disease is probably the highest among bacterial infections and also results in considerable loss of time and productivity.

Dental caries may be defined as the localized destruction of tooth tissue by bacterial action. Dissolution of the hydroxyapatite crystals seems to precede the loss of organic components of both enamel and dentine. Demineralization is thought to be caused by acids resulting from the bacterial fermentation of dietary carbohydrates. Not all surfaces of the tooth are afflicted equally; areas that are protected from cleansing, for example, the fissures and areas between the teeth, are much more susceptible to decay.

1. Immunity to Caries

The concept of immunity to caries depends on the demonstration that caries is a bacterial infection. Although vaccination against dental caries was attempted in the 1930s, the real impetus for development of vaccination came with the demonstration, using germ-free animals, that caries could not occur in the absence of bacteria regardless of diet and that specific bacteria were needed.

The tooth sits in a unique position between the secretory and systemic immune systems. The majority of the tooth surface would seem to be accessible to saliva, although the most caries-susceptible sites around the gingival margin and between the teeth are bathed in crevicular fluid (Figure 4). (Shillitoe and Lehner, 1972). Antibodies in crevicular fluid are derived largely from serum, although the local contribution, particularly of IgG, is up to ∓20% of the total antibody content (Brandtzaeg, 1972).

Both serum and secretory systems have been examined for natural immunity in humans, and for the protective effects in vaccination experiments in animal models. Induction of antibodies in both immune systems might be necessary to achieve effective protection by immunological methods.

2. Causative Bacteria

Streptococci, lactobacilli, and *Actinomyces* species all have been shown to be able to cause caries in animal models. In humans, by far the strongest association is with *Streptococcus mutans*. This organism can produce copious amounts of extra polysaccharide from sucrose, much of which is insoluble in water (or saliva). *Streptococcus mutans* is also very

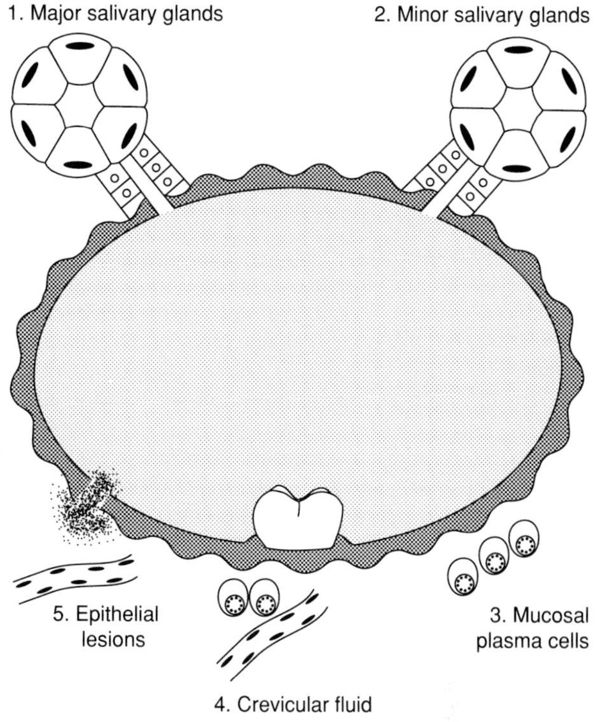

Figure 4 Source of immunoglobulins bathing the teeth. Modified from Lehner, T. (1992). Immunology of Oral Diseases, 3rd ed. p. 12. Blackwell Scientific Publications, Oxford.

to date, including rats, hamsters, monkeys, and gerbils.

In the absence of detectable caries, the number of *S. mutans* in plaque is very low, but in carious lesions the numbers are raised substantially in nearly all subjects (Huis in't Veld *et al.*, 1979). However, some lesions apparently can develop in the absence of *S. mutans*, particularly in fissures. In addition, large numbers of *S. mutans* in plaque do not necessarily lead to the initiation of caries.

3. Natural Immunity to Caries in Humans

The question of natural immunity requires the comparison of subjects with low caries experience with those with high caries experience in the absence of carious lesions. Several studies have compared low caries with rampant caries, but these studies confuse the question of natural immunity with that of an immune response to the caries process.

Subjects with low caries experience have significantly raised serum IgG antibody titers against whole cells of *S. mutans* compared with subjects with high caries experience (Figure 5; Challacombe and Lehner, 1976). This relationship seems to be specific to *S. mutans* and has not been found with strains of *Streptococcus sanguis, Streptococcus salivarius, Lactobacillus casei, Lactobacillus acidophilus,* or *Actinomyces viscosus* (Challacombe and Lehner, 1976). Serum IgG antibodies against the surface protein antigen I/II also are raised in subjects with low caries experience (Challacombe *et al.*, 1984). This protein has been used in immunization experiments in animals; inhibition studies indicate that antigen I/II is a major antigenic component of the *S. mutans* cell wall. (Czerkinsky *et al.*, 1983). IgG antibodies against antigen

I/II are mainly of the IgG1 subclass, whereas those against whole cells of *S. mutans* are mainly IgG1 and IgG2 (Challacombe *et al.*, 1986). These studies are consistent with the interpretation that serum IgG antibody contributes to protection against caries in humans.

4. Immune Responses That Follow Dental Caries

Raised serum IgG antibody titers against *S. mutans* are found in subjects with carious lesions (Figure 5) compared with those without. This raised antibody titer seems to be specific to *S. mutans,* thus further implicating this bacterium in the pathogenesis of caries (Challacombe and Lehner, 1976; Challacombe, 1980). These findings are consistent with the view that infection with *S. mutans* and the development of carious lesions is associated with a rise in specific antibodies against *S. mutans,* as was confirmed in longitudial studies (Challacombe, 1980), and are similar to findings in most infective diseases in which a rise in antibodies after infection is common.

Salivary antibody levels appear to be more variable than serum antibodies. The secretion rate of antibodies has been considered in few studies, although the great variation in salivary secretion rates is well known. No consistent patterns have emerged; raised levels of salivary IgA antibodies against *S. mutans* have not been found in subjects with low caries experience, and may reflect cumulative caries experience rather than protection (Challacombe and Lehner, 1976).

5. Genetic Factors

Genetic factors long have been thought to play a role in caries resistance. Evidence has been found of genetically related immune factors in association with caries. In a study of caries-prone and low caries subjects using streptococcal antigen I/II, specific helper factor was found to be released optimally by a dosage between 1 and 10 ng antigen I/II from lymphocytes of low caries subjects, but the optimal dosage for caries-prone subjects was 1000 ng (Lehner, 1982). This marked difference in responses supports the suggestion that caries-resistant and caries-prone subjects differ in their ability to mount and maintain serum antibody responses to *S. mutans*. The response to antigenic stimulation using antigen I/II was related to the HLA status of the subjects (Figure 6). HLA-DRw6-positive subjects generally showed an optimal response at a low dose, whereas subjects who showed an optimal response at the high antigen dose were found to be HLA-DRw6 negative. These findings suggest that the ability to respond to very small amounts of streptococcal antigen may be the reason for the high levels of antibody against *S. mutans* in low-caries subjects. However, the immunoregulation of such responses is complex, and this area requires further study.

6. Immunization against Dental Caries

Theoretically, local or systemic immunization might lead to protection against dental caries. With respect to local immunization, the rat has been used extensively as a model. Several groups have shown that the induction of salivary antibodies may be related to a reduction in caries (Smith *et al.*, 1979; McGhee and Michalek, 1981). Salivary IgA antibodies in humans may be induced by ingestion of capsules filled with *S. mutans* organisms (Mestecky *et al.*, 1978). No extended studies have been performed to see the effect of such antibody on caries. At present, longterm immunization seems

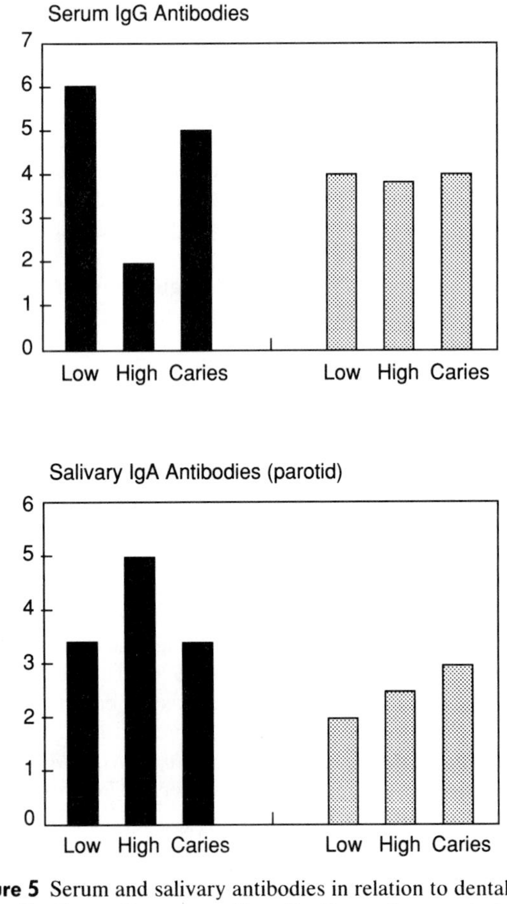

Figure 5 Serum and salivary antibodies in relation to dental caries. ■, antibodies to *S. mutans;* □, antibodies to *S. sanguis;* low, low DMF group; high, high DMF group; caries, group with carious lesions.

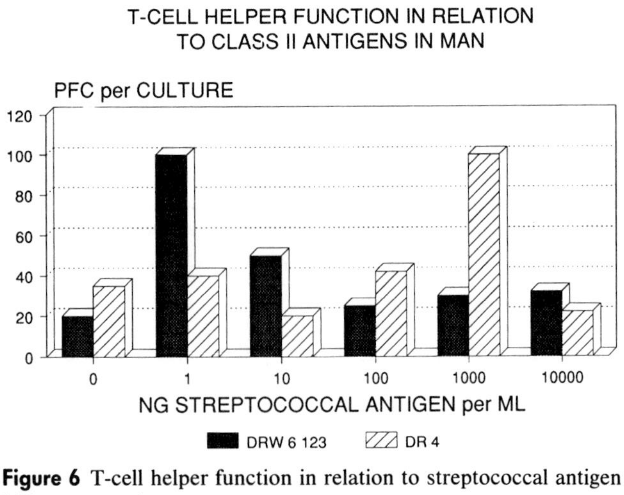

Figure 6 T-cell helper function in relation to streptococcal antigen I/II concentration.

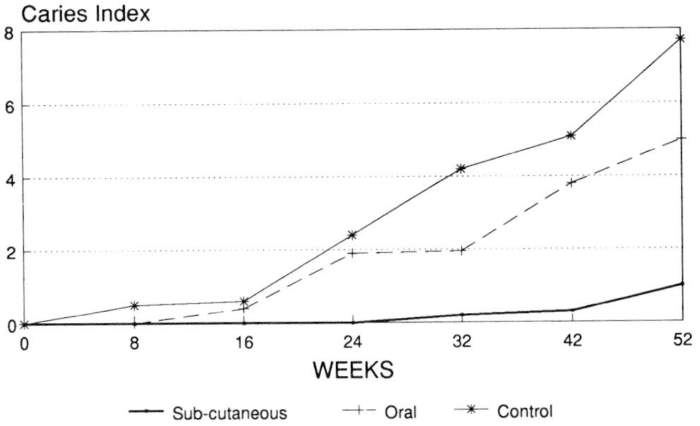

Figure 7 Reduction in caries by immunization with *Streptococcus mutans* antigens. Weeks 0–24 oral immunization; subcutaneous immunization at week 0.

to be necessary since the salivary antibody response is short lived. Salivary antibodies may prove to be effective since a reduction in *S. mutans* numbers has been reported in such immunized subjects (Cole *et al.*, 1984).

Successful systemic immunization against dental caries in monkeys was reported first in 1969. Since then, Lehner and colleagues (1976,1980) have described many experiments in the rhesus monkey model, and have demonstrated unequivocally that caries can be reduced by immunization. In early experiments, animals were immunized subcutaneously with whole cells of *S. mutans* in Freund's incomplete adjuvant; reduction in caries on the order of 75–80% was seen. Antibodies were detected in both serum and saliva, but the reduction in caries correlated best with serum antibodies against *S. mutans*. Passive transfer experiments in the monkey (Lehner *et al.*, 1978) have confirmed that serum IgG antibodies may be effective in reducing caries.

Subsequently, purified antigens from *S. mutans* also have been shown to be effective in reducing caries in the monkey (Figure 7). These antigens include glucosyltransferase and antigen I/II (Lehner *et al.*, 1980), as well as other protein antigens. Immunization with antigen I/II elicits serum IgG antibodies, skin delayed hypersensitivity, and a reduction of caries equivalent to that seen with immunization with whole cells of *S. mutans* (Lehner *et al.*, 1980). These studies suggest that vacc: tion of humans is a very real possibility.

An additional exciting possibility in caries prevention is passive immunization. Lehner and colleagues have shown that a monoclonal antibody against antigen I/II may inhibit the colonization of *S. mutans* in the oral cavity of humans and monkeys (Ma and Lehner, 1990). Given a suitable delivery system for monoclonal antibodies into humans, this method could be useful in reducing caries, and overcomes some of the objections to systemic therapy.

E. Immunology of Periodontal Diseases

1. Classification

Periodontal diseases can be divided into at least four clinical entities (Table V). Gingivitis is a reversible inflammation of the gingivae and can be considered an inflammatory reaction to the presence of plaque. Plaque contains many bacterial species; currently, the consensus is that gingivitis represents a nonspecific response to bacterial toxins and antigens.

Marked advances have been made in the past two decades in understanding the host responses that play a critical role in determining the course of periodontal infections. These advances have been facilitated greatly by additional knowledge of the microflora associated with different periodontal diseases. *Porphyromonas (Bacteroides) gingivalis* appears to be the major etiological organism associated with adult periodontitis, *Actinobacillus actinomycetemcomitans* is associated with localized juvenile periodontitis, and *Prevotella (Bacteroides) intermedia* and spirochaetes are associated with acute necrotizing ulcerative gingivitis. In addition, *Capnocytophaga* species have been associated with periodontal disease in immunocompromised hosts (Genco and Slots, 1984). Long-term epidemiological studies (Loe *et al.*, 1986) suggest that, even in subjects with gingivitis, only 10–15% eventually develop severe periodontal disease, clearly suggesting a role for host factors in the progression of periodontal diseases.

2. Adult Periodontitis

Not all cases of gingivitis ultimately develop periodontitis (Figure 8), but gingivitis always seems to precede periodontal disease. The hypothesis of four stages in the development of periodontal lesions (Page and Schroeder, 1982) was based primarily on histopathological findings and generally has been accepted (Figure 9).

1. The initial lesion is essentially gingivitis, localized to the gingival sulcus, and is reversible. Histologically, this condition is characterized by a polymorphonuclear leukocyte infiltration in response to plaque. This infiltrate has been shown in experimental gingivitis to develop within 2–4 days of plaque accumulation. Since serum antibodies against a variety of plaque bacteria can be detected (Genco and Slots, 1984), this initial lesion could be caused by activation of complement by the alternative pathway by plaque components or by the classical pathway by antibodies.
2. The early lesion is still essentially reversible and is characterized by a replacement of the polymorphonuclear infiltrate with lymphocytes, which may constitute some 75% of the cellular infiltration. At this stage, few plasma cells are seen. Most of the lymphocytes are T cells, with a small proportion of B cells, depending on the site examined.
3. The established lesion exists 2–3 wk after plaque accumulation. The distinguishing histopathological feature is the predominant plasma cell infiltrate. Many of the B cells seen in the early lesion are assumed to have been transformed by plaque antigens. Most of the plasma cells are IgG isotype. At this stage, the junctional epithelium may extend apically into the connective tissue, with an associated loss of collagen. Pocket formation occurs by a deepening of the gingival sulcus. Circulating systemic lympho-

Table V Classification of Periodontal Diseases[a]

Gingivitis		Periodontal diseases	
Acute	Chronic	Adult periodontitis	Periodontitis with systemic disease
Acute necrotizing gingivitis (ANUG)	Chronic marginal gingivitis	Early onset periodontitis	Down's syndrome, diabetes, cyclical neutropenia, Papillon-Lefevre syndrome, HIV infection
Acute herpetic gingivostomatitis	Plasma cell gingivitis	Prepubertal periodontitis	Necrotizing ulcerative periodontitis
Traumatic gingivitis	Desquamative gingivitis (Dermatoses)	Generalized	Refractory periodontitis
Physical (Toothbrushing)	HIV-associated gingivitis	Localized	
Chemical (Aspirin burn)	Drug-induced gingivitis (e.g., Phenytoin)	Juvenile periodontitis	
Leukemia		Generalized	
		Localized	
		Rapidly progressing periodontis	

[a] Reprinted with permission from the Proceedings of the World Workshop in Clinical Periodontics. Concensus Report, pp. I23–I24. Princeton, New Jersey (1989). American Academy of Periodontology, Chicago, Illinois.

cytes sensitized to plaque bacteria can be detected (Ivanyi and Lehner, 1970).

4. The advanced lesion marks the transition from a chronic established lesion to a destructive state. The host factors responsible for this transition have not been established fully, but evidence suggests that this stage of the disease is specific. *Porphyromonas* (*Bacteroides*) *gingivalis* has been associated strongly with this condition. Undoubtedly, the host immune responses play a critical role also. Histopathological features include pocket formation, ulceration of the pocket epithelium, destruction of the collagenous periodontal ligament, and, significantly, resorption of bone. These features eventually lead to mobility and loss of the teeth. The dense infiltration of plasma cells, lymphocytes, and macrophages now extends apically and is progressive.

3. Mechanisms of Damage in Periodontal Diseases

a. Bacterial invasion. Bacteria have been reported to invade the gingivae in gingivitis, in adult periodontitis (Saglie *et al.*, 1982), in acute ulcerative gingivitis (Listgarten, 1965), and in juvenile periodontitis (Gillett and Johnson, 1982). Bacterial invasion of the periodontal tissues could be an important component of the pathogenesis of periodontal disease, although bacterial toxins or the immune reaction to toxins could account equally for most of the damage seen.

b. Tissue destruction. Extensive studies have been made of the capabilities of periodontopathic bacteria to produce tissue damaging factors. *Porphyromonas gingivalis* shows an impressive ability to produce toxins or enzymes that are active against many substrates, including collagen, epithelial cells, and fibroblasts, and can stimulate bone resorption (Genco and Slots, 1984). No doubt, therefore, these organisms could inhibit most host responses marshalled against them.

c. Healing and fibrosis. An attractive hypothesis for the destructive phase of periodontal disease is that bacterial toxins or the reactions to them inhibit normal healing and repair, and that this inhibition leads to progressive damage to the periodontium (Figure 9). The role of macrophages, for example, in fibrosis and repair, has received little attention although they are important cells in tissue repair. Activated macrophages produce fibroblast activating factors that stimulate the fibroblasts into active proliferation (Wahl and Wahl,

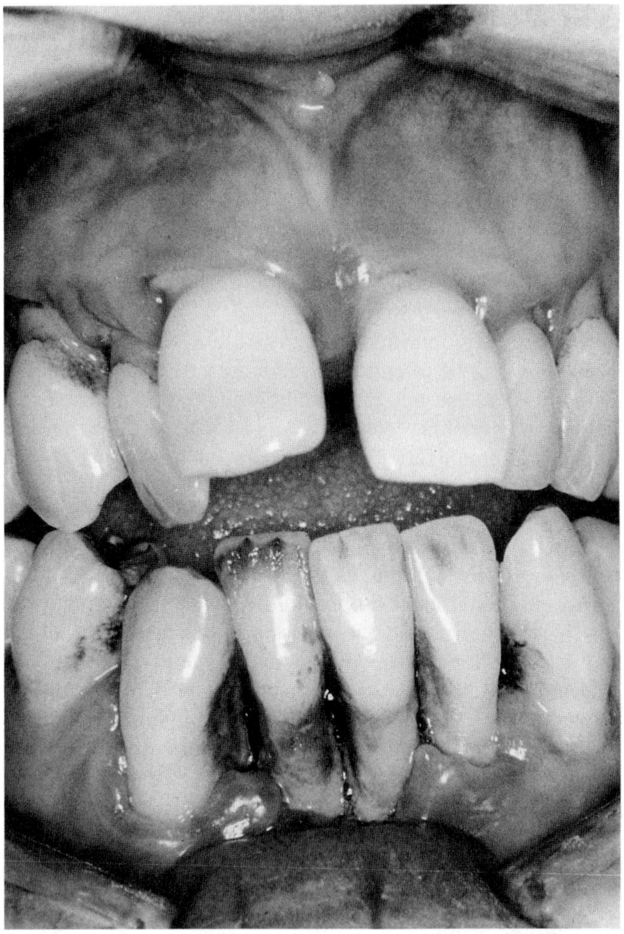

Figure 8 Anterior teeth showing loss of soft tissue attachment and underlying bone, with heavy plaque, and calculus deposits in adult periodontitis.

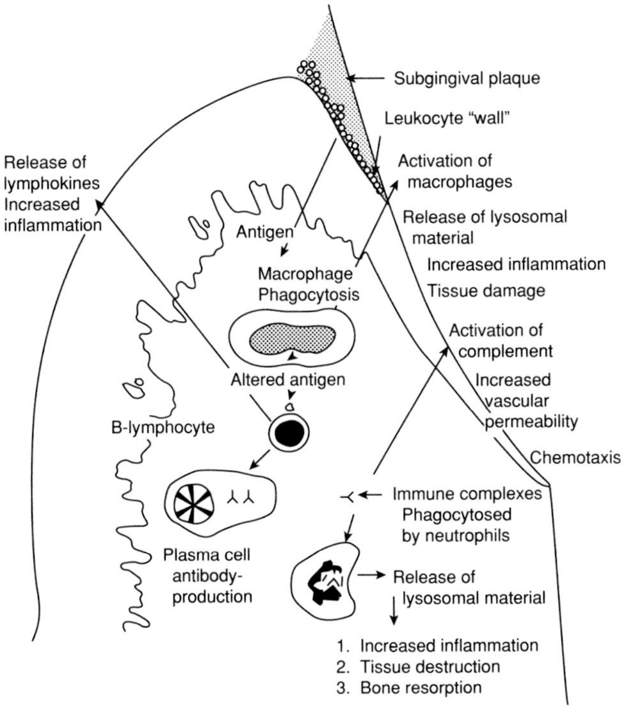

Figure 9 Hypothesis of periodontal aetiology. Reprinted with permission from Linde (1989).

1981). Fibroblast function also is affected by lymphocytes in inflammatory lesions, since the latter produce a chemotactic factor for fibroblasts (Postlethwaite *et al.,* 1976). Macrophages and lymphocytes therefore produce factors that recruit fibroblasts to the area of inflammation, stimulate their proliferation, and, thus, indirectly stimulate collagen production with replacement of lost collagen. Bacterial factors that interfere with this normal repair could have a profound effect on disease activity.

4. Serum Antibodies to Periodontal Bacteria

a. Adult periodontitis. Many studies have examined the presence of antibodies against periodontopathic bacteria in the serum of patients with periodontal disease (Genco and Slots, 1984). Most of these studies have found raised antibodies against *P. gingivalis* in patients with adult periodontitis in comparison with controls (Mouton *et al.,* 1981; Taubman *et al.,* 1982). *Prevotella intermedia* has not been associated immunologically with adult periodontitis, but has been implicated in acute necrotizing gingivitis (Dzink *et al.,* 1985). Overall, the immunological findings confirm bacteriological findings and support the association of *P. gingivalis* with adult periodontitis.

b. Juvenile periodontitis. This disease is associated strongly with the bacterium. *A. actinomycetemcomitans* (Genco and Slots, 1984). In addition, antibodies against *A. actinomycetemcomitans* have been found in all patients with juvenile periodontitis at levels significantly greater than in controls (Genco *et al.,* 1980). This *Actinobacillus* species produces a powerful leukotoxin (Taichman *et al.,* 1982); neutralizing activity against this toxin is present in the serum of patients with juvenile periodontitis (Tsai *et al.,* 1981). An interesting finding in this disease is the demonstration that many patients have depressed neutrophil chemotaxis and phagocytosis. Some 75% of patients with the classical localized disorder appear to suffer from a peripheral blood neutrophil chemotactic abnormality (Cianciola *et al.,* 1977). Neutrophil migration through the gingival crevice appears to be abnormal. These findings suggest a role for neutrophils in normal protection and suggest that, in juvenile periodontitis, this function is depressed, allowing for the overgrowth of organisms, particularly those such as *A. actinomycetemcomitans* that produce leukotoxic factors.

F. Immunology of Salivary Gland Diseases: Sjögren's Syndrome

Sjögren's syndrome (SS) is by far the most common immunologically based disease affecting the salivary glands. This condition is probably the second most prevalent collagen disease after rheumatoid arthritis (RA). SS is a chronic inflammatory disease with involvement of many systems and is characterized by a triad of dry eyes (keratoconjunctivitis sicca), dry mouth (xerostomia), and a connective tissue or collagen disease. The association of dry eyes and dry mouth, in the absence of a connective tissue disease, is known as the sicca syndrome. In secondary SS, the most commonly associated connective tissue disease is RA, but systemic lupus erythematosus, scleroderma, dermatomyositis, polyarteritis, primary biliary cirrhosis, and idiopathic thrombocytopenic purpura may be associated. SS affects females nine times more frequently than males, and is seen especially in the elderly. A dry mouth is the presenting symptom in the majority of patients.

A subdivision of Sjögren's syndrome has been described in which patients suffer from xerostomia and primary generalized nodal osteoarthritis; the salivary glands of these individuals show nonspecific sialadenitis, in contrast to the focal lymphocytic infilatrate of primary Sjögrens syndrome. This condition has been called SOX syndrome (Challacombe *et al.,* 1991). Whether it is a genetically homogeneous group is not clear. Nonspecific chronic sialadenitis in the absence of osteoarthritis is a common cause of xerostomia.

1. Pathogenesis of SS

SS has many of the characteristics of a cell-mediated autoimmune disease. Histopathology shows a mononuclear cell infiltration of the salivary glands, with acinar destruction but sparing of the ducts. The lymphocytes appear to originate from an extrasalivary source. T-cell sensitization to salivary tissue may occur (Berry *et al.,* 1972). Lymphocytes and plasma cells occur in a perivascular distribution and the proportion of T lymphocytes increases as the lesions progress (Talal *et al.,* 1974). Intraductal cell proliferation forms compact epimyoepithelial islands. Patients with primary SS show an increased association with HLA-DwA3 (84%) and HLA-B8 (Chused *et al.,*1977). IgG, IgA, or IgM autoantibodies against ductal cell ribonucleoproteins called SSA(Ro) and SSB(La), which appear to be dimers of 52 and 65 kDa, are found in Sjögrens syndrome but do not appear to be responsible for tissue destruction (Moutsopoulos and Zerva, 1990) and do not correlate with focal lymphocytic sialadenitis. A possible association with Epstein–Barr virus infection has been claimed (Gaston *et al.,* 1990; Syrjanen *et al.,* 1990), Talal *et al.* (1990) have found that sera from many cases of primary Sjögrens syndrome react with the retroviral p24 antigen. The significance of these findings remains to be determined.

Rheumatoid factor occurs in 52–100% of patients, even in the absence of RA, and antinuclear antibody is found in 60% of patients (Beck, 1961). Other autoantibodies, for example, to thyroglobulin gastric parietal cells and mitochondria, are seen often. B cells in some patients bear multiple classes of heavy chains, an abnormally that may be significant since, in a small proportion of patients, SS progresses to lymphoma.

III. ORAL MUCOSAL MANIFESTATIONS OF DISTANT IMMUNOLOGICAL DISEASES

A. Gastrointestinal Diseases

Celiac disease, ulcerative colitis, and Crohn's disease all can appear in the oral cavity. Frequently, the oral cavity can be the presenting site, although Crohn's disease can be limited to the oral cavity. Each of these gastroenteropathies can give rise to oral ulceration.

1. Celiac Disease

Some 25% of patients with celiac disease may give a history of oral ulceration. However, the converse is not true. Studies of the incidence of celiac disease in patients presenting with recurrent aphthous stomatitis found 2–4% on the basis of jejunal biopsy (Ferguson *et al.,* 1980). The oral ulcers of those patients with celiac disease often respond extremely well to correction of underlying hematological deficiencies, particularly folate and iron. The oral ulceration seems to be the result of the associated deficiencies rather than a direct response of the oral mucosa to the allergen. Cooper *et al.* (1980) have described adult female patients suffering from abdominal pain and chronic diarrhea who responded immediately to a gluten-free diet and in whom symptoms returned on gluten challenge. Oral uleration and macroglossia were described in several of these patients, but jejunal biopsies were normal, suggesting that oral signs and symptoms can be associated with gluten in the absence of celiac disease and that such oral symptoms are accompanied by varying abdominal problems.

2. Crohn's Disease

Many cases of oral Crohn's disease have been reported over recent years, with or without accompanying gastrointestinal Crohn's. Crohn's disease in the mouth may present either as thickened rubbery lips and cheeks with deep fissures and enlarged gingiva or as ulcers and epithelial tags in the buccal sulcus (Figure 10). In both these clinical manifestations, biopsy of the affected areas will show granulomata. A number of cases of swollen lips without any intraoral signs have been reported that also have been classified as oral Crohn's by some workers, although the term "cheilitis granulomatosa" would be more appropriate. The role of allergy to food or other substances has not been investigated fully, although some patients have been reported to be sensitive to cinnamon or sodium benzoate.

3. Ulcerative Colitis

Oral ulceration frequently is associated with ulcerative colitis and may be one of at least four types: (1) aphthous, (2) pyostomatitis necrotica, (3) pyostomatitis vegetans, or (4) hemorrhagic. The incidence of oral lesions in patients with ulcerative colitis is approximately 20%. The oral ulcers of groups 2, 3, and 4 are readily distinguishable from the more common types of aphthous ulceration. Unlike Crohn's disease, these lesions do not appear to occur in the oral cavity in the absence of any bowel symptoms.

4. Food Allergy and Oral Disease

Allergies to foods certainly may be manifest in the oral cavity. These sensitivities may present with a variety of oral signs and symptoms, including a perioral rash, swelling of the lips, oral pruritis, fissuring of the tongue, or oral ulceration (Challacombe, 1986). Aphthous ulceration affects approximately 10% of the population but food allergy or intolerance is unlikely to be responsible for more than a very small proportion of total cases, perhaps less than 1%. Overall, oral symptoms are most likely to be found in the atopic patient; in these subjects, allergy to foods should be entertained as a possible diagnosis in the absence of disease elsewhere.

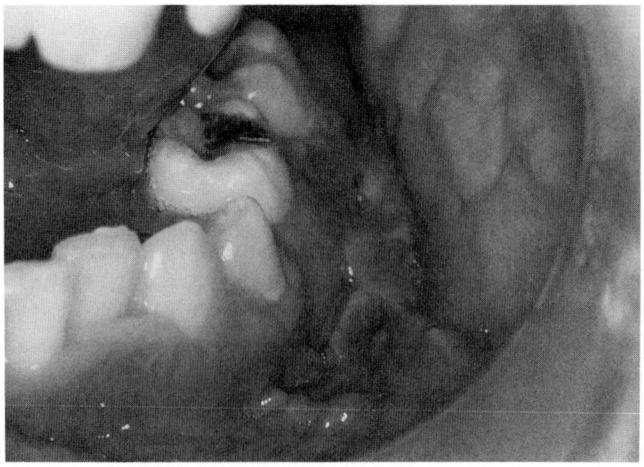

Figure 10 Ulceration in lower buccal sulcus associated with oral Crohn's disease. Note also folded appearance of buccal mucosa.

B. Dermatoses

1. Discoid Lupus Erythematosus

Traditionally, lupus erythematosus is classified into a chronic discoid type (DLE) and a systemic type (SLE). Both types may give rise to lesions within the oral mucosa. The buccal mucosa is involved most frequently and bilateral lesions are common. Classically, the lesions appear as atrophic erythematous areas surrounded by a keratotic border. Sometimes the lesions are more plaque like and may resemble lichen planus or leucoplakias. Skin lesions are found in approximately half the patients. Histologically, the epithelium always shows orthokeratosis and parakeratosis, and areas of moderate epithelial hyperplasia alternate with areas of epithelial atrophy. A rather deeply seated focal or perivascular accumulation of lymphocytes is seen. Although a genetic susceptibility exists in SLE, with an increased frequency of HLA-DR2 and DR3 in Caucasian populations, no such relationship has been established for DLE (Woodrow, 1988).

2. Pemphigus

Pemphigus is a potentially lethal chronic bullous disease of the stratified squamous mucosa and skin, occurring mainly in adults over the age of 60 but sometimes in young adults (Zegarelli and Zegarelli, 1977). This condition commonly affects the oral mucosa and may present orally. Histologically, acantholysis with intraepithelial bulla formation is present. Serum IgG, IgM, or sometimes IgA autoantibodies against intercellular substances of the suprabasilar epithelium of skin and mucosa are found in 95% of cases of pemphigus (Beutner *et al.*, 1968). The autoantibody titer is correlated with the severity of pemphigus, and antibody disappears as the lesions heal (Weissman *et al.*, 1978).

Serum from patients can produce the characteristic histological lesion in organ culture of the skin. Antibody can be demonstrated to be bound to the epidermal cells prior to the onset of acantholysis. Acantholysis may be caused by an autoantibody-induced release of autolytic enzymes from the damaged epithelial cells (Schiltz *et al.*, 1978). Using direct immunofluorescence, IgG antibodies bound to intercellular areas of epithelium in patients with pemphigus can be demonstrated (Beutner *et al.*, 1968). These autoantibodies are, therefore, likely to be the cause of the lesions. HLA associations have been reported, particularly in Jewish and Japanese populations. An increased incidence of HLA-A10 and HLA-DR4 is seen in pemphigus. An interesting finding is the association of pemphigus with an HLA-DQw1B allele (Sinha *et al.*, 1988).

3. Benign Mucous Membrane Pemphigoid

Benign mucous membrane pemphigoid (BMMP; cicatricial or ocular pemphigoid) is a disease giving rise to bullous lesions predominatly involving the mucous membranes rather than the skin. Most cases are detected in the fourth decade; the disease is much more frequent in females than in males (McCarthy, 1972). As in bullous pemphigoid, histopathological examination of the lesion shows subepithelial vesiculation and deposition of IgG, IgA, C_3, and C_4 in the basement membrane area. In contrast to bullous pemphigoid, serum autoantibodies against epithelial basement membrane are detected infrequently and are in low titer (Rogers *et al.*, 1982).

Intraorally, two variants of BMMP are seen. The most common consists of bullous lesions involving much of the nonkeratinized and occasionally the keratinized mucosa. The other type is a form of desquamating gingivitis and involves only the gingivae around the teeth. The gingivae are very erythematous and hyperemic. Small bullae may be formed in protected areas around the teeth.

4. Erythema Multiforme

Erythema multiforme is a mucocutaneous disease characterized by typical target skin lesions, with oral or ocular involvement in some cases and a marked tendency to recur. The condition mainly affects young adult males and has a seasonal incidence, being seen mainly in the spring or autumn.

The etiology of oral erythema multiforme has not been established, but many agents have been implicated. A wide range of drugs may be responsible, especially the barbiturates, phenylbutazone, sulfonamides, carbamazepine, and penicillin. The anticonvulsant drugs of the hydantoin and succinimide groups may cause a severe bullous form of erythema multiforme (Levantine and Almeyda, 1972). Certain infections such as herpes simplex, Mycoplasma, Histoplasma, and Trichomonas also may be associated with erythema multiforme (Shelley, 1967). The most common identifiable factor associated is a preceding herpes simplex virus infection, and this relationship is found in about 15% of patients (Lozada and Silverman, 1978). Herpes simplex virus usually is not isolated from the lesions nor is it demonstrable in biopsy specimens, but erythema multiforme can be induced by challenge with a vaccine of herpes simplex virus (Shelley, 1967). In the majority of instances, however, no causal factor is found; little evidence exists for an allergic cause. No abnormalities of immunoglobulin levels, lymphocyte transformation, or skin testing have been reported, but increased macrophage aggregation is seen (Krueger *et al.*, 1973). Immune complexes may activate the classical pathway of complement to initiate bulla formation (Safai *et al.*, 1977). Histologically, degenerative changes occur at the dermo-epidermal junction. Acanthosis occurs, with bullae either sub- or intraepithelially. The degenerating oral epithelium is strikingly eosinophilic and a lymphohistiocytic infiltration in the lamina propria is common (Lozada and Silverman, 1978).

References

Adinolfi, M., and Lehner, T. (1976). Acute phase proteins and C_9 in patients with Behcet's syndrome and aphthous ulcers. *Clin. Exp. Immunol.* **25,** 36–39.

Barnett, M. L. (1976). The nonkeratinocyte intraepithelial cell population in lichen planus. An ultrastructural characterization of cells in gingival lesions. *Oral Surg.* **41,** 338.

Beck, J. S. (1961). Variations in the morphological patterns of 'autoimmune' nuclear fluorescence. *Lancet* **i,** 1203–1205.

Behcet, M. (1937). Über rezidivierende Apthose durch ein Virus verursachte Geschwere am Mund, am Auge und an den Genitalien. *Dermatol. Wochenschr.* **105,** 1152–1157.

Berry, H., Bacon, P. A., and Davis, J. D. (1972). Cell mediated immunity in Sjögren's syndrome. *Ann. Rheum. Dis.* **31,** 298–302.

Beutner, E. H., Jordon, R. E., and Chorzelski, T. P. (1968). The immunopathology of pemphigus and bullous pemphigoid. *J. Invest. Dermatol.* **51,** 63–80.

Bhan, A. K., Harrist, T. J., Murphy, G. F., and Mihm, M. C., Jr. (1981). T cell subsets and Langerhans cells in lichen planus *in situ*. Characterization using monoclonal antibodies. *Br. J. Dermatol.* **105,** 617–622.

Biesbrock, A. R., Reddy, M. S., and Levine, M. J. (1991). Interaction of a salivary mucin–secretory immunoglobulin A complex with mucosal pathogens. *Infect. Immun.* **59,** 3492–3497.

Brandtzaeg, P. (1972). Local formation and transport of immunoglobulins. *In* "Host Resistance to Commensal Bacteria" (I. T. Macphee, ed.), pp. 116–150. Churchill Livingstone, Edinburgh.

Budtz-Jorgensen, E. (1973). Immune response to *Candida albicans* in monkeys with experimental candidiasis in the palate. *Scand. J. Dental Res.* **81,** 360–371.

Chajek, T., and Fainaru, M. (1975). Behcet's disease. Report of 41 cases and a review of the literature. *Medicine* **54,** 179–196.

Challacombe, S. J. (1980a). Serum and salivary antibodies to *Streptococcus mutans* in relation to the development and treatment of human dental caries. *Arch. Oral Biol.* **25,** 495–502.

Challacombe, S. J. (1980b). Passage of immunoglobulins from serum to the oral cavity. *In* "The Borderland between Caries and Periodontal Disease II" (T. Lehner and G. Cimasoni, ed.), pp. 51–67. Academic Press, San Diego.

Challacombe, S. J. (1983). Salivary antibodies and systemic tolerance in mice after oral immunisation with bacterial antigens. *Ann. N.Y. Acad. Sci.* **409,** 177–192.

Challacombe, S. J. (1987a). Oral manifestations of food allergy and intolerance. *In* "Food Allergy and Intolerance" (J. Brostoff and S. J. Challacombe, eds.), pp. 511–520. Bailliere Tindall, Eastbourne, England.

Challacombe, S. J. (1987b). The induction of secretory IgA responses. *In* "Food Allergy and Intolerance" (J. Brostoff and S. J. Challacombe, eds.), pp. 269–285. Bailliere Tindall, London.

Challacombe, S. J. (1991). Revised classification of HIV-associated oral lesions. *Brit. Dent. J.* **170,** 305–306.

Challacombe, S. J., and Lehner, T. (1976). Serum and salivary antibodies to cariogenic bacteria in man. *J. Dent. Res.* **55,** 139–148.

Challacombe, S. J., and Lehner, T. (1980). Salivary antibody responses in rhesus monkeys immunised with *Streptococcus mutans* by the oral, submucosal or subcutaneous routes. *Arch. Oral Biol.* **24,** 917–[redacted].

Challacombe, S. J., and Shirlaw, P. J. (1991). Oral ulceration: When to treat refer or ignore. *Dental Update* **52,** 368–373.

Challacombe, S. J., and Tomasi, T. B. (1980). Systemic tolerance and secretory immunity after oral immunisation. *J. Exp. Med.* **152,** 1459–1472.

Challacombe, S. J., Barkhan, P., and Lehner, T. (1977a). Haematological features and differentiation of recurrent oral ulceration. *Brit. J. Oral Surg.* **15,** 37–48.

Challacombe, S. J., Batchelor, J. R., Kennedy, L. A., and Lehner, T. (1977b). HLA antigens in recurrent oral ulceration. *Arch. Dermatol.* **113,** 1717–1719.

Challacombe, S. J., Russell, M. W., Hawkes, J. E., Bergmeier, L. A., and Lehner, T. (1978). Passage of immunoglobulins from plasma to the oral cavity in rhesus monkeys. *Immunology* **35,** 923–931.

Challacombe, S. J., Bergmeier, L. A., and Rees, A. S. (1984). Natural antibodies in man to a protein antigen from the bacterium *Streptococcus mutans* related to dental caries experience. *Arch. Oral Biol.* **29,** 179–184.

Challacombe, S. J., Greenhall, C., Biggerstaff, M., and Kemeny, D. M. (1986). ELISA detection of human IgG sub-class antibodies to *Streptococcus mutans*. *J. Immunol. Meth.* **87,** 95–102.

Challacombe, S. J., Panayi, G., Shirlaw, P. J., Hockey, K., and Morgan, P. R. (1991). SOX syndrome—Sialadenitis, osteoarthritis and xerostomia presenting as Sjögren's syndrome. *Clin. Exp. Rheumatol.* **9,** 75.

Challacombe, S. J., Rahman, D., Jeffery, H., Davis, S. S., and O'Hagan, D. T. (1992). Enhanced secretory IgA and systemic IgG antibody responses after oral immunization with biodegradable microparticles containing antigen. *Immunology* **76,** 164–168.

Chused, T. M., Kassan, S. S., Opelz, G., Moutzopozous, H. M., and Terasaki, P. I. (1977). Sjögren's syndrome associated with HLA-DW3. *N. Engl. J. Med.* **296,** 896–897.

Cianciola, L. J., Genco, R. J., Patters, M. R., McKenna, J., and Van Oss, C. J. (1977). Defective polymorphonuclear leukocyte function in human periodontal disease. *Nature (London)* **265,** 445–447.

Cole, M. F., Emilson, C. G., Hsu, D., and Bowen, W. H. (1984). Effect of personal immunization of humans with *Streptococcus mutans* on induction of salivary and antibodies and inhibition of experimental infection. *Infect. Immun.* **46,** 703–709.

Cooper, B. T., Holmes, G. K. T., Ferguson, R., Thompson, R. A., Auem, R. N., and Cooke, W. T. (1980). Gluten-sensitive diarrhoea without evidence of coeliac disease. *Gastroenterology* **79,** 801–806.

Crawford, J. M., Taubman, M. A., and Smith, D. J. (1975). Minor glands as a major source of secretory immuno globulins A in human oral cavity. *Science* **190,** 1206–1208.

Czerkinsky, C., Rees, A. S., Bergmeier, L. A., and Challacombe, S. J. (1983). The detection and specificity of class specific antibodies to whole bacterial cells using a sold phase radioimmunoassay. *Clin. Exp. Immunol.* **53,** 192–200.

Dawes, C., and Wood, C. M. (1973). The contribution of oral menu mucous gland secretions to the values of whole saliva in man. *Arch. Oral Biol.* **18,** 337–342.

Denman, A. M., Holton, W., Pelton, B. K., Palmer, R. G., Topper, R., and Smith–Burchenau, C. (1986). Viral aetiology of Behcet's syndrome in recent advances in Behcet's disease. (T. Lehner and C. G. Barnes, eds.), pp. 23–30. Royal Society of Medicine Services, London.

De Panfilis, G., Manara, G., Sansoni, P., and Allegra, F. (1983). T-cell infiltrate in lichen planus. Demonstration of activated lymphocytes using monoclonal antibodies. *J. Cut. Pathol.* **10,** 52–58.

Dockrell, H. M., and Greenspan, J. S. (1979). Histochemical identification of T cells in oral lichen planus. *Oral Surg.* **48,** 42–48.

Donatsky, O. (1976). Comparison of cellular and humoral immunity against streptococcal and adult oral mucosa antigens in relation to exacerbation of recurrent aphthous stomatitis. *Acta Pathol. Microbiol. Immunol. Scand.* **84,** 270–282.

Dzink, J. L., Tanner, A. C. R., Haffajee, A. D., and Socransky, S. S. (1985). Gram negative species associated with active destructive periodontal lesions. *J. Clin. Periodontol.* **12,** 648–659.

Eglin, R. P., Lehner, T., and Subak-Sharpe, J. H. (1982). Detection of RNA complementary to herpes simplex virus in mononuclear cells from patients with Behcet's syndrome and ROU. *Lancet* **ii,** 1356.

Eldridge, J. H., Staas, J. K., Meulbroek, J. A., McGhee, J. R., Tice, T. R., and Gilley, R. M. (1991). Biodegradable microspheres as a vaccine delivery system. *Mol. Immunol.* **28,** 287–294.

Emmings, F. G., Evans, R. T., and Genco, R. J. (1975). Antibody responses in the parotid fluid and serum of irus monkeys after local immunisation with *Streptococcus mutans*. *Infect. Immun.* **12,** 281–292.

Ferguson, M. M., Wray, D., Carmichael, H. A., Russell, R. I., and Lee, F. D. (1980). Coeliac disease associated with recurrent aphthae. *Gut* **21,** 223–226.

Gaston, J. S., Rowe, M., and Bacon, P. (1990). Sjögren's syndrome after infection by Epstein–Barr virus. *J. Rheumatol.* **17,** 558–561.

Genco, R. J., and Slots, J. (1984). Host response in periodontal diseases. *J. Dent. Res.* **63,** 441–451.

Genco, R. J., Slots, J., Mouton, C., and Murray, P. (1980). Systemic immune response to oral organisms. *In* "Anaerobic Bacteria: Selected Topics" (D. W. Lambe, R. J. Genco, and K. J. Mayberry-Carson, eds.), pp. 277–293. Plenum, New York.

Gillett, I. R., and Johnson, N. W. (1982). Bacterial invasion of the periodontium in a case of juvenile periodontitis. *J. Clin. Periodontol.* **9,** 93–100.

Hill, I. R., and Porter, P. (1974). Studies of bactericidal activity to *Escherichia coli* of porcine serum and colostral immunoglobulins and the role of lysozyme with secretory IgA. *Immunology* **26,** 1239–1250.

Huis in't Veld, J. H., van Palenstein Helderman, W. H., and Backer Dirks, O. (1979). *Streptococcus mutans* and dental caries in humans: A bacteriological and immunological study. *Antonie van Leevenhoek J. Microbiol. Serol.* **45,** 25–35.

Ivanyi, L., and Lehner, T. (1970). Stimulation of lymphocyte transformation by bacterial antigens in patients with periodontal disease. *Arch. Oral Biol.* **15,** 1089.

Krasse, B., Gahnberg, L., and Bratthall, D. (1988). Antibodies reacting with *Streptococcus mutans* in secretions from minor salivary glands in humans. *Adv. Exp. Med. Biol.* **107,** 349–354.

Krueger, G. G., Weston, W., Thorne, E., Mandel, M., and Jacobs, R. (1973). A phenomenon of macrophage aggregation in sera of patients with exfoliative erythrodermia, erythema multiforme and erythema nodosum. *J. Invest. Dermatol.* **60,** 282–285.

Lehner, T. (1978). Immunological aspects of recurrent oral ulceration and Behcet's syndrome. *J. Oral Pathol.* **7,** 424–430.

Lehner, T. (1982). Regulation of immune responses to streptococcal protein antigens in dental caries. *Immunol. Today* **3,** 73–77.

Lehner, T., and Barnes, C. G., eds. (1979). "Behcet's Syndrome." Academic Press, London.

Lehner, T., Wilton, J. M. A., and Ivanyi, L. (1972). Immunodeficiencies in chronic muco-cutaneous candidosis. *Immunology* **22,** 755–787.

Lehner, T., Challacombe, S. J., Wilton, J. M., and Caldwell, J. (1976). Cellular and humoral immune responses in vaccination against dental caries in monkeys. *Nature (London)* **264,** 69.

Lehner, T., Russell, M. W., Challacombe, S. J., Scully, E. M., and Hawkes, J. (1978). Passive immunisation with serum and immunoglobulin against dental caries in rhesus monkeys. *Lancet* **1,** 693–695.

Lehner, T., Russell, M. W., and Caldwell, J. (1980). Immunisation with a purified protein from *Streptococcus mutans* against dental caries in rhesus monkeys. *Lancet* **i,** 995–996.

Lehner, T., Welsh, K. I., and Batchelor, J. R. (1982). The relationship of HLA-B and DR phenotypes to Behcet's syndrome, recurrent oral ulceration and the class of immune complexes. *Immunology* **47(4),** 581–587.

Lehner, T., Lavery, E., Smith, R., van der Zee, R., Mizushima, Y., and Shinnick, T. (1991). Association between the 65-kilodalton heat shock protein, *Streptococcus sanguis,* and the corresponding antibodies in Behcet's syndrome. *Infect. Immun.* **59,** 1434–1441.

Leventine, A., and Almeyda, J. (1972). Drug reactions: 20 cutaneous reactions to anticonvulsants. *Brit. J. Dermatol.* **87,** 246–249.

Linde, J. (1989). Pathogenesis of plaque associated periodontal disease. *In* "Textbook of Clinical Periodoncology," 2nd Edition. p. 188. Munrsgaard, Coppenhagen.

Listgarten, M. A. (1965). Electron microscopic observations of the bacterial flora of acute necrotizing ulcerative gingivitis. *J. Periodontol.* **36,** 328–339.

Loe, H., Anerud, A., Boysen H., Monson, E. (1986). Natural history of periodontal disease in man. Rapid, moderate and no loss of attachment in Sri Lankan laborers 14 to < 6 years of age. *J. Clin. Perio.* **13,** 431–435.

Lozada, F., and Silverman, S. (1978). Erythema multiforme; Clinical characteristics and natural history in fifty patients. *Oral Surg. Oral Med. Oral Pathol.* **46,** 628–636.

Ma, J. K-C., and Lehner, T. (1990). Prevention of colonization of *Streptococcus mutans* by topical application of monoclonal antibodies in human subjects. *Arch. Oral Biol.* **35,** 115S–122S.

McCarthy, P. L. (1972). Benign mucous membrane pemphigoid. *Oral Surg. Oral Med. Oral Pathol.* **33,** 75–79.

McGhee, J. R., and Michalek, S. M. (1981). Immunobiology of dental caries: microbial aspects and local immunity. *Ann. Rev. Microbiol.* **35,** 595–638.

Matsumura, N., and Mizushima, Y. (1975). Leucocyte movement and colchicine treatment in Behcet's disease. *Lancet* **ii,** 813.

Matthews, J. B., Scully, C. M., and Potts, A. J. C. (1984). Oral lichen planus: An immuno-peroxidase study using monoclonal antibodies to lymphocyte subsets. *Br. J. Dermatol.* **III,** 587.

Medenica, M., and Lorincz, A. (1977). Lichen planus: An ultrastructural study. *Acta Derm. Venereol. (Stockh.)* **57,** 55–62.

Mestecky, J., McGhee, J. R., Arnold, R. R., Michalek, S. M., Prince, S. J., and Babb, J. C. (1978). Selective induction of an immune response in human external secretions by ingestion of bacterial antigen. *J. Clin. Invest.* **61,** 731–737.

Michalek, S. M., McGhee, J. R., and Babb, J. L. (1977). Effective immunity to dental caries: Dose dependent studies of secretory immunity by oral administration of *Streptococcus mutans* to rats. *Infect. Immun.* **19,** 217–223.

Miller, M. F., Garfunkel, A. A., Ram, C. C., and Ship, I. I. (1977). Inheritance patterns in recurrent aphthous ulcers: Twin and pedigree data. *Oral Surg.* **43,** 836–891.

Montgomery, P. C., Connell, K. M., Cohn, J., and Skandera, C. A. (1978). Remote site stimulation of secretory IgA antibodies following bronchial and gastric stimulation. *Adv. Exp. Med. Biol.* **107,** 113–122.

Mouton, C., Hammond, P. G., Slots, J., and Genco, R. J. (1981). Serum antibodies to oral *Bacteroides asaccharolyticus* (*Bacteroides gingivalis*): Relationship to age and periodontal disease. *Infect. Immun.* **31,** 182–192.

Moutsopoulos, H. M., and Zerva, L. V. (1990). Anti-Ro (SSA)/La (SSB) antibodies and Sjögren's syndrome. *Clin. Rheumatol.* **9,** 123–130.

Nair, P. N. R., and Schroeder, H. E. (1986). Duct-associated lymphoid tissue (DALT) of minor salivary glands and mucosal immunity. *Immunology* **57,** 171–175.

O'Hagan, D. T., Rahman, D., McGee, J. P., Jeffery, H., Davies, M. D., Williams, P., Davis, S. S., and Challacombe, S. J. (1991). Biodegradable microparticles as controlled release antigen delivery systems. *Immunology* **73,** 239–242.

Olson, R. G., Du Plessis, D., Barron, C., Schulz, E. J., Vihet, W. (1983). Lichen planus dermopathy. Demonstration of lichen planus specific epidermal antigen in affected patients. *J. Clin. Lab. Immun.* **10,** 103–106.

Page, R. C., and Schroeder, H. E. (1982). "Periodontitis in Man and Other Animals: A Comparative Review." Karger, Basel.

Postlethwaite, A. E., Snyderman, R., and Kang, A. H. (1976). The chemotactic attraction of fibroblasts to a lymphocyte-derived factor. *J. Exp. Med.* **144,** 1188–1203.

Ragaz, A., and Ackerman, A. B. (1981). Evolution, maturation, and regression of lesions of lichen planus, new observations and correlations of clinical and histological findings. *Am. J. Dermatopathol.* **3,** 5–11.

Rogers, R. S., Perry, H. O., Bean, S. F., and Jordan, R. E. (1982). Immunopathology of cicatricial pemphigoid: Studies of complement deposition. *J. Invest. Dermatol.* **68,** 39–43.

Russell, M. W., and Challacombe, S. J. (1976). Serum glucosyltransferase inhibiting antibodies and dental caries in rhesus monkeys immunized against *Streptococcus mutans. Immunology* **30,** 619–627.

Safai, B., Good, R. A., and Day, N. K. (1977). Erythema multiforme. Report of two cases and speculation on immune mechanisms involved in the pathogenesis. *Clin. Immunol. Immunopathol.* **7,** 379–385.

Saglie, R., Newman, M. G., Carranza, F. A., and Pattison, G. L. (1982). Bacterial invasion of gingiva in advanced periodontitis in humans. *J. Periodontol.* **53,** 217–222.

Sallay, K., Kulcsar, G., Nasz, I., Dan, P., and Geck, P. (1973). Adenovirus isolation from recurrent oral ulcers. *J. Periodontal.* **44,** 712–714.

Schiltz, J., Michel, B., and Papay, R. (1978). Pemphigus antibody interaction with human epidermal cells in culture. *J. Clin. Invest.* **62,** 778–788.

Shelley, W. B. (1967). Herpes simplex virus as a cause of erythema multiforme. *J. Am. Med. Assoc.* **201,** 153–156.

Shillitoe, E. J., and Lehner, T. (1972). Immunoglobulins and complement in crevicular fluid, serum and saliva. *Arch. Oral Biol.* **17,** 241–248.

Shimada, K., Kogure, M., Kawashima, T., and Nishioka, K. (1974). Reduction of complement in Behcet's disease and drug allergy. *Med. Biol.* **52,** 234–239.

Ship, I. I. (1965). Inheritance of aphthous ulcers in the mouth. *J. Dent. Res.* **44,** 837–844.

Sinha, A. A., Brautbar, C., Szafer, F., Friedmann, A., Tzfoni, E., Todd, A. E., Steinman, L., and McDeuitt, O. H. (1988). A newly characterised HLA-DQ allele associated with pemphigus vulgaris. *Science* **239,** 1026–1029.

Smith, D. J., Taubman, M. A., and Ebersole, J. L. (1979). Effect of oral administration of glucosyltransferase antigens on experimental dental caries. *Infect. Immun.* **26,** 82–89.

Spitler, L. E., Levin, A. S., and Fudenberg, H. H. (1974). Transfer factor. *Clin. Immunobiol.* **2,** 153–189.

Sun, A., Hsieh, R. P., Chu, C. T., and Wu, Y. C. (1991). Strong association of HLA-DRw9 in Chinese patients with recurrent oral ulcers. *J. Amer. Acad. Dermatol.* **24,** 195–198.

Syrjanen, S., Karja, V., Chang, F. J., Johansson, B., and Syrjanen, K. (1990). Epstein–Barr virus involvement in salivary gland lesions associated with Sjögren's syndrome. *ORL J. Otorhinolaryngol. Relat. Spec.* **52,** 254–259.

Taichman, N. S., McArthur, W. P., Tsai, C. C., Baehni, P. C., Shenker, B. J., Berthold, P., Evian, C., and Stevens, R. (1982). Leukocidal mechanisms of *Actinobacillus actinomycetemcomitans. In* "Host Parasite Interactions in Human Periodontal Disease" (R. J. Genco and S. E. Mergenhagen, eds.), pp. 261–269. American Society for Microbiology, Washington, D.C.

Talal, N., Sylvester, R. A., and Daniels, T. E. (1974). T and B lymphocytes in peripheral blood and tissue lesions in Sjögren's syndrome. *J. Clin. Invest.* **53,** 180–189.

Talal, N., Dauphinee, M. J., Dang, H., Alexander, S. S., Hart, D. J., and Garry, R. F. (1990). Detection of serum antibodies to retroviral proteins in patients with primary Sjögren's syndrome (autoimmune exocrinopathy). *Arthritis Rheum.* **33,** 774–781.

Taubman, M. A., Ebersole, J. L., and Smith, D. J. (1982). Association between systemic and local antibody in periodontal disease. *In* "Host-Parasite Interactions in Periodontal Disease" (R. J. Genco and S. E. Mergenhagen, eds.), pp. 283–298. American Society of Microbiology, Washington, D.C.

Thomas, D. W., Bagg, J., and Walker, D. M. (1990). Characterisation of the effector cells responsible for the *in vitro* cytotoxicity of blood leukocytes from aphthous ulcer patients for oral epithelial cells. *Gut* **31(3),** 294–299.

Tsai, C. C., McArthur, W. P., Baehni, P. C., Evian, C. C., Genco, J. R., and Taichman, S. N. (1981). Serum neutralizing activity against *Actinobacillus actinomycetemcomitans* leukotoxin in juvenile periodontitis. *J. Clin. Periodontol.* **8,** 338–348.

Valdimarrson, H., Higgs, J. M., Wells, R. S., Yamamura, M., Hobbs, J. R., and Holt, P. J. L. (1973). Immune abnormalities associated with chronic mucocutaneous candidiasis. *Cell. Immunol.* **6,** 348–361.

Wahl, S. M., and Wahl, L. M. (1981). Modulation of fibroblast growth and function by monokines and lymphokines. *Lymphokines* **2,** 179–201.

Weissman, V., Feuerman, E. J., Joshua, H., and Hazaz, B. (1978). The correlation between the antibody titres in sera of patients with pemphigus vulgaris and their clinical state. *J. Invest. Dermatol.* **71,** 107–109.

Williams, B. D., and Lehner, T. (1977). Immune complexes in Behcet's syndrome and recurrent oral ulceration. *Br. Med. J.* **1(6037),** 1387–1389.

Wilson, C. W. (1980). Food sensitivities, taste changes, aphthous ulcers and atopic symptoms in allergic disease. *Ann. Allergy* **44,** 302–307.

Woodrow, J. C. (1988). Immunogenetics of systemic lupus erythematosus. *J. Rheumatol.* **15,** 197–198.

Wray, D., Ferguson, M. M., Mason, D. K., Hutcheon, A. W., and Dagg, J. H. (1975). Recurrent aphthae: Treatment with vitamin B_{12}, folic acid and iron. *Br. Med. J.* **2,** 490–493.

Zegarelli, D. J., and Zegarelli, E. V. (1977). Intraoral pemphigus vulgaris. *Oral Surg.* **44,** 384–393.

50

Immunobiology of the Tonsils and Adenoids

Joel M. Bernstein • Noboru Yamanaka • David Nadal

I. INTRODUCTION

The palatine tonsils and the nasopharyngeal tonsil (adenoid) are lymphoepithelial tissues located in strategic areas of the oral pharynx and nasopharynx, respectively. These immunocompetent tissues represent the first line of defense against ingested or inhaled foreign proteins such as bacteria, viruses, or food antigens. Tonsillectomy and adenoidectomy are the most common major operations performed on children under general anesthesia in the United States (Paradise and Bluestone, 1976). However, the indications for tonsillectomy and adenoidectomy have been complicated by the controversy over the benefits of extracting a chronically infected tissue and the possible harm this operation may cause by eliminating an important source of local mucosal defense in the host. The information necessary to make a rational decision in resolving this controversy can be obtained by understanding the immunological potential of the normal tonsils and adenoids and by comparing these functions with the changes that occur in the chronically diseased tonsil and adenoid. This chapter reviews the distribution of immunocompetent cells in various locations of the palatine tonsil and nasopharyngeal tonsil, and compares their numbers and function in aging and chronic infection. Further, the role of the tonsils and adenoids as part of the common mucosal immune system is reviewed. Finally, the palatine tonsil as a potential source of autoimmunity in other parts of the body is discussed briefly.

II. IMMUNOLOGICAL CYTOARCHITECTURE OF THE TONSILS AND ADENOIDS

The palatine tonsil and nasopharyngeal tonsil have a characteristic lymphoid architecture that includes a reticular epithelium, a follicular region or primary and secondary germinal centers that are covered with mantle zones, and extrafollicular regions. The immunocompetent cells that are present in these various regions of the tonsil have been studied thoroughly by many investigators using specific polyclonal and monoclonal antibodies directed against specific epitopes of lymphocytes (Brandtzaeg *et al.*, 1979; Surjan *et al.*, 1978; Stein *et al.*, 1980; Surjan, 1980; Yamanaka *et al.*, 1983b,1992; Brandtzaeg, 1984,1987; Harabuchi *et al.*, 1985; Bernstein *et al.*, 1988).

Figure 1 summarizes the immunological cytoarchitecture of the palatine tonsil. The principal route of antigen uptake occurs in palatine tonsils in their crypts and in the nasopharyngeal tonsils in their furrows. In the human palatine tonsil, 10–20 crypts markedly increase the surface exposure for antigen uptake (Junqueira and Carneiro, 1980). Cells that may be important in antigen uptake, microfold (M) cells, are present that are also present in Peyer's patches of the small bowel (Owen and Nemanic, 1978). In addition, many HLA-DR-positive cells exist deep in the crypt that also may be important in antigen uptake (Brandtzaeg, 1984,1987). Other important cells involved in antigen transport are macrophages, interdigitating cells (ICs) that are present in the extrafollicular areas (Tew *et al.*, 1982), and follicular dendritic cells (FDCs) that are primarily present in the germinal centers (Heinen *et al.*, 1984; Tew *et al.*, 1989).

Using specific monoclonal antibodies directed against receptors on the surface of antigen-presenting cells (APCs), our laboratory has demonstrated the distribution and location of APCs in the nasopharyngeal tonsil (Bernstein *et al.*, 1991). MAC387 and CD68 were used to identify cells of the monocyte–macrophage series, S-100 antibody was used to identify interdigitating cells, and antibody directed against the C3b receptor defined antigen-retaining reticulum in germinal centers. Quantification of the cells was done in the four compartments of the nasopharyngeal tonsils, namely, the crypt epithelium, the extrafollicular zones, the mantle zone, and the germinal center. Table I summarizes the average percentage of PCAs in the compartments of the nasopharyngeal tonsil. Figure 2(a–g) demonstrates different types of APCs in the nasopharyngeal tonsil compartments.

Thymus-derived (T) cells characteristically occupy the extrafollicular zones, but the helper–inducer T lymphocytes are also present in the germinal centers (Yamanaka *et al.*, 1983b). B cells are primarily present in the germinal center and mantle zone, but also may be found in the reticular epithelium. Using the fluorescence activated cell sorter (FACS), we measured the percentages of various T-cell subsets and different types of B cells in the palatine tonsil and adenoid. These data are summarized in Table II and are compared with the lymphocyte subpopulations in the autologous peripheral blood. The average percentage of T and B cells in the palatine tonsils, respectively, is 42% and 52%. In the peripheral blood, 67% of lymphocytes are T cells and 14% are B cells. $CD4^{+}Leu8^{+}$ cells represent suppressor–inducer cells, whereas $CD4^{+}Leu8^{-}$ cells represent helper–

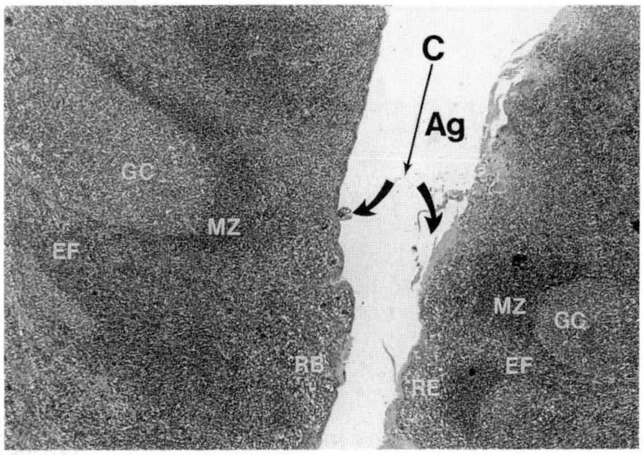

Figure 1 High power photomicrograph of the morphology of the tonsil surrounding a crypt (C). Antigen (Ag) enters the crypt and is taken up by cells of the reticular epithelium (RE). Antigen-presenting cells in this region consist of Langerhans cells, macrophages, and perhaps M cells. These cells then transport antigen to T cells in the extrafollicular zone (EF). In addition, antigen presentation to cells in the mantle zone (MZ) may stimulate memory cells with surface IgD and IgM to switch to more mature clones of B cells possessing IgA and IgG. Finally, specific dendritic cells in the germinal center (GC) may be responsible for antigen presentation to B cells in this area.

inducer cells (Lanier *et al.*, 1983). The helper–inducer cells represent the majority of cells found in the palatine tonsil, whereas the suppressor–inducer T cells are more abundant in the peripheral blood.

Using immunohistological localization of immunoglobulins, various investigators have studied the distribution of immunoglobulin-bearing cells in the palatine tonsils (Surjan *et al.*, 1978; Brandtzaeg *et al.*, 1978,1979; Brandtzaeg, 1984,1987,1991; Bernstein 1990; Nadal *et al.*, 1992). Actively Ig-secreting cells, or plasma cells, constitute no more than 2% of the total cells in the palatine tonsil and nasopharyngeal tonsils (Nadal *et al.*, 1992). IgG appears to be the predominant immunoglobulin. The ratio of IgA to IgM differs according to the methods of study used. Studying the cytoplasmic staining of immunocytes, Brandtzaeg and his colleagues have suggested that the number of IgA immunocytes is significantly greater than that of IgM immunocytes (Brandtzaeg, 1984,1987). However, using the ELISPOT technique, which specifically identifies cells that are secreting immunoglobulins actively, our laboratory has found that the numbers for IgA- and IgM-secreting cells are similar (Nadal *et al.*, 1992). However, IgA secretion in the palatine tonsils is significantly greater than in the lymph node (Woloschak *et al.*, 1986), suggesting that the palatine tonsil has characteristics of a mucosal immune system.

Table I Average Percentage of Antigen Presenting Cells in Compartments of Nasopharyngeal Tonsil[a]

	Antibody			
	MAC387	CD68	S-100	C3b
Crypt epithelium	6.1 ± 5.7 ↔	0.39 ± 1.13[b]	0.47 ± 0.86	0.01 ± 0.01
Extrafollicular zone	5.4 ± 2.3	4.4 ± 3.6	2.4 ± 1.5	0.01 ± 0.02
Mantle zone	0.17 ± 0.19	0.99 ± 2.4	0.05 ± 0.08	11.0 ± 7.8
Germinal center	0.66 ± 1.2 ↔	2.5 ± 1.3[c]	0.09 ± 0.24	42.0 ± 6.1

[a] MAC387 and CD68 are monoclonal antibodies that stain for macrophage cells. However, the distribution of CD68 is significantly different than that of MAC387 in the crypt epithelium and in the germinal center. CD68 in the germinal centers is believed to represent tingible macrophages.
[b] $p < 0.01$
[c] $p < 0.01$

Figure 2 (A) Immunohistochemical staining with MAC387 shows staining of macrophages (arrow) in the crypt of the nasopharyngeal tonsil (APAAP × 25, alkaline phosphatase–antialkaline phosphatase). C, Crypt. (B) Immunohistochemical staining with MAC387 in the extrafollicular zone of the nasopharyngeal tonsil (APAAP × 10). gc, germinal center. These cells appear to be confined to the extrafollicular area and are not found in the germinal center. They most likely represent macrophages, although they also may represent interdigitating cells. (C) Immunohistochemical localization of CD68 cells in the extrafollicular zone of the nasopharyngeal tonsil. These cells are few in the crypt epithelium, but the cells are found mainly in the extrafollicular zone (APAAP × 10). (D) Immunohistochemical localization of CD68 cells in the germinal center of the nasopharyngeal tonsil (APAAP × 10). mz, Mantle zone. Many cells are found in the follicle of the nasopharyngeal tonsil. These cells represent tingible macrophages. (E) Immunohistochemical localization of cells staining with S100 in the extrafollicular zone of the nasopharyngeal tonsil (APAAP × 10). These cells most likely represent interdigitating cells and are found mainly in the extrafollicular zone and not in the germinal center. (F) Immunohistochemical localization of C3b receptor on the follicular dendritic cells (FDC) of the nasopharyngeal germinal center (APAAP × 10). These cells stain for the complement receptor in the germinal center. (G) High powered photomicrograph of C3b labeling (arrow) of the dendritic processes of FDCs showing the antigen retaining reticulum (ARR) (APAAP × 49).

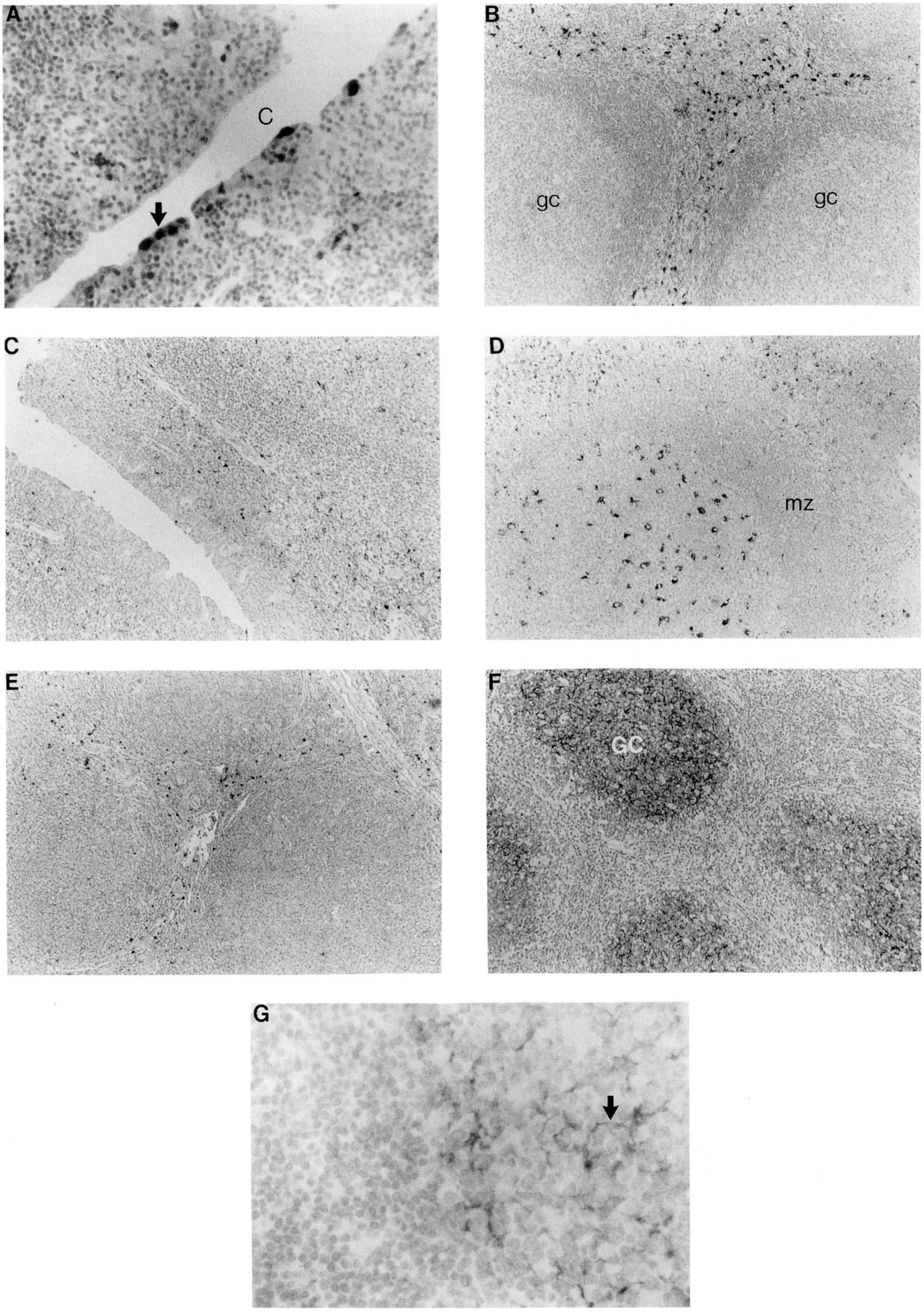
A
C
B
gc
gc
C
D
mz
E
F
GC
G

Table II Lymphocyte Subsets in Palatine Tonsils and Peripheral Blood[a]

	Peripheral blood		Palatine tonsils	
	Total lymphocytes (%)	B cells (%)	Total lymphocytes (%)	B cells (%)
IgD	2.5	22	1.2	8
IgG	2.1	18	31.0	73
IgA	0.318	5	7.3	20
IgM	9.7	88	19.9	43
CD19 (Total B)	14		52	
CD3 (Total T)	67		42	
CD4	35		32	
CD8	29		9	
$CD3^+$ Leu 8^+	30		10	
$CD3^+$ Leu 8^-	7		21	

[a] Samples were from 46 patients undergoing tonsillectomy. The predominant immunoglobulin in the palatine tonsils is IgG and represents 73% of the B cells, whereas the predominant immunoglobulin in B cells in the peripheral blood is IgM. The peripheral blood possesses a majority of T lymphocytes, whereas the average number of B cells in the tonsil is 52%. The ratio of T helper to T suppressor cells in the palatine tonsil is significantly greater than the ratio in the peripheral blood. $CD3^+Leu8^+$ cells, which represent suppressor inducer cells, are greater in the peripheral blood, whereas $CD3^+$ $Leu8^-$ cells, which represent helper inducer cells, are greater in the palatine tonsils.

The mantle zones of the tonsils appear to be very specific for early clones of B cells possessing both IgM and IgD on their surfaces (Yamanaka *et al.*, 1992). On the other hand, in the germinal center, IgD is found rarely whereas IgG and IgM are frequent, suggesting that significant switching of early clones of B cells to more mature B cells occurs in the germinal center (Brandtzaeg, 1987). Further, IgA and IgG immunocytes also are located in the crypt epithelium and in the extrafollicular zones (Figure 3A,B). A summary of the distribution of the cellular immunoglobulin isotypes in the human palatine tonsil is presented in Figure 4.

The production of J chain by different types of B cells in the palatine tonsil was studied by the Brandtzaeg laboratory and was shown to represent a very important concept with respect to the relationship between normal and diseased tonsils (Brandtzaeg *et al.*, 1979). A summary of J-chain expression by tonsillar immunoglobulin-producing cells in health and disease is shown in Figure 5.

This brief summary of the immunological cytoarchitecture of the palatine and nasopharyngeal tonsil suggests that these structures possess all the elements required of a mucosal immune system. Bacterial, viral, or food antigen can be adsorbed selectively by macrophages, HLA-positive cells, and M cells in the crypts of these lymphoepithelial tissues. Further, the antigens can be transported to T cells in the extrafollicular area by ICs and to B cells in the germinal centers by FDCs. Early clones of B cells in the mantle zone, which have surface IgM and IgD, may be memory cells that can be stimulated to switch into more mature clones of B cells, including IgG- and IgA-secreting cells. With proper stimulation by interleukins from T-helper cells in the follicular zone, B cells may mature into memory cells or into immunoglobulin-synthesizing plasma cells (Tew *et al.*, 1989). These plasma cells then are distributed in the extrafollicular zone and in the crypt epithelium, and the immunoglobulins are secreted into the crypt. Therefore, the tonsil plays an important role in maintaining the normal microbiological flora in the crypts of the tonsils and in the furrows of the adenoids, at least in the healthy person. Finally, B cells that possess J chain may mature into IgM and IgA plasma cells that secrete J-chain-bearing immunoglobulins. The nasopharyngeal tonsil, which possesses secretory component (SC), will function as a true secretory immune system. In contrast, the palatine tonsil, which possesses either stratified squamous epithelium or simple cuboidal epithelium as in the crypt, will secrete IgA into the crypt lumen but also may be the source of dimeric J-chain-positive IgA B cells for other areas of the upper respiratory system, such as the parotid gland, the lacrimal gland, the nasal mucosa, and the middle ear mucosa in otitis media (Brandtzaeg, 1984,1987).

Cell–cell interaction in the palatine tonsil has been studied by a number of investigators (Perry *et al.*, 1991; Tsubota *et al.*, 1991). For example, a series of molecules that play a crucial role in adhesion and signal transduction have been reported. These molecules are designated, in general, adhesion molecules. Immunohistochemical analysis showed vitronectin, fibronectin, and laminin, as well as other surface-associated adhesions, to be present on tonsillar lymphocytes. Further, interleukin 6 (IL-6), an important mediator of B-cell maturation, has been demonstrated in palatine tonsils and seems to be associated with the macrophage in the palatine tonsil (Sugiyama, 1991). Moreover, B cells with IL-6 receptors have been demonstrated in the tonsil. In addition, this cytokine may induce the proliferation and differentiation of cytotoxic T cells.

The microvasculature of the human palatine tonsil and its

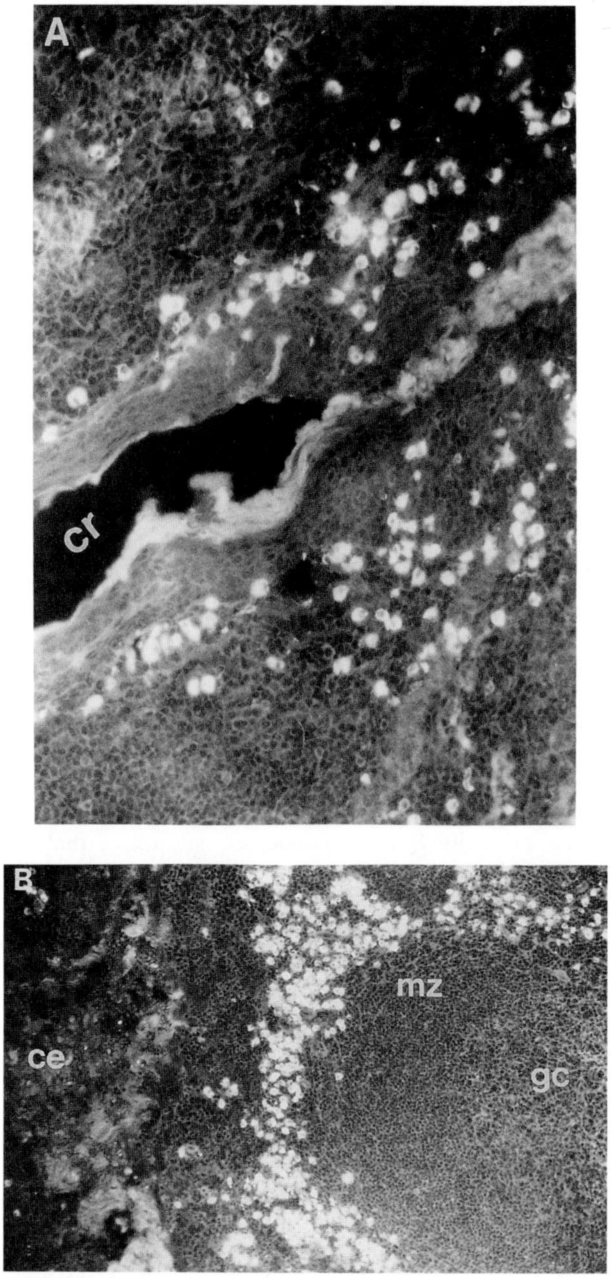

Figure 3 (A) Immunohistological localization of IgA using FITC conjugated anti-immunoglobulin A antibody. cr, Crypt. IgA plasma cells are found in the lamina propria underlying the crypt epithelium and in the interfollicular areas (APAAP × 25). (b) Immunohistological localization of IgG immunocytes in the tonsillar tissue. mz, Mantle zone; gc, germinal center; ce, crypt epithelium. Multiple immunocytes possessing IgG are seen in the interfollicular area. Virtually no IgG is seen in the mantle zone, and lacy staining between the cells is seen in the germinal center (APAAP × 16).

role in homing of lymphocytes has been studied by investigators at the University of London (Perry *et al.*, 1991). This selective process is thought to be mediated in part by the lymphocyte function-associated antigen 1 (LFA-1) that is

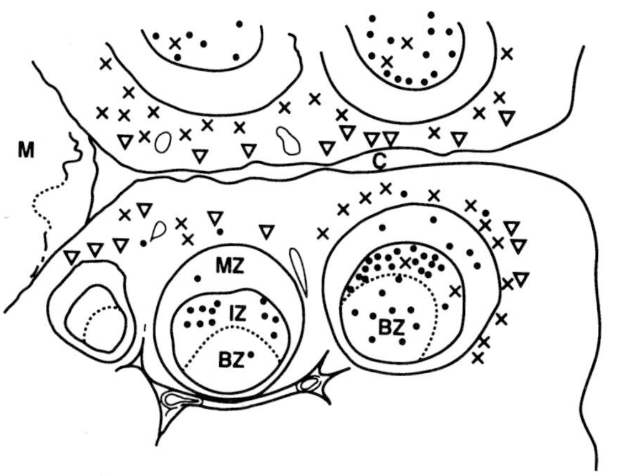

Figure 4 Diagram of the distribution of immunocytes found in the human palatine tonsil in 46 cases. IgM and IgG immunocytes are found in the germinal centers. A few IgM positive immunocytes are found in the mantle zone. IgG and IgA immunocytes are found primarily in the extrafollicular zones and in the crypt epithelium. MZ, Mantle zone; IZ, intermediate zone; B2, basal zone; M, medulla; C, crypt; ●, IgM-positive cells; X, IgG-positive cells; ▽, IgA-positive cells.

expressed on the surface of lymphocytes and by its ligand, the intercellular adhesion molecule-1 (ICAM-1), that is expressed on the endothelium. Localization of ICAM-1 was confined predominantly to the endothelium, with greatest expression seen on the high endothelial venules (HEV) in both the extrafollicular and the intraepithelial locations of the human palatine tonsil. LFA-1-expressing lymphocytes were seen in both intra- and extravascular locations, especially in the extrafollicular T-cell region close to the HEV. The increased expression of LFA-1 on the large number of tonsillar lymphocytes, in conjunction with the up-regulated expression of ICAM-1 on the HEV, suggests that the latter functions as a promoter of lymphocyte extravasation into tonsillar tissue.

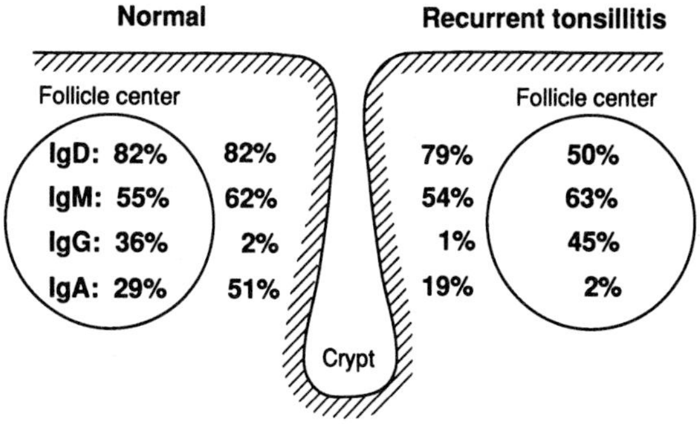

Figure 5 Schematic representation of average J-chain positivity shown by intra- and extrafollicular Ig-producing immunocytes of various isotypes, as indicated. A significant decrease in the J-chain positive IgA cells is seen in the follicle and in the extrafollicular area in recurrent tonsillitis. Reprinted with permission from Brandtzaeg (1987).

In summary, the palatine and nasopharyngeal tonsils represent strategically located lymphoepithelial tissues that harbor all the immunocompetent cells and molecules necessary for the exhibition of a local immune response. Inasmuch as normal human lungs lack organized bronchus-associated lymphoid tissue (BALT; Brandtzaeg, 1991), which is prominent in certain animal species (Scicchitano *et al.*, 1987), the major source of B-cell precursors in the upper respiratory tract of humans appears to be the lymphoid tissue of Waldeyer's ring, dominated by the palatine tonsil.

III. PALATINE TONSILS AND NASOPHARYNGEAL TONSIL AS LOCAL IMMUNE SYSTEMS

Tonsillar lymphocytes have the capacity to produce specific antibodies against a number of pathogens and other foreign proteins (Rynell-Dagoo, 1976; Harabuchi *et al.*, 1989; J. M. Bernstein and G. Rich, unpublished data). The predominant antibody isotype synthesized and released by both tonsillar lymphocytes and adenoidal lymphocytes is IgG. The observations of considerable interest, however, are that tonsillar and adenoidal lymphocytes exhibit specific activity against respiratory syncytial virus (RSV), an agent associated with upper airway disease, as well as *Streptococcus pneumoniae, Haemophilus influenzae,* and beta hemolytic *Streptococcus* Group A. Various cow milk antigens, including casein and β-lactoglobulin, induce specific T-cell responses in tonsillar lymphocytes (J. M. Bernstein and G. Rich, unpublished data). Further, adenoidal lymphocytes are capable of synthesizing specific IgG, IgA, and IgM antibody against RSV virus, both spontaneously and when stimulated with the virus (Soh *et al.*, 1991). In contrast, adenoidal lymphocytes exposed to the polyclonal B-cell mitogens, the lipopolysaccharide (LPS) from *Escherichia coli,* and purified protein derivative (PPD) demonstrate only a poor response (Rynnel-Dagoo, 1978; Meistrup-Larsen *et al.*, 1980). Exposure of adenoid lymphocytes to *H. influenzae in vitro* has been demonstrated to elicit higher responses when the cells are obtained from subjects apparently free from immediately preceding nasopharyngeal exposure to the same pathogen than when the cells are derived from individuals currently colonized with this bacterium (Harabuchi *et al.*, 1989). In our studies using RSV, the predominant immunoglobulin secreted was IgG (So *et al.*, 1991).

The results of these functional studies provide evidence that both the tonsils and adenoids are engaged continuously in local immune responses to viral and bacterial pathogens that have a tropism to the nasopharynx, oropharynx, and respiratory mucosa. In this regard, the clinical otolaryngologist must consider that tonsillectomy and adenoidectomy may result in the reduction of local immune competence against various pathogens and allergens, as suggested in a previous study detecting the fall of specific antibody titers against polio virus in nasopharyngeal washings (Ogra, 1971).

IV. TONSILS AS A SOURCE OF IMMUNOCOMPETENT CELLS FOR OTHER AREAS OF THE UPPER RESPIRATORY TRACT

The existence of a protective local immune system that functions fairly independently of systemic immunity was proposed by Besredka (1919) when he demonstrated that, after oral immunization with killed Shiga bacillus, rabbits were protected against fatal dysentery irrespective of a serum antibody titer (Besredka, 1919). The interest in local immunity was revived significantly in the 1960s when Tomasi *et al.* (1963) reported that the predominant immunoglobulin in external body fluids was IgA. In 1974, a common epithelial transport model was proposed for dimeric IgA and pentameric IgM by Brandtzaeg (1974). The joining J chain had been identified a few years earlier as a unique polypeptide shared by these two immunoglobulin polymers (Mestecky *et al.*, 1971).

All secretory sites of adults normally contain a remarkable predominance of IgA-producing immunocytes, including plasma cells and their immediate precursors. Although these immunocytes are particularly common in the intestinal mucosa, they also exist in the lacrimal gland, nasal mucosa, parotid gland, mammary gland, and the middle ear mucosa in otitis media and chronic otitis media with effusion. A relatively large proportion of the IgA2 subclass has been reported for the IgA immunocytes present in secretory sites in the colon (Conley and Bartelt, 1984), whereas the tonsils possess primarily IgA1 immunocytes, suggesting that the source of the IgA B cells may be different for these two mucosal systems (Kett *et al.*, 1986). The source of the B cells that reach the nasal mucosa, middle ear, or parotid gland could be chiefly the lymphoid tissue of Waldeyer's ring. Therefore, tonsils and adenoids have been suggested as sources of dimeric J-chain-positive IgA B cells. Therefore the tonsils would, indeed, play a role as a "Peyer's patch" of the upper respiratory tract and seed the upper respiratory mucosa with J-chain-positive IgA B cells. This concept has been demonstrated by Brandtzaeg (1987). Data from our laboratory support the concept that the tonsil may play such a role (Bernstein *et al.*, 1988). *Streptococcus mutans,* a common bacterial organism associated with dental caries, is never found in the mucosa of the middle ear or the nose. However, B cells with specific surface antibody against this organism can be found at these sites (Figure 6A,B). The tonsils and/or adenoids have been suggested to be the source of B cells with specific surface immunoglobulin directed against an organism that is not present in the middle ear or nasal mucosa. Thus, a specific B cell arising from the tonsil or adenoid lymphoid tissue may migrate to an adjacent site in the upper respiratory mucosa.

The IgD-expressing lymphocytes present in the mantle zone of tonsillar lymph follicles, for the most part, bear IgM on their surface. These cells are considered to be memory cells that follow antigen-driven proliferation. Retained surface IgD is apparently a marker of early memory clones, whereas persistent secondary stimulation seems to result in

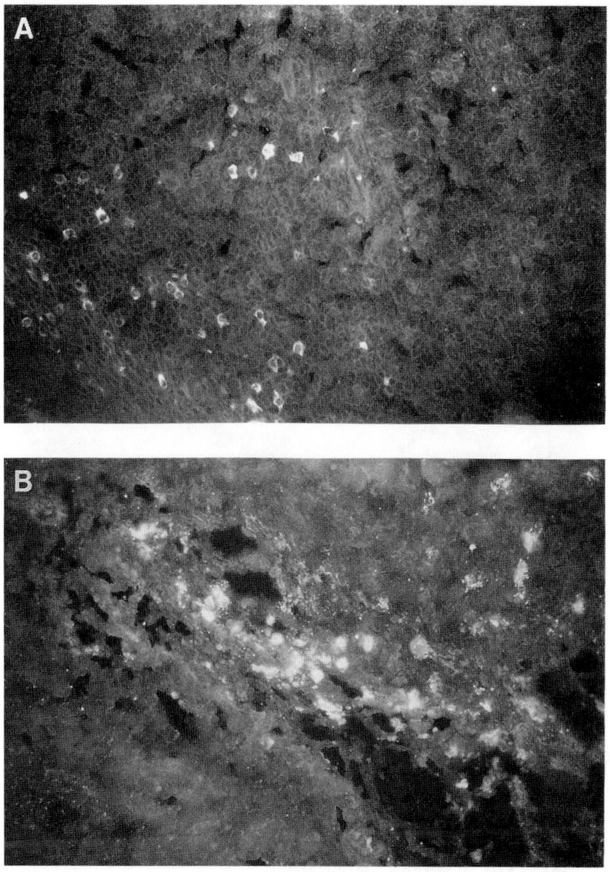

Figure 6 (A) Immunocytes in the extrafollicular zone of the tonsil staining positive for antibody specific for *Streptococcus mutans* (APAAP × 25). (B) Immunohistological localization of *S. mutans* in the middle ear mucosa using fluorescent conjugated antiserum specific for *S. mutans*. Multiple immunocytes are present in the middle ear mucosa. *Streptococcus mutans* is virtually never found in the middle ear. This result is an example of seeding of specific tonsillar B cells that have been stimulated with *S. mutans* and have migrated to a distant area of the upper respiratory tract mucosa (APAAP × 25).

IgD-negative mature memory clones with the potential to produce antibody of higher affinity such as IgG and IgA (Brandtzaeg *et al.*, 1979). As previously mentioned, cells with concomitant production of IgA and J chain are common in the extrafollicular area, but less common in the germinal center. This observation indicates that extensive isotype switching takes place in the early phase of clonal proliferation and differentiation of tonsillar B cells.

Such a clonal development of tonsillar IgA would strengthen the potential of palatine tonsil to act as a putative precursor source for the secretory IgA system similar to BALT and gut-associated lympoid tissue (GALT). Since a substantial number of B cells terminate in the extrafollicular region with concomitant production of IgA and J chain, precursors committed to this phenotype are likely to evade the tonsils and migrate to mucosal glandular tissue. The observation that *in vitro* stimulation of tonsillar lymphocytes with an alimentary antigen (β-lactoglobulin) results mainly in generation of IgA immunocytes from tonsillar lymphoid cells supports the idea that these cells are integrated with the secretory immune system (Paganelli and Levinsky, 1981).

Circumstantial evidence indicates that tonsillar B cells with a potential for J-chain expression may contribute to the secretory immune system in glandular tissue of the upper respiratory tract. Moreover, the fact that nasal IgA antibodies show relatively broad specificity supports the theory that they are products of B-cell clones at an early phase of maturation (Brandtzaeg, 1984). Therefore, the normal tonsil and adenoid, in addition to playing an important role in immune exclusion, also appear to be a source of dimeric J-chain-positive IgA, which is the critical secretory antibody for the mucosa of the upper respiratory tract.

Most important for clinicians is an understanding of events during the disease state. If alterations in the normal immunoglobulin function appear in diseased states of the tonsil, and immune exclusion and immune regulation are dysfunctional, the tonsil will not serve adequately as a first line of defense. As is suggested in subsequent discussion, the tonsil actually may be harmful to the organism, as in the case of autoimmunity associated with focal tonsillitis.

V. IMMUNOLOGICAL CYTOARCHITECTURE OF THE PALATINE AND NASOPHARYNGEAL TONSIL WITH AGE AND INFLAMMATORY DISEASE

Using the technique of image analysis, a quantitative study of the distribution of lymphoid cells in the tonsillar compartments in relation to infection and age has been undertaken (Yamanaka *et al.*, 1992). The distribution of lymphoid cells in the mantle zone, germinal center, extrafollicular area, and subepithelial area of the tonsil was evaluated quantitatively by image analysis in 90 subjects, aged 3 to 66 years. The number of immunoglobulin-positive cells in the tonsil decreased with advancing age in all compartments. This inverse correlation with age was statistically significant for IgD-, IgM-, and IgG-positive cells (Figure 7). The overall change of each T-cell subset with age was smaller than that of immunoglobulin-positive cells. An age-related marked decline was seen for $CD4^+$ cells only in the subepithelial area. KI-67-positive cells, which represent cells undergoing active division, were found mainly in the germinal centers. These cells also diminished in numbers with advancing age. Patients with frequent episodes of tonsillitis demonstrated a significant increase of IgD-positive cells and IgG-positive cells in extrafollicular and subepithelial compartments, and a decrease of $CD4^+$ cells in the germinal center and subepithelial areas. These results suggest that tonsillar involution with age is associated immunologically in all compartments with a decrease in immunoglobulin cells and cells undergoing active division, as demonstrated by KI-67-positive cells (Goding and Burn, 1981).

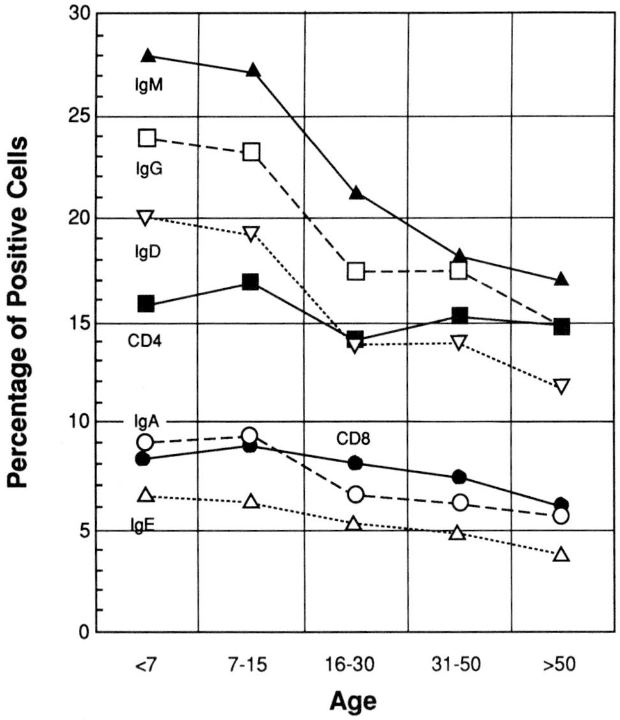

Figure 7 Using the technique of image analysis, a quantitative study of the distribution of lymphoid cells in relation to age is shown. IgM (▲), IgG (□), and IgD (▽) are decreased significantly with advancing age of the tonsil. IgA (○) and IgE (△) remain about the same with increased age, as do CD4 (■) and CD8(●) T cells.

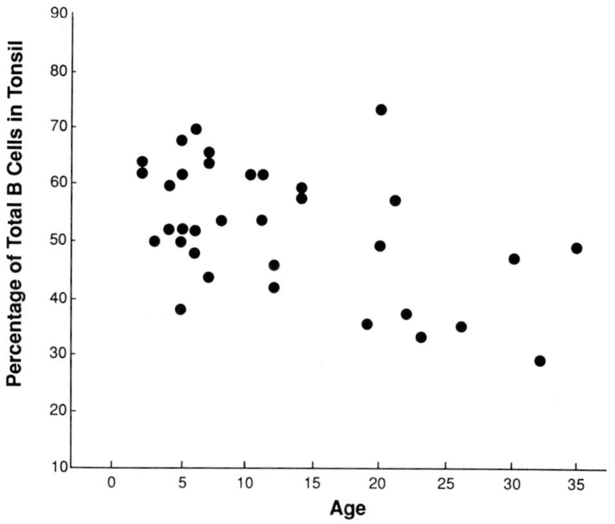

Figure 8 Regression analysis of CD19 (B cells) in the tonsil with increasing age. A highly significant inverse correlation (R^2 = 0.45582) is seen between the number of B cells in the tonsil and age.

On the basis of many other investigations, researchers generally agree that an altered immunological function occurs in the palatine tonsils with age and infection (Bernstein *et al.*, 1988; Brandtzaeg, 1984, 1987; Siegel, 1978; Siegel *et al.*, 1982; Surjan *et al.*, 1978; Surjan, 1980). Using FACS analysis with the monoclonal antibody against CD19, a statistically significant decrease of B cells with age was demonstrated (Figure 8). In addition, a decrease in the number of M cells, which are important APCs in the crypt epithelium, has been suggested (Brandtzaeg, 1987). The most extensive treatise on the immunopathology of tonsillar tissue has been presented by Brandtzaeg (1984,1987). Altered antigen uptake and altered B-cell activity are major problems that may occur in chronic tonsillitis and in the aging tonsil. This altered immunological function may contribute to recurrence of tonsillitis and thereby lead to a vicious cycle. The microenvironmental conditions that best enhance tonsillar proliferation of J-chain-positive IgA B cells may depend on appropriate antigen presentation by M cells found in the reticular crypt epithelium and on particular subsets of regulatory T cells. The putative role of tonsils as precursor sources for the secretory immune system thus is jeopardized by tonsillar disease. Our laboratory has demonstrated that IgD expression in the mantle zone decreases with increased episodes of tonsillitis (Bernstein *et al.*, 1988). Further, marked reduction in IgG immunocytes occurs with many episodes of recurrent tonsillitis. Moreover, HLA-DR-positive cells decrease significantly in the mantle zone; a similar trend is observed in the other compartments. As demonstrated in Figure 3, a significant decrease in J-chain expression by IgA-positive cells occurs in both the follicle and the extrafollicular regions in the tonsils of patients with recurrent tonsillitis, particularly in the germinal center (Brandtzaeg, 1984,1987).

VI. DISTRIBUTION AND ENGRAFTMENT PATTERNS OF HUMAN TONSILLAR MONONUCLEAR CELLS AND IMMUNOGLOBULIN-SECRETING CELLS IN MICE WITH SEVERE COMBINED IMMUNODEFICIENCY: THE ROLE OF EPSTEIN–BARR VIRUS

As mentioned already, the tonsils and adenoids seem the ideal source for lymphocytes seeding into the mucosa of the respiratory tract. The distribution and engraftment of human lymphocytes injected into mice with severe combined immunodeficiency (SCID) are not well understood. In our laboratory, human tonsillar mononuclear cells (hu-TMC) were injected intraperitoneally into SCID mice (Nadal *et al.*, 1991c). The hu-TMC–SCID mouse "chimeras" subsequently were tested for the appearance and distribution of human lymphocytes tagged with H33342 and of immunoglobulin-secreting cells in various systemic and mucosal immunocompetent tissues. This testing was performed by fluorescence microscopy of tissue sections for cells supravitally stained before transfer and by an ELISPOT assay using cells isolated from murine organs. Most importantly, engraftment of hu-TMCs proved to be dependent on the presence of anti-Epstein–Barr virus (EBV) antibody in the donor. hu-TMCs engrafted in decreas-

Table III Human Immunoglobulin-Secreting Cells in Donors and in SCID Mice Showing Engraftment of Human Tonsillar Mononuclear Cells[a,b,c]

	Donors anti-EBV positive			Donors anti-EBV negative		
	IgG	IgA	IgM	IgG	IgA	IgM
Donors	716.8 ± 261.5	126.9 ± 27.8	163.3 ± 24.5	946.5 ± 253.4	131.4 ± 26.1	167.5 ± 53.7
Murine tissue[d]						
Peritoneum	375.9 ± 187.5	64.1 ± 50.2	1403.5 ± 584.0	5.7 ± 5.7	0.3 ± 0.3	0
Liver	238.1 ± 115.8	67.4 ± 29.1	818.4 ± 348.4	1.3 ± 0.9	3.3 ± 3.3	0.1 ± 0.1
Spleen	43.8 ± 19.8	13.9 ± 6.9	197.6 ± 69.3	1.3 ± 0.6	0.1 ± 0.1	0
Bone marrow	10.9 ± 3.6	2.2 ± 0.9	45.4 ± 17.9	1.3 ± 0.5	0.1 ± 0.1	0.7 ± 0.7
Lung	155.2 ± 58.0	32.1 ± 12.2	448.6 ± 219.8	1.4 ± 1.1	1.0 ± 0.5	0.3 ± 0.3
Intestine	0	0	0	0	0	0

[a] IgM-positive cells are predominant in all the murine tissues studied. Also, only donors who were anti-EBV positive had cells that could be engrafted in the SCID mouse. A predilection exists for engraftment in the respiratory tract mucosa, whereas no engraftment occurs in the intestinal mucosa.

[b] SCID mice were injected and sacrificed as described elsewhere. Enumeration of human immunoglobulin-secreting cells (hu-ISC) was done by ELISPOT.

[c] Values are given as mean ± SEM of isotype specific hu-ISC per 10^5 mononuclear cells.

[d] Cell suspensions from murine tissue were enriched for human cells.

ing numbers in the following systemic organs: peritoneum liver, spleen, and bone marrow. Among mucosal tissues tested, hu-TMCs were seen in the lungs but not in the intestines. The engraftment of hu-TMCs in the lung was more extensive than that in the spleen. These studies demonstrate that hu-TMCs engrafted in a variety of murine tissues. The striking presence of hu-TMCs in the lungs compared with the intestines suggests selective engraftment among distinct mucosal tissues (Table III). Further, note that not only are these transferred cells in SCID mice viable and produce immunoglobulin, but they also produce specific antibody against RSV (Nadal *et al.*, 1991a) after intraperitoneal immunization with an activated RSV. These data demonstrate for the first time that hu-TMC–SCID mice will respond to immunization with a viral antigen (Table IV). In other experiments, 5–11 weeks later, 29.4% (10/34) of mice injected with hu-TMCs from EBV-seropositive donors, but none of 34 animals receiving hu-TMCs from EBV-seronegative donors, developed intraabdominal or intraperitoneal tumors ($p = 0.002$) (Nadal *et al.*, 1991b). By *in situ* hybridization using α satellite DNA from human chromosome 17, all tumors resulting after cell transfer from EBV-seropositive donors were identified to be of human origin. Histologically, the tumors resembled large cell lymphomas. EBV genome was detected by *in situ* hybridization and EBV nuclear antigen by immunofluorescence in these tumors. The tumors were poly- or oligoclonal and stained for human IgG, IgM, and, less frequently, IgA and IgD. Human IL-6 was detected in the serum of most of the animals with human lymphomas, but not in any animals without human lymphoma.

Table IV Human Immunoglobulin-Secreting Cells Recovered from Human Tonsillar Mononuclear Cell–SCID Mice Immunized with Respiratory Syncytial Virus[a]

	Positive for RSV-specific hu-ASC[b]			Negative for RSV-specific hu-ASC[c]		
Tissue	IgG	IgA	IgM	IgG	IgA	IgM
Peritoneum	2370 ± 1130	681 ± 615	16961 ± 6799	5237 ± 492	275 ± 216	568 ± 396
Nonmucosal						
Liver	1211 ± 449	722 ± 358	10083 ± 4426	6168 ± 4638	643 ± 466	2073 ± 1977
Spleen	268 ± 117	154 ± 84	2419 ± 807	1008 ± 683	123 ± 56	68 ± 29
Bone marrow	89 ± 37	25 ± 11	558 ± 212	183 ± 80	13 ± 7	10 ± 7
Mucosal						
Lung	1255 ± 618	361 ± 146	5467 ± 2646	3028 ± 1137	360 ± 232	488 ± 299
Intestine	0	0	0	0	0	0

[a] A predilection exists for IgM cells to engraft in the murine tissue. Further, engraftment only occurs in the mucosa of the lung, suggesting the tonsils preferentially engraft to respiratory mucosa rather than to intestinal mucosa.

[b] RSV, Respiratory syncytial virus; hu-ASC, human antibody-secreting cells; $n = 13$.

[c] $n = 4$.

In summary, these observations suggest that a distinct distribution pattern of lymphocytes from human tonsils exists for the respiratory tract. Tonsillar lymphocytes can engraft efficiently into these immunodeficient mice. Further, an immunospot assay to detect human immunoglobulin-secreting cells in cell preparations from various murine organs enriched for human cells strongly indicated that, after engraftment, the cells are not only viable but also functional. Interestingly the relative isotype distribution of human immunoglobulin-secreting cells in engrafted animals shows significant differences from the isotype distribution in the donor-cell suspensions (Table III). Engraftment of hu-TMCs shows an increase of the IgM human immunoglobulin-secreting cell population and a significant decrease in the IgG immunoglobulin population. Analysis of cells isolated from human tonsils also has demonstrated a high death rate of germinal center-derived B cells, which have a high percentage of IgG isotype. The results observed in the SCID mouse experiments may reflect a fast death rate of IgG B cells derived from tonsillar germinal centers. The observations summarized from these experiments also suggest that human tonsillar lymphocytes from EBV-positive children and young adults give rise to large cell lymphomas of human origin when transferred into SCID mice.

VII. TONSIL AS A SOURCE OF AUTOANTIBODY

The concept that altered antigens in the squamous epithelium of the palatine tonsil may serve as a source of autoantibody for diseases of the palms and soles long has been considered (Andrew *et al.*, 1935). Further, several renal diseases, including IgA nephropathy and glomerulonephritis, have been associated with inflammatory diseases of the upper respiratory tract (Miura *et al.*, 1984). In light of modern immunology, secondary disorders caused by focal infection of the tonsils may be considered in the category of autoimmune diseases. The final section of this chapter addresses the relationship between the palatine tonsils and autoimmunity as it may affect the skin.

Pustulosis palmaris et plantaris (PPP) is a chronic recurring disorder of the palms and soles characterized by sterile intraepidermal pustules (Ofuji *et al.*, 1958; Thomsen and Osterbye, 1973; Noda and Ura, 1983). PPP affects women slightly more frequently than men, between the ages of 30 and 60 years. The disease is characterized by numerous pustules and erythematous patches on the palmo-plantar skin (Figure 9; Uehara, 1983; Undeutsch, 1972; Uehara and Ofuji, 1974). The disease tends to have unpredictable excerbations that often occur during periods of acute aggravation of infected foci in the tonsil. The most popular pathogenic theory for PPP is focal infection of the tonsil (Andrew *et al.*, 1935; Thomsen and Osterbye, 1973). Further, several investigators have shown that PPP clears after tonsillectomy (Yamanaka *et al.*, 1983a,1989).

The primary histological change in PPP is a spongiotic vesicle located deep within the epidermis (Figure 10a–d). Mononuclear cells are observed mostly in the involved epidermis and adjacent dermis. As the upper pole of the vesicle comes into contact with the stratum corneum, neutrophils begin to invade the epidermis and gather at the roof of the vesicle. When the vesicle moves upward, neutrophils further accumulate in the vesicle and the eruption becomes completely pustular. The deposition of all major immunoglobulin classes—IgG, IgM, and IgA—or complement fraction C3 in the pustules and intercellular spaces around pustules in patients with PPP has been demonstrated (Husby *et al.*, 1973). These findings, in addition to the fact that the pustulation of PPP takes place only when direct contact between the blister and the stratum corneum occurs, suggests that *in vivo* formation of antigen–antibody complexes in the stratum corneum of lesions of PPP may activate complement via the classical pathway and release chemical mediators such as chemotactic factors, which then trigger the migration of neutrophils at the subcorneal areas of the blisters (Krogh and Tonder, 1970; Tagami and Ofuji, 1978). The proteolytic enzymes thus are released from neutrophils and may cause destruction of the stratum corneum, resulting in the formation of pustules.

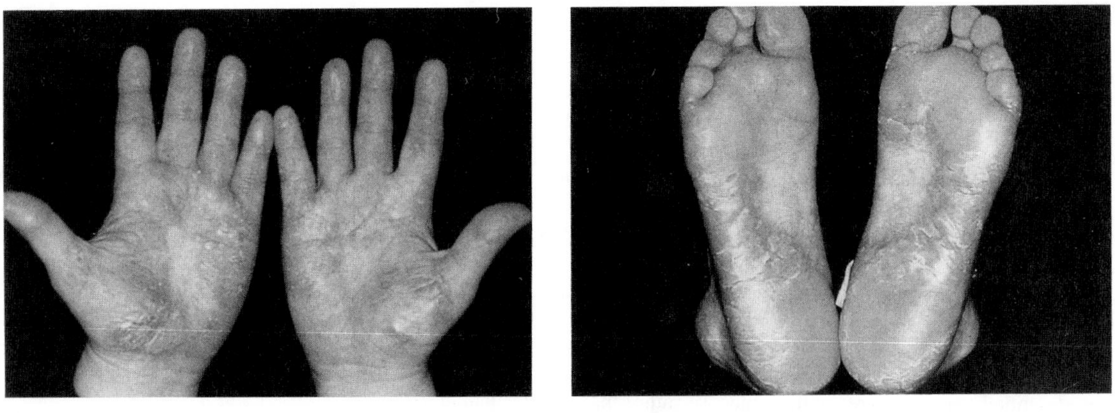

Figure 9 Typical skin lesions of pustulosis palmaris et plantaris (PPP). The disease is characterized by numerous pustules and erythematous patches on palmo-plantar skin.

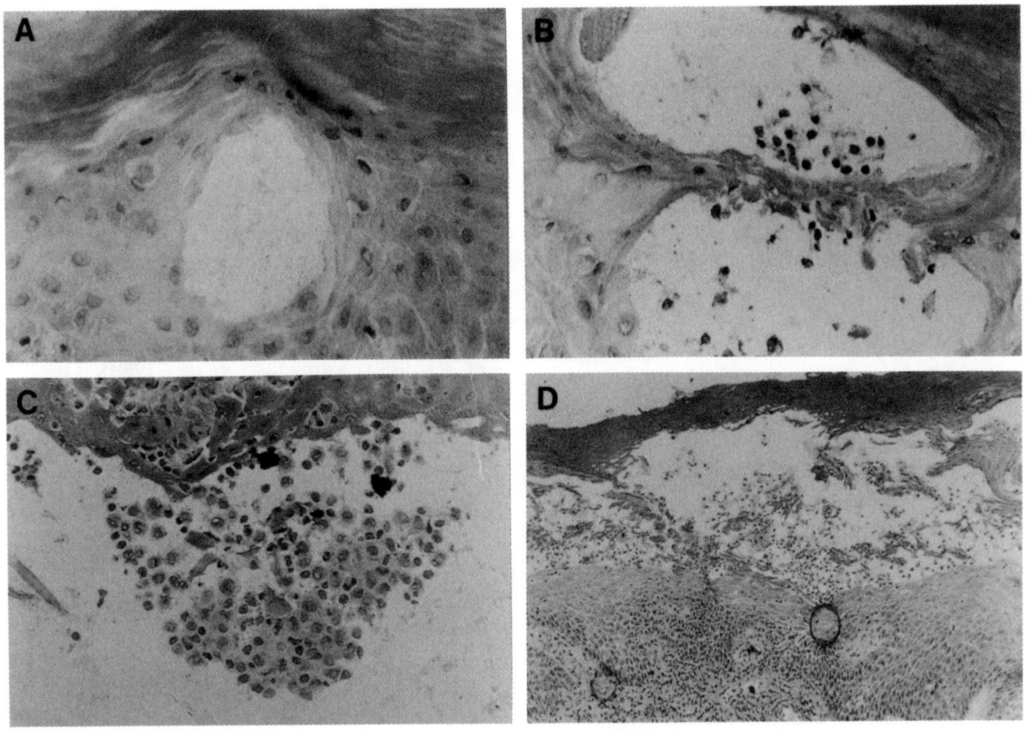

Figure 10 Histopathogenesis of PPP. (A) A spongionic vesicle; (B) mononuclear cells in the involved epidermis and adjacent dermis; (C) neutrophils gather at the center of the roof of the vesicle; (D) the eruption becomes pustular.

The immunopathological hypothesis relating the tonsils to PPP may be related to the structure of the crypt epithelium of the tonsil. The structure of the palatine tonsil, as mentioned earlier, is characterized by numerous crypts and lymphoid follicles. The tonsillar crypts have primary and secondary branches that markedly increase the surface of the tonsil and appear to be the entrance for foreign antigens such as bacteria and viruses that invade the tonsil and provoke an immune response in the tonsil (Maeda and Mogi, 1982). Ono and co-workers (1983b) have demonstrated the presence of a substance resembling the epidermal keratinous layer in the crypt epithelium of tonsil by light and electron microscopic examination. Ultrastructurally, the crypt epithelium contains tonofibrils, and even a structure with a keratin pattern in the upper layer, mixed with parakeratosis. Macrophage-like cells can phagocytose this horny cell-like substance. As shown in Figure 11, keratin-like cells and substances are observed diffusely in the lymphoepithelial symbiosis (LES) and intermingle with mononuclear cells. Therefore, an immune reaction against keratinous substances is very likely to take place in the deep crypt of the tonsil. Yamanaka and co-workers (1983a) demonstrated the presence of considerable numbers of helper T cells in LES; Harabuchi and co-workers (1985) reported the majority of the cells in the site to have membrane or cytoplasmic staining with anti-OKT9 antibody (Figure 12), which recognizes the transferrin receptor on the proliferating cells (Goding and Burn, 1981). These findings, in addition to the presence of a T-dependent response to skin antigen in the tonsils and blast formation of tonsillar lymphocytes but not in peripheral lymphocytes in response to skin extract (Tanaka *et al.*, 1983) strongly support the possibility of naturally occurring immune reactions of tonsillar lymphocytes against keratinous antigens common to both skin and crypt epithelium.

Advances in immunological techniques have made it possible to analyze soluble immune complexes and have brought new insight to the pathogenesis of many disorders with unknown etiology. Attempts to understand the pathophysiological relationship between PPP and the tonsil have been made by investigating immune complexes in the sera of patients with PPP. Yamanaka and co-workers (1983a) reported the presence of circulating immune complexes in the sera of patients with PPP using the $C1_q$-binding assay. Patients in whom a high serum level of immune complexes decreased after tonsillectomy had a remarkable subsequent improvement in their skin lesions.

Using anti-C3 solid-phase enzyme-linked immunosorbent assay (ELISA), soluble immune complexes in the sera of 60 patients with PPP and 20 healthy controls were analyzed. The immune complex level in healthy controls was 1.35 ± 0.2 (S.E.M.) μg aggregated human gammaglobulin equivalent (AHGeq)/ml and 7.12 ± 1.36(S.E.M.) μg AHGeq/ml in patients with PPP ($p < 0.05$). In this study, 35% of patients with PPP were positive for immune complexes. The patient population was classified into four groups according to the outcome of skin lesions more than 6 months after tonsillectomy—healed group, markedly improved group, moderately improved group, and unchanged group. The positive rate of

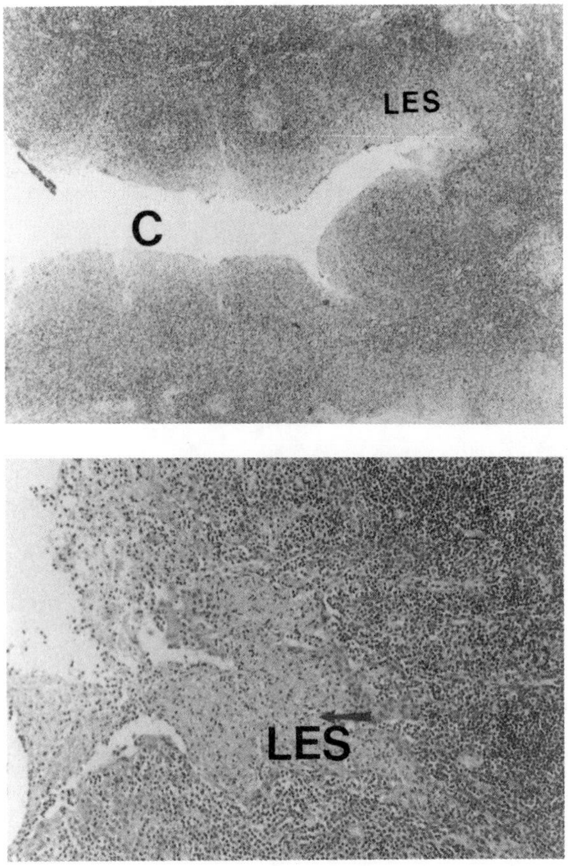

Figure 11 The structure of the lympho-epithelial symbiosis (LES) of the crypt of the tonsil. At the tip of crypt, the epithelium becomes sparse and mixes with mononuclear cells (arrow). C, Crypt.

immune complexes in each group is shown in Figure 13. In a longitudinal study, 62% of patients with PPP had a decrease of immune complex levels to less than 5 μg AHGeq/ml within 6 months of tonsillectomy. Since the immune complex levels in those patients with PPP who showed marked or moderate improvements in skin lesions after tonsillectomy fell to the almost normal range following this procedure, the tonsils may play an important role as a pathogenic focus that releases certain components of immune complexes or even whole immune complexes.

Antikeratin antibodies of the IgG and IgM classes are a constant feature in the sera of patients with PPP (Okamoto *et al.*, 1980; Yamanaka *et al.*, 1989). To clarify the role of antikeratin antibody in the pathogenesis of PPP as well as the relationship between tonsil and the formation of antikeratin antibody, a longitudinal study of antikeratin antibody level after tonsillectomy was performed and compared with the antibody level in individuals who showed no improvement after tonsillectomy.

Solid-phase ELISA on serum samples from 50 patients with PPP and 20 healthy volunteers was used to evaluate antikeratin antibodies. The periods of follow-up for the patients with PPP after tonsillectomy ranged from 6 to 24 months. As shown in Figure 14, the IgM antikeratin antibody level was significantly higher in the healed group and in the markedly improved group, as well as in the moderately improved group, than in the healthy control group. In addition, patients in the healed group and the markedly improved group showed significantly higher IgM antikeratin antibody levels than did those in the unchanged group ($p < 0.05$). With respect to IgG antikeratin antibody, only the moderately improved group showed a significantly higher level than the healthy control group ($p < 0.01$) (Figure 15). These results strongly suggest that IgM antikeratin antibody may play a

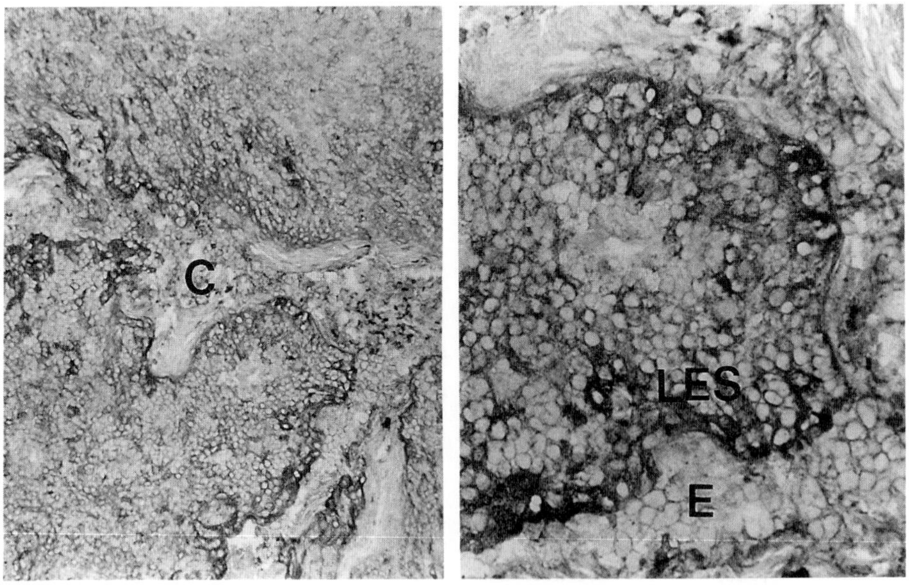

Figure 12 Immunohistology of crypt epithelium stained by OKT9 antibody. The majority of cells in the LES show membrane or cytoplasmic staining. C, Crypt; E, crypt epithelium; LES, lympho-epithelial symbiosis.

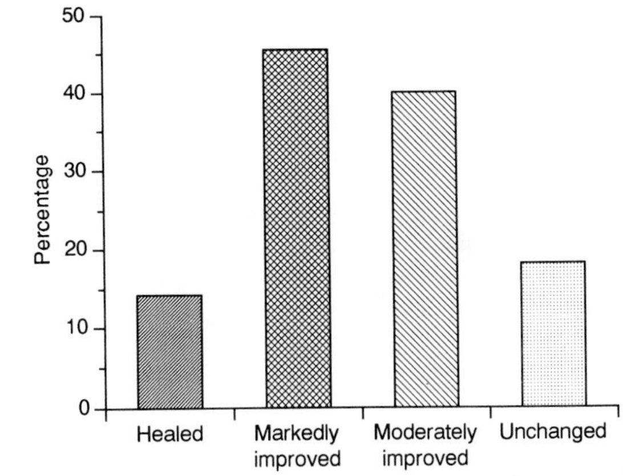

Figure 13 The positive rate of soluble immune complexes in the sera of patients with PPP. Immune complex levels more than 3.0 μg AHG eq/ml is set as positive.

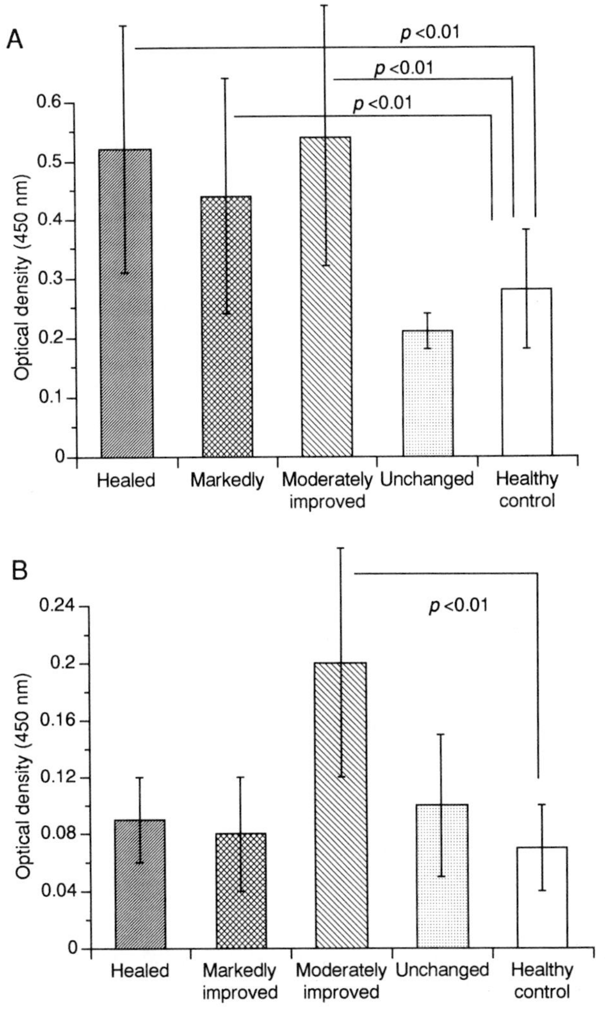

Figure 14 Anti-keratin antibody level in each group classified by the improvement of skin lesions after tonsillectomy. (A) IgM anti-keratin antibody. (B) IgG anti-keratin antibody.

more important role in the formation of pustules in patients who are free of skin lesions or show marked improvement in skin lesions after tonsillectomy, and support the concept that PPP is a tonsil-related immunological disorder.

EBV infects and transforms only human B cells. The tonsil is well known to be a B-cell dominant lymphoid organ (Yamanaka *et al.*, 1992). Further, some investigators have reported that EBV is associated with recurrent tonsillitis (Veltri *et al.*, 1976). In addition, EBV-transformed lymphocytes derived from peripheral blood or bone marrow secrete autoantibodies against various cellular components (Fong *et al.*, 1982; Robinson and Stevens, 1984). The possibility of autoantibody production by tonsillar lymphocytes infected with EBV has been analyzed. Tonsillar lymphocytes obtained from 15 patients with PPP were infected with EBV. Subsequently, transformed cell lines were obtained after incubation for 2–4 wk. Antibody activity against cultured cell line (Hep2)-derived human squamous cell carcinoma was evaluated by indirect immunofluorescence. Culture supernatant reacted with various cellular antigens of Hep2 cells in 4 of 15 patients with PPP. The immunofluorescence patterns were positive for nuclear envelope and cytoskeletal filaments, speckled nuclei, and nucleoli (Figure 14). Note that these autoantibodies were secreted only after EBV transformation. Other investigators (Garzelli *et al.*, 1984; Uhlig *et al.*, 1985) have reported that EBV-transformed lymphocytes produce autoantibodies reactive with various cellular antigens and with antigens in multiple organs, which may play an important role in the pathogenesis of autoimmune diseases. Thus, EBV may even be a trigger in the development of autoantibodies directed against squamous epithelium. The data described in this section, in addition to the anatomical location of the tonsil, show that the palatine tonsil is susceptible to viral and bacterial infections and strongly suggest the tonsil as a source of autoantibody against a number of organ systems.

In conclusion, focal tonsillitis caused by viruses or bacteria may produce altered antigens in the crypts of the tonsil. Both cell-mediated and humoral immunity directed against these altered antigens may produce immune complex disease directed against similar antigens in other parts of the body such as the skin, mesangium of the kidney, and perhaps the costoclavicular joints. Tonsillectomy is a surgical procedure that may reduce the severity of these diseases markedly and, in some cases, abrogate the disease completely (Ono, 1977; and Ono *et al.*, 1983a).

VIII. SUMMARY

This chapter has summarized the immunological characteristics of the lymphoid tissue of the tonsils and adenoids. The mucosa of the upper respiratory tract is protected by a secretory immune system that is under complex immunoregulatory control. B cells with the potential for J-chain expression are stimulated initially in organized mucosa-associated lymphoid tissue in the nasopharyngeal and palatine tonsil. Thereafter they migrate through lymph and blood to glandular sites, such as the paranasal sinuses and other mucosa of the

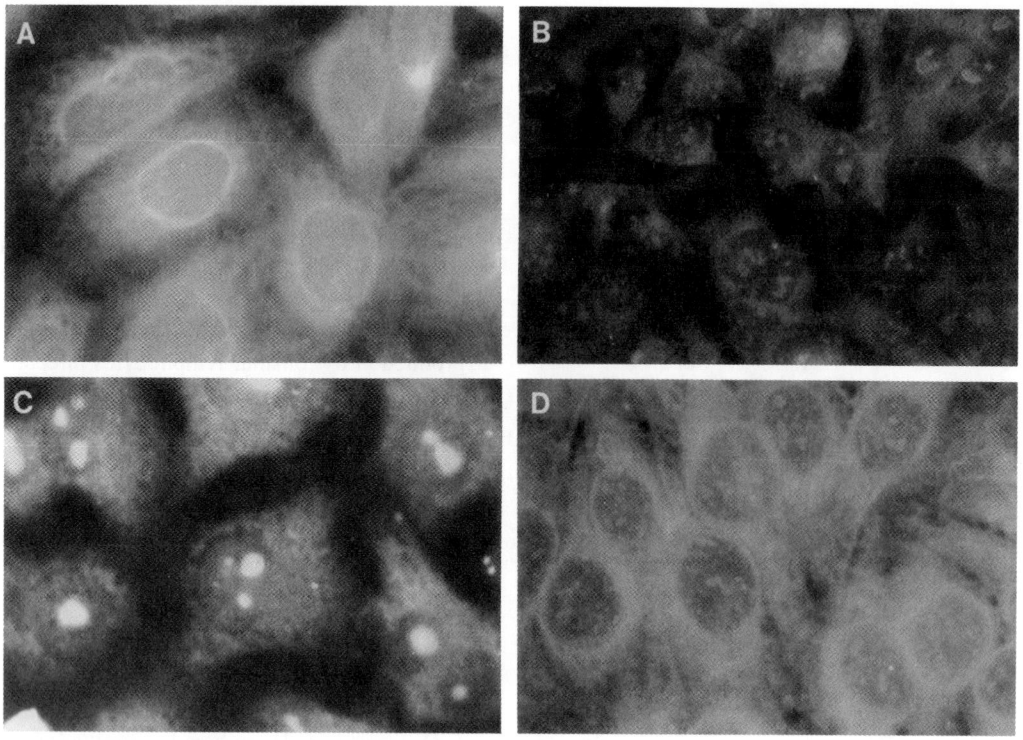

Figure 15 Autoantibodies to various cellular antigens secreted from Epstein–Barr virus (EBV)-transformed tonsillar lymphocytes. Cultures from EBV-transformed tonsillar lymphocytes originated from patients with PPP show positive reaction (A) with nuclear envelope and cytoskeletal filaments, (B) with speckled nuclei and nucleoli, (C) with nucleoli and with speckled nuclei, and (D) with cytoskeletal filaments.

upper respiratory tract, where they differentiate into plasma cells. Normal human lungs lack BALT, which is prominent in certain animal species. Therefore, the major source of B-cell precursors in the upper respiratory tract in humans appears to be the lymphoid tissue of Waldeyer's ring, dominated by the palatine tonsil. The reticular tonsillar crypt epithelium contains macrophages and dendritic cells that may transport antigen to the extrafollicular T-cell areas and the B-cell follicles. Interdigitating APCs are present in the extrafollicular zone and often are surrounded by T lymphocytes that are mainly of the $CD4^+$ (helper) phenotype. Tonsils, therefore, appear to be able to mount both primary and secondary T-cell responses. The preferential production of IgA1 in the upper respiratory tract suggests that the nasopharyngeal and palatine tonsil are responsible for the B cells that colonize the upper respiratory tract.

The capacity of palatine tonsils to generate J-chain-expressing B cells is significantly reduced in children afflicted with recurrent tonsillitis. A consequence of this reduction may be reduced maintenance of early memory B-cell clones that contribute to secretory immunity of the upper respiratory and digestive tract. Aging and chronic inflammation appear to effect APCs as well as B cells in the palatine and nasopharyngeal tonsil. These facts are not necessarily indications for removal of tonsils and adenoids, although chronically infected and aging tonsils may not be able to perform their immunological function in many cases. Work from our laboratory has been reviewed that demonstrates that human tonsillar lymphocytes can engraft SCID mice and produce viable cells that may release specific immunoglobulin against viruses. Finally, the tonsils may play a role in certain autoimmune diseases of the skin and kidney. For the clinician who removes these organs, an understanding of the immunological potential of the tonsils and adenoids is imperative so a wise decision can be made for the maintenance of maximum health of the child or adult.

References

Andrew, G. C., and Machacek, G. F. (1935). Pustular bacterids of the hands and feet. *Arch. Dermatol. Symphilol.* **32,** 837–847.

Bernstein, J. M. (1990). Immunobiology of the tonsils and adenoids. *In* "Instructional Courses" (J. Johnson, A. Blitzer, R. Ossoff, and J. Thomas, eds.), pp. 3–20. Mosby Yearbook, St. Louis, Missouri.

Bernstein, J. M., Scheeren, R., Schoenfeld, E., and Albini, B. (1988). The distribution of immunocompetent cells in the compartments of the palatine tonsils in bacterial and viral infections of the upper respiratory tract. *Acta. Otolaryngol.* (*Stockh.*) (*Suppl. 1*) **454,** 153–162.

Bernstein, J. M., Sendor, S., and Wactawski-Wende, J. (1991). Antigen presenting cells (APC) in the nasopharyngeal tonsil: A quantitative immunochemical study. Paper presented at the Second International Symposium on Tonsils, Pavia, Italy. September, 1991.

Besredka, A. (1919). De la vaccination contre les estats est typhoides par la boie buccale. *Ann. Inst. Pasteur* **33,** 883–903.

Brandtzaeg, P. (1974). Presence of J-chain in human immunocytes in man. *Nature* (*London*) **252,** 418–420.

Brandtzaeg, P. (1984). Immune functions of human nasal mucosa and tonsils in health and disease. *In* "Immunology of the Lung and Upper Respiratory Tract" (J. Bienenstock, ed.), pp. 28–95. McGraw-Hill, New York.

Brandtzaeg, P. (1987). Immune functions and immunopathology of the palatine and nasopharyngeal tonsils. *In* "Immunology of the Ear" (J. M. Bernstein and P. L. Ogra, eds.), pp. 63–106. Raven Press, New York.

Brandtzaeg, P. (1991). Immunology and immunopathology of the tonsils. Paper presented at the Second International Symposium on Tonsils, Pavia, Italy. September, 1991.

Brandtzaeg, P., Surjan, L., and Berdal, P. (1978). Immunoglobulin systems of human tonsils I. Control subjects of various ages: Quantification of IgE-producing cells, tonsillar morphometry, and serum Ig-concentrations. *Clin. Exp. Immunol.* **31,** 367–381.

Brandtzaeg, P., Gjeruldsen, S., Korsrud, F., and Bakline, K. (1979). The human secretory immune system shows striking heterogeneity with regard to involvement of J-chain positive IgD immunocytes. *J. Immunol.* **122,** 503–510.

Conley, M., and Bartelt, M. (1984). *In vitro* regulation of IgA subclass synthesis. II. The source of IgA_2 plasma cells. *J. Immunol.* **133,** 2312–2316.

Fong, S., Vaughan, J. H., Tsoukas, C. D., and Carson, D. A. (1982). Selective induction of autoantibody secretion in human bone marrow by Epstein–Barr virus. *J. Immunol.* **129,** 1941–1945.

Garzelli, C., Taub, F. E., Scharff, J. E., Prabkakar, B. S., Ginsberg-Fellner, F., and Notkins, A. L. (1984). Epstein–Barr virus-transformed lymphocytes produce monoclonal autoantibodies that react with antigens in multiple organs. *J. Virol.* **52,** 722–725.

Goding, J. W., and Burn, G. F. (1981). Monoclonal antibody OKT9 recognizes the receptor for transferrin on human acute lymphocytic leukemia cells. *J. Immunol.* **127,** 1256–1258.

Harabuchi, Y., Yamanaka, N., and Kataura, A. (1985). Immunohistological identification of B cell differentiation in human tonsillar follicles by using monoclonal antibodies. *Tohoku J. Exp. Med.* **147,** 21–31.

Harabuchi, Y., Hamamoto, N., Shirasaki, H., Asakura, K., and Matsuyama, H. (1989). Specific immune response of the adenoids to a respiratory antigen. *Am. J. Otolaryngol.* **10,** 138–142.

Heinen, E., Lilet-Leclerc, G., Mason, D., Stein, H., Boniver, J., Radoux, D., Kinet-Dendel, C., and Simar, L. J. (1984). Isolation of follicular dendritic cells from human tonsils and adenoids. II. Immunocytochemical characterization. *Eur. J. Immunol.* **14,** 267–273.

Husby, G., Rajka, G., and Larsen, T. E. (1973). Immunofluorescence studies in pustulosis palmoplantaris. *Acta. Derm. Venereol.* (*Stockh.*) **53,** 123–126.

Junqueira, L., and Carneiro, J. (1980). "Basic Histology." Lang Medical Publishing, Los Altos, California.

Kett, L., Brandtzaeg, P., Radl, J., and Haaijman, J. (1986). Different subclass distribution of IgA producing cells in human lymphoid organs and various secretory tissues. *J. Immunol.* **136,** 3631–3635.

Krogh, H. K., and Tonder, O. (1970). Subcorneal pustular dermatosis: Pathogenetic aspects. *Br. J. Dermatol.* **83,** 429–435.

Lanier, L. L., Engelman, E. G., Gatenby, P., Babcock, G. F., Warner, N. L., and Herzenberg, L. A. (1983). Correlation of functional properties of human lymphoid cell subsets and surface marker phenotypes using multiparameter analysis and flow cytometry. *Immunol. Rev.* **74,** 143–160.

Maeda, S., and Mogi, M. (1982). Microcrypt extensions of tonsillar crypts. *Ann. Otol. Rhinol. Laryngol.* **91,** 1–8.

Meistrup-Larson, K., Mogensen, H., Helweg-Larson, K., Pirmin H., Anderson, V., Ryguard, J., and Sorensen, H. (1980). Studies on lymphoid cells of adenoid tissue and relation to clinical findings. *O.R.L.* **42,** 158–170.

Mestecky, J., *et al.* (1971). Immunoglobulin and secretory immunoglobulin A: Evidence for a common polypeptide chain different from light changes. *Nature* (*London*) **170,** 1163–1165.

Miura, M., Tomino, Y., Suga, T., Endoh, M., Nomoto, Y., and Sakai, H. (1984). Increase of proteinuria and/or microhematuria following upper respiratory tract infections in patients with IgA nephropathy. *Tokai J. Exp. Clin. Med.* **9,** 139–145.

Nadal, D., Albini, B., Schläpfer, E., Chen, C., Brodsky, L., and Ogra, P. L. (1991a). Tissue distribution of mucosal antibody producing cells specific for respiratory syncytial virus in severe combined immunodeficiency (SCID) mice engrafted with human tonsils. *Clin. Exp. Immunol.* **85,** 358–364.

Nadal, D., Albini, B., Schläpfer, E., Bernstein, J. M., and Ogra P. L. (1992). Role of Epstein–Barr virus and interleukin-6 in the development of lymphomas of human origin in SCID mice engrafted with human tonsillar mononuclear cells. *J. Gen. Virol.* **73,** 113–121.

Nadal, D., Albini, B., Chen, C., Schläpfer, E., Bernstein, J. M., and Ogra P. L. (1991c). Distribution and engraftment patterns of human tonsillar mononuclear cells in mice with severe combined immunodeficiency. The role of Epstein–Barr virus. *Int. Arch. Allerg. Appl. Immunol.* **95,** 341–351.

Nadal, D., Soh, N., Schläpfer, E., Bernstein, J. M., and Ogra P. L. (1992b). Distribution characteristics of immunoglobulin secreting cells in adenoids. Relationship to age and disease. *Int. J. Pediatr. Otorhinolaryngol.* **24,** 121–130.

Noda, Y., and Ura, M. (1983). Pustulosis palmaris et plantaris due to tonsillar focal infections *Acta Otolaryngol.* (*Stockh.*) *Suppl.* **401,** 22–30.

Ofuji, S., Matsubara, T., and Watanabe, S. (1958). On pustulosis palmaris et plantaris. *Acta Dermatol.* **53,** 385–389.

Ogra, P. L. (1971). Effect of tonsillectomy and adenoidectomy on nasopharyngeal antibody response to polio virus. *N. Engl. J. Med.* **284,** 59–64.

Okamoto, H., Danno, K., and Ofuji, S. (1980). Anti-keratin layer antibody in pustulosis palmaris et plantaris. *Nishinihon J. Dermatol.* **43,** 301–305.

Ono, T. (1977). Evaluation of tonsillectomy as a treatment for pustulosis palmaris et plantaris. *J. Dermatol.* (*Tokyo*) **4,** 163–168.

Ono, T., Jono, M., Kito, M., *et al.* (1983a). Evaluation of tonsillectomy as a treatment for Pustulosis palmaris et plantaris. *Acta Otolaryngol.* (*Stockh.*) **401,** 12–16.

Ono, T., Jono, M., and Kageshita, T. (1983b). Morphological and immunological studies on Pustulosis palmaris et plantaris, especially on its focal infection theory. *Acta Otolaryngol.* (*Stockh.*) *Suppl.* **401,** 17–21.

Owen, R., and Nemanic, P. (1978). Antigen processing structures of the mammalian intestinal tract: A SEM of lymphoepithelial organs. *Scan. Electron. Microsc.* **2,** 367–378.

Paganelli, R., and Levinsky, R. (1981). Differences in specific antibody response of human tonsillar cells to an oral and a parenteral antigen. *Scand. J. Immunol.* **14,** 353–358.

Paradise, J., and Bluestone, C. (1976). Toward rational indications for tonsil and adenoid surgery. *Hosp. Pract.* **11,** 79–87.

Perry, M., Mustaf, Y., and Brown, K. (1991). The microvasculature of the human palatine tonsil and its role in homing of lymphocytes. Paper presented at the Second International Symposium on Tonsils, Pavia, Italy. September, 1991.

Robinson, J. E., and Stevens, K. C. (1984). Production of autoantibodies cellular antigens by human B cells transformed by Epstein–Barr virus. *Clin. Immunol. Immunopathol.* **33,** 339–350.

Rynnel-Dagoo, B. (1976). The immunological function of the adenoid. *Acta Otolaryngol.* **82,** 196–198.

Rynnel-Dagoo, B. (1978). Polyclonal activation to immunoglobulin secretion in human adenoid lymphocytes induced from bacteria in nasopharynx in vitro. *Clin. Exp. Immunol.* **34,** 402–410.

Scicchitano, R., Ernst, E., and Bienenstock, P. (1987). Respiratory tract lymphoid tissue and other affector cells. *In* "Immunology of the Ear" (J. M. Bernstein and P. L. Ogra, eds.), pp. 107–134. Raven Press, New York.

Siegel, G. (1978). Description of age-depending cellar changes in the human tonsil. *O.R.L.* **40,** 160–171.

Siegel, G., Linse, R., and Macheleidt, S. (1982). Factors of tonsillar involution: Age-dependent changes in B-activation and Langerhans' cell density. *Arch. Otorhinolaryngol.* **236,** 261–269.

Soh, N., Nadal, D., Schläpfer, E., Bernstein, J. M., and Ogra P. (1991). Immunological response of adenoidal lymphocytes to respiratory syncytial virus. *Ann. Otol. Rhinol. Laryngol.* **101,** 848–853.

Stein, H., Bonk, A., Tolksdorf, G., Lennert, K., Rodt, H., and Gerdes, J. (1980). Immunohistologic analysis of the organization of normal lymphoid tissue and non-Hodgkin's lymphomas. *J. Histochem. Cytochem.* **28,** 746–760.

Sugiyama, N. (1991). Influences of IL6 on proliferation and differentiation of tonsillar lymphocytes and detection of IL6 producing cells in tonsil. Paper presented at the Second International Symposium on Tonsils, Pavia, Italy. September, 1991.

Surjan, L. (1980). Reduced lymphoid activation in repeatedly inflamed human tonsils. *Acta Otolaryngol.* **89,** 187–194.

Surjan, L., Brandtzaeg, P., and Burdall, P. (1978). Immunoglobulin systems of human tonsils. II. Patients with chronic tonsillitis or tonsillar hyperplasia: Quantification of Ig-producing cells, tonsillar morphometry and serum Ig concentrations. *Clin. Exp. Immunol.* **31,** 382–390.

Tagami, H., and Ofuji, S. (1978). A leukotactic factor in the stratum corneum of Pustulosis palmaris et plantaris: A possible mechanism for the formation on intra-epidermal sterile pustules. *Acta Dermatol.* (*Stockh.*) **58,** 401–408.

Tanaka, N., Ichino, Y., Ikawa, T., and Ishiwawa, T. (1983). Immunological study of pustulosis palmaris et plantaris—Blastoid transformation of tonsil and peripheral blood lymphocytes by stimulation with human skin extract. *Acta Otolaryngol.* (*Stockh.*) *Suppl.* **401,** 68–74.

Tew, J., Thornbacke, J., and Steinman, R. M. (1982). Dendritic cells in the immune response. *J. Reticuloendothel. Soc.* **31,** 371–380.

Tew, J., Kosco, M., and Szakal, A. (1989). An alternative antigen pathway. *Immunol. Today* **10,** 229–231.

Thomsen, K., and Osterbye, P. (1973). Pustolosis palmaris et plantaris. *Br. J. Dermatol.* **89,** 293–302.

Tomasi, T., and Zigelbaum, S. (1963). The selective occurrence of IgA in certain body fluids. *J. Clin. Invest.* **42,** 1552–1560.

Tsubota, H., Ohguro, S., and Kataura, A. (1991). The role of integrin in tonsils. Paper presented at the Second International Symposium on Tonsils, Pavia, Italy. September, 1991.

Uehara, M. (1983). Pustulosis palmaris et plantaris-A review of clinical features and aggravating factors. *Acta Otolaryngol.* (*Stockh.*) *Suppl.* **401,** 7–11.

Uehara, M., and Ofuji, S. (1974). The morphogenesis of pustulosis palmaris et plantaris. *Arch. Dermatol.* **109,** 518–525.

Uhlig, H., Rutter, H., and Dernick, R. (1985). Self-reactive B lymphocytes detected in young adults, children and newborn after *in vitro* infection with Epstein–Barr virus. *Clin. Exp. Immunol.* **62,** 75–84.

Veltri, R. W., Sprinkle, P. M., and McClung, J. E. (1976). Epstein–Barr virus associated with episodes of recurrent tonsillitis. *Arch. Otolaryngol.* **101,** 552–556.

Woloschak, G., Liarakos, C., and Tomasi T. (1986). Identification of the major immunoglobulin heavy chain poly A RNA in murine lymphoid tissues. *Mol. Immunol.* **23,** 645–653.

Yamanaka, N., and Kataura, A. (1984). Viral infections associated with recurrent tonsillitis. *Acta Otolaryngol.* (*Stockh.*) *Suppl.* **416,** 30–37.

Yamanaka, N., Sambe, S., and Kataura, A. (1983a). A conceptual understanding of pustulosis palmaris et plantaris as an immune complex disease due to focal tonsillar infection. *Acta Otolaryngol.* (*Stockh.*) *Suppl.* **401,** 31–35.

Yamanaka, N., Sambe, S., Harabuchi, Y., and Kataura, A. (1983b). Immunological study of tonsil. Distribution of T cell subsets. *Acta Otolaryngol.* (*Stockh.*) **96,** 509–516.

Yamanaka, N., Shido, F., and Kataura, A. (1989). Tonsillectomy-induced changes in anti-keratin antibodies in patients with pustulosis palmaris et plantaris: A clinical correlation. *Acta Otolaryngol.* (*Stockh.*) **246,** 109–112.

Yamanaka, N., Matsuyama, H., Harabuchi, Y., and Kataru, A. (1992). Distribution of lymphoid cells in tonsillar compartments in relation to infection and age. *Acta Otolaryngol.* (*Stockh.*) **112,** 128–137.

Section H

Mammary Gland

Section Editor: M. E. Lamm

(Chapters 51 and 52)

51

Immunological Components of Milk: Formation and Function

Randall M. Goldblum • Armond S. Goldman

I. INTRODUCTION

Among the external secretions, milk is unique in its complexity and high concentrations of mucosal immune products. This chapter explores the nature of that uniqueness and attempts to explain its basis. Throughout the chapter, we emphasize human milk since it differs significantly from that of other nonprimate species. However, because bovine milk commonly is consumed by humans, particularly infants and children, we contrast human and bovine milk when major differences are known. The immunological outcomes of breast-feeding in the infant are discussed in Chapter 52.

The high degree of complexity of human milk, relative to the other external secretions, apparently has evolved to provide key factors for the nutritional, metabolic, and immunological needs of the infant. If the lactating woman is nourished adequately, her milk will contain essentially all the nutrients required by the infant for at least the first 6 months of life. In addition, many immunological factors are present in human milk, presumably to protect the lactating mammary gland and the nursing infant from pathogenic microorganisms. The immunological constituents of milk must enhance the probability that maternally derived nutrients will be transferred to the infant without contamination or degradation, so they can be used optimally for the growth and development of the infant.

Another source of complexity of human milk is the dynamic change in composition that occurs during lactation. In this sense, milk is really a series of secretions that is produced as lactation progresses and the infant matures. An interesting speculation is that the changes in milk composition are timed to respond to changing needs of the infant, whose own mucosal immune system is developing rapidly.

In trying to understand the function of the immunological factors in milk, we must recognize that the *in vivo* fate and functions have been demonstrated to date for a limited number of the factors. In particular, limited information exists concerning the distribution, survival, and function of immunological factors within the infant.

Finally, evidence suggests that the immunological impact on the infant of the feeding of human milk may not be totally passive in nature. Some milk factors may interact with factors produced by the infant, whereas others may act as stimuli for the development of the infant's own mucosal immune system. Thus, milk may be part of a dynamic mother–infant interaction that supports the newborn infant's growth and immunological development to a level that enhances the chances of survival in the extrauterine environment.

II. ANATOMY, CELL BIOLOGY, AND PHYSIOLOGY OF MILK PRODUCTION

A. General Features

The human mammary gland is a compound tubuloalveolar organ. The glandular secretions empty into ducts that coalesce as they course through the stroma of the breast toward the nipple. During pregnancy, the number and size of the alveolar clusters increase until, at parturition, 70% of the gland is composed of parenchymal tissue. The process of lactation is modulated by hormones including prolactin, insulin, and growth hormone. The release of some of these hormones, particularly prolactin, is triggered by a neurosensory–endocrine pathway that is initiated by nursing. The autocrine and paracrine events that control lactation remain poorly defined.

B. Secretory Pathways

Four pathways exists for the secretion of milk components. The first one is responsible for secretion of many of the aqueous components of milk including casein, α-lactalbumin, and lactose. Caseins, after translation, are transferred to the Golgi apparatus, where they are phosphorylated or glycosylated. As these proteins pass from the terminal cisternae of the Golgi compartment into secretory vesicles, their concentration increases to the millimolar range, causing aggregation of the casein molecules into micelles (Morr *et al.*, 1971). The secretory vesicles migrate to the apical membrane, fuse with it, and release their contents by exocytosis. One prominent milk protein, α-lactalbumin, forms a complex with the enzyme galactosyltransferase in the Golgi, where the complex catalyze the synthesis of lactose. The osmotic activity of this disaccharide draws water and presumably ions into the Golgi, providing the driving force for fluid secretion.

The second or apocrine pathway is responsible for secretion of milk fat. The substrate for milk fat synthesis derives from two sources. Fatty acids are synthesized from glucose by mammary alveolar cells that contain fatty acid synthetase. These fatty acids have somewhat shorter chain lengths (10–16 carbons) than those synthesized in adipose tissue because of the presence of a mammary gland-specific enzyme called thioesterase II. In addition, plasma triacylglycerols are cleaved within the mammary gland by the enzyme lipoprotein lipase. The resulting fatty acids are transported into the mammary alveolar cells, where they are reesterified with glycol to make the neutral fat molecules that coalesce to form milk fat globules. Alveolar cells have a columnar shape with copious endoplasmic reticulum surrounding the nucleus in the basal region. During milk secretion, the Golgi apparatus and secretory vesicles become more numerous toward the apical pole. Abundant cytoplasmic lipid droplets enlarge as they move toward the luminal end of the cell. As they press into the apical plasma membrane, the droplets are released into the milk as membrane-bound milk fat globules (Moyer-Mileur and Chan, 1989). Other globules that are formed during this process contain fewer lipids but larger amounts of other cytoplasmic constituents (Patton and Huston, 1985).

The third pathway transports certain small molecules including sodium, potassium, chloride, and glucose across the apical membrane of the cell. The secretion of the monovalent ions is effected by the electrical gradient across this membrane.

The fourth pathway transfers proteins and possible other substances from the interstitial space to the lumen using receptors and intracellular vesicles. This mechanism will be considered in the description of the formation of secretory IgA (SIgA) in milk via polymeric immunoglobulin receptors.

Finally, in addition to soluble components, certain cells and cellular membranes enter human colostrum and milk. Epithelial cells or their membranes are shed directly into milk. Most B cells that home to the mammary gland remain sessile, whereas many T cells, macrophages, and neutrophils that have entered the lamina propria pass through the intercellular junctions of alveolar cells into the milk (Brandtzaeg, 1983). The mechanisms that attract the leukocytes to the mammary gland and trigger the migration of those cells into the milk are considered in a subsequent section.

C. *Milk Ejection*

Milk secretions are stored in the alveoli and small ducts until they are ejected during nursing. Epithelial cells of the alveoli and ductules are surrounded by contractile basket-like epithelial cells. The ejection of milk from the breast is mediated by neuroendocrine events that culminate in the contraction of those myoepithelial cells. As a result of stimulation of sensory nerves at the nipple and areola during nursing, oxytocin is released from the hypothalamus into the posterior lobe of the pituitary gland and then into the peripheral circulation. Oxytocin triggers myoepithelial cells to contract, forcing milk into the larger ducts and finally through the orifice of the nipple.

III. COMPOSITION OF MILK

A. *Cellular Elements in Milk*

Human milk from early in lactation differs from most other external secretions because it contains viable leukocytes. The concentration of leukocytes is highest in colostrum and declines rapidly during the first months of lactation. Table I displays estimates of the numbers of neutrophils, macrophages, and lymphocytes in human milk during the first months of lactation. These numbers are based on morphological characterisitics. However, distinguishing neutrophils from macrophages in human milk is difficult because the morphology of both cells is dominated by the large amount of lipid-containing vesicles in the cytoplasm (Smith and Goldman, 1968). The mechanism by which maternal leukocytes enter the milk is poorly understood. However, one potentially important clue to this process is the finding that essentially all these cells have surface markers or physiological features of activated cells. Since most of the surface markers of activation on milk leukocytes are also present on leukocytes found in sites of inflammation, and are known to be important in homing and egress of leukocytes from the vascular compartment, the mechanism of migration of leukocytes into the milk may be similar to that involved in inflammation. Although the array and mechanisms of production of inflammatory mediators in the lactating mammary gland are not well understood, several cytokines that may be involved in leukocyte migration have been detected in human milk, as described in later sections of this chapter. The following sections discuss our current knowledge of the morphology and *in vitro* function of the milk leukocytes.

1. Macrophages

Macrophages may have been first photographed in human milk by the French microscopist Alfred Donné (1844). How-

Table I Estimated Mean (std) Concentration ($\times 10^9$/ml) of Leukocytes in Human Milk by Phase of Lactation[a]

	2–3 days	4 wk	24 wk	52 wk
Macrophages/neutrophils	3.6 (2.7)	0.06 (0.12)	0.04 (0.09)	<0.01
Lymphocytes	0.2 (0.1)	0.02 (0.03)	0.01 (0.02)	<0.01

[a] Adapted with permission from Goldman *et al.* (1982).

ever, little attention was paid to the cells in milk until Smith and Goldman (1968) described milk cells with the morphology and phagocytic activity consistent with activated macrophages. The concentration of macrophages in early milk is usually greater than that of their counterparts in peripheral blood, the monocytes.

More recent studies have demonstrated that the milk macrophages are more motile than their counterparts in blood (Özkaragöz *et al.*, 1988; Mushtaha *et al.*, 1989) and display a pattern of surface markers associated with activation (Keeney *et al.*, 1993). These cells also actively produce toxic oxygen radicals (Tsuda *et al.*, 1984). Attributing other activities to the milk macrophages is difficult since most studies of milk leukocytes have used unseparated cells. The role of the milk macrophage *in vivo* has not been established.

2. Polymorphonuclear Leukocytes

Early in lactation, the concentration of neutrophils in milk approaches that in peripheral blood (Table I). Neutrophils in human milk have been demonstrated to be phagocytic (Smith and Goldman, 1968). However, the adherence, response to chemotactic factors, and motility of these cells are less than those of neutrophils from peripheral blood (Thorpe *et al.*, 1986; Özkaragöz *et al.*, 1988). Studies of surface markers suggest that some of these functional features may be the result of prior activation of the neutrophils (Keeney *et al.*, 1993). Activation of neutrophils may occur during the process of egression from the vascular space, may relate to the process by which large numbers of milk globules are engulfed by neutrophils in milk, or may be the result of exposure to cytokines demonstrated to exist in milk (see subsequent text).

3. Lymphocytes

Although the concentration of lymphocytes in human milk is small relative to that in peripheral blood, these cells are consistently present in milk obtained during the first few months of lactation. Approximately 80% of milk lymphocytes are T cells (Wirt *et al.*, 1992). The precise distribution of T-cell subpopulations in milk lymphocytes is controversial, since different investigators have reported numbers of $CD4^+$ and $CD8^+$ cells similar to those in peripheral blood (Keller *et al.*, 1986), a $CD8^+$-cell predominance (Richie *et al.*, 1982), or moderate increase in the proportion of $CD8^+$ cells relative to peripheral blood (Wirt *et al.*, 1992). These differences may be the result of selection of certain subsets during the fractionation of milk or of the analytic limitations of direct fluorescent microscopy. These problems were avoided in the last study by using flow cytometry of unfractionated milk (Wirt *et al.*, 1992). As in the case for other milk leukocytes, the increased display of certain surface phenotypic markers, including CD45RO, CD25 (IL-2R), and HLA-DR, suggests that the T lymphocytes are activated memory cells (Wirt *et al.*, 1992).

Milk lymphocytes can be activated to proliferate using mitogens, but their responses are weaker than those of peripheral blood T cells (Parmely *et al.*, 1976; Goldblum *et al.*, 1981). The spectrum of antigen-specific responses, as measured by proliferation, is thought to differ from that of peripheral blood lymphocytes from the same donor (Parmely *et al.*, 1976), but the T-cell receptor repertoire of milk T lymphocytes has not been investigated. Although evidence exists for the production of interferon (Emodi and Just, 1974; Keller *et al.*, 1981; Bertotto *et al.*, 1990) and monocyte chemotactic factor (Keller *et al.*, 1981), the full array of cytokines produced by milk cells has not been determined.

B. Particulate Structure of Milk

In addition to viable cells, several different types of particles are suspended in human milk, including casein micelles, globules packed with lipid, and globular structures containing less lipid but more cytoplasmic structures (Patton and Huston, 1985). With low speed centrifugation, some of these particles sediment with the cells whereas many of the membrane-bound lipid-filled particles rise to the surface and coalesce. Understanding this particulate structure of milk may be important, since several studies suggest that some host defense factors are compartmentalized within these structures. For instance, centrifugation of human milk causes the concentration of lysozyme to increase approximately fivefold over the value obtained by sampling milk prior to centrifugation (Goldblum *et al.*, 1975). Crago *et al.* (1979) demonstrated that some of the SIgA antibodies in human milk are contained in lipid-filled particles. Little is known about the direct effects on host defenses of the particles suspended in human milk, although some of them may be neutrophil activators (Keeney *et al.*, 1992) or may interfere with the attachment of enterobacteria to epithelial cells (Schroten *et al.*, 1992).

C. Soluble Factors in Milk

1. Proteins and Peptides

a. Immunoglobulins and Ig transport fragments. The major class of immunoglobulins in human milk is IgA. In contrast, mature cow's milk contains predominantly IgG. The structure and function of SIgA, which makes up at least 80% of the milk IgA, is discussed in Chapters 7 and 11, respectively. Chapter 21 considers the distribution and characteristics of the cells that produce immunoglobulins within the mammary gland. The demonstration of a very high density of IgA1- and IgA2-producing cells in the lactating mammary gland (Brandtzaeg, 1983) helps explain why human colostrum and milk contain the highest concentrations of SIgA of any secretions. The high proportion of SIgA in human milk of the IgA2 isotype (~40%) relative to plasma (10%) also must be related to the isotype distribution of these cells in the mammary gland. These findings also provide evidence that most of the IgA secreted into the milk is produced locally within the breast, rather than transported from the plasma.

The mechanism of antigenic sensitization and migration of IgA-committed B cells into the mammary gland is considered in several earlier chapters. Briefly, current evidence indicates that many of the IgA antibody responses detected in human milk originate from antigenic stimulation at specialized mucosal sites in the intestinal and respiratory tracts

(Goldblum *et al.*, 1975; Roux *et al.*, 1977). IgA-committed B cells emerging from mucosal sites, such as Peyer's patches in the small intestine, migrate preferentially to other mucosal sites, including the lactating mammary gland. Migration to the mammary gland is under hormonal regulation (Weisz-Carrington *et al.*, 1978). The wide array of specific antibodies found in human milk suggests that some of these cells are derived from memory B cells rather than from recent antigenic exposure. In the breast, B cells mature into plasma cells, the predominant product of which is polymeric IgA.

As in other secretory mucosae, transport of immunoglobulins into colostrum and milk is accomplished predominantly by the polymeric immunoglobulin receptor (PIgR). Chapter 10 describes in detail the mechanism by which PIgR mediates specific binding, endocytosis, and transcellular transport of immunoglobulins. Proteolytic cleavage of PIgR at the apical membrane of the mammary alveolar cell releases the polymeric IgA molecule, covalently complexed to a fragment of PIgR termed secretory component (SC). This complex is called SIgA.

Some of the PIgR molecules are transported and cleaved by the epithelial cells without any attached immunoglobulin. The resulting proteolytic fragment, free SC, is also present in high concentrations in human milk. The function of free secretory component has not been established clearly. One study (Wilson and Christi, 1991) suggests that these molecules may be able to inhibit the enzyme phospholipase A_2, a function that could reduce inflammatory reactions along mucosal surfaces as well as, perhaps, the fluid accumulation produced by some intestinal pathogens (Peterson and Ochoa, 1989).

From this brief outline of the immunogenesis of SIgA, we can deduce that this system is well adapted for the production, and secretion into milk, of specific antibodies against pathogenic microorganisms to which the mother's mucosal immune system has been exposed. Since the mother–infant pair normally shares many environmental exposures, this system may be ideal for protecting the infant from potential pathogens entering the environment. As indicated in Chapter 52, several epidemiological studies have shown that the presence in milk of specific SIgA antibodies against enteric pathogens diminishes the incidence or severity of diarrhea caused by bacterial and viral organisms.

Immunoglobulins of the other major isotypes also are found in human milk, although at lower concentrations than in plasma. IgM in milk is in its typical pentameric form, although some of the molecules have noncovalently attached SC, suggesting that IgM is transported into the milk via the PIgR. However, the binding of free SC in milk could generate the same complexes. The antibody specificity of IgM in milk has not been tested extensively, but seems to parallel that of IgA when examined. The presence of IgM antibodies with attached SC should be considered when designing studies of SIgA in human milk, since detection systems based on anti-SC antibodies also may detect secretory IgM (Mellander *et al.*, 1985).

In cow milk, IgG is the major isotype. However, only small amounts of each of the subclasses of IgG have been detected in human milk. The relative proportion of IgG4 is greater in milk than in serum, suggesting that more of this isotype may be produced locally or selectively transported by the interstitium (Keller *et al.*, 1983). This hypothesis has not been borne out in a more recent investigation (Mehta *et al.*, 1991). Nonetheless, the total amount of IgG4 is so low that attributing biological functions to this or the other IgG isotypes will be difficult.

The concentration of IgD in human milk is very low, even relative to serum concentrations (Keller *et al.*, 1984). IgE is essentially absent from human milk (Underdown *et al.*, 1976).

Antibodies against a large number of microbes and specific antigens have been detected in human milk. Table II provides a summary of some of these specificities. This list should not be considered complete or thought to imply functional significance of the presence of antibodies of particular specificity, since it respresents a summary of studies from groups with particular interest in the antigens tested.

The stability of the immunoglobulins in human milk has been the subject of a number of studies, most of which have concentrated on SIgA. The majority of the IgA molecules in postnatal milk seems to be intact, based on Western blots using anti-α chain antibodies as developing reagents (Cleveland *et al.*, 1991). Thus, during active lactation, little degradation must occur within the mammary gland. Following the fate of the SIgA within the infant is difficult. Fecal excretion of SIgA has been examined in low birth weight and full-term infants (Schanler *et al.*, 1986; Prentice *et al.*, 1987; Davidson and Lönnerdal, 1987). The finding that SIgA excretion in the

Table II Antimicrobial SIgA Antibodies Detected in Human Milk

Bacteria and bacterial toxins	Viruses	Parasites/fungi
Enteric		
Clostridium difficile	Polio viruses	*Giardia lamblia*
Escherichia coli	Rotaviruses	*Candida albicans*
Klebsiella pneumoniae		
Salmonella sp.		
Shigella sp.		
Vibrio cholerae		
Respiratory		
Haemophilus influenzae	Respiratory syncytial virus	
Streptococcus pneumoniae	Influenza viruses	

feces was 30 times higher in low birth weight infants receiving human milk than in similar infants fed cow milk formulas strongly suggested that a portion of the ingested milk survived the whole gastrointestinal tract. However, when expressed as a proportion of the SIgA fed, approximately 9% of the SIgA was recovered as SIgA (Schanler *et al.*, 1986).

The function of mucosal immunoglobulins is discussed in detail in Chapter 11. Of potential importance for milk immunoglobulins is the amplification of the effect of other milk defense factors by IgA. For instance, some of the lactoferrin in milk is found complexed with IgA (Arnold *et al.*, 1977). These complexes may have enhanced activity since they can be targeted to surfaces of pathogenic microorganisms where lactoferrin could function to chelate selectively the iron needed by the microorganism for growth. Microorganisms that are resistant to the lytic action of lysozyme may become more susceptible in the presence of SIgA and complement (Adinolfi *et al.*, 1966). Galactosyltransferase enzyme also complexes tightly with IgA, although the functional significance of these complexes is not known (McGuire *et al.*, 1989).

b. Lysozyme. Lysozyme, a 12-kDa single polypeptide, catalyzes the hydrolysis of β1–4 linkages between *N*-acetylmuramic acid and 2-acetylamino-2-deoxy-D-glucose groups in bacterial cell walls, leading to direct lysis of susceptible bacteria, predominantly those without an extensive cell wall. As indicated earlier, interaction with IgA and complement may expand the antimicrobial range of activity of this secretory enzyme.

The quantity of lysozyme supplied to the infant each day are presented in Table III. Although the concentration varies during lactation the amount delivered appears to remain relatively constant for at least the first 4 months (Butte *et al.*, 1984). These concentrations are among the highest of any secretion (Jolles and Jolles, 1967).

The relative stability of lysozyme against acid denaturation and tryptic digestion makes it well suited to function in the gastrointestinal tract of the recipient infant. However, the fate of the ingested lysozyme is not clear. Low birth weight infants who are fed human milk excrete about eight times more lysozyme in their stool than do cow milk-fed infants (Schanler *et al.*, 1986).

c. Lactoferrin. Lactoferrin is the whey protein with the highest concentration in human milk. The daily amount of lactoferrin ingested by the infant at various stages of lactation are shown in Table III. A gradual decline is seen in the amount transferred to the infant, beginning soon after initiation of lactation.

A single chain glycoprotein of 79 kDa, lactoferrin consists of two globular lobes, each with two domains surrounding a binding cleft for an atom of ferric iron and a bicarbonate ion. The major function of lactoferrin is the chelation of iron. In that respect, apolactoferrin robs the siderophilins of microorganisms of iron that is essential for their growth (Spik *et al.*, 1978). The lactoferrin in human milk is well suited for this role, since 90% of the molecules are devoid of iron (Fransson and Lönnerdal, 1980). Several other functions have been suggested for lactoferrin. The finding of a specific receptor for lactoferrin on the mucosa of the upper bowel suggested that lactoferrin might enhance the uptake of milk iron by the infant (Davidson and Lönnerdal, 1988). The low degree of iron saturation in milk lactoferrin makes this function seem unlikely, unless iron was transferred from other compartments during the digestion process. Some evidence also suggests that lactoferrin has trophic effects on enterocytes (Nichols *et al.*, 1987) and may inhibit complement activity (Kijlstra and Jeurissen, 1982).

Few studies have been done on the disposition of milk lactoferrin in the infant. One study was carried out on infants with enterostomies, which allowed the gut contents to be recovered before entering the colon (Hambreus *et al.*, 1989). The results indicated that 9–32% of the ingested lactoferrin could be recovered from this site. Low birth weight infants fed a human milk preparation excreted almost 200 times more lactoferrin in their stool than similar infants fed a cow milk-based formula (Schanler *et al.*, 1986). However, only 3% of the ingested lactoferrin was recovered in the fecal sample. In addition, a major portion of the excreted lactoferrin was partially digested, resulting in molecules of unknown activity (Goldman *et al.*, 1990). Infants fed human milk also had a larger amount of lactoferrin and lactoferrin fragments in their urine (Goldblum *et al.*, 1989); the molecular sizes of those fragments were similar to those in the stools (Goldman *et al.*, 1990). Another study using stable isotope methods also suggested that some lactoferrin derived from the milk may

Table III Quantity (mg/kg/D) of Immune Factors [mean (Std)] Provided by Human Milk[a]

Factor	Phase of lactation (age of infants in months) 1	2	3	4
Lactoferrin	275 (75)	190 (80)	167 (70)	120 (25)
SIgA	130 (50)	105 (40)	88 (3)	77 (35)
Lysozyme	4 (3)	5 (3)	4.9 (1.5)	6 (2)

[a] Data modified from Butte *et al.* (1984).

be absorbed intact from the intestinal tract and then excreted into the urinary tract (Hutchens *et al.*, 1991). If this occurs, the absorbed lactoferrin must be cleared rapidly since human milk ingestion does not increase the serum concentration of lactoferrin (Schanler *et al.*, 1986).

d. Complement components. Many of the components of the classical and alternative complement pathway have been detected in human milk (Ballow *et al.*, 1974; Nakajima *et al.*, 1977). However, with the exception of C3, the concentrations of these factors are very low. The activity of the complement system in human milk is not likely to be great, although interactions with other milk constituents may allow some function (Adinolfi *et al.*, 1966).

e. Bioactive peptides. Several cytokines have been quantified by immunoassays in human milk, including interleukin-1β (IL-1β; Munoz *et al.*, 1990), tumor necrosis factor α (TNF-α; Mushtaha *et al.*, 1989; Rudloff *et al.*, 1992a) and IL-6 (Saito *et al.*, 1991; Rudloff *et al.*, 1992b). The functions of these factors in the infant remain to be elucidated. However, studies of the leukocytes in the milk suggest that some of these cytokines may be active (Söder, 1987; Mushtaha *et al.*, 1989). Of special interest is the finding that incubation of peripheral blood leukocytes with human milk causes monocytes and neutrophils to become activated. Further, addition of neutralizing antibodies against human TNFα abrogated the activating effects of milk on monocytes (Mushtaha *et al.*, 1989).

Some fragments of casein, the β-casomorphines, which are created during proteolysis of casein in the gastrointestinal tract, are biologically active (Teschenmacher, 1987). β-Casomorphines not only have endorphin effects but may be immunoregulatory as well (Parker *et al.*, 1984).

Several different isoforms of prolactin have been demonstrated in human milk that apparently are produced by posttranslational modifications in the mammary gland. Although the function of each of these isoforms is not delineated, the basic protein molecule has been found to influence the development of T cells in animal model systems (Chikanza and Panay, 1991; Gala, 1991; Rovensky *et al.*,1991) and to enhance the formation of specific antibodies in serum and milk (Ijaz *et al.*, 1990).

The array of growth factors in human milk includes epidermal growth factor (EGF), insulin, transforming growth factor β (TGF-β; Hooton *et al.*, 1991), and mammary gland derived growth factor (Kidwell *et al.*, 1987). Some of these factors have been postulated to aid in the postnatal development of the mucosal barriers of the intestinal and respiratory tracts. However, the *in vivo* effects of these factors are not well characterized.

2. Carbohydrates and Glycoconjugates

a. Lactobacillus growth factors. Human milk contains high levels of a growth-promoting activity for *Lactobacillus bifidus* var. *Pennsylvania* (György *et al.*, 1974). This activity, which is essentially absent from cow milk, is generated by oligosaccharides (György *et al.*, 1974), glycopeptides, and proteins (Nichols *et al.*, 1975; Bezkorovainy *et al.*, 1979). Similar activity associated with caseins also may be the result of oligosaccharide moieties on that protein (Bezkorovainy and Topouzian, 1981). The role of these factors in host defense may be related to the predominance of *Lactobacillus* in the bacterial flora in the colon of infants fed human milk. The large amount of acetic acid produced by these organisms suppresses the growth of enteropathogens.

b. Oligosaccharides and glycoconjugates. Human milk is rich in oligosaccharides that appear to be formed in the mammary epithelium by the same galactosyltransferases that glycosylate proteins and peptides, using lactose as the acceptor molecule. Various biological activities have been attributed to the whole group of oligosaccharides (Holmgren *et al.*, 1981) and, more recently, to individually characterized moieties, including fucosylated oligosaccharides that inhibit the hemagglutinin activity of the classical strain of *Vibrio cholerae* (Holmgren *et al.*, 1983) and protect against the heat-stable toxin of *Escherichia coli* (Newburg *et al.*, 1990). Mannose-containing glycoproteins and glycolipids interfere with the fimbria-mediated binding of *E. coli* (Holmgren *et al.*, 1987; Wold *et al.*, 1990). The attachment of *Haemophilus influenzae* and *Streptococcus pneumoniae* to epithelial cells is inhibited by saccharides containing the disaccharide subunit *N*-acetylglucosamine (1–3)-β-galactose (Andersson *et al.*, 1986). These units may exist as free oligosaccharide or in glycoproteins or peptides. In any case, molecules with these structures may act as false receptors for the lectin-like adherence structures on the microorganism and thereby protect the infant from colonization or infection with these pathogens. Although an *in vivo* role for these oligosaccharides is suggested by animal models (Otnaess and Svennerholm, 1982; Cleary *et al.*, 1983; Ashkanazi *et al.*, 1992) few human studies have been done that pertain to this question.

3. Lipids

a. Unsaturated fatty acids and monoglycerides. Free fatty acids and monoglycerides are produced by the digestion of milk triglycerides by bile salt-stimulated lipases or lipoprotein lipases in human milk. In addition, the lingual and gastric lipase activities of the recipient infant are active on the milk triglycerides (Hosmosh, 1990). The lipid products have several host defense activities including disruption of enveloped viruses (Stock and Frances, 1940; Welch *et al.*, 1979; Issacs *et al.*, 1986; Thromar *et al.*, 1987), which may prevent coronavirus infection in the intestinal tract (Resta *et al.*, 1985). The fatty acids and monoglycerides also may provide some defense against intestinal parasites such as *Giardia lamblia* (Gillin *et al.*, 1983,1985; Hernell *et al.*, 1987).

b. α-Tocopherol and β-carotene. Two vitamins found in human milk (Chapell *et al.*, 1985) also may have host defense activity. High levels of α-tocopherol in milk may serve as an antioxidant, but additionally this vitamin is known to stimulate the development of immunity (Tengerdy *et al.*, 1981; Bendich *et al.*, 1986). β-Carotene, another potent antioxidant, is present in high concentrations in the mammary gland at parturition. This agent is released from the tissue into milk during the first few days of lactation (Chapell *et al.*, 1985). As a result of the ingestion of α-tocopherol and β-carotene in human milk, the blood levels of these two agents rise substantially in the recipient infant (Chapell *et al.*, 1985; Ostrea *et al.*, 1986). These and other agents in human milk may regulate inflammatory responses and immune functions of the infant.

IV. OVERVIEW OF THE FUNCTION OF HUMAN MILK IN HOST PROTECTION AND CONCLUSIONS

Despite the identification and quantification in human milk of many factors that have the potential to protect the lactating breast and the recipient infant, little currently is known about how these factors function *in vivo*. Progress in this area has been limited by the types of studies that can be carried out in human infants and by the large species differences in milk composition and function that make experimental animal studies difficult to apply to humans. However, certain patterns of factors may provide clues to unique *in vivo* function of human milk.

A. Production of Immune Factors by the Breast Is Regulated

In contrast to many mucosal glands, which function on a continuous basis, the mammary gland secretion of immune factors is restricted largely to periods of lactation. The factors that regulate the onset, quality, and quantity of the human milk are only partially understood. Prolactin and other lactogenic hormones are essential for the onset and maintenance of lactation. An array of growth factors including EGF, insulin, and mammary gland derived growth factors that are concentrated in human milk (Kidwell *et al.*, 1987) also may play a role in these processes.

B. Immune Factors in Milk May Prevent Infection without Causing Inflammation

The same proximity of the mucosal surfaces to the external environment that leads to extensive exposure to microorganisms and other antigens allows the mucosal immune system to defend against infections without the need for the extensive inflammatory and phagocytic responses that are typical of the systemic defenses. Thus, if factors in milk can reduce the adherence, colonization, or growth of microorganisms in the infant's respiratory or intestinal tract, the incidence or severity of infection would decrease correspondingly without producing much physiological abnormality in the infant. We have hypothesized previously that a characteristic of the immune system in human milk is the absence of phlogistic factors and the presence of agents with anti-inflammatory activity (Goldman *et al.*, 1986). Demonstrations that infants who receive mother's milk that contains specific antibodies against an enteric pathogen still have culture-proven infections but less diarrhea than those receiving milk without those antibodies (Glass *et al.*, 1983; also see Chapter 52) are in keeping with this hypothesis. In that respect, the lower morbidity of breast-fed infants infected with rotavirus was not found to be related to the levels of specific antibodies in the milk (Duffy *et al.*, 1986). This result suggests that other agents, including anti-inflammatory factors, may be responsible for some of the protection against certain pathogens.

C. Long-Term Effects of Breast Feeding

Several studies suggest that breast feeding may have effects that last much longer than the breast-feeding period. For instance, breast-fed infants have a lower incidence of juvenile diabetes mellitus (Mayer *et al.*, 1988; Hamman *et al.*, 1988) and Crohn's disease (Koletzko *et al.*, 1989) than those fed formulas. Retrospective analysis also suggests a diminished risk of lymphomas after breast-feeding (Davis *et al.*, 1988). Whether these long-term effects are the result of mucosal immune factors in human milk is unclear. However, speculating that breast-feeding alters the development of the infant's immune system or protects against certain infections during a critical developmental period, thereby preventing illnesses that become manifest later in life, is interesting.

References

Adinolfi, M., Glynn, A. A., Linsay, M., *et al.* (1966). Serological properties of ηA antibodies to *Escherichia coli* present in human colostrum. *Immunology* **10,** 517–526.

Andersson, B., Porras, O., Hanson, L. Å., Lagergard, T., and Svanborg-Eden, C. (1986). Inhibition of attachment of *Streptococcus pneumoniae* and *Haemophilus influenzae* by human milk and receptor oligosaccharides. *J. Infect. Dis.* **153,** 232–237.

Arnold, R. R., Cole, M. F., and McGhee, J. R. (1977). A bactericidal effect for human milk lactoferrin. *Science* **197,** 263–265.

Ashkenazi, S., Newburg, D. S., and Cleary, T. G. (1992). The effect of human milk on the adherence of enterohemorrhagic *E. coli* to rabbit intestinal cells. *In* "Immunology of Milk and the Neonate" (J. Mestecky, C. Blair, and P. L. Ogra, eds.), pp. 173–177. Plenum Press, New York.

Ballow, M., Fang, F., Good, R. A., and Day, N. K. (1974). Developmental aspects of complement components in the newborn. The presence of complement components and C3 proactivator (properdin factor B) in human colostrum. *Clin. Exp. Immunol.* **18,** 257–266.

Bendich, A., Gabriel, E., and Machlin, L. J. (1986). Dietary vitamin E requirement for optimum immune responses in the rat. *J. Nutr.* **116,** 675–681.

Bertotto, A., Gerli, R., Fabietti, G., Crupi, S., Arcangeli, C., Scalise, F., and Vacarro, R. (1990). Human breast milk T cells display the phenotype and functional characteristics of memory T cells. *Eur. J. Immunol.* **20,** 1877–1880.

Bezkorovainy, A., and Topouzian, N. (1981). *Bifidobacterium bifidus* var. *pennsylvanicus* growth promoting activity of human milk casein and its derivatives. *Int. J. Biochem.* **13,** 585–590.

Bezkorovainy, A., Grohlich, D., and Nichols, J. H. (1979). Isolation of a glycopeptide fraction with *Lactobacillus bifidus* subspecies *pennsylvanicus* growth-promoting activity from whole human milk casein. *Am. J. Clin. Nutr.* **32,** 1428–1432.

Brandtzaeg, P. (1983). The secretory immune system of lactating human mammary glands compared with other exocrine organs. *Ann. N.Y. Acad. Sci.* **409,** 353–381.

Butte, N. F., Goldblum, R. M., Fehl, L. M., Loftin, K., Smith, E. O., Garza, C., and Goldman, A. S. (1984). Daily ingestion of immunologic components in human milk during the first four months of life. *Acta Paediatr. Scand.* **73,** 296–301.

Chapell, J. E., Francis, T., and Clandinin, M. T. (1985). Vitamin A and E content of human milk at early stages of lactation. *Early Hum. Dev.* **11,** 157–167.

Chikanza, I. C., and Panay, G. S. (1991). Hypothalamic-pituitary mediated modulation of immune function: Prolactin as a neuroimmune peptide. *Br. J. Pharm.* **30,** 203–207.

Cleary, T. G., Chambers, J. P., and Pickering, L. K. (1983). Protection of suckling mice from the heat-stable enterotoxin of *Escherichae coli* by human milk. *J. Infect. Dis.* **148,** 1114–1119.

Cleveland, M. G., Bakos, M-A., Pyron, D. L., Rajaraman, S., and Goldblum, R. M. (1991). Characterization of secretory component in amniotic fluid: Identification of new forms of secretory IgA. *J. Immunol.* **147,** 181–188.

Crago, S. S., Prince, S. J., Pretlow, T. G., McGhee, J. R., and Mestecky, J. (1979). Human colostral cells. I. Separation and characterization. *Clin. Exp. Immunol.* **38(3),** 585–597.

Davidson, L. A., and Lönnerdal, B. (1987). The persistence of human milk proteins in the breast-fed infant. *Acta Paediatr. Scand.* **76,** 733–740.

Davidson, L. A., and Lönnerdal, B. (1988). Specific binding of lactoferrin to brush-border membrane: Ontogeny and effect of glycan chain. *Am. J. Physiol.* **254,** G580–G585.

Davis, M. K., Savitz, D. A., and Grauford, B. (1988). Infant feeding in childhood cancer. *Lancet* **2,** 365–368.

Donné: (1844–1845). Cours de Microscopie, Vol 1. et Atlas No. 1. Baillière, Paris.

Duffy, L. C., Reipenhoff-Talty, M., Byers, T. E., La Scolea, M. A., Zeilezny, M. A., Dryja, D. M., and Ogra, P. L. (1986). Modulation of rotavirus enteritis during breast-feeding. *Am. J. Dis. Child.* **140,** 1164–1168.

Emodi, G., and Just, M. (1974). Interferon production by lymphocytes in human milk. *Scand. J. Immunol.* **3,** 157–160.

Fransson, G. B., and Lönnerdal, B. (1980). Iron in human milk. *Pediatrics* **96,** 380–384.

Gala, R. R. (1991). Prolactin and growth hormone in the regulation of the immune system. *Proc. Soc. Exp. Biol. Med.* **198,** 513–527.

Gillin, F. D., Reiner, D. S., and Wang, C-S. (1983). Human milk kills parasitic protozoa. *Science* **221,** 1290–1292.

Gillin, F. D., Reiner, D. S., and Gault, M. J. (1985). Cholate-dependent killing of *Giardia lamblia* by human milk. *Infect. Immun.* **47,** 619–622.

Glass, R. I., Svennerholm, A-M., Stoll, B. J., Khan, M. R., Hossain, K. M., Huq, M., and Holmgren, J. (1983). Protection against cholera in breast-fed children by antibodies in breast milk. *N. Engl. J. Med.* **308,** 1389–1392.

Goldblum, R. M., Ahlstedt, S., Carlsson, B., Hanson, L. A., Jodal, U., Lidin Janson, G., and Sohl, A. (1975). Antibody forming cells in human colostrum after oral immunization. *Nature (London)* **257,** 797–799.

Goldblum, R. M., Garza, C., Johnson, C. A., Harris, R., Nichols, B. L., and Goldman, A. S. (1981). Human milk banking I. Effects of container upon immunologic factors in mature milk. *Nutr. Res.* **1,** 449–459.

Goldblum, R. M., Schanler, R. J., Garza, C., and Goldman, A. S. (1989). Human milk feeding enhances the urinary excretion of immunologic factors in low birth weight infants. *Pediatr. Res.* **25,** 184–188.

Goldman, A. S., Garza, C., Nichols, B. L., and Goldblum, R. M. (1982). Immunologic factors in human milk during the first year of lactation. *J. Pediatr.* **100,** 563–567.

Goldman, A. S., Thorpe, L. W., Goldblum, R. M., and Hanson, L. Å. (1986). Anti-inflammatory properties of human milk. *Acta Paediatr. Scand.* **75,** 689–695.

Goldman, A. S., Garza, C., Schanler, R. J., and Goldblum, R. M. (1990). Molecular forms of lactoferrin in stool and urine from infants fed human milk. *Pediatr. Res.* **27,** 252–255.

György, P., Jeanloz, R. W., Von Nicolai, H., and Zilliken, F. (1974). Undialyzable growth factors for *Lactobacillus bifidus* var. *pennsylvanicus*. *Eur. J. Biochem.* **43,** 29–33.

Hambreus, L., Hjorth, G., Kristiansson, B., Hedlund, H., Andersson, H., Lönnerdal, B., and Sjöberg, L.-B. (1989). Lactoferrin content in feces in illeostomy-operated children fed human milk. *In* "Milk Proteins" (C. A. Barth and E. Schlimme, eds.), pp. 72–75. Steinkopff Verlag, Darmstadt, Germany.

Hamman, R. F., Gay, E. C., Lezotte, D. C., Savitz, D. A., and Klingensmith, G. J. (1988). Reduced risk of IDDM among breast fed children. The Colorado IDDM Registry. *Diabetes* **37,** 1625–1632.

Hamosh, M. (1990). Lingual and gastric lipases. *Nutrition* **6,** 421–428.

Hernell, O., Ward, H., Blackberg, L., and Pereira, M. E. (1987). Killing of Giardia Lamblia by human milk lipases: An effect mediated by lipolysis of milk lipids. *J. Infect. Dis.* **153,** 715–720.

Holmgren, J., Svennerholm, A-M., and Ahren, C. (1981). Nonimmunoglobulin fraction of human milk inhibits bacterial adhesion (hemagglutination) and enterotoxin binding of *Escherichia coli* and *Vibrio cholerae*. *Infect. Immun.* **33,** 136–141.

Holmgren, J., Svennerholm, A-M., and Lindblad, M. (1983). Receptor-like glycocompounds in human milk that inhibit classical and El Tor *Vibrio cholerae* cell adherence (hemagglutination). *Infect. Immun.* **39,** 147–154.

Holmgren, J., Svennerholm, A-M., Lindblad, M., and Strecker, G. (1987). Inhibition of bacterial adhesion and toxin binding by glycoconjugate and oligosaccharide receptor analogues in human milk. *In* "Human Lactation 3: The Effects of Human Milk on the Recipient Infant" (A. S. Goldman, S. A. Atkinson, and L. Å. Hanson, eds.), pp. 251–259. Plenum Press, New York.

Hooton, J. W. L., Pabst, H. F., Spady, D. W., and Paetkau, V. (1991). Human colostrum contains an activity that inhibits the production of IL-2. *Clin. Exp. Immunol.* **86,** 520–524.

Hutchens, T. W., Henry, J. F., Yip, T-T., Hachey, D. L., Schanler, R. J., Motil, K. J., and Garza, C. (1991). Origin of intact lactoferrin and its DNA-binding fragments found in the urine of human milk-fed preterm infants. Evaluation of stable isotopic enrichment. *Pediatr. Res.* **29,** 243–250.

Ijaz, M. K., Dent, D., and Babiuk, L. A. (1990). Neuroimmunomodulation of the *in vivo* anti-rotavirus humoral immune response. *J. Neuroimmunol.* **26,** 159–171.

Issacs, C. E., Thormar, H., and Pessolano, T. (1986). Membrane-disruptive effect of human milk: Inactivation of enveloped viruses. *J. Infect. Dis.* **154,** 966–971.

Jolles, J., and Jolles, P. (1967). Human tear and human milk lysozymes.. *Biochemistry* **6,** 411–417.

Keeney, S. E., Schmalstieg, F. C., Palkowetz, K. H., Binh-Minh, L., and Goldman, A. S. (1993). Activated neutrophils and nutraphil activators in human milk: Increased expression of CD11B and decreased expression of L-Selectin. *J. Leuk. Biol.* **54,** 97–104.

Keller, M. A., Kidd, R. M., Bryson, Y. J., Turner, J. L., and Carter, J. (1981). Lymphokine production by human milk lymphocytes. *Infect. Immun.* **32,** 632–636.

Keller, M. A., Heiner, D. C., Kidd, R. M., and Myers, A. S. (1983). Local production of IgG4 in human colostrum. *J. Immunol.* **130,** 1654–1657.

Keller, M. A., Heiner, D. C., Myers, A. S., and Reisinger, D. M. (1984). IgD—A mucosal immunoglobulin? *Pediatr. Res.* **18,** 258A.

Keller, M. A., Faust, J., Rolewic, L. J., and Stewart, D. D. (1986). T cell subsets in human milk. *J. Pediatr. Gastroenterol. Nutr.* **5,** 439–443.

Kidwell, W. R., Salomon, D. D., and Mohavam, S. (1987). Production of growth factors by normal human mammary cells in culture. *In* "Human Lactation 3: The Effects of Human Milk on the Recipient Infant" (A. S. Goldman, S. A. Atkinson, and L. Å. Hanson, eds.), pp. 227–239. Plenum Press, New York.

Kijlstra, A., and Jeurissen, S. H. M. (1982). Modulation of classical C3 convertase of complement by tear lactoferrin. *Immunology* **47,** 263–270.

Koletzko, S., Sherman, P., Corey, M., Griffiths, A., and Smith, C. (1989). Role of infant feeding practices in development of Crohn's disease in childhood. *Br. Med. J.* **298,** 1617–1618.

McGuire, E. J., Kerlin, R., Cebra, J. J., and Roth, S. (1989). A human milk galactosyltransferase is specific for secreted, but not plasma, IgA. *J. Immunol.* **143,** 2933–2938.

Mayer, E. J., Hamman, R. F., Gay, E. C., Lezotte, D. C., Savitz, D. A., and Klingensmith, G. J. (1988). Reduced risk of IDDM among breast fed children. The Colorado IDDM Registry. *Diabetes* **37,** 1625–1632.

Mehta, P. D., Issacs, C. E., and Coyle, P. K. (1991). Immunoglobulin G subclasses in human colostrum and milk. *In* "Immunology of Milk and the Neonate" (J. Mestecky, C. Blair, and P. Ogra, eds.), pp. 223–226. Plenum Press, New York.

Mellander, L., Calsson, B., Jalil, F., Soderstrom, T., and Hanson, L. A. (1985). Secretory IgA antibody response against PYexcheria coli antiens in finfants in relation to exposure. *J. Pediatr.* **107,** 430–433.

Morr, C. V., Josephson, R. V., Jenness, R., and Manning, R. B. (1971). Composition and properties of submicellar casein complexes in colloidal phosphate-free skim milk. *J. Dairy Sci.* **54,** 1555–1563.

Moyer-Mileur, L., and Chan, G. M. (1989). Milk membranes-origin, content, changes during lactation and nutritional importance. *In* "Textbook of Gastroenterology and Nutrition in Infancy" (E. Lebenthal, ed.), pp. 151–155. Raven Press, New York.

Munoz, C., Endres, S., van der Meer, J., Schlesinger, L., Arevalo, M., and Dinarello, C. (1990). Interleukin-1β in human colostrum. *Res. Immunol.* **141,** 501–513.

Mushtaha, A. A., Schmalstieg, F. C., Hughes, T. K., Rajaraman, S., Rudloff, H. E., and Goldman, A. S. (1989). Chemokinetic agents for monocytes in human milk: Possible role of tumor necrosis factor-α. *Pediatr. Res.* **25,** 629–633.

Nakajima, S., Baba, A. S., and Tamura, N. (1977). Complement system in human colostrum. *Int. Arch. Allergy Appl. Immunol.* **54,** 428–423.

Newburg, D. S., Pickering, L. K., McCluer, R. H., and Cleary, T. G. (1990). Fucosylated oligosaccharides of human milk protect suckling mice from heat-stable enterotoxin of *Escherichia coli*. *J. Infect. Dis.* **162,** 1075–1080.

Nichols, B. L., McKee, K. S., Henry, J. F., and Putnam, M. (1987). Human lactoferrin stimulates thymidine incorporation into DNA of rat crypt cells. *Pediatr. Res.* **21,** 563–567.

Nichols, J. H., Bezkorovainy, A., and Paque, R. (1975). Isolation and characterization of several glycoproteins from human colostral whey. *Biochim. Biophys. Acta* **412,** 99–108.

Ostrea, E. A., Jr., Balun, J. E., Winkler, R., and Porter, T. (1986). Influence of breast-feeding on the restoration of the low serum concentration of vitamin E and β-carotene in the newborn infant. *Am. J. Obstet. Gynecol.* **154,** 1014–1017.

Otnaess, A-B., and Svennerholm, A-M. (1982). Non-immunoglobulin fraction of human milk protects against enterotoxin-induced intestinal fluid secretion. *Infect. Immun.* **35,** 738–740.

Özkaragöz, F., Rudloff, H. E., Rajaraman, S., Mushtaha, A. A., Schmalstieg, F. C., and Goldman, A. S. (1988). The motility of human milk macrophages in collagen gels. *Pediatr. Res.* **23,** 449–452.

Parker, F., Migliore-Samour, D., Floch, F., Zerial, A., Werner, G. H., Jolles, J., Casaretto, M., Zahn, H., and Jolles, P. (1984). Immunostimulating hexapeptide from human casein: Amino acid sequence, synthesis, and biological properties. *Eur. J. Biochem.* **145,** 677–682.

Parmely, M. J., Beer, A. E., and Billingham, R. E. (1976). *In vitro* studies on the T-lymphocyte population of human milk. *J. Exp. Med.* **144,** 358–370.

Patton, S., and Huston, G. (1985). Isolation of fat globules from human milk. *In* "Human Lactation: Milk Components and Methodologies" (R. G. Jensen and M. C. Neville, eds.), p. 81. Plenum Press, New York.

Peterson, J. W., and Ochoa, L. G. (1989). Role of prostaglandins and cAMP in the secretory effects of cholera toxin. *Science* **245,** 857–859.

Prentice, A., Ewing, G., Roberts, S. B., Lucas, A., MacCarthy, A., Jarjou, L. M. A., and Whitehead, R. G. (1987). The nutritional role of breast milk IgA and lactoferrin. *Acta Paediatr. Scand.* **76,** 592–598.

Resta, S., Luby, J. P., Rosenfeld, C. R., and Siegel, J. D. (1985). Isolation and propagation of a human enteric coronavirus. *Science* **229,** 978–981.

Richie, E. R., Bass, R., Meistrich, M. L., and Dennison, D. K. (1982). Distribution of T lymphocyte subsets in human colostrum. *J. Immunol.* **129,** 1116–1119.

Roux, M. E., McWilliams, M., Phillips-Quagliata, J. M., Weisz-Carrington, P., and Lamm, M. E. (1977). Origin of IgA-secreting plasma cells in the mammary gland. *J. Exp. Med.* **146,** 1311–1322.

Rovensky, J., Vigas, M., Mare, K. J., Blazickova, S., Korcakova, L., and Vyletetelkova, L. (1991). Evidence for immunomodulation properties of prolactin in *in vitro* and *in vivo* situations. *Int. J. Immunopharmacol.* **13,** 267–272.

Rudloff, H. E., Schmalstieg, F. C., Jr., Mushtaha, A. A., Palkowetz, K. H., Liu, S. K., and Goldman, A. S. (1992a). Tumor necrosis factor-α in human milk. *Pediatr. Res.* **31,** 29–33.

Rudloff, H. E., Schmalstieg, F. C., Jr., Palkowetz, K. H., Paskiewicz, E. J., and Goldman, A. S. (1993b). Interleukin-6 (IL-6) in human milk. *J. Reprod. Immunol.* **23,** 13–20.

Saito, S., Maruyama, M., Kato, Y., Moriyama, I., and Ichijo, M. (1991). Detection of IL-6 in human milk and its involvement in IgA production. *J. Reprod. Immunol.* **20,** 267–276.

Schanler, R. J., Goldblum, R. M., Garza, C., and Goldman, A. S. (1986). Enhanced fecal excretion of selected immune factors in very low birth weight infants fed fortified human milk. *Pediatr. Res.* **20,** 711–715.

Schroten, H., Hanisch, F. G., Plogmann, R., Hacker, J., Uhlenbruck, G., Nobisbosch, R., and Wahn, V. (1992). Inhibition of adhesion of s-fimbriated *Escherichia coli* to buccal epithelial cells by human milk fat globule membrane components: A novel aspect of protective function of mucins in inoimmunoglobulin fraction. *Infect. Imm.* **60,** 2893–2899.

Smith, C. W., and Goldman, A. S. (1968). The cells of human colostrum. I. *In vitro* studies of morphology and functions. *Pediatr. Res.* **2,** 103–109.

Söder, O. (1987). Isolation of interleukin-1 from human milk. *Int. Arch. Allergy Appl. Immunol.* **83,** 19–23.

Spik, G., Cheron, A., Montreuil, J., and Dolby, J. M. (1978). Bacteriostasis of a milk-sensitive strain of *Escherichia coli* by immunoglobulins and iron-binding proteins in association. *Immunology* **35,** 663–671.

Stock, C. C., and Francis, T., Jr. (1940). The inactivation of the virus of epidemic influenza by soaps. *J. Exp. Med.* **71,** 661–681.

Tengerdy, R. P., Mathias, M. M., and Nockels, C. F. (1981). Vitamin E, immunity and disease resistance. *In* "Diet and Resistance to Disease" (M. Phillips and A. Baetz, eds.), pp. 27–42. Plenum Press, New York.

Teschemacher, H. (1987). β-Casomorphins: Do they have physiological significance? *In* "Human Lactation 3: The Effects of Human Milk on the Recipient Infant" (A. S. Goldman, S. A. Atkinson, and L. Å. Hanson, eds.), pp. 213–225. Plenum Press, New York.

Thorpe, L. W., Rudloff, H. E., Powell, L. C., and Goldman, A. S. (1986). Decreased response of human milk leukocytes to chemoattractant peptides. *Pediatr. Res.* **20,** 373–377.

Thromar, H., Isaacs, C. E., Brown, H. R., Barshatzky, M. R., and Pessolano, T. (1987). Inactivation of enveloped viruses and killing of cells by fatty acids and monoglycerides. *J. Am. Soc. Microbiol.* **32,** 27–31.

Tsuda, H., Takeshige, K., Shibata, Y., and Minakami, S. (1984). Oxygen metabolism of human colostral macrophages. *J. Biochem.* **95,** 1237–1245.

Underdown, B. J., Knight, A., and Papsin, F. R. (1976). The relative paucity of IgE in human milk. *J. Immunol.* **116,** 1435–1438.

Weisz-Carrington, P., Roux, M. E., McWilliams, M., Philips-Quaglita, J. M., and Lamm, M. E. (1978). Hormonal induction of the secretory immune system in the mammary gland. *Proc. Natl. Acad. Sci. U.S.A.* **75,** 2928–2932.

Welsh, J. K., Arsenakis, M., Coelen, R. J., and May, J. T. (1979). Effect of antiviral lipids, heat, and freezing on the activity of viruses in human milk. *J. Infect. Dis.* **140,** 332–338.

Wirt, D. P., Adkins, L. T., Palkowetz, K. H., Schmalstieg, F. C., and Goldman, A. S. (1992). Activated-memory T lymphocytes in human milk. *Cytometry* **13,** 282–290.

Wilson, T., and Christi, D. L. (1991). Gravidin, an endogenous inhibitor of phospholipase A2 activity, is a secretory component of IgA. *Biochem. Biophys. Res. Commun.* **176,** 447–452.

Wold, A., Mestecky, J., Tomana, M., Kobata, A., Ohbayashi, H., Endo, T., and Svanborg-Eden, C. (1990). Secretory IgA carries oligosaccharide receptors for *Escherichia coli* type 1 fimbrial lectin. *Infect. Immun.* **58,** 3073–3077.

52

Immunologic Effects of Breast-Feeding on the Infant

B. Carlsson • L. Å. Hanson

I. BREAST-FEEDING AND OTHER MODES OF FEEDING OF THE INFANT

No one would deny that breast-feeding is the natural mode of feeding of the human offspring. Most of us believe that it is only in modern times that neonates and young infants have been fed with foods and fluids other than human milk. However, this is not so. King Ashurrbanipal (7th century B.C.) may have been the first artificially fed infant to have been recorded in history. Writings from ancient India (B.C. 1500–A.D. 700) prescribed delayed onset of breastfeeding and so did the Greek physician Soranus (approximately A.D. 100) who claimed that the maternal milk was unwholesome for the first 20 days of lactation (Fildes, 1986).

Before describing the immunological consequences of breast-feeding for the infant it is necessary to define breast-feeding and to indicate to what extent infants really are breastfed.

Exclusive or complete breastfeeding will be used when nothing but maternal milk is given, not even water, which may be contaminated. *Partial breast-feeding* will include those who receive any other fluid or food in addition to the human milk.

A. The Time of Onset of Breast-Feeding

It is remarkable that the prescription of the ancient authors still seems to be in effect. Thus, in traditional societies (e.g., in Pakistan) the onset of breast-feeding is still delayed, with less than 50% of the infants being breast-fed at 48 hours of life (Hanson *et al.*, 1986; Ashraf *et al.*, 1992). Instead they are given various other foods and fluids, such as ghutti (cleared butter) and honey and herb extracts advised more than a thousand years ago (Fildes, 1986).

B. Prevalence and Duration of Breast-Feeding

The prevalence of breast-feeding decreased in industrialized countries to very low levels in the 1950s and 1960s, in parallel with the development of commercial formulas and the concept that the antibodies of human milk were of no importance since they were not resorbed by the breast-fed infant (Vahlqvist, 1958). With the increased understanding of the many nutritional and immunological advantages of breast-feeding a change in attitude has occurred that has resulted in a continuous increase both of direct onset of breast-feeding at birth and of the prevalence and duration of breast-feeding in some Western societies.

Breast-feeding is believed to be very common in traditional societies in the Third World. However, all infants in a large study in Lahore, Pakistan, received the initial traditional foods and fluids before breast-feeding started (Ashraf *et al.*, 1992). After that, only 9% were breast-fed exclusively after the first few days of life. About 70% were breast-feeding partially at 12 months of age (Ashraf *et al.*, 1992). Those infants not breast-feeding were found mainly in the upper middle class, in which commercial formulas were used widely. In contrast, such formulas were rarely given among the poor mothers, almost 100% of whom gave their infants water or buffalo milk in a bottle instead, usually in addition to breast-feeding. During the hot season, the infants were given more water under the misconception that breast-fed infants then require extra fluid. As a consequence, almost no exclusively breast-fed infants are found during this period, when diarrheal diseases are most common, the defense provided by the maternal milk is most needed, and other fluids more often may be contaminated (Ashraf *et al.*, 1992). Several studies have shown that no extra fluid is required for a breast-fed infant, even in a hot and dry climate (Ashraf *et al.*, 1992).

C. Effects of the Mode of Feeding on the Microbial Flora of the Infant

At birth, the newborn is exposed immediately to numerous microorganisms of different species, among which potential pathogens also may be included. Already in the first few days after parturition, many anaerobic as well as aerobic bacteria have colonized the gut.

The intestinal flora has been shown to differ in breast-fed and non-breast-fed infants (Ørskov and Biering-Sörensen, 1975; Raibaud, 1988; Balmer and Wharton, 1989). Pakistani infants, delivered both vaginally and by caesarian section, were colonized already from the first day of life, whereas some Swedish infants still had no demonstrable enterobacterial strains on the fifth day of life. The Swedish infants were colonized mainly only by one type of aerobic gram-negative bacterium whereas the Pakistani infants frequently carried strains of several types. In Pakistani infants, *Proteus, Klebsiella, Enterobacter,* and *Citrobacter* were significantly more common in non-breast-fed than in breast-fed babies; *Escherichia coli* was found significantly earlier in breast-fed than in non-breast-fed infants (Hanson *et al.,* 1989a; Adlerberth *et al.,* 1991).

Aerobic gram-negative bacteria from the intestine of breast-fed infants also have been demonstrated to be more sensitive to the bactericidal effects of antibodies than bacteria from formula-fed infants (Gothefors *et al.,* 1975), suggesting a decrease of virulence of the bacteria. Similar conclusions might be drawn from observations of the effect of breast-feeding on newborns colonized artificially by a harmless *E. coli* 083 strain during the first week of life (Lódinova-Zadnikóva *et al.,* 1991). The *E. coli* 083 strains from breast-fed infants more often carried type 1 fimbriae, which do not seem to be virulence factors (Wold *et al.,* 1990). Breast-feeding favored colonization by the type 1 fimbriated 083 strain (Lódinova-Zadnikóva *et al.,* 1991).

II. EFFECTS OF BREAST-FEEDING ON HOST DEFENSE COMPONENTS OF THE INFANT

A. Immunoglobulins

We have found that the newborn, already at birth, has secretory IgA and IgM (SIgA and SIgM) antibodies in saliva, against both *E. coli* and poliovirus antigens (Mellander *et al.,* 1984,1986). Such antibodies are present in newborns of healthy mothers as well as of mothers with hypogammaglobulinemia and IgA deficiency who lack IgA or IgM, supporting the idea that these antibodies are produced by the fetus (Mellander *et al.,* 1986; Hahn-Zoric *et al.,* 1992). We have proposed that the antigenic stimulus for the fetus could be anti-idiotypic antibodies that come from the mother (Mellander *et al.,* 1986). We were able to demonstrate such anti-anti-poliovirus antibodies in the immunoglobulin preparations given to the immunodeficient mothers, as well as in human milk (Hanson *et al.,* 1989b; M. Hahn-Zoric, 1993). If our assumption is correct, antibodies passively received by the fetus from the mother before birth via placenta or after birth via the milk can prime the immune system of the offspring actively in addition to conferring passive protection on the baby. In animal experiments, such an effect of anti-idiotypic antibodies has been demonstrated against bacterial as well as viral antigens when anti-antibodies were given directly to the newborn mouse or, via the mother animal, reached the offspring through the milk (Stein and Söderström, 1984; Okamoto *et al.,* 1989). The exposure of the mother to microbes is likely to direct her immune response and influence her levels of corresponding idiotypes and anti-idiotypes, which will be transferred to the fetus and infant, presumably both by serum and by milk. Presently, however, little is known about the factors that determine whether stimulation or inhibition of the immune response will result.

In preterm infants, serum immunoglobulin levels were higher in formula-fed infants than in breast-fed infants. For IgA, this difference was demonstrated from 7 weeks of age and for IgG, from 11 weeks (Savilahti *et al.,* 1983). Full-term infants showed similar patterns (Saarinen *et al.,* 1979; Savilahti *et al.,* 1987). In saliva, SIgA levels have been demonstrated to be higher in breast-fed than in formula-fed infants, although possible contamination from the milk was not excluded (Roberts and Freed, 1977). Other studies have shown no influence on serum IgA by the mode of feeding, but an increase of SIgA was seen in the stool and urine of breast-fed infants compared with formula-fed controls (Schanler *et al.,* 1986).

Human milk also contains considerable numbers of lymphocytes, granulocytes, and macrophages, especially during early lactation. Most of the milk lymphocytes are T cells, many of which carry the CDw29 marker of memory T cells (Bertotto *et al.,* 1990,1991). Such memory T cells could support the production of the wide diversity of milk SIgA antibodies, but also might have an effect on the breast-fed offspring. A positive tuberculin reaction has been observed temporarily in breast-fed infants of tuberculin-positive mothers (Mohr 1973; Ogra *et al.,* 1977; Schlesinger and Covelli, 1977).

Some, but not all, studies show no impairment of titers of milk IgA antibodies against various microbes by undernutrition (Cruz *et al.,* 1982,1985; Miranda *et al.,* 1983). However, a study by Herías *et al.* 1993 demonstrated a decreased milk SIgA concentration as well as decreased antibody affinity as a result of undernutrition, which could be an effect of undernutrition on T cells (Chandra, 1979a).

B. Vaccine Responses

In another study, we noticed that breast-fed infants had significantly higher serum and saliva antibodies against diphtheria and tetanus toxoids and poliovirus than did formula-fed infants after the first two vaccine doses (Hahn-Zoric *et al.,* 1990). The SIgA responses in saliva and IgM in stool samples were significantly higher at 3–4 months of age, whereas the serum IgG antibody response to diphtheria toxoid and the neutralizing antibodies against poliovirus were higher at 20–40 months of age. Similar results were found after immunization of infants using a *Haemophilus influenzae* type b conjugate vaccine; breast-fed babies were shown to have significantly higher serum antibody levels than formula-fed infants (Pabst and Spady, 1990). The purified protein derivative (PPD) reaction was stronger after immunization with *Bacillus* Calmette-Guerin (BCG) in breast-fed than in formula-fed infants (Pabst *et al.,* 1989). The possibility that the mother's milk enhances vaccine response might be of clinical relevance and suggests that the immunoglobulins in human milk may not merely provide the neonate with passive immunity but also may actively stimulate the lymphoid system of the breast-fed infants. Experimental data indicate that human milk contains anti-idiotypic antibodies (Hanson *et al.,* 1989b; M. Hahn-Zoric, 1993).

C. Other Components

Several molecules that are known to be responsible for inducing inflammation, for example, IgM and IgG antibodies, complement, and coagulation factors, are found at low levels in, or are almost absent from, human milk. In contrast, milk seems to be a rich source of other factors that block inflammation (Goldman *et al.*, 1986). The SIgA antibodies, present in high concentration in milk, as well as the milk oligosaccharides or glycoconjugates, which may be structurally similar to epithelial receptors for microbes, have the capacity to block the binding of microbes to mucosal epithelia, thus preventing infection in the newborn (Holmgren *et al.*, 1981; Andersson *et al.*, 1983,1986; Lagreid *et al.*, 1986; Lagreid and Kolstø Otnaess, 1987).

We have explored whether human milk components have the capacity to prevent the release of cytokines from various cells induced by exposure to lipopolysaccharides (LPS). This ability is of interest since these molecules are known to have striking effects, for example, on epithelial cells, making them produce cytokines such as interleukin 1 (IL-1), IL-6, and tumor necrosis factor α (TNFα). We have found that lactoferrin isolated from human milk can block LPS-induced IL-6 release from a human macrophage and a human colonic epithelium cell line (Hanson et al., 1991b; I. Mattsby Baltzer, A. Roseanu, I. Engberg, C. Motas, and L. Å. Hanson, unpublished data). Such activities of human milk components may help prevent the release of IL-6 or other cytokines in the newborn being colonized with gram-negative bacteria. Such a release might induce symptoms and catabolic effects, for instance, possibly explaining some of the early weight loss of neonates. Whether the prevention of cytokine release in mucosal membranes can have consequences for the immune response of the infant still must be explored. However, TNFα has been demonstrated in milk (Goldman *et al.*, 1991; Rudloff *et al.*, 1992). Breast-feeding has been suggested to stimulate the maturation of the immune system in the newborn; part of this stimulation may be caused by TNFα in human milk, which might up-regulate the expression of secretory component on epithelial cells or of Class I and II major histocompatibility complex (MHC) molecules on macrophages, or perhaps enhance maturation of monocytes or T lymphocytes (Goldman *et al.*, 1991).

Human milk also contains numerous components such as lysozyme, lipids, and antioxidants that prevent neutrophil chemotaxis, granular release, and production of free radicals (Goldman *et al.*, 1986). Such activities are likely to add to the well-being of the infant by depressing or preventing inflammatory reactivity. Epidermal growth factor (EGF), which is present in considerable amounts in milk, probably plays a role in the regulation of the development of the gastrointestinal tract of the newborn (Bines and Walker, 1991; Koldovsky *et al.*, 1991). The existence of analogous inhibitors of virus receptors also may be important in infections by viruses such as the human immunodeficiency virus (HIV). A factor in the macromolecular fraction of human milk has been demonstrated that inhibits binding of HIV epitope-specific monoclonal antibodies and HIV envelope glycoprotein gp120 to recombinant CD4 receptor molecules. The role this factor plays in HIV infection, as well as its chemical character, remains to be investigated (Newburg *et al.*, 1992).

III. EFFECTS OF BREAST-FEEDING ON INFECTIONS IN THE INFANT

A. Gastroenteritis

Extensive studies support the notion that breast-feeding is of importance in minimizing infant mortality and morbidity from diarrhea. In the 18th and 19th centuries, observers in Sweden noted that infant mortality due to diarrhea was strikingly increased during the summer months when mothers were not breast-feeding (Brändström, 1984). Feachem and Koblinsky (1984) reviewed the literature and concluded that the risk of dying from diarrhea was increased 25-fold in non-breast-fed infants compared with exclusively breast-fed infants. Infants who are breast-fed also suffer from fewer episodes of diarrhea than those who are not breast-fed (Feacham and Koblinsky, 1984; Cunningham *et al.*, 1991; F. Jalil, A. Mahmud, R. N. Ashraf, S. Zaman, J. Karlberg, L. Å. Hanson, and B. S. Lindblad, unpublished data). Clinical studies that are meant to demonstrate protection by breast-feeding often are disrupted by several confounding factors that influence the outcome (Victora, 1990). The late start of breast-feeding and the often unrecognized extra food or water given to the breast-fed infant in traditional societies often have not been considered. This oversight may have led to an underestimation of the protective value of breast-feeding (Hanson *et al.*, 1986). However, in Brazil, breast-feeding clearly was shown to protect against death in diarrhea, especially in the first few months of life (Victora *et al.*, 1987). Partial weaning was followed by an increased risk, and infants who were weaned completely were at the greatest risk.

In a field study in Lahore, Pakistan, significant protection against diarrhea by breast-feeding was demonstrated during the first 3 months for the upper middle class, for 6 months in the urban slum, and for 12–24 months for village and periurban slum inhabitants (F. Jalil, A. Mahmud, R. N. Ashraf, S. Zaman, J. Karlberg, L. Å. Hanson, and B. S. Lindblad, unpublished results). The protection was seen especially during the hot season, when diarrhea is more prevalent and the infectious dose presumably is higher. The efficacy of the protection was, in early life, as high as 70–80% in the two poorest groups (village and periurban slum) and ~40% in the upper middle class (Ashraf *et al.*, 1992). Even partial breast-feeding, which is the predominant mode of feeding in this area, can protect infants to a surprisingly high degree.

Few studies have been able to define the protective role and the importance of specific host defense components in maternal milk. However, the protection against diarrhea caused by *Vibrio cholerae*, enterotoxigenic *E. coli*, and *Campylobacter* in breast-fed infants has been shown to relate to the presence of special milk IgA antibodies against each of these pathogens in mother's milk (Glass *et al.*, 1983; Cruz *et al.*, 1988; Ruiz-Palacios *et al.*, 1990). Other milk components such as lactoferrin and receptor analogs could be important as well, but this has not been demonstrated.

B. Septicemia and Other Infections

Breast-feeding does not only seem to protect against gastroenteritis, but evidence also exists of protection against septicemia during early infancy (Winberg and Wessner, 1971; Narayanan *et al.*, 1981). In a study of neonatal septicemia in Lahore, Pakistan, an odds ratio of 18 was found for protection even by partial breast-feeding compared with feeding with animal milk (Ashraf *et al.*, 1991). Finding evidence for protection against lower respiratory tract infections has been more difficult but some positive studies have been presented (Victora *et al.*, 1987; Wright *et al.*, 1989; Howie *et al.*, 1990). Protection has not been demonstrated in all investigations, and a preliminary analysis of the prevalence of respiratory infections in our study in Pakistan to date has not shown a correlation to the mode of feeding (F. Jalil, *et al.*, unpublished data).

Certain investigations have indicated that breast-feeding protects against otitis media (Saarinen, 1982; Aniansson *et al.*, 1990) and necrotizing enterocolitis (Lucas and Cole, 1990). The latter authors estimate that breast-feeding could prevent as many as 500 cases of necrotizing enterocolitis a year in the United Kingdom, of which about 100 infants otherwise would die.

IV. EFFECTS OF BREAST-FEEDING ON ALLERGY IN THE INFANT AND CHILD

Atopic allergies are becoming increasingly common. Allergies to foods are especially prevalent in infancy and early childhood. Much interest has been directed toward breast-feeding as a possible way to prevent allergy.

A. Breast-Feeding and the Serum and Secretory Antibody Response to Food Proteins in the Infant

Salivary SIgA antibodies previously have been shown to be found in the neonate and increase rapidly on antigenic exposure (Mellander *et al.*, 1984,1985). Even the premature infant can respond with SIgA antibodies against cow's milk proteins in saliva (Roberton *et al.*, 1986). Breast-fed infants show significantly lower salivary SIgA anti-bovine casein than cow's milk-fed infants (Renz *et al.*, 1989). Infants without any risk factors for atopic allergy have significantly higher levels of such salivary SIgA antibodies after being fed cow's milk than do those with risk factors who were fed similarly.

Prolonged breast-feeding leaves infants with significantly lower serum IgG, IgM, and IgA levels than non-breast-fed infants (Savilahti *et al.*, 1987). Serum IgG antibodies against cow's milk proteins increased most in those infants given cow's milk formula before the age of 1 month. Fully weaned and partially breast-fed infants had similar increased levels (Tainio *et al.*, 1988). Exclusively breast-fed infants also produced antibodies against cow's milk, perhaps because of the presence of cow's milk proteins in the maternal milk (e.g., Machtinger and Moss, 1986) or because of the exposure to anti-idiotypic antibodies via the placenta or the maternal milk (Mellander *et al.*, 1986; Hanson *et al.*, 1989b; Hahn-Zoric *et al.*, 1990,1992,1993).

The appearance of anti-food antibodies was analyzed in infants breast-fed by mothers on a normal diet, on a diet free of the allergens of egg and cow's milk, or restricted with respect to the intake of these foods from week 28 of pregnancy to delivery. The babies of the mothers on the allergen-free diet curiously had significantly higher IgG, IgA, and IgM antibodies against ovalbumin and gluten, but not against β-lactoglobulin (Fälth-Magnusson *et al.*, 1988). In another similar study in which the diet restriction for one group of mothers included egg, cow's milk, and fish during the first 3 months of lactation, the only significant difference among the breast-fed infants from the two groups was that fewer infants in the diet group than the non-diet group had IgE antibodies against eggwhite and cow's milk proteins. IgE antibodies also appeared during exclusive breast-feeding (Hattevig *et al.*, 1990).

B. Antibodies in Human Milk in Relation to the Maternal Diet

Enteric exposure of the mother to foods may, via the enteromammaric pathway, result in SIgA antibodies against these foods in her milk. Mothers with cow's milk as a regular component of the diet had higher levels of SIgA antibodies against cow's milk proteins in their milk than did those who did not regularly drink cow's milk (Cruz *et al.*, 1981). Oral exposure to a cowpea protein induced a milk SIgA antibody response in lactating mothers who did not have any prevaccination titer. However, in the few individuals who had such titers, a decrease was seen instead after eating the cowpeas (Cruz and Hanson, 1986). In another study, no differences were seen in milk IgG and IgA antibody levels against β-lactoglobulin, ovalbumin, and gliadin between atopic and nonatopic mothers at 1 week of lactation. Also no differences were seen in antibody levels between mothers on a cow's milk- and egg-free diet and mothers on a normal diet during pregnancy (Fälth-Magnusson, 1989).

Obviously, we currently do not know how oral exposure to a food protein may affect the milk antibody level. Perhaps antibody responses in the milk partly originate from the influx of memory cells into the lactating gland. One finding to support such a view is the presence of such a wide array of different antibody specificities at one time in the maternal milk, many more than the mother is likely to produce against antigens to which she has been exposed recently (Hanson and Brandtzaeg, 1989). Further, the relative affinities of these milk antibodies are often high and do not increase by vaccination, suggesting the presence of already mature antibody responses (Roberton *et al.*, 1988; Dahlgren *et al.*, 1989).

C. Breast-Feeding and the Prevention of Allergy

Several studies have investigated the possibility that breast-feeding can prevent the development of atopic disease in the infant. Some of these studies have concerned risk families with a heredity predisposition to atopic diseases. In some investigations, the role of maternal avoidance diets has been analyzed.

Chandra and Hamed (1991) compared the incidence of atopic allergy in high risk children at 12 and 18 months of age; the infants were given a whey hydrolysate, conventional cow's milk formula, soy-based formula, or exclusively human milk. Atopic dermatitis and other allergic symptoms were significantly less common among those breast-fed or given the hydrolysate than among those given soy or cow's milk formula.

In an interesting study, Machtinger and Moss (1986) presented data that suggested that the risk of developing cow's milk allergy for the breast-fed infant may relate to the antibody content of the maternal milk. The milk of the mothers of children developing allergy had significantly lower total IgA and IgG antibodies against casein and whole cow's milk than did the milk of mothers whose children did not become allergic. These observations agree with those of Casimir *et al.* (1989) who studied IgG antibodies against β-lactoglobulin in maternal milk.

Some studies have noted that a maternal avoidance diet during late pregnancy has decreased atopic manifestations during infancy in high risk families (Chandra, 1979b; Zieger *et al.*, 1989). However, no difference in occurrence of allergy in breast-fed infants was found in a study of mothers on or off a diet of cow's milk and egg avoidance from week 28 of pregnancy to delivery (Fälth-Magnusson and Kjellman, 1987). Even at the 5-yr follow-up including 95% of the 209 initial children, no difference was found between the infants breast-fed by mothers in the diet and non-diet groups (Fälth-Magnusson and Kjellman, 1992). In another prospective study with maternal avoidance of egg, cow's milk, and fish during the first 3 months of lactation, a significantly lower incidence of atopic dermatitis was noted (Hattevig *et al.*, 1989). Reinvestigating the children at the age of 4 years showed that those in the diet group still had a cumulative incidence and a current prevalence of atopic dermatitis that was significantly lower than that of the non-diet group (Sigurs *et al.*, 1992). Other allergic manifestations did not differ, but the numbers of positive skin prick tests and specific serum IgE antibody reactions were significantly lower among the children in the diet group. A third study tried a low and a high intake of eggs and cow's milk for 171 atopic mothers during the last 3 months of pregnancy. All infants were breast-fed for at least 3 months. Investigating the infants at 18 months of age showed no difference between the diet groups with respect to occurrence of atopic disease (Lilja *et al.*, 1989). These authors assumed that genetic factors rather than allergen exposure were important in the development of allergy.

The question of the role of early introduction of cow's milk to breast-fed infants in the risk of developing allergy also has been analyzed. In a study assigning 250 infants to be given either cow's milk or a whey hydrolysate for 1–4 days before the onset of breast-feeding, IgG antibodies showed priming by the cow's milk exposure and IgE antibodies increased significantly (Schmitz *et al.*, 1991). Going back to detailed feeding records, Gustafsson *et al.* (D. Gustafsson, T. Löwhagen, and K. Andersson, unpublished data) could show that whether or not the neonates had been given early cow's milk formula supplementation before breast-feeding started did not affect the prevalence of atopic disease in the early teens.

The risk of developing food allergy does not seem to be higher in premature infants than full-term infants, even if the premature infants were breast-fed for a shorter period of time than the full-term infants (de Martino *et al.*, 1989).

V. CONCLUSIONS

The time of onset, the duration, and the rate of breast-feeding vary widely in different cultural settings. This variation has striking consequences for the infants, since the maternal milk is so important for the host defense of the newborn. The immunodeficiency that is secondary to lack of breast-feeding may be the most common in the world.

Breast-feeding influences the bacterial colonization, since it delays the appearence and decreases the virulence and number of the types of microbes that colonize the gut of the neonate. Human milk also contains several components that seem to counteract inflammatory activities. The protective effects of breast-feeding have been demonstrated against infections such as diarrhea, septicemia, and respiratory tract infections. Breast-feeding seems to enhance vaccine responses, possibly because of the effect of anti-idiotypic antibodies present in the milk. Breast-feeding also may decrease the risk of development of allergy in the infant.

Acknowledgments

We thank Ms. A.-C. Malmefeldt for typing the manuscript. Our own studies referred to in this chapter were supported by the Swedish Agency for Research Cooperation with Developing Countries, the Swedish Medical Research Council (No. 215), and the Ellen, Walter, and Lennart Hesselman Foundation.

References

Adlerberth, I., Carlsson, B., de Man, P., Jalil, F., Khan, S. R., Larsson, P., Mellander, L., Svanborg-Edén, C., Wold, A. E., and Hanson, L. Å. (1991). Intestinal colonization with Enterobacteriaceae in Pakistani and Swedish hospital delivered infants. *Acta Paediatr. Scand.* **80,** 602–610.

Andersson, B., Fahmén, J., Frejd, T., Leffler, H., Magnusson, G., Noori, G., and Svanborg-Edén, C. (1983). Identification of an active disaccharide unit of glycoconjugate receptor for pneumococci attaching to human pharyngeal cells. *J. Exp. Med.* **158,** 559–570.

Andersson, B., Porras, O., Hanson, L. Å., Lagergård, T., and Svanborg-Edén, C. (1986). Inhibition of attachment of *Streptococ-*

cus pneumoniae and *Haemophilus influenzae* by human milk and receptor oligosaccharides. *J. Infect. Dis.* **153,** 232–237.

Aniansson, B., Andersson, B., Alm, B., Larsson, P., Nylén, O., Pettersson, H., Rignér, P., Svanborg, M., and Svanborg-Edén, C. (1990). Protection of breastfeeding against bacterial colonization of the nasopharynx: A pilot study. *In* "Human Lactation 4: Breastfeeding, Nutrition, Infections and Infant Growth in Developed and Emerging Countries" (S. A. Atkinson, L. Å. Hanson, and R. K. Chandra, eds.), pp. 195–205. ARTS Biomedical Publishers, St. Johns, Newfoundland.

Ashraf, R. N., Jalil, F., Zaman, S., Karlberg, J., Khan, S. R., Lindblad, B. S., and Hanson, L. Å. (1991). Breastfeeding and protection against neonatal sepsis in a high risk population. *Arch. Dis. Child.* **66,** 488–490.

Ashraf, R., Jalil, F., Khan, S. R., Zaman, S., Karlberg, J., Lindblad, B. S., and Hanson, L. Å. (1993). Early child health in Lahore, Pakistan V. Feeding patterns in 0-24 months old children. *Acta Paediatr. Scand. Suppl.* **390,** 47–61.

Balmer, S. E., and Wharton, B. A. (1989). Diet and faecal flora in the newborn: Breastmilk and infant formula. *Arch. Dis. Child.* **64,** 1672–1677.

Bertotto, A., Gerli, R., Fabietti, G., Crupi, S., Arcangeli, C., Scalise, F., and Vaccaro, R. (1990). Human breast milk T lymphocytes display the phenotype and functional characteristics of memory T cells. *Eur. J. Immunol.* **20,** 1877–1880.

Bertotto, A., Castellucci, G., Scalise, F., Tognellini, R., and Vaccaro, R. (1991). "Memory" T cells in human breast milk. *Acta Paediatr. Scand.* **80,** 98–99.

Bines, J. E., and Walker, W. A. (1991). Growth factors and the development of neonatal host defense. *In* "Immunology of Milk and the Neonate" (J. Mestecky, C. Blair, and P. L. Ogra, eds.), pp. 31–39. Plenum Press, New York.

Brändström, A. (1984). The loveless mothers. Acta Universitalis Umaniensis, Umeå. *Studies in the Humanities* **62.** (in Swedish with English summary)

Casimir, G. J. A., Duchateau, J., Cuvelier, P., and Vis, H. L. (1989). Maternal immune status against β-lactoglobulin and cow milk allergy in the infant. *Ann. Allergy* **63,** 517–519.

Chandra, R. K. (1979a). Nutritional deficiencies and susceptibility to infection. *Bull. WHO* **57,** 167–177.

Chandra, R. K. (1979b). Prospective studies of the effect of breastfeeding on incidence of infection and allergy. *Acta Paediatr. Scand.* **68,** 691–694.

Chandra, R. K., and Hamed, A. (1991). Cumulative incidence of atopic disorders in high risk infants fed whey hydrolysate, soy and conventional cow milk formula. *Ann. Allergy* **67,** 129–132.

Cruz, J. R., and Hanson, L. Å. (1986). Specific milk immune response of rural and urban Guatemalan women to oral immunization with a food protein. *J. Pediatr. Gastroent. Nutr.* **5,** 450–454.

Cruz, J. R., Garcia, B., Urrutia, J. J., Carlsson, B., and Hanson, L. Å. (1981). Food antibodies in milk from Guatemalan women. *J. Pediatr.* **99,** 600–602.

Cruz, J. R., Carlsson, B., Garcia, B., Gebre-Medhin, M., Gothefors, L., Urrutia, J. J., and Hanson, L. Å. (1982). Studies of human milk III. Secretory IgA quantities and antibody levels against *Escherichia coli* in colostrum and milk samples from underpriviledged mothers. *Pediatr. Res.* **16,** 272–276.

Cruz, J. R., Carlsson, B., Hofvander, Y., Holme, D., and Hanson, L. Å. (1985). Studies of human milk II. Concentration of antibodies against *Salmonella* and *Shigella* in milk of women from different populations and the daily intake by their breast-fed infants. *Acta Paediatr. Scand.* **74,** 338–341.

Cruz, J. R., Gil, L., Cano, P., Caceres, P., and Pareja, G. (1988). Breastmilk anti-*Escherichia coli* heat-labile toxin IgA antibodies protect against toxin-induced infantile diarrhoea. *Acta Paediatr. Scand.* **77,** 658–662.

Cunningham, A. S., Jelliffe, D. B., and Jelliffe, E. F. P. (1991). Breastfeeding and health in the 1980s. A global epidemiologic review. *J. Pediatr.* **118,** 659–666.

Dahlgren, U., Carlsson, B., Jalil, F., MacDonald, R., Mascart-Lémone, F., Nilsson, K., Roberton, D., Sennhauser, F., Wold, A., and Hanson, L. Å. (1989). Induction of the mucosal immune response. *Curr. Top. Microbiol. Immunol.* **146,** 156–161.

de Martino, M., Donzelli, G. P., Galli, L., Scarano, E., de Marco, A., Rapisardi, G., Vecchi, C., and Vierucci, A. (1989). Food allergy in preterm infants fed human milk. *Biol. Neonate* **56,** 301–305.

Fälth-Magnusson, K. (1989). Breast milk antibodies to foods in relation to maternal diet, maternal atopy and the development of atopic disease in the baby. *Int. Arch. Allergy Appl. Immunol.* **90,** 297–300.

Fälth-Magnusson, K., and Kjellman, N. I. M. (1987). Development of atopic disease in babies whose mothers were receiving exclusion diet during pregnancy—A randomized study. *J. Allergy Clin. Immunol.* **80,** 868–875.

Fälth-Magnusson, K., and Kjellman, N. I. M. (1993). Allergy prevention by maternal elimination diet during late pregnancy—A five-year follow-up of a randomized study. *J. Allergy Clin. Immunol.*

Fälth-Magnusson, K., Kjellman, N. I. M., and Magnusson, K.-E. (1988). Antibodies IgG, IgA and IgM to food antigens during the first 18 months of life in relation to feeding and development of atopic disease. *J. Allergy Clin. Immunol.* **81,** 743–749.

Feachem, R. G., and Koblinsky, M. A. (1984). Interventions for the control of diarrhoeal diseases among young children: Promotion of breast-feeding. *Bull. WHO* **62,** 271–291.

Fildes, F. (1986). "Breast, Bottles & Babies. A History of Breastfeeding." Edinburgh University Press, Edinburg.

Glass, R. E., Svennerholm, A. M., Stoll, B. J., Khan, M. R., Hossein, K. M. B., Huq, M. I., and Holmgren, J. (1983). Protection against cholera in breast-fed children by antibodies in breast-milk. *N. Engl. J. Med.* **308,** 1389–1392.

Goldman, A. S., Thorpe, L. W., Goldblum, R. M., and Hanson, L. Å. (1986). An hypothesis: Anti-inflammatory properties of human milk. *Acta Paediatr. Scand.* **75,** 689–695.

Goldman, A. S., Rudloff, H. E., and Schmalstieg, F. C. (1991). Are cytokines in human milk? *In* "Immunology of Milk and the Neonate" (J. Mestecky, C. Blair, and P. L. Ogra, eds.), pp. 93–97. Plenum Press, New York.

Gothefors, L., Olling, S., and Winberg, J. (1975). Breastfeeding and biological properties of fecal *E. coli* strains. *Acta Paediatr. Scand.* **64,** 807–811.

Hahn-Zoric, M. Fulconis, F., Minoli, I., Moro, G., Carlsson, B., Böttiger, M., Räihä, N., and Hanson, L. Å. (1990). Antibody responses to parenteral and oral vaccines are impaired by conventional and low protein formulas as compared to breastfeeding. *Acta Paediatr. Scand.* **79,** 1137–1142.

Hahn-Zoric, M., Carlsson, B., Björkander, J., Osterhaus, A. D. M. E., Mellander, L., and Hanson, L. Å. (1992). Presence of non-maternal antibodies in newborns of mothers with antibody deficiencies. *Pediatr. Res.* **32,** 150–154.

Hahn-Zoric, M., Carlsson, B., Jeansson, S., Ekre, O., Osterhaus, A.D.M.E, Roberton, D. M., and Hanson, L. Å. (1993). Anti-idiotypic antibodies to poliovirus in commercial immunoglobulin preparations, human serum, and milk. *Pediatr. Res.* **33,** 475–480.

Hanson, L. Å., and Brandtzaeg, P. (1989). The mucosal defense system. *In* "Immunologic Disorders in Infants and Children" (E. R. Stiehm, ed.), 3d Ed., p. 116–155. Saunders, Philadelphia.

Hanson, L. Å., Adlerberth, I., Carlsson, B., Jalil, F., Karlberg, J., Lindblad, B. S., Mellander, L., Khan, S. R., Hasan, R., Sheikh, A. K., and Söderström, T. (1986). Breastfeeding in reality. *In* "Human Lactation 2: Maternal and Environmental Factors." (M.

Hamosh and A. S. Goldman, eds.), pp. 1–12. Plenum Press, New York.

Hanson, L. Å., Adlerberth, I., Carlsson, B., Dahlgren, U., Hahn-Zoric, M., Jalil, F., Khan, S. R., Larsson, P., Midtvedt, T., Roberton, D., Svanborg-Edén, C., and Wold, A. (1989a). Colonization with Enterobacteriacae and the immune response, especially in the neonate. *In* "The Regulatory and Protective Role of the Normal Microflora" (R. Grubb, T. Midtvedt, and E. Norin, eds.), pp. 59–69. Stockholm Press, New York.

Hanson, L. Å., Carlsson, B., Ekre, H. P., Hahn-Zoric, M., Osterhaus, A. D. M. E., and Roberton, D. (1989b). Immunoregulation of mother–fetus/newborn; A role for anti-idiotypic antibodies? *Acta Paediatr. Scand. Suppl.* **351,** 38–41.

Hanson, L. Å., Ashraf, R. N., Carlsson, B., Mattsby Baltzer, I., Motas, C., Hahn-Zoric, M., Mata, L., Herías, V., Cruz, J. R., Lindblad, B. S., Karlberg, J., and Jalil, F. (1992). Breastfeeding, infections and immunology. *In* "Nutritional Immunology" (R. K. Chandra, ed.). pp. 45–60. ARTS Biomedical Publishers and Distributors, St. John's, Newfoundland, Canada.

Hanson, L. Å., Ashraf, R. N., Hahn-Zoric, M., Carlsson, B., Herías, V., Wiedermann, U., Dahlgren, U., Motas, C., Mattsby Baltzer, I., Gonzales-Cossio, T., Cruz, J. R., Karlberg, J., Lindblad, B. S., and Jalil, F. (1991b). Breast milk: Role in neonatal host defense *In* "Immunophysiology of the Gut" (A. Walker, P. K. Harmatz, B. K. Wershil, eds.). Academic Press, San Diego. pp. 248–268.

Hattevig, G., Kjellman, B., Sigurs, N., Björksten, B., and Kjellman, N. I. M. (1989). The effect of maternal avoidance of eggs, cow's milk and fish during lactation upon allergic manifestations in infants. *Clin. Exp. Allergy* **19,** 27–32.

Hattevig, G., Kjellman, B., Sigurs, N., Grodzinsky, E., Hed, J., and Björksten, B. (1990). The effect of maternal avoidance of eggs, cow's milk and fish during lactation on the development of IgE, IgG and IgA antibodies in infants. *J. Allergy Clin. Immunol.* **85,** 108–115.

Herías, M. V., Cruz, J. R., González-Cossio, T., Nave, F., Carlsson, B., and Hanson, L. Å. (1993). The effect of caloric supplementation on milk IgA antibody titres and avidities in undernourished Guatemalan mothers. *Pediatr. Res.* **82,** 552–556.

Holmgren, J., Svennerholm, A.-M., and Åhrén, C. (1981). Non-immunoglobulin fraction of human milk inhibits bacterial adhesion (hemagglutination and enterotoxin binding of *Escherichia coli* and *Vibrio cholerae*. *Infect. Immun.* **33,** 136–141.

Howie, P. W., Forsyth, J. S., Ogston, S. A., Clark, A., and Florey, C. V. (1990). Protective effect of breastfeeding against infection. *Br. Med. J.* **300,** 11–16.

Koldovsky, O., Britton, J., Davis, D., Davis, T., Grimes, J., Kong, W., Rao, R., and Schaudies, P. (1991). The developing gastrointestinal tract and milk-bone epidermal growth factor. *In* "Immunology of Milk and the Neonate" (J. Mestecky, C. Blair, and P. L. Ogra, eds.), pp. 99–106. Plenum Press, New York.

Lagreid, A., and Kolstø Otnaess, A.-B. (1987). Trace amounts of ganglioside GM1 in human milk inhibit enterotoxins from *Vibrio cholerae* and *Escherichia coli*. *Life Sci.* **4,** 55–62.

Lagreid, A., and Kolstø Otnaess, A.-B., and Fuglesang, J. (1986). Human and bovine milk: Comparison of ganglioside composition and enterotoxin-inhibitory activity. *Pediatr. Res.* **20,** 416–421.

Lilja, G., Danneus, A., Foucard, T., Graff-Lonnevig, V., Johansson, S. G. O., and Öman, H. (1989). Effects of maternal diet during late pregnancy and lactation on the development of atopic diseases in infants up to 18 months of age—*In vivo* results. *Clin. Exp. Allergy* **19,** 473–479.

Lodinóva-Zadnikóva, R., Slavikóva, M., Tlaskalóva-Hógenóva, H., Adlerberth, I., Hanson, L. Å., Wold, A., Carlsson, B., Svanborg, C., and Mellander, L. (1991). The antibody response in breastfed and formula-fed infants after artificial colonization of the intestine with *Escherichia coli* O83. *Pediatr. Res.* **29,** 396–399.

Lucas, A., and Cole, T. J. (1990). Breast milk and neonatal necrotizing enterocolitis. *Lancet* **336,** 1519–1523.

Machtinger, S., and Moss, R. (1986). Cow's milk allergy in breast-fed infants: The role of allergen and maternal secretory IgA antibody. *J. Allergy Clin. Immunol.* **77,** 341–347.

Mellander, L., Carlsson, B., and Hanson, L. Å. (1984). Appearance of secretory IgM and IgA antibodies to *Escherichia coli* in saliva during early infancy and childhood. *J. Pediatr.* **104,** 564–568.

Mellander, L., Carlsson, B., Jalil, F., Söderström, T., and Hanson, L. Å. (1985). Secretory IgA antibody response against *Escherichia coli* antigens in infants in relation to exposure. *J. Pediatr.* **107,** 430–433.

Mellander, L., Carlsson, B., and Hanson, L. Å. (1986). Secretory IgA and IgM antibodies to *E. coli* O and poliovirus type 1 antigens occur in amniotic fluid, meconium and saliva from newborns. A neonatal immune response without antigenic exposure—A result of anti-idiotypic induction? *Clin. Exp. Immunol.* **63,** 555–561.

Miranda, R., Saravia, N. G., Ackerman, R., Murphy, N., Berman, S., and McMurray, D. N. (1983). Effect of maternal nutritional status on immunologic substances in human colostrum and milk. *Am. J. Clin. Nutr.* **37,** 632–640.

Mohr, J. (1973). The possible induction and/or acquisition of cellular hypersensitivity associated with ingestion of colostrum. *J. Pediatr.* **82,** 1062–1064.

Narayanan, I., Prakash, K., and Gujral, V. V. (1981). The value of human milk in the prevention of infection in the high-risk low-birth-weight infant. *J. Pediatr.* **99,** 496–498.

Newburg, D. S., Viscidi, R. P., Ruff, A., and Yolken, R. H. (1992). A human milk factor inhibits binding of human immunodeficiency virus to the CD4 receptor. *Pediatr. Res.* **31,** 22–28.

Ogra, S. S., Weintraub, D., and Ogra, P. L. (1977). Immunologic aspects of human colostrum and milk. III. Fate and absorption of cellular and soluble components in the gastrointestinal tract of the newborn. *J. Immunol.* **119,** 245–248.

Okamoto, Y., Tsutsumi, H., Kumar, N. S., and Ogra, P. L. (1989). Effect of breastfeeding on the development of idiotype antibody response to F glycoprotein of respiratory syncytial virus in infant mice after post-partum maternal immunization. *J. Immunol.* **142,** 2507–2512.

Ørskov, F., and Biering-Sörensen, K. (1975). *Escherichia coli* serogroups in breast-fed and bottlefed infants. *Acta Pathol. Microbiol. Immunol. Scand. B* **83,** 25–30.

Pabst, H. F., and Spady, D. W. (1990). Effect of breast-feeding on antibody response to conjugate vaccine. *Lancet* **336,** 269–270.

Pabst, H. F., Grace, M., Godel, J., Cho, H., and Spady, D. W. (1989). Effect of breast-feeding on immune response to BCG vaccination. *Lancet* **I,** 295–297.

Raibaud, P. (1988). Factors controlling the bacterial colonization of the neonatal intestine. *In* "Biology of Human Milk" (L. Å. Hanson, ed.), pp. 205–219. Raven Press, New York.

Renz, H., Brehler, C., Petzoldt, S., Prinz, H., and Rieger, C. H. L. (1989). Breastfeeding modifies production of SIgA cow's milk antibodies in infants. *Acta Paediatr. Scand.* **80,** 149–154.

Roberton, D. M., Forrest, P. J., Frangoulis, E., Jones, C. L., and Mermelstein, N. (1986). Early induction of secretory immunity in neonates' breastmilk. *Arch. Dis. Child.* **3,** 489–494.

Roberton, D., Carlsson, B., Coffman, K., Hahn-Zoric, M., Jalil, F., Jones, C., and Hanson, L. Å. (1988). Avidity of IgA antibody to *Escherichia coli* polysaccharide and diphtheria toxin in breastmilk from Swedish and Pakistani mothers. *Scand. J. Immunol.* **28,** 783–789.

Roberts, S. A., and Freed, D. L. (1977). Neonatal IgA secretion enhanced by breastfeeding. *Lancet* **II,** 1131.

Rudloff, H. E., Schmalstieg, F. C., Mustaha, A. A., Palkowetz, K. H., Liu, K. S., and Goldman, A. S. (1992). Tumor necrosis factor-α in human milk. *Pediatr. Res.* **31,** 29–33.

Ruiz-Palacios, G. M., Calva, J. J., and Pickering, L. K. (1990). Protection of breastfed infants against *Campylobacter* diarrhoea by antibodies in human milk. *J. Pediatr.* **116,** 707–713.

Saarinen, U. M. (1982). Prolonged breastfeeding as prophylaxis for recurrent otitis media. *Acta Paediatr. Scand.* **71,** 567–571.

Saarinen, U. M., Pelkonen, P., and Siimes, M. A. (1979). Serum immunoglobulin A in healthy infants: An accellerated postnatal increase in formula-fed, compared to breast-fed infants. *J. Pediatr.* **95,** 410–416.

Savilahti, E., Järvenpää, A. L., and Räihä, N. (1983). Serum immunoglobulins in preterm infants: Comparison of human milk and formula feeding. *Pediatrics* **72,** 312–317.

Savilahti, E., Salmenperä, L., Tainio, V.-M., Halme, H., Perheentupa, J., and Siimes, M. A. (1987). Prolonged exclusive breastfeeding results in low serum concentrations of immunoglobulins G, A and M. *Acta Paediatr. Scand.* **76,** 1–6.

Schanler, R. J., Goldblum, R. M., Garza, C., and Goldman, A. S. (1986). Enhanced fecal excretion of selected immune factors in very low birth weight infants fed fortified human milk. *Pediatr. Res.* **20,** 711–716.

Schlesinger, J. J., and Covelli, H. D. (1977). Evidence for transmission of lymphocyte response to tuberculine by breast-feeding. *Lancet* **II,** 529–532.

Schmitz, J., Digeon, B., Castany, C., Gibert, E., Dupoy, D., Leroux, B., Robillard, M., Gailing, M. O., and Strobel, S. (1991). Abstract ESPGAN.

Sigurs, N., Hattevig, G., and Kjellman, B. (1992). Maternal avoidance of eggs, cow's milk, and fish during lactation: Effect on allergic manifestations, skin prick tests and specific IgE antibodies in children at age 4 years. *Pediatrics* **89,** 735–739.

Stein, K. E., and Söderström, T. (1984). Neonatal administration of idiotype or anti-idiotype primes for protection against *E. coli* K13 infection in mice. *J. Exp. Med.* **160,** 1001–1011.

Tainio, V.-M., Savilahti, E., Arjomaa, P., Salmenperä, L., Perheentupa, J., and Siimes, M. A. (1988). Plasma antibodies to cow's milk are increased by early weaning and consumption of unmodified milk, but production of plasma IgA and IgM cow's milk antibodies is stimulated even during exclusive breastfeeding. *Acta Paediatr. Scand.* **77,** 807–811.

Vahlqvist, B. (1958). The transfer of antibodies from mother to offspring. *Adv. Pediatr.* **10,** 305–338.

Victora, C. G. (1990). Case-control studies of the influence of breastfeeding on child morbidity and mortality: Methodological issues. *In* "Human Lactation 4: Breastfeeding, Nutrition, Infection and Infant Growth in Developed and Emerging Countries" (S. A. Atkinson, L. Å. Hanson, and R. K. Chandra, eds.), pp. 405–418. ARTS Biomedical, St John's, Newfoundland.

Victora, C. G., Vaughan, J. P., Lombardi, C., Fuchs, S. M., Gigante, L. P., Smith, P. G., Noble, L. C., Texeira, A. M. B., Moreira, L. B., and Barros, F. C. (1987). Evidence for protection by breastfeeding against infant deaths from infectious diseases in Brasil. *Lancet* **II,** 319–322.

Winberg, J., and Wessner, G. (1971). Does breastmilk protect against septicemia in the newborn? *Lancet* **I,** 1091–1094.

Wold, A., Mestecky, J., Tomana, M., Kobata, A., Ohbayashi, H., Endo, T., and Svanborg-Edén, C. (1990). Secretory IgA carries oligosaccharide receptors for *Escherichia coli* type 1 fimbrial lectin. *Infect. Immun.* **58,** 3073–3077.

Wright, A. L., Holberg, C. J., Martinez, F. D., Morgan, W. J., and Taussig, L. M. (1989). Breast-feeding and lower respiratory tract illness in the first year of life. *Br. Med. J.* **299,** 946–949.

Zieger, R. S., Heller, S., Mellon, M., Forsythe, A. B., O'Connor, R., Hamburger, R. N., and Schatz, M. (1989). Effect of combined maternal and infant food-allergen avoidance on development of atopy in early infancy: A randomized study. *J. Allergy Clin. Immunol.* **84,** 72–89.

Section I

Genitourinary Tract

Section Editor: M. E. Lamm

(Chapters 53 through 58)

53

IgA Nephropathy and Related Diseases

Steven N. Emancipator • Michael E. Lamm

IgA nephropathy (IgAN) is defined as a form of glomerulonephritis in which immunoglobulins of the IgA isotype predominate or codominate in the glomerular deposits. The clinical and pathological features of both primary and secondary forms are well documented in several comprehensive reviews (Clarkson *et al.*, 1977; D'Amico *et al.*, 1985; Clarkson, 1987; D'Amico, 1987; Julian, 1988; Emancipator and Lamm, 1989; Sakai *et al.*, 1990; Emancipator, 1992; Schena, 1990) and will be presented here only briefly. We consider, in some detail, evidence for increased production of IgA, increased entry of antigen into the systemic circulation, and impaired clearance of aggregates containing IgA, whether immune or nonimmune in nature. In each of these categories of pathogenesis, we consider the potential contribution of the mucosal immune system. We conclude that, although several distinct mechanisms may underlie the pathogenesis of IgAN, the mucosal immune system is likely to figure prominently in each. Hence, we consider IgAN a consequence of a defective or inadequate mucosal immune system. Particularly, dysregulated specific responses to a variety of antigens, possibly multiple in an individual patient, are thought to lead to a set of conditions that favors glomerular deposition of immune complexes that contain IgA.

I. DISEASE PRESENTATION

A. Clinical Features

Although variable, the signs and symptoms of IgAN allow the grouping of cases into three syndromes that incorporate hematuria, proteinuria, hypertension, and renal insufficiency to varying degrees (reviewed in Emancipator, 1992). Hematuria may be evident to the naked eye (gross) or microscopic, and episodic or continuous. Proteinuria, ranging from a few hundred milligrams per day to frank nephrosis, is usually but not inevitably present. Acute or chronic renal failure may be observed, but is not common. Overall, the disease usually first becomes manifest during the second or third decade of life and is more prevalent in males by a factor of two or three. The most common syndrome is episodic macrohematuria associated with low-level (<1 g/24 hr) proteinuria (Clarkson *et al.*, 1977; D'Amico *et al.*, 1985). This pattern, typically observed in young males, also may feature bouts of acute hypertension or acute renal failure, and most often accompanies acute respiratory or gastrointestinal infections. The tendency for progression to glomerulosclerosis and chronic renal failure in this group, accounting for approximately 60% of all patients worldwide, is low (10%) over a sustained follow-up period (10–20 yr).

Microscopic hematuria, usually persistent but sometimes intermittent, is a somewhat less common presentation (Clarkson *et al.*, 1977; D'Amico *et al.*, 1985). Among these patients, many also have proteinuria in excess of 1 g/day. The proportion of all IgAN patients represented by such proteinuric patients varies geographically. In regions in which "major" signs or symptoms such as acute renal failure, gross hematuria, or substantial proteinuria are required before a renal biopsy is done, virtually all microhematuric patients have moderate or heavy proteinuria. Where persistent microhematuria is itself an indication for renal biopsy, roughly 30% of microhematuria patients have proteinuria exceeding 1 g/day.

Chronic renal insufficiency, frequently with hypertension, is the third syndrome. These patients, presumably with an earlier occult onset of disease, form the smallest group (10% of all patients) and often manifest proteinuria or hematuria on diagnosis as well.

B. Pathologic Features

In some 60% of cases, mesangial proliferation is observed in the biopsy of a patient with IgAN (reviewed by Emancipator and Lamm, 1989; Emancipator, 1992). This condition is defined as some combination of matrix expansion and cell proliferation confined to the mesangial compartment of the glomerulus, without compromise of capillary lumina. Mild or minimal mesangial change or focal endocapillary proliferation and matrix expansion, that is, lesions causing narrowing of some capillaries superimposed on an established mesangial proliferative pattern, occurs in roughly 15% of patients. The spectrum from mild mesangial to focal proliferative change to diffuse endocapillary proliferation (in which most capillaries are occluded by lesions) occurs in association with endogenous or foreign antigens complexed with specific antibody; such circulating immune complexes are implicated etiologically for glomerulonephritis in general (reviewed by Germuth and Rodriguez, 1973; McCluskey, 1992). In experimental animal models, the extent of the histological lesions is related to the amount and duration of circulating immune complexes, as well as to their character. Moreover, a correlation exists in patients between the histological pattern of injury and the level and frequency of detection of circulating immune complexes (reviewed by Germuth and Rodriguez, 1973; Hill, 1992; Silva, 1992). Therefore, the degree of proliferation and matrix expansion in immune complex glomerulonephritis may be viewed as an expression of the integral of immune complex load over time. In this context, note that immunoglobulins aggregated on a nonimmune basis and rheumatoid factor complexes share most of the biological properties of antigen–antibody complexes. "Immune complex glomerulonephritis" is a term that embraces these alternative immune aggregates. In any case, immune aggregates are likely to be related to the pathogenesis of glomerulonephritis; injection of aggregates into animals evokes disease (reviewed in Clarkson, 1987; Rifai, 1987; Emancipator, 1992).

Immunofluorescence detects the accumulation of Ig and activated complement components within diseased glomeruli in IgAN (reviewed by Emancipator, 1992). These deposits, electron dense by traditional transmission electron microscopy, also can be identified by immunoelectron microscopy (Dysart *et al.*, 1983; Doi *et al.*, 1984; Mathews *et al.*, 1985; Tanaka, 1986; Nakajima *et al.*, 1987). The complexes contain IgA as the predominant Ig, by definition, with IgG or IgM associated in most cases. Alternative pathway (B, D, H, C3, C5–9, and properdin) but not classical pathway (C1, C4, C2) complement components are almost invariably present in the mesangium (reviewed by Emancipator, 1992), another indication of the primacy of IgA, which does not activate the classical pathway. The deposits tend to be associated with reactive changes in the contractile mesangial cells, as predicted by the mesangial cell hypertrophy and hyperplasia seen by light microscopy. A significant proportion of cases also reveals deposits in the glomerular capillary walls, subendothelial or subepithelial; these patients typically exhibit segmental endocapillary proliferation by light microscopy. Overall, the correlation among light, electron, and immunofluorescence microscopy is excellent in IgAN.

Glomeruli in individual patients with IgAN may vary widely in appearance. The severity of morphological changes may differ from glomerulus to glomerulus and among the several segments in a particular glomerulus. Moreover, the elements of these changes—cellular hyperplasia, cellular hypertrophy, and expansion of extracellular matrix—occur independently. Hence, glomeruli with proliferation may be interposed with glomeruli with matrix expansion or both within one biopsy. This variation is consistent with the episodic clinical pattern, in which the severity may vary from time to time. A sample at a static time point, such as a biopsy, reveals lesions with different chronicity, presumably evoked by distinct "showers" of immune aggregates. Variation in immunohistology, for example, the extent of IgG or IgM co-deposits, classical complement components, and the extent and site of capillary wall deposits, are likely to be explained on a similar basis: the deposits represent a time-averaged view of the isotype repertoire, antigen load, and complementactivation capacity of the immune complexes generated.

The remaining 10% of IgAN patients reveal glomerular abnormalities that run the gamut of glomerular disease, including membranoproliferative, membranous, crescentic, and sclerotic. In some cases, overlap of two independent glomerular diseases has been invoked to explain the findings. Because IgAN is defined on the basis of the predominant Ig isotype deposited, IgAN can be expected to represent a microcosm of glomerular disease in general. Finally, note that tubulointerstitial nephritis and arteriolar changes also are observed frequently in IgAN patients (reviewed by Emancipator, 1992). These lesions may not derive from the glomerular injury, are of uncertain pathogenic significance, and often are observed in other forms of proliferative glomerulonephritis. They will not be considered further since no clear relation to a mucosal immune response is recognized.

II. PRIMARY IMMUNOLOGICAL ALTERATIONS IN IgA NEPHROPATHY

A. General Observations

The concentration of IgA in the serum of patients with IgAN is frequently (50%) increased relative to age-matched normal controls or patients with other glomerulonephritides, often 2- or 3-fold (Lopez-Trascasa *et al.*, 1980; Egido *et al.*, 1982a,1987a; Schena *et al.*, 1986; Williams *et al.*, 1987; van Es *et al.*, 1988; Peterman *et al.*, 1991). The IgA is polyclonal, but several investigators have reported that the percentage of J-chain-linked oligomers is elevated markedly in patients over controls (Kupor *et al.*, 1975; Lopez-Trascasa *et al.*, 1979; Woodroffe *et al.*, 1980; Stachura *et al.*, 1981; Lesavre *et al.*, 1982; Endoh *et al.*, 1984; Czerkinsky *et al.*, 1986; Hernando *et al.*, 1986; van Es *et al.*, 1988; Nagura, 1989; Jones *et al.*, 1990; Waldo, 1990; Chen *et al.*, 1991; Peterman *et al.*, 1991). Congruent with the renal deposits, IgA1 predominates over IgA2 in patient serum, as it does normally. The increased IgA may be immunologically specific because marked increases in the levels of circulating immune complexes containing IgA frequently are present and these complexes contain different antigens (Kupor *et al.*, 1975; Tung *et al.*, 1978; Lopez-Trascasa *et al.*, 1979; McKenzie *et al.*, 1980; Woodroffe *et al.*, 1980; Cairns *et al.*, 1981; Kauffmann *et al.*, 1981; Mustonen *et al.*, 1981; Stachura *et al.*, 1981; Coppo *et al.*, 1982a,1984; Lesavre *et al.*, 1982; Tomino *et al.*, 1982a,b,c; Hall *et al.*, 1983; Sancho *et al.*, 1983; van der Woude *et al.*, 1983; Endoh *et al.*, 1984; Nagy *et al.*, 1984,1988; Czerkinsky *et al.*, 1986; Hale *et al.*, 1986; Hernando *et al.*, 1986; Russell *et al.*,1986; Schena *et al.*, 1986; Drew *et al.*, 1987; Fornasieri *et al.*, 1987; Laurent *et al.*, 1987; Yap *et al.*, 1987; Rostoker *et al.*, 1989a,1991). IgG synthesis and immune aggregate content are heightened during disease exacerbation as well (Russell *et al.*, 1986; Schena *et al.*, 1986). Moreover, IgG1 and IgG3 are represented disproportionately in the circulating complexes and renal deposits, whereas serum IgG2 and IgM levels are decreased in patients with IgAN

(Aucouturier *et al.*, 1989; Rostoker *et al.*, 1989b). These observations also are consistent with an immune abnormality.

Studies *in vitro* suggest that at least part of the increment in circulating IgA results from increased production. Although not all observers agree, peripheral blood lymphocytes from patients with IgAN produce significantly more IgA during culture than do lymphocytes from control groups, whether resting or after mitogen stimulation. The frequency of B cells bearing surface IgA in the circulation and in culture, resting or mitogen stimulated, is also higher in patients relative to controls (Nomoto *et al.*, 1979; Sakai *et al.*, 1979b; Cosio *et al.*, 1982; Egido *et al.*, 1982b,1983a,c; Fornasieri *et al.*, 1982; Cagnoli *et al.*, 1985; Linné and Wasserman, 1985; Feehally *et al.*, 1986; Hale *et al.*, 1986; Schena *et al.*, 1986; Waldo *et al.*, 1986; Lai *et al.*, 1987; Chen *et al.*, 1991). Parallel alterations of B-cell function, *in vivo* and *in vitro*, have been reported in first-degree relatives of patients with IgAN, consonant with recognition of multiply affected individuals within several pedigrees of familial IgAN (Sakai *et al.*, 1979b; Egido *et al.*, 1985,1987a,b; Julian *et al.*, 1985; Waldo *et al.*, 1986; Waldo and Cochran, 1987; Waldo, 1992).

Some evidence suggests that IgAN patients' T cells are the site of the primary defect and that the B-cell dysfunction is largely secondary (Sakai, 1987,1988). Perhaps the most compelling support for a primary defect in T cells arises from *in vitro* experiments by the Sakai group. This group reported that B cells from patients function normally when cultured with histocompatible normal T cells, but that normal B cells reveal derangements similar to those just described when cultured with IgAN patient T cells (Sakai *et al.*, 1979a,b; Sakai, 1987). Defects in T-cell function and in the distribution of T-cell subsets have been described by a number of laboratories (Sakai *et al.*, 1979a,1982; Chatenoud and Bach, 1981; Cosio *et al.*, 1982; Egido *et al.*, 1982a,b,1983a,b,c; Woo *et al.*, 1982; Adachi *et al.*, 1983; Cagnoli *et al.*, 1985; Feehally *et al.*, 1986; Hale *et al.*, 1986; Waldo *et al.*, 1986). This concept also might explain discrepancies in some of the *in vitro* studies; use of IgAN patient unfractionated peripheral blood lymphocytes, which include T cells, or use of mitogens that are T-cell directed would favor observations of abnormal Ig production by patient B cells if the primary defect were in the T-cell population. Indeed, T cells from patients and first-degree relatives do respond aberrantly to a variety of stimuli, whereas lipopolysaccharide (LPS) stimulation of patient B cells appears normal.

Although a primary derangement in T-cell function seems plausible in IgAN, the evidence is limited and circumstantial. In fact, until a specific sequence of events leading to IgAN can be identified, even the concept of IgAN as an immunological disease remains somewhat speculative. More cogently, no confidence exists that all IgAN patients share the same pathogenic mechanism; IgAN may be a syndrome that develops via several distinct mechanisms, not all of which are necessarily immunological in nature. Notwithstanding these cautions, concluding that at least a percentage of IgAN patients suffers from an immunological disease does seem reasonable. Elucidation of the nature and character of the disease remains a priority.

B. The Mucosal Immune System and the Genesis of IgA Nephropathy

Focus on the mucosal immune system as an element in the genesis of IgAN began almost simultaneously with the recognition of IgAN as a clinicopathological entity some 25 years ago. Collectively, mucosal sites are rich in IgA-producing cells because of a high density of plasma cells and a disproportionately high fraction of IgA-producing plasma cells (Lamm, 1976; Underdown and Schiff, 1986; Mestecky and McGhee, 1987). Indeed, the gut and upper airways account for most of the total body content of IgA (Vaerman and Heremans, 1970; Craig and Cebra, 1975; Rothberg *et al.*, 1978). Moreover, the body's synthetic rate of IgA well exceeds that of all other Ig classes combined (Mestecky, 1988). Although the marrow and spleen are significant sources of IgA as well, and this IgA contributes significantly to the pool of IgA in serum, evidence exists that mucosally derived T cells can exert major regulatory influences on these sites (Pabst and Binns, 1981; Alley *et al.*, 1986; Pabst *et al.*, 1987). Hence, even IgA produced in extramucosal regions may, broadly speaking, be "mucosal."

In an attempt to identify the source of IgA in the glomerular deposits, some investigators have studied the properties of the IgA in glomeruli or in the circulating immune complexes. Initially, the presence of J chain within glomerular deposits in association with IgA was offered as evidence of a mucosal origin (Dobrin *et al.*, 1975; Lopez-Trascasa *et al.*, 1979; André *et al.*, 1980; Egido *et al.*, 1980; Béné *et al.*, 1982; Coppo *et al.*, 1982b; Donini *et al.*, 1982; Tomino *et al.*, 1982c; Komatsu *et al.*, 1983; Lomax-Smith *et al.*, 1983; Monteiro *et al.*, 1984; Waldherr *et al.*, 1983). Although Monteiro *et al.* (1984) eluted 300-kDa IgA-containing J chain from renal deposits, thereby demonstrating that at least some deposited IgA is a J-chain-linked dimer, the source of the IgA was not elucidated because both mucosal and extramucosal plasma cells produce J-chain-containing IgA oligomers. Moreover, IgM, which also contains J chain, frequently is co-deposited in glomeruli in patients with IgAN.

The subclass distribution of the deposited IgA also has been considered. Serum IgA, thought to be derived largely from marrow and other nonmucosal sites, is mostly IgA1, whereas secretory IgA derived from mucosal plasma cells contains considerable IgA2. Recognition that, in IgAN the renal deposits, elevations in serum IgA (oligomeric or not) and circulating immune complexes all are associated with IgA1 rather than IgA2 was cited by several groups as testimony to an extramucosal source of the renal IgA (Shigematsu *et al.*, 1980; Tomino *et al.*, 1981; Rambausek *et al.*, 1982; Hall *et al.*, 1983; Lomax-Smith *et al.*, 1983; Czerkinsky *et al.*, 1986; Conley and Delacroix, 1987; Béné and Faure, 1988; van den Wall Bake *et al.*, 1988). However, a substantial proportion of mucosal IgA is in fact IgA1, even predominating over IgA2 in some mucosal locations, particularly in the airways and small bowel. Moreover, certain categories of antigens may induce IgA1 (or IgA2) antibodies preferentially. Therefore, the source of the IgA cannot be identified reliably from its subclass distribution (Lamm, 1976; Underdown and

Schiff, 1986; Mestecky and McGhee, 1987; Rifai, 1987; Mestecky, 1988). The predominance of λ light chains in both renal deposits and IgA from mucosal versus nonmucosal sources was cited to support a mucosal origin for the IgA (Béné and Faure, 1988; Faure *et al.*, 1990; Chen *et al.*, 1991). Again, this argument is circumstantial and subject to reinterpretation if κ/λ ratios in mucosal sites other than tonsil and small bowel should resemble the marrow, where κ chains predominate, more closely.

A second line of evidence implicating the mucosal immune system in the genesis of IgAN derives from the antigens identified within the glomerular deposits and circulating immune complexes. The constellation of such antigens is large, ranging from "inert" proteins, glycoproteins, saccharides, and nucleic acids to infectious microorganisms and autoantigens. The inert antigens identified are nearly all dietary components; the infectious organisms identified to date are all trophic for mucosal sites since they invade the body via the airways or intestinal tract (Kupor *et al.*, 1975; Tung *et al.*, 1978; Lopez-Trascasa *et al.*, 1979; McKenzie *et al.*, 1980; Woodroffe *et al.*, 1980; Cairns *et al.*, 1981; Kauffmann *et al.*, 1981; Mustonen *et al.*, 1981; Stachura *et al.*, 1981; Coppo *et al.*, 1982a,1984; Lesavre *et al.*, 1982; Tomino *et al.*, 1982a,b,c,1987; Hall *et al.*, 1983; Sancho *et al.*, 1983; van der Woude *et al.*, 1983; Endoh *et al.*, 1984; Nagy *et al.*, 1984,1988,1989; Czerkinsky *et al.*, 1986; Hale *et al.*, 1986; Russell *et al.*, 1986; Schena *et al.*, 1986; Drew *et al.*, 1987; Fornasieri *et al.*, 1987; Laurent *et al.*, 1987; Sato *et al.*, 1987; Yap *et al.*, 1987; Nagura, 1989; Rostoker *et al.*, 1989a,1991).

A third and probably significant line of evidence derives from the close temporal relationship between acute "viral" syndromes, usually respiratory, and the onset or exacerbation of IgAN, particularly among macrohematuric patients (reviewed by Emancipator *et al.*, 1985; van Es *et al.*, 1988). Temporal associations also are recognized between dietary intake of gluten and the frequency and severity of hematuric episodes in IgAN (Coppo *et al.*, 1986; DelPrato *et al.*, 1988; Rostoker *et al.*, 1990a).

In a fourth line of evidence, Béné *et al.* (1984,1986,1991b) and Westberg *et al.* (1983) have studied tonsillar and, to a more limited degree, gut and scleral plasma cells in patients with nephritis and in controls. Although the tonsils are not a purely mucosal lymphoid tissue, tonsils and gut from IgAN patients reveal similar changes in the ratio of IgG : IgA plasma cells and similar abnormalities in Ig secretion by isolated cells in culture relative to normal controls and glomerulonephritic patients without IgA deposits. Yasumori (1990) reported that patients with IgAN have an increase in serum IgA associated with an increase in salivary secretory IgA levels relative to controls. The increase in salivary IgA is seen in all forms of glomerulonephritis, suggesting that polyclonal B-cell activation leads to increased IgA in general (Rostoker *et al.*, 1990b; Yasumori, 1990). However, patients with IgAN have a low ratio of salivary to serum IgA relative to individuals with non-IgA glomerulonephritis. Some patients with IgAN also have abnormally low secretory IgA in jejunal secretions. In addition, serum levels of secretory IgA are elevated in IgAN patients with hematuria (Yasumori, 1990). Therefore, perturbations in the mucosal immune system may exist in patients with IgAN with respect to transepithelial transport. A newly recognized deficiency in the production of J chain by lamina propria plasmacytes in intestinal biopsies of patients with IgAN relative to healthy individuals (J. Feehally, personal communication) predicts such diminished transepithelial transport, and may prove important in the genesis of IgAN.

Some of the most compelling evidence considers specific immune responses to mucosal immunization with tetanus toxoid in patients with IgAN. Waldo (1992) reported that patients with IgAN develop higher serum IgG antibody levels after mucosal immunization and a greater increase in specific IgG after boosting, relative to controls. These patients had lower levels of specific serum IgA than controls and did not increase specific IgA titers after boosting, despite increased IgA responses of peripheral blood mononuclear cells after mitogen stimulation. Indeed, patients with IgAN who had elevated IgA anti-poliovirus titers in serum manifested suppression of specific IgA after oral poliovirus challenge; parallel abnormalities were observed in cells from these patients *in vitro* (Waldo and Cochran, 1987). Patients also had increased total serum IgA not specific for poliovirus relative to controls, further supporting a dysregulation of IgA synthesis. Other vaccination studies also support a more vigorous immune response, particularly of the mucosal immune system, in patients with IgAN (Endoh *et al.*, 1984; Leinikki *et al.*, 1987; van Es *et al.*, 1988), as well as in first-degree relatives (Waldo and Cochran, 1987; Waldo, 1992). Abnormalities in serum IgA levels, particularly polymeric IgA1 and IgA associated with complement (i.e., conglutinin-binding IgA), are accentuated in IgAN patients during mucosal infections (van Es *et al.*, 1988; Jones *et al.*, 1990). Although these data further emphasize the contribution of mucosal immune responses to alterations in circulating IgA, they again do not pinpoint these alterations as the source of the glomerular deposits.

When all the evidence is considered, we believe it favors a mucosal source of the IgA aggregates in the kidney and in the circulation. Admittedly, however, despite the abundant data implicating the mucosal immune system in the pathogenesis of IgAN, little direct evidence supports such a link.

III. ENHANCED MUCOSAL PENETRABILITY BY ANTIGEN

The aforementioned increases in polyclonal IgA, and perhaps IgG, production have been viewed as the result of a dysregulated immune system, systemic or mucosal. However, an equally plausible scenario posits increased penetration of mucosal surfaces by antigen, perhaps in the face of a normally regulated immune response. The enhanced exposure of mucosa-associated lymphoid tissue (MALT) to antigen would evoke a heightened immune response, and would favor elevated levels of immune complexes within the body proper, including the mucosae. Such immune complexes could gain access to the circulation and ultimately could lodge in the kidney.

Data in support of specific mechanisms by which increased antigen penetration could occur are limited. As already mentioned, various dietary and airway antigens, complexes of those antigens with specific antibody, or specific antibodies are present in the blood of patients with IgAN in excess of the levels found in normals (Kupor *et al.*, 1975; Tung *et al.*, 1978; Lopez-Trascasa *et al.*, 1979; McKenzie *et al.*, 1980; Woodroffe *et al.*, 1980; Cairns *et al.*, 1981; Kauffmann *et al.*, 1981; Mustonen *et al.*, 1981; Stachura *et al.*, 1981; Coppo *et al.*, 1982a,1984; Lesavre *et al.*, 1982; Tomino *et al.*, 1982a,b,c,1987; Hall *et al.*,1983; Sancho *et al.*, 1983; van der Woude *et al.*, 1983; Endoh *et al.*, 1984; Nagy *et al.*, 1984, 1988; Czerkinsky *et al.*, 1986; Hale *et al.*, 1986; Russell *et al.*, 1986; Schena *et al.*, 1986; Drew *et al.*, 1987; Fornasieri *et al.*, 1987; Laurent *et al.*, 1987; Sato *et al.*, 1987; Yap *et al.*, 1987; Rostoker *et al.*, 1989a,1991). Although increased titers of antibodies specific for a variety of "mucosal" antigens also are seen in glomerulonephritides other than IgAN (Rostoker *et al.*, 1991), the presence of dietary antigens appears limited to IgAN patients, as are titers for some specific antibodies.

Increased antigen penetration consequent to a general failure of the mucosal barrier is encountered infrequently in IgAN patients, even during exacerbations of hematuria associated with increased dietary antigens in serum (Davin *et al.*, 1988; Jenkins *et al.*, 1988; Rostoker *et al.*, 1989a,1990a; Davin and Mahieu, 1992). The majority (75%) of patients with IgAN have normal or borderline high degrees of intestinal absorption of materials such as cellobiose and ^{51}Cr-labeled EDTA. These observations argue against a general intrinsic defect in mucosal surfaces. Moreover, these data also render two other hypotheses less likely: infectious injury to mucosal epithelium and immune-mediated injury to the mucosa (Emancipator and Lamm, 1989).

The increase in circulating dietary antigens without a general increase in gut permeability could be the result of a defect in immune inhibition of the uptake of macromolecules by the gut. Since specific secretory antibody in the lumen can interfere with the transport of macromolecules across the lining, defects in the secretion of specific antibodies could increase such transit (Cunningham-Rundles *et al.*, 1978; Walker and Bloch, 1983; Cunningham-Rundles, 1990,1991). Such defects would, in principle, include IgA deficiency, specific immune tolerance for penetrating antigens, inappropriate or inadequate differentiation or distribution of stimulated MALT B lymphocytes, impaired IgA transport across mucosal epithelium, or accelerated degradation of IgA within mucosal lumina. IgA deficiency is not likely in IgAN, since heightened or normal IgA production is characteristic *in vitro* and *in vivo*. Specific tolerance for selected antigens could occur; however, since a causal antigen is not known in any patient and may be multiple in a given patient, this issue cannot be evaluated. Dichotomy between secreted and systemic IgA levels is recognized (Cunningham-Rundles, 1990,1991). However, a defect in the secretion of selected specific IgA antibodies with a coexisting generation of systemic antibody of the same specificity, required to generate pathogenic immune complexes, seems improbable. Impaired differentiation or homing of MALT lymphocytes in general is also doubtful, since none of a significant sample of patients with IgAN had decrements in mucosal IgA plasma cells (Westberg *et al.*, 1983; Béné *et al.*, 1984,1986,1991b). Nonetheless, all these possibilities remain because small differences beyond the resolution of currently available assays could, over a long period of time and a large surface area as manifested in the mucosae, result in significant differences in the proportion and amounts of antigen and antibody in various parts of the body.

Perhaps more intriguing and plausible, impaired polymeric Ig receptor-mediated transport of IgA across the mucosa merits discussion. Salivary IgA is increased relative to other proteins in all glomerulonephritides, but the salivary content of secretory IgA is decreased selectively in patients with IgAN (Rostoker *et al.*, 1990b; Yasumori, 1990). Hematuric IgAN patients have increased secretory IgA in serum. During normal transport of IgA across exocrine epithelium, dimeric IgA is attached to the external domain of the polymeric Ig receptor; the receptor, in turn, is cleaved proteolytically at the junction of its external and transmembrane domains at the apical surface of the cell. Increased secretory IgA in serum, with decreased secretory IgA in secretions, could result from proteolytic release of secretory component at the basolateral surface of mucosal epithelium, related either to misdirection of IgA within the epithelial cell or to altered localization of the relevant plasma membrane endopeptidase. Although glomerular deposits do not contain appreciable secretory IgA in patients with primary IgAN (reviewed by Emancipator *et al.*, 1985), increased mucosal penetration by antigen favored by relatively small shifts in polymeric Ig receptor-mediated IgA transport could lead to increased antigen-specific antibody responses of mixed isotype in both mucosal and extramucosal sites. In this scenario, even if the IgA deposited in glomeruli were derived from marrow or splenic plasma cells, disease could be related to defective mucosal immunity. On the other hand, permeation of the mucosal defenses by antigen need not represent an actual defect in mucosal immunity. Rather, an antigen load could increase suddenly, generating a transient period of antigen excess that could overwhelm local immunity for a time. Although this sequence of events would, in a sense, represent a failure of the mucosal immune system, it would nonetheless be physiological. Moreover, repetition of such a scenario with differing "novel" antigens over a period of time might prove noxious, particularly in individuals such as patients with IgAN, with a tendency toward an especially robust immune response (Endoh *et al.*, 1984; Leinikki *et al.*, 1987; Waldo and Cochran, 1987; van Es *et al.*, 1988; Waldo, 1992). Finally, defective trans-mucosal transport of IgA antibody consequent to the diminished synthesis of J chain observed in the gut lamina propria of patients with IgAN (J. Feehally, personal communication) could favor increased penetration of the gut wall by antigen.

Of interest is the recognition that intraepithelial neutralization of mucosal pathogens by specific IgA antibody can occur, for example, if the transcytotic pathway of IgA intersects the cellular pathway followed by the synthesis and assembly of viral components (Mazanec *et al.*, 1992). Misdirection of IgA-containing vesicles might allow greater mucosal penetration by virus, viral antigens, or IgA immune complexes. Indeed, a parallel mechanism could be operative for inert macromolecules, if pinocytotic vesicles containing luminally derived antigens normally intersect with transcytotic vesicles containing specific IgA. Subversion of this system provides another mechanism by which mucosal penetration by antigen might occur.

IV. DEFECTIVE CLEARANCE OF IMMUNE COMPLEXES

A. Mononuclear Phagocyte System

Immune complexes in the circulation typically are taken up by cells of the mononuclear phagocyte (reticuloendothelial) system (Arend and Mannik, 1971; Mannik and Arend, 1971; Haakenstad and Mannik, 1974; Mannik and Jimenez, 1979), primarily in the liver and spleen (Mannik *et al.*, 1971). Fixed phagocytes can remove particles nonspecifically (Biozzi *et al.*, 1953; Normann, 1974). In addition, these cells bear a high density of receptors for immunoglobulin Fc regions and for complement components (reviewed by Cornacoff *et al.*, 1983; Medof *et al.*, 1983). Thus, uptake of particulates coated with antibody or complement (opsonized) is more efficient (Mannik *et al.*, 1971; Mannik and Jimenez, 1979). Impaired phagocyte function is, therefore, a potential contributor to immune complex disease, including glomerulonephritis (Haakenstad and Mannik, 1976; Germuth *et al.*, 1977,1982). With respect to this possibility, many variables must be considered that are related to the nature of the antigen and the host immune response.

Factors such as the chemical nature of the antigen, its electrostatic charge and catabolic rate, and the quantity and quality of the responding antibody (including isotype distribution and avidity) influence the molecular weight, electrostatic charge, and tissue distribution of the resultant complexes and, therefore, their rate of clearance (Haakenstad and Mannik, 1976; Germuth *et al.*,1977,1982; Finbloom *et al.*, 1981; Gauthier *et al.*, 1982; Isaacs and Miller, 1982; Gallo *et al.*, 1983; Mannik *et al.*, 1983). In human glomerulonephritis, however, these factors cannot be evaluated completely since the causal antigens have not been identified.

The study of immune complexes containing IgA involves its own distinct factors (Rifai and Mannik, 1983,1984). The presence of IgA within an immune lattice can influence its clearance kinetics in relation to mechanisms that depend on cellular immune adherence receptors (Waxman *et al.*, 1986). These receptors bind to activation fragments of the third component of complement with a higher affinity than Fc receptors have for Ig, and they promote uptake of immune complexes containing appropriate C3 polypeptides. Also, when inserted into immune complexes, C3b promotes binding to erythrocytes via one of these receptors (CR1). The erythrocyte then can transport such complexes efficiently to phagocytes in the spleen and liver without allowing the complexes to circulate freely in the interval (Cornacoff *et al.*, 1983; Medof *et al.*, 1983). Interestingly, when IgA is present, it seems to inhibit complement fixation by IgG in the same immune lattice (Waldo and Cochran, 1989). Hence, the presence of IgA in an immune complex may subvert immune adherence receptor-dependent mechanisms, and may impair the clearance of the complexes by phagocytes. For example, in baboons, immune complexes containing IgA do not bind erythrocytes as well as immune complexes containing only IgG antibody; IgG complexes contain relatively more complement (Waxman *et al.*, 1986). The IgA immune complexes are, nevertheless, taken out of circulation more quickly, presumably because they are free in solution rather than bound to erythrocytes and are distributed more widely, with relatively higher concentrations in organs other than liver and spleen, for example, the kidney and lungs. Hence, intercalation of IgA into an immune lattice may increase renal deposition. Deficient selective CR1 uptake of IgA-containing complexes cannot be ascribed to increased alternative versus classical pathway complement activation, since particles opsonized via alternative pathway activation by zymosan bind readily to primate erythrocytes (Cornacoff *et al.*, 1983; Medof *et al.*, 1983).

B. Other Mechanisms

In rodents, immune complexes containing polymeric IgA can be transported actively across hepatocytes by the same polymeric Ig receptor-dependent mechanism that normally applies to free polymeric IgA (Nagura *et al.*, 1981; Peppard *et al.*, 1981; Socken *et al.*, 1981; Brown *et al.*, 1982; Delacroix *et al.*, 1982; Mestecky *et al.*, 1989). In humans, biliary epithelial cells rather than hepatocytes support this function, but this process is relatively inefficient (Mestecky *et al.*, 1989; Rifai *et al.*, 1989). When radiolabeled model IgA immune complexes are injected into primates, the liver and, secondarily, the spleen manifest the most uptake in scintillographic studies in humans (Rifai *et al.*, 1989; Roccatello *et al.*, 1989,1992) and in direct γ counting of tissue samples in baboons (Waxman *et al.*, 1986). Fixed phagocytes appear to account for clearance of the aggregates, as outlined earlier, with little radiolabeled IgA excreted into bile. However, the observation that epithelial cells can transport immune complexes containing oligomeric IgA efficiently from the basolateral (lamina propria) surface to the apical (luminal) surface may be germane to elucidating the mechanism of clearance (Kaetzel *et al.*, 1991). The vast number and incessant activity of secretory epithelial cells may represent a critical, topographically diffuse mechanism for ridding the body of locally formed IgA immune complexes. A defect in this transport system, such as the deficient production of J chain reported in IgAN patients by Feehally and associates (J. Feehally, personal communication), would promote systemic accumulation of IgA immune complexes and, perhaps, mesangial IgA deposits.

Three clinical investigations from two separate laboratories failed to observe significant intestinal or bronchial uptake of model IgA immune complexes from the circulation (Rifai *et al.*, 1989; Roccatello *et al.*, 1989,1992). However, because a given cell would take up only a small amount of complexes, a widely disseminated mass of involved cells might not be recognized by the scintillographic imaging techniques employed. Moreover, traditional methods of measuring removal of radioactivity from the circulation over many hours cannot resolve the contribution by a particular organ.

The relative mass of the liver versus spleen makes hepatic clearance more significant than splenic clearance of IgA immune complexes, despite a greater amount of IgA binding per unit tissue in spleen. Similarly, in humans, the relative number of erythrocytes favors greater cumulative binding of C3b-containing immune complexes to erythrocytes than to circulating phagocytes, despite a lower number of CR1 receptors per red cell (Cornacoff *et al.*, 1983; Medof *et al.*, 1983). In analogous fashion, fewer immune complexes per cell may be cleared from the lamina propria by enterocytes and bronchial epithelial cells but this clearance, nevertheless, translates into more total transport when the aggregate number of cells in the body is considered. Evaluation of the potential excretion of IgA-containing immune complexes, particularly locally and perhaps from the circulation, by secretory epithelium *in vivo* is warranted in terms of our need to comprehend both normal "excretory" immune function and the pathogenesis of IgAN.

Although secretory component-mediated hepatobiliary transport of polymeric IgA is inefficient in humans relative to rodents (Mestecky *et al.*, 1989; Rifai *et al.*, 1989), hepatocytes may take up and catabolize IgA via the asialoglycoprotein receptor (Mestecky *et al.*, 1989). Although the extent to which hepatobiliary transport applies to circulating IgA immune complexes is not clear, indications are that this mechanism does operate in human liver (Mestecky *et al.*, 1989; Rifai *et al.*, 1989). Another potential mechanism for removal of IgA relates to erythrocyte binding independent of CR1. Approximately 40% of patients with IgAN exhibit an increase in such binding. The mechanism by which this binding occurs and its biological significance are uncertain (Matsuda *et al.*, 1988).

C. Role of Defective Clearance and Relation to the Mucosal Immune System

Studies addressing the issues just described for IgA immune complexes do not answer the specific question of a possible defect in clearance in patients with IgAN. Logically, a difference between controls and patients with IgAN in the rates of clearance of soluble macromolecular aggregates that contain IgA is more relevant to the pathogenesis of the disease than the previously reported defective clearance of IgG-coated erythrocytes (Lawrence *et al.*, 1983; Nicholls and Kincaid-Smith, 1984; Solomon *et al.*, 1984; Roccatello *et al.*, 1985). The relative clearance rates of complexes that contain only IgG compared with those with pure or admixed IgA might not relate to the pathogenesis of IgAN, given the central role of the IgA component in the immune complexes in this disease. The fate of IgA-containing complexes emerges as a potentially critical factor in the genesis of IgAN (Nagura, 1989), but results of studies in patients with human IgAN conflict (Rifai *et al.*, 1989; Roccatello *et al.*, 1989,1992). The discrepancy between the two laboratories that have addressed this issue directly could result from differences in the preparation, and therefore the character, of the model IgA aggregates. Alternatively, the discrepancy might reflect the fact that the differences between patients and controls, although statistically significant in one laboratory, are small and close to the limit of detection by current methods. Small differences, even if not statistically significant or measurable at present, nonetheless might prove critical in the chronic time-frame operative in IgAN. Particularly, the extensive mass and continuous activity of the intestinal epithelium might translate into a significant difference in the total excretion of local IgA immune complexes between IgAN patients and controls. Defects in polymeric Ig receptor-mediated excretion of mucosal immune complexes (Kaetzel *et al.*, 1991), perhaps in concert with defects in polymeric Ig receptor-mediated transport of free oligomeric IgA antibody, would favor accumulation of IgA immune complexes in the circulation and ultimately in the kidney.

As already discussed, under physiological circumstances an abrupt increase in the concentration of antigen intraluminally or intraepithelially could lead to transiently increased permeability of that antigen, whether it is a novel environmental or infectious agent or an antigen to which the host is already immune through prior exposure. Under these circumstances, small soluble immune complexes in response to antigen excess would form with the first available antibody. Locally formed IgA complexes with oligomeric IgA should be cleared efficiently by the overlying epithelium (Kaetzel *et al.*, 1991). However, complexes with monomeric IgA or IgG would be removed by this mechanism only if they also contained oligomeric IgA (C. Kaetzel, J. Robinson, and M. Lamm, unpublished observations). Small immune complexes formed under extreme antigen excess are less likely to contain both oligomeric and monomeric antibody in the same complex, since only one or two antibody molecules would be present. Small complexes of antigen with IgG or monomeric IgA but without oligomeric IgA would escape clearance by the mucosal epithelium and therefore would become concentrated within the lamina propria. Alternately, complexes that contain oligomeric IgA with relatively less J chain could develop in patients with IgAN (J. Feehally, personal communication), similarly less susceptible to clearance by the mucosal epithelium. These complexes could gain access to the circulation and deposit in glomeruli. As the mucosal immune response adapted to the new level of antigen exposure by making more antibody, free antibody (predominantly IgA) also would gain access to the circulation. At this point, the free IgA could deposit on top of the previously deposited glomerular immune complexes, adding appreciably more IgA. This sequence of events explains well the generation within the kidney of the mixed IgA and IgG isotypes considered particularly pathogenic in IgAN (reviewed by Emancipator and Lamm, 1989; Emancipator, 1990,1992). If this sequence of events actually occurs, it clearly relates the mucosal immune system to the pathogenesis of IgAN.

V. CONCLUDING PERSPECTIVES

The preceding discussion clearly shows that the source (mucosal or extramucosal) and the nature (immune complexes or nonimmune aggregates) of the IgA deposited in the mesangium in IgAN are still controversial. We favor a view of IgAN as a form of serum sickness in which mucosally derived antigens elicit local mucosal antibody synthesis, thereby generating pathogenic immune complexes. Although much of the evidence for either perspective is circumstantial, the unambiguous facets all support this view; some of the arguments advanced in favor of a mucosal source render extramucosal sources less likely (Béné and Faure, 1988). Moreover, the evidence cited to favor a bone marrow origin of the IgA deposits, that is, predominance of IgA1 not exclusively found as oligomers linked by J chain (van den Wall Bake *et al.*, 1988), does not necessarily argue against a mucosal source. Although dietary antigens and infectious agents interacting with mucosal epithelium certainly can gain access to extramucosal lymphoid tissue, mucosal lymphocytes would be exposed initially. Moreover, extramucosal sites of Ig synthesis, including the marrow, tend to produce more IgG and IgM relative to IgA than do mucosal sites.

Similar reasoning favors the concept that IgA aggregates are immune complexes. The renal deposits and the circulating IgA aggregates are acid dissociable. The eluted IgA, once fractionated, does not self-aggregate (Monteiro *et al.*, 1984). Although anti-Ig antibodies, including IgA rheumatoid factors and IgG specific for the constant domain of Fab fragments of IgA, have been invoked, no predictive value for diagnosis or severity of IgAN is associated with such antibodies (Czerkinsky *et al.*, 1986; Sinico *et al.*, 1986,1988; Jackson *et al.*, 1987; Jackson, 1988; Schena *et al.*, 1988; van Es *et al.*, 1988). Presumably, therefore, at least one non-Ig component is required for IgA or mixed-isotype dissociable immune aggregate formation. Although Ig-binding proteins such as lectins, which can bind glycosyl side chains of Ig (DelPrato *et al.*, 1988; Emancipator *et al.*, 1992), and extracellular matrix proteins such as collagen or fibronectin (reviewed in Jennette

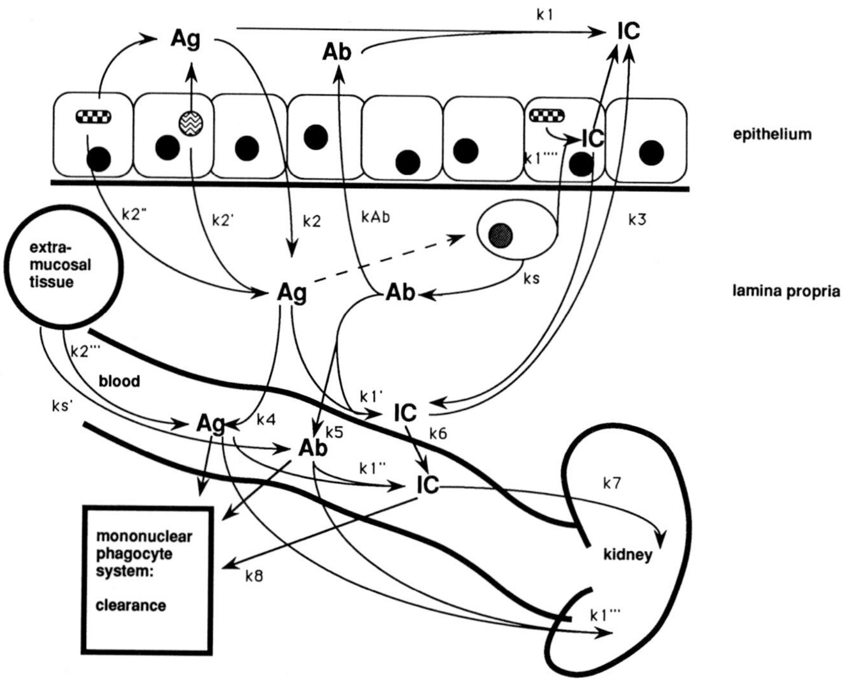

Figure 1 Some of the theoretically possible events related to the genesis of IgAN are schematized. Antigen (Ag) may combine with antibody (Ab) to generate immune complexes (IC) in the lumen, in the extracellular fluid in the mucosal lamina propria, in the circulation, or *in situ* in the glomeruli; these rate constants are denoted k_1, $k_{1'}$, $k_{1''}$, and $k_{1'''}$, respectively, since the formation rates vary in differing environments. Although mucosal immune responses to local antigens are emphasized, the scheme also can apply to antigen, antibody, and IC that enter the blood and tissues from other sites. Entry of antigen via the rate constants k_2, $k_{2'}$, $k_{2''}$, and $k_{2'''}$ consider penetration of mucosa by antigen (k_2), production of antigens within the mucosa such as autoantigens or products of microorganisms ($k_{2'}$, $k_{2''}$), and entry into the blood from an extramucosal source ($k_{2'''}$). Free antigen in the lamina propria also may enter the general circulation (k_4). Antibody synthesized by mucosal (k_s) or extramucosal ($k_{s'}$) plasma cells is subject to transport by the polymeric Ig receptor (k_{Ab}) if the antibody is a J-chain-containing oligomer; combination with antigen to form IC in various sites (k_1–$k_{1''''}$); or entry into the blood (k_5). ICs formed in the lamina propria may enter the blood (k_6) or, if they contain at least some J chain-linked oligomeric Ig, may be excreted actively by the overlying epithelium (k_3). Circulating ICs can be removed by the mononuclear phagocyte system or by other clearance mechanisms (k_8) or be deposited in glomeruli (k_7). Of course, free antigen and antibody in the circulation also are subject to catabolic removal (constants not shown). Within this complicated scheme, a number of possibilities for the genesis of IgAN can be accommodated. Within an individual patient, one or perhaps a few of these mechanisms might apply, but different patients could incorporate features in distinct portions of the scheme. For reasons explained in the text, we favor the dominance of mucosally related antigen (k_2, $k_{2'}$, $k_{2''}$) combining with local antibody to generate ICs ($k_{1'}$). Whatever the specific mechanisms, virtually all the possible pathways relate to mucosal function in some way.

et al., 1991) theoretically could promote aggregation of immunologically nonspecific Ig, innumerable antigens could elicit formation of complexes with specific antibodies. Many diverse mucosally related antigens have been implicated (Kupor *et al.*, 1975; Tung *et al.*, 1978; Lopez-Trascasa *et al.*, 1979; McKenzie *et al.*, 1980; Woodroffe *et al.*, 1980; Cairns *et al.*, 1981; Kauffmann *et al.*, 1981; Mustonen *et al.*, 1981; Stachura *et al.*, 1981; Coppo *et al.*, 1982a,1984; Lesavre *et al.*, 1982; Tomino *et al.*, 1982a,b,c; Hall *et al.*, 1983; Sancho *et al.*, 1983; van der Woude *et al.*, 1983; Endoh *et al.*, 1984; Nagy *et al.*, 1984,1988; Czerkinsky *et al.*, 1986; Hale *et al.*, 1986; Russell *et al.*, 1986; Schena *et al.*, 1986; Drew *et al.*, 1987; Fornasieri *et al.*, 1987; Laurent *et al.*, 1987; Yap *et al.*, 1987; Rostoker *et al.*, 1989a). Moreover, in the broad sense, dietary lectins or mucosal pathogen- or commensal-derived Ig-binding proteins or lectins are, themselves, potential immunogens. Aside from the issue of whether the glomerular aggregates represent immune complexes, several distinct mechanisms promoting renal deposition can be envisioned. Possibilities are summarized in Figure 1.

Several investigators, noting the diversity of features among patients with IgAN, have proposed that IgAN is a syndrome rather than a disease. This argument presupposes that different patient groups have distinct defects and pathogeneses and, therefore, distinct diseases. Perhaps several individual diseases, all with the common syndrome of IgAN, signal a primary defect in one of the pathways in Figure 1. Perusal of this scheme, however, reveals that mucosal function impacts a majority of the mechanisms considered. Therefore, various insufficiencies of mucosal defense could promote the development of IgAN.

A body of literature focusing on genetic risk has prompted speculation that IgAN is a polygenic disease (reviewed by Emancipator, 1992). In this context, immunoregulatory, transport, and cytokine genes all could impact upon elements of Figure 1. Except for aberrant regulation of Ig synthesis, data exist that contradict proposed defects in many of the pathways considered. Reports affirming defects often have borderline statistical significance or modest biological differences. We already have discussed the possibility that small quantitative differences over protracted time in a chronic disease such as IgAN could result in large differences in the accumulation of IgA deposits. Similarly, small shifts in the rate constants of multiple pathways in the overall scheme of Figure 1 could synergize to give a large shift in the overall rate of deposition versus clearance. Does this represent the polygenic origin postulated for IgAN?

A simple imbalance between production and clearance of immune complexes probably cannot account entirely for the development of IgAN (van Es *et al.*, 1988; Waldo, 1990; Julian *et al.*, 1991). Despite high levels of circulating IgA immune complexes, comparable to or in excess of levels seen in IgAN, patients with human immunodeficiency virus (HIV) infections rarely have glomerular deposits of IgA (Kenouch *et al.*, 1990; Béné *et al.*, 1991a; Schoeneman *et al.*, 1992). Indeed, IgAN associated with HIV has been recognized only recently, despite many renal biopsies of HIV-infected patients over several years. What factors, beyond the relative rates of production and clearance of IgA immune complexes, might apply to the development of this syndrome? Is the IgA produced by plasma cells from IgAN patients somehow different? Does the antigen component target IgA immune complexes to the mesangium in individuals at risk for IgAN (Emancipator *et al.*, 1992)? Is the mesangium of IgAN patients somehow different (Nagura, 1989)? Although such questions are emerging, their importance and relationship to the more established issues discussed earlier are speculative.

In conclusion, the pathogenesis of IgAN and the role of the mucosal immune system in the process are not yet clear. Nevertheless, we strongly favor the view that the glomerular IgA deposits represent complexes of mucosal antigens combined with antibodies synthesized by mucosal plasma cells that reached the circulation and were not cleared by the mononuclear phagocyte system or other mechanisms for elimination. This hypothesis, therefore, ascribes a major and central role in the genesis of IgAN to the mucosal immune system.

References

Adachi, M., Yodoi, J., Masuda, T., Takatsuki, T., and Uchino, H. (1983). Altered expression of lymphocyte Fcα receptor in selective IgA deficiency and IgA nephropathy. *J. Immunol.* **131,** 1246–1251.

Alley, C. D., Kiyono, H., and McGhee, J. R. (1986). Murine bone marrow IgA responses to orally administered sheep erythrocytes. *J. Immunol.* **136,** 4414–4419.

André, C., Berthoux, F. C., André, F., Gillon, J., Genin, C., and Sabatier, J. C. (1980). Prevalence of IgA2 deposits in IgA nephropathies: A clue to their pathogenesis. *N. Engl. J. Med.* **303,** 1343–1346.

Arend, W. P., and Mannik, M. (1971). Studies on antigen-antibody complexes. II. Quantification of tissue uptake of soluble complexes in normal and complement-depleted rabbits. *J. Immunol.* **107,** 63–75.

Aucouturier, P., Monteiro, R. C., Noel, L. H., Preud'homme, J. L., and Lesavre, P. (1989). Glomerular and serum immunoglobulin G subclasses in IgA nephropathy. *Clin. Immunol. Immunopathol.* **51,** 338–347.

Béné, M. C., and Faure, G. (1988). Mesangial IgA in IgA nephropathy arises from the mucosa. *Am. J. Kidney Dis.* **12,** 406–409.

Béné, M. C., Faure, G., and Duheille, J. (1982). IgA nephropathy: Characterization of the polymeric nature of mesangial deposits by *in vitro* binding of free secretory component. *Clin. Exp. Immunol.* **47,** 527–534.

Béné, M. C., Hurault de Ligny, B., Sirbat, D., Faure, G., Kessler, M., and Duheille, J. (1984). IgA nephropathy: Dimeric IgA-secreting cells are present in episcleral infiltrate. *Am. J. Clin. Nephrol.* **82,** 608–611.

Béné, M. C., Hurault de Ligny, B., Faure, G., Kessler, M., and Duheille, J. (1986). Histoimmunological discrepancies in primary IgA nephropathy and anaphylactoid purpura sustain relationships between mucosa and kidney. *Nephron* **43,** 214–216.

Béné, M. C., Canton, P., Amiel, C., May, T., and Faure, G. (1991a). Absence of mesangial IgA in AIDS: A postmortem study. *Nephron* **58,** 240–241.

Béné, M. C., Hurault de Ligny, B., Kessler, M., and Faure, G. (1991b). Confirmation of tonsillar anomalies in IgA nephropathy: A multicenter study. *Nephron* **58,** 425–428.

Biozzi, G., Benacerraf, B., and Halpern, B. N. (1953). Quantitative study of the granulopectic activity of the reticuloendothelial system. II. A study of the kinetics of the granulopectic activity of the R.E.S. in relation to the dose of carbon injected. Relationship between the weight of the organs and their activity. *Br. J. Exp. Pathol.* **34,** 441–457.

Brown, T. A., Russell, M. W., and Mestecky, J. (1982). Hepatobiliary transport of IgA immune complexes: Molecular and cellular aspects. *J. Immunol.* **128,** 2183–2186.

Cagnoli, L., Beltrandi, E., Pasquali, S., Biasi, R., Casadei-Maldini, M., Rossi, L., and Zucchelli, P. (1985). B and T cell abnormalities in patients with primary IgA nephropathy. *Kidney Int.* **28,** 646–651.

Cairns, S. A., London, A., and Mallick, N. P. (1981). Circulating immune complexes following food: Delayed clearance in idiopathic glomerulonephritis. *J. Clin. Lab. Immunol.* **6,** 121–126.

Chatenoud, L., and Bach, M. A. (1981). Abnormalities of T-cell subsets in glomerulonephritis and systemic lupus erythematosus. *Kidney Int.* **20,** 267–274.

Chen, N., Nusbaum, P., and Halbwachs-Mecarelli, L. (1991). Light-chain composition of serum IgA1 and *in vitro* IgA1 production in IgA nephropathy. *Nephrol. Dial. Transplant.* **6,** 846–850.

Clarkson, A. R., ed. (1987). "IgA Nephropathy." Martinus Nijhoff, Boston.

Clarkson, A. R., Seymour, A. E., Thompson, A. J., Haynes, W. D. G., Chan, Y-L., and Jackson, B. (1977). IgA nephropathy: A syndrome of uniform morphology, diverse clinical features, and uncertain prognosis. *Clin. Nephrol.* **8,** 459–471.

Conley, M. E., and Delacroix, D. L. (1987). Intravascular and mucosal immunoglobulin A: Two separate but related systems of immune defense? *Ann. Intern. Med.* **106,** 892–899.

Coppo, R., Basolo, B., Martina, G., Rollino, C., DeMarchi, M., Giacchino, F., Mazzucco, G., Messina, M., and Piccoli, G. (1982a). Circulating immune complexes containing IgA, IgG and IgM in patients with primary IgA nephropathy and with Henoch–Schoenlein nephritis. Correlation with clinical and histologic signs of activity. *Clin. Nephrol.* **18,** 230–239.

Coppo, R., Basolo, B., Mazzucco, G., Bulzomi, M. R., Roccatello, D., Messina, M., Barbiano, G., Martina, G., Rollino, C., and Piccoli, G. (1982b). IgA_1 and IgA_2 in circulating immune complexes and in renal deposits of Berger's and Schönlein–Henoch glomerulonephritis. *Proc. Eur. Dial. Transplant Assoc.* **19,** 648–654.

Coppo, R., Basolo, B., Piccoli, G., Mazzucco, G., Bulzomi, M. R., Roccatello, D., De Marchi, M., Carbonara, A. O., and Barbiano di Belgiojoso, G. (1984). IgA_1 and IgA_2 immune complexes in primary IgA nephropathy and Henoch–Schönlein nephritis. *Clin. Exp. Immunol.* **57,** 583–590.

Coppo, R., Basolo, B., Rollino, C., Roccatello, D., Martina, G., Amore, A., Bongiorno, G., and Piccoli, G. (1986). Mediterranean diet and primary IgA nephropathy. *Clin. Nephrol.* **26,** 72–82.

Cornacoff, J. B., Hebert, L. A., Smead, W. L., VanAman, M. E., Birmingham, D. J., and Waxman, F. J. (1983). Primary erythrocyte-immune complex-clearing mechanism. *J. Clin. Invest.* **71,** 236–247.

Cosio, F. G., Lam, S., Folami, A. O., Conley, M. E., and Michael, A. F. (1982). Immune regulation of immunoglobulin production in IgA nephropathy. *Clin. Immunol. Immunopathol.* **23,** 430–436.

Craig, S. W., and Cebra, J. J. (1975). Rabbit Peyer's patches, appendix and popliteal lymph node B-lymphocytes: A comprehensive analysis of their membrane immunoglobulin components and plasma cell precursor potential. *J. Immunol.* **114,** 492–502.

Cunningham-Rundles, C. (1990). Genetic aspects of immunoglobulin A deficiency. *Adv. Hum. Genet.* **19,** 235–266.

Cunningham-Rundles, C. (1991). Dietary antigens and immunologic disease in humans. *Rheum. Dis. Clin. North Am.* **17,** 287–307.

Cunningham-Rundles, C., Brandeis, W., and Good, R. (1978). Milk precipitins, circulating immune complexes and IgA deficiency. *Proc. Natl. Acad. Sci. U.S.A.* **75,** 3387–3389.

Czerkinsky, C. M., Koopman, W. J., Jackson, S., Collins, J. S., Crago, S. S., Schrohenloer, R. E., Julian, B. A., Galla, J. H., and Mestecky, J. (1986). Circulating immune complexes and immunoglobulin A rheumatoid factor in patients with mesangial immunoglobulin A nephropathies. *J. Clin. Invest.* **77,** 1931–1938.

D'Amico, G. (1987). The commonest glomerulonephritis in the world: IgA nephropathy. *Q. J. Med.* (*New Ser.*) **64,** 709–727.

D'Amico, G., Imbasciati, E., Barbiano di Belgioioso, G., Bertoli, S., Fogazzi, G., Ferrario, F., Fellin, G., Ragni, A., Colasanti, G., Minetti, L., and Ponticelli, C. (1985). Idiopathic IgA mesangial nephropathy. Clinical and histological study of 374 patients. *Medicine* **64,** 49–60.

Davin, J. C., and Mahieu, P. R. (1992). Sequential measurements of intestinal permeability to [^{51}Cr]EDTA in children with Henoch-Schönlein purpura nephritis. *Nephron* **60,** 498–499.

Davin, J. C., Forget, P., and Mahieu, P. R. (1988). Increased intestinal permeability to (^{51}Cr) EDTA is correlated with IgA immune complex-plasma levels in children with IgA-associated nephropathies. *Acta Paediatr. Scand.* **77,** 118–124.

Delacroix, D. L., Hodgson, H. J. F., McPherson, A., Dive, C., and Vaerman, J. P. (1982). Selective transport of polymeric immunoglobulin A in bile. *J. Clin. Invest.* **70,** 230–241.

Delprato, S., Rostoker, G., Pilatte, Y., and Lagrue, G. (1988). IgA antigliadin antibodies detected by ELISA are not an artifact due to lectin-like activity of gliadin. *J. Immunol. Meth.* **112,** 147.

Dobrin, R. S., Knudson, F. E., and Michael, A. F. (1975). The secretory immune system and renal disease. *Clin. Exp. Immunol.* **21,** 318–328.

Doi, T., Kanatsu, K., Nagai, H., Kohrogi, N., and Hamashima, Y. (1984). Immunoelectron microscopic studies of IgA nephropathy. *Nephron* **36,** 246–251.

Donini, U., Casanova, S., Zini, N., and Zucchelli, P. (1982). The presence of J chain in mesangial immune deposits of IgA nephropathy. *Proc. Eur. Dial. Transplant Assoc.* **19,** 655–662.

Drew, P. A., Nieuwhof, W. N., Clarkson, A. R., and Woodroffe, A. J. (1987). Increased concentration of serum IgA antibody to pneumococcal polysaccharides in patients with IgA nephropathy. *Clin. Exp. Immunol.* **67,** 124–129.

Dysart, N. K., Sisson, S., and Vernier, R. L. (1983). Immunoelectron microscopy of IgA nephropathy. *Clin. Immunol. Immunopathol.* **29,** 254–270.

Egido, J., Sancho, J., Mampaso, F., Lopez-Trascasa, M., Sanchez-Crespo, M., Blasco, R., and Hernando, L. (1980). A possible common pathogenesis of the mesangial IgA glomerulonephritis in patients with Berger's Disease and Schönlein–Henoch Syndrome. *Proc. Eur. Dial. Transplant Assoc.* **17,** 660–666.

Egido, J., Blasco, R., Sancho, J., Illescas, M., and Hernando, L. (1982a). Abnormalities of immune regulation in patients with IgA mesangial glomerulonephritis (Berger's Disease). *Proc. Eur. Dial. Transplant Assoc.* **19,** 642–647.

Egido, J., Blasco, R., Sancho, J., Lozano, L., Sanchez-Crespo, M., and Hernando, L. (1982b). Increased rates of polymeric IgA synthesis by circulating lymphoid cells in IgA mesangial glomerulonephritis. *Clin. Exp. Immunol.* **47,** 309–316.

Egido, J., Blasco, R., and Sancho, J. (1983a). Immunoregulation abnormalities in patients with IgA nephropathy. *Ann. N.Y. Acad. Sci.* **409,** 817–818.

Egido, J., Blasco, R., Sancho, J., and Lozano, L. (1983b). T-cell dysfunctions in IgA nephropathy: Specific abnormalities in the regulation of IgA synthesis. *Clin. Immunol. Immunopathol.* **26,** 201–212.

Egido, J., Blasco, R., Sancho, J., Lozano, L., and Gutierrez-Millet, V. (1983c). Immunological studies in a familial IgA nephropathy. *Clin. Exp. Immunol.* **54,** 532–538.

Egido, J., Blasco, R. A., Sancho, J., and Hernando, L. (1985). Immunological abnormalities in healthy relatives of patients with IgA nephropathy. *Am. J. Nephrol.* **5,** 14–20.

Egido, J., Garcia-Hoyo, R., Lozano, L., Gonzalez-Cabrero, J., de Nicolas, R., and Hernando, L. (1987a). Immunological studies in familial and sporadic IgA nephropathy. *Sem. Nephrol.* **7,** 311–314.

Egido, J., Julian, B. A., and Wyatt, R. J. (1987b). Genetic factors in primary IgA nephropathy. *Nephrol. Dial. Transplant.* **2,** 134–139.

Emancipator, S. N. (1990). Immunoregulatory factors in the pathogenesis of IgA nephropathy. *Kidney Int.* **38,** 1216–1229.

Emancipator, S. N. (1992). Primary and secondary forms of IgA nephritis, Schönlein–Henoch syndrome. *In* "Pathology of the Kidney" (R. H. Heptinstall, ed.), 4th Ed., Vol. I, pp. 389–476. Little, Brown, Boston.

Emancipator, S. N., and Lamm, M. E. (1989). Biology of disease: IgA nephropathy: Pathogenesis of the most common form of glomerulonephritis. *Lab. Invest.* **60,** 168–183.

Emancipator, S. N., Gallo, G. R., and Lamm, M. E. (1985). IgA nephropathy: perspectives on pathogenesis and classification. *Clin. Nephrol.* **24,** 161–179.

Emancipator, S. N., Rao, C. S., Amore, A., Coppo, R., and Nedrud, J. G. (1992). Macromolecular properties that promote mesangial binding and mesangiopathic nephritis. *J. Am. Soc. Nephrol.* **2,** S149–S158.

Endoh, M., Suga, T., Miura, M., Tomino, Y., Nomoto, Y., and Sakai, H. (1984). *In vivo* alteration of antibody production in patients with IgA nephropathy. *Clin. Exp. Immunol.* **57,** 564–570.

Faure, G. C., Tang, J. G., Molé, C., and Béné, M. C. (1990). Plasma cells producing lambda light chains are predominant in human gut and tonsils. An immunohistomorphometric study. *Am. J. Clin. Pathol.* **12,** 315–320.

Feehally, J., Beattie, T. J., Brenchley, P. E. C., Coupes, B. M., Mallick, N. P., and Postlethwaite, R. J. (1986). Sequential study of the IgA system in relapsing IgA nephropathy. *Kidney Int.* **30,** 924–931.

Finbloom, D. S., Magilavy, D. B., Hartford, J. B., Rifai, A., and Plotz, P. H. (1981). The influence of antigen on immune complex behavior in mice. *J. Clin. Invest.* **68,** 214–224.

Fornasieri, A., Sinico, R., Fiorini, G., Goldaniga, D., Colasanti, G., Vendemia, F., Gibelli, A., and D'Amico, G. (1982). T-lymphocyte subsets in primary and secondary glomerulonephritis. *Proc. Eur. Dial. Transplant Assoc.* **19,** 635–641.

Fornasieri, A., Sinico, R. A., Maldifassi, P., Bernasconi, P., Vegni, M., and D'Amico, G. (1987). IgA anti-gliadin antibodies in IgA mesangial nephropathy (Berger's Disease). *Br. Med. J.* **295,** 78–80.

Gallo, G. R., Caulin-Glaser, T., Emancipator, S. N., and Lamm, M. E. (1983). Nephritogenicity and differential distribution of glomerular immune complexes related to immunogen charge. *Lab. Invest.* **48,** 353–362.

Gauthier, V. J., Mannik, M., and Striker, G. E. (1982). Effect of cationized antibodies in preformed immune complexes on deposition and persistence in renal glomeruli. *J. Exp. Med.* **156,** 766–777.

Germuth, F. G., Jr., and Rodriguez, E. (1973). "Immunopathology of the Renal Glomerulus." Little, Brown, Boston.

Germuth, F. G., Jr., Taylor, J. J., Siddiqui, S. Y., and Rodriguez, E. (1977). Imune complex disease, VI. Some determinants of the varieties of glomerular lesions in the chronic bovine serum albumin–rabbit system. *Lab. Invest.* **37,** 162–169.

Germuth, F. G., Jr., Rodriguez, E., and Wise, O'L. (1982). Passive immune complex glomerulonephritis in mice. III. Clearance kinetics and properties of circulating complexes. *Lab. Invest.* **46,** 515–519.

Haakenstad, A. O., and Mannik, M. (1974). Saturation of the reticuloendothelial system with soluble immune complexes. *J. Immunol.* **112,** 1939–1948.

Haakenstad, A. O., and Mannik, M. (1976). The disappearance kinetics of soluble immune complexes prepared with reduced and alkylated antibodies and with intact antibodies in mice. *Lab. Invest.* **35,** 283–292.

Hale, G. M., McIntosh, S. L., Hiki, Y., Clarkson, A. R., and Woodroffe, A. J. (1986). Evidence for IgA-specific B cell hyperactivity in patients with IgA nephropathy. *Kidney Int.* **29,** 718–724.

Hall, R. P., Stachura, I., Cason, J., Whiteside, T. L., and Lawley, T. J. (1983). IgA-containing circulating immune complexes in patients with IgA nephropathy. *Am. J. Med.* **74,** 56–63.

Hernando, P., Egido, J., de Nicolas, R., and Sancho, J. (1986). Clinical significance of polymeric and monomeric IgA complexes in patients with IgA nephropathy. *Am. J. Kidney Dis.* **8,** 410–416.

Hill, G. S. (1992). Systemic lupus erythematosus and mixed connective-tissue disease. *In* "Pathology of the Kidney" (R. H. Heptinstall, ed.), 4th Ed., Vol. I, pp. 871–950. Little, Brown, Boston.

Isaacs, K., and Miller, F. (1982). Role of antigen size and charge in immune complex glomerulonephritis. I. Active induction of disease with dextran and its derivatives. *Lab. Invest.* **47,** 198–205.

Jackson, S. (1988). Immunoglobulin-antiimmunoglobulin interactions and immune complexes in IgA nephropathy. *Am. J. Kidney Dis.* **12,** 425–429.

Jackson, S., Montgomery, R. I., Mestecky, J., Julian, B. A., Galla, J. H., and Czerkinsky, C. (1987). Antibodies directed at Fab of IgA in the sera of normal individuals and IgA nephropathy patients. *Adv. Exp. Biol. Med.* **216B,** 1537–1544.

Jenkins, D. A. S., Bell, G. M., Ferguson, A., and Lambie, A. T. (1988). Intestinal permeability in IgA nephropathy. *Nephron* **50,** 390.

Jennette, J. C., Wieslander, J., Tuttle, R., and Falk, R. J. (1991). Serum IgA-fibronectin aggregates in patients with IgA nephropathy and Henoch–Schönlein purpura: diagnostic value and pathogenic implications. The Glomerular Disease Collaborative Network. *Am. J. Kidney Dis.* **18,** 466–471.

Jones, C. L., Powell, H. R., Kincaid-Smith, P., and Roberton, D. M. (1990). Polymeric IgA and immune complex concentrations in IgA-related renal disease. *Kidney Int.* **38,** 323–331.

Julian, B. A. (Ed.) (1988). IgA Nephropathy: A National Symposium *Am. J. Kidney Dis.* **12.**

Julian, B. A., Quiggins, P. A., Thompson, J. S., Woodford, S. Y., Gleason, K., and Wyatt, R. J. (1985). Familial IgA nephropathy: Evidence of an inherited mechanism of disease. *N. Engl. J. Med.* **312,** 202–208.

Julian, B. A., Cannon, V. R., Waldo, F. B., and Egido, J. (1991). Macroscopic hematuria and proteinuria preceding renal IgA deposition in patients with IgA nephropathy. *Am. J. Kidney Dis.* **17,** 472–479.

Kaetzel, C. S., Robinson, J. K., Chintalacharuvu, K. R., Vaerman, J.-P., and Lamm, M. E. (1991). The polymeric immunoglobulin receptor (secretory component) mediates transport of immune complexes across epithelial cells: A local defense function for IgA. *Proc. Natl. Acad. Sci. U.S.A.* **88,** 8796–8800.

Kauffmann, R. H., Van Es, L. A., and Daha, M. R. (1981). The specific detection of IgA immune complexes. *J. Immunol. Meth.* **40,** 117–129.

Kenouch, S., Delahousse, M., Méry, J. P., and Nochy, D. (1990). Mesangial IgA deposits in two patients with AIDS-related complex. *Nephron* **54,** 338–340.

Komatsu, N., Nagura, H., Watanabe, K., Nomoto, Y., and Kobayashi, K. (1983). Mesangial deposition of J chain-linked polymeric IgA in IgA nephropathy. *Nephron* **33,** 61–64.

Kupor, L. R., Mullins, J. D., and McPhaul, J. J. (1975). Immunopathologic findings in idiopathic renal hematuria. *Arch. Intern. Med.* **135,** 1204–1211.

Lai, K. N., Lai, F. M., Chiu, S. H., Chan, Y. M., Tsao, G. S. W., Leung, K. N., and Lam, C. W. K. (1987). Studies of lymphocyte subpopulations and immunoglobulin production in IgA nephropathy. *Clin. Nephrol.* **28,** 281–287.

Lamm, M. E. (1976). Cellular aspects of immunoglobulin A. *Adv. Immunol.* **22,** 223–290.

Laurent, J., Branellec, A., Heslan, J.-M., Rostoker, G., Bruneau, C., Andre, C., Intrator, L., and Lagrue, G. (1987). An increase in circulating IgA antibodies to gliadin in IgA mesangial glomerulonephritis. *Am. J. Nephrol.* **7,** 178–183.

Lawrence, S., Pussell, B. A., and Charlesworth, J. A. (1983). Mesangial IgA nephropathy: Detection of defective reticulophagocytic function *in vivo*. *Clin. Nephrol.* **16,** 280–283.

Leinikki, P. O., Mustonen, J., and Pasternack, A. (1987). Immune response to oral polio vaccine in patients with IgA glomerulonephritis. *Clin. Exp. Immunol.* **68,** 33–38.

Lesavre, P. H., Digeon, M., and Bach, J. F. (1982). Analysis of circulating IgA and detection of immune complexes in primary IgA nephropathy. *Clin. Exp. Immunol.* **48,** 61–69.

Linné, T., and Wasserman, J. (1985). Lymphocyte subpopulations and immunoglobulin production in IgA nephropathy. *Clin. Nephrol.* **23,** 109–111.

Lomax-Smith, J. D., Zabrowarny, L. A., Howarth, G. S., Seymour, A. E., and Woodroffe, A. J. (1983). The immunochemical characterization of mesangial IgA deposits. *Am. J. Pathol.* **113,** 359–364.

Lopez-Trascasa, M., Egido, J., Sancho, J., and Hernando, L. (1979). Evidence of high polymeric IgA levels in serum of patients with Berger's Disease and its modification with phenytoin treatment. *Proc. Eur. Dial. Transplant Assoc.* **16,** 513–519.

Lopez-Trascasa, M., Egido, J., Sancho, J., and Hernando, L. (1980). IgA glomerulonephritis (Berger's Disease): Evidence of high serum levels of polymeric IgA. *Clin. Exp. Immunol.* **42,** 247–254.

McCluskey, R. T. (1992). Immunologic aspects of renal disease. *In* "Pathology of the Kidney" (R. H. Heptinstall, ed.), 4th Ed., Vol. I, pp. 169–260. Little, Brown, Boston.

McKenzie, P. E., Gormly, A. A., Clarkson, A. R., Seymour, A. E., Kwitko, A. O., Shearman, D. J. C., and Woodroffe, A. J. (1980). Gut-derived antigens and immune complexes in IgA nephropathy. *Aust. N. Z. J. Med.* **10,** 126–128.

Mannik, M., and Arend, W. P. (1971). Fate of preformed immune complexes in rabbits and rhesus monkeys. *J. Exp. Med.* **134,** 19s–31s.

Mannik, M., and Jimenez, R. A. H. (1979). The mononuclear phagocyte system (MPS) and immune complex diseases. *In* "Immunopathology: Proceedings of the 6th International Convocation on Immunology" (F. Milgrom and B. Albini, eds.), pp. 212–216. Karger, Basel.

Mannik, M., Arend, W. P., Hall, A. P., and Gilliland, B. C. (1971). Studies on antigen-antibody complexes. I. Elimination of soluble complexes from rabbit circulation. *J. Exp. Med.* **133,** 713–739.

Mannik, M., Agodoa, L. Y. C., and David, K. A. (1983). Rearrangement of immune complexes in glomeruli leads to persistence and development of electron-dense deposits. *J. Exp. Med.* **157,** 1516–1527.

Mathews, D. C., Bell, J. A., Dowling, J. P., and Kincaid-Smith, P. S. (1985). Immunoelectron microscopic localization of glomerular IgA deposits using a postembedding method with a protein A-colloidal gold probe. *Ultrastruc. Pathol.* **8,** 43–48.

Matsuda, S., Waldo, F. B., Czerkinsky, C., Moldoveanu, Z., and Mestecky, J. (1988). Binding of IgA to erythrocytes from patients with IgA nephropathy. *Clin. Immunol. Immunopathol.* **48,** 1–9.

Mazanec, M. B., Kaetzel, C. S., Lamm, M. E., Fletcher, D., and Nedrud, J. G. (1992). Intracellular neutralization of virus by IgA antibodies. *Proc. Natl. Acad. Sci. U.S.A.* **89,** 6901–6905.

Medof, M. E., Lam, T., Prince, G. M., and Mold, C. (1983). Requirement for human red blood cells in inactivation of C3b in immune complexes and enhancement of binding to spleen cells. *J. Immunol.* **130,** 1336–1340.

Mestecky, J. (1988). Immunobiology of IgA. *Am. J. Kidney Dis.* **12,** 378–383.

Mestecky, J., and McGhee, J. R. (1987). Immunoglobulin A (IgA): Molecular and cellular interactions involved in IgA biosynthesis and immune response. *Adv. Immunol.* **40,** 153–245.

Mestecky, J., Moldoveanu, Z., Tomana, M., Epps, J. M., Thorpe, S. R., Phillips, J. O., and Kulhavy, R. (1989). The role of the liver in catabolism of mouse and human IgA. *Immunol. Invest.* **18,** 313–324.

Monteiro, R. C., Halbwachs-Mecarelli, L., Berger, J., and Lesavre, P. (1984). Characteristics of eluted IgA in primary IgA nephropathy. *Contrib. Nephrol.* **40,** 107–111.

Mustonen, J., Pasternack, A., Helin, H., Rilva, A., Penttinen, K., Wager, O., and Harmoinen, A. (1981). Circulating immune complexes, the concentration of serum IgA and the distribution of HLA antigens in IgA nephropathy. *Nephron* **29,** 170–175.

Nagura, H. (1989). IgA nephropathy and mucosal immune system. *Tokai J. Exp. Clin. Med.* **14,** 1–4.

Nagura, H., Smith, P. D., Nakane, P. K., and Brown, W. R. (1981). IgA in human bile and liver. *J. Immunol.* **126,** 587–595.

Nagy, J., Uj, M., Szëcs, G., Trinn, C., and Burger, T. (1984). Herpes virus antigens and antibodies in kidney biopsies and sera of IgA glomerulonephritis. *Clin. Nephrol.* **21,** 259–262.

Nagy, J., Scott, H., and Brandtzaeg, P. (1988). Antibodies to dietary antigens in IgA nephropathy. *Clin. Nephrol.* **29,** 275–279.

Nagy, J., Srov, I., Sámik, J., Trinn, C., Kun, L., Burger, T., and Sarov, B. (1989). IgA and IgG antibodies to *Chlamydia* in IgA nephropathy as well as in mesangiocapillary and membranous glomerulonephritis. *Orv. Hetil.* **130,** 1530–1537.

Nakajima, M., Hirota, T., Kusumoto, K., Taira, K., and Kamitsuji, H. (1987). Immunoelectron microscopic study of glomerular lesions using a postembedding method with a protein A-gold complex. *Nephron* **46,** 182–187.

Nicholls, K., and Kincaid-Smith, P. (1984). Defective *in vivo* Fc- and C3b-receptor function in IgA nephropathy. *Am. J. Kidney Dis.* **4,** 128–134.

Nomoto, Y., Sakai, H., and Arimori, S. (1979). Increase of IgA-bearing lymphocytes in peripheral blood from patients with IgA nephropathy. *Am. J. Clin. Pathol.* **71,** 158–160.

Normann, S. J. (1974). Kinetics of phagocytosis. II. Analysis of *in vivo* clearance with demonstration of competitive inhibition between similar and dissimilar foreign particles. *Lab. Invest.* **31,** 161–169.

Pabst, R., and Binns, R. M. (1981). *In vivo* labelling of the spleen and mesenteric lymph nodes with fluorescein isothicyoanate for lymphocyte migration studies. *Immunology* **44,** 321–329.

Pabst, R., Binns, R. M., and Reynolds, J. D. (1987). Peyer's patches export lymphocytes throughout the lymphoid system in sheep. *J. Immunol.* **139,** 3981–3985.

Peppard, J., Orlans, E., Payne, A. W. R., and Andrew, E. (1981). The elimination of circulating complexes containing IgA by excretion in the bile. *Immunology* **42,** 83–90.

Peterman, J. H., Julian, B. A., Kirk, K. A., and Jackson, S. (1991). Selective elevation of monomeric IgA1 in IgA nephropathy patients with normal renal function. *Am. J. Kidney Dis.* **18,** 313–319.

Rambausek, M., Seelig, H. P., Andrassy, K., Waldherr, R., Lenhard, V., and Ritz, E. (1982). Clinical and serological features of mesangial IgA glomerulonephritis. *Proc. Eur. Dial. Transplant Assoc.* **19,** 663–668.

Rifai, A. (1987). Experimental models for IgA-associated nephritis. *Kidney Int.* **31,** 1–7.

Rifai, A., and Mannik, M. (1983). Clearance kinetics and fate of mouse IgA immune complexes prepared with monomeric or dimeric IgA. *J. Immunol.* **130,** 1826–1832.

Rifai, A., and Mannik, M. (1984). Clearance of circulating IgA immune complexes is mediate by a specific receptor on Kupffer cells in mice. *J. Exp. Med.* **160,** 125–137.

Rifai, A., Schena, F. P., Montinaro, V., Mele, M., D'Addabbo, A., Nitti, L., and Pezzullo, J. C. (1989). Clearance kinetics and fate of macromolecular IgA in patients with IgA nephropathy. *Lab. Invest.* **61,** 381–388.

Roccatello, D., Coppo, R., Piccoli, G., Cordonnice, D., Martina, G., Rollino, C., Picciotto, G., Sena, L. M., and Amoroso, A. (1985). Circulating Fc-receptor blocking factors in IgA nephropathies. *Clin. Nephrol.* **23,** 159–168.

Roccatello, D., Picciotto, G., Coppo, R., Piccoli, G., Molino, A., Cacace, G., Amore, A., Amoroso, A., Quattrocchio, G., and Sena, L. M. (1989). Clearance of polymeric IgA aggregates in humans. *Am. J. Kidney Dis.* **14,** 354–360.

Roccatello, D., Picciotto, G., Ropolo, R., Coppo, R., Quattrocchio, G., Cacace, G., Molino, A., Amoroso, A., Baccega, M., Isidoro, C., Cardosi, R., Sena, L. M., and Piccoli, G. (1992). Kinetics and fate of IgA–IgG aggregates as a model of naturally occurring immune complexes in IgA nephropathy. *Lab. Invest.* **66,** 86–95.

Rostoker, G., Delprato, S., BenMaadi, A., Petit-Phar, M., Andre, C., Laurent, J., Lang, P., Weil, B., and Lagrue, G. (1989a). Signification des anticorps IgA antigliadine au cours des glomérulonéphrites primitives avec dépôts mésangiaux d'IgA. *Ann. Med. Interne* **140,** 571–574.

Rostoker, G., Pech, M.-A., del Prato, S., Petit-Phar, M., BenMaadi, A., Dubert, J.-M., Lang, P., Weil, B., and Lagrue, G. (1989b). Serum IgG subclasses and IgM imbalances in adult IgA mesangial glomerulonephritis and idiopathic Henoch–Schoenlein purpura. *Clin. Exp. Immunol.* **75,** 30–34.

Rostoker, G., Chaumette, M. T., Wirquin, E., Delchier, J. C., Petit-Phar, M., Andre, C., Weil, B., and Lagrue, G. (1990a). IgA mesangial nephritis, IgA antigliadin antibodies, and coeliac disease. *Lancet* **336,** 824–825.

Rostoker, G., Pech, M.-A., Petit-Phar, M., BenMaadi, A., Cholin, S., Lang, P., Dubert, J.-M., Weil, B., and Lagrue, G. (1990b). Mucosal immunity in primary glomerulonephritis. I. Evaluation of salivary IgA subclasses and components. *Nephron* **54,** 42–46.

Rostoker, G., Petit-Phar, M., Delprato, S., Terzidis, H., Lang, P., Dubert, J. M., Weil, B., and Lagrue, G. (1991). Mucosal immunity in primary glomerulonephritis: II. Study of the serum IgA subclass repertoire to food and airborne antigens. *Nephron* **59,** 561–566.

Rothberg, R. M., Rieger, C. H. L., Kraft, S. C., and Lustig, J. V. (1978). Development of humoral antibody following the infestion of soluble protein antigen by passively immunized animals. *In* "Secretory Immunity and Infection" (J. R. McGhee, J. Mestecky, and J. L. Babb, eds), pp. 123–132. Plenum Press, New York.

Russell, M. W., Mestecky, J., Julian, B. A., and Galla, J. H. (1986). IgA-associated renal diseases: antibodies to environmental antigens in sera and deposition of immunoglobulins and antigen in glomeruli. *J. Clin. Immunol.* **6,** 74–86.

Sakai, H. (1987). Lymphocyte function in IgA nephropathy. *In* "IgA Nephropathy" (A. R. Clarkson, ed.), pp. 176–187. Martinus Nijhoff, Boston.

Sakai, H. (1988). Cellular immunoregulatory aspects of IgA nephropathy. *Am. J. Kidney Dis.* **54,** 532–538.

Sakai, H., Nomoto, Y., and Arimori, S. (1979a). Decrease of IgA specific suppressor T cells activity in patients with IgA nephropathy. *Clin. Exp. Immunol.* **38,** 243–248.

Sakai, H., Nomoto, Y., Arimori, S., Komori, K., Inouye, H., and Tsuji, K. (1979b). Increase of IgA bearing peripheral blood lymphocytes in families of patients with IgA nephropathy. *Am. J. Clin. Pathol.* **72,** 452–456.

Sakai, H., Endoh, M., Tomino, Y., and Nomoto, Y. (1982). Increase of IgA specific helper T cells in patients with IgA nephropathy. *Clin. Exp. Immunol.* **50,** 77–82.

Sakai, H., Sakai, O., and Nomoto, Y. (1990). "Pathogenesis of IgA Nephropathy." Harcourt Brace Jovanovich Japan, Tokyo.

Sancho, J., Egido, J., Rivera, F., and Hernando, L. (1983). Immune complexes in IgA nephropathy: Presence of antibodies against diet antigens and delayed clearance of specific polymeric IgA immune complexes. *Clin. Exp. Immunol.* **54,** 194–202.

Sato, M., Takayama, K., Wakasa, M., and Koshikawa, S. (1987). Estimate of circulating immune complexes following oral challenge with cow's milk in patients with IgA nephropathy. *Nephron* **47,** 43–48.

Schena, F. P. (1990). A retrospective analysis of the natural history of primary IgA nephropathy worldwide. *Am. J. Med.* **89,** 209–215.

Schena, F. P., Mastrolitti, G., Fracasso, A. R., Pastore, A., and Ladisa, N. (1986). Increased immunoglobulin-secreting cells in the blood of patients with active idiopathic IgA nephropathy. *Clin. Nephrol.* **26,** 163–168.

Schena, F. P., Pastore, A., Sinico, R. A., Montinaro, V., and Fornasieri, A. (1988). Polymeric IgA decreases the capacity of serum to solubilize circulating immune complexes in patients with primary IgA nephropathy. *J. Immunol.* **141,** 125–130.

Schoeneman, M. J., Ghali, V., Lieberman, K., and Reisman, L. (1992). IgA nephritis in a child with human immunodeficiency virus: A unique form of human immunodeficiency virus-associated nephropathy? *Pediatr. Nephrol.* **6,** 46–49.

Shigematsu, H., Kobayashi, Y., Tateno, S., and Tsukada, M. (1980). Ultrastructure of acute glomerular injury in IgA nephritis. *Arch. Pathol. Lab. Med.* **104,** 303–307.

Silva, F. G. (1992). Acute postinfectious glomerulonephritis and glomerulonephritis complicating persistent bacterial infection. *In* "Pathology of the Kidney" (R. H. Heptinstall, ed.), 4th Ed., Vol. I, pp. 297–388. Little, Brown, Boston.

Sinico, R. A., Fornasieri, A., Oreni, N., Benuzzi, S., and D'Amico, G. (1986). Polymeric IgA rheumatoid factor in idiopathic IgA mesangial nephropathy (Berger's disease). *J. Immunol.* **137,** 536–541.

Sinico, R. A., Fornasieri, A. Maldifassi, P., Colasanti, G., and D'Amico, G. (1988). The clinical significance of IgA rheumatoid factor in idiopathic IgA mesangial nephropathy (Berger's disease). *Clin. Nephrol.* **30,** 182–186.

Socken, D. J., Simms, E. S., Nagy, B. R., Fisher, M. M., and Underdown, B. J. (1981). Secretory component-dependent hepatic transport of IgA antibody-antigen complexes. *J. Immunol.* **127,** 316–319.

Solomon, L. R., Rawlinson, V. I., Howarth, S., and Mallick, N. P. (1984). Reticuloendothelial function in glomerulonephritis. *Nephron* **37,** 54–59.

Stachura, I., Singh, G., and Whiteside, T. L. (1981). Immune abnormalities in IgA nephropathy (Berger's Disease). *Clin. Immunol. Immunopathol.* **20,** 373–388.

Tanaka, M. (1986). Immunoelectron microscopic studies of IgA nephropathy in children. *Hokkaido Igaku Zasshi* **61,** 83–93.

Tomino, Y., Endoh, M., Nomoto, Y., and Sakai, H. (1981). Immunoglobulin A_1 in IgA nephropathy. *N. Engl. J. Med.* **305,** 1159–1160.

Tomino, Y., Endoh, M., Nomoto, Y., and Sakai, H. (1982a). Specificity of eluted antibody from renal tissues of patients with IgA nephropathy. *Am. J. Kidney Dis.* **1,** 276–284.

Tomino, Y., Sakai, H., Endoh, M., Kaneshige, H., and Nomoto, Y. (1982b). Detection of immune complexes in polymorphonuclear leukocytes by double immunofluorescence in patients with IgA nephropathy. *Clin. Immunol. Immunopathol.* **24,** 63–71.

Tomino, Y., Sakai, H., Miura, M., Endoh, M., and Nomoto, Y. (1982c). Detection of polymeric IgA in glomeruli from patients with IgA nephropathy. *Clin. Exp. Immunol.* **49,** 419–425.

Tomino, Y., Sakai, H., Hashimoto, K., and Tanaka, S. (1987). Antigenic heterogeneity in patients with IgA nephropathy. *Sem. Nephrol.* **7,** 294–296.

Tung, K. S. K., Woodroffe, A. J., Ahlin, T. D., Williams, R. C., Jr., and Wilson, C. B. (1978). Application of the solid phase C1q and Raji cell radioimmune asays for the detection of circulating immune complexes in glomerulonephritis. *J. Clin. Invest.* **62,** 61–72.

Underdown, B. J., and Schiff, J. M. (1986). Immunoglobulin A: strategic defense initiative at the mucosal surface. *Ann. Rev. Immunol.* **4,** 389–417.

Vaerman, J. P., and Heremans, J. F. (1970). Origin and molecular size of IgA in the mesenteric lymph of the dog. *Immunology* **18,** 27–38.

van den Wall Bake, A. W. L., Daha, M. R., Radl, J., Haaijman, J. J., van der Ark, A., Valentijn, R. M., and van Es, L. A. (1988). The bone marrow as production site of the IgA deposited in the kidneys of patients with IgA nephropathy. *Clin. Exp. Immunol.* **72,** 321–325.

van der Woude, F. J., Hoedemaeker, P. J., van der Giessen, M., de Graeff, P. A., de Monchy, J., The, T. H., and van der Hem, G. K. (1983). Do food antigens play a role in the pathogenesis of some cases of human glomerulonephritis? *Clin. Exp. Immunol.* **51,** 587–594.

van Es, L. A., van den Wall Bake, A. W. L., Valentijn, R. M., and Daha, M. R. (1988). Composition of IgA-containing circulating immune complexes in IgA nephropathy. *Am. J. Kidney Dis.* **12,** 397–401.

Waldherr, R., Seelig, H. P., Rambausek, M., Andrassy, K., and Ritz, E. (1983). Deposition of polymeric IgA in idiopathic mesangial IgA glomerulonephritis. *Klin. Wochenschr.* **61,** 911–915.

Waldo, F. B. (1990). Role of IgA in IgA nephropathy. *J. Pediatr.* **116,** S78–S85.

Waldo, F. B. (1992). Systemic immune response after mucosal immunization in patients with IgA nephropathy. *J. Clin. Immunol.* **12,** 21–26.

Waldo, F. B., and Cochran, A. M. (1987). Systemic immune response to oral polio immunization in patients with IgA nephropathy. *J. Clin. Lab. Immunol.* **28,** 109–114.

Waldo, F. B., and Cochran, A. M. (1989). Mixed IgA-IgG aggregates as a model of immune complexes in IgA nephropathy. *J. Immunol.* **142,** 3841–3846.

Waldo, F. B., Beischel, L., and West, C. D. (1986). IgA synthesis by lymphocytes from patients with IgA nephropathy and their relatives. *Kidney Int.* **29,** 1229–1233.

Walker, W. A., and Bloch, K. J. (1983). Intestinal uptake of macromolecules: *In vitro* and *in vivo* studies. *Ann. N.Y. Acad. Sci.* **409,** 593–602.

Waxman, F. J., Hebert, L., Cosio, F. G., Smead, W. L., VanAman, M. E., Taguiam, J. M., and Birmingham, D. J. (1986). Differential binding of immunoglobulin A and immunoglobulin G1 immune complexes to primate erythrocytes *in vivo*. *J. Clin. Invest.* **77,** 82–89.

Westberg, N. G., Baklien, K., Schmekel, B., Gillberg, R., and Brandtzaeg, P. (1983). Quantitation of immunoglobulin-producing cells in small intestinal mucosa of patients with IgAN nephropathy. *Clin. Immunol. Immunopathol.* **26,** 442–445.

Williams, D. G., Perl, S. J., Knight, J. F., and Harada, T. (1987). Immunoglobulin production *in vitro* in IgA nephropathy and Henoch–Schönlein purpura. *Sem. Nephrol.* **7,** 322–324.

Woo, K. T., Tan, Y. O. Lau, Y. K., Ng, S. L., Chew, T. S., Chan, S. H., and Lim, C. H. (1982). Suppressor cell function in IgA nephritis. *Aust. N. Z. J. Med.* **12,** 208–210.

Woodroffe, A. J., Gormly, A. A., McKenzie, P. E., Wootton, A. M., Thompson, A. J., Seymour, A. E., and Clarkson, A. R. (1980). Immunologic studies in IgA nephropathy. *Kidney Int.* **18,** 366–374.

Yap, H. K., Sakai, R. S., Woo, K. T., Lim, C. H., and Jordan, S. C. (1987). Detection of bovine serum albumin in the circulating IgA immune complexes of patients with IgA nephropathy. *Clin. Immunol. Immunopathol.* **43,** 395–402.

Yasumori, R. (1990). Measurement of secretory IgA in salivary juice and the localization of secretory IgA in duodenal mucosa in patients with IgA nephropathy. *Nippon Jinzo Gakkai Shi* **32,** 171–181.

54

Mucosal Immunity in the Female and Male Reproductive Tracts

Margaret B. Parr · Earl L. Parr

I. INTRODUCTION

Mucosal immunity in the female and male reproductive tracts is uniquely adapted to serve the particular requirements of reproduction. This immune system reacts against microorganisms and helps maintain an aseptic environment in the genital tracts during most stages of the reproductive process. At the same time, the system fails to react against the antigens of sperm, the zona pellucida, and the early embryo, and thereby avoids inhibiting reproduction. A consequence of this adaptation is that mucosal immunity in the genital tracts differs in significant ways from that in the intestine. In particular, several basic characteristics of mucosal immunity in the intestine are absent or inconspicuous in the genital tracts, including antigen-transporting epithelial cells, mucosal lymphoid nodules, homing, and a preponderance of IgA in secretions. A consideration of these differences is a major focus of this chapter.

Progress in several important clinical and public health issues cannot be made without a better understanding of mucosal immunology in the genital tracts. For example, effective vaccination to protect the genital tracts against sexually transmitted diseases, including acquired immunodeficiency syndrome (AIDS), probably will require activation of local immune mechanisms in the mucosa (Archibald *et al.*, 1987; Forrest, 1991; Ward, 1993). Similarly, considerable interest has arisen in the development of vaccines that stimulate local secretory immunity against sperm for short- or intermediate-term immunocontraception (E. L. Parr and M. B. Parr, 1993). A need to understand better the immunologically mediated infertility that occurs in a few individuals of both sexes as a result of IgA antisperm antibody in the genital tracts also exists (Bronson *et al.*, 1984).

Finally, we would like to emphasize, as did Schumacher (1980), that remarkable variation in the structure and function of the mammalian reproductive system occurs from one stage of the reproductive process to another, as well as among species. Caution, therefore, is necessary when correlating immunological results with reproductive function and when extending results from one species to another.

II. FEMALE REPRODUCTIVE TRACT

A. Efferent Limb of Mucosal Immunity

The main elements of secretory immunity in the genital tract appear to be secretory component (SC) in epithelial cells, IgA plasma cells in the underlying stroma, and immunoglobulins (SIgA and IgG) in luminal fluids. In the following sections, we summarize available information concerning these immune elements in the oviduct, uterus, and vagina of several species. We also discuss the pathways of immunoglobulin movement across the mucosa of those organs.

1. Secretory Component, Plasma Cells, and Immunoglobulins

In humans, SC and IgA plasma cells in the female genital tract have been the subject of numerous investigations. These studies have shown that the isthmus and ampulla of the oviduct contain SC on the luminal epithelium and IgA plasma cells in the stroma, suggesting that the oviduct is a potential site for mucosal immunity in the genital tracts of women (Tourville *et al.*, 1970; Kutteh *et al.*, 1988,1990). Specific observations are not available for the preampulla of the oviduct, in which plasma cells and interstitial immunoglobulins are most concentrated in the mouse oviduct (E. L. Parr and M. B. Parr, 1985). The body and fundus of the uterus contain SC and IgA in glandular epithelia and IgA in the glandular lumina (Tourville *et al.*, 1970; Vaerman and Ferin, 1974; Rebello *et al.*, 1975; Kelly and Fox, 1979; Kutteh *et al.*, 1988). However, IgA plasma cells are rare or absent, suggesting that serum may be an important source of IgA for secretion in this part of the uterus. The endocervix, which in humans is lined by columnar epithelium and contains numerous glands, exhibits SC on the luminal and glandular epithelia and contains many IgA plasma cells (Rebello *et al.*, 1975; Kutteh *et al.*, 1988). These observations suggest that the endocervix is likely to be a focal point for mucosal immunity in the genital tract of women (Ingerslev, 1981). The ectocervix, on the other hand, is similar to the vagina; it is lined by stratified squamous epithelium, lacks glands and SC, and shows few subepithelial IgA plasma cells.

Several studies have shown that both IgA and IgG are present in cervicovaginal fluids and that IgG appears to be the predominant immunoglobulin, but the reported ratios of IgG to IgA vary from approximately 2:1 to 10:1 (Chordirker and Tomasi, 1963; Masson *et al.*, 1969; Schumacher, 1973,1980; Tjokronegoro and Sirisinha, 1975; Coughlan and Skinner, 1977; Jalanti and Isliker, 1977; Usala *et al.*, 1989). One report indicates that the predominant immunoglobulin in these secretions is IgA with characteristics of secretory IgA (Waldman *et al.*, 1972a). The reasons for these differences are not entirely clear, but note that many technical problems are involved in obtaining accurate measurements of immunoglobulins in genital tract secretions. The recovery of sufficient quantities of secretions uncontaminated by serum or tissue fluids is difficult, and methods for extraction of immunoglobulins from mucus have not been standardized and may be ineffective (Schumacher, 1980; Ingerslev, 1981). Other problems include the use of 7 SIgA standards for measurement of 11 SIgA (Schumacher, 1980), as well as the variability of immunoglobulin concentrations in cervicovaginal mucus during the menstrual cycle (Schumacher, 1980; Sullivan *et al.*, 1984; Suzuki *et al.*, 1984).

Measurements of immunoglobulins in human uterine fluid also indicate that IgG is the predominant immunoglobulin present (Schumacher *et al.*, 1979). Nevertheless, the uterus may be the primary source of IgA in cervicovaginal fluids, since the concentration of IgA in vaginal fluid from hysterectomized women was only about 10% of normal (Jalanti and Isliker, 1977). Also, SC has not been detected in human vaginal epithelium. On the other hand, the concentration of IgA in vaginal fluid of three hysterectomized women appeared to be normal (Waldman *et al.*, 1972a). The IgG in vaginal fluid appears to be derived locally from the vaginal mucosa, since its concentration in intact and hysterectomized women is the same (Waldman *et al.*, 1972a; Jalanti and Isliker, 1977).

In mice, the preampulla of the oviduct, which is the short initial segment composed of the fimbria and infundibulum, contains some IgA plasma cells in the stroma. IgA and IgG are present in the luminal epithelium and interstitial space (M. B. Parr and E. L. Parr, 1985; E. L. Parr and M. B. Parr, 1986; Parr *et al.*, 1988b). These immune features are not observed in the remainder of the oviduct. Many IgA plasma cells are found in the uterine horns and body, where they are concentrated around the endometrial glands (Bernard *et al.*, 1981; Rachman *et al.*, 1983,1984; M. B. Parr and E. L. Parr, 1985). SC is also present on the glandular epithelium and, to a lesser extent, on the luminal epithelium (E. L. Parr and M. B. Parr, unpublished data). These observations suggest that the preampulla of the oviduct and the horns and body of the uterus are important sites of IgA secretion into luminal fluids of the genital tract. The mouse cervix and vagina are similar because both are lined by stratified squamous epithelium, lack glands, and contain few IgA plasma cells (M. B. Parr and E. L. Parr, 1985). The mouse cervix is, thus, quite different from the human endocervix. The uterine horns and body in mice and the endocervix in women appear to be the main regions of the genital tract involved in IgA secretion in these species.

Both IgA and IgG have been detected in murine uterine and vaginal fluids that were uncontaminated by serum or tissue fluids (E. L. Parr and M. B. Parr, 1990; Thapar *et al.*, 1990a). Neither the antibody concentrations nor the IgA:IgG ratios in these fluids have been reported. Most of the IgA in vaginal fluid appears to come from the uterus, since specific IgA titers in vaginal fluids of hysterectomized mice were only about 5% of those in controls. Titers of IgG, on the other hand, increased to some extent in vaginal fluids of hysterectomized mice, indicating that IgG readily crosses the vaginal mucosa (E. L. Parr and M. B. Parr, 1990).

The number of IgA plasma cells in the murine genital tract changes during the estrous cycle. These cells are most numerous at proestrus and estrus (Rachman *et al.*, 1983), and their numbers increase further between days 1 and 5 of pregnancy (Bernard *et al.*, 1981; M. B. Parr and E. L. Parr, 1985; Rachman *et al.*, 1986). The increased number of plasma cells at estrus may be caused by the action of estradiol (Canning and Billington, 1983), whereas the additional rise that occurs during early pregnancy may be caused, at least in part, by the action of progesterone on an estrogen-primed uterus (M. B. Parr and E. L. Parr, 1986a). Also, migration of radiolabeled lymphoblasts from the mesenteric lymph node to the genital tract is maximal during proestrus and estrus (McDermott *et al.*, 1980).

In rats, the luminal and glandular epithelial cells of uterine horns contain IgA (Mitchell, 1986) and SC (Parr and Parr, 1989a), but the occurrence of IgA plasma cells in the endometrium is controversial. These cells were reported by Wira and colleagues (Wira *et al.*, 1980), but were not detected in other studies (Mitchell, 1986; Parr and Parr, 1989a). No studies have been done on SC or IgA in the oviduct, but SC is present in the mucous epithelial cells lining the cervix and vagina at diestrus and proestrus (Parr and Parr, 1989a). Uterine and vaginal fluids contain SC, IgA, and IgG (Wira and Sandoe, 1977; Sullivan and Wira, 1981; Wira and Sullivan, 1985).

Less is known about secretory immunity in the genital tracts of other species. Plasma cells containing IgA or IgG have been reported in the genital tracts of the monkey (Miller *et al.*, 1992), pig (Hussein *et al.*, 1981,1983a,b), horse (Kenney and Khaleel, 1975; Mitchell *et al.*, 1982; Widders *et al.*, 1985b; Waelchli and Winder, 1987), and hamster (Roig de Vargas-Linares, 1968). Immunoglobulins A and G have been detected in reproductive tract secretions in the monkey (Yang and Schumacher, 1979; Miller *et al.*, 1992), cow (Wilkie *et al.*, 1972), horse (Widders *et al.*, 1985a), and rabbit (Symons and Herbert, 1971; McAnulty and Morton, 1978), and SC is present in equine endometrial glands (Widders *et al.*, 1985b).

2. Transfer of Immunoglobulins into the Lumen of the Genital Tract

The vaginal fluids of all species studied contain IgA and IgG. The pathways followed by these immunoglobulins to reach the vaginal lumen may be of some relevance to mucosal immunity. Studies of hysterectomized humans and mice suggest that much of the IgA in vaginal fluid is derived from the uterus (Jalanti and Isliker, 1977; E. L. Parr and M. B. Parr, 1990). SC has been demonstrated in the mucous layer of the vaginal epithelium at diestrus and proestrus in rats (Parr and Parr, 1989a) and mice (E. L. Parr and M. B. Parr, unpublished data), but the possibility that it might mediate direct transport of IgA across vaginal epithelium at these stages has not been evaluated. The hysterectomy studies cited earlier also suggest that IgG passes directly across the vaginal mucosa, since its concentration in vaginal fluid is the same in hysterectomized and intact individuals. However, the pathway of IgG movement across the vaginal epithelium is not entirely understood. Tracer studies indicate that proteins can enter the intercellular channels in the basal layers of the monkey vaginal epithelium, but are blocked at the granular layer in the superficial part of the epithelium (King, 1983,1985). Similarly, IgG has been localized in the intercellular spaces of the mouse vaginal epithelium at diestrus, but whether the immunoglobulin penetrates the tight junctions joining the superficial mucous cells is not clear (E. L. Parr and M. B. Parr, unpublished data). Therefore, whether IgG reaches vaginal fluid by slow leakage through the intercellular permeability barrier or by an intracellular transport pathway is currently unknown. In either case, the stage of the reproductive cycle, through its effect on the structure of the epithelial layer, is likely to influence the rate of IgG movement across the epithelium.

Immunoglobulins A and G are also present in the luminal fluids of the oviduct and uterus in several species. In rats and mice, and probably in other species as well, these organs are lined by simple columnar epithelial cells that are joined by functional tight junctions (Parr, 1980b; Parr *et al.*, 1988b; Tung *et al.*, 1988), suggesting that immunoglobulins are transported from the stroma into the lumen of these organs primarily by an intracellular route. In the mouse, IgA, IgG, and intravenously administered protein tracers have been demonstrated in the luminal epithelium covering the villi in the preampulla of the oviduct and in luminal and glandular epithelial cells in the uterine horns (Parr, 1980ab; E. L. Parr and M. B. Parr, 1986; Parr *et al.*, 1988b; Tung *et al.*, 1988). IgA presumably is taken into the epithelial cells by receptor-mediated endocytosis, the receptor being SC, whereas IgG may be present in these or other vesicles in proportion to its concentration in the interstitial fluid.

B. Afferent Limb of Mucosal Immunity

1. Langerhans Cells and Lymphocytes in the Epithelium

Infection or local immunization in the genital tract can elicit immune responses (Strauss, 1961; Omran and Hulka, 1971; Waldman *et al.*, 1972b; Wilkie *et al.*, 1972; Ogra and Ogra, 1973; Yang and Schumacher, 1979; Widders *et al.*, 1986; Parr *et al.*, 1988a), but the pathways of antigen uptake and the sites of antigen recognition remain to be clarified. A major advance in our understanding of antigen recognition in the lower part of the female genital tract has come with reports that Langerhans cells (LCs) are present in the stratified epithelium of the murine vagina and cervix (Young, 1985; Young *et al.*, 1985; Young and Hosking, 1986; Lin *et al.*, 1988; Parr and Parr, 1991; Parr *et al.*, 1991a,b). LCs have been studied extensively in the epidermis, where they function as antigen-presenting cells for T lymphocytes in conjunction with major histocompatibility complex (MHC) molecules (Stingl *et al.*, 1989). Results of *in vivo* and *in vitro* studies suggest that LCs capture antigen within the epidermis and carry it to the draining lymph nodes, where T lymphocytes become activated, multiply, and differentiate into immune helpers or effectors (Stingl *et al.*, 1989).

LCs in the mouse vagina and cervix are immunophenotypically similar to epidermal LCs; they exhibit NLDC-145, Ia, F4/80, and CD45 surface antigens and contain ATPase and LC granules (Parr and Parr, 1991; Parr *et al.*, 1991b). Moreover, LCs take up luminal proteins by endocytosis during late metestrus and diestrus when the vaginal epithelium is most permeable (Figures 1 and 2; M. B. Parr and E. L. Parr, 1990; Parr *et al.*, 1991a). The presence of LCs in the vaginal and cervical epithelia, close to the lumen, indicates a significant potential for local antigen processing in the lower part of the female genital tract.

Interestingly, LCs in the vagina and cervix also have been shown to phagocytose epithelial cells undergoing apoptosis or programmed cell death (Young *et al.*, 1985; Parr *et al.*, 1991b). This activity may be unique to LCs in the genital tract because epidermal LCs are considered to be nonphagocytotic and only weakly pinocytotic (Stingl *et al.*, 1989). Death of

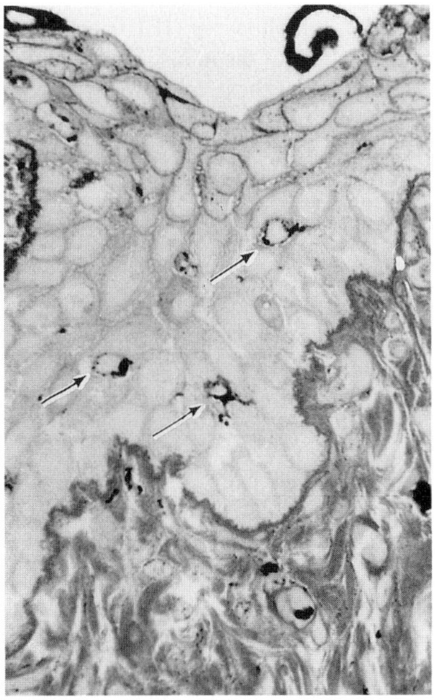

Figure 1 Mouse vagina at early metestrus, 2 hr after intravaginal administration of horseradish peroxidase. The tracer is located between epithelial cells, in three dendritic LCs (arrows) in the epithelium, and in the stroma. ×500. (Reproduced with permission from Parr *et al.*, 1991a.)

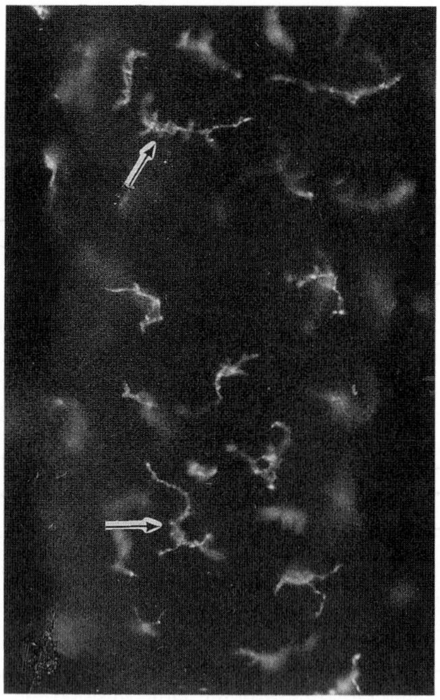

Figure 2 Fluorescent labeling of Ia antigen on dendritic LCs (arrows) in an isolated sheet of epithelium from the mouse vagina. ×200.

vaginal epithelial cells and phagocytosis of the dead cells by LCs may play a role in the extensive tissue remodeling that occurs in the vagina and cervix during the estrous cycle.

Intraepithelial T lymphocytes (IELs) are also present in the stratified epithelium of the mouse vagina and cervix (Parr and Parr, 1991). Whether these cells are involved in the afferent or efferent limb of mucosal immunity, or both, is not known. The cells are Thy1 positive (Figure 3) and either CD4 or CD8 positive, and are more numerous at diestrus than at any other stage in the estrous cycle (Parr and Parr, 1991). The latter observation suggests an influx of T cells into the vaginal epithelium during each estrous cycle when the epithelium is thinnest and most permeable to protein tracers. The IELs occasionally are seen in contact with LCs, although the functional significance of this association remains speculative (Parr and Parr, 1991; Parr *et al.*, 1991b). Knowing whether IELs in the genital tract are involved in the cell-mediated protective effects that have been reported in chlamydial and herpesvirus infections would be most interesting (McDermott and Svedsmith, 1989; Ramsey and Rank, 1991).

As in the mouse, LCs and IELs are present in the human vagina and cervix (Figueroa and Carosi, 1981; Becker *et al.*, 1985; Hawthorn *et al.*, 1988). Moreover, the cells are most concentrated in the transformation zone of the cervix, where they are ideally situated to guard the entrance to the uterus (Morris *et al.*, 1983; Edwards and Morris, 1985; Roncalli *et al.*, 1988). In the cervix, cell contacts are observed between LCs and several other cell types, including IELs, capillary endothelium in the subepithelial connective tissue, and "hugging cells" (possibly macrophages) that are applied closely to the stromal side of the basement membrane. The uterus and oviduct also contain IELs that are mainly of the T cytotoxic/suppressor subtype (Morris *et al.*, 1986; Kamat and Issacson, 1987; Otsuki, 1989). Additionally, IELs have been identified in the uterine epithelium of the rat (Sawicki *et al.*, 1988), cow (Vander-Wielen and King, 1984), sheep (Lee *et al.*, 1988), and pig (King, 1988).

2. Antigen Uptake

One of the most important aspects of the afferent limb of the immune system in the genital tract is the movement of antigen from the lumen into the mucosa. Early studies suggested that the vaginal stratified epithelium was permeable to various proteins (see M. B. Parr and E. L. Parr, 1990, for references). Studies have demonstrated that proteins can cross the epithelium of the murine cervix and vagina during diestrus and early pregnancy and, to a lesser extent, at proestrus and metestrus; however, proteins do not cross the epithelium at estrus (M. B. Parr and E. L. Parr, 1990). When proteins cross the cervicovaginal epithelium, they are taken up by epithelial LCs and by stromal cells that resemble dendritic cells, fibroblasts, or macrophages. The observations suggest that the mouse vagina and cervix sample antigens from the external environment during certain stages of the reproductive cycle and early pregnancy. This sampling may lead to immune responses. In contrast, the block against antigen uptake at estrus would minimize sensitization to sperm and seminal fluid proteins at the time of mating.

Proteins do not appear to cross the uterine epithelium from the lumen to the endometrial stroma. Specialized antigen-transporting epithelial cells have not been reported in the

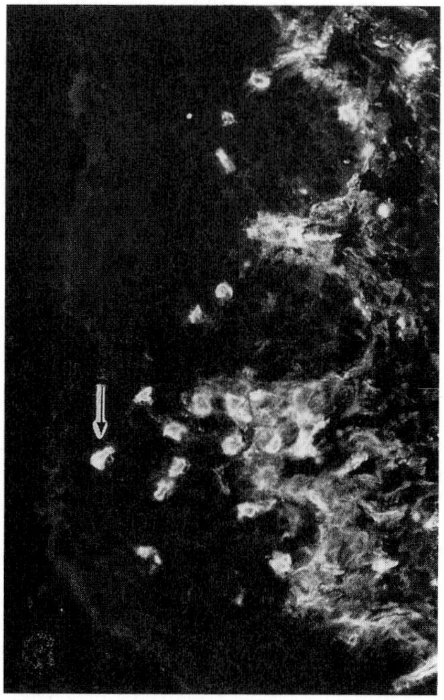

Figure 3 Fluorescent labeling of Thy1 on IELs (arrow) in the mouse vagina. L, Lumen. ×200.

uterus or in any other part of the female reproductive tract. Proteins in the luminal fluid can be taken into uterine epithelial cells by endocytosis at certain stages, but such proteins are channeled into the lysosome system for digestion and do not appear to be released into the stroma (Parr and Parr, 1978; Parr, 1980b; M. B. Parr and E. L. Parr, 1986b; Tung *et al.*, 1988). Some investigators have reported that proteins injected into the uterine lumen were detected later in the stroma, but these results seem likely to be due to epithelial damage caused by the use of sutures to prolong retention of tracers or to other nonphysiological conditions in the uterine lumen (Parr, 1980b).

3. Stromal Lymphoid Cells and Nodules

The precursors of IgA plasma cells in the intestine and respiratory tract are believed to originate mainly in the mucosal lymphoid nodules of those organs (Mestecky, 1987; Scicchitano *et al.*, 1988). Thus, another important aspect of the afferent limb of mucosal immunity in the female genital tract is that mucosal lymphoid nodules containing B lymphocytes are far less abundant in the genital tract than in the intestinal and respiratory mucosae. Extensive histological examinations of mouse oviduct, uterus, and vagina have never revealed mucosal lymphoid nodules (M. B. Parr and E. L. Parr, 1985; Parr *et al.*, 1988a; E. L. Parr and M. B. Parr, unpublished observations). In humans, lymphoid nodules are rare in the endometrium (Schumacher, 1980): those that have been reported were mainly aggregates of T lymphocytes; germinal centers and mantle zones containing B lymphocytes were present only in a few specimens (Morris *et al.*, 1985; Bulmer *et al.*, 1988). The low numbers of B cells in human endometrial lymphoid nodules may be related to lack of antigen stimulation, since the Peyer's patches of neonatal animals also contain mainly T lymphocytes (Morris *et al.*, 1985). A few lymphoid nodules have been reported in the human oviduct and cervix, but not in the vagina (Edwards and Morris, 1985; Otsuki, 1989). Since B cells are rare in the mouse and human female genital tracts, IgA plasma cells in those tracts are likely to be derived mainly from other sources, such as genital lymph nodes or other mucosal tissues. The significance of mucosal lymphoid nodules for local immunity in the human female tract requires clarification, but the few that are present may be the residue of previous responses to invasive microorganisms. In sheep, lymphoid nodules were observed in 3 of the 24 uteri examined (Lee *et al.*, 1988).

In addition to lacking lymphoid nodules, the stroma of the normal murine vagina and cervix contains few individual T lymphocytes and no B lymphocytes (Parr and Parr, 1991). Information concerning the occurrence of T lymphocytes in the stroma of murine uterine horns and oviducts is not available, but a few stromal T cells have been observed in the rat uterus (Head and Gaede, 1986). The stroma of the human cervix contains numerous T cells, but such cells are infrequent in vaginal stroma (Edwards and Morris, 1985). The endometrial stroma contains T cells that are mainly of the $CD8^+$ phenotype, both individually and in occasional aggregates (Morris *et al.*, 1985; Kamat and Issacson, 1987; Bulmer *et al.*, 1988); B cells are relatively common in the stroma of the oviduct (Morris *et al.*, 1986).

4. Biological Significance

The biological function of the female reproductive tract requires that the mucosal surface of the tract be exposed to sperm and seminal fluid proteins. These substances stimulate immune responses if they are administered parenterally in females. Antisperm antibodies in luminal fluids of the female genital tract cause reduced fertility (Bronson *et al.*, 1984). Thus, an effective mechanism is needed to prevent sperm and seminal fluid proteins in the luminal compartment of the female tract from stimulating the immune system. The evidence reviewed earlier indicates that, at the time of mating, the luminal epithelium of the genital tract functions as a barrier that prevents luminal proteins from reaching immune cells or lymphatic vessels in the tissues. Although other immune suppressive mechanisms may be involved as well, this barrier function of the luminal epithelium is likely to be fundamentally important to reproduction. In mice and rats, the epithelium of the oviduct and uterus constitutes a barrier to protein movement at all stages of the reproductive cycle and early pregnancy, whereas the vaginal epithelium is a barrier mainly at the time of mating. Thus, in the absence of damage to the epithelial layer, the available evidence indicates that local mucosal immunization in the female genital tract with noninvasive antigens would stimulate immune responses mainly when the antigens are applied to the vaginal mucosa at nonestrous stages. Invasive microorganisms, of course, may trigger immune responses whenever they penetrate the epithelial barrier.

C. Role of Mucosal Immunity in Protection against Infections

1. Antibodies to Microorganisms

Local secretory immunity generally is considered to be important in protecting mucosal surfaces against invading microorganisms (Waldman and Ganguly, 1974), but few reports demonstrate this characteristic in the genital tract. In women, cervicovaginal fluids contain antibodies against microorganisms (Schumacher, 1980). Studies of women with genital tract infections involving herpes simplex virus 2 (HSV-2) or *Chlamydia trachomatis* have revealed inverse relationships between specific SIgA antibody titers in cervicovaginal secretions and the number of disease organisms present (Brunham *et al.*, 1983; Merriman *et al.*, 1984). Similarly, the susceptibility of women to *Escherichia coli* urinary tract infections is correlated inversely with the titers of specific IgA antibodies against *E. coli* in their vaginal fluids (Stamey *et al.*, 1978). Data on the local immune response to genital papillomaviruses have been reviewed by Roche and Crum (1991).

In mice, one of the many mammalian species in which insemination occurs directly into the uterine lumen, bacteria are introduced into the uterine horns at the time of mating. These bacteria are cleared from the uterus during the next 2–3 days, before embryos arrive for implantation (E. L. Parr and M. B. Parr, 1985). We have observed IgA and IgG bound to many bacteria in the uterine lumen on the morning after mating, as well as IgA bound to bacteria in the vagina of normal mice (E. L. Parr and M. B. Parr, 1985; M. B. Parr and E. L. Parr, 1985). The uterine fluid of normal mice also contains antibodies against most of the bacterial species that were cultured from the vagina (E. L. Parr and M. B. Parr, 1988b).

Specific antibodies in luminal fluids of the reproductive tract may protect against infections by several mechanisms. For example, immunoglobulins may inhibit binding of microorganisms to the endometrial epithelium, a step that is thought to be required for infection of mucosal surfaces (Williams and Gibbons, 1972; Fubara and Freter, 1973; Abraham and Beachey, 1985). These antibodies may cause agglutination and thus reduce the number of organisms available to bind to the epithelium (Bellamy *et al.*, 1975; Steele *et al.*, 1975), and may opsonize organisms for phagocytosis. Opsonization is mediated by IgG and perhaps also by IgA when the latter is combined with small amounts of IgG (Goldstein *et al.*, 1983). Opsonization would be augmented by C3, which is bound to some of the uterine bacteria in mice (E. L. Parr and M. B. Parr, 1988) and is secreted by luminal epithelial cells (Sundstrom *et al.*, 1990). Since we have observed phagocytosis of bacteria by neutrophils in the mouse uterine lumen after mating (E. L. Parr and M. B. Parr, 1985b), evidently this process plays a role in returning the uterine lumen to an aseptic state after mating. Finally, secretory IgA may mediate local killing of bacteria by antibody-dependent cellular cytotoxicity (Tagliabue *et al.*, 1984).

2. Importance of IgA Relative to IgG

Whether IgA is more important than IgG in protecting the female genital tract against bacterial and viral infections is not yet clear. On the one hand, IgA may be intrinsically more effective than an equivalent amount of IgG against certain infections in the intestine and respiratory tract (Fubara and Freter, 1973; Taylor and Dimmock, 1985; Bessen and Fischetti, 1988), and IgA antibody against sperm has a greater contraceptive effect than an equivalent amount of IgG antisperm antibody in human immunological infertility (Parr and Parr, 1993). On the other hand, available data indicate that the concentration of IgG in human cervicovaginal mucus may be higher than that of IgA (Schumacher, 1980). IgG appears to be protective against vaginal HSV-2 infection, since parenteral immunization with glycoprotein D of HSV-2 or with mixtures of membrane glycoproteins from HSV-1 and HSV-2, which presumably generates mainly IgG antibody in the genital tract, protects guinea pigs against vaginal challenge with HSV-2 (Berman *et al.*, 1984; Meignier *et al.*, 1987; Sanchez-Pescador *et al.*, 1988; Mishkin *et al.*, 1991). Given the diversity of organisms that can infect the female reproductive tract, the issue of which immunoglobulin class is more protective, or whether humoral immunity is more important than cellular immunity, may depend as much on the specific pathogen involved as on any fundamental immunological considerations. Thus, the development of immunization strategies that protect the human female tract from its diverse pathogens probably will require an integrated understanding of both mucosal immunology in the female tract and the infectious processes of the organisms.

D. Immunization to Elicit Mucosal Immunity

Immunization that produces secretory immunity in the female reproductive tract against sperm or sexually transmitted disease organisms could have important practical applications, but methods to stimulate vigorous sustained IgA responses at this site are not yet well established. Investigators have attempted to elicit secretory immunity in the genital tract using three routes of immunization: local mucosal immunization in the genital tract, remote mucosal immunization in the intestine, and local parenteral immunization in the pelvis.

1. Local Mucosal Immunization

Local mucosal immunization in the intestine or respiratory tract can be an effective way to stimulate secretory immune responses at those sites, but local immunization in the female reproductive tract under physiological conditions elicits little or no specific antibody generation in genital tract secretions. An early indication of this is the observation that intravaginal (ivag) immunization of mice with spermatozoa had no effect on fertility, whereas parenteral immunization with sperm significantly reduced fertility (Bell, 1969). Subsequent studies of immunization in the human and rabbit uterine lumen with horse ferritin, sperm, or horseradish peroxidase failed to detect immune responses in the reproductive tract (Vaerman and Ferin, 1974; McAnulty and Morton, 1978; Moretti-Rojas *et al.*, 1990), although specific antibody was detected in the human tract after intrauterine immunization with killed influenza virus (Ogra and Ogra, 1973). Other reports indicating that immune responses are detectable in the reproductive tract after intrauterine immunization have involved nonphysiological conditions, such as the use of ligatures to close the cervical end of the uterus after immunization or the mixture of antigen with an adjuvant (Menge and Lieberman, 1974; Lande *et al.*, 1981; Lande, 1986; Wira and Sandoe, 1989). The sutures and adjuvants are likely to damage the uterine epithelium, thus allowing antigen to reach lymphoid cells and lymphatic vessels in the stroma. Comparative studies have demonstrated that antibody titers in luminal fluids of the monkey and mouse female tract after ivag immunization are low in comparison with titers produced by systemic immunization (Yang and Schumacher, 1979; Parr *et al.*, 1988a; Thapar *et al.*, 1990b,1991). Adjuvants, including aluminum hydroxide and lipid A, increased local immune responses to ivag immunization with large doses of horse ferritin in mice, but the specific IgA titers observed in vaginal fluid were only slightly higher than those obtained by parenteral immunization with single small doses of ferritin; the IgG titers were lower (Thapar *et al.*, 1990a).

The relatively weak immune responses after local immunization in the uterus or vagina with noninvasive antigens are probably caused by the inability of the antigen to penetrate the luminal epithelium and by the rapid loss of antigen from the genital tract. Immune responses to ivag immunization in mice might be higher if the animals were immunized at diestrus or during early pregnancy, when penetration of proteins across the vaginal epithelium was maximal (M. B. Parr and E. L. Parr, 1990). Edwards (1960) reported that vaginal immunization of rabbits with sperm during early pregnancy gave stronger immune responses than similar immunization at estrus. Responses also might be increased by the use of bioadhesive microspheres and absorption enhancing agents, which promote the retention and absorption of proteins on mucosal surfaces (Illum *et al.*, 1990).

In contrast to protein antigens, invasive microorganisms may penetrate the epithelium of the reproductive tract. McDermott and colleagues (McDermott *et al.*, 1984,1987,1990; McDermott and Svedsmith, 1989) have studied vaginal HSV-2 infection in mice, using a viral strain isolated from humans and adapted to mice. The virus causes lethal neurological illness in mice after ivag inoculation, but an attenuated strain causes only a transient vaginal infection and is incapable of lethal neurological spread. Importantly, ivag inoculation with the attenuated virus induces protective immunity to subsequent lethal challenge with wild-type virus (McDermott *et al.*, 1984). The basis of this immunity has been investigated and appears to involve T lymphocytes (McDermott and Svedsmith, 1989); the possible protective role of specific antiviral IgA and IgG antibodies in genital tract secretions is not yet clear. Note that infection of the female genital tract can be markedly dependent on the stage of the reproductive process. For example, ivag infection with HSV-2 is increased in pregnant or progesterone-treated adult mice (Baker and Plotkin, 1978), and genital infection of mice with *C. trachomatis* requires pre-treatment with a progestagen (Tuffrey *et al.*, 1986).

2. Remote Mucosal Immunization

The hypothesis of a common mucosal immune system predicts that presentation of antigen in the intestine will stimulate local B lymphocytes that ultimately will migrate as IgA plasmablasts to other mucosal sites (Scicchitano *et al.*, 1988). Migration of lymphoblasts from the mesenteric lymph node to the mouse female genital tract has been demonstrated by McDermott *et al.* (1980), suggesting that immunization in the intestine, which has specialized antigen-transporting epithelial cells and abundant mucosal lymphoid tissue, effectively might generate immune responses in the genital tract. This relationship has been illustrated by several studies. Specific IgA antibodies in mouse uterine washings were produced by two oral immunizations with a live influenza vaccine (Briese *et al.*, 1987). Oral vaccination of guinea pigs with HSV-1 developed protection against intravaginal challenge with HSV-2, presumably because of the antigenic similarity of the two viruses (Sturn and Schneweis, 1978). A live oral chlamydial vaccine proved to be effective against both ocular and vaginal challenge with the homologous organism in guinea-pigs (Nichols *et al.*, 1978), and against pulmonary and vaginal challenge in mice (La Scolea *et al.*, 1991). Oral immunization of rats with spermatozoa caused reduced fecundity (Allardyce, 1984). However, oral immunization of mice with a large dose of horse ferritin (5 mg) without adjuvant caused no detectable IgA response in vaginal washings, although it did prime the mice for vaginal boosting (Parr *et al.*, 1988a). The IgA titer in mouse vaginal fluid after oral–vaginal immunization was approximately equal to that produced by a single parenteral immunization with ferritin in Freund's complete adjuvant. Oral immunization with a large dose of horse ferritin also caused a detectable IgA, but not IgG, response in uterine fluid (E. L. Parr and M. B. Parr, 1990). The magnitude of this IgA response was not greater than that produced by several other routes of immunization.

In general, secretory immune responses in the intestine are developed most effectively by replicating microorganisms (Mestecky, 1987). Most nonreplicating antigens do not stimulate vigorous immune responses in the intestine (Waldman and Ganguly, 1974; Fuhrman and Cebra, 1981; Nicklin and Miller, 1983; Elson and Ealding, 1984; Dahlgren *et al.*, 1986), perhaps because of digestion of antigens in the intestine, complexing with pre-existing antibodies, or failure to penetrate the mucus layer covering the epithelium (Mestecky, 1987). Despite these limitations, the advantages of oral vaccination to generate IgA immune responses in the genital tract are obvious. Further investigation of this procedure is warranted. One approach to improving immunization in the intestine involves the use of antigen-containing microparticles, which are transported across M cells into Peyer's patches (Eldridge *et al.*, 1990). Another approach uses an antigen-expressing organism that can colonize the intestine, for example, a genetically engineered *Salmonella* strain (Curtiss, 1993).

3. Local Nonmucosal Immunization

Parenteral immunization generally is associated with serum IgG responses and little secretory IgA. However, a few reports have suggested that parenteral immunization in the vicinity of a mucosal organ can elicit significant IgA secretion by that mucosa (reviewed by Thapar *et al.*, 1990b). We immunized female mice at two parenteral sites in the pelvis: the subserous space and the presacral space. Immunization at these pelvic sites, either with horse ferritin adsorbed to aluminum hydroxide or with a Quil A immunostimulating complex (ISCOM) containing sheep erythrocyte membrane proteins, caused higher and better sustained IgA titers in vaginal fluid than parenteral immunization at nonpelvic sites. All parenteral immunizations, both in the pelvis and elsewhere, generated similar IgG titers in vaginal fluid (Thapar *et al.*, 1990b,1991).

The immunological basis of IgA responses in the female reproductive tract after parenteral immunization in the pelvis is not well understood, but such responses are most likely to be generated in the iliac or para-aortic lymph nodes that drain the reproductive tract (Thapar *et al.*, 1990b). Lymph nodes that drain large mucosal tissues such as the lungs and female genital tract may differ from peripheral lymph nodes that drain nonmucosal tissues. Such differences could arise because of unique antigen-presenting cells or cytokines entering mucosa-associated nodes from the mucosae. A striking difference between peripheral and mucosa-associated lymph nodes has been demonstrated (Daynes *et al.*, 1990). T helper cells from mouse peripheral lymph nodes produced interleukin 2 (IL-2) almost exclusively, whereas those from mucosa-associated nodes produced mainly IL-4. Interestingly, IL-4 has been shown to induce IgM-positive B cells to express IgA *in vitro* (Kunimoto *et al.*, 1988; Harriman *et al.*, 1989).

III. MALE REPRODUCTIVE TRACT

A. Efferent Limb of Mucosal Immunity

The mucosal immune system in the male urogenital tract has been studied in the rat, mouse, and human. Both IgA and IgG are found in seminal fluids of normal men (Chordirker and Tomasi, 1963; Hermann and Hermann, 1969; Uehling, 1971; Tauber *et al.,* 1975). IgA or SIgA sperm agglutinins are present in seminal fluids of men with autoimmunity to spermatozoa. SIgA with antisperm activity also has been found in the genital tracts of some vasectomized men (see Parr and Parr, 1987b, for references). The origin of secretory immunoglobulins in seminal fluids is not precisely known. Prostatic fluids contain IgA; studies of split human ejaculates have suggested that seminal fluid immunoglobulins may originate either in the prostate (Rumke, 1974; Hekman and Rumke, 1976) or in the seminal vesicles (Uehling, 1971). The human prostate contains a few IgA plasma cells (Ablin *et al.,* 1972; Doble *et al.,* 1990), IgG in the basal part of the epithelial cells, and both IgA and IgG in secretory granules in the lumen of the prostatic ducts (Ablin *et al.,* 1972). These studies suggest that secretory epithelial cells in the prostate contribute at least some of the immunoglobulins in human seminal fluid.

In rats, SC has been demonstrated by immunolabeling at several sites in the male urogenital tract, including the ejaculatory ducts, excretory ducts of several accessory glands, and urethral glands in the pelvic and bulbous portions of the urethra (Figures 4 and 5; Parr and Parr, 1989b). Pale staining of SC also was detected in epithelial cells of the ventral prostate gland. Plasma cells containing IgA were observed only in the urethral glands in the wall of the bulbous urethra. These results suggest that IgA may be transported into the urogenital tract from the ventral prostate as well as at several sites distal to the production of seminal fluid and spermatozoa. Locally synthesized IgA may be available in the urethral glands, but serum appears to be the main source of IgA for transport into the rat urogenital tract at other sites where SC was demonstrated (Parr and Parr, 1989b). Similarly, immunolabeling in the urogenital tract of the male mouse showed SC in the excretory ducts of the ventral prostate and in the urethral glands in the pelvic and bulbous urethrae (E. L. Parr and M. B. Parr, unpublished observations), as well as IgA in plasma cells in the urethral glands (Parr and Parr, 1989b).

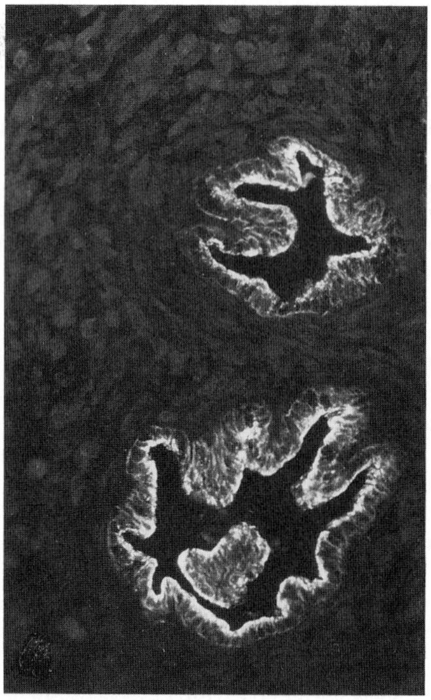

Figure 4 Fluorescent labeling of SC in the excretory ducts of the dorso-lateral prostate glands in the rat male genital tract. SC is localized at the basolateral borders of the epithelial cells and in the apical portions of many cells. ×170. (Reproduced with permission from Parr and Parr, 1989b.)

B. Afferent Limb of Mucosal Immunity

The afferent limb of mucosal immunity in the male genital tract remains unexplored. Data are not available concerning local immunization at the mucosal surface, presumably because the mucosa of the male genital tract is relatively inaccessible and parts of it are washed frequently by urine. Similarly, no direct studies of antigen transport across the epithelium of the male tract have been reported, but the epithelium is likely normally to be an effective barrier to noninvasive antigens because sperm are antigenic and antisperm immunity in males causes infertility (Bronson *et al.,* 1984). Studies of the fate of invasive microorganisms, such as human immunodeficiency virus (HIV), in the male urogenital tract would be of great interest.

Mucosal lymphoid nodules appear to be rare in the human male genital tract (El-Demiry and James, 1988). During our immunohistological studies of the male tract in mice and rats, we only rarely observed aggregates of lymphoid cells (E. L. Parr and M. B. Parr, unpublished observations). However, IELs have been reported in the human epididymis (Wang and Holstein, 1983; Ritchie *et al.,* 1984), and ductus deferens (El-Demiry and James, 1988), and from the tubuli recti of the testes to the ductus deferens in monkeys and rats (Dym and Romrell, 1975). The role of these cells in mucosal defense is unknown. Lymphoid cells, including macrophages, neutrophils, and lymphocytes, are normally present in seminal fluids of fertile men (El-Demiry *et al.,* 1986; Wolff and Anderson, 1988; Harrison *et al.,* 1991).

C. Role of Mucosal Immunity in Protection against Infections

The functions of mucosal immunity in the male genital tract are poorly documented. Bacteria isolated from prostatic fluid of patients with prostatitis were coated with IgA and IgG antibodies (Drach and Kohnen, 1977). Prostatitis and nonspecific urethritis may be accompanied by abnormally

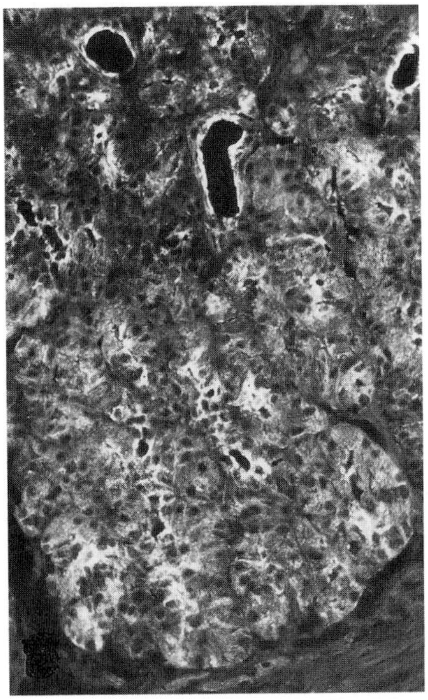

Figure 5 Fluorescent labeling of SC in the acini and ducts of the urethral glands in the bulbous portion of the urethra in the male rat genital tract. × 190. (Reproduced with permission from Parr and Parr, 1989b.)

high local levels of IgA. Seminal fluid immunoglobulins normally may prevent harmful effects of vaginal bacteria on spermatozoa (Uehling, 1971). Plasma cells containing IgA or IgM were observed in the human prostate and were most numerous in patients with previous prostatitis, suggesting local response to bacterial stimuli (Bene *et al.,* 1988). Also of interest is that sperm-agglutinating antibodies in seminal fluid are mainly of the IgA class (Friberg, 1974). These antibodies cause infertility and thus have clinical significance (Bronson *et al.,* 1984). Collectively, these observations suggest that IgA in seminal fluid may play a role in protecting the male urogenital tract against infection, and that it occasionally may be involved in immunologically mediated infertility.

Acknowledgments

Experimental results from our laboratory that were included in this chapter were supported by NIH Grant HD-17337 and the World Health Organization.

References

Ablin, R. J., Soanes, W. A., and Gonder, M. J. (1972). *In vivo* bound immunoglobulin in the human prostate-their identification and possible significance. *Zeit. Immunitaetsforsch.* **144,** 233–241.

Abraham, S. N., and Beachey, E. H. (1985). Host defenses against adhesion of bacteria to mucosal surfaces. *In* "Advances in Host Defense Mechanisms" (J. I. Gallin and A. S. Fauci, ed.), pp. 63–88. Raven Press, New York.

Allardyce, R. A. (1984). Effect of ingested sperm on fecundity in the rat. *J. Exp. Med.* **159,** 1548–1553.

Archibald, D. W., Witt, D. J., Craven, D. E., Vogt, M. W., Hirsch, M. S., and Essex, M. (1987). Antibodies to human immunodeficiency virus in cervical secretions from women at risk for AIDS. *J. Infect. Dis.* **156,** 240–241.

Baker, D. A., and Plotkin, S. A. (1978). Enhancement of vaginal infection in mice by herpes simplex virus type II with progesterone. *Proc. Soc. Exp. Biol. Med.* **158,** 131–134.

Becker, J., Behem, J., Lioning, T., Reichart, P., and Geerlings, H. (1985). Quantitative analysis of immunocompetent cells in human normal oral and uterine cervical mucosa, oral papillomas and leukoplasias. *Arch. Oral Biol.* **30,** 257–264.

Bell, E. B. (1969). Immunological control of fertility in the mouse: A comparison of systemic and intravaginal immunization. *J. Reprod. Fertil.* **18,** 183–190.

Bellamy, J. E. C., Knop, J., Steele, E. J., Chaicumpa, W., and Rowley, D. (1975). Antibody cross-linking as a factor in immunity to cholera in infant mice. *J. Infect. Dis.* **132,** 181–188.

Bene, M. C., Studer, A., and Faure, G. (1988). Immunoglobulin-producing cells in human prostate. *Prostate* **12,** 113–117.

Berman, R. W., Gregory, T., Crase, D., and Lasky, L. A. (1984). Protection from genital herpes simplex virus type 2 infection by vaccination with cloned type 1 glycoprotein D. *Science* **227,** 1490–1492.

Bernard, O., Rachman, F., and Bennett, D. (1981). Immunoglobulins in the mouse uterus before implantation. *J. Reprod. Fertil.* **63,** 237–240.

Bessen, D., and Fischetti, V. A. (1988). Passive acquired mucosal immunity to group A streptococci by secretory immunoglobulin A. *J. Exp. Med.* **167,** 1945–1950.

Briese, V., Pohl, W.-D., Noack, K., Tischner, H., and Waldman, R. H. (1987). Influenza specific antibodies in the female genital tract of mice after oral administration of live influenza vaccine. *Arch. Gynecol.* **240,** 153–157.

Bronson, R. A., Cooper, G. W., and Rosenfeld, D. L. (1984). Sperm antibodies: Their role in infertility. *Fert. Steril.* **42,** 171–183.

Brunham, R. C., Kuo, C.-C., Cles, L., and Holmes, K. K. (1983). Correlation of host immune response with quantitative recovery of *Chlamydia trachomatis* from the human endocervix. *Infect. Immun.* **39,** 1491–1494.

Bulmer, J. N., Lunny, D. P., and Hagin, S. V. (1988). Immunohistochemical characterization of stromal leukocytes in nonpregnant human endometrium. *Am. J. Reprod. Immunol. Microbiol.* **17,** 83–90.

Canning, M. B., and Billington, W. D. (1983). Hormonal regulation of immunoglobulin and plasma cells in the mouse uterus. *J. Endocrinol.* **97,** 419–424.

Chordirker, W. B., and Tomasi, T. B. J.(1983). Gammaglobulins: quantitative relationships in human serum and non-vascular fluids. *Science* **142,** 1080–1081.

Coughlan, B. M., and Skinner, G. R. B. (1977). Immunoglobulin concentrations in cervical mucus in patients with normal and abnormal cervical cytology. *Br. J. Obstet. Gynecol.* **84,** 129–134.

Curtiss, R. (1993). Immunogen construction: Recombinant vectors. *In* "Scientific Basis of Fertility Regulation" (P. M. Johnson, and D. Griffin, ed.), pp. 489–476. Oxford University Press, Oxford.

Dahlgren, U. I. H., Ahlstedt, S., and Hanson, L. Å. (1986). Origin and kinetics of IgA, IgG and IgM antibodies in primary and secondary responses of rats. *Scand. J. Immunol.* **23,** 273–278.

Daynes, R. A., Arano, B. A., Dowell, T. A., Huang, K., and Dudley, D. (1990). Regulation of murine lymphokine production *in vivo.* III. The lymphoid tissue microenvironment exerts regulatory influences over T helper cell function. *J. Exp. Med.* **171,** 979–996.

Doble, A., Walker, M. M., Harris, J. R. W., Taylor-Robinson, D., and Witherow, R. O. N. (1990). Intraprostatic antibody deposition in chronic abacterial prostatitis. *Brit. J. Urol.* **65,** 598–605.

Drach, G. W., and Kohnen, P. W. (1977). Prostatitis. *In* "Prostatitis" (M. Tannenbaum, ed.), pp. 157–170. Lea and Febiger, Philadelphia.

Dym, M., and Romrell, L. J. (1975). Intra-epithelial lymphocytes in the male reproductive tract of rats and rhesus monkeys. *J. Reprod. Fertil.* **42,** 1–7.

Edwards, J. N. T., and Morris, H. B. (1985). Langerhan's cells and lymphocyte subsets in the female genital tract. *Br. J. Obstet. Gynaecol.* **92,** 974–982.

Edwards, R. G. (1960). Antigenicity of rabbit semen, bull semen and egg yolk after intravaginal or intramuscular injection of female rabbits. *J. Reprod. Fertil.* **1,** 385–401.

El-Demiry, M., and James, K. (1988). Lymphocyte subsets and macrophages in the male genital tract in health and disease. *Eur. Urol.* **14,** 226–235.

El-Demiry, M. I. M., Young, H., Elton, R. A., Hargreave, T. B., James, K., and Chisholm, G. D. (1986). Leukocytes in the ejaculate from fertile and infertile men. *Br. J. Urol.* **58,** 715–720.

Eldridge, J. H., Hammond, C. J., Meulbroek, J. A., Staas, J. K., Gilley, R. M., and Tice, T. R. (1990). Controlled vaccine release in the gut-associated lymphoid tissues. I. Orally administered biodegradable microspheres target the Peyers' Patches. *J. Controlled Release* **11,** 205–214.

Elson, C. O., and Ealding, W. (1984). Generalized systemic and mucosal immunity in mice after mucosal stimulation with cholera toxin. *J. Immunol.* **132,** 2736–2741.

Figueroa, J., and Carosi, I. (1981). An ultrastructural and morphometric study of Langerhans cells in normal human exocervix. *J. Anat.* **131,** 669–682.

Forrest, B. D. (1991). Women, HIV, and mucosal immunity. *Lancet* **337,** 835–836.

Friberg, J. (1974). Immunological studies on human sperm agglutinating seminal fluid. *Acta Obstet. Gynecol. Scand. Suppl.* **36,** 65–72.

Fubara, E. S., and Freter, R. (1973). Protection against enteric bacterial infection by secretory IgA antibodies. *J. Immunol.* **111,** 395–403.

Fuhrman, J. A., and Cebra, J. J. (1981). Special features of the priming process for a secretory IgA response: B cell priming with cholera toxin. *J. Exp. Med.* **153,** 534–544.

Goldstein, S. N., Tsai, A., Kemp, C. J., and Fanger, M. W. (1983). Role of IgA antibody in phagocytosis by human polymorphonuclear leukocytes. *Ann. N.Y. Acad. Sci.* **71,** 203–210.

Harriman, G. R., Kunimoto, D. Y., and Strober, W. (1989). IgA B cell differentiation. *Immunol. Invest.* **18,** 17–28.

Harrison, P. E., Barratt, C. L. R., Robinson, A. J., Vessopoulos, E., and Cooke, I. D. (1991). Detection of white blood cell populations in the ejaculates of fertile men. *J. Reprod. Immunol.* **19,** 95–98.

Hawthorn, R., Murdoch, J., MacLean, A., and Mackie, R. (1988). Langerhan's cells and subtypes of human papillomavirus in cervical intraepithelial neoplasia. *Brit. Med. J.* **297,** 643–646.

Head, J. R., and Gaede, S. D. (1986). Ia antigen expression in the rat uterus. *J. Reprod. Immunol.* **9,** 137–153.

Hekman, A., and Rumke, R. (1976). Seminal antigens and autoimmunity. *In* "Human Semen and Fertility Regulation in Men" (E. S. E. Hafez, ed.), pp. 245–257. Mosby, St. Louis, Missouri.

Herrmann, W. P., and Hermann, G. (1969). Immunoelectrophoretic and chromatographic demonstration of IgG, IgA and fragments of γ globulin in the human seminal fluid. *Int. J. Fertil.* **14,** 211–215.

Hussein, A. M., Bourne, F. J., and Newby, T. J. (1981). The female reproductive tract immune system. VII. Proportions of immunoglobulins synthesized in vitro by tissues of the female reproductive tract. *Sudan J. Vet. Res.* **3,** 87–90.

Hussein, A. M., Newby, T. J., and Bourne, F. J. (1983a). Immunohistochemical studies of the local immune system in the reproductive tract of the sow. *J. Reprod. Immunol.* **5,** 1–15.

Hussein, A. M., Newby, T. J., Stokes, C. R., and Bourne, F. J. (1983b). Quantitation and origin of immunoglobulins A, G or M in the secretions and fluids of the reproductive tract of the sow. *J. Reprod. Immunol.* **5,** 17–26.

Illum, L., Farraj, N., Davis, S. S., and Johansen, B. R. (1990). Investigation of the nasal absorption of biosynthetic human growth hormone in sheep-use of a bioadhesive microsphere delivery system. *Int. J. Pharmacol.* **63,** 207–211.

Ingerslev, H. J. (1981). Antibodies against spermatozoal surface-membrane antigens in female infertility. *Acta Obstet. Gynecol. Scand., Suppl.* **100,** 1–52.

Jalanti, R., and Isliker, H. (1977). Immunoglobulin in human cervicovaginal secretions. *Int. Arch. Allergy Appl. Immunol.* **53,** 402–408.

Kamat, B. R., and Issacson, P. G. (1987). The immunocytochemical distribution of leukocyte subpopulations in human endometrium. *Am. J. Pathol.* **127,** 66–73.

Kelly, J. K., and Fox, H. (1979). The local immunological defense system of the human endometrium. *J. Reprod. Immunol.* **1,** 39–45.

Kenney, R. M., and Khaleel, S. A. (1975). Bacteriostatic activity of the mare uterus: A progress report on immunoglobulins. *J. Reprod. Fertil. Suppl.* **23,** 357–358.

King, B. F. (1983). The permeability of nonhuman primate vaginal epithelium: A freeze-fracture and tracer-perfusion study. *J. Ultrastruct. Res.* **83,** 99–110.

King, B. F. (1985). Ultrastructural localization of acid phosphatase in nonhuman primate vaginal epithelium. *Cell Tissue Res.* **239,** 249–252.

King, G. J. (1988). Reduction in uterine intra-epithelial lymphocytes during early gestation in pigs. *J. Reprod. Immunol.* **14,** 41–46.

Kunimoto, D. Y., Harriman, G. R., and Strober, W. (1988). Regulation of IgA differentiation in CH 12 LX B cells by lymphokines. *J. Immunol.* **141,** 713–720.

Kutteh, W. H., Hatch, K. D., Blackwell, R. E., and Mestecky, J. (1988). Secretory immune system of the female reproductive tract: I. Immunoglobulins and secretory component-containing cells. *Obstet. Gynecol.* **71,** 56–60.

Kutteh, W. H., Blacwell, R. E., Gore, H., Kutteh, C. C., Carr, B. R., and Mestecky, J. (1990). Secretory immune system of the female reproductive tract. II. Local immune system in normal and infected fallopian tube. *Fertil. Steril.* **54,** 51–55.

Lande, I. J. M. (1986). Systemic immunity developing from intrauterine antigen exposure in the nonpregnant rat. *J. Reprod. Immunol.* **9,** 57–66.

Lande, I. J. M., Head, J. R., and Billingham, R. E. (1981). Immune reactivity induced by antigenic exposure in the rat uterus. *Trans. Proc.* **8,** 1256–1259.

La Scolea, L. J. J., Cui, Z., Kopti, S., Fisher, J., and Ogra, P. L. (1991). Prevention of pulmonary and genital chlamydia infection by oral immunization. *In* "Vaccines for Sexually Transmitted Diseases" (A. Mehus and R. E. Spier, ed.), pp. 86–91. Butterworths, London.

Lee, C. S., Gogolin-Ewens, K., and Brandon, M. R. (1988). Identification of a unique lymphocyte subpopulation in the sheep uterus. *Immunology* **63,** 157–164.

Lin, X., Huang, T., and Zhang, S. (1988). Langerhans cells in mouse vaginal epithelium—Variations in relation to keratinization. *Arch. Dermatol. Res.* **280,** 451–453.

McAnulty, P., and Morton, D. (1978). The immune response of the genital tract of the female rabbit following systemic and local immunization. *J. Clin. Lab. Immunol.* **1,** 255–260.

McDermott, M. R., and Svedsmith, C. H. (1989). T lymphocytes in genital lymph nodes protect mice from intravaginal infection with herpes simplex virus type 2. *J. Infect. Dis.* **159,** 460–466.

McDermott, M. R., Clark, D. A., and Bienenstock, J. (1980). Evidence for a common mucosal immunologic system. II. Influence of the estrous cycle on B immunoblast migration into genital and intestinal tissues. *J. Immunol.* **124,** 2536–2539.

McDermott, M. R., Smiley, B. J., Brais, P. L. J., Rudzroga, H., and Bienenstock, J. (1984). Immunity in the female genital tract after intravaginal vaccination of mice with an attenuated strain of herpes simplex virus type 2. *J. Virol.* **51,** 247–253.

McDermott, M. R., Brais, P. L. J., Goettsche, G. C., Evelgh, M. J., and Goldsmith, C. H. (1987). Expression of immunity to intravaginal herpes simplex virus type 2 infection in the genital tract and associated lymph nodes. *Arch. Virol.* **93,** 51–68.

McDermott, M. R., Brais, L. J., and Evelegh, M. J. (1990). Mucosal and systemic antiviral antibodies in mice inoculated intravaginally with herpes simplex virus type 2. *J. Gen. Virol.* **71,** 1497–1504.

Masson, P. L., Heremans, J. F., and Ferin, J. (1969). Clinical importance of the biochemical changes in the female genital tract. I. Studies on the proteins of cervical mucus. *Int. J. Fertil.* **14,** 1–7.

Meignier, B., Jourdier, T. M., Norrild, B., Pereira, L., and Roizman, B. (1987). Immunization of experimental animals with reconstituted glycoprotein mixtures of herpes simplex virus 1 and 2: Protection against challenge with virulent virus. *J. Infect. Dis.* **155,** 921–930.

Menge, A. C., and Lieberman, M. E. (1974). Antifertility effects of immunoglobulins from uterine fluids of semen-immunized rabbits. *Biol. Reprod.* **10,** 422–428.

Merriman, H., Woods, S., Winter, C., Fohnlander, A., and Corey, L. (1984). Secretory IgA antibody in cervicovaginal secretions from women with genital infection due to herpes simplex virus. *J. Infect. Dis.* **149,** 505–510.

Mestecky, J. (1987). The common mucosal immune system and current strategies for induction of immune responses in external secretions. *J. Clin. Immunol.* **7,** 265–276.

Miller, C. J., Kang, D. W., Marthas, M., Moldoveanu, Z., Kiyono, H., Marx, P., Eldridge, J. H., Mestecky, J., and McGhee, J. R. (1992). The genital secretory immune response to chronic SIV infection: A comparison between intravenously and genitally inoculated rhesus macaques. *Clin. Exp. Immunol.* **88,** 520–526.

Mishkin, E. M., Fahey, J. R., Kino, Y., Klein, R. J., Abramovitz, A. S., and Mento, S. J. (1991). Native herpes simplex virus glycoprotein-D vaccine—Immunogenicity and protection in animal models. *Vaccine* **9,** 147–153.

Mitchell, B. S. (1986). The localization of immunoglobulins in the non-pregnant rat uterus. *J. Anat.* **146,** 237.

Mitchell, G., Liu, I. K., Perryman, L. E., Stabenfeldt, G. H., and Hughes, J. P. (1982). Preferential production and secretion of immunoglobulins by equine endometrium—A mucosal immune system. *J. Reprod. Fertil. Suppl.* **32,** 161–168.

Moretti-Rojas, I., Rojas, F. J., Leisure, M., Stone, S. C., and Asch, R. H. (1990). Intrauterine inseminations with washed human spermatozoa does not induce formation of antisperm antibodies. *Fertil. Steril.* **53,** 180–182.

Morris, H. H. B., Gatter, K. C., Stein, H., and Mason, D. Y. (1983). Langerhans' cells in human cervical epithelium: An immunohistochemical study. *Br. J. Obstet. Gynaecol.* **90,** 400–411.

Morris, H., Edwards, J., Tiltman, A., and Emms, M. (1985). Endometrial lymphoid tissue: An immunohistological study. *J. Clin. Pathol.* **38,** 644–652.

Morris, H., Emms, M., Visser, T., and Timme, A. (1986). Lymphoid tissue of the normal fallopian tube—A form of mucosal-associated lymphoid tissue (MALT)? *Int. Soc. Gynecol. Pathol.* **5,** 11–22.

Nichols, R. L., Murray, E. S., and Nisson, P. E. (1978). Use of enteric vaccines in protection against chlamydial infections of the genital tract and the eye of guinea pigs. *J. Infect. Dis.* **138,** 742–746.

Nicklin, S., and Miller, K. (1983). Local and systemic immune responses to intestinally presented antigen. *Int. Arch. Allergy Appl. Immunol.* **42,** 87–90.

Ogra, P., and Ogra, S. (1973). Local antibody response to poliovaccine in the human female genital tract. *J. Immunol.* **110,** 1307–1311.

Omran, K., and Hulka, J. (1971). Infertility associated with induced local antibody secretion against sperm in the bovine uterine cervix. *Int. J. Fertil.* **16,** 195–199.

Otsuki, Y. (1989). Lymphatics and lymphoid tissue of the fallopian tube: Immunoelectronmicroscopic study. *Anat. Rec.* **225,** 288–289.

Parr, E. L., and Parr, M. B. (1985). Secretory immunoglobulin binding to bacteria in the mouse uterus after mating. *J. Reprod. Immunol.* **8,** 71–82.

Parr, E. L., and Parr, M. B. (1986). Uptake of immunoglobulins and other proteins from serum into epithelial cells of the mouse uterus and oviduct. *J. Reprod. Immunol.* **9,** 339–354.

Parr, E. L., and Parr, M. B. (1988a). Binding of C3 to bacteria in the mouse uterus after mating. *J. Reprod. Immunol.* **12,** 315–319.

Parr, E. L., and Parr, M. B. (1988b). Anti-bacterial IgA and IgG in mouse uterine luminal fluids, vaginal washings, and serum. *J. Reprod. Immunol.* **13,** 65–72.

Parr, E. L., and Parr, M. B. (1990). A comparison of antibody titres in mouse uterine fluid after immunization by several routes, and the effect of the uterus on antibody titres in vaginal fluid. *Reprod. Fertil.* **89,** 619–625.

Parr, E. L., and Parr, M. B. (1993). Local immunization for antifertility immunity. *In* "Scientific Basis of Fertility Regulation" (P. M. Johnson, and D. Griffin, ed.), pp. 441–458. Oxford University Press, Oxford.

Parr, E., Parr, M., and Thapar, M. (1988a). A comparison of specific antibody responses in mouse vaginal fluid after immunization by several routes. *J. Reprod. Immunol.* **14,** 165–176.

Parr, E., Tung, H. N., and Parr, M. B. (1988b). Endocytosis in the epithelial cells of the mouse oviduct. *Am J. Anat.* **181,** 393–400.

Parr, M. B. (1980a). Endocytosis at the basal and lateral membranes of rat uterine epithelial cells during early pregnancy. *J. Reprod. Fertil.* **60,** 95–99.

Parr, M. B. (1980b). Endocytosis in the uterine epithelium during early pregnancy. *Prog. Reprod. Biol.* **7,** 81–91.

Parr, M., and Parr, E. L. (1978). Uptake and fate of ferritin in the uterine eipthelium of the rat during early pregnancy. *J. Reprod. Fertil.* **52,** 183–188.

Parr, M., and Parr, E. (1985). Immunohistochemical localization of immunoglobulins A, G. and M in the mouse female genital tract. *J. Reprod. Fertil.* **74,** 361–370.

Parr, M. B., and Parr, E. L. (1986a). The effects of estradiol-17β and progesterone on the number of plasma cells in uteri of ovariectomized mice. *J. Reprod. Fertil.* **77,** 91–97.

Parr, M. B., and Parr, E. L. (1986b). Endocytosis in the rat uterine epithelium at implantation. *Ann. N.Y. Acad. Sci.* **476,** 110–121.

Parr, M. B., and Parr, E. L. (1989a). Immunohistochemical investigation of secretory component and immunoglobulin A in the genital tract of the female rat. *J. Reprod. Fertil.* **85,** 105–113.

Parr, M. B., and Parr, E. L. (1989b). Immunohistochemical localization of secretory component and immunoglobulin A in the urogenital tract of the male rodent. *J. Reprod. Fertil.* **85,** 115–124.

Parr, M. B, and Parr, E. L. (1990). Antigen recognition in the female reproductive tract: I. Uptake of intraluminal protein tracers in the mouse vagina. *J. Reprod. Immunol.* **17,** 101–114.

Parr, M. B., and Parr, E. L. (1991). Langerhans cells and T lymphocyte subsets in the murine vagina and cervix. *Biol. Reprod.* **44,** 491–498.

Parr, M. B., Kepple, L., and Parr, E. L. (1991a). Antigen recognition in the female reproductive tract: II. Endocytosis of horseradish peroxidase by Langerhans cells in the murine vaginal epithelium. *Biol. Reprod.* **45,** 261–265.

Parr, M. B., Kepple, L., and Parr, E. L. (1991b). Langerhans cells phagocytose vaginal epithelial cells undergoing apoptosis during the murine estrous cycle. *Biol. Reprod.* **45,** 252–260.

Rachman, F., Casimiri, V., Psychoyos, A., and Bernard, O. (1983). Immunoglobulins in the mouse uterus during the oestrous cycle. *J. Reprod. Fertil.* **69,** 17–21.

Rachman, F., Casimiri, V., and Bernard, O. (1984). Maternal immunoglobulins G, A, and M in mouse uterus and embryo during the post implantation periods. *J. Reprod. Immunol.* **6,** 39–47.

Rachman, F., Casimiri, V., Psychoyos, A., and Bernard, O. (1986). Influence of the embryo on the distribution of maternal immunoglobulins in the mouse uterus. *J. Reprod. Fertil.* **77,** 257–264.

Ramsey, K. H., and Rank. R. G. (1991). Resolution of chlamydial genital infection with antigen-specific lymphocyte-T lines. *Infect. Immun.* **59,** 925–931.

Rebello, R., Green, F. H. Y., and Fox, H. (1975). A study of the secretory immune system of the female genital tract. *Brit. J. Obstet. Gynaecol.* **82,** 812–816.

Ritchie, A. W. S., Hargreave, T. B., James, K., and Chisholm, G. A. (1984). Intra-epithelial lymphocytes in the normal epididymis. A mechanism for tolerance to sperm auto-antigens? *Br. J. Urol.* **56,** 79–83.

Roche, J. K., and Crum, C. P. (1991). Local immunity and the uterine cervix: Implications for cancer-associated viruses. *Cancer Immunol. Ummunother.* **33,** 203–209.

Roig de Vargas-Linares, C. E. (1968). Plasma cells in the hamster vagina: Cyclical and experimental variations. *J. Reprod. Fertil.* **15,** 389–394.

Roncalli, M., Sideri, M., Gie, P., and Servida, E. (1988). Immunophenotypic analysis of the transformation zone of human cervix. *Lab. Invest.* **58,** 141–149.

Rumke, P. (1974). The origin of immunoglobulins in semen. *Clin. Exp. Immunol.* **17,** 287–297.

Sanchez-Pescador, L., Burke, R. L., Ott, G., and Van Nest, B. (1988). The effect of adjuvants on the efficacy of a recombinant herpes simplex virus glycoprotein vaccine. *J. Immunol.* **141,** 1720–1727.

Sawicki, W., Choroszewska, A., Bem, W., and Strojny, P. (1988). Lymphocyte number and distribution in the rat uterine epithelium during estrous cycle and early pregnancy. *Cell Tissue Res.* **253,** 241–244.

Schumacher, G. F. B. (1973). Soluble proteins in cervical mucus. *In* "The Biology of the Cervix" (R. J. Blandau, and K. Moghissi, ed.), pp. 201-233. University of Chicago Press, Chicago.

Schumacher, G. F. B. (1980). Humoral immune factors in the female reproductive tract and their changes during the cycle. *In* "Immunological Aspects of Infertility and Fertility Regulation" (D. Dhindsa, and G. F. B. Schumacher, ed.), pp. 93–135. Elsevier/North Holland, New York.

Schumacher, G. F. B., Holt, J. A., and Reale, F. (1979). Approaches to the analysis of human endometrial secretions. *In* "Approaches to the Analysis of Human Endometrial Secretions" (F. K. Beller, and G. F. B. Schumacher, ed.), pp. 115–130. Elsevier/North Holland, New York.

Scicchitano, R., Stanisz, A., Ernst, P., and Bienenstock, J. (1988). A common mucosal immune system revisited. *In* "Migration and Homing of Lymphoid Cells" (A. J. Husband, ed.), pp. 1–34. CRC Press, Boca Raton, Florida.

Stamey, T. A., Wehner, N., Mihara, G., and Condy, M. (1978). The immunologic basis of recurrent bacteriuria: Role of cervicovaginal antibody in enterobacterial colonization of the introital mucosa. *Medicine* **57,** 47–56.

Steele, E. J., Chaicumpa, W., and Rowley, D. (1975). Further evidence for cross-linking as a protective factor in experimental cholera. Properties of antibody fragments. *J. Immunol. Meth.* **132,** 175–180.

Stingl, G., Tschachler, E., Groh, V., Wolff, K., and Hauser, C. (1989). The immune functions of epidermal cells. *In* "Immune Mechanisms in Cutaneous Disease" (D. A. Norris, ed.), pp. 3–72. Marcel Dekker, New York.

Strauss, E. (1961). Occurrence of antibody in human vaginal mucus. *Proc. Soc. Exp. Biol. Med.* **106,** 617–621.

Sturn, B., and Schneweis, K.-E. (1978). Protective effect of an oral infection with herpes simplex virus type 1 against subsequent genital infections with herpes simplex virus type 2. *Med. Microbiol. Immunol.* **165,** 119–128.

Sullivan, D. A., and Wira, C. R. (1981). Estradiol regulation of secretory component in the female reproductive tract. *J. Steroid Biochem.* **15,** 439–444.

Sullivan, D. A., Richardson, G. S., MacLaughlin, D. T., and Wira, C. R. (1984). Variations in the levels of secretory component in human uterine fluid during the menstrual cycle. *J. Steroid Biochem.* **20,** 509–513.

Sundstrom, S. A., Komm, B. S., Ponce-de-Leon, H., Yi, Z., Teuscher, C., and Lyttle, C. R. (1990). Estrogen regulation of tissue-specific expression of complement C3. *J. Biol. Chem.* **264,** 16941–16947.

Suzuki, M., Ogawa, M., Tamada, T., Nagura, H., and Watanabe, K. (1984). Immunohistochemical localization of secretory component and IgA in the human endometrium in relation to menstrual cycle. *Acta Histochem. Cytochem.* **17,** 223–229.

Symons, D. B. A., and Herbert, J. (1971). Incidence of immunoglobulins in fluids of the rabbit genital tract and the distribution of IgG-globulin in the tissues of the female tract. *J. Reprod. Fert.* **24,** 55–62.

Tagliabue, A., Boraschi, D., Villa, L., Keren, D. F., Lowell, G. F., Rappuoli, R., and Nencioni, L. (1984). IgA-dependent cell-mediated activity against enteropathogenic bacteria: Distribution, specificity, and characterization of the effector cells. *J. Immunol.* **133,** 988–992.

Tauber, P. F., Zaneveld, L. T. D., Propping, D., and Schumacher, G. F. B. (1975). Components of human split ejaculates. I. Spermatozoa, fructose, immunoglobulin, albumin, lactoferrin, transferrin, and other plasma proteins. *J. Reprod. Fertil.* **43,** 249–267.

Taylor, H. P., and Dimmock, N. J. (1985). Mechanism of neutralization of influenza virus by secretory IgA is different from that of monomeric IgA or IgG. *J. Exp. Med.* **161,** 198–209.

Thapar, M., Parr, E. L., and Parr, M. B. (1990a). The effect of adjuvants on antibody titers in mouse vaginal fluid after intravaginal immunization. *J. Reprod. Immunol.* **17,** 207–216.

Thapar, M., Parr, E. L., and Parr, M. B. (1990b). Secretory immune responses in mouse vaginal fluid after pelvic, parenteral, or vaginal immunization. *Immunology* **70,** 121–125.

Thapar, M. A., Parr, E. L., Bozzola, J. J., and Parr, M. B. (1991). Secretory immune responses in the mouse vagina after parenteral or intravaginal immunization with an immunostimulating complex (ISCOM). *Vaccine* **9,** 129–133.

Tjokronegoro, A., and Sirisinha, S. (1975). Quantitative analysis of immunoglobulins and albumin in secretion of female reproductive tract. *Fertil. Steril.* **26,** 413–417.

Tourville, D. R., Ogra, S. S., Lippes, J., and Tomasi, T. B. (1970). The human female reproductive tract: Immunohistological localization of γA, γG, γM secretory "piece" and lactoferrin. *Am. J. Obstet. Gynecol.* **108,** 1102–1108.

Tuffrey, M., Falder, P., Gale, J., and Taylor-Robinson, D. (1986). Salpingitis in mice induced by human strains of *Chlamydia trachomatis*. *Br. J. Exp. Pathol.* **67,** 605–616.

Tung, H. N., Parr, E. L., and Parr, M. B. (1988). Endocytosis in mouse uterine luminal and glandular epithelial cells during early pregnancy. *Am. J. Anat.* **182,** 120–129.

Uehling, D. T. (1971). Secretory IgA in seminal plasma. *Fertil. Steril.* **22,** 769–773.

Usala, S. J., Usala, F. O., Hariski, R., Holt, J. A., and Schumacher, G. F. B. (1989). IgG and IgA content of vaginal fluid during the menstrual cycle. *J. Reprod. Med.* **34,** 292.

Vaerman, J. P., and Ferin, J. (1974). Local immunological response of the vagina, cervix, and endometrium. *Acta Endocrinol. Suppl.* **194,** 281–301.

Vander-Wielen, A. L., and King, G. J. (1984). Intraepithelial lymphocytes in the bovine uterus during the oestrous cycle and early gestation. *J. Reprod. Fertil.* **70,** 457–462.

Waelchli, R. O., and Winder, N. C. (1987). Immunohistochemical evaluation of the equine endometrium during the oestrous cycle. *Equine Vet. J.* **19,** 299–302.

Waldman, R. H., and Ganguly, R. (1974). Immunity to infections on secretory surfaces. *J. Infect. Dis.* **130,** 419–440.

Waldman, R. H., Cruz, J. M., and Rowe, D. S. (1972a). Immunoglobulin levels to *Candida albicans* in human cervicovaginal secretions. *Clin. Exp. Immunol.* **10,** 427–434.

Waldman, R. H., Cruz, J. M., and Rowe, D. S. (1972b). Intravaginal immunization of humans with *Candida albicans. J. Immunol.* **109,** 662–664.

Wang, Y. F., and Holstein, A. F. (1983). Intraepithelial lymphocytes and macrophages in the human epididymis. *Cell Tissue Res.* **233,** 517–521.

Ward, M. (1993). The development of an anti-chlamydia vaccine. *In* "Scientific Basis of Fertility Regulation" (D. Griffin and P. M. Johnson, ed.), pp. 409–425. Oxford University Press, Oxford.

Widders, P. R., Stokes, C. R., David, J. S., and Bourne, F. J. (1985a). Effect of cycle stage on immunoglobulin concentration in reproductive tract secretions of the mare. *J. Reprod. Immunol.* **7,** 233–242.

Widders, P. R., Stokes, C. R., David, J. S., and Bourne, F. J. (1985b). Immunohistological studies of the local immune system in the reproductive tract of the mare. *Res. Vet. Sci.* **38,** 88–95.

Widders, P. R., Stokes, C. R., David, J. S., and Bourne, F. J. (1986). Specific antibody in the equine genital tract following local immunisation and challenge infection with contagious equine metritis organism (*Taylorella equigenitalis*). *Res. Vet. Sci.* **40,** 54–58.

Wilkie, B., Duncan, J., and Winter, A. (1972). The origin, class and specificity of immunoglobulins in bovine cervico-vaginal mucus: Variation with parenteral immunization and local infection with *Vibrio fetus. J. Reprod. Fertil.* **31,** 359–365.

Williams, R. C., and Gibbons, R. J. (1972). Inhibition of bacterial adherence by secretory immunoglobulin A: A mechanism of antigen disposal. *Science* **177,** 697–699.

Wira, C. R., and Sandoe, C. P. (1977). Sex steroid hormone regulation of IgA and IgG in rat uterine secretions. *Nature* (*London*) **268,** 534–535.

Wira, C. R., and Sandoe, C. P. (1989). Effect of uterine immunization and oestradiol on specific IgA and IgG antibodies in uterine, vaginal and salivary secretions. *Immunology* **68,** 24–30.

Wira, C. R., and Sullivan, D. A. (1985). Estradiol and progesterone regulation of immunoglobulin A and G and secretory component in cervicovaginal secretions of the rat. *Biol. Reprod.* **32,** 90–95.

Wira, C. R., Hyde, E., Sandoe, C. P., Sullivan, D., and Spencer, S. (1980). Cellular aspects of the rat uterine IgA response to estradiol and progesterone. *J. Steroid Biochem.* **12,** 451–459.

Wolff, H., and Anderson, D. J. (1988). Immunohistologic characterization and quantitation of leukocyte subpopulations in human semen. *Fertil. Steril.* **49,** 497–504.

Yang, S., and Schumacher, G. (1979). Immune response after vaginal application of antigens in the rhesus monkey. *Fertil. Steril.* **32,** 588–598.

Young, W. G. (1985). Epithelial kinetics affect Langerhans' cells of mouse vaginal epithelium. *Acta Anat.* **123,** 131–136.

Young, W. G., and Hosking, A. R. (1986). Langerhans cells in murine vaginal epithelium affected by oestrogen and topical vitamin A. *Acta Anat.* **125,** 59–64.

Young, W. G., Newcomb, G. M., and Hosking, A. R. (1985). The effect of atrophy, hyperplasia and keratinization accompanying the estrous cycle on Langerhans' cells in mouse vaginal epithelium. *Am. J. Anat.* **174,** 173–186.

55

Immunologically Mediated Male and Female Reproductive Failure

R. A. Bronson • F. M. Fusi

I. INTRODUCTION

Spermatozoa possess a variety of unique tissue-specific antigens not present in the individual during fetal life, when immune self-recognition takes place and tolerance toward self occurs. Since spermatogenesis is not initiated until puberty, antigens unique to spermatozoa are not included in that recognition process; their physiological development must proceed in a milieu that limits their exposure to the male immune system to avoid generating an immune response.

Spermatozoa also have an unusual relationship with the immune system of women, whose bodies they periodically invade, as foreigners, after coitus. However, after their intravaginal deposition, spermatozoa may pass through various compartments of the female reproductive tract that are capable of mounting an immune response without eliciting the formation of sperm-directed antibodies. That the mechanisms that prevent these pathological immune responses can be impaired is attested to by the long-standing clinical association of infertility in men and women with the presence of humoral antisperm antibodies.

In this chapter, we review the mechanisms that normally prevent the development of immunity to spermatozoa and describe conditions that may abrogate those defenses. Evidence is presented that the local immune system of the reproductive tracts of both men and women can participate in immunologically mediated infertility. Increasing evidence also has been accumulated that antisperm antibodies alter sperm function, both in terms of their ability to populate the female reproductive tract and in terms of gamete interactions.

II. MECHANISMS THAT PREVENT IMMUNITIES TO SPERMATOZOA

The first line of defense against the development of a sperm-specific autoimmune response in men is the blood–testis barrier between Sertoli cells (Table I). The tight junctions between Sertoli cells divide the seminiferous tubules into adluminal and basal compartments, excluding the passage of lymphocytes and high molecular weight proteins such as immunoglobulins and complement (Hamilton, 1975; Gilula *et al.*, 1976). In addition, the Sertoli cells form an immunological barrier by actively phagocytosing and degrading sperm and residual products of spermatogenesis that would be a major source of antigenic stimulation if absorbed. Only approximately one-fifth of sperm produced leave the testis; the remaining four-fifths are resorbed (Johnson *et al.*, 1983). Additionally, Sertoli cells probably produce immunoregulatory factors since they secrete transferrin, which has been shown to inhibit lymphocyte blastogenesis and complement-mediated cell lysis (Skinner *et al.*, 1984). The barrier between the reproductive system and the immune system is less effective in the rete testis and the ductus efferentes so these sites are more accessible to cellular immune components, as demonstrated in mice by the ability of sperm-sensitized activated T lymphocytes, transferred to recipient males, to react with autoantigens in this region as well as in the vas deferens (Tung *et al.*, 1987). Conversely, dilution of sperm antigens in the rete testis (Jones, 1977) and its poor vascularization (Kormana and Reijonen, 1976) may limit the interchange between intraluminal and intravascular compartments.

In females, the absence of an immune response to spermatozoa after coitus has been ascribed to several factors. First, except when ovulatory cervical mucus is present, spermatozoa are confined to the vagina; even when cervical mucus allows the passage of spermatozoa, the majority of sperm-containing semen is expelled. The human vagina is lined with a thick stratified squamous epithelium that retards the passage of spermatozoa into the vascular system (Shearer and Rabson, 1984) and has only a limited number of plasma cells beneath its epithelial surface (Haas and Beer, 1986). However, this area is not an immunologically privileged site, as suggested by the study of Ogra and Ogra (1973), who observed that intravaginal as well as intrauterine immunization with poliovirus type I resulted in the appearance of secretory IgA antibody against poliovirus in the genital tract.

In addition to the barrier mechanisms that limit the contact of sperm antigens with both male and female immune systems, an active semen-related immunosuppression appears to exist. Several lines of evidence have been presented for the existence of immunosuppressive factors within the seminal fluid. Seminal plasma inhibits the ability of T and B lymphocytes to proliferate in response to mitogen or antigen challenge (Lord *et al.*, 1977; Marcus *et al.*, 1978), impairs antibody-dependent cell-mediated cytotoxicity (James and

Table I Factors Limiting an Antisperm Immune Response in the Male

Tight junctions between Sertoli cells
T suppressor/T helper ratio
Immunoregulatory factors
Effects of seminal plasma
Inhibition of T and B lymphocyte proliferation by mitogens and target antigens
Block of antibody-dependent cell-mediated cytotoxicity
Inhibition of NK and T cytotoxic lymphocyte recognition of tumors and polymorphonuclear leukocytes (PMNs)
Inhibition of macrophage and PMN phagocytosis
Inhibition of the action of complement
Block of the Fc portion of IgG ?
Effects of spermatozoa
Immunosuppression
Inhibition of B lymphocyte antibody production through activation of C3a

Szymaniesc, 1985), and blocks the recognition of tumor cells or virally infected cells by natural killer (NK) and cytotoxic T lymphocytes (Marcus *et al.*, 1984; Witkin, 1984). In addition, seminal fluid inhibits phagocytosis by macrophages and polymorphonuclear leukocytes (PMNs; Witkin, 1986) and the action of complement (Tarter and Alexander, 1984). Soluble receptors for IgG (FcγRIII) have been detected in human seminal plasma (Thaler *et al.*, 1989), raising the possibility of their role in blocking antibody-mediated sperm damage by binding to the Fc portion of the immunoglobulin molecule. Spermatozoa also have been demonstrated to be immunosuppressive, as judged by their ability to induce tolerance *in vitro* in an autologous system (Hurtenbach *et al.*, 1980). Since they are able to induce the activation of complement by the alternative pathway (Witkin *et al.*, 1983), spermatozoa may modulate the immune response via C3a, which suppresses antibody production by B lymphocytes *in vitro* (Morgan, 1987).

Evidence also exists for active cellular immunosuppressive activity in the male reproductive system and in semen. T suppressor lymphocytes have been detected in the interstitium of the testis and in the submucosal regions of epididymis (El-Demiry and James, 1988). The ratio of T suppressor to T helper lymphocytes in semen indicates the prevalence of suppressing activity (Witkin, 1988). In the female, a dominance in the activity of T suppressor lymphocytes may exist. In mice, after their intravaginal exposure to sperm, an increase in the weight of the draining lymph nodes occurs that is not followed by antibody production, suggesting that a suppressive response may be stimulated in the lymph nodes (Beer and Billingham, 1978). Hill *et al.* (1987a) observed, in clear follicular fluid aspirated from follicles of women undergoing oocyte retrieval for *in vitro* fertilization, that the $CD4^+ : CD8^+$ T lymphocyte ratio, which is usually 2:1 in peripheral blood, is decreased dramatically in follicular fluid to 1:25, with a clear predominance of suppressor cells. T suppressor ($CD8^+$) cells, which may function in the induction of immune tolerance, also were found in the intraepithelial spaces of fallopian mucosa (Kutteh *et al.*, 1990).

III. PATHOPHYSIOLOGY OF THE PRODUCTION OF ANTISPERM ANTIBODIES

Evidence exists in humans, as well as in other species, that both the male and the female reproductive tracts are able to participate in mucosal immunity and to secrete antibodies, primarily secretory IgA, locally (Ogra and Ogra, 1973; Mestecky and McGhee, 1987; Parr and Parr, 1990; Wira and Stern, 1990).

In women, subepithelial plasma cells have been identified in the fallopian tube, endocervix, ectocervix, and vagina (Kutteh *et al.*, 1988,1990). Approximately two-thirds of the immunoglobulin-positive cells contained IgA and J chain, indicating that they produce polymeric IgA. Secretory component (SC)-producing epithelial cells were found in the fallopian tube and endocervix. In addition, although the IgA1-containing plasma cells predominated in all tissues examined (except vagina), the relative proportion of IgA2 plasma cells was found to be increased compared with tissues such as bone marrow and spleen (Kutteh *et al.*, 1988). The number of plasma cells of all classes, including IgG and IgM, also was found to be 6- to 10-fold higher in infected fallopian tubes than in normal tubes, suggesting that a local immune system is functioning in the female genital tract (Kutteh *et al.*, 1990).

In addition, the local immune response may not be restricted geographically, since migration of lymphocytes between different mucosae can occur (McGhee and Mestecky, 1990). IgA precursor cells may populate remote secretory sites, including the uterus and the cervix, that differ from the initial site of immunization. Heremans and Bazin (1971) found plasma cells producing secretory IgA directed against specific antigens in nonlymphatic organs after oral immunization of mice with sheep red blood cells.

Evidence of lymphocyte trafficking in humans is suggested by the presence of specific secretory IgA antibodies against *Streptococcus mutans* in saliva and tears after their ingestion in gelatin capsules (Arnold *et al.*, 1976). The intragastric immunization of women with polio vaccine also results in the presence of antiviral IgA antibodies in both uterine and vaginal secretions (Ogra and Ogra, 1973).

Evidence also has been presented that an IgE-mediated allergic response to seminal plasma proteins may occur in vagina, leading to a chronic vulvovaginitis (Chang, 1976; Witkin, 1987) and perhaps to anaphylaxis (Halpern *et al.*, 1967). Skin testing with antigens indicated that this allergy is caused by hypersensitization to seminal plasma proteins, not by sperm cells (Halpern *et al.*, 1967). Although increased levels of IgE have been associated with infertility (Mathur *et al.*, 1981), no evidence has been presented for immunological infertility caused by specific antisperm IgE antibodies. The production of secretory IgA appears to be the most important local immune response to spermatozoa.

That the male reproductive tract can participate in a local

immune response to infections has been suggested by the finding that total IgA concentration is greater in the prostatic secretions than that of IgG or IgM. Total IgA in the presence of prostatitis has been found to be greater than total IgA in men with urinary tract infection. More than 50% of the total prostatic fluid IgA contains SC, suggesting local production or active transport from serum by prostatic epithelium. In prostatitis caused by *E. coli*, 90% of total IgA and IgG is *E. coli* specific. *Escherichia coli*-specific IgA concentration is 40 times higher in prostatic fluid than in serum, providing further circumstantial evidence that active IgA transport occurs in the prostate (Fowler and Mariano, 1982).

A mixture of IgA and IgG antisperm antibodies is observed in ejaculates of men with autoimmunity to sperm. Antisperm IgG is derived primarily as a transudate from serum, and its presence in the ejaculate correlates with the titer of circulating antisperm antibodies (Rumke, 1974). The local production of antisperm IgA in the male genital tract has been suggested both by its detection in semen although absent from serum and by the presence of antisperm antibodies with unique regional binding specificities on the spermatozoan surface that differ from those present in serum. In a study of 856 matched serum and semen samples, immunoglobulins primarily of the IgA class were detected on the sperm surface in 15% of cases (Pavia *et al.*, 1987). Hellstrom *et al.* (1988) also have demonstrated the presence of IgA on sperm despite its absence in serum, as detected by immunobead binding.

Since IgA is transported locally across mucosal surfaces through its association with SC, which is produced by epithelial cells, the finding of SC in association with IgA on the sperm surface is presumptive evidence for its local secretion, although not necessarily its local production (Parslow *et al.*, 1985; Meinertz *et al.*, 1990). Meinertz *et al.* (1990,1991) have detected SC, utilizing a mixed agglutination reaction (MAR) test, on the surface of spermatozoa in men with autoimmunity to sperm.

Additional evidence for the involvement of local mucosal immunity in the production of antisperm antibodies comes from an analysis of IgA subclasses. Whereas monomeric IgA1 predominates in serum, immunoglobulins of the IgA2 class, in addition to IgA1, are present in mucosal secretions such as tears, saliva, and colostrum (Crago *et al.*, 1983; Delacroix *et al.*, 1983).

Using mouse monoclonal antibodies directed against the two different subclasses of human IgA (IgA1 and IgA2), and subsequently using immunobeads coated with anti-mouse immunoglobulins, Bronson and Cooper (1988) showed that a preponderance of IgA1 exists in the ejaculates of men with antisperm autoimmunity, although a wide variation was noted in the ratio of IgA1 to IgA2 among different patients. The varying proportion of antisperm IgA subclasses in different men might be a reflection of varying etiologies or different routes of immunization.

Conditions that result in an alteration in the balance between the exposure of the male or female immune system to sperm antigen and immunosuppresive factors may lead to antisperm antibody production (Table II).

Vasectomy is associated with autoimmunity to spermatozoa in 60–70% of men (Alexander and Anderson, 1979), perhaps mediated by the absorption of an increased amount of sperm antigens that cannot be balanced by immunosuppressive factors. Testicular trauma (Haensch, 1973), torsion (Mastrogiacomo *et al.*, 1982), biopsy (Hjort *et al.*, 1974), and tumors (Guazziero *et al.*, 1985) also have been associated with the production of antisperm antibodies. Witkin and Toth (1983) have presented evidence that genital tract infections, which can act as adjuvants for immune activation, are associated with antisperm antibody production. Nongonococcal urethritis, particularly urethritis resulting from *Chlamydia*, has been associated with antisperm autoantibodies (Shamanesh *et al.*, 1986). Even unilateral obstruction of the vas deferens may be responsible for antisperm antibody production (Hendry *et al.*, 1982). In addition, congenital obstruction of the vas deferens, seen in cystoc fibrosis, has been associated with the appearance of antisperm antibodies (D'Cruz *et al.*, 1991).

Other possible causes of sperm antibody formation are related to the failure of immunosuppressive mechanisms. A decrease in the number or activity of T suppressor cells in the male genital tract or in semen has been postulated to play a role in the production of antisperm antibodies by B lymphocytes and plasma cells. In fact, men who underwent a vasectomy and whose semen contained antibody-labeled spermatozoa showed predominantly helper cells in their ejaculates (Witkin, 1988). In addition, the lack of immunosuppressive factors in the seminal plasma or the diminution of Fcγ receptors or their inactivity might induce an immune response in both men and women. Abnormal expression of antigens by spermatozoa or display of certain immunodomi-

Table II Summary of the Conditions Associated with the Production of Antisperm Antibodies

Men	Women
Disruptions of the blood–testis barrier Vasectomy Testicular traumas Tumors Biopsy Torsion Genital tract infections Obstructions Cystic fibrosis	Factors depending on spermatozoa or seminal plasma Decrease of T suppressor lymphocyte activity? Genital tract infections (adjuvant action by bacteria) Oral or anal sex
Failure of the mechanisms of immunosuppression Decrease of T suppressor lymphocyte activity Lack of immunosuppressive factors in the seminal plasma?	
Abnormal expression of antigens on the sperm surface?	
Gastrointestinal exposure to spermatozoa (homosexuals)	

nant antigens also has been proposed to cause lymphocyte activation (Mathur *et al.*, 1983,1988). An abnormal decrease in number or activity of T suppressor lymphocytes or an adjuvant action by bacteria in the female reproductive tract could, in theory, play a role in antisperm antibody production. Studies performed using immunoblot analysis of sperm antigen extracts showed that upper genital tract infections in women appear to be associated with the production of antisperm antibodies directed against antigens different from those involved in idiopathic immune infertility (Cunningham *et al.*, 1991).

A different pathogenesis of autoimmunity to spermatozoa has been suggested for homosexual men and for women who engage in oral and anal intercourse. Under experimental conditions, the rectal introduction of spermatozoa in rabbits elicits a systemic immune response (Richards *et al.*, 1984); gastric administration to rats of homologous spermatozoa results in an antisperm antibody production associated with decreased fertility (Allardyce, 1984). In humans, a higher prevalence of antisperm antibodies has been described in homosexual men than in heterosexual men from infertile couples (Witkin and Sonnabend, 1983, Bronson *et al.*, 1983; Table III). In 40–50% of homosexual men, antisperm antibodies can be detected in serum (Wolff and Schill, 1985). Bronson *et al.* (1983) observed a higher prevalence of antisperm antibodies of the IgM class relative to IgG and IgA in sera of homosexual men than in sera of autoimmune men from infertile couples. These researchers proposed that these differences might reflect differences in the etiology of autoimmunity to sperm in the two groups. Intrarectal ejaculation in cases of sodomy may lead to altered processing of antigens, since the single layer columnar epithelium of the rectum is much more permeable than the thick epithelium of the vagina. In addition, the population of B lymphocytes and plasma cells in the gastrointestinal tract is different from that present in the reproductive tract (Mestecky and McGhee, 1987), and the reactivity of these cells with sperm antigens might be different. Several lines of evidence have been presented that the large intestine is an organ in which plasma cells producing the IgA2 subclass of antibodies prevail (Kett *et al.*, 1986; Crago *et al.*, 1984). Intrarectal deposition of spermatozoa has been postulated to result in the stimulation of IgM- or IgA2-producing cells, which might then home to the genital tract, leading to the production of antisperm antibodies of this isotype and subclass within semen rather than to the production of those present in immune infertile men (e.g., IgA1 and IgG).

IV. PATHOGENESIS OF INFERTILITY DUE TO ANTISPERM ANTIBODIES

Immunity to spermatozoa is not an all-or-nothing phenomenon, that is, the effects of antibodies on fertility depend on their titer, the class of immunoglobulin produced, the affinity for specific epitopes displayed by spermatozoa, the nature of the antigens involved, and other associated phenomena, such as the time between ejaculations.

Antisperm antibodies can affect the mechanisms of transport of spermatozoa within the female genital tract, can alter sperm capacitation or the acrosome reaction, can interfere with egg fertilization, or can have postfertilization effects on the zygote and pre-implantation early embryo.

A. Sperm Transport

As a first step in their passage through the human female genital tract, spermatozoa must penetrate and progress through cervical mucus to gain entry into the uterus and fallopian tubes. The association between abnormal or inhibited mucus penetration and the presence of antisperm antibodies was reported first when Fjallbrant (1969) demonstrated that antisperm antibodies, obtained from infertile patients or from immunized rabbits, are able to inhibit *in vitro* penetration of human cervical mucus by human spermatozoa.

Sperm penetration through cervical mucus *in situ* is evaluated clinically by means of the postcoital test, which in summary consists of the evaluation of number and motility of spermatozoa present in the cervical mucus 8–12 hr after intercourse at the time of ovulation. The results of a postcoital test depend on mucus quality, particularly sialic acid biochemistry (Lutjen *et al.*, 1984); sperm concentration in semen (Jette and Glass, 1972); the pattern of sperm motility (Mortimer *et al.*, 1986); and the proportion of spermatozoa labeled with antibodies (Bronson *et al.*, 1984a).

Many studies have demonstrated that antisperm antibodies affect sperm penetration into and motility within cervical mucus (Alexander, 1984; Bronson *et al.*, 1984a; Haas, 1986). The greater the proportion of antibody-bound sperm, the

Table III Comparison of Incidence of Antisperm Antibodies in Sera of Homosexual Men and Men from Infertile Couples Suspected of Immunological Infertility

	Number of serum samples	Antibody-negative sera (%)	Antibody-positive sera (%)	
			High levels[a]	Low levels
Homosexual males	60	21.7	50	28.3
Heterosexual infertile males	180	45.6	25.3	31.1

[a] More than 40% of spermatozoa bind immunobeads following preincubation with sera diluted at 1:4.

fewer sperm are able to enter and pass through cervical mucus; when all spermatozoa are coated with antibodies, seeing motile spermatozoa in the mucus is uncommon (Bronson *et al.*, 1984a). Hence, these men should be considered functionally oligospermic, despite normal sperm concentration in semen. Antisperm IgG and IgA have been found in the cervical mucus after its liquefaction with bromelain (Clarke *et al.*, 1984a). Kremer and Jager (1980) suggested that antibodies of the IgA class were responsible for the shaking of antibody-labeled spermatozoa within cervical mucus. These investigators postulated that IgA was attached via SC to glycoproteins of the cervical mucus. Later, Jager *et al.* (1981a) showed that IgG also induces a shaking phenomenon, suggesting that other mechanisms are involved, and implicated the Fc region of the immunoglobulin molecule. Disulfide exchanges between sulfhdryl residues of sperm-bound immunoglobulins and glycoprotein molecules of mucin have been suggested to lead to impairment of motility of antibody-labeled sperm within cervical mucus (Bronson *et al.*, 1984a). The fact that monoclonal antibodies raised in mice (Bronson and Cooper, 1987) and polyclonal antibodies raised in rabbits (Fjallbrant, 1969) impair the ability of human spermatozoa to penetrate cervical mucus suggests that this effect is not species specific. Studies performed using an IgA1 protease derived from *Neisseria gonorrhoeae* demonstrated that the pretreatment of IgA-coated spermatozoa with this protease improved their mucus-penetrating ability (Bronson and Cooper, 1988). This protease cleaves a single peptide bond of the heavy chain of IgA1, liberating the Fc portion of the molecule (Plaut, 1983). The fact that IgA-labeled (but not IgG-labeled) spermatozoa treated with this protease show an improved ability to penetrate into and sustain motility within cervical mucus, although they remain coated with IgA Fab (Bronson *et al.*, 1987a; Table IV), suggests that the failure of cervical mucus penetration might not be related to the Fab portion of antibodies, nor to sperm surface antigens, but to the Fc portion. Alternatively, the effect might be caused by a different activity of univalent rather than multivalent IgA. However, these findings confirmed the earlier data presented by Jager *et al.* (1981b), which demonstrated that spermatozoa exposed to Fab preparations of antisperm IgA are able to penetrate cervical mucus, in contrast to those exposed to the intact immunoglobulins. On this basis, we can postulate that human cervical mucus possesses a receptor for the Fc portion of the immunoglobulin molecule. Monoclonal antibodies raised against spermatozoa from several species including humans (Anderson *et al.*, 1987), directed against epitopes present on the surface of live sperm, impaired human sperm penetration through a column of bovine cervical mucus whereas monoclonal antibodies directed against subsurface epitopes did not (Bronson and Cooper, 1987).

A correlation also has been observed between the regional specificity of antisperm antibodies to the spermatozoan surface and their ability to impair penetration of cervical mucus. Binding of IgG and IgA immunoglobulins to the tail tip of spermatozoa is not associated with an alteration of their mucus-penetrating ability (Bronson *et al.*, 1984b). In contrast, sperm-head directed antibodies, mainly those of the IgA class, as well as antibodies of both IgA and IgG classes directed against antigens on the principal piece of the sperm tail severely impair the ability of spermatozoa to penetrate mucus (Wang *et al.*, 1985).

Both the immunoglobulin class and the regional specificity of antibodies are important for the second mechanism of sperm transport impairment, that is, complement-mediated immobilization. IgG and IgM immunoglobulins are able to activate the complement cascade, which results in target cell lysis. Whereas a single molecule of IgM is necessary to lyse

Table IV Percentage of Spermatozoa Antibody-Bound by IgA and IgG before and after Treatment with IgA1 Protease[a]

	Preprotease				Postprotease			
	Iga		IgG		IgA		IgG	
Semen sample number	Head	Tail	Head	Tail	Head	Tail	Head	Tail
1	100	100	ND[b]	ND			ND	ND
2	100	21	ND	ND	29	9	ND	ND
3	100	80	ND	ND	15	ND	ND	ND
4	100	100	8	49	29	43	11	71
5	100	100	ND	43	29	70	ND	43
6	100	100	64	100	39	99	35	100
7	80	100	ND	50	4	46	ND	ND
8	74	26	11	30	ND	1	7	32
9	100	60	100	100	86	60	96	50
10	ND	100	30	100	ND	13	25	100
11	ND	ND	100	30	ND	ND	100	30

[a] Adapted with permission from Bronson *et al.* (1987a).
[b] ND, None detected.

a red blood cell, approximately 1000 molecules of IgG are required (Humphrey and Dourmashkin, 1965). IgA does not activate the classical complement pathway. Complement proteins have been found in several secretions of the female genital tract, for example, those of the cervix (Price and Boettcher, 1979), uterus (Lint, 1980), fallopian tubes (Yang *et al.*, 1983), and ovarian follicle (Schumacher, 1980; Clarke *et al.*, 1984b; D'Cruz *et al.*, 1990). Price and Boettcher (1979), using hemolysis of red blood cells exposed to anti-red blood cell antibodies, showed that the complement activity in cervical mucus is much lower than that in serum (10%). This observation may explain why complement-mediated sperm immobilization within cervical mucus does not take place immediately after sperm penetration into the cervical mucus, but requires 4–8 hr. The regional specificity of antibody binding to the spermatozoan surface is also an important factor in complement-mediated immobilization. IgG antibodies directed against the head, the distal one-fifth of the sperm tail principal piece, or the tail end piece were found to be ineffective in promoting complement-mediated loss of sperm motility, whereas a high degree of sperm immobilization was observed when IgG binding occurred on a majority of the principal piece of the sperm tail or when IgM labeled the tail end piece (Bronson *et al.*, 1982b). Hence, the amount of antibody, its location, and its isotype all play a role in sperm immobilization.

An accessory mechanism of interference with fertilization by antisperm antibodies may be antibody-dependent cell-mediated cytotoxicity (ADCC). Macrophages that populate the female genital tract may interact with the Fc portion of immunoglobulins or with C3 fixed by IgG and IgM antibodies and phagocytosis may be promoted, as demonstrated by the lysis of ^{111}In-labeled spermatozoa by peritoneal macrophages when spermatozoa were covered with specific antibodies (London *et al.*, 1985).

B. Sperm Capacitation and Acrosome Reaction

Fresh ejaculated spermatozoa are not able to penetrate oocytes and must undergo a series of calcium-dependent biochemical and structural changes before they become capable of fusing with the egg plasma membrane. First, spermatozoa must undergo plasma membrane modifications termed capacitation, which render them able to undergo the acrosome reaction. This latter process consists of loss of the plasma membrane of the rostral portion of the spermatozoan head, shedding of the acrosomal cap (a modified secretory granule situated over this region of the sperm head), and exposure of the inner acrosomal membrane (Yanagimachi, 1988). Only acrosome-reacted sperm can penetrate the zona pellucida and fuse with the egg plasma membrane. The release of the acrosomal contents—which consist of the enzymes acrosin, a trypsin-like protease, and hyaluronidase—plays a role in spermatozoan passage through the cumulus oophorus and the zona pellucida, allowing its contact with the oolemma, the egg plasma membrane. Evidence has been presented that antisperm antibodies may induce a premature acrosome reaction (Lansford *et al.*, 1988) which may alter the ability of sperm to penetrate the zona, so their fertilizing life-span may be shortened (Wolf, 1989). Bronson *et al.* (1987b), demonstrated that antisperm antibodies of the IgG class directed against the rostral portion of the head, in the presence of complement, are able to increase the number of acrosome-reacted spermatozoa, as detected by ultrastructural studies. Other antibodies might have an opposite effect on the acrosome reaction, since a monoclonal antisperm antibody has been reported to block the calcium ionophore-induced acrosome reaction (Wolf, 1989).

C. Sperm–Egg Interaction

Antisperm antibodies directed against antigens involved in the interaction between the male and the female gametes may alter fertilization by affecting the ability of spermatozoa to bind to the zona pellucida as well as the fusion between the spermatozoan and egg plasma membranes.

Several lines of evidence have been presented that indicate that antisperm antibodies may interfere with sperm recognition of the zona pellucida, in other mammals and in humans. During the process of fertilization, spermatozoa bind to species-specific receptors on the zona pellucida. In mice, several monoclonal antibodies are able to inhibit the binding of spermatozoa to zona pellucida (Saling and Lakosky, 1985). In guinea pigs, autoantibodies induced by vasectomy block zona binding and *in vitro* fertilization (Huang *et al.*, 1981). A specific autoantigen, RSA-1, was demonstrated in the rabbit to be involved in zona recognition by the ability of specific antisera to block fertilization (O'Rand, 1981). In a series of experiments performed with donor spermatozoa exposed to sera containing antisperm antibodies, Bronson *et al.* (1982a) showed that the presence of these antibodies on the sperm surface interferes with their recognition of salt-stored zonae pellucidae of oocytes obtained from human ovaries that had been removed surgically. When the titer of antisperm antibodies was lowered by absorption of these sera with spermatozoa before their exposure to test sperm, a partial recovery of zona binding ability could be observed. These experiments also suggested that the isotype of antisperm antibody bound to the head may be important in determining the degree of impairment of sperm zona binding, since IgA was more inhibitory than IgG. In addition, the total immunoglobulin labeling of the sperm surface appeared to be an important prognostic factor: when 100% of spermatozoa were antibody labeled, the impairment of zona binding was more evident. A similar experiment using live oocytes obtained by follicular aspiration for *in vitro* fertilization confirmed these findings for the effect of antisperm antibodies (Tsukui *et al.*, 1986). Further studies, performed using salt-stored human zonae pellucidae (Yanagimachi *et al.*, 1979) that were bisected to allow each egg to act as its own control, have demonstrated that antibodies directed against the sperm head can affect zona binding (Mahoney *et al.*, 1990), but not in every case. This result suggests that the zona binding impairment depends on the antigens against which antibodies are directed, that is, whether these antigens are the functional epitopes of a zona receptor ligand.

Many studies also have been performed on the effect of antisperm antibodies on sperm–oolemmal fusion, using the ability of zona-free hamster oocytes to be penetrated by capacitated human spermatozoa. Yanagimachi *et al.* (1976) reported that hamster eggs removed from their vestments (the cumulus oophorus and the zona pellucida) could be penetrated by acrosome-reacted sperm of several species, including humans. Several investigators have shown that homologous antibodies can affect the penetration of hamster oocytes by human spermatozoa (Alexander, 1984; Dor *et al.*, 1981; Requeda *et al.*, 1983; Haas *et al.*, 1985; Abdel-Latif *et al.*, 1986). In some studies, the inhibitory properties were found to be retained by IgG fractions of antisera (Haas *et al.*, 1980; Alexander, 1984). In one study, the Fab fractions from three antisera also were found to be inhibitory (Menge *et al.*, 1984). In apparent contrast with these findings, Bronson *et al.* (1981) found that some sera containing antisperm antibodies promote the penetration of zona-free hamster eggs by human spermatozoa after enhancing their oolemmal adhesion. These observations were confirmed by Aitken *et al.* (1987,1988), who showed that purified IgG from sera of patients containing antisperm antibodies can promote human sperm penetration of zona-free hamster eggs, inhibit penetration, or be inactive. Bronson *et al.* (1990a) observed that, when antisperm antibodies promoted penetration, the number of oolemmal-adherent antibody-labeled sperm was increased greatly (Table V). However, once these antibody-labeled sperm adhered to the oolemma, their chance of penetrating the egg was the same as that of antibody-free spermatozoa from the same ejaculate. This finding suggests that the promotion of egg penetration by antisperm antibodies is caused solely by their promotion of sperm–oolemmal binding. Evidence has been presented that Fcγ receptors, present on the oolemma of both hamster (Bronson *et al.*, 1990b) and human (Bronson *et al.*, 1991) oocytes, may account for the increased adherence of antibody-labeled sperm to eggs. Zona-free hamster eggs, preincubated with IgG Fc to occupy oolemmal Fcγ receptors, bound fewer IgG-labeled spermatozoa than unexposed eggs. Via Fab preparations of monoclonal antibodies directed against FcγRI, FcγRII, and FcγRIII, all three receptors were demonstrated to be present on the oolemma of unfertilized human eggs; their ability to bind human and murine IgG-Fc was shown also (Bronson *et al.*, 1991). The promotion of oolemmal binding of spermatozoa coated with antisperm antibodies via the interaction of oolemmal Fc receptors and the Fc portion of immunoglobulins could lead to a higher number of sperm penetrations. This mechanism could result *in vivo* in polyspermic fertilization of oocytes, diminishing the chances of reproductive success, since polyploid embryos exhibit diminished preimplantation growth potential and a higher rate of spontaneous abortion (Hassold *et al.*, 1980).

Conversely, in cases in which the penetration of oocytes is inhibited by antisperm antibodies, these antibodies are likely to be directed against fertilization antigens that play a role in sperm–egg plasma membrane fusion. Antibodies directed against the rabbit antigens RSA-1, 2, and 3, which also cross-react with human spermatozoa, block penetration of zona-free hamster oocytes by these spermatozoa (O'Rand and Irons, 1984). Naz *et al.* (1984) have identified a 23-kDa sperm membrane glycoprotein (FA-1) and have demonstrated that a monoclonal antibody directed against FA-1 completely blocks the fertilization of zona-free hamster oocytes by human spermatozoa. The monoclonal antibody MH61, raised against human spermatozoa and reacting mainly with capacitated and acrosome-reacted sperm (being barely reactive with fresh sperm), was found to inhibit the penetration of hamster eggs by human spermatozoa almost completely (Okabe *et al.*, 1990).

Evidence that peptides containing the Arg–Gly–Asp sequence (RGD), a recognition sequence involved in many cell–cell adhesion mechanisms (Ruoslahti and Piershbacher, 1986), interfere with oolemmal adhesion and sperm penetration of hamster oocytes (Bronson and Fusi, 1990a,b), suggests that this sequence also is involved in the binding of spermatozoa by the oolemma. The presence of RGD-binding moieties on the oolemma of hamster (Bronson and Fusi, 1990a) and human (Fusi *et al.*, 1991) oocytes, and the detection of RGD-containing proteins such as fibronectin, vitronectin, and laminin on the surface of capacitated human spermatozoa (Fusi *et al.*, 1992a,c). might indicate that these molecules are involved in sperm–oolemmal interaction. Antisperm antibodies directed against these glycoproteins, either from infertile couples or produced experimentally, could inhibit pentration of hamster and human eggs by spermatozoa.

Table V Effects of Different Antisperm IgG, Directed against the Sperm Head, on the Ability of Human Spermatozoa to Adhere to and Penetrate Zona-Free Hamster Eggs

Serum number	Number of eggs	Mean oolemmal adherent sperm (range)	Eggs penetrated (%)	Penetrating sperm per egg
1	15	33 (12–64)	67	1.4
2	29	55 (27–85)	93	2.9
3	27	71 (43–121)	100	8.2
4	28	78 (49–112)	100	5.2
5	27	110 (68–152)	100	6.5
6	29	140 (92–184)	100	8.2
Control	29	25 (13–41)	78	1.7

Preliminary evidence for this idea comes from experiments in which *in vitro* exposure of human spermatozoa to monoclonal and polyclonal antifibronectin antibodies partially inhibits their binding to and penetration of hamster oocytes (Fusi and Bronson, 1991; Table VI).

Retrospective and prospective analysis of fertilization data from programs performing *in vitro* fertilization provide another means of assessing the possible effects of antisperm antibodies on fertilization. Clarke and associates (1985b,1986) have shown that fertilization could be achieved at higher frequences in women with humoral antisperm antibodies when culture medium was supplemented with nonimmune serum in place of the patient serum. These data suggest that the presence of antisperm antibodies in the *in vitro* fertilization culture medium results in an impairment of fertilization. Immunoglobulins of the IgA class appeared to be more effective in impairing fertilization than those of the IgG class. A more critical examination of the results of *in vitro* fertilization in women with immunities to sperm has revealed both a diminished fertilization rate and a diminished embryonic cleavage rate, resulting ultimately in a diminished chance of pregnancy (Vasquez-Levin *et al.*, 1991). In this study, bovine serum albumin was used in the culture medium in lieu of patient serum if significant levels of serum antisperm antibodies were present. In these women, 44% of eggs were fertilized in 50 cycles compared with 75% for the bovine serum albumin controls. The percentage of high-quality embryos was 49% in the immunologically infertile group compared with 75% for the control subjects. Clinical pregnancies occurred in 10 individuals of the former group, compared with 18 in the latter. Although the results are promising because they illustrate that significant pregnancy rates can be achieved in these couples despite the presence of antisperm antibodies, these results suggest that these antibodies cannot be eliminated from the egg by washing, hence impairing fertilization, or that the antibodies may be cytotoxic to the egg.

Clarke *et al.* (1985a) and De Almeida *et al.* (1989) studied the relationship between antisperm antibodies in the ejaculates of men with autoimmunity to sperm and human *in vitro* fertilization. Both groups found that, when more than 80% of spermatozoa were labeled with head-directed IgA or a combination of IgA and IgG, a low fertilization rate of human oocytes was seen. In another study, Junk *et al.* (1986) suggested that fertilization rates were affected adversely if the autoimmunity against spermatozoa was caused by associated IgG and IgA antibodies, whereas impairment was less evident when only IgG or IgA was present. These researchers concluded that inhibition of fertilization may be caused by a synergistic effect of both classes of antibodies. Although these studies are suggestive, the analysis of the effects of antisperm antibodies on *in vitro* fertilization is quite difficult. In effect, the small number of patients makes a serious statistical analysis difficult because the association of nonimmunological factors relating to egg quality and sperm penetrating ability may bias the results in a group.

D. Effects of Antisperm Antibodies on Reproduction after Fertilization

Evidence that spermatozoa share antigenic specificities with fertilized ova and cleaving embryos has been demonstrated by several authors in several mammalian species. In guinea pigs (Behrman and Otani, 1963; Otani *et al.*, 1963; Kiddy and Rollins, 1973) and in rabbits (Sawada and Behrman, 1966), researchers have shown that immunization with spermatozoa had little effect on fertilization but resulted in a much greater incidence of postfertilization embryonic losses. Menge (1970), using rabbits, demonstrated that isoimmunization of females with sperm or testis, but not seminal plasma, resulted in an impaired chance of embryonic survival to term. In addition, a reduction in the survival of fertilized eggs transferred to immunized pseudo-pregnant females was observed in relation to those transferred to nonimmunized controls. Subsequently, the same authors (Menge and Lieberman, 1974; Menge *et al.*, 1974) found that antisperm IgA obtained from the uterus of rabbits immunized with homologous spermatozoa led to degenerative changes in morulas and blastocysts when cultured *in vitro* in its presence, whereas antisperm IgG did not. Menge and Naz (1988) suggested three mechanisms by which antisperm antibodies can affect embryo survival.

The first mechanism consists of the possibility that sperm surface antigens are incorporated into the zygotic membrane at fertilization. Fertilization involves the fusion of sperm and oolemma plasma membranes, leading to a mixture of anti-

Table VI Effects of Anti-Fibronectin Antibodies on the Adhesion and Penetration of Zona-Free Hamster Eggs by Human Spermatozoa

Antibody	Eggs penetrated (%)	Penetrating sperm per egg	Number of oolemmal adherent sperm
Mouse anti-FN Monoclonal Antibody	6.6	0.06 ($p = 0.001^a$)	26.2 ± 7.5 ($p = 0.005^a$)
Rabbit anti-FN Polyclonal Antibody	16.6	0.16 ($p = 0.001^a$)	27.9 ± 5.4 ($p = 0.005^a$)
Control[b]	89	1.24	45.4 ± 9.4
Antibody-Free Medium	100	1.45	56.9 ± 12.4

[a] Student *t* test of anti-fibronectin antibody versus the MOPC21-containing control.
[b] Control consisted of MOPC21, a mouse myeloma IgG protein.

gens. In rabbits, O'Rand (1977) presented evidence that sperm antigens were transferred to eggs after fertilization. Gaunt (1983) showed the same phenomenon in rats, using a monoclonal antibody directed against a single antigen, and demonstrated that the incorporated antigen was no longer present on the zygote plasma membrane after the first cleavage division. In humans, Wiley *et al.* (1987) demonstrated that some antisperm antibodies present in sera of infertile couples could react with hamster oocytes penetrated by human spermatozoa, as judged by complement-dependent lysis, but not with unpenetrated oocytes, suggesting that antigens could be transferred to the oolemma at the time of fertilization.

The second mechanism proposed is that similar epitopes are present on spermatozoa and embryos. Several common antigens have been found, including the nervous system antigens NS-4 and NS-7 (Solter and Schachner, 1976; Chaffee and Schachner, 1978). Oncofetal antigens also have been observed on both sperm and embryos, for example, teratocarcinoma antigen OTT6050 (Webb, 1980), PCCC4 (Gachelin *et al.*, 1977) PYS-2 (Artzt *et al.*, 1976), and F-9 (Artzt *et al.*, 1973). Antibodies raised against teratocarcinoma cells, mainly those directed against F-9 (Hamilton *et al.*, 1979; Johnson *et al.*, 1979), have been reported to induce both infertility and preimplantation loss (Hamilton *et al.*, 1979). Different antigens, such as the TLX antigen (Anderson *et al.*, 1989) commonly found on trophoblasts, also have been found on sperm surfaces after capacitation.

Another proposed mechanism to account for postfertilization reproductive loss mediated by antisperm antibodies is an indirect effect of antibodies on embryo development. The release of lymphokines, monokines, interleukins, and tumor necrosis factors from women sensitized to sperm after their exposure to semen could affect embryo development. Several studies, in fact, have demonstrated that those substances are cytotoxic to preimplanting embryos (Faikih *et al.*, 1987; Hill *et al.*, 1987b). However, despite laboratory data, no clear clinical evidence has been found in humans for an association between perinidatory early pregnancy loss and immunities to spermatozoa.

V. SUMMARY

Antisperm antibodies are able to interfere, through several mechanisms, with all stages of human fertilization, and may exhibit postfertilization effects on embryonic growth as well. Antisperm antibodies of the IgA class appear to be particularly able to affect reproductive outcome of patients sensitized to spermatozoa, suggesting that the local immune response could be important in infertile couples. Several of the mechanisms responsible for these effects appear to involve specific antigens, whereas others (particularly those impairing sperm transport) may be related to the Fc portion of the immunoglobulin molecule. Hence, the determination of the epitopes specifically involved in binding of spermatozoa to the zona pellucida and in sperm–oolemmal interaction appears to be a necessary step in the assessment of the reproductive prognosis of these individuals.

Spermatozoa must traverse the female reproductive tract, a part of the greater common mucosal immune system, to reach the oocyte. That the interaction of gametes occurs therein suggests that aberrant local immunological responses could play a significant role in human infertility. Increasing knowledge of the normal regulation of immunoglobulin production and secretion within the genital tracts of men and women, as well as of the response of the mucosal immune system of the reproductive tracts to microbial pathogens, will allow us to substantiate this thesis.

References

Abdel-Latif, A., Mathur, S., Rust, P. F., Fredericks, C. M., Abdel-Aal, H., and Williamson, H. O. (1986). Cytotoxic sperm antibodies inhibit sperm penetration of zona-free hamster eggs. *Fertil. Steril.* **45,** 542–549.

Aitken, R. J., Hulme, M. J., Henderson, C. T., Hargreave, T., and Ross, A. (1987). Analysis of the surface labelling characteristics of human spermatozoa and the interaction with anti-sperm antibodies. *J. Reprod. Fertil.* **80,** 473–485.

Aitken, R. J., Parslow, J. M., Hargreave, T. B., and Hendry, W. F. (1988). Influence of antisperm antibodies on human sperm function. *Br. J. Urol.* **62,** 367–373.

Alexander, N. J. (1984). Antibodies to human spermatozoa impede sperm penetration of cervical mucus or hamster eggs. *Fertil. Steril.* **41,** 433–439.

Alexander, N. J., and Anderson, D. J. (1979). Vasectomy: Consequences of autoimmunity to sperm antigens. *Fertil. Steril.* **32,** 253–259.

Allardyce, R. A. (1984). Effect of ingested sperm on fecundity in the rat. *J. Exp. Med.* **159,** 1548–1551.

Anderson, D. J., Johnson, P. M., Alexander, N. J., Jones, W. R., and Griffin, P. D. (1987). Monoclonal antibodies to human trophoblast and sperm antigens: Report of two WHO-sponsored workshops, June 30, 1986- Toronto, Canada. *J. Reprod. Immunol.* **10,** 231–257.

Anderson, D. J., Michaelson, J. S., and Johnson, P. M. (1989). Trophoblast/leukocyte-common antigen is expressed by human testicular germ cells and appears on the surface of acrosome reacted sperm. *Biol. Reprod.* **41,** 285–293.

Arnold, R., Mestecky, J., and McGhee, J. R. (1976). Naturally occurring secretory immunoglobulin A antibodies to *Streptococcus mutans* in human colostrum and saliva. *Infect. Immunol.* **14,** 355–362.

Artzt, K., Dubois, P. H., Bennet, D., Condamine, H., Babinet, C., and Jacob, F. (1973). Surface antigens common to mouse cleavage embryos and primitive teratocarcinoma cells in culture. *Proc. Natl. Acad. Sci. U.S.A.* **70,** 2988–2992.

Artzt, K., Hamburger, L., and Jakob, H. (1976). Embryonic surface antigens: A "quasi-endodermal" teratoma antigen. *Dev. Biol.* **51,** 152–157.

Beer, A. E., and Billingham, R. E. (1978). Immunoregulatory aspects of pregnancy. *Fed. Proc.* **37,** 2374–2379.

Behrman, S. J., and Otani, Y. (1963). Transvaginal immunization of the guinea pig with homologous testis and epidydimal sperm. *Int. J. Fertil.* **8,** 829–834.

Bronson, R. A., and Cooper, G. W. (1987). Effect of sperm-reactive monoclonal antibodies on the cervical mucus penetrating ability of human spermatozoa. *Am. J. Reprod. Immunol. Microbiol.* **14,** 59–61.

Bronson, R. A., and Cooper, G. W. (1988). Documentation of IgA1 and IgA2 antisperm antibodies within seminal fluid. *Am. J. Reprod. Immunol.* **18,** 7–10.

Bronson, R. A., and Fusi, F. (1990a). Evidence that an Arg-Gly-Asp (RGD) sequence plays a role in mammalian fertilization. *Biol. Reprod.* **43,** 1019–1025.

Bronson, R. A., and Fusi, F. (1990b). Sperm-oolemmal interaction: role of the RGD adhesion peptide. *Fertil. Steril.* **36,** 778–783.

Bronson, R. A., Cooper, G. W., and Rosenfeld, D. L. (1981). Ability of antibody-bound sperm to penetrate zona-free hamster eggs. *Fertil. Steril.* **36,** 778–783.

Bronson, R. A., Cooper, G. W., and Rosenfeld, D. L. (1982a). Sperm-specific isoantibodies and autoantibodies inhibit the binding of human sperm to the human zona pellucida. *Fertil. Steril.* **38,** 724–729.

Bronson, R. A., Cooper, G. W., and Rosenfeld, D. L. (1982b). Correlation between regional specificity of antisperm antibodies to the spermatozoan surface and complement-mediated sperm immobilization. *Am. J. Reprod. Immunol.* **2,** 222–225.

Bronson, R. A., Cooper, G. W., Rosenfeld, D. W., Gold, J., Kaplan, M., and Brody, N. (1983). Comparison of antisperm antibodies in homosexual and infertile men with autoimmunity to spermatozoa. Paper presented at the 30th Annual Meeting of the Society for Gynecologic Investigation, March 17–20. Washington, D.C.

Bronson, R. A., Cooper, G. W., and Rosenfeld, D. L. (1984a). Autoimmunity to spermatozoa: Effect on sperm penetration of cervical mucus as reflected by postcoital testing. *Fertil. Steril.* **41,** 609–614.

Bronson, R. A., Cooper, G. W., and Rosenfeld, D. L. (1984b). Sperm antibodies: Their role in infertility. *Fertil. Steril.* **42,** 171–183.

Bronson, R. A., Cooper, G. W., Rosenfeld, D. L., Gilbert, J. V., and Plaut, A. G. (1987a). The effect of an IgA1 protease on immunoglobulins bound to the sperm surface and sperm cervical mucus penetrating ability. *Fertil. Steril.* **47,** 985–991.

Bronson, R. A., Cooper, G. W., and Phillips, D. M. (1987b). Effects of sperm-reactive antibodies and complement on the ultrastructure of human spermatozoa. *Ann. N.Y. Acad. Sci.* **513,** 574–576.

Bronson, R. A., Fusi, F., Cooper, G. W., and Phillips, D. M. (1990a). Antisperm antibodies induce polyspermy by promoting adherence of human sperm to zona-free hamster eggs. *Hum. Reprod.* **5,** 690–696.

Bronson, R. A., Fleit, H. B., and Fusi, F. (1990b). Identification of an oolemmal Fc receptor: Its role in promoting binding of antibody-labelled human sperm to zona-free hamster eggs. *Am. J. Reprod. Immunol.* **23,** 87–92.

Bronson, R. A., Fusi, F. M., and Fleit, H. B. (1992). Monoclonal antibodies indentify Fcγ Receptors on unfertilized human oocytes but not spermatozoa. *J. Reprod. Immunol.* **49,** 887–896.

Chaffee, J. K., and Schachner, M. (1978). NS-7 (nervous system antigen-7): A cell surface antigen of mature brain, kidney and spermatozoa shared by embryonal tissues and transformed cells. *Dev. Biol.* **62,** 185–192.

Chang, T. W. (1976). Familial allergic seminal vulvovaginitis. *Am. J. Obstet. Gynecol.* **126,** 442–444.

Clarke, G. N. (1988). Sperm antibodies and human fertilization. *Am. J. Reprod. Immunol. Microbiol.* **17,** 65–71.

Clarke, G. N., Stojanoff, A., Cauchi, M. N., McBain, J. C., Speirs, A. L., and Johnston, W. I. H. (1984a). Detection of antispermatozoal antibodies of IgA class in cervical mucus. *Am. J. Reprod. Immunol.* **5,** 61–65.

Clarke, G. N., Hsieh, C., Koh, S. H., and Cauchi, M. N. (1984b). Sperm antibodies, immunoglobulins and complement in human follicular fluid. *Am. J. Reprod. Immunol.* **5,** 179–182.

Clarke, G. N., Lopata, A., McBain, J. C., Baker, H. W. G., and Johnston, W. I. H. (1985a). Effect of sperm antibodies in males in human in vitro fertilization (IVF). *Am. J. Reprod. Immunol. Microbiol.* **8,** 62–66.

Clarke, G. N., McBain, J. C., Lopata, A., and Johnston, W. I. H. (1985b). In vitro fertilization results for women with sperm antibodies in plasma and follicular fluid. *Am. J. Reprod. Immunol. Microbiol.* **8,** 130–131.

Clarke, G. N., Lopata, A., and Johnston, W. I. H. (1986). Effect of sperm antibodies in females on human in vitro fertilization. *Fertil. Steril.* **46,** 435–441.

Crago, S. S., Kutteh, W. H., Prince, S. J., Radl, J., Haaijman, J. J., and Mestecky, J. (1983). Distribution of IgA1 and IgA2 subclasses in human tissue: correlation with the presence of J-chain. *Ann. N.Y. Acad. Sci.* **409,** 803–812.

Crago, S. S., Kutteh, W. H., Allansmith, M. R., Radl, J., Haaijman, J. J. and Mestecky, J. (1984). Distribution of IgA1, IgA2 and J chain containing cells in human tissue. *J. Immunol.* **132,** 16–18.

Cunningham, D. S., Fulgham, D. L., Rayl, D. L., Hansen, K. A., and Alexander, N. J., (1991). Antisperm antibodies to sperm surface antigens in women with genital tract infection. *Am. J. Obstet. Gynecol.* **164,** 791–796.

D'Cruz, O. J., Haas, G. G., and Lambert, H. (1990). Evaluation of antisperm complement-dependent immune mediators in human ovarian follicular fluid. *J. Immunol.* **144,** 3841–3848.

D'Cruz, O. J., Haas, G. G., de La Rocha, R., and Lambert, H. (1991). Occurrence of serum antisperm antibodies in patients with cystic fibrosis. *Fertil. Steril.* **56,** 519–527.

DeAlmeida, M., Gazagne, I., Jeulin, C., Herry, M., Belaisch-Allart, J., Frydman, R., Jouannet, P., and Testart, J. (1989). In vitro processing of sperm with autoantibodies and in vitro fertilization results. *Hum. Reprod.* **4,** 49–53.

Delacroix, D. L., Elkon, K. B., and Vaerman, J. P. (1983). IgA size and IgA subclass distribution in serum and secretions. *Ann. N.Y. Acad. Sci.* **409,** 812–827.

Dor, J., Rudak, E., and Aitken, R. J. (1981). Antisperm antibodies: Their effect on the process of fertilization studied in vitro. *Fertil. Steril.* **35,** 535–541.

El-Demiry, M., and James, K. (1988). Lymphocyte subsets and macrophages in the male genital tract in health and disease. *Eur. J. Urol.* **14,** 226–245.

Faikih, H., Baggett, B., Holtz, G., Tsang, K., Lee, J., and Williamson, H. (1987). Interleukin I: A possible role in the infertility associated with endometriosis. *Fertil. Steril.* **47,** 213–217.

Fjallbrant, B. (1969). Cervical mucus penetration by human spermatozoa treated with anti-spermatozoal antibodies from rabbit and man. *Acta Obstet. Gynecol. Scand.* **48,** 71–77.

Fowler, J. E., and Mariano, M. (1982). Immunologic response of the prostate to bacteria and bacterial prostatitis. II. Antigen specific immunoglobulin in prostatic fluid. *J. Urol.* **128,** 105–115.

Fusi, F. M., and Bronson, R. A. (1992a). Sperm surface fibronectin, expression following capacitation. *J. Androl.* **13,** 28–35.

Fusi, F. M., Vignali, M., Busacca, M., and Bronson, R. A. (1992b). Evidence for the presence of an integrin cell adhesion receptor on the oolemma of unfertilized human oocytes. *Mol. Reprod. Develop.* **31,** 215–222.

Fusi, F. M., Lorenzetti, I., Vignali, M., and Bronson, R. A. (1992c). Sperm surface proteins following capacitation: expression of vitronectin on the equatorial segment and laminin on the sperm tail. *J. Androl.* **13,** 488–497.

Gachelin, G., Kemler, R., Kelly, F., and Jacob, F. (1977). PCC4, a new cell surface antigen common to multipotential embryonal carcinoma cells, spermatozoa, and mouse early embryo. *Dev. Biol.* **57,** 199–209.

Gaunt, S. J. (1983). Spreading of a sperm surface antigen within the plasma membrane of the egg after fertilization in the rat. *J. Embryol. Exp. Morphol.* **75,** 259–270.

Gilula, N. B., Fawcett, D. W., and Aoki, A., (1976). The Sertoli cell occluding junctions and gap junctions in mature and developing mammalian testis. *Dev. Biol.* **50,** 142–148.

Guazziero, S., Lembo, A., Ferro, G., Artibani, W., Merlo, F., Zanchetta, R., and Pagano, F. (1985). Sperm antibodies and infertility in patients with testicular cancer. *Urology* **26,** 139–144.

Haas, G. G. (1986). The inhibitory effect of sperm-associated immunoglobulins on cervical mucus penetration. *Fertil. Steril.* **46,** 334–337.

Haas, G. G., and Beer, A. E. (1986). Immunologic influences on reproductive biology: Sperm gametogenesis and maturation in the male and female genital tract. *Fertil. Steril.* **46,** 753–765.

Haas, G. G., Sokoloski, J. E., and Wolf, D. P. (1980). The interfering effect of human IgG antisperm antibodies on human sperm penetration of zona-free hamster eggs. *Am. J. Reprod. Immunol. Microbiol.* **1,** 40–43.

Haas, G. G., Ausmanas, M., Culp, L., Tureck, R. W., and Blasco, L. (1985). The effect of immunoglobulin occurring on human sperm in vivo on the human sperm/hamster ova penetration assay. *Am. J. Reprod. Immunol. Microbiol.* **7,** 109–112.

Haensch, R. (1973). Spermatozoen-Autoimmunphaenomene bei Genitaltraumen und Verschlubbazoospermie. *Andrologia* **5,** 147–151.

Halpern, B. N., Ky, T., and Robert, B. (1967). Clinical and immunological study of an exceptional case of reaginic type sensitization to human seminal fluid. *Immunology* **12,** 247–254.

Hamilton, D. W. (1975). Structure and function of the epithelium lining the ductuli efferentes, ductus epididymis and ductus deferens. *In* "Handbook of Physiology" (R. O. Greep, and A. B. Astwood, eds.), p. 259. American Physiological Society, Washington, D.C.

Hamilton, M. S., May, R. D., Beer, A. E., and Vitetta, E. S. (1979). The influence of immunization of female mice with F-9 teratocarcinoma cells on their reproductive performance. *Transplant. Proc.* **11,** 1069–1072.

Hassold, T. J., Chan, N., Funkhauser, S., Jooss, T., Manuel, R., Matsuura, J., Matsuyama, A., Wilson, C., Yamane, T. A., and Jacobss, P. A. (1980). A cytogenetic study of 1000 human abortions. *Ann. Hum. Genet.* **44,** 151–178.

Hellstrom, W. J. G., Overstreet, J. W., Samuels, S. J., and Lewis, E. I. (1988). The relationship pf circulating antisperm antibodies to sperm surface antibodies in infertile men. *J. Urol.* **140,** 1039–1044.

Hendry, W. F., Parslow, J., Stedronska, J., and Wallace, D. M. A. (1982). The diagnosis of unilateral testicular obstruction in subfertile males. *Br. J. Urol.* **54,** 774–777.

Heremans, J. F., and Bazin, H. (1971). Antibodies induced by local antigenic stimulation of mucosal surfaces. *Ann. N.Y. Acad. Sci.* **190,** 268–275.

Hill, J. A., Barbieri, R. L., and Anderson, D. J. (1987a). Detection of T8 (suppressor/cytotoxic) lymphocytes in human ovarian follicular fluid. *Fertil. Steril.* **47,** 114–117.

Hill, J. A., Florina, H., and Anderson, D. J. (1987b). Products of activated lymphocytes and macrophages inhibit mouse embryo development. *J. Immunol.* **139,** 2250–2254.

Hjort, T., Husted, S., and Linnet-Jepsen, P. (1974). The effect of testis biopsy on autosensitization against spermatozoal antigens. *Clin. Exp. Immunol.* **18,** 201–209.

Huang, T. T. F., Tung, K. S. K., and Yanagimachi, R. (1981). Autoantibodies from vasectomized guinea pigs inhibit fertilization in vitro. *Science* **213,** 1267–1269.

Humphrey, J. H., and Dourmashkin, R. R. (1965). Electron microscopic studies on immune cell lysis. *In* "CIBA Foundation Symposium: Complement," (G. E. W. Wolstenholme and J. Knight, eds.) p. 175–189. Little, Brown, Boston.

Hurtenbach, U., Morgenstern, F., and Bennet, D. (1980). Induction of tolerance in vitro by autologous murine testicular cells. *J. Exp. Med.* **151,** 827–838.

Jager, S., Kremer, J., Kuiken, J., Van Slochteren-Draaisma, T., Mulder, I., and DeWilde-Janssen, I. W. (1981a). Induction of the shaking phenomenon by pretreatment of spermatozoa with sera containing antispermatozoal antibodies. *Fertil. Steril.* **36,** 784–791.

Jager, S., Kremer, J., Kuiken, J., and Mulder, I. (1981b). The significance of the Fc part of antispermatozoal antibodies for the shaking phenomenon in the sperm-cervical mucus contact. *Fertil. Steril.* **36,** 792–797.

James, K., and Szymaniesc, S. (1985). Human seminal plasma is a potent inhibitor of natural killer cell activity in vitro. *J. Reprod. Immunol.* **8,** 61–76.

Jette, N. T., and Glass, R. H. (1972). Prognostic value of the postcoital test. *Fertil. Steril.* **23,** 29–36.

Johnson, L., Petty, C. S., and Neaves, W. B. (1983). Further quantification of human spermatogenesis: Germ cell loss during postprophase of meiosis and its relationship to daily sperm production. *Biol. Reprod.* **29,** 207–213.

Johnson, M. H., Chakraabarty, J., Hanyside, A. H., Willison, K., and Stern, P. (1979). The effect of prolonged decompaction on the development of the preimplantation mouse embryo. *J. Embryol. Exp. Morphol.* **54,** 241–261.

Jones, R. C. (1977). The nature of the barrier to autoimmunity in the excurrent ducts of the mammalian testes. *In* "Immunological Influences on Human Fertility" (B. Boettcher, ed.), p. 67–85. Academic Press, New York.

Junk, S. M., Matson, P. L., Yovich, Y. M., Bootsma, B., and Yovich, J. L. (1986). The fertilization of human oocytes by spermatozoa from men with antispermatozoal antibodies in semen. *J. in Vitro Fert. Embryo Transfer.* **3,** 350–352.

Kett, K., Brandtzaeg, D., and Radl, J. (1986). Different subclass distribution of IgA-producing cells in human lymphoid organs and various secretory tissues. *J. Immunol.* **136,** 3631–3635.

Kiddy, C. A., and Rollins, R. M. (1973). Infertility in female guinea pigs injected with testis. *Biol. Reprod.* **8,** 545–549.

Kormana, M., and Reijonen, K. (1976). Microvascular structure of the human epididymis. *Am. J. Anat.* **145,** 23–41.

Kremer, J., and Jager, S. (1980). Characteristics of anti-spermatozoal antibodies responsible for the shaking phenomena with special regard to immunoglobulin class and antigen-reactive sites. *Int. J. Androl.* **3,** 143–152.

Kutteh, W. H., Hatch, K. D., Blackwell, R. E., and Mestecky, J. (1988). Secretory immune system of the female reproductive tract: I. Immunoglobulin and secretory component-containing cells. *Obst. Gynecol.* **71,** 56–60.

Kutteh, W. H., Blackwell, R. E., Gore, H., Kutteh, C. C., Carr, B. R., and Mestecky, J. (1990). Secretory immune system of the female reproductive tract. II. Local immune system in normal and infected fallopian tube. *Fertil. Steril.* **54,** 51–55.

Lansford, B., Haas, G. G., DeBault, L. E., and Wolf, D. P. (1988). Effect of antisperm antibodies on the acrosomal reactivity of human sperm. *In* "The American Fertility Society Program and Abstracts," 44th Annual Meeting, Atlanta, October 10–13, p. 522.

Lint, T. F. (1980). Complement. *In* "Immunological Aspects of Infertility and Fertility Regulation," D. F. Dhindsa and G. F. B. Schmacher, eds.), pp. 13–21. Elsevier/North-Holland, New York.

London, S. N., Haney, A. F., and Weinberg, J. B. (1985). Macrophages and infertility: Enhancement of human macrophage-mediated sperm killing by antisperm antibodies. *Fertil. Steril.* **43,** 274–278.

Lord, E. K., Senabaugh, G. F., and Stites, D. P. (1977). Immunosoppressive activity of human seminal plasma: I. Inhibition of in vitro lymphocyte activation. *J. Immunol.* **118,** 1706–1711.

Lutjen, P. J., McBain, J. C., and Trounson, A. O. (1984). Biochemical aspects of spermatozoal cervical mucus interaction. *Proc. Fertil. Soc. Aust.* **3,** 26–34.

McGhee, J. R., and Mestecky, J. (1990). In defense of mucosal surfaces. *Infert. Dis. Clin. North Am.* **4,** 315–341.

Mahoney, M. C., Alexander, N. J., and Bronson, R. A. (1991). Inhibition of human sperm-zona pellucida tight binding in the presence of antisperm antibody positive polyclonal patient sera. *J. Reprod. Immunol.* **19,** 287–290.

Marcus, Z. H., Freisheim, J. H., and Houk, J. L. (1978). In vitro studies in reproductive immunology: I. Suppression of cell-mediated immune response by human spermatozoa and fractions isolated from human seminal plasma. *Clin. Immunol. Immunopathol.* **9,** 318–323.

Marcus, Z. H., Misgav, N., and Zacut, H. (1984). Inhibition of natural killer cell activity by a fraction of human seminal plasma. *IRCS Med. Sci.* **12,** 897–903.

Mastrogiacomo, I., Zanchetta, R., Graziotti, P., Betterle, C., Scrufari, P., and Lembo, A. (1982). Immunological and clinical study in patients after spermatic cord torsion. *Andrologia* **14,** 25–29.

Mathur, S., Williamson, H. O., Baker, E. R., and Fudenberg, H. H. (1981). Immunoglobulin E levels and antisperm antibody titers in infertile couples. *Am. J. Obstet. Gynecol.* **140,** 923–930.

Mathur, S., Williamson, H. O., Genco, P. V., Koopman, W. R., Jr., Rust, P. F., and Fudenberg, H. H. (1983). Sperm immunity in infertile couples: Antibody titers are higher against the husband's sperm than to sperm from controls. *Am. J. Reprod. Immunol.* **3,** 18–22.

Mathur, S., Chao, L., Goust, J., Milroy, G. T., Woodley-Miller, C., Caldwell, J. Z., Daru, J., and Williamson, H. O. (1988). Special antigens on sperm from autoimmune infertile men. *Am. J. Reprod. Immunol.* **17,** 5–13.

Meinertz, H., Linnet, L., Fogh-Anderson, P., and Hjort, T. (1990). Antisperm antibodies and fertility after vasovasostomy. *Fertil. Steril.* **54,** 315–321.

Meinertz, H., Linnet, L., Wolf, H., and Hjort, T. (1991). Antisperm antibodies on epididymal spermatozoa. *Am. J. Reprod. Immunol.* **25,** 158–162.

Menge, A. C. (1970). Immune reactions and infertility. *J. Reprod. Fertil.* (*Suppl.*) **10,** 171–186.

Menge, A. C., and Lieberman, M. E. (1974). Antifertility effects of immunoglobulins from uterine fluids of semen-immunized rabbits. *Biol. Reprod.* **10,** 422–428.

Menge, A. C., and Naz, R. K. (1988). Immunologic reactions involving sperm cells and preimplantation embryos. *Am. J. Reprod. Immunol. Microbiol.* **18,** 17–20.

Menge, A. C., Rosenberg, A., and Burkons, D. M. (1974). Effects of uterine fluids and immunoglobulins from semen-immunized rabbits on rabbit embryos cultured in vitro. *Proc. Soc. Exp. Biol. Med.* **145,** 371–378.

Menge, A. C., Mangione, C. M., Dietrich, J. W., and Black, C. S. (1984). Effect of antisperm antibodies in serum and cervical mucus on the capacity of human sperm to penetrate zona-free hamster ova. *Arch. Androl.* **12,** 83–88.

Mestecky, J., and McGhee, J. R. (1987). Immunoglobulin A (IgA): Molecular and cellular interactions involved in IgA biosynthesis and immune response. *Adv. Immunol.* **40,** 153–245.

Morgan, E. L. (1987). The role of prostaglandin in C3a-mediated suppression of human in vitro polyclonal antibody responses. *Clin. Immunol. Immunopathol.* **44,** 1–11.

Mortimer, D., Pandya, I. J., and Sawers, R. S., (1986). Relationship between sperm motility characteristics and sperm penetration into cervical mucus in vitro. *J. Reprod. Fertil.* **78,** 93–102.

Naz, R. K., Alexander, N. J., Isahakie, M., and Hamilton, M. S. (1984). Monoclonal antibody to a human germ cell membrane glycoprotein that inhibits fertilization. *Science* **225,** 342–344.

Ogra, P. L., and Ogra, S. S. (1973). Local antibody response to poliovaccine in the human female genital tract. *J. Immunol.* **110,** 1307–1311.

Okabe, M., Nagira, M., Kawai, Y., Matzno, M. S., Mimura, T., and Mayumi, T. (1990). A human sperm antigen possibly involved in binding and/or fusion with zona-free hamster eggs. *Fertil. Steril.* **54,** 1121–1126.

O'Rand, M. G. (1977). The presence of sperm specific isoantigens on the egg following fertilization. *J. Exp. Zool.* **202,** 267–293.

O'Rand, M. G. (1981). Inhibition of fertility and sperm-zona binding by antiserum to the rabbit sperm membrane auto-antigen RSA-1. *Biol. Reprod.* **25,** 621–628.

O'Rand, M. G., and Irons, G. P. (1984). Monoclonal antibodies to rabbit sperm autoantigens. II. Inhibition of human sperm penetration of zona-free hamster eggs. *Biol. Reprod.* **30,** 731–736.

Otani, Y., Behrman, S. J., Porter, C. W., and Nakayama, M. (1963). Reduction of fertility in immunized guinea pigs. *Int. J. Fertil.* **8,** 835–839.

Parr, E. L., and Parr, M. B. (1990). A comparison of antibody titres in mouse uterus found after immunization by several routes, and the effect of the uterus on titres in vaginal fluid. *J. Reprod. Fertil.* **89,** 619–625.

Parslow, J. M., Poulton, T. A., Bassee, G. M., and Hendry, W. F. (1985). The clinical relevance of classes of immunoglobulins on spermatozoa from infertile and vasovasostomized males. *Fertil. Steril.* **43,** 621–625.

Pavia, C. S., Stites, D. P., and Bronson, R. A. (1987). Reproductive Immunology. *In* "Basic and Clinical Immunology" (D. P. Stites, J. D. Stobo, and J. V. Wells, eds.), pp. 619–633. Appleton and Lange, Norwalk, Connecticut.

Plaut, A. G. (1983). The IgA1 proteases of bacteria. *Ann. Rev. Microbiol.* **37,** 603–665.

Price, R. J., and Boettcher, B. (1979). The presence of complement in human cervical mucus and its possible relevance to infertility in women with complement-dependent sperm immobilizing antibodies. *Fertil. Steril.* **32,** 61–67.

Requeda, E., Charron, J., Roberts, K. D., Chapdelaine, A., and Bleau, G. (1983). Fertilizing capacity and sperm antibodies in vasostomized men. *Fertil. Steril.* **39,** 197–203.

Richards, J. M., Bedford, J. M., and Witkin, S. S. (1984). Rectal insemination modifies immune responses in rabbits. *Science* **224,** 390–392.

Rumke, P. (1974). Origin of immunoglobulin in semen. *Clin. Exp. Immunol.* **12,** 287–297.

Ruoslahti, E., and Piershbacher, M. D. (1986). Arg-Gly-Asp: A versatile cell recognition signal. *Cell* **44,** 517–518.

Saling, P. M., and Lakoski, K. A. (1985). Mouse sperm antigens that participate in fertilization. II. Inhibition of sperm penetration through the zona pellucida using monoclonal antibodies. *Biol. Reprod.* **33,** 527–536.

Sawada, Y., and Behrman, S. J. (1966). Reduction of fertility in rabbits by isoimmunization: Mechanism of action. *Proc. Fifth World Congr. Exc. Med. Found.* **133,** 758–764.

Schumacher, G. F. B. (1980). Humoral immune factors in the female reproductive tract and their changes during the cycle. *In* "Immunological Aspects of Infertility and Fertility Regulation" (D. S. Dhindsa and G. F. B. Schumacher, eds.), p. 93. Elsevier/North-Holland, New York.

Shahmanesh, M., Stedronska, J., and Hendry, W. F. (1986). Antispermatozoal antibodies in men with urethritis. *Fertil. Steril.* **46,** 308–311.

Shearer, G. M., and Rabson, A. S. (1984). Semen and AIDS. *Nature (London)* **308,** 230–231.

Skinner, M. K., Cosand, W. L., and Griswold, M. D. (1984). Purification and characterization of testicular transferrin secreted by rat Sertoli cells. *Biochem. J.* **218,** 313–320.

Solter, D., and Schachner, M. (1976). Brain and sperm cell surface antigens (NS-4) on preimplantation mouse embryo. *Dev. Biol.* **52,** 98–104.

Tarter, T. H., and Alexander, N. J. (1984). Complement-inhibiting activity of seminal plasma. *Am. J. Reprod. Immunol.* **6,** 28–31.

Thaler, C. J., Faulk, W. P., and McIntyre, J. A., (1989). Soluble antigens of IgG gamma receptors in human seminal plasma. *J. Immunol.* **143,** 1937–1939.

Tsukui, S., Noda, Y., Yano, J., Fukuda, A., and Mori, T. (1986). Inhibition of sperm penetration through human zona pellucida by antisperm antibodies. *Fertil. Steril.* **46,** 92–96.

Tung, K. S. K., Yule, T. D., Mahi-Brown, C. A., and Listrom, M. B. (1987). Distribution of histopathology and Ia positive cells in actively induced and passively tranferred experimental autoimmune orchitis. *J. Immunol.* **138,** 752–759.

Vasquez-Levin, M., Kaplan, P., Guzman, I., Grunfeld, L., Garrisi, G. J., and Navot, D., (1991). The effect of female antisperm antibodies on in vitro fertilization, early embryonic development and pregnancy outcome. *Fertil. Steril.* **56,** 84–90.

Wang, C., Gordon Baker, H. W., Jennings, M. G., Burger, H. G., and Lutjen, P. (1985). Interaction between human cervical mucus and sperm surface antibodies. *Fertil. Steril.* **44,** 484–488.

Webb, C., (1980). Characterization of antisera against mouse teratocarcinoma OTT6050: Molecular species recognized on embryoid bodies, preimplantation embryos and sperm. *Dev. Biol.* **76,** 203–214.

Wiley, L. M., Obasaju, M. F., Overstreet, J. W., Cross, N. L., Hanson, F. W., and Chang, R. J., (1987). Detection of antisperm antibodies: Their localization to human sperm antigens that are transferred to the surface of zona-free hamster oocytes during the sperm penetration assay. *Fertil. Steril.* **48,** 292–298.

Wira, C. R., and Stern, J. E. (1992). Endocrine regulation of the mucosal immune system in the female reproductive tract: Control of IgA, IgG and secretory component during the reproductive cycle, at implantation and throughout pregnancy. *In* "Hormones and Fetal Pathophysiology" (J. R. Pasqualini and R. Scholler, eds.). pp. 343–367. Marcel Decker, New York.

Witkin, S. S. (1984). Suppressor T lymphocytes and cross-reactive sperm antigens in human semen. *AIDS Res.* **1,** 339–345.

Witkin, S. S. (1986). Selective activation of functional suppressor cells by human seminal fluid. *Clin. Exp. Immunol.* **64,** 364–369.

Witkin, S. S. (1987). Immunology of recurrent vaginitis. *Am. J. Reprod. Immunol.* **15,** 34–37.

Witkin, S. S. (1988). Mechanisms of active suppression of the immune response to spermatozoa. *Am. J. Reprod. Immunol. Microbiol.* **17,** 61–64.

Witkin, S. S., and Sonnabend, J. (1983). Immune response to spermatozoa in homosexual men. *Fertil. Steril.* **39,** 337–342.

Witkin, S. S., and Toth, A. (1983). Relationship between genital tract infections, sperm antibodies in seminal fluid, and infertility. *Fertil. Steril.* **40,** 805–808.

Witkin, S. S., Richards, J. M., and Bedford, J. M. (1983). Influence of epididymal maturation on the capacity of hamster and rabbit spermatozoa for complement activation. *J. Reprod. Fertil.* **69,** 517–521.

Wolf, D. P. (1989). Acrosomal status quantitation in human sperm. *Am. J. Reprod. Immunol.* **20,** 106–113.

Wolff, H., and Schill, W. B. (1985). Antisperm antibodies in infertile and homosexual men: Relationship to serologic and clinical findings. *Fertil. Steril.* **44,** 673–677.

Yanagimachi, R. (1988). Sperm-egg fusion. *In* "Current Topics in Membranes and Transport" (F. Bronner, ed.), pp. 3–43. Academic Press, Orlando, Florida.

Yanagimachi, R., Yanagimachi, H., and Rogers, B. J. (1976). The use of zona-free animal ova as a test-system for the assessment of the fertilizing capacity of human spermatozoa. *Biol. Reprod.* **15,** 471–476.

Yanagimachi, R., Lopata, A., Odom, C. B., Bronson, R. A., Mahi, C. A., and Nicolson, G. L. (1979). Retention of biologic characteristics of zona pellucida in highly concentrated salt solution: The use of salt stored eggs for assessing the fertilizing capacity of spermatozoa. *Fertil. Steril.* **31,** 562.

Yang, S. L., Schumacher, G. F. B., Broer, K. A., and Holt, J. A. (1983). Specific antibodies and immunoglobulins in the oviductal fluid of the rhesus monkey. *Fertil. Steril.* **39,** 359–369.

56

Endocrine Regulation of Mucosal Immunity: Effect of Sex Hormones and Cytokines on the Afferent and Efferent Arms of the Immune System in the Female Reproductive Tract

Charles R. Wira • Jan Richardson • Rao Prabhala

I. INTRODUCTION

Optimal immune protection at mucosal surfaces is dependent on the secretory immune system, which responds to both viral and bacterial pathogens (for reviews see Heremans, 1974; Mestecky and McGhee, 1987). Characterized by the presence of secretory IgA and IgG (Ogra *et al.*, 1981; Brandtzaeg and Prydz, 1984), immune protection is dependent on T and B lymphocytes, monocytes, and macrophages, as well as on other antigen-presenting cells that monitor the external environment and respond to antigenic challenge (McDermott and Bienenstock, 1979; Underdown and Schiff, 1986). After the recognition of antigen, immune protection is conferred through humoral and cell-mediated components of the mucosal immune system which respond by cytotoxic mechanisms (Shen and Fanger, 1981), the production of specific antibodies (Williams and Gibbons, 1972; Heremans, 1974), and phagocytosis (Fanger *et al.*, 1983) to destroy potential pathogens or exclude them from gaining access to the body.

Within the female reproductive tract, the mucosal immune system has evolved to protect against potential pathogens without compromising fetal survival (Harbour and Blalock, 1989; Wira and Stern, 1992). Periodically exposed to allogeneic sperm and to a fetal–placental unit that is immunologically distinct, the mucosal immune system within the uterus, cervix, and vagina is controlled precisely by the female sex hormones to optimize both maternal and fetal survival (Wira and Sandoe, 1977; Schumacher, 1980; Sullivan *et al.*, 1984). Depending on the site analyzed and the reproductive state (endocrine balance), immunocompetency of the female reproductive tract may be enhanced or suppressed to meet maternal and fetal needs (Wira and Stern, 1992).

Despite the effectiveness of immune protection, sexually transmitted diseases (STD) represent a major global health problem that threatens both adult and newborn (Cates, 1986; Piot *et al.*, 1988). The limited success achieved in controlling gonorrhea, herpes simplex virus 2, pelvic inflammatory disease, group B *Streptococcus*, *Chlamydia*, and human immunodeficiency virus (HIV), the causative agent of acquired immunodeficiency syndrome (AIDS) (Peterman and Curran, 1986; McDonough, 1987), demonstrates the need for a better understanding of the elements of the secretory immune system in the female reproductive tract and the ways in which the endocrine system regulates immune function at these sites.

Previous studies have shown that both oral and reproductive tract immunization can lead to the presence of specific antibodies in uterine and vaginal secretions. Ogra and Ogra (1973) demonstrated that inactivated poliovirus, given orally or deposited locally into the uterus or vagina of women, generated IgG antibodies in uterine and cervicovaginal secretions. In contrast, when horseradish peroxidase was placed in the uterus, no antibody response was detected (Vaerman and Ferin, 1974). Several studies focusing on vaginal and cervical deposition of antigen have demonstrated local antibody production in the lower genital tract (Kerr, 1955; Bell and Wolf, 1967; Yang and Schumacher, 1979; Parr *et al.*, 1988). That gastrointestinal, intrauterine, and pelvic immunization lead to the accumulation of antibodies in genital tract secretions (Wira and Sandoe, 1987,1989; Wira and Prabhala, 1992) also shows that specific IgA and IgG antibodies in uterine, cervical, and vaginal secretions are derived from distal and local (genital tract) exposure to antigen. Despite this progress, much remains to be learned about the mechanisms by which immune protection is conferred within the reproductive tract and the ways in which sex hormones and selected cytokines regulate immune events at mucosal surfaces.

Implicit in the ability of the female reproductive tract to respond to local antigen exposure is the requirement that antigen-presenting cells recognize and present antigen to T lymphocytes (Ziegler and Unanue, 1981; Weinberger *et al.*, 1981). At other sites in the body, for example, macrophages (Rosenthal and Shevach, 1973) as well as B lymphocytes (Ashwell *et al.*, 1984), dendritic cells (Steinman and Nussenzweig, 1980), keratinocytes (Gaspari and Katz, 1988), Langerhans cells (Aiba and Katz, 1991), and epithelial cells have been shown to present antigen. Antigen presentation is characterized by the internalization and processing of exogenous antigen to immunogenic fragments, which then are presented in combination with major histocompatibility complex (MHC) Class II molecules to T lymphocytes. These events, in turn, lead to the production of cytokines that mediate cellular and humoral immune responses (Balkwill and Burke, 1989). Despite the absence of aggregated follicles similar to Peyer's patches in the gastrointestinal tract, the reproductive tract contains B lymphocytes, macrophages, and dendritic cells as well as epithelial cells that are potentially capable of presenting antigen. Within the reproductive tract, endometrial cells of the uterus express MHC Class II molecules that are under estradiol and cytokine control (Head and Gaede, 1986; Tabibzadeh *et al.*, 1986a,b). The identification of interferon γ (IFNγ) receptors in the uterus (Tabibzadeh, 1990), interleukin 1 (IL-1) and IL-6 production by uterine cells (Takacs *et al.*, 1988; Tabibzadeh *et al.*, 1989), and the important observation that estradiol stimulates IFNγ mRNA production by lymphocytes (Fox *et al.*, 1991) provide evidence for the complex interactions that exist between hormones and cytokines in the regulation of mucosal immunity in the female reproductive tract.

In this chapter, we present studies from our laboratory that define the roles of steroid hormones in regulating the efferent (response) arm of the mucosal immune system in the female reproductive tract. We include our most recent findings that demonstrate that the afferent (inductive) arm of the immune system exists in the female reproductive tract and is controlled by sex hormones and cytokines. Particular attention is paid to the mechanisms by which hormones and cytokines exert their effects, during the reproductive cycle as well as after exogenous hormone administration. The data presented in this chapter indicate that the regulation of reproductive tract mucosal immunity is the result of a precise interplay between sex hormones and cytokines. Further, they indicate that sex hormones and cytokines, working together, are major contributors to the maintenance of immune function. Finally, these studies emphasize that immune function and its regulatory control within the fallopian tube, uterus, cervix, and vagina are separate and distinct, and that each site must be analyzed in the context of the unique contributions it makes to procreation and to maternal and fetal protection.

II. SEX HORMONE AND GLUCOCORTICOID REGULATION OF MUCOSAL IMMUNITY

Figure 1 shows results from our laboratory in 1977 that demonstrated that IgA and IgG levels in uterine secretions change markedly in intact rats during the reproductive cycle; higher levels are measured at the time of ovulation than at any other stage of the cycle (Wira and Sandoe, 1977). These observations led to the conclusion that estradiol and progesterone are the principle hormones responsible for regulating IgA and IgG in uterine secretions. As seen in Figure 2, when ovariectomized rats were treated with estradiol, IgA and IgG levels in uterine secretions were elevated relative to saline controls (Wira and Sandoe, 1980). We unexpectedly found that IgA and IgG levels in cervicovaginal secretions were controlled hormonally. Unlike the uterus, however, levels here were lowered in response to hormone treatment (Wira and Sullivan, 1985). These responses are separate and distinct, since uterine ligation had no effect on the hormone response of IgA and IgG to estradiol treatment. We also found that the uterine response was specific for estradiol, that progesterone blocks estradiol-stimulated increases in uterine

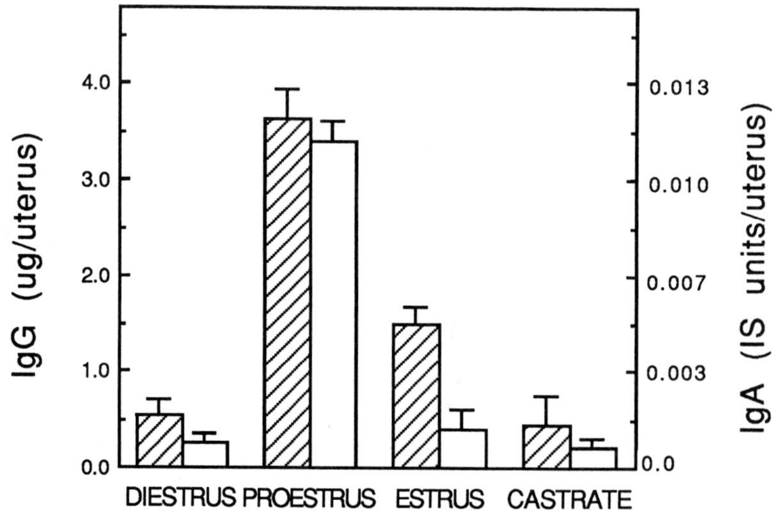

Figure 1 Immunoglobulin A and G levels in uterine secretions of adult female rats at various stages of the estrous cycle and following castration. Values represent the mean ± SEM of 5–8 rats per group. IgG values (open bars) are expressed as μg per uterus, IgA results (hatched bars) as immunocytoma serum (IS) units, where 1.0 IS unit is defined as a concentration of 1 mg lyophilized immunocytoma serum in 1 ml distilled water. Values of IgA and IgG at proestrus and IgA at estrus are significantly different from those measured during diestrus and following castration ($P < 0.01$). No significant differences were measured in serum samples. Adapted with permission from Wira and Sandoe (1977).

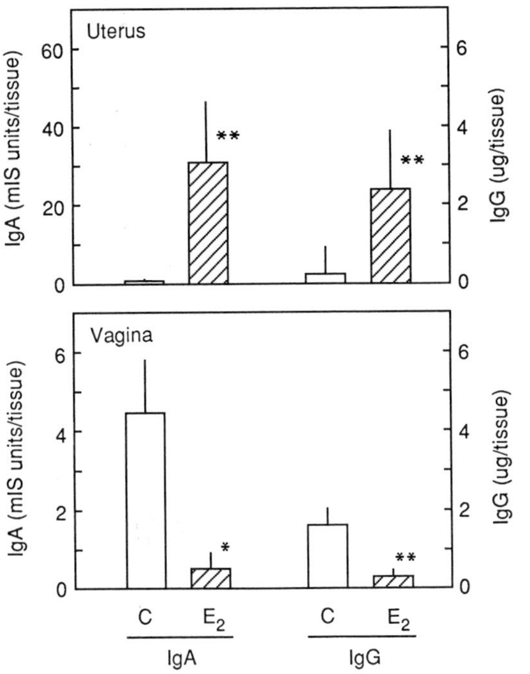

Figure 2 The influence of estradiol on immunoglobulin A and G levels in uterine (*top*) and vaginal (*bottom*) secretions. Ovariectomized rats were injected with estradiol (E_2; 1 μg/day) or saline (C) for 3 days prior to sacrifice 24 hr after the third injection. Each bar represents the mean value of 5–7 animals per group. The vertical line on each bar represents the standard error (SE). *, Significantly ($P < 0.05$) different from control (saline); **, significantly ($P < 0.01$) different from control. Reprinted with permission from Wira and Sandoe (1987b).

IgA and IgG, and that progesterone either alone or with estradiol inhibits cervicovaginal levels of IgA and IgG.

Since IgA is transported into secretions at mucosal surfaces by secretory component (SC), the external domain of the polymeric IgA receptor (for review, see Mestecky and McGhee, 1987), studies were undertaken to determine whether SC is also under hormonal control. As seen in Figure 3, when estradiol was given to ovariectomized rats for 3 days, SC levels increased sharply, in parallel with IgA in uterine secretions (Sullivan *et al.,* 1983). In contrast, SC levels in cervicovaginal secretions were reduced markedly in response to estradiol treatment (Wira and Sullivan, 1985). Subsequent studies showed that, whereas IgA of blood origin enters uterine tissues within 2–4 hr of each injection of estradiol, IgA movement from tissue to lumen takes place only after uterine epithelial cells produce SC in response to estradiol or IFNγ (Prabhala and Wira, 1991).

An apparent paradox involving the time required for estradiol to exert a stimulatory effect on uterine SC levels was resolved when animals were ovariectomized on day 2 of diestrus, just after estradiol had been released by the ovary. Under these conditions, uterine SC levels increased within 16 hr of hormone stimulation (Wira and Stern, 1985). Since the earliest response occurs approximately 3 days after estradiol is given to ovariectomized rats, these findings indicate that, when uterine tissues are deprived hormonally by ovariectomy, more time is required for hormones to exert their actions on cell growth.

To examine the mechanisms by which estradiol exerts its effect on uterine SC, uteri from saline- and estradiol-treated rats were incubated with actinomycin D (Figure 4) and cycloheximide (not shown). SC accumulation in the incubation media was inhibited, suggesting that hormonal regulation of uterine SC is mediated through mRNA and protein synthesis (Wira *et al.,* 1984). We used the SC cDNA probe (Banting *et al.,* 1989) to measure rat uterine SC mRNA levels in the presence or absence of estradiol. As seen in Table I, when ovariectomized rats were treated with estradiol daily for 3 days, SC mRNA levels increased after the second and third injection of estradiol (Morganielli *et al.,* 1991). Although preliminary, these findings suggest that estradiol increases uterine SC levels by increasing SC mRNA levels in uterine tissues. In other studies (not shown), we have found that SC mRNA levels in vaginal tissues are lowered in response to hormone treatment. Studies are currently underway to deter-

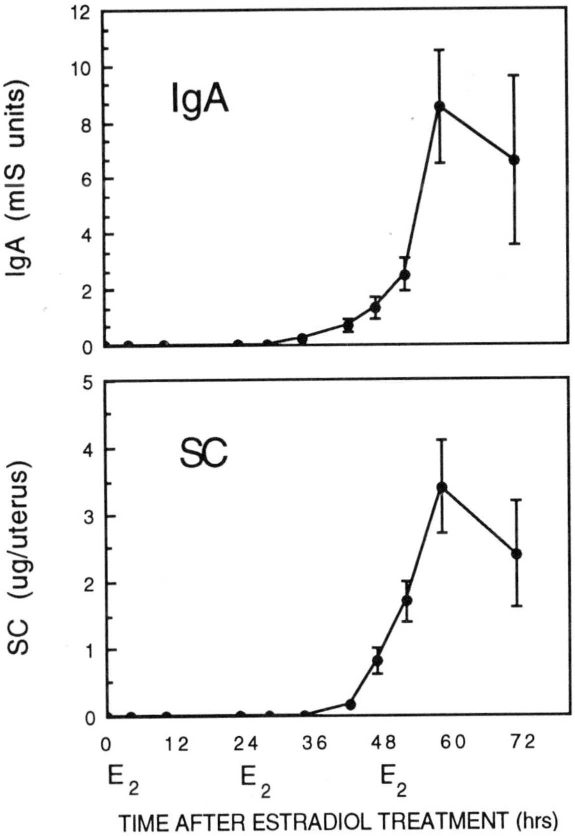

Figure 3 Time course of the effect of 1, 2, or 3 estradiol treatments on secretory component (SC) (*bottom*) and IgA (*top*) content in uterine secretions of ovariectomized rats. Animals were injected with either estradiol (E_2; 2 μg/day) or saline (controls; indicated as 0 time point). Each value equals the mean ± SE of 4 (E_2) or 12 (saline) determinations. The levels of IgA are reported as immunocytoma (IS) units, as previously described (Wira and Sandoe, 1980). Reprinted with permission from Sullivan *et al.* (1983).

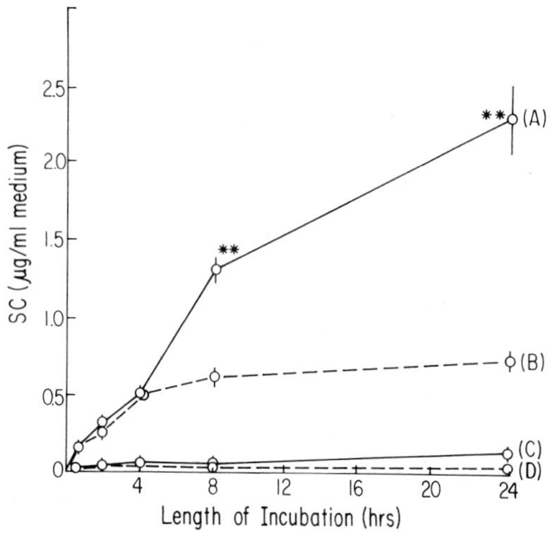

Figure 4 Antagonism by actinomycin D of the estradiol-induced increase in uterine secretory component (SC) *in vitro*. After 3 days of *in vivo* estradiol (1 μg/day) or saline treatment of ovariectomized rats (4 animals per group), uterine horns were divided and were placed either in incubation medium or in medium with actinomycin D (20 μg/ml). The curves shown are as follows: (A) estradiol; (B) estradiol/actinomycin D; (C) saline; (D) saline/actinomycin D. Numbers represent the mean ± SE of samples taken at the indicated time point. **, Significantly greater than the value from estradiol-treated uteri in actinomycin D-containing media. Reprinted with permission from Wira *et al.* (1984).

mine whether estradiol influences synthesis or stability of SC mRNA in reproductive tract tissues.

To examine the role of other steroid hormones in regulating SC and IgA levels in uterine secretions, ovariectomized animals were treated with estradiol, progesterone, or dexamethasone, a synthetic glucocorticoid. As seen in Figure 5, dexamethasone and progesterone, given with estradiol for 3 days, had pronounced inhibitory effects on uterine IgA levels. In contrast, dexamethasone, unlike progesterone, had no effect on SC levels (Sullivan *et al.,* 1983). These findings indicate that glucocorticoids influence mucosal immune responses to estradiol in the female reproductive tract in a different way than progesterone.

To examine more fully the role of glucocorticoids in influencing mucosal immune responses, dexamethasone was given to ovariectomized animals for 1, 2, and 3 days. As seen in Figure 6, IgA levels in serum were significantly higher in dexamethasone-treated rats than in saline-treated rats (Wira *et al.,* 1990). In contrast, IgA levels in salivary (and vaginal, not shown) secretions were lowered in animals treated with dexamethasone. In other studies (not shown), we found that dexamethasone raises specific IgA antibodies in serum and lowers antibody levels in secretions after Peyer's patch priming and uterine boosting with sheep red blood cell (SRBC) antigen. This result suggests that glucocorticoids cause a redistribution of IgA from mucosal surfaces to serum, possibly to enhance systemic immune protection. To determine whether glucocorticoids influence SC levels in serum, animals were treated with dexamethasone for 1, 2, or 3 days (Wira and Rossoll, 1991). Under these conditions, SC levels in serum increased significantly with dexamethasone treatment. Our finding that SC in serum is associated with polymeric IgA suggests that, by increasing serum SC levels, dexamethasone may be decreasing SC-mediated clearance of IgA from blood into bile. In other studies, we found that dexamethasone stimulates SC production by rat hepatocytes (Wira and Colby, 1985), suggesting that serum SC, which has a molecular mass of 29 and 27 kDa, may be of liver origin. Additional studies are needed to identify the origins of serum SC and to determine whether IgA antibodies in serum after dexamethasone stimulation exert a protective effect against systemic antigenic challenge.

III. ROUTES OF IMMUNIZATION AND HORMONALLY STIMULATED ANTIBODIES IN MUCOSAL SECRETIONS

To identify the origins of antibodies and the role of hormones in regulating their presence in reproductive tract secretions, adult female rats were immunized via Peyer's patches (pp), intraperitoneally (ip), and subcutaneously (sc), and boosted 6 days later with SRBC, a known T cell-dependent antigen. Uterine secretions were collected from uterine-ligated animals after each rat had gone through two normal estrous cycles. As seen in Figure 7, when animals were immunized pp or ip, specific anti-SRBC IgA antibodies were found in uterine and cervicovaginal secretions (Wira and Sandoe, 1987). IgG antibodies were found in uterine but not in cervicovaginal secretions. In contrast, sc immunization resulted in a weak uterine IgG antibody response but failed to elicit an IgA response.

The role of estradiol in the accumulation of specific antibodies in reproductive tract secretions is shown in Figure 8. After priming (pp) and boosting (pp) with SRBC, little antibody was found in ovariectomized animals that received saline. With estradiol treatment, IgA and IgG antibodies in-

Table I Effect of Estradiol on Secretory Component mRNA Levels in Uterine Tissues of Ovariectomized Rats[a]

	Estradiol treatment on day			
	0	1	2	3
SC mRNA (area/slot)	±	+	+ + +	+ + +

[a] RNA was extracted from uteri of rats (7–12 animals/group) treated with estradiol (1 μg/day) for 1, 2, or 3 days prior to sacrifice 24 hr later. Control animals received saline for 3 days. RNA was extracted essentially by homogenization in RNA extraction buffer as described by Sambrook *et al.* (1989). Poly(A) + RNA was isolated on oligo(dT)-cellulose. Poly(A) + RNA (50μg) was used for slot blot analysis and probed with ^{32}P-labeled secretory component (SC) cDNA, kindly provided by G. Banting. Hybridization signals for each group were quantified by densitometry. Amount of SC mRNA: ±very low; +low; + +medium; + + +high.

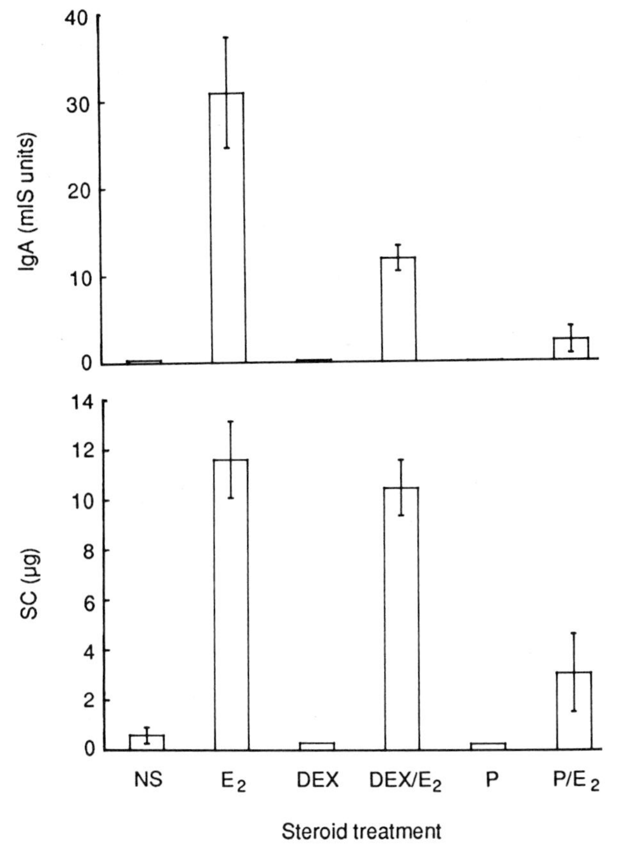

Figure 5 Antagonism by dexamethasone and progesterone of the uterine secretory component (SC) (*bottom*) and IgA (*top*) responses to estradiol. Ovariectomized rats with uterine ligations received saline (NS), dexamethasone (DEX; 1 mg/day), or progesterone (P; 2 mg/day) approximately 30 min before an injection of saline or estradiol (E_2; 1 µg/day). Animals were killed 24 hr after the third injection. Numbers represent the mean ± SE of 5–6 values. Reprinted with permission from Sullivan *et al.* (1983).

creased in uterine secretions relative to control animals. To study the effectiveness of the uterus in responding to antigenic challenge, ovariectomized rats were immunized by placing SRBC directly into the uterine lumen (Wira and Sandoe, 1989). As seen in Figure 8, uterine (ut/ut) immunization resulted in pronounced IgA and IgG antibody responses in the immunized horns that were 20- to 30-fold (IgA) and 2- to 5-fold (IgG) greater than those seen after pp/pp immunization. In contrast to pp/pp immunization, estradiol administered for 3 days had no effect on uterine antibody levels at the end of the immunization procedure. In other studies, we found that intraperitoneal immunization with SRBC leads to uterine antibody responses that, similar to those seen with pp immunization, are dependent on estradiol for genital tract antibody accumulation (Wira and Prabhala, 1992).

Of particular interest in our uterine immunization studies is that, as a consequence of placing SRBC in the uterine lumen, specific antibodies appear in the contralateral (nonimmunized) uterine horn, in vaginal secretions, in serum, and in saliva. These studies demonstrate for the first time that, in addition to being an inductive site for humoral immune responses, the reproductive tract provides immunological information to other mucosal surfaces in the form of IgA and IgG antibodies that may be distributed systemically through the blood. The implication of these findings is that antigen challenge in the reproductive tract may result in immune protection at other sites of the body.

As part of our uterine immunization studies, we analyzed IgA in uterine secretions by high performance liquid chromatography (HPLC) and found that all IgA antibodies existed as dimers. We then examined the possibility that SC was responsible for the accumulation of IgA in uterine secretions. As seen in Figure 9, in the absence of estradiol, SC levels increased in uterine secretions in response to uterine immunization with SRBC. When analyzed by HPLC, SC consisted of free SC and SC bound to IgA anti-SRBC antibodies (Wira *et al.*, 1991). Western blot analysis demonstrated that SRBC-stimulated SC consists of two major bands (75 and 76 kDa) and a third minor band (30 kDa). The major bands are identical to those seen in bile and in uterine fluid from nonimmunized animals (Whittemore *et al.*, 1990). Our conclusion from these studies was that, in addition to stimulating a local anti-

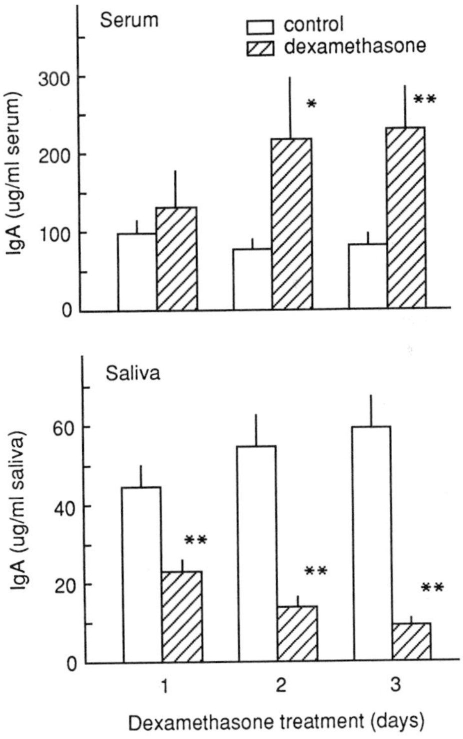

Figure 6 Time course of the effect of dexamethasone on the levels of IgA in serum (*top*) and saliva (*bottom*). Ovariectomized rats were treated with dexamethasone (1 mg/day; hatched bars) or saline (0.1 ml; open bars) for 1, 2, or 3 days. Then, 24 hr after the last injection, saliva and serum were collected and analyzed for IgA. Bars represent the mean ± SE of 7–8 animals/group. *Significantly ($P < 0.01$) different from control groups; **significantly ($P < 0.001$) different from control groups. Reprinted with permission from Wira *et al.* (1990).

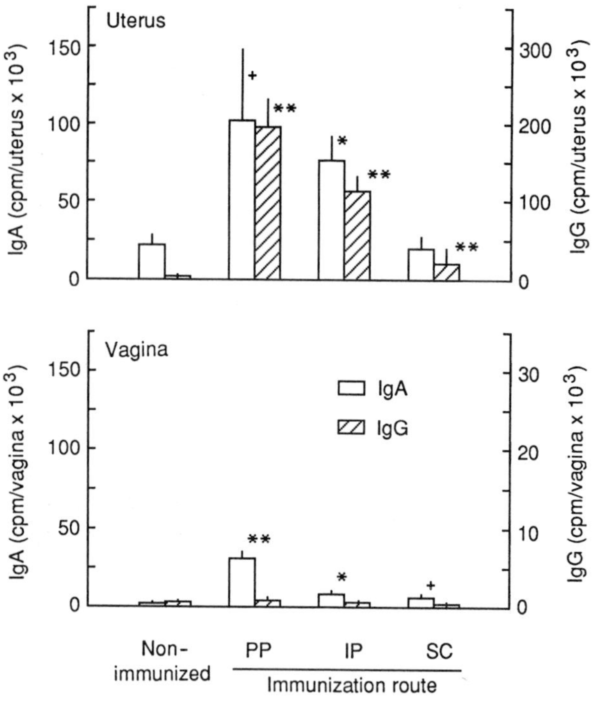

Figure 7 Influence of route of immunization on the presence of specific IgA (open bars) and IgG (hatched bars) antibodies in uterine (*top*) and vaginal (*bottom*) secretions. Intact female rats were immunized with sheep red blood cells (SRBC) injected into PP, i.p., or s.c. and were boosted via the same route 6 days later. All animals had uteri ligated at the uterocervical junction at the time of primary immunization. Animals (7–8 per group) went through at least two normal 4-day estrous cycles before sacrifice 7–9 days after secondary immunization. Bars represent the mean ± SE values of 7–8 animals per group. ⁺, Significantly greater ($P < 0.05$) than control (nonimmunized) group; *, significantly greater ($P < 0.01$) than control; **, significantly greater ($P < 0.001$) than control. Reprinted with permission from Wira and Sandoe (1987).

body response, SRBC antigen also stimulates the production of SC, which may be responsible for the transport of polymeric IgA into uterine secretions.

IV. INFLUENCE OF CYTOKINES ON GENITAL TRACT HUMORAL IMMUNITY

To examine the possibility that IFNγ might be involved in regulating SC production in the rat uterus, IFNγ was placed in the uterine lumen of ovariectomized rats. As seen in Figure 10, increasing doses of IFNγ increased SC levels in uterine secretions. This response was specific for IFNγ because IFNα/β at the same dose (5000 Units) had no effect on uterine SC levels (Prabhala and Wira, 1991). These studies build on the important observation by Sollid *et al.* (1987) that, when IFNγ was added to the incubation media of human colon carcinoma cells (HT29), SC expression increased. These results led to the proposal that epithelial cell-mediated SC IgA transport might respond to cytokine stimulation (Kvale *et al.*, 1988). To test this hypothesis with normal cells, we ovariectomized rats and treated them with IFNγ or estradiol. As seen in Figure 11, when animals received IFNγ alone, SC but not IgA levels increased in the uterine lumen. Since tissue IgA levels are known to be low in the absence of estradiol (Sullivan and Wira, 1983), animals were treated with estradiol for 2 days prior to sacrifice 4 hr after the second injection. This time interval of estradiol exposure previously has been shown to increase tissue levels of monomeric and polymeric IgA without increasing either SC or IgA levels in uterine secretions (Sullivan and Wira, 1983,1984). In contrast, when estradiol was given to IFNγ-treated animals, IgA levels increased in uterine secretions relative to those in animals that

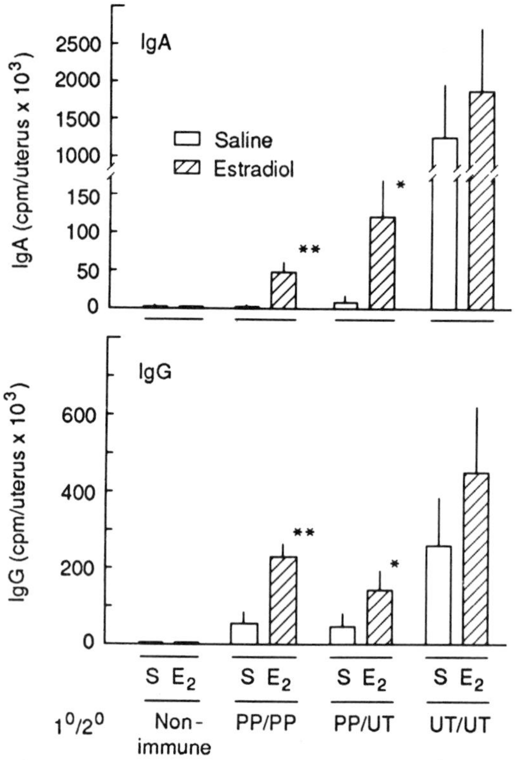

Figure 8 Influence of estradiol and route of immunization on the presence of anti-SRBC-specific IgA (*top*) and IgG (*bottom*) antibodies in uterine secretions. Ovariectomized animals were immunized with SRBC injected into Peyer's patches (PP) or instilled intraluminally into one uterine horn (UT). Animals were immunized (primary, day 0) via the Peyer's patches and boosted (secondary, day 13) either via the Peyer's patches (PP/PP) or the uterus (PP/UT), or were immunized and boosted by placing SRBC directly into the uterine lumen (UT/UT). Nonimmunized animals were sham-operated at the time of primary and secondary immunization. Animals were injected with 0.1 ml saline (S) or estradiol (E_2; 1.0 μg/day) for 3 days prior to killing 24 hr after the last injection on day 26 after primary immunization. Bars represent the mean ± SE values of samples taken from 5–6 animals/group. *, Significantly ($P < 0.05$) greater than saline-treated immunized controls, **, significantly ($P < 0.01$) greater than saline-treated immunized controls. Reprinted with permission from Wira and Sandoe (1989).

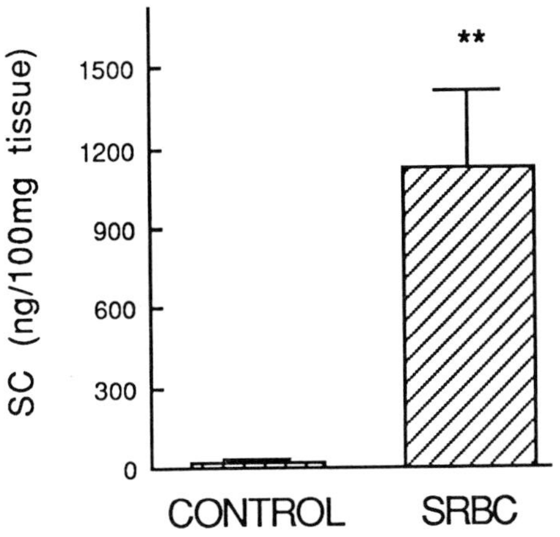

Figure 9 Influence of uterine immunization and boost on the presence of secretory component (SC) in uterine secretions. Ovariectomized animals were immunized with SRBC (20 μl/horn) instilled intraluminally into both uterine horns. Animals were immunized (primary, day 0), boosted (secondary, day 13) in the same uterine horn, and killed on day 26. Nonimmunized animals received 20 μl of PBS in each uterine horn at the time of primary and secondary immunization. After injection of SRBC or PBS into the lumen, uteri were ligated at the uterocervical junction. On the day of boost, SRBC or PBS was injected into the oviductal ends of immunized horns and then ligated. Bars represent the mean ± SE of 6 animals per group. **, Significantly more than nonimmune or contralateral controls ($P < 0.01$). Reprinted with permission from Wira *et al.* (1991).

received either estradiol or IFNγ alone. These findings demonstrate that stimulation of uterine SC by IFNγ increases the movement of IgA from tissue to lumen. These results also represent our most direct evidence to date that some IgA in uterine secretions is of serum origin.

In light of our finding that intrauterine-instilled IFNγ (5000 Units) had a stimulatory effect on uterine SC levels, animals were treated with 10,000 Units of IFNγ. Unexpectedly, we found that SC responses in the uterine lumen to 10,000 Units were significantly lower than those to 5000 Units of IFNγ (Prabhala and Wira, 1991). To examine the possibility that IFNγ might have effects beyond the uterus, spleen cells from rats that received 5000 or 10,000 Units of IFNγ/uterus were analyzed for their responsiveness to B- and T-cell mitogens. As seen in Figure 12, IFNγ (5000 Units) had a marked stimulatory effect on spleen cell mitogenesis in response to concanavalin A (ConA), phytohemagglutinin (PHA), and lipopolysaccharide (LPS). In contrast, when 10,000 Units were placed in the uterine lumina of ovariectomized rats, the response to mitogens was significantly lower than that seen in animals that received 5000 Units. In other studies (not shown), we found that 5000 Units given sc to ovariectomized rats had no effect on spleen cell mitogenesis. These findings indicate that intrauterine exposure to IFNγ results in a signal that is sent from the genital tract to the spleen and influences both B- and T-cell mitogenesis. Further, we find that the magnitude of this response, similar to that seen in the reproductive tract, is dependent on the dose of IFNγ administered as well as the location (intrauterine vs subcutaneous) of IFNγ administration.

In other studies, we examined the possibility that other cytokines may be involved in IgA movement into uterine secretions. Since IL-6 is synthesized by stromal cells in the uterine endometrium (Tabibzadeh *et al.*, 1989), we instilled IL-6 into the uteri of ovariectomized rats. As seen in Table II, IL-6 had a pronounced stimulatory effect on both SC and IgA accumulation within the uterine lumen. What remains unclear is whether IL-6 increased the movement of IgA from serum into uterine tissues and stimulated SC production, or whether IL-6 influenced the terminal differentiation of IgA-lymphoid cells in the reproductive tract into plasma cells, which then synthesized IgA for transport into uterine secretions.

V. REGULATION OF CELL-MEDIATED IMMUNITY AND ANTIGEN PRESENTATION BY SEX HORMONES AND CYTOKINES

Several studies have shown that immune cells are present throughout the female reproductive tract. Bulmer *et al.* (1988,1991), for example, reported that macrophages, B cells, and T cells are present in the human endometrium and that numbers vary during the menstrual cycle depending on the region of endometrium analyzed. Others have found that lymphocyte numbers remain unchanged whereas macrophage numbers increase during the latter part (secretory phase) of the cycle (Morris *et al.*, 1985; Kamat and Isaacson, 1987). In an attempt to determine whether T-cell numbers

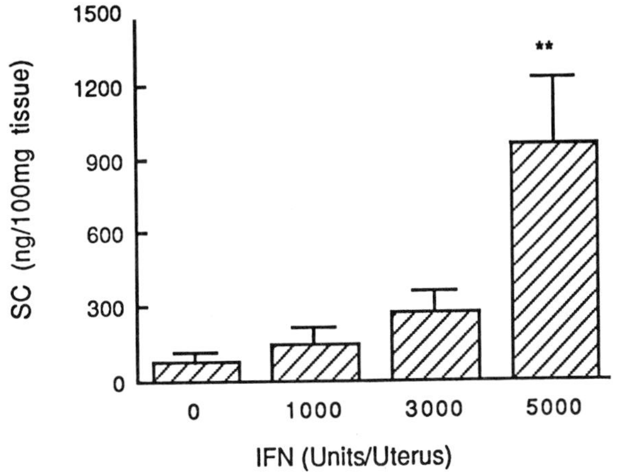

Figure 10 Effect of increasing doses of IFNγ on uterine lumina secretory component (SC) levels. Ovariectomized rats received 20 μl of IFNγ (1000, 3000, or 5000 Units/uterus) in each uterine horn. Control animals were given PBS by the same route. Animals were sacrificed and uterine secretions collected for analysis of SC levels 7 days after intrauterine instillation of IFNγ. Each bar represents the mean ± SE of 6 animals per group. **, Significantly ($P < 0.01$) greater than the control group. Reprinted with permission from Prabhala and Wira (1991).

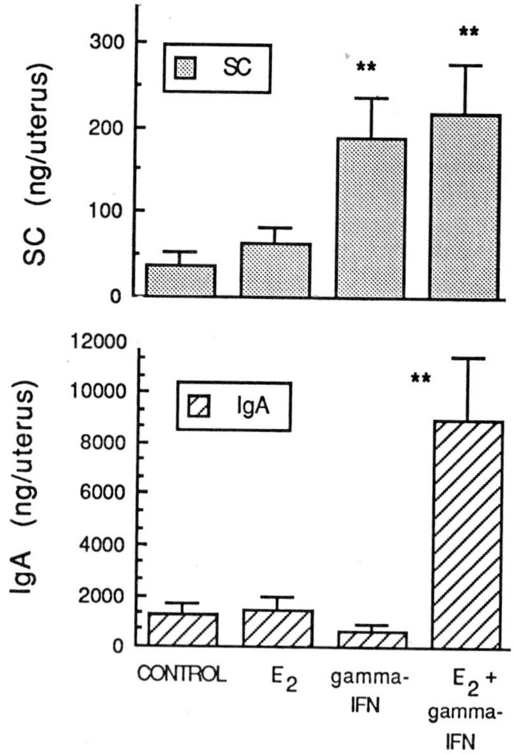

Figure 11 The effect of IFNγ and estradiol on secretory component (SC) (*top*) and IgA (*bottom*) levels in the uterine lumen of ovariectomized animals. PBS or IFNγ (5000 Units/uterus) was placed in the uterine lumen. Animals were given, systemically, either saline (0.1 ml) or estradiol (2 μg/day) daily for the last 2 days prior to sacrifice 4–6 hr after the second injection on day 7. Bars represent the mean ± SE of 6 animals per group. **, Significantly ($P < 0.01$) greater than control values. Reprinted with permission from Prabhala and Wira (1991).

in the female reproductive tract vary with the stage of the reproductive cycle and are influenced by endocrine balance, studies were undertaken to measure T-cell numbers in the rat uterus. As seen in Table III, when analyzed by flow cytometry, significant numbers of total T lymphocytes (Ti) and T-helper lymphocytes (Th) were found in the uteri of intact rats at the proestrous stage of the reproductive cycle. In contrast, cell numbers were reduced at estrus and were either low or not detectable at diestrus. This information indicates that these cells, in addition to B lymphocytes and macrophages (not shown), are present in the uterus in greatest numbers when estradiol levels are known to be highest in serum (at proestrus).

To determine whether estradiol influences the presence of lymphocytes at intraepithelial sites in the uterus, ovariectomized animals were treated with hormone for 3 days prior to histological analysis. As seen in Figure 13A, very few intraepithelial lymphocytes and polymorphonuclear leukocytes (1 ± 0.4 cells/uterine section) were found in uterine tissues in the absence of estradiol (Prabhala and Wira, 1991). In response to estradiol (13B), increased numbers of lymphocytes (17 ± 2 cells/uterine section) and polymorphonuclear leukocytes (5.7 ± 0.5 cells/uterine section) were found adjacent to the basement membrane region of epithelial cells. When IFNγ (5000 Units) was placed in the uterine lumen (13C), intraepithelial and subepithelial lymphocytes (37 ± 6 cells/uterine section) and polymorphonuclear leukocytes (23 ± 7.5 cells/uterine section) increased significantly beyond levels seen with estradiol. In contrast, IFNα/β administered at the same dose (13D) had no effect on either lymphocyte or polymorphonuclear leukocyte numbers. In other studies, Itohara *et al.* (1990) demonstrated that γ/δ intraepithelial cells are present in the female reproductive tract. Haas *et al.* (1990) reported that γ/δ intraepithelial lymphocytes are present in greatest numbers at the proestrous stage of the reproductive cycle. Our findings that estradiol and IFNγ increase intraepithelial lymphocytes and polymorphonuclear leukocytes demonstrate that these cells are responsive to sex hormones and cytokines, and suggest that immune functions of γ/δ cells, including immunosurveillance (Raulet, 1989), cytotoxicity (Ferrini *et al.*, 1987), and cytokine production (Christmas and Meager, 1990), may be regulated hormonally in the female reproductive tract. Additional studies are needed to identify the mechanisms through which estradiol and IFNγ exert their stimulatory effects on immune cell migration into the female reproductive tract.

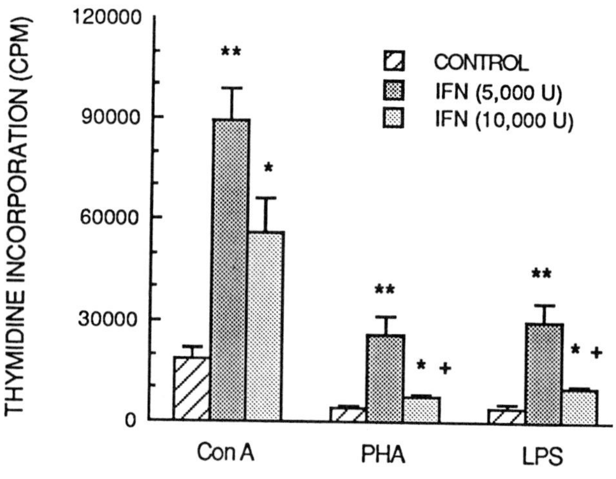

Figure 12 Mitogenic response of isolated spleen cells from ovariectomized rats treated with varying doses of IFNγ. Ovariectomized rats were given IFNγ (5000 or 10000 Units/uterus) or PBS (20 μl/horn) by intrauterine instillation. Seven days later, animals (6/group) were sacrificed and spleens were collected. Splenocytes were prepared from pooled spleens and incubated either with ConA (1 μg/ml), PHA (5 μg/ml), or LPS (10 μg/ml) for 3 days. [^{3}H]Thymidine was added to culture wells for the last 24 hr of each incubation. Each bar represents the mean ± SE minus background (cpm/well in the absence of mitogen) of 6 animals per group. **, Significantly ($P < 0.01$) greater than control values; *, significantly ($P < 0.03$) greater than control values; $^+$, significantly ($P < 0.03$) lower than 5000 Unit IFNγ values. Reprinted with permission from Prabhala and Wira (1991).

Table II Influence of IL-6 on Secretory Component and IgA Levels in Uterine Secretions[a]

	SC (ng/100 mg tissue)	IgA (ng/100 mg tissue)
Control	±	±
IL-6[b]	+ + +	+ + +

[a] IL-6 (1000 Units/20 μl PBS/uterine horn) or PBS (20 μl/uterine horn) was placed in the uterine lumina of ovariectomized rats 7 days prior to sacrifice. Collection of uterine secretions was as described elsewhere (Prabhala and Wira, 1991). Amount of SC or IGA: ±very low; +low; + +medium; + + +high.

[b] Significantly ($p < 0.01$) greater than controls.

In preliminary studies, to determine whether cells in the female reproductive tract are able to present antigen, purified uterine epithelial cells were isolated from the uteri of rats at the proestrous stage of the reproductive cycle. Epithelial cells were prepared as described previously (McCormack and Glasser, 1980) and following preincubation to remove macrophages, cells were incubated with sensitized T lymphocytes prepared from the lymph nodes of animals immunized by footpad injections with ovalbumin (OVA) antigen. As seen in Figure 14, when epithelial cells were incubated with T lymphocytes in the presence of OVA, they were able to present antigen to sensitized T lymphocytes. Lymphocyte proliferation, measured as [^{3}H]thymidine incorporation, was significantly greater than that seen when epithelial cells or lymphocytes were incubated with OVA or when epithelial cells and lymphocytes were incubated together in the absence of OVA. Studies are underway to verify that uterine epithelial cells used in antigen presentation studies are free of macrophages, which are known to enter uterine tissues in increasing numbers at proestrus (Head and Gaede, 1986b). In a parallel study (Figure 14), stromal cells were prepared from the uteri of proestrous rats. When incubated under the conditions described for epithelial cells, stromal cells were able to present antigen to sensitized T lymphocytes. Based on our preliminary findings of macrophages, B lymphocytes, and dendritic cells in the uterine stroma and the recognition that these cells present antigen at other sites in the body, these cells are likely to be responsible for antigen presentation in our studies. To the best of our knowledge, this demonstration is the first that uterine cells present antigen and thereby initiate an immune response in the reproductive tract.

In other studies, we undertook to determine whether antigen presentation varies with the stage of the reproductive cycle. When uterine cells from proestrous, estrous, and diestrous rats were incubated with sensitized T lymphocytes in the presence of OVA, cells from proestrous rats presented antigen more efficiently than did cells from either estrous or diestrous animals. We have treated ovariectomized rats with estradiol (1 μg/day for 3 days) and found that antigen presentation is increased markedly in response to hormone treatment relative to saline controls. As a part of these studies, we found that antigen presentation by uterine cells is MHC Class II restricted. Further, Class II expression on uterine cells is hormonally dependent, that is, expression is elevated at proestrus relative to estrus and diestrus in the reproductive cycle. In other studies (not shown), we have found that IFNγ placed in the uterine lumen of ovariectomized rats increases MHC Class II expression on uterine luminal epithelial cells. Further, intrauterine instillation of IFNγ or IL-6 enhanced antigen presentation by uterine cells. Studies are currently underway to define more clearly the mechanisms by which antigen presentation is regulated by sex hormones and cytokines.

VI. CONCLUSIONS

The results presented indicate that the secretory immune system in the female reproductive tract is fully immunocompetent and able to respond to antigenic challenge. Moreover, our findings indicate that the recognition of antigen (afferent arm) and the response to antigenic challenge (efferent arm) of the immune system in the uterus are regulated precisely by sex hormones, cytokines, and glucocorticoids. Our present understanding of the multiple levels at which hormones and cytokines interact with the secretory immune system is presented schematically in Figure 15. In response to antigen, uterine cells are capable of presenting antigen to sensitized T cells. When estradiol is given systemically, or is present as a normal consequence of the reproductive cycle, antigen presentation that is Class II restricted is enhanced. An increase in antigen presentation also occurs when IFNγ or IL-6 is placed in the uterus. In light of the findings that IL-6 and IFNγ are produced by cells in the reproductive tract, our studies indicate that enhancement of the afferent arm of the immune system occurs in response to sex hormones and

Table III Presence of T Lymphocytes in Uterine Tissues at Various Stages of the Estrous Cycle[a]

	Estrous cycle stage		
	Proestrus	Estrus	Diestrus
Total (T_l)	+ + +	+ +	±
Helper (Th)	+ +	+	±

[a] T lymphocytes/gm tissue (× 10^5). Each value represents the mean ± SE of 2–4 animals/group. Uterine cells were prepared by endometrial scraping and needle aspiration (16–22 g) to prepare isolated cells. Endometrial cells were incubated with W3/25 (T helper) and W3/13 (T total) monoclonal antibodies before analysis by flow cytometer. Number of T cells: ±very low; +few; + +some; + + +many.

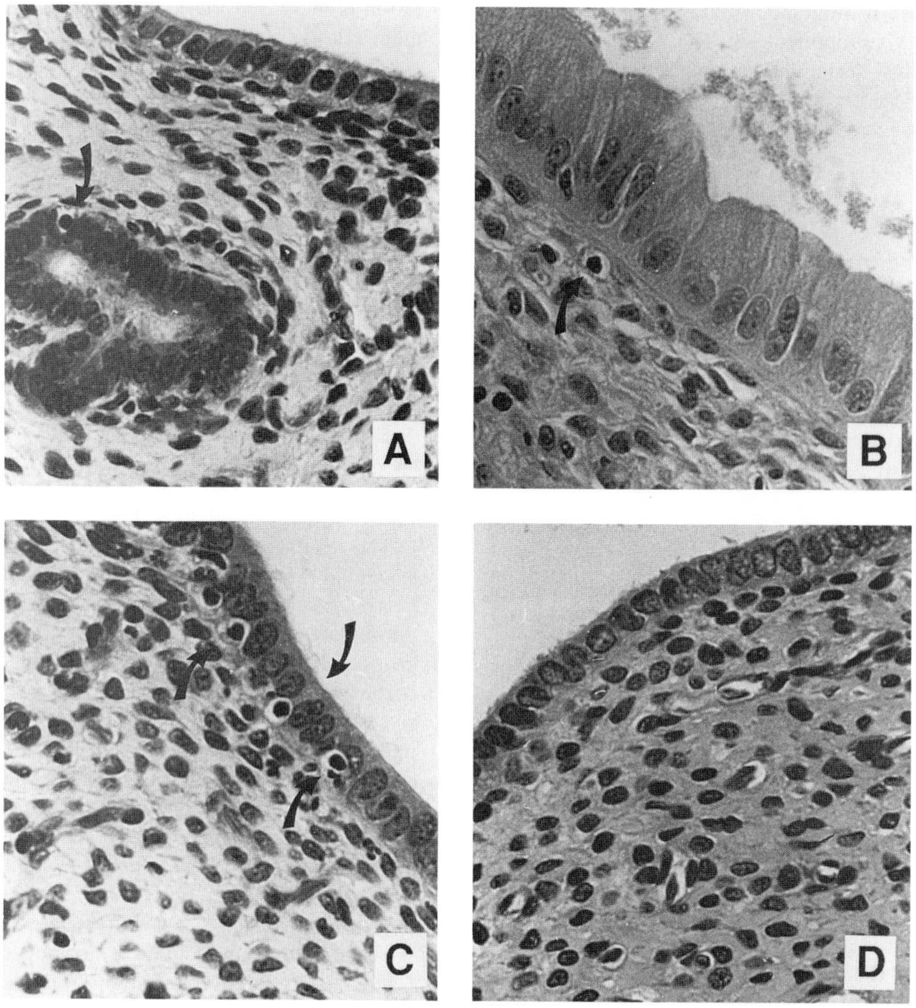

Figure 13 Light microscopic appearance of intraepithelial lymphocytes and epithelial cells in uteri from rats after treatment with interferons and/or estradiol. Ovariectomized rats were given a single dose of either IFNγ (5000 Units/uterus), IFNα/β (5000 Units/uterus), or PBS (20 μl/horn) by intrauterine instillation 7 days prior to sacrifice. Rats were injected subcutaneously either with estradiol (2 μg/0.1 ml/day) or saline (0.1 ml/day) for 3 days prior to sacrifice 24 hr after the third injection on day 7. Uteri were fixed to Bouin's solution, sectioned, and stained with hematoxylin and eosin. Uterine sections were prepared from rats as follows: (A) saline-treated controls; (B) estradiol treatment; (C) intrauterine instillation of IFNγ; and (D) intrauterine IFNα/β. Arrows indicate the locations of intra- and subepithelial lymphocytes. $\times$1860. Reprinted with permission from Prabhala and Wira (1991).

cytokines, and that antigen presentation during the reproductive cycle may be a reflection of an interaction that exists between these two groups of immune regulators. From a physiological standpoint, differential control of the afferent arm might result in immune protection from antigenic challenge during the reproductive cycle that would be enhanced prior to and following ovulation to protect against potential pathogens, and would be suppressed at the time of fertilization when the female is exposed to allogeneic antigens of paternal origin.

Also shown in Figure 15 is the effect of estradiol on the movement of T cells, B cells, macrophages, and intraepithelial lymphocytes into reproductive tract tissues. This influx of cells into the reproductive tract, in addition to eosinophils and neutrophils (not shown), is controlled precisely during the reproductive cycle and is under hormonal control. Movement of these cells and the mechanisms involved in their selective infiltration, however, remain to be established.

An unexpected finding in our study was that IFNγ placed in the uterine lumen had a stimulatory effect on spleen B- and T-cell responses to mitogens. Since an identical dose of IFNγ (5000 Units) given subcutaneously had no effect, we conclude that factors other than leakage of IFNγ from the uterine lumina are involved in spleen cell responses. These studies suggest that, in response to IFNγ, macrophages or dendritic cells (Head and Billingham, 1986) may move from the reproductive tract into the spleen or lymph nodes to influence mitogenesis. This possibility is supported further by the finding that IFNγ enhances the activation and migration of dendritic cells from the heart and respiratory tract to the spleen (Larsen *et al.,* 1990). Studies are needed to determine whether immune cells in the reproductive tract migrate to distal sites and to define the role of sex hormones and cytokines in influencing this process.

Our earlier studies have demonstrated that the efferent arm of the immune system in the female reproductive tract is under hormonal control. As seen in Figure 15, estradiol and progesterone control the levels of IgA, IgG, and SC in uterine as well as in cervicovaginal secretions. These findings led us to the conclusion that endocrine balance during the reproductive cycle, at implantation and throughout pregnancy (Wira and Stern, 1992), results in separate and distinct changes in the mucosal immune system that are unique to the uterus, cervix, and vagina. In several studies, we focused on the origin(s) of specific IgA and IgG antibodies and determined that antibodies in reproductive tract secretions are derived from both the gastrointestinal and the reproductive tracts. On examining the role of hormone balance in antibody levels in reproductive tract secretions, we found that estradiol stimulates the accumulation of gastrointestinally derived antibodies in uterine secretions. We also found that animals respond locally to uterine antigenic challenge. In addition to accumulating at the site of antigenic challenge, IgA and IgG antibodies accumulate in the nonimmunized uterine horn, in vaginal secretions, in serum, and in saliva. These studies demonstrate that, in addition to receiving antibodies from distal sites, the reproductive tract shares immunological information with other mucosal surfaces.

On further examination of the uterine immune response, we found that antigen, IFNγ, and IL-6 stimulate SC production by uterine epithelial cells. This study suggests that antigenic control of uterine SC may be mediated by IFNγ and IL-6, which act to stimulate SC production and IgA transport.

In conclusion, our studies demonstrate that the female reproductive tract is an inductive site for mucosal immune responses and that the mucosal immune system in the uterus, cervix, and vagina is regulated by estradiol, progesterone, and selected cytokines, including IFNγ and IL-6. By ob-

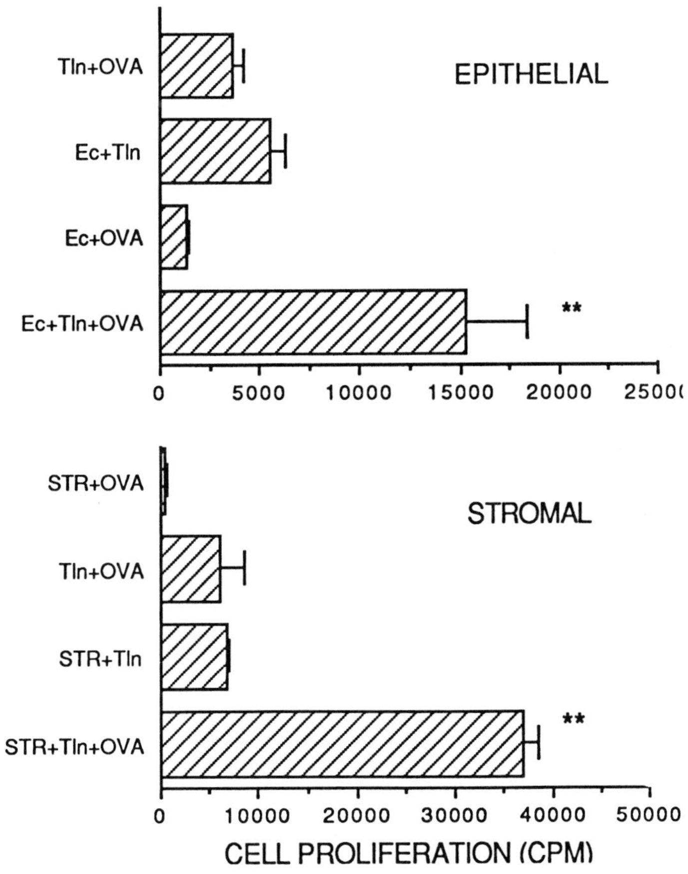

Figure 14 Antigen presentation by uterine luminal epithelial cells (Ec; *top*) and stromal cells (STR; *bottom*) to antigen-primed lymph node T lymphocytes (Tln). Epithelial cells (10^5) and/or primed T lymphocytes (5×10^5) were incubated with ovalbumin (OVA; 1000 μg/ml) for 18 hr. T lymphocytes were isolated on Ficoll–Hypaque and allowed to proliferate for 72 hr prior to incubation for 24 hr with [^{3}H]thymidine (1 μCi/well). **, Significantly greater ($P < 0.01$) than controls. Reprinted with permission from Wira and Prabhala (1992).

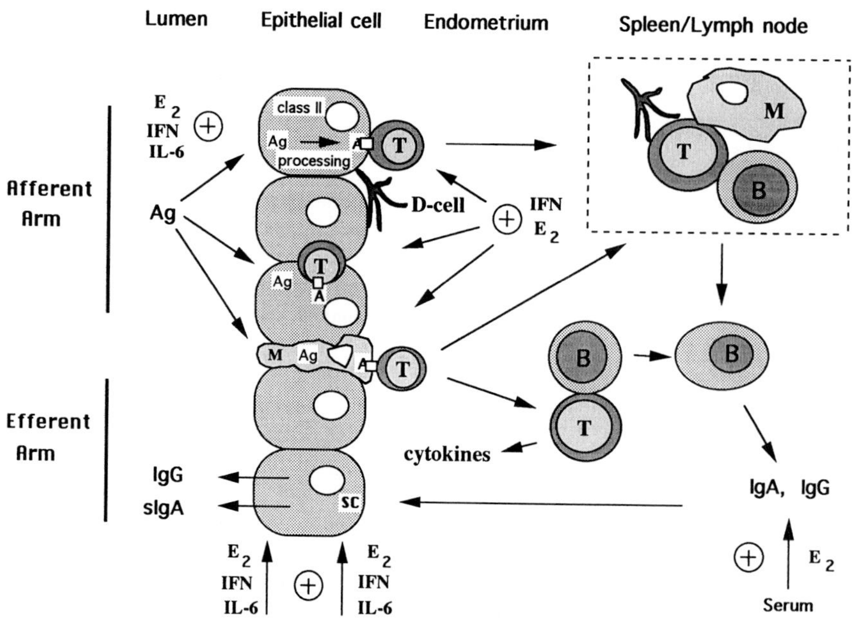

Figure 15 Possible sites of action at which sex hormones and cytokines exert an influence on the afferent and efferent arms of the secretory immune system in the uterus of the rat. E_2, estradiol; IFN, interferon-γ; IL-6, interleukin 6; T, T lymphocyte; B, B lymphocyte; M, macrophage; D, dendritic cell; SC, secretory component; SIgA, secretory IgA; Ag, antigen; A, processed antigen.

taining a clearer understanding of the interrelationships between sex hormones, cytokines, and glucocorticoids as they influence mucosal immunity in the female reproductive tract, valuable information should become available for the development of appropriate immunoprophylaxis to regulate fertility and control sexually transmitted diseases.

Acknowledgments

The studies from the author's laboratory reported in this chapter were supported by NIH Grants A1-13541 and AI-07363 and by NCI Grant CA 23108. We express our appreciation to Edie Coates for typing this manuscript.

References

Aiba, S., and Katz, S. I. (1991). The ability of cultured Langerhans cells to process and present protein antigens is MHC-dependent. *J. Immunol.* **146,** 2479–2487.

Ashwell, J. D., DeFranco, A. L., Paul, W. E., and Schwartz, R. H. (1984). Antigen presentation by resting B cells. Radiosensitivity of the antigen-presenting function and two distinct pathways of T cell activation. *J. Exp. Med.* **158,** 881–905.

Balkwill, F. R., and Burke, F. (1989). The cytokine network. *Immunol. Today* **10,** 299–304.

Banting, G., Broke, B., Braghetta, P., Luzio, J. P., and Stanley, K. K. (1989). Intracellular targetting signals of polymeric immunoglobulin receptors are highly conserved between species. *FEBS Lett.* **254,** 177–183.

Bell, E. B., and Wolf, B. (1967). Antibody synthesis *in vitro* by the rabbit vagina against diptheria toxoid. *Nature (London)* **214,** 423–424.

Brandtzaeg, P., and Prydz, H. (1984). Direct evidence for an integrated function of J-chain and secretory component in epithelial transport of immunoglobulins. *Nature (London)* **311,** 71–73.

Bulmer, J. N., Lunny, D. P., and Hagin, S. V. (1988). Immunohistochemical characterization of stromal leucocytes in nonpregnant human endometrium. *Am. J. Reprod. Immunol. Microbiol.* **17,** 83–90.

Bulmer, J. N., Longfellow, M., and Ritson, A. (1991). Leukocytes and resident blood cells in endometrium. *Ann. N.Y. Acad. Sci.* **622,** 57–68.

Cates, W., Jr. (1986). Priorities for sexually transmitted diseases in the late 1980's and beyond. *Sex. Trans. Dis.* **13,** 114–117.

Christmas, S. E., and Meager, A. (1990). Production of interferon-γ and tumor necrosis factor-α by human T-cell clones expressing different forms of the receptor. *Immunology* **71,** 486–492.

Fanger, M. W., Goldstine, S. N., and Shen, L. (1983). Cytofluorographic analysis of receptors for IgA on human polymorphonuclear cells and monocytes and the correlation of receptor expression with phagocytosis. *Mol. Immunol.* **20,** 1019–1027.

Ferrini, S., Bottino, C., Biassoni, R., Poggi, R., Sehaly, R. P., Moretta, L., and Moretta, M. (1987). Characterization of CD3+4-8- clones expressing the putative T-cell receptor. *J. Exp. Med.* **166,** 277–282.

Fox, H. S., Bond, B. L., and Parslow, T. G. (1991). Estrogen regulates the IFN-γ promoter. *J. Immunol.* **146,** 4362–4367.

Gaspari, A. A., and Katz, S. I. (1988). Induction and functional characterization of class II MHC (Ia) antigens on murine karatinocytes. *J. Immunol.* **140,** 2956–2963.

Haas, W., Kaufman, S., and Martinez, C. (1990). The development and function of T-cells. *Immunol. Today* **11,** 340–343.

Harbour, D. V., and Blalock, J. E. (1989). Lymphocytes and lymphocytic hormones in pregnancy. *Prog. Neuroendocrinol. Immunol.* **2,** 55–63.

Head, J. R., and Billingham, R. E. (1986). Concerning the immunology of the uterus. *Am. J. Reprod. Immunol. Microbiol.* **10,** 76–81.

Head, J. R., and Gaede, S. D. (1986). Ia antigen expression in the rat uterus. *J. Reprod. Immunol.* **9,** 137–153.

Heremans, J. F. (1974). Immunoglobulin A. *In* "The Antigens" (M. Sela, ed.), pp. 365–522. Academic Press, New York.

Itohara, S., Farr, A. G., Lafaille, J. J., Bonneville, M., Takagaki, Y., Haas, W., and Tonegawa, S. (1990). Homing of a thymocyte subset with homogeneous T-cell receptors to mucosal epithelia. *Nature (London)* **343,** 754–757.

Kamat, B. R., and Isaacson, P. G. (1987). The immunocytochemical distribution of leukocytic subpopulations in human endometrium. *Am. J. Pathol.* **127,** 66–73.

Kerr, W. R. (1955). Vaginal and uterine antibodies in cattle with particular reference to *Brucella abortus. Brit. Vet. J.* **111,** 169.

Kvale, D., Brandtzaeg, P., and Lovhaug, D. (1988). Up-regulation of the expression of secretory component and HLA molecules in a human colonic cell line by tumor necrosis factor-α and γ-interferon. *Scand. J. Immunol.* **28,** 351–357.

Larsen, C. P., Morris, P. J., and Austyn, J. M. (1990). Migration of dendritic leukocytes from cardiac allografts into host spleens: A novel pathway for initiation of rejection. *J. Exp. Med.* **171,** 307–314.

McCormack, S. A., and Glasser, S. R. (1980). Differential response of individual uterine cell types from immature rats treated with estradiol. *Endocrinology* **106,** 1634–1649.

McDermott, M. R., and Bienenstock, J. (1979). Evidence for a common mucosal immunologic system. I. Migration of B immunoblasts into intestinal, respiratory and genital tissues. *J. Immunol.* **122,** 1892–1898.

McDonough, P. G. (1987). Cd4 (T4+) Lymphocytes in semen of healthy heterosexual men: Implications for the transmission of AIDS. *Fertil. Steril.* **48,** 703–704.

Mestecky, J., and McGhee, J. R. (1987). Immunoglobulin A (IgA): Molecular and cellular interactions involved in IgA biosynthesis and immune response. *Adv. Immunol.* **40,** 153–245.

Morganielli, C., Rossoll, R., and Wira, C. R. (1991). Estrogen induced expression of mRNA for secretory component in the rat uterus. *FASEB J.* **5,** 1694A.

Morris, H., Edwards, J., Tiltman, A., and Emms, M. (1985). Endometrial lymphoid tissue: an immunohistological study. *J. Clin. Pathol.* **38,** 644–652.

Ogra, P. L., and Ogra, S. S. (1973). Local antibody response to poliovaccine in the human female genital tract. *J. Immunol.* **110,** 1307–1311.

Ogra, P. L., Yamanaka, T., and Losonsky, G. A. (1981). Local immunologic defenses in the genital tract. *In* "Reproductive Immunology" (N. Fleicher, ed.), pp. 381–39. Liss, New York.

Parr, E. L., Parr, M. B., and Thapar, M. (1988). A comparison of specific antibody responses in mouse vaginal fluid after immunization by various routes. *J. Reprod. Immunol.* **14,** 165–176.

Peterman, T. A., and Curran, J. W. (1986). Sexual transmission of human immunodeficiency virus. *J. Am. Med. Assoc.* **256,** 2222–2226.

Piot, P., Plummer, F. A., Mhalu, F. S., Lamboray, J. L., Chin, J., and Mann, J. M. (1988). AIDS: An international perspective. *Science* **239,** 573–579.

Prabhala, R. H., and Wira, C. R. (1991). Cytokine regulation of the mucosal system. *In vivo* stimulation by interferon-γ of secretory component and IgA in uterine secretions and proliferation of lymphocytes from spleen. *Endocrinology* **129,** 2915–2923.

Raulet, D. H. (1989). The structure, function and molecular genetics of the T-cell receptor. *Ann. Rev. Immunol.* **7,** 175–207.

Rosenthal, A. S., and Shevach, E. M. (1973). Function of macrophages in antigen recognition by guinea pig T-lymphocytes. *J. Exp. Med.* **138,** 1194–1212.

Sambrook, J., Fritsch, E. F., and Maniatis, T. (1989). "Molecular Cloning," 2d Ed. Cold Spring Harbor Laboratory Press, Cold Spring Harbor, New York.

Schumacher, G. F. B. (1980). Humoral immune factors in the female reproductive tract and their changes during the cycle. *In* "Immunological Aspects of Infertility and Fertility Control" (D. Dindsa and G. Schumacher, eds.), pp. 93–141. North Holland/Elsevier, New York.

Shen, L., and Fanger, M. W. (1981). Secretory IgA antibodies synergize with IgG in promoting ADCC by human polymorphonuclear cells, monocytes and lymphocytes. *Cell. Immunol.* **59,** 75–81.

Sollid, L. M., Kvale, D., Brandtzaeg, P., Markussen, G., and Thorsby, E. (1987). Interferon-γ enhances expression of secretory component, the epithelial receptor for polymeric immunoglobulins. *J. Immunol.* **138,** 4303–4306.

Steinman, R. M., and Nussenzweig, M. C. (1980). Dendritic cells: Features and functions. *Immunol. Rev.* **53,** 127–147.

Sullivan, D. A., and Wira, C. R. (1983). Hormonal regulation of immunoglobulins in the rat uterus: Uterine response to a single estradiol treatment. *Endocrinology* **112,** 260–268.

Sullivan, D. A., and Wira, C. R. (1984). Hormonal regulation of immunoglobulins in the rat uterus: Uterine response to multiple estradiol treatments. *Endocrinology* **114,** 650–658.

Sullivan, D. A., Underdown, B. J., and Wira, C. R. (1983). Steroid hormone regulation of free secretory component in the rat uterus. *Immunology* **49,** 379–386.

Sullivan, D. A., Richardson, G. S., McLaughlin, D. T., and Wira, C. R. (1984). Variations in the levels of secretory component in human uterine fluid during the menstrual cycle. *J. Steroid Biochem.* **20,** 509–513.

Tabibzadeh, S. S. (1990). Evidence of T cell activation and potential cytokine action in human endometrium. *J. Clin. Endocrinol. Metab.* **71,** 645–649.

Tabibzadeh, S. S., Bettica, A., and Gerber, M. A. (1986a). Variable expression of Ia antigens in human endometrium and in chronic endometritis. *Am. J. Clin. Pathol.* **86,** 153–160.

Tabibzadeh, S. S., Gerber, M. A., and Satyaswaroop, P. G. (1986b). Induction of HLA-DR antigen expression in human endometrial cells *in vitro* by recombinant gamma-interferon. *Am. J. Pathol.* **125,** 90–96.

Tabibzadeh, S. S., Santhahnam, U., Sehgal, P. B., and May, L. T. (1989). Cytokine-induced production of IFN-β2/IL-6 by freshly explanted human endometrial stromal cells: Modulation by estradiol-17β. *J. Immunol.* **142,** 3134–3139.

Takacs, L., Kovacs, E. J., Smith, R. S., Young, H. A., and Dvum, S. K. (1988). Detection of IL-1 and IL-1 gene expression by *in situ* hybridization: Tissue localization of IL-1 mRNA in normal c57BL/6 mouse. *J. Immunol.* **141,** 3081–3095.

Underdown, B. J., and Schiff, J. M. (1986). Immunoglobulin A: Strategic defense initiative at the mucosal surface. *Ann. Rev. Immunol.* **4,** 389–417.

Vaerman, J.-P., and Férin, J. (1974). Local immunological response in the vagina, cervix and endometrium. *Acta Endocrinol.* **194,** 281–305.

Weinberger, O., Herrmann, S., Mescher, M. F., Benacerraf, B., and Burakaff, S. J. (1981). Antigen presenting cell function in induction of helper T cells for cytotoxic T-lymphocyte responses: Evidence for antigen processing. *Proc. Natl. Acad. Sci. U.S.A.* **78,** 1796–1799.

Whittemore, S. L., Bodwell, J. E., and Wira, C. R. (1990). Characterization of secretory component from rat uterine fluid. *In* "Advances in Mucosal Immunology" (T. T. MacDonald, S. J. Challacombe, P. W. Bland, C. R. Stokes, R. V. Heatley, and

A. M. Mowat, eds.), pp. 602–605. Kluwer Academic Publishers, Boston.

Williams, C. R., and Gibbons, R. J. (1972). Inhibition of bacterial adherence by secretory immunoglobulin A: A mechanism for antigen disposal. *Science* **177,** 697–699.

Wira, C. R., and Colby, E. B. (1985). Regulation of secretory component by glucocorticoids in primary cultures of rat hepatocytes. *J. Immunol.* **134,** 1744–1748.

Wira, C. R., and Prabhala, R. H. (1992). The female reproductive tract as an inductive site for immune responses: Effect of estradiol and antigen on antibody and secretory component levels in uterine and cervico-vaginal secretions following various routes of immunization. (1993). *In* "Local Immunity in Reproductive Tract Tissues." P. D. Griffin, and P. M. Johnson, eds.), Oxford University Press, New York. World Health Organization, Geneva, Switzerland. pp. 271–293.

Wira, C. R., and Rossoll, R. M. (1991). Glucocorticoid regulation of the humoral immune system. Dexamethasone stimulation of secretory component in serum, saliva, and bile. *Endocrinology* **128,** 835–842.

Wira, C. R., and Sandoe, C. P. (1977). Sex steroid hormone regulation of IgG and IgA in rat uterine secretions. *Nature (London)* **268,** 534–536.

Wira, C. R., and Sandoe, C. P. (1980). Hormone regulation of immunoglobulins: Influence of estradiol on IgA and IgG in the rat uterus. *Endocrinology* **106,** 1020–1026.

Wira, C. R., and Sandoe, C. P. (1987a). Specific IgA and IgG antibodies in the female reproductive tract: Effects of immunization and estradiol on expression of this response *in vivo*. *J. Immunol.* **138,** 4159–4164.

Wira, C. R., and Sandoe, C. P. (1987b). Origin of IgA and IgG antibodies in the female reproductive tract: Regulation of the genital response by estradiol. *In* (J. Mestecky, J. R. McGhee, J. Bienenstock, and P. L. Ogra, eds.). Recent Advances in Mucosal Immunology; Part A: Cellular Interactions. pp. 403–412. New York, Plenum Press.

Wira, C. R., and Sandoe, C. P. (1989). Effect of uterine immunization and oestradiol on specific IgA and IgG antibodies in uterine, vaginal, and salivary secretions. *Immunology* **68,** 24–30.

Wira, C. R., and Stern, J. E. (1985). Rapid effect of ovarian hormones on secretory component (SC) in uterine secretions of the rat: Involvement of RNA synthesis in SC production. *Protides Biol. Fluids* **32,** 255–257.

Wira, C. R., and Stern, J. E. (1992). Endocrine regulation of the mucosal immune system in the female reproductive tract: Control of IgA, IgG, and secretory component during the reproductive cycle, at implantation, and throughout pregnancy. *In* "Hormones and Fetal Pathophysiology" (J. R. Pasqualini and R. Scholler, eds.), pp. 343–367. Marcel Dekker, New York.

Wira, C. R., and Sullivan, D. A. (1985). Estradiol and progesterone regulation of IgA, IgG and secretory component in cervico-vaginal secretions of the rat. *Biol. Reprod.* **32,** 90–95.

Wira, C. R., Stern, J. E., and Colby, E. B. (1984). Estradiol regulation of secretory component in the uterus of the rat: Evidence for involvement of RNA synthesis. *J. Immunol.* **133,** 2624–2628.

Wira, C. R., Sandoe, C. P., and Steele, M. G. (1990). Glucocorticoid regulation of the humoral immune system: I. *In vivo* effects of dexamethasone on IgA and IgG in serum and at mucosal surfaces. *J. Immunol.* **144,** 142–146.

Wira, C. R., Bodwell, J. E., and Prabhala, R. H. (1991). *In vivo* response of secretory component in the rat uterus to antigen, interferon-γ and estradiol. *J. Immunol.* **146,** 1893–1899.

Yang, S.-L., and Schumacher, G. F. B. (1979). Immune response after vaginal application of antigens in the rhesus monkey. *Fertil. Steril.* **32,** 588–598.

Ziegler, K., and Unanue, E. R. (1981). Identification of a macrophage antigen-processing event required for Ia region-restricted antigen presentation to T-lymphocytes. *J. Immunol.* **127,** 1869–1875.

57

Mucosal Immunopathophysiology of HIV Infection

Phillip D. Smith

I. INTRODUCTION

Despite major advances in medical science and public health measures, the world has witnessed the emergence of a new and devastating infectious disease—the acquired immunodeficiency syndrome (AIDS). Indeed, as the 21st century approaches, this disease has reached pandemic proportions. In the United States alone, 315,390 persons have been reported to have AIDS, of whom 194,354 have died (Centers for Disease Control, 1993). Worldwide, up to 20 million persons are predicted to acquire asymptomatic infection with the causative agent of AIDS, human immunodeficiency virus (HIV), by the year 2000. Accentuating the magnitude of this global epidemic is the absence of an effective cure for HIV infection, which eventually leads to death in 100% of cases. Thus, AIDS is having an enormous impact on individuals and, consequently, on whole societies in developed and developing nations.

The magnitude of the AIDS epidemic and the absence of a curative antiviral agent underscore the need for an effective vaccine against HIV. Since most homosexual and heterosexual transmission of the virus involves passage across mucosal surfaces, such a vaccine will need to induce protective or neutralizing factors at mucosal membranes. Designing this vaccine will require a detailed understanding of the mucosal events that occur in HIV disease. Accordingly, the goal of this chapter is to integrate into a common hypothesis the known and presumed immunopathophysiological events that occur in the mucosa during HIV infection. Divided into early-, intermediate-, and late-phase events, this chapter describes how these events predispose the host to the mucosal manifestations of HIV disease.

II. EARLY PHASE MUCOSAL EVENTS IN HIV INFECTION

A. HIV Entry

The gastrointestinal tract plays a critical role in the pathogenesis of HIV disease. At the outset, the distal colon serves as the most likely portal of entry for HIV in homosexual men, who constitute the majority of persons infected with HIV in developed countries. Many homosexual men have trauma-induced (Sohn and Ribilotti, 1977) or infection-associated (Quinn *et al.*, 1981; Surawicz *et al.*, 1986) erosions, breaks, and tears of the rectal mucosa. After inoculation, these lesions provide the virus direct access to the microcirculation of the rectal mucosa (Figure 1, Step 1).

In homosexual men without mucosal changes in the distal colon, however, HIV may enter the host through membranous microfold (M) cells (Figure 1, Step 2). Present throughout the intestinal tract, but with increased frequency in the distal colon (O'Leary and Sweeney, 1986), these specialized epithelial cells bind macromolecules and microorganisms, including viruses such as poliovirus and reovirus (Wolf *et al.*, 1981; Sicinski *et al.*, 1990), to their apical surface and transport them by a nondegradative process to their basal surface (Owen, 1977). The intact macromolecule or microorganism then is delivered by exocytosis to interdigitating mononuclear cells in the underlying lymphoid aggregate, where accessory cells take up, process, and present the antigens to lymphocytes within the aggregate. In this regard, studies in a mouse model of M-cell uptake indicate that murine M cells are capable of taking up and transporting HIV to underlying lymphoid aggregates (Amerongen *et al.*, 1991). Studies to determine the role of human M cells as a potential route of entry for HIV are currently in progress. The mucosa of the upper gastrointestinal tract, including tonsillar M cells, also could play a role in the postnatal transmission of HIV in colostrum and milk from mother to infant (Van de Perre *et al.*, 1991). In hemophiliacs and persons using illicit intravenous drugs, the virus is inoculated directly into the circulation (Figure 1, Step 3).

B. HIV Infection of $CD4^+$ Cells

After entry into the host, the initial event in the interaction between HIV and lymphoid cells is binding of the envelope glycoprotein 120 (gp120) on the virus to the cell-surface CD4 molecule, which serves as receptor for the virus (Klatzman *et al.*, 1984a,b). The viral envelope then fuses to the cell plasma membrane, and the virus is internalized (Stein *et al.*, 1987). Alternatively, studies of HIV infection of cells *in vitro* (Homsy *et al.*, 1989) suggest that the virus also might enter monocytes and macrophages by a mechanism involving FcγRIII (CD16) receptor-mediated uptake of HIV–antibody complexes. In this connection, the increased expression of FcγRIII receptors on circulating monocytes and tissue macrophages in patients with AIDS could contribute to HIV

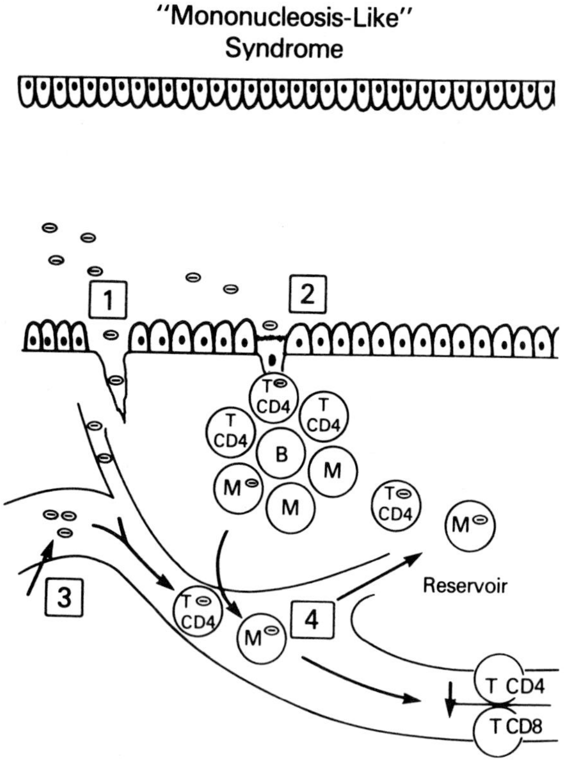

Figure 1 Early phase immunopathophysiological events in the mucosa in HIV infection. Adapted with permission from Smith *et al.* (1992b).

infection of mononuclear phagocytes (Allen *et al.*, 1990). For virus entering the host through mucosal breaks, CD4-bearing cells could be infected in the microcirculation of the mucosa and then be distributed via the systemic circulation to tissues, including the gastrointestinal mucosa, throughout the body (Figure 1, Step 4).

For virus entering the host through M cells, however, mononuclear cells in the underlying lymphoid aggregate are likely to be potential targets for HIV infection. Lymphocytes leave the lymphoid aggregate, migrating via the lymphatics to the mesenteric lymph nodes and via the thoracic duct to the systemic circulation. A mechanism involving homing receptors on mucosa-derived lymphocytes and organ-specific molecules on lamina propria endothelial cells then directs these antigen-reactive lymphocytes to the mucosal lamina propria and epithelium (Jalkanen *et al.*, 1986). Thus, lymphocytes stimulated at one site in the gastrointestinal tract eventually are distributed to distant mucosal sites, thereby providing a potential mechanism by which mononuclear cells, at least lymphocytes, infected with HIV in the rectum could distribute to the lamina propria throughout the gastrointestinal tract (Figure 1, Step 4).

Several days to weeks after inoculation, sufficient quantities of virus trigger a humoral immune response and seroconversion. At the time of HIV seroconversion, the first manifestation of HIV infection is experienced as an acute mononucleosis-like illness (Cooper *et al.*, 1985). Varying degrees of this syndrome appear to occur in a majority of newly infected persons. Among the clinical features of the syndrome are the "early" gastrointestinal symptoms of HIV infection, including diarrhea, nausea, and anorexia. The pathophysiology of the syndrome is unknown but could involve the local or systemic release of cytokines such as interleukin 1 (IL-1) and tumor necrosis factor (TNF), which have important roles in mediating acute febrile responses. Although controversial, the increased levels of these cytokines in HIV-infected patients could be generated, in part, by the ability of HIV-1 and its envelope glycoprotein (gp120) to stimulate mononuclear cell production of IL-1 (Wahl *et al.*, 1989) and TNF-α (Wright *et al.*, 1988; Voth *et al.*, 1990; Riekmann *et al.*, 1991). Acute symptomatic HIV infection is associated with expression of high titers of cytopathic virus followed by a rapid and spontaneous decline in the viral burden (Clark *et al.*, 1990; Daar *et al.*, 1991). The mononucleosis-like syndrome associated with seroconversion is transient and the patient recovers, at least symptomatically.

III. INTERMEDIATE PHASE MUCOSAL EVENTS IN HIV INFECTION

A. Reduction in Mucosal $CD4^+$ (Helper/Inducer) Lymphocytes

The migration of HIV-infected lymphocytes from the rectal mucosa to distant mucosal sites, either randomly or via a homing mechanism, provides one potential explanation for the presence of HIV-infected mononuclear cells throughout the gastrointestinal tract. Accordingly, HIV has been identified in mononuclear cells in the mucosa of the esophagus (Smith *et al.*, 1993) duodenum (Ulrich *et al.*, 1989; Jarry *et al.*, 1990), ileum (Harriman *et al.*, 1989), colon, and rectum (Fox *et al.*, 1989). Similar to the low level of HIV infection in mononuclear cells in the circulation ($\leq 1/100$ $CD4^+$ cells) (Schnittman *et al.*, 1989), the frequency of HIV-infected cells in the gastrointestinal tract lamina propria is also low ($\leq 1/100$ mononuclear cells; P. D. Smith, personal observations). Moreover, HIV-infected cells are detected in only one-third of intestinal biopsy specimens from HIV-infected persons (Fox *et al.*, 1989; Ulrich *et al.*, 1989; Jarry *et al.*, 1990). Although the frequency of HIV-infected $CD4^+$ cells is low in the circulation and the mucosa, these infected cells are likely to contribute to the progressive reduction in the total number of $CD4^+$ cells by a mechanism in which fusion of uninfected $CD4^+$ cells with viral components or budding virus expressed on HIV-infected $CD4^+$ cells causes the formation of multinucleated giant cells and lysis of the uninfected cells (Lifson *et al.*, 1986; Yolffe *et al.*, 1987).

The apparent removal of giant syncytia by the reticuloendothelial system and the lysis of $CD4^+$ cells fused to HIV-infected cells lead to a progressive decline in the number of $CD4^+$ lympohcytes. The decline in the number of $CD4^+$ T cells in comparison to the relatively constant number of $CD8^+$ (suppressor/cytotoxic) T cells is reflected in a progressive reduction in the ratio of $CD4^+$ to $CD8^+$ cells in the circulation. A corresponding reduction in the number of $CD4^+$ T cells also occurs in intestinal mucosa (Figure 2, Step 5) (Rodgers

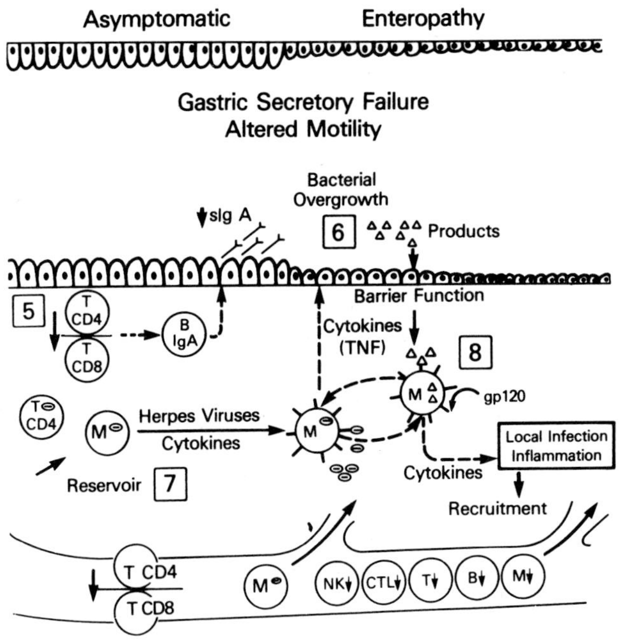

Figure 2 Intermediate phase immunopathophysiological events in the mucosa in HIV infection. Adapted with permission from Smith *et al.* (1992b).

et al., 1986; Budhraja *et al.*, 1987; Ellakany *et al.*, 1987). Since $CD4^+$ T cells play a critical role in providing helper and inducer function for many immune responses, the reduction in the ratio of $CD4^+$ to $CD8^+$ cells in the gastrointestinal mucosa suggests that the immune function of the mucosa is impaired also.

In addition to causing the selective depletion of $CD4^+$ lymphocytes, HIV impairs certain functions of these cells. For example, $CD4^+$ T cells from AIDS patients have a reduced ability to respond to soluble antigens, such as tetanus toxoid and *Candida albicans* (Lane *et al.*, 1985a; Giorgi *et al.*, 1987). In light of the role of $CD4^+$ T cells in regulating IgA class-specific immunoglobulin production (Elson *et al.*, 1979; Richman *et al.*, 1981), the reduced number and function of $CD4^+$ T cells could affect the switch of IgM- to IgA-bearing B cells in the lymphoid aggregates of the intestinal mucosa (Kawanishi *et al.*, 1983a) as well as the terminal differentiation of IgA-bearing to IgA-secreting B cells (Kawanishi *et al.*, 1983b). From this perspective, the observations by Kotler *et al.* (1984b) that AIDS patients have a reduced number of IgA-bearing plasma cells in the intestinal mucosa are particularly relevant. Thus, a reduction in the number and function of mucosal $CD4^+$ cells ultimately could contribute to a dysregulation in the generation and function of IgA-secreting cells. In support of the latter result are observations of a reduced IgA class-specific antibody response to HIV, which we have detected in intestinal fluids (Janoff *et al.*, 1989) and others have detected in saliva (Jackson, 1990).

In addition to specific secretory antibody responses, nonspecific host defense mechanisms such as gastric acid secretion and intestinal peristalsis play an important role in protecting intestinal mucosa against ingested organisms (Giannella *et al.*, 1973; Vantrappon *et al.*, 1977). Several studies (Lake-Bakaar *et al.*, 1988a,b) have shown that some AIDS patients, however, have an impaired capacity to secrete gastric acid, resulting in an increase in fasting gastric pH and a reduction in stimulated gastric acid secretion. The presence of circulating antiparietal cell antibodies in approximately 50% of these patients suggests an autoimmune mechanism. In addition to dysfunction in acid secretion, preliminary studies (Reeves-Darby *et al.*, 1991) indicate that some HIV-infected patients also exhibit a dysfunction in intestinal motility, manifesting as markedly abnormal migrating motor complexes.

B. Intestinal Bacteria

Colonization of the proximal small intestine by increased numbers of bacteria reflects an alteration in the delicate balance between host defense mechanisms and enteric microrganisms. In HIV-infected persons, impaired secretory antibody responses in conjunction with gastric secretory failure and intestinal dysmotility could predispose the host to increased numbers of intestinal bacteria (Figure 2, Step 6). In this regard, we (Smith *et al.*, 1988) and others (Budhraja *et al.*, 1987) have detected 4.5×10^4–10^5 bacteria/ml intestinal fluid in the proximal small intestine in AIDS patients with diarrhea. Although aerobes predominated or were equivalent in number to anaerobes, these levels of bacteria represent an increase over the number of bacteria (10^3 bacteria/ml) generally accepted as the upper limit of normal in the proximal small intestine. Increased numbers of bacteria in the small intestine, particularly anaerobes, play an etiological role in some malabsorption syndromes. Accordingly, low-grade bacterial overgrowth could contribute to the malabsorption and diarrhea that is common in patients with AIDS before such patients manifest full-blown opportunistic viral and parasitic intestinal infections.

C. HIV Reservoir

In addition to gut-associated lymphoid tissues as a site for immunosuppression, the gastrointestinal tract also may serve as a reservoir for HIV-infected mononuclear cells. The indentification of a cellular DNA binding protein that represses HIV-1 transcription in *in vitro* studies (Kato *et al.*, 1991) raises the intriguing possibility that local production of this factor may play a role in promoting latent HIV infection in mononuclear cells in the mucosa. As previously discussed, approximately one-third of HIV-infected persons have detectable HIV in their intestinal mucosa. Our identification of HIV in biopsy specimens from the esophagus in 36% of HIV-infected patients with esophageal symptoms (Smith *et al.*, 1993) indicates that, in symptomatic persons, HIV infects the mucosa of the esophagus as often as it infects the mucosa of the intestine. Although the frequency of HIV-infected $CD4^+$ cells within the mucosa appears to be similar to that in the circulation, the large number of mononuclear cells within the mucosa (making it the largest lymphoid organ in the body) would allow the alimentary canal to act as a major reservoir for HIV (Figure 2, Step 7).

In light of its potential role as a reservoir for HIV, the gastrointestinal tract is also likely to be a site for the expression of HIV from HIV-infected mononuclear cells. Two factors that stimulate expression of HIV *in vitro,* herpes-group viruses (Gendelman *et al.,* 1986) and certain cytokines (Rosenberg and Fauci, 1990 and Koyanagi *et al.,* 1988), may be present in the gastrointestinal mucosa of persons at risk for HIV infection or with AIDS (Figure 2, Step 7). Among the herpes-group viruses, herpes simplex virus is the most common cause of nongonococcal proctitis in sexually active homosexual males (Goodell *et al.,* 1983; Quinnan *et al.,* 1984) and is an important cause of esophagitis (Smith *et al.,* 1993) and proctitis (Siegal *et al.,* 1981) in patients with AIDS. Another herpes group virus, cytomegalovirus, causes subclinical infection in more than 90% of HIV-seronegative homosexual men (Drew *et al.,* 1981) and is a common cause of serious disease in virtually any organ of the gastrointestinal tract in patients with AIDS (Smith *et al.,* 1992a). The relevance of these pathogens to gastrointestinal tract HIV infection lies in their ability to activate transcription of latent HIV in HIV-infected cells. In the case of herpes simplex virus, this event probably occurs by a *trans*-acting factor encoded by the virus (Mosca *et al.,* 1987a,b); in the case of cytomegalovirus, the immediate-early gene region of the virus is likely to be responsible (Davis *et al.,* 1987). These factors stimulate HIV expression *in vitro* by activating the single promoter located within the 5′-long terminal repeat (LTR), which directs HIV transcription. Coincident with herpes-group virus stimulation of HIV expression, HIV stimulation of herpes-group virus (cytomegalovirus) expression has been demonstrated *in vitro* (Skolnik *et al.,* 1988), raising the possibility that bidirectional viral up-regulation may occur *in vivo* in tissues such as the gastrointestinal tract where mononuclear cells could be infected, albeit infrequently, by both viruses.

In addition to herpes-group viruses, cytokines also activate mononuclear cells, thereby stimulating the expression of HIV from cells that are infected latently or are producing low levels of HIV (Figure 2, Step 7). Granulocyte-macrophage colony-stimulating factor (Folks *et al.,* 1987; Perno *et al.,* 1989), interleukin 6 (Poli *et al.,* 1990a), and TNF (Poli *et al.,* 1990b; Mellors *et al.,* 1991) are capable of stimulating HIV expression in mononuclear cell lines and primary cells by a mechanism that is likely to involve the transcriptional regulation of HIV. TNF, for example, induces HIV expression from infected cells *in vitro* by an autocrine and paracrine mechanism (Rosenberg and Fauci, 1990), probably by induction of cellular factors that bind to the nuclear factor kB, thereby stimulating the HIV enhancer that induces HIV expression (Osborn *et al.,* 1989).

Within the gastrointestinal mucosa, these cytokines could play a particularly important role in the regulation of HIV expression. Infectious processes such as cytomegalovirus colitis have been shown to be associated with the expression of TNF within the colonic mucosa (Smith *et al.,* 1992c). Thus, local production of TNF and other inflammatory cytokines capable of up-regulating HIV expression (Clouse *et al.,* 1989) could obviate the requirement that both viruses be present in the same cell to induce HIV transcription.

During the intermediate phase of mucosal events in HIV infection, the patient begins to re-experience gastrointestinal symptoms, most commonly diarrhea. The diarrhea may occur initially in the absence of detectable pathogens, a condition referred to as the "AIDS enteropathy" (Kotler *et al.,* 1984a). The intestinal mucosa in this setting has been reported to show structural and functional alterations, including low-grade small bowel atrophy, a maturational defect in enterocytes, and decreased mucosal enzyme activities. Small bowel atrophy and defects in enterocyte maturation could contribute to a reduction in normal mucosal surface area. Factors that may play an etiological role in these alterations include mucosal HIV, which has been identified in the lamina propria of patients with these changes (Ulrich *et al.,* 1989), and increased numbers of certain intestinal bacteria (Budhraja *et al.,* 1987; Smith *et al.,* 1988) or their products, such as deconjugated bile salts. In addition, cytokines currently are being investigated for their ability to alter electrolyte transport mechanisms in mucosal epithelium. In this respect, we showed that the increased levels of TNF produced by activated alveolar macrophages during endotoxin administration (P. D. Smith, A. F. Suffridini, J. B. Allen, J. E. Parillo, and S. M. Wahl, unpublished data) are associated with local changes in lung permeability (Suffridini *et al.,* 1992). Thus, HIV, luminal bacteria, and cytokines are potential factors that might contribute to changes in the structure and function of mucosal epithelium.

D. Macrophage Activation

The structural and functional changes in the intestinal mucosa described in this chapter are associated with increased mucosal permeability to luminal materials, including bacterial products (Lichtman *et al.,* 1991). Since cell wall turnover is a characteristic of many gram-negative microorganisms (Doyle *et al.,* 1988), one product of potential significance is the surface protein shed by such bacteria. We have used *Helicobacter pylori,* a noninvasive mucosal bacterial pathogen, to show that surface proteins from gram-negative bacteria can be absorbed across the mucosal epithelium and can serve as chemoattractants for monocytes and neutrophils (Mai *et al.,* 1992). These chemotactic products are also potent activators of monocytes and macrophages, causing the release of increased amounts of inflammatory cytokines, such as TNF and interleukin 1, and toxic products, such as oxygen radicals (Mai *et al.,* 1991). Interestingly, the single reported case of invasive *H. pylori* gastritis was in a patient with AIDS (Meiselman *et al.,* 1988). Although *H. pylori* actually may infect HIV-infected persons less frequently than seronegative persons (Francis *et al.,* 1990), products from other enteric bacteria could function as pro-inflammatory factors similar to *H. pylori* surface proteins. One such product, lipopolysaccharide (LPS), is a potent activator of macrophages and can stimulate HIV-infected cell-line monocytes to express HIV as well (Pomerantz *et al.,* 1990). However, LPS induction of HIV expression has not been reproduced in primary monocytes infected with the virus (Kornbluth *et al.,* 1989; Bernstein *et al.,* 1991) and, to date, has not been investigated in tissue macrophages. Viruses and their products also can stimulate macrophages. For example, cytomegalovirus (Smith *et al.*, 1992c) is similar to influenza A (Gong *et al.*, 1991) in its ability to prime monocytes and macrophages for increased inducible TNF production. In addition, HIV is capable of activating monocytes (Allen *et al.*, 1990; Allen *et al.*, 1991), and HIV envelope gp120 is capable of stimulating monocytes and macrophages to produce increased amounts of inflammatory cytokines and prostaglandins (Wahl *et al.*, 1989) and B cells to produce TNF (Riekmann *et al.*, 1991). Thus, luminal bacteria and viruses or their products are potential activators of macrophages, leading to the production of increased amounts of cytokines and soluble inflammatory mediators (Figure 2, Step 8) that could, in turn, promote and perpetuate the chronic inflammation that characterizes mucosal histopathology in HIV-infected persons (Smith *et al.*, 1988).

IV. LATE PHASE MUCOSAL EVENTS IN HIV INFECTION

A. Lymphoid Cell Responses

After a period that may last from weeks to months or even years, the late phase of HIV infection emerges. By this point, increasing numbers of circulating natural killer cells, cytotoxic lymphocytes, T lymphocytes, B lymphocytes, and monocytes have impaired functions (Fauci, 1988; Meltzer *et al.*, 1990). Those functions that are impaired in circulating lymphoid cells have not been investigated yet in mucosal lymphoid cells. Nevertheless, mucosal lymphoid cell function probably becomes impaired as well (Figure 3, Step 9), since circulating lymphoid cells traffic through and populate the mucosa.

B. Opportunistic Infections

Impaired cellular immune responses, in conjunction with gastric secretory failure, altered intestinal motility, and impaired local IgA responses, predispose the gastrointestinal tract in HIV disease to a wide spectrum of opportunistic pathogens (Janoff and Smith, 1988). We define opportunistic gastrointestinal pathogens as those infectious agents that consistently cause severe, chronic, or frequent gastrointestinal disease in persons with compromised immune function (Smith and Janoff, 1988). Nonopportunistic pathogens are those that usually cause acute treatable gastrointestinal disease (Smith and Janoff, 1988) in immunocompromised as well as immunocompetent persons. The opportunistic and nonopportunistic pathogens that cause enteric infection in HIV-infected persons include the viral, fungal, bacterial, and protozoan agents listed in Table I.

Among the first pathogens that herald the late phase of the gastrointestinal manifestations of HIV disease is *C. albicans*. The presence of oral candidiasis in persons at risk for AIDS signals the likelihood of concomitant HIV infection, since 60% of such persons ultimately develop an AIDS-related infection or Kaposi's sarcoma within 2 yr (Klein *et al.*, 1984).

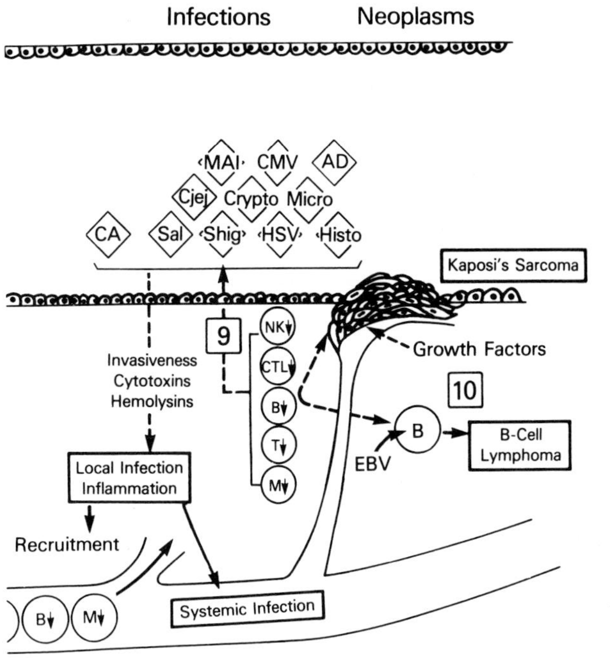

Figure 3 Late phase immunopathophysiological events in the mucosa in HIV infection. Adapted with permission from Smith *et al.* (1992b).

Candida albicans is a typical opportunistic pathogen by virtue of the fact that, in immunosuppressed HIV-infected persons, it frequently causes severe chronic disease of the oral cavity and esophageal mucosa whereas, in immunocompetent persons, it is a common nonpathogenic commensal of the gastrointestinal tract. Further, the striking similarity among isolates of *C. albicans* that cause mucosal disease in AIDS patients and isolates present in healthy persons, which we reported (Whelan *et al.*, 1990), suggests that candidiasis in patients with AIDS is not caused by a unique or particularly virulent strain, but is the consequence of a defect in local cell-mediated host defense mechanisms.

The many enteric infections that may develop during late phase mucosal events in HIV infection have been reviewed (Kotler, 1989; Smith *et al.*, 1992a). One or more of these pathogens can be identified in the majority of AIDS patients with gastrointestinal symptoms (Smith *et al.*, 1988; Laughon *et al.*, 1988), in contrast to the previously held notion that the majority of HIV-infected persons with diarrhea had AIDS enteropathy. In fact, increasing numbers of persons diagnosed initially as having AIDS enteropathy have been found on further analysis to have one of the more recently appreciated enteric pathogens, such as *Enterocytozoon bieneusi* (microsporidia; Kotler *et al.*, 1990) and adenovirus (Janoff *et al.*, 1991).

C. Mucosal Neoplasms

Malignant neoplasia of the gastrointestinal tract occurs in approximately 12% of patients with AIDS (Danzig *et al.*, 1991). Kaposi's sarcoma is the most common of such neoplasias, occurring in 60% of AIDS patients with gastrointestinal malignancies (Danzig *et al.*, 1991). Lesions begin as small

Table I Enteric Pathogens in HIV Disease

Pathogen	Viral	Protozoal	Fungal	Bacterial
Opportunistic	Cytomegalovirus Herpes simplex Adenovirus	*Cryptosporidia* *Isospora belli* *Enterocytozoon bieneusi*	*Candida albicans* Histoplasma capsulatum	*Mycobacterium avium-intracellulare* *Salmonella* sp. *Shigella flexneri* *Campylobacter jejuni*
Nonopportunistic	Rotavirus Norwalk agent	*Giardia lamblia* *Entamoeba histolytica*		*Mycobacterium* Spirochetes

papules that progress into multifocal vascular nodules because of the proliferation of a mixed cell population, in particular spindle-like cells with neovascularization. Gastrointestinal Kaposi's sarcoma is present in 40–50% of patients with skin involvement (Friedman *et al.*, 1985). Involvement of the small and large intestine is nearly always asymptomatic (Friedman *et al.*, 1985), whereas lesions in the esophagus that involve the sphincters or epiglottis may cause dysphagia (Eisner and Smith, 1990).

In contrast to the association between opportunistic infections and declining immune function (Lane *et al.*, 1985b; Smith *et al.*, 1988), Kaposi's sarcoma is not necessarily related to the degree of HIV-induced immunosuppression (Lane *et al.*, 1985b). *In vitro* studies (Nakamura *et al.*, 1988; Ensoli *et al.*, 1990) suggest that HIV-infected mononuclear cells release a transactivator of transcription (Tat) protein and certain cytokines (i.e., TNF) that stimulate proliferation of Kaposi's sarcoma-derived spindle cells (Figure 3, Step 10). Spindle cells produce, in turn, several growth factors (IL-1, IL-6, basic fibroblast growth factor) that stimulate their own growth as well as the growth of other cells, such as cells of vascular and lymphatic origin, within the Kaposi lesion (Salahuddin *et al.*, 1988; Ensoli *et al.*, 1989; Miles *et al.*, 1990). Oncostatin M, another growth factor produced by Kaposi's sarcoma cells and activated T cells (Nair *et al.*, 1992; Miles *et al.*, 1992), appears to be the most potent mitogen for spindle-cell growth, acting in an autocrine and paracrine loop. Thus, the presence of HIV-infected $CD4^+$ T cells and increased levels of cytokines in the gastrointestinal mucosa, as discussed earlier, could play an important role in the development of gastrointestinal Kaposi's sarcoma.

Lymphoma is the second most common malignancy of the gastrointestinal tract in patients with AIDS. Occurring in approximately 35% of AIDS patients with gastrointestinal malignancy (Danzig *et al.*, 1991), the lymphoma is usually non-Hodgkin's. In contrast to Kaposi's sarcoma, gastrointestinal lymphoma often produces obstruction or pain. Latent and replicating Epstein–Barr virus (EBV) DNA has been detected in lymphomas in patients with AIDS and other lymphoproliferative disorders (Katz *et al.*, 1989). Infection with EBV is common in AIDS patients (Quinnan *et al.*, 1984). The virus is capable of replicating in mucosal epithelial cells (Lemon *et al.*, 1977; Sixbey *et al.*, 1984); thus, in the setting of impaired EBV-specific cytotoxic T-cell responses (Rickenson, 1986; Figure 3, Step 9), lymphoproliferative lesions in the gastrointestinal tract could represent the outgrowth of EBV-transformed B cells (Figure 3, Step 10), similar to that reported in severe combined immunodeficient (SCID) mice inoculated with peripheral blood leukocytes from EBV-seropositive donors (Rowe *et al.*, 1991).

In summary, a sequence of interrelated immunological events in the gastrointestinal mucosa is a major complication of HIV infection. Over time, these events lead to local immunosuppresion, predisposing the gastrointestinal tract to the acquisition of opportunistic infections and the development of certain neoplasms. Understanding the immunopathophysiology of the mucosal events in HIV infection should facilitate the development of more effective therapies for the gastrointestinal complications of AIDS and, eventually, of an effective vaccine against HIV.

References

Allen, J. B., McCartney-Francis, N., Smith, P. D., Simon, G., Gartner, S., and Wahl, S. M. (1990). Expression of interleukin 2 receptors by monocytes from patients with acquired immunodeficiency syndrome and induction of monocyte interleukin 2 receptors by human immunodeficiency virus in vitro. *J. Clin. Invest.* **85,** 192–199.

Allen, J. B., Wong, H. L., Guyre, P. M., Simon, G. L., and Wahl, S. M. (1991). Association of circulating FcγRIII-receptor positive monocytes in AIDS patients with elevated levels of transforming growth factor-β. *J. Clin. Invest.* **87,** 1773–1779.

Amerongen, H. M., Weltzin, R., Farnet, C. M., Michetti, P., Haseltine, W. A., and Neutra, M. R. (1991). Transepithelial transport of HIV-1 by intestinal M cells: A mechanism for transmission of AIDS. *J. Acquir. Immune Defic. Synd.* **4,** 760–765.

Bernstein, M. S., Tong-Starksen, S. E., and Locksley, R. M. (1991). Activation of human monocyte-derived macrophages with lipopolysaccharide decreases human immunodeficiency virus replication in vitro at the level of gene expression. *J. Clin. Invest.* **88,** 540–545.

Budhraja, M., Levendoglu, H., Kocka, F., Mangkornkanok, M., and Sherer, R. (1987). Duodenal mucosal T cell subpopulation and bacterial cultures in acquired immune deficiency syndrome. *Am. J. Gastroenterol.* **82,** 427–431.

Centers for Disease Control (1992). "HIV Disease Surveillance Report: Year-end edition." United States Public Health Service, Department of Health and Human Services, Washington, D.C.

Clark, S. J., Saag, M. S., Decker, W. D., Campbell-Hill, S., Roberson, J. L., Veldkamp, P. J., Kappes, J. C., Hahn, B. H., and Shaw, G. M. (1990). High titers of cytopathic virus in plasma of patients with symptomatic primary HIV-1 infection. *N. Engl. J. Med.* **324,** 954–960.

Clouse, K. A., Robbins, P. B., Fernie, B., Ostrove, J. M., and Fauci, A. S. (1989). Viral antigen stimulation of the production of human monokines capable of regulating HIV-1 expression. *J. Immunol.* **143,** 470–475.

Cooper, A. D., Gold, J., MacLean, P., Donovan, B., Finlayson, R., and Barnes, T. G. (1985). Acute AIDS retrovirus infection—Definition of a clinical illness associated with seroconversion. *Lancet* **2,** 537–540.

Daar, E. S., Moudgil, T., Meyer, R. D., and Ho, D. D. (1991). Transient high levels of viremia in patients with primary human immunodeficiency virus type 1 infection. *N. Engl. J. Med.* **324,** 961–964.

Danzig, J. B., Brandt, L. J., Reinus, J. F., and Klein, R. S. (1991). Gastrointestinal malignancy in patients with AIDS. *Am. J. Gastroenterol.* **86,** 715–718.

Davis, M. G., Kenney, S. C., Kamine, J., Pagano, J. S., and Huang, E. S. (1987). Immediate early gene region of human cytomegalovirus trans-activates the promoter of human immunodeficiency virus. *Proc. Natl. Acad. Sci. U.S.A.* **84,** 8641–8646.

Doyle, R. J., Chaloupka, J., and Vinter, V. (1988). Turnover of cell walls in microorganisms. *Microbiol. Rev.* **52,** 554–567.

Drew, W. L., Mintz, L., Miner, R. C., Sands, M., and Katterer, B. (1981). Prevalence of cytomegalovirus infection in homosexual men. *J. Infect. Dis.* **143,** 188–192.

Ellakany, S., Whiteside, T. L., Schade, R. R., and Van Thiel, D. H. (1987). Analysis of intestinal lymphocyte subpopulations in patients with acquired immunodeficiency syndrome (AIDS) and AIDS-related complex. *J. Clin. Pathol.* **87,** 356–364.

Elson, C. O., Heck, J. A., and Strober, W. (1979). T-cell regulation of murine IgA synthesis. *J. Exp. Med.* **149,** 632–643.

Ensoli, B., Nakamura, S., Salahuddin, S. Z., Biberfield, P., Larsson, L., Beaver, B., Wong-Staal, F., and Gallo, R. C. (1989). AIDS-Kaposi's sarcoma-derived cells express cytokines with autocrine and paracrine growth effects. *Science* **243,** 223–226.

Ensoli, B., Barillari, G., Salahuddin, S. Z., Gallo, R. C., and Wong-Staal, F. (1990). Tat protein of HIV-1 stimulates growth of cells derived from Kaposi's sarcoma lesions of AIDS patients. *Nature (London)* **345,** 84–86.

Fauci, A. S. (1988). The human immunodeficiency virus: Infectivity and mechanisms of pathogenesis. *Science* **239,** 617–622.

Folks, T. M., Justament, J., Kinter, A., Dinarello, C. A., and Fauci, A. S. (1987). Cytokine-induced expression of HIV-1 in a chronically infected promonocyte cell line. *Science* **238,** 800–802.

Fox, C. H., Kotler, D. P., Tierney, A. R., Wilson, C. S., and Fauci, A. S. (1989). Detection of HIV-1 RNA in the lamina propria of patients with AIDS and gastrointestinal disease. *J. Infect. Dis.* **159,** 467–471.

Francis, N. D., Logan, R. P. H., Walker, M. M., Polson, R. J., Boylston, A. W., Pinching, A. J., Harris, J. R. W., and Baron, J. H. (1990). *Campylobacter pylori* in the upper gastrointestinal tract of patients with HIV-1 infection. *J. Clin. Pathol.* **43,** 60–62.

Friedman, S. L., Wright, T. L., and Altman, D. F. (1985). Gastrointestinal Kaposi's sarcoma in patients with acquired immunodeficiency syndrome. Endoscopic and autopsy findings. *Gastroenterology* **89,** 102–108.

Gendelman, H. E., Phelps, W., Feigenbaum, L., Ostrove, J. M., Adachi, A., Howley, P. M., Khoury, G., and Ginsberg, H. S. (1986). Transactivation of the human immunodeficiency virus long terminal repeat sequence by DNA viruses. *Proc. Natl. Acad. Sci. U.S.A.* **83,** 9759–9763.

Giannella, R. A., Broitman, S. A., and Zamchek, N. (1973). Influence of gastric acidity on bacterial and parasitic enteric infections. A perspective. *Ann. Intern. Med.* **78,** 271–276.

Giorgi, J. V., Fahey, J. L., Smith, D. C., Hultin, L. E., Cheng, H. L., Mitsuyasu, R. T., and Detels, R. V. (1987). Early effects of HIV on CD4 lymphocytes *in vivo*. *J. Immunol.* **138,** 3725–3730.

Gong, J. H., Sprenger, H., Hinder, F., Bender, A., Schmidt, A., Horch, S., Nain, M., and Gemsa, D. (1991). Influenza A virus infection of macrophages. Enhanced tumor necrosis factor-α (TNF-α) gene expression and lipopolysaccharide triggered TNF-α release. *J. Immunol.* **147,** 3507–3513.

Goodell, S. E., Quinn, T. C., Mkrtichian, E., Schuffler, M. D., Holmes, K. K., and Corey, L. (1983). Herpes simplex virus proctitis in homosexual men. Clinical, sigmoidoscopic, and histopathologic features. *N. Engl. J. Med.* **308,** 868–871.

Harriman, G. R., Smith, P. D., Horne, M. K., Fox, C. H., Koenig, S., Lack, E. E., Lane, H. C., and Fauci, A. S. (1989). Vitamin B12 malabsorption in patients with acquired immunodeficiency syndrome. *Arch. Intern. Med.* **149,** 2039–2041.

Homsy, J., Meyer, M., Tateno, M., Clarkson, C., and Levy, J. A. (1989). The Fc and not CD4 receptor mediates antibody enhancement of HIV infection in human cells. *Science* **244,** 1357–1360.

Jackson, S. (1990). Secretory and serum IgA are inversely altered in AIDS patients. *In* "Advances in Mucosal Immunology" (T. T. MacDonald, S. J. Challacombe, P. W. Bland, C. R. Stokes, R. V. Heatley, and A. McMowat, eds.), pp. 665–668. Kluwer Academic Publishers, London.

Jalkanen, S., Reichert, R. A., Gallatin, W. M., Bargatze, R. F., Weissman, I. L., and Butcher, E. C. (1986). Human lymphocyte and lymphoma homing receptors. *Immunol. Rev.* **91,** 39–60.

Janoff, E. N., and Smith, P. D. (1988). Perspectives on gastrointestinal infections in AIDS. *Gastroenterol. Clin. North Am.* **17,** 451–463.

Janoff, E. N., Wahl, S. M., and Smith, P. D. (1989). Antibodies to human immunodeficiency virus-1 (HIV) in the small intestine are primarily IgG, not IgA. *Gastroenterology* **96,** 236A.

Janoff, E. N., Orenstein, J. M., Manischewitz, J. F., and Smith, P. D. (1991). Adenovirus colitis in the acquired immunodeficiency syndrome. *Gastroenterology* **100,** 976–979.

Jarry, A., Cartez, A., Rene, E., Muzeau, F., and Brousse, N. (1990). Infected and immune cells in the gastrointestinal tract of AIDS patients. An immunohistochemical study of 127 cases. *Histopathology* **16,** 133–140.

Kato, H., Horikoshi, M., and Roeder, R. G. (1991). Repression of HIV-1 transcription by a cellular protein. *Science* **251,** 1476–1479.

Katz, B. Z., Raab-Traub, N., and Miller, G. (1989). Latent and replicating forms of Epstein-Barr virus DNA in lymphomas and lymphoproliferative diseases. *J. Infect. Dis.* **160,** 589–598.

Kawanishi, H., Saltzman, L., and Strober, W. (1983a). Mechanisms regulating IgA class-specific immunoglobulin production in murine gut-associated lymphoid tissues. I. T cells derived from Peyer's patches that switch SIgM B cells to SIgA B cells in vitro. *J. Exp. Med.* **157,** 433–450.

Kawanishi, H., Saltzman, L., and Strober, W. (1983b). Mechanisms regulating IgA class-specific immunoglobulin production in murine gut-associated lymphoid tissues II. Terminal differentiation of postswitch SIgA-bearing Peyer's patch B cells. *J. Exp. Med.* **158,** 649–669.

Klatzman, D., Barre-Sinoussi, F., Nugeyere, M. T., Dauguet, C., Vilmer, E., Griscelli, C., Brun-Vezinet, F., Rouzioux, C., Gluckman, J. C., Chermann, J.-C., and Montagmer, L. (1984a). Selective tropism of lymphadenopathy associated virus (LAV) for helper-inducer lymphocytes. *Science* **225,** 39.

Klatzman, D., Champagne, E., Chamaret, S., Gruest, J., Guetard, D., Hercend, T., Gluckman, J.-C., and Montagnier, L. (1984b). T lymphocyte T4 molecule behaves as the receptor for the human retrovirus LAV. *Nature (London)* **312,** 767.

Klein, R. S., Harris, C. A., Small, C. B., Moll, B., Lesser, M., and Friedland, G. H. (1984). Oral candidiasis in high-risk patients as the initial manifestation of the acquired immunodeficiency syndrome. *N. Engl. J. Med.* **311,** 354–358.

Kornbluth, R. S., Oh, P. S., Munis, J. R., Cleveland, P. H., and

Richman, D. D. (1989). Interferons and bacterial lipopolysaccharide protect macrophages from productive infection by human immunodeficiency virus *in vitro*. *J. Exp. Med.* **169,** 1137–1151.

Kotler, D. P. (1989). Intestinal and hepatic manifestations of AIDS. *Adv. Intern. Med.* **34,** 43–72.

Kotler, D. P., Gaetz, H. P., Lange, M., Klein, E. B., and Holt, P. R. (1984a). Enteropathy associated with the acquired immunodeficiency syndrome. *Ann. Intern. Med.* **101,** 421–428.

Kotler, D. P., Scholes, J. V., and Tierney, A. R. (1984b). Intestinal plasma cell alterations in acquired immunodeficiency syndrome. *Dig. Dis. Sci.* **32,** 129–138.

Kotler, D. P., Francisco, A., Clayton, F., Scholes, J. V., and Orenstein, J. M. (1990). Small intestinal injury and parasitic diseases in AIDS. *Ann. Intern. Med.* **113,** 444–449.

Koyanagi, Y., O'Brien, W. A., Zhao, W. A., Golde, D. W., Gasson, J. C., and Chen, I. S. Y. (1988). Cytokines alter production of HIV-1 from primary mononuclear phagocytes. *Science* **241,** 1673–1675.

Lake-Bakaar, G., Quadros, E., Beidas, S., Elsakr, M., Tom, W., Wilson, D. E., Dincsoy, H. O., Cohen, P., and Straus, E. W. (1988a). Gastric secretory failure in patients with the acquired immunodeficiency syndrome (AIDS). *Ann. Intern. Med.* **109,** 502–504.

Lake-Bakaar, G., Tom, W., Lake-Bakaar, D., Gupta, N., Beidas, S., Elsakr, M., and Straus, E. (1988b). Gastropathy and ketoconazole malabsorption in the acquired immunodeficiency syndrome (AIDS). *Ann. Intern. Med.* **109,** 471–473.

Lane, H. C., Depper, J. M., Greene, W. C., Whalen, G., Waldman, T. A., and Fauci, A. S. (1985a). Qualitative analysis of immune function in patients with the acquired immunodeficiency syndrome. Evidence for a selective defect in soluble antigen recognition. *N. Engl. J. Med.* **313,** 79–84.

Lane, H. C., Masur, H., Gelmann, E. P., Longo, D. L., Steis, R. G., Chused, T., Whalen, G., Edgar, L. C., and Fauci, A. S. (1985b). Correlation between immunologic function and clinical subpopulations of patients with the acquired immune deficiency syndrome. *Am. J. Med.* **78,** 417–422.

Laughon, B. E., Druckman, D. A., Vernon, A., Quinn, T. C., Polk, B. F., Modlin, J. F., Yolken, R. H., and Bartlett, J. G. (1988). Prevalence of enteric pathogens in homosexual men with and without acquired immunodeficiency syndrome. *Gastroenterology* **94,** 984–993.

Lemon, S. M., Hutt, L. M., Shaw, J. E., Li, J. L. H., and Pagano, J. S. (1977). Replication of EBV in epithelial cells during infectious mononucleosis. *Nature (London)* **268,** 268–270.

Lichtman, S. N., Keku, J., Schwab, J. H., and Sartor, R. B. (1991). Evidence for peptidoglycan absorption in rats with experimental small bowel bacterial overgrowth. *Infect. Immun.* **59,** 555–562.

Lifson, J. D., Reyes, G. R., McGrath, M. S., Stein, B. S., and Engleman, E. G. (1986). AIDS retrovirus induced cytopathology: Giant cell formation and involvement of CD4 antigen. *Science* **232,** 1123–1127.

Mai, U. E. H., Perez-Perez, G. I., Wahl, L. M., Wahl, S. M., Blaser, M. J., and Smith, P. D. (1991). Soluble surface proteins from *Helicobacter pylori* activate monocytes/macrophages by a lipopolysaccharide-independent mechanism. *J. Clin. Invest.* **87,** 894–900.

Mai, U. E. H., Perez-Perez, G. I., Allen, J. B., Wahl, S. M., Blaser, M. J., and Smith, P. D. (1992). Surface proteins from *Helicobacter pylori* exhibit chemotactic activity for human leukocytes and are present in gastric mucosa. *J. Exp. Med.* **175,** 517–525.

Meiselman, M. S., Miller-Catchpole, R., Christ, M., and Randal, E. (1988). *Campylobacter pylori* gastritis in the acquired immunodeficiency syndrome. *Gastroenterology* **95,** 209–212.

Mellors, J. W., Griffith, B. P., Oritz, M. A., Landry, M. L., and Ryan, J. L. (1991). Tumor necrosis factor-alpha/cachectin enhances human immunodeficiency virus type 1 replication in primary macrophages. *J. Infect. Dis.* **163,** 78–82.

Meltzer, M. S., Skillman, D. R., Gomatos, P. J., Kalter, D. C., and Gendelman, H. E. (1990). Role of mononuclear phagocytes in the pathogenesis of human immunodeficiency virus infection. *Ann. Rev. Immunol.* **8,** 169–194.

Miles, S. A., Rezai, A. R., Salazar-Gonzalez, J. F., Meyden, M. V., Stevens, R. H., Logan, D. M., Mitsuyasu, R. T., Taga, T., Hirano, T., Kishimoto, T., and Martinez-Maza, O. (1990). AIDS Kaposi sarcoma-derived cells produce and respond to interleukin 6. *Proc. Natl. Acad. Sci. U.S.A.* **87,** 4068–4072.

Miles, S. A., Martinez-Maza, O., Rezai, A., Magpantay, L., Kishimoto, T., Nakamura, S., Radka, S. F., and Linsley, P. S. (1992). Oncostatin M as a potent mitogen for AIDS-Kaposi's sarcoma-derived cells. *Science* **225,** 1432–1434.

Mosca, J. D., Bednarik, D. P., Raj, N. B. K., Rosen, C. A., Sodroski, J. G., Haseltine, W. A., Hayward, G. S., and Pitha, P. M. (1987a). Activation of human immunodeficiency virus by herpes virus infection: Identification of a region within the long terminal repeat that responds to a trans-activating factor encoded by herpes simplex virus I. *Proc. Natl. Acad. Sci. U.S.A.* **84,** 7408–7412.

Mosca, J. D., Bednarik, D. P., Raj, N. B. K., Rosen, C. A., Sodroski, J. G., Haseltine, W. A., and Pitha, P. M. V. (1987b). Herpes simplex virus type-1 can reactivate transcription of latent human immunodeficiency virus. *Nature (London)* **325,** 67–70.

Nair, B. C., DeVico, A. L., Nakamura, S., Copeland, T. D., Chen, Y., Patel, A., O'Neil, T., Oroszlan, S., Gallo, R. C., and Sarngadharan, M. G. (1992). Identification of a major growth factor for AIDS-Kaposi's sarcoma cells as Oncostatin M. *Science* **255,** 1430–1432.

Nakamura, S., Salahuddin, S. Z., Biberfeld, P., Ensoli, B., Markham, P. D., Wong-Stael, F., and Gallo, R. C. (1988). Kaposi's sarcoma cells: Long-term culture with growth factor from retrovirus-infected CD4+ T cells. *Science* **242,** 426–430.

O'Leary, A. D., and Sweeney, E. C. (1986). Lymphoglandular complexes of the colon: Structure and distribution. *Histopathology* **10,** 267–283.

Osborn, L., Kunkel, S., and Nabel, G. J. (1989). Tumor necrosis factor alpha and interleukin 1 stimulate the human immunodeficiency virus enhancer by activation of the nuclear factor kB. *Proc. Natl. Acad. Sci. U.S.A.* **86,** 2336–2340.

Owen, R. L. (1977). Sequential uptake of horseradish peroxidase by lymphoid follicle epithelium of Peyers's patches in the normal unobstructed mouse intestine: An ultrastructural study. *Gastroenterology* **72,** 440–451.

Perno, C.-F., Yarchoan, R., Cooney, D. A., Hartman, N. R., Webb, D. S. A., Hao, Z., Mitsuya, H., Johns, D. G., and Broder, S. (1989). Replication of human immunodeficiency virus in monocytes. Granulocyte–macrophage colony-stimulating factor (GM-CSF) potentiates viral production yet enhances the antiviral effect mediated by 3′-azido-2′3′-dideoxythymidine (AZT) and other dideoxynucleoside congeners of thymidine. *J. Exp. Med.* **169,** 933–951.

Poli, G., Bressler, P., Kinter, A., Duh, E., Timmer, W. C., Rabson, A., Justement, S., Stanley, S., and Fauci, A. S. (1990a). Interleukin 6 induces human immunodeficiency virus expression in infected monocytic cells alone and in synergy with tumor necrosis factor alpha by transcriptional and post-transcriptional mechanisms. *J. Exp. Med.* **172,** 151–158.

Poli, G., Kinter, A., Justement, J. S., Kehrl, J. H., Bressler, P., Stanley, S., and Fauci, A. S. (1990b). Tumor necrosis factor alpha functions in an autocrine manner in the induction of human immunodeficiency virus expression. *Proc. Natl. Acad. Sci. U.S.A.* **87,** 782–785.

Pomerantz, R. J., Feinberg, M. B., Trono, D., and Baltimore, D.

(1990). Lipopolysaccharide is a potent monocyte/macrophage-specific stimulator of human immunodeficiency virus type 1 expression. *J. Exp. Med.* **172,** 253–261.

Quinn, T. C., Corey, L., Chaffee, R. G., Schuffler, M. D., Brancato, F. P., and Holmes, K. K. (1981). The etiology of anorectal infections in homosexual men. *Am. J. Med.* **71,** 395–406.

Quinnan, G. V., Masur, H., Rook, A. H., Armstrong, G., Frederick, W., Epstein, J., Manischewitz, J. F., Macher, A. M., Jackson, L., Ames, J., Smith, H. A., Parker, M., Pearson, G. R., Panilo, J., Mitchell, C., and Straus, S. (1984). Herpesvirus infections in the acquired immune deficiency syndrome. *J. Am. Med. Assoc.* **252,** 72–77.

Reeves-Darby, V. G., Mathias, J. R., and Clench, M. H. (1991). Abnormal gastrointestinal motility in patients with human immunodeficiency virus 1 (HIV-1). *Gastroenterology* **100,** 608A.

Reikmann, P., Poli, G., Fox, C. H., Kehrl, J. H., and Fauci, A. S. (1991). Recombinant gp120 specifically enhances tumor necrosis factor-α production and Ig secretion in B lymphocytes from HIV-infected individuals but not from seronegative donors. *J. Immunol.* **147,** 2922–2927.

Richman, L. K., Graeff, A. S., Yarchoan, R., and Strober, W. (1981). Simultaneous induction of antigen-specific IgA helper T cells and IgG suppressor T cells in the murine Peyer's patch after protein feeding. *J. Immunol.* **128,** 2079–2083.

Rickenson, A. B. (1986). Cellular immune responses to the virus infection. *In* "The Epstein–Barr Virus: Recent Advances" (M. A. Epstein and B. G. Achong, eds.), p. 75. William Heinemann Medical Books, London.

Rodgers, V. D., Fassett, R., and Kagnoff, M. F. (1986). Abnormalities in intestinal mucosal T cells in homosexual populations including those with the lymphadenopathy syndrome and acquired immunodeficiency syndrome. *Gastroenterology* **90,** 552–558.

Rosenberg, Z. F., and Fauci, A. S. (1990). Immunopathogenic mechanisms of HIV infection: Cytokine induction of HIV expression. *Immunol. Today* **11,** 176–180.

Rowe, M., Young, L. S., Crocker, J., Stokes, H., Henderson, S., and Rickinson, A. B. (1991). Epstein-Barr virus (EBV)-associated lymphoproliferative disease in the SCID mouse model: Implications for the pathogenesis of EBV-positive lymphomas in man. *J. Exp. Med.* **173,** 147–158.

Salahuddin, S. Z., Nakamura, S., Biberfeld, ■., Kaplan, M. H., Markham, P. D., Larsson, L., Gallo, R. C. (1988). Angiogenic properties of Kaposi's sarcoma-derived cells after long-term culture in vitro. *Science* **242,** 430–433.

Schnittman, S. M., Psallidopoulos, M. C., Lane, H. C., Thompson, L., Baseler, M., Massari, F., Fox, C. H., Salzman, N. P., and Fauci, A. S. (1989). The reservoir for HIV-1 in human peripheral blood is a T cell that maintains expression of CD4. *Science* **245,** 305–308.

Sicinski, P., Rowinski, J., Warchol, J. B., Jarzabek, Z., Gut, W., Szczygiel, B., Bielecki, K., and Koch, G. (1990). Poliovirus type 1 enters the human host through intestinal M cells. *Gastroenterology* **98,** 56–58.

Siegal, F. P., Lopez, C., Hammer, G. S., Brown, A. E., Kornfield, S. J., Gold, J., Hassett, J., Hirschman, S. Z., Cunningham-Rundles, C., Adelsberg, B. R., Parham, D. M., Siegal, M., Cunningham-Rundles, S., and Armstrong, D. (1981). Severe acquired immunodeficiency in male homosexuals, manifested by chronic perianal ulcerative herpes simplex lesions. *N. Engl. J. Med.* **305,** 1439–1444.

Sixbey, J. W., Nedrud, J. G., Raab-Traub, N., Hanes, R. A., and Pagano, J. S. (1984). Epstein–Barr virus replication in oropharyngeal epithelial cells. *N. Engl. J. Med.* **310,** 1225–1230.

Skolnik, P. R., Kosloff, B. R., and Hirsch, M. S. (1988). Bidirectional interactions between human immunodeficiency virus type 1 and cytomegalovirus. *J. Infect. Dis.* **157,** 508–514.

Smith, P. D., and Janoff, E. N. (1988). Infectious diarrhea in human immunodeficiency virus infection. *Gastroenterol. Clin. North Am.* **17,** 587–598.

Smith, P. D., Lane, H. C., Gill, V. J., Manischewitz, J. F., Quinnan, G. V., Fauci, A. S., and Masur, H. (1988). Intestinal infections in patients with the acquired immunodeficiency syndrome. Etiology and response to therapy. *Ann. Intern. Med.* **108,** 328–333.

Smith, P. D., Eisner, M. S., Manischewitz, J. F., Gill, V. J., Masur, H., and Fox, C. F. (1993). Esophageal disease in AIDS is associated with pathological processes rather than mucosal HIV. *J. Infect. Dis.* **167,** 547–552.

Smith, P. D., Quinn, T. C., Strober, W., Janoff, E. N., and Masur, H. (1992a). Gastrointestinal infections of AIDS. *Ann. Intern. Med.* **116,** 63–77.

Smith, P. D., Saini, S. S., Manischewitz, J. F., Raffeld, M., and Wahl, S. M. (1992c). Cytomegalovirus induction of tumor necrosis factor-α by human monocytes/macrophages. *J. Clin. Invest.* **90,** 1642–1648.

Smith, P. D., and Mai, U. E. H. (1992b). Immunopathophysiology of gastrointestinal disease in HIV infection. *Gastroenterol. Clin. North Am.* **21,** 331–345.

Sohn, N., and Ribilotti, J. G. (1977). The gay bowel syndrome. A review of colonic and rectal conditions in 200 male homosexuals. *Am. J. Gastroenterol.* **67,** 478–484.

Stein, B. S., Gowda, S. D., Lifson, J. D., Penhallow, R. C., Benseh, K. G., and Engleman, E. G. (1987). pH-independent HIV entry into CD4 positive T cells via virus envelope fusion to the plasma membrane. *Cell* **49,** 659–668.

Suffridini, A. F., Shelhamer, J. H., Newmann, R. D., Brenner, M. Baltaro, R. J., and Parillo, J. E. (1992). Pulmonary effects of intravenous endotixin administration to normal humans. *Am. Rev. Resp. Dis.* **145,** 1398–1408.

Surawicz, C. M., Goodell, S. E., Quinn, T. C., Roberto, P. L., Corey, L., Holmes, K. K., Schuffler, M. D., and Stamm, W. E. (1986). Spectrum of rectal biopsy abnormalities in homosexual men with intestinal symptoms. *Gastroenterology* **91,** 651–659.

Ullrich, R., Zeitz, M., Heise, W., L'age, M., Hoffken, G., and Riecker, E. O. (1989). Small intestinal structure and function in patients infected with human immunodeficiency virus (HIV): Evidence for HIV-induced enteropathy. *Ann. Intern. Med.* **3,** 15–21.

Van de Perre, P., Simonon, A., Msellati, P., Hittmana, D. G., Vaira, D., Bazubogira, A., Van Goethem, C., Stevens, A. M., Karita, E., Sondag-Thull, D., Dabis, F., and Lepage, P. (1991). Postnatal transmission of human immunodeficiency virus type 1 from mother to infant. A prospective cohort study in Kigoli, Rwanda. *N. Engl. J. Med.* **325,** 593–598.

Vantrappen, G., Janssens, J., Hellemans, J., and Ghoos, X. (1977). The interdigestive motor complex of normal subjects and patients with bacterial overgrowth of the small intestine. *J. Clin. Invest.* **59,** 1158–1166.

Voth, R., Rossol, S., Klein, K., Hess, G., Schütt, K. H., Schröder, H. C., Zum Büschenfelde, K.-H. M., and Müller, W. E. G. (1990). Differential gene expression of IFN-α and tumor necrosis factor-α in peripheral blood mononuclear cells from patients with AIDS related complex and AIDS. *J. Immunol.* **144,** 970–975.

Wahl, S. M., Corcoran, M. L., Pyle, S. W., Arthur, L. O., Harel-Bellan, A., and Farrar, W. L. (1989). Human immunodeficiency virus glycoprotein (gp 120) induction of monocyte arachidonic acid metabolites and interleukin 1. *Proc. Natl. Acad. Sci. U.S.A.* **86,** 621–625.

Whelan, W. L., Kirsch, D. R., Kwon-Chung, K. J., Wahl, S. M., and Smith, P. D. (1990). *Candida albicans* in patients with the acquired immunodeficiency syndrome: Absence of a novel or hypervirulent strain. *J. Infect. Dis.* **162,** 513–518.

Wolf, J. L., Rubin, D. H., Finberg, R., Kauffman, R. S., Sharpe, A. H., Frier, J. S., and Fields, B. N. (1981). Intestinal M cells: A pathway for entry of reovirus into the host. *Science* **212,** 471–472.

Wright, S. C., Jewett, A., Mitsuyasu, R., and Bonavida, B. (1988). Spontaneous cytotoxicity and tumor necrosis factor production by peripheral blood monocytes from AIDS patients. *J. Immunol.* **141,** 99–104.

Yolffe, B., Lewis, D. E., Petrie, B. L., Noonan, C. A., Melnick, J. L., and Hollinger, F. B. (1987). Fusion as a mediator of cytolysis in mixtures of uninfected $CD4^+$ lymphocytes and cells infected by human immunodeficiency virus. *Proc. Natl. Acad. Sci. U.S.A.* **84,** 1429–1433.

58

Genital Tract Infection: Implications in the Prevention of Maternal and Fetal Disease

Debra A. Tristram · Pearay L. Ogra

I. INTRODUCTION

The incidence of sexually transmitted diseases (STDs) has risen markedly worldwide in the past decade (Antal, 1987; Johnson *et al.*, 1989; Brunham and Plummer, 1990). The acquisition of the human immunodeficiency virus (HIV) and development of acquired immunodeficiency syndrome (AIDS), widespread drug abuse, and prostitution for drugs or money have resulted in the resurgence of many STDs once thought to be controlled in developed nations. Since most species of organisms responsible for STDs are not capable of survival outside the human host and must be transmitted by direct human contact, STDs characteristically are restricted to a sexually active population, with a peak incidence between the ages of 15 and 34, and to newborns of women in this population. Although the incidence of AIDS in the homosexual population has decreased largely because of alterations in high-risk behavior, AIDS has continued to rise at an alarming rate in the heterosexual and drug-abusing populations of many countries [Morbidity and Mortality Weekly Reports (MMWR), 1991a,b; World Health Organization (WHO), 1991]. Although these HIV-positive individuals are not the only reservoir for STDs, they have become a major source. Clearly current strategies for disease containment are insufficient; other modalities, including immunization, are needed desperately to prevent the widespread continued increase of STDs.

Sexually transmitted agents long have been recognized to be responsible for many acute genital infections, but only recently has a wider role been established for these agents in the epidemiology of prolonged maternal and infant morbidity and mortality. Although men can have long-term complications from STDs, they are often more symptomatic early in the infection cycle and, thus, may seek care before the infection becomes deeply established. Women, on the other hand, are more susceptible to infection and may be asymptomatic in the early stages of infection. Thus, they may be less likely to seek health care and more likely to transmit disease to other sexual partners. In addition to causing widespread infections, STDs have a major impact on reproductive health: infertility has been linked to some genital infections (e.g., *Chlamydia* and *Mycoplasma* species) and maternal–fetal transmission of genital organisms remains a common cause of fetal and infant morbidity and mortality. Since pregnant women, regardless of their socioeconomic status, are likely to seek medical attention at or near the time of delivery, they constitute a reasonable target population for intervention. A significant decrease in infant morbidity (and possibly fetal and infant mortality) might be achieved if STDs could be controlled better in women of child-bearing age. The unique immune system of the pregnant and lactating female has been demonstrated in the past to provide temporary protection against a host of agents to which the mother has been exposed previously. Perhaps advantage could be taken of maternal immunity to provide additional protection for the infant at the time of delivery and for the mother during her subsequent years of sexual activity. The immunology of the male and female genital tracts (Chapter 54), lactation (Chapters 51 and 52), and mucosal response to viral and bacterial pathogens are discussed in detail elsewhere in this volume. Hence, this chapter provides a brief overview of the local female immune response to several common STDs and the possible impact of controlling these infections on maternal and child health.

II. DEFENSE MECHANISMS OF THE FEMALE GENITAL TRACT

The entire mucosal surface of the female genital tract, including the vagina, cervix, endometrium, fallopian tubes, and oviduct, is bathed in protective secretions. Among the various sections of the genital tract, these secretions differ in their biochemical and biological functions. The vaginal secretions represent a mixture of contaminants from the secretory products of the fallopian tubes, cervix, and endometrium, as well as small amounts of secretions produced by the Skene's and Bartholin's glands. Although plasma cells of the IgG type have been observed infrequently in the vaginal mucosa (Blandau and Moghissi, 1983), neither IgA- nor IgM-containing cells have been detected in the subepithelial regions of the vaginal mucosa (Tourville *et al.*, 1970). Secretory component (SC), the nonimmunglobulin portion associated with secretory IgA, has been found in vaginal secretions in a free form rather than associated with the superficial epithelial layers and apical glands typically found in the cervix and other portions of the upper female genital tract. Free SC, as well as the IgA and IgM detected in vaginal secretions, has been suggested to be a contaminant from the upper genital tract, particularly from the cervical mucosa (Moghissi, 1970). However, Lai and colleagues were able to demonstrate that vaginal explants from the mucocutaneous regions of the vaginal epithelium were capable of producing IgA and SC (Lai *et al.*, 1973). Although hemolytic complement activity or fluorescent localization of the components of complement in the vagina has not been observed, the synthesis of C3 in the vaginal mucosa has been noted using labeled amino acids (Lai *et al.*, 1973). Clearly the presence of antibody and the ability to generate complement components in the lower tract in proximity to the entry of most pathogens would be advantageous, whether or not these components are produced locally or migrate from the upper genital tract.

In contrast to the vaginal secretions, the cervical secretions contain significant amounts of IgG and IgA; the ratio of IgA to IgG is greater than that observed in serum (Moghissi and Neuhaus, 1962). IgM, although present, is found in much smaller amounts (Moghissi and Neuhaus, 1962). During the menstrual cycle, these immunoglobulins undergo considerable variation in concentration; IgG and IgA are highest at the beginning and end of the cycle and decrease toward midcycle. Hence, midcycle has the least immunoglobulin and the most favorable (thinnest) cervical mucus to allow penetration of sperm. Unfortunately, microorganisms also can gain access to the upper genital tract at midcycle and may, in part, be responsible for the increased incidence of STDs in the second portion of the menstrual cycle. The content of IgA and IgG in the cervical mucus ranges from 0.05 to 1.4 mg/ml and 0.1 to 6 mg/ml, respectively, whereas IgM is present to a lesser degree. Immunoglobulin content is not altered by oral contraceptive agents, although hormones have been found to have other influences on pathogen growth and host immunity (Schumacher, 1973a,b). Most of this immunoglobulin appears to be produced by the IgA- and IgG-containing plasma cells (Blandau and Moghissi, 1983; Hulka and Omran, 1969; Lippes *et al.*, 1970; Rebello *et al.*, 1975; Tjokonegoro and Sirisinha, 1975), and cells staining positive for SC (Lippes *et al.*, 1970) in the human endocervix. Note that studies of cervical biopsy tissues from infertile women demonstrate significantly higher numbers of IgA-containing plasma cells than tissues from parous women; antispermatozoal antibodies of the three major immunoglobulin classes have been detected in cervical mucus (Clarke, 1984). Additionally, women with genital infections, compared with women without infection, exhibit increased numbers of IgA-positive cells in this region of the genital tract (Waldman *et al.*, 1972). However, the numbers of IgG- and IgM-containing plasma cells in the two groups are comparable (Hutcheson *et al.*, 1974). From these and other studies, we know that secretory IgA in the genital tract is produced in response to foreign antigens, both human sperm and infectious agents, and seems to function in the genital tract as it does on other mucosal surfaces (reviewed by Mestecky and McGhee, 1987; Tomasi, 1989).

All major immunoglobulin classes have been demonstrated in human endometrial secretions. IgG-containing cells are slightly greater in number than IgA-containing cells, similar to the endocervical immunohistology (Lippes *et al.*, 1970). IgM is demonstrated infrequently in the human endometrium during the proliferative, secretory, and decidual phases (Lippes *et al.*, 1970). Most of the immunoglobulin appears to be distributed in the stroma between the glands and along the basement membranes of the glandular epithelium. During the early proliferative phase, IgA- and IgG-staining plasma cells have been located in the endometrium. SC has been identified in the apical glands during the secretory and proliferative phases (Tourville *et al.*, 1970).

Lymphoid tissues, although not as numerous as in other branches of the mucosa-associated lymphoid tissue (MALT), have been demonstrated in the female genital tract. Many segments of the female genital tract contain glandular epithelium and possess varying amounts of organized lymphoid tissue or lymphocytes diffusely scattered in the subepithelial regions. Although the uterus has not been demonstrated to possess organized lymphoid tissue, the endocervix has been reported to contain lymphoid aggregates that are analogous to the Peyer's patches of the small intestine (Blandau and Moghissi, 1983). As mentioned, the cervix contains numbers of lymphocytes and plasma cells, whereas the vagina has minimal to no collections of epithelial or subepithelial lymphoidal tissue. Little published information is available regarding the presence of T cells, T-cell subpopulations, or possible *in vitro* correlates of cellular immunity in the female genital tract. However, sufficient data are available regarding the fate of allogeneic transplants in the uterus in several animal models (Beer and Billingham, 1971,1975). Histoincompatible grafts are rejected uniformly, so the uterus appears to possess a significant degree of T cell-mediated immunocompetence. However, during pregnancy the fetus, despite the presence of incompatible antigens, is not rejected (reviewed by Scott, 1991). This response appears to be local, since pregnancy per se does not increase the survival of orthotopic skin grafts. Suppressor subpopulations of T lymphocytes have been suggested to predominate in the fetal environment and at the transplantation site of the embryo in the uterus. This possibility is supported by observations that fetal blood possesses a higher proportion of suppressor T lymphocytes (Olding and Oldstone, 1974). Another hypothesis is that effector lymphocytes may be inhibited by an increase in the level of a "blocking factor," as observed in the tumor immunity systems (Hellstrom and Hellstrom, 1971; Scott, 1991). Although clearly for the fetus to be undisturbed by the maternal immune response is a survival advantage, some systemic impairment of maternal immunity is evidenced by more severe primary varicella infection, occasionally resulting in death of the mother from severe pneumonia. Whether or not these phenomena are mediated by maternal or fetal suppressor T-cell activity is unknown. More recent studies (see subsequent discussion) have demonstrated that local lymphocytes are capable of proliferation in response to infectious agents, and that lymphocyte reactivity may be, in part, responsible for immunocompetence against some infectious agents in the genital tract.

III. INFECTIOUS AGENTS AND THE MUCOSAL IMMUNE RESPONSE

Most STD organisms first contact the host mucosal surface in the genital tract. Attachment must take place here before a cycle of infection can occur; the host has the first encounter with the invading pathogen at this site as well. Maternal infection is correlated most often with subsequent fetal or newborn infection, but maternal colonization with STD organisms can affect the fetus or newborn even if maternal infection has not yet been established. A partial list of important sexually transmitted female genital tract pathogens associated with fetal and neonatal disease is presented in Table I.

Although each specific sexually transmitted organism elicits a unique host response, some common features are shared by the mucosal immune response in the genital tract and the mucosal immune responses at other mucosal surfaces (i.e., the respiratory tract and the gastrointestinal tract, collectively called the MALT). Unlike the other mucosal surfaces of the MALT, the female genital tract undergoes a series of continual and well-defined developmental changes from the onset of menarche to the appearance of menopause. In addition, these tissues are exquisitely sensitive to changes in the hormonal milieu of the host during the menstrual cycle and pregnancy and lactation. A large number of nonspecific and specific factors plays an important role in providing a broad-range barrier to the penetration of environmental pathogens across the genital mucosa, in a manner similar to those of the respiratory and intestinal tracts (see Table II). Often, these cells and their products acting in concert are successful; often they are not. In the case of a pregnant female, the health and well-being of both the mother and the fetus are dependent on the maternal immune system to provide adequate protection against infection.

IV. SPECIFIC PATHOGENS AND THE ROLE OF THE FEMALE IMMUNE RESPONSE

Microorganisms applied to the genital tract, either by natural infection or by experimental application, have been demonstrated to produce a local and systemic immune response in human and other mammalian species (see Table III). These and other studies clearly demonstrate immunological reactivity in the genital tract. The discussion that follows focuses on some specific pathogens that are transmitted by sexual contact, with emphasis on local or systemic immune re-

Table I Microorganisms Transmitted by Sexual Contact and Their Association with Neonatal Disease

Association with significant disease	Mode of acquisition
Strong	
Bacteria	
Chlamydia trachomatis	Passage through colonized or infected birth canal; ascending infection
Neisseria gonorrhoeae	
Streptococcus group B	
Treponema pallidum[a]	Transplacental
Fungi	
Candida albicans	Passage through birth canal
Viruses	
Cytomegalovirus[a]	Transplacental; maternal secretions
Hepatitis B	Infected secretions; aspirated maternal blood
Herpes simplex[a]	Infected secretions; ascending infection
Human immunodeficiency virus[a]	Transplacental infection; secretions and maternal blood; virus in breast milk
Human papilloma virus	Infected secretions
Rare	
Protozoa	
Trichomonas vaginalis	Passage through brith canal
Possible	
Mycoplasma	
Mycoplasma hominis[a]	Transplacental
Ureaplasma urealyticum[a]	Passage through birth canal

[a] Can also cause fetal infection, birth defects, abortion, and/or stillbirth.

Table II Factors with a Potential Role in the Local Defense Mechanisms of the Genital Tract

	Soluble	Mechanism of action	Cellular	Mechanism of action
Nonspecific	Vaginal secretions Cervical mucus soluble proteins mucin Endometrial secretions uteroglobulin lactoferrin lysozyme other proteins Oviductal fluid Follicular fluid	Natural barrier; inhibition of growth; nonspecific binding of organisms; impairment of organism motility; masking of receptors; digestion of organism glycoproteins or glycolipids	Intact skin and mucosa	Barrier; when damaged may release products involved in cell recruitment; antigen presentation by certain epithelial and endothelial cells possible
			Phagocytes macrophages PMNs	Nonspecific phagocytosis and intracellular lysis of invading organism; macrophages also participate in generation specific responses by antigen presentation
	Hormones	Alteration of host cell receptor expression		
			NK cells	Infected cell cytotoxicity
	Prostaglandins	Alterations in vascular permeability and coagulation		
	Leukotrienes	Recruitment of cells to site of infection		
Immunologically specific	Immunoglobulins			
	mucosal antibody	Inhibition of attachment of invading microorganisms	CTL	Direct lysis of infected cells
	circulating antibody	Opsonization; ADCC; neutralization	ADCC	Lysis of cells coated with specific antibody
	Complement			
	Soluble mediators of cellular immunity—interferon	Prevention of intracellular infections through uninfected neighboring cells		

sponses that are potentially capable of conferring protection to the mother and her offspring.

A. Neisseria gonorrhoeae

Neisseria gonorrhoeae is a pathogen of the mucosal surface, causing the majority of its infections in the genitourinary tract. Humans are the primary reservoir. Many laboratory animals have some inherent resistance to infection; hence, studies of host–pathogen interactions have been hampered by lack of a suitable host and sample material. Uncomplicated gonococcal infections manifest as urethritis in males and endocervical infection in women. A pregnant woman with gonococcal disease can transmit the organism to her offspring, causing a spectrum of diseases from mild conjunctivitis to invasive gonococcal infection (Gutman and Holmes, 1990). Although local and systemic antibody responses, both IgG and IgA, are produced during infection, little is known about the ability of antibody to prevent or modify the course of disease in adults or in newborns.

Infection with *N. gonorrhoeae* occurs in two stages: attachment and invasion. The initial attachment brings the gonococcus and the host cell in close proximity and is thought to be mediated by nonspecific factors such as surface charge, hydrophobic/hydrophilic interactions, and pH (Watt and Ward, 1980). This interaction allows the more specific attachment structures—pili and outer membrane proteins (OMP)—to interact with host receptors (McGee *et al.*, 1978). By studying human fallopian cell cultures, several investigators have demonstrated that gonococci adhere to nonciliated epithelial cells and subsequently are endocytosed (Ward *et al.*, 1974; McGee *et al.*, 1978). Intracellular replication and excretion of the organisms into the lamina propria sets up a submucosal infection. An OMP (PI) appears to facilitate entry into the host cell after the initial attachment is established (Blake, 1985).

Polymorphonuclear leukocytes are attracted locally in response to gonococcal infection, but their role in host immunity is currently in question. Gonococcal antibody is known to be opsonic, and facilitates the uptake of gonococci by polymorphonuclear leukocytes. However, evidence suggests that intracellular oxidative neutrophil systems may be relatively inefficient at lysis of *N. gonorrhoeae* (Casey *et al.*, 1979,1980,1983; Parsons *et al.*, 1981,1982,1985,1986; Veale *et al.*, 1977,1979) but that nonoxidative systems may contribute to the intraphagosomal lysis of gonococci (Casey *et al.*, 1986). Observations by Shafer *et al.* concur with the speculation that, although gonococci may be eliminated more effectively *in vivo* than in *in vitro* study systems, the relative

Table III Evidence of Local and Systemic Immune Responses to Natural Infection or Artificially Applied Sexually Transmitted Disease Antigens in the Genital Tract of Humans and Other Mammalian Species

	Species	Site	Immunogen	Host response	Protection	References
Bacterial						
Chlamydia	human, mouse	cervix	live organism	specific IgA and IgG	partial	Rank, *et al.* (1979); Schlachter *et al.* (1983); Cui *et al.* (1991)
	guinea pig		inactivated organism	specific IgA	partial	Rank *et al.* (1990)
				lymphocyte activation	partial	Rank *et al.* (1990)
	human	systemic	whole organism	specific immunoglobulin	partial	Katz *et al.* (1987); Rank *et al.* (1988)
N. gonorrhoeae	human	cervix	whole organism	specific IgG, IgM, and IgA	yes—serovar specific	Buchanan *et al.* (1980)
		male urethra	whole organism	specific IgG, IgM, and IgA	yes—serovar specific	Kearns *et al.* (1973a,b) McMillan *et al.* (1979a); Tramont *et al.* (1980)
		vaginal washings	pili, LPS, and outer membrane proteins	specific IgA and IgG	partial	Lammel *et al.* (1985); Ison *et al.* (1986)
		systemic	whole organism	specific Ig	partial	Lammel *et al.* (1985); Ison *et al.* (1986)
Viruses						
CMV	human	systemic	whole organism	specific Ig, lymphocyte transformation	yes	Plotkin *et al.* (1976,1984); Stern (1984)
		systemic	subunit	lymphocyte transformation	yes, but declines	Plotkin *et al.* (1990)
HSV	human	cervix	whole organism	CMI, specific Ig	partial	Shore *et al.* (1976,1977)
	human, mouse	systemic	whole organism, glycoproteins	specific Ig (ADCC, CDC, neutralizing antibody)	partial	Kohl *et al.* (1978); Balachandran *et al.* (1982); Sullender *et al.* (1987)

inefficiency of intracellular neutralization and killing of gonococci may contribute to the spread of disease, both within and outside the genital tract (Shafer and Rest, 1989).

As in most mucosal infections, the function of local antibody is thought to be prevention of attachment and subsequent infection of the host mucosa (Mestecky and McGhee, 1987). Urethral exudates from men with gonococcal infection have demonstrated that all three antibody classes are produced in response to infection (Kearns *et al.*, 1973a,b; McMillan *et al.*, 1979a). In women, vaginal washings after infection with gonococci have been shown to contain both IgG and IgA antibody against pili, lipopolysaccharide (LPS), and the OMPs implicated in attachment (Lammel *et al.*, 1985; Ison *et al.*, 1986). Although IgG and IgA specific for gonococci have been demonstrated, production of specific IgM has not been well documented (O'Reilly *et al.*, 1976; McMillan *et al.*, 1979b; Ison *et al.*, 1986). Despite the formation of these local antibodies, little is known about their functional activity. Antibody directed against pili and outer membrane complexes altered the ability of the gonococci to attach to epithelial cells *in vitro* (Tramont *et al.*, 1980), whereas mucosal antibody produced after vaccination of male volunteers could inhibit attachment, requiring larger inocula to achieve infection (Tramont *et al.*, 1980). This result suggests that local antibody can modify colonization.

Since antibody apears to be the most effective means for the prevention and control of gonococcal infections, immunization would be a reasonable means of stimulating host antibody production. Repeat infection with a homologous gonococcus strain is unusual, but infection with heterologous strains can and probably does occur frequently. Buchanan and colleagues (1980) demonstrated that women with salpingitis developed antibody and protection against the original infecting serotypes. Systemic antibody response seems to be much stronger than the mucosal response, according to data from several investigators (Lammel *et al.*, 1985; Ison *et al.*, 1986). Whether or not this result reflects less local antibody production or the formation of antibody–antigen immune complexes that prevent antibody detection by present methods, as suggested by Ison (1988), is unknown. Further characterization of the gonococcus-specific antibody responses has involved identification of the major antigens that stimulate a specific antibody response. These include pili, OMPs (PI, PII, and PIII), and LPS, all constituents of the gonococcal surface (Tramont *et al.*, 1980; Lammel *et al.*, 1985; Ison *et al.*, 1986). Although antibody directed against pili would be desirable to prevent attachment of the organism to the host epithelial surface, the remarkable strain variation in pili limits their usefulness as a sole agent in vaccine candidates. A similar problem has been encountered for LPS and protein II (PII). Studies also suggest that antibodies against PII may block the interactions of the gonococcus with host neutrophils (Elkins and Rest, 1990). PIII, although a highly conserved OMP, can induce a polyclonal antibody response to its antigenic determinants that has been demonstrated to inhibit the effects of PI-induced antibodies *in vitro* and in animal hosts (Buchanan and Arko, 1977; Rice *et al.*, 1985,1986; Blake *et al.*, 1988). These blocking antibodies have been implicated in the earlier failure of OMP preparations to protect against subsequent infection. In fact, one such preparation administered to individuals with a history of previous gonococcal infection induced a quantitative decrease in opsonic antibody and bactericidal antibody after immunization that was below that of the preimmunization sera (Arminjon *et al.*, 1987).

To date, PI appears to have the most potential as a vaccine candidate, but must be purified from other outer membrane components. Fortunately, although some antigenic diversity exists among different *N. gonorrhoeae* strains producing PI, the differences fall into two major immunological and biological groups: PIA and PIB (Sandstrom *et al.*, 1982). Antibodies, both polyclonal and monoclonal, directed against PI are opsonic and bactericidal, and can prevent the *in vitro* invasion of gonococci into cell cultures (Joiner *et al.*, 1985; Virji *et al.*, 1986,1987). However, the vehicle of antigen administration to animals has a marked effect on the *in vivo* development of antibody response. Wetzler and colleagues (1988) utilized a chromatographically prepared PI vaccine composed of PIA– and PIB–alum adjuvant and found minimal opsonic and bactericidal antibody production. However, the opposite was noted when PI was inserted into liposomes (Wetzler *et al.*, 1988). A small but significant quantity of PIII may have contaminated this vaccine preparation and generated antibodies against this immunogen. The clinical significance of these results remains unknown since this study did not employ subsequent challenge of the immunized animals with virulent organisms.

Currently, a suitable vaccine for the prevention or modification of gonococcal disease remains elusive. Studies focusing on outer membrane components show the most promise (Heckels *et al.*, 1989,1990), but have not met with complete success yet. Meanwhile, the gonococcus itself has begun to develop considerable antibiotic resistance in certain parts of the world, making management of disease more difficult and development of a vaccine more critical. Although maternal and neonatal disease constitute only a small percentage of the total number of gonococcal infections reported yearly, effective maternal vaccination would help reduce the pool of infected and transmitting partners.

B. Chlamydia

Chlamydial infections of the genital tract are a major health problem in both developed and developing countries (Schachter and Grossman, 1990). Infection rates can reach as high as 30% among sexually active teenagers in the United States. Urethritis and cervicitis are common and often can be asymptomatic in females, contributing to additional spread of infection prior to treatment. More serious infection of the upper genital tract in women can lead to involuntary sterility. In addition, a pregnant woman infected with *Chlamydia* can transmit the organism to her offspring, producing conjunctivitis and pneumonia. In Third World nations, where STDs are more common, serious infections such as trachoma and lymphogranuloma venereum can be transmitted by other chlamydial serovars. Hence, effective control strategies must target both the asymptomatic carrier and the symptomatic patient. To date, a vaccine has not been developed, yet information regarding host response to infection through study of natural human infection and infection in animal models has led to several exciting prospects.

Nonspecific host defenses that can inactivate chlamydial elementary bodies *in vitro* have been identified, but the extent of their contribution to prevention or eradication of chlamydial infection *in vivo* is unknown. Biochemical inactivators are present in seminal plasma, and reduce the infectivity of several chlamydial serovars in cell culture (Mardh *et al.*, 1980; Hanna *et al.*, 1981). Spermine, cupric chloride, and zinc chloride inhibit the elementary bodies of serovar F. Although the specific mode of action for these compounds is unknown, they could be used in the future as adjuncts to preventive or therapeutic measures used to control *Chlamydia trachomatis* infection.

Hormones also affect the growth of *C. trachomatis* in cell culture. Cortisol has variable effects on *C. trachomatis* serovars: preincubation of tissue culture cells prior to inoculation with *Chlamydia* inhibits the growth of serovar L2 whereas postinoculation incubation with cortisol enhances the growth of L2 (Bushell and Hobson, 1978; Reed and Hann, 1980). Estrogens have no effect on the binding of elementary bodies to cell cultures; incubation of tissue culture with estrogens nearly doubles the numbers of infectious bodies recoverable from the tissue culture (Sugarman and Agbor, 1986). This estrogen effect has been exploited by researchers using animal models to increase the yield of infectious organisms and may also may explain, in part, the increased susceptibility of women using oral contraceptive agents to this organism. Progesterone, testosterone, and other hormones do not appear to have any effect on the growth of *C. trachomatis*.

Chlamydia can induce the production of interferon γ (IFNγ), most likely because, as an obligate intracellular parasite, this organism causes alterations in the cell surface membrane of the cell it has parasitized. In the mouse model, IFNγ induction rapidly follows intravenous injection of elementary bodies. Infected cell cultures, HeLa cells, and L cells also produce IFNγ in response to several chlamydial serovars. Both human and mouse IFNγ can inhibit various stages of chlamydial intracellular growth in *in vitro* cell cultures (Hanna *et al.*, 1967; Kazar *et al.*, 1971; Rothermel *et al.*, 1983; de la Maza *et al.*, 1985,1986; Shemer and Sarov, 1985). However, *in vivo* human correlates of tissue culture and animal models for *Chlamydia*-induced IFNγ production are lacking.

In addition to these biochemical mechanisms capable of chlamydial inhibition, a number of cellular mechanisms can inhibit or destroy *Chlamydia* elementary bodies. However, whether these responses are completely nonspecific or require the participation of specific antisera is questionable. *In vitro* studies by Yong *et al.* (1982,1986) and Zvillich and Sarov (1985) have shown that polymorphonuclear leukocytes (PMNs) rapidly take up elementary bodies and degrade them, but the role of specific or nonspecific human sera was not investigated in this phenomenon. Enhancement of chemiluminescent responses of PMNs to elementary bodies was noted with the addition of *Chlamydia* serovar-specific sera but not group-specific sera (Soderlund *et al.*, 1984), whereas the same response using L2 elementary bodies is enhanced with human sera, regardless of whether or they contain serovar-specific antibody (Hammerschlag *et al.*, 1985). Clearly PMNs do interact with *Chlamydia*, but their role in disease control is not clarified.

Lymphocytes, monocytes, and macrophages also interact with *Chlamydia in vitro*. L2 elementary bodies, when incubated with peripheral blood lymphocytes, have decreased infectivity but can replicate in macrophages (Manor and Sarov, 1986). An increased production of nonspecific immunoglobulin is stimulated by cocultivation of *Chlamydia* L2 elementary bodies (live or formalin fixed) with human peripheral blood lymphocytes, regardless of the donor's previous exposure to *Chlamydia*, and probably represents nonimmune polyclonal responses to chlamydial antigen (Bard and Levitt, 1984). Further studies by Bard have revealed that about 50% of the B lymphocytes so exposed bind elementary bodies whereas less than 10% of the T cells do so (Bard and Levitt, 1986). However, although binding was not assessed, an increase in nonspecific T-cell proliferative response to concanavalin A (ConA) was noted by Rank *et al.* in the peripheral blood lymphocytes of guinea pigs immunized subcutaneously with live or UV-inactivated *C. trachomatis* (Rank *et al.*, 1990). However, this treatment appeared to have little effect on the resulting genital chlamydial infection when immunized guinea pigs were challenged subsequently.

Although several nonspecific host responses to *C. trachomatis* antigen exist, specific immune responses, both cell-mediated and specific antibody-dependent, are more likely to modify infection or to confer immunity against reinfection. Several groups of investigators have documented the production of serovar-specific antibody, particularly in women who experienced upper genital tract infection (salpingitis, endometritis). However, little correlation appears to exist between the intensity of the humoral immune response and resistance to reinfection. More important is the role of local antibody, particularly IgA, in resistance to or modification of infection of the genital tract.

The antibody response to *C. trachomatis* has been well documented (Rank *et al.*, 1979; Monnickendam and Pearce, 1983; Schachter *et al.*, 1983; Monnickendam, 1988). Although humoral antibodies are generated in *C. trachomatis* infection (IgG, IgM, IgA), their role in subsequent protection is partial or transitory, at best (Katz *et al.*, 1987; Rank *et al.*, 1988). However, in the mouse model, passive immunization with polyclonal and certain monoclonal antibodies against *Chlamydia psittaci* antigens was shown to decrease the rate of placental infection and spontaneous abortion (Buzoni-Gatel *et al.*, 1990). This study suggests that antibodies directed against the proper immunogen can be protective. Immunotype- or serovar-specific antibodies are protective in the owl monkey (Nichols *et al.*, 1973) and the guinea pig model (Murray and Charbonnet, 1971; Murray *et al.*, 1973; Murray, 1977) and in cell culture (Peeling *et al.*, 1984; Lucero and Kuo, 1985) but local secretory antibody appears to play a more important role in protection against infection than humoral antibody, as has been demonstrated by numerous investigators (Murray and Charbonnet, 1971; Murray *et al.*, 1973; Nichols *et al.*, 1973; Howard *et al.*, 1976; Alani *et al.*,

1977; Murray, 1977; McComb *et al.*, 1979; Richmond *et al.*, 1980; Brunham *et al.*, 1983; Cui *et al.*, 1989,1991). Most recently, studies in our laboratory have demonstrated that oral administration of live *Chlamydia* can decrease or eliminate cervical shedding of *Chlamydia* on subsequent challenge intravaginally with live organisms (Cui *et al.*, 1991). In addition, a marked booster effect was noted in antibody responses, both locally at the site of rechallenge and in the serum (see Figures 1 and 2). However, the local and humoral antibody responses appear to decline with time, allowing reinfection to take place as demonstrated in the guinea pig model (Rank *et al.*, 1988) and by clinical observation of human disease (Katz *et al.*, 1987). Despite this decline in immunity with time, vaccination might be used to protect a delivering infant from subsequent *C. trachomatis* infection. Theoretically, one could vaccinate the pregnant female orally with live (Cui *et al.*, 1991) or inactivated (Rank *et al.*, 1990) organism to stimulate local IgA production, which might prevent subsequent colonization of the infant by decreasing or preventing colonization of the mother's genital tract. Pregnant mice, when immunized orally with live *C. trachomatis,* were capable of producing *Chlamydia*-specific IgA in the milk (Z. Cui, personal communication), but the potential protective effect of specific IgA was not investigated by *Chlamydia* challenge in this case. Approximately 30% and 15% of infants exposed to maternal *Chlamydia* acquire conjunctivitis and pneumonia, respectively, in the United States (Frommell *et al.*, 1979; Schachter *et al.*, 1986); local *Chlamydia*-specific maternal secretory IgA (or IgG or IgM) antibody, passively acquired by the infant in passage through the birth canal or through suckling, may be one of the factors explaining why these percentages are not significantly greater.

The importance of prevention of this most common STD is clearly evident, but attempts to develop an effective vaccine against *Chlamydia* have been only partially successful to date. Further careful investigation of the host immune responses will be necessary before control of this STD through immunization can be achieved.

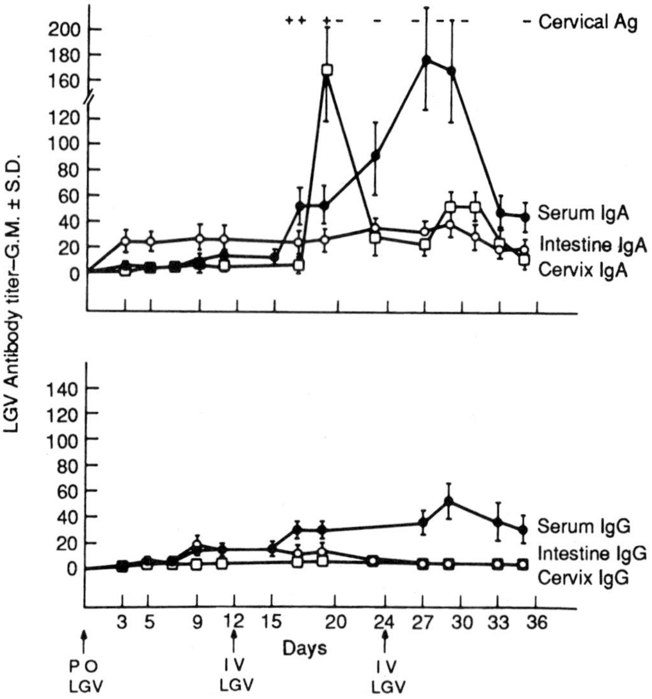

Figure 2 Immunization with *Chlamydia trachomatis* LGV-434-II administered intragastrically in BALB/c mice and the effect of direct intravaginal (IV) challenge on the kinetics of IgA and IgG antibody responses. Ag, Antigen; PO, intragastric; GM, geometric mean; SD, standard deviation. Reprinted with permission from Cui *et al.* (1991) and the American Society for Microbiology.

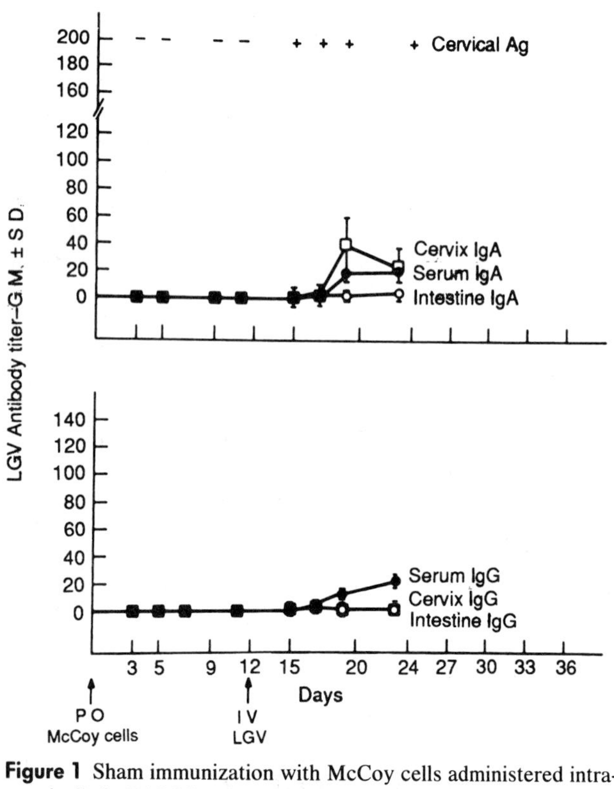

Figure 1 Sham immunization with McCoy cells administered intragastrically in BALB/c mice and the effect of direct intravaginal (IV) *Chlamydia trachomatis* LGV-434-II challenge on the kinetics of IgA and IgG antibody responses. Ag, Antigen; PO, intragastric; GM, geometric mean; SD, standard deviation. Reprinted with permission from Cui *et al.* (1991) and the American Society for Microbiology.

C. Herpes Simplex Virus Infections

Genital herpes simplex virus (HSV) infections have significant morbidity in adults, but rarely cause death in the immunologically normal host. In sharp contrast is neonatal HSV infection, with its concomitant high mortality and frequency of subsequent neurological sequelae in survivors despite antiviral therapy (Whitley, 1990). Both type 1 (10% of total cases of neonatal HSV) and type 2 have been recovered from infected infants. Interestingly, although primary maternal HSV infection at the time of delivery has nearly 50% risk of viral acquisition by vaginal delivery of the infant, recurrent maternal genital HSV carries less than 5% risk for the infant at the time of vaginal delivery. Although the reasons for these differences have been explored, the role of maternal immunity in the prevention of HSV transmission to the delivering infant is far from understood.

Herpesviruses are acquired by direct exposure of the mucous membranes to viral particles, with subsequent establishment of infection. From this local entry portal, virus can disseminate in the immunocompromised host or the neonate (who has a relative immunodeficiency compared with an adult). Thus, the local immune response should play a role in the prevention of recurrent attacks. However, members of the Herpesviridae family have the unique ability to establish latency within the host, most likely within immunoprivileged sites (such as the lumbosacral ganglia following genital HSV infection), and hence are sequestered from the host's local immune response until reactivation of the virus. When infected with HSV, the host has both nonspecific and specific immune responses similar to those activated during other STDs. Although the initial and secondary host immune responses to HSV infection are under careful investigation, mechanisms that maintain latency and control subsequent events initiated during recurrences are poorly understood and hamper attempts at effective control through vaccination.

Local and systemic immunological reactivity against HSV seems to have relevance in the moderation and eradication of infectious viral particles. Studies have demonstrated that maternal and cord blood samples possess similar levels of IgG class antibodies with antiviral activity that mediate neutralization and antibody-dependent cell-mediated cytotoxicity (ADCC) (Shore *et al.*, 1976,1977). Maternal ADCC has been shown to pass to the neonate (Shore *et al.*, 1976,1977; Kohl *et al.*, 1978). However, human cord blood monocytes have less ability to generate the ADCC response than adult leukocytes (Shore *et al.*, 1977). Kohl and colleagues found a difference between adherent (macrophages) and nonadherent (lymphocyte) populations in cord blood once these populations were separated from each other (Kohl *et al.*, 1981b). These researchers proposed that cell separation also may have removed some inhibitory factors, and altered the results of their studies (Kohl *et al.*, 1981a; Kohl, 1984). Subsequently, their group found that the route of birth, vaginal delivery compared with caesarian section, had marked effects on ADCC of cord mononuclear cells; cells from infants delivered by caesarian section had much lower ADCC activity than those from infants delivered vaginally (Frazier *et al.*, 1982). Cellular cytotoxicity and peripheral blood mononuclear leukocyte ADCC was decreased in the first months of life (Kohl, 1984), but cord blood PMNs had ADCC similar to that of adult PMNs (Kohl *et al.*, 1981b). These findings may help explain the sensitivity of the newborn to the devastating effects of HSV infection, particularly if the mother has not experienced previous HSV infection and has not generated neutralizing and ADCC antibody to provide to her infant.

Since HSV is such a devastating disease in the neonatal period despite antiviral therapy, significant impetus exists to find alternative methods of protection for the exposed infant. Although cell-mediated immune responses to HSV are clearly important in limiting viral activity and in resolution of infection, HSV-specific antibody is an important adjunct in host immunity against this viral pathogen. Although the role of humoral antibodies is not entirely clear in humans, evidence suggests that maternal antibody against HSV is important in decreasing dissemination in neonates and in promoting recovery from HSV infections in some studies (Yeager *et al.*, 1980; Sullender *et al.*, 1987), but not in others (Whitley *et al.*, 1980). Newer tests using antibody response to gG glycoprotein are thought to be type specific for HSV-2 (Lee *et al.*, 1985,1986; Sullender *et al.*, 1988). These tests will allow clearer analysis of human HSV antibody responses without the problems of cross-reactivity with antibody against HSV-1, a problem common to many earlier assays. The data regarding the role of antibody in HSV disease are clearer in animal studies, in which passive prophylaxis of animals with hyperimmune sera against HSV can decrease the severity of induced infection, particularly lethal central nervous system infection (Evans *et al.*, 1946; Cheever and Daikos, 1950; Luyet *et al.*, 1975; Baron *et al.*, 1976; Davis *et al.*, 1979). Irradiated mice were not protected despite hyperimmune serum administration, indicating that an irradiation-sensitive arm of the host immune system is also important in the immune response to HSV (Davis *et al.*, 1979). Immunosuppressed mice also do not produce appreciable antibody, nor do they demonstrate cell-mediated activity toward HSV-1 infection (Worthington *et al.*, 1980). Whether these issues can be clarified in human studies remains to be seen.

The viral glycoproteins appear to be the most potent inducers of humoral antibody. Five surface glycoproteins (gA,gB,gC,gD, and gE) are the principal immunogens identified to date (Spear, 1976; Ruyechan *et al.*, 1979). Such antibodies are involved in ADCC and viral neutralization; antibodies against gB, gC, and gD mediate ADCC (Norrild *et al.*, 1979; Sethi, 1983) and complement-dependent cytotoxicity of HSV-infected cells (Kohl *et al.*, 1981a). High titers of neutralizing antibodies against HSV are generated by purified gD; monoclonal antibodies directed against this glycoprotein can limit infectious spread of induced HSV infection in mice (Cohen *et al.*, 1972,1984; Eisenberg *et al.*, 1982). Passive transfer of monoclonal antibodies against the principal glycoproteins inducing ADCC but not neutralization still could confer protection against HSV challenge in mice (Balachandran *et al.*, 1982). Similar studies have been conducted in the naturally HSV-exposed neonate, showing that passive transfer of HSV-specific antibody may prevent or moderate the disease in exposed infants (Yeager *et al.*, 1980; Nahmias, 1983; Prober *et al.*, 1987; Sullender *et al.*, 1987). Unfortunately, the prospect of a useful vaccine against HSV-2 to provide protection for mothers and their infants is far from realized.

D. Cytomegaloviruses

Cytomegaloviruses (CMV) are also members of the herpesvirus family. These common viral agents infect many animal species including humans (Weller, 1971). At present,

CMV is the leading cause of congenital and perinatal viral disease in infants (Reynolds *et al.*, 1973; Stagno *et al.*, 1975; Pass *et al.*, 1981; Stagno, 1990). Although many exposed infants have mild to no obvious disease, congenitally infected infants can have severe manifestations including deafness and multiple organ system involvement (Kumar *et al.*, 1973; Reynolds *et al.*, 1974; Stagno *et al.*, 1977,1981; Alford *et al.*, 1990; Stagno, 1990). Additionally, infants infected *in utero* can continue to shed virus from the urine for more than 5 yr and from the nasopharynx for 2–4 yr (Stagno *et al.*, 1975,1984; Pass *et al.*, 1980). Hence, prevention of this disease in susceptible pregnant females would be beneficial to their infants. CMV, like HSV, can produce recurrences; asymptomatic shedding from the cervix, urinary tract, and pharynx is not uncommon in women. In postpartum women, the breast appears to be a common site of reactivation; more than 30% of seropositive females intermittently excrete CMV in their milk during the first year after delivery (Stagno *et al.*, 1980; Dworsky *et al.*, 1983).

Like HSV infections, primary CMV infection of the pregnant woman is much more likely to cause fetal or neonatal infection than recurrent infection. Both antibody- and specific cell-mediated immunity appear to have a role in protection against CMV. Indirect evidence for the efficacy of specific CMV antibody in disease prevention and modulation comes from studies of renal transplant patients (Syndman *et al.*, 1987). A reduction in the incidence of symptomatic CMV infection was noted in renal transplant patients given prophylaxis with high titer CMV immunoglobulin, although the overall incidence of CMV remained the same. Stern *et al.* noted that women with strong lymphocyte proliferative responses to CMV during primary infection delivered infants without infections, whereas 60% of their female patients without such responses delivered infected infants (Stern, 1984). Maternal immunity also seems to modify the severity of neonatal infection (Stagno *et al.*, 1982,1986), a result that has led to attempts to immunize the nonimmune population to control congenital CMV infection with a live attenuated strain of CMV (Plotkin *et al.*, 1976,1984; Stern, 1984). However, immunity appears to dissipate with time; antibody and lymphocyte transformation reactions to CMV disappeared in half the vaccinees over an 8-yr period (Stern, 1984). Additional issues regarding reactivation of viral vaccine strains, latency, and oncogenic potential of such live vaccines have not been answered adequately (Stagno, 1990). These problems, in conjunction with the issue of waning immunity, make the development and use of subunit vaccines much more attractive than live vaccines (Plotkin *et al.*, 1990). Whether or not this new vaccine, or another like it, will reduce the incidence of congenital CMV infections as effectively as vaccination of susceptible populations with rubella vaccine curbed congenital rubella syndrome in the 1960s remains to be seen.

E. Genital Mycoplasmas

Unlike the previously discussed STDs, the roles of genital mycoplasmas and other bacterial commensals of the vagina in adverse pregnancy outcome and infant morbidity and mortality are less clearly established. Genital mycoplasmas have been implicated in the development of chorioamnionitis, preterm labor, and low birth weight infants (Cassell *et al.*, 1986; Driscoll, 1986; Gravett and Eschenbach, 1986; Kass *et al.*, 1986; Hillier *et al.*, 1988; Liepmann *et al.*, 1988; Watts *et al.*, 1989). *Ureaplasma urealyticum* has been implicated in the development of neonatal pneumonia and chronic lung disease of the premature infant (Quinn *et al.*, 1985; Cassell *et al.*, 1988; Wang *et al.*, 1988; Waites *et al.*, 1989), although the pathogenesis has not been clarified entirely. Depending on the study population, as many as 80% of pregnant women have been noted to be colonized with *U. urealyticum* in their genital tracts at some point during pregnancy (Harrison, 1986). However, only a small subset of exposed premature infants develops chronic lung disease (bronchopulmonary dysplasia, BPD) and the multiple factors involved in the generation of BPD will be difficult to evaluate. Clearly *Ureaplasma* and *Mycoplasma* species produce phospholipases, particularly A_2, which may contribute to relative surfactant deficiency in the sick premature infant, despite surfactant replacement therapy. Clearly this avenue of research must be pursued to assess the maternal response to these organisms and to clarify their role in neonatal pneumonia.

Mycoplasma hominis, a less common isolate in pregnant women than *U. urealyticum*, has been recovered occasionally from multiple sites in infants and children (McDonald and Moore, 1988). Meningitis (Wealthall, 1975; Mardh, 1983; McDonald and Moore, 1988; Waites *et al.*, 1988), pericardial effusion (Miller *et al.*, 1982), and sepsis (Unsworth *et al.*, 1985) all have been documented with *M. hominis* as the only organism recovered from these sites. However, a prevalence study of *M. hominis* and other genital mycoplasmas as agents in sepsis and meningitis in young infants failed to recover these agents from the blood or cerebral spinal fluid in nearly 200 cases, whereas 6 *M. hominis* and 9 *U. urealyticum* isolates were recovered from the urinary tract, indicating colonization of the infants with these organisms (Likitnukul *et al.*, 1986).

Despite evidence to suggest the role of genital mycoplasmas in maternal and neonatal disease, very little is known about the local host response to these organisms. Humoral antibody responses have been documented for most *Mycoplasma* species in human and animal hosts, but a direct relationship between the level of circulating antibody and resistance to mycoplasmal infection is not always obvious. Although little or no data are available on the local antibody responses to genital mycoplasmas in humans, some data from a mouse model of genital tract infection suggest that specific IgG and IgM are produced in the genital tract (Taylor-Robinson, 1988). However, although IgA would be speculated to be present, it could not be confirmed (Taylor-Robinson, 1988). Additionally, resistance to reinfection appeared to correlate with the presence or absence of local IgG (P. Furr and D. Taylor-Robinson, unpublished data). As the role of mycoplasmas is better defined in the neonate, a clearer cause and effect relationship may be established between carriage of genital mycoplasmas by the mother and her ability to transmit the organisms to her offspring.

V. SUMMARY

The evidence presented thus far indicates that the mucosal surfaces of the female genital tract are able to mount a locally induced specific antibody and specific cell-mediated immune response. The local antibody response appears to be independent of the serum antibody response and is associated mostly (but not exclusively) with secretory IgA immunoglobulin and locally reactive lymphocyte populations. The precise origin of cells responsible for cell-mediated immunity is unknown. Data suggest that the sparse amount of IgA immunocompetent tissue observed in the female genital tract may be derived largely from immunoreactive cells from the gastrointestinal tract, particularly Peyer's patches. Additional data regarding the immune response of the breast suggest that a similar population of antigen-primed IgA-producing cells from the gastrointestinal tract migrates to the female breast and secretes specific IgA into the milk. Thus, antigen exposure in the gut-associated lymphoid tissue produces a sharing of immune experience at all mucosal surfaces, with particular enhancement at the surface of secondary exposure which, in this case, is the genital tract. Reduction of female genital tract colonization by pathogens through immunization programs may be able to reduce the incidence of transmission of the offending organisms to the neonate's mucosal surfaces. The neonate's own immune system, although not as active against certain organisms that require cytotoxic responses, also is capable of a broad range of immunological responses. Hence, the exploitation of antigen-sensitized precursor cells in the gastrointestinal tract of the mother by oral priming with genital pathogens (or antigenically reactive components of the pathogens, such as OMPs) may provide protection against genital pathogens in the near future. This benefit would be dual: not only could the infection rate and subsequent morbidity and mortality in newborns be decreased, but it may be possible to reduce the rampant spread of STDs through such immunization programs in the ensuing decade.

References

Alani, M. D., Darougar, S., Burns, D. C. M., Thin, R. N., and Dunn, H. (1977). Isolation of *Chlamydia trachomatis* from the male urethra. *Br. J. Vener. Dis.* **53,** 88–92.

Alford, C. A., Stagno, S., Pass, R. F., and Britt, W. J. (1990). Congenital and perinatal cytomegalovirus infections. *Rev. Infect. Dis.* **12,** S745–S753.

Antal, G. (1987). The epidemiology of sexually transmitted diseasea in the tropics. *In* "Clinical Tropical Medicine and Communicable Diseases, Vol. I" (A. O. Osoba, ed.), pp. 1–16. Balliere Tindall, London.

Arminjon, P., Cadoz, M., Morse, S. A., Rock, J. P., and Sarafin, S. K. (1987). Bactericidal and opsonic activities of sera from individuals immunized with a gonococcal protein I vaccine. *Abstracts Ann. Meet.* **118.**

Balachandran, N., Bacchetti, S., and Rawls, W. E. (1982). Protection against lethal challenge of BALB/c mice by passive transfer of monoclonal antibodies to five glycoproteins of herpes simplex virus type 2. *Infect. Immun.* **37,** 1132–1139.

Bard, J., and Levitt, D. (1984). *Chlamydia trachomatis* stimulates human peripheral blood B lymphocytes to proliferate and secrete polyclonal immunoglobulin in vitro. *Infect. Immun.* **43,** 84–92.

Bard, J., and Levitt, D. (1986). *Chlamydia trachomatis* (L2 serovar) binds to distinct subpopulations of human peripheral blood leukocytes. *Clin. Immunol. Immunopathol.* **38,** 150–160.

Baron, S., Worthington, M., Williams, J., and Gaines, J. W. (1976). Postexposure serum prophylaxis of neonatal herpes simplex virus infection of mice. *Nature* (*London*) **261,** 505–508.

Beer, A., and Billingham, R. E. (1971). Immunobiology of mammalian reproduction. *Adv. Immunol.* **14,** 1–84.

Beer, A., and Billingham, R. E. (1975). Host responses to intrauterine tissue, cellular and fetal allografts. *J. Reprod. Fertil.* (*Suppl.*) **21,** 59–88.

Blake, M. S. (1985). Implications of the active role of gonococcal porins in disease. *In* "The Pathogenic *Neisseria,* Vol. II" (G. K. Schoolnik, ed.), pp. 251–258. American Society of Microbiology, Washington, D.C.

Blake, M. S., Lytton, E. J., Seiff, M. E., and Gotschlich, E. C. (1988). Studies on gonococcal protein III. *In* "Host Cell Interaction" (M. A. Horowitz, ed.), pp. 85–97. Liss, New York.

Blandau, R. J., and Moghissi, K. (1983). "The Biology of the Cervix." University of Chicago Press, Chicago.

Brunham, R. C., and Plummer, F. A. (1990). A general mode of sexually transmitted disease epidemiology and its implications for control. *Med. Clin. North Am.* **74,** 1339–1352.

Brunham, R. C., Kuo, C. C., Cles, L., and Holmes, K. K. (1983). Correlation of host immune response with quantitative recovery of *Chlamydia trachomatis* from the human endocervix. *Infect. Immun.* **39,** 1491–1494.

Buchanan, T. M., and Arko, R. J. (1977). Immunity to gonococcal infection induced by vaccination with isolated outer mmbranes of Neisseria gonorrhoeae in guinea pigs. *J. Infect. Dis.* **135,** 879–884.

Buchanan, T. M., Eschenbach, D. A., Knapp, D. A., and Holmes, K. K. (1980). Gonococcal salpingitis is less likely to recur with *Neisseria gonorrhoeae* of the same outer membrane antigenic type. *Am. J. Obstet. Gynecol.* **138,** 978–980.

Bushell, A. C., and Hobson, D. (1978). Effect of cortisol on the growth of *Chlamydia trachomatis* in McCoy cells. *Infect. Immun.* **21,** 946–953.

Buzoni-Gatel, D., Bernard, F., Andersen, A., and Rodolakis, A. (1990). Protective effect of polyclonal and monoclonal antibodies against abortion in mice infected by *Chlamydia psittaci. Vaccine* **8,** 342–352.

Casey, S. G., Veale, D. R., and Smith, H. (1979). Demonstration of intracellular growth of gonococci in human phagocytes using spectinomycin to kill extracellular organisms. *J. Gen. Microbiol.* **113,** 395–398.

Casey, S. G., Veale, D. R., and Smith, H. (1980). Intracellular survival of *Neisseria gonorrhoeae* in human uretheral exudate. *FEMS Microbiol. Lett.* **8,** 97–100.

Casey, S. G., Veale, D. R., and Smith, H. (1983). Cytotoxicity of *Neiserria gonorrhoeae* for human peripheral blood phagocytes. *J. Gen. Microbiol.* **129,** 1097–1102.

Casey, S. G., Shafer, W. M., and Spitznagel, J. K. (1986). *Neisseria gonorrhoeae* survives intraleukocyte oxygen-independent antimicrobial capabilities of anaerobic and aerobic granulocytes in the presence of pyocin lethal for extracellular gonococci. *Infect. Immun.* **52,** 384–389.

Cassell, G. H., Waites, K. B., Gibbs, R. S., and Davis, J. K. (1986). Role of *Ureaplasma urealyticum* in amnionitis. *Pediatr. Infect. Dis.* **5,** S247–S252.

Cassell, G. H., Crouse, D. T., Waites, K. B., Rudd, P. T., and Davis, J. K. (1988). Does *Ureaplasma urealyticum* cause respiratory disease in newborns? *Pediatr. Infect. Dis.* **7,** 535–541.

Cheever, F. S., and Daikos, G. (1950). Studies on the protective effect of gamma globulin against herpes simplex infections in mice. *J. Immunol.* **65,** 135–142.

Clarke, G. N. (1984). Detection of antispermatozoal antibodies of IgG, IgA and IgM immunoglobulin class in cervical mucus. *Am. J. Reprod. Immunol.* **6,** 195–204.

Cohen, G. H., Ponce de Leon, M., and Nichols, C. (1972). Isolation of a herpes simplex virus-specific antigenic fraction which stimulates the production of neutralising antibody. *J. Virol.* **10,** 1021–1027.

Cohen, G. H., Dietzschold, B., Ponce de Leon, M., Long, D., Golub, E. A., Varrichio, A., Pereira, L., and Eisenberg, R. J. (1984). Localisation and synthesis of an antigenic determinant of herpes simplex virus glycoprotein D that stimulates production of neutralising antibody. *J. Virol.* **49,** 102–108.

Cui, Z.-D., LaScolea, L. J., Fisher, J., and Ogra, P. L. (1989). Immunoprophylaxis of *Chlamydia trachomatis* lymphogranuloma venereum pneumonitis in mice by oral immunization. *Infect. Immun.* **57,** 739–744.

Cui, Z.-D., Tristram, D. A., LaScolea, L. J., Kwiatkowski, T. J., Kopti, S., and Ogra, P. L. (1991). Induction of antibody response to *Chlamydia trachomatis* in the genital tract by oral immunization. *Infect. Immun.* **59,** 1465–1469.

Davis, W. B., Taylor, J. A., and Oakes, J. E. (1979). Ocular infection wih herpes simplex virus type I: Prevention of acute herpetic encephalitis by systemic administration of virus specific antibody. *J. Infect. Dis.* **140,** 534–542.

de la Maza, L. M., Peterson, E. M., Fennie, C. W., and Czarniecki, C. W. (1985). The anti-chlamydial and anti-proliferative activities of recombinant murine interferon-gamma are not dependent on tryptophan concentrations. *J. Immunol.* **135,** 4198–4200.

de la Maza, L. M., Plunkett, M., Peterson, E. M., and Czarniecki, C. W. (1986). Inhibition of *C. trachomatis* by recombinant Mu-IFN-gamma. *In* "Chlamydial Infections" (D. Oriel, G. Ridgway, J. Schachter, D. Taylor-Robinson, and M. Ward, eds.), pp. 441–444. Cambridge University Press, Cambridge.

Driscoll, S. G. (1986). Chorioamnionitis: Perinatal morbidity and mortality. *Pediatr. Infect. Dis.* **5,** S273–S275.

Dworsky, M. E., Yow, M., Stagno, S., Pass, R. F., and Alford, C. A. (1983). Cytomegalovirus infection of breast milk and transmission in infancy. *Pediatrics* **72,** 295–299.

Eisenberg, R. J., Ponce de Leon, M., Pereira, L., Long, D., and Cohen, G. H. (1982). Purification of glycoprotein gD of herpes simplex virus types 1 and 2 by use of monoclonal antibodies. *J. Virol.* **41,** 1099–1105.

Elkins, C., and Rest, R. F. (1990). Monoclonal antibodies to outer membrane protein PII block interactions of *Neisseria gonorrhoeae* with human neutrophils. *Infect. Immun.* **58,** 1078–1084.

Evans, C. A., Slavin, H. B., and Berry, G. P. (1946). Studies on herpetic infections in mice. IV. The effect of specific antibodies on the progression of the virus within the nervous system of young mice. *J. Exp. Med.* **84,** 429–434.

Frazier, J. P., Kohl, S., Pickering, L. K., and Loo, L. S. (1982). The effect of route of delivery on neonatal natural killer cytotoxicity and antibody-dependent cellular cytotoxicity to herpes simplex virus-infected cell. *Pediatr. Res.* **16,** 558–560.

Frommell, G. T., Rothenberg, R., Wang, S., and McIntosh, K. (1979). Chlamydial infections of mothers and their newborns. *J. Pediatr.* **95,** 28–32.

Gravett, M. G., and Eschenbach, D. A. (1986). Possible role of Ureaplasma urealyticum in preterm premature rupture of the fetal membranes. *Pediatr. Infect. Dis.* **5,** S253–S257.

Gutman, L. T., and Holmes, K. K. (1990). Gonococcal infection. *In* "Infectious Diseases of the Fetus and Newborn Infant" (J. S. Remington and J. O. Klein, ed.), 3d Ed., pp. 848–865. Saunders, Philadelphia.

Hammerschlag, M. R., Suntharalingam, K., and Fikrig, S. (1985). The effect of *Chlamydia trachomatis* on luminol-dependent chemiluminescence of human polymorphonuclear leukocytes: requirements for oposonization. *J. Infect. Dis.* **151,** 1045–1051.

Hanna, L., Merigan, T. C., and Jawetz, E. (1967). Effect of interferon on TRIC agents and induction of interferon by TRIC agents. *Am. J. Ophthalmol.* **63,** 1115–1119.

Hanna, L., Keshishyan, H., Brooks, G. F., Stites, D. P., and Jawetz, E. (1981). Effect of seminal plasma on *Chlamydia trachomatis* L B-1 in cell culture. *Infect. Immun.* **32,** 404–406.

Harrison, H. R. (1986). Cervical colonization with *Ureaplasma urealyticum* and pregnancy outcome: Prospective studies. *Pediatr. Infect. Dis.* **5,** S266–S269.

Heckels, J. E., Fletcher, J. N., and Virji, M. (1989). The potential effect of immunization with outer-membrane protein I from *Neisseria gonorrhoeae*. *J. Gen. Microbiol.* **135,** 2269–2276.

Heckels, J. E., Virji, M., and Tinsley, C. R. (1990). Vaccination against gonorrhoea: The potential protective effect of immunization with a synthetic peptide containing a conserved epitope of gonococcal outer membrane protein IB. *Vaccine* **8,** 225–230.

Hellstrom, I., and Hellstrom, K. E. (1971). Neonatally induced allograft tolerance may be mediated by serum born factors. *Nature (London)* **230,** 161–162.

Hillier, S. L., Martius, J., Krohn, M., Kiviat, N., Holmes, K. K., and Eschenbach, D. A. (1988). A case-control study of chorioamnionic infection and histologic chorioamnionitis in prematurity. *N. Engl. J. Med.* **319,** 972–978.

Howard, L., O'Leary, M., and Nichols, R. (1976). Animal model studies of genital chlamydial infections: Immunity to reinfection with guinea pig inclusion conjunctivitus agent in the urethra and eye of male guinea pigs. *Br. J. Vener. Dis.* **52,** 261–265.

Hulka, J. P., and Omran, K. F. (1969). The uterine cervix as a potential local antibody secretor. *Am. J. Obstet. Gynecol.* **104,** 440–442.

Hutcheson, R. B., Anderson, T. D., and Holborow, E. J. (1974). Cervical plasma cell population in infertile patients. *Br. Med. J.* **3,** 783–784.

Ison, C. A. (1988). Immunology of gonorrhea. *In* "Immunology of Sexually Transmitted Diseases" (D. J. M. Wright, ed.), pp. 95–116. Kluwer Academic Publishers, Dordrecht, The Netherlands.

Ison, C. A., Hadfield, S. G., Bellinger, C. M., Dawson, S. G., and Glynn, A. A. (1986). The specificity of serum and local antibodies in female gonorrhea. *Clin. Exp. Med.* **65,** 198–205.

Johnson, R. E., Nahmias, A. J., Magder, L. S., Lee, F. K., Brooks, C. A., and Snowden, C. B. (1989). A seroepidemiologic survey of the prevalence of herpes simplex virus type 2 infection on the United States. *N. Engl. J. Med.* **321,** 7–12.

Joiner, K. A., Warren, K. A., Tam, M., and Frank, M. M. (1985). Monoclonal antibodies directed against gonococcal protein I vary in bacterial activity. *J. Infect. Dis.* **148,** 1025.

Kass, E. H., Lin, J.-S., and McCormack, W. M. (1986). Low birth weight and maternal colonization with genital mycoplasmas. *Pediatr. Infect. Dis.* **5,** S279–281.

Katz, B. P., Batteiger, B. E., and Jones, R. B. (1987). Effect of prior sexually transmitted disease on the isolation of *Chlamydia trachomatis*. *Sex. Transm. Dis.* **14,** 160–164.

Kazar, J., Gillmore, J. D., and Gordon, F. B. (1971). Effect of interferon and interferon inducers on infections with a nonviral intracellular microorganism, *Chlamydia trachomatis*. *Infect. Immun.* **3,** 825–832.

Kearns, D. H., O'Reilly, R. L., Lee, L., and Welch, B. G. (1973a). Secretory IgA antibodies in the uretheral exudate of men with uncomplicated uretheritis due to *Neisseria gonorrhoeae*. *J. Infect. Dis.* **127,** 99–101.

Kearns, D. H., Sibert, G. B., O'Reilly, R., Lee, L., and Logan, L. (1973b). Paradox of the immune response to uncomplicated gonococcal urethritis. *N. Engl. J. Med.* **289,** 1170–1174.

Kohl, S. (1984). The immune response of the neonate to herpes simplex virus infection. *In* "Immunobiology of Herpes Simplex Virus Infection" (B. T. Rouse and C. Lopez, ed.), pp. 121–130. CRC Press, Boca Raton, Florida.

Kohl, S., Shaban, S. S., Starr, S. E., Wood, P. A., and Nahmias, A. J. (1978). Human neonatal and maternal monocyte-macrophage and lymphocyte-mediated antibody-dependent cytotoxicity in cells infected either herpes simplex. *J. Pediatr.* **93,** 206–210.

Kohl, S., Lawman, M. J., Rouse, B. T., and Cahall, D. J. (1981a). Effect of herpes simplex virus infection on murine antibody-dependent cellular cytotoxicity and natural killer cytotoxicity. *Infect. Immun.* **31,** 704.

Kohl, S., Frazier, J. P., Pickering, L. K., and Loo, L. S. (1981b). Normal function of neonatal polymorphonuclear leukocytes in antibody-dependent cellular-cytotoxicity to herpes simplex virus-infected cells. *J. Pediatr.* **98,** 783–785.

Kumar, M. L., Nankervos, G. A., and Gold, E. (1973). Inapparant congenital cytomegalovirus infection, a follow-up study. *N. Engl. J. Med.* **288,** 1370–1372.

Lai, A., Fat, R. F. M., Suurmond, D., and VanFurth, R. (1973). In vitro synthesis of immunoglobulins, secretory component and complement in normal and pathological skin and adjacent mucous membranes. *Clin. Exp. Med.* **14,** 377–395.

Lammel, C. J., Sweet, R. L., Rice, P. A., Knapp, J. S., Schoolnik, G. K., Heilbron, D. C., and Brooks, G. F. (1985). Antibody-antigen specificity in the immune response to infection with *Neisseria gonorrhoeae. J. Infect. Dis.* **152,** 990–1001.

Lee, F. K., Coleman, R. M., Pereira, L., Bailey, P. D., Tatsune, M., and Nahmias, A. J. (1985). Detection of herpes simplex virus type 2-specific antibody with glycoprotein G. *J. Clin. Microbiol.* **22,** 641–644.

Lee, F. K., Pereira, L., Griffin, C., Reid, E., and Nahmias, A. J. (1986). A novel glycoprotein for detection of herpes simplex type 1 specific antibodies. *J. Virol. Meth.* **14,** 111–118.

Liepmann, M.-F., Wattre, P., Dewilde, A., Papierok, G., and Delacour, M. (1988). Detection of antibodies to *Ureaplasma urealyticum* in pregnant women by enzyme-linked immunosorbent assay using membrane antigen and investigation of the significance of the antibodies. *J. Clin. Microbiol.* **26,** 2157–2160.

Likitnukul, S., Kusmiesz, H., Nelson, J. D., and McCracken, G. H. (1986). Role of genital mycoplasmas in young infants with suspected sepsis. *J. Pediatr.* **109,** 971–974.

Lippes, J., Ogra, S., Tomasi, T. B., and Tourville, D. R. (1970). Immunohistological localization of G, A, M, secretory piece and lactoferrin in the human female genital tract. *Contraception* **1,** 163–183.

Lucero, M. E., and Kuo, C. C. (1985). Neutralization of *Chlamydia trachomatis* cell culture infection by serovar-specific monoclonal antibodies. *Infect. Immun.* **50,** 595–597.

Luyet, F., Samra, D., Soneji, A., and Marks, M. (1975). I. Passive immunization in experimental herpesvirus hominis infection of newborn mice. *Infect. Immun.* **12,** 1258–1263.

McComb, D. E., Nichols, R. L., Semine, D. Z., Evrard, J. R., Alpert, S., Crockett, V. A., Rosner, B., Zinner, S. H., and McCormack, W. M. (1979). *Chlamydia trachomatis* in women: Antibody in cervical secretions as a possible indicator of genital infection. *J. Infect. Dis.* **139,** 628–633.

McDonald, J. C., and Moore, D. L. (1988). *Mycoplasma hominis* meningitis in a premature infant. *Pediatr. Infect. Dis.* **7,** 795–798.

McGee, Z. A., Melly, M. A., Gregg, C. R., Horn, R. G., Taylor-Robinson, D., Jonhson, A. P., and McCutchan, J. A. (1978). Virulence factors of gonococci: Studies using human fallopian tube organ cultures. *In* "Immunobiology of *Neisseria gonorrhoeae*" (G. F. Brooks, E. C. Gotschlich, K. K. Holmes, W. D. Sawyer, and F. E. Young, ed.), pp. 258–262. American Society of Microbiology, Washington, D.C.

McMillan, A., McNeillage, G., and Young, H. (1979a). Antibodies to *Neisseria gonorrhoeae*. A study of the uretheral exudates of 232 men. *J. Infect. Dis.* **140,** 89–95.

McMillan, A., McNeillage, G., Young, H., and Bain, S. S. R. (1979b). Secretory antibody response of the cervix to infection with *Neisseria gonorrhoeae. Br. J. Vener. Dis.* **55,** 265–270.

Manor, E., and Sarov, I. (1986). Fate of *Chlamydia trachomatis* in human monocytes and monocyte-derived macrophages. *Infect. Immun.* **54,** 90–95.

Mardh, P. (1983). *Mycoplasma hominis* infection of the central nervous system of newborn infants. *Sex. Transm. Dis.* **10,** 331–333.

Mardh, P.-A., Colleen, S., and Sylwan, J. (1980). Inhibitory effect on the formation of chlamydial inclusions in McCoy cells by seminal fluid and some of its components. *Invest. Urol.* **17,** 510–513.

Mestecky, J., and McGhee, J. R. (1987). Immunoglobulin A (IgA): Molecular and cellular interactions involved in IgA biosynthesis and immune response. *Adv. Immunol.* **40,** 153–245.

Miller, T. C., Baman, S. I., and Albers, W. H. (1982). Massive pericardial effusion due to *Mycoplasma hominis* in a newborn. *Am. J. Dis. Child.* **136,** 271–272.

Moghissi, K. S. (1970). Human fallopian tube fluid. I. Protein composition. *Fertil. Steril.* **21,** 821–829.

Moghissi, K. S., and Neuhaus, O. W. (1962). Composition and properties of human cervical mucus. II. Immunoelectrophoretic studies of the proteins. *Am. J. Obstet. Gynecol.* **83,** 149–155.

Monnickendam, M. A. (1988). Chlamydial genital infections. *In* "Immunology of Sexually Transmitted Diseases" (D. J. M. Wright, ed.), pp. 117–161. Kluwer Academic Publishers, Dordrecht, The Netherlands.

Monnickendam, M. A., and Pearce, J. H. (1983). Immune responses and chlamydial infections. *Br. Med. Bull.* **39,** 187.

Morbidity and Mortality Weekly Reports (1991a). HIV/AIDS epidemic: The first 10 years. *Morbid. Mortal. Wkly. Rep.* **40,** 357.

Morbidity and Mortality Weekly Reports (1991b). Update: Acquired Immunodeficiency syndrome—United States 1981–1990. *Morbid. Mortal. Wkly. Rep.* **40,** 358–369.

Murray, E. (1977). Review of clinical epidemiological and immunological studies of guinea pig inclusion conjunctivitus infection in guinea pigs. *In* "Nongonococcal Urethritis and Related Infections" (K. K. Holmes and D. Hodson, eds.), pp. 199–204. American Society of Microbiologists, Washington, D.C.

Murray, E. S., and Charbonnet, L. T. (1971). Experimental conjunctival infection of guinea pigs with the guinea pig inclusion conjunctivitis organism. *In* "Trachoma and Related Disorders Caused by Chlamydial Agents" (R. L. Nichols, ed.), pp. 369–376. Excerpta Medica, Amsterdam.

Murray, E. S., Charbonnet, L. T., and MacDonald, A. B. (1973). Immunity to chlamydial infections of the eye. I. The role of circulatory and secretory antibodies in resistance to reinfection with guinea pig inclusion conjunctivitis. *J. Immunol.* **110,** 1518–1525.

Nahmias, A. J. (1983). Herpes simplex. *In* "Infectious Diseases of the Fetus and Newborn Infant" (J. S. Remington and J. O. Klein, ed.), pp. 156–190. Saunders, Philadelphia.

Nichols, R. L., Oertley, R. E., Fraser, C. E. O., MacDonald, A. B., and McComb, E. D. (1973). Immunity to chlamydial infections of the eye. VI. Homologous neutralization of trachoma infectivity for the owl-monkey conjunctiva by eye secretions from humans with trachoma. *J. Infect. Dis.* **127,** 429–432.

Norrild, B., Shore, S. L., and Nahmias, A. J. (1979). Herpes simplex virus glycoprotein antigens in immunocytolysis and their correlation with previously identified glycopeptides. *J. Virol.* **32,** 741–746.

Olding, L. B., and Oldstone, M. B. A. (1974). Lymphocytes from newborns abrogate mitosis of their mother's lymphocytes. *Nature (London)* **249,** 161–162.

O'Reilly, R. J., Lee, L., and Welch, B. G. (1976). Secretory IgA antibody response to *Neisseria gonorrhoeae* in the genital secretions of infected females. *J. Infect. Dis.* **133,** 113–125.

Parsons, N. J., Kwaasi, A. A., Turner, J. A., Veale, D. R., Perera, V. Y., Patel, P. V., Martin, P. M., and Smith, H. (1981). Investigation of the determinants of the survival of *Neisseria gonorrhoeae* within polymorphonuclear phagocytes. *J. Gen. Microbiol.* **127,** 103–112.

Parsons, N. J., Kwaasi, A. A., Perera, V. Y., Patel, P. V., Martin, P. M., and Smith, H. (1982). Outer membrane proteins of *Neisseria gonorrhoeae* associated with survival within human polymorphonuclear phagocytes. *J. Gen. Microbiol.* **128,** 3077–3081.

Parsons, N. J., Kwaasi, A. A., Patel, P. V., Nairn, C. A., and Smith, H. (1985). A determinant of resistance of *Neisseria gonorrhoeae* to killing by human phagocytes: An outer membrane lipoprotein of about 20 kDa with a high content of glutamic acid. *J. Gen. Microbiol.* **132,** 3277–3287.

Parsons, N. J., Kwaasi, A. A., Patel, P. V., Nairn, C. A., and Smith, H. (1986). Association of resistence of *Neisseria gonorrhoeae* to killing by human phagocytes with outer membrane proteins of about 20 kilodaltons. *J. Gen. Microbiol.* **131,** 601–610.

Pass, R. F., Stagno, S., Myers, G. J., and Alford, C. A. (1980). Outcome of symptomatic congenital cytomegalovirus infection: Results of long-term longitudinal follow-up. *Pediatrics* **66,** 758–762.

Pass, R. F., Dworsky, M. E., Whitley, R. J., August, A. M., Stagno, S., and Alford, C. A. (1981). Specific lymphocyte blastogenic responses in children with cytomegalovirus and herpes simplex virus infections acquired early in infancy. *Infect. Immun.* **34,** 166–69.

Peeling, R., Maclean, I. W., and Brunham, R. C. (1984). In vitro neutralization of *Chlamydia trachomatis* with monoclonal antibodies to an epitope on the major outer membrane protein. *Infect. Immun.* **46,** 484–488.

Plotkin, S. A., Farguhar, J., and Hornberger, E. (1976). Clinical trials of immunization with the Towne 125 strain of human cytomegalovirus. *J. Infect. Dis.* **134,** 470–475.

Plotkin, S. A., Smiley, M. L., Friedman, H. M., Starr, S. E., Fleisher, G. R., Wlodaver, C., Dafoe, D. C., Friedman, A. D., Grossman, R. A., and Barker, C. F. (1984). Prevention of cytomegalovirus disease by Towne strain live attenuated vaccine. *Birth Def.* **20,** 271–287.

Plotkin, S. A., Starr, S. E., Friedman, H. M., Gonczol, E., and Brayman, K. (1990). Vaccines for the prevention of human cytomegalovirus infection. *Rev. Infect. Dis.* **12,** S827–S838.

Prober, C. G., Sullender, W. M., Yasukawa, L. L., Au, D. S., Yeager, A. S., and Arvin, A. M. (1987). Low risk of herpes simplex virus infections in neonates exposed to the virus at the time of vaginal delivery to mothers with recurrent genital herpes simplex virus infections. *N. Engl. J. Med.* **316,** 240–244.

Quinn, P. A., Gillan, J. E., Markestad, T., St. John, M. A., Daneman, A., Lie, K. I., Li, H. C. S., Czegledy-Nagy, E., Klein, A., and Klein, M. (1985). Intrauterine infection with *Ureaplasma urealyticum* as a cause of fatal neonatal pneumonia. *Pediatr. Infect. Dis.* **4,** 538–543.

Rank, R. G., White, H. J., and Barron, A. L. (1979). Humoral immunity in the resolution of genital infection in female guinea pigs infected with the agent of guinea pig inclusion conjunctivitis. *Infect. Immun.* **26,** 573–579.

Rank, R. G., Batteiger, B. E., and Soderberg, L. S. F. (1988). Susceptibility of reinfection after a primary chlamydial genital infection. *Infect. Immun.* **56,** 2243–2249.

Rank, R. G., Battiger, B. E., and Soderberg, L. S. F. (1990). Immunization against chlamydial genital infection in guinea pigs with UV-inactivated and viable chlamydiae administered by different routes. *Infect. Immun.* **58,** 2599–2605.

Rebello, R., Green, F. H. Y., and Fox, H. (1975). A study of the secretory immune response of the female genital tract. *Br. J. Obstet. Gynaecol.* **82,** 812–816.

Reed, S. I., and Hann, W. D. (1980). The effect of cortisol on glycogen and fructose-1, 6-biphosphatase in baby hamster kidney cells infected with *Chlamydia trachomatis. Can. J. Microbiol.* **26,** 135–140.

Reynolds, D. W., Stagno, S., Hosty, T. S., Tiller, M., and Alford, C. A. (1973). Maternal cytomegalovirus excretion and perinatal infection. *N. Engl. J. Med.* **289,** 1–5.

Reynolds, D. W., Stagno, S., Stubbs, K. G., Dahle, A. J., Livingston, M. M., Saxon, S. S., and Alford, C. A. (1974). Inapparent congenital cytomegalovirus infection with elevated cord IgM levels: Causal relationship with auditory and mental deficiency. *N. Engl. J. Med.* **290,** 291–296.

Rice, P. A., Tam, M. R., and Blake, M. S. (1985). Immunoglobulin G antibodies in normal human serum directed against protein III block killing of serum-resistant *Neisseria gonorrhoeae* by immune human serum. *In* "The Pathogenic Neisseriae" (G. K. Schoolnik, ed.), pp. 427–430. American Society of Microbiology, Washington, D.C.

Rice, P. A., Vayo, H. E., Tam, M. R., and Blake, M. S. (1986). Immunoglobulin G antibodies directed against protein III block killing of serum resistant *Neisseria gonorrhoeae* by immune sera. *J. Exp. Med.* **164,** 1735.

Richmond, S. J., Milne, J. D., Hilton, A. L., and Caul, E. O. (1980). Antibodies to *Chlamydia trachomatis* in cervicvaginal secretions: Relation to serum antibodies and current chlamydial infection. *Sex. Transm. Dis.* **7,** 11–15.

Rothermel, C. D., Byrne, G. I., and Havell, E. A. (1983). Effect of interferon on the growth of *Chlamydia trachomatis* in mouse fibroblasts (L cells). *Infect. Immun.* **39,** 362–370.

Ruyechan, W. T., Morse, L. S., Knipe, D. M., and Roizman, B. (1979). Molecular genetics of herpes simplex virus. II. Mapping of the major viral glycoproteins and of the genetic loci specifying the social behavior of infected cells. *J. Virol.* **29,** 677–683.

Sandstrom, E. G., Chen, K. C., and Buchanan, T. M. (1982). Serology of *Neisseria gonorrhoeae:* Co-agglutination serogroups WI and WII/III correspond to different outer membrane protein molecules. *Infect. Immun.* **38,** 462–470.

Schachter, J. and Grossman, M. (1990). Chlamydia. *In* "Infections of the Fetus and Newborn Infant" (J. S. Remington and J. O. Klein, ed.), pp. 464–474. Saunders, Philadelphia.

Schachter, J., Cles, J. D., Ray, R. M., and Hesse, F. E. (1983). Is there immunity to chlamydial infections of the human gential tract? *Sex. Transm. Dis.* **10,** 123–125.

Schachter, J., Grossman, M., Sweet, R. L., Holt, J., Jordan, C., and Bishop, E. (1986). Prospective study of perinatal transmission of *Chlamydia trachomatis. J. Am. Med. Assoc.* **255,** 3374–3377.

Schumacher, G. F. B. (1973a). Soluble proteins of human cervical mucus. *In* "Cervical Mucus in Human Reproduction" (M. Elstein, K. S. Morghissi, and R. Borth, ed.), pp. 93–113. Scriptor, Copenhagen.

Schumacher, G. F. B. (1973b). Soluble proteins of cervical mucus. *In* "The Biology of the Cervix" (R. J. Blandau and K. S. Morghissi, ed.), pp. 201–233. University of Chicago Press, Chicago.

Scott, J. R. (1991). Immunologic disorders in pregnancy. *In* "Danforth's Obstetrics and Gynecology" (J. R. Scott, P. J. DiSaia, C. B. Hammond, and W. N. Spellacy, ed.), 6th Ed., pp. 461–491. Lippincott, Philadelphia.

Sethi, K. K. (1983). Effects of monoclonal antibodies directed against herpes simplex virus-specified glycoproteins on the generation of virus-specific and H-2 restricted cytotoxic T-lymphocytes. *J. Gen. Virol.* **64,** 2033–2038.

Shafer, W. M., and Rest, R. F. (1989). Interactions of gonococci with phagocytic cells. *Ann. Rev Microbiol.* **43,** 121–145.

Shemer, Y., and Sarov, I. (1985). Inhibition of growth of *Chlamydia trachomatis* by human gamma interferon. *Infect. Immun.* **48,** 592–596.

Shore, S. L., Black, C. M., Melewiez, F. M., Wood, P., and Nahmias, A. J. (1976). Antibody-dependent cell mediated cytotoxicity to target cells infected with type 1 and type 2 herpes simplex virus. *J. Immunol.* **116,** 194–201.

Shore, S. L., Milgrom, H., Wood, P., and Nahmias, A. J. (1977). Neonatal function of antibody-dependent cell-mediated cytotoxicity to target cells infected with herpes simplex virus. *Pediatrics* **59,** 22–28.

Soderlund, G., Dahlgren, C., and Kihlstrom, E. (1984). Interaction between human polymorphonuclear leukocytes and *Chlamydia trachomatis. FEMS Microbiol. Lett.* **22,** 21–25.

Spear, P. G. (1976). Membrane proteins specified by herpes simplex viruses. I. Identification of four glycoprotein precursors and their products in type I infected cells. *J. Virol.* **17,** 991–997.

Stagno, S. (1990). Cytomegalovirus. *In* "Infectious Diseases of the Fetus and Newborn Infant" (J. S. Remington and J. O. Klein, ed.), pp. 241–281. Saunders, Philadelphia.

Stagno, S., Reynolds, D. W., Tsiantos, A., Fucilld, D. A., Long, W., and Alford, C. A. (1975). Comparative, serial virologic and serologic studies of symptomatic and subclinical congenital and natally acquired cytomegalovirus infection. *J. Infect. Dis.* **132,** 568–577.

Stagno, S., Reynolds, D. W., Amos, C. S., Dahle, A. J., McCollister, F. P., Mohindra, I., Ermocilla, R., and Alford, C. A. (1977). Auditory and visual defects resulting from symptomatic and subclinical congenital cytomegalovirus and toxoplasma infections. *Pediatrics* **59,** 669–678.

Stagno, S., Reynolds, D. W., Pass, R. F., and Alford, C. A. (1980). Breast milk and the risk of cytomegalovirus infection. *N. Engl. J. Med.* **302,** 1073–1076.

Stagno, S., Brasfield, D., Brown, M. B., Cassell, G. H., Pifer, L. L., Whitley, R., and Tiller, R. E. (1981). Infant pneumonitis associated with cytomegalovirus, *Chlamydia, Pneumocystis,* and *Ureaplasma:* A prospective study. *Pediatrics* **68,** 322–329.

Stagno, S., Pass, R. F., Dworsky, M. E., Moore, E. G., Walton, P. D., and Alford, C. A. (1982). Congenital cytomegalovirus infection: The relative importance of primary and recurrent maternal infection. *N. Engl. J. Med.* **306,** 945–949.

Stagno, S., Cloud, G., Pass, R. F., Britt, W. J., and Alford, C. A. (1984). Factors associated with primary cytomegalovirus infection during pregnancy. *J. Med. Virol.* **13,** 347–353.

Stagno, S., Pass, R. F., Cloud, G., Britt, W. J., Henderson, R. E., Walton, P. D., Veren, D. A., Page, F., and Alford, C. A. (1986). Primary cytomegalovirus infection in pregnancy: Incidence, transmission to fetus, and clinical outcome. *J. Am. Med. Assoc.* **256,** 1904–1908.

Stern, H. (1984). Live cytomegalovirus vaccination of healthy volunteers: Eight-year follow-up studies. *Birth Def.* **20,** 263–269.

Sugarman, B., and Agbor, P. (1986). Estrogens and *Chlamydia trachomatis. Proc. Soc. Exp. Biol. Med.* **183,** 125–131.

Sullender, W. M., Miller, J. L., Yasukawa, L. L., Bradley, J. S., Black, S. B., Yeager, A. S., and Arvin, A. M. (1987). Humoral and cell-mediated immunity in neonates with herpes simplex virus infection. *J. Infect. Dis.* **155,** 28–37.

Sullender, W. M., Yasukawa, L. L., Schwartz, M., Pereira, L., Hensleigh, P. A., Prober, C. G., and Arvin, A. M. (1988). Type-specific antibodies to herpes simplex virus type 2 (HSV-2) glycoprotein G in pregnant women, infants exposed to maternal HSV-2 infections at delivery, and infants with neonatal herpes. *J. Infect. Dis.* **157,** 164–171.

Syndman, D. R., Werner, B. G., Heinze-Lacey, B., Berardi, V. P., *et al.* (1987). The use of cytomegalovirus immune globulin to prevent cytomegalovirus disease in renal transplant recipients. *N. Engl. J. Med.* **317,** 1049–1054.

Taylor-Robinson, D. (1988). Immunology of genital mycoplasmal infections. *In* "Immunology of Sexually Transmitted Diseases" (D. J. M. Wright, ed.), pp. 163–177. Kluwer Academic Publishers, Dordrecht, The Netherlands.

Tjokonegoro, A., and Sirisnha, S. (1975). Quantitative analysis of immunoglobulins and albumin in the secretion of the female reproductive tract. *Fertil. Steril.* **26,** 413–417.

Tomasi, T. B. (1989). Regulation of the mucosal IgA response—An overview. *Immunol. Invest.* **18,** 1–15.

Tourville, D. R., Ogra, S. S., Lippes, J., and Tomasi, T. B. J. (1970). The female reproductive tract: Immunohistologic localization of A, G, M, secretory "piece" and lactoferrin. *Am. J. Obstet. Gynecol.* **108,** 1102–1108.

Tramont, E. C., Ciak, J., Boslego, J., McChesney, D. C., Brinton, C. C., and Zollinger, W. (1980). Antigenic specificity of antibodies in vaginal secretion during infection with *Neisseria gonorrhoeae. J. Infect. Dis.* **140,** 23–31.

Unsworth, P. F., Taylor-Robinson, D., Shoo, E. E., and Furr, P. M. (1985). Neonatal mycoplasaemia: *Mycoplasma hominis* as a significant cause of disease? *J. Infect.* **10,** 163–8.

Veale, D. R., Sen, D., Penn, C. W., Finch, H., Smith, H., and Witt, K. (1977). Interactions of *Neiserria gonorrhoeae* with guinea pig defence mechanisms in subcutaneously implanted chambers. *FEMS Microbiol. Lett.* **1,** 3–6.

Veale, D. R., Goldner, M., Penn, C. W., Ward, J., and Smith, H. (1979). The intracellular survival and growth of gonococci in human phagocytes. *J. Gen. Microbiol.* **113,** 383–393.

Virji, M., Zak, M., and Heckles, J. E. (1986). Monoclonal antibodies to gonococcal outer membrane protein IB: Use in the investigation of the potential protective effect of antibodies directed against conserved and type-specific epitopes. *J. Gen. Microbiol.* **132,** 1621–1629.

Virji, M., Fletcher, J. N., Zak, K., and Heckels, J. E. (1987). The potential protective effect of monoclonal antibodies to gonococcal outer membrane protein IA. *J. Gen. Microbiol.* **133,** 2639.

Waites, K. B., Rudd, P. T., Crouse, D. T., Canupp, K. C., Nelson, K. G., Ramsey, C., and Cassell, G. H. (1988). Chronic *Ureaplasma urealyticum* and *Mycoplasma hominis* infections of the central nervous system. *Lancet* **1,** 17–22.

Waites, K. B., Crouse, D. T., Philips, J. B. I., Canupp, K. C., and Cassell, G. H. (1989). Ureaplasma pneumonia and sepsis associated with persistent pulmonary hypertension of the newborn. *Pediatrics* **83,** 79–85.

Waldman, R. H., Cruz, J. M., and Rowe, D. S. (1972). Immunoglobulin levels and antibody to *Candida albicans* in human cervicovaginal secretions. *Clin. Exp. Immunol.* **10,** 427–434.

Wang, E. E. L., Frayha, H., Watts, J., Hammerberg, O., Chernesky, M. A., Mahony, J. B., and Cassell, G. H. (1988). Role of *Ureaplasma urealyticum* and other pathogens in the development of chronic lung disease of prematurity. *Pediatr. Infect. Dis.* **7,** 547–551.

Ward, M. E., Watt, P. J., and Robertson, N. J. (1974). The human fallopian tube: A laboratory model for gonococcal infection. *J. Infect. Dis.* **129,** 650–659.

Watt, P. J., and Ward, M. E. (1980). Adherence of *Neisseria gonorrhoeae* and other *Neisseria* species to mammalian cells. *In* "Receptors, Recognition and Bacterial Adherence" (E. H. Beachey, ed.), Vol. B6, pp. 251–288. Chapman and Hill, London.

Watts, D. H., Eschenbach, D. A., and Kenny, G. E. (1989). Early postpartum endometritis: The role of bacteria, genital mycoplasmas, and *Chlamydia trachomatis*. *Obstet. Gynecol.* **73,** 52–59.

Wealthall, S. R. (1975). Mycoplasma meningitis in infants with spina bifida. *Dev. Med. Child. Neurol.* **17,** 117–22.

Weller, T. H. (1971). The cytomegaloviruses: Ubiquitous agents with protean clinical manifestations. Second of 2 parts. *N. Engl. J. Med.* **285,** 267–274.

Wetzler, L. M., Blake, M. S., and Gotschlich, E. C. (1988). Characterization and specificity of antibodies to protein I of *Neisseria gonorrhoeae* produced by injection with various protein I-adjuvant preparations. *J. Exp. Med.* **168,** 1883–1897.

Whitley, R. J. (1990). Herpes simplex virus infections. *In* "Infectious Diseases of the Fetus and Newborn Infant" (J. S. Remington and J. O. Klein, ed.), pp. 282–305. Saunders, Philadelphia.

Whitley, R. J., Nahmais, A. J., Vistine, A. M., Fleming, C. L., and Alford, C. A. (1980). The natural history of herpes simplex virus infection of the mother and newborn. *Pediatrics* **66,** 489–494.

World Health Organization (1991). In point of fact. *WHO Bull.* **74.**

Worthington, M., Coniffe, M. A., and Baron, S. (1980). Mechanism of recovery from systemic herpes simplex virus infection. I. Comparative effect of antibody and reconstruction of immune spleen cells on immunosuppressed mice. *J. Infect. Dis.* **142,** 163–167.

Yeager, A. S., Arvin, A. M., Urbani, L. J., and Kemp, J. A., 3rd (1980). Relationship of antibody to outcome in neonatal herpes simplex virus infections. *Infect. Immun.* **29,** 532–538.

Yong, E. C., Klebanoff, S. J., and Kuo, C.-C. (1982). Toxic effect of human polymorphonuclear leukocytes on *Chlamydia trachomatis*. *Infect. Immun.* **37,** 422–426.

Yong, E. C., Chi, E. Y., Chen, W.-J., and Kuo, C.-C. (1986). Degradation of *Chlamydia trachomatis* in human polymorphonuclear leukocytes: An ultrastructural study of peroxidase-positive phagolysosomes. *Infect. Immun.* **53,** 427–431.

Zvillich, M., and Sarov, I. (1985). Interaction between human polymorphonuclear leukocytes and *Chlamydia trachomatis* elementary bodies: Electron microscopy and chemiluminescent response. *J. Gen. Microbiol.* **131,** 2627–2635.

Index